The Biomedical Engineering Handbook
Third Edition

Biomedical Engineering Fundamentals

The Electrical Engineering Handbook Series

Series Editor
Richard C. Dorf
University of California, Davis

Titles Included in the Series

The Handbook of Ad Hoc Wireless Networks, Mohammad Ilyas
The Avionics Handbook, Cary R. Spitzer
The Biomedical Engineering Handbook, Third Edition, Joseph D. Bronzino
The Circuits and Filters Handbook, Second Edition, Wai-Kai Chen
The Communications Handbook, Second Edition, Jerry Gibson
The Computer Engineering Handbook, Vojin G. Oklobdzija
The Control Handbook, William S. Levine
The CRC Handbook of Engineering Tables, Richard C. Dorf
The Digital Signal Processing Handbook, Vijay K. Madisetti and Douglas Williams
The Electrical Engineering Handbook, Third Edition, Richard C. Dorf
The Electric Power Engineering Handbook, Leo L. Grigsby
The Electronics Handbook, Second Edition, Jerry C. Whitaker
The Engineering Handbook, Third Edition, Richard C. Dorf
The Handbook of Formulas and Tables for Signal Processing, Alexander D. Poularikas
The Handbook of Nanoscience, Engineering, and Technology, William A. Goddard, III,
   Donald W. Brenner, Sergey E. Lyshevski, and Gerald J. Iafrate
The Handbook of Optical Communication Networks, Mohammad Ilyas and
   Hussein T. Mouftah
The Industrial Electronics Handbook, J. David Irwin
The Measurement, Instrumentation, and Sensors Handbook, John G. Webster
The Mechanical Systems Design Handbook, Osita D.I. Nwokah and Yidirim Hurmuzlu
The Mechatronics Handbook, Robert H. Bishop
The Mobile Communications Handbook, Second Edition, Jerry D. Gibson
The Ocean Engineering Handbook, Ferial El-Hawary
The RF and Microwave Handbook, Mike Golio
The Technology Management Handbook, Richard C. Dorf
The Transforms and Applications Handbook, Second Edition, Alexander D. Poularikas
The VLSI Handbook, Wai-Kai Chen

The Biomedical Engineering Handbook
Third Edition

Edited by
Joseph D. Bronzino

Biomedical Engineering Fundamentals

Medical Devices and Systems

Tissue Engineering and Artificial Organs

The Biomedical Engineering Handbook
Third Edition

Biomedical Engineering Fundamentals

Edited by
Joseph D. Bronzino

Trinity College
Hartford, Connecticut, U.S.A.

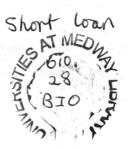

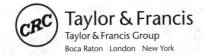

Taylor & Francis
Taylor & Francis Group
Boca Raton   London   New York

A CRC title, part of the Taylor & Francis imprint, a member of the
Taylor & Francis Group, the academic division of T&F Informa plc.

Published in 2006 by
CRC Press
Taylor & Francis Group
6000 Broken Sound Parkway NW, Suite 300
Boca Raton, FL 33487-2742

© 2006 by Taylor & Francis Group, LLC
CRC Press is an imprint of Taylor & Francis Group

No claim to original U.S. Government works
Printed in the United States of America on acid-free paper
10 9 8 7 6 5 4 3 2 1

International Standard Book Number-10: 0-8493-2121-2 (Hardcover)
International Standard Book Number-13: 978-0-8493-2121-4 (Hardcover)
Library of Congress Card Number 2005054864

Library of Congress Cataloging-in-Publication Data

Biomedical engineering fundamentals / edited by Joseph D. Bronzino.
     p. cm. -- (The electrical engineering handbook series)
  Includes bibliographical references and index.
  ISBN 0-8493-2121-2 (alk. paper)
  1. Biomedical engineering. I Bronzino, Joseph D., 1937- II. Title. III. Series.

R856.B513 2006
610.28--dc22   2005054864

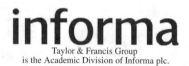
informa
Taylor & Francis Group
is the Academic Division of Informa plc.

Visit the Taylor & Francis Web site at
http://www.taylorandfrancis.com

and the CRC Press Web site at
http://www.crcpress.com

Introduction and Preface

During the past five years since the publication of the Second Edition — a two-volume set — of the *Biomedical Engineering Handbook*, the field of biomedical engineering has continued to evolve and expand. As a result, this Third Edition consists of a three-volume set, which has been significantly modified to reflect the state-of-the-field knowledge and applications in this important discipline. More specifically, this Third Edition contains a number of completely new sections, including:

- Molecular Biology
- Bionanotechnology
- Bioinformatics
- Neuroengineering
- Infrared Imaging

as well as a new section on ethics.

In addition, all of the sections that have appeared in the first and second editions have been significantly revised. Therefore, this Third Edition presents an excellent summary of the status of knowledge and activities of biomedical engineers in the beginning of the 21st century.

As such, it can serve as an excellent reference for individuals interested not only in a review of fundamental physiology, but also in quickly being brought up to speed in certain areas of biomedical engineering research. It can serve as an excellent textbook for students in areas where traditional textbooks have not yet been developed and as an excellent review of the major areas of activity in each biomedical engineering subdiscipline, such as biomechanics, biomaterials, bioinstrumentation, medical imaging, etc. Finally, it can serve as the "bible" for practicing biomedical engineering professionals by covering such topics as historical perspective of medical technology, the role of professional societies, the ethical issues associated with medical technology, and the FDA process.

Biomedical engineering is now an important vital interdisciplinary field. Biomedical engineers are involved in virtually all aspects of developing new medical technology. They are involved in the design, development, and utilization of materials, devices (such as pacemakers, lithotripsy, etc.) and techniques (such as signal processing, artificial intelligence, etc.) for clinical research and use; and serve as members of the healthcare delivery team (clinical engineering, medical informatics, rehabilitation engineering, etc.) seeking new solutions for difficult healthcare problems confronting our society. To meet the needs of this diverse body of biomedical engineers, this handbook provides a central core of knowledge in those fields encompassed by the discipline. However, before presenting this detailed information, it is important to provide a sense of the evolution of the modern healthcare system and identify the diverse activities biomedical engineers perform to assist in the diagnosis and treatment of patients.

Evolution of the Modern Healthcare System

Before 1900, medicine had little to offer the average citizen, since its resources consisted mainly of the physician, his education, and his "little black bag." In general, physicians seemed to be in short supply, but the shortage had rather different causes than the current crisis in the availability of healthcare professionals. Although the costs of obtaining medical training were relatively low, the demand for doctors' services also was very small, since many of the services provided by the physician also could be obtained from experienced amateurs in the community. The home was typically the site for treatment and recuperation, and relatives and neighbors constituted an able and willing nursing staff. Babies were delivered by midwives, and those illnesses not cured by home remedies were left to run their natural, albeit frequently fatal, course. The contrast with contemporary healthcare practices, in which specialized physicians and nurses located within the hospital provide critical diagnostic and treatment services, is dramatic.

The changes that have occurred within medical science originated in the rapid developments that took place in the applied sciences (chemistry, physics, engineering, microbiology, physiology, pharmacology, etc.) at the turn of the century. This process of development was characterized by intense interdisciplinary cross-fertilization, which provided an environment in which medical research was able to take giant strides in developing techniques for the diagnosis and treatment of disease. For example, in 1903, Willem Einthoven, a Dutch physiologist, devised the first electrocardiograph to measure the electrical activity of the heart. In applying discoveries in the physical sciences to the analysis of the biologic process, he initiated a new age in both cardiovascular medicine and electrical measurement techniques.

New discoveries in medical sciences followed one another like intermediates in a chain reaction. However, the most significant innovation for clinical medicine was the development of x-rays. These "new kinds of rays," as their discoverer W.K. Roentgen described them in 1895, opened the "inner man" to medical inspection. Initially, x-rays were used to diagnose bone fractures and dislocations, and in the process, x-ray machines became commonplace in most urban hospitals. Separate departments of radiology were established, and their influence spread to other departments throughout the hospital. By the 1930s, x-ray visualization of practically all organ systems of the body had been made possible through the use of barium salts and a wide variety of radiopaque materials.

X-ray technology gave physicians a powerful tool that, for the first time, permitted accurate diagnosis of a wide variety of diseases and injuries. Moreover, since x-ray machines were too cumbersome and expensive for local doctors and clinics, they had to be placed in healthcare centers or hospitals. Once there, x-ray technology essentially triggered the transformation of the hospital from a passive receptacle for the sick to an active curative institution for all members of society.

For economic reasons, the centralization of healthcare services became essential because of many other important technological innovations appearing on the medical scene. However, hospitals remained institutions to dread, and it was not until the introduction of sulfanilamide in the mid-1930s and penicillin in the early 1940s that the main danger of hospitalization, that is, cross-infection among patients, was significantly reduced. With these new drugs in their arsenals, surgeons were able to perform their operations without prohibitive morbidity and mortality due to infection. Furthermore, even though the different blood groups and their incompatibility were discovered in 1900 and sodium citrate was used in 1913 to prevent clotting, full development of blood banks was not practical until the 1930s, when technology provided adequate refrigeration. Until that time, "fresh" donors were bled and the blood transfused while it was still warm.

Once these surgical suites were established, the employment of specifically designed pieces of medical technology assisted in further advancing the development of complex surgical procedures. For example, the Drinker respirator was introduced in 1927 and the first heart–lung bypass in 1939. By the 1940s, medical procedures heavily dependent on medical technology, such as cardiac catheterization and angiography (the use of a cannula threaded through an arm vein and into the heart with the injection of radiopaque dye) for the x-ray visualization of congenital and acquired heart disease (mainly valve disorders due to rheumatic fever) became possible, and a new era of cardiac and vascular surgery was established.

Following World War II, technological advances were spurred on by efforts to develop superior weapon systems and establish habitats in space and on the ocean floor. As a by-product of these efforts, the development of medical devices accelerated and the medical profession benefited greatly from this rapid surge of technological finds. Consider the following examples:

1. Advances in solid-state electronics made it possible to map the subtle behavior of the fundamental unit of the central nervous system — the neuron — as well as to monitor the various physiological parameters, such as the electrocardiogram, of patients in intensive care units.
2. New prosthetic devices became a goal of engineers involved in providing the disabled with tools to improve their quality of life.
3. Nuclear medicine — an outgrowth of the atomic age — emerged as a powerful and effective approach in detecting and treating specific physiologic abnormalities.
4. Diagnostic ultrasound based on sonar technology became so widely accepted that ultrasonic studies are now part of the routine diagnostic workup in many medical specialties.
5. "Spare parts" surgery also became commonplace. Technologists were encouraged to provide cardiac assist devices, such as artificial heart valves and artificial blood vessels, and the artificial heart program was launched to develop a replacement for a defective or diseased human heart.
6. Advances in materials have made the development of disposable medical devices, such as needles and thermometers, as well as implantable drug delivery systems, a reality.
7. Computers similar to those developed to control the flight plans of the *Apollo* capsule were used to store, process, and cross-check medical records, to monitor patient status in intensive care units, and to provide sophisticated statistical diagnoses of potential diseases correlated with specific sets of patient symptoms.
8. Development of the first computer-based medical instrument, the computerized axial tomography scanner, revolutionized clinical approaches to noninvasive diagnostic imaging procedures, which now include magnetic resonance imaging and positron emission tomography as well.
9. A wide variety of new cardiovascular technologies including implantable defibrillators and chemically treated stents were developed.
10. Neuronal pacing systems were used to detect and prevent epileptic seizures.
11. Artificial organs and tissue have been created.
12. The completion of the genome project has stimulated the search for new biological markers and personalized medicine.

The impact of these discoveries and many others has been profound. The healthcare system of today consists of technologically sophisticated clinical staff operating primarily in modern hospitals designed to accommodate the new medical technology. This evolutionary process continues, with advances in the physical sciences such as materials and nanotechnology, and in the life sciences such as molecular biology, the genome project and artificial organs. These advances have altered and will continue to alter the very nature of the healthcare delivery system itself.

Biomedical Engineering: A Definition

Bioengineering is usually defined as a basic research-oriented activity closely related to biotechnology and genetic engineering, that is, the modification of animal or plant cells, or parts of cells, to improve plants or animals or to develop new microorganisms for beneficial ends. In the food industry, for example, this has meant the improvement of strains of yeast for fermentation. In agriculture, bioengineers may be concerned with the improvement of crop yields by treatment of plants with organisms to reduce frost damage. It is clear that bioengineers of the future will have a tremendous impact on the qualities of human life.

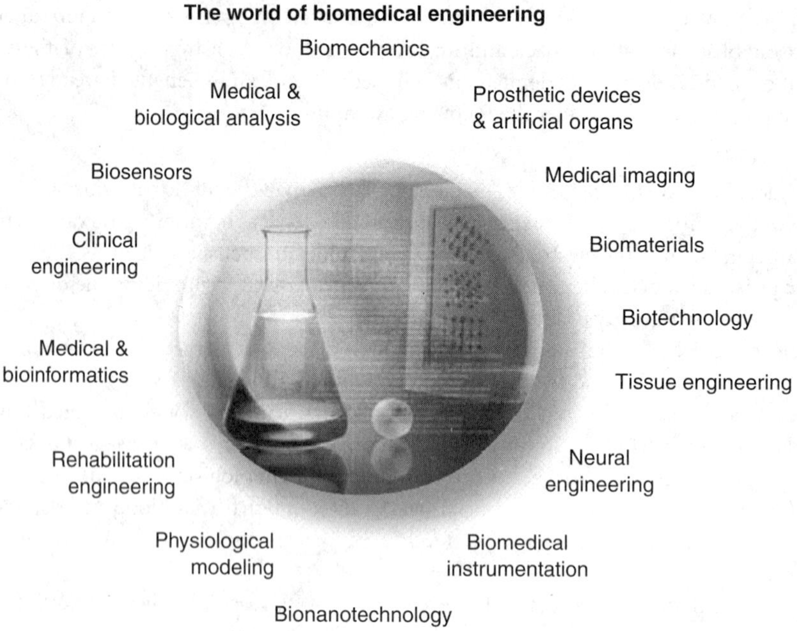

The world of biomedical engineering

Biomechanics

Medical &
biological analysis

Prosthetic devices
& artificial organs

Biosensors

Medical imaging

Clinical
engineering

Biomaterials

Biotechnology

Medical &
bioinformatics

Tissue engineering

Rehabilitation
engineering

Neural
engineering

Physiological
modeling

Biomedical
instrumentation

Bionanotechnology

FIGURE 1   The world of biomedical engineering.

The potential of this specialty is difficult to imagine. Consider the following activities of bioengineers:

- Development of improved species of plants and animals for food production
- Invention of new medical diagnostic tests for diseases
- Production of synthetic vaccines from clone cells
- Bioenvironmental engineering to protect human, animal, and plant life from toxicants and pollutants
- Study of protein–surface interactions
- Modeling of the growth kinetics of yeast and hybridoma cells
- Research in immobilized enzyme technology
- Development of therapeutic proteins and monoclonal antibodies

   Biomedical engineers, on the other hand, apply electrical, mechanical, chemical, optical, and other engineering principles to understand, modify, or control biologic (i.e., human and animal) systems, as well as design and manufacture products that can monitor physiologic functions and assist in the diagnosis and treatment of patients. When biomedical engineers work within a hospital or clinic, they are more properly called clinical engineers.

Activities of Biomedical Engineers

The breadth of activity of biomedical engineers is now significant. The field has moved from being concerned primarily with the development of medical instruments in the 1950s and 1960s to include a more wide-ranging set of activities. As illustrated below, the field of biomedical engineering now includes many new career areas (see Figure 1), each of which is presented in this handbook. These areas include:

- Application of engineering system analysis (physiologic modeling, simulation, and control) to biologic problems
- Detection, measurement, and monitoring of physiologic signals (i.e., biosensors and biomedical instrumentation)

- Diagnostic interpretation via signal-processing techniques of bioelectric data
- Therapeutic and rehabilitation procedures and devices (rehabilitation engineering)
- Devices for replacement or augmentation of bodily functions (*artificial organs*)
- Computer analysis of patient-related data and clinical decision-making (i.e., medical informatics and artificial intelligence)
- Medical imaging, that is, the graphic display of anatomic detail or physiologic function
- The creation of new biologic products (i.e., *biotechnology* and *tissue engineering*)
- The development of new materials to be used within the body (biomaterials)

Typical pursuits of biomedical engineers, therefore, include:

- Research in new materials for implanted artificial organs
- Development of new diagnostic instruments for blood analysis
- Computer modeling of the function of the human heart
- Writing software for analysis of medical research data
- Analysis of medical device hazards for safety and efficacy
- Development of new diagnostic imaging systems
- Design of telemetry systems for patient monitoring
- Design of biomedical sensors for measurement of human physiologic systems variables
- Development of expert systems for diagnosis of disease
- Design of closed-loop control systems for drug administration
- Modeling of the physiological systems of the human body
- Design of instrumentation for sports medicine
- Development of new dental materials
- Design of communication aids for the handicapped
- Study of pulmonary fluid dynamics
- Study of the biomechanics of the human body
- Development of material to be used as replacement for human skin

Biomedical engineering, then, is an interdisciplinary branch of engineering that ranges from theoretical, nonexperimental undertakings to state-of-the-art applications. It can encompass research, development, implementation, and operation. Accordingly, like medical practice itself, it is unlikely that any single person can acquire expertise that encompasses the entire field. Yet, because of the interdisciplinary nature of this activity, there is considerable interplay and overlapping of interest and effort between them. For example, biomedical engineers engaged in the development of biosensors may interact with those interested in prosthetic devices to develop a means to detect and use the same bioelectric signal to power a prosthetic device. Those engaged in automating the clinical chemistry laboratory may collaborate with those developing expert systems to assist clinicians in making decisions based on specific laboratory data. The possibilities are endless.

Perhaps a greater potential benefit occurring from the use of biomedical engineering is identification of the problems and needs of our present healthcare system that can be solved using existing engineering technology and systems methodology. Consequently, the field of biomedical engineering offers hope in the continuing battle to provide high-quality care at a reasonable cost. If properly directed toward solving problems related to preventive medical approaches, ambulatory care services, and the like, biomedical engineers can provide the tools and techniques to make our healthcare system more effective and efficient; and in the process, improve the quality of life for all.

Joseph D. Bronzino
Editor-in-Chief

Editor-in-Chief

Joseph D. Bronzino received the B.S.E.E. degree from Worcester Polytechnic Institute, Worcester, MA, in 1959, the M.S.E.E. degree from the Naval Postgraduate School, Monterey, CA, in 1961, and the Ph.D. degree in electrical engineering from Worcester Polytechnic Institute in 1968. He is presently the Vernon Roosa Professor of Applied Science, an endowed chair at Trinity College, Hartford, CT and President of the Biomedical Engineering Alliance and Consortium (BEACON), which is a nonprofit organization consisting of academic and medical institutions as well as corporations dedicated to the development and commercialization of new medical technologies (for details visit www.beaconalliance.org).

He is the author of over 200 articles and 11 books including the following: *Technology for Patient Care* (C.V. Mosby, 1977), *Computer Applications for Patient Care* (Addison-Wesley, 1982), *Biomedical Engineering: Basic Concepts and Instrumentation* (PWS Publishing Co., 1986), *Expert Systems: Basic Concepts* (Research Foundation of State University of New York, 1989), *Medical Technology and Society: An Interdisciplinary Perspective* (MIT Press and McGraw-Hill, 1990), *Management of Medical Technology* (Butterworth/Heinemann, 1992), *The Biomedical Engineering Handbook* (CRC Press, 1st ed., 1995; 2nd ed., 2000; Taylor & Francis, 3rd ed., 2005), *Introduction to Biomedical Engineering* (Academic Press, 1st ed., 1999; 2nd ed., 2005).

Dr. Bronzino is a fellow of IEEE and the American Institute of Medical and Biological Engineering (AIMBE), an honorary member of the Italian Society of Experimental Biology, past chairman of the Biomedical Engineering Division of the American Society for Engineering Education (ASEE), a charter member and presently vice president of the Connecticut Academy of Science and Engineering (CASE), a charter member of the American College of Clinical Engineering (ACCE), and the Association for the Advancement of Medical Instrumentation (AAMI), past president of the IEEE-Engineering in Medicine and Biology Society (EMBS), past chairman of the IEEE Health Care Engineering Policy Committee (HCEPC), past chairman of the IEEE Technical Policy Council in Washington, DC, and presently Editor-in-Chief of Elsevier's BME Book Series and Taylor & Francis' *Biomedical Engineering Handbook*.

Dr. Bronzino is also the recipient of the Millennium Award from IEEE/EMBS in 2000 and the Goddard Award from Worcester Polytechnic Institute for Professional Achievement in June 2004.

Contributors

James J. Abbas
Center for Rehabilitation
Neuroscience and
Rehabilitation Engineering
The Biodesign Institute
Arizona State University
Tempe, Arizona

Kai-Nan An
Biomedical Laboratory
Mayo Clinic
Rochester, Minnesota

Isabel Arcos
Alfred Mann Foundation for
Scientific Research
Sylmar, California

Gary J. Baker
Stanford University
Stanford, California

Berj L. Bardakjian
Institute of Biomaterials and
Biomedical Engineering
University of Toronto
Toronto, Ontario, Canada

Roger C. Barr
Department of Biomedical
Engineering
School of Engineering
Duke University
Durham, North Carolina

A. Barriskill
Neopraxis Pty. Ltd.
Lance Cove,
N.S.W., Australia

Pamela J. Hoyes Beehler
University of Texas-Arlington
Arlington, Texas

Edward J. Berbari
Indiana University-Purdue
University
Indianapolis, Indiana

R. Betz
Shriners Hospital for Children
Philadelphia, Pennsylvania

W.C. Billotte
University of Dayton
Dayton, Ohio

Joseph D. Bronzino
Trinity College and The
Biomedical Alliance and
Consortium
Hartford, Connecticut

K.J.L. Burg
Carolinas Medical Center
Charlotte, North Carolina

Thomas J. Burkholder
School of Applied Physiology
Georgia Institute of Technology
Atlanta, Georgia

Thomas R. Canfield
Argonne National Laboratory
Argonne, Illinois

Ewart R. Carson
Centre for Health Informatics
City University
London, U.K.

Fernando Casas
Department of Biomedical
Engineering
The Cleveland Clinic Foundation
Cleveland, Ohio

Andrea Caumo
San Raffaele Scientific Institute
Milan, Italy

K.B. Chandran
Department of Biomedical
Engineering
College of Engineering
University of Iowa
Iowa City, Iowa

Chih-Chang Chu
TXA Department
Cornell University
Ithaca, New York

Ben M. Clopton
Advanced Cochlear Systems
Snoqualmie, Washington

Claudio Cobelli
Department of Information
Engineering
University of Padova
Padova, Italy

Rory A. Cooper
School of Health and
Rehabilitation Sciences
University of Pittsburgh
Pittsburgh, Pennsylvania

Derek G. Cramp
School of Management
University of Surrey
Guildford, Surrey, U.K.

Ross Davis
Neural Engineering Clinic
Melbourne Beach, Florida
Alfred Mann Foundation for
    Scientific Research
Sylmar, California

Roy B. Davis, III
Motion Analysis Laboratory
Shriners Hospital for Children
Greenville, South Carolina

Peter A. DeLuca
Gait Analysis Laboratory
University of Connecticut
    Children's Medical Center
Hartford, Connecticut

Daniel J. DiLorenzo
BioNeuronics Corporation
Seattle, Washington

Philip B. Dobrin
Hines VA Hospital and Loyola
    University Medical Center
Hines, Illinois

Cathryn R. Dooly
University of Maryland
College Park, Maryland

Gary M. Drzewiecki
Department of Biomedical
    Engineering
Rutgers University
New Brunswick, New Jersey

Dominique M. Durand
Biomedical Engineering
    Department
Neural Engineering Center
Case Western Reserve University
Cleveland, Ohio

Jeffrey T. Ellis
Department for Bioengineering
    and Biosciences
Georgia Institute of Technology
Atlanta, Georgia

John D. Enderle
Biomedical Engineering
University of Connecticut
Storrs, Connecticut

Michael J. Furey
Mechanical Engineering
    Department
Virginia Polytechnic Institute
    and State University
Blacksburg, Virginia

Vijay K. Goel
Department of Biomedical
    Engineering
University of Iowa
Iowa City, Iowa

Wallace Grant
Engineering Science and
    Mechanics Department
Virginia Polytechnic Institute
    and State University
Blacksburg, Virginia

Daniel Graupe
University of Illinois
Chicago, Illinois

Robert J. Greenberg
Second Sight
Sylmar, California

Warren M. Grill
Department of Biomedical
    Engineering
Duke University
Durham, North Carolina

Robert E. Gross
Department of Neurosurgery
Emory University
Atlanta, Georgia

Alan R. Hargens
Department of Orthopedic
    Surgery
University of California-San
    Diego
San Diego, California

Kaj-Åge Henneberg
University of Montreal
Montreal, Quebec, Canada

Katya Hill
Assistive Technology Center
Edinboro University of
    Pennsylvania
Edinboro, Pennsylvania

Douglas Hobson
University of Pittsburgh
Pittsburgh, Pennsylvania

Robert M. Hochmuth
Department of Mechanical
    Engineering
Duke University
Durham, North Carolina

T. Houdayer
Neural Engineering Clinic
Melbourne Beach, Florida

Ben F. Hurley
Department of Kinesiology
College of Health and Human
    Performance
University of Maryland
College Park, Maryland

Sheik N. Imrhan
University of Texas-Arlington
Arlington, Texas

Fiacro Jiménez
Stereotaxic and Functional
    Neurosurgery Unit
Mexico City General Hospital
Mexico City, Mexico

Arthur T. Johnson
Engineering Department
Biological Resource
University of Maryland
College Park, Maryland

Christopher R. Johnson
Department of Computer Science
University of Utah
Salt Lake City, Utah

T. Johnston
Shriners Hospital for Children
Philadelphia, Pennsylvania

Richard D. Jones
Department of Medical Physics
    and Bioengineering
Christchurch Hospital
Christchurch, New Zealand

Kurt A. Kaczmarek
Department of Rehabilitation
    Medicine
Medical Science Center
University of Wisconsin
Madison, Wisconsin

J. Lawrence Katz
School of Dentistry
University of Missouri
Kansas City, Missouri

Jessica Kaufman
Department of Biomedical
    Engineering
Boston University
Boston, Massachusetts

Kenton R. Kaufman
Biomechanical Laboratory
Mayo Clinic
Rochester, Minnesota

J.C. Keller
University of Iowa
Iowa City, Iowa

Philip R. Kennedy
Emory University
Atlanta, Georgia

Gilson Khang
Department of Polymer Science
    and Technology
Chonbuk National University
Seoul, North Korea

Young Kon Kim
Inje University
Kyungnam, North Korea

Albert I. King
Biomaterials Engineering Center
Wayne State University
Detroit, Michigan

Catherine Klapperich
Department of Biomedical
    Engineering
Boston University
Boston, Massachusetts

George V. Kondraske
Electrical and Biomedical
    Engineering
Human Performance Institute
University of Texas-Arlington
Arlington, Texas

Roderic S. Lakes
University of Wisconsin-Madison
Madison, Wisconsin

Christopher G. Lausted
The Institute for Systems Biology
Seattle, Washington

Hai Bang Lee
Biomaterials Laboratory
Korea Research Institute of
    Chemical Technology
Yusung Taejon, North Korea

Jin Ho Lee
Department of Polymer Science
    and Engineering
Hannam University
Taejon, North Korea

Jack D. Lemmon
Department of Bioengineering
    and Bioscience
Georgia Institute of Technology
Atlanta, Georgia

John K-J. Li
Department of Biomedical
    Engineering
Rutgers University
Piscataway, New Jersey

Shu-Tung Li
Collagen Matrix, Inc.
Franklin Lakes, New Jersey

Baruch B. Lieber
Department of Mechanical and
    Aerospace Engineering
State University of
    New York-Buffalo
Buffalo, New York

Richard L. Lieber
Departments of Orthopedics and
    Bioengineering
University of California
La Jolla, California

Adolfo Llinás
Pontificia Universidad Javeriana
Bogota, Colombia

Marilyn Lord
Instrument Division
Medical Engineering and Physics
King's College Hospital
London, U.K.

Jaakko Malmivuo
Ragnar Granit Institute
Tampere University of Technology
Tampere, Finland

Vasilis Z. Marmarelis
Department of Biomedical
    Engineering
University of Southern California
Los Angeles, California

Kenneth J. Maxwell
BMK Consultants
North York, Ontario, Canada

Andrew D. McCulloch
Department of Bioengineering
University of
    California-San Diego
La Jolla, California

Evangelia Micheli-Tzanakou
Department of Biomedical
    Engineering
Rutgers University
Piscataway, New Jersey

Phil Mobley
Alfred Mann Foundation for
    Scientific Research
Sylmar, California

Anette Nievies
Department of Neurology
Robert Wood Johnson Medical
    School
New Brunswick, New Jersey

Abraham Noordergraaf
Cardiovascular Studies Unit
University of Pennsylvania
Philadelphia, Pennsylvania

Gerrit J. Noordergraaf
Department of Anesthesia and
    Resuscitation
St. Elisabeth Hospital
Tilburg, Netherlands

Johnny T. Ottesen
Department of Physics and
    Mathematics
University of Roskilde
Roskilde, Denmark

Sylvia Õunpuu
Center for Motion Analysis
University of Connecticut
    Children's Medical Center
West Hartford, Connecticut

Joseph L. Palladino
Department of Engineering
Trinity College
Hartford, Connecticut

Joon B. Park
Department of Biomedical
    Engineering
University of Iowa
Iowa City, Iowa

Sang-Hyun Park
Orthopedic Research Center
Orthopedic Hospital
Los Angeles, California

Mohamad Parnianpour
Department of IWSE
Ohio State University
Columbus, Ohio

Donald R. Peterson
University of Connecticut Health
    Center
Biodynamics Laboratory
Farmington, Connecticut

Roland N. Pittman
Medical College of Virginia
Richmond, Virginia

Robert Plonsey
Department of Biomedical
    Engineering
School of Engineering
Duke University
Durham, North Carolina

Chi-Sang Poon
Division of Health Sciences and
    Technology
Massachusetts Institute of
    Technology
Cambridge, Massachusetts

Aleksander S. Popel
Department of Biomedical
    Engineering
Johns Hopkins University
Baltimore, Maryland

Dejan B. Popović
Center for Sensory Motor
    Interaction
Aalborg University
Aalborg, Denmark
Faculty of Electrical Engineering
University of Belgrade
Belgrade, Serbia and Montenegro

Mirjana B. Popović
Center for Sensory Motor
    Interaction
Aalborg University
Aalborg, Denmark
Faculty of Electrical Engineering
University of Belgrade
Belgrade, Serbia and Montenegro

Charles J. Robinson
Clarkson University and the
    Syracuse VA Medical Center
Potsdam, New York

Barry Romich
Prentke Romich Company
Wooster, Ohio

Bradley J. Roth
Department of Physics
Oakland University
Rochester, Michigan

Yiftach Roth
New Advanced Technology Center
Sheba Medical Center
Tel-Hashomer, Israel

Carl F. Rothe
Department of Physiology
    Medical Science
Indiana University
Indianapolis, Indiana

Maria Pia Saccomani
Department of Information
    Engineering
University of Padova
Padova, Italy

Gert J. Scheffer
Department of Anesthesiology
University Medical Center
Nijmegen, Netherlands

Daniel J. Schneck
Virginia Polytechnic Institute and
    State University
Blacksburg, Virginia

Wil H.A. Schilders
Department of Mathematics and
    Informatics
Technical University
Eindhoven, Netherlands

Geert W. Schmid-Schönbein
Department of Bioengineering
University of
    California-San Diego
La Jolla, California

Joe Schulman
Alfred Mann Foundation for
    Scientific Research
Sylmar, California

S.W. Shalaby
Poly-Med, Inc.
Anderson, South Carolina

Artin A. Shoukas
Department of Biomedical
    Engineering
Johns Hopkins University School
    of Medicine
Baltimore, Maryland

B. Smith
Shriners Hospital for Children
Philadelphia, Pennsylvania

Susan S. Smith
Texas Women's University
Dallas, Texas

William M. Smith
University of
    Alabama-Birmingham
Birmingham, Alabama

Giovanni Sparacino
Department of Information
    Engineering
University of Padova
Padova, Italy

Alexander A. Spector
Biomedical Engineering
Johns Hopkins University
Baltimore, Maryland

Charles R. Steele
Applied Mechanical Division
Stanford University
Stanford, California

George D. Stetten
Department of Biomedical
  Engineering
Carnegie Mellon University
Pittsburgh, Pennsylvania

Karl Syndulko
UCLA School of Medicine
Los Angeles, California

William D. Timmons
EnteraTech, Inc.
Hilliard, Ohio

Gianna Maria Toffolo
Department of Information
  Engineering
University of Padova
Padova, Italy

Jason A. Tolomeo
Stanford University
Stanford, California

Roger Tran-Son-Tay
University of Florida
Gainesville, Florida

Elaine Trefler
University of Pittsburgh
Pittsburgh, Pennsylvania

Alan Turner-Smith
King's College Hospital
London, U.K.

Gregg Vanderheiden
University of Wisconsin
Madison, Wisconsin

Anthony Varghese
Institute of Mathematics and
  Its Applications
University of Minnesota
Minneapolis, Minnesota

Paul J. Vasta
Electrical and Biomedical
  Engineering
Human Performance Institute
University of Texas-Arlington
Arlington, Texas

Ana Luisa Velasco
Stereotaxic and Functional
  Neurosurgery Unit
Mexico City General Hospital
Mexico City, Mexico

Francisco Velasco
Stereotaxic and Functional
  Neurosurgery Unit
Mexico City General Hospital
Mexico City, Mexico

Marcos Velasco
Stereotaxic and Functional
  Neurosurgery Unit
Mexico City General Hospital
Mexico City, Mexico

David C. Viano
Wayne State University
Detroit, Michigan

Herbert F. Voigt
Biomedical Engineering
  Department
Boston University
Boston, Massachusetts

Cedric F. Walker
Department of Biomedical
  Engineering
Tulane University
New Orleans, Louisiana

Richard E. Waugh
Department of Pharmacology and
  Physiology
University of Rochester Medical
  Center
Rochester, New York

Jamés Wolfe
Alfred Mann Foundation for
  Scientific Research
Sylmar, California

Joyce Y. Wong
Department of Biomedical
Boston University
Boston, Massachusetts

Ajit P. Yoganathan
Department for Bioengineering
  and Bioscience
Georgia Institute of Technology
Atlanta, Georgia

Abraham Zangen
Department of Neurobiology
Weizmann Institute of Science
Rehovot, Israel

Deborah E. Zetes-Tolomeo
Stanford University
Stanford, California

Xiaohong Zhou
Medical Center
Duke University
Durham, North Carolina

Ying Zhu
Adow Innovation
Robbinsville, New Jersey

Contents

SECTION III Bioelectric Phenomena

William M. Smith

SECTION IV   Neuroengineering

Daniel J. DiLorenzo, Cedric F. Walker, Ross Davis

SECTION V   Biomaterials

Joyce Y. Wong

SECTION VI Biomechanics

Donald R. Peterson

SECTION VII Rehabilitation Engineering

Charles J. Robinson

SECTION VIII Human Performance Engineering

George V. Kondraske

SECTION IX   Ethics

Joseph D. Bronzino

I

Physiologic Systems

Herbert F. Voigt
Boston University

THE *BIOMEDICAL ENGINEERING HANDBOOK* is an ambitious project to identify and catalogue the many intersections of engineering and the life sciences. The Physiologic Systems section is an attempt to describe a number of systems that have benefited from joining engineering and physiologic approaches to understanding. The "systems approach" to biology and physiology has been one of engineering's gifts to the investigator of life's secrets. There are literally endless biological and physiological systems; however, those still await careful engineering analysis and modeling. Much has been done, but so much more remains to be done.

As Robert Plonsey so aptly put it, "While the application of engineering expertise to the life sciences requires an obvious knowledge of contemporary technical theory and its applications, it also demands an adequate knowledge and understanding of relevant medicine and biology. It has been argued that the most challenging part of finding engineering solutions to problems lies in the formulation of the solution in engineering terms. In Biomedical engineering, this usually demands a full understanding of the life science substrates as well as the quantitative methodologies."

In this section, careful selections of systems that have benefited from a system's approach are offered. Because of space limitations, we are unable to offer more. We trust that these selections will provide information that will enhance the sections that follow.

1

An Outline of Cardiovascular Structure and Function

Daniel J. Schneck
*Virginia Polytechnic Institute and
State University*

Because not every cell in the human body is near enough to the environment to easily exchange with it's mass (including nutrients, oxygen, carbon dioxide, and the waste products of metabolism), energy (including heat), and momentum, the physiologic system is endowed with a major highway network — organized to make available thousands of miles of access tubing for the transport to and from a different neighborhood (on the order of 10 μm or less) of any given cell whatever it needs to sustain life. This highway network, called the *cardiovascular system*, includes a pumping station, the heart; a working fluid, blood; a complex branching configuration of distributing and collecting pipes and channels, blood vessels; and a sophisticated means for both intrinsic (inherent) and extrinsic (autonomic and endocrine) control.

1.1   The Working Fluid: Blood

Accounting for about $8 \pm 1\%$ of total body weight, averaging 5200 ml, blood is a complex, heterogeneous suspension of formed elements — the *blood cells*, or *hematocytes* — suspended in a continuous, straw-colored fluid called *plasma*. Nominally, the composite fluid has a mass density of 1.057 ± 0.007 g/cm^3, and it is three to six times as viscous as water. The hematocytes (Table 1.1) include three basic types of cells: red blood cells (erythrocytes, totalling nearly 95% of the formed elements), white blood cells (leukocytes, averaging <0.15% of all hematocytes), and platelets (thrombocytes, on the order of 5% of all blood cells). Hematocytes are all derived in the active ("red") bone marrow (about 1500 g) of adults from undifferentiated **stem cells** called *hemocytoblasts*, and all reach ultimate maturity via a process called *hematocytopoiesis*.

TABLE 1.1 Hematocytes

Cell type	Number cells per mm³ blood[a]	Corpuscular diameter (μm)[a]	Corpuscular surface area (μm²)[a]	Corpuscular volume (μm³)[a]	Mass density (g/cm³)[a]	Percent water[a]	Percent protein[a]	Percent extractives[a,b]
Erythrocytes (red blood cells)	4.2–5.4 × 10⁶ ♀ 4.6–6.2 × 10⁶ ♂ (5 × 10⁶)	6–9 (7.5) Thickness 1.84–2.84 "Neck" 0.81–1.44	120–163 (140)	80–100 (90)	1.089–1.100 (1.098)	64–68 (66)	29–35 (32)	1.6–2.8 (2)
Leukocytes (white blood cells)	4,000–11,000 (7,500)	6–10	300–625	160–450	1.055–1.085	52–60 (56)	30–36 (33)	4–18 (11)
Granulocytes								
Neutrophils: 55–70% WBC (65%)	2–6 × 10³ (4,875)	8–8.6 (8.3)	422–511 (467)	268–333 (300)	1.075–1.085 (1.080)	—	—	—
Eosinophils: 1–4% WBC (3%)	45–480 (225)	8–9 (8.5)	422–560 (491)	268–382 (321)	1.075–1.085 (1.080)	—	—	—
Basophils: 0–1.5% WBC (1%)	0–113 (75)	7.7–8.5 (8.1)	391–500 (445)	239–321 (278)	1.075–1.085 (1.080)	—	—	—
Agranulocytes								
Lymphocytes: 20–35% WBC (25%)	1,000–4,800 (1875)	6.75–7.34 (7.06)	300–372 (336)	161–207 (184)	1.055–1.070 (1.063)	—	—	—
Monocytes: 3–8% WBC (6%)	100–800 (450)	9–9.5 (9.25)	534–624 (579)	382–449 (414)	1.055–1.070 (1.063)	—	—	—
Thrombocytes (platelets)	(1.4 ♂), 2.14 (♀) –5 × 10⁵ (2.675 × 10⁵)	2–4 (3) Thickness 0.9–1.3	16–35 (25)	5–10 (7.5)	1.04–1.06 (1.05)	60–68 (64)	32–40 (36)	Neg.

[a] Normal physiologic range, with "typical" value in parentheses.
[b] Extractives include mostly minerals (ash), carbohydrates, and fats (lipids).

The primary function of erythrocytes is to aid in the transport of blood gases — about 30 to 34% (by weight) of each cell consisting of the oxygen- and carbon dioxide-carrying protein hemoglobin ($64,000 \leq MW \leq 68,000$) and a small portion of the cell containing the enzyme carbonic anhydrase, which catalyzes the reversible formation of carbonic acid from carbon dioxide and water. The primary function of leukocytes is to endow the human body with the ability to identify and dispose of foreign substances such as infectious organisms) that do not belong there — agranulocytes (lymphocytes and monocytes) essentially doing the "identifying" and granulocytes (neutrophils, basophils, and eosinophils) essentially doing the "disposing." The primary function of platelets is to participate in the blood clotting process.

Removal of all hematocytes from blood centrifugation or other separating techniques leaves behind the aqueous (91% water by weight, 94.8% water by volume), saline (0.15 N) suspending medium called *plasma* — which has an average mass density of 1.035 ± 0.005 g/cm^3 and a viscosity $1\frac{1}{2}$ to 2 times that of water. Some 6.5 to 8% by weight of plasma consists of the plasma proteins, of which there are three major types — albumin, the globulins, and fibrinogen — and several of lesser prominence (Table 1.2).

The primary functions of albumin are to help maintain the osmotic (oncotic) transmural pressure differential that ensures proper mass exchange between blood and interstitial fluid at the capillary level and to serve as a transport carrier molecule for several hormones and other small biochemical constituents (such as some metal ions). The primary function of the globulin class of proteins is to act as transport carrier molecules (mostly of the α and β class) for large biochemical substances, such as fats (lipoproteins) and certain carbohydrates (muco- and glycoproteins) and heavy metals (mineraloproteins), and to work together with leukocytes in the body's immune system. The latter function is primarily the responsibility of the γ class of immunoglobulins, which have antibody activity. The primary function of fibrinogen is to work with thrombocytes in the formation of a blood clot — a process also aided by one of the most abundant of the lesser proteins, prothrombin (MW $\simeq 62,000$).

Of the remaining 2% or so (by weight) of plasma, just under half (0.95%, or 983 mg/dl plasma) consists of minerals (inorganic ash), trace elements, and electrolytes, mostly the cations sodium, potassium, calcium, and magnesium and the anions chlorine, bicarbonate, phosphate, and sulfate — the latter three helping as buffers to maintain the fluid at a slightly alkaline pH between 7.35 and 7.45 (average 7.4). What is left, about 1087 mg of material per deciliter of plasma, includes (1) mainly (0.8% by weight) three major types of fat, that is, cholesterol (in a free and esterified form), phospholipid (a major ingredient of cell membranes), and triglyceride, with lesser amounts of the fat-soluble vitamins (A, D, E, and K), free fatty acids, and other lipids, and (2) "extractives" (0.25% by weight), of which about two-thirds includes glucose and other forms of carbohydrate, the remainder consisting of the water-soluble vitamins (B-complex and C), certain enzymes, nonnitrogenous and nitrogenous waste products of metabolism (including urea, creatine, and creatinine), and many smaller amounts of other biochemical constituents — the list seeming virtually endless.

Removal from blood of all hematocytes and the protein fibrinogen (by allowing the fluid to completely clot before centrifuging) leaves behind a clear fluid called *serum*, which has a density of about 1.018 ± 0.003 g/cm^3 and a viscosity up to $1\frac{1}{2}$ times that of water. A glimpse of Table 1.1 and Table 1.2, together with the very brief summary presented above, nevertheless gives the reader an immediate appreciation for why blood is often referred to as the "river of life." This river is made to flow through the vascular piping network by two central pumping stations arranged in series: the left and right sides of the human heart.

1.2 The Pumping Station: The Heart

Barely the size of the clenched fist of the individual in whom it resides — an inverted, conically shaped, hollow muscular organ measuring 12 to 13 cm from base (top) to apex (bottom) and 7 to 8 cm at its widest point and weighing just under 0.75 lb (about 0.474% of the individual's body weight, or some 325 g) — the human heart occupies a small region between the third and sixth ribs in the central portion of the thoracic cavity of the body. It rests on the diaphragm, between the lower part of the two lungs, its

TABLE 1.2 Plasma

Constituent	Concentration range (mg/dl plasma)	Typical plasma value (mg/dl)	Molecular weight range	Typical value	Typical size (nm)
Total protein, 7% by weight	6400–8300	7245	21,000–1,200,000	—	—
Albumin (56% TP)	2800–5600	4057	66,500–69,000	69,000	15 × 4
α_1-Globulin (5.5% TP)	300–600	400	21,000–435,000	60,000	5–12
α_2-Globulin (7.5% TP)	400–900	542	100,000–725,000	200,000	50–500
β-Globulin (13% TP)	500–1230	942	90,000–1,200,000	100,000	18–50
γ-Globulin (12% TP)	500–1800	869	150,000–196,000	150,000	23 × 4
Fibrinogen (4% TP)	150–470	290	330,000–450,000	390,000	(50–60) × (3–8)
Other (2% TP)	70–210	145	70,000–1,000,000	200,000	(15–25) × (2–6)
Inorganic ash, 0.95% by weight	930–1140	983	20–100	—	—
					(Radius)
Sodium	300–340	325	—	22.98977	0.102 (Na^+)
Potassium	13–21	17	—	39.09800	0.138 (K^+)
Calcium	8.4–11.0	10	—	40.08000	0.099 (Ca^{2+})
Magnesium	1.5–3.0	2	—	24,30500	0.072 (Mg^{2+})
Chloride	336–390	369	—	35.45300	0.181 (Cl^-)
Bicarbonate	110–240	175	—	61.01710	0.163 (HCO_3^-)
Phosphate	2.7–4.5	3.6	—	95.97926	0.210 (HPO_4^{2-})
Sulfate	0.5–1.5	1.0	—	96.05760	0.230 (SO_4^{2-})
Other	0–100	80.4	20–100	—	0.1–0.3
Lipids (fats), 0.80% by weight	541–1000	828	44,000–3,200,000	= Lipoproteins	Up to 200 or more
Cholesterol (34% TL)	12–105 "free"	59	386.67	Contained mostly in intermediate to LDL β-lipoproteins; higher in women	
	72–259 esterified,	224			
	84–364 "total"	283			
Phospholipid (35% TL)	150–331	292	690–1,010	Contained mainly in HDL to VHDL α_1-lipoproteins	
Triglyceride (26% TL)	65–240	215	400–1,370	Contained mainly in VLDL α_2-lipoproteins and chylomicrons	
Other (5% TL)	0–80	38	280–1,500	Fat-soluble vitamins, prostaglandins, fatty acids	
Extractives, 0.25% by weight	200–500	259	—	—	—
Glucose	60–120, fasting	90	—	180.1572	0.86 D
Urea	20–30	25	—	60.0554	0.36 D
Carbohydrate	60–105	83	180.16–342.3	—	0.74–0.108 D
Other	11–111	61	—	—	—

base-to-apex axis leaning mostly toward the left side of the body and slightly forward. The heart is divided by a tough muscular wall — the interatrial-interventricular septum — into a somewhat crescent-shaped right side and cylindrically shaped left side (Figure 1.1), each being one self-contained pumping station, but the two being connected in series. The left side of the heart drives oxygen-rich blood through the aortic semilunar outlet valve into the *systemic circulation,* which carries the fluid to within a differential neighborhood of each cell in the body — from which it returns to the right side of the heart low in oxygen and rich in carbon dioxide. The right side of the heart then drives this oxygen-poor blood through the pulmonary semilunar (pulmonic) outlet valve into the *pulmonary circulation,* which carries the fluid to the lungs — where its oxygen supply is replenished and its carbon dioxide content is purged before it returns to the left side of the heart to begin the cycle all over again. Because of the anatomic proximity of the heart to the lungs, the right side of the heart does not have to work very hard to drive

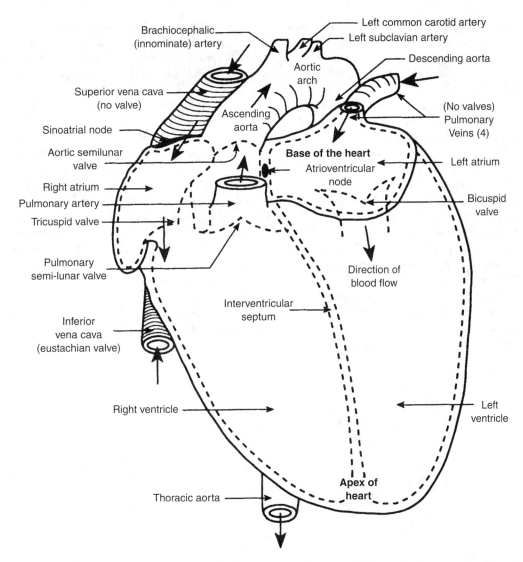

FIGURE 1.1 Anterior view of the human heart showing the four chambers, the inlet and outlet valves, the inlet and outlet major blood vessels, the wall separating the right side from the left side, and the two cardiac pacing centers — the **sinoatrial node** and the **atrioventricular node**. Boldface arrows show the direction of flow through the heart chambers, the valves, and the major vessels.

blood through the pulmonary circulation, so it functions as a low-pressure ($P \leq 40$ mmHg gauge) pump compared with the left side of the heart, which does most of its work at a high pressure (up to 140 mmHg gauge or more) to drive blood through the entire systemic circulation to the furthest extremes of the organism.

Each cardiac (heart) pump is further divided into two chambers: a small upper receiving chamber, or atrium (auricle), separated by a one-way valve from a lower discharging chamber, or ventricle, which is about twice the size of its corresponding atrium. In order of size, the somewhat spherically shaped left atrium is the smallest chamber — holding about 45 ml of blood (at rest), operating at pressures on the order of 0 to 25 mmHg gauge, and having a wall thickness of about 3 mm. The pouch-shaped right atrium is next (63 ml of blood, 0 to 10 mmHg gauge of pressure, 2-mm wall thickness), followed by the conical/cylindrically shaped left ventricle (100 ml of blood, up to 140 mmHg gauge of pressure, variable wall thickness up to 12 mm) and the crescent-shaped right ventricle (about 130 ml of blood, up to 40 mmHg gauge of pressure, and a wall thickness on the order of one-third that of the left ventricle, up to about 4 mm). All together, then, the heart chambers collectively have a capacity of some 325 to 350 ml, or about 6.5% of the total blood volume in a "typical" individual — but these values are nominal, since the organ alternately fills and expands, contracts, and then empties as it generates a *cardiac output*.

During the 480-msec or so filling phase — diastole — of the average 750-msec cardiac cycle, the inlet valves of the two ventricles (3.8-cm-diameter tricuspid valve from right atrium to right ventricle; 3.1-cm-diameter bicuspid or mitral valve from left atrium to left ventricle) are open, and the outlet valves (2.4-cm-diameter pulmonary valve and 2.25-cm-diameter aortic semilunar valve, respectively) are closed — the heart ultimately expanding to its end-diastolic-volume (EDV), which is on the order of 140 ml of blood for the left ventricle. During the 270-msec emptying phase — systole — electrically induced vigorous contraction of **cardiac muscle** drives the intraventricular pressure up, forcing the one-way inlet valves closed and the unidirectional outlet valves open as the heart contracts to its end-systolic-volume (ESV), which is typically on the order of 70 ml of blood for the left ventricle. Thus the ventricles normally empty about half their contained volume with each heart beat, the remainder being termed the *cardiac reserve volume*. More generally, the difference between the *actual* EDV and the *actual* ESV, called the *stroke volume* (SV), is the volume of blood expelled from the heart during each systolic interval, and the ratio of SV to EDV is called the *cardiac ejection fraction*, or *ejection ratio* (0.5–0.75 is normal, 0.4–0.5 signifies mild cardiac damage, 0.25–0.40 implies moderate heart damage, and <0.25 warms of severe damage to the heart's pumping ability). If the stroke volume is multiplied by the number of systolic intervals per minute, or heart (HR), one obtains the total cardiac output (CO):

$$CO = HR \times (EDV - ESV) \qquad (1.1)$$

Dawson [1991] has suggested that the cardiac output (in milliliters per minute) is proportional to the weight W (in kilograms) of an individual according to the equation

$$CO - 224W^{3/4} \qquad (1.2)$$

and that "normal" heart rate obeys very closely the relation

$$HR = 229W^{-1/4} \qquad (1.3)$$

For a "typical" 68.7-kg individual (blood volume = 5200 ml), Equation 1.1, Equation 1.2, and Equation 1.3 yield CO = 5345 ml/min, HR = 80 beats/min (cardiac cycle period = 754 msec) and SV = CO/HR = $224W^{3/4}/229W^{-1/4}$ = $0.978W$ = 67.2 ml/beat, which are very reasonable values. Furthermore, assuming this individual lives about 75 years, his or her heart will have cycled over 3.1536 billion times, pumping a total of 0.2107 billion liters of blood (55.665 million gallons, or 8134 quarts per day) — all of it emptying into the circulatory pathways that constitute the vascular system.

1.3   The Piping Network: Blood Vessels

The vascular system is divided by a microscopic capillary network into an upstream, high-pressure, efferent arterial side (Table 1.3) — consisting of relatively thick-walled, viscoelastic tubes that carry blood away from the heart — and a downstream, low-pressure, afferent venous side (Table 1.4) — consisting of correspondingly thinner (but having a larger caliber) elastic conduits that return blood back to the heart. Except for their differences in thickness, the walls of the largest arteries and veins consist of the same three distinct, well-defined, and well-developed layers. From innermost to outermost, these layers are (1) the thinnest *tunica intima*, a continuous lining (the vascular **endothelium**) consisting of a single layer of simple

TABLE 1.3 Arterial System[a]

Blood vessel type	(Systemic) typical number	Internal diameter range	Length Range[b]	Wall thickness	Systemic volume	(Pulmonary) typical number	Pulmonary volume
Aorta	1	1.0–3.0 cm	30–65 cm	2–3 mm	156 ml	—	—
Pulmonary artery	—	2.5–3.1 cm	6–9 cm	2–3 cm	—	1	52 ml
Wall morphology: Complete tunica adventitia, external elastic lamina, tunica media, internal elastic lamina, tunica intima, subendothelium, endothelium, and vasa vasorum vascular supply							
Main branches	32	5 mm–2.25 cm	3.3–6 cm	≃2 mm	83.2 ml	6	41.6 ml
(Along with the aorta and pulmonary artery, the largest, most well-developed of all blood vessels)							
Large arteries	288	4.0–5.0 mm	1.4–2.8 cm	≃1 mm	104 ml	64	23.5 ml
(A well-developed tunica adventitia and vasa vasorum, although wall layers are gradually thinning)							
Medium arteries	1152	2.5–4.0 mm	1.0–2.2 cm	≃0.75 mm	117 ml	144	7.3 ml
Small arteries	3456	1.0–2.5 mm	0.6–1.7 cm	≃0.50 mm	104 ml	432	5.7 ml
Tributaries	20,736	0.5–1.0 mm	0.3–1.3 cm	≃0.25 mm	91 ml	5184	7.3 ml
(Well-developed tunica media and external elastic lamina, but tunica adventitia virtually nonexistent)							
Small rami	82,944	250–500 μm	0.2–0.8 cm	≃125 μm	57.2 ml	11,664	2.3 ml
Terminal branches	497,664	100–250 μm	1.0–6.0 mm	≃60 μm	52 ml	139,968	3.0 ml
(A well-developed endothelium, subendothelium, and internal elastic lamina, plus about two to three 15-μm-thick concentric layers forming just a very thin tunica media; no external elastic lamina)							
Arterioles	18,579,456	25–100 μm	0.2–3.8 mm	≃20–30 μm	52 ml	4,094,064	2.3 ml
Wall morphology: More than one smooth muscle layer (with nerve association in the outermost muscle layer), a well-developed internal elastic lamina; gradually thinning in 25- to 50-μm vessels to a single layer of smooth muscle tissue, connective tissue, and scant supporting tissue							
Metarterioles	238,878,720	10–25 μm	0.1–1.8 mm	≃5–15 μm	41.6 ml	157,306,536	4.0 ml
(Well-developed subendothelium; discontinuous contractile muscle elements; one layer of connective tissue)							
Capillaries	16,124,431,360	3.5–10 μm	0.5–1.1 mm	≃0.5–1 μm	260 ml	3,218,406,696	104 ml
(Simple endothelial tubes devoid of smooth muscle tissue; one-cell-layer-thick walls)							

[a] Vales are approximate for a 68.7-kg individual having a total blood volume of 5200 ml.

[b] Average uninterrupted distance between branch origins (except aorta and pulmonary artery, which are total length).

TABLE 1.4 Venous System

Blood vessel type	(Systemic) Typical number	Internal diameter range	Length range	Wall thickness	Systemic volume	(Pulmonary) Typical number	Pulmonary volume
Postcapillary venules	4,408,161,734	8–30 μm	0.1–0.6 mm	1.0–5.0 μm	166.7 ml	306,110,016	10.4 ml
(Wall consists of thin endothelium exhibiting occasional pericytes (pericapillary connective tissue cells) which increase in number as the vessel lumen gradually increases)							
Collecting venules	160,444,500	30–50 μm	0.1–0.8 mm	5.0–10 μm	161.3 ml	8,503,056	1.2 ml
(One complete layer of pericytes, one complete layer of veil cells (veil-like cells forming a thin membrane), occasional primitive smooth muscle tissue fibers that increase in number with vessel size)							
Muscular venules	32,088,900	50–100 μm	0.2–1.0 mm	10–25 μm	141.8 ml	3,779,136	3.7 ml
(Relatively thick wall of smooth muscle tissue)							
Small collecting veins	10,241,508	100–200 μm	0.5–3.2 mm	$\simeq$30 μm	329.6 ml	419,904	6.7 ml
(Prominent tunica media of continuous layers of smooth muscle cells)							
Terminal branches	496,900	200–600 μm	1.0–6.0 mm	30–150 μm	206.6 ml	34,992	5.2 ml
(A well-developed endothelium, subendothelium, and internal elastic lamina; well-developed tunica media but fewer elastic fibers than corresponding arteries and much thinner walls)							
Small veins	19,968	600 μm–1.1 mm	2.0–9.0 mm	$\simeq$0.25 mm	63.5 ml	17,280	44.9 ml
Medium veins	512	1–5 mm	1–2 cm	$\simeq$0.50 mm	67.0 ml	144	22.0 ml
Large veins	256	5–9 mm	1.4–3.7 cm	$\simeq$0.75 mm	476.1 ml	48	29.5 ml
(Well-developed wall layers comparable to large arteries but about 25% thinner)							
Main branches	224	9.0 mm–2.0 cm	2.0–10 cm	$\simeq$1.00 mm	1538.1 ml	16	39.4 ml
(Along with the vena cava and pulmonary veins, the largest, most well-developed of all blood vessels)							
Vena cava	1	2.0–3.5 cm	20–50 cm	$\simeq$1.50 mm	125.3 ml	—	—
Pulmonary veins	—	1.7–2.5 cm	5–8 cm	$\simeq$1.50 mm	—	4	52 ml

Wall morphology: Essentially the same as comparable major arteries but a much thinner tunica intima, a much thinner tunica media, and a somewhat thicker tunica adventitia; contains a vasa vasorum

Total systemic blood volume: 4394 ml — 84.5% of total blood volume; 19.5% in arteries (~3:2 large:small), 5.9% in capillaries, 74.6% in veins (~3:1 large:small); 63% of volume is in vessels greater than 1 mm internal diameter.

Total pulmonary blood volume: 468 ml — 9.0% of total blood volume; 31.8% in arteries, 22.2% in capillaries, 46% in veins; 58.3% of volume is in vessels greater than 1 mm internal diameter; remainder of blood in heart, about 338 ml (6.5% of total blood volume).

squamous (thin, sheetlike) endothelial cells "glued" together by a polysaccharide (sugar) intercellular matrix, surrounded by a thin layer of subendothelial connective tissue interlaced with a number of circularly arranged elastic fibers to form the subendothelium, and separated from the next adjacent wall layer by a thick elastic band called the *internal elastic lamina*, (2) the thickest *tunica media*, composed of numerous circularly arranged elastic fibers, especially prevalent in the largest blood vessels on the arterial side (allowing them to expand during systole and to recoil passively during diastole), a significant amount of smooth muscle cells arranged in spiraling layers around the vessel wall, especially prevalent in medium-sized arteries and arterioles (allowing them to function as control points for blood distribution), and some interlacing collagenous connective tissue, elastic fibers, and intercellular mucopolysaccharide substance (extractives), all separated from the next adjacent wall layer by another thick elastic band called the *external elastic lamina*, and (3) the medium-sized *tunica adventitia*, an outer vascular sheath consisting entirely of connective tissue.

The largest blood vessels, such as the aorta, the pulmonary artery, the pulmonary veins, and others, have such thick walls that they require a separate network of tiny blood vessels — the vasa vasorum — just to service the vascular tissue itself. As one moves toward the capillaries from the arterial side (see Table 1.3), the vascular wall keeps thinning, as if it were shedding 15-μm-thick, onion-peel-like concentric layers, and while the percentage of water in the vessel wall stays relatively constant at 70% (by weight), the ratio of elastin to collagen decreases (actually reverses) — from 3 : 2 in large arteries (9% elastin, 6% collagen, by weight) to 1 : 2 in small tributaries (5% elastin, 10% collagen) — and the amount of smooth muscle tissue increases from 7.5% by weight of large arteries (the remaining 7.5% consisting of various extractives) to 15% in small tributaries. By the time one reaches the capillaries, one encounters single-cell-thick endothelial tubes — devoid of any smooth muscle tissue, elastin, or collagen — downstream of which the vascular wall gradually "reassembles itself," layer-by-layer, as it directs blood back to the heart through the venous system (Table 1.4).

Blood vessel structure is directly related to function. The thick-walled large arteries and main *distributing branches* are designed to withstand the pulsating 80 to 130 mmHg blood pressures that they must endure. The smaller elastic *conducting vessels* need only operate under steadier blood pressures in the range 70 to 90 mmHg, but they must be thin enough to penetrate and course through organs without unduly disturbing the anatomic integrity of the mass involved. Controlling arterioles operate at blood pressures between 45 and 70 mmHg but are heavily endowed with smooth muscle tissue (hence their being referred to as *muscular vessels*) so that they may be actively shut down when flow to the capillary bed they service is to be restricted (for whatever reason), and the smallest capillary *resistance vessels* (which operate at blood pressures on the order of 10 to 45 mmHg) are designed to optimize conditions for transport to occur between blood and the surrounding interstitial fluid. Traveling back up the venous side, one encounters relatively steady blood pressures continuously decreasing from around 30 mmHg all the way down to near zero, so these vessels can be thin-walled without disease consequence. However, the low blood pressure, slower, steady (time-dependent) flow, thin walls, and larger caliber that characterize the venous system cause blood to tend to "pool" in veins, allowing them to act somewhat like reservoirs. It is not surprising, then, that at any given instant, one normally finds about two-thirds of the total human blood volume residing in the venous system, the remaining one-third being divided among the heart (6.5%), the microcirculation (7% in systemic and pulmonary capillaries), and the arterial system (19.5 to 20%).

In a global sense, then, one can think of the human cardiovascular system — using an electrical analogy — as a voltage source (the heart), two capacitors (a large venous system and a smaller arterial system), and a resistor (the microcirculation taken as a whole). Blood flow and the dynamics of the system represent electrical inductance (inertia), and useful engineering approximations can be derived from such a simple model. The cardiovascular system is designed to bring blood to within a capillary size of each and every one of the more than 10^{14} cells of the body — but *which* cells receive blood at any given time, *how much* blood they get, the *composition* of the fluid coursing by them, and related physiologic considerations are all matters that are not left up to chance.

1.4   Cardiovascular Control

Blood flows through organs and tissues either to nourish and sanitize them or to be itself processed in some sense — for example, to be oxygenated (pulmonary circulation), stocked with nutrients (splanchnic circulation), dialyzed (renal circulation), cooled (cutaneous circulation), filtered of dilapidated red blood cells (splenic circulation), and so on. Thus any given vascular network normally receives blood according to the metabolic needs of the region it perfuses and/or the function of that region as a blood treatment plant and/or thermoregulatory pathway. However, it is not feasible to expect that our physiologic transport system can be "all things to all cells all of the time" — especially when resources are scarce and/or time is a factor. Thus the distribution of blood is further prioritized according to three basic criteria (1) how essential the perfused region is to the maintenance of life itself (e.g., we can survive without an arm, a leg, a stomach, or even a large portion of our small intestine but not without a brain, a heart, and at least one functioning kidney and lung, (2) how essential the perfused region is in allowing the organism to respond to a life-threatening situation (e.g., digesting a meal is among the least of the body's concerns in a "fight or flight" circumstance), and (3) how well the perfused region can function and survive on a decreased supply of blood (e.g., some tissues — like striated skeletal and smooth muscle — have significant anaerobic capability; others — like several forms of connective tissue — can function quite effectively at a significantly decreased metabolic rate when necessary; some organs — like the liver — are larger than they really need to be; and some anatomic structures — like the eyes, ears, and limbs — have duplicates, giving them a built-in redundancy).

Within this generalized prioritization scheme, control of cardiovascular function is accomplished by mechanisms that are based either on the inherent physicochemical attributes of the tissues and organs themselves — so-called intrinsic control — or on responses that can be attributed to the effects on cardiovascular tissues of other organ systems in the body (most notably the **autonomic nervous system** and the **endocrine system**) — so-called extrinsic control. For example, the accumulation of wastes and depletion of oxygen and nutrients that accompany the increased rate of metabolism in an active tissue both lead to an *intrinsic* relaxation of local **precapillary sphincters** (rings of muscle) — with a consequent widening of corresponding capillary entrances — which reduces the local resistance to flow and thereby allows more blood to perfuse the active region. On the other hand, the *extrinsic* innervation by the autonomic nervous system of smooth muscle tissues in the walls of arterioles allows the central nervous system to completely shut down the flow to entire vascular beds (such as the cutaneous circulation) when this becomes necessary (such as during exposure to extremely cold environments).

In addition to prioritizing and controlling the *distribution* of blood, physiologic regulation of cardiovascular function is directed mainly at four other variables: cardiac output, blood pressure, blood volume, and blood composition. From Equation 1.1 we see that cardiac output can be increased by increasing the heart rate (a **chronotropic** effect), increasing the end-diastolic volume (allowing the heart to fill longer by delaying the onset of systole), decreasing the end-systolic volume (an **inotropic** effect), or doing all three things at once. Indeed, under the extrinsic influence of the sympathetic nervous system and the adrenal glands, HR can triple — to some 240 beats/min if necessary — EDV can increase by as much as 50% — to around 200 ml or more of blood — and ESV and decrease a comparable amount (the cardiac reserve) — to about 30 to 35 ml or less. The combined result of all three effects can lead to over a sevenfold increase in cardiac output — from the normal 5 to 5.5 l/min to as much as 40 to 41 l/min or more for very brief periods of strenuous exertion.

The control of blood pressure is accomplished mainly by adjusting at the arteriolar level the downstream resistance to flow — an increased resistance leading to a rise in arterial backpressure, and vice versa. This effect is conveniently quantified by a fluid-dynamic analogue to Ohm's famous $E = IR$ law in electromagnetic theory, voltage drop E being equated to fluid pressure drop ΔP, electric current I corresponding to flow — cardiac output (CO) — and electric resistance R being associated with an analogous vascular "peripheral resistance" (PR). Thus one may write

$$\Delta P = (CO)(PR) \tag{1.4}$$

Normally, the total systemic peripheral resistance is 15 to 20 mmHg/l/min of flow but can increase significantly under the influence of the vasomotor center located in the medulla of the brain, which controls arteriolar muscle tone.

The control of blood volume is accomplished mainly through the excretory function of the kidney. For example, antidiuretic hormone (ADH) secreted by the pituitary gland acts to prevent renal fluid loss (excretion via urination) and thus increases plasma volume, whereas perceived extracellular fluid overloads such as those which result from the peripheral vasoconstriction response to cold stress lead to a sympathetic/adrenergic receptor-induced renal diuresis (urination) that tends to decrease plasma volume — if not checked, to sometimes dangerously low dehydration levels. Blood composition, too, is maintained primarily through the activity of endocrine hormones and enzymes that enhance or repress specific biochemical pathways. Since these pathways are too numerous to itemize here, suffice it to say that in the body's quest for **homeostasis** and stability, virtually nothing is left to chance, and every biochemical end can be arrived at through a number of alternative means. In a broader sense, as the organism strives to maintain life, it coordinates a wide variety of different functions, and central to its ability to do just that is the role played by the cardiovascular system in transporting mass, energy, and momentum.

Defining Terms

Atrioventricular (AV) node: A highly specialized cluster of neuromuscular cells at the lower portion of the right atrium leading to the interventricular septum; the AV node delays sinoatrial, (SA) node-generated electrical impulses momentarily (allowing the atria to contract first) and then conducts the depolarization wave to the bundle of His and its bundle branches.

Autonomic nervous system: The functional division of the nervous system that innervates most glands, the heart, and smooth muscle tissue in order to maintain the internal environment of the body.

Cardiac muscle: Involuntary muscle possessing much of the anatomic attributes of skeletal voluntary muscle and some of the physiologic attributes of involuntary smooth muscle tissue; SA node-induced contraction of its interconnected network of fibers allows the heart to expel blood during systole.

Chronotropic: Affecting the periodicity of a recurring action, such as the slowing (bradycardia) or speeding up (tachycardia) of the heartbeat that results from extrinsic control of the SA node.

Endocrine system: The system of ductless glands and organs secreting substances directly into the blood to produce a specific response from another "target" organ or body part.

Endothelium: Flat cells that line the innermost surfaces of blood and lymphatic vessels and the heart.

Homeostasis: A tendency to uniformity or stability in an organism by maintaining within narrow limits certain variables that are critical to life.

Inotropic: Affecting the contractility of muscular tissue, such as the increase in cardiac *power* that results from extrinsic control of the myocardial musculature.

Precapillary sphincters: Rings of smooth muscle surrounding the entrance to capillaries where they branch off from upstream metarterioles. Contraction and relaxation of these sphincters close and open the access to downstream blood vessels, thus controlling the irrigation of different capillary networks.

Sinoatrial (SA) node: Neuromuscular tissue in the right atrium near where the superior vena cava joins the posterior right atrium (the sinus venarum); the SA node generates electrical impulses that initiate the heartbeat, hence its nickname the cardiac "pacemaker."

Stem cells: A generalized parent cell spawning descendants that become individually specialized.

Acknowledgments

The author gratefully acknowledges the assistance of Professor Robert Hochmuth in the preparation of Table 1.1 and the Radford Community Hospital for their support of the Biomedical Engineering Program at Virginia Tech.

References

Bhagavan, N.V. 1992. *Medical Biochemistry*. Boston, Jones and Bartlett.

Beall, H.P.T., Needham, D., and Hochmuth, R.M. 1993. Volume and osmotic properties of human neutrophils. *Blood* 81: 2774–2780.

Caro, C.G., Pedley, T.J., Schroter, R.C., and Seed, W.A. 1978. *The Mechanics of the Circulation*. New York, Oxford University Press.

Chandran, K.B. 1992. *Cardiovascular Biomechanics*. New York, New York University Press.

Frausto da Silva, J.J.R. and Williams, R.J.P. 1993. *The Biological Chemistry of the Elements*. New York, Oxford University Press/Clarendon.

Dawson, T.H. 1991. *Engineering Design of the Cardiovascular System of Mammals*. Englewood Cliffs, NJ, Prentice-Hall.

Duck, F.A. 1990. *Physical Properties of Tissue*. San Diego, Academic Press.

Kaley, G. and Altura, B.M. (Eds.). *Microcirculation*, Vol. I (1977), Vol. II (1978), Vol. III (1980). Baltimore, University Park Press.

Kessel, R.G. and Kardon, R.H. 1979. *Tissue and Organs — A Text-Atlas of Scanning Electron Microscopy*. San Francisco, WH Freeman.

Lentner, C. (Ed.). 1984. *Geigy Scientific Tables, vol 3: Physical Chemistry, Composition of Blood, Hematology and Somatometric Data*, 8th ed. New Jersey, Ciba-Geigy.

Lentner, C. 1990. *Heart and Circulation*, 8th ed., Vol. 5. New Jersey, Ciba-Geigy.

Schneck, D.J. 1990. *Engineering Principles of Physiologic Function*. New York, New York University Press.

Tortora, G.J. and Grabowski, S.R. 1993. *Principles of Anatomy and Physiology*, 7th ed. New York, HarperCollins.

2

Endocrine System

Derek G. Cramp
University of Surrey

Ewart R. Carson
City University-London

2.1 Introduction

The body, if it is to achieve optimal performance, must possess mechanisms for sensing and responding appropriately to numerous biologic cues and signals in order to control and maintain its internal environment. This complex role is effected by the integrative action of the endocrine and neural systems. The endocrine contribution is achieved through a highly sophisticated set of communication and control systems involving signal generation, propagation, recognition, transduction, and response. The signal entities are chemical messengers or hormones that are distributed through the body mainly by the blood circulatory system to their respective target sites, organs, or cells, to modify their activity in some fashion.

Endocrinology has a comparatively long history, but real advances in the understanding of endocrine physiology and mechanisms of regulation and control began in the late 1960s with the introduction of sensitive and relatively specific analytical methods; these enabled low concentrations of circulating hormones to be measured reliably, simply, and at relatively low cost. The breakthrough came with the development and widespread adoption of competitive protein binding and radioimmunoassays that superseded existing cumbersome bioassay methods. Since then, knowledge of the physiology of individual endocrine glands and of the neural control of the pituitary gland and the overall feedback control of the endocrine system has progressed and is growing rapidly. Much of this has been accomplished by applying to endocrinological research the methods developed in cellular and molecular biology and recombinant DNA technology. At the same time, theoretical and quantitative approaches using mathematical modeling to complement experimental studies have been of value in gaining a greater understanding of endocrine dynamics.

2.2   Endocrine System: Hormones, Signals, and Communication between Cells and Tissues

Hormones are chemical messengers synthesized and secreted by specialized endocrine glands to act locally or at a distance, having been carried in the bloodstream (classic endocrine activity) or secreted into the gut lumen (lumocrine activity) to act on target cells that are distributed elsewhere in the body. Probably, to be more correct three actions should be defined, namely: endocrine action when the hormone is distributed in circulation binds to distant target cells; paracrine action in which the hormone acts locally by diffusing from its source to target cells in close proximity; and autocrine action when the hormone acts upon the cell that actually produced it.

Hormones are chemically diverse, physiologically potent molecules that are the primary vehicle for intercellular communication with the capacity to override the intrinsic mechanisms of normal cellular control. They can be classified broadly into four groups according to their physicochemical characteristics (1) steroid hormones, (2) peptide and protein hormones, (3) those derived from amino acids, principally the aromatic amino acid tyrosine, and (4) the eicosanoids (fatty acid derivatives).

1. *Steroids* are lipids, more specifically, derivatives of cholesterol produced by chemical modification. Examples include the sex steroids such as testosterone and the adrenal steroids such as cortisol. The first and rate-limiting step in the synthesis of all steroid hormones is the conversion of cholesterol to pregnenolone, which is formed on the inner membrane of cell mitochondria then transferred to the endoplasmic reticulum for further enzymatic transformations that yield the steroid hormones. Newly synthesized steroid hormones are rapidly secreted from the cell, so an increase in secretion reflects an accelerated rate of synthesis. Lipid-derived molecules, like the steroid hormones, are hydrophobic, so to improve their solubility they have to be carried in the circulation bound to specific transport proteins, though to a limited extent there is low-affinity, nonspecific binding to plasma proteins, such as plasma albumen. Binding capability and production clearance rates affect their half-life, which is comparatively long, and the rate of elimination. Steroid hormones are typically eliminated, following enzymatic inactivation in the liver, by excretion in urine and bile.

2. *Peptide and protein hormones* are synthesized in the cellular endoplasmic reticulum and then transferred to the Golgi apparatus where they are packaged into secretory vesicles for export. They can then be secreted either by regulated secretion or by constitutive secretion. In the former case, the hormone is stored in secretory granules and released in "bursts" when appropriately stimulated. This process enables cells to secrete a large amount of hormone over a short period of time. However, in the second case, the hormone is not stored within the cell, but rather it is released from the secretory vesicles as it is synthesized. As products of posttranslational modification of RNA-directed protein synthesis, they vary considerably in size, encompassing a range from that of peptides as short as three amino acids to large, multiple subunit glycoproteins. Several protein hormones are synthesized as prohormones, then subsequently modified by proteolysis to yield their active form. In other cases, the hormone is originally embedded within the sequence of a larger precursor, the active molecule being released by proteolytic cleavage of the parent molecule. The peptide and protein hormones are essentially hydrophilic and are therefore able to circulate in the blood in the free state; their half-life tends to be very short, of the order of a few minutes only.

3. *Amino acid derivatives*: There are two groups of hormones derived from the amino acid tyrosine; namely, thyroid hormones which are basically a "double" tyrosine ring incorporating three or four iodine atoms and the catecholamines that include epinephrine and norepinephrine that have the capability of functioning as both hormones and neurotransmitters. However, the two groups have highly different half-lives in the circulation, the thyroid hormones being of the order of several days, being inactivated by intracellular deiodinases, while that of the catecholamines is a few minutes only. Two other amino acids are involved in hormone synthesis: tryptophan, which is the precursor of both serotonin and the pineal hormone melatonin and glutamic acid, which is the precursor of histamine.

4. *Eicosanoids* are comprised of a large group of molecules derived from polyunsaturated fatty acids, the principal groups of the class being the prostaglandins, prostacyclins, leukotrienes, and thromboxanes. The specific eicosanoids which are synthesized by the cell is determined by a complex enzyme system within the cell following stimulation. Arachadonic acid released through the action of various lipases from cell plasma membrane lipids is the precursor for these hormones. All these hormones are rapidly metabolized and are active for a few seconds only.

2.2.1   A System View

The endocrine and nervous systems are physically and functionally linked by a specific region of the brain called the hypothalamus, which lies immediately above the pituitary gland, to which it is connected by an extension called the pituitary stalk. The integrating function of the hypothalamus is mediated by cells that possess the properties of both nerve and processes that carry electrical impulses and on stimulation can release their signal molecules into the blood. Each of the hypothalamic neurosecretory cells can be stimulated by other nerve cells in higher regions of the brain to secrete specific peptide hormones or release factors into the adenohypophyseal portal vasculature. These hormones can then specifically stimulate or suppress the secretion of a second hormone from the anterior pituitary. Figure 2.1 and Table 2.1 show, in schematic and descriptive form, respectively, details of the major endocrine glands of the body and the endocrine pathways.

The pituitary hormones in the circulation interact with their target tissues, which, if endocrine glands, are stimulated to secrete further (third) hormones that feedback to inhibit the release of the pituitary hormones. It will be seen from Figure 2.1 and Table 2.1 that the main targets of the pituitary are the adrenal cortex, the thyroid, and the gonads. These axes provide good examples of the control of pituitary hormone release by negative-feedback inhibition; for example, adrenocorticotropin (ACTH), luteinizing hormone (LH), and follicle-stimulating hormone (FSH) are selectively inhibited by different steroid hormones, as is thyrotropin (thyroid stimulating hormone [TSH]) release by the thyroid hormones.

In the case of growth hormone (GH) and prolactin, the target tissue is not an endocrine gland and thus does not produce a hormone; then the feedback control is mediated by inhibitors. Prolactin is under dopamine inhibitory control, whereas hypothalamic releasing and inhibitory factors control GH release. The two posterior pituitary (neurohypophyseal) hormones, oxytocin and vasopressin, are synthesized in the supraoptic and paraventricular nuclei and are stored in granules at the end of the nerve fibers in the posterior pituitary. Oxytocin is subsequently secreted in response to peripheral stimuli from the cervical stretch receptors or the suckling receptors of the breast. In a like manner, antidiuretic hormone (ADH, vasopressin) release is stimulated by the altered activity of hypothalamic osmoreceptors responding to changes in plasma solute concentrations.

It will be noted that the whole system is composed of several endocrine axes with the hypothalamus, pituitary, and other endocrine glands together forming a complex hierarchical regulatory system. There is no doubt that the anterior pituitary occupies a central position in the control of hormone secretion and, because of its important role, was often called the "conductor of the endocrine orchestra." However, the release of pituitary hormones is mediated by complex feedback control (discussed in the following sections), so the pituitary should be regarded as having a permissive role rather than having the overall control of the endocrine system.

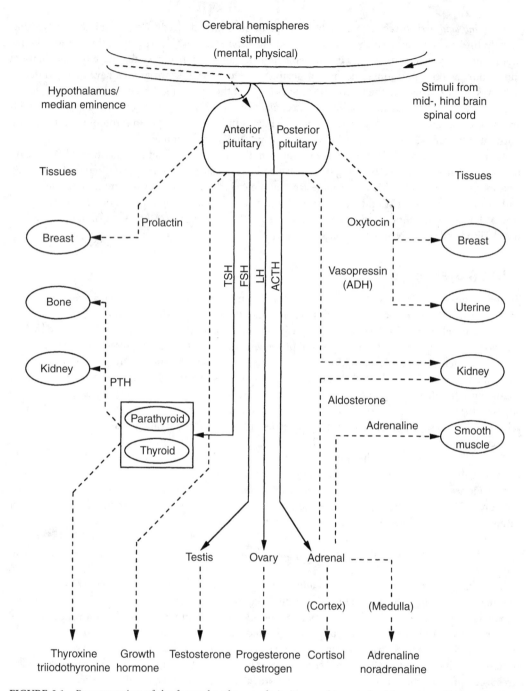

FIGURE 2.1 Representation of the forward pathways of pituitary and target gland hormone release and action: ——— tropic hormones; – – – – tissue-affecting hormones.

2.3 Hormone Action at the Cell Level: Signal Recognition, Signal Transduction, and Effecting a Physiological Response

The ability of target glands or tissues to respond to hormonal signals depends on the ability of the cells to recognize the signal. This function is mediated by specialized proteins or glycoproteins in or on the cell

TABLE 2.1   Main Endocrine Glands and the Hormones They Produce and Release

Gland	Hormone	Chemical characteristics
Hypothalamus/median eminence	Thyrotropin-releasing hormone (TRH)	Peptides
	Somatostatin	
	Gonadotropin-releasing hormone	Amine
	Growth hormone-releasing hormone	
	Corticotropin-releasing hormone	
	Prolactin inhibitor factor	
Anterior pituitary	Thyrotropin (TSH)	Glycoprotiens
	Luteinizing hormone	
	Follicle-stimulating hormone (FSH)	Proteins
	Growth hormones	
	Prolactin	
	Adrenocorticotropin (ACTH)	
Posterior pituitary	Vasopressin (antidiuretic hormone, ADH)	
	Oxytocin	Peptides
Thyroid	Triidothyronine (T3)	Tyrosine derivatives
	Thyroxine (T4)	
Parathyroid	Parathyroid hormone (PTH)	Peptide
Adrenal cortex	Cortisol	Steroids
	Aldosterone	
Adrenal medulla	Epinephrine	Catecolamines
	Norepinephrine	
Pancreas	Insulin	Proteins
	Glucagon	
	Somatostatin	
Gonads		
Testes	Testosterone	Steroids
Ovaries	Oestrogen	
	Progesssterone	

TABLE 2.2   Summary of Location of Receptor, Associated Classes of Hormones, and Their Principle Mechanism of Action

Location of receptors	Classes of hormones	Principal mechanism of action
Plasma membrane (cell surface)	Proteins and peptides, catecholamines and eicosanoids	Generation of second messengers that primarily modulate the activity of intracellular enzymes
Intracellular (cytoplasm and/or nucleus)	Steroids and thyroid hormones	Modification of RNA-directed protein synthesis and the transcriptional activity of responsive genes

plasma membrane that are specific for a particular hormone, able to recognize it, bind it with high affinity, and react when very low concentrations are present. Recognition of the hormonal signal and activation of the cell surface receptors initiates a flow of information to the cell interior, which triggers a chain of intracellular events in a preprogrammed fashion that produces a characteristic response. It is useful to classify the site of such action of hormones into two groups (see Table 2.2): those which act at the cell surface without, generally, traversing the cell membrane and those which actually enter the cell before effecting a response. In the study of this multistep sequence, two important events can be readily studied, namely, the binding of the hormone to its receptor, and activation of cytoplasmic effects. These events, such as receptor activation and signal generation, are an active area of research.

One technique employed in an attempt to elucidate the intermediate steps has been to use ineffective mutant receptors, which when assayed are either defective in their hormone-binding capabilities or in effector activation and thus unable to transduce a meaningful signal to the cell. However, the difficulty with these studies has been to distinguish receptor-activation and signal-generation defects from hormone-binding and effector activation defects. A parallel technique is to explore the use of agonists, which are molecules that behave like the "normal" hormone, bind the receptor and induce all the postreceptor events that yield a physiological effect. Natural hormones are themselves agonists and, in many cases, more than one distinct hormone can bind to the same receptor. For a given receptor, different agonists can have dramatically different potencies. The corollary to this is to explore the use of antagonists, that is molecules that bind the receptor and block-binding of the agonist, but fail to trigger intracellular signaling events. Hormone antagonists have obvious pharmaceutical potential in clinical endocrinology.

The peptide and protein hormones circulate at very low concentrations relative to other proteins in the blood plasma. These low concentrations are reflected in the very high affinity and specificity of the receptor sites, which permit recognition of the relevant hormones amid the prolusion of protein molecules in the circulation. Adaptation to a high concentration of a signal ligand in a time-dependent reversible manner enables cells to respond to changes in the concentration of a ligand instead of to its absolute concentration. The number of receptors in a cell is not constant; synthesis of receptors may be induced or repressed by other hormones or even by their own hormones. Adaptation can occur in several ways. Ligand binding can inactivate a cell surface receptor either by inducing its internalization and degradation or by causing the receptor to adopt an inactive conformation. Alternatively, it may result from the changes in one of the nonreceptor proteins involved in signal transduction following receptor activation. Down regulation is the name given to the process whereby a cell decreases the number of receptors in response to intense or frequent stimulation and can occur by degradation or more temporarily by phosphorylation and sequestration. Up regulation is the process of increasing receptor expression either by other hormones or in response to altered stimulation.

2.3.1 Structure of Cell Surface Receptors

Cell surface receptors are integral membrane proteins and, as such, have regions that contribute to three basic domains:

- *Extracellular domains*: Some of the residues exposed to the outside of the cell interact with and bind the hormone — another term for these regions is the ligand-binding domain.
- *Transmembrane domains*: Hydrophobic stretches of amino acids are "comfortable" in the lipid bilayer and serve to anchor the receptor in the membrane.
- *Cytoplasmic or intracellular domains*: Tails or loops of the receptor that are within the cytoplasm react to hormone binding by interacting in some way with other molecules, leading to generation of second messengers. Cytoplasmic residues of the receptor are thus the effector region of the molecule.

Several distinctive variations in receptor structure have been identified; some receptors being simple, single-pass proteins, many growth factor receptors take this form. Others, such as the receptor for insulin, have more than one subunit. Another class, which includes the beta-adrenergic receptor, is threaded through the membrane seven times.

Receptor molecules are neither isolated nor fixed in one location of the plasma membrane. In some cases, other integral membrane proteins interact with the receptor to modulate its activity. Some types of receptors cluster together in the membrane after binding hormone. Finally, as elaborated in the following sections, interaction of the hormone-bound receptor with other membrane or cytoplasmic proteins is the key to generation of second messengers and transduction of the hormonal signal.

2.3.2 Fate of the Hormone–Receptor Complex

Normal cell function depends upon second messenger cascades being transient events. Indeed, a number of cancers are associated with receptors that continually stimulate second messenger systems. One important part of negative regulation on hormone action is that cell surface receptors are internalized. In many cases, internalization is stimulated by hormone binding. Internalization occurs by endocytosis through structures called coated pits. The resulting endosomes may fuse with lysosomes, leading to destruction of the receptor and hormone. In other cases, it appears that the hormone dissociates and the receptor is recycled by fusion of the endosome back into the plasma membrane.

2.4   Hormones Acting at the Cell Surface

Most peptide and protein hormones are hydrophilic and thus unable to traverse the lipid-containing cell membrane and must therefore act through activation of receptor proteins on the cell surface. When these receptors are activated by the binding of an extracellular signal ligand, the ligand–receptor complex initiates a series of protein interactions within or adjacent to the inner surface of the plasma membrane, which in turn brings about changes in intracellular activity. This can happen in one of two ways. The first involves the so-called second messenger, by altering the activity of a plasma membrane-bound enzyme, which in turn increases (or sometimes decreases) the concentration of an intracellular mediator. The second involves activation of other types of cell surface receptors, which leads to changes in the plasma membrane electrical potential and the membrane permeability, resulting in altered transmembrane transport of ions or metabolites. If the hormone is thought of as the "first messenger," cyclic adenosine monophosphate (cAMP) can be regarded as the "second messenger," capable of triggering a cascade of intracellular bio-chemical events that can lead either to a rapid secondary response such as altered ion transport, enhanced metabolic pathway flux, steroidogenesis or to a slower response such as DNA, RNA, and protein synthesis resulting in cell growth or cell division.

2.4.1   Second Messenger Systems

Currently, four second messenger systems are recognized in cells, as summarized in Table 2.3. Note that not only do multiple hormones utilize the same second messenger system, but a single hormone can utilize more than one system. Understanding how cells integrate signals from several hormones into a coherent biological response remains a challenge.

The cell surface receptors for peptide hormones are linked functionally to a cell membrane-bound enzyme that acts as the catalytic unit. This receptor complex consists of three components (1) the receptor itself which recognizes the hormone, (2) a regulatory protein called a G-protein that binds guanine nucleotides and is located on the cytosolic face of the membrane, and (3) adenylate cyclase, which catalyzes the conversion of adenosine triphosphate (ATP) to cAMP. As the hormone binds at the receptor site, it is coupled through a regulatory protein, which acts as a transducer, to the enzyme adenyl cyclase, which catalyzes the formation of cAMP from ATP. The G-protein consists of three subunits, which in the unstimulated state form a heterotrimer to which a molecule of guanine diphosphate (GDP) is bound. Binding of the hormone to the receptor causes the subunit to exchange its GDP for a molecule of guanine triphosphate (GTP), which then dissociates from the subunits. This in turn decreases the affinity of

TABLE 2.3   Second Messenger/Examples of Hormones Which Utilize This System

Second messenger	Examples of dependent hormones
Cyclic AMP	Epinephrine and norepinephrine, glucagon, luteinizing hormone, follicle stimulating hormone, thyroid stimulating hormone, calcitonin, parathyroid hormone, antidiuretic hormone
Protein kinase	Insulin, growth hormone, prolactin, oxytocin, erythropoietin, various growth factors
Calcium ions and phosphoinositides	Epinephrine and norepinephrine, angiotensin II, antidiuretic hormone, gonadotrophin releasing hormone, thyroid releasing hormone
Cyclic GMP	Atrial natriuretic hormone, nitric oxide

the receptor for the hormone and leads to its dissociation. The GTP subunit not only activates adenylate cyclase, but also has intrinsic GTPase activity and slowly converts GTP back to GDP, thus allowing the subunits to reassociate and so regain their initial resting state. There are hormones, such as somatostatin, that possess the ability to inhibit AMP formation but still have similarly structured receptor complexes. The G-protein of inhibitory complexes consists of an inhibitory subunit complexed with a subunit thought to be identical to the subunits of the stimulatory G-protein. However, it appears that a single adenylate cyclase molecule can be simultaneously regulated by more than one G-protein enabling the system to integrate opposing inputs.

The adenylate cyclase reaction is rapid, and the increased concentration of intracellular cAMP is short-lived, since it is rapidly hydrolyzed and destroyed by the enzyme cAMP phosphodiesterase, which terminates the hormonal response. The continual and rapid removal of cAMP and free calcium ions from the cytosol makes for both the rapid increase and decrease of these intracellular mediators when the cells respond to signals. Rising cAMP concentrations affect cells by stimulating cAMP-dependent protein kinases to phosphorylate-specific target proteins.

Phosphorylation of proteins leads to conformational changes that enhance their catalytic activity, thus providing a signal amplification pathway from hormone to effector. These effects are reversible because phosphorylated proteins are rapidly dephosphorylated by protein phosphatases when the concentration of cAMP falls. A similar system involving cyclic GMP, although less common and less well studied, plays an analogous role to that of cAMP. The action of thyrotropin-releasing hormone (TRH), parathyroid hormone (PTH), and epinephrine is catalyzed by adenyl cyclase, and this can be regarded as the classic reaction.

2.4.1.1 Calcium Ion and Phosphoinositide Second Messenger Systems

However, there are variant mechanisms. In the phosphatidylinositol-diacylglycerol (DAG)/inositol tri-phosphate (EP3) system, some surface receptors are coupled through another G-protein to the enzyme phospholipase C, which cleaves the membrane phospholipid to form DAG and IP3 or phospholipase D which cleaves phosphatidyl choline to DAG via phosphatidic acid. DAG causes the calcium, phospholid-dependent protein kinase C to translocate to the cell membrane from the cytosolic cell compartment to become 20 times more active in the process. IP3 mobilizes calcium from storage sites associated with the plasma and intracellular membranes thereby contributing to the activation of protein kinase C as well as other calcium-dependent processes. DAG is cleared from the cell either by conversion to phosphatidic acid, which may be recycled to phospholipid, or it may be broken down to fatty acids and glycerol. The DAG derived from phosphatidylinositol usually contains arachidonic acid esterified to the middle carbon of glycerol. Arachidonic acid is the precursor of the prostaglandins and leuk-otrienes, which are biologically active eicosanoids. Thyrotropin and vasopressin modulate an activity of phospholipase C that catalyzes the conversion of phosphatidylinositol to diacylglycerol and inositol, 1,4,5-triphosphate, which act as the second messengers. They mobilize bound intracellular calcium and activate a protein kinase, which in turn alters the activity of other calcium-dependent enzymes within the cell.

Increased concentrations of free calcium ions affect cellular events by binding to and altering the molecular conformation of calmodulin; the resulting calcium ion–calmodulin complex can activate many different target proteins, including calcium ion-dependent protein kinases. Each cell type has a charac-teristic set of target proteins that are so regulated by cAMP-dependent kinases and calmodulin that it will respond in a specific way to an alteration in cAMP or calcium ion concentrations. In this fashion, cAMP or calcium ions act as second messengers in such a way as to allow the extracellular signal not only to be greatly amplified but, just as importantly, also to be made specific for each cell type.

2.4.1.2 Protein Kinase Second Messenger Systems

The hormone binds to domains exposed on the cell's surface, resulting in a conformational change that activates kinase domains located in the cytoplasmic regions of the receptor. In many cases, the receptor phosphorylates itself as part of the kinase activation process. The activated receptor phosphorylates a variety of intracellular targets, many of which are enzymes that become activated or are inactivated upon phosphorylation. The receptors for several protein hormones are themselves protein kinases, which are switched on by binding of hormone. The kinase activity associated with such receptors results in phosphorylation of tyrosine residues on other proteins. Insulin is an example of a hormone whose receptor is a tyrosine kinase.

The action of the important hormone insulin that regulates glucose metabolism depends on the activation of the enzyme tyrosine kinase catalyzing the phosphorylation of tyrosyl residues of proteins. This effects changes in the activity of calcium-sensitive enzymes, leading to enhanced movement of glucose and fatty acids across the cell membrane and modulating their intracellular metabolism. The binding of insulin to its receptor site has been studied extensively; the receptor complex has been isolated and characterized. It was such work that highlighted the interesting aspect of feedback control at the cell level down-regulation: the ability of peptide hormones to regulate the concentration of cell surface receptors. After activation, the receptor population becomes desensitized, or "down-regulated"; leading to a decreased availability of receptors and thus a modulation of transmembrane events.

As with cAMP second messenger systems, activation of receptor tyrosine kinases leads to rapid modulation in a number of target proteins within the cell. Interestingly, some of the targets of receptor kinases are protein phosphatases, which, upon activation by receptor tyrosine kinase, become competent to remove phosphates from other proteins and alter their activity. Again, a seemingly small change due to hormone binding is amplified into a multitude of effects within the cell.

In some cases, binding of hormone to a surface receptor induces a tyrosine kinase cascade, even though the receptor is not itself a tyrosine kinase. The growth hormone receptor is one example of such a system — the interaction of growth hormone with its receptor leads to activation of cytoplasmic tyrosine kinases, with results conceptually similar to that seen with receptor kinases.

2.5   Hormones Acting within the Cell

Receptors for steroid and thyroid hormones are located inside target cells, in the cytoplasm or nucleus, and function as ligand-dependent transcription factors. That is to say, the hormone–receptor complex binds to promoter regions of responsive genes and stimulate or sometimes inhibit transcription from those genes. Thus, the mechanism of action of these hormones is to modulate gene expression in target cells. By selectively affecting transcription from a battery of genes, the concentration of those respective proteins are altered, which clearly can change the phenotype of the cell.

2.5.1   Structure of Intracellular Receptors

Steroid and thyroid hormone receptors are members of a large group of transcription factors. In some cases, multiple forms of a given receptor are expressed in cells, adding to the complexity of the response. All of these receptors are composed of a single polypeptide chain that has three distinct domains: the amino-terminus, involved in activating or stimulating transcription by interacting with components of the transcriptional machinery; the DNA-binding domain responsible for binding of the receptor to specific DNA sequences; and the carboxy-terminus or ligand-binding domain, which binds hormone. In addition to these three core domains, two other important regions of the receptor protein are a nuclear localization sequence, which targets the protein to nucleus, and a dimerization domain, responsible for latching two receptors together in a form capable of binding DNA.

2.5.2   Hormone–Receptor Binding and Interactions with DNA

Steroid hormones are small hydrophobic molecules derived from cholesterol that are solubilized by binding reversibly to specify carrier proteins in the blood plasma. Once released from their carrier proteins, they readily pass through the plasma membrane of the target cell and bind, again reversibly, to steroid hormone receptor proteins in the cytosol. This is a relatively slow process when compared to protein hormones. The latter second messenger-mediated phosphorylation–dephosphorylation reactions modify enzymatic processes rapidly with the physiological consequences becoming apparent in seconds or minutes and are as rapidly reversed. Nuclear-mediated responses, on the other hand, lead to transcription/translation-dependent changes that are slow in onset and tend to persist since reversal is dependent on degradation of the induced proteins. The protein component of the steroid hormone–receptor complex has an affinity for DNA in the cell nucleus, where it binds to nuclear chromatin and initiates the transcription of a small number of genes. These gene products may, in turn, activate other genes and produce a secondary response, thereby amplifying the initial effect of the hormone. Each steroid hormone is recognized by a separate receptor protein, but this same receptor protein has the capacity to regulate several different genes in different target cells. This, of course, suggests that the nuclear chromatin of each cell type is organized so that only the appropriate genes are made available for regulation by the hormone–receptor complex. The thyroid hormone triiodothyronine (T3) also acts, though by a different mechanism than the steroids, at the cell nucleus level to initiate genomic transcription. The hormonal activities of GH and prolactin influence cellular gene transcription and translation of messenger RNA by complex mechanisms.

2.6 Endocrine System: Some Other Aspects of Regulation and Control

2.6.1 Control of Endocrine Activity

The physiologic effects of hormones depend largely on their concentration in blood and extracellular fluid. Almost inevitably, disease results when hormone concentrations are either too high or too low, and precise control over circulating concentrations of hormones is therefore crucial. The concentration of hormone as seen by target cells is determined by three factors:

- Rate of production: the synthesis and secretion of hormones are the most highly regulated aspect of endocrine control, which is mediated by feedback circuits, as described in the following sections
- Rate of delivery: a blood-flow-dependent factor
- Rate of degradation and elimination

2.6.2 Feedback Control of Hormone Production

From the foregoing sections it is clear that the endocrine system exhibits complex molecular and metabolic dynamics, which involve many levels of control and regulation. At lower levels within this hierarchy, there is inherent feedback and control within the dynamics of metabolic processes themselves. Superimposed upon this there are also complex patterns of feedback and control that result from the effects of enzymes that catalyze such metabolic reactions. However, our focus here is the higher level of feedback and control resulting from hormonal dynamics. Hormones are chemical signals released from a hierarchy of endocrine glands and propagated through the circulation to a hierarchy of cell types. The integration of this system depends on a series of what systems engineers call "feedback loops"; feedback is a reflection of mutual dependence of the system variables: variable x affects variable y, and y affects x. Further, it is essentially a closed-loop system in which the feedback of information from the system output to the input has the capacity to maintain homeostasis. A diagrammatic representation of the ways in which hormone action is controlled is shown in Figure 2.2. One example of this control structure arises in the context of the thyroid hormones. In this case, TRH, secreted by the hypothalamus, triggers the anterior pituitary into the production of TSH. The target gland is the thyroid, which produces T3 and thyroxine (T4). The complexity of control includes both direct and indirect feedback of T3 and T4, as outlined in Figure 2.2, together with TSH feedback on to the hypothalamus.

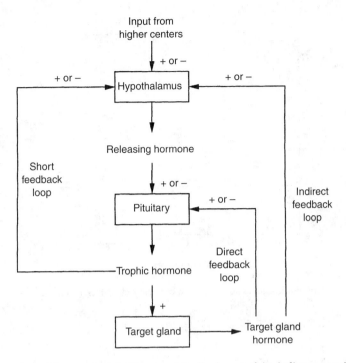

FIGURE 2.2 Illustration of the complexity of hormonal feedback control (+ indicates a positive or augmenting effect; − indicates a negative or inhibiting effect).

2.6.3 Negative Feedback

If an increase in y causes a change in x, which in turn tends to decrease y, feedback is said to be negative; in other words, the signal output induces a response that feeds back to the signal generator to decrease its output. Simply, negative feedback is seen when the output of a pathway inhibits inputs to the pathway. This is the most common form of control in physiologic systems, and examples are many. For instance, as mentioned earlier, the anterior pituitary releases trophic or stimulating hormones that act on peripheral endocrine glands such as the adrenals or thyroid or to gonads to produce hormones that act back on the pituitary to decrease the secretion of the trophic hormones. These are examples of what is called long-loop feedback (see Figure 2.2). (Note: the adjectives long and short reflect the spatial distance or proximity of effector and target sites.) The trophic hormones of the pituitary are also regulated by feedback action at the level of their releasing factors. Ultrashort-loop feedback is also described. There are numerous examples of short-loop feedback as well, the best being the reciprocal relation between insulin and blood glucose concentrations, as depicted in Figure 2.3. In this case, elevated glucose concentration (and positive rate of change, implying not only proportional but also derivative control) has a positive effect on the pancreas, which secretes insulin in response. This has an inhibiting effect on glucose metabolism, resulting in a reduction of blood glucose toward a normal concentration; in other words, classic negative-feedback control.

Feedback loops are also involved extensively to regulate secretion of hormones in the hypothalamic-pituitary axis. An important example of a negative-feedback loop is seen in control of thyroid hormone secretion. The thyroid hormones thyroxine and triiodothyronine (T4 and T3) are synthesized and secreted by thyroid glands and affect metabolism throughout the body. The negative-feedback control sequence in this system is: neurones in the hypothalamus secrete TRH, which stimulates cells in the anterior pituitary to secrete TSH. The released TSH binds to receptors on epithelial cells in the thyroid gland, stimulating synthesis and secretion of thyroid hormones, which affect probably all cells in the body. However, when the blood concentrations of thyroid hormones increase above a certain threshold, TRH-secreting neurons

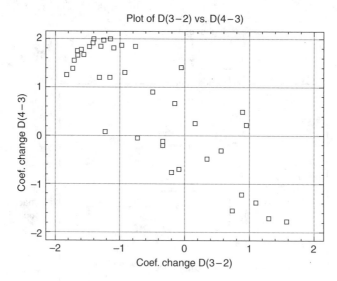

FIGURE 2.3   The interaction of insulin as an illustration of negative feedback within a hormonal control system.

in the hypothalamus are inhibited and stop secreting TRH. Inhibition of TRH secretion leads to shutoff of TSH secretion, which leads to shutoff of thyroid hormone secretion. As thyroid hormone levels decay below the threshold, negative feedback is relieved, TRH secretion starts again, leading to TSH secretion.

2.6.4   Positive Feedback

If increase in y causes a change in x, which tends to increase y, feedback is said to be positive; in other words, a further signal output is evoked by the response it induces or provokes. This is intrinsically an unstable system, but there are physiologic situations where such control is valuable. In the positive feedback situation, the signal output will continue until no further response is required. Suckling provides an example; stimulation of nipple receptors by the suckling child provokes an increased oxytocin release from the posterior pituitary with a corresponding increase in milk flow. Removal of the stimulus causes cessation of oxytocin release.

2.6.5   Pulsatile and Rhythmic Endocrine Control

An important consequence of feedback control and the limited physical half-life of hormones is that a pulsatile pattern of secretion and thus of hormone concentrations is seen over time for virtually all hormones, with variations in pulse characteristics that reflect specific physiologic states. In addition to these short-term pulses, longer-term temporal oscillations or endocrine rhythms are also commonly observed and undoubtedly important in both normal and pathologic states. Many hormone functions exhibit rhythmicity in the pulsatile release of hormones.

The most readily recognizable is the approximately 24-h cycle (circadian or diurnal rhythm). For instance, blood sampling at frequent intervals has shown that ACTH is secreted episodically, each secretory burst being followed 5 to 10 min later by cortisol secretion. These episodes are most frequent in the early morning, with plasma cortisol concentrations highest around 7 to 8 A.M. and lowest around midnight. ACTH and cortisol secretion vary inversely, and the parallel circadian rhythm is probably due to a cyclic change in the sensitivity of the hypothalamic feedback center to circulating cortisol. Longer cycles are also known, for example, the infradian menstrual cycle.

It is clear that such inherent rhythms are important in endocrine communication and control, suggesting that its physiologic organization is based not only on the structural components of the system but also on the dynamics of their interactions. The rhythmic, pulsatile nature of release of many hormones is a means whereby time-varying signals can be encoded, thus allowing large quantities of information to be transmitted and exchanged rapidly in a way that small, continuous changes in threshold levels would not allow.

2.6.6 Coda

Inevitably, our brief exposition has been able to touch upon an enormous subject only by describing some of the salient features of this fascinating domain, but it is hoped that it may nevertheless stimulate a further interest. However, not surprisingly, the endocrinology literature is massive both in terms of the number of books and texts and an ever-increasing number of journals. It is suggested that anyone wishing to read further may initially start from one of the many excellent textbooks and go on from there.

Further Reading

Alberts B. Johnson, Lewis, Raff, and Roberts, Walter. 2002. *Molecular Biology of the Cell*, 4th ed. Garland Science. ISBN 0815340729.

Goodman H.M. 1994. *Basic Medical Endocrinology*, 2nd ed. Raven Press.

Greenspan F.S. and Gardner D.G. (Eds.) 2003. Basic and Clinical Endocrinology (Lange). Appleton and Lange. ISBN 0071402977.

Krauss G. 2003. *Biochemistry of Signal Transduction and Regulation*, 3rd ed. Wiley. ISBN 3527305912.

Larsen P.R., Kronenberg H.M., Melmed S., Polonsky K.S., Wilson J.D., and Foster D.W. (Eds.) 2002. *Williams Textbook of Endocrinology*, 10th ed. W.B. Saunders. ISBN 0721691846.

Martin C.R. (Ed.) 1995. *Dictionary of Endocrinology and Related Biomedical Sciences.* Oxford University Press. ISBN 0195060334.

O'Malley B.W., Birnbaumer L., and Hunter T. (Eds.) 1998. *Hormones and Signaling* (Vol. 1). Academic Press.

Timiras P.S., Quay W.D., and Vernadakis A. (Eds.) 1995. *Hormones and Aging.* CRC Press. ISBN 0849324467.

3

Nervous System

Evangelia Micheli-Tzanakou
Rutgers University

Anette Nievies
Robert Wood Johnson Medical School

Nervous system unlike other organ systems is primarily concerned with signals, information encoding and processing, and control rather than manipulation of energy. It acts like a communication device whose components use substances and energy in processing signals and in reorganizing them, choosing and commanding as well as in developing and learning. A central question that is often asked is how nervous systems work and what governs the principles of their operation. In an attempt to answer this question, we, at the same time, ignore other fundamental questions such as anatomical or neurochemical and molecular aspects. We rather concentrate on relations and transactions between neurons and their assemblages in the nervous system. We deal with neural signals (encoding and decoding), the evaluation and weighting of incoming signals, and the formulation of outputs. A major part of this chapter is devoted to higher aspects of the nervous system such as memory and learning rather than individual systems such as vision and audition, which are treated extensively elsewhere [1]. Finally, some known abnormalities of the nervous system including Parkinson's and Alzheimer's disease, epilepsy, and the phantom limb sensation, and pain are the subjects we deal with.

3.1 Definitions

Nervous systems can be defined as organized assemblies of nerve cells as well as nonnervous cells. Nerve cells or neurons are specialized in the generation, integration, and conduction of incoming signals from the outside world or from other neurons and deliver them to other excitable cells or to *effectors* such as muscle cells. Nervous systems are easily recognized in higher animals, but not in the lower species, since the defining criteria are difficult to apply.

A central nervous system (CNS) can be easily distinguished from a peripheral nervous system (PNS), since it contains most of the motor and the nucleated parts of neurons that innervate muscles and other effectors. The PNS contains all the sensory nerve cell bodies with some exceptions, plus local *plexuses*, local *ganglia*, and peripheral axons that make up the *nerves*. Most sensory axons go all the way into the central nervous system while the remaining relay in peripheral plexuses. Motor axons originating in the CNS innervate effector cells.

The nervous system has two major roles: first, to regulate, acting homeostatically, in restoring some conditions of the organism after some external stimulus and second, to act to alter a preexisting condition by replacing it or modifying it. In both cases — regulation or initiation of a process — learning can be superimposed. In most species, learning is more or less an adaptive mechanism, combining and timing species-characteristic acts, with a large degree of evolution toward perfection.

The nervous system is a complex structure for which realistic assumptions have led to irrelevant oversimplifications. One can break down the nervous system into four components: sensory transducers, neurons, axons, and muscle fibers. Each of these components gathers processes and transmits information impinging upon them from the outside world, usually in the form of complex stimuli. The processing is carried out by excitable tissues — neurons, axons, sensory receptors, and muscle fibers. Neurons are the basic elements of the nervous system. If, put in small assemblies or clusters, they form neuronal assemblies or neuronal networks communicating with each other either chemically via *synaptic junctions* or electrically via *tight* junctions. The main characteristics of a cell are the *cell body* or *soma*, which contains the *nucleus*, and a number of processes originating from the cell body called the *dendrites*, which reach out to the surroundings to make contacts with other cells. These contacts serve as the incoming information to the cell, while the outgoing information follows a conduction path, the axon. The incoming information is integrated in the cell body and generates the result of this at the *axon hillock*. There are two types of outputs that can be generated and therefore two types of neurons: those who generate *grated* potentials that attenuate with distance and those who generate *action* potentials. The action potential, travels through the axon, a thin long process that passively passes the action potential or rather a train of action potentials without attenuation (*all-or-none* effect). A series of action potentials is often called a *spike train*. A threshold built into the hillock, and depending on its level, allows or stops the generation of the spike train. Axons usually terminate on other neurons by means of *synaptic terminals* or *boutons* and have properties similar to those of an electric cable with varying diameters and speeds of signal transmission. Axons can be of two types, namely *myelinated* or *unmyelinated*. In the former the axon is surrounded by a thick fatty material, the myelin sheath, which is interrupted at regular intervals by gaps called the *nodes of Ranvier*. These nodes provide for the *saltatory* conduction of the signal along the axon. The axon makes functional connections with other neurons at synapses either on the cell body, the dendrites, or the axons. There exist two kinds of synapses: *excitatory* and *inhibitory* and as the name implies they either increase the *firing* frequency of the postsynaptic neurons or decrease it, respectively [5].

Sensory receptors are specialized cells that, in response to an incoming stimulus, generate a corresponding electrical signal, a graded receptor potential. Although the mechanisms by which the sensory receptors generate receptor potentials, are not exactly known, the most plausible scenario is that an external stimulus alters the membrane permeabilities. The receptor potential then is the change in intracellular potential relative to the *resting* potential.

It is important to notice here that the term receptor is used in physiology to refer not only to sensory receptors but in a different sense to proteins that bind neurotransmitters, hormones, and other substances with great affinity and specificity as a first step in starting up physiological responses. This receptor is often associated with nonneural cells that surround it and form a *sense organ*. The forms of energy converted by the receptors include mechanical, thermal, electromagnetic, and chemical energy. The particular form of energy to which a receptor is most sensitive is called its *adequate stimulus*. The problem of how receptors convert energy into action potentials in the sensory nerves has been the subject of intensive study. In the complex sense organs such as those concerned with hearing and vision there exist separate receptor cells and synaptic junctions between receptors and afferent nerves. In other cases such as the cutaneous sense organs, the receptors are specialized. Where a stimulus of constant strength is applied to a receptor repeatedly, the frequency of the action potentials in its sensor nerve declines over a period of time. This phenomenon is known as *adaptation*; if the adaptation is very rapid then the receptors are called *phasic*, otherwise as *tonic*.

Another important issue is the *coding* of sensory information. Action potentials are similar in all nerves although there are variations in their speed of conduction and other characteristics. But if the action potentials are the same in most cells, then what makes the visual cells sensitive to light and not to sound and the touch receptors sensitive to a sensation of touch and not of smell? And how can we tell if these sensations are strong or not? These sensations depend upon the specific part of the brain called the *doctrine of specific nerve energies* and has been questioned over time by several researchers. No matter where a particular sensory pathway is stimulated along its path of connecting to the brain, the sensation produced is always referred to the location of the receptor site. This is the principle of the *law of projections*. An example of this law is the "phantom limb" where an amputee of a limb is complaining about pain or an itching sensation in that limb. This phenomenon is discussed in a greater detail later on in the chapter.

3.2 Functions of the Nervous System

The basic unit of integrated activity is the *reflex arc*. This arc consists of a sense organ, an afferent neuron, one or more synapses in a central integrating station (or sympathetic ganglion), an efferent neuron, as well as, an effector. The simplest reflex arc is the *monosynaptic* one, which only has one synapse between the afferent and efferent neuron. With more than one synapses the reflex arc is called *polysynaptic*. In each of these cases, activity is modified by both spatial and temporal facilitation, occlusion, and other effects [2,3].

In mammals, the connection between afferent and efferent somatic neurons is found either in the brain or the spinal cord. The Bell–Magendie law dictates the fact that in the spinal cord the dorsal roots are sensory while the ventral roots are motor. The action potential message that is carried by an axon is eventually fed to a muscle, or to a secretory cell, or to the dendrite of another neuron. If an axon is carrying a graded potential, its output is too weak to stimulate a muscle, but it can terminate on a secretory cell or dendrite. The latter can have as many as 10,000 inputs. If the end point is a motor neuron, which has been found experimentally in the case of fibers from the primary endings, then there is a time lag between the time when a stimulus was applied and a response obtained from the muscle. This time interval is called the *reaction time* and in humans is approximately 20 msec for a stretch reflex. The distance from the spinal cord can be measured and since the conduction velocities of both the efferent and afferent fibers are known, another important quantity can be calculated, namely the *central delay*. This delay is the portion of the reaction time that was spent for conduction to and from the spinal cord. It has been found that muscle spindles also make connections that cause muscle contraction via polysynaptic pathways, while the afferents from secondary endings make connections that excite extensor muscles. When a motor neuron sends a burst of action potentials to its skeletal muscle, the amount of contraction depends largely on the discharge frequency, but on many other factors as well, such as the history of the load on the muscle and the load itself. *The stretch error* can be calculated from the desired motion minus the actual stretch. If this error is then fed back to the motor neuron, its discharge frequency is modified appropriately. This frequency modification corresponds to one of the three feedback loops that are available locally. Another loop corrects for overstretching beyond the point at which the muscle or tendon may tear. Since a muscle can only contract, it must be paired with another muscle (*antagonist*) in order to affect the return motion. Generally speaking, a flexor muscle is paired with an extension muscle that cannot be activated simultaneously. This means that the motor neurons that affect each one of these muscles are not activated at the same time. Instead when one set of motor neurons is active, the other is inhibited and vice versa. When a movement involves two or more muscles that normally cooperate by contracting simultaneously, the excitation of one causes facilitation of the other *synergistic* members via cross connections. All of these networks form feedback loops. An engineer's interpretation of how these loops work would be to assume dynamic conditions, as is the case in all parts of the nervous system. This has little value in dealing with stationary conditions, but it provides for an ability to adjust to changing conditions.

The nervous system, as mentioned in the introduction, is a control system of processes that adjust both internal and external operations. As humans we have experiences that change our perception of events in our environment. The same is true for higher animals that besides having an internal environment, the status of which is of major importance, also share an external environment of utmost richness and variety. Objects and conditions that have direct contact with the surface of an animal directly affect the future of the animal. Information about changes at some point provides a prediction of possible future. The amount of information required to represent changing conditions increases as the required temporal resolution of detail increases. This creates a vast amount of data to be processed by any finite system. Considering the fact that the information reaching sensory receptors is too extensive and redundant, as well as modified by external interference (noise), the nervous system has a tremendously difficult task to accomplish. Enhanced responsiveness to a particular stimulus can be produced by structures that either increase the energy converging on a receptor or increase the effectiveness of coupling of a specific type of stimulus to the receptor. Different species have sensory systems that respond to stimuli that are important to them for survival. Often one nervous system responds to conditions that are not sensed by another nervous system [4,5]. The transduction, processing, and transmission of signals in any nervous system, produces a survival mechanism for an organism but only after these signals have been further modified by effector organs. Although the nerve impulses that drive a muscle as explained earlier are discrete events, a muscle twitch takes much longer to happen, a fact that allows for responses to overlap and produce a much smoother output. Neural control of motor activity of skeletal muscle is accomplished entirely by the modification of the muscle excitation, which involves changes in velocity, length, stiffness, and heat production. The importance of accurate timing of inputs, and the maintenance of this timing across several synapses, is obvious in sensory pathways of the nervous system. Cells are located next to other cells that have overlapping or adjacent receptive or motor fields. The dendrites provide important and complicated sites of interactions as well as channels of variable effectiveness for excitatory inputs, depending on their position relative to the cell body. Among the best examples are the cells of the medial superior olive in the auditory pathway. These cells have two major dendritic trees extending from opposite poles of the cell body. One receives synaptic inhibitory input from the ipsilaterial cochlear nucleus and the other from the contralateral, which normally is an excitatory input. These cells deal with the determination of the azimuth of a sound. When a sound is present at the contralateral side, most cells are excited while ipsilateral sounds cause inhibition. It has been shown that the cells can go from complete excitation to full inhibition with a difference of only a few hundred milliseconds in arrival time of the two inputs.

The question then arises: how does the nervous system put together the signals available to it so that a determination of our output takes place? To arrive at an understanding of how the nervous system intergrates incoming information at a given moment of time, we must understand that the processes that take place depend both on cellular forms and a topological architecture as well as on the physiological properties that relate input to output. That is, we have to know the *transfer* functions or *coupling* functions. Integration depends on the weighting of inputs. One of the important factors determining weighting is the area of synaptic contact. The extensive dendrites are the primary integrating structures. Electronic spread is the means of mixing, smoothing, attenuating, delaying, and summing postsynaptic potentials. The spatial distribution of input is often not random but systematically restricted. Also, the wide variety of characteristic geometries of synapses is, no doubt, important not just for the weighting of different combinations of inputs. When repeated stimuli are presented at various intervals at different junctions, higher amplitude synaptic potentials are generated, if the intervals between them are not too short or too long. This increase in amplitude is due to a phenomenon called *facilitation*. If the response lasts longer than the interval between impulses, so that the second response rises from the residue of the first, then it is called *temporal summation*. If in addition, the response increment due to the second stimulus is larger than the previous one, then it is facilitation. Facilitation is an important function of the nervous system and is found in quite different forms and durations ranging from a few milliseconds to tenths of seconds. Facilitation may grade from forms of sensitization to learning, especially at long intervals. A special case is the so-called *posttetanic potentiation* which is the result of high frequency stimulation for long periods of time (about 10 sec). The latter is an interesting case since, no effects can be seen during stimulation but afterward any test stimulus at various intervals creates a marked increase in response up to many times more than the "tetanic" stimulus. *Antifacilitation*, is the phenomenon where a decrease of response from the neuron is observed at certain junctions, due to successive impulses. Its mechanism is less understood than facilitation. Both facilitation and antifacilitation may be observed on the same neuron but when different functions are performed.

3.3   Representation of Information in the Nervous System

Whenever information is transferred between different parts of the nervous system some communication paths have to be established, and some parameters of impulse firing relevant to communication must be set up. Since what is communicated is nothing more than impulses — spike trains — the only basic variables in a train of events are the number of and the interval between spikes. With respect to that, the nervous system acts like a pulse coded analog device since the intervals are continuously graded. There exists a distribution of interval lengths between individual spikes, which in any sample can be expressed by the shape of the interval histogram. If one examines different examples, it will be seen that their distributions markedly differ. Some histograms look like Poisson distributions, some others exhibit Gaussian or bimodal shapes. The coefficient of variation — expressed as the standard deviation over the mean — in some cases is constant while in others it varies. Some other properties depend on the sequence of longer and shorter intervals than the mean. Some neurons show no linear dependence, some others positive or negative correlations of successive intervals. If stimulus is delivered and a discharge from the neuron is observed, a *poststimulus time histogram* can be used using the onset of the stimulus as a reference point and average many responses in order to reveal certain consistent features of temporal patterns. Coding of information can then be based on the average frequency, which can represent relevant gradations of the input. Mean frequency is the code in most cases, although no definition of it has been given with respect to measured quantities such as averaging time, weighting functions, and forgetting functions. Characteristic transfer functions have been found that suggest that there are several distinct coding principles in addition to the mean frequency. Each theoretically possible code becomes a candidate code as long as there exists some evidence that is readable by the system under investigation. So, one has to first test for the availability of the code by imposing a stimulus that is considered normal. After a response has been observed, the code is considered to be available. If the input is changed to different levels of one parameter and changes are observed at the postsynaptic level, the code is called *readable*. However, only if both are formed in the same preparation and no other parameter is available and readable, can the code be said to be the *actual* code employed. Some such parameters are:

- Time of firing
- Temporal pattern
- Number of spikes in the train
- Variance of interspike intervals
- Spike delays or latencies
- Constellation code

The latter is a very important one, especially when used in conjunction with the concept of *receptive fields* of units in different sensory pathways. The unit receptors do not need to have highly specialized abilities to permit encoding of a large number of distinct stimuli. Receptive fields are topographic and overlap extensively. Any given stimulus will excite a certain constellation of receptors and is therefore encoded in the particular set that is activated. A large degree of uncertainty prevails and requires the brain to operate probabilistically. In the nervous system there exists a large amount of *redundancy* although neurons might have different thresholds. It is questionable, however, if these units are entirely equivalent although they share parts of their receptive fields. The nonoverlapping parts might be of importance and critical to sensory function. On the other hand, redundancy does not necessarily mean unspecified or random connectivity. It rather allows for greater sensitivity and resolution, improvement of signal to noise ratio, while at the same time it provides stability of performance.

Integration of large numbers of converging inputs to give a single output can be considered as an averaging or probabilistic operation. The "decisions" made by a unit depend on its inputs or some intrinsic states and on its reaching a certain threshold. This way every unit in the nervous system can make a decision, when it changes from one state to a different one. A theoretical possibility also exists that a mass of randomly connected neurons may constitute a trigger unit and that activity with a sharp threshold can spread through such a mass redundancy. Each part of the nervous system and in particular the receiving side can be thought of as a filter. Higher-order neurons do not merely pass that information on, but instead, they use convergence from different channels, as well as divergence of the same channels and other processes, in order to modify incoming signals. Depending on the structure and coupling functions of the network, what gets through is determined. Similar networks exist at the output side. They also act as filters, but since they formulate decisions and commands with precise *spatiotemporal* properties they can be thought of as *pattern generators*.

3.4   Lateral Inhibition

Our discussion will be incomplete without the description of a very important phenomenon in the nervous system. This phenomenon called *lateral inhibition* is used by the nervous system to improve spatial resolution and contrast. The effectiveness of this type of inhibition decreases with distance. In the retina, for example, lateral inhibition is used extensively in order to improve contract. As the stimulus approaches a certain unit, it first excites neighbors of the recorded cell. Since these neighbors inhibit that unit, its response is a decreased firing frequency. If the stimulus is exactly over the recorded unit, this unit is excited and fires above its normal rate and as the stimulus moves out again the neighbors are excited while the unit under consideration fires less. If we now examine the output of all the units as a whole and at once, while half of the considered array is stimulated the other half is not, we will notice that at the point of discontinuity of the stimulus going from stimulation to nonstimulation, the firing frequencies of the two halves have been differentiated to the extreme at the stimulus edge, which has been enhanced. The neuronal circuits responsible for lateral shifts are relatively simple. Lateral inhibition can be considered to give the negative of the second spatial derivative of the input stimulus. A second layer of neurons could be constructed to perform this spatial differentiation on the input signal to detect only the edge. It is probably lateral inhibition that explains the psychophysical illusion known as *Mach bands*. It is probably the same principle that operates widely in the nervous system to enhance the sensitivity to contrast in the visual system in particular and in all other modalities in general. Through the years different models have been developed in order to describe lateral inhibition mathematically and various methods of analysis have been employed. These models include both one-dimensional examination of the phenomenon and two-dimensional treatment, where a two-dimensional array is used as a stimulus. This two-dimensional treatment is justified since most of the sensory receptors of the body form two-dimensional maps (receptive fields). In principle, if a one-dimensional lateral inhibition system is linear, one can extend the analysis to two dimensions by means of superposition. The objective is the same as that of the nervous system: to improve image sharpness without introducing too much distortion. This technique requires storage of each picture element (pixel) and lateral "inhibitory" interactions between adjacent pixels. Since a picture may contain millions of pixels, high-speed computers with large-scale memories are required.

At a higher level, similar algorithms can be used to evaluate decision-making mechanisms. In this case, many inputs from different sensory systems are competing for attention. The brain evaluates each one of the inputs as a function of the remaining ones. One can picture a decision-making mechanism resembling a "locator" of stimulus peaks. The final output depends on what weights are used at the inputs of a push–pull mechanism. Thus a decision can be made depending on the weights an individual's brain is applying to the incoming information about the situation under consideration. The most important information is heavily weighted while the rest is either totally masked or weighted very lightly.

3.5   Higher Functions of the Nervous System

3.5.1   Human Perception and Pattern Recognition

One way of understanding the human perception is to study the mechanisms of information processing in the brain. The recognition of patterns of sensory input is one function of the brain, a task accomplished by neuronal circuits, the *feature extractors*. Although such neuronal information is more likely to be processed globally, by a large number of neurons, in animals, single-unit recording is one of the most powerful tools in the hands of a physiologist. Most often, the concept of the *receptive field* is used as a method of understanding the sensory information processing. In the case of the visual system we would call the receptive field a well-defined region of the visual field, which when stimulated will change the firing rate of a neuron in the visual pathway. The response of the neuron will usually depend on the distribution of light in the receptive field. Therefore, the information collected by the brain from the outside world is transformed into spatial as well as temporal patterns of neural activity.

The question often asked is how do we perceive and recognize faces, objects, and scenes. Even in those cases where only noisy representations exist, we are still able to make some inference as to what the pattern represents. Unfortunately in humans, single-unit recording, as mentioned earlier is impossible. As a result, one has to use other kinds of measurements, such as evoked potentials (EPs) or functional imaging techniques such as functional magnetic resonance imaging (fMRI), and positron emission tomography (PET). Although physiological in nature, EPs are still far away from giving us information at the neuronal level. However, all these methods have been used extensively as a way of probing the human (and animal) brains because of their noninvasive character. EPs can be considered to be the result of integrations of the neuronal activity of many neurons somewhere in the brain. These gross potentials can be used as a measure of the response of the brain to sensory inputs.

The question then arises: Can we use this response to influence the brain in producing patterns of activity that we want? None of the efforts of the past closed that loop. How do we explain then the phenomenon of selective attention by which we selectively direct our attention to something of interest and discard the rest? And what happens with the evolution of certain species that change appearance according to their everyday needs? All of these questions tend to lead to the fact that somewhere in the brain there is a loop where previous knowledge or experience is used as a feedback to the brain itself. This feedback modifies the ability of the brain to respond in a different way to the same stimulus the next time it is presented. In a way then, the brain creates mental "images" independent of the stimulus, which tend to modify the representation of the stimulus in the brain [1].

This section describes some efforts in which different methods have been used in trying to address the difficult task of feedback loops in the brain. However, no attempt will be made to explain or even postulate where these feedback loops might be located. If one considers the brain as a huge set of neural networks, then one question has been debated for many years: what is the role of the individual neuron in the net and what is the role of each network in the global processes of the brain? More specifically, does the neuron act as an analyzer or a detector of specific features or does it merely reflect the characteristic response of a population of cells of which it happens to be a member? What invariant relationships exist between sensory input and the response of a single neuron and how much can be "read" about the stimulus parameters from the record of a single EP? In turn, then, how much feedback can one use from a single EP in order to influence the stimulus and how successful can that influence be? Many physiologists express doubts that simultaneous observations of large number of individual neuronal activities can be readily interpreted. In other words, can then, a feedback process influence and modulate the stimulus patterns so that they appear as being optimal? If this were proven to be true, it would mean that we can reverse the pattern recognition process and instead of recognizing a pattern we would be able to create a pattern from a vast variety of possible patterns. It would be like creating a link between our brain and a computer, equivalent to a brain–computer system network. Figure 3.1 is a schematic representation of such a process involved in what we call the feedback loop of the system. The *pattern recognition device* (PRD) is connected to an ALOPEX system (a computer algorithm and an image processor in this case) and faces a display

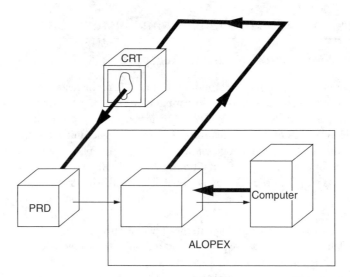

FIGURE 3.1   An ALOPEX system. The stimulus is presented on the cathode ray tube (CRT). The observer or any pattern recognition device (PRD) faces the CRT; the subject's response is sent to the ALOPEX interface unit where it is recorded and integrated and the final response is sent to the computer. The computer calculates the values of the new pattern to be presented on the CRT according to the ALOPEX algorithm and the process continues until the desired pattern appears on the CRT. At this point the response is considered to be optimal and the process stops.

monitor where different intensity patterns can be shown. In this figure, thin arrows represent response information and heavy arrows represent detailed pattern information generated by the computer and relayed by an ALOPEX system to the monitor. ALOPEX is a set of algorithms described in detail elsewhere in this Handbook. If this kind of arrangement is used for the determination of visual-receptive fields of neurons, then the PRD is nothing more than the brain of the experimental animal or human. This way the neuron under investigation does its own selection of the best stimulus or trigger feature, and reverses the role of the neuron from being a feature extractor to becoming a feature generator as mentioned earlier. The idea is to find the response of the neuron to a stimulus and use this response as a positive feedback in the directed evaluation of the initially random pattern. Thus, the cell filters out the key trigger features from the stimulus and reinforces them with the feedback.

As a generalization of this process we might consider that a neuron, N, receives a visual input from a pattern, P, which is transmitted in a modified form P' to an analyzer neuron AN (or even a complex of such neurons) as shown in Figure 3.2. The analyzer responds with a scalar variable, R, that is then fed back to the system and the pattern is modified accordingly. The process continues in small steps (iterations) until there is an almost perfect correlation between the original pattern (template) and the one that the neuron, N, indirectly created. This integrator sends the response back to the original modifier. The integrator need not be a linear one. It could take any nonlinear form, a fact that is a more realistic representation of the visual cortex. We can envision the input patterns as templates preexisting in the memory of the system, a situation that might come about with visual experience. For a "naive" system, any initial pattern will do. As experience is gained the patterns become less random. If one starts with a pattern that has some resemblance to one of the preexisting patterns, evolution will take its course. In nature, there might exist a mechanism similar to that of ALOPEX [1]. By filtering the characteristics that are most important for the survival of the species, changes would be triggered. *Perception*, therefore, could be considered to be an interaction between sensory inputs and past experience in the form of templates stored in the memory bank of the perceiver and is specific to the perceiver's needs. These templates are modifiable with time and adjusted accordingly to the input stimuli. With this approach the neural nets and ensembles of nets generate patterns that describe their thinking and memory properties. Thus, the normal flow of information is *reversed* and controls the afferent systems.

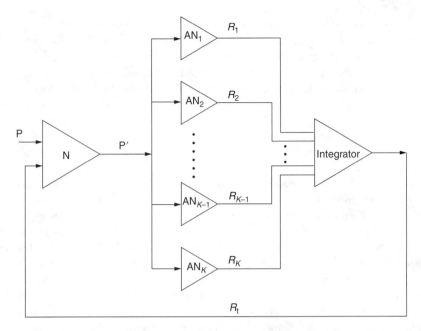

FIGURE 3.2 Schematic representation of the ALOPEX "inverse" pattern recognition scheme. Each neuron represents a feature analyzer, which responds to the stimulus with a scalar quantity R called the *response*. R is then fed back to the system and the pattern is modified accordingly. This process continues until there is an almost perfect correlation between the desired output and the original pattern.

Perception processes as well as feature extraction or suppression of images or objects can be ascribed to specific neural mechanisms due to some sensory input, or even due to some "wishful thinking" of the PRD. If it is true that the association cortex is affecting the sensitivity of the sensory cortex, then an ALOPEX mechanism is what one needs to close the loop for memory and learning.

3.5.2 Memory and Learning

If we try to define what memory is, we will face the fact that memory is not a single mental faculty but it is rather composed of multiple abilities mediated by separate and distinct brain systems. Memory for a recent event can be expressed *explicitly* as a conscious recollection, or *implicitly*, as a facilitation of test performance without conscious recollection. The major distinction between these two memories is that explicit or *declarative* memory depends on limbic and diencephalic structures and provides the basis for recollection of events, while implicit or *nondeclarative* memory, supports skills and habit learning, single conditioning, and the well-researched phenomenon of *priming* [7].

Declarative memory refers to memory of recent events and is usually assessed by tests of recall or recognition for specific single items. When the list of items becomes longer, a subject not only learns about each item on the list but also makes associations about what all these items have in common, that is, the subject learns about the category that the items belong to. Learning leads to changes that increase or decrease the effectiveness of impulses arriving at the junctions between neurons and the cumulative effect of these changes constitutes memory. Very often a particular pattern of neural activity leads to a result that occurs some time after that activity has ended. Learning then requires some means of relating the activity that is to be changed to the evaluation that can be made only by the delayed consequence. This phenomenon in physics is called *hysteresis* and refers to any modifications of future actions due to past actions. *Learning* then could be defined as change in any neuronal response resulting from previous experiences due to an external stimulus. *Memory* in turn, would be the maintenance of these changes over time. The collection of neural changes representing memory is commonly known as the *engram* and a major part of recent work has been to identify and locate engrams in the brain, since specific parts of the nervous system are capable of specific types of learning. The view of memory that has recently emerged is that, information storage is tied to specific processing areas that are engaged during learning. The brain is organized so that separate regions of the neocortex simultaneously carry out computations on specific features or characteristics of the external stimulus, no matter how complex that stimulus might be. If the brain learns specific properties or features of the stimulus then we talk about the *nonassociative memory*. Associated with this type of learning is the phenomenon of *habituation* in which, if the same stimulus is presented repeatedly, the neurons respond less and less, while the introduction of a new stimulus increases the sensitization of the neuron. If learning includes two related stimuli then we talk about associative learning. This type of learning can be of two types: classical conditioning and operant conditioning. The former deals with relationships among stimuli while the latter deals with the relationship of the stimulus to the animal's own behavior. In humans, there exist two types of memory: short- and long-term memories. The best way to study any physiological process in humans (especially memory) is to study its pathology. The study of amnesia has provided strong evidence of distinguishing between these types of memory. Amnesic patients can keep a short list of numbers in mind for several minutes if they pay attention to the task. The difficulty comes when the list becomes longer, especially if the amount to be learned exceeds the brain capacity of what can be held in immediate memory. It could be that this happens because more systems have to be involved and that temporary information storage may occur within each brain area where stable changes in synaptic efficacy can eventually develop. *Plasticity* within existing pathways can account for most of the observations and short-term memory occurs too quickly for it to require any major modifications of neuronal pathways. The capacity of long-term memory requires the integrity of the medial temporal and diencephalic regions, in conjunction with neurons for storage of information. Within the domain of long-term memory amnesic patients demonstrate intact learning and retention of certain motor, perceptual and cognitive skills, and intact priming effects. These patients do not exhibit any learning deficits but have no conscious awareness of prior study sessions or recognition of previously presented stimuli.

Priming effects can be tested by presenting words and then providing either the first few letters of the word or the last part of the word for recognition by the patient. Normal subjects, as expected, perform better than amnesic subjects. But if these patients are instructed to "read" the incomplete word instead of memorizing it, then they perform as well as the normal. Also, amnesic patients perform well if words are cued by category names. Thus, priming effects seem to be independent of the processes of recall and recognition memory, which is also observed in normal subjects. All these evidences support the notion that the brain has organized its memory functions around fundamentally different information storage systems. In perceiving a word, a preexisting array of neurons is activated that have concurrent activities that produce perception and priming is one of these functions.

Memory is not fixed immediately after learning, but continues to grow toward stabilization over a period of time. This stabilization is called *consolidation of memory*. Memory consolidation is a *dynamic* feature of long-term memory, especially the declarative memory, but is neither an automatic process with fixed lifetime nor is it determined at the time of learning. It is rather a process of reorganization of stored information. As time passes, some not yet consolidated memories fade out by remodeling the neural circuitry that is responsible for the original representation or by establishing new representations, since the original one might be forgotten.

The problems of learning and memory are studied continuously and with increased interest these years, especially because artificial systems such as Neural Networks can be used to mimic functions of the nervous system.

3.6 Abnormalities of the Nervous System

3.6.1 Parkinson's Disease

Parkinson's disease is a slowly progressive neurodegenerative disease of the CNS (central nervous system) first described in 1817 by James Parkinson. The incidence rates ranges from 4.5 to 21/100,000 individuals per year. At least 750,000,000 people are affected in the United States alone. Although most patients affected are over 60 years of age, as many as 10% may be less than 40.

Parkinson's disease occurs due to degeneration of the substantia nigra, a part of the brain involved in motor control, whose cells secretes the neurotransmitter dopamine to other movement-control centers known as the basal ganglia. The basal ganglia circuitry, which utilizes other neurotransmitters like gamma-aminobutyric acid and serotonin among others, is therefore affected. It is due to these other neurotransmitters that patients may develop nonmotor symptoms later in the disease. Some of these symptoms include cognitive problems, psychiatric disorders (e.g., depression), sleep disorders (e.g., restless leg syndrome, rapid eye movement (REM), behavior disorder), and autonomic nervous system dysfunction among others [8].

A minority of patients may have a genetic disorder. Those patients know of other family members, throughout the different generations, with Parkinson's disease. But what causes the degeneration in the substantia nigra in the majority of the patients is still unknown. Multiple reports were published in the late 1970s and early 1980s of patients who developed parkinsonism induced by MPTP (1-methyl-4-phenyl-1,2,3,6-tetrahydropyridine), a contaminant of illicit narcotics. Some other culprits include manganese, carbon monoxide, pesticides, antidopaminergic therapy, but these are implicated only in very few cases.

The diagnosis is made clinically when the characteristic motor deficits appear. These include tremor, bradykinesia (slowed movements), rigidity, and postural instability. The tremor occurs at rest. It occasionally begins with an alternating opposition of the fingers and thumb called "pill-rolling" tremor. The characteristic frequency of the Parkinsonian tremor is of 3 to 5 cycles/sec. Symptoms usually begin on one side of the body and slowly progresses over years to decades to include the other side.

The various pharmacological treatments currently available are designed to affect the dopaminergic system. The "gold standard" is levodopa. However, long-term use of levodopa leads to motor complications, mainly dyskinesias or chorea (involuntary, uncontrolled movements of the body). Dopamine agonists appear to delay the onset of dyskinesias for a few years. Currently under study are a few nondopaminergic drugs with the hope of improving motor symptoms, avoid motor complications, and delay neurodegeneration [10].

3.6.2 Alzheimer's Disease

Alzheimer's disease (AD) it is the most common form of dementia among elders. It is named after Alois Alzheimer, who described both the clinical features and pathologic changes in 1906. Like Parkinson's disease, it is also a progressive neurodegenerative disease. The prevalence in the United States in patients above age 65 is 10.3%, rising to 47% in those over the age of 80.

Alzheimer's disease is primarily the result of degeneration or death of nerve cells in the cerebral cortex and in areas that usually control functions such as memory, personality, logical thinking, and other. As the nerve cells become withered and small, they cause the enlargement of the ventricles of the brain. Recent events are not remembered, the individual is not able to perform calculations or make plans and decisions. Abrupt personality changes alarm family members and friends thus disabling the person from functioning normally.

The etiology of the majority of the cases still remains unknown, although it appears to be depending on multiple factors. Familial AD, although rare, can be inherited. The patients in this group have an earlier onset (age 30 to 60) than the common form of AD. The one risk factor for the more common form is a protein involved in cholesterol transport known as apolipoprotein E (apoE). The allele frequency of an isoform of apoE (apoE4) was found to be 40% in either familial or common form AD compared to 15% in patients without AD [11].

Alzheimer's disease is characterized by atrophy of the cerebral cortex, usually more severe in the frontal, parietal, and temporal lobes. The most characteristic microscopic findings are the senile plaques and neurofibrillary tangles. These are mostly found throughout the cerebral cortex and hippocampus. The activity of choline acetyltransferase, the biosynthetic enzyme of acetylcholine, has a 50 to 90% reduction in the cerebral cortex and hippocampus in AD. Therefore, cholinergic neurons are largely affected.

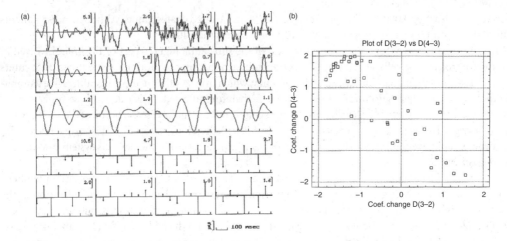

FIGURE 3.3   (a) A normal waveform (leftmost column) and three pathological waveforms. The 6th octave wavelet and residual signals (2nd and 3rd rows) and their Wavelet Coefficients (4th and 5th rows respectively). Vertical tickmarks indicate the vertical scale of the plots. (b) Scatter plot of D_{3-2} vs. D_{4-3}. In the scatter plot, the upper leftmost grid and its immediate right and down neighbors indicate an acceptable range of coefficient changes for the $(N_{70}\text{-}P_{100}\text{-}N_{130})$ complex of the pattern reversal VEP, analyzed by B-spline wavelets.

Amyloid-beta (AB) is the major substance implicated in the progression of AD. Large amounts of this peptide due to overproduction, lack of degradation, or other factors lead to the formation of senile plaques. Their presence may trigger the release of cytochrome C, which is associated with *apoptosis* (cell death) and neurodegeneration. (Parkinson's disease, also involves amyloids that aggregate and participate in the direct or indirect loss of synapses and neurons.) Other studies point to excessive amounts of glutamate in the extracellular fluid. Their presence are thought to very rapidly inhibit the transport of molecules from the cell body to the end terminal of the axon, therefore leading to the loss of synapses — the end result of AD. Thus, chemical synaptic input is stopped and the ability of the person to perform certain functions is greatly inhibited.

Since the only definite way to diagnose AD is through histopathology, clinicians can diagnose possible or probable AD depending on signs and symptoms until a brain autopsy confirms the diagnosis. Some of the symptoms include progressive worsening of memory and other cognitive functions and cognitive loss impairing social or occupational functioning and causing a significant decline from a previous level of functioning. The current therapies used for AD include cholinesterase inhibitors, estrogen, nonsteroidal anti-inflammatory drugs, and vitamin E.

A physiological approach in determining the relative severity of the pathological changes in the associative cortex is the use of EPs, mainly visual. These recordings account for the clinical finding of diminished visual interpretation skills with normal visual acuity. The most important finding and consistent abnormality with flash visual evoked potentials (VEPs) is the delayed latency of the P_{100} component and at the same time an increase in its amplitude. The later VEP peaks may also be delayed in patients with AD. Sophisticated analysis with B-spline wavelets was performed on data collected from 40 subjects, 14 of them suffering from a degenerative disease like AD. The scatter plot of Figure 3.3, shows that the VEP complex $(N_{70}\text{-}P_{100}\text{-}N_{130})$ in the delta–theta and alpha bands yields a negative wavelet coefficient D_{3-2} in the $[-2, -1]$ region, a positive D_{4-3} in the region $[1, 2]$, and a negative third coefficient in the sixth octave, standing for an alpha discharge, is observed for normal waveforms. Any deviations from these findings may be interpreted as abnormal behavior.

3.6.3   Epilepsy

This is a disease that affects 1% of the world's population and is characterized by a sudden malfunction of the brain. The malfunctioning might reappear and reflects the clinical signs of extensive activity of neurons in synchrony. Two types of epilepsy have been identified: *generalized* and *focal*. The former involves the whole brain while the latter involves specific smaller well-defined regions of the brain. Symptoms associated with epilepsy include impairment of consciousness, autonomic or sensory symptoms, motor phenomena as well as psychic symptoms.

When antiepileptic medication stops affecting the patient's symptoms, surgery is recommended. However, the gold standard of the exact localization of the epileptic focus is to use electroencephalography (EEG). Depending on the individual occurrence of seizures, EEG analysis has been proven very valuable. It would be even more valuable if it could give a reliable prediction of when a seizure might occur, a fact that would be of enormous importance to the individual suffering from epilepsy. As in many other nervous system disorders, our knowledge of epilepsy comes from animal models. Despite the fact that there exists an enormous amount of literature on the subject, the main mechanisms (both physiological and chemical) are still not well understood.

A lot of work is still needed, especially in terms of understanding the content of EEGs using both linear and nonlinear techniques, the latter used lately more often. So far, research with nonlinear methods of analysis can, at best, predict a seizure only a few seconds before it happens and none of these methods have been adopted clinically.

3.6.4 Phantom Limb Sensation/Pain

Phantom limb pain (PLP) is a term that describes a class of painful phenomena that affect individuals who have undergone a traumatic amputation of a limb. These individuals experience painful sensations that are perceived to be originating from the amputated limb. In subjects with PLP the painful sensations are generated in the higher cortical areas of the CNS. This is in contrast to the normal condition in which pain signals originate in the PNS and are then passed to the higher processing centers where these signals are perceived as pain. The fact that PLP is centrally generated means that traditional pain treatments are relatively ineffective in the long-term treatment of PLP, since these treatments act on the pathway between the PNS and the CNS to stop the transmission of painful stimuli.

It has been observed that chronic PLP can lead to significant impairment in areas of daily living. Of the sufferers of PLP, 18% were unable to work, 33.5% report that PLP interferes with their ability to work, 82% have sleep disorders, 43% report that PLP impairs their social activities, and 45% of patients report an impairment in their daily activities.

Work performed in our laboratories utilized fMRI to test the hypothesis that there exists a neural construct such that higher-processing areas in the brain responsible for integrating motor, somatosensory, and visual information into a unified somatic perception expect certain cohesive patterns of input from the lower areas of the brain. More specifically, these areas expect that somatosensory and visual feedback is consistent and that it agrees with motor output. Under normal conditions these expectations are typically met. When a part of the body is amputated, however, the motor cortex is still capable of issuing motor commands to the missing limb but there is erroneous somatosensory and a complete lack of visual feedback. This inconsistency in information pertaining to the limb results in higher-processing centers receiving patterns of input that are not consistent with the neural construct. It is hypothesized that upon receiving patterns of inconsistent information the higher-associative areas that comprise the hypothetical neural construct conclude that things are not as they should be with the missing limb and that this conclusion leads to the perception of pain originating from the missing limb. One would expect that, if the hypothesis is correct, there might be found a conflict recognition center, or a region or regions of the brain that are active in response to somatosensory sensory conflict. The insula is an area of the brain that is known to be a center of multimodal sensory integration and an area whose activity is correlated with various types of pain. For these reasons, the insula is an area of great interest in the search for the hypothetical conflict recognition center.

The fMRI was used to investigate patterns of neural activation in normal subjects and amputees during experiments involving the movement and visual monitoring of intact and phantom limbs. With amputees, visual feedback was manipulated to bring visual and motor activity into closer agreement. In the normal experiments visual feedback was manipulated to create disagreement between visual and motor activity.

If the hypothesis were correct one would expect to see different patterns of activation when the motor and sensory systems are in agreement as opposed to when they are not.

Work by other laboratories support the role of insula as an integrator of information, a region associated with various forms of pain and discomfort and a region whose activity has been found to correlate with conditions being other than what they should be according to the individual. It is suggested here that it is the identification that things are not as they should be that leads to the perception of pain and that this process is mediated, in part, by the insula.

References

[1] Micheli-Tzanakou, E. (2000). *Supervised and Unsupervised Pattern Recognition: Feature Extraction and Computational Intelligence,* CRC Press, Boca Raton, FL.

[2] McMahon, T.A. (1984). *Muscles, Reflexes and Locomotion,* Princeton University Press, Princeton, NJ.

[3] Hartzell, H.C. (1981). "Mechanisms of slow postsynaptic potentials," *Nature,* 291, 593.

[4] Cowan, W.M. and Cuenod, M. (Eds.), (1975). *Use of Axonal Transport for Studies of Neuronal Connectivity,* Elsevier, Amsterdam, pp. 217–248.

[5] Shepherd, G.M. (1978). "Microcircuits in the nervous system," *Sci. Am.* (Feb.), 238(2), pp. 93–103.

[6] Deutsch, S. and Micheli-Tzanakou, E. (1987). *Neuroelectric Systems,* New York University Press.

[7] Partridge, L.D. and Partridge, D.L. (1993). *The Nervous System: Its Function and Interaction with the World,* MIT Press, Cambridge, MA.

[8] Ganong, W.F. (1989). *Review of Medical Physiology,* 14th ed., Appleton and Lange, Norwalk, CT.

[9] Deutsch, S. and Deutsch, A. (1993). *Understanding the Nervous System: An Engineering Perspective,* IEEE Press, Piscataway, NJ.

[10] Watts, R.L. and Koller, W.C. (Eds.), (1997). *Movement Disorders Neurologic Principles and Practice.* New York, McGraw-Hill.

[11] Rowland, L.P. (Ed.) (2000). *Merritt's Textbook of Neurology,* 10th ed., Lippincott Williams & Wilkins, Pennsylvania.

[12] Ostrowsky, K., Magnin, M., Ryvlin, P., Isnard, J., Guenot, M., and Mauguiere, F. (2002). "Representation of pain and somatic sensation in the human insula: a study of responses to direct electrical cortical stimulation," *Cereb. Cortex,* 12, 376–385.

4

Vision System

George D. Stetten
Carnegie Mellon University

David Marr, an early pioneer in computer vision, defined vision as extracting "... from images of the external world, a description that is useful for the viewer and not cluttered with irrelevant information" [Marr, 1982]. Advances in computers and video technology in the past decades have created the expectation that artificial vision should be realizable. The nontriviality of the task is evidenced by the continuing proliferation of new and different approaches to computer vision without any observable application in our everyday lives. Actually, computer vision is already offering practical solutions in industrial assembly and inspection, as well as for military and medical applications; so it seems we are beginning to master some of the fundamentals. However, we have a long way to go to match the vision capabilities of a 4-year-old child. In this chapter, we explore what is known about how nature has succeeded at this formidable task — that of interpreting the visual world.

4.1 Fundamentals of Vision Research

Research into biologic vision systems has followed several distinct approaches. The oldest is psychophysics, in which human and animal subjects are presented with visual stimuli and their responses recorded. Important early insights also were garnered by correlating clinical observations of visual defects with known neuroanatomic injury. In the past 50 years, a more detailed approach to understanding the mechanisms of vision has been undertaken by inserting small electrodes deep within the living brain to monitor the electrical activity of individual neurons and by using dyes and biochemical markers to track the anatomic course of nerve tracts. This research has led to a detailed and coherent, if not complete, theory of a visual system capable of explaining the discrimination of form, color, motion, and depth. This theory has been confirmed by noninvasive radiologic techniques that have been used recently to study the physiologic responses of the visual system, including positron emission tomography [Zeki et al., 1991] and functional magnetic resonance imaging [Belliveau et al., 1992; Cohen and Bookheimer, 1994], although these noninvasive techniques provide far less spatial resolution and thus can only show general regions of activity in the brain.

4.2   A Modular View of the Vision System

4.2.1   The Eyes

Movement of the eyes is essential to vision, not only allowing rapid location and tracking of objects but also preventing stationary images on the retina, which are essentially invisible. Continual movement of the image on the retina is essential to the visual system.

The eyeball is spherical and therefore free to turn in both the horizontal and vertical directions. Each eye is rotated by three pairs of mutually opposing muscles, innervated by the oculomotor nuclei in the brainstem. The eyes are coordinated as a pair in two useful ways: turning together to find and follow objects and turning inward to allow adjustment for parallax as objects become closer. The latter is called convergence.

The optical portion of the eye, which puts an image on the retina, is closely analogous to a photographic or television camera. Light enters the eye, passing through a series of transparent layers — the cornea, the aqueous humor, the lens, and the vitreous body — to eventually project on the retina.

The cornea, the protective outer layer of the eye, is heavily innervated with sensory neurons, triggering the blink reflex and tear duct secretion in response to irritation. The cornea is also an essential optical element, supplying two thirds of the total refraction in the eye. Behind the cornea is a clear fluid, the aqueous humor, in which the central aperture of the iris, the pupil, is free to constrict or dilate. The two actions are accomplished by opposing sets of muscles.

The lens, a flexible transparent object behind the iris, provides the remainder of refraction necessary to focus an image on the retina. The ciliary muscles surrounding the lens can increase the lens' curvature, thereby decreasing its focal length and bringing nearer objects into focus. This is called accommodation. When the ciliary muscles are at rest, distant objects are in focus. There are no contradictory muscles to flatten the lens. This depends simply on the elasticity of the lens, which decreases with age. Behind the lens is the vitreous humor, consisting of a semigelatinous material filling the volume between the lens and the retina.

4.2.2   The Retina

The retina coats the back of the eye and is therefore spherical, not flat, making optical **magnification** constant at 3.5 degrees of scan angle per millimeter. The retina is the neuronal front end of the visual system, the image sensor. In addition, it accomplishes the first steps in edge detection and color analysis before sending the processed information along the optic nerve to the brain. The retina contains five major classes of cells, roughly organized into layers. The dendrites of these cells each occupy no more than 1 to 2 mm^2 in the retina, limiting the extent of spatial integration from one layer of the retina to the next.

First come the receptors, which number approximately 125 million in each eye and contain the light-sensitive pigments responsible for converting photons into chemical energy. Receptor cells are of two general varieties: rods and cones. The cones are responsible for the perception of color and they function only in bright light. When the light is dim, only rods are sensitive enough to respond. Exposure to a single photon may result in a measurable increase in the membrane potential of a rod. This sensitivity is the result of a chemical cascade, similar in operation to the photomultiplier tube, in which a single photon generates a cascade of electrons. All rods use the same pigment, whereas three different pigments are found in three separate kinds of cones.

Examination of the retina with an otoscope reveals its gross topography. The yellow circular area occupying the central 5 degrees of the retina is called the macula lutea, within which a small circular pit called the fovea may be seen. Detailed vision occurs only in the fovea, where a dense concentration of cones provides visual activity to the central 1° of the visual field.

On the inner layer of the retina one finds a layer of ganglion cells, whose axons make up the optic nerve, the output of the retina. They number approximately 1 million, or less than 1% of the number of receptor cells. Clearly, some data compression has occurred in the space between the receptors and the ganglion cells. Traversing this space are the bipolar cells, which run from the receptors through the retina to the ganglion cells. Bipolar cells exhibit the first level of information processing in the visual system; namely, their response to light on the retina demonstrates "center/surround" **receptive fields**. By this I mean that a small dot on the retina elicits a response, while the area surrounding the spot elicits the opposite response. If both the center and the surround are illuminated, the net result is no response. Thus bipolar cells respond only at the border between dark and light areas. Bipolar cells come in two varieties, on-center and off-center, with the center respectively brighter or darker than the surround.

The center response of bipolar cells results from direct contact with the receptors. The surround response is supplied by the horizontal cells, which run parallel to the surface of the retina between the receptor layer and the bipolar layer, allowing the surrounding area to oppose the influence of the center. The amacrine cells, a final cell type, also run parallel to the surface but in a different layer, between the bipolar cells and the ganglion cells, and are possibly involved in the detection of motion.

Ganglion cells, since they are triggered by bipolar cells, also have center/surround receptive fields and come in two types, on- and off-center. On-center ganglion cells have a receptive field in which illumination of the center increases the firing rate and a surround where it decreases the rate. Off-center ganglion cells display the opposite behavior. Both types of ganglion cells produce little or no change in firing rate when the entire receptive field is illuminated, because the center and surround cancel each other. As in many other areas of the nervous system, the fibers of the optic nerve use frequency encoding to represent a scalar quantity.

Multiple ganglion cells may receive output from the same receptor, since many receptive fields overlap. However, this does not limit overall spatial resolution, which is maximum in the fovea, where two points separated by 0.5 min of arc may be discriminated. This separation corresponds to a distance on the retina of 2.5 mm, which is approximately the center-to-center spacing between cones. Spatial resolution falls off as one moves away from the fovea into the peripheral vision, where resolution is as low as 1 degree of arc.

Several aspects of this natural design deserve consideration. Why do we have center/surround receptive fields? The ganglion cells, whose axons make up the optic nerve, do not fire unless there is meaningful information, that is, a border, falling within the receptive field. It is the edge of a shape we see rather than its interior. This represents a form of data compression. Center/surround receptive fields also allow for relative rather than absolute measurements of color and brightness. This is essential for analyzing the image independent of lighting conditions. Why do we have both on- and off-center cells? Evidently, both light and dark are considered information. The same shape is detected whether it is lighter or darker than the background.

4.2.3 Optic Chiasm

The two optic nerves, from the left and right eyes, join at the optic chiasm, forming a hemidecussation, meaning that half the axons cross while the rest proceed uncrossed. The resulting two bundles of axons leaving the chiasm are called the optic tracts. The left optic tract contains only axons from the left half of each retina. Since the images are reversed by the lens, this represents light from the right side of the visual field. The division between the right and left optic tracts splits the retina down the middle, bisecting the fovea. The segregation of sensory information into the contralateral hemispheres corresponds to the general organization of sensory and motor centers in the brain.

Each optic tract has two major destinations on its side of the brain (1) the superior colliculus and (2) the lateral geniculate nucleus (LGN). Although **topographic mapping** from the retina is scrambled within the optic tract, it is reestablished in both major destinations so that right, left, up, and down in the image correspond to specific directions within those anatomic structures.

4.2.4 Superior Colliculus

The superior colliculus is a small pair of bumps on the dorsal surface of the midbrain. Another pair, the inferior colliculus, is found just below it. Stimulation of the superior colliculus results in contralateral eye movement. Anatomically, output tracts from the superior colliculus run to areas that control eye and neck movement. Both the inferior and superior colliculi are apparently involved in locating sound. In the bat, the inferior colliculus is enormous, crucial to that animal's remarkable echolocation abilities. The superior colliculus processes information from the inferior colliculus, as well as from the retina, allowing the eyes to quickly find and follow targets based on visual and auditory cues.

Different types of eye movements have been classified. The saccade (French, for "jolt") is a quick motion of the eyes over a significant distance. The saccade is how the eyes explore an image, jumping from landmark to landmark, rarely stopping in featureless areas. Nystagmus is the smooth pursuit of a moving image, usually with periodic backward saccades to lock onto subsequent points as the image moves by. Microsaccades are small movements, several times per second, over 1 to 2 min of arc in a seemingly random direction. Microsaccades are necessary for sight; their stabilization leads to effective blindness.

4.2.5 Lateral Geniculate Nucleus

The thalamus is often called "the gateway to the cortex" because it processes much of the sensory information reaching the brain. Within the thalamus, we find the LGN, a peanut-sized structure that contains a single synaptic stage in the major pathway of visual information to higher centers. The LGN also receives information back from the cortex, so-called reentrant connections, as well as from the nuclei in the brainstem that control attention and arousal.

The cells in the LGN are organized into three pairs of layers. Each pair contains two layers, one from each eye. The upper two pairs consist of parvocellular cells (P cells) that respond with preference to different colors. The remaining lower pair consists of magnocellular cells (M cells) with no color preference but with transient responses that contribute to motion perception (Figure 4.1). The topographic mapping is identical for all six layers; that is, passing through the layers at a given point yields synapses responding to

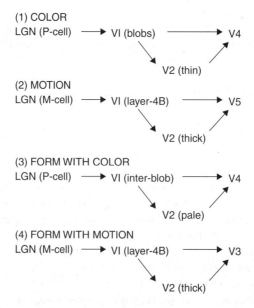

FIGURE 4.1   Visual pathways to cortical areas showing the separation of information by type. The lateral geniculate nucleus (LGN) and areas V1 and V2 act as gateways to more specialized higher areas.

a single area of the retina. Axons from the LGN proceed to the primary visual cortex in broad bands, the optic radiations, preserving this topographic mapping and displaying the same center/surround response as the ganglion cells.

4.2.6 Area V1

The LGN contains approximately 1.5 million cells. By comparison, the primary visual cortex, or striate cortex, which receives the visual information from the LGN, contains 200 million cells. It consists of a thin (2-mm) layer of gray matter (neuronal cell bodies) over a thicker collection of white matter (myelinated axons) and occupies a few square inches of the occipital lobes. The primary visual cortex has been called area 17 from the days when the cortical areas were first differentiated by their **cytoarchitectonics** (the microscopic architecture of their layered neurons). In modern terminology, the primary visual cortex is often called visual area 1, or simply V1.

Destroying any small piece of V1 eliminates a small area in the visual field, resulting in scotoma, a local blind spot. Clinical evidence has long been available that a scotoma may result from injury, stroke, or tumor in a local part of V1. Between neighboring cells in V1's gray matter, horizontal connections are at most 2 to 5 mm in length. Thus, at any given time, the image from the retina is analyzed piecemeal in V1. Topographic mapping from the retina is preserved in great detail. Such mapping is seen elsewhere in the brain, such as in the somatosensory cortex [Mountcastle, 1957]. Like all cortical surfaces, V1 is a highly convoluted sheet, with much of its area hidden within its folds. If unfolded, V1 would be roughly pear shaped, with the top of the pear processing information from the fovea and the bottom of the pear processing the peripheral vision. Circling the pear at a given latitude would correspond roughly to circling the fovea at a fixed radius.

The primary visual cortex contains six layers, numbered 1 through 6. Distinct functional and anatomic types of cells are found in each layer. Layer 4 contains neurons that receive information from the LGN. Beyond the initial synapses, cells demonstrate progressively more complex responses. The outputs of V1 project to an area known as visual area 2 (V2), which surrounds V1, and to higher visual areas in the occipital, temporal, and parietal lobes as well as to the superior colliculus. V1 also sends reentrant projections back to the LGN. Reentrant projections are present at almost every level of the visual system [Edelman, 1978; Felleman and Essen, 1991].

Cells in V1 have been studied extensively in animals by inserting small electrodes into the living brain (with surprisingly little damage) and monitoring the individual responses of neurons to visual stimuli. Various subpopulations of cortical cells have thus been identified. Some, termed simple cells, respond to illuminated edges or bars at specific locations and at specific angular orientations in the visual field. The angular orientation must be correct within 10 to 20° for the particular cell to respond. All orientations are equally represented. Moving the electrode parallel to the surface yields a smooth rotation in the orientation of cell responses by about 10 degrees for each 50 mm that the electrode is advanced. This rotation is subject to reversals in direction, as well as "fractures," or sudden jumps in orientation.

Other cells, more common than simple cells, are termed complex cells. Complex cells respond to a set of closely spaced parallel edges within a particular receptive field. They may respond specifically to movement perpendicular to the orientation of the edge. Some prefer one direction of movement to the other. Some complex and simple cells are end-stopped, meaning they fire only if the illuminated bar or edge does not extend too far. Presumably, these cells detect corners, curves, or discontinuities in borders and lines. End-stopping takes place in layers 2 and 3 of the primary visual cortex. From the LGN through the simple cells and complex cells, there appears to be a sequential processing of the image. It is probable that simple cells combine the responses of adjacent LGN cells and that complex cells combine the responses of adjacent simple cells.

A remarkable feature in the organization of V1 is **binocular convergence**, in which a single neuron responds to identical receptive fields in both eyes, including location, orientation, and directional sensitivity to motion. It does not occur in the LGN, where axons from the left and right eyes are still segregated into different layers. Surprisingly, binocular connections to neurons are present in V1 at birth. Some binocular neurons are equally weighted in terms of responsiveness to both eyes, while others are more sensitive to one eye than to the other. One finds columns containing the latter type of cells in which one eye dominates, called ocular dominance columns, in uniform bands approximately 0.5-mm wide everywhere in V1. Ocular dominance columns occur in adjacent pairs, one for each eye, and are prominent in animals with forward-facing eyes, such as cats, chimpanzees, and humans. They are nearly absent in rodents and other animals whose eyes face outward.

The topography of orientation-specific cells and of ocular dominance columns is remarkably uniform throughout V1, which is surprising because the receptive fields near the fovea are 10 to 30 times smaller than those at the periphery. This phenomenon is called magnification. The fovea maps to a greater relative distance on the surface of V1 than does the peripheral retina, by as much as 36-fold [Daniel and Whitteridge, 1961]. In fact, the majority of V1 processes only the central 10° of the visual field. Both simple and complex cells in the foveal portion can resolve bars as narrow as 2 min of arc. Toward the periphery, the resolution falls off to 1° of arc.

As an electrode is passed down through the cortex perpendicular to the surface, each layer demonstrates receptive fields of characteristic size, the smallest being at layer 4, the input layer. Receptive fields are larger in other layers due to lateral integration of information. Passing the electrode parallel to the surface of the cortex reveals another important uniformity to V1. For example, in layer 3, which sends output fibers to higher cortical centers, one must move the electrode approximately 2 mm to pass from one collection of receptive fields to another that does not overlap. An area approximately 2 mm across thus represents the smallest unit piece of V1, that is, that which can completely process the visual information. Indeed, it is just the right size to contain a complete set of orientations and more than enough to contain information from both eyes. It receives a few tens of thousands of fibers from the LGN, produces perhaps 50,000 output fibers, and is fairly constant in cytoarchitectonics whether at the center of vision, where it processes approximately 30 min of arc, or at the far periphery, where it processes 7 to 8° of arc.

The topographic mapping of the visual field onto the cortex suffers an abrupt discontinuity between the left and right hemispheres, and yet our perception of the visual scene suffers no obvious rift in the midline. This is due to the corpus collousum, an enormous tract containing at least 200 million axons, that connects the two hemispheres. The posterior portion of the corpus collousum connects the two halves of V1, linking cells that have similar orientations and whose receptive fields overlap in the vertical midline. Thus a perceptually seamless merging of left and right visual fields is achieved. Higher levels of the visual system are likewise connected across the corpus collousum. This is demonstrated, for example, by the clinical observation that cutting the corpus collousum prevents a subject from verbally describing objects in the left field of view (the right hemisphere). Speech, which normally involves the left hemisphere, cannot process visual objects from the right hemisphere without the corpus collousum.

By merging the information from both eyes, V1 is capable of analyzing the distance to an object. Many cues for depth are available to the visual system, including occlusion, parallax (detected by the convergence of the eyes), optical focusing of the lens, rotation of objects, expected size of objects, shape based on perspective, and shadow casting. **Stereopsis**, which uses the slight difference between images due to the parallax between the two eyes, was first enunciated in 1838 by Sir Charles Wheatstone and it is probably the most important cue [Wheatstone, 1838]. Fixating on an object causes it to fall on the two foveas. Other objects that are nearer become outwardly displaced on the two retinas, while objects that are farther away become inwardly displaced. About 2° of horizontal disparity is tolerated, with fusion by the visual system into a single object. Greater horizontal disparity results in double vision. Almost no vertical displacement (a few minutes of arc) is tolerated. Physiologic experiments have revealed a particular class of complex cells in V1 that are disparity tuned. They fall into three general classes. One class fires only when the object is at the fixation distance, another only when the object is nearer, and a third only when it is farther away [Poggio and Talbot, 1981]. Severing the corpus collousum leads to a loss of stereopsis in the vertical midline of the visual field.

When the inputs to the two retinas cannot be combined, one or the other image is rejected. This phenomenon is known as retinal rivalry and can occur in a piecewise manner or can even lead to blindness in one eye. The general term amblyopia refers to the partial or complete loss of eyesight not caused by abnormalities in the eye. The most common form of amblyopia is caused by strabismus, in which the eyes are not aimed in a parallel direction but rather are turned inward (cross-eyed) or outward (wall-eyed). This condition leads to habitual suppression of vision from one of the eyes and sometimes to blindness in that eye or to alternation, in which the subject maintains vision in both eyes by using only one eye at a time. Cutting selected ocular muscles in kittens causes strabismus, and the kittens respond by alternation, preserving functional vision in both eyes. However, the number of cells in the cortex displaying binocular responses is greatly reduced. In humans with long-standing alternating strabismus, surgical repair making the eyes parallel again does not bring back a sense of depth. Permanent damage has been caused by the subtle condition of the images on the two retinas not coinciding. This may be explained by the Hebb model for associative learning, in which temporal association between inputs strengthens synaptic connections [Hebb, 1961].

Further evidence that successful development of the visual system depends on proper input comes from clinical experience with children who have cataracts at birth. Cataracts constitute a clouding of the lens, permitting light, but not images, to reach the retina. If surgery to remove the cataracts is delayed until the child is several years old, the child remains blind even though images are restored to the retina. Kittens and monkeys whose eyelids are sown shut during a critical period of early development stay blind even when the eyes are opened. Physiologic studies in these animals show very few cells responding in the visual cortex. Other experiments depriving more specific elements of an image, such as certain orientations or motion in a certain direction, yield a cortex without the corresponding cell type.

4.2.7 Color

Cones, which dominate the fovea, can detect wavelengths between 400 and 700 nm. The population of cones in the retina can be divided into three categories, each containing a different pigment. This was established by direct microscopic illumination of the retina [Marks et al., 1964; Wald, 1974]. The pigments have a bandwidth on the order of 100 nm, with significant overlap, and with peak sensitivities at 560 nm (yellow–green), 530 nm (blue–green), and 430 nm (violet). These three cases are commonly known as red, green, and blue. Compared with the auditory system, whose array of cochlear sensors can discriminate thousands of different sonic frequencies, the visual system is relatively impoverished with only three frequency parameters. Instead, the retina expends most of its resolution on spatial information. Color vision is absent in many species, including cats, dogs, and some primates, as well as in most nocturnal animals, since cones are useless in low light.

By having three types of cones at a given locality on the retina, a simplified spectrum can be sensed and represented by three independent variables, a concept known as trichromacy. This model was developed by Thomas Young and Hermann von Helmholtz in the 19th century before neurobiology existed and does quite well at explaining the retina [Young, 1802; Helmholtz, 1889]. The model is also the underlying basis for red–green–blue (RGB) video monitors and color television [Ennes, 1981]. Rods do not help in discriminating color, even though the pigment in rods does add a fourth independent sensitivity peak.

Psychophysical experimentation yields a complex, redundant map between spectrum and perceived color, or hue, including not only the standard red, orange, yellow, green, and blue but hues such as pink, purple, brown, and olive green that are not themselves in the rainbow. Some of these may be achieved by introducing two more variables: saturation, which allows for mixing with white light, and intensity, which controls the level of color. Thus three variables are still involved: hue, saturation, and intensity.

Another model for color vision was put forth in the 19th century by Ewald Hering [1864]. This theory also adheres to the concept of trichromacy, espousing three independent variables. However, unlike the

Young–Helmholtz model, these variables are signed; they can be positive, negative, or zero. The resulting three axes are red–green, yellow–blue, and black–white. The Hering model is supported by the physiologic evidence for the center/surround response, which allows for positive as well as negative information. In fact, two populations of cells, activated and suppressed along the red–green and yellow–blue axes, have been found in monkey LGN. Yellow is apparently detected by a combination of red and green cones.

The Hering model explains, for example, the perception of the color brown, which results only when orange or yellow is surrounded by a brighter color. It also accounts for the phenomenon of **color constancy**, in which the perceived color of an object remains unchanged under differing ambient light conditions provided background colors are available for comparison. Research into color constancy was pioneered in the laboratory of Edwin Land [Land and McCann, 1971]. As David Hubel says, "We require color borders for color, just as we require luminance borders for black and white" [Hubel, 1998]. As one might expect, when the corpus collousum is surgically severed, color constancy is absent across the midline.

Color processing in V1 is confined to small circular areas, known as blobs, in which double-opponent cells are found. They display a center/surround behavior based on the red–green and yellow–blue axes but lack orientation selectivity. The V1 blobs were first identified by their uptake of certain enzymes, and only later was their role in color vision discovered [Livingstone and Hubel, 1984]. The blobs are especially prominent in layers 2 and 3, which receive input from the P cells of the LGN.

4.2.8 Higher Cortical Centers

How are the primitive elements of image processing so far discussed united into an understanding of the image? Beyond V1 are many higher cortical centers for visual processing, at least 12 in the occipital lobe and others in the temporal and parietal lobes. Area V2 receives axons from both the blob and interblob areas of V1 and performs analytic functions such as filling in the missing segments of an edge. V2 contains three areas categorized by different kinds of stripes: thick stripes which process relative horizontal position and stereopsis, thin stripes which process color without orientations, and pale stripes which extend the process of end-stopped orientation cells.

Beyond V2, higher centers have been labeled V3, V4, V5, etc. Four parallel systems have been delineated [Zeki, 1992], each system responsible for a different attribute of vision, as shown in Figure 4.1. This is obviously an oversimplification of a tremendously complex system.

Corroborative clinical evidence supports this model. For example, lesions in V4 lead to achromatopsia, in which a patient can only see gray and cannot even recall colors. Conversely, a form of poisoning, carbon monoxide chromatopsia, results when the V1 blobs and V2 thin stripes selectively survive exposure to carbon monoxide thanks to their rich vasculature, leaving the patient with a sense of color but not of shape. A lesion in V5 leads to akinetopsia, in which objects disappear.

As depicted in Figure 5.1, all visual information is processed through V1 and V2, although discrete channels within these areas keep different types of information separate. A total lesion of V1 results in the perception of total blindness. However, not all channels are shown in Figure 4.1, and such a "totally blind" patient may perform significantly better than expected if they were truly behind when forced to guess between colors or between motions in different directions. The patient with this condition, called blindsight, will deny being able to see anything [Weiskrantz, 1990].

Area V1 preserves retinal topographic mapping and shows receptive fields, suggesting a piecewise analysis of the image, although a given area of V1 receives sequential information from disparate areas of the visual environment as the eyes move. V2 and higher visual centers show progressively larger receptive fields and less-defined topographic mapping but more specialized responses. In the extreme of specialization, neurobiologists joke about the "grandmother cell," which would respond only to a particular face. No such cell has yet been found. However, cortical regions that respond to faces in general have been found in the temporal lobe. Rather than a "grandmother cell," it seems that face-selective neurons are members of ensembles for coding facts [Gross and Sergen, 1992].

Defining Terms

Binocular convergence: The response of a single neuron to the same location in the visual field of each eye.

Color constancy: The perception that the color of an object remains constant under different lighting conditions. Even though the spectrum reaching the eye from that object can be vastly different other objects in the field of view are used to compare.

Cytoarchitectonics: The organization of neuron types into layers as seen by various staining techniques under the microscope. Electrophysiologic responses of individual cells can be correlated with their individual layer.

Magnification: The variation in amount of retinal area represented per unit area of V1 from the fovea to the peripheral vision. Even though the fovea takes up an inordinate percentage of V1 compared with the rest of the visual field, the scale of the cellular organization remains constant. Thus the image from the fovea is, in effect, magnified before processing.

Receptive field: The area in the visual field that evokes a response in a neuron. Receptive fields may respond to specific stimuli such as illuminated bars or edges with particular directions of motion, etc.

Stereopsis: The determination of distance to objects based on relative displacement on the two retinas because of parallax.

Topographic mapping: The one-to-one correspondence between location on the retina and location within a structure in the brain. Topographic mapping further implies that contiguous areas on the retina map to contiguous areas in the particular brain structure.

References

Belliveau J.H., Kwong K.K. et al. 1992. Magnetic resonance imaging mapping of brain function: human visual cortex. *Invest. Radiol.* 27: S59.

Cohen M.S. and Bookheimer S.Y. 1994. Localization of brain function using magnetic resonance imaging. *Trends Neurosci.* 17: 268.

Daniel P.M. and Whitteridge D. 1961. The representation of the visual field on the cerebral cortex in monkeys. *J. Physiol.* 159: 203.

Edelman G.M. 1978. Group selection and phasic reentrant signalling: a theory of higher brain function. In G.M. Edelman and V.B. Mountcastle (Eds.), *The Mindful Brain*, pp. 51–100, Cambridge, MIT Press.

Ennes H.E. 1981. NTSC color fundamentals. In *Television Broadcasting: Equipment, Systems, and Operating Fundamentals.* Indianapolis, Howard W. Sams & Co.

Felleman D.J. and Van Essen D.C. 1991. Distributed hierarchical processing in the primate cerebral cortex. *Cereb. Cortex* 1: 1.

Gross C.G. and Sergen J. 1992. Face recognition. *Curr. Opin. Neurobiol.* 2: 156.

Hebb D.O. 1961. *The Organization of Behavior.* New York, John Wiley & Sons.

Helmholtz H. 1889. *Popular Scientific Lectures.* London, Longmans.

Hering E. 1864. *Outlines of a Theory of Light Sense.* Cambridge, Harvard University Press.

Hubel D.H. 1998. *Eye, Brain, and Vision.* New York, Scientific American Library.

Land E.H. and McCann J.J. 1971. Lightness and retinex theory. *J. Opt. Soc. Am.* 61: 1.

Livingstone M.S. and Hubel D.H. 1984. Anatomy and physiology of a color system in the primate visual cortex. *J. Neurosci.* 4: 309.

Marks W.B., Dobelle W.H., and MacNichol E.F. 1964. Visual pigments of single primate cones. *Science* 143: 1181.

Marr D. 1982. *Vision.* San Francisco, WH Freeman.

Mountcastle V.B. 1957. Modality and topographic properties of single neurons of cat's somatic sensory cortex. *J. Neurophysiol.* 20: 408.

Poggio G.F. and Talbot W.H. 1981. Mechanisms of static and dynamic stereopsis in foveal cortex of the rhesus monkey. *J. Physiol.* 315: 469.

Wald G. 1974. Proceedings: visual pigments and photoreceptors — review and outlook. *Exp. Eye Res.* 18: 333.

Weiskrantz L. 1990. The Ferrier Lecture: outlooks for blindsight: explicit methodologies for implicit processors. *Proc. R. Soc. Lond. B* 239: 247.

Wheatstone S.C. 1838. Contribution to the physiology of vision. *Philosoph. Trans. R. Soc. Lond.* Vol. 128, pp. 371–394.

Young T. 1802. The Bakerian Lecture: on the theory of lights and colours. *Philosoph. Trans. R. Soc. Lond.* 92: 12.

Zeki S. 1992. The visual image in mind and brain. *Sci. Am.* September, 69.

Zeki S., Watson J.D., Lueck C.J. et al. 1991. A direct demonstration of functional specialization in human visual cortex. *J. Neurosci.* 11: 641.

Further Reading

An excellent introductory text about the visual system is *Eye, Brain, and Vision*, by Nobel laureate, David H. Hubel (1995, Scientific American Library, New York). A more recent general text with a thorough treatment of color vision, as well as the higher cortical centers, is *A Vision of the Brain*, by Semir Zeki (1993, Blackwell Scientific Publications, Oxford).

Other useful texts with greater detail about the nervous system are *From Neuron to Brain*, by Nicholls, Martin, Wallace, and Kuffler (3rd ed., 1992, Sinauer Assoc., Sunderand Mass.), *The Synaptic Organization of the Brain*, by Shepherd (4th ed., 1998, Oxford Press, New York), and *Fundamental Neuroanatomy*, by Nauta and Feirtag (1986, Freeman, New York).

A classic text that laid the foundation of computer vision by *Vision*, by David Marr (1982, Freeman, New York). Other texts dealing with the mathematics of image processing and image analysis are *Digital Image Processing*, by Pratt (1991, Wiley, New York), and *Digital Imaging Processing and Computer Vision*, by Schalkoff (1989, Wiley, New York).

Two books dealing with perceptual issues are *Visual Perception: Physiology, Psychology and Ecology*, by Bruce, Green, and Georgeson (3rd ed., 1996, Psychology Press, Hove, East Sussex.) and *Sensation and Perception*, by Goldstein (6th ed., 2001, Wadsworth Publishing).

5
Auditory System

Ben M. Clopton
Advanced Cochlear Systems

Herbert F. Voigt
Boston University

5.1 Overview

Human hearing arises from airborne waves alternating 50 to 20,000 times a second about the mean atmospheric pressure. These pressure variations induce vibrations of the tympanic membrane, movement of the middle-ear ossicles connected to it, and subsequent displacements of the fluids and tissues of the cochlea in the inner ear. Biomechanical processes in the cochlea analyze sounds to frequency-mapped vibrations along the basilar membrane, and approximately 3,500 inner hair cells modulate transmitter release and spike generation in 30,000 spiral ganglion cells whose proximal processes make up the auditory nerve. This neural activity enters the central auditory system and reflects sound patterns as temporal and spatial spike patterns. The nerve branches and synapses extensively in the cochlear nuclei, the first of the central auditory nuclei. Subsequent brainstem nuclei pass auditory information to the medial geniculate and auditory cortex (AC) of the thalamocortical system.

We extract more information from sound than from any other sense. Although primates are described as "visual" animals, speech and music carry more of our cultural and societal meaning than sight or other senses, and we suffer more from deafness than with other sensory losses. Highly effective adaptations of auditory processing occur in many animals including insects, amphibians, birds, cetaceans, and bats for prey acquisition, predator avoidance, intraspecies signaling, and other tasks. This chapter surveys current understanding of the hearing process.

5.2 The Peripheral Auditory System

5.2.1 The External and Middle Ear

As shown in Figure 5.1, ambient sounds are collected by the pinna, the visible portion of the external ear, and guided to the middle ear by the external auditory meatus, or ear canal. Sounds are filtered due to the

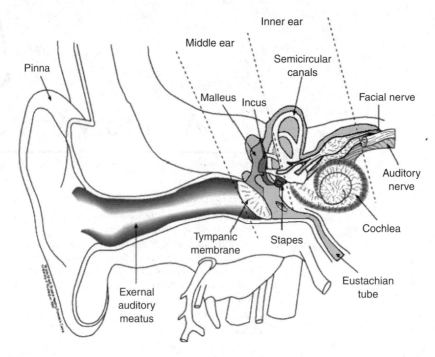

FIGURE 5.1   The peripheral auditory system showing the external-ear structures (pinna and external meatus), the middle ear, and the inner ear. (Courtesy of Virginia Merrill Bloedel Hearing Research Center, Seattle, Washington.)

geometry of the pinna and sound shadowing effects of the head. In species with movable pinnae selective scanning of the auditory environment is possible for high frequencies [Geisler, 1998; Kinsler et al., 1999].

The bounding interface between the external and middle ear is the tympanic membrane. Pressure variations across the membrane move three ossicles, the malleus (hammer) connected to the membrane, the incus (anvil), and the stapes (stirrup) whose footplate is a piston-like structure fitting into the oval window, an opening to the fluid-filled cavities of the inner ear. Ligaments and muscles suspend the middle-ear ossicles so that they move freely. If sound reaches fluids of the inner ear directly, 99.9% of the energy is reflected [Wever and Lawrence, 1954], a 30-dB loss due to the mismatch in acoustic impedance between air and inner-ear fluids. Properties of the external meatus, middle-ear cavity, tympanic membrane, and middle-ear ossicles shape the responsiveness of a species to different frequencies.

The eustachian tube is a bony channel lined with soft tissue extending from the middle ear to the nasopharynx. In humans it is often closed, except during swallowing, and provides a means by which pressure is equalized across the tympanic membrane. The function is clearly observed with changes in altitude or barometric pressure. A second function of the eustachian tube is to aerate the tissues of the middle ear.

The volume of the air-filled middle-ear cavity inversely determines the stiffness of the tympanic membrane at low frequencies. A reduction of low-frequency impedance for some desert rodents with large middle-ear cavities [Ravicz and Rosowski, 1997] enhances detection of predators at a distance. On the other hand, the mass of the middle-ear ossicles dominates impedance at high frequencies and is related to head mass [Nummela, 1995]. For this reason small mammals generally have good high-frequency hearing, often extending above 60 kHz. As sound frequency increases, impedances decrease due to eardrum stiffness and increase due to ossicular mass leaving a middle range where sound transmission to the inner ear is most efficient, limited only by resistive forces [Geisler, 1999], resonances of the cavities, and mechanical advantages provided by the tympanic membrane, ossicles, and oval window.

Since the ear canal and middle-ear cavities are, or approximate, closed volumes, they support quarter-wavelength resonances. The human meatus has a broad resonance between 3 and 4 kHz, enhancing sound pressure at the membrane by 12 dB [Weiner and Ross, 1946; von Békésy, 1950]. This will be modified by obstructing the meatus with headphones or a hearing aid and must be considered in system designs.

The head and external and middle-ear structures impose a transfer function on sound pressure at the tympanic membrane [Bateau, 1967; Blauert, 1997]. The monaural (single-ear) head-related transfer function (HRTF) is a function of sound-source azimuth and elevation relative to pressure waveforms at the tympanic membrane. It is complex, affecting both sound amplitudes and phases over their spectrum. Sound localization, highly dependent on binaural hearing, involves a binaural HRTF combining the left and right monaural HRTFs. Since the structures determining these functions vary, individualized HRTFs combined with head-position sensing are important for computer synthesis of realistic three-dimensional sound experiences delivered through headphones [Wightman and Kistler, 1989]. For some source locations, even the shadowing effects of the torso produce HRTF cues [Algazi et al., 2002].

Since the acoustic impedance of the atmospheric source is much less than that of the aqueous medium of the inner ear, a very inefficient energy transfer would exist without the external and middle ears. The ossicles form an impedance transformer with a mechanical advantage that passes the acoustic signal at the tympanic membrane to inner-ear fluids with low loss. Essentially air-based sounds of low-pressure and high-volume velocity are transformed to fluid displacements in the inner ear having high-pressure and low-volume velocity. Two important mechanisms promote this transfer: the area of the tympanic membrane is about 20 times that of the footplate of the stapes, and the lengths of the malleus and incus form a lever advantage from the eardrum to oval window of about 1.3 in humans [Wever and Lawrence, 1954; Geisler, 1998]. The hydraulic piston due to the areal ratio contributes about 26 dB to counteract the impedance mismatch, and the lever mechanism about 2.3 dB. These concepts of middle-ear mechanisms hold at frequencies below about 2 kHz, but the tympanic membrane does not behave as a piston at higher frequencies and can support multiple modes of vibration. Second, the mass of the ossicles becomes significant contributing to resonances. Third, connections between the ossicles are not lossless, and their stiffness cannot be ignored. Fourth, pressure variations in the middle-ear cavity can change the stiffness of the tympanic membrane, as do reflexive contractions of middle-ear muscles, especially in response to intense sounds. Fifth, the cavity of the middle ear produces resonances at acoustic frequencies. All of these factors produce variations in high-frequency acoustic transmission from the external to the inner ear specific to individuals, species, and conditions.

5.2.2 The Inner Ear

The acoustic portion of the mammalian inner ear is a spiral structure, the cochlea (snail), containing a central core, the modiolus, where fibers of the auditory nerve collect. The nerve fibers arise from spiral ganglion cells (SGCs) whose somas form the spiral ganglion in a bony canal around the modiolus. Around the modiolus spiral three fluid-filled chambers or scalae, the scala vestibule (SV), the scala media (SM), and the scala tympani (ST) as shown in Figure 5.2. At the base of the cochlea the stapes footplate displaces fluid in the SV through the oval window. At the other end of the spiral, the apex of the cochlea, the SV and the ST communicate through the helicotrema. Both are filled with perilymph, similar to extracellular fluid. The SM spirals between them and is filled with endolymph, a medium high in K+ and low in Na+ due to active processes in the stria vascularis lining the lateral wall. A positive potential of 80 mV is maintained in the SM by the metabolically driven ionic pumps of the stria vascularis. The SM is separated from the SV by Reissner's membrane, which is impermeable to ions. The SM is separated from the ST by the basilar membrane (BM) with a length of about 31 mm over 2.5 spiral turns in human [Wever and Lawrence, 1954]. Resting on the BM is the organ of Corti consisting of one row of inner hair cells (IHCs) that transduce acoustic signals into neural signals, three rows of outer hair cells (OHCs) that play an active role in the biomechanics of the cochea, cells that support the hair cells, and the tectorial membrane overlying the stereocilia of the hair cells.

Stapes displacements for tones above behavioral threshold are very small, estimates of 0.0001 nm being common [Geisler, 1998]. This can be compared to 0.1 nm for the diameter of a hydrogen atom.

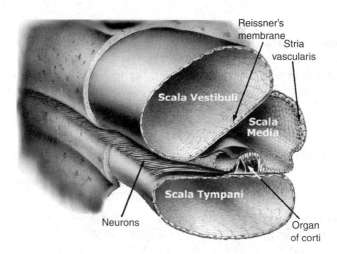

FIGURE 5.2   A cross-sectional representation of one turn of the cochlea.

The structures of the inner ear transform these infinitesimal movements to neural discharges that underlie the detection of sounds.

5.2.2.1   The Basilar Membrane

The cochlear partition (BM and organ of Corti) provides the primary passive mechanical filter function of the inner ear. Alternating fluid displacements at the footplate of the stapes induce pressure differences across the partition from its base near the oval window to its apex near the helicotrema. The cochlear partition has graded mechanical properties favoring rapid movement to high frequencies near the base and slower movement to low frequencies near the apex resulting in a traveling wave motion in that order. The membrane's width varies as it traverses the cochlear duct, narrower at its basal end than at its apical end. It is stiffer at the base than at the apex, with stiffness varying by about two orders of magnitude. Pressure relief is provided for the incompressible fluids of the inner ear by the round window, a membrane-covered opening from the ST to the middle-ear cavity. A transient pressure increase (condensation) at the stapes displaces its footplate inward, a traveling wave is initiated along the BM, pressure is increased in the ST, and a compensatory outward displacement of the round window membrane occurs. A rarefaction causes the round window membrane to move inward toward the ST.

Sound decomposition into its frequency components is a major function of the cochlea. Georg von Békésy observed the traveling wave on the cochlear partitions of cadavers under stroboscopic light synchronized to high-intensity, low-frequency tones. The traveling wave reached a maximum displacement along the BM depending on the frequency of the tone indicating a roughly logarithmic mapping of increasing frequencies from the apex to the base. His experiments on the peripheral auditory system are collected in a book [von Békésy, 1950], and he was awarded the 1961 Nobel Prize in medicine for his research.

Movements of the BM are very small, in the nanometer range or less for normal hearing, and a new technique increased measurement resolution to this level [Johnstone and Boyle, 1967]. The Mössbauer technique uses Doppler shift in γ emissions from a small radioactive particle placed on the moving tissue being observed. In 1971, Rhode published Mössbauer measurements of tuning in the basal region of the living cochlea. These tuning curves were remarkably sharp (Q_{10} of 7 to 8) for pure tones at low intensities, but they degraded to broad tuning at high intensities. The slopes of the tuning curve are much greater at the high-frequency edge than at the low-frequency edge. In the absence of an explanation using passive models, these and subsequent observations came to implicate active tuning processes in the cochlea, sometimes called the "cochlear amplifier."

Measurements using laser interferometer techniques now allow displacement resolutions of less than a nanometer [Mammano and Ashmore, 1995] and have aided investigations of the cochlea's active tuning

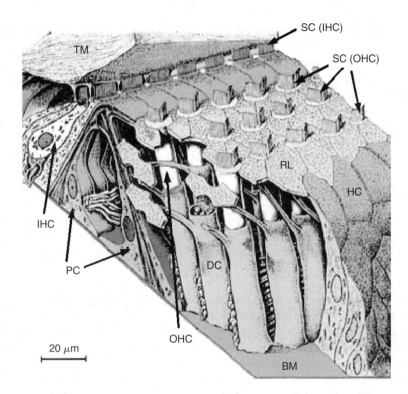

FIGURE 5.3 A depiction of the organ of Corti and its cellular structures. TM: tectorial membrane elevated to show stereocilia, PC: inner and outer pillar cells, DC: Deiter's cells, RL: reticular lamina, SC (IHC): one row of stereocilia for IHCs, SC (OHC): three rows of stereocilia for OHCs, HC: Hensen's cells. Other abbreviations are as used in text. Synapses from SGCs are seen at the bottoms of IHCs with efferent axons to OHCs seen in the tunnel and passing between Deiters' cells.

mechanisms. It has been discovered that the cochlear amplifier operates primarily in the basal, high-frequency regions and is highly compressive, that is, large increases in high-frequency tone intensity cause small increases in the maximum displacement of the BM [Geisler, 1998].

5.2.2.2 The Organ of Corti

As shown in Figure 5.3, the organ of Corti is comprised of supporting cells, the hair cells themselves, and the tectorial membrane. The ciliated ends of both OHCs and IHCs are rigidly fixed by supporting cells, for example, Deiters cells form the reticular lamina, a rigid plate holding the upper ends of the OHCs. Pillar cells form a rigid triangular tunnel whose upper surface extends the reticular lamina. The reticular lamina and upper ends of the pillar cells and other support cells form a barrier to ions, thereby isolating the endolymph of the SM from the perilymph of the ST surrounding the lower parts of the hair cells.

Both IHCs and OHCs have precise patterns of stereocilia at the end held within the rigid plate formed by supporting cells. The tectorial membrane overlies the stereocilia, but while those of OHCs contact the tectorial membrane, the stereocilia of the IHCs do not. At the end opposite the stereocilia, IHCs synapse with the distal processes of SGCs. The proximal processes of SGCs are generally myelinated and form most of the auditory nerve. The nerve is laid down as these fibers collect from the apex and base in an orderly spiral manner. The nerve retains the frequency map of the BM, that is, it is tonotopically organized, a characteristic that carries through much of the auditory system.

5.2.2.2.1 Inner Hair Cells

The IHCs lie in a single row on the modiolar side of the organ of Corti and number between 3000 and 4000 in human [Nadol, 1988]. The IHCs' stereocilia are of graded, increasing length from the modiolar side of the cell. Early in ontogeny, a kinocilium is positioned next to the longest stereocilia, and excitation of hair cells occurs from ciliary displacement in that direction further opening membrane channels to potassium and depolarizing the cell [Hudspeth, 1987]. The positive potential in the endolymph of the SM drives K+ ions through the gating mechanism of IHC stereocilia to the negative intracellular potential. Displacement in the other direction reduces channel opening and produces a relative hyperpolarization [Hudspeth and Corey, 1977]. These changes in intracellular potential modulate transmitter release through vesicle exocytosis at the base of the IHCs. The transmitter is related to glutamate but not glutamate itself [Gleich et al., 1990].

The IHCs are not attached to the tectorial membrane, so their response is thought to be responsive to fluid velocity over their stereocilia rather than direct displacement. Hair cells in some species exhibit frequency tuning when isolated [Crawford and Fettiplace, 1985], but mammalian hair cells do not. The tuning of the mammalian auditory system arises from the motions of the cochlear partition, and this is transferred to the IHCs and to the rest of the auditory system through their connection to SGCs. The nature of membrane channels and molecular mechanisms in auditory hair cells is being examined using a number of techniques [Hudspeth, 2000; Ashmore and Mammano, 2001].

5.2.2.2.2 Outer Hair Cells

There are about 12,000 OHCs in the human cochlea [Nadol, 1988]. They have primarily *efferent* innervation, a puzzling arrangement for many years since the cochlea was a "sensory organ." The discovery of cochlear tuning that was not readily explainable from passive mechanical properties shifted attention to the OHCs where research, over the last few decades, has focused on their cellular and molecular mechanisms.

It was discovered that electrical stimulation of isolated OHCs produced lengthening or shortening [Brownell et al., 1985]. It is generally accepted that the motility of OHCs counters viscous drag from fluids and cells of the cochlear partition. Through their contact to the tectorial membrane they sense the subnanometer displacements of the BM and feedback, in phase, to augment them. This positive feedback occurs at auditory frequencies and is responsible for cochlear amplification. It occurs, or is most obvious, at low sound intensities, so it is responsible for the incredible sensitivity of the ear and for the nonlinear compression of the dynamic range of intensity coding. It was also observed that iontophoretic application of acetylcholine to the synaptic end of OHCs causes them to shorten. Efferents to OHCs release acetylcholine and thereby modulate the mechanical properties of the cochlea. The OHCs appear to affect the response of the auditory system in several ways. They enhance the tuning characteristics of the system to sinusoidal stimuli, decreasing thresholds and narrowing the filter's bandwidth, and they likely influence the damping of the BM dynamically by actively changing its stiffness.

Before the role of OHCs was determined it was observed that sounds could be measured in the meatus, both spontaneously and in response to other sounds [Wilson, 1986]. In humans they tend to contain spectrally narrow components and vary across individuals. OHCs are strongly implicated as the source for these emissions because sounds in the opposite ear affect them (presumably through the efferent system) and aspirin, known to affect OHCs, reduces them [Geisler, 1998]. As with most positive-feedback systems, spontaneous oscillation is suggested. Otoacoustic emissions are becoming important in the clinical evaluation of cochlear function for their potential signaling of cochlear pathologies.

5.2.2.3 Spiral Ganglion Cells and the Auditory Nerve

The auditory nerve of the human contains about 30,000 afferent fibers. Most (93%) are heavily myelinated and arise from Type I SGCs whose distal processes synapse on IHCs. The rest are from smaller, more lightly myelinated Type II SGCs. Each IHC has, on average, a number of Type I SCCs that synapse with it, 8 in the human and 18 in the cat. In contrast, each Type II SGC contacts OHCs at a rate of about 10 to 60 cells per fiber. The tonotopically organized nerve (low-frequency fibers in the center and high-frequency fibers in the outer layers) exits the modiolus and enters the internal auditory meatus of the temporal bone on its path to the cochlear nuclei.

Discharge spike patterns from the nerve have typically been characterized with repeated tone bursts varied in frequency and intensity [Kiang, 1965]. Three views of the data are commonly used:

1. The temporal pattern of response to a tone burst is summarized in a peristimulus time histogram (PSTH). Auditory neurons may discharge only a few times during a brief tone burst, but if a histogram of spike events is synchronized to the onset of repeated tone bursts, a PSTH results that is more statistically representative of the neuron's response. Discharge patterns from the nerve have a primary-like pattern (see Figure 5.5).

2. A rate-level function of spike counts vs. intensity at one tonal frequency has a threshold level, where counts rise from quiet levels, and a maximum rate, often a plateau holding for further increases in intensity. The range from threshold to the maximum, or saturation, level is called the dynamic range for sound-intensity signaling by response rate changes. A spontaneous rate of discharge, ranging from 50 spikes per second to less than 10, is usually measured for subthreshold stimulus levels.

3. Fiber responses are also characterized with tuning curves, a plot of thresholds for stimulus intensity vs. frequency. Tuning curves for auditory nerve fibers have a minimum intensity (maximum sensitivity) at a characteristic frequency (CF).

Sounds are coded in nerve discharges in two major ways: the level of discharge activity within the fiber population reflects the spectrum of sounds (labeled-line or place coding), and the temporal pattern of discharges in a fiber is partially synchronized to the cycle-by-cycle timing of frequencies near its CF (temporal synchrony coding). Furthermore, complex sounds undergo nonlinear interactions in the cochlea, an example being two-tone suppression where the introduction of a new tone reduces both the discharge rate and synchrony of a fiber to CF tones [Geisler, 1998].

While these coding mechanisms were discovered with tones, Sachs and Young [1979] found that the spectra of lower-intensity vowel sounds are represented as corresponding tonotopic rate peaks in nerve activity, but for higher intensities this place code is lost as discharge rates saturate. At high intensities, spike synchrony to frequencies near CF continue to signal the relative spectral content of vowels, a temporal code. These results hold for high-spontaneous-rate fibers (over 15 spikes sec), which are numerous. Less common, low-spontaneous-rate fibers (<15 spikes sec) appear to maintain the rate code at higher intensities, suggesting different coding roles for these two fiber populations. Furthermore, it has more recently been argued that these results from the cat do not represent the human cochlea. When vowels are spectrally scaled to match the cat's cochlea, the rate code appears to remain at high intensities [Recio et al., 2002].

5.3 The Central Auditory System

The central auditory system consists of the cochlear nuclei; groups of brainstem nuclei including the superior olivary complex (SOC) , nuclei of the lateral lemniscus (LL), and inferior colliculus (IC); and the auditory thalamocortical system consisting of the medial geniculate in the thalamus and multiple areas of the cerebral cortex. Figure 5.4 schematically indicates the nuclear levels and pathways. Efferent pathways are not shown. Page constraints prevent us from providing uniform detail for all levels of the auditory system.

5.3.1 Cochlear Nuclei

Many studies have focused on the anatomy and physiology of the cochlear nucleus (CN) revealing a wealth of information. It can be subdivided into three regions, the anteroventral CN (AVCN) anterior to the nerve entry, the posteroventral CN (PVCN), and the dorsal CN (DCN), each with one or more distinctive neuron types and connections. The axon from each Type I SGC in the nerve branches to each of the three divisions in an orderly manner so that tonotopic organization is maintained. Neurons with

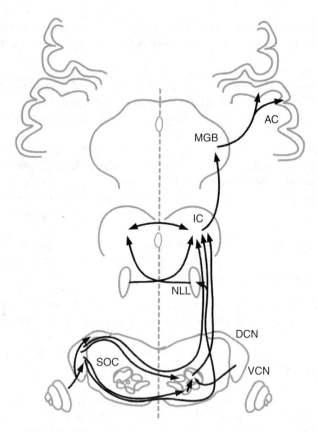

FIGURE 5.4 Schematic of the auditory system. Some of the major pathways and connections have been represented. The system is bilaterally symmetrical (midline as dashed line), paths are crossed and shown for one side in most cases for clarity.

common morphologic classifications are found in all three divisions, especially granule cells, which tend to receive connections from Type II SGCs.

Morphologic categories based on shapes of dendritic trees and somas include spherical bushy cells in the anterior part of the AVCN, both globular bushy cells and spherical bushy in posterior AVCN, stellate cells throughout the AVCN and in the lower layers of the DCN, octopus cells (asymmetrical dendritic tree resembling an octopus) in the PVCN, and fusiform and giant cells in DCN. In AVCN spherical bushy cells receive input from one Type I ganglion cell through a large synapse formation containing end bulbs of Held, while the globular cells receive inputs from a few afferent fibers. The AVCN is tonotopically organized, and neurons having similar CFs form layers called "isofrequency laminae" [Bourk et al., 1981], an organization repeated with variation through most auditory nuclei. The DCN is structurally the most intricate of the CN subnuclei having four or five layers in many species giving it a "cortical" structure comparable to the cerebellum [see Young, 1998; Oertel and Young, 2004]. Extracellular recording techniques, including simultaneous recording from pairs of physiologically identified DCN units and responses to tones and noise has allowed the development of conceptual models of DCN neuronal circuitry in cat [Young and Brownell, 1976; Voigt and Young, 1980, 1990; Young and Davis, 2002] and gerbil [Davis and Voigt, 1997]. Although some differences between the two species have been noted, these may well be explained by a similar underlying neural circuit model whose parameters are somewhat species specific (as opposed to completely different neuronal architectures) [Davis and Voigt, 1997].

Intracellular recording in slice preparation has identified the membrane characteristics of CN neuronal types [Bal and Oertel, 2001; Manis, 1990]. Some of these characteristics have been confirmed *in vivo* [Hancock and Voigt, 2002]. The diversity of neuronal morphologic types, their participation in local

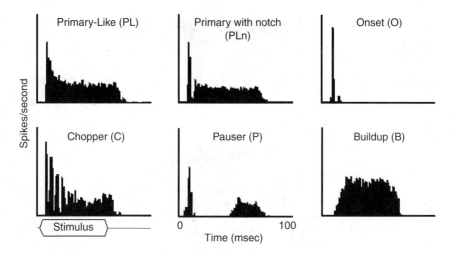

FIGURE 5.5   PSTH categories obtained for neural spike activity in the nerve and cochlear nuclei in response to brief tone bursts (stimulus envelope shown in lower left). Discharges in the nerve have the PL pattern while the others are associated with regions of the VCN and DCN and with specific morphological types.

circuits, and the emerging knowledge of their membrane biophysics are motivating detailed modeling [Babalian et al., 2003].

5.3.1.1   Spike Discharge Patterns

Tone bursts at a cell's CF and 40 dB above threshold produce PSTHs with shapes distinctive to different nuclear subdivisions and even different morphologic types. PSTH patterns provide insight into sound features exciting auditory neurons. Figure 5.5 illustrates the major PSTH pattern types obtained from the auditory nerve and CN. Auditory nerve fibers and spherical bushy cells in AVCN have primary-like patterns in their PSTHs, an elevated spike rate after tone onset, falling to a slowly adapting level until the tone burst ends. Globular bushy cells may have primary-like, pri-notch (primary-like with a brief notch after onset), or chopper patterns. Stellate cells have nonprimary-like patterns. Onset response patterns, one or a few brief peaks of discharge at onset with little or no discharges afterward, are observed in the PVCN from octopus cells. Chopper, pauser, and buildup patterns are observed in many cells of the DCN. For most CN neurons, these patterns are not necessarily stable over different stimulus intensities; a primary-like pattern may change to a pauser pattern and then to a chopper pattern as intensity is raised [Young, 1984].

Because central neurons often have inhibitory inputs, some stimuli reduce discharge probabilities, and so threshold tuning curves are extended to response-field maps. Figure 5.6 shows three response-field patterns, but many variations have been observed on these. Fibers and neurons with primary-like PSTHs generally have response maps with only an excitatory region (Figure 5.6a) although controls must be used to identify two-tone suppression. The lower edges of this region approximate the threshold-tuning curve. Octopus cells often have very broad tuning curves and extended response maps, as suggested by their frequency-spanning dendritic trees. More complex response maps are observed for some neurons, such as those in the DCN. Inhibitory regions alone, a frequency–intensity area of suppressed spontaneous discharge rates, or combinations of excitatory and inhibitory regions have been observed. Some neurons are excited only within islands of frequency–intensity combinations, demonstrating a CF but having no response to high-intensity or wide-band sounds [Spirou et al., 1999]. Response maps in the DCN containing both excitatory and inhibitory regions have been shown to arise from a convergence of inputs from neurons with only excitatory or inhibitory regions in their maps [Young and Voigt, 1981].

Categorization of CN neurons increasingly depends on many measures: cellular morphology, PSTH and response-field response patterns tones, responses to wide-band stimuli and binaural stimuli, membrane channel physiology, afferent and efferent connectivity, and molecular expressions and

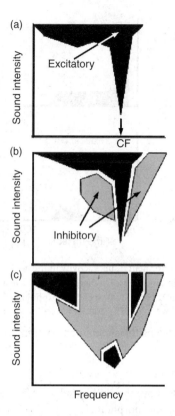

FIGURE 5.6 Response-field maps characteristic of auditory-nerve fibers (a) and central neurons. Two-tone suppression in the cochlea, not due to inhibitory synapses, may resemble panel b maps. Maps are extracted from discharge rates sampled over the stimulus intensity–frequency parameter space. The inhibitory areas represent decreases in spontaneous or evoked discharge rates by tone bursts of the frequency and intensity under test.

responses [Spirou et al., 1999; Fujino and Oertel, 2001]. Beyond mere cellular categorization, information processing in the CN is being discovered as the functions of neuronal circuits are dissected.

Principal neurons of cats [Spirou and Young, 1991] and gerbils [Parsons et al., 2001] have shown to be sensitive to spectral notches like those appearing in HRTFs. These notches, whose center frequency changes with elevation, are thought to be cues for sounds localized in the median plane, where interaural time and intensity cues are absent. Thus, part of the function of the DCN may be to aide in median plane sound localization. The DCN, however, integrates these spectral cues with information from the somato-sensory and vestibular systems, as well as from descending auditory pathways. The DCN shows signs of both long-term potentiation (LTP) and long-term depression (LTD) of some of its synapses, providing the infrastructure for learning [see Oertel and Young, 2004]. Whether these learning mechanisms are used exclusively during development (e.g., when we need to learn to associate specific spectral notch frequencies with specific median plane locations) or if they function in adults navigating within their acoustic environments remains a topic of intense interest.

In addition to the contributions to our understanding of CN function gained through anatomy, physiology, pharmacology, and behavioral approaches, computational modeling of the neuronal circuitry of the CN has also contributed to our understanding of CN function. Auditory nerve models have provided the front ends to CN models [Carney, 1993]. Single CN neurons [Kim et al., 1994, Hewitt and Meddis, 1995] as well as neural populations have been modeled [Voigt and Davis, 1996; Hancock and Voigt, 1999]. A major reason for computational modeling of the neuronal circuitry is to verify the behavior of the model, compare it to the known physiology, and to predict behavior of the model to novel stimuli [see Hancock et al., 1997; Nelkin et al., 1997].

5.3.2 Superior Olivary Complex

The SOC contains ten or more subdivisions in some species. It is the first major site at which connections from the two ears converge and is therefore a center for binaural processing that underlies sound localization. There are large differences in the subdivisions between mammalian groups such as bats, primates, cetaceans, and burrowing rodents that utilize vastly different binaural cues. Binaural cues to the locus of sounds include interaural level differences (ILDs), interaural time differences (ITDs), and detailed spectral differences for multispectral sounds due to head and pinna filtering characteristics. These are summarized in the binaural HRTF [Tollin and Yin, 2001].

The medial superior olive (MSO) and lateral superior olive (LSO) process ITDs and ILDs, respectively. A neuron in the MSO receives projections from spherical bushy cells of the CN from both sides and thereby the precise timing and tuning cues of nerve fibers passed through the large synapses mentioned. The temporal accuracy of the pathways and the comparison precision of MSO neurons permit the discrimination of changes in ITD of a few tens of microseconds. MSO neurons project to the ipsilateral IC through the LL. Globular bushy cells of the CN project to the medial nucleus of the trapezoid body (MNTB) on the contralateral side, where they synapse on one and only one neuron in a large, excitatory synapse, the calyx of Held. MNTB neurons send inhibitory projections to neurons of the LSO on the same side, which also receives excitatory input from spherical bushy cells and probably other neurons in the AVCN on the same side [Doucet and Ryugo, 2003]. Sounds reaching the ipsilateral side will excite discharges from an LSO neuron, while those reaching the contralateral side will inhibit its discharge. The relative balance of excitation and inhibition is a function of ILD resulting in this cue being encoded in LSO discharge rates.

One of the subdivisions of the SOC, the dorsomedial periolivary nucleus (DMPO), is a source of efferent fibers that reach the contralateral cochlea in the crossed olivocochlear bundle (COCB). Neurons of the DMPO receive inputs from collaterals of globular bushy cell axons of the contralateral ACVN that project to the MNTB and from octopus cells on both sides. The functional role of the feedback from the DMPO to the cochlea is not well understood.

5.3.3 Nuclei of the Lateral Lemniscus

The LL consists of ascending axons from the CN and LSO. The nuclei of the lateral lemniscus (NLL) lie within this tract, and some, such as the dorsal nucleus LL (DNLL), are known to process binaural information [Burger and Pollak, 2001], but less is known about these nuclei as a group than others, partially due to their relative inaccessibility.

5.3.4 Inferior Colliculi

The IC are paired structures lying on the surface of the upper brainstem. Each colliculus has a large central nucleus, the ICC, a surface cortex, and paracentral nuclei. Each colliculus receives afferents from a number of lower brainstem nuclei, projects to the medial geniculate body (MGB) through the brachium, and communicates with the other colliculus through a commissure. The ICC is the major division and has distinctive isofrequency laminae formed from cells with disk-shaped dendritic trees and afferent fibers. The terminal endings of afferents form fibrous layers between laminae. The remaining neurons in the ICC are stellate cells that have dendritic trees spanning laminae. Axons from these two cell types make up much of the ascending ICC output.

Both monaural and binaural information converge at the IC through direct projections from the CN and from the SOC and NLL. Crossed CN inputs and those from the ipsilateral MSO are excitatory. Inhibitory synapses in the ICC arise from the DNLL, mediated by gamma-amino-butyric acid (GABA), and from the ipsilateral LSO, mediated by glycine [Faingold et al., 1991].

These connections provide an extensive base for identifying sound direction at this midbrain level, but due to their convergence, it is difficult to determine what binaural processing occurs at the IC as opposed to being passed from the SOC and NLL. Many neurons in the IC respond differently depending on binaural parameters. Varying ILDs for clicks or high-frequency tones often indicate that contralateral sound is excitatory. Ipsilateral sound may have no effect on responses to contralateral sound, classifying the cell as E0, or it may inhibit responses, in which case the neuron is classified as EI, or maximal excitation may occur for sound at both ears, classifying the neuron as EE. Neurons responding to lower frequencies are influenced by ITDs, specifically the phase difference between sinusoids at the ears. Spatial receptive fields for sounds are not well documented in the mammalian IC, but barn owls, who use the sounds of prey for hunting at night, have sound-based spatial maps in the homologous structure [Knudsen and Knudsen, 1983; Bala et al., 2003]. In mammals and owls the superior colliculus, situated just rostral to the IC and largely visual in function, has spatial auditory receptive field maps.

5.3.5 Thalamocortical System

5.3.5.1 Medial Geniculate

The MGB and AC form the auditory thalamocortical system. As with other sensory systems, extensive projections to and from the cortical region exist in this system. The MGB has three divisions, the ventral, dorsal, and medial. The ventral division is the largest and has the most precise tonotopic organization. Almost all its input is from the ipsilateral ICC through the brachium of the IC. Its large bushy cells have dendrites oriented so as to lie in isofrequency layers, and the axons of these neurons project to the AC.

5.3.5.2 Auditory Cortex

As suggested previously, it is inaccurate to view central auditory pathways as a frequency-mapped sensory conduit to higher centers. The auditory system, indeed the entire brain operates to ensure survival by promoting effective behaviors and storing experience in memory for future decisions. In essence, audition identifies critical sound events and associates them with appropriate responses. This is evident in many observations at the cerebral cortex, but examples for bats and human speech suggest the range and complexity of processing in auditory pathways.

5.3.5.2.1 Bat Cortex

Bats of the suborder Microchiroptera use echos from cries they emit to locate and capture prey, usually insects. A well-studied species, the mustached bat (Pteronotus parnellii) emits brief sounds with a fundamental continuous frequency (CF) around 30 kHz with a short downward frequency-modulated (FM) sweep at the end. This cry has strong harmonics, so much of the returning energy is at multiples of the fundamental. This CF–FM sound is just one strategy used by various Microchiroptera, but the role of the AC in the mustached bat has been extensively studied. Figure 5.7 shows responsive regions in this bat's cortex. In an expanded region of a tonotopic map is the Doppler-shifted CF (DSCF) area with responses to the second harmonic of the 30-kHz chirp the bat emits. Cochlear specializations in this bat's inner ear greatly emphasize frequency resolution in the 60-kHz region. Specifically, returning CF sounds are mapped so precisely that the Doppler shift produced by insect wing flutters will cause the site of maximum activity to vary. Another area, the CF/CF area, compares the frequency of the returning CF signal with that of the emitted signal, a cue for the relative velocity of the prey. The FM–FM region responds to the time difference between the emitted and returning FM cry components as a cue to the distance of the prey [Suga, 1990].

To illustrate the variation in cortical function, it is noted that other species of bats process sound differently in their auditory cortices. The pallid bat uses echolocation for obstacle avoidance and passive listening to locate prey [Razak and Fuzessery, 2002]. As with the mustached bat, echolocation uses frequencies above 30 kHz, but prey location uses frequencies below 20 kHz, and neuron responses differ accordingly over the tonotopic map at cortex.

5.3.5.2.2 Human Cortex

The understanding and production of speech has evolved in human-ancestral primates over the last two hundred thousand years and are mediated by the primary AC and surrounding areas. The primary AC is tonotopically organized, but surrounding areas implicated in higher-level language functions are not

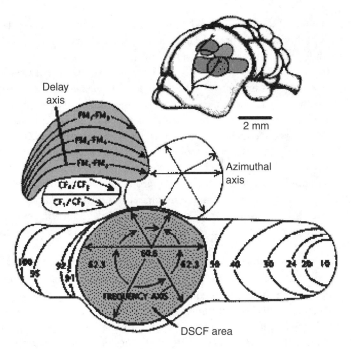

FIGURE 5.7 Auditory cortical areas of the mustached bat showing selective processing in different cortical areas for the emitted and returning components of the CF-FM echolocation cry. (Adapted from Suga [1990]. *Sci. Am.* 262: 60–68.)

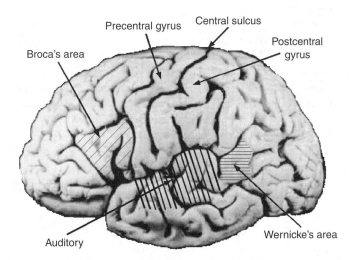

FIGURE 5.8 Cortical areas in human involved with hearing and language. The auditory areas are located on the temporal lobe, the primary area (A1) being on the dorsal surface within the Sylvan sulcus (not visible). Broca and Wernicke's areas are involved with the production and understanding of language.

easily analyzed. Studies of stroke and injury have helped differentiate the roles of these areas. In most individuals these functions are limited to the left side of the brain.

Figure 5.8 shows the major regions of auditory and language processing relative to common cortical landmarks. The primary auditory area is on the upper surface of the temporal lobe (not shown), but supplementary areas are located on the lateral temporal lobe. Broca's area is located in the posterior portion of the frontal lobe near the auditory regions in the temporal lobe. Wernicke's area is in the posterior part of the temporal lobe. Regions surrounding these also participate in language, but it is difficult to define many of the functions involved because they involve mixtures of speech production and understanding with subtle grammatical and logical relationships.

Two clinical conditions arising from stroke or injury have been studied extensively, Broca's and Wernicke's aphasias. Damage to Broca's area will often lead to labored but generally correct speech production, but spoken sentences with complex grammars will not be understood. The concept that Broca's area provides short-term working memory for the comparison of sentence components has been suggested. In contrast, patients with damage to Wernicke's area will often speak effortlessly but with many lexical errors, and they generally do not understand sentences spoken by others. Wernicke's area, once thought to underlie "speech comprehension" is now considered a link between areas for concept and meaning with those for word choice and grammar. Wernicke's area is often grouped with the supramarginal gyrus (SMG) just above it. A third clinical syndrome, conduction aphasia, results from damage to neural pathways linking Wernicke's to the SMG and Broca's area. Speech production and understanding is less affected in conduction aphasia, but it has distinctive features including an inability to repeat sentences accurately and difficulty in naming things.

Significant variations arise over the range of clinical damage to cortical and white matter surrounding these areas, especially the SMG, and if tissue damage is restricted to a small area, the aphasia may be transient. Auditory input at the cortical level goes far beyond tonotopic organization to complexities of language, and when it is absent other sensory input may take over. An example of the generality of function is the disruption of signing by a deaf patient during electrical stimulation of these areas during awake brain surgery for temporal lobe epilepsy [Corina et al., 1999]. Tissues normally involved with understanding and producing speech switch to visual cues with deafness.

5.4 Pathologies

Hearing loss results from conductive and neural deficits. Conductive hearing loss due to attenuation in the outer or middle ear often can be alleviated by amplification provided by hearing aids and may be subject to surgical correction. Sensorineural loss due to the absence of IHCs results from genetic deficits, biochemical insult, and exposure to intense sound, or aging (presbycusis). For some cases of sensorineural loss, partial hearing function can be restored with the cochlear prosthesis, direct electrical stimulation of remaining SGCs using small arrays of electrodes inserted into the ST (see chapter on cochlear implants) As of 2004, an estimated 70,000 people have received cochlear implants.

Lesions of the nerve and central structures occur due to trauma, tumor growth, and vascular accidents. These may be subject to surgical intervention to prevent further damage and promote functional recovery. In patients having no auditory nerve due to tumor removal, direct electrical stimulation of the CN has been used to provide auditory sensation.

5.5 Further Topics

In a brief survey it is not possible to cover many important topics for the auditory system. Excellent books treat these in detail. A great deal of attention has been and is being paid to plasticity in neural and behavioral mechanisms of hearing [Parks et al., 2004]. Likewise, little has been said about perceptual mechanisms and the techniques for assessing the behavioral limits of hearing [Hartmann, 1998].

References

Algazi V.R., Duda R.O., Duraiswami R., Gumerov N.A., and Tang Z. (2002). Approximating the head-related transfer function using simple geometric models of the head and torso. *J. Acoust. Soc. Am.* 112: 2053–2064.

Ashmore J.F. and Mammano F. (2001). Can you still see the cochlea for the molecules? *Curr. Opin. Neurobiol.* 11: 449–454.

Babalian A.L., Ryugo D.K., and Rouiller E.M. (2003). Discharge properties of identified cochlear nucleus neurons and auditory nerve fibers in response to repetitive electrical stimulation of the auditory nerve. *Exp. Brain Res.* 153: 452–460.

Bal R. and Oertel D. (2001). Potassium currents in octopus cells of the mammalian cochlear nucleus. *J. Neurophysiol.* 86: 2299–2311.

Bala A.D.S., Spitzer M.W., Takahashi T.T. (2003). Prediction of auditory spatial acuity from neuronal images on the owl's auditory space map. *Nature* 424: 771–773.

Batteau D.W. (1967). The role of the pinna in human localization. *Proc. R. Soc. London, Ser. B* 168: 158–80.

Blauert J.P. (1997). *Spatial Hearing.* Cambridge: MIT Press.

Bourk T.R., Mielcarz J.P., and Norris B.E. (1981). Tonotopic organization of the anteroventral cochlear nucleus of the cat. *Hear. Res.* 4: 215.

Brownell W.E., Bader C.R., Bertrand D., and de Ribaupierre Y. (1985). Evoked mechanical responses of isolated cochlear outer hair cells. *Science* 227: 194–196.

Burger R.M. and Pollak G.D. (2001). Reversible inactivation of the dorsal nucleus of the lateral lemniscus reveals its role in the processing of multiple sound sources in the inferior colliculus of bats. *J. Neurosci.* 21: 4830–4843.

Carney L.H. (1993). A model for the responses of low-frequency auditory nerve fibers in cat. *J. Acoust. Soc. Am.* 93: 401–417.

Corina D.P., McBurney S.L., Dodrill C., Hinshaw K., Brinkley J., and Ojeman G. (1999). Functional roles of Broca's area and SMG: evidence from cortical stimulation mapping in a deaf signer. *NeuroImage* 10: 570–581.

Crawford A.C. and Fettiplace R. (1985). The mechanical properties of ciliary bundles of turtle cochlear hair cells. *J. Physiol.* 364: 359.

Davis K.A. and Voigt H.F. (1997). Evidence of stimulus-dependent correlated activity in the dorsal cochlear nucleus of decerebrate gerbils. *J. Neurophysiol.* 78: 229–247.

Doucet J.R. and Ryugo D.K. (2003). Axonal pathways to the lateral superior olive labeled with biotinylated dextran amine injections in the dorsal cochlear nucleus of rats. *J. Comp. Neurol.* 461: 452–465.

Faingold C.L., Gehlbach G., and Caspary D.M. (1991). Functional pharmacology of inferior colliculus neurons. In: *Neurobiology of Hearing: The Central Auditory System.* Altschuler R.A., Bobbin R.P., Clopton B.M., and Hoffman D.W. (Eds.), New York: Raven Press, pp. 223–251.

Fujino K. and Oertel D. (2001). Cholinergic modulation of stellate cells in the mammalian ventral cochlear nucleus. *J. Neurosci.* 21: 7372–7383.

Geisler C.D. (1998). *From Sound to Synapse: Physiology of the Mammalian Ear.* New York: Oxford University Press.

Gleich O., Johnstone B.M., and Robertson D. (1990). Effects of L-glutamate on auditory afferent activity in view of proposed excitatory transmitter role in the mammalian cochlea. *Hear. Res.* 45: 295–312,

Hancock K.E. and Voigt H.F. (1999). Wideband inhibition of dorsal cochlear nucleus type IV units in cat: a computational model. *Ann. Biomed. Eng.* 27: 73–87.

Hancock K.E. and Voigt H.F. (2002). Intracellularly labeled fusiform cells in dorsal cochlear nucleus of the gerbil. I. Physiological response properties. *J. Neurophysiol.* 87: 2505–2519.

Hancock K.E., Davis K.A., and Voigt H.F. (1997). Modeling inhibition of type II units in the dorsal cochlear nucleus. *Biol. Cybern.* 76: 419–428.

Hartmann W.M. (1998). *Signals, Sound, and Sensation.* New York: Springer-Verlag.

Hewitt M.J. and Meddis R. (1995). A computer model of dorsal cochlear nucleus pyramidal cells: Intrinsic membrane properties. *J. Acoust. Soc. Am.* 97(4):2405–2413.

Hudspeth A.J. (1987). Mechanoelectrical transduction by hair cells in the acousticolateralis sensory system. *Ann. Rev. Neurosci.* 6: 187.

Hudspeth A.J. (2000). Sensory transduction in the ear. In: *Principles of Neural Science.* Chapter 31, Kandel E.R., Schwartz J.H., and Jessell T.M. (Eds.), New York: McGraw-Hill, pp. 614–624.

Hudspeth A.J. and Corey D.P. (1977). Sensitivity, polarity, and conductance change in the response of vertebrate hair cells to controlled mechanical stimuli. *Proc. Natl Acad. Sci. USA* 74: 2407.

Johnstone B.M. and Boyle A.J.F (1967). Basilar membrane vibration examined with the Mössbauer technique. *Science* 158: 390–391.

Kiang N.Y.-S., Watanabe T., Thomas E.C., and Clark L.F. (1965). *Discharge Patterns of Single Fibers in the Cat's Auditory Nerve.* MIT Press, Cambridge.

Kim D.O., Ghosal S., Khant S.L. and Parham K. (1994). A computational model with ionic conductances for the dorsal cochlear nucleus (DCN) fusiform cell. *J. Acoust. Soc. Am.* 96: 1501–1514.

Kinsler L.E., Frey A.R., Coppens A.B., and Sanders J.V. (1999). *Fundamentals of Acoustics.* New York: Wiley.

Knudsen E.I. and Knudsen P.F. (1983). Space-mapped auditory projections from the inferior colliculus to the optic tectum in the barn owl. *J. Comp. Neurol.* 218: 187–196.

Mammano F. and Ashmore J.F. (1995). A laser interferometer for sub nanometre measurements in the cochlea. *J. Neurosci. Meth.* 60: 89–94.

Manis P.B. (1990). Membrane properties and discharge characteristics of guinea pigs dorsal cochlear nucleus neurons studied *in vitro*. *J. Neurosci.* 10: 2338–2351.

Nadol J.B. Jr. (1988). Comparative anatomy of the cochlea and auditory nerve in mammals. *Hear. Res.* 34: 253.

Nelkin I., Kim P.J., and Young E.D. (1997). Linear and nonlinear spectral integration in type IV neurons of the dorsal cochlear nucleus. II. Predicting responses with the use of nonlinear models. *J. Neurophysiol.* 78: 800–811.

Nummela S. (1995). Scaling of the mammalian middle ear. *Hear. Res.* 85: 18–30.

Oertel D. and Young E.D. (2004). What's a cerebellar circuit doing in the auditory system? *Trends Neurosci.* 27: 104–110.

Parks T.N., Rubel E.W., Popper A.N., Fay R.R. (Eds.) (2004). *Plasticity of the Auditory System.* Springer Handbook of Auditory Research, New York: Springer-Verlag, 23: 323.

Parsons J.E., Lim E., and Voigt H.F. (2001). Type III units in the gerbil dorsal cochlear nucleus may be spectral notch detectors. *Ann. Biomed. Eng.* 29: 887–896.

Ravicz M.E. and Rosowski J.J. (1997). Sound-power collection by the auditory periphery of the Mongolian gerbil Meriones unguiculatus: III. Effect of variations in middle-ear volume. *J. Acoust. Soc. Am.* 101: 2135–2147.

Razak K.A. and Fuzessery Z.M. (2002). Functional organization of the pallid bat auditory cortex: emphasis on binaural organization. *J. Neurophysiol.* 87: 72–86.

Recio A., Rhode W.S., Kiefte M., and Kluender K.R. (2002). Responses to cochlear normalized speech stimuli in the auditory nerve of cat. *J. Acoust. Soc. Am.* 111:2213–2218.

Rhode W.S. (1971). Observations of the vibration of the basilar membrane in squirrel monkeys using the Mössbauer technique. *J. Acoust. Soc. Am.* 49: 1218–1231.

Sachs M.B. and Young E.D. (1979). Encoding of steady-state vowels in the auditory nerve: representation in terms of discharge rate. *J. Acoust. Soc. Am.* 66: 470.

Spirou G.A. and Young E.D. (1991). Organization of dorsal cochlear nucleus type IV unit response maps and their relationship to activation by band-limited noise. *J. Neurophysiol.* 66: 1750–1768.

Spirou G.A., Davis K.A., Nelken I. and Young E.D. (1999). Spectral integration by Type II interneurons in dorsal cochlear nucleus. *J. Neurophysiol.* 82: 48–663, 1999.

Suga N. (1990). Biosonar and neural computation in bats. *Sci. Am.* 262: 60–68.

Tollin D.J. and Yin T.C.T (2001). Investigation of spatial location coding in the lateral superior olive using virtual space stimulation. In *Physiological and Psychophysical Bases of Auditory Function.* Houtsma A.J.M., Kohlrausch A., Prijs V.F., and Schoonhoven R. (Eds.), Maastricht: Shaker Publishing, pp. 236–243.

Voigt H.F. and Davis K.A. (1996). Computer simulations of neural correlations in the dorsal cochlear nucleus. In: *Cochlear Nucleus: structure and function in relation to modeling.* Ainsworth W.A. (Ed.), London: JAI Press, pp. 351–375.

Voigt H.F. and Young E.D. (1980). Evidence of inhibitory interactions between neurons in the dorsal cochlear nucleus. *J. Neurophysiol.* 44: 76–96.

Voigt H.F. and Young E.D. (1990). Cross-correlation analysis of inhibitory interactions in dorsal cochlear nucleus. *J. Neurophysiol.* 64: 1590–1610.

von Békésy G. (1960). *Experiments in Hearing.* New York: McGraw-Hill.

Weiner F.M. and Ross D.A. (1946). The pressure distribution in the auditory canal in a progressive sound field. *J. Acoust. Soc. Am.* 18: 401–408.

Wever E.G. and Lawrence M. (1954). *Physiological Acoustics.* Princeton: Princeton University Press.

Wightman F.L. and Kistler D.J. (1989). Headphone simulation of free-field listening. II: Psychophysical validation. *J. Acoust. Soc. Am.* 85: 868–878.

Wilson P.J. (1986). Otoacoustic emissions and tinnitus. *Scand. Audiol. Suppl.* 25: 109–119.

Young E.D. (1984). Response characteristics of neurons of the cochlear nuclei. In: *Hearing Science: Recent Advances.* C.I. Berlin (Ed.), San Diego, California: College-Hill Press.

Young E.D. (1998). The cochlear nucleus. In: *Synaptic Organization of the Brain.* Shepard G.M. (Ed.), New York: Oxford Press, pp. 121–157.

Young E.D. and Brownell W.E. (1976). Responses to tones and noise of single cells in dorsal cochlear nucleus of unanesthetized cats. *J. Neurophysiol.* 39: 282–300.

Young E.D. and Davis K.A. (2002). Circuitry and function of the dorsal cochlear nucleus. In: *Integrative Functions in the Mammalian Auditory Pathway.* Oertel D., Fay R.R., and Popper A.N. (Eds.), New York: Springer-Verlag.

Young E.D. and Voigt H.F. (1981). The internal organization of the dorsal cochlear nucleus. In: *Neuronal Mechanisms in Hearing,* Syka J. and Aitkin L. (Eds), New York: Plenum Press. pp. 127–133.

6

Gastrointestinal System

Berj L. Bardakjian
University of Toronto

6.1   Introduction

The primary function of the gastrointestinal system (Figure 6.1) is to supply the body with nutrients and water. The ingested food is moved along the alimentary canal at an appropriate rate for digestion, absorption, storage, and expulsion. To fulfill the various requirements of the system, each organ has adapted one or more functions. The esophagus acts as a conduit for the passage of food into the stomach for trituration and mixing. The ingested food is then emptied into the small intestine, which plays a major role in the digestion and absorption processes. The chyme is mixed thoroughly with secretions and it is propelled distally (1) to allow further gastric emptying, (2) to allow for uniform exposure to the absorptive mucosal surface of the small intestine, and (3) to empty into the colon. The vigor of mixing and the rate of propulsion depend on the required contact time of chyme with enzymes and the mucosal surface for efficient performance of digestion and absorption. The colon absorbs water and electrolytes from the chyme, concentrating and collecting waste products that are expelled from the system at appropriate times. All of these motor functions are performed by contractions of the muscle layers in the gastrointestinal wall (Figure 6.2).

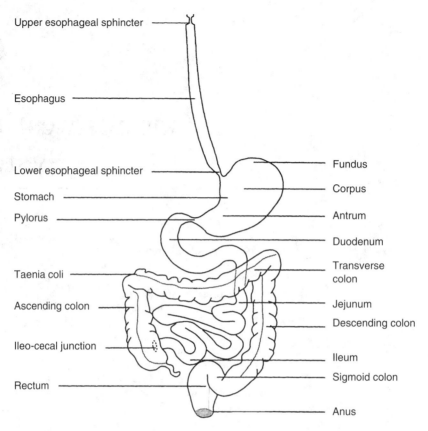

FIGURE 6.1 The gastrointestinal tract.

6.2 Gastrointestinal Electrical Oscillations

6.2.1 Main Features

Gastrointestinal motility is governed by myogenic, neural, and chemical control systems. The myogenic control system is manifest by rhythmic depolarizations of the smooth muscle cells, which constitute electrical oscillations called the electrical control activity (ECA) or slow waves [Daniel and Chapman, 1963]. The properties of this myogenic system and its electrical oscillations dictate to a large extent the contraction patterns in the stomach, small intestine, and colon [Szurszewski, 1987]. The ECA controls the contractile excitability of smooth muscle cells since the cells may contract only when depolarization of the membrane voltage exceeds an excitation threshold. The normal spontaneous amplitude of ECA depolarization does not exceed this excitation threshold except when neural or chemical excitation is present. The myogenic system affects the frequency, direction, and velocity of the contractions. It also affects the coordination or lack of coordination between adjacent segments of the gut wall. Hence, the electrical activities in the gut wall provide an electrical basis for gastrointestinal motility.

In the distal stomach, small intestine, and colon, there are intermittent bursts of rapid electrical oscillations, called the electrical response activity (ERA) or spike bursts. The ERA occurs during the depolarization plateaus of the ECA if a cholinergic stimulus is present and it is associated with muscular contractions (Figure 6.3). Thus, neural and chemical control systems determine whether contractions will occur or not, but when contractions are occurring, the myogenic control system (Figure 6.4) determines the spatial and temporal patterns of contractions.

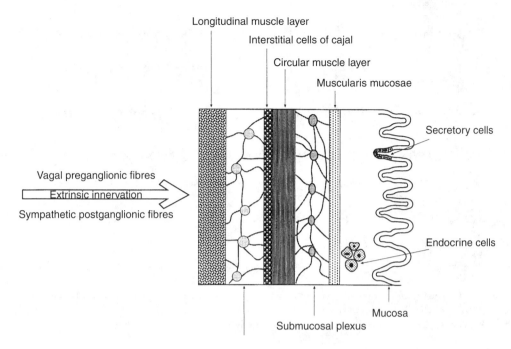

FIGURE 6.2   The layers of the gastrointestinal wall.

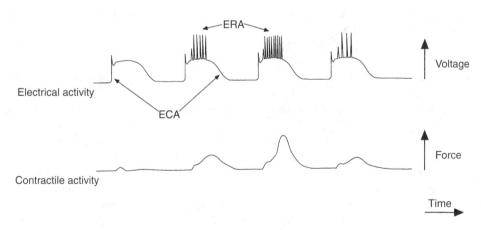

FIGURE 6.3   The relationships between ECA, ERA, and muscular contractions. The ERA occurs in the depolarized phase of the ECA. Muscular contractions are associated with the ERA, and their amplitude depends on the frequency of response potentials within an ERA burst.

There is also a cyclical pattern distally propagating ERA that appears in the small intestine during the fasted state [Szurszewski, 1969], called the migrating motility complex (MMC). This pattern consists of four phases [Code and Marlett, 1975]: Phase I has little or no ERA, phase II consists of irregular ERA bursts, phase III consists of intense repetitive ERA bursts where there is an ERA burst on each ECA cycle, and phase IV consists of irregular ERA bursts but is usually much shorter than phase II and may not be always present. The initiation and propagation of the MMC is controlled by enteric cholinergic neurons in the intestinal wall (Figure 6.2). The propagation of the MMC may be modulated by inputs from extrinsic nerves or circulating hormones [Sarna et al., 1981]. The MMC keeps the small intestine clean of residual food, debris, and desquamated cells.

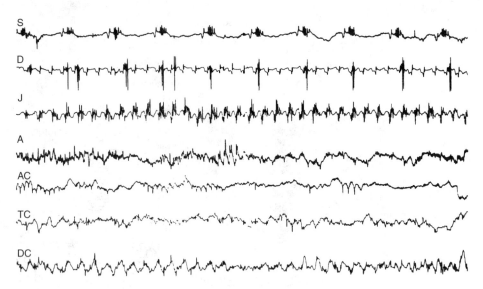

FIGURE 6.4   The Gastrointestinal ECA and ERA, recorded in a conscious dog from electrode sets implanted sub-serosally on stomach (S), duodenum (D), jejunum (J), proximal ascending colon (A), distal ascending colon (AC), transverse colon (TC), and descending colon (DC), respectively. Each trace is of 2 min duration.

6.2.2   Intercellular Communication

Interstitial cells of Cajal (ICC) pace gastrointestinal smooth muscle by initiating slow waves in both longitudinal and circular muscle layers, and they appear to be preferred sites for reception of neurotransmitters [Ward et al., 2001; Sanders et al., 2002; Daniel, 2004]. ICC of the myenteric plexus play a crucial role in pacing slow waves and contractions while intramuscular ICC appear to play a role in receiving neural messages [Ward et al., 2001; Sanders et al., 2002]. Coupling between ICC and smooth muscle networks is essential for entrainment of ECA to obtain coordinated muscle contraction. Gap junctions play an important role in intercellular communication since they provide direct electrical and metabolic coupling between cytoplasm of neighboring cells [Chanson and Spray, 1995], but cells are also coupled by a variety of other structures [Daniel et al., 1976; Huizinga et al., 1992]. ICC may be coupled to smooth muscle by gap junctions as found at the inner border of the circular muscle layer in the canine colon [Berezin et al., 1988], but at other sites, such as between ICC and the muscle layers of the mouse small intestine, gap junctions were not found; however, there was an abundance of close apposition junctions [Thuneberg, 1982]. Within certain muscle layers no gap junctions can be recognized by electron microscopic techniques such as in the longitudinal muscle of the intestine and colon of a variety of species [Zamir and Hanani, 1990; Liu et al., 1998]. In such tissues, close apposition junctions are always observed. Such contacts may contain small groups of connexons, which would allow electrical and metabolic communication although it could not be identified as a gap junction; only a large aggregate of connexons can be recognized as a gap junction by electron microscopy. Nevertheless, electrical communication other than purely resistive is likely to occur.

One type of conspicuous contact is the peg-and-socket junction, where an extrusion of one cell forms a peg, which penetrates a neighboring cell and fits into an intrusion that forms a socket with an intracellular gap of 20 nm. This extrusion can be up to 10 μm long, undergo a 90° bend upon entering a cell, and be up to 1.5 μm in diameter [Thuneberg et al., 1998]. The abundance of these structures in areas of no demonstrable gap junctions and their absence in areas that have many gap junctions suggest that they may provide an intercellular communication pathway other than a direct low-resistance pathway as provided by a gap junction.

Daniel [2004] reviewed communication between ICC and gastrointestinal smooth muscle and he considered structural, theoretical, and experimental difficulties with the possible role of gap junctions in pacing and in neurotransmission. Furthermore, he considered the following alternate possibilities for transmission of ICC pacing and neural messages (a) The production of an electric field potential in narrow clefts between cells, such as in close apposition junctions, which was shown to be sufficient to allow electrical coupling [Sperelakis et al., 1977; Vigmond and Bardakjian, 1995; Sperelakis, 2002; Sperelakis and McConnell, 2002; Sperelakis and Ramasamy, 2002] and (b) Potassium accumulation in the narrow clefts, such as in peg-and-socket junctions, which was shown to facilitate electrical coupling without gap junctions [Sperelakis et al., 1984; Vigmond and Bardakjian, 2000].

6.2.3 Coupled Nonlinear Oscillators

There is an extensive literature on the mathematical modeling of the generation of oscillations, their coupling, their entrainment, and frequency pulling [Fitzhugh, 1961; Pavlidis, 1973; Plant and Kim, 1976; Winfree, 1980; Ermentrout and Kopell, 1984; Grasman, 1984; Rinzel, 1987; Sherman and Rinzel, 1991; Bardakjian and Diamant, 1994]. The entrainment of coupled oscillators is governed by both intrinsic oscillator properties and coupling mechanisms. The theory of second-order relaxation oscillators, as "traditionally" formulated was qualitative in nature. Two types of oscillators were described (a) Van der Pol type oscillators [Van der Pol and Van der Mark, 1928], which were generalized [Fitzhugh, 1961] to exhibit neuronal-like features and (b) Winfree-type oscillators [Winfree, 1980, 1989], which focused on rate processes of phase and amplitude of oscillation and they were helpful in elucidating the nature of "phase-resetting" phenomena in biological oscillators. Furthermore, quantitative fourth-order models of the Hodgkin-Huxley type [Hodgkin and Huxley, 1952; Plant and Kim, 1976] have been described that closely reproduce neuronal transmembrane voltages. However, development of these quantitative oscillator models requires a full biophysical description of ionic transport mechanisms through membrane channels, pumps, and exchangers. A simpler alternative is the leaky integrate-and-fire model [Stein, 1967], which can only reproduce basic spiking behavior and it is mostly useful for investigation of large networks where the focus is not on individual cells.

On the other hand, the mapped clock oscillator (MCO) [Bardakjian and Diamant, 1994] is a multiportal generalization of the Winfree-type oscillator that is quantitative in nature and exhibits refractory properties. Its parameters are the coefficients of the Fourier series representation of the intrinsic transmembrane voltage oscillation. Hence, they can be obtained directly from the Fourier analysis of the biologically measured intrinsic waveform of the isolated oscillator (e.g., in experiments where segments of an organ are isolated from each other by transaction). Each oscillator consists of, first, a dynamic nonlinearity represented by two nonlinear simultaneous differential equations that govern the state variables of the system and, second, a static nonlinearity that maps the two state variables onto the observable output. The dynamic nonlinearity represents the clock mechanism of the oscillator. The values of its state variables can be modified by three input "portals," each of which correspond to a different type of coupling pathway (gap junctions, field effects, and membrane receptors). The static nonlinearity represents the cellular membrane. This mapper can be changed to represent the waveform of the specific cell being modeled. The MCO can represent transmembrane voltage oscillations in different systems (e.g., neurons, cardiac cells, gastrointestinal muscle, and pancreatic beta cells).

6.3 A Historical Perspective

6.3.1 Minute Rhythms

Alvarez and Mahoney [1922] reported the presence of a rhythmic electrical activity (which they called "action currents") in the smooth muscle layers of the stomach, small intestine, and colon. Their data was acquired from cat (stomach and small intestine), dog (stomach, small intestine, and colon), and rabbit (small intestine and colon). They also demonstrated the existence of frequency gradients in excised stomach and bowel. Puestow [1933] confirmed the presence of a rhythmic electrical activity (which he called "waves of altered electrical potential") and a frequency gradient in isolated canine small intestinal segments. He also demonstrated the presence of an electrical spiking activity (associated with muscular contractions) superimposed on the rhythmic electrical activity. He implied that the rhythmic electrical activity persisted at all times, whereas the electrical spike activity was of an intermittent nature. Bozler [1938, 1939, 1941] confirmed the occurrence of an electrical spiking activity associated with muscular contractions both *in vitro* in isolated longitudinal muscle strips from guinea pig (colon and small intestine) and rabbit (small intestine), and *in situ* in exposed loops of small intestine of anesthetized cat, dog, and rabbit as well as in cat stomach. He also suggested that the strength of a spontaneous muscular contraction is proportional to the frequency and duration of the spikes associated with it.

The presence of two types of electrical activity in the smooth muscle layers of the gastrointestinal tract in several species had been established [Milton and Smith, 1956; Bulbring et al., 1958; Burnstock et al., 1963; Daniel and Chapman, 1963; Bass, 1965; Gillespie, 1962; Duthie, 1974; Christensen, 1975; Daniel, 1975; Sarna, 1975a]. The autonomous electrical rhythmic activity is an omnipresent myogenic activity [Burnstock et al., 1963] whose function is to control the appearance in time and space of the electrical spiking activity (an intermittent activity associated with muscular contractions) when neural and chemical factors are appropriate [Daniel and Chapman, 1963]. Neural and chemical factors determine whether or not contractions will occur, but when contractions are occurring, the myogenic control system determines the spatial and temporal patterns of contractions.

Isolation of a distal segment of canine small intestine from a proximal segment (using surgical transection or clamping) had been reported to produce a decrease in the frequency of both the rhythmic muscular contractions [Douglas, 1949; Milton and Smith, 1956] and the electrical rhythmic activity [Milton and Smith, 1956] of the distal segment, suggesting frequency entrainment or pulling of the distal segment by the proximal one. It was demonstrated [Milton and Smith, 1956] that the repetition of the electrical spiking activity changed in the same manner as that of the electrical rhythmic activity, thus confirming a one-to-one temporal relationship between the frequency of the electrical rhythmic activity, the repetition rate of the electrical spiking activity, and the frequency of the muscular contractions (when all are present at any one site). Nelson and Becker [1968] suggested that the electrical rhythmic activity of the small intestine behaves like a system of coupled relaxation oscillators. They used two forward coupled relaxation oscillators, having different intrinsic frequencies, to demonstrate frequency entrainment of the two coupled oscillators. Uncoupling of the two oscillators caused a decrease in the frequency of the distal oscillator simulating the effect of transection of the canine small intestine.

The electrical rhythmic activity in canine stomach [Sarna et al., 1972], canine small intestine [Nelson and Becker, 1968; Diamant et al., 1970; Sarna et al., 1971], human small intestine [Robertson–Dunn and Linkens, 1974], human colon [Bardakjian and Sarna, 1980], and human rectosigmoid [Linkens et al., 1976] has been modeled by populations of coupled nonlinear oscillators. The interaction between coupled nonlinear oscillators is governed by both intrinsic oscillator properties and coupling mechanisms.

6.3.2 Hour Rhythms

The existence of periodic gastric activity in the fasted state in both dog [Morat, 1882] and man [Morat, 1893] has been reported. The occurrence of a periodic pattern of motor activity, comprising bursts of contractions alternating with "intervals of repose," in the gastrointestinal tracts of fasted animals was noted early in the 20th century by Boldireff [1905]. He observed that (1) the bursts recurred with a periodicity of about 1.5 to 2.5 h, (2) the amplitude of the gastric contractions during the bursts were larger than those seen postprandially, (3) the small bowel was also involved, and (4) with longer fasting periods, the bursts occurred less frequently and had a shorter duration. Periodic bursts of activity were also observed in (1) the lower esophageal sphincter, [Cannon and Washburn, 1912], and (2) the pylorus [Wheelon and Thomas, 1921]. Further investigation of the fasting contractile activity in the upper small intestine was undertaken in the early 1920s with particular emphasis on the coordination between the stomach and duodenum [Wheelon and Thomas, 1922; Alvarez and Mahoney, 1923]. More recently, evidence was obtained [Itoh et al., 1978] that the cyclical activity in the lower esophageal sphincter noted by Cannon and Washburn [1912] was also coordinated with that of the stomach and small intestine.

With the use of implanted strain gauges, it was possible to observe contractile activity over long periods of time and it was demonstrated that the cyclical fasting pattern in the duodenum was altered by feeding [Jacoby et al., 1963]. The types of contractions observed during fasting and feeding were divided into four groups [Reinke et al., 1967; Carlson et al., 1972]. Three types of contractile patterns were observed in fasted animals (1) quiescent interval, (2) a shorter interval of increasing activity, and (3) an interval of maximal activity. The fourth type was in fed animals and it consisted of randomly occurring contractions of varying amplitudes. With the use of implanted electrodes in the small intestine of fasted dogs, Szurszewski [1969] demonstrated that the cyclical appearance of electrical spiking activity at each electrode site was due to the migration of the cyclical pattern of quiescence, increasing activity, and maximal electrical activity down the small intestine from the duodenum to the terminal ileum. He called this electrical pattern the migrating myoelectric complex (MMC). Grivel and Ruckebusch [1972] demonstrated that the mechanical correlate of this electrical pattern, which they called the migrating motor complex, occurs in other species such as sheep and rabbits. They also observed that the velocity of propagation of the maximal contractile activity was proportional to the length of the small intestine. Code and Marlett [1975] observed the electrical correlate of the cyclical activity in dog stomach that was reported by Morat [1882; 1893] and they demonstrated that the stomach MMC was coordinated with the duodenal MMC.

The MMC pattern has been demonstrated in other mammalian species [Ruckebusch and Fioramonti, 1975; Ruckebusch and Bueno, 1976], including humans. Bursts of distally propagating contractions have been noted in the gastrointestinal tract of man [Beck et al., 1965], and their cyclical nature was reported by Stanciu and Bennet [1975]. The MMC has been described in both normal volunteers [Vantrappen et al., 1977; Fleckenstein, 1978; Thompson et al., 1980; Kerlin and Phillips, 1982; Rees et al., 1982] and in patients [Vantrappen et al., 1977; Thompson et al., 1982; Summers et al., 1982].

6.3.3 Terminology

A nomenclature to describe the gastrointestinal electrical activities has been proposed to describe the minute rhythm [Sarna, 1975b] and the hour rhythm [Carlson et al., 1972; Code and Marlett, 1975].

Control cycle is one depolarization and repolarization of the transmembrane voltage. Control wave (or slow wave) is the continuing rhythmic electrical activity recorded at any one site. It was assumed to be generated by the smooth muscle cells behaving like a relaxation oscillator at that site. However, recent evidence [Hara et al., 1986; Suzuki et al. 1986; Barajas–Lopez et al., 1989; Serio et al., 1991] indicates that it is generated by a system of interstitial cells of Cajal (ICC) and smooth muscle cells at that site. ECA is the totality of the control waves recorded at one or several sites. Response Potentials (or spikes) are the rapid oscillations of transmembrane voltage in the depolarized state of smooth muscle cells. They are associated with muscular contraction and their occurrence is assumed to be in response to a control cycle when acetylcholine is present. ERA is the totality of the groups of response potentials at one or several sites.

Migrating motility complex (MMC) is the entire cycle, which is composed of four phases. Initially, the electrical and mechanical patterns were referred to as the migrating myoelectric complex and the migrating motor complex, respectively. Phase I is the interval during which fewer than 5% of ECA have associated ERA and no or very few contractions are present. Phase II is the interval when 5 to 95% of the ECA has associated ERA, and intermittent contractions are present. Phase III is the interval when more than 95% of ECA have associated ERA and large cyclical contractions are present. Phase IV is a short and waning interval of intermittent ERA and contractions. Phases II and IV are not always present and are difficult to characterize, whereas phases I and III are always present. MMC cycle time is the interval from the end of one phase III to the end of a subsequent phase III at any one site. Migration time is the time taken for the MMC to migrate from the upper duodenum to the terminal ileum.

6.4   The Stomach

6.4.1   Anatomical Features

The stomach is somewhat pyriform in shape with its large end directed upward at the lower esophageal sphincter and its small end bent to the right at the pylorus. It has two curvatures, the greater curvature which is four to five times as long as the lesser curvature, and it consists of three namely, regions: the fundus, the corpus (or body), and the antrum, respectively. It has three smooth muscle layers. The outermost layer is the longitudinal muscle layer, the middle is the circular muscle layer, and the innermost is the oblique muscle layer. These layers thicken gradually in the distal stomach toward the pylorus, which is consistent with stomach function since trituration occurs in the distal antrum. The size of the stomach varies considerably among subjects. In an adult male, its greatest length when distended is about 25 to 30 cm and its widest diameter is about 10 to 12 cm [Pick and Howden, 1977].

   The structural relationships of nerve, muscle, and interstitial cells of Cajal in the canine corpus indicated a high density of gap junctions indicating very tight coupling between cells. Nerves in the corpus are not located close to circular muscle cells but are found exterior to the muscle bundles, whereas ICCs have gap junction contact with smooth muscle cells and are closely innervated [Daniel and Sakai, 1984].

6.4.2   Gastric ECA

In the canine stomach, the fundus does not usually exhibit spontaneous electrical oscillations, but the corpus and antrum do exhibit such oscillations. In the intact stomach, the ECA is entrained to a frequency of about 5 cpm (about 3 cpm in humans) throughout the electrically active region with phase lags in both the longitudinal and circumferential directions [Sarna et al., 1972]. The phase lags decrease distally from corpus to antrum.

   There is a marked intrinsic frequency gradient along the axis of the stomach and a slight intrinsic frequency gradient along the circumference. The intrinsic frequency of gastric ECA in isolated circular muscle of the orad and midcorpus is the highest (about 5 cpm) compared to about 3.5 cpm in the rest of the corpus, and about 0.5 cpm in the antrum. Also, there is an orad to aborad intrinsic gradient in resting membrane potential, with the terminal antrum having the most negative resting membrane potential, about 30 mV more negative than the fundal regions [Szurszewski, 1987]. The relatively depolarized state of the fundal muscle may explain its electrical inactivity since the voltage-sensitive ionic channels may be kept in a state of inactivation. Hyperpolarization of the fundus to a transmembrane voltage of -60 mV produces fundal control waves similar to those recorded from mid and orad corpus.

   The ECA in canine stomach was modeled [Sarna et al., 1972] using an array of 13 bidirectionally coupled relaxation oscillators. The model featured (1) an intrinsic frequency decline from corpus to the pylorus and from greater curvature to the lesser curvature, (2) entrainment of all coupled oscillators at a frequency close to the highest intrinsic frequency, and (3) distally decreasing phase lags between the entrained oscillators. A simulated circumferential transection caused the formation of another frequency plateau aboral to the transection. The frequency of the orad plateau remained unaffected while that of the aborad plateau was decreased. This is consistent with the observed experimental data.

6.4.3   The Electrogastrogram

In a similar manner to other electrophysiological measures such as the electrocardiogram (EKG) and the electroencephalogram (EEG), the electrogastrogram (EGG) was identified [Stern and Koch, 1985; Chen and McCallum, 1994]. The EGG is the signal obtained from cutaneous recording of the gastric myoelectrical activity by using surface electrodes placed on the abdomen over the stomach. Although the first EGG was recorded in the early 1920s [Alvarez, 1922], progress *vis-à-vis* clinical applications has been relatively slow, in particular when compared to the progress made in EKG, which also started in the early 1920s. Despite many attempts made over the decades, visual inspection of the EGG signal has not led to the identification of waveform characteristics that would help the clinician to diagnose functional or organic diseases of the stomach. Even the development of techniques such as time–frequency analysis [Qiao et al., 1998] and artificial neural network-based feature extraction [Liang et al., 1997; Wang et al., 1999] for computer analysis of the EGG did not provide clinically relevant information about gastric motility disorders. It has been demonstrated that increased EGG frequencies (1) were seen in perfectly healthy subjects [Pffafenbach et al., 1995] and (2) did not always correspond to serosally recorded tachygastria in dogs [Mintchev and Bowes, 1997]. As yet, there is no effective method of detecting a change in the direction or velocity of propagation of gastric ECA from the EGG.

6.5 The Small Intestine

6.5.1 Anatomical Features

The small intestine is a long hollow organ, which consists of the duodenum, jejunum, and ileum, respectively. Its length is about 650 cm in humans and 300 cm in dogs. The duodenum extends from the pylorus to the ligament of Treitz (about 30 cm in humans and dogs). In humans, the duodenum forms a C-shaped pattern, with the ligament of Treitz near the corpus of the stomach. In dogs, the duodenum lies along the right side of the peritoneal cavity, with the ligament of Treitz in the pelvis. The duodenum receives pancreatic exocrine secretions and bile. In both humans and dogs, the jejunum consists of the next one third whereas the ileum consists of the remaining two thirds of the intestine. The major differences between the jejunum and ileum are functional in nature, relating to their absorption characteristics and motor control. The majority of sugars, amino acids, lipids, electrolytes, and water are absorbed in the jejunum and proximal ileum, whereas bile acids and vitamin B12 are absorbed in the terminal ileum.

6.5.2 Small Intestinal ECA

In the canine small intestine, the ECA is not entrained throughout the entire length [Diamant and Bortoff, 1969a; Sarna et al., 1971]. However, the ECA exhibits a plateau of constant frequency in the proximal region whereby there is a distal increase in phase lag. The frequency plateau (of about 20 cpm) extends over the entire duodenum and part of the jejunum. There is a marked intrinsic frequency gradient in the longitudinal direction with the highest intrinsic frequency being less than the plateau frequency. When the small intestine was transected *in vivo* into small segments (15 cm long), the intrinsic frequency of the ECA in adjacent segments tended to decrease aborally in an exponential manner [Sarna et al., 1971]. A single transection of the duodenum caused the formation of another frequency plateau aboral to the transection. The ECA frequency in the orad plateau was generally unaffected, while that in the aborad plateau was decreased [Diamant and Bortoff, 1969b; Sarna et al., 1971]. The frequency of the aborad plateau was either higher than or equal to the highest intrinsic frequency distal to the transection, depending on whether the transection of the duodenum was either above or below the region of the bile duct [Diamant and Bortoff, 1969b].

The ECA in canine small intestine was modeled using a chain of 16 bidirectionally coupled relaxation oscillators [Sarna et al., 1971]. Coupling was not uniform along the chain, since the proximal oscillators were strongly coupled and the distal oscillators were weakly coupled. The model featured (1) an exponential intrinsic frequency decline along the chain, (2) a frequency plateau which is higher than the highest intrinsic frequency, and (3) a temporal variation of the frequencies distal to the frequency plateau region. A simulated transection in the frequency plateau region caused the formation of another frequency plateau aboral to the transection, such that the frequency of the orad plateau was unchanged whereas the frequency of the aborad plateau decreased.

The ECA in human small intestine was modeled using a chain of 100 bidirectionally coupled relaxation oscillators [Robertson-Dunn and Linkens, 1976]. Coupling was nonuniform and asymmetrical. The model featured (1) a piecewise linear decline in intrinsic frequency along the chain, (2) a piecewise linear decline in coupling similar to that of the intrinsic frequency, (3) forward coupling which is stronger than backward coupling, and (4) a frequency plateau in the proximal region, which is higher than the highest intrinsic frequency in the region.

6.5.3 Small Intestinal MMC

The MMCs in canine small intestine have been observed in intrinsically isolated segments [Sarna et al., 1981; 1983], even after the isolated segment has been stripped of all extrinsic innervation [Sarr and Kelly, 1981] or removed in continuity with the remaining gut as a Thiry Vella loop [Itoh et al., 1981]. This intrinsic mechanism is able to function independently of extrinsic innervation, since vagotomy [Weisbrodt et al., 1975; Ruckebusch and Bueno, 1977] does not hinder the initiation of the MMC. The initiation of the small intestinal MMC is controlled by integrative networks within the intrinsic plexuses utilizing nicotinic and muscarinic cholinergic receptors [Ormsbee et al., 1979; El-Sharkawy et al., 1982].

When the canine small intestine was transected into four equal strips [Sarna et al., 1981, 1983], it was found that each strip was capable of generating an independent MMC that would appear to propagate from the proximal to the distal part of each segment. This suggested that the MMC could be modeled by a chain of coupled relaxation oscillators. The average intrinsic periods of the MMC for the four segments were reported to be 106.2, 66.8, 83.1, and 94.8 min, respectively. The segment containing the duodenum had the longest period, while the subsequent segment containing the jejunum had the shortest period. However, in the intact small intestine, the MMC starts in the duodenum and not the jejunum. Bardakjian et al. [1981, 1984] have demonstrated that both the intrinsic frequency gradients and resting level gradients have major roles in the entrainment of a chain of coupled oscillators. In modeling the small intestinal MMC with a chain of four coupled oscillators, it was necessary to include a gradient in the intrinsic resting levels of the MMC oscillators (with the proximal oscillator having the lowest resting level) in order to entrain the oscillators and allow the proximal oscillator to behave as the leading oscillator [Bardakjian and Ahmed, 1992].

6.6 The Colon

6.6.1 Anatomical Features

In humans, the colon is about 100 cm in length. The ileum joins the colon approximately 5 cm from its end, forming the cecum, which has a worm-like appendage — the appendix. The colon is sacculated and the longitudinal smooth muscle is concentrated in three bands (the taeniae). It lies in front of the small intestine against the abdominal wall and it consists of the ascending (on the right side), transverse (across the lower stomach), and descending (on the left side) colon. The descending colon becomes the sigmoid colon in the pelvis as it runs down and forward to the rectum. Major functions of the colon are (1) to absorb water, certain electrolytes, short chain fatty acids, and bacterial metabolites; (2) to slowly propel its luminal contents in the caudad direction; (3) to store the residual matter in the distal region; and (4) to rapidly move its contents in the caudad direction during mass movements [Sarna, 1991]. In dogs, the colon is about 45 cm in length and the cecum has no appendage. The colon is not sacculated, and the longitudinal smooth muscle coat is continuous around the circumference [Miller et al., 1968]. It lies posterior to the small intestine and it consists mainly of ascending and descending segments with a small transverse segment. However, functionally it is assumed to consist of three regions, each of about 15 cm in length, representing the ascending, transverse, and descending colon, respectively.

6.6.2 Colonic ECA

In the human colon, the ECA is almost completely phase-unlocked between adjacent sites as close as 1 to 2 cm apart and its frequency (about 3 to 15 cpm) and amplitude at each site vary with time [Sarna et al., 1980]. This results in short duration contractions that are also disorganized in time and space. The disorganization of ECA and its associated contractions is consistent with the colonic function of extensive mixing, kneading, and slow net distal propulsion [Sarna, 1991]. In the canine colon, the reports about the intrinsic frequency gradient were conflicting [Vanasin et al., 1974; Shearin et al., 1978; El-Sharkawy, 1983].

The human colonic ECA was modeled [Bardakjian and Sarna, 1980] using a tubular structure of 99 bidirectionally coupled nonlinear oscillators arranged in 33 parallel rings where each ring contained three oscillators. Coupling was nonuniform and it increased in the longitudinal direction. The model featured (1) no phase-locking in the longitudinal or circumferential directions, (2) temporal and spatial variation of the frequency profile with large variations in the proximal and distal regions and small variations in the middle region, and (3) waxing and waning of the amplitudes of the ECA, which was more pronounced in the proximal and distal regions. The model demonstrated that the "silent periods" occurred because of the interaction between oscillators and they did not occur when the oscillators were uncoupled. The model was further refined [Bardakjian et al., 1990] such that when the ECA amplitude exceeded an excitation threshold, a burst of ERA was exhibited. The ERA bursts occurred in a seemingly random manner in adjacent sites because (1) the ECA was not phase-locked and (2) the ECA amplitudes and waveshapes varied in a seemingly random manner.

6.7 Epilogue

The ECA in stomach, small intestine, and colon behaves like the outputs of a population of coupled nonlinear oscillators. The populations in the stomach and the proximal small intestine are entrained, whereas those in the distal small intestine and colon are not entrained. There are distinct intrinsic frequency gradients in the stomach and small intestine but their profile in the colon is ambiguous.

The applicability of modeling of gastrointestinal ECA by coupled nonlinear oscillators has been reconfirmed [Daniel et al., 1994] and a novel nonlinear oscillator, the mapped clock oscillator, was proposed [Bardakjian and Diamant, 1994] for modeling the cellular ECA. The oscillator consists of two coupled components: a clock, which represents the interstitial cells of Cajal and a mapper, which represents the smooth muscle transmembrane ionic transport mechanisms [Skinner and Bardakjian, 1991]. Such a model accounts for the mounting evidence supporting the role of the interstitial cells of Cajal as a pacemaker for the smooth muscle transmembrane voltage oscillations [Hara et al., 1986; Suzuki et al., 1986; Barajas–Lopez et al., 1989; Serio et al., 1991; Sanders, 1996; Sanders et al., 2002; Daniel, 2004].

Modeling of the gastrointestinal ECA by populations of coupled nonlinear oscillators [Bardakjian, 1987] suggests that gastrointestinal motility disorders associated with abnormal ECA can be effectively treated by (1) electronic pacemakers to coordinate the oscillators, (2) surgical interventions to remove regional ectopic foci, and (3) pharmacotherapy to stimulate the oscillators. Electronic pacing has been demonstrated in canine stomach [Kelly and LaForce, 1972; Sarna and Daniel, 1973; Bellahsene et al., 1992] and small intestine [Sarna and Daniel, 1975c; Becker et al., 1983]. Also, pharmacotherapy with prokinetic drugs such as Domperidone and Cisapride has demonstrated improvements in the coordination of the gastric oscillators.

Acknowledgments

The author would like to thank his colleagues Dr. Sharon Chung and Dr. Karen Hall for providing biological insight.

References

Alvarez, W.C. 1922. The electrogastrogram and what it shows. *J. Am. Med. Assoc.*, 78: 1116–1119.
Alvarez, W.C. and Mahoney, L.J. 1922. Action current in stomach and intestine. *Am. J. Physiol.*, 58: 476–493.

Alvarez, W.C. and Mahoney, L.J. 1923. The relations between gastric and duodenal peristalsis. *Am. J. Physiol.*, 64: 371–386.

Barajas-Lopez, C., Berezin, I., Daniel, E.E., and Huizinga, J.D. 1989. Pacemaker activity recorded in interstitial cells of Cajal of the gastrointestinal tract. *Am. J. Physiol.*, 257: C830–C835.

Bardakjian, B.L. 1987. Computer models of gastrointestinal myoelectric activity. *Automedica*, 7: 261–276.

Bardakjian, B.L. and Ahmed, K. 1992. Is a peripheral pattern generator sufficient to produce both fasting and postprandial patterns of the migrating myoelectric complex (MMC)? *Dig. Dis. Sci.*, 37: 986.

Bardakjian, B.L. and Diamant, N.E. 1994. A mapped clock oscillator model for transmembrane electrical rhythmic activity in excitable cells. *J. Theor. Biol.*, 166: 225–235.

Bardakjian, B.L. and Sarna, S.K. 1980. A computer model of human colonic electrical control activity (ECA). *IEEE Trans. Biomed. Eng.*, 27: 193–202.

Bardakjian, B.L. and Sarna, S.K. 1981. Mathematical investigation of populations of coupled synthesized relaxation oscillators representing biological rhythms. *IEEE Trans. Biomed. Eng.*, 28: 10–15.

Bardakjian, B.L., El-Sharkawy, T.Y., and Diamant, N.E. 1984. Interaction of coupled nonlinear oscillators having different intrinsic resting levels. *J. Theor. Biol.*, 106: 9–23.

Bardakjian, B.L., Sarna, S.K., and Diamant, N.E. 1990. Composite synthesized relaxation oscillators: Application to modeling of colonic ECA and ERA. *Gastrointest. J. Motil.*, 2: 109–116.

Bass, P. 1965. Electric activity of smooth muscle of the gastrointestinal tract. *Gastroenterology*, 49: 391–394.

Beck, I.T., McKenna, R.D., Peterfy, G., Sidorov, J., and Strawczynski, H. 1965. Pressure studies in the normal human jejunum. *Am. J. Dig. Dis.*, 10: 437–448.

Becker, J.M., Sava, P., Kelly, K.A., and Shturman, L. 1983. Intestinal pacing for canine postgastrectomy dumping. *Gastroenterology*, 84: 383–387.

Bellahsene, B.E., Lind, C.D., Schirmer, B.D., et al. 1992. Acceleration of gastric emptying with electrical stimulation in a canine model of gastroparesis. *Am. J. Physiol.*, 262: G826–G834.

Berezin, I., Huizinga, J.D., and Daniel, E.E. 1988. Interstitial cells of Cajal in the canine colon: a special communication network at the inner border of the circular muscle. *J. Comp. Neurol.* 273: 42–51.

Boldireff, W.N. 1905. Le travail periodique de l'appareil digestif en dehors de la digestion. *Arch. Des. Sci. Biol.*, 11: 1–157.

Bozler, E. 1938. Action potentials of visceral smooth muscle. *Am. J. Physiol.*, 124: 502–510.

Bozler, E. 1939. Electrophysiological studies on the motility of the gastrointestinal tract. *Am. J. Physiol.*, 127: 301–307.

Bozler, E. 1941. Action potentials and conduction of excitation in muscle. *Biol. Symposia*, 3: 95–110.

Bulbring, E., Burnstock, G., and Holman, M.E. 1958. Excitation and conduction in the smooth muscle of the isolated taenia coli of the guinea pig. *J. Physiol.*, 142: 420–437.

Burnstock, G., Holman, M.E., and Prosser, C.L. 1963. Electrophysiology of smooth muscle. *Physiol. Rev.*, 43: 482–527.

Cannon, W.B. and Washburn, A.L. 1912. An explanation of hunger. *Am. J. Physiol.*, 29: 441–454.

Carlson, G.M., Bedi, B.S., and Code, C.F. 1972. Mechanism of propagation of intestinal interdigestive myoelectric complex. *Am. J. Physiol.*, 222: 1027–1030.

Chanson, M. and Spray, D.C. 1995. Electrophysiology of gap junctional communication. In: *Pacemaker Activity and Intercellular Communication*. Huizinga, J.D. (Ed.), CRC Press, Baton Rouge, FL.

Chen, J.Z. and McCallum, R.W. 1994. *Electrogastrography: Principles and Applications*. Raven Press, New York.

Christensen, J. 1975. Myoelectric control of the colon. *Gastroenterology*, 68: 601–609.

Code, C.F. and Marlett, J.A. 1975. The interdigestive myoelectric complex of the stomach and small bowel of dogs. *J. Physiol.*, 246: 289–309.

Daniel, E.E. 1975. Electrophysiology of the colon. *Gut*, 16: 298–329.

Daniel, E.E. 2004. Communication between interstitial cells of Cajal and gastrointestinal muscle. *Neurogastroenterol. Motil.*, 16: 118–122.

Daniel, E.E. and Chapman, K.M. 1963. Electrical activity of the gastrointestinal tract as an indication of mechanical activity. *Am. J. Dig. Dis.*, 8: 54–102.

Daniel, E.E. and Sakai, Y. 1984. Structural basis for function of circular muscle of canine corpus. *Can. J. Physiol. Pharmacol.,* 62: 1304–1314.

Daniel, E.E., Duchon, D.G., Garfield, R.E., Nichols, M., Malhorta, S.K., and Oki, M. 1976. Is the nexus necessary for cell-to-cell coupling of smooth muscle. *Mem. Biol.,* 28: 207–239.

Daniel, E.E., Bardakjian, B.L., Huizinga, J.D., and Diamant, N.E. 1994. Relaxation oscillators and core conductor models are needed for understanding of GI electrical activities. *Am. J. Physiol.,* 266: G339–G349.

Diamant, N.E. and Bortoff, A. 1969a. Nature of the intestinal slow wave frequency gradient. *Am. J. Physiol.,* 216: 301–307.

Diamant, N.E. and Bortoff, A. 1969b. Effects of transection on the intestinal slow wave frequency gradient. *Am. J. Physiol.,* 216: 734–743.

Douglas, D.M. 1949. The decrease in frequency of contraction of the jejunum after transplantation to the ileum. *J. Physiol.,* 110: 66–75.

Duthie, H.L. 1974. Electrical activity of gastrointestinal smooth muscle. *Gut,* 15: 669–681.

El-Sharkawy, T.Y. 1983. Electrical activity of the muscle layers of the canine colon. *J. Physiol.,* 342: 67–83.

El-Sharkawy, T.Y., Markus, H., and Diamant, N.E. 1982. Neural control of the intestinal migrating myoelectric complex: a pharmacological analysis. *Can. J. Physiol. Pharm.,* 60: 794–804.

Ermentrout, G.B. and Kopell, N. 1984. Frequency plateaus in a chain of weakly coupled oscillators. *SIAM J. Math. Anal.,* 15: 215–237.

Fitzhugh, R. 1961. Impulses and physiological states in theoretical models of nerve membranes. *Biophys. J.,* 1: 445–466.

Fleckenstein, P. 1978. Migrating electrical spike activity in the fasting human small intestine. *Dig. Dis. Sci.,* 23: 769–775.

Gillespie, J.S. 1962. The electrical and mechanical responses of intestinal smooth muscle cells to stimulation of their extrinsic parasympathetic nerves. *J. Physiol.,* 162: 76–92.

Grasman, J. 1984. The mathematical modeling of entrained biological oscillators. *Bull. Math. Biol.,* 46: 407–422.

Grivel, M.L. and Ruckebusch, Y. 1972. The propagation of segmental contractions along the small intestine. *J. Physiol.,* 277: 0 611–625.

Hara, Y.M., Kubota, M., and Szurszewski, J.H. 1986. Electrophysiology of smooth muscle of the small intestine of some mammals. *J. Physiol.,* 372: 501–520.

Hodgkin, A.L. and Huxley, A.F.A. 1952. A quantitative description of membrane current and its application to conduction and excitation in nerve. *J. Physiol.,* 117: 500–544.

Huizinga, J.D., Liu, L.W.C., Blennerhassett, M.G., Thuneberg, L., and Molleman, A. 1992. Intercellular communication in smooth muscle. *Experientia,* 48: 932–941.

Itoh, Z., Honda, R., Aizawa, I., Takeuchi, S., Hiwatashi, K., and Couch, E.F. 1978. Interdigestive motor activity of the lower esophageal sphincter in the conscious dog. *Dig. Dis. Sci.,* 23: 239–247.

Itoh, Z., Aizawa, I., and Takeuchi, S. 1981. Neural regulation of interdigestive motor activity in canine jejunum. *Am. J. Physiol.,* 240: G324–G330.

Jacoby, H.I., Bass, P., and Bennett, D.R. 1963. *In vivo* extraluminal contractile force transducer for gastrointestinal muscle. *J. Appl. Physiol.,* 18: 658–665.

Kelly, K.A. and LaForce, R.C. 1972. Pacing the canine stomach with electric stimulation. *Am. J. Physiol.,* 222: 588–594.

Kerlin, P. and Phillips, S. 1982. The variability of motility of the ileum and jejunum in healthy humans. *Gastroenterology,* 82: 694–700.

Liang, J., Cheung, J.Y., and Chen, J.D.Z. 1997. Detection and deletion of motion artifacts in electrogastrogram using feature analysis and neural networks. *Ann. Biomed. Eng.,* 25: 850–857.

Linkens, D.A., Taylor, I., and Duthie, H.L. 1976. Mathematical modeling of the colorectal myoelectrical activity in humans. *IEEE Trans. Biomed. Eng.,* 23: 101–110.

Liu, L.W.C., Farraway, L.A., Berezin, I., and Huizinga, J.D. 1998. Interstitial cells of Cajal: mediators of communication between longitudinal and circular muscle cells of canine colon. *Cell Tissue Res.*, 294: 69–79.

Miller, M.E., Christensen, G.C., and Evans, H.E. 1968. *Anatomy of the Dog*, W.B. Saunders, Philadelphia.

Milton, G.W. and Smith, A.W.M. 1956. The pacemaking area of the duodenum. *J. Physiol.*, 132: 100–114.

Mintchev, M.P. and Bowes, K.L. 1997. Do increased electrogastrographic frequencies always correspond to internal tachygastria? *Ann. Biomed. Eng.*, 25: 1052–1058.

Morat, J.P. 1882. Sur l'innervation motrice de l'estomac. *Lyon. Med.*, 40: 289–296.

Morat, J.P. 1893. Sur quelques particularites de l'innervation motrice de l'estomac et de l'intestin. *Arch. Physiol. Norm. Path.*, 5: 142–153.

Nelson, T.S. and Becker, J.C. 1968. Simulation of the electrical and mechanical gradient of the small intestine. *Am. J. Physiol.*, 214: 749–757.

Ormsbee, H.S., Telford, G.L., and Mason, G.R. 1979. Required neural involvement in control of canine migrating motor complex. *Am. J. Physiol.*, 237: E451–E456.

Pavlidis, T. 1973. *Biological Oscillators: Their Mathematical Analysis.* Academic Press, New York.

Pffafenbach, B., Adamek, R.J., Kuhn, K., and Wegener, M. 1995. Electrogastrography in healthy subjects. Evaluation of normal values: influence of age and gender. *Dig. Dis. Sci.*, 40: 1445–1450.

Pick, T.P. and Howden, R. 1977. *Gray's Anatomy*, Bounty Books, New York.

Plant, R. E. and Kim, M. 1976. Mathematical description of a bursting pacemaker neuron by a modification of the Hodgkin-Huxley equations. *Biophys. J.*, 16: 227–244.

Puestow, C.B. 1933. Studies on the origins of the automaticity of the intestine: the action of certain drugs on isolated intestinal transplants. *Am. J. Physiol.*, 106: 682–688.

Qiao, W., Sun, H.H., Chey, W.Y., and Lee, K.Y. 1998. Continuous wavelet analysis as an aid in the representation and interpretation of electrogastrographic signals. *Ann. Biomed. Eng.*, 26: 1072–1081.

Rees, W.D.W., Malagelada, J.R., Miller, L.J., and Go, V.L.W. 1982. Human interdigestive and postprandial gastrointestinal motor and gastrointestinal hormone patterns. *Dig. Dis. Sci.*, 27: 321–329.

Reinke, D.A., Rosenbaum, A.H., and Bennett, D.R. 1967. Patterns of dog gastrointestinal contractile activity monitored in vivo with extraluminal force transducers. *Am. J. Dig. Dis.*, 12: 113–141.

Rinzel, J. 1987. A formal classification of bursting mechanisms in excitable cells. In *Mathematical Topics in Population Biology, Morphogenesis, and Neurosciences*, Teramoto, E. and Yamaguti, M. (Eds.), Lecture Notes in Biomathematics, vol. pp. 71:Springer-Verlag, Berlin, 267–281.

Robertson-Dunn, B. and Linkens, D.A. 1974. A mathematical model of the slow wave electrical activity of the human small intestine. *Med. Biol. Eng.*, 12: 750–758.

Ruckebusch, Y. and Bueno, L. 1976. The effects of feeding on the motility of the stomach and small intestine in the pig. *Br. J. Nutr.*, 35: 397–405.

Ruckebusch, Y. and Bueno, L. 1977. Migrating myoelectrical complex of the small intestine. *Gastroenterology*, 73: 1309–1314.

Ruckebusch, Y. and Fioramonti, S. 1975. Electrical spiking activity and propulsion in small intestine in fed and fasted states. *Gastroenterology*, 68: 1500–1508.

Sanders, K.M. 1996. A case for interstitial cells of Cajal as pacemakers and mediators of neurotransmission in the gastrointestinal tract. *Gastroenterology*, 111: 492–515.

Sanders, K.M., Ordog, T., and Ward, S.M. 2002. Physiology and pathophysiology of the interstitial cells of Cajal: From bench to bedside. IV. Genetic and animal models of GI motility disorders caused by loss of interstitial cells of Cajal. *Am. J. Physiol. Gastrointest. Liver Physiol.*, 282: G747–G756.

Sarna, S.K. 1975a. Models of smooth muscle electrical activity. In: *Methods in Pharmacology*, Daniel, E.E. and Paton, D.M. (Eds.), Plenum Press, New York, pp. 519–540.

Sarna, S.K. 1975b. Gastrointestinal electrical activity: terminology. *Gastroenterology*, 68: 1631–1635.

Sarna, S.K. 1991. Physiology and pathophysiology of colonic motor activity. *Dig. Dis. Sci.*, 6: 827–862.

Sarna, S.K. and Daniel, E.E. 1973. Electrical stimulation of gastric electrical control activity. *Am. J. Physiol.*, 225: 125–131.

Sarna, S.K. and Daniel, E.E. 1975. Electrical stimulation of small intestinal electrical control activity. *Gastroenterology*, 69: 660–667.

Sarna, S.K., Daniel, E.E., and Kingma, Y.J. 1971. Simulation of slow wave electrical activity of small intestine. *Am. J. Physiol.*, 221: 166–175.

Sarna, S.K., Daniel, E.E., and Kingma, Y.J. 1972. Simulation of the electrical control activity of the stomach by an array of relaxation oscillators. *Am. J. Dig. Dis.*, 17: 299–310.

Sarna, S.K., Bardakjian, B.L., Waterfall, W.E., and Lind, J.F. 1980. Human colonic electrical control activity (ECA). *Gastroenterology*, 78: 1526–1536.

Sarna, S.K., Stoddard, C., Belbeck, L., and McWade, D. 1981. Intrinsic nervous control of migrating myoelectric complexes. *Am. J. Physiol.*, 241: G16–G23.

Sarna, S., Condon, R.E., and Cowles, V. 1983. Enteric mechanisms of initiation of migrating myoelectric complexes in dogs. *Gastroenterology*, 84: 814–822.

Sarr M.G. and Kelly, K.A. 1981. Myoelectric activity of the autotransplanted canine jejunoileum. *Gastroenterology*, 81: 303–310.

Serio, R., Barajas-Lopez, C., Daniel, E.E., Berezin, I., and Huizinga, J.D. 1991. Pacemaker activity in the colon: Role of interstitial cells of Cajal and smooth muscle cells. *Am. J. Physiol.*, 260: G636–G645.

Shearin, N.L., Bowes, K.L., and Kingma, Y.J. 1978. *In vitro* electrical activity in canine colon. *Gut*, 20: 780–786.

Sherman, A. and Rinzel, J. 1991. Model for synchronization of pancreatic beta-cells by gap junction coupling. *Biophys. J.*, 59: 547–559.

Skinner, F.K. and Bardakjian, B.L. 1991. A barrier kinetic mapping unit. Application to ionic transport in gastric smooth muscle. *Gastrointest. J. Motil.*, 3: 213–224.

Stanciu, C. and Bennett, J.R. 1975. The general pattern of gastroduodenal motility: 24 hour recordings in normal subjects. *Rev. Med. Chir. Soc. Med. Nat. Iasi.*, 79: 31–36.

Stern, R.M. and Koch, K.L. 1985. *Electrogastrography: Methodology, Validation, and Applications.* Praeger Publishers, New York.

Sperelakis, N. 2002. An electric field mechanism for transmission of excitation between myocardial cells. *Circ. Res.*, 91: 985–987.

Sperelakis, N. and Mann, J.E. 1977. Evaluation of electric field change in the cleft between excitable cells. *J. Theor. Biol.*, 64: 71–96.

Sperelakis, N. and McConnell, K. 2002. Electric field interactions between closely abutting excitable cells. *IEEE Eng. Med. Biol. Mag.*, 21: 77–89.

Sperelakis, N., and Ramasamy, L. 2002. Propagation in cardiac and smooth muscle based on electric field transmission at cell junctions: an analysis by Pspice. *IEEE Eng. Med. Biol. Mag.*, 21: 177–190.

Sperelakis, N., LoBrocco, B., Mann, J.E., and Marshall, R. 1984. Potassium accumulation in intercellular junctions combined with electric field interaction for propagation in cardiac muscle. *Innov. Technol. Biol. Med.*, 6: 24–43.

Stein, R.B. 1967. Some models of neuronal variability. *Biophys. J.*, 7: 37–68.

Summers, R.W., Anuras, S., and Green, J. 1982. Jejunal motility patterns in normal subjects and symptomatic patients with partial mechanical obstruction or pseudo-obstruction. In: *Motility of the Digestive Tract*, Weinbeck, M. (Ed.), Raven Press, New York, pp. 467–470.

Suzuki, N., Prosser, C.L., and Dahms, V., 1986. Boundary cells between longitudinal and circular layers: Essential for electrical slow waves in cat intestine. *Am. J. Physiol.*, 280: G287–G294.

Szurszewski, J.H. 1969. A migrating electric complex of the canine small intestine. *Am. J. Physiol.*, 217: 1757–1763.

Szurszewski, J.H. 1987. Electrical basis for gastrointestinal motility. In: *Physiology of the Gastrointestinal Tract*, Johnson, L.R. (Ed.), Raven Press, New York, chap. 12.

Thompson, D.G., Wingate, D.L., Archer, L., Benson, M.J., Green, W.J., and Hardy, R.J. 1980. Normal patterns of human upper small bowel motor activity recorded by prolonged radiotelemetry. *Gut*, 21: 500–506.

Thunberg, L. 1982. Interstitial cells of Cajal: intestinal pacemaker cells. *Adv. Anat. Embryol. Cell. Biol.,* 71: 1–130.

Thunberg, L., Rahnamai, M.A., and Riazi, H. 1998. The peg-and-socket junction: an alternative to the gap junction in coupling of smooth muscle cells. *Neurogastroenterol. Motil.,* 10.

Van der Pol, B. and Van der Mark, J. 1928. The heart considered as a relaxation oscillator and an electrical model of the heart. *Phil. Mag.,* 6: 763–775.

Vanasin, B., Ustach, T.J., and Schuster, M.M. 1974. Electrical and motor activity of human and dog colon in vitro. *Johns Hopkins Med. J.,* 134: 201–210.

Vantrappen, G., Janssens, J.J., Hellemans, J., and Ghoos, Y. 1977. The interdigestive motor complex of normal subjects and patients with bacterial overgrowth of the small intestine. *J. Clin. Invest.,* 59: 1158–1166.

Vigmond, E.J. and Bardakjian, B.L. 1995. The effect of morphological interdigitation on field coupling between smooth muscle cells. *IEEE Trans. Biomed. Eng.,* 42: 162–171.

Vigmond, E.J., Bardakjian, B.L., Thunberg, L., and Huizinga, J.D. 2000. Intercellular coupling mediated by potassium accumulation in peg-and-socket junctions. *IEEE Trans. Biomed. Eng.,* 47: 1576–1583.

Wang, Z., He, Z., and Chen, J.D.Z. 1999. Filter banks and neural network-based feature extraction and automatic classification of electrogastrogram. *Ann. Biomed. Eng.,* 27: 88–95.

Ward, S.M. and Sanders, K.M. 2001. Interstitial cells of Cajal: Primary targets of enteric motor innervation. *Anat. Rec.,* 262: 125–135.

Weisbrodt, N.W., Copeland, E.M., Moore, E.P., Kearly, K.W., and Johnson, L.R. 1975. Effect of vagotomy on electrical activity of the small intestine of the dog. *Am. J. Physiol.,* 228: 650–654.

Wheelon, H. and Thomas, J.E. 1921. Rhythmicity of the pyloric sphincter. *Am. J. Physiol.,* 54: 460–473.

Wheelon, H. and Thomas, J.E. 1922. Observations on the motility of the duodenum and the relation of duodenal activity to that of the pars pylorica. *Am. J. Physiol.,* 59: 72–96.

Winfree, A.T. 1980. *The Geometry of Biological Time,* Springer-Verlag, New York.

Winfree, A.T. 1989. Electrical instability in cardiac muscle: Phase singularities and rotors. *J. Theor. Biol.,* 138: 353–405.

Zamir, O. and Hanani, M. 1990. Intercellular dye-coupling in intestinal smooth muscle: are gap junctions required for intercellular coupling. *Experientia,* 46: 1002–1005.

7

Respiratory System

Arthur T. Johnson
University of Maryland

Christopher G. Lausted
The Institute for Systems Biology

Joseph D. Bronzino
Trinity College

As functioning units, the lung and heart are usually considered as a single complex organ, but because these organs contain essentially two compartments — one for blood and one for air — they are usually separated in terms of the tests conducted to evaluate heart or pulmonary function. This chapter focuses on some of the physiologic concepts responsible for normal function and specific measures of the lung's ability to supply tissue cells with enough oxygen while removing excess carbon dioxide.

7.1 Respiration Anatomy

The respiratory system consists of the lungs, conducting airways, pulmonary vasculature, respiratory muscles, and surrounding tissues and structures (Figure 7.1). Each plays an important role in influencing respiratory responses.

7.1.1 Lungs

There are two lungs in the human chest; the right lung is composed of three incomplete divisions called lobes, and the left lung has two, leaving room for the heart. The right lung accounts for 55% of total gas volume and the left lung for 45%. Lung tissue is spongy because of the very small (200–300×10^{-6} m diameter in normal lungs at rest) gas-filled cavities called **alveoli**, which are the ultimate structures for gas exchange. There are 250–350 million alveoli in the adult lung, with a total alveolar surface area of 50–100 m^2 depending on the degree of lung inflation [Johnson, 1991].

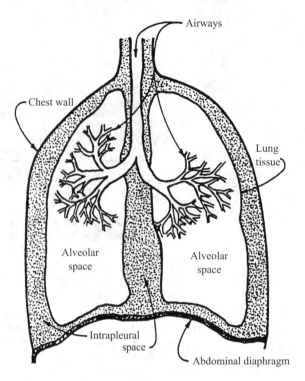

FIGURE 7.1   Schematic representation of the respiratory system.

7.1.2 Conducting Airways

Air is transported from the atmosphere to the alveoli beginning with the oral and nasal cavities, through
the pharynx (in the throat), past the glottal opening, and into the trachea or windpipe. Conduction of air
begins at the larynx, or voice box, at the entrance to the trachea, which is a fibromuscular tube 10–12 cm
in length and 1.4–2.0 cm in diameter [Kline, 1976]. At a location called the carina, the trachea terminates
and divides into the left and right bronchi. Each bronchus has a discontinuous cartilaginous support in its
wall. Muscle fibers capable of controling airway diameter are incorporated into the walls of the bronchi,
as well as in those of air passages closer to the alveoli. Smooth muscle is present throughout the respiratory
bronchiolus and alveolar ducts but is absent in the last alveolar duct, which terminates in one to several
alveoli. The alveolar walls are shared by other alveoli and are composed of highly pliable and collapsible
squamous epithelium cells.

The bronchi subdivide into subbronchi, which further subdivide into bronchioli, which further subdivide, and so on, until finally reaching the alveolar level. Table 7.1 provides a description and dimensions
of the airways of adult humans. A model of the geometric arrangement of these air passages is presented
in Figure 7.2. It will be noted that each airway is considered to branch into two subairways. In the adult
human there are considered to be 23 such branchings, or generations, beginning at the trachea and ending
in the alveoli.

Movement of gases in the respiratory airways occurs mainly by bulk flow (convection) throughout
the region from the mouth to the nose to the fifteenth generation. Beyond the fifteenth generation, gas
diffusion is relatively more important. With the low gas velocities that occur in **diffusion**, dimensions of
the space over which diffusion occurs (alveolar space) must be small for adequate oxygen delivery into the
walls; smaller alveoli are more efficient in the transfer of gas than are larger ones. Thus animals with high
levels of oxygen consumption are found to have smaller-diameter alveoli compared with animals with low
levels of oxygen consumption.

TABLE 7.1 Classification and Approximate Dimensions of Airways of Adult Human Lung (Inflated to about 3/4 of TLC)[a]

Common name	Numerical order of generation	Number of each	Diameter, mm	Length, mm	Total cross-sectional area, cm²	Description and comment
Trachea	0	1	18	120	2.5	Main cartilaginous airway; partly in thorax
Main bronchus	1	2	12	47.6	2.3	First branching of airway; one to each lung; in lung root; cartilage
Lobar bronchus	2	4	8	19.0	2.1	Named for each lobe; cartilage
Segmental bronchus	3	8	6	7.6	2.0	Named for radiographical and surgical anatomy; cartilage
Subsegmental bronchus	4	16	4	12.7	2.4	Last generally named bronchi; may be referred to as medium-sized bronchi; cartilage
Small bronchi	5–10	1,024[b]	1.3[b]	4.6[b]	13.4[b]	Not generally named; contain decreasing amounts of cartilage. Beyond this level airways enter the lobules as defined by a strong elastic lobular-limiting membrane
Bronchioles	11–13	8,192[b]	0.8[b]	2.7[b]	44.5[b]	Not named; contain no cartilage, mucus-secreting elements, or cilia. Tightly embedded in lung tissue
Terminal bronchioles	14–15	32,768[b]	0.7[b]	2.0[b]	113.0[b]	Generally 2 or 3 orders so designated; morphology not significantly different from orders 11–13
Respiratory bronchioles	16–18	262,144[b]	0.5[b]	1.2[b]	534.0[b]	Definite class; bronchiolar cuboidal epithelium present, but scattered alveoli are present giving these airways a gas exchange function. Order 165 often called first-order respiratory bronchiole; 17, second-order; 18, third-order
Alveolar ducts	19–22	4,194,304[b]	0.4[b]	0.8[b]	5,880.0[b]	No bronchial epithelium; have no surface except connective tissue framework; open into alveoli
Alveolar sacs	23	8,388,608	0.4	0.6	11,800.0	No reason to assign a special name; are really short alveolar ducts
Alveoli	24	300,000,000	0.2			Pulmonary capillaries are in the septae that form the alveoli

[a] The number of airways in each generation is based on regular dichotomous branching. [b] Numbers refer to last generation in each group.

Source: Used with permission from Suki, B. and Bates, J.H.T. 1991. *J. Appl. Physiol.* 71: 826–833 and Weibel, E.R. 1963. New York, Academic Press; adapted by Comroe [1965].

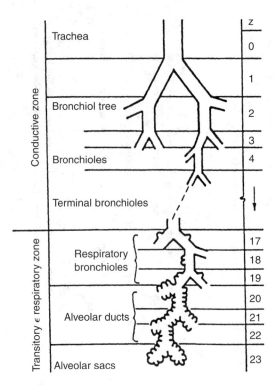

FIGURE 7.2   General architecture of conductive and transitory airways. In the conductive zone air is conducted to and from the lungs while in the respiration zone, gas exchange occurs. (Used with permission from Weibel [1963].)

7.1.3   Alveoli

Alveoli are the structures through which gases diffuse to and from the body. To ensure that gas exchange occurs efficiently, alveolar walls are extremely thin. For example, the total tissue thickness between the inside of the alveolus to pulmonary capillary blood plasma is only about 0.4×10^{-6} m. Consequently, the principal barrier to diffusion occurs at the plasma and red blood cell level, not at the alveolar membrane [Ruch and Patton, 1966]. Molecular diffusion within the alveolar volume is responsible for mixing of the enclosed gas. Due to small alveolar dimensions, complete mixing probably occurs in less than 10 msec, fast enough that alveolar mixing time does not limit gaseous diffusion to or from the blood [Astrand and Rodahl, 1970].

   Of particular importance to proper alveolar operation is a thin surface coating of surfactant. Without this material, large alveoli would tend to enlarge and small alveoli would collapse. It is the present view that surfactant acts like a detergent, changing the stress–strain relationship of the alveolar wall and thereby stabilizing the lung [Johnson, 1991].

7.1.4   Pulmonary Circulation

There is no true pulmonary analogue to the systemic arterioles, since the **pulmonary circulation** occurs under relatively low pressure [West, 1977]. Pulmonary blood vessels, especially capillaries and venules, are very thin walled and flexible. Unlike systemic capillaries, pulmonary capillaries increase in diameter, and pulmonary capillaries within alveolar walls separate adjacent alveoli with increases in blood pressure or decreases in alveolar pressure. Flow, therefore, is significantly influenced by elastic deformation. Although pulmonary circulation is largely unaffected by neural and chemical control, it does respond promptly to hypoxia.

There is also a high-pressure systemic blood delivery system to the bronchi that is completely independent of the pulmonary low-pressure ($\sim$3330 N/m^2) circulation in healthy individuals. In diseased states, however, bronchial arteries are reported to enlarge when pulmonary blood flow is reduced, and some arteriovenous shunts become prominent [West, 1977].

Total pulmonary blood volume is approximately 300–500 cm^3 in normal adults, with about 60–100 cm^3 in the pulmonary capillaries [Astrand and Rodahl, 1970]. This value, however, is quite variable, depending on such things as posture, position, disease, and chemical composition of the blood [Kline, 1976].

Since pulmonary arterial blood is poor in oxygen and rich in carbon dioxide, it exchanges excess carbon dioxide for oxygen in the pulmonary capillaries, which are in close contact with alveolar walls. At rest, the transit time for blood in the pulmonary capillaries is computed as

$$t = V_c / \dot{V}_c$$

where t is blood transmit time, sec; V_c is capillary blood volume, m^3; $\dot{V}_c$ is total capillary blood flow (cardiac output, m^3/sec); and is somewhat less than 1 sec, while during exercise it may be only 500 msec or even less.

7.1.5 Respiratory Muscles

The lungs fill because of a rhythmic expansion of the chest wall. The action is indirect in that no muscle acts directly on the lung. The diaphragm, the muscular mass accounting for 75% of the expansion of the chest cavity, is attached around the bottom of the thoracic cage, arches over the liver, and moves downward like a piston when it contracts. The external intercostal muscles are positioned between the ribs and aid **inspiration** by moving the ribs up and forward. This, then, increases the volume of the thorax. Other muscles are important in the maintenance of thoracic shape during breathing. For details, see Ruch and Patton [1966] and Johnson [1991].

Quiet **expiration** is usually considered to be passive; that is, pressure to force air from the lungs comes from elastic expansion of the lungs and chest wall. During moderate to severe exercise, the abdominal and internal intercostal muscles are very important in forcing air from the lungs much more quickly than would otherwise occur. Inspiration requires intimate contact between lung tissues, pleural tissues (the **pleura** is the membrane surrounding the lungs), and chest wall and diaphragm. This is accomplished by reduced intrathoracic pressure (which tends toward negative values) during inspiration.

Viewing the lungs as an entire unit, one can consider the lungs to be elastic sacs within an airtight barrel — the thorax — which is bounded by the ribs and the diaphragm. Any movement of these two boundaries alters the volume of the lungs. The normal breathing cycle in humans is accomplished by the active contraction of the inspiratory muscles, which enlarges the thorax. This enlargement lowers intrathoracic and interpleural pressure even further, pulls on the lungs, and enlarges the alveoli, alveolar ducts, and bronchioli, expanding the alveolar gas and decreasing its pressure below atmospheric. As a result, air at atmospheric pressure flows easily into the nose, mouth, and trachea.

7.2 Lung Volumes and Gas Exchange

Of primary importance to lung functioning is the movement and mixing of gases within the respiratory system. Depending on the anatomic level under consideration, gas movement is determined mainly by diffusion or convection.

Without the thoracic musculature and rib cage, as mentioned above, the barely inflated lungs would occupy a much smaller space than they occupy *in situ*. However, the thoracic cage holds them open. Conversely, the lungs exert an influence on the thorax, holding it smaller than should be the case without the lungs. Because the lungs and thorax are connected by tissue, the volume occupied by both together is between the extremes represented by relaxed lungs alone and thoracic cavity alone. The resting volume VR, then, is that volume occupied by the lungs with glottis open and muscles relaxed.

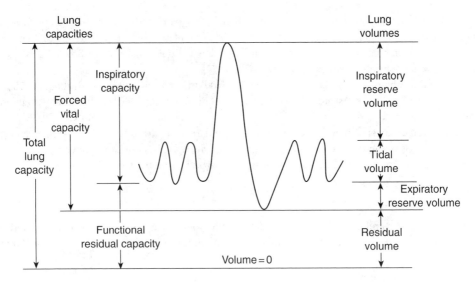

FIGURE 7.3   Lung capacities and lung volumes.

Lung volumes greater than resting volume are achieved during inspiration. Maximum inspiration is represented by inspiratory reserve volume (IRV). IRV is the maximum additional volume that can be accommodated by the lung at the end of inspiration. Lung volumes less than resting volume do not normally occur at rest but do occur during exhalation while exercising (when exhalation is active). Maximum additional expiration, as measured from lung volume at the end of expiration, is called expiratory reserve volume (ERV). Residual volume is the amount of gas remaining in the lungs at the end of maximal expiration.

Tidal volume VT is normally considered to be the volume of air entering the nose and mouth with each breath. Alveolar **ventilation** volume, the volume of fresh air that enters the alveoli during each breath, is always less than tidal volume. The extent of this difference in volume depends primarily on the anatomic **dead space**, the 150- to 160-ml internal volume of the conducting airway passages. The term dead is quite appropriate, since it represents wasted respiratory effort; that is, no significant gas exchange occurs across the thick walls of the trachea, bronchi, and bronchiolus. Since normal tidal volume at rest is usually about 500 ml of air per breath, one can easily calculate that because of the presence of this dead space, about 340–350 ml of fresh air actually penetrates the alveoli and becomes involved in the gas exchange process. An additional 150–160 ml of stale air exhaled during the previous breath is also drawn into the alveoli.

The term volume is used for elemental differences of lung volume, whereas the term capacity is used for combination of lung volumes. Figure 7.3 illustrates the interrelationship between each of the following lung volumes and capacities:

1. *Total lung capacity (TLC)*: The amount of gas contained in the lung at the end of maximal inspiration.
2. *Forced vital capacity (FVC)*: The maximal volume of gas that can be forcefully expelled after maximal inspiration.
3. *Inspiratory capacity (IC)*: The maximal volume of gas that can be inspired from the resting expiratory level.
4. ***Functional residual capacity (FRC)***: The volume of gas remaining after normal expiration. It will be noted that FRC is the same as the resting volume. There is a small difference, however, between resting volume and FRC because FRC is measured while the patient breathes, whereas resting volume is measured with no breathing. FRC is properly defined only at end-expiration at rest and not during exercise.

TABLE 7.2   Typical Lung Volumes for Normal, Healthy Males

Lung volume	Normal values	
Total lung capacity (TLC)	6.0×10^{-3} m^3	(6,000 cm^3)
Residual volume (RV)	1.2×10^{-3} m^3	(1,200 cm^3)
Vital capacity (VC)	4.8×10^{-3} m^3	(4,800 cm^3)
Inspiratory reserve volume (IRV)	3.6×10^{-3} m^3	(3,600 cm^3)
Expiratory reserve volume (ERV)	1.2×10^{-3} m^3	(1,200 cm^3)
Functional residual capacity (FRC)	2.4×10^{-3} m^3	(2,400 cm^3)
Anatomic dead volume (V_D)	1.5×10^{-4} m^3	(150 cm^3)
Upper airways volume	8.0×10^{-5} m^3	(80 cm^3)
Lower airways volume	7.0×10^{-5} m^3	(70 cm^3)
Physiologic dead volume (V_D)	1.8×10^{-3} m^3	(180 cm^3)
Minute volume ($\dot{V}_e$) at rest	1.0×10^{-4} m^3/sec	(6,000 cm^3/min)
Respiratory period (T) at rest	4 sec	
Tidal volume (V_T) at rest	4.0×10^{-4} m^3	(400 cm^3)
Alveolar ventilation volume (V_A) at rest	2.5×10^{-4} m^3	(250 cm^3)
Minute volume during heavy exercise	1.7×10^{-3} m^3/sec	(10,000 cm^3/min)
Respiratory period during heavy exercise	1.2 sec	
Tidal volume during heavy exercise	2.0×10^{-3} m^3	(2,000 cm^3)
Alveolar ventilation volume during exercise	1.8×10^{-3} m^3	(1,820 cm^3)

Source: Adapted and used with permission from Forster et al. [1986].

These volumes and specific capacities, represented in Figure 7.3, have led to the development of specific tests (that will be discussed below) to quantify the status of the pulmonary system. Typical values for these volumes and capacities are provided in Table 7.2.

7.3   Perfusion of the Lung

For gas exchange to occur properly in the lung, air must be delivered to the alveoli via the conducting airways, gas must diffuse from the alveoli to the capillaries through extremely thin walls, and the same gas must be removed to the cardiac atrium by blood flow. This three-step process involves (1) alveolar ventilation, (2) the process of diffusion, and (3) ventilatory **perfusion**, which involves pulmonary blood flow. Obviously, an alveolus that is ventilated but not perfused cannot exchange gas. Similarly, a perfused alveolus that is not properly ventilated cannot exchange gas. The most efficient gas exchange occurs when ventilation and perfusion are matched.

There is a wide range of ventilation-to-perfusion ratios that naturally occur in various regions of the lung [Johnson, 1991]. Blood flow is somewhat affected by posture because of the effects of gravity. In the upright position, there is a general reduction in the volume of blood in the thorax, allowing for larger lung volume. Gravity also influences the distribution of blood, such that the perfusion of equal lung volumes is about five times greater at the base compared with the top of the lung [Astrand and Rodahl, 1970]. There is no corresponding distribution of ventilation; hence the ventilation-to-perfusion ratio is nearly five times smaller at the top of the lung (Table 7.3). A more uniform ventilation-to-perfusion ratio is found in the supine position and during exercise [Jones, 1984b].

Blood flow through the capillaries is not steady. Rather, blood flows in a halting manner and may even be stopped if intraalveolar pressure exceeds intracapillary blood pressure during diastole. Mean blood flow is not affected by heart rate [West, 1977], but the highly distensible pulmonary blood vessels admit more blood when blood pressure and cardiac output increase. During exercise, higher pulmonary blood pressures allow more blood to flow through the capillaries. Even mild exercise favors more uniform perfusion of the lungs [Astrand and Rodahl, 1970]. Pulmonary artery systolic pressures increases from 2670 N/m^2 (20 mmHg) at rest to 4670 N/m^2 (35 mmHg) during moderate exercise to 6670 N/m^2 (50 mmHg) at maximal work [Astrand and Rodahl, 1970].

TABLE 7.3   Ventilation-to-Perfusion Ratios from the Top to
Bottom of the Lung of Normal Man in the Sitting Position

Percent lung volume, %	Alveolar ventilation rate, cm^3/sec	Perfusion rate, cm^3/sec	Ventilation-to-perfusion ratio
	Top		
7	4.0	1.2	3.3
8	5.5	3.2	1.8
10	7.0	5.5	1.3
11	8.7	8.3	1.0
12	9.8	11.0	0.90
13	11.2	13.8	0.80
13	12.0	16.3	0.73
13	13.0	19.2	0.68
	Bottom		
13	13.7	21.5	0.63
100	84.9	100.0	

Source: Used with permission from West [1962]. *J. Appl. Physiol.* 17:
893–898.

7.4   Gas Partial Pressure

The primary purpose of the respiratory system is gas exchange. In the gas-exchange process, gas must
diffuse through the alveolar space, across tissue, and through plasma into the red blood cell, where it
finally chemically joins to hemoglobin. A similar process occurs for carbon dioxide elimination.

As long as intermolecular interactions are small, most gases of physiologic significance can be considered
to obey the ideal gas law:

$$pV = nRT$$

where p is pressure; N/m^2; V is volume of gas, m^3; n is number of moles, mol; R is gas constant,
$(N \times m)/(mol \times K)$; and T is the absolute temperature, K.

The ideal gas law can be applied without error up to atmospheric pressure; it can be applied to a
mixture of gases, such as air, or to its constituents, such as oxygen or nitrogen. All individual gases in a
mixture are considered to fill the total volume and have the same temperature but reduced pressures. The
pressure exerted by each individual gas is called the **partial pressure** of the gas.

Dalton's law states that the total pressure is the sum of the partial pressures of the constituents of a
mixture:

$$p = \sum_{i=1}^{N} p_i$$

where p_i is the partial pressure of the ith constituent, N/m^2 and N is the total number of constituents.

Dividing the ideal gas law for a constituent by that for the mixture gives

$$\frac{P_i V}{PV} = \frac{n_i R_i T}{nRT}$$

so that

$$\frac{p_i}{p} = \frac{n_i R_i}{nR}$$

TABLE 7.4 Molecular Masses, Gas Constants, and Volume Fractions for Air and Constituents

Constituent	Molecular mass, kg/mol	Gas constant, $N \cdot m/(mol \cdot K)$	Volume fraction in air, m^3/m^3
Air	29.0	286.7	1.0000
Ammonia	17.0	489.1	0.0000
Argon	39.9	208.4	0.0093
Carbon dioxide	44.0	189.0	0.0003
Carbon monoxide	28.0	296.9	0.0000
Helium	4.0	2078.6	0.0000
Hydrogen	2.0	4157.2	0.0000
Nitrogen	28.0	296.9	0.7808
Oxygen	32.0	259.8	0.2095

Note: Universal gas constant is $8314.43\ N \cdot m/kg \cdot mol \cdot K$.

which states that the partial pressure of a gas may be found if the total pressure, mole fraction, and ratio of gas constants are known. For most respiratory calculations, p will be considered to be the pressure of 1 atmosphere, $101\ kN/m^2$. Avogadro's principle states that different gases at the same temperature and pressure contain equal numbers of molecules:

$$\frac{V_1}{V_2} = \frac{nR_1}{nR_2} = \frac{R_1}{R_2}$$

Thus

$$\frac{p_i}{p} = \frac{V_i}{V}$$

where V_i/V is the volume fraction of a constituent in air and is therefore dimensionless. Table 7.4 provides individual gas constants, as well as volume fractions, of constituent gases of air.

Gas pressures and volumes can be measured for many different temperature and humidity conditions. Three of these are body temperature and pressure, saturated (**BTPS**); ambient temperature and pressure (**ATP**); and standard temperature and pressure, dry (**STPD**). To calculate constituent partial pressures at STPD, total pressure is taken as barometric pressure minus vapor pressure of water in the atmosphere:

$$p_i = (V_i/V)(p - pH_2O)$$

where p is total pressure, kN/m^2; pH_2O is vapor pressure of water in atmosphere, kN/m^2; and V_i/V as a ratio does not change in the conversion process.

Gas volume at STPD is converted from ambient condition volume as

$$V_i = V_{amb}[273/(273 + \Theta)][(p - pH_2O)/101.3]$$

where V_i is volume of gas i corrected to STPD, m^3; V_{amb} is volume of gas i at ambient temperature and pressure, m^3; Θ is ambient temperature, °C; p is ambient total pressure, kN/m^2; and pH_2O is the vapor pressure of water in the air, kN/m^2.

Partial pressures and gas volumes may be expressed in BTPS conditions. In this case, gas partial pressures are usually known from other measurements. Gas volumes are converted from ambient conditions by

$$V_i = V_{amb}[310/(273 + \Theta)][(p - pH_2O)/p - 6.28]$$

Table 7.5 provides gas partial pressure throughout the respiratory and circulatory systems.

TABLE 7.5   Gas Partial Pressures (kN/m^2) Throughout the Respiratory and
Circulatory Systems

Gas	Inspired air[a]	Alveolar air	Expired air	Mixed venous blood	Arterial blood	Muscle tissue
H_2O	—	6.3	6.3	6.3	6.3	6.3
CO_2	0.04	5.3	4.2	6.1	5.3	6.7
O_2	21.2	14.0	15.5	5.3	13.3	4.0
$N2$[b]	80.1	75.7	75.3	76.4	76.4	76.4
Total	101.3	101.3	101.3	94.1	101.3	93.4

[a] Inspired air considered dry for convenience.
[b] Includes all other inert components.
   Source: Used with permission from Astrand and Rodahl [1970].

7.5   Pulmonary Mechanics

The respiratory system exhibits properties of resistance, compliance, and inertance analogous to the electrical properties of resistance, capacitance, and inductance. Of these, inertance is generally considered to be of less importance than the other two properties.

Resistance is the ratio of pressure to flow:

$$R = P/V$$

where R is resistance, $N \times sec/m^5$; P is pressure, N/m^2; and V is the volume flow rate, m^3/sec.

Resistance can be found in the conducting airways, in the lung tissue, and in the tissues of the chest wall. Airways exhalation resistance is usually higher than airways inhalation resistance because the surrounding lung tissue pulls the smaller, more distensible airways open when the lung is being inflated. Thus airways inhalation resistance is somewhat dependent on lung volume, and airways exhalation resistance can be very lung-volume-dependent [Johnson, 1991]. Respiratory tissue resistance varies with frequency, lung volume, and volume history. Tissue resistance is relatively small at high frequencies but increases greatly at low frequencies, nearly proportional to $1/f$. Tissue resistance often exceeds airway resistance below 2 Hz. Lung tissue resistance also increases with decreasing volume amplitude [Stamenovic et al., 1990].

Compliance is the ratio of lung volume to lung pressure:

$$C = V/P$$

where C is compliance, m^5/N; V is lung volume/m^3; and P is the pressure, N/m^2.

As the lung is stretched, it acts as an expanded balloon that tends to push air out and return to its normal size. The static pressure–volume relationship is nonlinear, exhibiting decreased static compliance at the extremes of lung volume [Johnson, 1991]. As with tissue resistance, dynamic tissue compliance does not remain constant during breathing. Dynamic compliance tends to increase with increasing volume and decrease with increasing frequency [Stamenovic et al., 1990].

Two separate approaches can be used to model lung tissue mechanics. The traditional approach places a linear viscoelastic system in parallel with a plastoelastic system. A linear viscoelastic system consists of ideal resistive and compliant elements and can exhibit the frequency dependence of respiratory tissue. A plastoelastic system consists of dry-friction elements and compliant elements and can exhibit the volume dependence of respiratory tissue [Hildebrandt, 1970]. An alternate approach is to utilize a nonlinear viscoelastic system that can characterize both the frequency dependence and the volume dependence of respiratory tissue [Suki and Bates, 1991].

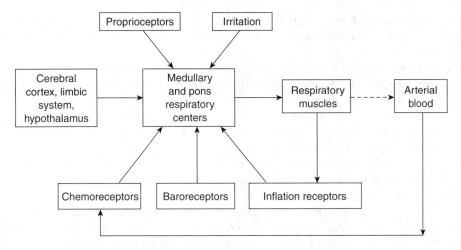

FIGURE 7.4   General scheme of respiratory control.

Lung tissue hysteresivity relates resistance and compliance:

$$\omega R = \eta / C_{\text{dyn}}$$

where ω is frequency, rad/sec; R is resistance, N $\times$ sec/m^5; η is hysteresivity, unitless; and C_{dyn} is the dynamic compliance, m^5/n.

Hysteresivity, analogous to the structural damping coefficient used in solid mechanics, is an empirical parameter arising from the assumption that resistance and compliance are related at the microstructural level. Hysteresivity is independent of frequency and volume. Typical values range from 0.1 to 0.3 [Fredberg and Stamenovic, 1989].

7.6 Respiratory Control

Control of respiration occurs in many different cerebral structures [Johnson, 1991] and regulates many things (Hornbein, 1981). Respiration must be controled to produce the respiratory rhythm, ensure adequate gas exchange, protect against inhalation of poisonous substances, assist in maintenance of body pH, remove irritations, and minimize energy cost. Respiratory control is more complex than cardiac control for at least three reasons:

1. Airways airflow occurs in both directions
2. The respiratory system interfaces directly with the environment outside the body
3. Parts of the respiratory system are used for other functions, such as swallowing and speaking

As a result, respiratory muscular action must be exquisitely coordinated; it must be prepared to protect itself against environmental onslaught, and breathing must be temporarily suspended on demand.

All control systems require sensors, controllers, and effectors. Figure 7.4 presents the general scheme for respiratory control. There are **mechanoreceptors** throughout the respiratory system. For example, nasal receptors are important in sneezing, apnea (cessation of breathing), bronchodilation, bronchoconstriction, and the secretion of mucus. Laryngeal receptors are important in coughing, apnea, swallowing, bronchoconstriction, airway mucus secretion, and laryngeal constriction. Tracheobronchial receptors are important in coughing, pulmonary hypertension, bronchoconstriction, laryngeal constriction, and mucus production. Other mechanoreceptors are important in the generation of the respiratory pattern and are involved with respiratory sensation.

Respiratory **chemoreceptors** exist peripherally in the aortic arch and carotic bodies and centrally in the ventral medulla oblongata of the brain. These receptors are sensitive to partial pressures of CO_2 and O_2 and to blood pH.

The respiratory controller is located in several places in the brain. Each location appears to have its own function. Unlike the heart, the basic respiratory rhythm is not generated within the lungs but rather in the brain and is transmitted to the respiratory muscles by the phrenic nerve.

Effector organs are mainly the respiratory muscles, as described previously. Other effectors are muscles located in the airways and tissues for mucus secretion. Control of respiration appears to be based on two criteria (1) removal of excess CO_2 and (2) minimization of energy expenditure. It is not the lack of oxygen that stimulates respiration but increased CO_2 partial pressure that acts as a powerful respiratory stimulus. Because of the buffering action of blood bicarbonate, blood pH usually falls as more CO_2 is produced in the working muscles. Lower blood pH also stimulates respiration.

A number of respiratory adjustments are made to reduce energy expenditure during exercise: respiration rate increases, the ratio of inhalation time to exhalation time decreases, respiratory flow waveshapes become more trapezoidal, and expiratory reserve volume decreases. Other adjustments to reduce energy expenditure have been theorized but not proven [Johnson, 1991].

7.7   The Pulmonary Function Laboratory

The purpose of a pulmonary function laboratory is to obtain clinically useful data from patients with respiratory dysfunction. The pulmonary function tests (PFTs) within this laboratory fulfill a variety of functions. They permit (1) quantification of a patient's breathing deficiency, (2) diagnosis of different types of pulmonary diseases, (3) evaluation of a patient's response to therapy, and (4) preoperative screening to determine whether the presence of lung disease increases the risk of surgery.

Although PFTs can provide important information about a patient's condition, the limitations of these tests must be considered. First, they are nonspecific in that they cannot determine which portion of the lungs is diseased, only that the disease is present. Second, PFTs must be considered along with the medical history, physical examination, x-ray examination, and other diagnostic procedures to permit a complete evaluation. Finally, the major drawback of some PFTs is that they require a full patient cooperation and for this reason these tests cannot be conducted on critically ill patients. Consider some of the most widely used PFTs: spirometry, body **plethysmography**, and diffusing capacity.

7.7.1   Spirometry

The simplest PFT is the spirometry maneuver. In this test, the patient inhales to TLC and exhales forcefully to residual volume. The patient exhales into a displacement bell chamber that sits on a water seal. As the bell rises, a pen coupled to the bell chamber inscribes a tracing on a rotating drum. The spirometer offers very little resistance to breathing; therefore, the shape of the spirometry curve (Figure 7.5) is purely a function of the patient's lung compliance, chest compliance, and airway resistance. At high lung volumes, a rise in intrapleural pressure results in greater expiratory flows. However, at intermediate and low lung volumes, the expiratory flow is independent of effort after a certain intrapleural pressure is reached.

Measurements made from the spirometry curve can determine the degree of a patient's ventilatory obstruction. FVC, forced expiratory volumes (FEVs), and forced expiratory flows (FEFs) can be determined. The FEV indicates the volume that has been exhaled from TLC for a particular time interval. For example, FEV0.5 is the volume exhaled during the first half-second of expiration, and FEV1.0 is the volume exhaled during the first second of expiration; these are graphically represented in Figure 7.5. Note that the more severe the ventilatory obstruction, the lower are the timed volumes (FEV0.5 and FEV1.0). The FEF is a measure of the average flow (volume/time) over specified portions of the spirometry curve and is represented by the slope of a straight line drawn between volume levels. The average flow over the first quarter of the forced expiration is the FEF0–25%, whereas the average flow over the middle 50% of

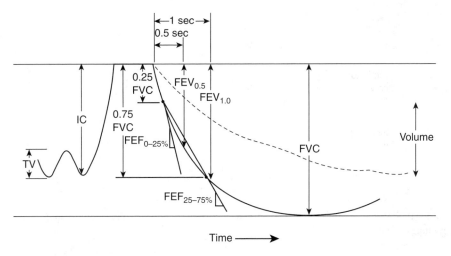

FIGURE 7.5 Typical spirometry tracing obtained during testing; inspiratory capacity (IC), tidal volume (TV), forced vital capacity (FVC), forced expiratory volume (FEV), and forced expiratory flows. Dashed line represents a patient with obstructive lung disease; solid line represents a normal, healthy individual.

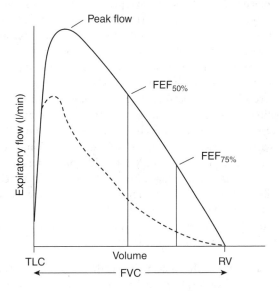

FIGURE 7.6 Flow-volume curve obtained from a spirometry maneuver. Solid line is a normal curve; dashed line represents a patient with obstructive lung disease.

the FVC is the FEF25–75%. These values are obtained directly from the spirometry curves. The less steep curves of obstructed patients would result in lower values of FEF0–25% and FEF25–75% compared with normal values, which are predicted on the basis of the patient's sex, age, and height. Equations for normal values are available from statistical analysis of data obtained from a normal population. Test results are then interpreted as a percentage of normal.

Another way of presenting a spirometry curve is as a flow-volume curve. Figure 7.6 represents a typical flow-volume curve. The expiratory flow is plotted against the exhaled volume, indicating the maximum flow that may be reached at each degree of lung inflation. Since there is no time axis, a time must mark the FEV0.5 and FEV1.0 on the tracing. To obtain these flow-volume curves in the laboratory, the patient usually exhales through a **pneumotach**. The most widely used pneumotach measures a pressure drop

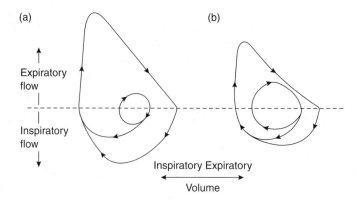

FIGURE 7.7 Typical flow-volume loops. (a) Normal flow-volume loop. (b) Flow-volume loop of patient with obstructive lung disease.

across a flow-resistive element. The resistance to flow is constant over the measuring range of the device; therefore, the pressure drop is proportional to the flow through the tube. This signal, which is indicative of flow, is then integrated to determine the volume of gas that has passed through the tube.

Another type of pneumotach is the heated-element type. In this device, a small heated mass responds to airflow by cooling. As the element cools, a greater current is necessary to maintain a constant temperature. This current is proportional to the airflow through the tube. Again, to determine the volume that has passed through the tube, the flow signal is integrated.

The flow-volume loop in Figure 7.7 is a dramatic representation displaying inspiratory and expiratory curves for both normal breathing and maximal breathing. The result is a graphic representation of the patient's reserve capacity in relation to normal breathing. For example, the normal patient's tidal breathing loop is small compared with the patient's maximum breathing loop. During these times of stress, this tidal breathing loop can be increased to the boundaries of the outer ventilatory loop. This increase in ventilation provides the greater gas exchange needed during the stressful situation. Compare this condition with that of the patient with obstructive lung disease. Not only is the tidal breathing loop larger than normal, but also the maximal breathing loop is smaller than normal. The result is a decreased ventilatory reserve, limiting the individual's ability to move air in and out of the lungs. As the disease progresses, the outer loop becomes smaller, and the inner loop becomes larger.

The primary use of spirometry is in detection of obstructive lung disease that results from increased resistance to flow through the airways. This can occur in several ways:

1. Deterioration of the structure of the smaller airways that results in early airways closure.
2. Decreased airway diameters caused by bronchospasm or the presence of secretions increases the airway's resistance to airflow.
3. Partial blockage of a large airway by a tumor decreases airway diameter and causes turbulent flow.

Spirometry has its limitations, however. It can measure only ventilated volumes. It cannot measure lung capacities that contain the residual volume. Measurements of TLC, FRC, and RV have diagnostic value in defining lung overdistension or restrictive pulmonary disease; the body plethysmograph can determine these absolute lung volumes.

7.7.2 Body Plethysmography

In a typical plethysmograph, the patient is put in an airtight enclosure and breathes through a pneumotach. The flow signal through the pneumotach is integrated and recorded as tidal breathing. At the end of a normal expiration (at FRC), an electronically operated shutter occludes the tube through which the patient is breathing. At this time the patient pants lightly against the occluded airway. Since there is no

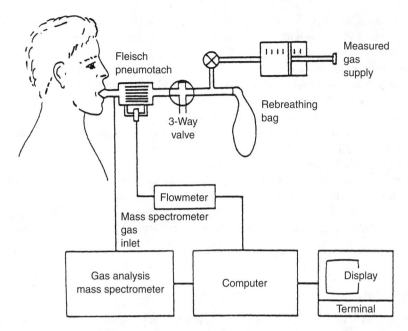

FIGURE 7.8 Typical system configuration for the measurement of rebreathing pulmonary diffusing capacity.

flow, pressure measured at the mouth must equal alveolar pressure. But movements of the chest that compress gas in the lung simultaneously rarify the air in the plethysmograph, and vice versa. The pressure change in the plethysmograph can be used to calculate the volume change in the plethysmograph, which is the same as the volume change in the chest. This leads directly to determination of FRC.

At the same time, alveolar pressure can be correlated to plethysmographic pressure. Therefore, when the shutter is again opened and flow rate is measured, airway resistance can be obtained as the ratio of alveolar pressure (obtainable from plethysmographic pressure) to flow rate [Carr and Brown, 1993]. Airway resistance is usually measured during panting, at a nominal lung volume of FRC and flow rate of ± 1 l/sec.

Airway resistance during inspiration is increased in patients with asthma, bronchitis, and upper respiratory tract infections. Expiratory resistance is elevated in patients with emphysema, since the causes of increased expiratory airway resistance are decreased driving pressures and the airway collapse. Airway resistance also may be used to determine the response of obstructed patients to bronchodilator medications.

7.7.3 Diffusing Capacity

So far the mechanical components of airflow through the lungs have been discussed. Another important parameter is the diffusing capacity of the lung, the rate at which oxygen or carbon dioxide travel from the alveoli to the blood (or vice versa for carbon dioxide) in the pulmonary capillaries. Diffusion of gas across a barrier is directly related to the surface area of the barrier and inversely related to the thickness. Also, diffusion is directly proportional to the solubility of the gas in the barrier material and inversely related to the molecular weight of the gas.

Lung diffusing capacity (Dl) is usually determined for carbon monoxide but can be related to oxygen diffusion. The popular method of measuring carbon monoxide diffusion utilizes a rebreathing technique in which the patient rebreathes rapidly in and out of a bag for approximately 30 sec. Figure 7.8 illustrates the test apparatus. The patient begins breathing from a bag containing a known volume of gas consisting of 0.3–0.5% carbon monoxide made with heavy oxygen, 0.3–0.5% acetylene, 5% helium, 21% oxygen, and a balance of nitrogen. As the patient rebreathes the gas mixture in the bag, a modified **mass spectrometer** continuously analyzes it during both inspiration and expiration. During this rebreathing procedure, the carbon monoxide disappears from the patient-bag system; the rate at which this occurs is a function of the lung diffusing capacity.

The helium is inert and insoluble in lung tissue and blood, and equilibrates quickly in unobstructed patients, indicating the dilution level of the test gas. Acetylene, on the other hand, is soluble in blood and is used to determine the blood flow through the pulmonary capillaries. Carbon monoxide is bound very tightly to hemoglobin and is used to obtain diffusing capacity at a constant pressure gradient across the alveolar-capillary membrane.

Decreased lung diffusing capacity can occur from the thickening of the alveolar membrane or the capillary membrane as well as the presence of interstitial fluid from edema. All these abnormalities increase the barrier thickness and cause a decrease in diffusing capacity. In addition, a characteristic of specific lung diseases is impaired lung diffusing capacity. For example, fibrotic lung tissue exhibits a decreased permeability to gas transfer, whereas pulmonary emphysema results in the loss of diffusion surface area.

Defining Terms

Alveoli: Respiratory airway terminals where most gas exchange with the pulmonary circulation takes place.
BTPS: Body temperature (37°C) and standard pressure (1 atm), saturated (6.28 kN/m^2).
Chemoreceptors: Neural receptors sensitive to chemicals such as gas partial pressures.
Dead space: The portion of the respiratory system that does not take part in gas exchange with the blood.
Diffusion: The process whereby a material moves from a region of higher concentration to a region of lower concentration.
Expiration: The breathing process whereby air is expelled from the mouth and nose. Also called exhalation.
Functional residual capacity: The lung volume at rest without breathing.
Inspiration: The breathing process whereby air is taken into the mouth and noise. Also called inhalation.
Mass spectrometer: A device that identifies relative concentrations of gases by means of mass-to-charge ratios of gas ions.
Mechanoreceptors: Neural receptors sensitive to mechanical inputs such as stretch, pressure, irritants, and so on.
Partial pressure: The pressure that a gas would exert if it were the only constituent.
Perfusion: Blood flow to the lungs.
Plethysmography: Any measuring technique that depends on a volume change.
Pleura: The membrane surrounding the lung.
Pneumotach: A measuring device for airflow.
Pulmonary circulation: Blood flow from the right cardiac ventricle that perfuses the lung and is in intimate contact with alveolar membranes for effective gas exchange.
STPD: Standard temperature (0°C) and pressure (1 atm), dry (moisture removed).
Ventilation: Airflow to the lungs.

References

Astrand, P.O. and Rodahl, K. 1970. *Textbook of Work Physiology.* New York, McGraw-Hill.
Carr, J.J. and Brown, J.M. 1993. *Introduction to Biomedical Equipment Technology.* Englewood Cliffs, NJ, Prentice-Hall.

Fredberg, J.J. and Stamenovic, D. 1989. On the imperfect elasticity of lung tissue. *J. Appl. Physiol.* 67: 2408–2419.

Hildebrandt, J. 1970. Pressure–volume data of cat lung interpreted by plastoelastic, linear viscoelastic model. *J. Appl. Physiol.* 28: 365–372.

Hornbein, T.F. (Ed.) 1981. *Regulation of Breathing.* New York, Marcel Dekker.

Johnson, A.T. 1991. *Biomechanics and Exercise Physiology.* New York, John Wiley & Sons.

Jones, N.L. 1984. Normal values for pulmonary gas exchange during exercise. *Am. Rev. Respir. Dis.* 129:544–546.

Kline, J. (Ed.) 1976. *Biologic Foundations of Biomedical Engineering.* Boston, Little, Brown.

Parker, J.F. Jr. and West, V.R. (Eds.) 1973. *Bioastronautics Data Book.* Washington, NASA.

Ruch, T.C. and Patton, H.D. (Eds.) 1966. *Physiology Biophysics.* Philadelphia, Saunders.

Stamenovic, D., Glass, G.M., Barnas, G.M., and Fredberg, J.J. 1990. Viscoplasticity of respiratory tissues. *J. Appl. Physiol.* 69: 973–988.

Suki, B. and Bates, J.H.T. 1991. A nonlinear viscoelastic model of lung tissue mechanics. *J. Appl. Physiol.* 71: 826–833.

Weibel, E.R. 1963. *Morphometry of the Human Lung.* New York, Academic Press.

West, J. 1962. Regional differences in gas exchange in the lung of erect man. *J. Appl. Physiol.* 17: 893–898.

West, J.B. (Ed.) 1977. *Bioengineering Aspects of the Lung.* New York, Marcel Dekker.

Further Reading

Fredberg, J.J., Jones, K.A., Nathan, A., Raboudi, S., Prakash, Y.S., Shore, S.A., Butler, J.P., and Sieck, G.C. 1996. Friction in airway smooth muscle: mechanism, latch, and implications in asthma. *J. Appl. Physiol.* 81: 2703–2712.

Hantos, Z., Daroczy, B., Csendes, T., Suki, B., and Nagy, S. 1990. Modeling of low-frequency pulmonary impedance in dogs. *J. Appl. Physiol.* 68: 849–860.

Hantos, Z., Daroczy, B., Suki, B., and Nagy, S. 1990. Low-frequency respiratory mechanical impedance in rats. *J. Appl. Physiol.* 63: 36–43.

Hantos, Z., Petak, F., Adamicza, A., Asztalos, T., Tolnai, J., and Fredberg, J.J. 1997. Mechanical impedance of the lung periphery. *J. Appl. Physiol.* 83: 1595–1601.

Maksym, G.N. and Bates, J.H.T. 1997. A distributed nonlinear model of lung tissue elasticity. *J. Appl. Physiol.* 82: 32–41.

Petak, F., Hall, G.L., and Sly, P.D. 1998. Repeated measurements of airway and parenchymal mechanics in rats by using low frequency oscillations. *J. Appl. Physiol.* 84: 1680–1686.

Thorpe, C.W. and Bates, J.H.T. 1997. Effect of stochastic heterogeneity on lung impedance during acute bronchoconstriction: a model analysis. *J. Appl. Physiol.* 82: 1616–1625.

Yuan, H., Ingenito, E.P., and Suki, B. 1997. Dynamic properties of lung parenchyma: mechanical contributions of fiber network and interstitial cells. *J. Appl. Physiol.* 83: 1420–1431.

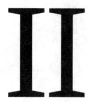

Physiological Modeling, Simulation, and Control

Joseph L. Palladino
Trinity College

THE COMPLEXITIES OF PHYSIOLOGICAL SYSTEMS often lead to the creation of new models to aid in the understanding of measured experimental data and to predict new features of the system under study. Models may serve to compactly summarize known system properties, including biomechanical, chemical, and electrical phenomena. Experiments performed on the model yield new information that casts light on unknown mechanisms underlying these properties and stimulate the formulation of new questions and the design of new experiments. Further, such quantitative description often leads to a better understanding of the physical mechanisms underlying both normal and altered (diseased) system performance. Ultimately, modeling may facilitate clinical diagnosis of system failure at an early stage of disease development.

Models begin conceptually; for example, the concept that a blood vessel behaves as a fluid-filled pipe. Concepts may be developed into physical models, for example, using a latex tube to describe a blood vessel, upon which experiments are performed. Often, concepts are realized as mathematical models, whereby the concept is described by physical laws, transformed into a set of mathematical equations, and solved via computer. Simulations, distinct from models, are descriptions that mimic the physiological system. The quantitative nature of physiological models allows them to be employed as components of systems for the study of physiological control, illustrated in several of this section's chapters.

Chapter 8 describes the iterative process of physiological modeling and presents three recent, widely different, modeling approaches in cardiovascular dynamics. The first is a compact model of the canine left ventricle. Its modular design permits application to study the greater human cardiovascular system, or the specific study of flow during closed chest CPR. Next, a large-scale, distributed muscle model shows how mechanical description of muscle structure can predict a molecular mechanism responsible for heart muscle's complex mechanical function, that is, structure predicts function. Finally, an approach for predicting ventricular hypertrophy based on cardiac function is presented, with function predicting structure.

Chapter 9 shows how compartmental models may be used to describe physiological systems, for example, pharmacokinetics. The production, distribution, transport, and interaction of exogenous materials, such as drugs or tracers, and endogenous materials, such as hormones, are described. Examples of both linear and nonlinear compartmental models are presented, as well as parameter estimation, optimal experiment design, and model validation.

Chapter 10 demonstrates the importance of cardiovascular modeling in designing closed-loop drug delivery systems, such as intravenous infusion pumps for pharmacological agents. The chapter begins with an extensive review of segmental and transmission line models of the arterial system and time-varying elastance descriptions of the left ventricle. The author makes an argument for employing nonlinear cardiovascular-linked pharmacological models to aid in controller design since data from these models can improve, and reduce the number of, animal and human experiments, and can be used to simulate human conditions not easily produced in animals.

Chapter 11 presents models used to study the continual interaction of the respiratory mechanical system and pulmonary gas exchange. Traditionally, the respiratory system is described as a chemostat — ventilation increases with increased chemical stimulation. Alternatively, the author proposes that quantitative description of the "respiratory central pattern generator," a network of neuronal clusters in the brain, is a much more sophisticated and realistic approach. Study of this dynamic, optimized controller of a nonlinear plant is interesting from both physiological and engineering perspectives, the latter due to applications of these techniques for new, intelligent control system design.

Chapter 12 introduces the use of neural network techniques and their application in modeling physiological control systems. As their name implies, neural networks are computational algorithms based upon the computational structure of the nervous system, and are characterized as distributed processing and adaptive. Neural networks have been used to describe the control of arm movements with electrical stimulation and the adaptive control of arterial blood pressure.

Chapter 13 surveys methods of system identification in physiology, the process of extracting models or model components from experimental data. Identification typically refers to model specification or model estimation, where unknown parameters are estimated within the specified model using experimental data and advanced computational techniques. Estimation may be either parametric, where algebraic or difference equations represent static or dynamic systems, or nonparametric, where analytical (convolution), computational (look-up tables), or graphical (phase-space) techniques characterize the system. This chapter closes with a recent hybrid modular approach.

Chapter 14 shows how modeling can propose mechanisms to explain experimentally observed oscillations in the cardiovascular system. A control system characterized by a slow and delayed change in resistance due to smooth muscle activity is presented. Experiments on this model show oscillations in the input impedance frequency spectrum, and flow and pressure transient responses to step inputs consistent with experimental observations. This autoregulation model supports the theory that low-frequency oscillations in heart rate and blood pressure variability spectra (Mayer waves) find their origin in the intrinsic delay of flow regulation.

Chapter 15 presents models to describe the control of human movement, primarily the dynamics of human extremities. Presented are the challenges associated with description of the extremities as rigid bodies using laws of mechanics such as D'Alembert's principle, the Newton–Euler method, and the LaGrange equations. Analytic limb models are presented first, described by sets of ordinary differential equations. Next, the complexities of limb movement control are described by nonanalytic models, for example an expert system denoted "artificial reflex control," learning algorithms and fuzzy logic. Finally, hybrid controller models combining analytic and nonanalytic techniques are discussed.

Chapter 16 describes physiological models of the fast eye movement, or saccade, that enables the eye to move quickly from one image to another. This common eye movement is encountered when scanning from the end of one line of printed text to the start of another. Early quantitative models helped define important characteristics of saccades. Increasingly complex models of the oculomotor plant were derived using improved models of the rectus eye muscle. Finally, application of system control theory and simulation methods led to a saccade generator model in close agreement with experimental data.

Chapter 17 adopts a comparative approach using biological scaling laws to compare the cardiovascular systems of different mammals. Allometry, the change of proportions with increase of size, and dimensional analysis is used to develop allometric relations for important cardiovascular parameters such as stroke volume, peripheral resistance, and heart efficiency. Optimal cardiovascular design is also discussed.

Chapter 18 presents a biomedical analysis of cardiopulmonary resuscitation. This work begins by characterizing open and closed chest techniques. The authors then review the broad range of adjuvant techniques, such as MAST augmented or impulse CPR. The chapter proposes a modeling based approach suggesting that CPR as a technique should reestablish cardiac valvular function to be effective.

8

Modeling Strategies and Cardiovascular Dynamics

Joseph L. Palladino
Trinity College

Gary M. Drzewiecki
Rutgers University

Abraham Noordergraaf
University of Pennsylvania

8.1 Introduction

A model, in the broad sense, is a representation of something, be it a physical or cerebral representation. In the sciences, models often begin as conceptual interpretations of experimental observations (Figure 8.1). Experimental observations (stage 1) lead to a qualitative concept (stage 2) and additional questions, which then require additional experiments (stage 3). At some point, sufficient knowledge is gained that quantitative representations, or models, arise (stage 4). Such models may take the form of physical models, for example, where a network of elastic tubes represent the arterial circulation. Commonly in medicine, the term model refers to an animal model, with the assumption that a particular animal's physiology is similar to that of a human.

This chapter focuses on mathematical models, where equations of motion are developed and solved to describe the physiological system of interest. In physics and chemistry, a multitude of experimental observations can be captured in a small number of concepts, often referred to as laws. A law is a statement of the relation between quantities, which, as far as is known, is invariable within a range of conditions. For example, Ohm's law expresses the ratio between the voltage difference across and the current through an object as a constant. In physiology, experimental observations can likewise be ordered by relating them to natural laws, if expanded with features peculiar to living beings, such as control phenomena,

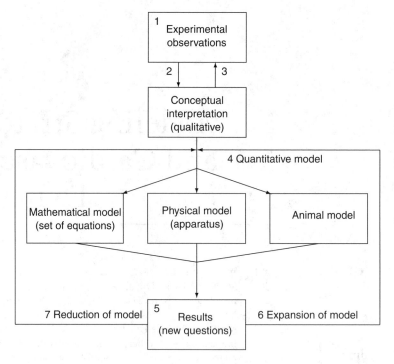

FIGURE 8.1   A schematic depicting the iterative inter-relationships between models and experiments. Stages 1 to 7 are described in the text.

especially homeostasis. The life sciences guide application of these natural laws. Common natural laws originally developed for inanimate materials must also be rewritten for living materials. In such complex systems, several laws may play their part, and the process is then referred to as development of a model. Model design, therefore, must meet stringent requirements and serves to rein in undisciplined speculation. Modeling attempts to identify the mechanism(s) responsible for experimental observations and is fundamentally distinct from simulation, in which anything that reproduces the experimental data is acceptable.

A successful mathematical model provides guidance to new experiments, which may modify or generalize the model, in turn suggesting additional new experiments. This iterative process is illustrated in Figure 8.1. The quest for understanding of a body of experimental observations leads to a tentative conceptual interpretation, which is transformed into quantitative statements by invoking established natural laws. The resulting mathematical model consists of a set of equations, which are solved, generally with the aid of a computer. The equation solutions (stage 5) are quantitative statements about experimental observations, some of which were not part of the original body of experiments, extending knowledge about the system under study. Consequently, new experiments become specified, adding to the store of experimental data. The enlarged body of experimental observations may cause modification in the investigator's conceptual interpretation, which in turn may give reason to modify the model. This iterative process should weed out flawed experiments and misconceptions in the mathematical model. If the entire effort is successful, a comprehensive, quantitative, and verified interpretation of the relevant experimental observations will result. Sometimes, the resulting model is expanded (stage 6) to incorporate new discoveries. Alternatively, the model may be systematically reduced (stage 7) to eliminate minor features, and is often then used as a building block for incorporation into a larger-scale system model. Model reduction is based on understanding, allowing intelligent separation of major and minor effects. Model simplification, on the other hand, implies arbitrary action based on intuition.

The iterative process in model building was described by Popper in 1959 [1]. He points out that no model is perfect, in fact, he proposes that models must exhibit "falsifiability." Clearly, models possess the inherent danger of refinement beyond which no new information is gained. Another potential pitfall is the balance between experiments and model development. Collecting experimental data without a framework of understanding, or postulating model results without experimental verification may be equally hazardous. Model refinement may continue until its complexity increases without any increase in knowledge. Kuhn takes this idea one step further, proposing that scientific developments sometimes stagnate until a "revolution" occurs [2]. One recent example is the study of wave transmission in blood vessels. For many years, investigators focused on description of a single tube, with limited results. It was only when the novel approach of including arterial branching arose that a wide range of previously unexplained experimental observations could be understood [3,4]. For example, experiments showed that the arterial flow pulse decreases moving away from the heart, as expected for a passive network. The arterial pressure pulse, however, increases, seemingly in violation of energy conservation. This paradox was explained via wave reflection in the new (revolutionary) branching model.

The first case study of this chapter outlines the development of a model of left ventricular pumping. The model is devised from canine experiments and represents the left ventricle as a time, volume, and outflow-dependent pressure generator. In the course of model development, a new analytical method of measuring ventricular elastance emerges, with the potential of clarifying issues with previous elastance measurements. One application is a slight model expansion to study the cardiac pump theory of cardiopulmonary resuscitation (CPR).

A major challenge in the biosciences today is integration of a large body of molecular level information, with the ultimate goal of understanding organ function. Two different, novel modeling approaches to this goal are next presented. The first shows how a model based on muscle structure can predict a molecular mechanism responsible for muscle's mechanical properties (function). The second presents an approach for predicting ventricular hypertrophy (structure) based on cardiac metabolic function. Due to space constraints, discussion is limited to the main points; however, details are available in the original research papers cited.

8.2 Modeling Heart Dynamics

8.2.1 Introduction

Mechanical performance of the heart, more specifically the left ventricle, is typically characterized by estimates of ventricular elastance. The heart is an elastic bag that stiffens and relaxes with each heartbeat. Elastance is a measure of stiffness, classically defined as the differential relation between pressure and volume:

$$E_v = \frac{dp_v}{dV_v} \tag{8.1}$$

Here, p_v and V_v denote ventricular pressure and volume, respectively. For any instant in time, ventricular elastance E_v is the differential change in pressure with respect to volume. Mathematically, this relation is clear. Measurement of E_v is much less clear.

Equation 8.1 was estimated using the ratio of finite changes in ventricular pressure and volume [5]:

$$E_v = \frac{\Delta p_v}{\Delta V_v} \tag{8.2}$$

This approach leads to physically impossible results. For example, before the aortic valve opens, the left ventricle is generating increasing pressure while there is not yet any change in volume. The ratio in Equation 8.2 gives an infinite elastance when the denominator is zero. Integration of Equation 8.1 leads

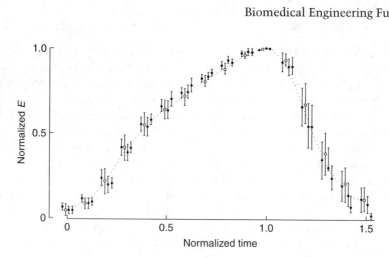

FIGURE 8.2 Time-varying ventricular elastance curves measured using the definition in Equation 8.3. Measured elastance curves are distinctive in shape. (Adapted from Suga, H. and Sagawa, K. 1974. Instantaneous pressure–volume relationship under various end-diastolic volume. *Circ. Res.* 35: 117–126.)

to time-varying elastance definitions of the form

$$E_v(t) = \frac{p_v(t)}{V_v(t) - V_d} \tag{8.3}$$

an equation with extensive application [6,7]. In this equation, V_d is a dead volume that remains constant. Now all other terms are allowed to be varying with time. Ventricular elastance measured in this way leads to elastance curves as depicted in Figure 8.2. These curves show wide variation, as suggested by the large error bars. The distinctive asymmetric shape leads to a puzzle. Equation 8.3 shows that under isovolumic conditions ventricular pressure p_v must have the same shape as elastance $E_v(t)$. However, experiments show that isovolumic pressure curves are symmetric, unlike Figure 8.2. A further complication is the requirement of ejecting beats for measuring $E_v(t)$, which requires not only the heart but also a circulation. Ventricular pressure is a strong function of both volume contained and time

$$p_v = p_v(V_v, t) \tag{8.4}$$

Hence, an incremental change in pressure requires

$$\Delta p_v = \frac{\partial p_v}{\partial V_v} \Delta V_v + \frac{\partial p_v}{\partial t} \Delta t \tag{8.5}$$

which leads to

$$\frac{\Delta p_v}{\Delta V_v} = \frac{\partial p_v}{\partial V_v} + \frac{\partial p_v}{\partial t} \frac{\Delta t}{\Delta V_v} \tag{8.6}$$

$\Delta t / \Delta V_v$ in the second term of the right-hand side is equal to $-1/Q_v$, inverse ejection outflow. Consequently, elastance definitions such as Equation 8.2 and Equation 8.3 are not measures purely of ventricular elastance but also include arterial effects. This may explain why such models have difficulty in accurately predicting flow [8]. Consequently, a new measure of the heart's mechanical properties was developed.

8.2.2 Left Ventricular Dynamics

A new ventricle model was developed using isolated canine heart experiments [10,11]. Experiments began with measurement of isovolumic ventricular pressure [10]. For each experiment, the isolated left ventricle was filled with an initial volume (end-diastolic) and the aorta was clamped to prevent outflow of blood. The ventricle was stimulated and the generated ventricular pressure was measured and recorded. The ventricle was then filled to a new end-diastolic volume and the experiment repeated. As in the famous experiments of Otto Frank [12], isovolumic pressure is directly related to filling.

These isovolumic pressure curves were then described by the following equation. Ventricular pressure p_v is a function of time t and ventricular volume V_v according to

$$p_v = a(V_v - b)^2 + (cV_v - d)\left[\frac{(1 - e^{-(t/\tau_c)^\alpha})e^{-((t-t_b)/\tau_r)^\alpha}}{(1 - e^{-(t_p/\tau_c)^\alpha})e^{-((t_p-t_b)/\tau_r)^\alpha}} \right] \tag{8.7}$$

or written more compactly,

$$p_v(t, V_v) = a(V_v - b)^2 + (cV_v - d)f(t) \tag{8.8}$$

where $f(t)$ is the activation function in square brackets in Equation 8.7. The function $f(t)$ describes the time course of active force generation, a product of contraction and relaxation exponentials related to myofilament crossbridge bond formation and detachment, respectively, and is given by

$$f(t) = \begin{cases} \dfrac{(1 - e^{-(t/\tau_c)^\alpha})}{(1 - e^{-(t_p/\tau_c)^\alpha})e^{-((t_p-t_b)/\tau_r)^\alpha}}, & 0 \le t \le t_b \\[3ex] \dfrac{(1 - e^{-(t/\tau_c)^\alpha})e^{-((t-t_b)/\tau_r)^\alpha}}{(1 - e^{-(t_p/\tau_c)^\alpha})e^{-((t_p-t_b)/\tau_r)^\alpha}}, & t_b < t < 1 \end{cases} \tag{8.9}$$

t_b is derived from α, τ_c, τ_r, and t_p [11]. The constants a, b, c, d, t_p, τ_c, τ_r, and α were experimentally derived. Figure 8.3 shows a set of isovolumic pressure curves computed for a normal canine left ventricle.

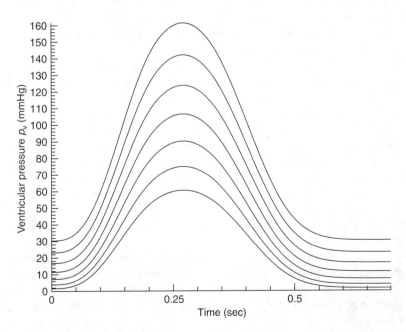

FIGURE 8.3 Isovolumic canine ventricular pressure curves described by Equation 8.8. Initial volumes range from 25 to 50 ml.

TABLE 8.1 Ventricle Model Quantities
Measured from Animal Experiments and Adapted
for the Human Analytical Model

Constant	Canine (measured)	Human (adapted)
a	0.003 (mmHg/ml^2)	0.0007
b	1.0 (ml)	20.0
c	3.0 (mmHg/ml)	2.5
d	20.0 (mmHg)	80.0
τ_c	0.164 (sec)	0.264
t_p	0.271 (sec)	0.371
τ_r	0.199 (sec)	0.299
t_b	0.233 (sec)	0.258
α	2.88	2.88

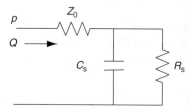

FIGURE 8.4   Equivalent systemic arterial load. Circuit elements are described in the text.

Equation 8.8 depicts the ventricle as a time- and volume-dependent pressure generator. The term to the left of the plus sign (including constants a and b) describes the ventricle's passive elastic properties. a is a measure of diastolic ventricular elastance. b corresponds to diastolic volume at zero pressure. The term to the right (including c and d) describes its active elastic properties, arising from the active generation of force in the underlying heart muscle. c and d are directly related to volume-dependent and -independent components of actively developed pressure, respectively. Representative model quantities derived from canine experiments are given in Table 8.1. This model was adapted to describe the human left ventricle using quantities in the right-hand column [11].

The most widely used arterial load is the three-element modified windkessel shown in Figure 8.4. The model appears as an electrical circuit due to its origin prior to the advent of the digital computer. Z_0 is the characteristic impedance of the aorta, in essence the aorta's flow resistance. C_s is transverse arterial compliance and describes the stretch of the arterial system in the radial direction. R_s is the peripheral resistance, describing the systemic arteries' flow resistance downstream of the aorta. The left ventricle model was coupled to this reduced arterial load model and allowed to eject blood. Model parameter values for a normal arterial load are given in Table 8.2. Figure 8.5 shows results for a normal canine left ventricle ejecting into a normal arterial system. The solid curves (left ordinate) describe ventricular pressure p_v and root aortic pressure as functions of time. Root arterial pulse pressure is about 120/65 mmHg. The dashed curve (right ordinate) shows ventricular outflow. The ventricle was filled with an end-diastolic volume of 45 ml and it ejected 30 ml (stroke volume), giving an ejection fraction of 66%, which is about normal for this size animal.

The same ventricle may be coupled to a pathological arterial system, for example, one with doubled peripheral resistance R_s. As expected, increased peripheral resistance raises arterial pulse pressure (to 140/95 mmHg) and impedes the ventricle's ability to eject blood (Figure 8.6). The ejection fraction decreases to 50% in this experiment. Other experiments, such as altered arterial stiffness, may be performed. The model's flexibility allows description of heart pathology as well as changes in blood vessels. This one equation (Equation 8.8) with one set of measured parameters is able to describe the wide range of hemodynamics observed experimentally [11].

TABLE 8.2 Representative Systemic Arterial Model
Element Values

Model element	Symbol	Control value
Characteristic aorta impedance	Z_0	0.1 mmHg sec/ml
Systemic arterial compliance	C_S	1.5 ml/mmHg
Peripheral arterial resistance	R_S	1.0 mmHg sec/ml

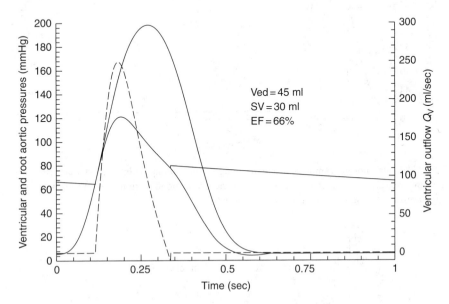

FIGURE 8.5 Ventricular and root aortic pressures (solid curves, left ordinate) and ventricular outflow (dashed curve, right ordinate) computed using the model of Equation 8.8 for a normal canine left ventricle pumping into a normal arterial circulation. The topmost solid curve corresponds to a clamped aorta (isovolumic). This ventricle has initial volume of 45 ml and pumps out 30 ml, for an ejection fraction of 66%, about normal.

Since ventricular pressure is now defined as an analytical function (Equation 8.7), ventricular elastance, E_v, defined in the classical sense as $\partial p_v / \partial V_v$, may be calculated as

$$E_v(t, V_v) = 2a(V_v - b) + c\left[\frac{(1 - e^{-(t/\tau_c)^\alpha})e^{-((t - t_b)/\tau_r)^\alpha}}{(1 - e^{-(t_p/\tau_c)^\alpha})e^{-((t_p - t_b)/\tau_r)^\alpha}} \right] \tag{8.10}$$

or

$$E_v(t, V_v) = 2a(V_v - b) + cf(t) \tag{8.11}$$

Figure 8.7 shows ventricular elastance curves computed using Equation 8.10. Elastance was computed for a wide range of ventricular and arterial states, including normal and pathological ventricles, normal and pathological arterial systems, and isovolumic and ejecting beats. These elastance curves are relatively invariant and cluster in two groups — either a normal or a weakened ventricle contractile state. Consequently, this new measure of elastance may now effectively assess the health of the heart alone, separate from blood vessel pathology.

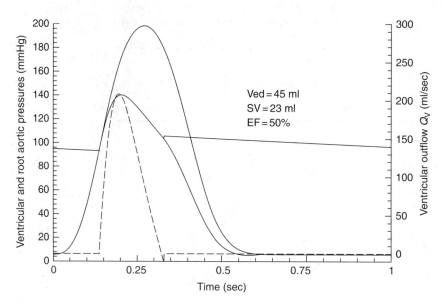

FIGURE 8.6 The same normal canine ventricle of Figure 8.5 now pumping into an arterial system with doubled peripheral (flow) resistance. As expected, increased resistance, corresponding to narrowed vessels, leads to increased arterial pulse pressure. Ejection fraction is reduced from 66 to 50%.

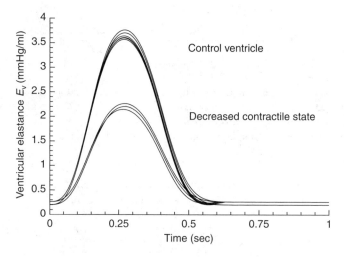

FIGURE 8.7 Ventricular elastance curves computed using the new analytical function of Equation 8.10. Elastance curves computed in this way are representative of the ventricle's contractile state.

8.2.3 The Ejection Effect

Experiments show that when the left ventricle ejects blood, ventricular pressure is somewhat different than expected. As depicted in Figure 8.8, early during ejection the ventricle generates less pressure than expected, denoted pressure *deactivation*. Later in systole the heart generates greater pressure, denoted *hyperactivation*. These two variations with flow have been termed the *ejection effect* [13]. The ejection effect was incorporated into Equation 8.8 by adding a flow-dependent term:

$$p_v(t, V_v, Q_v) = a(V_v - b)^2 + (cV_v - d)F(t, Q_v) \qquad (8.12)$$

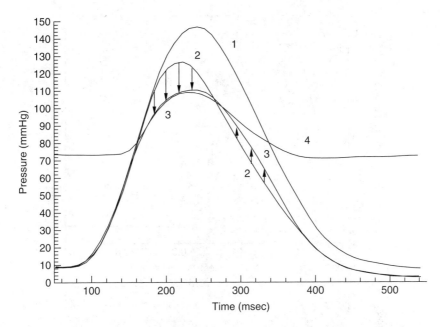

FIGURE 8.8 The ejection effect, showing that early during blood ejection (systole) the heart generates somewhat less pressure than expected, denoted *deactivation* (down arrows). Later in systole, the heart generates greater pressure, denoted *hyperactivation*. Curves 1 and 2 are ventricular pressures for initial and ejected volumes, respectively. Curve 3 is the measured ejecting pressure curve. Curve 4 is root aortic pressure.

with F replacing the time function f in Equation 8.8:

$$F(t, Q_v) = f(t) - k_1 Q_v(t) + k_2 Q_v^2(t - \tau), \quad \tau = \kappa t \quad\quad (8.13)$$

and k_1, k_2, and κ are additional model constants. The ventricle is now depicted as a time-, volume- and flow-dependent pressure generator. Figure 8.9 shows computed pressures and flows for this formulation (top), compared to the results minus the ejection effect (below). The ejection effect tends to change the shape of both pressure and flow curves to more closely resemble experimental curves.

Addition of the ejection effect modifies the computed ventricular elastance curves, as depicted in Figure 8.10. All curves are computed using the new function of Equation 8.10. The dashed curve, minus the ejection effect, is symmetric, as in Figure 8.7. Addition of the ejection effect (solid) makes ventricular elastance asymmetrically skewed to the right, much like the measured curves depicted in Figure 8.2 using the time-varying elastance definition of Equation 8.3. As expected, the mechanical process of ejecting blood has a direct effect on the heart's elastance.

The left ventricle model of Equation 8.8 was used to describe each of the four chambers of the human heart, depicted in Figure 8.11 [14]. This complete model of the circulatory system displays a broad range of cardiovascular physiology with a small set of equations and parameters. Figure 8.12 shows computed left and right ventricle work loops for a normal heart ejecting into a normal (control) circulatory system, depicted by solid curves. Figure 8.12 also shows the same two work loops for a weakened left ventricle (dashed curves). As expected, the left ventricle work loop is diminished in size. This work loop also shifts to the right on the volume axis. Since the weaker ventricle ejects less blood, more remains to fill the heart more for the subsequent beat (EDV of 194 instead of 122 ml). This increased filling partially compensates for the weakened ventricle via Starling's law.

Changing only one model constant, c, in Equation 8.8 is sufficient to vary chamber contractile state. For example, Table 8.3 shows examples of congestive heart failure, resulting from decreases in c for the left ventricle and for the right ventricle. Decreasing left ventricular contractile state to one third of the control

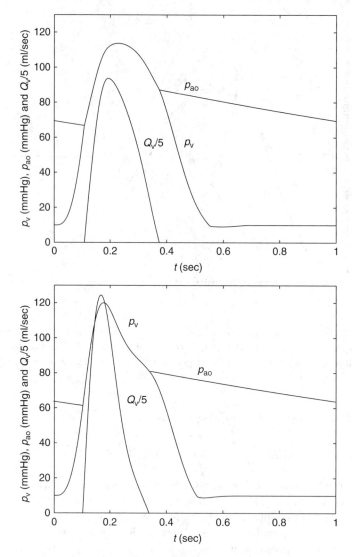

FIGURE 8.9 The ejection effect incorporated in the ventricle model (top) with the uncorrected ventricular pressure and outflow curves for the same conditions (below) for comparison. Ventricular outflow Q_v is normalized by 1/5 to use the same numeric scale as for ventricular pressure.

value ($c = 1.0$) lowers left ventricular ejection fraction from 53 to 25%, and root aortic pulse pressure decreases from 133/70 to 93/52 mmHg. Left ventricular stroke volume decreases less, from 64 to 48 ml, since it is compensated by the increased left end-diastolic volume (194 ml) via Starling's law. Decreasing left ventricular contractile state produces left congestive heart failure. Consequently, pulmonary venous volume increases from 1347 to 1981 ml (not shown), indicating pulmonary congestion for this case.

Similar changes are noted when the right ventricle's contractile state is halved ($c = 0.5$). The right ventricular ejection fraction drops from 46 to 24%, root pulmonary artery pulse pressure decreases from 49/15 to 29/12 mmHg, and right stroke volume decreases from 64 to 44 ml, with an increased end-diastolic volume of 164 ml, from 141 ml. Conversely, c can be increased in any heart chamber to depict administration of an inotropic drug. Although not plotted, pressures, flows, and volumes are available at any circuit site, all as functions of time.

Changes in blood vessel properties may be studied alone or in combination with altered heart properties. Other system parameters such as atrial performance, as well as other experiments, may be examined. The

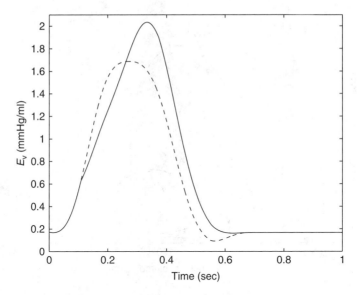

FIGURE 8.10 Ventricular elastance curves computed using Equation 8.10 without (dashed) and with the ejection effect (solid).

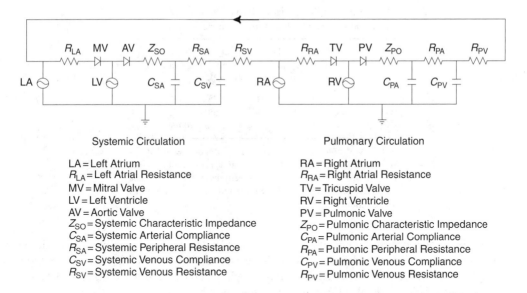

Systemic Circulation

LA = Left Atrium
R_{LA} = Left Atrial Resistance
MV = Mitral Valve
LV = Left Ventricle
AV = Aortic Valve
Z_{SO} = Systemic Characteristic Impedance
C_{SA} = Systemic Arterial Compliance
R_{SA} = Systemic Peripheral Resistance
C_{SV} = Systemic Venous Compliance
R_{SV} = Systemic Venous Resistance

Pulmonary Circulation

RA = Right Atrium
R_{RA} = Right Atrial Resistance
TV = Tricuspid Valve
RV = Right Ventricle
PV = Pulmonic Valve
Z_{PO} = Pulmonic Characteristic Impedance
C_{PA} = Pulmonic Arterial Compliance
R_{PA} = Pulmonic Peripheral Resistance
C_{PV} = Pulmonic Venous Compliance
R_{PV} = Pulmonic Venous Resistance

FIGURE 8.11 Application of the canine left ventricle model to hemodynamic description of the complete human cardiovascular system. (Adapted from Palladino, J.L., Ribeiro, L.C., and Noordergraaf, A., 2000. IOS Press, Amsterdam, pp. 29–39.)

modular form of this model allows its expansion for more detailed studies of particular sites in the circulatory system.

8.2.4 Predictive Power: Application to CPR

The left ventricle may be described as a time-, volume- and flow-dependent pressure generator. A small number of experimentally derived parameters is sufficient to describe the wide range of observed cardiovascular dynamics. This approach links experiment and theory, leading to new ideas and experiments.

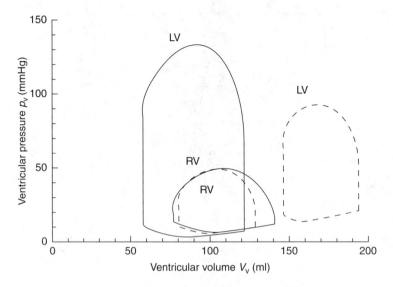

FIGURE 8.12 Computed work loops for the left and right ventricles under control conditions (solid curves) and for the case of a weakened left ventricle (dashed curves).

TABLE 8.3 Cardiovascular Performance for a Normal Heart, and Weakened Left and Right Ventricles

	SV (ml)		EDV (ml)		EF (%)		p_{AO}	p_{PU}
	LV	RV	LV	RV	LV	RV	(mmHg)	
Control	64	64	122	141	53	46	133/70	49/15
Weak LV	48	48	194	129	25	38	93/52	49/21
Weak RV	44	44	102	164	49	24	109/59	29/12

Note: SV denotes stroke volume, EDV denotes end-diastolic volume, EF is ejection fraction and p_{AO} and p_{PU} are root aorta and root pulmonary artery pressures, respectively, for the left (LV) and right (RV) ventricles. Note that SV left and right are equal under all conditions.

This ventricle model permits computation of ventricular elastance, and may resolve difficulties with previous time-varying elastance definitions. Work is currently underway to devise a new measure of cardiovascular health using this model. In essence, it is thought that the magnitude of the observed ejection effect for a particular heart should be directly related to its health.

The ventricle model of Equation 8.12 was expanded to study closed-chest CPR [15]. The left ventricle was filled by a constant pressure source, and was coupled to the three-element modified windkessel arterial load, with mitral and aortic valves. Equation 8.12 includes a new term, $p_e(t)$, the external pressure applied directly to the ventricle during asystole and application of CPR:

$$p_v(V_v, t, Q_v) - p_e(t) = a(V_v - b)^2 + (cV_v - d)F(t, Q_v) \qquad (8.14)$$

The main results of this predictive study are twofold. First, the normal circulation, including the mitral and aortic valves, can effectively circulate blood (with a reduced stroke volume) via external compression. This result supports the cardiac pump theory proposed by Kouwenhoven et al. [16]. Second, if the valves are removed or made incompetent no significant net flow is circulated, for either the normally beating ventricle, or the asystolic ventricle subjected to external compressions. The small (8 ml/sec) net outflow observed in both cases results from the venous pressure contributed by the constant pressure filling source. Sloshing of blood (large net backflow) is evident with each beat. As a result, net downstream circulation is ineffective [15].

8.3 Modeling Muscle Dynamics

8.3.1 Introduction

Description of muscle contraction has essentially evolved into two separate approaches — lumped whole muscle models and specialized crossbridge models of the sarcomere. The former seek to interpret muscle's complex mechanical properties with a single set of model elements. Muscle experiments measure muscle force and length subjected to isometric (fixed length) conditions, isotonic (fixed load) conditions, and transient analysis where either length or load is rapidly changed.

Muscle force generation is believed to arise from the formation of crossbridge bonds between thick and thin myofilaments within the basic building block of muscle, the sarcomere. These structures, in the nanometer to micrometer range, must be viewed by electron microscopy or x-ray diffraction, limiting study to fixed, dead material. Consequently, muscle contraction at the sarcomere level must be described by models that integrate metabolic and structural information.

Mayow [17] proposed that muscle contraction arises from changes in its constituent elastic fibers as a by-product of respiration, introducing the concept of muscle as an elastic material that changes due to metabolic processes. Weber [18] viewed muscle as an elastic material, or spring, whose stiffness depends on whether it is in a passive or active state. In 1890, Chauveau and Laulanié [19,20] also considered muscle as an elastic spring with time-dependent stiffness, and proposed that velocity of shortening plays a role in force production. Fick [21] and Blix [22] refuted a purely elastic description on thermodynamic grounds, finding that potential energy stored during stretching a strip of muscle was less than the sum of energy released during shortening as work and heat. Blix also noticed that at the same muscle length, muscle tension produced during stretch was greater than that during release. Tension would be the same during stretch and release for a simple spring. Further, Blix reported that he was unable to describe stress relaxation and creep in muscle with a viscoelastic model.

Hill [23] coupled the spring with a viscous medium, thereby reintroducing viscoelastic muscle models, after noticing that external work done accelerating an inertial load was inversely related to shortening velocity. A two-element viscoelastic model is objectionable on mechanical grounds: in series (Maxwell body), length is unbounded for a step change in force; in parallel (Voight body), force is infinite for a step change in length. Further, Fenn [24] reported that energy released by the muscle differs for isometric or shortening muscle. Subsequently, Hill [25] developed the *contractile element*, embodied as an empirical hyperbolic relation between muscle force and shortening velocity. The contractile element was combined with two standard springs, denoted the parallel and series elastic elements. Current whole muscle models have, in general, incorporated Hill's contractile element, an empirically derived black-box force generator, in networks of traditional springs and dashpots [26]. Since model elements are not directly correlated to muscle structure, there is no logical reason to stop at three elements — models with at least nine have been proposed [27].

This approach can be criticized on the following grounds: there exists little, if any, correlation between model elements and muscle anatomical structures. No single model has been shown to comprehensively describe different muscle-loading conditions, for example, isometric, isotonic, and so on. Models tend to focus on description of a single type of experiment, and are typically based on a force–velocity relation measured under specific loading conditions. These models give little or no insight into the mechanism of contraction at the sarcomere level. Energy considerations, including the fundamental necessity of a biochemical energy source, have been ignored.

Crossbridge models focus on mechanics at the sarcomere level. Prior to actual observation of cross-bridge bonds, Huxley [28] proposed a model whereby contractile force is generated by the formation of crossbridge bonds between myofilaments. This model was subsequently shown unable to describe muscle's transient mechanical properties. Extension of Huxley's ideas to multiple-state crossbridges has been very limited in scope, for example, the Huxley and Simmons [29] two-state model does not include crossbridge attachment, detachment or filament sliding, but rather describes only the mechanics of a single set of overlapping actin and myosin filaments. In general, crossbridge models dictate bond attachment and detachment by probability or rate functions. This approach has shifted emphasis away from muscle mechanics toward increasingly complex rate functions [30].

8.3.2 Distributed Muscle Model

A large-scale, distributed muscle model was developed based on ultrastructural kinetics and possessing direct anatomic and physiologic relevance [31]. This model describes all of muscle's fundamental mechanical properties with a single set of assumptions: isometric and isotonic contractions and force transients resulting from rapid changes in muscle length during contraction. Variations in muscle properties with current loading conditions arise from the dynamic model structure, rather than adaptation of a particular force–velocity curve to describe the contractile element, or of a particular bond attachment or detachment function as for previous models. The following assumptions define the model:

- The sarcomere consists of overlapping thick and thin filaments connected by crossbridge bonds, which form during activation and detach during relaxation.
- The mass of the myofilaments is taken into account.
- Crossbridge bonds have viscoelastic properties [29] and thus may exhibit stress relaxation and creep.
- In passive muscle, thick filaments exist in stable suspension at the center of the sarcomere, which contributes to the muscle's passive elastic properties [32].
- Calcium ions serve as a trigger, which allows bond formation between filaments. Bonds formed are stretched via biochemical energy, thereby converting chemical to potential energy and developing force. This stretching results from crossbridge motion [29].
- The number of bonds formed depends upon the degree of thick–thin filament overlap [33].
- Asynchrony in bond formation and unequal numbers of bonds formed in each half sarcomere, as well as mechanical disturbances such as shortening and imposed length transients, cause movement of thick with respect to thin filaments. Since myofilament masses are taken into account these movements take the form of damped vibrations. Such vibrations occur with a spectrum of frequencies due to the distributed system properties.
- When the stress in a bond goes to zero the bond detaches [29].
- Myofilament motion and bond stress relaxation lead to bond detachment and therefore produce relaxation.

Crossbridge bonds are described as linear viscoelastic material, each represented by a three-element spring-dashpot model (Figure 8.13). During activation, the attached crossbridge head rotates, stretching the bond and generating force. A passive sarcomere is mechanically represented as myofilament masses interconnected by a matrix of permanently attached passive viscoelastic bonds. During activation, dynamically attached active bonds are formed as calcium ion and energy (ATP) allows.

The sarcomere model is extended to a muscle fiber by taking N sarcomeres in series each with M parallel pairs of active bonds. The model currently consists of 50 series sarcomeres, each with 50 parallel pairs of crossbridges. Bond formation is taken to be distributed in two dimensions due to muscle's finite electrical propagation speed and the finite diffusion rate of calcium ions from the sarcoplasmic reticulum. The large set of resulting differential equations (5300) is solved by digital computer. Since the instantaneous number of crossbridge bonds, and therefore the model system equations, is continuously changing, the resulting model is strongly nonlinear and time-varying, despite its construction from linear, time-invariant components. Crossbridge bonds are added in a raster pattern due to the distributed system properties. After all bonds have been added, no further conditions are imposed. Crossbridge bonds subsequently

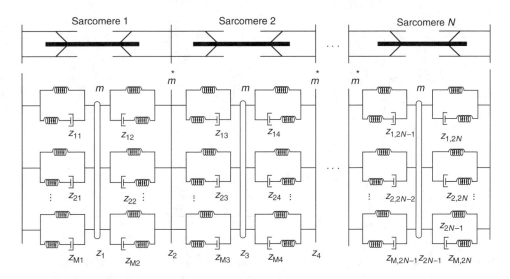

FIGURE 8.13 Schematic representation of a muscle fiber composed of N series sarcomeres each with M parallel pairs of active, viscoelastic bonds. Each bond is described by a three-element viscoelastic model. (Adapted from Palladino, J.L. and Noordergraaf, A. 1998. Springer-Verlag, New York, pp. 33–57.)

detach simply from the small internal movements of myofilaments. Consequently, the model relaxes without separate assumptions.

This model was subjected to a wide range of loading conditions. A single set of model parameters is sufficient to describe the main features of isometric, isotonic, and quick release and stretch experiments. The model is sensitive to mechanical disturbances, consistent with experimental evidence from muscle force curves [34], aequorin measurements of free calcium ion [35], and high-speed x-ray diffraction studies [36]. The model is also consistent with sarcomere length feedback studies [29] where reduced internal motion delays relaxation.

The outermost curve of Figure 8.14 depicts an isometric contraction computed from the muscle fiber model. At each Δt available bonds are attached, adding their equations to the model, and force is generated via bond stretching. For the twitch contractions in Figure 8.14 and Figure 8.15, bonds are attached from $t = 0$ to 0.5 sec. Since bond formation is not perfectly symmetrical, due to the raster attachment pattern, small force imbalances within thick–thin units develop, leading to small myofilament motions that tend to detach bonds as their force goes to zero. Consequently, at each Δt of solution, bonds are added during activation and detach continuously. Despite this very dynamic state, Figure 8.14 shows that the net isometric fiber force generated smoothly rises during muscle activation. Peak isometric force of 250 nN is in close agreement with recent experimental measurements on isolated guinea pig myocytes [34].

The time of peak force corresponds to the end of bond attachment. Physiologically, this point is associated with a lack of available bond attachment sites. This may be due to lack of calcium ion for the release of steric inhibition of actin–myosin interaction by troponin/tropomyosin, lack of myosin heads in a state necessary for attachment, or some other mechanism. Force relaxation then results simply from bond detachment due to the same internal myofilament motion mechanism. Net force smoothly recovers to the resting force level, in contrast to the dynamic motions of individual bonds and myofilaments. Surprisingly, this smooth relaxation occurs without the added feature of crossbridge recycling, that is, bond reattachment after detachment.

Transient response to quick length change is a critical test of any muscle model. This distributed model predicts that rapid length changes enhance system vibration and thereby promote bond detachment and muscle relaxation, underlying muscle's force deactivation phenomenon. Figure 8.14 also shows force deactivation following quick release during an otherwise isometric twitch contraction. This particular release corresponds to 0.2% of sarcomere length over 10 msec. Quick release corresponding to 2% of

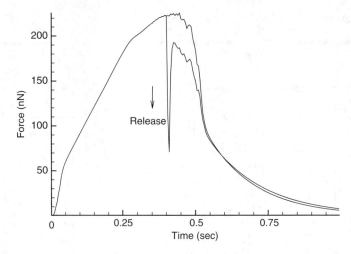

FIGURE 8.14 Outermost curve describes an isometric contraction computed from the distributed muscle fiber model. Also plotted is force computed during a quick release experiment, showing significant force deactivation. (Adapted from Palladino, J.L. and Noordergraaf, A. 1998. Springer-Verlag, New York, pp. 33–57.)

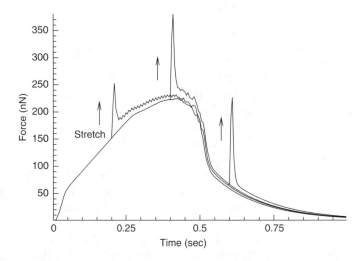

FIGURE 8.15 Quick stretches computed from the distributed muscle fiber model. (Adapted from Palladino, J.L. and Noordergraaf, A. 1998. Springer-Verlag, New York, pp. 33–57.)

sarcomere length applied during 10 msec was sufficient to bring fiber force to zero (not shown). Slower releases produce less force deactivation. These curves compare favorably with quick release transients measured on whole muscle strips and more recent experiments on isolated frog myocytes [37,38], and for ferret papillary muscles [39].

Figure 8.15 shows quick stretches computed for the distributed fiber model. Stretches corresponding to 0.2% of sarcomere length were performed over 10 msec. Curves show rapid force overshoot, followed by rapid recovery and slow recovery back to the isometric force levels. Quick stretch response is in agreement with classic studies on muscle strip and recent studies on ferret papillary muscles [39].

8.3.3 Reduced Muscle Model

The large-scale distributed muscle model can be reduced to a compact model analogous to the ventricle model previously presented (Equation 8.8). Muscle fibers (cells), or strips, can be described as force

TABLE 8.4 Model
Constant Values and Units

Constant	Value	Unit
a	2	mN/mm^2
b	8	mm
c	20	mN/mm
d	160	mN
τ_c	0.264	sec
τ_r	0.299	sec
t_p	0.371	sec
t_b	0.258	sec
α	2.88	—

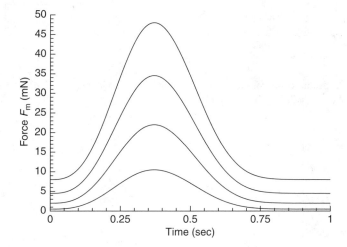

FIGURE 8.16 Isometric contractions for muscle strip computed from Equation 8.15 for different initial muscle lengths $l_m = 8.5, 9.0, 9.5$, and 10.0 mm (topmost).

generators that are time, muscle length, and velocity of shortening dependent:

$$f_m(t, \ell_m) = a(\ell_m - b)^2 + (c\ell_m - d)f(t) \tag{8.15}$$

where f_m is muscle force and ℓ_m is muscle length. The model parameters a, b, c, and d are determined from muscle strip experiments, as is the activation function $f(t)$. $f(t)$ has the same form as in Equation 8.9. Model constant values are presented in Table 8.4. t_b is derived from α, τ_c, τ_r, and t_p [40]. Muscle elastance, E_m, may now be defined as $\partial f_m / \partial l_m$. This muscle strip model was subjected to a wide range of loading conditions.

Figure 8.16 shows isometric force curves computed from the muscle model for initial muscle lengths $l_m = 8.5$ to 10.0 mm. The curve shapes and magnitudes compare favorably with experimental curves in the literature, for example [41].

Figure 8.17 shows computed isotonic contractions for different fixed loads. Although not shown, this muscle model exhibits an inverse relation between isotonic load and amount of shortening, and a direct relation between initial length and shortening (Starling's law). Results are also consistent with experiments, for example [42].

Figure 8.18 shows computed initial muscle shortening velocity plotted as a function of isotonic load, which resembles Hill's hyperbolic force–length relation for tetanized skeletal muscle. This curve closely resembles the experimental $F - v$ curves of Brady from cardiac twitch contractions [43].

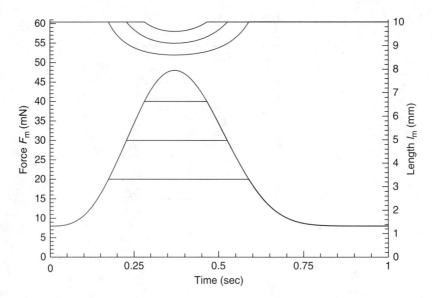

FIGURE 8.17   Isotonic contractions for muscle strip computed from Equation 8.15 for three intermediate and one isometric load. Top shows muscle length (right y-axis).

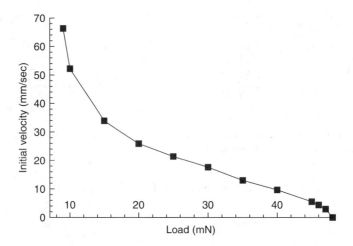

FIGURE 8.18   Initial muscle shortening velocity computed as a function of isotonic load.

Muscle force transients arising from rapid (but small) changes in muscle length during otherwise isometric contractions may be described by expanding the model as the ventricle model was expanded to incorporate the ejection effect:

$$f_{\mathrm{m}}(t, \ell_{\mathrm{m}}, v_{\mathrm{m}}) = a(\ell_{\mathrm{m}} - b)^2 + (c\ell_{\mathrm{m}} - d)F(t, v_{\mathrm{m}}) \tag{8.16}$$

with muscle velocity of lengthening or shortening, v_{m}, and F replacing the time function f in Equation 8.15:

$$F(t, v_{\mathrm{m}}) = f(t) - k_1 v_{\mathrm{m}}(t) + k_2 v_{\mathrm{m}}^2(t - \tau), \quad \tau = \kappa t \tag{8.17}$$

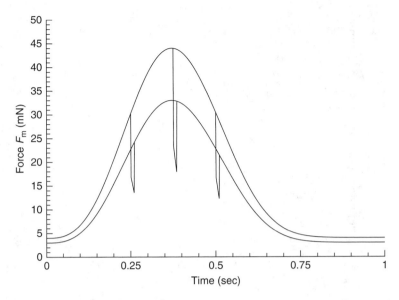

FIGURE 8.19 Quick releases of 10% of muscle length over 10 msec computed from the reduced muscle model (Equation 8.16) at three different times during contraction.

and k_1, k_2, and κ are additional model constants. In summary, muscle is a time-, length- and velocity-dependent force generator. Figure 8.19 shows computed quick releases of 10% of muscle length over 10 msec for three different times during otherwise isometric contractions. The outer envelope of force depicts isometric force at the initial length, and the inner at the new released length. As for muscle, developed force is initially much less than expected, a result of deactivation, and subsequently recovers via hyperactivation. Figure 8.20 shows the inverse experiment with computed quick stretches. Initial transient force is higher than expected, with subsequent quick drop and then isometric recovery. These results compare favorably with muscle experiments in the literature [43].

8.3.4 Predictive Power: Muscle Contraction

The idea for this distributed muscle fiber model arose in 1990 [44]. At that time, muscle fibers were assumed to be functionally similar to muscle strips. Recently, experiments on isolated muscle fibers show this to be the case. Predictions from the model have recently been borne out, for example, the magnitude of computed peak isometric force compared to that measured on isolated guinea pig myocytes [34]. Peak isometric stress measured on isolated rabbit myocytes (5.4 mN/mm^2) is very close to peak stress from rabbit papillary muscle strips (6.4 mN/mm^2) [45]. The distributed model generates peak isometric stress of 2.5 mN/mm^2. Other muscle phenomena measured on the isolated fiber include: a quadratic force–length relation [45], inotropic changes in contractile state [37], quick release and stretch [37,39], and isotonic contractions [46], all in agreement with model predictions.

Physiological modeling strives to create a framework that integrates experimental observations. A great strength of modeling is its capacity for predicting new experiments and physiological phenomena (Figure 8.1). The distributed muscle fiber model predicts that mechanical external vibration of muscle should enhance its internal vibration and promote bond detachment and therefore relaxation. To test this hypothesis, ultrasound was used to vibrate muscle. A single millisecond pulse of ultrasound delivered to the *in vivo* frog heart during systole was observed to reduce developed aortic pressure [47,48]. Experiments were designed to eliminate heating effects. Ultrasound pulses applied late in the twitch had particularly strong effects. After peak muscle force is generated, bond attachment ends so detachment via vibration has no mechanism for recovery. This force (pressure) deactivation was

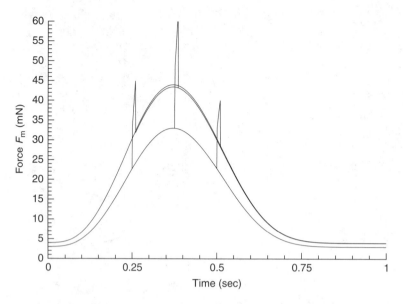

FIGURE 8.20 Quick stretches of 10% of muscle length over 10 msec computed using Equation 8.16.

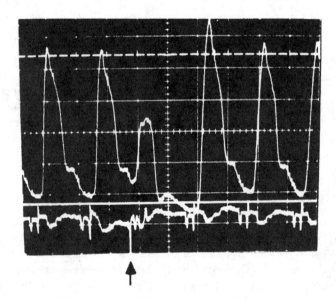

FIGURE 8.21 Premature ventricular contraction following ultrasound irradiation, during diastole, of the *in vivo* frog heart. The top trace is aortic pressure and below is the ECG. A lithotripter pulse of 20 MPa, 5 msec duration, is delivered at the vertical arrow. (Adapted from Dalecki, D., Raeman, C.H., Child, S.Z., and Carstensen, E.L. 1997. *Ultrasound Med. Biol.* 23: 275–285.)

reproducible and not permanently damaging as beats without irradiation produced normal pressure magnitudes and time courses. A mechanical effect is likely since moving the heart slightly out of the ultrasound beam produced no deactivation effect, despite having the same electrical environment. Ultrasound delivered during diastole was found to produce a premature ventricular contraction, as depicted in Figure 8.21, an unexpected result. These experiments suggest that medical ultrasound may have strong effects on living tissues, and demonstrates how modeling can lead to the discovery of new physiological phenomena.

8.4 Modeling Heart Function during Hypertrophy

8.4.1 Integration of Micro- and Macro-Dynamics

Modeling methodology often relies on the availability of structural parameters that have been determined from prior physical and quantitative experimentation. Alternatively, it is of vital interest to understand how a given structure arises, that is, to understand nature's design. To accomplish this, it is necessary to allow the system to adapt to its external functional demands. Due to adaptive processes, a biological system may be undergoing synthesis and desynthesis simultaneously. The balance of these opposing mechanisms results in a structure that meets the system's current functional demand. The advantage of this type of modeling approach is that it obviates measurement of every parameter. This enables the physiological modeler to provide theoretical insight outside the realm of conventional experimentation.

Often models become increasingly complex in the attempt to study smaller levels of structural detail. Ultimately, there may be a minimum level of structure at which the function is known and relatively constant, for example, a cell or a cardiac sarcomere. This structure is denoted the *micro-unit*. The assembly of such units comprises the biological system and is denoted the *macro-unit*. The macro-unit function may also be known, characterized, for example, by ventricular pressure and flow. It is the arrangement and interaction of multiple micro-units that introduces complexity in modeling. To resolve this problem, the micro-unit function is integrated while structure is varied to identify structural rules. The resulting rules are usually simple and thereby offer a special advantage to the integrative approach.

The concept of integrating micro-level function to solve for the macro-level of physiological function and overall geometry has been discussed earlier by Taylor and Weibel [49]. These researchers stated in qualitative terms that an organ system achieves "a state of structural design commensurate to functional needs resulting from regulated morphogenesis, whereby the formation of structural elements is regulated to satisfy but not exceed the requirements of the functional system." This process has been termed symorphosis.

8.4.2 Integrative Modeling

In its simplest form, this method matches function at two different levels of structure. A match is achieved by varying the macro-structure until energy utilization of the system is minimized. Structural variation can be accomplished analytically, or in the case of discontinuous or nonlinear functions by means of a computer. Energy is then minimized in terms of the micro-unit. Since the time frame for the adaptive process tends to be long, it may be difficult to accumulate experimental results. Alternatively, it would be difficult to design an "integrative experiment" whereby the macro-structure is actually altered. For example, it is not easy to add or subtract selected cardiac myocytes to or from an intact cardiac ventricle without trauma to the animal. Usually, the same heart is observed over long time periods for its response to various external loading conditions. A theoretical approach can overcome some of these difficulties.

Integrative modeling begins by identifying a minimal level of structure at which its function is known. For an organ, this could be at the cellular level or, even lower, at the molecular level. The function of interest must be defined in terms of a physical quantity, such as electrical, mechanical, chemical, and so on. The physical quantity of interest may also be time dependent, but the function of the micro-unit must be independent of change in the geometry of the macro-structure. For normal physiological conditions, this rule is valid, but it may break down in the case of a disease process. Pathological conditions further require an analysis of how the micro-unit function alters with time, for example, how myocyte function deteriorates over time in heart failure. The dimensions of the micro-unit must be defined. Since the micro-unit is chosen to be the smallest structural element, its mean dimensions are often treated as constants.

The macro-unit, for example, the structure at the organ level, consists of a group of organized micro-dynamic units. Macro-unit function must be defined in terms of the physical quantities of interest. The physical quantities at the two structural levels must be of the same type, for example, myocyte force and ventricular wall tension define force at different structural levels. Once the macro-function is defined, it must be independent of variation in the macro-structure, that is, unchanged by the adaptive process over long time periods. Since the macro-function is important to the survival of the animal, it may be independent of a disease process as well. This is generally true until structural changes cannot accommodate the deterioration of micro-function at a sufficiently rapid pace.

The organization of the micro-units defines the macro-structure. If the structure is a simple geometry that models the anatomic shape, analytical expressions can be obtained. Use of the actual anatomical shape forces the modeling to be computational. Once the geometry is prescribed, the physical equilibrium equations can be derived that relate the micro-function to the macro-function. This is accomplished by mathematically integrating the micro-function over the entire geometry, hence the name integrative modeling. For example, the myocardial force is integrated over the ventricle in order to relate it to wall tension. The final equations contain the geometric dimensions of the model and are unknowns at the onset.

8.4.3 Energy Considerations

The micro-unit is the smallest building block employed to assemble the overall structure. The dimensions of the micro-unit therefore represent the limit of resolution for any physical quantity computed from the model. Of particular interest is the energy required by the micro-unit. When the micro-unit is fixed in dimensions, on average, it provides a gauge of energy consumption that is size independent. While the macro-unit is varied in size, the effect on the energy at the micro-unit level can then be observed. Energy considerations for biological systems are typically more complex than for standard engineering systems. For example, care must be taken to include the energy required for the basal tissue metabolism as well as the energy consumption necessary to accomplish functional tasks. This differs from a nonliving structure where only physical energy considerations suffice.

The final analysis solves for the dimensions of the macro-structure, accomplished by examining the micro-unit energy consumption, while the dimensions are varied. A solution is then obtained by solving for a zero derivative of energy with respect to each dimension and minimum in energy. Specific problems may require variance from the above procedure. For example, additional information may be available to assist in finding the solution or in placement of physiological constraints. This is particularly useful when a completely analytical approach is not possible. Lastly, it is not always necessary to obtain the solution relative to the micro-unit energy. Energy was chosen here because of its generality to all systems, but other physical quantities may be used. Whichever quantity is chosen it must be evaluated for the smallest functional unit. Ultimately, the resulting dimensions represent the optimal solution for the structure in terms of its smallest functional building block. These integrative modeling concepts are illustrated in the next section in a study of cardiac hypertrophy.

8.4.4 Predictive Power: Cardiac Hypertrophy

Current thinking dictates that the left ventricle attempts to normalize its peak wall stress values during systole and diastole by altering its dimensions [50]. There are several reasons to doubt the validity of this concept. First, anatomical locations of systolic and diastolic stress transducers have not been identified. Second, the value of wall stress cannot be determined from basic physical knowledge. Instead, wall stress is assumed to be regulated by an unknown mechanism. Last, this theory cannot explain ventricular size alterations due to metabolic disturbance, as opposed to a mechanical disturbance. Alternatively, integrative modeling is applied to the problem of cardiac hypertrophy.

It was hypothesized that cardiac size can be determined from energetics at the sarcomere level of structure, that is, the micro-unit [51]. The cardiac sarcomere was redefined as a *sarcounit* (Figure 8.22), a constant volume structure capable of axial stress generation. The function of the sarcounit was defined by its active and passive stress–length curves (Figure 8.23), with the active function corresponding to maximal activation. Maximal stress was modulated by a periodic time function, which was zero during diastole.

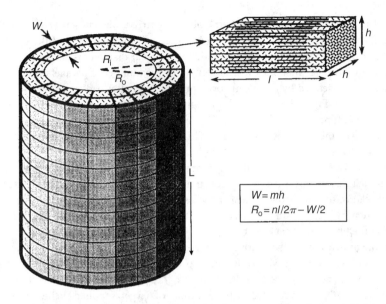

FIGURE 8.22 Cardiac sarcounit (upper right) and structural arrangement to form a cylindrical left ventricle. (Adapted from Drzewiecki, G.M., Karam, E., Li, J.K.-J., and Noordergraaf, A. 1992. *Am. J. Physiol.* 263: H1054–H1063.)

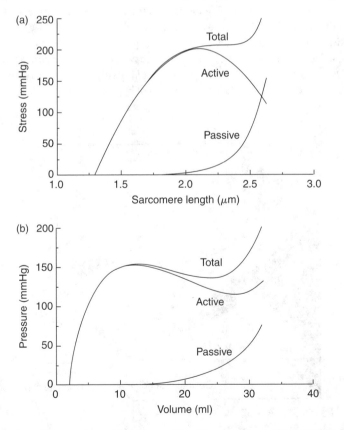

FIGURE 8.23 (a) Active and passive stress–length curves describing the sarcounit. (b) Active and passive pressure–volume curves for the initial cylindrical left ventricle model. (Adapted from Drzewiecki, G.M, Karam, E., and Welkowitz, W. 1989. *J. Theor. Biol.* 139: 465–486.)

A cylindrical approximation to the geometry of the ventricle was chosen (Figure 8.22). Thus, its structure was described by the length, diameter (D), and wall thickness (W) of the cylinder [52]. The sarcounits were arranged in series and parallel so that ventricular diameter is determined by the number of series units and ventricular wall thickness and length by the number of parallel units.

Macro-function was defined by the mean aortic pressure and afterload impedance, using a modified windkessel arterial load. Preload was treated as a constant filling pressure in series with a constant flow resistance. Ventricular function was then equated with micro-function by integrating the stress and length of the sarcounits over the cylindrical structure. This yielded ventricular pressure and volume at any instant of time for given sarcounit stress and length at the corresponding time (Figure 8.23). Heart rate was allowed to vary as necessary to maintain constant mean aortic pressure. The sarcounit energetics were evaluated from the rate of myocardial oxygen consumption (MVO_2). MVO_2 was computed by assuming a proportional relationship with the area of the stress–length loop of the sarcounit per unit time. All quantities were then computed numerically, allowing several cycles to achieve steady state. Each quantity was measured at the final steady-state beat.

To solve for the dimensions of the ventricle, ventricular diameter and wall thickness were varied while evaluating all quantities, including MVO_2. Results show that MVO_2 is minimized only at a specific shape of the cylinder, or W/D ratio (Figure 8.24). Additionally, the level of MVO_2 varied with the overall size of the ventricle. When MVO_2 is also equated with the amount of oxygen supplied by the coronary circulation, a unique solution for left ventricular size and shape is obtained.

The above model was further employed to study observed patterns of cardiac hypertrophy. First, the initial size of the ventricle was consistent with that of a normal dog. Second, a pressure overload was created by raising mean aortic pressure. The model was then used to recompute ventricular size for the new afterload condition. Results show the classic wall thickening and increased wall thickness-to-diameter ratio (W/D), consistent with observed *concentric hypertrophy*. Third, volume overload was imposed by elevating cardiac output. In this case, the model predicted an increase in diameter with relatively little increase in the W/D ratio, referred to as *eccentric hypertrophy*. Lastly, the sarcomere function was impaired and its effect on the ventricle evaluated. An eccentric form of hypertrophy resulted. The diameter-to-length

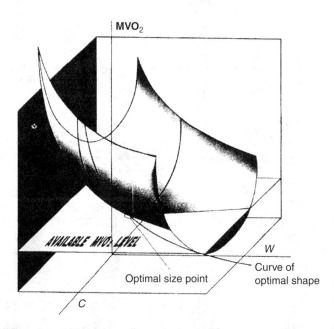

FIGURE 8.24   Sarcounit myocardial oxygen consumption (MVO_2) vs. the circumference (C) and wall thickness (W) of the ventricle model. (Adapted from Drzewiecki, G.M., Karam, E., Li, J.K.-J., and Noordergraaf, A. 1992. *Am. J. Physiol.* 263: H1054–H1063.)

ratio was found to increase along with the degree of myocardial dysfunction [53]. This was consistent with observations that show the ventricle assuming a progressively more spherical shape with further myocardial failure [54].

In conclusion, modeling by means of integrating micro- and macro-function was applied to the study of cardiac hypertrophy. This approach matches the functional information available at two different levels of structure. The ability to predict macro-structure dimensions is a result of achieving this match. The cardiac growth model suggests the conclusion that the ventricular shape can be determined by the regulation of a single quantity, MVO_2, at the sarcomere level. This modeling approach is more general than the wall stress theory as it can predict growth response to metabolic anomaly, as well as to mechanical overloads. As a primary benefit, this approach permits theoretical analysis that may be impractical to realize experimentally.

8.5   Summary

This chapter presents modeling as a tool to identify and quantify the mechanism(s) responsible for observed phenomena in physiology, illustrated with recent examples from cardiovascular dynamics. The rather strict rules to which the modeling process is subject generally lead to the formulation of new, specific experiments, thereby broadening the pool of experimental data, and the database for modeling. On occasion, this process leads to areas of experimentation and the development of concepts originally judged to lie outside the scope of the original problem definition. Consequently, successful modeling aids in deepening a researcher's insight and breadth of view.

References

[1] Popper, K.R. 1959. *The Logic of Scientific Discovery*, Basic Books, New York, NY.

[2] Kuhn, T.S. 1996. *The Structure of Scientific Revolutions* (3rd ed.), University of Chicago Press, Chicago, IL.

[3] Noordergraaf, A. 1969. Hemodynamics. In: *Biological Engineering*, H.P. Schwan (Ed.), Chap 3, Chap. 5, McGraw-Hill, New York.

[4] Noordergraaf, A. 1978. *Circulatory System Dynamics*. Academic Press, New York.

[5] Kennish, A., Yellin, E., and Frater, R.W. 1975. Dynamic stiffness profiles in the left ventricle. *J. Appl. Physiol.* 39: 665.

[6] Suga, H. 1971. Left ventricular pressure–volume ratio in systole as an index of chronic complete heart block in dogs. *Jpn. Heart J.* 12: 153–160.

[7] Sagawa, K. 1987. The ventricular pressure–volume diagram revisited. *Circ. Res.* 43: 677–687.

[8] Campbell, K.B., Ringo, J.A., Knowlen, G., Kirkpatrick, R., and Schmidt, S.L. 1986. Validation of optional elastance–resistance left ventricular pump models. *Am. J. Physiol.* 251: H382–H397.

[9] Suga, H. and Sagawa, K. 1974. Instantaneous pressure–volume relationship under various end-diastolic volume. *Circ. Res.* 35: 117–126.

[10] Mulier, J.P. 1994. Ventricular Pressure as a Function of Volume and Flow. Ph.D. dissertation, University of Leuven, Belgium.

[11] Palladino, J.L., Mulier, J.P., and Noordergraaf, A. 1997. Closed-loop circulation model based on the Frank mechanism. *Surv. Math. Ind.* 7: 177–186.

[12] Frank, O. 1895. Zur Dynamik des Herzmuskels. *Z. Biol.* (Munich) 32: 370 [Eng. transl., see C.B. Chapman and E. Wasserman, *Am. Heart J.* 58: 282–317, 467–478 1959].

[13] Danielsen, M., Palladino, J.L., and Noordergraaf, A. 2000. The left ventricular ejection effect. In: *Mathematical Modelling in Medicine*, J.T. Ottesen and M. Danielsen, Eds., IOS Press, Amsterdam, pp. 13–27.

[14] Palladino, J.L., Ribeiro, L.C., and Noordergraaf, A. 2000. Human circulatory system model based on Frank's mechanism. In: *Mathematical Modelling in Medicine*, J.T. Ottesen and M. Danielsen, Eds., IOS Press, Amsterdam, pp. 29–39.

[15] Noordergraaf, G.J., Dijkema, T.J., Kortsmit, J.P.M., Schilders, W.H.A., Scheffer, G.J., and Noordergraaf, A. 2005. Modeling in cardiopulmonary resuscitation: pumping the heart. *Cardiovasc. Eng.*, 5(3): 104–118.

[16] Kouwenhoven, W.B., Jude, J.R., and Knickerbocker, G.G. 1960. Closed chest cardiac massage. *JAMA* 173: 1064–1067.

[17] Mayow, J. 1907. On muscular motion and animal spirits, fourth treatise. In: *Medical–Physical Works*, Alembic Club Reprint no. 17, published by the Alembic Club.

[18] Weber, E. 1846. *Handwörterbuch der Physiologie*. Vol. 3B. R. Wagner, Ed., Vieweg, Braunschweig.

[19] Chauveau, A. 1890. L'élasticité active du muscle et l'énergie consacreé à sa création dans le cas de contraction statique. *C.R. Acad. Sci.* 111: 19, 89.

[20] Laulanié, F. 1890. Principes et problèmes de la thermodynamique musculaire d'après les récents traveaux de *M. Chauveau*. Rev. Vét. 15: 505.

[21] Fick, A. 1891. Neue Beitrage zur Kentniss von der Wärmeentwicklung im Muskel. *Pflügers Arch.* 51, 541.

[22] Blix, M. 1893. Die Länge und die Spannung des muskels. *Skand. Arch. Physiol.* 4: 399.

[23] Hill, A.V. 1922. The maximum work and mechanical efficiency of human muscles, and their most economical speed. *J. Physiol.* 56: 19.

[24] Fenn, W.O. 1923. Quantitative comparison between energy liberated and work performed by isolated sartorius muscle of the frog. *J. Physiol.* 58: 175–203.

[25] Hill, A.V. 1939. The heat of shortening and dynamic constants of muscle. *Proc. R. Soc. Lond. (B)* 126: 136.

[26] Montevecchi, F.M. and Pietrabissa, R. 1987. A model of multicomponent cardiac fiber. *J. Biomech.* 20: 365–370.

[27] Parmley, W.W., Brutsaert, D.L., and Sonnenblick, E.H. 1969. Effect of altered loading on contractile events in isolated cat papillary muscle. *Circ. Res.* 24: 521.

[28] Huxley, A.F. 1957. Muscle structure and theories of contraction. *Prog. Biophys.* 7: 255–318.

[29] Huxley, A.F. and Simmons, R.M. 1973. Mechanical transients and the origin of muscle force. *Cold Spring Harbor Symp. Quant. Biol.* 37: 669–680.

[30] Eisenberg, E., Hill, T.L., and Chen, Y. 1980. Cross-bridge model of muscle contraction. *Biophys. J.* 29: 195–227.

[31] Palladino, J.L. and Noordergraaf, A. 1998. Muscle contraction mechanics from ultrastructural dynamics. In: *Analysis and Assessment of Cardiovascular Function*, G.M. Drzewiecki and J.K.-J. Li, Eds., Springer-Verlag, New York, chap. 3, pp. 33–57.

[32] Winegrad, S. 1968. Intracellular calcium movements of frog skeletal muscle during recovery from tetanus. *J. Gen. Physiol.* 51: 65–83.

[33] Gordon, A., Huxley, A., and Julian, F. 1966. The variation in isometric tension with sarcomere length in vertebrate muscle fibers. *J. Physiol.* 184: 170–192.

[34] White, E., Boyett, M.R., and Orchard, C.H. 1995. The effects of mechanical loading and changes of length on single guinea-pig ventricular myocytes. *J. Physiol.* 482: 93–107.

[35] Allen, D.G. and Blinks, J.R. 1978. Calcium transients in aequorin-injected frog cardiac muscle. *Nature* 273: 509–513.

[36] Huxley, H.E., Simmons, R.M., Faruqi, A.R., Kress, M., Bordas, J., and Koch, M.H.J. 1983. Changes in the X-ray reflections from contracting muscle during rapid mechanical transients and their structural implications. *J. Mol. Biol.* 169: 469–506.

[37] Brandt, P.W., Colomo, F., Poggesi, C., and Tesi, C. 1993. Taking the first steps in contraction mechanics of single myocytes from frog heart. In: *Mechanism of Myofilament Sliding in Muscle Contraction*, H. Sugi and G.H. Pollack, Eds., Plenum Press, NY.

[38] Colomo, F., Poggesi, C., and Tesi, C. 1994. Force responses to rapid length changes in single intact cells from frog heart. *J. Physiol.* 475: 347–350.

[39] Kurihara, S. and Komukai, K. 1995. Tension-dependent changes of the intracellular Ca^{++} transients in ferret ventricular muscles. *J. Physiol.* 489: 617–625.

[40] Palladino, J.L., Danielsen, M., and Noordergraaf, A. 2000. An analytical description of heart muscle. *Proceedings of 30th IEEE Northeast Bioengineering Conference.*

[41] Sonnenblick, E.H. 1962. Force–velocity relations in mammalian heart muscle. *Am. J. Physiol.* 202: 931

[42] Brutsaert, D.L., Claes, V.A., and Sonnenblick, E.H. 1971. Effects of abrupt load alterations on force–velocity–length and time relations during isotonic contractions of heart muscle: load clamping. *J. Physiol.* 216: 319.

[43] Brady, A.J. 1966. Onset of contractility in cardiac muscle. *J. Physiol.* 184: 560.

[44] Palladino, J.L. 1990. Models of Cardiac Muscle Contraction and Relaxation. Ph.D. dissertation, University of Pennsylvania, Philadelphia. Univ. Microforms, Ann Arbor, MI.

[45] Bluhm, W.F., McCulloch, A.D., and Lew, W.Y.W. 1995. Technical note: active force in rabbit ventricular myocytes. *J. Biomech.* 28: 1119–1122.

[46] Parikh, S.S., Zou, S.-Z., and Tung, L. 1993. Contraction and relaxation of isolated cardiac myocytes of the frog under varying mechanical loads. *Circ. Res.* 72: 297–311.

[47] Dalecki, D., Carstensen, E.L., Neel, D.S., Palladino, J.L., and Noordergraaf, A. 1991. Thresholds for premature ventricular contractions in frog hearts exposed to lithotripter fields. *Ultrasound Med. Biol.* 17: 341–346.

[48] Dalecki, D., Raeman, C.H., Child, S.Z., and Carstensen, E.L. 1997. Effects of pulsed ultrasound on the frog heart: III. The radiation force mechanism. *Ultrasound Med. Biol.* 23: 275–285.

[49] Taylor, C.R. and Weibel, E.R. 1981. Design of the mammalian respiratory system I: problem and strategy, *Resp. Physiol.*, 44: 1–10.

[50] Grossman, W. 1980. Cardiac hypertrophy: useful adaptation or pathologic process? *Am. J. Med.* 69: 576–584.

[51] Drzewiecki, G.M., Karam, E., Li, J.K.-J., and Noordergraaf, A. 1992. Cardiac adaptation of sarcomere dynamics to arterial load: a model of hypertrophy. *Am. J. Physiol.* 263: H1054–H1063.

[52] Drzewiecki, G.M, Karam, E., and Welkowitz, W. 1989. Physiological basis for mechanical time-variance in the heart: special consideration of non-linear function. *J. Theor. Biol.* 139: 465–486.

[53] Drzewiecki, G., Li, J.K.-J., Knap, B., Juznic, S., Juznic, G., and Noordergraaf, A. 1996. Cardiac hypertrophy and shape — a noninvasive index? *J. Cardiovasc. Diag. Proced.* 13: 193–198.

[54] Juznic, S.C.J.E., Juznic, G., and Knap, B. 1997. Ventricular shape: spherical or cylindrical? In: *Analysis and Assessment of Cardiovascular Function*, G. Drzewiecki and J. Li, Eds., Springer-Verlag, New York, pp. 156–171.

9

Compartmental Models of Physiologic Systems

Claudio Cobelli
Giovanni Sparacino
Maria Pia Saccomani
Gianna Maria Toffolo
University of Padova

Andrea Caumo
San Raffaele Scientific Institute

9.1 Introduction

Compartmental models are a class of dynamic, that is, differential equation, models derived from mass balance considerations, which are widely used for quantitatively studying the kinetics of materials in physiologic systems. Materials can be either exogenous, such as a drug or a tracer, or endogenous, such as a substrate or a hormone, and kinetics include processes such as production, distribution, transport, utilization, and substrate–hormone control interactions.

Compartmental modeling was first formalized in the context of isotopic tracer kinetics. Over the years it has evolved and grown as a formal body of theory [Carson et al. 1983; Godfrey, 1983; Jacquez 1996; Cobelli et al., 2000].

Compartmental models have been widely employed for solving a broad spectrum of physiologic problems related to the distribution of materials in living systems in research, diagnosis, and therapy both at whole-body, organ, and cellular level. Examples and references can be found in books [Gibaldi and Perrier, 1982; Carson et al., 1983; Jacquez, 1996; Cobelli et al., 2000; Carson and Cobelli, 2001] and reviews [Carson and Jones, 1979; Cobelli, 1984; Cobelli and Caumo, 1998]. Purposes for which compartmental models have been developed include:

- Identification of system structure, that is, models to examine different hypotheses regarding the nature of specific physiologic mechanisms.
- Estimation of unmeasurable quantities, that is, estimating internal parameters and variables of physiologic interest.
- Simulation of the intact system behavior where ethical or technical reasons do not allow direct experimentation on the system itself.
- Prediction and control of physiologic variables by administration of therapeutic agents, that is, models to predict an optimal administration of drug in order to keep one or more physiologic variables within desirable limits.
- Cost/effectiveness optimization of dynamic clinical tests, that is, models to obtain maximal information from the minimum number of blood samples withdrawn from a patient.
- Diagnosis, that is, models to augment quantitative information from laboratory tests and clinical symptoms, thus improving the reliability of diagnosis.
- Teaching, that is, models to aid in the teaching of many aspects of physiology, clinical medicine, and pharmacokinetics.

The use of compartmental models of physiologic systems has been greatly facilitated by the availability of specific software packages for PC [SAAMII, 1998; AdaptII, 1997], which can be used both for simulation and identification.

9.2   Definitions and Concepts

Let us start with some definitions. A *compartment* is an amount of material that acts as though it is well-mixed and kinetically homogeneous. A *compartmental model* consists of a finite number of compartments with specified interconnections among them. The interconnections represent fluxes of material which physiologically represent transport from one location to another or a chemical transformation, or both, or control signals. An example of a simple two-compartment model is illustrated in Figure 9.1 where the compartments are represented by circles and the interconnections by arrows.

Given the introductory definitions, it is useful before explaining *well-mixed* and *kinetic homogeneity* to consider possible candidates for compartments. Consider the notion of a compartment as a physical space. Plasma is a candidate for a compartment; a substance such as plasma glucose could be a compartment.

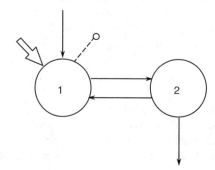

FIGURE 9.1   A two-compartment model. The substance enters *de novo* compartment 1 (arrow entering a compartment from "outside") and irreversibly leaves from compartment 2 (arrow leaving a compartment to the "outside"). Material exchanges occur between compartments 2 and 1 and compartments 1 and 2 and are represented by arrows. Compartment 1 is the accessible compartment; test input and measurement (output) are denoted by a large arrow and a dashed line with a bullet, respectively.

Zinc in bone could be a compartment also as could thyroxine in the thyroid. In some experiments, different substances could be followed in plasma: plasma glucose, lactate, and alanine provide examples. Thus in the same experiment, there can be more than one plasma compartment, one for each of the substances being studied. This notion extends beyond plasma. Glucose and glucose-6-phosphate could be two different compartments inside a liver cell. Thus a physical space may actually represent more than one compartment.

In addition, one must distinguish between compartments that are accessible and nonaccessible for measurement. Researchers often try to assign physical spaces to the nonaccessible compartments. This is a very difficult problem that is best addressed once one realizes that the definition of a compartment is actually a theoretical construct, which may in fact lump material from several different physical spaces in a system; to equate a compartment with a physical space depends upon the system under study and assumptions about the model.

With these notions of what might constitute a compartment, it is easier to define the concepts of well-mixed and kinetic homogeneity. What *well-mixed* means is that any two samples taken from the compartment at the same time would have the same concentration of the substance being studied and therefore be equally representative. Thus the concept of well-mixed relates to uniformity of information contained in a single compartment.

Kinetic homogeneity means that every particle in a compartment has the same probability of taking the pathways leaving the compartment. Since, when a particle leaves a compartment, it does so because of metabolic events related to transport and utilization, it means that all particles in the compartment have the same probability of leaving due to one of these events.

The notion of a compartment, that is, lumping material with similar characteristics into collections that are homogeneous and behave identically, is what allows one to reduce a complex physiologic system into a finite number of compartments and pathways. The required number of compartments depends both on the system being studied and on the richness of the experimental configuration. A compartmental model is clearly unique for each system studied, since it incorporates known and hypothesized physiology and biochemistry. It provides the investigator with insights into the system structure and is as good as the assumptions that are incorporated in the model.

9.3 The Compartmental Model

9.3.1 Theory

Figure 9.2 represent the ith compartment of an n-compartment model; $q_i \geq 0$ denotes the mass of the compartment. The arrows represent fluxes into and out of the compartment: the input flux into the compartment from outside the system, for example, *de novo* synthesis of material and exogenous test

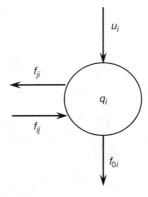

FIGURE 9.2   The ith compartment of an n-compartment model.

input, is represented by $u_i \geq 0$; the flux to the environment and therefore out of the system by f_{0i}; the flux from compartment i to j by f_{ji}, and the flux from compartment j to i by f_{ij}. All fluxes are greater than or equal to zero. The general equations for the compartmental model are obtained by writing the mass balance equation for each compartment:

$$\dot{q}_i = \sum_{\substack{j=1 \\ j \neq i}}^{n} f_{ij} - \sum_{\substack{j=1 \\ j \neq i}}^{n} f_{ji} - f_{0i} + u_i, \quad q_i(0) = q_{i0} \tag{9.1}$$

The input fluxes u_i are generally constant or functions of only time. The fluxes f_{ji}, f_{ij}, and f_{0i} can be functions of $q_1, \ldots, q_n$ and sometimes also of time (for the sake of simplicity, we will ignore this dependence). It is always possible to write:

$$f_{ij}(\mathbf{q}) = k_{ij}(\mathbf{q})q_j \tag{9.2}$$

where $\mathbf{q} = [q_1, \ldots, q_n]^{\mathrm{T}}$ is the vector of the compartmental masses. As a result, Equation 9.1 can be written as:

$$\dot{q}_i = \sum_{\substack{j=1 \\ j \neq i}}^{n} k_{ij}(\mathbf{q})q_j - \left(\sum_{\substack{j=1 \\ j \neq i}}^{n} k_{ji}(\mathbf{q}) + k_{0i}(\mathbf{q}) \right) q_i + u_i, \quad q_i(0) = q_{i0} \tag{9.3}$$

The k_{ij}'s are called *fractional transfer coefficients*. Equation 9.3 describes the generic *nonlinear* compartmental model. If the k_{ij}'s do not depend on the compartmental masses q_i's, the model becomes *linear*.

Defining $k_{ii}(\mathbf{q}) = -\left(\sum_{\substack{j=1 \\ j \neq i}}^{n} k_{ji}(\mathbf{q}) + k_{0i}(\mathbf{q}) \right)$ we can now write Equation 9.3 as:

$$\dot{q}_i = \sum_{j=1}^{n} k_{ij}(\mathbf{q})q_j + u_i, \quad q_i(0) = q_{i0} \tag{9.4}$$

and the model of the whole system as

$$\dot{\mathbf{q}} = \mathbf{K}(\mathbf{q})\mathbf{q} + \mathbf{u}, \quad \mathbf{q}(0) = \mathbf{q}_0 \tag{9.5}$$

where $\mathbf{K}$ is the $n \times n$ *compartmental matrix* (hereafter, let us drop the dependence on $\mathbf{q}$, for simplicity of notation) and $\mathbf{u} = [u_1, \ldots, u_n]^{\mathrm{T}}$ is the vector of input fluxes into the compartments from outside the system.

For the linear case, $\mathbf{K}$ is constant and one has:

$$\dot{\mathbf{q}} = \mathbf{K}\mathbf{q} + \mathbf{u}, \quad \mathbf{q}(0) = \mathbf{q}_0 \tag{9.6}$$

The entries of the compartmental matrix $\mathbf{K}$, for both the nonlinear 9.5 and the linear 9.6 model, satisfy

$$k_{ii} \leq 0, \quad \text{for all } i \tag{9.7}$$

$$k_{ij} \geq 0, \quad \text{for all } i \neq j \tag{9.8}$$

$$\sum_{i=1}^{n} k_{ij} = \sum_{\substack{i=1 \\ i \neq j}}^{n} k_{ij} + k_{jj} = -k_{0j} \leq 0, \quad \text{for all } j \tag{9.9}$$

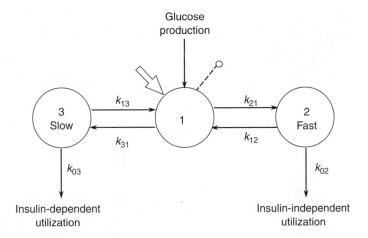

FIGURE 9.3   The linear compartmental model of glucose kinetics by Cobelli et al. [1984b].

K is thus a (column) diagonally dominant matrix. This is a very important property, and in fact the stability properties of compartmental models are closely related to the diagonal dominance of the compartmental matrix. For instance for the linear model, Equation 9.6, one can show that all eigenvalues have nonpositive real parts and that there are no purely imaginary eigenvalues: this means that all solutions are bounded and if there are oscillations they are damped. The qualitative theory of linear and nonlinear compartmental models have been reviewed in Jacquez and Simon [1993], where some stability results on nonlinear compartmental models are also presented.

9.3.2   The Linear Model

The linear model, Equation 9.6, has become very useful in applications due to an important result: the kinetics of a tracer in a constant steady-state system, linear or nonlinear, are linear with constant coefficients. An example is shown in Figure 9.3 where the three-compartment model by Cobelli et al. [1984b] for studying tracer glucose kinetics in steady state at the whole-body level is depicted. Linear compartmental models in conjunction with tracer experiments have been extensively used in studying distribution of materials in living systems both at whole-body, organ and cellular level. Examples and references can be found in Carson et al. [1983], Jacquez [1996], and Cobelli et al. [2000], Carson and Cobelli [2001].

An interesting application of linear compartmental models at the organ level is in describing the exchange of materials between blood, interstitial fluid, and cell of a tissue from multiple tracer indicator dilution data. Compartmental models provide a finite difference approximation in the space dimension of a system described by partial differential equations, which may be easier resolvable from the data. These models are discussed in Jacquez [1996] and an example of a model describing glucose transport and metabolism in the human skeletal muscle can be found in Saccomani et al. [1996].

9.3.3   The Nonlinear Model

Almost all the biological models are nonlinear dynamic systems, including for example saturation or threshold processes. In particular, nonlinear compartmental models, Equation 9.5, are frequently found in biomedical applications. For such models the entries of **K** are functions of **q**, most commonly k_{ij} is a function of only few components of **q**, often q_i or q_j. Examples of k_{ij} function of q_i or q_j are the Hill and

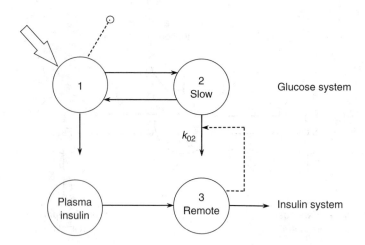

FIGURE 9.4 The nonlinear compartmental model of insulin control on glucose distribution and metabolism by Caumo and Cobelli [1993]. The dashed line denotes a control signal.

the Langmuir nonlinearities described respectively by:

$$k_{ij}(q_j) = \frac{\alpha q_j(t)^{h-1}}{\beta + q_j(t)^h} \tag{9.10}$$

$$k_{ij}(q_i) = 1 - \frac{q_i}{\gamma} \tag{9.11}$$

where α, β, γ are positive reals, and h is a positive integer. For $h = 1$, Equation 9.10 turns into the widely used Michaelis–Menten equation.

Other interesting examples arise in describing substrate–hormone control systems. For instance the model of Figure 9.4 has been proposed [Caumo and Cobelli, 1993; Vicini et al., 1997] to describe the control of insulin on glucose distribution and metabolism during a glucose perturbation which brings the system out of steady state. The model assumes compartmental descriptions for glucose and insulin kinetics, interacting via a control signal, which emanates from the remote insulin compartment and affects the transfer rate coefficient, k_{02}, responsible for insulin-dependent glucose utilization. In this case one has:

$$k_{02}(q_3) = \delta + q_3 \tag{9.12}$$

where δ is a constant.

Additional examples and references on nonlinear compartmental models can be found in Carson et al. [1983], Godfrey [1983], Jacquez [1996], and Carson and Cobelli [2001].

9.3.4 Use in Simulation and Indirect Measurement

Models such as those described by Equation 9.5 can be used for *simulation*. Assuming that both the matrix **K** and initial state **q**(0) are known, it is possible to predict the behavior of the state vector **q** for any possible input function **u**.

A major use of compartmental models is in the *indirect measurement* of physiologic parameters and variables. For instance, given data obtained from m compartments which are accessible to measurement (usually m is a small fraction of the total number of compartments n), the model is used to estimate not directly measurable parameters and predict quantities related to nonaccessible compartments. In this case **K** is unknown and input–output experiments are performed to generate data to determine **K**. These data can be usually described by a linear algebraic equation

$$\mathbf{y} = \mathbf{Cq} \tag{9.13}$$

where $\mathbf{y} = [y_1, \ldots, y_m]^T$ is the vector of the m model outputs and $\mathbf{C}$ is the $m \times n$ observation matrix. If model outputs are concentrations, the entries of $\mathbf{C}$ are the inverse of the volumes of the m compartments accessible to measurement. Real data are noisy, thus an error term $\mathbf{v}$ is usually added to $\mathbf{y}$ in Equation 9.13 to describe the actual measurements $\mathbf{z}$

$$\mathbf{z} = \mathbf{y} + \mathbf{v} \tag{9.14}$$

$\mathbf{v}$ is usually given a probabilistic description, for example, errors are assumed to be independent and often Gaussian. Equation 9.13 and Equation 9.14 together with Equation 9.5 or Equation 9.6 define the compartmental model of the system, that is, the model structure and the input–output experimental configuration.

The identification techniques described in the following section are aimed to determine the entries of $\mathbf{K}$ (and often also those of $\mathbf{C}$) from the data vector $\mathbf{z}$ of Equation 9.14.

9.4 A Priori Identifiability

Let us assume that a compartmental model structure has been postulated to describe the physiologic system, that is, the number of compartments and the connections among them have been specified. This is the most difficult step in compartmental model building.

The structure can reflect a number of facts: there may be some a priori knowledge about the system, which can be incorporated in the structure; one can make specific assumptions about the system, which are reflected in the structure; by testing via simulation one can arrive at a structure that is needed to fit the data. The result at this stage is a nonlinear, Equation 9.5, or linear, Equation 9.6, where parameters of the compartmental matrix $\mathbf{K}$ and those of the observation matrix $\mathbf{C}$, Equation 9.13, are usually unknown. Before performing the experiment or, if the experiment was already completed, before numerically estimating the model parameters from the experimental data, the following question arises: does the data contain enough information to unequivocally estimate (e.g., via least squares or maximum likelihood) all the unknown parameters of the postulated model structure? This question, set in the ideal context of error-free model structure and noise-free measurements, is usually referred to as the a priori *global identifiability*. Despite its theoretical nature, it is an essential, but often overlooked, prerequisite for model parameter estimation from real data. In particular, if it turns out in such an ideal context that some model parameters are not identifiable from the data, there is no way that the parameters can be identified in a real situation, with errors in the model structure and noise in the data.

A priori identifiability thus examines whether, given the ideal noise-free data $\mathbf{y}$, Equation 9.13, and the error-free compartmental model structure, Equation 9.5 or Equation 9.6, it is possible to make unique estimates of all the unknown model parameters. A model can be *uniquely (globally) identifiable* — that is all its parameters have one solution — or *nonuniquely (locally) identifiable* — that is, one or more of its parameters has more than one but a finite number of possible values — or *nonidentifiable* — that is, one or more of its parameters has an infinite number of solutions. For instance, the model of Figure 9.1 is uniquely identifiable, while that of Figure 9.3 is *nonidentifiable*.

A priori identifiability is also crucial in qualitative experiment design [Saccomani and Cobelli, 1992], which studies the input–output configuration necessary to ensure unique estimation of the unknown parameters. In fact, it allows to distinguish among those experiments that cannot succeed and those that might and, among the latter, may help in determining the minimal input-output configuration to ensure estimation of the unknown parameters. This is of particular relevance for physiological systems, where the number and sites of application of inputs and outputs are severely constrained by ethical and technical reasons.

The identifiability problem is in general a difficult task, since it requires to solve a system of nonlinear algebraic equations with a number of terms and nonlinearity degree increasing with the model order. For linear compartmental models various specific methods, for example, based on transfer function, similarity transformation and graph topology, have been developed [Cobelli and DiStefano, 1980; Walter, 1982; Carson et al., 1983; Godfrey, 1983; Jacquez, 1996]. Explicit identifiability results on catenary and mamillary compartmental models [Cobelli et al., 1979] and on the three-compartmental model [Norton, 1982] are available. The introduction of computer algebraic algorithms has allowed to considerably simplifying the complexity of the problem [Audoly et al., 1998].

For nonlinear compartmental models the problem is more difficult and very few results are available, for example, based on the similarity transformation [Chappell and Godfrey, 1992] and on the output series expansion [Pohjanpalo, 1978]. When applied to large models, these methods involve nonlinear algebraic equations difficult to be solved, even by resorting to symbolic algebraic manipulative languages (e.g., Reduce, Maple). Given the relevance of identifiability of nonlinear models in biological studies, the above difficulties have stimulated new approaches to study global identifiability based on differential algebra tools. In particular, the introduction of concepts of differential algebra has been an important factor for addressing identifiability of nonlinear (compartmental and noncompartmental) models previously thought to be intractable [Ollivier, 1990; Ljung and Glad, 1994; Audoly et al., 2001]. However, the construction of an efficient algorithm still remains a difficult task. Recently a new differential algebra algorithm to test identifiability of nonlinear models with given initial conditions has been developed [Saccomani et al., 2003]. This algorithm integrates the different strategies proposed before and broadens their domain of applicability. In particular, it is a very useful tool for biological and physiological systems that often exhibit nongeneric initial conditions, for example, a model of radiotracer kinetics is characterized by zero initial conditions.

From the above considerations, it follows that if a model is a priori uniquely identifiable, then identification techniques can be used to estimate from the noisy data $\mathbf{z}$, Equation 9.14, the numerical values of the unknown parameters. Conversely, if a model is either a priori nonuniquely identifiable or nonidentifiable, numerical estimation may lead to parametric values which are ambiguous and thus not informative about the biological system under study; this is particularly critical when dealing with physiological systems where a different numerical estimate can characterize a pathological from a normal state. In this case, to solve the problem, different strategies can be used, for example, derivation of bounds for nonidentifiable parameters [DiStefano, 1983], model reparametrization (parameter aggregation), incorporation of additional knowledge, or design of a more informative experiment. An example on the use of some of these approaches for dealing with the nonidentifiable model of glucose kinetics of Figure 9.3 is given in Cobelli and Toffolo [1987].

In conclusion, a priori unique identifiability is a prerequisite for well posedness of parameter estimation and for reconstructability of state variables in compartments not accessible to measurement. It is a necessary but not sufficient condition to guarantee successful estimation of model parameters from real input–output data.

9.5 Parameter Estimation

Given an uniquely identifiable compartmental model, one can proceed by estimating the values of the unknown parameters from the experimental data. Assuming, for the sake of simplicity, that the model is linear and that only one output variable is observed, that is, $m = 1$, by integrating Equation 9.6 one can obtain the explicit solution for the model output, that is, $y(t) = g(t, \boldsymbol{\theta})$, where $\boldsymbol{\theta}$ is a p-dimension vector which contains the p unknown parameters of the model. For instance, if the model of Figure 9.1 is used to describe the kinetics of a tracer after the administration of a pulse of known amplitude D (i.e., $u(t) = D\delta(t)$ and $q_1(0) = q_2(0) = 0$), the vector $\boldsymbol{\theta}$ is a 4-dimension vector containing the fractional transfer coefficients k_{01}, k_{12}, k_{21}, and the volume V of the accessible compartment, while the accessible tracer concentration profile $y(t)$ is

$$y(t) = g(t, \boldsymbol{\theta}) = \frac{D}{V} \left(\frac{k_{21} + k_{01} + \sqrt{(k_{12} + k_{21} + k_{01}) + 4k_{12}k_{01}}}{2\sqrt{(k_{12} + k_{21} + k_{01}) + 4k_{12}k_{01}}} e^{-(k_{12}+k_{21}+k_{01}+\sqrt{(k_{12}+k_{21}+k_{01})+4k_{12}k_{01}})t} \right.$$

$$\left. + \frac{k_{12} + k_{01} + \sqrt{(k_{12} + k_{21} + k_{01}) + 4k_{12}k_{01}}}{2\sqrt{(k_{12} + k_{21} + k_{01}) + 4k_{12}k_{01}}} e^{-(k_{12}+k_{21}+k_{01}-\sqrt{(k_{12}+k_{21}+k_{01})+4k_{12}k_{01}})t} \right)$$

$$(9.15)$$

In practical cases, experimental data are collected at N discrete time instants $t_1, \ldots, t_N$, so that discrete time measurements $y(t_k) = g(t_k, \boldsymbol{\theta})$ are available. Letting $\mathbf{z} = [z(t_1), \ldots, z(t_N)]^T$ to denote the vector of the noisy samples of the output, according to Equation 9.14 one has:

$$\mathbf{z} = \mathbf{g}(\boldsymbol{\theta}) + \mathbf{v} \tag{9.16}$$

where $\mathbf{g}(\boldsymbol{\theta}) = [g(t_1, \boldsymbol{\theta}), \ldots, g(t_N, \boldsymbol{\theta})]^T$, while $\mathbf{v} = [v(t_1), \ldots, v(t_N)]^T$ denotes the vector of the (additive) measurement error samples. Moreover, explicit solution of Equation 9.5 or Equation 9.6 is often non available. Thus $\mathbf{g}(\boldsymbol{\theta})$ is obtained by numerical integration of Equation 9.5 or Equation 9.6.

Estimates of $\boldsymbol{\theta}$ can be determined by several methods. These methods can be divided in two major categories. In the so-called Fisher estimation approach, only the data vector $\mathbf{z}$ of Equation 9.16 is supplied to the estimator in order to estimate the unknown model parameters $\boldsymbol{\theta}$. The second approach, known as the Bayes estimation approach, takes into account not only $\mathbf{z}$ but also some statistical information that is a priori available on the unknown parameter vector $\boldsymbol{\theta}$.

9.5.1 Fisher Approach

In the Fisher approach, parameter estimates can be obtained by nonlinear least squares or maximum likelihood together with their precision, such as, a measure of a posteriori or numerical identifiability. Details and references on parameter estimation of physiologic system models can be found in Carson et al. [1983] and Landaw and DiStefano [1984]. Weighted nonlinear least squares is mostly used, in which an estimate $\hat{\boldsymbol{\theta}}$ of the model parameter vector $\boldsymbol{\theta}$ is determined as

$$\hat{\boldsymbol{\theta}} = \arg \min_{\boldsymbol{\theta}} [\mathbf{z} - \mathbf{g}(\boldsymbol{\theta})]^T \mathbf{W} [\mathbf{z} - \mathbf{g}(\boldsymbol{\theta})] \tag{9.17}$$

where $\mathbf{W}$ is a $N \times N$ matrix of weights. In order to numerically solve Equation 9.17, both direct and gradient-type search methods are implemented in estimation schemes.

A correct knowledge of the error structure is needed in order to have a correct summary of the statistical properties of the estimates. This is a difficult task. Measurement errors are usually independent, and often a known distribution, for example, Gaussian, is assumed. Many properties of least squares hold approximately for a wide class of distributions if weights are chosen optimally, that is, equal to the inverse of the variances of the measurement errors, or at least inversely proportional to them if variances are known up to a proportionality constant, that is, $\mathbf{W}^{-1}$ is equal or proportional to $\boldsymbol{\Sigma}_\mathbf{v}$, the $N \times N$ covariance matrix of the measurement error $\mathbf{v}$. Under these circumstances, an asymptotically correct approximation of the covariance matrix of the estimation error $\tilde{\boldsymbol{\theta}} = \boldsymbol{\theta} - \hat{\boldsymbol{\theta}}$ can be used to evaluate the precision of parameter estimates:

$$\text{cov}(\tilde{\boldsymbol{\theta}}) \cong \sigma^2 (\mathbf{S}^T \mathbf{W} \mathbf{S})^{-1} \tag{9.18}$$

where matrix $\mathbf{S}$ is the $N \times p$ Jacobian matrix of $\mathbf{g}(\boldsymbol{\theta})$ calculated at $\hat{\boldsymbol{\theta}}$ and σ^2 is the scale factor (possibly estimated a posteriori) such that $\boldsymbol{\Sigma}_\mathbf{v} = \sigma^2 \mathbf{W}^{-1}$. The approximation of Equation 9.18 becomes exact for a sufficiently large sample size and decreasing variances of the measurement error. If measurement errors are Gaussian, then this approximation is the Cramer–Rao lower bound (inverse of the Fisher information matrix), that is, the optimally weighted least squares estimator is equivalent to the maximum likelihood estimator. Care must be taken in not using lower-bound variances as true parameter variances. Several factors corrupt these variances, for example, inaccurate knowledge of error structure, limited data set. Monte Carlo studies are needed to assess robustness of Cramer–Rao lower bound in specific practical applications.

To examine the quality of model predictions to observed data, in addition to visual inspection, various statistical tests on residuals are available to check for presence of systematic misfitting, nonrandomness of the errors, and accordance with assumed experimental noise. Model order estimation, that is, number of compartments in the model, is also relevant here, and for linear compartmental models, criteria such as F-test, and those based on the parsimony principle such as the Akaike and Schwarz criteria, can be used if measurement errors are Gaussian.

9.5.2 Bayes Approach

Bayes estimators assume that the parameter vector is the realization of a random vector $\boldsymbol{\theta}$, the a priori probability distribution of which $p_{\boldsymbol{\theta}}(\boldsymbol{\theta})$ is available, for example, from preliminary population studies. Starting from the knowledge of both the model of Equation 9.16 and the probability distribution of the noise vector $\mathbf{v}$, one can calculate the likelihood function $p_{z|\boldsymbol{\theta}}(\mathbf{z}|\boldsymbol{\theta})$ (i.e., the probability distribution of the measurement vector in dependence of the parameter vector). From $p_{\boldsymbol{\theta}}(\boldsymbol{\theta})$ and $p_{z|\boldsymbol{\theta}}(\mathbf{z}|\boldsymbol{\theta})$, the a posteriori probability distribution $p_{\boldsymbol{\theta}|z}(\boldsymbol{\theta}|\mathbf{z})$ (i.e., the probability distribution of the parameter vector given the data vector) can be determined by exploiting the Bayes theorem:

$$p_{\boldsymbol{\theta}|z}(\boldsymbol{\theta}|\mathbf{z}) = \frac{p_{z|\boldsymbol{\theta}}(\mathbf{z}|\boldsymbol{\theta})p_{\boldsymbol{\theta}}(\boldsymbol{\theta})}{\int p_{z|\boldsymbol{\theta}}(\mathbf{z}|\boldsymbol{\theta})p_{\boldsymbol{\theta}}(\boldsymbol{\theta})\, d\boldsymbol{\theta}} \qquad (9.19)$$

From the function of Equation 9.19 several estimators can be defined. For instance, the Maximum a Posteriori (MAP) estimate is found by determining the value of $\boldsymbol{\theta}$, which renders $p_{\boldsymbol{\theta}|z}(\boldsymbol{\theta}|\mathbf{z})$ maximum, while the Mean Square (MS) estimate is defined as the expected value of θ, given the data vector:

$$\hat{\boldsymbol{\theta}} = \mathrm{E}[\boldsymbol{\theta}|\mathbf{z}] = \int \boldsymbol{\theta} p_{\boldsymbol{\theta}|z}(\boldsymbol{\theta}|\mathbf{z})\, d\boldsymbol{\theta} \qquad (9.20)$$

When $\mathbf{v}$ and $\boldsymbol{\theta}$ are uncorrelated and Gaussian, both the MS and MAP estimates are given by

$$\hat{\boldsymbol{\theta}} = \arg \min_{\boldsymbol{\theta}}[\mathbf{z} - \mathbf{g}(\boldsymbol{\theta})]^{\mathrm{T}}\Sigma_{\mathbf{v}}^{-1}[\mathbf{z} - \mathbf{g}(\boldsymbol{\theta})] + [\boldsymbol{\theta} - \boldsymbol{\mu}_{\boldsymbol{\theta}}]^{\mathrm{T}}\Sigma_{\boldsymbol{\theta}}^{-1}[\boldsymbol{\theta} - \boldsymbol{\mu}_{\boldsymbol{\theta}}] \qquad (9.21)$$

where $\boldsymbol{\mu}_{\boldsymbol{\theta}}$ and $\Sigma_{\boldsymbol{\theta}}$ are, respectively, the a priori expected value (size p) and covariance matrix (size $p \times p$) of vector $\boldsymbol{\theta}$. The concepts previously considered in the Fisher approach, that is, determination of a confidence interval of the parameter estimates and choice of model order, can be addressed in the Bayes approach as well. Bayes estimation can be of relevant interest, since when statistical information on the unknown parameters of the model is a prior available and exploited, a possibly significant improvement in the parameter estimates precision with respect to Fisher estimation can be obtained, see for example, Cobelli et al. [1999] and Sparacino et al. [2000] for an example of application. However, in most cases the handling of $p_{\boldsymbol{\theta}|z}(\boldsymbol{\theta}|\mathbf{z})$ and its integration in Equation 9.20 is analytically intractable and the sophisticate but computationally demanding numerical simulation techniques called Markov chain Monte Carlo must be used to determine Bayesian parameter estimates and their confidence intervals, see for example, Pillonetto et al. [2002] and Magni et al. [2001] for two recent applications.

9.5.3 Population Approaches

So far, even if homogenous experimental data sets in M different individuals were available, for example, because the same input–output experiment to identify a compartmental model with a given structure was repeated in M homogenous individuals, model identification in each individual is attacked independently. In the literature, alternative parameter estimation approaches, called "population" approaches, have also been devised to identify simultaneously the M individual models starting from the ensemble of the M sets of experimental data. Both deterministic and Bayesian approaches are available [Beal and Sheiner, 1982; Steimer et al., 1984; Davidian and Giltinan, 1995; Sheiner and Wakefield, 1999; Lunn et al., 2002]. Albeit complicated, both theoretically and algorithmically, they are particularly appealing when only few or particularly noisy data are available for each of the subjects under study, as it often happens in pharmacokinetic/pharmacodynamic research or epidemiological studies. In fact, thanks to the fact that "poor" individual data sets can borrow strength from the others, population parameter estimation approaches often allow to achieve results more satisfactory than standard single-subject parameter estimation approaches, see for example, the compartmental model applications recently made in Vicini et al. [1998], Vicini and Cobelli [2001], and Bertoldo et al. [2004].

9.6 Optimal Experiment Design

At this point one has a compartmental model structure, a description of the measurement error, and a numerical value of the parameters together with the precision with which they can be estimated. It is now appropriate to address the optimal experiment design issue. The rationale of optimal experiment design is to act on design variables such as number of test input and outputs, form of test inputs, number of samples and sampling schedule, and measurement errors so as to maximize, according to some criterion, the precision with which the compartmental model parameters can be estimated [DiStefano, 1981; Carson et al., 1983; Landaw and DiStefano, 1984; Walter and Pronzato, 1990].

In the Fisher approach, the Fisher information matrix J, which is the inverse of the lower bound of the covariance matrix, is treated as a function of the design variables and usually the determinant of J (this is called D-optimal design) is maximized in order to maximize precision of parameter estimates, and thus numerical identifiability.

The optimal design of sampling schedules, that is, the determination of the number and location of discrete-time points where samples are collected, has received much attention as it is the variable which is less constrained by the experimental situation. Theoretical and algorithmic aspects have been studied, and software is available, for both the single- and multioutput case [DiStefano, 1981; Cobelli et al., 1985; Landaw and DiStefano, 1984]. Optimal sampling schedules are usually obtained in an iterative manner: one starts with the model obtained from pilot experiments and the program computes optimal sampling schedules for subsequent experimentation. An important result for single-output linear compartmental models is that D-optimal design usually consists of independent replicates at P distinct time points, where P is the number of parameters to estimate.

Optimal sampling schedule design has been shown for example, to improve precision as compared to schedules designed by intuition or other convention and to optimize the cost effectiveness of a dynamic clinical test by reducing the number of blood samples withdrawn from a patient without significantly deteriorating their precision [Cobelli and Ruggeri, 1989; 1991].

The optimal input design problem has been relatively less studied, but some results are available on optimal equidose rectangular inputs (including the impulse) for parameter estimation in compartmental models [Cobelli and Thomaseth, 1987; 1988a, b].

In a Bayes estimation context, optimal experiment design is a more difficult task (see [Walter and Pronzato, 1990] for a survey). Applications have thus been less than those with a Fisher approach, also because the numerical implementation of the theoretical results is much more demanding.

Finally, some results on optimal experiment design in a population parameter estimation context have also been recently presented [Hooker et al., 2003].

9.7   Validation

Validation involves assessing whether or not the compartmental model is adequate for its purpose. This is a difficult and highly subjective task in modeling of physiologic systems, because intuition and understanding of the system play an important role. It is also difficult to formalize related issues such as model credibility, that is, the use of the model outside its established validity range. Some efforts have been made however to provide some formal aids for assessing the value of models of physiologic systems [Carson et al., 1983; Cobelli et al., 1984a]. A set of validity criteria have been explicitly defined, such as empirical, theoretical, pragmatic and heuristic validity, and validation strategies have been outlined for two classes of models, broadly corresponding to simple and complex models. This operational classification is based on a priori identifiability and leads to clearly defined strategies as both complexity of model structure and extent of available experimental data are taken into account. For simple models quantitative criteria based on identification, for example, a priori identifiability, precision of parameter estimates, residual errors, can be used in addition to physiologic plausibility. In contrast with simple models, complex simulation models are essentially incomplete, as there will naturally be a high degree of uncertainty with respect to both structure and parameters. Therefore validation will necessarily be based on less solid grounds. The following aids have been suggested: increasing model testability through model simplification; improved experimental design and model decomposition; adaptive fitting based on qualitative and quantitative feature comparison and time-course prediction; model plausibility.

References

Adapt II User's Guide. 1997. Biomedical Simulation Resource, University of Southern California, Los Angeles.

Audoly, S., D'Angio', L., Saccomani, M.P., and Cobelli, C. 1998. Global identifiability of linear compartmental models. A computer algebra algorithm. *IEEE Trans. Biom. Eng.* 45: 36–47.

Audoly, S., Bellu, G., D'Angio', L., Saccomani, M.P., and Cobelli, C. 2001. Global identifiability of nonlinear models of biological systems. *IEEE Trans. Biom. Eng.* 48: 55–65.

Beal, S.L. and Sheiner, L.B. 1982. Estimating population kinetics. *Crit. Rev. Biomed. Eng.* 8: 195–222.

Bertoldo, A., Sparacino, G., and Cobelli, C. 2004. "Population" approach improves parameter estimation of kinetic models from dynamic PET data. *IEEE Trans. Med. Imag.*, 23: 297–306.

Carson, E.R. and Jones, E.A. 1979. The use of kinetic analysis and mathematical modeling in the quantitation of metabolic pathways *in vivo*: application to hepatic anion metabolism. *New Engl. J. Med.* 300: 1016–1027 and 1078–1986.

Carson, E.R., Cobelli, C., and Finkelstein, L. 1983. *The Mathematical Modelling of Metabolic and Endocrine Systems.* John Wiley & Sons, New York.

Carson, C. and Cobelli, C. 2001. *Modeling Methodology for Physiology and Medicine*, Academic Press (Biomedical Engineering Series).

Caumo, A. and Cobelli, C. 1993. Hepatic glucose production during the labelled IVGTT: estimation by deconvolution with a new minimal model. *Am. J. Physiol.* 264: E829–E841.

Chappell, M.J. and Godfrey, K.R. 1992. Structural identifiability of the parameters of a nonlinear batch reactor model. *Math. Biosci.* 108: 245–251.

Cobelli, C. and Caumo, A. 1998. Using what is accessible to measure that which is not: necessity of model of system. *Metabolism*, 47: 1009.

Cobelli, C., Lepschy, A., and Romanin Jacur, G. 1979. Identifiability results on some constrained compartmental systems. *Math. Biosci.* 47: 173–196.

Cobelli, C. and DiStefano III, J.J. 1980. Parameter and structural identifiability concepts and ambiguities: a critical review and analysis. *Am. J. Physiol.* 239: R7–R24.

Cobelli, C. 1984. Modeling and identification of endocrine-metabolic systems. Theoretical aspects and their importance in practice. *Math. Biosci.* 72: 263–289.

Cobelli, C., Carson, E.R., Finkelstein, L., and Leaning, M.S. 1984a. Validation of simple and complex models in physiology and medicine. *Am. J. Physiol.* 246: R259–R266.

Cobelli, C., Toffolo, G., and Ferrannini, E. 1984b. A model of glucose kinetics and their control by insulin. Compartmental and noncompartmental approaches. *Math. Biosci.* 72: 291–315.

Cobelli, C., Ruggeri, A., DiStefano III, J.J., and Landaw, E.M. 1985. Optimal design of multioutput sampling schedules: software and applications to endocrine-metabolic and pharmacokinetic models. *IEEE Trans. Biom. Eng.* 32: 249–256.

Cobelli, C. and Thomaseth, K. 1987. The minimal model of glucose disappearance: optimal input studies. *Math. Biosci.* 83: 127–155.

Cobelli, C. and Toffolo, G. 1987. Theoretical aspects and practical strategies for the identification of unidentifiable compartmental systems. In *Identifiability of Parametric Models*, Walter, E., Ed., Pergamon, Oxford, pp. 85–91.

Cobelli, C. and Thomaseth, K. 1988a. On optimality of the impulse input for linear system identification. *Math. Biosci.* 89: 127–133.

Cobelli, C. and Thomaseth, K. 1988b. Optimal equidose inputs and role of measurement error for estimating the parameters of a compartmental model of glucose kinetics from continuous-and discrete-time optimal samples. *Math. Biosci.* 89: 135–147.

Cobelli, C., Saccomani, M.P., Ferrannini, E., DeFronzo, R.A., Gelfand, R., and Bonadonna, R.C. 1989. A compartmental model to quantitate *in vivo* glucose transport in the human forearm. *Am. J. Physiol.* 257: E943–E958.

Cobelli, C. and Ruggeri, A. 1989. Optimal design of sampling schedules for studying glucose kinetics with tracers. *Am. J. Physiol.* 257: E444–E450.

Cobelli, C. and Ruggeri, A. 1991. A reduced sampling schedule for estimating the parameters of the glucose minimal model from a labelled IVGTT. *IEEE Trans. Biom. Eng.* 38: 1023–1029.

Cobelli, C., Caumo A., and Omenetto, M. 1999. Minimal model SG overestimation and SI underestimation: improved accuracy by a Bayesian two-compartment model. *Am. J. Physiol.* 277: E481–488.

Cobelli, C., Foster, D.M., and Toffolo, G. *Tracer Kinetics in Biomedical Research: From Data to Model*. Plenum Publishing Corp., 2000.

Davidian, M. and Giltinan, D. 1995. *Nonlinear Models for Repeated Measurement Data*. Chapman and Hall, New York.

DiStefano III, J.J. 1981. Optimized blood sampling protocols and sequential design of kinetic experiments. *Am. J. Physiol.* 9: R259–R265.

DiStefano III, J.J. 1983. Complete parameter bounds and quasi identifiability conditions for a class of unidentifiable linear systems. *Math. Biosci.* 65: 51–68.

Gibaldi, M. and Perrier, D. 1982. *Pharmacokinetics*. 2nd ed., Marcel Dekker, New York.

Godfrey, K. 1983. *Compartmental Models and Their Application*. Academic Press, London.

Hooker, A.C., Foracchia, M., Dodds, M.G., and Vicini, P. 2003. An evaluation of population D-optimal designs via pharmacokinetic simulations. *Ann. Biomed. Eng.* 31: 98–111.

Jacquez, J.A. 1996. *Compartmental Analysis in Biology and Medicine*. 3rd ed., Biomedware, Ann Arbor, MI.

Jacquez, J.A. and Simon, C.P. 1993. Qualitative theory of compartmental systems. *Siam. Rev.*, 35: 43–79.

Landaw, E.M. and DiStefano III, J.J. 1984. Multiexponential, multicompartmental, and noncompartmental modeling. II. Data analysis and statistical considerations. *Am. J. Physiol.* 246: R665–R677.

Ljung, L. and Glad, T. 1994. On global identifiability for arbitrary model parametrizations. *Automatica*, 30: 265–276.

Lunn, D.J., Best, N., Thomas, A., Wakefield, J., and Spiegelhalter, D. 2002. Bayesian analysis of population PK/PD models: general concepts and software. *J. Pharmacokinet. Pharmacodynam.* 29: 271–307.

Magni, P., Bellazzi, R., Nauti, A., Patrini, C., and Rindi, G. 2001. Compartmental model identification based on an empirical Bayesian approach: the case of thiamine kinetics in rats. *Med. Biol. Eng. Comput.* 39: 700–706.

Norton, J.P. 1982. An investigation of the sources of non-uniqueness in deterministic identifiability. *Math. Biosci.* 60: 89–108.

Ollivier, F. 1990. Le problème l'identifiabilité structurelle globale: étude théorique, méthodes effectives et bornes de complexité. Thèse de Doctorat en Science, École Polytechnique.

Pillonetto, G., Sparacino, G., Magni, P., Bellazzi, R., and Cobelli, C. 2002. Minimal model S(I)=0 problem in NIDDM subjects: nonzero Bayesian estimates with credible confidence intervals. *Am. J. Physiol. Endocrinol. Metab.* 282: E564–E573.

Pohjanpalo, H. 1978. System identifiability based on the power series expansion of the solution. *Math. Biosci.* 41: 21–33.

SAAM II User Guide 1998. SAAM Institute FL-20, University of Washington, Seattle, WA.

Saccomani, M.P. and Cobelli, C. 1992. Qualitative experiment design in physiological system identification. *IEEE Contr. Syst. Mag.* 12: 18–23.

Saccomani, M.P., Bonadonna, R., Bier, D.M., De Fronzo, R.A., and Cobelli, C. 1996. A model to measure insulin effects on glucose transport and phosphorylation in muscle: a three-tracer study. *Am. J. Physiol.* 33: E170–E185.

Saccomani, M.P., Audoly, S., and D'Angio', L. 2003. Parameter identifiability of nonlinear systems: the role of initial conditions. *Automatica* 39: 619–632.

Sheiner, L. and Wakefield, J. Population modelling in drug development. 1999. *Stat. Meth. Med. Res.* 8: 183–193.

Sparacino, G., Tombolato, C., and Cobelli, C. 2000. Maximum-likelihood versus maximum a posteriori parameter estimation of physiological system models: the C-peptide impulse response case study. *IEEE Trans. Biom. Eng.* 47: 801–811.

Steimer, J.L., Mallet, A., Golmard, J.L., and Boisvieux, J.F. 1984. Alternative approaches to estimation of population pharmacokinetic parameters: comparison with the nonlinear mixed-effect model. *Drug Metab. Rev.* 15: 265–292.

Vicini, P., Sparacino, G., Caumo, A., and Cobelli, C. 1997. Estimation of hepatic glucose release after a glucose perturbation by nonparametric stochastic deconvolution. *Comp. Meth. Progr. Biomed.* 52: 147.

Vicini, P., Barrett, P.H., Cobelli, C., Foster, D.M., and Schumitzky, A. 1998. Approaches to population kinetic analysis with application to metabolic studies. *Adv. Exp. Med. Biol.* 445: 103–113.

Vicini, P. and Cobelli, C. 2001. The iterative two-stage population approach to IVGTT minimal modeling: improved precision with reduced sampling. Intravenous glucose tolerance test. *Am. J. Physiol. Endocrinol. Metab.* 280: E179–E186.

Walter, E., and Pronzato, L. 1990. Qualitative and quantitative experiment design for phenomenological models — a survey. *Automatica* 26: 195–213.

Walter, E. 1982. *Identifiability of State Space Models.* Springer-Verlag, Berlin.

10

Cardiovascular Models and Control

Fernando Casas
The Cleveland Clinic Foundation

William D. Timmons
EnteraTech, Inc.

This chapter reviews cardiovascular (CV) modeling for use in controller design, especially for closed-loop drug delivery systems (IV infusions of vasodilators, inotropes, anesthetics, neoplastic agents, and so on) and other pharmacologic applications. This first section describes the advantages and disadvantages of employing CV models for design and control and presents a brief history of CV modeling. The next section describes the basic principles and techniques for modeling the CV system, as well as the uptake, distribution, and action of cardio- and vasoactive pharmaceuticals. The chapter ends with a sample of modeling applications. A short, annotated bibliography follows the reference section for those interested in further reading.

10.1 Advantages and Disadvantages of Desktop Patients

More and more industries are coming to rely on computer simulations to increase productivity and decrease costs as well as to increase reliability and safety of resulting products. The defense, automotive, and aerospace industries come most quickly to mind, but the medical field is rapidly gaining ground in this area, too. Recent ARPA initiatives for defense technology conversion are probably most responsible for the recent surge in computer-aided health care. Today, computerized simulators teach medical students everything from basic anatomy to techniques in radial keratotomy, and skilled surgeons design, evaluate, and practice new and risky procedures without ever cutting into a single patient. Thanks to the ARPA initiative, telesurgery will soon be viable, so that in the near future, surgeons may operate on patients from half a world away. From the calculation of simple-dosage regimens to the design of sophisticated blood pressure controllers, cardiovascular medicine also benefits from this technology. CV models can be used to prove initial feasibility, reduce development time, decrease costs, and increase reliability and safety of cardiovascular devices and therapeutics.

The increasing speed and decreasing costs of computers are having an enormous impact on controller design. There is a veritable explosion in the number of control designs as well as the theory to go with them. The ready availability of powerful computer workstations and sophisticated engineering design packages (e.g., MATLAB, LabView, MATRIXx) allow for the interactive design of high-performance, robust controllers. Engineers can tweak a controller or perturb a system, then immediately assess the effect. When combined with modern visualization techniques, these tools allow one to readily see problems and solutions that might otherwise have taken years to find and solve. Furthermore, such capabilities allow for exhaustive testing and debugging, so that the transition from the workbench to the field becomes smooth. Many companies and agencies have reported flawless transitions from the simulator to the field, most notably NASA, with its many satellites and probes that have had to work right the first time. Various companies are using simulations to improve or correct equipment and systems already in the field. A recent example is BAE Automated Systems Inc. of Dallas, Texas, which is using simulations to help debug and correct the troubled baggage system at the new Denver International Airport [Geppert, 1994].

The risk of failure or the fear of malpractice often precludes the design and evaluation of controllers in live humans, so that devices and treatments are often tested on computer and animal models first. In the past, animals have been the preferred choice, but this approach is continually being reevaluated. Whereas most researchers readily agree that animal experimentation has been and will continue to be necessary for the advancement of medical science, most would welcome methods and procedures that might reduce or even eliminate the use of animals. Furthermore, animals are rarely perfect models of human diseases and conditions. Thus, there has been and will continue to be a demand for alternative models and procedures. Tissue cultures are beginning to fill some of this need, and it is likely that computer modeling and simulation may also fill this need.

Desktop patients, if used to complement animal studies, can actually increase the reliability and applicability of certain animal tests, while also reducing the number of required experiments. In certain instances, computer modeling may be the only way to test a device prior to human use, since some human conditions are extremely difficult if not impossible to reproduce in animals. Indeed, as computers become more powerful and models become better, it may be that some day computers will be used in place of certain animal and human trials. Meanwhile, computer models can be used to (1) demonstrate feasibility, (2) increase confidence in controller designs by complementing animal studies, (3) help design better animal and clinical experiments, and (4) reduce the number of required animal and human experiments.

The disadvantage of using computer simulation is that available models will almost certainly need to be tailored to the application at hand. Since there is generally no predefined method for modeling or for modifying an existing model, the accuracy and reliability of the resulting model will depend heavily on the skill of the modeler, the appropriateness of the modifications, and the model's intended scope. Furthermore, modeling typically requires a good understanding of the physics of the problem, and this in turn requires supporting data and experimentation. Thus, modifications to include new pharmaceuticals may be problematic, since their mechanisms may only be poorly understood. And, even if supporting data are available, if a basic model does not yet exist, a significant time commitment may be required to develop one. Despite this up-front cost, model development may save tremendous time and costs later in the development process.

Fortunately, there are a large number of CV models to pick from, and experienced modelers can determine which, if any, is best for a given application. Once determined, the model can usually be converted easily to a form compatible with the development platform. Once converted, model integrity and suitability must be checked. Modifications can then be made, after which the model integrity must again be checked to ensure that it has not been compromised. Once a model is obtained and suitably modified, adequate thought must be given to program flow. Ideally, program flow should be designed such that the controller code is the same for real time and for simulation. This may be facilitated by treating all facets of data acquisition as part of the controlled system, instead of as part of the controller.

With this approach, all software for I/O and calibration would be bundled separately from the controller software. Windows-based systems facilitate this separation even further by allowing the controller and plant software to be compiled and run as two separate programs.

Other issues that must be considered involve the practical aspects of computer simulation. Even if a well-designed and validated model exists, many factors can affect the accuracy of the simulation. Stiffness, machine precision, program coding, integration method, step size, and even computer language can affect the results. Probably more insidious than all these factors is the operation of the model in regions outside its scope. This happens most often in large, complex programs when a variable takes on values outside its intended range. For example, a sudden increased cardiac preload may shift the end diastolic volume of the heart into a nonlinear region of the diastolic pressure-volume relationship. If the nonlinear behavior is not included in the model, misleading results might be produced. Finally, even in the best commercial code (let alone home-brewed code), bugs may affect simulation accuracy. For example, many commercial simulation packages are particularly poor at handling discrete events (such as a bolus infusion of a drug) when variable step-size algorithms are used to integrate continuous time models [Gustafsson, 1993].

10.2   History of Cardiovascular Modeling

William Harvey in the early 17th century was probably the first to clearly and convincingly demonstrate the role of the heart as a pump which caused the blood to flow in a unidirectional closed circuit through the systemic and pulmonary circulations. Prior to Harvey, the Galenic viewpoint from the 2d century ad predominated, namely, that the blood ebbed to and fro in the veins to provide nutrition to the rest of the body, that the arteries (from the Greek arteria, meaning windpipe) carried air, that the lungs cooled the heart and removed sooty impurities from new blood as it entered from the intestines, and that the heart contained pores to allow spirit or gaseous exchange across the septum [Acierno, 1994].

It was Stephen Hales in his Statistical Essays nearly a century later who considered arterial elasticity and postulated its buffering effect on the pulsatile nature of blood flow [Hales, 1733]. He likened the depulsing effect to the fire engines of his day, in which a chamber with an air-filled dome ("inverted globe") acted to cushion the bolus from the inlet water pump so that "a more nearly equal spout" flowed out the nozzle. This analogy became the basis of the first modern cardiovascular models and antedated the ARPA movement by quite a few decades! In the translation from English to German, Hales's inverted globe became a windkessel (air kettle); his idea later became known as the Windkessel theory when it was more formally developed and propounded by the German physiologist Otto Frank (of the Frank–Starling law of the heart) near the beginning of our century [Noordergraaf, 1978].

Frank was initially a strong proponent of the Windkessel theory, and his work spawned the interest of many subsequent investigators and led to a proliferation of modified Windkessel-type models. A critical review of these early models can be found in Aperia [1940]. The development of the analog computer shortly after World War II lead to another burst in CV modeling, based on more sophisticated segmental and transmission line theories. Grodins [1959] was probably one of the first to use these new machines to simulate cardiovascular hemodynamics. Interestingly, another early analog computer model, PHYSBE [McLeod, 1966], became a popular benchmark that is still used today to evaluate computers and simulation languages. About the mid-1970s, the advent of the inexpensive digital computer led to another revolution in CV modeling, which has continued to the present with ever-increasingly detail and scope. As Rideout [1991] observed, model complexity seems to have been limited only by computer technology. If this trend continues, we can expect to see highly detailed models emerging within the next few years as parallel computers become economical.

The major criticism of the pure Windkessel theory is that it does not allow for finite wave propagation and reflection in the arteries. Whereas blood flow in the arterial vasculature is more properly formulated in terms of space and time, the Windkessel theory ignores spacial considerations and instead lumps all the vasculature into a single point, or compartment, in space. Attempts to correct this shortcoming include adding inertial and damping factors as well as collapsible components. In addition, the great arteries can be partitioned into sections to produce segmental models, or, when electrical network theory is invoked, transmission line models. Frank himself realized that the Windkessel theory was flawed, and so he too added modifications to include traveling waves and reflections [Noordergraaf, 1978; Milnor, 1989; Rideout, 1991].

Despite its flaws, the pure Windkessel theory is still useful as a teaching tool because of its simplicity and clear, intuitive imagery. Furthermore, as mean pressure accounts for approximately 90% of the power in the arterial pressure waveform, it performs surprisingly well and displays many of the interesting phenomena seen in the vasculature. Add to this the fact that the equations are readily extended to include spacial effects (the segmental and transmission line models), and one can see why the theory has persisted into the late 20th century. Of course, one must keep in mind that any of these approaches is only an approximation; the segmental and transmission line approaches are in many ways only a mathematical convenience that allows one to fit an arbitrarily high-order model to observed data. These approaches do not necessarily lend themselves to extrapolations and predictions regarding the physiology.

Even before Frank, there was great interest in the pure mathematics of blood flow in distensible vessels. Many a famous mathematician and scientist explored wave propagation, reflection, and pressure-flow relations in blood vessels, including: Bernoulli, Euler, Young (of Young's modulus), Poiseuille, Navier and Stokes, the Weber brothers, Resal, Moens and Korteweg, Lamb, and Witzig; more recent investigators including Morgan and Kiely, and Womersley and McDonald [Noordergraaf, 1978; Fung, 1984; Milnor, 1989]. Womersley and McDonald's students continue to be influential in cardiovascular modeling today. Early studies of theoretical hemodynamics greatly influenced the field of fluid mechanics and paved the way for modern pulse-wave propagation and reflection models of the vasculature. These models are treated in the texts by Noordergraaf [1978], Fung [1985], Li [1987], and Milnor [1989].

The hydrodynamic pulse-wave CV models are not without criticisms either. For example, they are limited to short segments of the arterial or venous tree for which input and terminal impedances must be supplied. This restriction makes them currently impractical for the analysis of long-acting pharmaceutical agents and their feedback effects on the cardiovascular system. Pharmaceuticals with vaso- and cardio-active effects usually require the tracking of drug concentrations throughout the body, which, for these models, would require an exceedingly large number of components and would result in huge programs requiring large computers, with the simulations invariably being slow and cumbersome. Furthermore, numerical techniques such as the finite-element method must be used to solve many of the hydrodynamic equations, which over extended periods might incur significant round-off and integration errors. Nevertheless, this approach will certainly form the basis of future pharmacologically linked CV models as faster and more sophisticated computers and algorithms are developed.

Because of the current shortfall in computational technology, most pharmacologic simulations requiring a CV model employ simplified or reduced-order models mentioned earlier. Besides the segmental and transmission line approaches, purely black box models are also used. The reduced segmental and transmission line models are probably most appropriate for simulations of fast-acting CV pharmaceuticals, whereas compartmental models (see Chapter 9) are more appropriate for slower-acting drugs.

The distinction between segmental and transmission line models has become increasingly blurred, especially as elements of both are often combined into the same model. Transmission line models were used as early as 1905 by Frank, although Westerhof and Noordergraaf [1969] were probably most influential in promoting the transmission line approach. As a result, these models are often called Westkessel models. They employ black box, two-terminal circuits (Westkessel terminations) to reproduce the input impedances of lumped vascular trees. Segmental models, however, are generally three terminal circuits, with two terminals representing inertial flows and viscous resistances and the third representing the compliance of the segment with respect to an external reference (typically atmospheric pressure). The segmental approach is described in more detail below.

As mentioned above, reduction in model order is typically achieved by combining segmental and transmission line models. The idea here is to represent critical, nonlinear components by segments, while the less critical, more linear components are lumped together and represented by Westkessel terminations.

Unfortunately, the black box Westkessel sections lose their physiologic meaning, which may present a problem in certain applications.

The highly simplified black box models are even worse in this regard. They are less concerned with the physiology than with the input-output relationships of the system and typically employ linear dynamics fit to observed patient responses. Though easy to implement, once defined, physiologically relevant per-turbations may be difficult to produce. Furthermore, these models should not be used to infer properties or behaviors outside the range of the data sets. This is a potentially crippling drawback, especially when designing and evaluating CV controllers. However, if the goal is to generate clinically observed behaviors irrespective of the pathophysiology, then these models make an excellent choice.

Another potential drawback, which applies to both simplified and reduced-order models, is the loss of phenomena associated with pulse propagation and its effects on cardiac-arterial coupling and energetics. These effects are usually considered minor from a pharmacologic point of view, but their omission may lead to potentially serious design flaws when the resulting controller is used in certain patient populations. For example, isolated systolic hypertension (ISH) significantly contributes to strokes and heart disease in the elderly, and O'Rourke [1993] suggests that the therapy of choice, as well as the goal of treatment, should be different for ISH than for diastolic and mean arterial hypertension. It may be prudent, then, for control applications aimed at this population to be evaluated on more detailed models.

10.3 Cardiovascular Modeling

In this section, the concepts behind the segmental CV approach are described. Neurohumoral controls are also briefly discussed, as is the inclusion of pharmacokinetics and pharmacodynamics for drug uptake, distribution, and action.

10.3.1 An Idealized Segment of Artery

A short segment of artery can be modeled by an elastic, isobaric chamber attached to a rigid inlet and outlet tube (Figure 10.1). The ability of the chamber to store fluid depends on its compliance, C, which is defined as

$$C = \frac{dV_c}{dP_c} \tag{10.1}$$

where V_c is total segment (chamber) volume and P_c is chamber pressure. Many modelers prefer to use the reciprocal of compliance (termed stiffness, S, or elastance, E). Here, viscoelastic (stress relaxation) effects are assumed negligible, so that compliance is not an explicit function of time. Thus, compliance

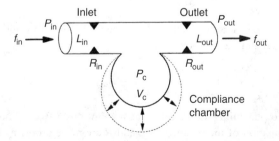

FIGURE 10.1   Idealized segment of artery approximated by an elastic, isobaric chamber attached to a rigid inlet and outlet tube. P_{in}, P_{out}, and P_c are inlet, outlet, and chamber pressures; f_{in} and f_{out} are flows; L_{in} and L_{out} are inertances; R_{in} and R_{out} are viscous resistances to flow; and V_c is total segment (chamber) volume. Compliance C is defined in the text.

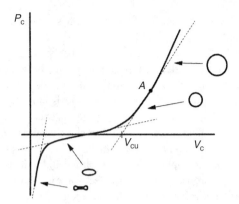

FIGURE 10.2   Static pressure–volume (P–V) relationship of a segment of artery.

becomes an instantaneous variable which can be obtained from the experimentally determined, steady-state pressure–volume (P–V) relationship of the segment. Furthermore, model order can now be reduced, as pressure can be mathematically represented as an empirical function of volume, either by a piecewise linear approximation, a polynomial quotient, or some other function fit to the P–V relationship. A typical P–V curve is illustrated in Figure 10.2, along with its piecewise linear approximation.

In arteries, pressure is usually positive with small oscillations about a nominal operating point (point A in Figure 10.2). Hence the piecewise linear approximation can be reduced to a single line with constant slope $1/C$:

$$P_c = \frac{(V_c - V_{cu})}{C} \tag{10.2}$$

where V_{cu} is the unstressed volume (the idealized zero-pressure volume intercept). Of course, if pressure fluctuates outside this region, then additional straight-line sections should be included.

Assuming that blood is incompressible and newtonian, that the flow profile is parabolic and unchanging with axial distance along a straight rigid tube, then flow (poisenillean) is linearly proportional to the pressure gradient across the ends of the tube. Hence, flow into and out of the chamber in Figure 10.1 may be calculated given P_{in} and P_{out} (the inlet and outlet pressures); P_c; L_{in} and L_{out} (the inertances due to fluid mass); and R_{in} and R_{out} (the resistances due to viscous drag)

$$L_{in}\frac{df_{in}}{dt} + R_{in}f_{in} = P_{in} - P_c$$
$$L_{out}\frac{df_{out}}{dt} + R_{out}f_{out} = P_c - P_{out} \tag{10.3}$$

where f_{in} and f_{out} are the flows into and out of the segment. Volume can now be calculated from the difference between the inlet and outlet flows:

$$\frac{dV_c}{dt} = f_{in} - f_{out} \tag{10.4}$$

P_c, V_c, f_{in}, and f_{out} can now be uniquely determined at any time given P_{in}, P_{out}, and the initial conditions of the segment. Determination of the parameters L and R are more problematic. They can be derived analytically, although probably because the modeling assumptions are not completely correct, an empirical fit generally produces better segmental properties.

The simplified segmental structure can be represented as an RLC circuit as shown in Figure 10.3a. Tsitlik et al. [1992] remind us that each capacitor should contain a residual charge to simulate the respective

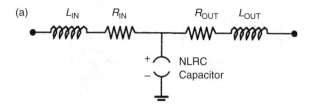

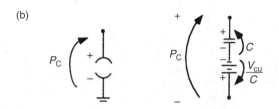

FIGURE 10.3   (a) The idealized segment of artery from Figure 10.1 as an RLC circuit. (b) The nonlinear residual charge capacitor in (a). (After Tsitlik J.E. et al. 1992. *Ann. Biomed. Eng.* 20: 595.)

segment's unstressed volume (V_{cu}). This can be achieved most easily by inserting a battery between a standard capacitor and ground (Figure 10.3b) [Tsitlik et al., 1992]. Or, if the unstressed volume for the segment remains constant (say, because the pharmacologic drug of interest has little effect on it), then the unstressed volume (and the battery) can be eliminated by subtracting it from the total vascular blood volume. The segment will then contain the stressed volume only (V_c-V_{cu}), so that an ordinary capacitor will suffice (again assuming operation near point A on the P–V curve).

10.3.2   An Idealized Segment of Vein

In most of the venous circulation, the pressure inside the vessels is greater than the external pressure, so that the pressure-flow relationship is like that in the arteries. However, in the vena cava, in certain organs such as the lungs and during certain procedures such as resuscitation or measurement of blood pressure using a cuff, venous collapse may occur [Fung, 1984]. Thus, in contrast to an artery in which only one condition normally exists, two additional conditions must be considered for a vein.

The first condition occurs when the inlet and outlet transmural pressures are positive. [Transmural pressure is defined as the pressure gradient across the vessel wall ($P_{inside}-P_{outside}$).] In this instance, the vein can be treated as discussed above for an artery. A second condition occurs when the inlet and outlet transmural pressures are negative. In this instance, the vein will collapse, and flow will stop or be greatly reduced.

The third condition occurs when the inlet transmural pressure is positive and the outlet transmural pressure is negative. In this instance, blood flows into the chamber but not out because the outlet will be collapsed. As blood flows in, the pressure inside rises until it exceeds the external pressure, forcing the outlet open and allowing blood to flow out. But, as blood flows out, the internal pressure decreases, so that the outlet transmural pressure may become negative again, collapsing the outlet, and commencing the next cycle. This cycling is called flutter, and the collapsing at the outlet, choking. Besides flutter, a limited steady-state flow is also possible if the outlet is not completely choked off [Fung, 1984]. Limited flow is the predominant (and likely the only) effect occurring under physiologic conditions [Noordergraaf, 1978].

Purmutt et al. [1962] described this effect as a vascular waterfall. Water flowing over a falls depend only on conditions at the top, not on the length of the drop. In 1994 Holt used the term flow regulator for this effect in his seminal work on the collapsible penrose tube, and Conrad in 1969 called it a negative impedance conduit [Noordergraaf, 1978]. Starling in 1915 also made use of this concept when he used a collapsible tube, now known as a Starling resistor, to control peripheral resistance in his heart–lung

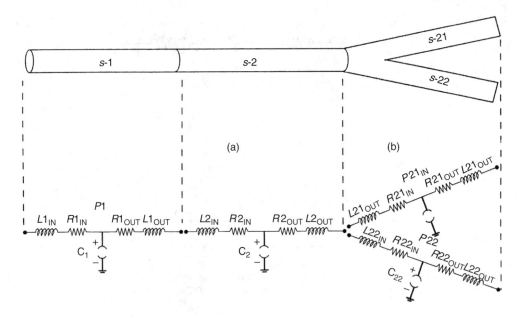

FIGURE 10.4   (a) A segmented, arbitrary length of vessel. (b) The equivalent RLC circuit.

preparations. Once flutter was found to be absent in the human physiology, Brower in 1970, Brower and Noordergraaf in 1973, and Griffiths in 1975 developed simplified equations of the pressure–flow relationship [Noordergraaf, 1978]. Snyder and Rideout [1969] also developed a model of collapsible vein. They employed a two-line approximation of the $P-V$ curve — one for the uncollapsed region and one for the collapsed region. Then, based on modifications of the Navier–Stokes equations for an elliptical tube (the cross-sectional shape of a collapsing vessel), and assuming a flat flow profile, they were able to relate flow to pressure and volume in terms of nonlinear inertances, resistances, and compliances in Equation 10.2 and Equation 10.3. They also included the effects of gravity and external pressures in the model.

10.3.3   Arterial and Venous Trees

By using the output of one segment as the input to a second, and the output of the second as the input to a third, and so on, differential equations for arbitrary lengths of vessel can be constructed (Figure 10.4a). This method also allows bifurcations to be added. Another approach can be used to derive these same equations. First, partial differential equations are formulated to define flow along the desired length of vessel. The spacial differentials are then changed to finite differences, leaving only time derivatives [Noordergraaf, 1978].

Similar to an arterial section, the resulting lumped model of the vascular tree can be represented as an electrical circuit if desired (Figure 10.4b), and nearby resistors and inductances can be combined to form Γ, T, or PI sections. A similar approach can be used for the venous circulation. To prevent ringing and other problems due to sudden impedance changes, it is often useful to add intermediate segments to taper the impedances between the heart and the capillaries [Rideout, 1991]. That is, the impedances of the large arteries should be tapered to match the higher resistive impedances of the arterioles and capillary beds and then reduced back again from the capillary beds to the large veins.

Arterial and venous branching can be roughly grouped by vessel size (large, medium, and small arteries, arterioles, capillaries, etc.) or by organ system (heart, head, legs, liver, fat, skin, muscle, etc.). Vessel grouping is useful when the model needs to track drug concentrations at whole-body effector sites, such as nitroprusside concentration in the systemic arteriolar and venous compartments. Organ grouping is useful when the model needs to track drug concentrations in certain organs, such as insulin in the liver,

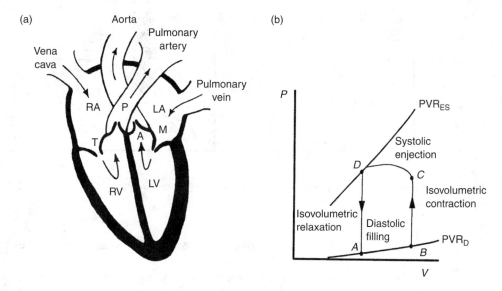

FIGURE 10.5 (a) The chambers and valves of the heart. LV, left ventricle; RV, right ventricle; LA, left atrium; RA, right atrium; M, mitral valve; A, aortic valve; T, tricuspid valve; P, pulmonary valve. (b) The left ventricular cardiac cycle in the P–V plane. See text.

glucose in the pancreas, or antineoplastic agents in diseased tissues. Note that within each organ, the flows can be broken down further by vessel size or by regional or conceptual intraorgan blood flows. Once the desired organs and vessels are described, Westkessel-type impedances can be used for the rest of the vasculature.

10.3.4 Models of the Heart

The heart is a muscular pump with four chambers intimately linked into one organ (Figure 10.5a). Nevertheless, in modeling the heart, each chamber is usually modeled independently of the others. Each is typically set up as an elastic compartment with inertance and resistance similar to an artery or vein (see above). The differences are (1) that valves are included to constrain flow to one direction, and (2) that elastance (the inverse of compliance) is treated as a time-varying parameter.

The valves are straightforward and are often implemented as ideal diodes (for electrical circuit models) or as IF-THEN-ELSE statements (for algorithmic models) to keep all flows nonnegative. Defects in the valves can be added to simulate heart defects (e.g., leaky diodes for regurgitation). Other types of heart defects are just as easily simulated. For example, Blackstone et al. [1976] placed an impedance between the atrial chambers to simulate a septal opening.

Mathematical representation of the time-varying elastance is more complicated and is generally based on the characterization of the cardiac work cycle in the pressure-volume plane. In the P–V diagram in Figure 10.5b, the time course of the left ventricular cardiac cycle proceeds as follows.

During diastolic filling (A to B), ventricular pressure is below atrial and aortic pressures, so the mitral valve (between the left atrium and the left ventricle) is open, and the aortic valve (between the left ventricle and the aorta) is closed. Blood therefore flows from the atrium into the ventricle, based on the pressure gradient and the inertances and resistances of the inlet. Note that the pressure gradient will decrease as the ventricle fills due to the passive compliance of the chamber and the drop in pressure in the atrium.

After diastole, the ventricle is stimulated to contract so that pressure rises above the atrial pressure, closing the mitral valve. In this state, pressure is too low for the aortic valve to open, so that both valves are closed and no blood flow occurs. Meanwhile, the ventricle continues to contract, raising ventricular

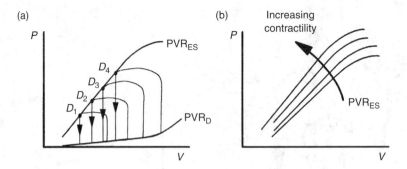

FIGURE 10.6   (a) Heart cycles with varying preload and afterload. (b) The end-systolic P–V curve with increasing contractility of the heart.

pressure. This period (B to C) is termed isovolumetric contraction. Here, the muscle contraction can be thought of as decreasing the compliance of the chamber.

Once ventricular pressure exceeds the pressure in the aorta, the aortic valve opens and systolic ejection commences (C to D). Blood flows out from the ventricle into the aorta based on the pressure gradient, the inertances, and the resistances of the outlet. The muscle continues to contract until the cardiac action potentials have run their course.

As the muscle begins to relax, pressure will drop until it falls below the aortic pressure. At this time, the aortic valve closes, and again blood flow ceases. Meanwhile, the ventricle continues to relax, decreasing the ventricular pressure. This period (D to A) is termed isovolumetric relaxation. Here, muscle relaxation can be thought of as increasing the compliance of the chamber. Finally, ventricular pressure falls below atrial pressure, the mitral valve opens, and the cycle begins anew.

Suga and Sagawa [1972, 1974] identified and characterized several key properties of the time-varying compliance in the pressure-volume plane. In their experiments, they varied preload, afterload, stroke volume, cardiac contractility, and heart rate for both ejecting beats (heart valves patent) and isovolumic beats (heart valves sewn shut). Four observations should be noted. First, the P–V point at the end of systole (Figure 10.6a, points D_1–D_4) nearly always lies along the static P–V curve for activated myocardium. Second, the end systolic P–V curve is unaffected by changes in preload and afterload (Figure 10.6a); however, it is affected by changes in cardiac contractility (Figure 10.6b). Third, t_{max}, the time to end systole (point D), is also unaffected by changes in preload and afterload; however, it is affected by changes in cardiac contractility and heart rate. And fourth, the ventricular filling phase allows the static P–V curve for relaxed myocardium, as expected. There are some deviations from these observations, but over normal ranges these behaviors are fairly reliable [Sunagawa and Sagawa, 1982; Maughan et al., 1984].

Based on these observations, a continuum of static P–V relationships can be visualized as spanning the space between the fully relaxed and the fully contracted curves, say, as a linear combination of the two. The active curve at any time could then be construed as a function of the activity level of the myocardium, α, which itself could be a function of time and t_{max}, and which would range from zero (inactive) to one (fully active):

$$\mathrm{PVR}(\alpha(t, t_{max})) = \alpha(t, t_{max}) \cdot \mathrm{PVR_{ES}} + (1 - \alpha(t, t_{max})) \cdot \mathrm{PVR_D} \tag{10.5}$$

Here, PVR (pressure–volume relationship) is the active P–V curve, and $\mathrm{PVR_{ES}}$ and $\mathrm{PVR_D}$ are the end systolic and diastolic P–V curves, respectively. Using this approach, the $\mathrm{PVR_{ES}}$ curve would be parameterized in terms of the inotropic state of the myocardium, and t_{max} would be a function of inotropic state and heart rate.

Suga and Sagawa [1972] originally approximated the two curves, $\mathrm{PVR_{ES}}$ and $\mathrm{PVR_D}$, with two straight lines that intersected in a common point on the volume axis (V_d, the unstressed, or dead, volume). This was a reasonable approximation, since, in their original experiments, the nonlinear portions of the P–V curves were not encountered. Based on this approach, the elastance E as a function of time becomes greatly simplified:

$$E(t) = \frac{P(t)}{V(t) - V_d} \quad (10.6)$$

With this formulation, $\alpha(t, t_{max})$ maps to $E(t)$ by the relation

$$E(t) = \alpha(t, t_{max}) \cdot E_{max} + (1 - \alpha(t, t_{max})) \cdot E_{min} \quad (10.7)$$

where E_{min} and E_{max} are the minimum and maximum elastances. E_{max} sets the inotropic state, and E_{min} sets the diastolic filling curve. A later modification allowed each curve to have its own dead volume [Sunagawa and Sagawa, 1982].

A common definition of $\alpha(t, t_{max})$ is a squared sine wave, time scaled and shifted to fit its first half-period into the systolic time interval, and zeroed elsewhere, for example, see Martin et al. [1986]. Another common definition uses the first half-period of a sine wave, time-scaled and shifted to fit into the systolic interval. It is sometimes clipped and sometimes modified with a second harmonic to skew the waveform, for example, see Rideout [1991]. Still others have approximated $\alpha(t, t_{max})$ as a square wave [Warner, 1959], a triangle wave [McLeod, 1966; Katona et al., 1967], a sum of charging and discharging exponentials [Sun and Chiaramida, 1992], and even as a sum of gaussian (bell-shaped) exponentials [Chung et al., 1994].

Pulsations can likewise be added to the other heart chambers, although the shape of the elastance curves are somewhat different [Sunagawa and Sagawa, 1982]. In the left ventricle, $E(t)$ appears more like a skewed sine wave while $V_d(t)$ is fairly constant during ejection; in the right ventricle, $E(t)$ appears more like a squared sine wave with a larger E_{max}, while $V_d(t)$ varies continuously throughout the systolic period; in the right atrium, $E(t)$ and $V_d(t)$ behave as in the right ventricle. A common simplification of this relationship was employed by Leaning et al. [1983]. They used the same function for each chamber's elastance (in this case a sine wave), but with a different E_{min}, E_{max}, and t_{max} for each, as well as a different time shift to contract them when appropriate, for example, the atria prior to the ventricles. As is common, they also made V_d constant, though each chamber was provided with a different value.

Since the activation function is typically time-scaled to fit within the heart period, the effect of a changing heart rate, say, due to neural reflexes, can be explored. However, this requires that the heart period itself be partitioned into diastolic and systolic intervals. Various partitioning schemes exist. For the left ventricle, some fix the duration of systole [Grodins, 1959] or set it to a percentage of the heart period, with diastole taking up the rest of the period [Rideout, 1991]. A general clinic rule allocates one-third to systole and two-thirds to diastole. However, Beneken and DeWit [1967], after summarizing several publications, suggest that ventricular systole is better approximated by one-fifth the heart period plus 0.16 sec. Likewise, they determined the duration of atrial systole as 9/100 the heart period plus 0.1 sec. These formulae have gained considerable popularity, for example, see Leaning et al. [1983] and Rideout [1991].

In many drug-delivery applications, the time constants of interest are on the order of minutes to hours. In these situations, a pulsatile heart is not needed and can be traded advantageously for a mean flow model. Mean flow models are based either on the Frank–Starling law of the heart or on the pulsatile model above. In the Frank–Starling approach, a family of flow curves is constructed based on experimental observations of the heart under various conditions of preload and afterload (Figure 10.7) [Sagawa, 1967]. These are then used to calculate stroke volume for each beat. In the other approach, the stroke volume is derived analytically from the equations of the pulsatile heart [Rideout, 1991]. When using the Frank-Starling law, attenuation factors are used to impose the effects of inotropic state and heart rate. Examples of nonpulsatile heat models include those by Sagawa [1967], Greenway [1982], Möller et al. [1983], and Tham et al. [1990]. The Guyton–Coleman model [Guyton et al., 1972, 1980] is also nonpulsatile heart, though it uses a very different approach (see below).

Some models of the uptake and distribution of slow-acting drugs do not explicitly use a heart, or, for that matter, a circulation. These fall under the category of purely compartmental models. In these

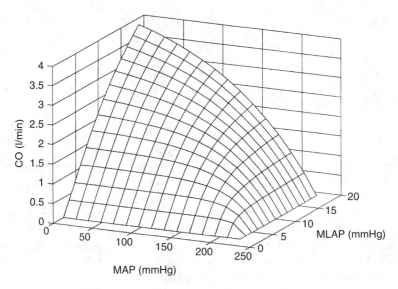

FIGURE 10.7   The Frank-Starling law of the heart; 3-D of Sagawa's [1967] left-ventricle equation for a 10-kg dog; CO, cardiac output; MAP, mean arterial pressure; MLAP, mean left arterial pressure.

models, the heart and circulation are subsumed into an assumption that each compartment in the model is uniformly mixed (see Chapter 9).

10.3.5   Models of Combined Heart and Circulation

Whole-body CV models couple a model of the heart to models of the vasculature. The complexity of the coupling depends on the particular need and can give rise to nonpulsatile left side (*left side* meaning the systemic circulation) only, nonpulsatile left and right side (*right side* meaning the pulmonary circulation), and pulsatile left and right side models [Rideout, 1991].

Left-side-only models are justified when the pharmaceutical agents of interest have little effect on the pulmonary circulation. In these cases, the right side is considered a follower circuit and hence can be eliminated to provide computational savings. Even if the agents of interest to affect the pulmonary circulation, an occamistic left-side-only model may still suffice. This approach may work for two reasons: either the model order is high enough that the right-side effects are inadvertently captured in the left-side model, or the drug effects are essentially the same on both sides. Keep in mind that these models have limited scope and hence should be used with care.

As an example of the modeling considerations for drug delivery, consider the following two drugs: propranolol, a beta blocker; and sodium nitroprusside (SNP), a vasodilator. Propranolol has a time constant on the order of 33 min, primarily affects the heart, and has only minor effects on the pulmonary circulation (although it may constrict the airways) [Ewy and Bressler, 1992; Gilman et al., 1993]. Hence, for propranolol, a nonpulsatile left-side-only model should be adequate for controller design. SNP, however, has a transport delay of 0.5 min and a time constant between 0.25 and 0.50 min. It affects the arterioles, the venous unstressed volume, and venous compliance. It also significantly decreases pulmonary wedge pressure [Ewy and Bressler, 1992; Gilman et al., 1993; Greenway, 1982]. Hence, for SNP, a nonpulsatile model is questionable, though it may be adequate. Furthermore, a two-sided model should be used, since SNP may have a significant effect on the pulmonary circulation. Greenway's [1982] two-sided nonpulsatile model seems to function adequately, although other investigators have switched to two-sided pulsatile models, for example, see Yu et al., 1990.

Interestingly, Martin et al. [1986] may have finessed the field of nonpulsatile models by overcoming the speed limitations associated with pulsatile models. They did this by solving the pulsatile model equations

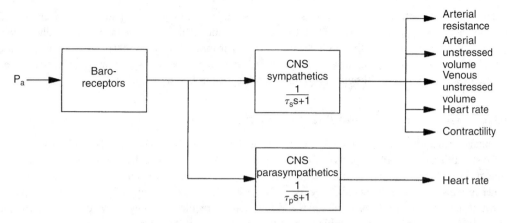

FIGURE 10.8 Baroreceptor firing rate is passed through a low-pass filter representing the CNS and then mapped back to changes in heart rate, contractility, vascular resistances, and vascular unstressed volumes.

semi-analytically, and were thus able to significantly reduce simulation time. Their model currently makes an attractive choice for studying and designing automated drug-delivery systems.

Despite the emphasis here on nonlinear CV-based modeling, probably the most used model for the design of blood pressure controllers is the model by Slate and Sheppard [1982]. It is based on a linear, first-order impulse response of the effects of nitroprusside on mean arterial blood pressure. The model includes a recirculation effect, as well as an occasionally observed nonlinear reflex (possibly due to the chemoreceptors). It has gained wide acceptance probably because of its simplicity. Nevertheless, it has severe limitations: it lumps the effects of the primary neural and humoral reflexes as well as the patient drug sensitivity into one gain; it does not account for the effect of changing cardiac output on drug transport; and it is not easily extended to include additional drugs or disease states.

10.3.6 Neural and Humoral Control

Once the heart and vasculature are linked, neural and hormonal controls need to be added. These include the baroreflex, the chemoreflex, the renin-angiotensin reflex, capillary fluid shift, autoregulation, stress relaxation, and renal–body-fluid balance (water intake and urine output).

Baroreceptors monitor the pressure in the carotid sinuses, the aortic arch, and other large systemic arteries and increase their firing rate when the pressure increases. Their response is nonlinear and depends on whether they are exposed to mean pressure only, pulsatile pressure only, or a combination of both. Katona et al. [1967] developed a model of baroreceptor feedback that has become the basis for many CV neural control models. The output of the baroreceptor model is often passed through a low pass filter representing the CNS and then mapped back to changes in heart rate, contractility, vascular resistances, and vascular unstressed volumes through the sympathetic and parasympathetic nervous systems (Figure 10.8), for example, see Yu et al. [1990].

In addition to baroreceptors, chemoreceptors may also mediate a strong CV response, especially when systemic arterial pressure falls below 80 mmHg [Guyton et al., 1972; see also Dampney, 1994]. This reflex, through the CNS, increases cardiac activity and peripheral resistance. Strangely, few models include this effect, although Slate and Sheppard [1982] may have inadvertently included it in their simplified black box model.

The renin-angiotensin reflex is mediated hormonally through the kidneys. When pressure falls below normal, renin is secreted into the blood stream by the kidneys, which then causes the release of free angiotensin. Angiotensin causes marked vasoconstriction and thus increases peripheral resistance and arterial pressure. This reflex is often included in models because it plays an important role in many forms of hypertension and heart failure.

The other CV control reflexes are only sometimes included, although these and others are elucidated and modeled by Guyton et al. [1972, 1980]. In his elaborate model, there are five main empirically derived physiologic function blocks with many subcomponents. The model has nearly 400 parameters and is quite remarkable in its scope. Given current computer technology, however, it is somewhat cumbersome for drug delivery applications, although it promises to have great utility in the future.

10.3.7 Combined CV and Pharmacologic Models

For pharmacologic control studies, CV models readily lend themselves to the calculation of drug uptake and distribution to the various parts of the body (pharmacokinetics). Once the transport model has been built, models of drug action (pharmacodynamics) then need to be linked and related back to the CV model. Other models must also be linked if necessary. For example, models of inhalational anesthetic uptake, distribution, and effect on the respiratory and CV systems require not only a CV and pharmacologic model but also a lung model. Combined models such as these are known as multiple models, a term coined by Rideout's group [Beneken and Rideout, 1968; Rideout, 1991]. Again, the time course of the agents and their effects on the heart and circulation determine whether a pulsatile or nonpulsatile model is needed, as well as the requisite level of vascular detail.

To calculate drug uptake and transport, mass balance equations can be set up for each segment and compartment in the CV model. Additional compartments, such as a tissue or an effects compartment, can also be added (see Chapter 9). For example, given a particular compartment (or segment), the mass of drug in the compartment is calculated as follows:

$$\frac{dq_i}{dt} = f_{in,i}c_{i-1} - f_{out,i}c_i \tag{10.8}$$

where i identifies the compartment, q is the mass of drug, c is its concentration, f_{in} is the rate of blood flow into the compartment (normally equal to the flow out of the previous compartment), and f_{out} is the rate of blood flow out of the compartment. The instantaneous concentration in any compartment can then be calculated based on drug mass and total volume of the compartment (stressed plus unstressed volumes);

$$c_i = \frac{q_i}{V_i} \tag{10.9}$$

Once the concentration is known at the effector site, a pharmacodynamic model is used to describe its action. Saturation may need to be built into the effect, as well as a possible threshold concentration. Hill's sigmoidal equation can accommodate both:

$$EFF = \frac{c_e^n}{c_{50}^n + c_e^n} \tag{10.10}$$

where EFF is the normalized pharmacologic effect ($0 \le EFF \le 1$), c_e is the concentration at the effector site, c_{50} is the half-matrix concentration, and n parameterizes the steepness of the sigmoid. Hill's equation becomes the Michaelis–Menten equation when $n = 1$.

Once calculated, the drug effect can be used to modify the parameters in the CV model, much like the neural and humoral reflexes. Resistances, compliances (including the unstressed volumes) of each segment, neural and humoral feedback gains, heart rate, and contractility are all typically modified by drugs. For example, sodium nitroprusside causes vasodilation and blood pooling; therefore it would be made to primarily increase the compliance and unstressed volume of the veins, as well as to decrease arteriolar (peripheral) resistance [Greenway, 1982; Yu et al., 1990].

10.3.8 Modeling Applications

Stand-alone CV models and their development have been somewhat disconnected from other modeling applications, in particular artificial cardiovascular assist devices. Models of ventricular assist devices (VADs), total artificial hearts (TAHs), and other blood pumping devices such as cardio pulmonary bypass (CPB) pumps usually concentrate on describing the behavior and performance of the device itself. Computer modeling packages exist for designing rotary pumps as well as for testing their hydraulic performance using computational fluid dynamics (CFD). Additional computer modeling software is available for designing automatic control strategies. With the advent of increased computer processing power, the next modeling step is to integrate all these components into a comprehensive desktop patient where cardiovascular pathologies could be simulated along with the mechanical assist device, its control architecture, and its behavior with changing vascular dynamics and pharmacological effects.

Currently, modeling techniques are being used in academia, medical research, and industry. Some of their uses include describing the behavior and predicting the performance of VADs and TAHs along with their respective control strategies [Fu, 1997; Veres, 1997; Xu, 1997; Golding, 1998; Zhou, 1999; Vitale, 2001; Casas, 2004], description of not only systemic dynamics but also pulmonary venous function [Thomas, 1997], understanding of the mechanical interdependences of cardiac muscle and their implications in cardiac pathologies and treatments [McCulloch, 2001; Guccione, 2003], modeling of blood pressure and regulation of heart rate [Zhang, 2001], and effects of pharmacological treatments in cardiovascular pathologies [Popovic, 2004].

An example of simulation techniques used in the development of VADs and TAHs is presented in [Vitale, 2001] where a comprehensive dynamic model of the Cleveland Clinic Foundation — Foster Miller Technologies MagScrew blood pump was used to find the maximum device efficiency by optimizing the magnetic pitch of the noncontacting magnetic thread of the driver system. This model and corresponding numerical simulation incorporated and considered blood pump operating conditions and physiological factors such as inlet and outlet pressures and device beat rate, magnetic field strength of MagScrew and motor magnets at different dimensions, mechanical factors such as plunger motion, friction within the actuation mechanism, and electrical factors such as actuator motor bridge path resistances and supply voltages.

Results from this modeling effort not only provided information on peak efficiency operating conditions but also provided insight into other device parameters such as motor current and MagScrew forces, among others important variables, keys to the design process, and understanding of experimental tests results.

10.4 Conclusions

For designing controllers to automate cardiovascular therapeutics, the nonlinear, cardiovascular-linked pharmacologic models are well worth the added effort and time needed to construct and interface them to the design platform. Not only can they help prove initial feasibility, but they can also speed up the overall design process. For example, they can be used for interactive controller design; they can be used to design improved animal and human experiments, which can potentially reduce the total number of experiments; and they can be used to simulate human conditions that are not easily produced in animals.

The reduced compartmental and combined segmental and transmission line models are probably the most practical model form at this time given current computer technology. However, as computer technology grows, we can expect to see increasingly detailed pharmacologic models that include additional cardiovascular features such as pulse wave propagation and reflection as well as multiple short- and long-term neurohumoral feedback loops.

Acknowledgments

Dr. Casas acknowledges support from grant K01HL073076 from the National Institutes of Health and the National Heart, Lung, and Blood Institute.

The authors recognize the following individuals for their help in preparing the first edition of this work: Mr. S. Kumar for help in collecting the references; Ms. O. Huynh for help in preparing the figures; and Dr. S.E. Rittgers for his comments on the text.

References

Acierno L.J. 1994. *The History of Cardiology*, Pearl River, NY, Parthenon.

American Society for Artificial Internal Organs (ASAIO) Abstracts for the 50th Anniversary Conference. Washington, DC, USA, June 17–19, 2004. *ASAIO J.* 50: 111–186.

Aperia A. 1940. Hemodynamical studies. *Scand. Arch. Physiol.* 83: 1.

Beneken J.E.W. 1963. Investigation on the regulatory system of the blood circulation. In A. Noordergraaf, G.N. Jager and N. Westerhof (Eds.), *Circulatory Analog Computers*, pp. 16–28, Amsterdam, North-Holland.

Beneken J.E.W. 1972. Some computer models in cardiovascular research. In D.H. Bergel (Ed.), *Cardiovascular Fluid Dynamics*, vol. 1, pp. 173–223, New York, Academic Press.

Beneken J.E.W. and DeWit B. 1967. A physical approach to hemodynamic aspects of the human cardio-vascular system. In E.B. Reeve and A.C. Guyton (Eds.), *Physical Bases of Circulatory Transport*, pp. 1–45, Philadelphia, W.B. Saunders.

Beneken J.E.W. and Rideout V.C. 1968. The use of multiple models in cardiovascular system studies: transport and perturbation methods. *IEEE Trans. BME* 15: 281.

Blackstone E.H., Gupta A.K., and Rideout V.C. 1976. Cardiovascular simulation study of infants with transposition of the great arteries after surgical correction. In L. Dekker (Ed.), *Simulation of Systems*, pp. 599–608, Amsterdam, North-Holland.

Carson E.R., Cobelli C., and Finkelstein L. 1983. *The Mathematical Modeling of Metabolic and Endocrine Systems*, New York, John Wiley & Sons.

Casas F., Orozco A., Smith W.A., De Abreu-García J.A., and Durkin J. 2004. A fuzzy system cardio pulmonary bypass rotary blood pump controller. *Exp. Syst. Appl.* 26: 357–361.

Chung D.C., et al. 1994. A mathematical model of the canine circulation. In B.W. Patterson (Ed.), *Modeling and Control in Biomedical Systems: Proceedings of the IFAC Symposium*, pp. 109–112, Galveston Tex.

Dampney R.A.L. 1994. Functional organization of central pathways regulating the cardiovascular system. *Physiol. Rev.* 74: 323.

Dick D.E. and Rideout V.C. 1965. Analog simulation of left heart and arterial dynamics. *Proceedings of 18th ACEMB*, p. 78, Philadelphia.

Ewy G.A. and Bressler R. 1992. *Cardiovascular Drugs and the Management of Heart Disease*, 2nd ed., New York, Raven Press.

Frank O. 1899. Die Grundform des arteriellen Pulses. *Z. Biol.* 37: 483.

Fu M., Xu L., Medvedev A., Smith W.A. and Golding L.A. 1997. Design of a DSP controller for an innovative ventricular assist system. *ASAIO J.* 43: M615–M619.

Fung Y.C. 1984. *Biodynamics: Circulation*, New York, Springer-Verlag.

Geppert L. 1994. Faults & failures. *IEEE Spectrum* 31: 17.

Gilman A.G., Rall T.W., Nies A.S., et al. 1993. *Goodman and Gilman's The Pharmacological Basis of Therapeutics*, 8th ed., New York, McGraw-Hill.

Golding L., Medvedev A., Massiello A., Smith W., Horvath D. and Kasper R. 1998. Cleveland Clinic continuous flow blood pump: progress in development. *Artif. Organs* 22: 447–450.

Greenway C.V. 1982. Mechanisms and quantitative assessment of drug effects on cardiac output with a new model of the circulation. *Pharm. Rev.* 33: 213.

Grodins F.S. 1959. Integrative cardiovascular physiology: a mathematical synthesis of cardiac and blood vessel hemodynamics. *Q. Rev. Biol.* 34: 93.

Guccione J.M., Salahieh A., Moonly S.M., Kortsmit J., Wallace A.W. and Ratcliffe M.B. 2003. Myosplint decreases wall stress without depressing function in the failing heart: a finite element model study. *Ann. Thorac. Surg.* 76: 1171–1180 (discussion 1180).

Gustafsson K. 1993. Stepsize selection in implicit Runge-Kutta methods viewed as a control problem. *Proceedings of 12th IFAC World Congress* 5: 137.

Guyton A.C. 1980. *Arterial Pressure and Hypertension*, Philadelphia, W.B. Saunders.

Guyton A.C., Coleman T.G., Cowley A.W., et al. 1972. Systems analysis of arterial pressure regulation and hypertension. *Ann. Biomed. Eng.* 1: 254.

Hales S. 1733. *Statical Essays: Containing Haemastaticks*, vol. 2, London, Innys and Manby (Pfizer Laboratories, 1981).

Isaka S. and Sebald A.V. 1993. Control strategies for arterial blood pressure regulation. *IEEE Trans. BME.* 40: 353–363.

Katona P.G. 1988. Closed loop control of physiological variables. *Proceedings of 1st IFAC Symposium on Modelling Control Biomed Systems*, Venice.

Katona P.G., Barnett G.O. and Jackson W.D. 1967. Computer simulation of the blood pressure control of the heart period. In P. Kezdi (Ed.), *Baroreceptors and Hypertension*, pp. 191–199, Oxford, Pergamon Press.

Kono A., Maughan W.L., Sunagawa K., et al. 1984. The use of left ventricular end-ejection pressure and peak pressure in the estimation of the end-systolic pressure–volume relationship. *Circulation* 70: 1057.

Kosaka R., Sankai Y., Jikuya T., Yamane T., and Tsutsui T. 2004. Resonant frequency control for artificial heart using online parameter identification. *Artif. Organs.* 28: 921–6.

Leaning M.S., Pullen H.E., Carson E.R., et al. 1983. Modelling a complex biological system: the human cardiovascular system — 1. Methodology and model description. *Trans. Inst. Meas. Contr.* 5: 71.

Li J.K.-J. 1987. *Arterial System Dynamics*, New York, New York University Press.

Linkens D.A. and Hacisalihzade S.S. 1990. Computer control systems and pharmacological drug administration: a survey. *J. Med. Eng. Tech.* 14: 41.

Martin J.F., Schneider A.M., Mandel J.E., et al. 1986. A new cardiovascular model for real-time applications. *Trans. Soc. Comp. Sim.* 3: 31.

Maughan W.L., Sunagawa K., Burkhoff D., et al. 1984. Effect of arterial impedance changes on the end-systolic pressure-volume relation. *Circ. Res.* 54: 595.

McCulloch A.D. and Mazhari R. 2001. Regional myocardial mechanics: integrative computational models of flow — function relations. *J. Nucl. Cardiol.* 8: 506–519.

McDonald D.A. 1974. *Blood Flow in Arteries*, 2nd ed., Baltimore, Williams & Wilkins.

McLeod J. 1966. PHYSBE — a physiological simulation benchmark experiment. *Simulation* 7: 324.

Melchior F.M., Srinivasan R.S., and Charles J.B. 1992. Mathematical modeling of human cardiovascular system for simulation of orthostatic response. *Am. J. Physiol.* 262 (*Heart Circ. Physiol.* 31): H1920.

Middleman S. 1972. *Transport Phenomena in the Cardiovascular System*, New York, John Wiley & Sons.

Milnor W.R. 1989. *Hemodynamics*, 2nd ed., Baltimore, Williams & Wilkins.

Möller D., Popović D., and Thiele G. 1983. *Modeling, Simulation and Parameter-Estimation of the Human Cardiovascular System*, Friedr, Braunschweig, Vieweg & Sohn.

Noordergraaf A. 1978. *Circulatory System Dynamics*, New York, Academic Press.

O'Rourke M.F. 1982. *Arterial Function in Health and Disease*. New York, Churchill Livingstone.

O'Rourke M.F. 1993. Hypertension and the conduit and cushioning functions of the arterial tree. In M.E. Safar and M.F. O'Rourke (Eds.), *The Arterial System in Hypertension*, pp. 27–37, the Netherlands, Kluwer Academic Pub.

Popovic Z.B., Khot U.N., Novaro G.M., Casas F., Greenberg N.L., Garcia M.J., Francis G.S., and Thomas J.D. 2005. Effects of sodium nitroprusside in aortic stenosis associated with severe heart failure: pressure-volume loop analysis using a numerical model. *Am. J. Physiol. Heart Circ. Physiol.* 288(1): H416–23. Epub 2004 Sep 2.

Purmutt S., Bromberger-Barnea B. and Bane H.N. 1962. Alveolar pressure, pulmonary venous pressure, and the vascular waterfall. *Med. Thorac.* 19:239.

Reesink K., Dekker A., van der Nagel T., Blom H., Soemers C., Geskes G., Maessen J., and van der Veen E. 2004. Physiologic-insensitive left ventricular assist predisposes right-sided circulatory failure: a pilot simulation and validation study. *Artif. Organs* 28: 933–9.

Rideout V.C. 1991. *Mathematical and Computer Modeling of Physiological Systems*, Englewood Cliffs, NJ, Prentice-Hall (now distributed by Medical Physics Pub., Madison, WI).

Sagawa K. 1967. Analysis of the ventricular pumping capacity as a function of input and output pressure loads. In E.B. Reeve and A.C. Guyton (Eds.), *Physical Bases of Circulatory Transport*, pp. 141–149, Philadelphia, W.B. Saunders.

Sagawa K. 1973. Comparative models of overall circulatory mechanics. In J.H.U. Brown and J.F. Dickson III (Eds.), Advances in Biomedical Engineering, vol. 3, pp. 1–95, New York, Academic Press.

Slate J.B. and Sheppard L.C. 1982. Automatic control of blood pressure by drug infusion. *IEE Proceedings*, Pt. A 129: 639.

Snyder M.F. and Rideout V.C. 1969. Computer simulation studies of the venous circulation. *IEEE Trans. BME* 16: 325.

Suga H. and Sagawa K. 1972. Mathematical interrelationship between instantaneous ventricular pressure-volume ratio and myocardial force-velocity relation. *Ann. Biomed. Eng.* 1: 160.

Suga H. and Sagawa K. 1974. Instantaneous pressure volume relationships and their ratio in the excised, supported canine left ventricle. *Circ. Res.* 35: 117.

Sun Y. and Chiaramida S. 1992. Simulation of hemodynamics and regulatory mechanisms in the cardiovascular system based on a nonlinear and time-varying model. *Simulation* 59: 28.

Sunagawa K. and Sagawa K. 1982. Models of ventricular contraction based on time-varying elastance. *Crit. Rev. Biomed. Eng.* 9: 193.

Tham R.Q.Y., Sasse F.J., and Rideout V.C. 1990. Large-scale multiple model for the simulation of anesthesia. In D.P.F. Moller (Ed.), *Advanced Simulation in Biomedicine*, pp. 173–195, New York, Springer-Verlag.

Thomas J.D., Zhou J., Greenberg N., Bibawy G., McCarthy P.M., and Vandervoort P.M. 1997. Physical and physiological determinants of pulmonary venous flow: numerical analysis. *Am. J. Physiol.* 272: H2453–H2465.

Tsitlik J.E., Halperin H.R., Popel A.S., et al. 1992. Modeling the circulation with three-terminal electrical networks containing special nonlinear capacitors. *Ann. Biomed. Eng.* 20: 595.

Veres J.P., Golding L.A., Smith W.A., Horvath D. and Medvedev A. 1997. Flow analysis of the Cleveland Clinic centrifugal pump. *ASAIO J.* 43: M778–M781.

Vitale N. 2001. Optimization of screw pitch in a screw driven reciprocating pulsatile ventricle assist device. *Proceedings of 27th Annual Northeast Bioengineering Conference* in Storrs, CT, March 31–April 1.

Westenskow D.R. 1986. Automating patient care with closed-loop control. *MD Comput.* 3: 14.

Westerhof N. and Noordergraaf A. 1969. Reduced models of the systemic arteries. *Proceedings of 8th International Conference on Medical Engineering*, Chicago.

Xu L., Wang F., Fu M., Medvedev A., Smith W.A., and Golding L.A. 1997. Analysis of a new PM motor design for a rotary dynamic blood Pump. *ASAIO J.* 43: M559–M564.

Yu C., Roy R.J., and Kaufman H. 1990. A circulatory model for combined nitroprusside-dopamine therapy in acute heart failure. *Med. Prog. Tech.* 16: 77.

Zhang R., Behbehani K., Crandall C.G., Zuckerman J.H., and Levine B.D. 2001. Dynamic regulation of heart rate during acute hypotension: new insight into baroreflex function. *Am. J. Physiol. Heart Circ. Physiol.* 280: H407–H419.

Zhou J., Armstrong G.P., Medvedev A.L., Smith W.A., Golding L.A., and Thomas J.D. 1999. Numeric modeling of the cardiovascular system with a left ventricular assist device. *ASAIO J.* 45: 83–89.

Further Information

The text by Rideout [1991] has a particularly good tutorial on cardiovascular modeling and even includes ACSL source code. McDonald's [1974] and Noordergraaf's [1978] texts are classics, thoroughly reviewing cardiovascular physiology and the physical principles useful in modeling it. More recent texts on the cardiovascular system with a bioengineering slant include those by Milnor [1989], Li [1987], and Fung [1984]. Also, Guyton's 1980 text provides a detailed review of his model and its application for the analysis of hypertension and is well worth reading. Along this same line, Safar and O'Rourke's [1993] text, as well as O'Rourke's earlier work [1982], are also worth reading and provide many insights into hypertension and cardiovascular modeling. Melchior, Srinivasan, and Charles [1992] also present an overview of cardiovascular modeling, though with an emphasis on orthostatic response.

For historical interest, The History of Cardiology by Acierno [1994] provides fascinating reading, going back beyond even the early Greeks. In more recent history, a review of early CV models (early 1900s up to 1940) can be found in Aperia's monograph (1940), and a review of the post-World War II era models (late 1950s to early 1970s) that set the tone for almost all modern CV models can be found in Sagawa [1973].

For those interested in pharmacologic modeling, along with examples using the CV system, Carson, Cobelli, and Finkelstein's 1983 text is a good source. Middleman's 1972 text specifically targets in transport in the CV system, but it is somewhat dated. The current understanding of the anatomic and functional organization of the neurohumoral regulation pathways can be found in Dampney [1994].

For a survey of blood pressure controllers, the reader is referred to the recent article by Isaka and Sebald [1993]. Linkens and Hacisalihzade [1990], Katona [1988], and Westenskow [1986] also survey blood pressure controllers as well as other CV control applications. Further examples of modeling applications incorporating assist devices could be found in ASAIO [2004], Kosaka [2004], and Reesink [2004].

11
Respiratory Models and Control

Chi-Sang Poon
Massachusetts Institute of Technology

The respiratory system is a complex neurodynamical system. It exhibits many interesting characteristics that are akin to other physiologic control systems. However, the respiratory system is much more amenable to modeling analysis than many other systems for two reasons. First, the respiratory system is dedicated to a highly specific physiologic function, namely, the exchange of O_2 and CO_2 through the motor act of breathing. This physiologic function is readily distinguishable from extraneous disturbances arising from behavioral and other functions of the respiratory muscles. Second, the respiratory control system is structurally well organized, with well-defined afferent and efferent neural pathways, peripheral controlled processes, and a central controller. The functional and structural specificity of the respiratory system — and the diverse neurodynamic behaviors it represents — make it an ideal model system to illustrate the basic principles of physiologic control systems in general.

Like any closed-loop system, the behavior of the respiratory control system is defined by the continual interaction of the controller and the peripheral processes being controlled. The latter include the respiratory mechanical system and the pulmonary gas exchange process. These peripheral processes have been extensively studied, and their quantitative relationships have been described in detail in previous reviews. Less well understood is the behavior of the respiratory controller and the way in which it processes afferent inputs. A confounding factor is that the controller may manifest itself in many different ways, depending on the modeling and experimental approaches being taken. Traditionally, the respiratory control system has been modeled as a closed-loop *feedback/feedforward regulator* whereby homeostasis of arterial blood gas and pH is maintained. Alternatively, the respiratory controller may be viewed as a *central pattern generator* in which rhythmic respiratory activity is produced in response to phasic afferent feedback. Finally, there is increasing evidence that the respiratory controller may function as an *adaptive self-tuning regulator* which optimizes breathing pattern and ventilation according to certain performance measure.

Each modeling approach reveals a separate "law" of a multifaceted controller. However, these control laws must be somehow related to one another because they are governed by the same neural network that forms the respiratory controller. It is therefore instructive to examine not only how the various models work but also how they might be fit together to encompass the myriad of response behaviors of the respiratory control system.

11.1 Structure of the Respiratory Control System

The respiratory control system is a nonlinear, multioutput, delayed-feedback dynamic system which is constantly being perturbed by unknown physiologic and pathologic disturbances (Figure 11.1). Rhythmic respiratory activity is produced by a respiratory central pattern generator (RCPG) which consists of a network of neuronal clusters in the medulla oblongata and pons areas of the brain stem. The RCPG forms the kernel of the respiratory controller. The control problem is defined by the characteristics of the controlled processes (plants) and the control objective.

11.1.1 Chemical Plant

11.1.1.1 Pulmonary Gas Exchange

The chemical plant is propelled by the ventilation of the lung, $\dot{V}_E$ which determines the alveolar PCO_2 and PO_2 according to the following mass-balance equations:

$$V_L CO_2 \cdot \frac{d}{dt} P_A CO_2 = \dot{V}_E \left(1 - \frac{V_D}{V_T}\right)(P_I CO_2 - P_A CO_2) + 863 \dot{V} CO_2 \tag{11.1}$$

$$V_L O_2 \cdot \frac{d}{dt} P_A O_2 = \dot{V}_E \left(1 - \frac{V_D}{V_T}\right)(P_I O_2 - P_A O_2) - 863 \dot{V} O_2 \tag{11.2}$$

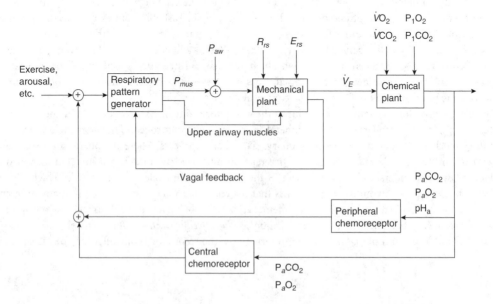

FIGURE 11.1   Block diagram of the respiratory control system.

The input–output relationships of the chemical plants are subject to several endogenous and exogenous disturbances. For example, increases in the metabolic production of CO_2 during muscular exercise, PCO_2 in the inspired air, and respiratory dead space during rebreathing — all contribute to an increase in CO_2 load to the lung. The added CO_2 is eliminated by an increase in pulmonary ventilation, but the effectiveness of the control action in restoring P_ACO_2 varies considerably with the type of disturbance. The input–output sensitivity $S_{pco_2} \neq \delta P_A CO_2 / \delta \dot{V}_E$ of the plant is highest with metabolic CO_2 load and lowest with inhaled CO_2 load, whereas the plant dynamics is slowest with dead space load.

In pulmonary disease the efficiency of the plant in removing CO_2 is further decreased because of pulmonary ventilation/perfusion maldistribution [Poon, 1987a]. Another source of disturbance is metabolic acidosis and alkalosis which alter arterial blood gas tensions and pH through acid–base buffering in blood. All these disturbances interact nonlinearly with the plant and are not directly sensed. How does the controller cope with such variety of disturbances effectively if its only means is to alter $\dot{V}_E$? Not surprisingly, the controller responds quite differently to the various forms of CO_2 disturbance and their combinations [Oren et al., 1981; Juratsch et al., 1982; Poon and Greene, 1985; Poon, 1989a, b, 1992b; Sidney and Poon, 1995].

11.1.1.2 Chemosensory Feedback

The peripheral (arterial) chemoreceptors response to changes in $P_a CO_2$ may be modeled by linear first-order dynamics [Bellville et al., 1979]

$$\tau_p \cdot \frac{d}{dt} A_p = -A_p + G_p [P_a CO_2 (t - T_p) - I_p] \tag{11.3}$$

where τ_p, G_p, I_p, are the time constant, gain, threshold of the peripheral chemoreceptor, and T_p is the lung-to-chemoreceptor transit delay of blood flow. Similarly, the central (intracranial) chemoreceptor is responsive to brain tissue PCO_2

$$A_c = G_c \{P_b CO_2 - I_c\} \tag{11.4}$$

where the brain tissue PCO_2 is given by

$$V_b CO_2 \cdot \frac{d}{dt} P_b CO_2 = \dot{Q}_b \{P_a CO_2 (t - T_c) - P_b CO_2\} + \frac{\dot{M}_b CO_2}{K CO_2} \tag{11.5}$$

and the cerebral blood flow [Vis and Folgering, 1980] is given by

$$\dot{Q}_b(t) = \dot{Q}_0 + \Delta \dot{Q}_b(t) \tag{11.6}$$

$$\tau_b \cdot \frac{d}{dt} \Delta \dot{Q}_b = -\Delta \dot{Q}b + G_b \cdot P_a CO_2 (t - T_c) \tag{11.7}$$

The central chemoreceptor normally has a greater sensitivity than the peripheral chemoreceptors (which may be silenced by hyperoxia). Their combined effects are presumably additive at low to moderate stimulation levels [Heeringa et al., 1979] but may become progressively saturated at higher levels [Eldridge et al., 1981]. The peripheral chemoreceptors have a shorter response time constant and delay than the central chemoreceptor, presumably due to their proximity to the lung and arterial blood gases. They are generally thought to be more responsive to rapid changes in blood chemistry; although the central chemoreceptor may also contribute substantially to the transient respiratory response to breath-to-breath fluctuations in chemical input during eupneic breathing in wakefulness [Bruce et al., 1992].

The dynamic response of the peripheral chemoreceptors to $P_a O_2$ may be modeled in a similar fashion but the steady-state response is hyperbolic [Cunningham et al., 1986]. Furthermore, hypoxia and hypercapnia have a multiplicative effect on carotid chemoreceptor discharge [Fitzgerald and Lahiri, 1986], although the effect of changes in pH is presumably additive [Cunningham et al., 1986]. Prolonged hypoxia has a depressant effect on central respiratory neurons [Neubauer et al., 1990] which may offset the stimulatory effect of peripheral chemosensitivity.

Inputs from the peripheral chemoreceptors are temporally gated throughout the respiratory cycle. Stimuli are effective only if they are delivered during the second half of the inspiratory or expiratory cycle [Hildebrandt, 1977; Teppema et al., 1985; Eldridge and Millhorn, 1986]. The effect of such stimuli on medullary respiratory neurons is excitatory during the inspiratory phase and inhibitory during the expiratory phase [Lipski and Voss, 1990]. The gating effect may be modeled by a gated time function

$$A_{epg} = \text{gate}\{A_p(t)\} \tag{11.8}$$

where gate $\{\cdot\}$ is a windowing function which reflects the phasic activity of peripheral chemoreceptor inputs.

The intrinsic transient delay and nonlinearity in the transduction of chemical signals are undesirable from an automatic control perspective. On the other hand, they may represent neural preprocessing in the sensory nervous system. Such transformations in the feedback path may have important bearing on the controller's ability to achieve the control objective.

11.1.2 Mechanical Plant

11.1.2.1 Respiratory Mechanics

Pulmonary ventilation results from tidal expansion and relaxation of the lung. The equation of motion is:

$$R_{rs} \cdot \frac{dV}{dt} = -E_{rs} \cdot V + P_{aw}(t) - P_{mus}(t) \tag{11.9}$$

Both R_{rs} and E_{rs} may be nonlinear. The mechanical load of the respiratory muscles is increased by airway constriction or lung restriction in pulmonary disease, or by the imposition of external resistance and elastance which cause a back pressure P_{aw} at the airway opening. Increases in ventilatory load may elicit a compensatory response in P_{mus} so that $\dot{V}_E$ is largely restored [Poon, 1987b, 1989a, b] except under severe ventilatory loading. Reverse compensatory responses are observed during ventilatory unloading [Ward et al., 1982; Poon et al., 1987a, b].

11.1.2.2 Respiratory Muscles

The mechanical plant is propelled by the respiratory muscles which serve as a mechanical pump. Normally, P_{mus} is sustained by the inspiratory muscles (principally the diaphragm and, to a lesser extent, the external intercostal and parasternal muscles). During hyperpnea or with increased expiratory load the expiratory muscles may be recruited [Marroquin, 1991], as are accessory muscles which may contribute significantly to the generation of P_{mus} in paraplegics.

Paradoxically, the respiratory muscles may also act to reduce ventilation. During quiet breathing some postinspiratory inspiratory activity may persist during the early expiratory phase, retarding lung emptying [Poon et al., 1987b]. In disease states inspiratory activity may also be recruited during the expiratory phase to prevent lung collapse [Stark et al., 1987] or overinflation. The upper airways abductor muscles may be activated by the controller or higher brain centers to increase R_{rs} in disease states [Stark et al., 1987] or in sleep [Phillipson and Bowes, 1986]. In awake states, respiration may be interrupted by behavioral, emotional, or defensive activities which compete for the respiratory apparatus under cortical or somatic sensory commands.

The mechanical efficiency of the respiratory muscles is limited by the force-velocity and force-length relationships which may be modeled as linear "active" resistance and elastance, respectively [Milic-Emili and Zin, 1986]. Neuromechanical efficiency may be impaired in respiratory muscle fatigue or muscle weakness, resulting in diminished P_{mus} for any given neural drive.

Thus the respiratory pump is equipped with various types of actuators to regulate V_F in the face of many exogenous and endogenous mechanical disturbances. Such disturbances are detected by mechanoafferents originating in the lungs, thorax, and airways.

11.1.2.3 Mechanosensory Feedback

Among the various types of mechanoafferents, vagal slowly adapting pulmonary stretch receptors (SAR) input exerts the greatest influence on respiration by inhibiting inspiratory activity and facilitating expiratory activity (Hering-Breurer reflex). Vagal SAR volume feedback is crucial for the compensatory response of the RCPG to mechanical disturbances.

The SAR characteristic is liner at low lung volumes but may exhibit saturation nonlinearity at elevated volumes. Also, at any given lung volume SAR discharge increases with increasing rate of lung inflation [Pack et al., 1986]. To a first approximation vagal volume feedback may be modeled by

$$\text{vag}(t) = \text{sat}\{a_0 + a_1 V(t) + a_2 \dot{V}(t)\} \qquad (11.10)$$

where $\text{sat}\{\cdot\}$ is a saturation function; a_0 denotes tonic vagal activity [Phillipson, 1974]; and a_1, a_2 are sensitivity parameters.

11.1.3 Control Object

It is generally assumed that the prime function of respiration is to meet the metabolic demand by the exchange of O_2 and CO_2. The control problem is to accomplish this objective within some prescribed tolerance, subject to the physical as well as environmental constraints of the respiratory apparatus. Various models of the controller have been proposed as possible solutions to the control problem [Petersen, 1981], each representing a separate control strategy and degree of modeling abstraction. In what follows we provide a synopsis of the various modeling approaches and their physiologic significance.

11.2 Chemoreflex Models

The simplest controller model is a proportional controller [Grodins and Yamashiro, 1978; Cunningham et al., 1986]. In this approach attention is focused on the control of the chemical plant; the RCPG and the mechanical plant are lumped together to form a constant-gain controller. The control signal is taken to be $\dot{V}_E$, and the effects of the breathing pattern and vagal feedback are often neglected. Thus the controller is assumed to be a fixed relay station that regulates $\dot{V}_E$ via the chemoreflex loop. These simplification allow quantitative closed-loop analyses of the chemoreflex system.

11.2.1 Feedback Control

In the chemoreflex model the respiratory control system acts like a chemostat. This is consistent with the well-known experimental observation that ventilation increases with increasing chemical stimulation. The steady-state ventilatory response to CO_2 inhalation is given by:

$$\dot{V}_E = \alpha(P_a CO_2 - \beta) \qquad (11.11)$$

This empirical relationship is in agreement with the chemoreflex model which assumes that ventilatory output is proportional to the sum of chemosensory feedback:

$$\dot{V}_E = G_0(A_c + A_p) \qquad (11.12)$$

Equation 11.11 follows from the steady-state solutions to the model Equation 11.3 to Equation 11.7 and Equation 11.12, provided that the effect of changes in cerebral blood flow may be neglected. The effects of hypoxia and hypoxic–hypercapnic interaction may be modeled in a similar fashion by a hyperbolic relation [Cunningham et al., 1986].

A comprehensive model of the dynamical chemoreflex system is due to the classic work of Grodins and coworkers [1967]. The dynamical response to CO_2 is given by the transient solutions of the system equations. Equation 11.3 to Equation 11.7 and Equation 11.12. Under closed-loop conditions system dynamics is also influenced by the nonlinear dynamical response of the chemical plant, Equation 11.1, as well as CO_2 uptake in body tissues. Therefore, measurement of the CO_2 response curve, Equation 11.8, is often a slow and tedious procedure. Open-loop conditions may be achieved by dynamic forcing of end-tidal PCO_2 with servo-control of P_tCO_2 which obviates the nonlinearity and slow equilibration of the lung and other body tissue stores. This technique has been used to experimentally estimate the model parameters in normal and peripheral-chemoreceptor denervated subjects by means of system identification techniques [Bellville et al., 1979]. Another open-loop technique is the CO_2 rebreathing procedure [Read, 1967] which causes a metabolically induced ramp increase in P_aCO_2 and, hence, a similar increase in $\dot{V}_F$ by way of chemoreflex. The rebreathing technique is much simpler to use than dynamic end-tidal PCO_2 forcing and is therefore suitable for clinical applications. However, this technique may not accurately determine the steady-state CO_2 response, presumably because of the variability in cerebral blood flow induced by changing P_aCO_2. More reliable techniques using pulse-step [Poon and Olson, 1985] or step-ramp [Dahan, 1990] P_ICO_2 forcings have been proposed for rapid determination of the steady-state CO_2 response with minimal experimental requirements.

Stability of the chemoreflex model may be studied by linearization of the system about some nominal state. Instability may occur if the loop gain and phase shift exceed unity and 180°, respectively. This may explain the periodic breathing phenomena found in hypoxia or high altitude where peripheral chemoreceptor gain is increased and congestive heart failure in which transit delay is prolonged [Khoo et al., 1982]. However, chemical instability alone does not account for the periodic episodes in obstructive sleep apnea which may also be influenced by fluctuation in arousal state [Khoo et al., 1991]. A technique for estimation of chemoreflex loop gain using pseudorandom binary CO_2 forcing has been proposed [Ghazanshahi and Khoo, 1997].

11.2.2 Feedforward Control

The chemoreflex model provides a satisfactory explanation for the chemical regulation of ventilation as well as respiratory instability. However, it fails to explain a fundamental aspect of ventilatory control experienced by everyone in everyday life: the increase in ventilation during muscular exercise. Typically, $\dot{V}_E$ increases in direct proportion to the metabolic demand ($\dot{V}CO_2$, $\dot{V}O_2$) such that the outputs of the chemical plant, Equation 11.1 and Equation 11.2, are well regulated at constant levels from rest to exercise. As a result, homeostasis of arterial blood chemistry is closely maintained over a wide range of work rates. The dilemma is: if increases in metabolic rate are not accompanied by corresponding increases in chemical feedback, then what causes exercise hyperpnea?

One possible explanation of exercise hyperpnea is the so-called set-point hypothesis [Defares, 1964; Oren et al., 1981] which stipulates that P_aCO_2 and P_aO_2 are regulated at constant levels by the chemoreflex controller. However, a set point is not evident during hypercapnic and hypoxic challenges where the homeostasis of P_aCO_2 and P_aO_2 is readily abolished. Furthermore, to establish a set point the controller gain must be exceedingly high, but this is not found experimentally in the hypercapnic and hypoxic ventilatory sensitivities. Finally, from a control systems perspective a high gain controller is undesirable because it could drive the system into saturation or instability.

Another possible explanation of exercise hyperpnea is that the proportional controller may be driven by two sets of inputs: a chemical feedback component via the chemoreflex loop and a feedforward component induced by some exercise stimulus [Grodins and Yamashiro, 1978]. The "feedforward–feedback control" hypothesis offers a simple remedy of the chemoreflex model, but its validity can be verified only if the postulated "exercise stimulus" is identified. Unfortunately, although many such signals have been proposed as possible candidates [Wasserman et al., 1986], none of them has so far been unequivocally shown to represent a sufficient stimulus for exercise.

Among the variously proposed mechanisms of exercise hyperpnea, the "PCO_2 oscillation" hypothesis of Yamamoto [1962] has received widespread attention. According to this hypothesis, the controller may be responsive not only to the mean value of chemical feedback but also to its oscillatory waveform which is induced by the tidal rhythm of respiration. This hypothesis is supported by the experimental finding that alterations of the temporal relationship of the P_ACO_2 waveform could profoundly modulate the exercise hyperpnea response [Poon, 1992b].

Regardless of the origin (or even existence) of the exercise stimulus, there is evidence that exercise and chemical signals are processed by the controller in a multiplicative fashion [Poon and Greene, 1985; Poon, 1989a, b]. The input–output relationship of the controller may therefore be written as

$$\dot{V}_E = G_0(A_c + A_p)A_{ex} + G_{ex}A_{ex} \qquad (11.13)$$

Note that $\dot{V}_E$ vanishes when A_{ex} is reduced to zero, in agreement with the finding of Phillipson and colleagues [1981].

11.3   Models of Respiratory Central Pattern Generator

Although the chemoreflex model is useful in studying the closed-loop control of ventilation and the chemical plant, it is lacking as to the control of breathing pattern and the mechanical plant. Models of the RCPG are often studied under open-loop conditions with chemical feedbacks being held constant while vagal volume feedback is experimentally manipulated. Modeling and analysis of the RCPG in closed-loop form are difficult because the input-output relationships of the RCPG and the mechanism of pattern generation are poorly understood. Several modeling approaches have been used to characterize its behavior under specific conditions.

11.3.1   Phase-Switching Models

The breathing cycle consists of two distinct phases: inspiration and expiration. It is therefore natural to model each phase separately and then combine them with a model of phase switching (for review, see Younes and Remmers [1981]). Each phase is controlled by a separate "center" which generates ramp-like central inspiratory and expiratory activity, respectively. The resulting lung expansion and collapse are sensed by SAR, which causes the RCPG to switch from inspiration phase to expiration phase, or vice versa, when the volume–time relationship reaches some inspiratory or expiratory off-switch threshold. The off-switch mechanisms are dependent on both the threshold values and the corresponding volume-time histories. Also, inspiratory and expiratory off-switches may be mechanically linked, as suggested by the correlation between inspiratory and expiratory durations in consecutive breaths. Both the rate of rise of inspiratory activity and the inspiratory off-switch threshold increase with increasing chemical stimulation. Throughout the inspiratory phase, vagal volume feedback exerts graded and reversible inhibition on inspiratory activity until immediately before the inspiratory off-switch where inspiratory termination becomes irreversible [Younes et al., 1978]. Perturbations of the mechanical plant, such as increases in ventilatory load, alter respiratory rhythm by changing the volume–time profiles and off-switch thresholds (Figure 11.2). These effects are abolished by vagotomy such that the RCPG always oscillates with a fixed rhythm. Various neuronal models of phase switching have been proposed [Cohen and Feldman, 1977], and putative phase-switching neurons in the medulla have been identified [Oku et al., 1992].

The two-phase respiratory cycle may be expanded into three phases if the expiratory phase is subdivided into an early postinspiratory inspiratory phase (stage I) and a late expiration phase (stage II). Vagal feedback has differential effects on neural activities during the two stages of expiration [St. John and Zhou, 1990].

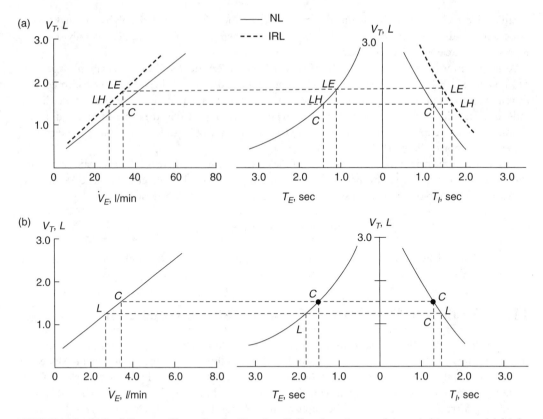

FIGURE 11.2 Stylized diagrams illustrating the Hey plots (*left*) and respiratory phase-switching curves (*right*) for subjects breathing normally (NL) or (a) under an inspiratory resistive load (IRL), (b) under an inspiratory elastic load (IEL) at rest or during exercise. In (a), IRL causes the normal operating point (C) to move to a new point *LE* if the inspirate is free of CO_2, or to a point *LH* if CO_2 is added. In (b), IEL moves the operating point to the same point *L* whether CO_2 is present in the inspirate. Thus, the consequence of load compensation is highly dependent on the background CO_2 and the type of load. Relative scales only are shown on all axes. (From Poon, C.-S. 1989a. *J. Appl. Physiol.* 66:2400; Poon, C.-S. 1989b. *J. Appl. Physiol.* 66:2391. With permission.)

An important link between RCPG and chemoreflex models is the Hey plot [Hey et al., 1966] which suggests that $\dot{V}_E$ and V_T are linearly related except when V_T approaches vital capacity. The slope of the Hey plot is altered by resistive loads but not elastic loads to ventilation (Figure 11.2).

11.3.2 Neural Network Models

Respiratory rhythmicity is an emergent property of the RCPG resulting from mutual inhibition of inspiratory and expiratory related neurons. A minimal model due to Duffin [1991] postulated the early-burst inspiratory (I) neurons and Bötzinger complex expiratory (E) neurons to be the mutually inhibiting pair. Adaptation of the I neurons (e.g., by calcium-activated potassium conductance) results in sustained relaxation oscillation in the network under constant chemical excitation. Both neuron groups are assumed to have monosynaptic inhibitory projections to bulbospinal inspiratory (I_R) output neurons (Figure 11.3). The model equations are:

$$T_t \frac{dx_t}{dt} - x_i = R_i - E_i + \sum C_n y_n$$

$$T_f \frac{dx_f}{dt} + x_f = R_f + C_f x_1$$

(11.14)

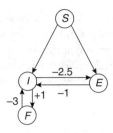

FIGURE 11.3   A minimal neural network model of RCPG. *I* and *E* denote respectively the early-burst inspiratory neurons and Bötzinger complex expiratory neurons; *F* is a fictive adaptation neuron; *S* is an excitation neuron or pacemaker cell. Not shown is the bulbospinal output neuron (I_g). Numbers denote connection strengths. (From Masakazu and coworkers [1998]. With permission.)

where $y_i \equiv g(x_i - H_i)$; $g(X) \equiv \max(0, X)$; T_i, R_i, E_i, H_i are respectively the membrane time constant, resting activity, excitation, and threshold of the *i*th neuron; C_{ij} is the connection strength between the *i*th and *j*th neurons; and x_1, x_2, x_3, x_f correspond respectively to the activities of the I, E, I_R neurons and a fictive (F) neuron which represents the adaptation effect.

The two-phase Duffin model may be extended to a three-phase pattern by incorporating other respiratory-related neurons. Richter and coworkers [Richter et al., 1986; Ogilvie et al., 1992] have proposed a three-phase RCPG model with mutual inhibition between I neurons and postinspiratory, late-inspiratory, and E neurons, all with adaptations. Botros and Bruce [1990] have described several variants of the Richter model with varying connectivity patterns, with and without adaptation.

Balis and coworkers [1994] proposed a RCPG model comprised of distributed populations of spiking neurons which are described by the Hodgkin–Huxley equations. Based on extensive spike-train analysis of neural recordings *in vivo*, the network connectivity differs from the Richter model in several essential ways. The model has been shown to mimic the normal and abnormal respiratory neural waveforms including the inspiratory ramp, inspiratory and expiratory off-switches, as well as apnea and apneusis. Rybak and colleagues [1997a, b] proposed a similar RCPG model that is modulated by both the membrane properties of the unit neuron and afferent feedback of the respiratory system.

11.3.3   Pacemaker and Hybrid Models

Respiratory rhythm may also originate from endogenous pacemaker cells. In neonatal rats, certain conditional bursting pacemaker neurons have recently been identified in a region of the ventrolateral medulla referred to as the pre-Botzinger complex [Smith et al., 1991]. Network oscillation by mutual inhibition is difficult in neonates because of immaturity of the GABAergic inhibitory system. During the postnatal developmental stage there may be progressive transformation from pacemaker to network oscillation with possibly some form of hybrid operation in the transition period [Smith, 1994]. A hybrid RCPG model composed of a neural network oscillator driven by a pacemaker cell (Figure 11.3) has been proposed [Matsugu et al., 1998].

11.3.3.1   Nonlinear Dynamics

An empirical (black-box) approach to studying rhythmic behavior is to model the oscillation as limit cycles of a nonlinear oscillator. A classic example of limit-cycle oscillation is the Van der Pol oscillator:

$$\ddot{V} = \epsilon \left\{ 1 - \left(\frac{V}{a}\right)^2 \right\} V - V \tag{11.15}$$

where ϵ and a are shape and amplitude parameters, respectively. This model has been shown to mimic the phase resetting and phase singularity properties of the RCPG [Eldridge et al., 1989] which are typical of any oscillator with isolated limit cycles. Similar properties are exhibited by a network oscillator model of RCPG [Ogilvie et al., 1992] which produces similar limit cycles.

Another property of nonlinear oscillators is that they may be entrained by (or phase-locked to) other oscillators that are coupled to them. The respiratory rhythm has been shown to be entrained by a variety of oscillatory inputs including locomotion, mechanical ventilation, blood gas oscillation, and musical rhythm.

A third property of nonlinear oscillators is that the limit-cycle trajectory may bifurcate and become quasiperiodic or chaotic when the system is perturbed by nonlinear feedback or other oscillatory sources. The resting respiratory rhythm is highly rhythmic in vagotomized animals but may become chaotic in normal humans [Donaldson, 1992] and vagi-intact animals [Sammon and Bruce, 1991] especially when lung volume is reduced [Sammon et al., 1993]. Both entrainment quasiperiodic and chaotic regimes have been demonstrated in a network oscillator model of the RCPG that is driven by periodic inputs [Matsugu et al., 1998]. The significance of nonlinear variations in respiratory pattern is discussed in a recent review [Bruce, 1996].

11.4 Optimization Models

All control systems are meant to accomplish certain (implicit or explicit) control objectives, it is perhaps too simplistic to assume that the sole objective of respiration is to meet the metabolic demand; a complex physiologic system may subserve multiple objectives that are vital to animal survival. One approach to understanding respiratory control is therefore to discover the innate control objective that fits the observed behavior of the controller.

11.4.1 Optimization of Breathing Pattern

Any given level of ventilation may be produced by a variety of breathing patterns ranging from deep-and-slow to shallow-and-rapid breathing. How is the breathing pattern set for each ventilatory level? Rohrer [1925] was among the first to recognize that respiratory frequency at rest may be chosen by the controller to minimize the work rate of breathing, a notion that was subsequently advanced by Otis and colleagues [1950]. Mead [1960] showed that the resting frequency may be determined more closely on the basis of optimal inspiratory pressure–time integral, a measure of the energy cost of breathing. Neither the work nor energy measure, however, correctly predicts the inspiratory flow pattern [Bretschger, 1925; Ruttimann and Yamamoto, 1972]; such discrepancy has led to the suggestion that the optimization criterion may consist of a weighted sum of work and energy expenditures [Bates, 1986] or some higher-order terms [Yamashiro and Grodins, 1971; Hämäläinen and Sipilä, 1984].

Similarly, the optimization principle has also been applied to the prediction of airway caliber and dead space volume [Widdicombe and Nadel, 1963] as well as end-expiratory lung volume and respiratory duty cycle [Yamashiro et al., 1975]. In most cases, the cost functions are generally found to be relatively flat in the resting state but may become much steeper during CO_2 or exercise stimulations [Yamashiro et al., 1975]. This may explain the observed variability of breathing pattern which is generally more pronounced at rest than during hyperpnea or ventilatory loading.

11.4.2 Optimization of Ventilation

The classical optimization hypothesis of Rohrer [1925] and Bretschger [1925] suggests that conservation of energy may be an important factor in the genesis of breathing pattern. It thus appears that the controller is charged with two opposing objectives: to meet the metabolic demand by performing the work of breathing, and to conserve energy by minimizing the work. How does the controller reconcile such conflict? One possible solution is to establish priority. In a hierarchical model of respiratory control, metabolic needs take priority over energetic needs. At the higher hierarchy (outer/chemical feedback loop) ventilatory output is set by feedforward/feedback proportional control of the chemical plant to meet the metabolic demand, whereas at the lower hierarchy (inner/vagal feedback loop) breathing pattern is optimized by the RCPG for efficient energy utilization by the mechanical plant at a ventilation set by the higher hierarchy.

A potential drawback of such a hierarchical system is that it is nonrobust to perturbations. Changes in ventilatory load, for example, would disrupt the ventilatory command from the feedforward signal. This is at variance with the experimental observation of a load compensation response of the controller which protects ventilation against perturbations of the mechanical plant at rest and during exercise [Poon et al., 1987a, b; Poon, 1989a, b]. Furthermore, if the prime objective of the controller were indeed to meet the metabolic demand (i.e., to maintain chemical homeostasis), then the hierarchical control system seems to perform quite poorly; it is well known that arterial chemical homeostasis is readily disrupted environmental changes.

Another form of conflict resolution is compromise. Poon [1983a, 1987] proposed that an optimal controller might counterbalance the metabolic needs versus energetic needs of the body, and the resulting compromise would determine the ventilatory response. The tug-of-war between the two conflicting control objectives may be represented by a compound optimization criterion which reflects the balance between the chemical and mechanical costs of breathing:

$$J = \begin{cases} J_c + J_m \\ \{\alpha(P_eCO_2 - \beta)\}^2 + \ln \dot{W} \end{cases} \tag{11.16}$$

The power (quadratic) form and logarithmic form for J_c and J_m correspond, respectively, to the classical Steven's law and Fechner–Weber law of sensory perception [Milsum, 1966]. Assuming that the work rate of breathing $\dot{W} \sim \dot{V}_j^2$, Equation 11.16 yields an optimal ventilatory response that conforms with the normal hypercapnic ventilatory response during CO_2 inhalation and the isocapnic ventilatory response during exercise [Poon, 1983a, 1987]. Furthermore, by generalizing Equation 11.16 to include other chemical and work rate components, it is possible to predict the normal ventilatory responses to hypoxia and acidosis [Poon, 1983a], mechanical loading [Poon, 1987b], as well as breathing pattern responses to chemical and exercise stimulation [Poon, 1983b].

The ventilatory optimization model [Poon, 1983a, b, 1987b] has several interesting implications. First, it provides a unified and coherent framework for describing the control of ventilation and control of breathing pattern with a common optimization criterion. Second, it offers a parsimonious explanation of exercise hyperpnea and ventilatory load compensation responses, without the need to invoke any putative exercise stimulus and load compensation stimulus. Third, it suggests that disruption of chemical homeostasis (e.g., during CO_2 inhalation) may represent an optimal response as much as maintenance of homeostasis during exercise.

Energetics of breathing is only one of many constraints that conflict with the metabolic cause of respiration. Another is the sensation of dyspnea which may be a limiting factor at high ventilatory levels [Oku et al., 1993]. A general optimization criterion may therefore include both energetic and dyspneic penalties as follows:

$$J = \{\alpha(P_aCO_2 - \beta)\}^2 + 2\ln \dot{V}_E + k\dot{V}_E^2 \tag{11.17}$$

where k is a weighting factor. At low to moderate ventilatory levels the energetic component (logarithmic term) dominates, and at high ventilatory levels the dyspneic component ($k \cdot \dot{V}_E^2$) dominates in counterbalancing the chemical component. In addition, the ventilatory apparatus may also be constrained by other factors such as behavioral and postural interference, which may further tip the balance of the optimization equation. It has been suggested that the periodic breathing pattern at extremely high altitudes may represent an optimal response for the conservation of chemical and mechanical costs of hypoxic ventilation [Ghazanshahi and Khoo, 1993].

11.4.3 Optimization of Neural Waveform

The neural output of the controller has been traditionally described in terms of measurable quantities such as breathing pattern and ventilation. A more accurate representation of the control signal is $P_{mus}(t)$ which drives the respiratory pump. The resulting continuous inspiratory and expiratory airflow, Equation 11.9, then determine V_E and all other ventilatory patterns. The control problem the RCPG must solve is how to optimize $P_{mus}(t)$ in order to deliver adequate ventilation without incurring excessive energy (or other) losses. It has been shown by Poon and colleagues [1992] that many interesting characteristics of the RCPG conform to a general optimal control law that calls for dynamic optimization of $P_{mus}(t)$.

The model of Poon and coworkers [1992] assumes a compound optimization criterion, Equation 11.16, with a mechanical penalty given by a weighted sum of the work rate of inspiration and expiration

$$\dot{W} = \dot{W}_t + \lambda \dot{W}_E \tag{11.18}$$

where

$$
\begin{aligned}
\dot{W} &= \frac{1}{T_T} \int_0^{T_1} \frac{P_{mus}(t)\dot{V}(t)}{[1 - P_{mus}(t)/P_{\max}]^n [1 - P_{mus}(t)/p_{\max}]^n}\,dt \\
\dot{W}_E &= \frac{1}{T_T} \int_{T_l}^{T_T} P_{mus}(t)\dot{V}(t)\,dt
\end{aligned}
\tag{11.19}
$$

The terms $P_{\max}$ and $\dot{P}_{\max}$ denote the limiting capacities of the inspiratory muscles, and n is an efficiency index. The optimal $P_{mus}(t)$ output is found by minimization of J subjects to the constraints set by the chemical and mechanical plants, Equation 11.1 and Equation 11.9. Because $P_{mus}(t)$ is generally a continuous time function with sharp phase transitions, this amounts to solving a difficult dynamic nonlinear optimal control problem with piecewise smooth trajectories. An alternative approach adopted by Poon and coworkers [1992] is to model $P_{mus}(t)$ as a biphasic function

$$
P_{mus}(t) = \begin{cases} a_0 + a_1 t + a_2 t & 0 \le t \le T_1 \\ P_{mus}(T_1) \exp\left[-\dfrac{(t - T_1)}{\tau} \right] & T_1 \le t \le T_T \end{cases}
\tag{11.20}
$$

where a_0, a_1, a_2, and t are shape parameters; T_1 is the duration of the inspiratory phase of neural activity. The optimal P_{mus} waveform is given by the set of optimal parameters $a_0^\star, a_1^\star, a_2^\star, t^\star, T_1^\star, T_T^\star$ that minimize Equation 11.16.

Poon and colleagues [1992] have shown that the dynamic optimization model predicts closely the $P_{mus}(t)$ trajectories under various conditions of ventilatory loading as well as respiratory muscle fatigue and weakness (Figure 11.4). In addition, the model also accurately predicts the ventilatory and breathing pattern responses to combinations of chemical and exercise stimulation and ventilatory loading [Poon et al., 1992], all without invocation of any putative exercise stimulus or load compensation stimulus. The generality of model predictions strongly supports the hypothesis that neural processing in the RCPG is governed by an optimization law.

11.5 Self-Tuning Regulator Models

Optimization models suggest an empirical objective function that might be obeyed by the controller. They do not, however, reveal the mechanism of such neural optimization. Priban and Fincham [1965] suggested that an optimal operating for arterial pH, PCO_2, and PO_2 might be achieved by a self-adaptive controller which seeks the optimal solution by a process of hill climbing. There is increasing evidence that the respiratory system is an adaptive control system [Poon, 1992a].

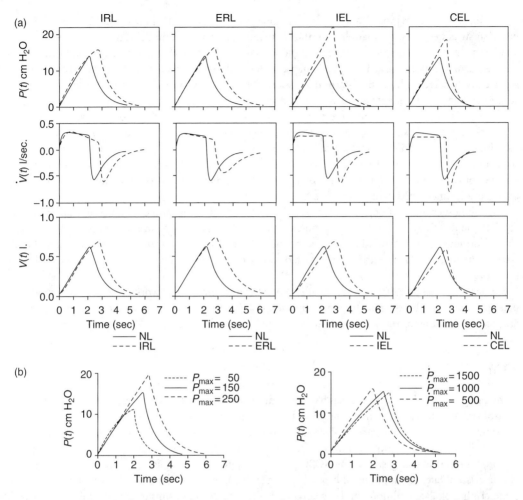

FIGURE 11.4 (a) Optimal waveforms for respiratory muscle driving pressure, $P(t)$; respiratory airflow, V; and respired volume, V, during normal breathing (NL) or under various types of ventilatory loads; IRL and ERL, inspiratory and expiratory resistive load; IEL and CEL, inspiratory and continuous elastic load. (b) Optimal waveforms for $P(t)$ under increasing respiratory muscle fatigue (amplitude limited; *upper* panel) and muscle weakness (rate limited; *lower* panel). (From Poon and coworkers [1992]. With permission.)

There are two basic requirements in any adaptive system. The first is that in order to adapt to changes, the system signals must be constantly fluctuating or persistently exciting. This should be readily satisfied by the respiratory system which is inherently oscillatory [Yamamoto, 1962] and chaotic [Donaldson, 1992; Sammon and Bruce, 1992]. Another requirement is that the system must be able to learn and then memorize the changes in the environment. Learning and memory in neuronal circuits are generally believed to result from synaptic modifications in the form of long-term or short-term potentiation which are mediated by NMDA receptors [Bliss and Collingridge, 1993]. Evidence for learning and memory in the RCPG is provided by the recent discoveries of both short-term potentiation [Fregosi, 1991; Wagner and Eldridge, 1991] and long-term potentiation [Martin and Mitchell, 1993] *in vivo*. Similar short and long-term memories have been identified recently in brain stem cardiorespiratory-related region *in vitro* [Zhou et al., 1997]. Also, neonatal mice which lack functional NMDA receptors have been found to suffer severe respiratory depression [Poon et al., 1994]. It has been shown that learning and memory in the brain are sufficient to achieve an optimal behavior characterized by the chemoreflex response and isocapnic exercise response [Poon, 1991].

One form of synaptic modification — correlation Hebbian learning [Sejnowski and Tesauro, 1989] — has been suggested to be compatible with the ventilatory optimization model [Poon, 1993, 1996; Young and Poon, 1998]. According to this neuronal model, variations in the chemical feedback and mechanical feedback signals converging at a Hebbian synapse in the RCPG may induce short-term potentiation if they are negatively correlated, or short-term depression if they are positively correlated. In other words, the controller gain may be adaptively increased or decreased depending on the coupling between the cause and effect of respiration. During exercise, ventilatory neural output and chemical feedback are strongly negatively correlated (since S_{pco_2} has a large negative value) so that the controller learns to increase its gain, G_0, in proportion to metabolic load. During CO_2 inhalation, $\dot{V}_E$ and P_aCO_2 are only weakly correlated (i.e., S_{pco_2} is small), and the controller gain remains unchanged. Such a neural controller is analogous to a self-tuning regulator [Åstrom and Wittenmark, 1975] which regulates the output by adaptive adjustment of system parameters.

Implicit in such a self-tuning regulator model is the assumption that afferent inputs may up- or down-regulate the RCPG by inducing synaptic potentiation or depression of neural transmission. Respiratory short- and long-term potentiation have been variously reported as indicated above. The possibility of synaptic depression was recently demonstrated in the nucleus tractus solitarius of the medulla [Zhou et al., 1997].

Similarly, it is possible that some form of synaptic learning might be at work in the RCPG to modulate pattern generation, thereby resulting in an optimal $P_{mus}(t)$. However, experimental and simulation data are presently lacking for verification of this conjecture.

11.6   Conclusion

Many empirical and functional models have been proposed to describe various aspects of the respiratory control system. The classical chemostat model is useful in describing chemoreflex responses but may be too simplistic to explain the variety of system responses to exercise input and mechanical disturbances. The recent discovery of various complex behaviors of the controller such as nonlinear dynamics, optimization, and learning suggest that the RCPG may be endowed with highly sophisticated computational characteristics. Such computational capability of the RCPG may be important for the maintenance of optimal physiologic conditions under changing environments. The computational problem — which amounts to dynamic optimal control of a nonlinear plant — is a very difficult one even by the standard of modern digital computers but seems to be solved by the RCPG from instant to instant with relative ease. This remarkable ability of the respiratory neural network is interesting from both biologic and engineering standpoints. Understanding how it works may shed light on not only the wisdom of the body [Cannon, 1932] but also on the design of novel intelligent control systems with improved speed, accuracy and economy.

Nomenclature

A_c, A_p	Activity of central, peripheral chemoreceptor
a, b	Slope and intercept of CO_2 response curve; l/min/mmHg, mmHg
J_c, J_m, J	Chemical, mechanical, and total costs of breathing
KCO_2	Solubility constant of CO_2 in blood; $mmHg^{-1}$
$MbCO_2$	Metabolic CO_2 production in brain tissues; l/min STPD
P_ACO_2, P_AO_2	Alveolar partial pressure of CO_2, O_2; mmHg
P_aCO_2, P_aO_2	Arterial partial pressure of CO_2, O_2; mmHg
P_bCO_2	Brain tissue PCO_2; mmHg
P_jCO_2, P_jO_2	Inspired partial pressure of CO_2, O_2; mmHg
P_{aw}	Airway pressure; cmH_2O
P_{mus}	Respiratory muscle driving pressure; cmH_2O

Q_b	Cerebral blood flow; l/min
RCPG	Respiratory central pattern generator
R_{rs}, E_{rs}	Total respiratory resistance, elastance; cmH_0/l/sec, cmH_2O/l
S_{pco_2}	Input–output sensitivity of chemical plant, $SP_ACO_2/S\dot{V}_F$ mmHg/l/min
T_j, T_F, T_T	Inspiratory, expiratory, and total respiration duration; sec
V	Lung volume above relaxation volume; l
V_bCO_2	Brain tissue store of CO_2; l
$\dot{V}CO_2, \dot{V}O_2$	Whole-body metabolic CO_2 production, O_2 consumption; l/min STPD
V_D/V_T	Ratio of respiratory dead space to tidal volume
$V_lCO_2; V_lO_2$	Lung tissue store of CO_2, $O2$; l
$\dot{V}_b$	Total ventilation of the lung; l/min BTPS
W	Work rate of breathing

References

Åstrom, K.J. and Wittenmark, B. 1975. On self-tuning regulators. *Automatica* 9: 185.

Bruce, E.N. 1996. Temporal variations in the pattern of breathing. *J. Appl. Physiol.* 80: 1079.

Balis, U.J., Morris, K.F., Koleski, J. et al. 1994. Simulations of a ventrolateral medullary neural network for respiratory rhythmogenesis inferred from spike train cross-correlation. *Biol. Cybern.* 70: 311.

Bates, J.H.T. 1986. The minimization of muscular energy expenditure during inspiration in linear models of the respiratory system. *Biol. Cybern.* 54: 195.

Bellville, J.W., Whipp, B.J., Kaufman, R.D. et al. 1979. Central and peripheral chemoreflex loop gain in normal and carotid body-resected subjects. *J. Appl. Physiol.* 46: 843.

Bliss, T.V.P. and Collingridge, G.L. 1993. A synaptic model of memory: long-term potentiation in the hippocampus. *Nature* 361: 31.

Botros, S.M. and Bruce, E.N. 1990. Neural network implementation of the three-phase model of respiratory rhythm generation. *Biol. Cybern.* 63: 143.

Bretschger, H.J. 1925. Die geschwindigkeitskurve der menschlichen atemluft. *Pflügers Arch für die Gesellsch. Physiol.* 210: 134.

Bruce, E.N., Modarreszadeh, M., and Kump, K. 1992. Identification of closed-loop chemoreflex dynamics using pseudorandom stimuli. In Y. Honda, Y. Miyamoto, K. Konno et al. (Eds.), *Control of Breathing and its Modeling Perspective*, pp. 137–142, New York, Plenum Press.

Cannon, W.B. 1932. *The Wisdom of the Body*, New York, Norton.

Cohen, M.I. and Feldman, J.L. 1977. Models of respiratory phase-switching. *Fed. Proc.* 36: 2367.

Cunningham, D.J.C., Robbins, P.A., and Wolff, C.B. 1986. Integration of respiratory responses to changes in alveolar partial pressures of CO_2 and O_2 and in arterial pH. In N.S. Cherniack and J.G. Widdicombe (Eds.), *Handbook of Physiology*, sec 3, *The Respiratory System*, Vol. 2, *Control of Breathing*, part 2, pp. 475–528, Washington, DC, American Physiological Society.

Dahan, A., Berkenbosch, A., DeGoede, J. et al. 1990. On a pseudo-rebreathing technique to assess the ventilatory sensitivity to carbon dioxide in man. *J. Physiol.* 423: 615.

Defares, J.G. 1964. Principles of feedback control and their application to the respiratory control system. In W.O. Fenn and H. Rahn (Eds.), *Handbook of Physiology*, sec. 3, Respiration, Vol. 1, pp. 649–680, Washington, DC, American Physiological Society.

Donaldson, G.C. 1992. The chaotic behavior of resting human respiration. *Respir. Physiol.* 88: 313.

Duffin, J. 1991. A model of respiratory rhythm generation. *NeuroReport* 2: 623.

Eldridge, F.L., Gill-Kumar, P., and Millhorn, D.E. 1981. Input–output relationships of central neural circuits involved in respiration in cats. *J. Physiol.* 311: 81.

Eldridge, F.L. and Millhorn, D.E. 1986. Oscillation, gating, and memory in the respiratory control system. In N.S. Cherniack and J.G. Widdicombe (Eds.), *Handbook of Physiology*, sec 3, *The Respiratory*

System, Vol. 2, *Control of Breathing*, part 2, pp. 93–134, Washington, DC, American Physiological Society.

Eldridge, F.L., Paydarfar, D., Wagner, P. et al. 1989. Phase resetting of respiratory rhythm: effect of changing respiratory "drive." *Am. J. Physiol.* 257: R271.

Fitzgerald, R.S. and Lahiri, S. 1986. Reflex responses to chemoreceptor stimulation. In N.S. Cherniack and J.G. Widdicombe (Eds.), *Handbook of Physiology*, sec 3, *The Respiratory System*, Vol. 2, *Control of Breathing*, part 1, pp. 313–362, Washington, DC, American Physiological Society.

Ghazanshahi, S.D. and Khoo, M.C.K. 1993. Optimal ventilatory patterns in periodic breathing. *Ann. Biomed. Eng.* 21: 517.

Ghazanshahi, S.D. and Khoo, M.C.K. 1997. Estimation of chemoreflex loop gain using pseudorandom binary CO_2 stimulation. *IEEE Trans. Biomed. Eng.* 44: 357.

Grodins, F.S., Buell, S.J., and Bart, A.J. 1967. Mathematical analysis and digital simulation of the respiratory control system. *J. Appl. Physiol.* 22: 260.

Grodins, F.S. and Yamashiro, S.M. 1978. *Respiratory Function of the Lung and its Control.* New York, Macmillan.

Hämäläinen, R.P. and Sipilä, A. 1984. Optimal control of inspiratory airflow in breathing. *Optimal Control Appl. Meth.* 5: 177.

Heeringa, J., Berkenbosch, A., de Goede, J. et al. 1979. Relative contribution of central and peripheral chemoreceptors to the ventilatory response to CO_2 during hyperoxia. *Respir. Physiol.* 37: 365.

Hey, E.N., Lloyd, B.B., Cunningham, D.J.C. et al. 1966. Effects of various respiratory stimuli on the depth and frequency of breathing in man. *Respir. Physiol.* 1: 193.

Hildebrandt, J.R. 1977. Gating: a mechanism for selective receptivity in the respiratory center. *Fed. Proc.* 36: 2381.

Juratsch, C.E., Whipp, B.J., Huntsman, D.J. et al. 1982. Ventilatory control during experimental maldistribution of $\dot{V}_A/\dot{Q}$ in the dog. *J. Appl. Physiol.* 52: 245.

Khoo, M.C.K, Kronauer, R.E., Strohl, K.P. et al. 1982. Factors including periodic breathing in humans: a general model. *J. Appl. Physiol.* 53: 644.

Khoo, M.C.K, Gottschalk, A, and Pack, A.I. 1991. Sleep induced periodic breathing and apnea: a theoretical study. *J. Appl. Physiol.* 70: 2014.

Lipski, J. and Voss, M.D. 1990. Gating of peripheral chemoreceptor input to medullary inspiratory neurons: role of Bötzinger complex neurons. In H. Acker, A. Trzebski, R.G. O'Regan et al. (Eds.), *Chemoreceptors and Chemoreceptor Reflexes*, pp. 323–329, New York, Plenum Press.

Marroquin, E. Jr. 1991. *Control of Respiration Under Simulated Airway Compression.* Thesis. Harvard-MIT Division of Health Sciences and Technology, Harvard Medical School, Boston.

Martin, P.A. and Mitchell, G.S. 1993. Long-term modulation of the exercise ventilatory response in goats. *J. Physiol.* 470: 601.

Masakazu, M., Duffin, J., and Poon, C.-S. 1998. Entrainment, instability, quasi-periodicity, and chaos in a compound neural oscillator. *J. Comput. Neurosci.* 5: 35.

Mead, J. 1960. Control of respiratory frequency. *J. Appl. Physiol.* 15: 325.

Milic-Emili, J. and Zin, W.A. 1986. Relationship between neuromuscular respiratory drive and ventilatory output. In P.T. Macklem and J. Mead (Eds.), *Handbook of Physiology*, sec 3, *The Respiratory System*, Vol. 3, *Mechanics of Breathing*, part 2, pp. 631–646, Washington, DC, American Physiological Society.

Milsum, J.H. 1966. *Biological Control Systems Analysis*, New York, McGraw-Hill.

Neubauer, J.A., Melton, J.E., and Edelman, N.H. 1990. Modulation of respiration during brain hypoxia. *J. Appl. Physiol.* 68: 441.

Oku, Y., Saidel, G.M., Altose, M.D. et al. 1993. Perceptual contributions to optimization of breathing. *Ann. Biomed. Eng.* 21: 509.

Ogilvie, M.D., Gottschalk, A., Anders, K. et al. 1992. A network model of respiratory rhythmogenesis. *Am. J. Physiol.* 263: R962.

Oku, Y., Tanaka, I., and Ezure, K. 1992. Possible inspiratory off-switch neurones in the ventrolateral medulla of the cat. *NeuroReport* 3: 933.

Oren, A., Wasserman, K., Davis, J.A. et al. 1981. Regulation of CO_2 set point on ventilatory response to exercise. *J. Appl. Physiol.* 51: 185.

Otis, A.B., Fenn, W.O., and Rahn, H. 1950. The mechanics of breathing in man. *J. Appl. Physiol.* 2: 592.

Pack, A.I., Ogilvie, M.D., Davies, R.O. et al. 1986. Responses of pulmonary stretch receptors during ramp inflations of the lung. *J. Appl. Physiol.* 61: 344.

Petersen, E.S. 1981. A survey of applications of modeling to respiration. In J.G. Widdicombe (Ed.), *International Review of Physiology. Respiratory Physiology III*, Vol. 23, pp. 261–326, Baltimore, University Park Press.

Phillipson, E.A. 1974. Vagal control of breathing pattern independent of lung inflation in conscious dogs. *J. Appl. Physiol.* 37: 183.

Phillipson, E.A. and Bowes, G. 1986. Control of breathing during sleep. In N.S. Cherniack and J.G. Widdicombe (Eds.), *Handbook of Physiology*, sec 3, *The Respiratory System*, Vol. 2, *Control of Breathing*, part 2, pp. 649–689, Washington, DC, American Physiological Society.

Phillipson, E.A., Duffin, J., and Cooper, J.D. 1981. Critical dependence of respiratory rhythmicity on metabolic CO_2 load. *J. Appl. Physiol.* 50: 45.

Poon, C.-S. 1983a. Optimal control of ventilation in hypoxia, hypercapnia and exercise. In B.J. Whipp and D.M. Wiberg (Eds.), *Modelling and Control of Breathing*, pp. 189–196, New York, Elsevier.

Poon, C.-S. 1983b. Optimality principle in respiratory control. *Proceedings of the Second American Control Conference*, pp. 36–40.

Poon, C.-S. 1987a. Estimation of pulmonary $\dot{V}/\dot{Q}$ distribution by inert gas elimination: state of the art. In C. Cobelli and L. Mariani (Eds.), *Modelling and Control in Biomedical Systems*, pp. 443–453, New York, Pergamon Press.

Poon, C.-S. 1987b. Ventilatory control in hypercapnia and exercise: optimization hypothesis. *J. Appl. Physiol.* 62: 2447.

Poon, C.-S. 1989a. Effects of inspiratory elastic load on respiratory control in hypercapnia and exercise. *J. Appl. Physiol.* 66: 2400.

Poon, C.-S. 1989b. Effects of inspiratory resistive load on respiratory control in hypercapnia and exercise. *J. Appl. Physiol.* 66: 2391.

Poon, C.-S. 1991. Optimization behavior of brainstem respiratory neurons: a cerebral neural network model. *Biol. Cybern.* 66: 9.

Poon, C.-S. 1992a. Introduction: optimization hypothesis in the control of breathing. In Y. Honda, Y. Miyamoto, K. Konno et al. (Eds.), *Control of Breathing and its Modeling Perspective*, pp. 371–384, New York, Plenum Press.

Poon, C.-S. 1992b. Potentiation of exercise ventilatory response by CO_2 and dead space loading. *J. Appl. Physiol.* 73: 591.

Poon, C.-S. 1993. Adaptive neural network that subserves optimal homeostatic control of breathing. *Ann. Biomed. Eng.* 21: 501.

Poon, C.-S. 1996. Self-tuning optimal regulation of respiratory motor output by Hebbian covariance learning. *Neural Networks*, 9: 1367.

Poon, C.-S. and Greene, J.G. 1985. Control of exercise hyperpnea during hypercapnia in humans. *J. Appl. Physiol.* 59: 792.

Poon, C.-S, Li, Y., Li, S.X. et al. 1994. Respiratory rhythm is altered in neonatal mice with malfunctional NMDA receptors. *FASEB J.* 8: A389.

Poon, C.-S, Lin, S.-L., and Knudson, O.B. 1992. Optimization character of inspiratory neural drive. *J. Appl. Physiol.* 72: 2005.

Poon, C.-S and Olson, R.J. 1985. A simple quasi-steady technique for accelerated determination of CO_2 response. *Fed. Proc.* 44: 832.

Poon, C.-S., Ward, S.A., and Whipp, B.J. 1987a. Influence of inspiratory assistance on ventilatory control during moderate exercise. *J. Appl. Physiol.* 62: 551.

Poon, C.-S., Younes, M., and Gallagher, C.G. 1987b. Effects of expiratory resistive load on respiratory motor output in conscious humans. *J. Appl. Physiol.* 63: 1837.

Priban, I.P. and Fincham, W.F. 1965. Self-adaptive control and the respiratory system. *Nature Lond.* 208: 339.

Read, D.J.C. 1967. A clinical method for assessing the ventilatory response to carbon dioxide. *Austral. Ann. Med.* 16: 20.

Richter, D.W., Ballantyne, D., and Remmers, J.E. 1986. How is the respiratory rhythm generated? A model. *News Physiol. Sci.* 1: 109.

Rohrer, F. 1926. Physilogie der Atembewegung. In A.T.J. Bethe, G. von Bergmann, G. Embden et al. (Eds.), *Handbuch der normalen und pathologischen Physiologie*, Vol. 2, pp. 70–127, Berlin, Springer-Verlag.

Ruttimann, U. and Yamamoto, W.S. 1972. Respiratory airflow patterns that satisfy power and force criteria of optimality. *Ann. Biomed. Eng.* 1: 146.

Rybak, I.A., Paton, J.F.R, and Schwaber, J.S. 1997a. Modeling neural mechanisms for genesis of respiratory rhythm and pattern: II. Network models of the central respiratory pattern generator. *J. Neurophysiol.* 77: 2007.

Rybak, I.A., Paton, J.F.R., and Schwaber, J.S. 1997b. Modeling neural mechanisms for genesis of respiratory rhythm and pattern: III. Comparison of model performances during afferent nerve stimulation. *J. Neurophysiol.* 77: 2027.

Sammon, M.P. and Bruce, E.N. 1991. Vagal afferent activity increases dynamical dimension of respiration in rats. *J. Appl. Physiol.* 70: 1748.

Sammon, M., Romaniuk, J.R., and Bruce, E.N. 1993. Bifurcations of the respiratory pattern associated with reduced lung volume in the rat. *J. Appl. Physiol.* 75: 887.

Sejnowski, T.J. and Tesauro, G. 1989. The Hebb rule for synaptic plasticity: algorithms and implementations. In JH Byrne and WO Berry (Eds.), *Neural Models of Plasticity*, pp. 94–103, New York, Academic Press.

Sidney, D.A. and Poon, C-S. 1995. Ventilatory responses of dead space and CO_2 breathing under inspiratory resistive load. *J. Appl. Physiol.* 78: 555.

Smith, J.C. 1994. A model for developmental transformations of the respiratory oscillator in mammals. *FASEB J.* 8: A394.

Smith, J.C., Ellenberger, H.H., Ballanyi, K. et al. 1991. Pre-Bötzinger complex: a brainstem region that may generate respiratory rhythm in mammals. *Science* 254: 726.

St. John, W.M. and Zhou, D. 1990. Discharge of vagal pulmonary receptors differentially alters neural activities during various stages of expiration in the cat. *J. Physiol.* 424: 1.

Stark, A.R., Cohlan, B.A., Waggener, T.B. et al. 1987. Regulation of end-expiratory lung volume during sleep in premature infants. *J. Appl. Physiol.* 62: 1117.

Teppema, L.J., Barts, P.W.J.A., and Evers, J.A.M. 1985. The effect of the phase relationship between the arterial blood gas oscillations and central neural respiratory activity on phrenic motoneurone output in cats. *Respir. Physiol.* 61: 301.

Vis, A. and Folgering, H. 1980. The dynamic effect of Pet_{CO_2} on vertebral bloodflow in cats. *Respir. Physiol.* 42: 131.

Wagner, P.G. and Eldridge, F.L. 1991. Development of short-term potentiation. *Respir. Physiol.* 83: 129.

Ward, S.A., Whipp, B.J., and Poon, C.-S. 1982. Density dependent airflow and ventilatory control during exercise. *Respir. Physiol.* 49: 267.

Wasserman, K., Whipp, B., and Casaburi, R. 1986. Respiratory control during exercise. In NS Cherniack and JG Widdicombe (Eds.), *Handbook of Physiology*, sec 3, *The Respiratory System*, Vol. 2, *Control of Breathing*, part 2, pp. 595–619, Washington, DC, American Physiological Society.

Widdicombe, J.G. and Nadel, J.A. 1963. Airway volume, airway resistance and work, and force of breathing — theory. *J. Appl. Physiol.* 35: 522.

Yamamoto, W.S. 1962. Transmission of information by the arterial blood stream with particular reference to carbon dioxide. *Biophys. J.* 2: 143.

Yamashiro, S.M., Daubenspeck, J.A., Lauritsen, T.N. et al. 1975. Total work rate of breathing optimization in CO_2 inhalation and exercise. *J. Appl. Physiol.* 38: 702.

Yamashiro, S.M. and Grodins, F.S. 1971. Optimal regulation of respiratory airflow. *J. Appl. Physiol.* 18: 863.

Younes M. and Remmers J.E. 1981. Control of tidal volume and respiratory frequency. In T.F. Hornbein (Ed.), *Regulation of Breathing*, part 1, pp. 621–671, New York, Marcel Dekker.

Younes, M., Remmers, J.E., and Baker, J. 1978. Characteristics of inspiratory inhibition by phasic volume feedback in cats. *J. Appl. Physiol.* 45: 80.

Young, D.L. and Poon, C.-S. 1998. Hebbian covariance learning: a nexus for respiratory variability, memory, and optimization? In R.L. Hughson, D.A. Cunningham, and J. Duffin (Eds.), *Advances in Modeling and Control of Ventilation*, pp. 73–83, New York, Plenum.

Zhou, Z., Champagnat, J., and Poon, C.-S. 1997. Phasic and long-term depression in brainstem nucleus tractus solitarius neurons: differing roles of AMPA receptor desensitization. *J. Neurosci.* 17: 5349.

12

Neural Networks for Physiological Control

James J. Abbas
Arizona State University

12.1 Introduction

This chapter is intended to provide a description of **neural network** control systems and of their potential for use in biomedical engineering control systems. Neural network techniques have been used by the engineering community in a variety of applications, with particular emphasis on solving pattern recognition and pattern classification problems [Grossberg, 1988a, b; Pao, 1988; Carpenter, 1989; Hecht-Nielsen, 1989; Sanchez-Sinencio and Lau, 1992; Zurada, 1992; Nerrand etal., 1993; Hagan et al., 1996]. More recently, there has been much research into the use of these techniques in control systems [Antsaklis, 1990; Miller et al., 1990b; White and Sofge, 1992]. Much of this research has been directed at utilizing neural network techniques to solve problems that have been inadequately solved by other control systems techniques. For example, neural networks have been used in adaptive control of nonlinear systems for which good models do not exist. The success of neural network techniques on this class of problems suggest that they may be particularly well suited for use in a wide variety of biomedical engineering applications. It should be emphasized that the field of neural network control is a relatively new area of research and that it is not intended to replace traditional engineering control. Rather, the focus has been on the integration of neural network techniques into control systems for use when traditional control systems alone are insufficient.

There are several textbooks available on neural networks that provide good presentations of the implementation and applications of neural network techniques [Simpson, 1990; Sanchez-Sinencio and Lau, 1992; Zurada, 1992; Hagan et al., 1996]. Recently, a few books have been published that review the application of neural network techniques to control systems problems [Miller et al., 1990b; White, 1992].

This chapter is intended to provide an introduction to neural network techniques and a guide to their application to biomedical control systems problems. The reader is referred to recently published textbooks and numerous journal articles for the specific information required to implement a given neural network control system.

12.2 Neural Network Basics

The term neural networks is used to refer to a class of computational algorithms that are loosely based upon the computational structure of the nervous system. There is a wide variety among various neural network algorithms, but the key features are that they have a set of inputs and a set of outputs, they utilize distributed processing, and they are adaptive. The basic idea is that computation is collectively performed by a group of distinct units, or neurons (sometimes referred to as processing elements), each of which receives inputs and performs its own local calculation. These units interact by providing inputs to each other via synapses and some units interact with the environment via input/output signals. The connectivity of various units determines the structure, or architecture, of the network. Adjustments to the strengths of the synapses (i.e., adjustments to the **synaptic weights**) modify the overall input–output properties of the network and are adjusted via a **learning algorithm**. The design of a neural network includes the specification of the neuron, the architecture, and the learning algorithm.

Most neural networks are based on a model of a neuron that captures the most basic features of real neurons: a neuron receives inputs from other neurons via synapses and the output from a neuron is a nonlinear function of a weighted summation of its inputs. There are many different sets of equations that capture these basic features; the following set of equations is commonly used:

$$y_i = \sum_{i=1}^{n} w_{ij} x_i$$

$$z_j = \frac{1}{(1 + e^{-m y_j})}$$

(12.1)

where y_j is the weighted summation of inputs to neuron j, x_i is the input from neuron i, n is the number of neurons providing synaptic input to neuron j, w_{ij} is the synaptic weight from neuron i to neuron j, z_j is the output from neuron j, and m is the slope of the sigmoidal output function. Note that in this set of equations, the output of a neuron is a static nonlinear function of the weighted summation of its inputs. Some commonly used variations on this model include: the use of different nonlinear output functions [Lippman, 1987], the use of recurrent inputs (i.e., past values of a neurons output would be included in the input summation) [Pineda, 1989; Williams and Zipser, 1989], and the use of dynamic neurons (i.e., Equation 12.1 would be a differential equation rather than an algebraic one) [Hopfield, 1982; Grossberg, 1988a; Carpenter, 1989]. The use of recurrent inputs and/or dynamic neuron models may be particularly important for applications in the control of dynamic systems because they provide the individual neurons with memory and temporal dynamics [Pineda, 1989].

Most applications use networks of neurons that are arranged in layers. The most commonly used architecture is a three layer network which has an input layer, a hidden layer and an output layer. A feedforward neural network architecture is one in which each neuron receives input from neurons in the previous layer. The number of neurons in each layer must be specified by the designer. There are some heuristic rules, but no solid theory, to guide the designer in specifying the number of neurons [Zurada, 1992]. Some commonly used variations on this architecture include: the use of only a single layer of neurons [Widrow, 1962; Kohonen, 1989], the use of bidirectional connections between layers [Carpenter, 1989], the use of intra-layer connections [Kohonen, 1989], the use of pruning techniques which cut some of the connections for greater efficiency [Zurada, 1992], and the use of heterogeneous networks in which more than one neuron model is used to describe the various neurons in the network [Hecht-Nielson, 1989].

A general form of a neural network learning algorithm is given by:

$$\Delta w_{ij} = f(\eta, z_i, z_j, e_{ij})$$

This equation states that the change in synaptic weight is a function of the learning rate (η), the activation of the presynaptic neuron (z_i), the activation of the postsynaptic neuron (z_j), and a training signal (e_{ij}). Several different learning algorithms have been developed [Grossberg, 1988a; Rumelhart and McClelland, 1988; Hinton, 1989; Fogel and sebald, 1990; Hecht-Nielsen, 1990], most of which fit into this general form, but may not use all of the terms. An example is Hebbian learning [Hebb, 1949; Brown et al., 1990] in which the change in weight is proportional to the product of the presynaptic activation and the postsynaptic activation. Often, gradient descent techniques are used to adjust the synaptic weights. The most commonly used learning algorithm, error backpropogation, uses an error gradient descent technique and passes the output error backwards through the network to determine the training signal for a given neuron [Rumelhart and McClleland, 1988; Vogl et al., 1988; Pineda, 1989]. Most of the commonly used learning algorithms are classified as supervised learning techniques because they use a specification of the desired output of the network to determine the output error of the network. Other learning algorithms, such as reinforcement learning (discussed below) can be used in situations when it is not possible to directly specify the desired output of the network.

In most engineering applications, the neural network is used to perform a nonlinear mapping from the space of network inputs to the space of network outputs. In addition to the internal specifications of the network discussed above, the engineer using a neural network must select the signals to be used as input to the network and the signals to be used as output from the network. Although this decision appears to be trivial, in many applications it is not. For applications in control systems, the selection of input and output signals is dependent upon how the neural network fits into the overall structure of the system. Several different options are described below.

12.3 Neural Network Control Systems

Neural networks have often been applied in control systems where, at a block diagram level, the neural network replaces one component of the control system. Typically, the motivation for utilizing the neural network lies in the ability to perform nonlinear mappings, in the ability to handle a wide range of model structures, and/or in the ability of the network to adapt. While there has been activity in the development of a theoretical framework for neural network control systems, most applications to-date have been heuristically-based to one degree or another [Miller et al., 1990b; Nguyen and Widrow, 1990; Farotimi et al., 1991; Wang et al., 1992; White and Sofge, 1992; Quinn and Espano Chied, 1993]. The field of neural network control has been described as bridging the gap between mathematically-based control systems engineering and heuristically-based artificial intelligence [Barto, 1990].

In designing a neural network control system, one must select the overall structure of the system and decide which components will utilize neural network algorithms. Several examples of control system structures are provided below, each of which utilizes one or more neural networks as described above. This section of the chapter provides a brief overview of some neural control systems that have potential for application in biomedical control systems. For excellent, thorough reviews of recent developments in neural network control systems, the reader is referred to Miller [1990b] and White and Sofge [1992].

12.3.1 Supervised Control

In this structure (Figure 12.1), the neural network is used to mimic, and eventually replace, an existing control system. Here, the neural network is used in a traditional feedback arrangement where it performs a mapping from the system outputs to the system inputs. The network would be trained using data collected from the actual system or a computer simulated model with the original controller active. The training signal for the network would be the difference between the output of the original controller and the

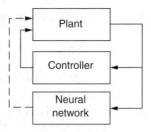

FIGURE 12.1   Supervised control system structure.

output of the network. After the network learns to adequately mimic the original controller, the training is completed. Thus, the synaptic weights would no longer be adapted, and the original control system would be replaced by the neural network. This type of an arrangement could be useful in situations where the neural network could perform the task less expensively or more efficiently than the original one. One situation would be when the original control system requires such heavy computation that it is impractical for real-time use on an affordable computer system. In this case, the neural network might be able to learn to perform the same (or functionally equivalent) operation more efficiently such that implementation on an affordable general purpose computer or on specialized neural network hardware would be practical. A second situation would be when the original control system is a human operator that might be either expensive or prone to error. In this case the neural network is acting as an adaptive expert system that learns to mimic the human expert [Werbos, 1990]. A third situation would be when the neural network could learn to perform the control using a different, and more easily measured, set of output variables [Barto, 1990]. This type of application would be particularly well-suited for biomedical applications in which an invasive measurement could be replaced by a non-invasive one.

12.3.2   Direct Inverse Control

In direct inverse control, (Figure 12.2), the neural network is used to compute an inverse model of the system to be controlled [Levin et al., 1991; Nordgren and Meckl, 1993]. In classical linear control techniques, one would find a linear model of the system then analytically compute the inverse model. Using neural networks, the network is trained to perform the inverse model calculations, that is, to map system outputs to system inputs. Biomedical applications of this type of approach include the control of arm movements using electrical stimulation [Lan et al., 1994] and the adaptive control of arterial blood pressure [Chen et al., 1997].

A variety of neural network architectures can be used in this direct inverse control system structure. A multi-layer neural network architecture with error **backpropagation** learning could be used off-line to learn an inverse model using a set of system input/output data. If on-line learning is desired, a feedforward model of the system can be trained while a feedback controller is active [Miyamoto et al., 1988; Miller, 1990a]. This technique, referred to as feedback error learning [Miyamoto et al., 1988], uses the control signal coming from the feedback controller as the training signal for the feedforward controller update. The idea used here is that if the feedforward control is inadequate, the feedback controller would be active and it would lead to updates in the feedforward controller. To achieve the rapid learning rates that would be desirable in on-line feedback error learning, typically single-layer networks have been used or the learning has been constrained to occur at one layer. This type of an approach is particularly useful in applications where on-line fine tuning of feedforward controller parameters is desired.

12.3.3   Model-Based Approaches to Control

Neural network approaches have been used as an alternative to other nonlinear techniques for modeling physiological systems [Chon et al., 1998]. Several neural network control systems have utilized model-based approaches in which the neural network is used to identify a forward nonlinear system

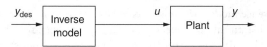

FIGURE 12.2 Direct inverse control system structure.

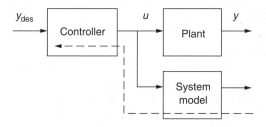

FIGURE 12.3 Backpropagating system output error through the system model.

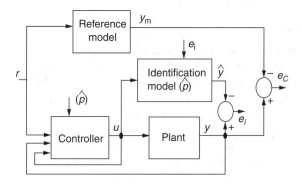

FIGURE 12.4 Indirect adaptive control system structure.

model. Often, these systems utilize neural network components in control system architectures that have been developed using linear or nonlinear components.

For many control applications, system output error can be readily measured but in order to adapt the controller parameters one needs to relate system output error to controller output (system input) error. One strategy would be to use the derivative of the system's output error with respect to its input to perform gradient descent adaptation of the controller parameters. However, there is no direct way of calculating the derivative of the system's output error with respect to its input and therefore it must be approximated. To implement such an approximation, a pair of multi-layer neural networks (Figure 12.3) have been used: one for identification of a forward model of the plant, and one for implementation of the controller [Barto, 1990]. The forward model is used to provide a means of computing the derivative of the model's output with respect to its input by backpropagating the error signal (the actual plant output tracking error) through the model of the plant to estimate the error in the control signal. The error in the control signal can then be backpropagated through the controller neural network. As described here, the backpropagation algorithm is used to minimize the output error of the system, which is a special case of maximization of utility. Although this is a very powerful technique with potential applications in a wide variety of nonlinear control problems, its primary limitation for many biomedical applications is the relatively slow training rate achieved by the backpropagation algorithm.

Neural networks have also been used in model reference adaptive control (MRAC) structures (Figure 12.4) [Naranedra and Parthasarathy, 1990; Narendra, 1992]. This approach builds upon established techniques for adaptive linear control and incorporates neural networks to address the problem of controlling nonlinear systems. The MRAC approach is directed at adapting the controlled system such that it behaves like a reference model, which is specified by the control system designer. In the structure shown in Figure 12.4, the identification model is a model of plant dynamics, the parameters of which are identified online using the identification error (the difference between the actual and the estimated plant outputs) as the training signal. The controller uses the estimates of the plant parameters, reference inputs, and system outputs to determine inputs to the system. In the neural network version of the control system structure, neural networks can be used for the identification of the system model, for the controller, or for both. Multi-layer neural networks using error backpropagation or a modified version of error back-propagation, termed dynamic backpropagation, have been used for adaptive control of nonlinear systems [Narendra and Parthasarathy, 1990; Narendra, 1992].

A third model-based approach is neural predictive control, which is a neural network version of nonlinear model predictive control [Trajanoski and Wach, 1998]. In this approach, the neural network is used for off-line identification of a system model, which is then used to design a nonlinear model predictive controller. This design may provide suitable control of nonlinear systems with time-delays and thus may be particularly useful in biomedical applications. Recent computer simulation studies have demonstrated positive results for control of insulin delivery [Trajanoski and Wach, 1998].

12.3.4 Adaptive Critics

All of the approaches to control discussed thus far have utilized supervised learning techniques. The training signal used for adaptation in these techniques is an error vector that gives the magnitude of the error in the system output signal and the direction in which it should change. For many complex, multi-variable control problems this type of system output error information is not readily available. The only measure available might be a scalar measure of system performance that is not directly related to the system outputs in a way that is understood by the control system designer. In such cases, a directed search of the control system parameter space could be performed in order to maximize (optimize) the scalar performance measure. Dynamic programming is a control systems engineering technique that has been used for optimal control of linear systems but these techniques are not well suited for large-scale systems or nonlinear systems. Neural networks have been used in an approach that is similar to dynamic programming in order to optimize system performance of large-scale nonlinear systems. These techniques, termed "adaptive critic methods," utilize a structure (Figure 12.5) in which a critic module provides an evaluation signal to the controller module. The controller module utilizes a **reinforcement learning algorithm** in order to optimize performance. The details of this class of neural network controllers are beyond the scope of this chapter, but descriptions and example applications are given in [Barto, 1990, 1992; Werbos, 1992].

Adaptive critic algorithms may be particularly useful in several biomedical engineering control systems where the relationship between system performance and measurable system outputs are ill-defined. While

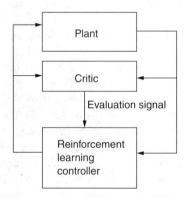

FIGURE 12.5   Adaptive critic control system structure.

these methods that use reinforcement learning may be attractive because they are general and do not require detailed information about the system, this increased generality comes at a cost of increased training times [Barto, 1990]. Supervised learning methods, when they can be used, can be more efficient than reinforcement learning methods.

12.3.5 Neurophysiologically Based Approaches

All neural network systems are based upon neurophysiological models to some degree, but in most cases this biological basis is very superficial, as is evident in the description given above. Computational neuroscience is a term used to describe the development of computational models of the nervous system [Koch and Segev, 1989; Schwartz, 1990; Bower, 1998]. Such models are intended to be used by neuroscientists in their basic science efforts to understand the functioning of the nervous system. There are several examples of neural network control system designs that have utilized models developed in the field of computational neuroscience [Bullock and Grossberg, 1988; Houk etal., 1990; Taga et al., 1991; Beer et al., 1993; Abbas, 1995]. These designs have extended the notion of "mimicking the nervous system" beyond what is used in most neural networks. The reasoning behind this approach is based upon a view that biological systems solve many problems that are similar to, or exactly the same as, those faced in many engineering applications and that by mimicking the biological system we may be able to design better engineering systems. This reasoning is similar to the motivation for much of the work in the neural network field and for the recent emphasis in biomimetic techniques in other engineering disciplines.

One approach to incorporating a stronger neurophysiological foundation has been to utilize an architecture for the overall control system that is based upon neurophysiological models, that is, mimicking the neurophysiological system at a block diagram level. This type of approach has led to the development of hierarchical control systems that are based upon the hierarchical structure of the human motor control system [Kawato et al., 1987; Srinivasan et al., 1992].

A second approach to incorporating a stronger neurophysiological foundation has been to utilize more realistic models of neurons and of their interconnections in the design of the neural network [Beer, 1990; Houk et al., 1990; Missler and Kamangar, 1995]. An example of this approach is the design of a coupled oscillator neural network circuit that is based upon the locomotor control system of the cockroach [Beer et al., 1992; Quinn and Espenschied, 1993]. In this neural network, some of the neurons are capable of endogenously oscillating due to intrinsic membrane currents and the network is heterogeneous, meaning that each neuron is not described by the same model. Most of the parameters of the models are fixed. This network has been shown to robustly generate patterns for statically-stable gaits at various speeds.

A biomedical control system that utilizes a neurophysiologically-based approach has been developed for use in Functional Neuromuscular Stimulation (FNS) systems [Abbas, 1995; Abbas and Chizeck, 1995]. FNS is a rehabilitation engineering technique that uses computer-controlled electrical stimuli to activate paralyzed muscle. The task of a control system is to determine appropriate stimulation levels to generate a given movement or posture. The neural network control system utilizes a block diagram structure that is based on hierarchical models of the locomotor control system. It also utilizes a heterogenous network of neurons, some of which are capable of endogenous oscillation. This network has been shown to provide rapid adaptation of the control system parameters [Abbas and Chizeck, 1995; Abbas and Triolo, 1997] and has been shown to exhibit modulation of reflex responses [Abbas, 1995].

12.4 Summary

This chapter presents an overview of the relatively new field of neural network control systems. A variety of techniques are described and some of the advantages and disadvantages of the various techniques are discussed. The techniques described here show great promise for use in biomedical engineering applications in which other control systems techniques are inadequate. Currently, neural network control systems lack the type of theoretical foundation upon which linear control systems are based, but recently there have been some promising theoretical developments. In addition, there are numerous examples of successful engineering applications of neural networks to attest to the utility of these techniques.

Defining Terms

Backpropagation: A technique used to determine the training signal used for adjusting the weights of a given neuron in a neural network.

Learning algorithm: An algorithm used to update the synaptic weights in a neural network.

Neural network: A term used to refer to a broad class of computational algorithms that are loosely based on models of the nervous system.

Reinforcement learning algorithms: Learning algorithms that utilize a system performance measure (that may or may not have a direct, known relationship to output error of the neural network) as a training signal for the neural network.

Supervised learning algorithms: Learning algorithms often used in neural networks that use the output error of the neural network as a training signal.

Synaptic weight: A scaling factor on the signal from one neuron in a network to another.

Acknowledgments

The author gratefully acknowledges the support of the National Science Foundation (NSF-BCS-9216697), The Whitaker Foundation, the School of Engineering at The Catholic University of America, and the Center for Biomedical Engineering at the University of Kentucky.

References

Abbas, J.J. 1995. Using neural models in the design of a movement control system. In *Computational Neuroscience*. J.M. Bower, Ed. pp. 305–310. Academic Press, New York.

Abbas, J.J. and Chizeck, H.J. 1995. Neural network control of functional neuromuscular stimulation systems. *IEEE Trans. Biomed. Eng.*, 42: 1117–1127.

Abbas, J.J. and Triolo, R.J. 1997. Experimental evaluation of an adaptive feedforward controller for use in functional neuromuscular stimulation systems. *IEEE Trans. Rehabil. Eng.*, 5: 12–22.

Antsaklis, P.J. 1990. Neural networks in control systems. *IEEE Control. Syst. Mag.*, 10: 3–5.

Barto, A.G. 1990. Connectionist learning for control: an overview. In *Neural Networks for Control*. W.T. Miller, R.S. Sutton, and P.J. Werbos, Eds. pp. 5–58. MIT Press, Cambridge, MA.

Barto, A.G. 1992. Reinforcement learning and adaptive critic methods. In *Handbook of Intelligent Control: Neural, Fuzzy and Adaptive Approaches*. D.A. White and D.A. Sofge, Eds. pp. 469–492. Van Nostrand Reinhold, New York.

Beer, R.D. 1990. *Intelligence as Adaptive Behavior: An Experiment in Computational Neuroethology*, Academic Press, Boston.

Beer, R.D., Chiel, H.J., Quinn, R.D., Espenschied, K.S., and Larsson, P. 1992. A distributed neural network architecture for hexapod robot locomotion. *Neural Comput.*, 4: 356–365.

Beer, R.D., Ritzmann, R.E., and McKenna, T. 1993. *Biological Neural Networks in Invertebrate Neuroethology and Robotics*, Academic Press, New York.

Bower, J.M. 1998. *Computational Neuroscience: Trends in Research*, Plenum Press, New York.

Brown, T.H., Kairiss, E.W., and Keenan, C.L. 1990. Hebbian synapses: biophysical mechanisms and algorithms. *Annu. Rev. Neurosci.*, 13: 475–511.

Bullock, D. and Grossberg, S. 1988. Neural dynamics of planned arm movements: emergent invariants and speed–accuracy properties during trajectory formation. In *Neural Networks and Natural Intelligence*. S. Grossberg, Ed. pp. 553–622. MIT Press, Cambridge, MA.

Carpenter, G. 1989. Neural network models for pattern recognition and associative memory. *Neural Networks*, 2: 243–258.

Chen, C.-T., Lin, W.-L., Kuo, T.-S., and Wang, C.-Y. 1997. Adaptive control of arterial blood pressure with a learning controller based on multilayer neural networks. *IEEE Trans. BME*, 44: 601–609.

Chon, K.H., Holstein-Rathlou, N.-H., Marsh, D.J., and Marmarelis, V.Z. 1998. Comparative nonlinear modeling of renal autoregulation in rats: volterra approach versus artificial neural networks. *IEEE Trans. Neural Networks*, 9: 430–435.

Farotimi, O., Dembo, A., and Kailath, T. 1991. A general weight matrix formulation using optimal control. *IEEE Trans. Neural Networks*, 2: 378–394.

Fogel, D. and Sebald, A.V. 1990. Use of evolutionary programming in the design of neural networks for artifact detection. *Proc. of IEEE/EMBS Conf.*, 12: 1408–1409.

Grossberg, S. 1988a. *Neural Networks and Natural Intelligence*, MIT Press, Cambridge, MA.

Grossberg, S. 1988b. Nonlinear neural networks: principles, mechanisms and architectures. *Neural Networks*, 1: 17–61.

Hagan, M.T., Demuth, H.B., and Beale, M. 1996. *Neural Network Design*, PWS Publishing Co., New York.

Hebb, D.O. 1949. *The Organization of Behavior, A Neuropsychological Theory*, John Wiley, New York.

Hecht-Nielson, R. 1989. *Neurocomputing*, Addison-Wesley, New York.

Hinton, G.E. 1989. Connectionist learning procedures. *Artif. Intell.*, 40: 185–234.

Hopfield. 1982. Neural networks and physical systems with emergent collective computational abilities. *Proc. Natl Acad. Sci. USA*, 79: 2554–2558.

Houk, J.C., Singh, S.P., Fisher, C., and Barto, A.G. 1990. An adaptive sensorimotor network inspired by the anatomy and physiology of the cerebellum. In *Neural Networks for Control*. W.T. Miller, R.S. Sutton, and P.J. Werbos, Eds. pp. 301–348. MIT Press, Cambridge, MA.

Kawato, M., Furukawa, K., and Suzuki, R. 1987. A hierarchical neural-network model for control and learning of voluntary movement. *Biol. Cybern.*, 57: 169–185.

Koch, C. and Segev, I. 1989. *Methods in Neuronal Modeling: From Synapses to Networks*, MIT Press, Cambridge, MA.

Kohonen, T. 1989. *Self-Organization and Associative Memory*, Springer-Verlag, New York.

Lan, N., Feng, H.Q., and Crago, P.E. 1994. Neural network generation of muscle stimulation patterns for control of arm movements. *IEEE Trans. Rehab. Eng.*, 2: 213–224.

Levin, E., Gewirtzman, R., and Inbar, G.E. 1991. Neural network architecture for adaptive system modeling and control. *Neural Networks*, 4: 185–191.

Lippman, R.P. 1987. An introduction to computing with neural nets. *IEEE Mag. Acoust., Signal Speech Proc.*, April: 4–22.

Miller, W.T., Hewes, R.P., Glanz, F.G., and Kraft, L.G.I.I.I. 1990a. Real-time dynamic control of an industrial manipulator using a neural-network-based learning controller. *IEEE Trans. Robotics Automation*, 6: 1–9.

Miller, W.T., Sutton, R.S., and Werbos, P.J. 1990b. *Neural Networks for Control*, MIT Press, Cambridge, MA.

Missler, J.M. and Kamangar, F.A. 1995. A neural network for pursuit tracking inspired by the fly visual system. *Neural Networks*, 8: 463–480.

Miyamoto, H., Kawato, M., Setoyama, T., and Suzuki, R. 1988. Feedback-error-learning neural network for trajectory control of a robotic manipulator. *Neural Networks*, 1: 251–265.

Narendra, K.S. 1992. Adaptive control of dynamical systems using neural networks. In *Handbook of Intelligent Control: Neural, Fuzzy and Adaptive Approaches*. D.A. White and D.A. Sofge, Eds. pp. 141–184. Van Nostrand Reinhold, New York.

Narendra, K.S. and Parthasarathy, K. 1990. Identification and control of dynamical systems using neural networks. *IEEE Trans. Neural Networks*, 1: 4–27.

Nerrand, O., Roussel-Ragot, P., Personnaz, L., Dreyfus, G., and Marcos, S. 1993. Neural networks and nonlinear adaptive filtering: unifying concepts and new algorithms. *Neural Comput.*, 5: 165–199.

Nguyen, D.H. and Widrow, B. 1990. Neural networks for self-learning control systems. *IEEE Contr. Syst. Mag.*, 10: 18–23.

Nordgren, R.E. and Meckl, P.H. 1993. An analytical comparison of a neural network and a model-based adaptive controller. *IEEE Trans. Neural Networks*, 4: 685–694.

Pao, Y.H. 1989. *Adaptive Pattern Recognition and Neural Networks*, Addison-Wesley, Reading, MA.

Pined, F.J. 1989. Recurrent backpropagation and the dynamical approach to adaptive neural computation. *Neural Comput.*, 1: 161–172.

Quinn, R.D. and Espenschied, K.S. 1993. Control of a hexapod robot using a biologically inspired neural network. In *Biological Neural Networks in Invertebrate Neuroethology and Robotics*. R.D. Beer, R.E. Ritzmann, and T. McKenna, Eds. pp. 365–382. Academic Press, New York.

Rumelhart, D.E. and McClelland, J.L. 1988. *Parallel Distributed Processing: Explorations in the Microstructure of Cognition*, MIT Press, Cambridge, MA.

Sanchez-Sinencio, E. and Lau, C. 1992. *Artificial Neural Networks: Paradigms, Applications and Hardware Implementations*, IEEE Press, New York.

Schwartz, E.L. 1990. *Computational Neuroscience*, MIT Press, Cambridge, MA.

Simpson. 1990. *Artificial Neural Systems*, Pergamon Press, New York.

Srinivasan, S., Gander, R.E., and Wood, H.C. 1992. A movement pattern generator model using artificial neural networks. *IEEE Trans. BME*, 39: 716–722.

Taga, G., Yamaguchi, Y., and Shimizu, H. 1991. Self-organized control of bipedal locomotion by neural oscillators in unpredictable environment. *Biol. Cybern.*, 65: 147–159.

Trajanoski, Z. and Wach, P. 1998. Neural predictive controller for insulin delivery using the subcutaneous route. *IEEE Trans. BME*, 45: 1122–1134.

Vogl, T.P., Mangis, J.K., Rigler, A.K., Zink, W.T., and Alkon, D.L. 1988. Accelerating the convergence of the back-propagation method. *Biol. Cybern.*, 59: 257–263.

Wang, H., Lee, T.T., and Graver, W.A. 1992. A neuromorphic controller for a three-link biped robot. *IEEE Trans. Syst. Man. Cyber.*, 22: 164–169.

Werbos, P.J. 1990. Overview of designs and capabilities. In *Neural Networks for Control*. W.T. Miller, R.S. Sutton, and P.J. Werbos, Eds. pp. 59–66. MIT Press, Cambridge, MA.

Werbos, P.J. 1992. Approximate dynamic programming for real-time control and neural modeling. In *Handbook of Intelligent Control: Neural, Fuzzy and Adaptive Approaches*. D.A. White and D.A. Sofge, Eds. pp. 493–526. Van Nostrand Reinhold, New York.

White, D.A. and Sofge, D.A. 1992. *Handbook of Intelligent Control: Neural, Fuzzy, and Adaptive Approaches*, Van Nostrand Reinhold, New York.

Widrow, B. 1962. Generalization and information storage in networks of adaline "neurons." In *Self-Organizing Systems*. M.C. Jovitz, T. Jacobi, and Goldstein, Eds. pp. 435–461. Spartan Books, Washington, D.C.

Williams, R.J. and Zipser, D. 1989. A learning algorithm for continually running fully recurrent neural networks. *Neural Comput.*, 1: 270–280.

Zurada, J.M. 1992. *Artificial Neural Systems*, West Publishing Co., New York.

Further Information

Very good introductions to the operation of neural networks are given in *Neural Network Design* by Hagan, Demuth, and Beale and in *Artificial Neural Systems* by J.M. Zurada.

Detailed descriptions of the neural network control systems described in this chapter are provided in *Neural Network Control Systems* edited by Miller, Sutton, and Werbos and *The Handbook of Intelligent Control* edited by White and Sofge.

For journal articles on neural network theory and applications, the reader is referred to *IEEE Transactions on Neural Networks*, *Neural Computation* (MIT Press), and *Neural Networks* (Pergamon Press).

For occasional journal articles on biomedical applications of neural networks, the reader is referred to *IEEE Transactions on Biomedical Engineering*, *IEEE Transactions on Rehabilitation Engineering*, and the *Annals of Biomedical Engineering*.

13

Methods and Tools for Identification of Physiologic Systems

Vasilis Z. Marmarelis

University of Southern California

The problem of system identification in physiology derives its importance from the need to acquire quantitative models of physiologic function (from the subcellular to the organ system level) by use of experimental observations (data). Quantitative models can be viewed as summaries of experimental observations that allow scientific inference and organize our knowledge regarding the functional properties of physiologic systems. Selection of the proper (mathematical or computational) form of the model is based on existing knowledge of the system's functional organization. System identification is the process by which the system model is determined from data. This modeling and identification problem is rather challenging in the general use of a physiologic system, where insufficient knowledge about the internal workings of the system or its usually confounding complexity prevents the development of an explicit model. The models may assume diverse forms (requiring equally diverse approaches) depending on the specific characteristics of the physiologic system (e.g., static/dynamic, linear/nonlinear) and the prevailing experimental conditions (e.g., noise contamination of data, limitations on experimental duration). This chapter will not address the general modeling issue, but rather it will concentrate on specific methods and tools that can be employed in order to accomplish the system identification task in most cases encountered in practice. Because of space limitations, the treatment of these system identification methods will be consistent with the style of a review article providing overall perspective and guidance while deferring details to cited references.

Since the complexity of the physiologic system identification problem rivals its importance, we begin by demarcating those areas where effective methods and tools currently exist. The selection among candidate models is made on the basis of the following key functional characteristics (1) static or dynamic; (2) linear or nonlinear; (3) stationary or nonstationary; (4) deterministic or stochastic; (5) single or multiple inputs and/or outputs; (6) lumped or distributed. These classification criteria do not constitute an exhaustive list but cover most cases of current interest. Furthermore, it is critical to remember that contaminating noise (be it systemic or measurement-related) is always present in an actual study, and experimental constraints often limit experimentation time and the type of data obtainable from the system. Finally, the computational requirements for a practicable identification method must not be extraordinary, and the obtained results (models) must be amenable to physiologic interpretation, in addition to their demonstrated predictive ability.

A critical factor in determining our approach to the system modeling and identification task is the availability and quality of prior knowledge about the system under study with respect to the mechanisms that subserve its function. It can be said in general that, if sufficient knowledge about the internal mechanisms subserving the function of a system is available, then the development of an explicit model from first (physical or chemical) principles is possible, and the system modeling and identification task is immensely simplified by reducing to an estimation problem of the unknown parameters contained in the explicit model. Although the ease of this latter task depends on the manner in which the unknown parameters enter in the aforementioned explicit model, as well as on the quality of the available data, it is typically feasible. Furthermore, the obtained model is amenable to direct and meaningful physiologic interpretation. Unfortunately, it is rare that such prior knowledge (of adequate quality and quantity) is available in systems physiology. It is far more common that only limited prior knowledge is available, relative to the customary complexity of physiologic systems, that prevents the development of an explicit model from first principles and necessitates the search for a model that is compatible with the available input–output data.

Thus, the system identification problem is typically comprised of two tasks:

1. *Model specification*: the selection or postulation of a model form suitable for the system at hand
2. *Model estimation*: the estimation of the unknown parameters or functions contained within the specified model, using experimental data

All prior knowledge about the system under study is utilized in the model specification task. This includes results from specially designed preliminary experiments, which can be used to establish, for instance, whether the system is static or dynamic, linear or nonlinear, and so on. The model estimation task, however, relies on the quality of the available data (e.g., spectral characteristics, noise conditions, data length) and may set specific data-collection requirements.

This chapter will focus on practicable methods to perform both the model specification and model estimation tasks for systems/models that are static or dynamic and linear or nonlinear. Only the stationary case will be detailed here, although the potential use of nonstationary methods will be also discussed briefly when appropriate. In all cases, the models will take deterministic form, except for the presence of additive error terms (model residuals). Note that stochastic experimental inputs (and, consequently, outputs) may still be used in connection with deterministic models. The cases of multiple inputs and/or outputs (including multidimensional inputs/outputs, e.g., spatio-temporal) as well as lumped or distributed systems, will not be addressed in the interest of brevity. It will also be assumed that the data (single input and single output) are in the form of evenly sampled time-series, and the employed models are in discrete-time form (e.g., difference equations instead of differential equations, discrete summations instead of integrals).

In pursuing the model specification task, two general approaches have developed: parametric and nonparametric. In the parametric approach, algebraic or difference equation models are typically used to represent the input–output relation for static or dynamic systems, respectively. These models are accordingly linear or nonlinear, and contain a (typically small) number of unknown parameters. The latter may be constant or time-varying depending on whether the system or model is stationary or nonstationary. The precise form of these parametric models (e.g., degree/order of equation) must be determined in order to complete the model specification task. This precise form is either postulated a priori or guided by the data (in which case it is intertwined with the model parameter estimation task) as outlined in the following section.

In the nonparametric approach, the input–output relation is represented either analytically (in convolutional form through Volterra–Wiener expansions where the unknown quantities are kernel functions), computationally (i.e., by compiling all input–output mapping combinations to look-up tables) or graphically (in the form of operational surfaces/subspaces in phase-space). The graphical representation, of course, is subject to the three-dimensional limitation for the purpose of visual inspection. The model specification requirements for the Volterra–Wiener formulation consist of the order of system nonlinearity and system memory, and, for the computational or graphical approach, they consist of defining the appropriate phase-space mapping dimensions, as discussed below. Of the nonparametric approaches, the Volterra–Wiener (kernel) formulation has been used more extensively in a nonlinear context and will be the focus of this review, since nonlinearities are ubiquitous in physiology. Note that the nonparametric model estimation task places certain requirements on the experimental input (i.e., sufficient coverage of the frequency bandwidth and amplitude range of interest in each application) in order to secure adequate probing of the system functional characteristics.

An important hybrid approach has also developed in recent years that makes use of block-structured or modular models. These models are composed of parametric and/or nonparametric components properly connected to represent reliably the input–output relation. The model specification task for this class of models is more demanding and may utilize previous parametric and/or nonparametric modeling results. A promising variant of this approach, which derives from the general Volterra–Wiener formulation, employs principal dynamic modes as a canonical set of filters to represent a broad class of nonlinear dynamic systems. Another variant of the modular approach that has recently acquired considerable popularity but will not be covered in this review is the use of artificial neural networks to represent input–output nonlinear mappings in the form of connectionist models. These connectionist models are often fully parametrized, making this approach affine to parametric modeling, as well.

The relations among these approaches (parametric, nonparametric, and modular) are of critical practical importance and the subject of several recent studies [Marmarelis, 1994, 1997]. Considerable benefits may accrue from the combined use of these approaches in a cooperative manner that aims at securing the full gamut of distinct advantages specific to each approach.

In the following sections, an overview of these methodologies will be presented and the relative advantages and disadvantages in practical applications will be briefly outlined. The ultimate selection of a particular methodology hinges upon the specific characteristics of the application at hand and the prioritization of objectives by the individual investigator. Two general comments are in order:

1. No single methodology is globally superior to all others, that is, excelling with regard to all criteria and under all possible circumstances. Judgment must be exercised in each individual case
2. The general system identification problem is not solvable in all cases at present, and challenging problems remain for future research

13.1 Parametric Approach

Consider the input and output time-series data, $x(n)$, respectively. If the system is static and linear, then we can employ the simplest (and most widely used) model of linear regression

$$y(n) = ax(n) + b + \varepsilon(n) \tag{13.1}$$

to represent the input–output relation for every n, where $\varepsilon(n)$ represents the noise or error term (or model residual) at each n. The unknown parameters (a, b) can be easily estimated through least-squares fitting, using a well-developed set of linear regression methods (e.g., ordinary least-squares or generalized least-squares depending on whether $\varepsilon(n)$ is a white sequence).

This model can be extended to multiple inputs $\{x_1, x_2, \ldots, x_k\}$ and outputs $\{y_i\}$ as

$$y_i(n) = a_1 x_1(n) + a_2 x_2(n) + \cdots + a_k x_k(n) + b + \varepsilon(n) \tag{13.2}$$

and well-developed multiple linear regression techniques exist that can be used for estimation of the unknown parameters $(a_1, a_2, \ldots, a_k, b)$ for each output y_i. Although these estimation methods are widely known and readily available in the literature — see, for instance, Eykhoff [1974] and Soderstrom and Stoica [1989] — they will be briefly reviewed at the end of this section.

In the event of nonstationarities, the regression coefficients (model parameters) will vary through time and can be estimated either in a piecewise stationary fashion over a sliding time window (batch processing) or in a recursive fashion using an adaptive estimation formula (recursive processing). The latter has been favored and extensively studied in recent years [Ljung and Soderstrom, 1983; Goodwin and Sin, 1984; Ljung, 1987], and it is briefly outlined at the end of this section.

If the system is static and nonlinear, then a nonlinear input–output relation

$$y(n) = \sum_{j=1}^{J} c_j P_j[x(n)] + \varepsilon(n) \tag{13.3}$$

can be used as a parametric model, where the $\{P_j\}$ functions represent a set of selected nonlinear functions (e.g., powers, polynomials, sinusoids, sigmoids, exponentials or any other suitable of functions over the range of x), and $\{c_j\}$ are the unknown parameters that can be easily estimated through linear regression — provided that the $\{P_j\}$ functions do not contain other unknown parameters in a nonlinear fashion. In the latter case, nonlinear regression methods must be used (e.g., the gradient steepest-descent method) that are well developed and readily available [Eykhoff, 1974; Ljung, 1987; Soderstrom and Stoica, 1989], although their use is far from problem-free or devoid of risk of misleading results (e.g., local minima or noise effects). Naturally, the choice of the $\{P_j\}$ functions is critical in this regard and may depend on the characteristics of the system or the type of available data.

These cases of static systems have been extensively studied to date but have only limited interest or applicability to actual physiologic systems, since the latter are typically dynamic — that is, the output value at time n depends also on input and/or output values at other previous times (lags). Note that the possible dependence of the present output value on previous output values can be also expressed as a dependence on previous input values. Thus, we now turn to the all-important case of dynamic systems.

For linear (stationary) dynamic systems, the discrete-time parametric model takes the form of an *auto-regressive moving average with exogenous variable* (ARMAX) equation:

$$\begin{aligned} y(n) = & \alpha_1 y(n-1) + \cdots + \alpha_k y(n-k) + \beta_0 x(n) + \beta_1 x(n-1) \\ & + \cdots + \beta_1 x(n-1) + w(n) + \gamma_1 w(n-1) + \cdots + \gamma_m w(n-m) \end{aligned} \tag{13.4}$$

where $w(n)$ represents a white noise sequence. This ARMAX model is a difference equation that expresses the present value of the output, $y(n)$, as a linear combination of k previous values of the output (AR part), l previous (and the present) values of the input (X part), and m previous (and the present) values of the white noise disturbance sequence (MA part) that compose the model residual (error). When $\gamma_i = 0$ for all $i = 1, \ldots, m$, the residuals form a white sequence, and the coefficients $(\alpha_1, \ldots, \alpha_k, \beta_0, \beta_1, \ldots, \beta_l)$ can be estimated through the ordinary least-squares procedure. However, if any γ_i is nonzero, then unbiased and consistent estimation requires generalized or extended least-squares procedures, similar to the one required for the multiple regression model of Equation 13.2 when $\varepsilon(n)$ is a nonwhite error sequence (reviewed at the end of the section).

Although the estimation of the ARMAX model parameters can be straightforward through multiple linear regression, the model specification task remains a challenge. The latter consists of determining the maximum lag values (k, l, m) in the difference Equation 13.4 from given input–output data, $x(n)$ and $y(n)$. A number of statistical procedures have been devised for this purpose (e.g., weighted residual variance, Akaike information criterion), all of them based on the prediction error for given model order (k, l, m) compensated properly for the remaining degrees of freedom (i.e., the total number of data minus the number of parameters). It is critical that the prediction error (typically, in mean-square sense) be evaluated on a segment of input–output data distinct from the one used for the estimation of the model parameters. Application of these criteria is repeated successively for ascending values of the model order (k, l, m), and the model specification process is completed when an extremum (minimum or maximum, depending on the criterion) is achieved [Soderstrom and Stoica, 1989].

For nonlinear (stationary) systems, the ARMAX model can be extended to the NARMAX model (nonlinear ARMAX) that includes nonlinear expressions of the variables on the right side of Equation 13.4 [Billings and Voon, 1984]. For instances, a second-degree multinomial NARMAX model of order $(k = 2, l = 1, m = 0)$ with additive white-noise residuals takes the form

$$\begin{aligned} y(n) = &\ \alpha_1 y(n-1) + \alpha_2 y(n-2) + \alpha_{1,1} y^2(n-1) + \alpha_{1,2} y(n-1)y(n-2) \\ &+ \alpha_{2,2} y^2(n-2) + \beta_0 x(n) + \beta_1 x(n-1) + \beta_{0,0} x^2(n) \\ &+ \beta_{0,1} x(n)x(n-1) + \beta_{1,1} x^2(n-1) + \gamma_{1,0} y(n-1)x(n) \\ &+ \gamma_{2,0} y(n-2)x(n) + \gamma_{1,1} y(n-1)x(n-1) \\ &+ \gamma_{2,1} y(n-2)x(n-1) + w(n) \end{aligned}$$
(13.5)

Clearly, the form of a NARMAX model may become rather unwieldy, and the model specification task (i.e., the form and degree of nonlinear terms, as well as the number of input, output, and noise lags involved in the model) is very challenging. Several approaches have been proposed for this purpose [Billings and Voon, 1984, 1986; Korenberg, 1988; Haber and Unbenhauen, 1990; Zhao and Marmarelis, 1994], and they are all rather involved computationally. However, if the structure of the NARMAX model is established, then the parameter estimation task is straightforward in a manner akin to multiple linear regression — since the unknown parameters enter linearly in the NARMAX model.

It is evident that all these multiple linear regression problems defined by Equation 13.2 to Equation 13.5 can be written in a vector form:

$$y(n) = \phi^T(n)\theta + \varepsilon(n)$$
(13.6)

where $\phi(n)$ represents the vector of all regression variables in each case, and θ denotes the unknown parameter vector. For a set of data points $(n = 1, \ldots, N)$, Equation 13.6 yields the matrix formulation

$$y = \Phi\theta + \varepsilon$$
(13.7)

The ordinary least-squares (OLS) estimate of θ

$$\hat{\theta}^{OLS} = [\Phi^T\Phi]^{-1}\Phi^T y$$
(13.8)

yields unbiased and consistent estimates of minimum variance, if $\varepsilon(n)$ is a white sequence; otherwise, the generalized least-squares (GLS) estimator

$$\hat{\theta}^{GLS} = [\Phi^T\Sigma^{-1}\Phi]^{-1}\Phi^T\Sigma^{-1} y$$
(13.9)

ought to be used to achieve minimum estimation variance, where Σ denotes the covariance matrix of ε. Practical complications arise from the fact that Σ is not a priori known and, therefore, must be either postulated or estimated from the data. The latter case, which is more realistic in actual applications, leads to an iterative procedure that may not be convergent or yield satisfactory results (i.e., start with an OLS estimate of θ; obtain a first estimate of ε and Σ; evaluate a first GLS estimate of θ; obtain a second estimate of ε and Σ; and iterate until the process converges to a final GLS estimate of θ). As an alternative to this iterative procedure, an estimate of the moving-average model of the residual term:

$$\varepsilon(n) = w(n) + \gamma_1 w(n-1) + \cdots + \gamma_m w(n-m) \tag{13.10}$$

may be obtained from initial OLS estimation, and the covariance matrix Σ may be estimated from Equation 13.10. Although this alternative approach avoids problems of convergence, it does not necessarily yield satisfactory results due to the dependence on the noise model estimation of Equation 13.10. Equivalent to this latter procedure is the residual whitening method, which amounts to prefiltering the data with the inverse of the transfer function corresponding to Equation 13.10 (prewhitening filter), prior to OLS estimation. Finally, the parameter vector may be augmented to include the coefficient $\{\gamma_i\}$ of the moving-average model of the residuals in Equation 13.10, leading to a pseudo-linear regression problem (since the estimates of $w(n)$ depend on $\hat{\theta}$) that is operationally implemented as an iterative extended least-squares (ELS) procedure [Ljung and Soderstrom, 1983; Billings and Voon, 1984, 1986; Ljung, 1987; Soderstrom and Stoica, 1989].

In the presence of nonstationarities, the parameter vector θ may vary through time, and its estimation may be performed either in a piecewise stationary manner (with segment-to-segment updates that may be obtained either recursively or through batch processing) or by introducing a specific parametrized time-varying structure for the parameters and augmenting the unknown parameter vector to include the additional parameters of the time-varying structure (e.g., a pth degree polynomial structure of time-varying model parameters will introduce p additional parameters for each time-varying term into the vector θ, that need be estimated from the data via batch processing).

Any batch processing approach folds back to the previously discussed least-squares estimation methods. However, the recursive approach requires a new methodological framework that updates continuously the parameter estimates on the basis of new data. This adaptive or recursive approach has gained increasing popularity in recent years, although certain important practical issues (e.g., speed of algorithmic convergence, effect of correlated noise) remain causes for concern in certain cases [Ljung and Soderstrom, 1983; Goodwin and Sin, 1984; Ljung, 1987]. The basic formulae for the recursive least-squares (RLS) algorithm are

$$\hat{\theta}(n) = \hat{\theta}(n-1) + \Psi(n)[y(n) - \phi^{\mathrm{T}}(n)\hat{\theta}(n-1)] \tag{13.11}$$

$$\Psi(n) = \gamma(n)P(n-1)\phi(n) \tag{13.12}$$

$$P(n) = P(n-1) - \gamma(n)P(n-1)\phi(n)\phi^{\mathrm{T}}(n)P(n-1) \tag{13.13}$$

$$\gamma(n) = [\phi^{\mathrm{T}}(n)P(n-1)\phi(n) + \alpha(n)]^{-1} \tag{13.14}$$

where the matrix $P(n)$, the vector $\Psi(n)$, and the scalar $\gamma(n)$ are updating instruments of the algorithm computed at each step n. Note that $\{\alpha(n)\}$ denotes a selected sequence of weights for the squared prediction errors in the cost function and is often taken to be unity. This recursive algorithm can be used for on-line identification of stationary or nonstationary systems. A critical issue in the nonstationary case is the speed of algorithmic convergence relative to the time-variation of the system/model parameters. Its initialization is commonly made as: $\hat{\theta}(0) = 0$ and $P(0) = c_0 I$, where c_0 is a large positive constant (to suppress the effect of initial conditions) and I is the identity matrix.

It is important to note that when output autoregressive terms exist in the model, the regression vector $\phi(n)$ is correlated with the residual $\varepsilon(n)$, and, thus, none of the aforementioned least-squares estimates of the parameter vector will converge to the actual value. This undesirable correlation weakens when the predicted output values are used at each step for the autoregressive lagged terms (closed-loop mode or one-step predictive model) instead of the observed output values (open-loop mode or global predictive model). To remedy this problem, the instrumental variable (IV) method has been introduced that makes use of a selected IV that is uncorrelated with the residuals but strongly correlated with the regression vector

$\phi(n)$ in order to evaluate the least-squares estimate [Soderstrom and Stoica, 1989]. The IV estimates can be computed in batch or recursive fashion.

In closing this section, we should note that a host of other estimation methods has been developed through the years and that these methods are operationally affine to the foregoing ones (e.g., prediction-error methods, stochastic approximation, gradient-based methods) or represent different statistical approaches to parameter estimation (e.g., maximum likelihood, bayesian approach) including the state-space formulation of the problem, that cannot be detailed here in the interest of space [for review, see Eykhoff, 1974; Goodwin and Payne, 1977; Ljung and Soderstrom, 1983; Goodwin and Sin, 1984; Ljung, 1987; Soderstrom and Stoica, 1989].

13.2 Nonparametric Approach

In the linear stationary case, the discrete-time nonparametric model takes the convolutional form:

$$y(n) = \sum_{m=0}^{M} h(m)x(n-m) + \varepsilon(n) \tag{13.15}$$

where $\varepsilon(n)$ is an output-additive error/noise term and $h(m)$ is the discrete impulse response of the linear time-invariant (stationary) system with memory extent M. For finite-memory systems (i.e., when $h(m)$ becomes negligible for $m > M$ and M is finite), the estimation of $h(m)$ from input–output data can be accomplished by multiple regression, since the model of Equation 13.15 retains the form of a parametric model with no autoregressive terms. Note that any stable ARMAX model can be put in the form of Equation 13.15, where $M \rightarrow \infty$ and $h(m)$ is absolute-summable. The estimation of $h(m)$ can be also accomplished in the frequency domain via discrete Fourier transforms (DFTs, implemented as FFTs), observing the fact that convolution turns into multiplication in the frequency domain. Particular attention must be paid to cases where the input DFT attains very small values to avoid numerical or estimation problems during the necessary division. In actual physiologic practice, many investigators have chosen to perform experiments with specific input waveforms to facilitate this identification task, that is, the use of an impulsive input of unit strength directly yields $h(m)$, or the use of sinusoidal inputs of various frequencies yields directly the values of the DFT of $h(m)$ at the corresponding frequencies (covering the entire frequency range of interest).

In the nonlinear stationary case, the most widely used methodology for nonparametric modeling is based on the Volterra functional expansions and Wiener's theory that employs a gaussian white noise (GWN) test input in conjunction with a modified (orthogonalized) Volterra functional expansion. Wiener's critical contribution is in suggesting that GWN is an effective test input for identifying non-linear systems of a very broad class and in proposing specific mathematical procedures for the estimation of the unknown system descriptors (kernels) from input–output data, as outlined below [for more details, see Schetzen, 1980; Rugh, 1981; Marmarelis and Marmarelis, 1987; Marmarelis, 2004].

The input–output relation of a causal nonlinear stationary system in discrete time is seen as a mapping of a vector comprised of the input past (and present) values onto the (scalar) present value of the output:

$$y(n) = F[x(n'), n - M \le n' \le n] \tag{13.16}$$

where M is the system memory and F is a fixed multivariate function representing this mapping — note that, in continuous time, F is a functional. If the system is nonstationary, the function F varies through time. If the function F is analytic and the system is stable, then a discrete-time Volterra series expansion exists of the form:

$$y(n) = \sum_{i=0}^{\infty} \sum_{m_1=0}^{M} \cdots \sum_{m_i=0}^{M} k_i(m_1, \ldots, m_i) x(n - m_1) \cdots x(n - m_i) \qquad (13.17)$$

This series converges for any stable system within the radius of convergence defined by the input ensemble. If the multivariate function F is not analytic but is continuous, then a finite-order Volterra model can be found that achieves any desirable degree of approximation (based on the Stone–Weierstrass theorem).

The multiple convolutions of the Volterra model involve kernel functions $\{k_i(m_1, \ldots, m_i)\}$ which constitute the descriptors of the system nonlinear dynamics. Consequently, the system identification task is to obtain estimates of these kernels from input–output data. These kernel functions are symmetric with respect to their arguments.

When a sinusoidal input is used, then the ith order Volterra functional (i.e., the i-tuple convolution in the Volterra model) gives rise to output harmonics of order $i, (i - 2), \ldots, (i - 2j)$ where j is the integer part $i/2$. When an impulse $A\delta(n)$ is used as input, then the ith order Volterra functional is contributing the term $A_i k_i(n, \ldots, n)$ to the output. This suggests that the Volterra kernels of a general system cannot be separated from each other and directly determined from input–output data, unless the Volterra expansion is of finite order. For a finite-order Volterra expansion, kernel estimation can be achieved through least-squares fitting procedures [Stark, 1968; Watanabe and Stark, 1975; Korenberg, 1988] or by use of specialized test inputs such as multiple impulses or step function [Schetzen, 1965; Stark, 1968; Shi and Sun, 1990] and sums of sinusoids of incommensurate frequencies [Victor et al., 1977], although the testing and analysis procedures can be rather laborious in those cases. The latter method yields estimates of the system kernels in the frequency domain at the selected input frequencies (and their harmonic/intermodulation frequencies) with increased accuracy but with limited frequency resolution.

The inability to estimate the Volterra kernels in the general case of an infinite series prompted Wiener to suggest the orthogonalization of the Volterra series when a GWN test input is used. The functional terms of the Wiener series are constructed on the basis of a Gram–Schmidt orthogonalization procedure requiring that the covariance between any two Wiener functionals be zero. The resulting Wiener series expansion takes the form:

$$y(n) = \sum_{i=0}^{\infty} G_i[h_i; x(n'), n' \leq n]$$

$$= \sum_{i=0}^{\infty} \sum_{j=0}^{i/2} \frac{(-1)^j i! P^j}{(i - 2j)! j! 2^j} \sum_{m_1} \cdots \sum_{m_i} h_i(m_1, \ldots, m_{i-2j}, l_1, l_1, \ldots, l_j, l_j)$$

$$x(n - m_1) \cdots x(n - m_{i-2j}) \qquad (13.18)$$

where $[i/2]$ is the integer part of $i/2$ and P is the power level of the GWN input. The set of Wiener kernels $\{h_i\}$ is, in general, different from the set of Volterra kernels $\{k_i\}$, but specific relations exist between the two sets [Marmarelis and Marmarelis, 1978; Marmarelis, 2004].

The Wiener kernels depend on the GWN input power level P (because they correspond to an orthogonal expansion), whereas the Volterra kernels are independent of any input characteristics. This situation can be likened to the coefficients of an orthogonal expansion of an analytic function being dependent on the interval of expansion. It is therefore imperative that Wiener kernel estimates be reported in the literature with reference to the GWN input power level that they were estimated with. When a complete set of Wiener kernels is obtained, then the complete set of Volterra kernels can be evaluated. Approximations of Volterra kernels can be obtained from Wiener kernels of the same order estimated with various input power levels. Complete Wiener or Volterra models can predict the system output to any given input.

When the Wiener or Volterra model is incomplete, the accuracy of the predicted output will be, in general, different for the two models and will depend on each specific input.

The orthogonality of the Wiener series allows decoupling of the various Wiener functionals and the estimation of the respective Wiener kernels from input–output data through cross-correlation [Lee and Schetzen, 1965]

$$h_i(m_1, \ldots, m_i) = \frac{1}{i! P^i} E[y_i(n) x(n - m_1) \cdots x(n - m_i)] \tag{13.19}$$

where $y_i(n)$ is the ith response residual

$$y_i(n) = y(n) - \sum_{j=0}^{i-1} G_j(n) \tag{13.20}$$

The simplicity and elegance of the cross-correlation technique led to its adoption by many investigators in modeling studies of nonlinear physiologic systems [Stark, 1968; McCann and Marmarelis, 1975; Marmarelis and Marmarelis, 1978; Marmarelis, 1987, 1989, 1994].

Since the ensemble average of Equation 13.19 is implemented in practice by time-averaging over a finite data-record, and since GWN is not physically realizable, many importance practical issues had to be explored in actual applications of the cross-correlation technique. To name but a few: the generation of appropriate quasi-white test signals (that adequately approximate the ideal and not physically realizable GWN); the choice of input bandwidth relative to the system bandwidth; the accuracy of the obtained kernel estimates as a function of input bandwidth and record length; the effect of extraneous noise and experimental imperfections. An extensive study of some of these practical considerations can be found in Marmarelis and Marmarelis [1978] and in Marmarelis [1979].

A broad class of effective quasi-white test signals (CSRS) has been introduced that can be easily generated on the computer and may follow any zero-mean symmetric (discrete or continuous) amplitude probability density function [Marmarelis, 1977]. The use of this type of test signal allows through analysis of kernel estimation errors via cross-correlation and the optimization of the input bandwidth B (for given record length N) on the basis of a total mean-square error (TMSE) criterion for the ith-order kernel estimate given by:

$$(\text{TMSE})_i = \frac{a_i}{B^4} + \frac{b_i B^{i-1}}{N} \tag{13.21}$$

where a_i and b_i are positive constants characteristic of the ith-order kernel [Marmarelis, 1979].

The cross-correlation technique results in considerable variance in the kernel estimates, unless very long data-records are available, because of the stochastic nature of the input. This has prompted the use of pseudo-random m-sequences [Ream, 1970; Billings and Fakhouri, 1981; Moller, 1983; Sutter, 1992] — which can reduce considerably the data-record requirements and yield improved estimation accuracy, provided that proper attention is given to certain problems in their high-order autocorrelation functions. To the same end, frequency-domain methods have been proposed for kernel estimation [Brillinger, 1970; French, 1976; Victor et al., 1977] yielding computational savings in some cases and offering a different perspective for the interpretation of results.

To reduce the requirements of long experimental data records and improve the kernel estimation accuracy, least-squares methods also can be used to solve the classical linear inverse problem described earlier in Equation 13.6, where the parameter vector θ includes all discrete kernel values of the finite Volterra model of Equation 13.17, which is linear in these unknown parameters (i.e., kernel values). Least-squares methods also can be used in connection with orthogonal expansions of the kernels to reduce the number of unknown parameters, as outlined below. Note that solution of this inverse problem via OLS requires inversion of a large square matrix with dimensions $[(M + I + 1)!/((M + 1)!I!)]$, where M is the kernel memory and I is the (maximum) nonlinear order of the Volterra model. Since direct inversion of this matrix may require considerable computing effort and be subject to conditioning problems, it is often expedient to solve this inverse problem by use of QR decomposition that offers certain computational and numerical advantages. One such implementation is Korenberg's exact orthogonalization method [Korenberg, 1988], which estimates the discrete kernel values through least-squares fitting of a sequence of orthogonal vectors built from input values in accordance with the Volterra expansion (effectively forming the Q orthogonal matrix of the QR decomposition). Other numerical methods also can be used for matrix inversion, depending on the requirements of each application. Likewise, a variety of orthogonal bases can be used for kernel expansion in order to obtain a more concise representation of the kernels in each particular application. The use of the Laguerre orthogonal basis typically results in reduction of the number of unknown parameters for most physiologic system kernels (due to their built-in exponential structure), with consequent improvement in estimation accuracy [Watanabe and Stark, 1975; Marmarelis, 1993, 2004]. Thus, if $\{b_j(m)\}$ is a complete orthonormal basis defined over the system memory $[O, M]$, then the ith-order Volterra kernel can be expanded as

$$k_i(m_1, \ldots, m_i) = \sum_{j_1} \cdots \sum_{j_i} c_i(j_1, \ldots, j_i) b_{j_1}(m_1) \cdots b_{j_i}(m_i) \tag{13.22}$$

Then the Volterra model of Equation 13.17 takes the form:

$$y(n) = \sum_i \left\{ \sum_{j_1} \cdots \sum_{j_i} c_i(j_1, \ldots, j_i) v_{j_1}(n) \cdots v_{j_i}(n) \right\} \tag{13.23}$$

where,

$$v_j(n) \sum_{m=0}^{M} b_j(m) x(n - m) \tag{13.24}$$

and the expansion coefficients $\{c_i(j_1, \ldots, j_i)\}$ of the unknown kernels can be estimated through multiple regression of $y(n)$ on the multinomial terms composed of the known functions $\{v_j(n)\}$. The kernel estimates are then reconstructed on the basis of Equation 13.22. This kernel estimation method has been shown to be far superior to the conventional cross-correlation technique in terms of estimation accuracy and robustness to noise or experimental imperfections [Marmarelis, 1993, 2004].

Based on this observation, a general model for the Volterra class of systems can be proposed that is comprised of a set of parallel linear filters with impulse response functions $\{b_j(m)\}$ whose outputs are fed into a multi-input static nonlinearity, $y = f(v_1, v_2, \ldots)$, to produce the system output. If was Wiener who first proposed the use of Laguerre functions (albeit in continuous-time form) for the set $\{b_j(m)\}$, since they are defined over the interval $[0, \infty)$ compatible with causal systems and can be generated in analog form — a fashionable model at the time — by a simple RC ladder network. He also suggested that the multi-input static nonlinearity be expanded in terms of orthogonal hermite functions to yield a system characterization in terms of the resulting Hermite expansion coefficients that are estimated through covariance computations. For a review of this approach, see Schetzen [1980]. This approach has been viewed as rather unwieldy and has not found many applications to date. However, the use of Laguerre expansions of kernels (in discrete time) in conjunction with least-squares fitting has been shown to be rather promising for practical kernel estimation from short and noisy data records [Marmarelis, 1993, 2004] and consequently suitable for experimental studies of physiologic systems.

The greatest obstacle to the broader use of the Volterra–Wiener approach has been the practical limitations in estimating high-order kernels due to two reasons (1) The amount of required computations increases geometrically with the order of estimated kernel; (2) kernel functions of more than three dimensions are difficult to inspect or interpret meaningfully. As a result, application of this approach has been limited to weakly nonlinear systems (second or third order).

A practical way of overcoming this limitation in the order of estimated kernels has been recently presented as a spin-off of studies on the relation between Volterra models and feedforward artificial neural networks [Marmarelis and Zhao, 1994; Marmarelis, 2004]. According to this approach, a perceptronlike network with polynomial activation functions is trained with the experimental data using a modified version of the back-propagation algorithm. The parameters of the resulting network can be subsequently converted to kernel estimates of arbitrary high order (although the network itself is a nonlinear model of the system on its own right). This alternative to current kernel estimation algorithms seems to hold significant promise, since it relaxes many of the requirements of existing methods (e.g., input whiteness and low-order models) at the only apparent cost of greater computing effort.

In the event of nonstationarities, the kernel become dependent on time, and their estimation can be accomplished either in a piecewise stationary manner (when the nonstationary is slow relative to the system dynamic bandwidth) or through truly nonstationary estimation methods. In the former case, the piecewise stationary estimates can be obtained over adjacent segments or using sliding (overlapping) windows along the time record. They can be subsequently displayed in a time-ordered sequence (revealing the time-varying pattern), under the assumption of system quasi-stationarity over the data segment or sliding window. Kernel estimation through truly nonstationary methods may be accomplished by (1) adaptive methods, employing the recursive least-squares formulae previously reviewed, which track changes in least-squares kernel estimates by continuous updating based on the output prediction error at each discrete step [Goodwin and Sin, 1984]; (2) ensemble-averaging methods, employing direct averaging of results obtained from many repetitions of identical experiments, which are rarely used because the latter is seldom feasible or practical in a physiologic experimental setting; (3) temporal expansion methods, employing explicit kernel expansions over time to avoid the experimental burden of the ensemble-averaging approach and the methodological constraints of adaptive methods, which utilize a single input–output data record to obtain complete nonstationary model representations under mild constraints [Marmarelis, 1981].

We note that the Volterra–Wiener approach has been extended to the case of nonlinear systems with multiple inputs and multiple outputs [Marmarelis and McCann, 1973; Marmarelis and Naka, 1974; Westwick and Kearney, 1992; Marmarelis, 2004] where functional terms are introduced, involving cross-kernels which measure the nonlinear interactions of the inputs as reflected on the output. This extension has led to a generalization for nonlinear systems with spatio-temporal inputs that has found applications to the visual system [Yasui et al., 1979; Citron et al., 1981]. Extension of the Volterra–Wiener approach to systems with spike (action potential) inputs encountered in neurophysiology also has been made, where the GWN test input is replaced by a Poisson process of impulses [Krausz, 1975]; this approach has found many applications including the study of the hippocampal formation in the brain [Sclabassi et al., 1988]. Likewise, the case of neural systems with spike outputs has been explored in the context of the Volterra–Wiener approach, leading to efficient modeling and identification methods [Marmarelis et al., 1986; Marmarelis and Orme, 1993; Marmarelis, 2004].

The mathematical relations between parametric (NARMAX) and nonparametric (Volterra) models have been explored, and significant benefits are shown to accrue from combined use [Zhao and Marmarelis, 1998]. These studies follow on previous efforts to relate certain classes of nonlinear differential equations with Volterra functional expansions in continuous time [Rugh, 1981; Marmarelis, 1989; Marmarelis, 2004].

Only brief mention will be made of the computational and graphical nonparametric methods of phase-space mappings. The computational method requires prior specification of the number of input and output lags that are needed to express the present output value as

$$y(n) = G[y(n-1), \ldots, y(n-k), x(n), x(n-1), \ldots, x(n-l)] \qquad (13.25)$$

where $G[\bullet]$ is an unknown function which maps the appropriate input–output vector $z(n) = [y(n-1), \ldots, y(n-k), x(n), \ldots, x(n-l)]$ onto the present value of the output $y(n)$. Then, using experimental data, we compile on the computer a list of correspondences between $z(n)$ and $y(n)$ in the form of an empirical model that can predict the output for a given z by finding the closest correspondence within the compiled list (look-up table) or using a properly defined interpolation scheme.

The graphical method is based on the notion that the mathematical model of a discrete-time finite-order (stationary) dynamic system is, in general, a multivariate function $f(\bullet)$ of the appropriate lagged values of the input–output variables

$$f[y(n), y(n-1), \ldots, y(n-k), x(n-1), \ldots, x(n-l)] = 0 \qquad (13.26)$$

This function (model) is a "constraint" among these input–output lagged (and present) values at each time instant n. The number of variables that partake in this relation and the particular form of $f(\bullet)$ are characteristic of the system under study. Therefore, in a geometric sense, the system (and its model) are represented by a subspace in a multidimensional space defined by the coordinate system of these variables. If one can define the appropriate space by choosing the relevant variables, then a model can be easily obtained by following the vector point corresponding to the data through time — provided that the input is such that the data cover the model subspace densely. If the input is ergodic, then sufficiently long observations will allow reliable estimation of the system model.

Although this is an old and conceptually straightforward idea, it has not been widely used (except in some recent studies of chaotic dynamics of autonomous systems, where no input variable exists) because several important practical issues must be addressed in its actual implementation, for example, the selection of the appropriate coordinate variables (embedding space) and the impracticality of representation in high-dimensional spaces. If a low-dimensional embedding space can be found for the system under study, this approach can be very powerful in yielding models of strongly nonlinear systems. Secondary practical issues are the choice of an effective test input and the accuracy of the obtained results in the presence of extraneous noise.

13.3 Modular Approach

The practical limitations in the use of Volterra–Wiener models for strongly nonlinear systems have led some investigators to explore the use of block-structured or modular models in the form of cascaded or parallel configurations of linear subsystems (L) and static nonlinearities (N). This model representation often provides greater insight into the functional organization of the system under study and facilitates that identification task by allowing separate estimation of the various component subsystems (L and N), thereby avoiding the computational burden associated with the dimensionality of high-order kernel functions. The advantages afforded by this approach can be had only when prior specification of the structure of the modular model is possible.

Simple cascade models (e.g., L–N, N–L, L–N–L) have been studied extensively, yielding estimates of the component subsystems with moderate computational effort [Marmarelis and Marmarelis, 1978; Billings and Fakhouri, 1982; Korenberg and Hunter, 1986; Shi and Sun, 1990]. Distinctive kernel relationships (e.g., between first-order and second-order kernels) exist for each type of cascade model, which can be used for validation of the chosen modular model on the basis of the kernel estimates obtained from the data — a task that is often referred to as structural identification. Thus, the combined use of the modular and nonparametric approaches may yield considerable benefits. This idea can be extended to more complicated modular structures entailing multiple parallel and cascaded branches [Chen et al., 1990; Korenberg, 1991]. The case of nonlinear feedback in modular models attracts considerable interest, because of its frequent and critical role in physiologic control and autoregulation. A case of weak nonlinear feedback in sensory systems has received thorough treatment [Marmarelis, 1991, 2004]. Naturally, the analysis becomes more complicated as the complexity of the modular model increases. Particular mention should be made of a rather complex model of parallel L–N–L cascades (usually called the S_m model) that covers a broad class of nonlinear systems [Billings and Fakhouri, 1981; Rugh, 1981].

A method for the development of a general model for the Volterra–Wiener class of systems, which assumes a modular form, was originally proposed by Wiener and his associates and is reviewed in Schetzen [1980]. A general modular model, comprised of parallel L–N cascades, also has been proposed by Korenberg [1991], and another, employing principal dynamic modes as a filterbank whose outputs feed into a multi-input static nonlinearity, has been recently proposed by Marmarelis [1997].

This latter general model evolved from the original Wiener modular model. It was first adapted to studies of neural systems that generate spikes (action potentials), whereby a threshold-trigger is placed at the output of the general modular model that obviates the use of high-order kernels and yields a parsimonious complete model [Marmarelis and Orme, 1993]. The importance of this development is found in that, ever since the Volterra–Wiener approach was applied to the study of spike-output neural systems, it had been assumed that a large number of kernels would be necessary to produce a satisfactory model prediction of the timing of output spikes, based on the rationale that the presence of a spike-generating mechanism constitutes a hard nonlinearity. Although this rationale is correct if we seek to reproduce the numerical binary values of the system output using a conventional Volterra–Wiener model, the inclusion of a threshold trigger in our modular model yields a compact and complete model (of possibly low order) that predicts precisely the timing of the output spikes [Marmarelis et al., 1986]. This also led to a search for the principal pathways of dynamic transformations of neural signals using eigen-decomposition of a matrix composed of the Laguerre expansion coefficients of the first- and second-order kernels [Marmarelis and Orme, 1993]. The estimation of these principal dynamic modes is accomplished via the aforementioned eigen-decomposition [Marmarelis, 1994] or through the training of a specific artificial neural network (a modified perceptron with polynomial activation functions) using a modified back-propagation algorithm [Marmarelis and Zhao, 1997]. The latter method holds great promise in providing a practical solution to the ultimate problem of nonlinear system identification, because it is not limited to low-order nonlinearities and does not place stringent requirements on the necessary input–output data, but it does retain a remarkable degree of robustness in the presence of noise.

The methodology employing Principal Dynamic Modes (PDM) holds great promise in addressing the long-standing problem of dimensionality in high-order nonlinear systems, as well as in the most challenging case of multiinput/multioutput systems, because of the compactness of representation that it achieves. Several recent applications of the PDM approach to a variety of physiological systems (neural, cardiovascular, renal, metabolic) have demonstrated this promise [for a comprehensive review, see Marmarelis, 2004].

Acknowledgment

This work was supported in part by Grant No. RR-01861 awarded to the Biomedical Simulations Resource at the University of Southern California from the National Center of Research Resources and the National Institute for Biomedical Imaging and Bioengineering of the National Institutes of Health.

References

Billings, S.A. and Fakhouri, S.Y. 1981. Identification of nonlinear systems using correlation analysis and pseudorandom inputs. *Int. J. Syst. Sci.* 11: 261.

Billings, S.A. and Fakhouri, S.Y. 1982. Identification of systems containing linear dynamic and static nonlinear elements. *Automatica* 18: 15.

Billings, S.A. and Voon, W.S.F. 1984. Least-squares parameter estimation algorithms for non-linear systems. *Int. J. Syst. Sci.* 15: 601.

Billings, S.A. and Voon, W.S.F. 1986. A prediction-error and stepwise-regression estimation algorithm for non-linear systems. *Int. J. Control* 44: 803.

Brillinger, D.R. 1970. The identification of polynomial systems by means of higher order spectra. *J. Sound Vib.* 12: 301.

Chen, H.-W, Jacobson, L.D., and Gaska, J.P. 1990. Structural classification of multi-input nonlinear systems. *Biol. Cybern.* 63: 341.

Citron, M.C., Kroeker, J.P., and McCann, G.D. 1981. Non-linear interactions in ganglion cell receptive fields. *J. Neurophysiol.* 46: 1161.

Eykhoff, P. 1974. *System Identification: Parameter and State Estimation.* New York, Wiley.

French, A.S. 1976. Practical nonlinear system analysis by Wiener kernel estimation in the frequency domain. *Biol. Cybern.* 24: 111.

Goodwin, G.C. and Payne, R.L. 1977. *Dynamic System Identification: Experiment Design and Data Analysis.* New York, Academic Press.

Goodwin, G.C. and Sin, K.S. 1984. *Adaptive Filtering, Prediction and Control.* Englewood Cliffs, NJ, Prentice-Hall.

Haber, R. and Unbenhauen, H. 1990. Structure identification of nonlinear dynamic systems — a survey of input/output approaches. *Automatica* 26: 651.

Korenberg, M.J. 1988. Identifying nonlinear difference equation and functional expansion representations: The fast orthogonal algorithm. *Ann. Biomed. Eng.* 16: 123.

Korenberg, M.J. 1991. Parallel cascade identification and kernel estimation for nonlinear systems. *Ann. Biomed. Eng.* 19: 429.

Korenberg, M.J. and Hunter, I.W. 1986. The identification of nonlinear biological systems: LNL cascaded models. *Biol. Cybern.* 55: 125.

Krausz, H.I. 1975. Identification of nonlinear systems using random impulse train inputs. *Biol. Cybern.* 19: 217.

Lee, Y.W. and Schetzen, M. 1965. Measurement of the Wiener kernels of a nonlinear system by cross-correlation. *Int. J. Control* 2: 237.

Ljung, L. 1987. *System Identification: Theory for the User.* Englewood Cliffs, NJ, Prentice-Hall.

Ljung, L. and Soderstrom, T. 1983. *Theory and Practice of Recursive Identification.* Cambridge, MA, MIT Press.

Marmarelis, V.Z. 1977. A family of quasi-white random signals and its optimal use in biological system identification: I. *Theor. Biol. Cybern.* 27: 49.

Marmarelis, V.Z. 1979. Error analysis and optimal estimation procedures in identification of nonlinear Volterra systems. *Automatica* 15: 161.

Marmarelis, V.Z. 1981. Practicable identification of nonstationary nonlinear systems. *Proc. IEE, Part D* 128: 211.

Marmarelis, V.Z. (Ed.). 1987. *Advanced Methods of Physiological System Modeling: Vol. I, Biomedical Simulations Resource.* Los Angeles, CA, University of Southern California.

Marmarelis, V.Z. (Ed.). 1989a. *Advanced Methods of Physiological System Modeling,* Vol. II. New York, Plenum.

Marmarelis, V.Z. 1989b. Identification and modeling of a class of nonlinear systems. *Math. Comput. Model.* 12: 991.

Marmarelis, V.Z. 1991. Wiener analysis of nonlinear feedback in sensory systems. *Ann. Biomed. Eng.* 19: 345.

Marmarelis, V.Z. 1993. Identification of nonlinear biological systems using Laguerre expansions of kernels. *Ann. Biomed. Eng.* 21: 573.

Marmarelis, V.Z. (Ed.). 1994a. *Advanced Methods of Physiological System Modeling,* Vol. III. New York, Plenum.

Marmarelis, V.Z. 1994b. Nonlinear modeling of physiological systems using principal dynamic modes. In V.Z. Marmarelis (Ed.), *Advanced Methods of Physiological Systems Modeling,* Vol. III. pp. 1–28, New York, Plenum.

Marmarelis, V.Z. 1997. Modeling methodology for nonlinear physiological systems. *Ann. Biomed. Eng.* 25: 239.

Marmarelis, V.Z. 2004. *Nonlinear Dynamic Modeling of Physiological Systems.* Wiley Interscience and IEEE Press, New York.

Marmarelis, P.Z. and Marmarelis, V.Z. 1978. *Analysis of Physiological Systems: The White-Noise Approach.* New York, Plenum. Russian translation: Mir Press, Moscow, 1981. Chinese translation: Academy of Sciences Press, Beijing, 1990.

Marmarelis, P.Z. and McCann, G.D. 1973. Development and application of white-noise modeling techniques for studies of insect visual nervous system. *Kybernetik* 12: 74.

Marmarelis, P.Z. and Naka, K.-I. 1974. Identification of multi-input biological systems. *IEEE Trans. Biomed. Eng.* 21: 88.

Marmarelis, V.Z., Citron, M.C., and Vivo, C.P. 1986. Minimum-order Wiener modeling of spike-output systems. *Biol. Cybern.* 54: 115.

Marmarelis, V.Z. and Orme, M.E. 1993. Modeling of neural systems by use of neuronal modes. *IEEE Trans. Biomed. Eng.* 40: 1149.

Marmarelis, V.Z. and Zhao, X. 1997. Volterra models and three-layer perceptions. *IEEE Trans. Neural Network* 8: 1421.

McCann, G.D. and Marmarelis, P.Z. (Eds.). 1975. *Proceedings of the First Symposium on Testing and Identification of Nonlinear Systems,* Pasadena, CA, California Institute of Technology.

Moller, A.R. 1983. Use of pseudorandom noise in studies of frequency selectivity: the periphery of the auditory system. *Biol. Cybern.* 47: 95.

Ream, N. 1970. Nonlinear identification using inverse repeat m-sequences. *Proc. IEEE* 117: 213.

Rugh, W.J. 1981. *Nonlinear System Theory: The Volterra/Wiener Approach.* Baltimore, MD, Johns Hopkins University Press.

Schetzen, M. 1965. Measurement of the kernels of a nonlinear system of finite order. *Int. J. Control* 2: 251.

Schetzen, M. 1980. *The Volterra and Wiener Theories of Nonlinear Systems.* New York, Wiley.

Sclabassi, R.J., Krieger, D.N., and Berger, T.W. 1988. A systems theoretic approach to the study of CNS function. *Ann. Biomed. Eng.* 16: 17.

Shi, J. and Sun, H.H. 1990. Nonlinear system identification for cascade block model: an application to electrode polarization impedance. *IEEE Trans. Biomed. Eng.* 37: 574.

Soderstrom, T. and Stoica, P. 1989. *System Identification.* London, Prentice-Hall International.

Stark, L. 1968. *Neurological Control Systems: Studies in Bioengineering.* New York, Plenum.

Sutter, E. 1992. A deterministic approach to nonlinear systems analysis. In R.B. Pinter and B. Nabet (Eds.), *Nonlinear Vision,* pp. 171–220, Boca Raton, FL, CRC Press.

Victor, J.D., Shapley, R.M., and Knight, B.W. 1977. Nonlinear analysis of retinal ganglion cells in the frequency domain. *Proc. Natl Acad. Sci. USA* 74: 3068.

Watanabe, A. and Stark, L. 1975. Kernel method for nonlinear analysis: identification of a biological control system. *Math. Biosci.* 27: 99.

Westwick, D.T. and Kearney, R.E. 1992. A new algorithm for identification of multiple input Wiener systems. *Biol. Cybern.* 68: 75.

Yasui, S., Davis, W., and Naka, K.I. 1979. Spatio-temporal receptive field measurement of retinal neurons by random pattern stimulation and cross-correlation. *IEEE Trans. Biomed. Eng.* 26: 263.

Zhao, X. and Marmarelis, V.Z. 1998. Nonlinear parametric models from Volterra kernels measurements. *Math. Comput. Model.* 27: 37.

14

Autoregulating Windkessel Dynamics May Cause Low Frequency Oscillations

Gary M. Drzewiecki
John K-J. Li
Rutgers University

Abraham Noordergraaf
University of Pennsylvania

14.1 Introduction

The control of blood flow is a process involving neural and metabolic mechanisms. It is widely accepted that neural processes accomplish short term control of blood precapillary flow resistance such that blood pressure and flow are regulated. While metabolic processes dominate in the long term [Guyton, 1963] they ultimately determine the regulated blood flow levels in the various tissues in accordance with metabolic demands. This is achieved locally by the precapillary sphincters that adjust the duration and number of capillaries open and which, in turn, determine the value of the peripheral resistance, R_s. Another theory suggests that it is the mechanical effect of pressure and flow that stimulates vascular smooth muscle to react. However experiments have shown that tissue blood flow and systemic circulation is directly related to its metabolic demand [Berne and Levy, 1977]. Experimental observations of low frequency flow oscillations can be found in studies of a single vascular bed as well as the entire systemic circulation. This differs from mechanical stimulation where researchers have employed a drug response. For example,

Kenner and Ono [1972] have observed what they termed flow autooscillations in the carotid and femoral arteries of the dog, following intravenous administration of acetylcholine. Similar oscillations in flow have been observed following the infusion of adenosine into the coronary circulation [Wong and Klassen, 1991]. These researchers attributed this response to opposing vasodilator and vasoconstrictor processes.

Other experimental evidence of low frequency resonance can be found in measurements of heart rate variability and blood pressure variability spectra [Chess et al., 1975; Akselrod et al., 1981; Pagani et al., 1986]. Experiments in animals have shown that low frequency oscillations persist following denervation [Rimoldi et al., 1990], during external constant cardiac pacing [Wang et al., 1995], and in animals and humans with an artificial heart [Yambe et al., 1993; Cooley et al., 1998]. To our knowledge, the origin of the low frequency resonance in the variability spectrum, the so-called Mayer waves [Mayer, 1876] is currently unexplained, although vasoregulatory dynamics has been proposed. The study by Yambe et al. [1993] revealed that the long waves were nearly 100% correlated with the periodicity of peripheral resistance.

Further autoregulatory instability has been observed in the pathological situation. For example, prominent low frequency oscillations have been observed during heart failure [Goldberger et al., 1984]. While it has been proposed that these oscillations follow the respiratory rate, they have been observed to occur at even lower frequencies.

With innervation intact, the circulation at rest maintains constant ventricular stroke volume and blood pressure, on average. In addition, the regulation of cardiac output is accomplished primarily through the control of peripheral resistance. Then, the slow changes in heart rate (f_h) are directly related to cardiac output (CO) and inversely to peripheral resistance (R_s), so that, $f_h \propto \text{CO} \propto 1/R_s$ [Berne and Levy, 1977]. This relationship is fundamental to the vascular theory of heart rate variation [Hering, 1924] and underscores the role of a time varying peripheral resistance. In this chapter, the dynamics of peripheral resistance control is examined analytically as an explanation of the very low frequency variation in heart rate.

14.2   Background

The control of blood flow resistance has been analyzed theoretically at both the organ and the microcirculatory level. Since metabolic demand of the tissue is related to oxygen uptake under aerobic conditions, Huntsman et al. [1978] developed a model for control of blood flow resistance for skeletal muscle based on this concept. In this study, it was found that the metabolic control considerably outweighed that of neural and myogenic. The time frame of observation was also important, where longer time periods emphasized the metabolic control factors. The model controlled flow by means of regulating the oxygen stored in the extra-vascular spaces. The control of peripheral resistance was affected by invoking the relationship between arterial diameter and oxygen tension. This model successfully predicted the large blood flow response following a brief occlusion.

The autoregulation response should ultimately arise from the action of multiple precapillary sphincters and resistance arterioles in the microcirculation. The control of flow in a microvascular model was analyzed by Mayrovitz et al. [1978]. This model included muscular arterial and venous vasomotion, capillary filtration and reabsorption, and lymph flow. Tissue pressure was assumed to be regulated and was used to provide the control pathway for the activation of the precapillary sphincter. Local flow was found to vary considerably with periodic sphincter activity. This model demonstrated that autoregulation of flow is likely to find its genesis at the microcirculatory level.

Although our knowledge of pulse propagation in the arterial system is extensive, it has been useful to approximate the relationship between pressure and flow in a single artery or vascular bed. Such approximations have been referred to as reduced arterial system models of which the three element Windkessel is the most widely employed [Westerhof et al., 1971; Noordergraaf, 1978]. This Windkessel model is modified here to study the effects of peripheral resistance.

The three element Windkessel model approximates the pulse propagation quality of the arterial system as a combination of an infinitely long tube, which is represented by its characteristic impedance, Z_0, in series with a parallel arrangement of a peripheral flow resistance, R_s, and a total arterial compliance, C_s. Within a single cardiac cycle, these three parameters are generally assumed to be constants [Toorop et al., 1987]. Recent studies have scrutinized this assumption. For example, the compliance has been shown to depend on the level of arterial pressure [Bergel, 1961]. Other studies have called into question the accuracy of the various methods employed to experimentally determine their values [Stergiopulos et al., 1995a]. This difficulty has been addressed by Quick et al. [1998] who showed that wave reflection imparts frequency dependence on the values of R_s and C_s.

The Windkessel model is often employed as a simplified load for the left ventricle. Under steady conditions and a fixed heart rate, this model is appropriate. But, given the case of varying ventricular function, the model responds inaccurately. The difficulty lies in the regulation of cardiac output, that is, autoregulation is not provided. To correct this problem, our group has employed an iterative procedure that permits R_s to change such that cardiac output is maintained [Drzewiecki et al., 1992]. This procedure, although providing autoregulation, does not account for the dynamics associated with this physiological mechanism.

In this chapter, the dynamics of autoregulation are incorporated into the modified Windkessel model. The frequency response of this autoregulating Windkessel is then predicted and compared with that of the standard three element model. The time response is also determined and discussed relative to the experimental observations in the literature. The stability of the model is also examined with respect to very low frequency oscillation in peripheral resistance.

The physical relationships that govern the Windkessel model are now reviewed. Time dependency is provided by the blood volume storage property of arterial compliance, C_s. The time derivative of peripheral arterial pressure, P_s, is proportional to the difference in blood flow into and out of the compliance, according to,

$$\frac{dP_s}{dt} = \left(Q - \frac{P_s - P_o}{R_s} \right) \frac{1}{C_s P_s} \tag{14.1}$$

where Q is the inflow. P_o accounts for the critical closing pressure [Alexander, 1977]. The input pressure, P, is then determined from the sum of pressure due to flow through the characteristic impedance and the pressure, P_s,

$$P = Q Z_o + P_s \tag{14.2}$$

The arterial compliance may be treated as a function of pressure also, accounting for large changes in blood pressure. The pressure dependence of compliance is then modeled by an exponential function [Liu et al., 1989; Li et al., 1990], as,

$$C_s = a\, e^{-bP_s} \tag{14.3}$$

where a and b are empirical constants evaluated from experimental data.

14.3 Modeling Methods

14.3.1 Steady Regulation

In this study, it will be assumed that the local tissue bed or whole animal is in a steady metabolic state. For this regulated condition, the level of blood flow is denoted Q_0, the peripheral resistance, R_{so}, and the pressure across it, P_{so}. The relation between these quantities reads,

$$P_{so} = R_{so} Q_0 \tag{14.4}$$

When the flow is disturbed, the value of the peripheral resistance is adjusted in an attempt to restore flow to Q_0. Since the control of flow is not ideal, the new steady flow condition is described by

$$P_s = R_{reg} Q \tag{14.5}$$

where R_{reg} is the new value of peripheral resistance. Applying the simplest form of control, which is also imperfect, it is assumed that the change in peripheral resistance is proportional to the change in flow, that is, linear proportional control. The change in peripheral resistance is then determined from the control equation,

$$\Delta R_s = R_{reg} - R_{so} = \frac{G(Q - Q_0)}{Q_0} \tag{14.6}$$

where G is defined as the autoregulatory gain.

14.3.2 Autoregulation Dynamics

There are two dynamic effects that must be accounted for to accurately model the physiological control mechanism. First, the change in peripheral resistance is delayed. This represents a delay from the time that the flow changes to when the vascular smooth muscle activity actually initiates the process of correcting the flow. This time delay in the change of peripheral resistance is denoted τ_Q. To account for this effect, the change in peripheral resistance determined from the steady value was written as $\Delta R_s(t - \tau_Q)$.

Physiologically, even when peripheral resistance adjusts, it cannot be changed instantaneously. To account for the slow change in resistance, a first-order rate equation was used to represent the slow action of vascular smooth muscle. Thus, the time dependent value of peripheral resistance was determined from the following,

$$\frac{dR_s}{dt} = \frac{1}{\tau_{sm}} \Delta R_s(t - \tau_Q) \tag{14.7}$$

where the time constant for smooth muscle action is τ_{sm}. This equation simply states that the rate of change of peripheral resistance with respect to time is proportional to desired change in resistance, ΔR_s.

The net effect of delay in autoregulation and smooth muscle response is to cause R_s to slowly approach its new control value, as defined by Equation 14.6.

14.3.3 Regulatory Limitations

If the actual blood flow differs significantly from Q_0, the regulatory error can be large. Since a linear model is being employed here, the value of R_s predicted by Equation 14.4 to Equation 14.7 may fall outside of the physiological range. Thus, the time dependent value of R_s was limited to maximum and minimum values of $1.6R_{so}$ and $0.4R_{so}$, respectively. These values correspond with maximal vasoconstriction and vasodilation. When the computations reveal that the limit has been reached, the limited value of resistance was then inserted into Equation 14.1 of the Windkessel model. Otherwise, the time dependent value obtained from Equation 14.7 was employed.

The two differential equations (Equation 14.1 and Equation 14.7) govern the time dependent characteristics of the autoregulating Windkessel model. They were integrated numerically by a computer. All parameters were evaluated for the canine systemic arterial system (Table 14.1).

TABLE 14.1 Parameters

Parameter	Value	Description
Z_0	0.25 mmHg/ml/sec	Characteristic impedance
C_s	0.50 ml/mmHg	Arterial compliance
R_{so}	3.10 mmHg/ml/sec	Basal peripheral resistance
a	3.0 ml/mmHg	Nonlinear compliance constant
b	0.02 mmHg^{-1}	Nonlinear compliance constant
G	5.0	Autoregulation gain
Q_0	27.0 ml/sec	Regulated flow level
τ_Q	5.0 sec	Flow delay time
τ_{sm}	3.0 sec	Smooth muscle time constant

14.4 Results

14.4.1 Autoregulation Curve

The standard experimental approach to measuring the autoregulation curve of a vascular bed has been to slowly vary input flow while recording pressure. Alternatively, one may alter pressure while measuring flow. In either case, the dependent variable stabilizes after several minutes. The set of final values results in the steady state autoregulation curve. This procedure was followed using the autoregulating Windkessel model (Figure 14.1). To reduce computation time, the time constants of the model were shortened. This does not affect the result, but simply shortens the time to reach steady state.

The model generated autoregulation curve shows three distinct segments. The low flow segment was found to be a line of slope $0.4R_{so}$, and corresponds with maximal vasodilation. There was no control of flow in this region either. The middle flow segment represents the autoregulatory range. The peripheral resistance was found to alter continuously in accordance with the feedback control relationship of Equation 14.6 in this region. The slope of this segment was also proportionate to the autoregulatory gain factor, G, of the model. A greater slope reflects tighter control of flow, but, as will be shown later, can lead to autoregulatory instability.

14.4.2 Input Impedance

The frequency response of the autoregulating Windkessel was determined by applying a small constant amplitude flow sinusoid as input while the mean flow is held fixed. The resulting sinusoidal pressure response was computed from the model. The response was evaluated for as many cycles as were needed to obtain a sinusoidal steady state. For frequencies much below the heart rate, this required up to 30 sec. The input impedance magnitude was then obtained by finding the ratio of the sinusoidal pressure and flow amplitudes over the range of frequencies. Phase was determined by finding the phase difference between the pressure and flow waves (Figure 14.2a,b). In order to compare these results with the conventional modified Windkessel, the input impedance was reevaluated when the autoregulatory gain is zero ($G = 0$) and is shown on the same graphs.

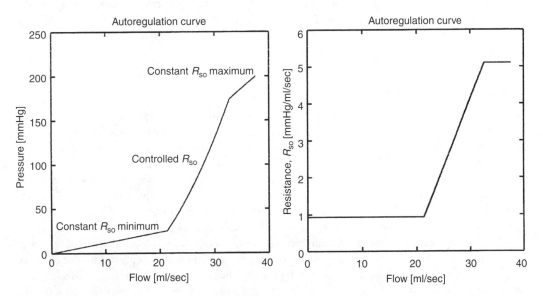

FIGURE 14.1 Pressure and flow relationship of the canine aorta obtained from the autoregulating Windkessel in the steady state. Flow regulation occurs in the range where the slope is steepest.

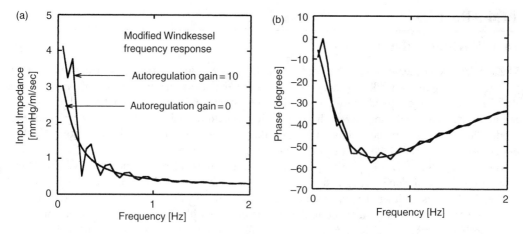

FIGURE 14.2 Input impedance magnitude (a) and phase (b) frequency spectrum obtained from the model. The oscillating curve represents active autoregulation. The smooth curve is the standard three-element Windkessel with constant peripheral resistance.

The high frequency impedance was found to be identical for both models. This might be expected, since autoregulation is slow compared with the heart rate. An unexpected result was that the impedance and phase were found to oscillate at about that of the modified Windkessel for frequencies near the heart rate. This oscillation was traced to the autoregulation delay time, τ_Q. The magnitude of these oscillations was found to increase further if the autoregulatory gain is increased. If the gain or the delay time was reduced to zero, the oscillations are eliminated. These oscillations in the frequency domain could have been predicted by referring to the Fourier transform of a delayed time function.

The very low frequency portion of the autoregulating impedance magnitude was higher in comparison with that of the unregulated Windkessel, where impedance approaches R_s at zero frequency. This can be explained by referring again to Figure 14.1. Instead of converging to R_s, the autoregulating impedance approaches the slope of the pressure–flow curve. That is because the sinusoidal response measures the dynamic variation about the flow control point, Q_0. This is not contradictory, since the mean pressure divided by the mean flow is simultaneously $R_s = R_{so}$, at this point. And, the derivative of pressure, dP/dQ, for a given flow, must be the slope of the autoregulation curve in the steady state.

14.4.3 Flow Step Response

The pressure was computed from the model given a step increase in flow above the control level. A flow step was initiated 2.0 sec from the beginning of the calculations (Figure 14.3). An immediate increase in pressure occurs. This coincided with the time dependent increase in blood volume that shifts into the compliance, C_s. The peripheral resistance did not change during this time due to flow delay. It remains at the control value of R_{so}. Five seconds later, the resistance begins to increase toward the new value required by Equation 14.4 and for autoregulation. Pressure increased nearly in proportion with resistance. The rate of change was determined by the time constant of smooth muscle response, τ_{sm}, and Equation 14.5. An equilibrium value was reached about 20 sec after the flow step occurred.

The above flow step response was repeated with a constant amplitude flow pulse added to the mean flow (Figure 14.4). A flow step was initiated 10 sec from the beginning of computations. The envelope of the pressure response follows that shown in Figure 14.3, but additionally permits the observation of systolic and diastolic pressures. It was found that the pulse pressure amplitude increases following the step. This was associated with the decrease in pressure dependent compliance due to elevated pressure (Equation 14.3).

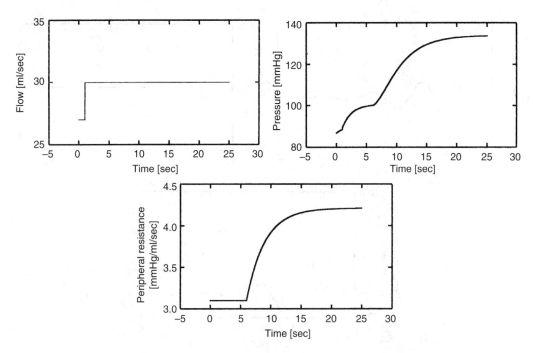

FIGURE 14.3 Flow step response of the model for steady levels of flow. The time responses of pressure and peripheral resistance are shown.

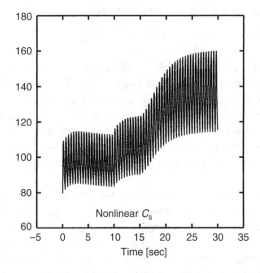

FIGURE 14.4 Flow step response as in Figure 14.3, but with the addition of constant pulsatile flow. The effect of nonlinear compliance is evident as the pulse pressure increases following the increase in mean flow.

14.4.4 Pressure Step Response

The flow was computed from the model following a step change in input pressure. The step change was initiated immediately by altering the initial condition for pressure from the steady state value of 83 to 90 mmHg (Figure 14.5).

The graphs for flow and resistance were found to be 180° out of phase. This was expected, since they are inversely proportional for constant pressure. Part of the initial increase in flow was due to transient

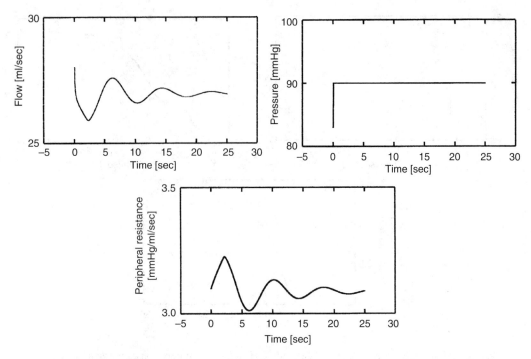

FIGURE 14.5 Pressure step response computed from the model ($\tau_Q = 2$, $\tau_{sm} = 5$, and $G = 10$). The step was produced by altering the initial condition for pressure at $t = 0$. Note that pressure and resistance are 180° out of phase. A damped resonant response is evident with a resonant frequency of ~0.1 Hz.

filling of the compliance, C_s. Flow was found to oscillate about its control value. This was reasonable since the control system consists of feedback with two time lags. Thus, the stability of control becomes a consideration. It was found that increasing τ_Q or the gain factor, G, led to unstable low frequency pressure oscillations. The smooth muscle time constant, τ_{sm}, was found to possess a damping effect and could be increased to eliminate oscillations. Thus, too rapid smooth muscle activation and accurate autoregulation were predicted to be a destabilizing influence on the circulation. Since the flow resistance was always limited to either maximal vasoconstriction or vasodilation, the amplitude of the oscillations was also constrained.

As another type of pressure step, an arterial occlusion was computed from the model. A 2 sec occlusion was applied by rapidly reducing the input pressure to zero and then restoring it to the preocclusion level. The initial effect was to cause a rapid negative flow (Figure 14.6). This represents blood volume decrease of the arterial compliance. The effect was brief since the outflow time constant is less than one second. Peripheral resistance was unchanged until the end of the occlusion due to autoregulation delay. Afterwards, it rapidly dropped to the minimal resistance level of complete vasodilation. When the occlusion was released, the flow rapidly increased. Initially, the flow was briefly high at positive values as the blood volume of the compliance was restored. Flow remained elevated to relieve the ischemia. Following a delay time, flow was then restored to its initial value prior to occlusion. This was done in an oscillatory manner.

14.4.5 Minimal Circuit Model

As in much of hemodynamic research, the Windkessel model, as well as others, have been portrayed in electrical circuit form. The autoregulating Windkessel described here cannot be simplified completely in circuit form. But, a useful approximation was designed. It was assumed that the time constants of autoregulation

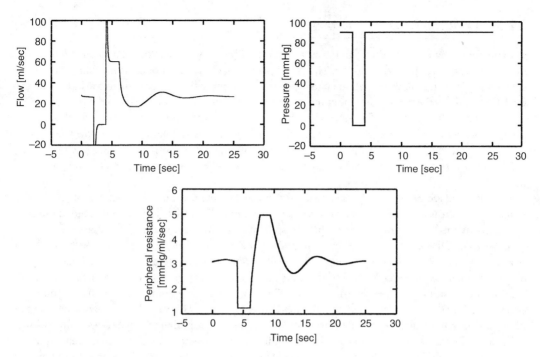

FIGURE 14.6 A vascular occlusion produced by reducing the input pressure to zero for 2 sec. The flow response transients are due to compliance effects. Flow increases to maximum value corresponding with complete vasodilation. A damped oscillatory response returns the flow and resistance to control levels.

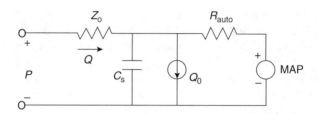

FIGURE 14.7 Simplified autoregulating Windkessel in electrical circuit form.

and smooth muscle activation are minimal. Then, autoregulation is immediate. Additionally, it was assumed that vasoconstriction and vasodilation are not limited. Under these conditions, the circuit model of Figure 14.7 can be used to approximate the autoregulating Windkessel. The constant current source represents the control value of autoregulated flow, Q_0. The resistance, R_{auto}, is the slope of the autoregulation line (Figure 14.1). When the actual flow, $Q = Q_0$, the average blood pressure is equal to the pressure source, MAP. Also, under this condition, $R_s = R_{so} = MAP/Q_0$. Note, that these expressions assume that the pressure drop across the characteristic impedance, Z_o, is negligible.

The impedance frequency spectrum was evaluated for the autoregulating circuit model. It was found to follow the result previously shown in Figure 14.2, with the exception of impedance oscillations. The predicted impedance was in error by the amount of the oscillation amplitude. On average, over a range of frequencies, the error was negligible. Hence, for steady state conditions, the minimal circuit model offers a simple solution to the autoregulating Windkessel. The transient step responses, as predicted by the complete model, cannot be reproduced by this simplified circuit model.

14.5 Discussion

The autoregulation curve described in the current model differs from physiological data only in the sense that it is a segmented linear description. This was due to the fact that the model assumed linear feedback regulation. The actual flow regulation system possesses nonlinearities not accounted for in the current model. Most researchers have found that the steady state pressure flow curve is sigmoidal [Folkow, 1953; Granger and Guyton, 1969]. Other researchers have expressed these nonlinearities as feedback gain that is flow dependent [Van Huis et al., 1985]. Still others have found that a linear pressure–flow relationship is a good approximation within the normal physiological range of blood pressure [Sagawa and Eisner, 1975]. In this case, the current model would be most accurate when flow is near Q_0 and blood pressure is near MAP.

The autoregulation curve has been shown to be affected by the carotid baroreflex function [Shoukas et al., 1984]. Increased carotid pressure leads to a decrease in peripheral resistance so that blood pressure can be maintained at a given cardiac output. In spite of the baroreceptor effect, these same researchers have shown that the steady state pressure-flow curve remains sigmoidal in shape. Thus, the concept of a steady state autoregulation curve applies just as well as when the baroreceptors are functional. The net effect of the baroreceptor response is to decrease the autoregulatory gain, as observed by a decrease in the slope of the steady state pressure-flow curve. This might be expected since pressure has the opposite effect on peripheral resistance to that of flow [Burattini et al., 1991]. This would have the added benefit of stabilizing the autoregulation system by preventing its gain from becoming too high (see stability below). Thus, since the autoregulating Windkessel does not incorporate this response, its primary value is in the analysis of peripheral vascular beds. And, provided that the autoregulatory gain is reduced to account for the baroreceptor effect, it can be applied to the systemic circulation.

The autoregulating Windkessel incorporates the critical closing pressure phenomenon [Alexander, 1977]. Critical closing causes the flow to cease at a slightly positive pressure, P_0. Debate over the mechanism that leads to P_0 continues. Since its value is typically small compared with systemic blood pressure, its value was set to zero here.

The low frequency impedance of the autoregulating Windkessel was found to be greater than that predicted by the modified Windkessel (Figure 14.2). The sinusoidal input impedance of a vascular bed has not been explored extensively below the frequency of the heart rate. Sipkema and Westerhof [1980] examined the low frequency range experimentally using an external sinusoidal pump. Under these conditions, it was found that the low frequency impedance approaches the slope of the autoregulation curve, as predicted by the autoregulating Windkessel. These researchers distinguish the low frequency impedance from peripheral resistance by defining it as a dynamic resistance.

Input impedance measurements have identified a variation in the frequency spectrum. While experimental studies have not provided an explanation for the origin of these variations, the current model ties them to autoregulation delay (τ_Q). The model predicts that the spectrum should follow an oscillatory pattern, particularly for frequencies at and below the heart rate. Moreover, the sinusoidal steady state may not be easily achieved experimentally. The model required over one minute duration to obtain the steady state response. The model further predicts an erratic or random variation in the impedance spectrum if the steady state was not obtained. Another explanation could be that the different vascular beds may possess slightly different delay times. When measured at the aorta, this may appear as impedance scatter. Other researchers have attributed the source of impedance variations to nonlinear vascular properties [Stergiopulos et al., 1995b].

The flow step response of the model follows experimental studies quite precisely [Braakman et al., 1983; Shoukas et al., 1984; Van Huis et al., 1985]. Others have observed experimentally an initial autoregulation delay and a slow adjustment of the vascular smooth muscle in response to a step in flow. The time constants of the model were determined in accordance with previous observations. The time course of the flow step response was similar for a single vascular bed and for the entire systemic circulation. Experimental measurements found no oscillations in response to a flow step for the systemic circulation [Shoukas et al., 1984]. Hence, employing a higher order model than was used here would be of little value.

But, *in vivo* measurements in organs have detected the presence of oscillations in the step flow response [Westerhof et al., 1983]. The amplitude of these oscillations were small. Modifying the model to include these higher order dynamics may be at the sacrifice of simplicity and was not considered in this study.

The flow step response examines the autoregulation control under open loop conditions. This procedure essentially forces the flow to a specific level independent of the tissue's metabolic demands. The results of this experiment provide information about the dynamics of the regulatory process. Alternatively, the pressure step response permits autoregulation to function under *in vivo* conditions and provides the closed loop response. Under these conditions, the autoregulating Windkessel shows a damped resonant flow response. This resonant behavior was linked to the time lag of flow regulation. Damping was provided by the slow smooth muscle function. Others have modeled the resonant behavior of autoregulation as a second-order control system that attempts to regulate blood pressure by adjusting the peripheral resistance [Burattini et al., 1987]. While this approach may achieve a similar response, the physiological mechanism differs from that employed in our model. Moreover, data obtained from the open loop flow response, supports the use of a time lag theory. In general, oscillations have been modeled and observed in other biological systems that possess time lags in their feedback pathways [An der Heiden, 1979]. It may be reasonable to expect that biology accomplishes flow autoregulation in a way similar to other types of homeostasis.

While the response to a vasoactive drug was not computed from the autoregulation model, it can be obtained by applying a step change in the time dependent value of R_s [Kenner and Ono, 1972]. In this case, the model also predicts that oscillatory flow will result. Hence, the model suggests, alternatively, that the origin of oscillations may be due to regulatory delays. This interpretation, though, does not rely on conventional control system analysis and does not involve the parasympathetic and sympathetic reflex pathways [Wong and Klassen, 1991].

The model predicted that autoregulation can be unstable for some parameter values. When the parameters were calibrated to match flow step experiments, the model produced a stable result. But, the pressure step can best be characterized as a damped low frequency resonance. Experimental evidence of very low frequency resonance can be found in measurements of the heart rate variability and blood pressure variability spectra [Chess et al., 1975; Akselrod et al., 1981; Pagani et al., 1986], following denervation [Rimoldi et al., 1990], during external constant cardiac pacing [Wang et al., 1995], and in animals with total artificial heart [Yambe et al., 1993]. This experimental observation that a nervous system is not necessary to produce such low frequencies in the cardiovascular system has been perplexing. So much so, that these oscillations have been referred to as the Mayer waves [Mayer, 1876], an observed but currently unexplained phenomenon. The autoregulation model provided here supports the theory that these low frequency oscillations find their origin in the intrinsic delay of flow regulation.

Model parameter values that lie outside the normal physiological range can further enhance autoregulatory instability. Abnormal values may occur in the pathological situation. Oscillations in pressure and flow were predicted by the model to lie well below heart rate, in the range below 0.1 Hz for the dog. For example, prominent low frequency oscillations have been observed during heart failure [Goldberger et al., 1984]. While it has been proposed that these oscillations follow the respiratory rate, they have been observed to occur at even lower frequencies. The autoregulating Windkessel model offers a possible explanation of the source of these oscillations given pathological conditions. It also suggests the possibility that they may be used to noninvasively monitor the condition of the autoregulatory system.

14.6   Conclusions

The autoregulating Windkessel was found to accurately reproduce the experimental flow step response of both vascular beds and the systemic circulation. The model further provided the steady-state pressure–flow autoregulation curve, in linearized form. The impedance spectrum was predicted to differ from that of the three element Windkessel for frequencies below the heart rate. For frequencies near zero, the impedance approached the slope of the pressure–flow autoregulation curve, as opposed to peripheral resistance. But, simultaneously, the average pressure divided by the average flow of the model yielded the usual value of peripheral resistance. The low frequency impedance spectrum was also predicted to contain oscillations that were traced to autoregulatory delay. This result provides an explanation of the variability obtained experimentally during multi-beat examination of the impedance spectrum. The pressure step response of the autoregulating Windkessel revealed a damped low frequency resonant behavior. The model parameters that cause increased autoregulatory gain and decreased damping were found to lead to sustained flow oscillations at frequencies well below the heart rate. This resonance explains the origin of very low frequencies observed in the heart rate variability spectrum referred to as the Mayer waves.

References

Akselrod, S., Gordon, D., Ubel, F.A., Shannon, D.C., and Cohen, R.J. 1981. Power spectrum analysis of heart rate fluctuation: a quantitative probe of beat-to-beat cardiovascular control. *Science* 213: 220–222.

Alexander, R.S. 1977. Critical closure reexamined. *Circ. Res.* 40: 531–535.

Bergel, D.H. 1961. The dynamic elastic properties of the arterial wall. *J. Physiol. (Lond.)* 156: 458–469.

Berne, R.M. and Levy, M.N. 1977. *Cardiovascular Physiology*, Mosby.

Braakman, R., Sipkema, P., and Westerhof, N. 1983. Steady state and instantaneous pressure–flow relationships: characterisation of the canine abdominal periphery. *Card. Res.* 17: 577–588.

Burattini, R., Borgdorff, P., Gross, D.R., Baiocco, B., and Westerhof, N. 1991. Systemic autoregulation counteracts the carotid baroreflex. *IEEE Trans. Biomed. Eng.* 38: 48–56.

Burattini, R., Reale, P., Borgdorff, P., and Westerhof, N. 1987. Dynamic model of the short-term regulation of arterial pressure in the cat. *Med. Biol. Eng. Comput.* 25: 269–276.

Chess, G.F., Tam, H.K., and Calarescu, F.R. 1975. Influence of cardiac neural inputs on rhythmic variations of heart period in the cat. *Am. J. Physiol.* 228: 775–780.

Cooley, R.L., Montano, N., Cogliati, C., Van de Borne, P., Richenbacher, W., Oren, R., and Somers, V.K. 1998. Evidence for a central origin of the low-frequency oscillation in the RR-interval variability. *Circulation* 98: 556–561.

Drzewiecki, G.M., Karam, E., Li, J.K.-J., and Noordergraaf, A. 1992. Cardiac adaptation from sarcomere dynamics to arterial load: a model of physiologic hypertrophy. *Am. J. Physiol.* 263: H1054–H1063.

Folkow, B. 1953. A study of the factors influencing the tone of denervated blood vessels perfused at various pressures. *Acta Physiol. Scand.* 27: 99–117.

Goldberger, A.L., Findley, L.J., Blackburn, M.R., and Mandell, A.J. 1984. Nonlinear dynamics in heart failure: implications of long-wavelength cardiopulmonary oscillations. *Am. Heart J.* 107: 612–615.

Granger, H.J. and Guyton, A.C. 1969. Autoregulation of the total systemic circulation following destruction of the nervous system in the dog. *Circ. Res.* 25: 379–388.

Guyton, A.C. 1963. *Circulatory Physiology: Cardiac Output and its Regulation.* Philadelphia, Saunders.

An der Heiden, U. 1979. Delays in physiological systems. *J. Math. Biol.* 8: 345–364.

Hering, H.E. 1924. Die Aenderung der Herzschlagzahl durch Aenderung des arteriellen Blutdruckes erfolgt auf reflectorischem Wege. *Pfluegers Arch. Gesamte Physiol. Menschen Tiere.* 206: 721.

Huntsman, L.L., Attinger, E.O., and Noordergraaf, A. 1978. Metabolic autoregulation of blood flow in skeletal muscle. In *Cardiovascular System Dynamics* (Baan, J., Noordergraaf, A., and Raines, J, Eds.), MIT Press, Cambridge, MA, pp. 400–414.

Kenner, T. and Ono, K. 1972. Analysis of slow autooscillations of arterial flow. *Pflugers Arch.* 331: 347–356.

Li, J.K.-J., Cui, T., and Drzewiecki, G.M. 1990. A nonlinear model of the arterial system incorporating a pressure-dependent compliance. *IEEE Trans. Biomed. Eng.* BME 37: 673–678.

Liu, Z., Ting, C.-T., Zhu, S., and Yin, F.C.P. 1989. Aortic compliance in human hypertension. *Hypertension* 14: 129–136.

Mayer, S. 1876. Studien zur physiologie des herzens und der blutgefasse. V. Uber spotane blut-druckschwankungen. *Akad. Wiss. Wien. Math-Nat.* 74: 281–307.

Mayrovitz, H.N., Wiedeman, M.P., and Noordergraaf, A. 1978. Interaction in the microcirculation. In *Cardiovascular System Dynamics* (Baan, J., Noordergraaf, A., and Raines, J., Eds.), MIT Press, pp. 194–204.

Noordergraaf, A. 1978. *Circulatory System Dynamics*. New York, Academic Press.

Pagani, M., Lombardi, F., Guzzetti, S., Rimoldi, O., Furlan, R., Pizzinelli, P., Sandrone, G., Malfatto, G., Dell'Orto, S., Piccaluga, E., Turiel, M., Baselli, G., Cerutti, S., and Malliani, A. 1986. Power spectral analysis of heart rate and arterial pressure variabilities as a marker of sympatho-vagal interaction in man and conscious dog. *Circ. Res.* 59: 178–192.

Quick, C.M., Berger, D.S., and Noordergraaf, A. 1998. Apparent arterial compliance. *Am. J. Physiol.* 274: H1393–H1403.

Rimoldi, O., Pierimi, S., Ferrari, A., Cerutti, S., Pagani, M., and Malliani, A. 1990. Analysis of short-term oscillations of R–R and arterial pressure in conscious dogs. *Am. J. Physiol.* 258: H967–H976.

Sagawa, K. and Eisner, A. 1975. Static pressure–flow relation in the total systemic vascular bed of the dog and its modification by the baroreceptor reflex. *Circ. Res.* 36: 406–413.

Shoukas, A.A., Brunner, M.J., Frankle, A.E., Greene, A.S., and Kallman, C.H. 1984. Carotid sinus baroreceptor reflex control and the role of autoregulation in the systemic and pulmonary arterial pressure–flow relationships of the dog. *Circ. Res.* 54: 674–682.

Sipkema, P. and Westerhof, N. 1980. Peripheral resistance and low frequency impedance of the femoral bed. In *Cardiac Dynamics* (Baan, J., Alexander, C., Arntzenius, A., and Yellin, E.L., Eds.), M Nijhoff, Boston, pp. 501–508.

Stergiopulos, N., Meister, J.-J., and Westerhof, N. 1995a. Evaluation of methods for estimation of total arterial compliance. *Am. J. Physiol.* 268: H1540–H1548.

Stergiopulos, N., Meister, J.-J., and Westerhof, N. 1995b. Scatter in input impedance spectrum may result from the elastic nonlinearity of the arterial wall. *Am. J. Physiol.* 269: H1490–H1495.

Toorop, G.P., Westerhof, N., and Elzinga, G. 1987. Beat-to-beat estimation of peripheral resistance and arterial compliance during pressure transients. *Am. J. Physiol.* 252: H1275–H1283.

Van Huis, G.A., Sipkema, P., and Westerhof, N. 1985. Instantaneous and steady-state pressure–flow relations of the coronary system in the canine beating heart. *Card. Res.* 19: 121–131.

Wang, M., Evans, J., and Knapp, C. 1995. Spectral patterns and frequency response characteristics of arterial pressure in heart paced dogs. *IEEE Trans. Biomed. Eng.* 42: 708–717.

Westerhof, N., Elzinga, G., and Sipkema, P. 1971. An artificial arterial system for pumping hearts. *J. Appl. Physiol.* 31: 776–781.

Wong, A.Y. and Klassen, G.A. 1991. Vasomotor coronary oscillations: a model to evaluate autoregulation. *Basic Res. Cardiol.* 86: 461–475.

Yambe, T., Nitta, S.-I., Sonobe, T., Naganuma, S., Kakinuma, Y., Kobayashi, S.-I., Nanka, S., Ohsawa, N., Akiho, H., Tanaka, M., Fukuju, T., Miura, M., Uchida, N., Sato, N., Mohri, H., Koide, S., Abe, K.-I., Takeda, H., and Yoshizawa, M. 1993. Origin of the rhythmical fluctuations in the animal without a natural heartbeat. *Artif. Organs* 17: 1017–1021.

15

External Control of Movements

Dejan B. Popović
Mirjana B. Popović
University of Belgrade and Aalborg
University

15.1 Introduction

The mechanical system being controlled is referred to as the **plant**. The configuration of the system at any instant in time comprises the plant **states**. The devices that power the system are called **actuators**. The signals driving the actuators are called **controls**. The **controller** encompasses processes by which the controls are generated. The time histories of the plant states in response to the control signals are referred to the system **trajectory**.

Controllers can be designed to function without sensors and therefore without knowledge of the actual plant trajectory (**open-loop control**, Figure 15.1a). **Reference-based open-loop controllers** precompute and store control signals, and execute the desired motor task in real time. To correct for disturbances and modeling errors a feedback controller with ongoing knowledge of the effects of the disturbances can be used. **Closed-loop system** (Figure 15.1b), or so-called *error-driven controllers* use feedback information from sensors measuring the states. Both controllers described require the full knowledge on the system parameters, desired trajectories of the system components, and allowed tracking errors. Operation of an open-loop or closed-loop controller can be simulated using analytic tools derived from mechanics and mathematics.

Nonanalytic control is a technique that attempts to mimic the organization found in biological systems. Nonanalytic control considers the system operation as a block box. Heuristics or machine intelligence or both are used to determine the mappings between inputs and outputs of the specific system operation that are adequate for the implementation of nonanalytic external control (Figure 15.1c).

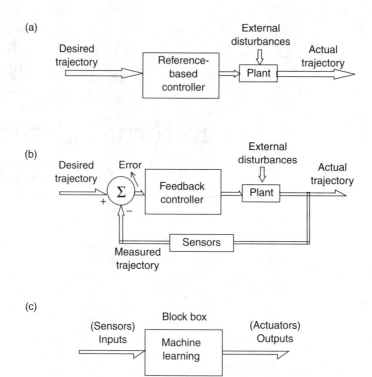

FIGURE 15.1   Open (a) and closed-loop (b) control systems. Nonanalytic model (c) for control of movements.

Control of movements in humans is a very complex task dealing with large-scale, nonlinear, time-variable, dynamically nondetermined, redundant system [1]. A dynamical system may change its states in a continuous way. Without an optimization criterion, all trajectories of a system are equivalent. The term trajectory has a broad meaning; it does refer to the way the system coordinates vary in the course of transition from the current to the next **state**. An optimization criterion assigns to each transition trajectory or a subset of trajectories, a value so that they can be arranged in the order of preference. In some cases, the trajectories of the dynamical system may be well-ordered so that a single solution stands in front. Such a trajectory is given the name the optimal solution. Instances when optimal solutions of control tasks exist, or can be analytically determined, are relatively rare although this term is used rather loosely in everyday life.

15.2   Biological Control of Movements

The skeletomotor system provides the structure and drives to move the body and limbs relative to the surroundings and to maintain the posture in space. The motor systems act on the environment by transforming neural information and metabolic energy into movement. Changes in external events or in the internal environment, signaled by the sensory systems, set up commands that are transmitted to the skeletal muscles by nerve impulses. The muscles convert the neural information into a command that transforms chemical into mechanical energy by generating a contractile force.

The control of movement and posture is achieved solely by adjusting the degree of contraction of skeletal muscles; however, this control requires that the motor systems be provided with a continuous flow of information about events from the periphery. Exteroceptors provide the motor systems with information about the spatial coordinates of the objects. Proprioceptors relay information about the position of the body vs. the vertical, the angles of the joints, the length and tension of muscles, and so on. Through proprioceptors, the motor systems gain access to information about the condition of the peripheral motor plant, the muscles and joints that have to be moved. The motor systems need information about the consequences of their actions. Both exteroceptors and proprioceptors provide this information, which can then be used to calibrate the next series of motor commands. Thus, motor mechanisms are intimately related to and functionally dependent upon sensory information.

The following three properties are especially important for the control (1) Muscles contract and relax slowly. Changes in muscle tension do not represent a simple one-to-one transformation of the firing patterns of motor neurons. The muscle filters the information contained in the temporal pattern of the spike train produced by motorneurons. Because of this filtering action, muscles faithfully reproduce only those signals that vary slowly. The ability of the muscular force to follow fluctuations is greatly diminished if the signals fluctuate rapidly. This indicates that it is necessary to alternate contraction in opposing muscle in order to produce fast change of the force; (2) Muscles have spring-like properties; thus, within limits, the tension exerted by muscles varies in proportion to length. Neural input is changing the muscles' resting length and stiffness. The actual change of muscle length depends on the neural drive and also on both initial lengths of the muscle and external loads; and (3) The motor systems need to control many muscles acting at the same joint simultaneously with muscles acting at different joints. Reaching while standing is an example of using many muscles to achieve a task. Bringing a segment of the hand to a desired position requires contraction of a group of muscles acting as prime movers (agonist muscles), yet antagonist muscles, which oppose the actions, must be controlled.

Mechanisms for control of posture: There are multiple definitions of posture [2–5]. When dealing with posture two functions emerge [6] (1) the antigravity operation. This function includes first the building up of the body segment configuration against gravity. A related function is the static and dynamic support provided by skeletal segments in contact with the support base to the moving segments; and (2) the interface for perception and action between the environment and the body. The orientation with respect to space of given segments such as head or trunk serves as a reference frame for the perception of the body movements with respect to space and for balance control. They also serve as a reference frame for the calculation of the target position in space and for the calculation of the trajectories for reaching the targets.

Quiet standing comprises some swaying of the body. During quiet standing, the gravity, ground reaction forces, and inertial forces produced by swaying are in equilibrium. The center of mass (CoM) is the point at the body where the resultant gravity force acts. The projection of the CoM to the base of support is called the center of gravity (CoG). The point of origin of the ground reaction force, the point through which the resultant ground reaction forces passes, is named the center of pressure (CoP). Maintaining posture is a process of continuous swaying of the body around the position of labile stability. Since the human body contains many segments that move relative to each other, CoM constantly changes its position; therefore, CoG constantly moves in the ground-contact plane. The central nervous system has to adjust the relative position of segments to prevent falling, that is, to control many muscles according to ensure dynamic equilibrium.

Mechanisms for control of walking: Walking is among the most highly automated movements of humans. The bipedal locomotion of humans is an unusually stable structure, although the mechanical structure is far from the favorable. All basic details of normal walking may be found in each and every able-bodied subject. Individual differences between subjects neither depend on the differences in the structure of walking, nor on the assembly of elements encountered, but only in the rhythms and amplitudes of the ratios between these elements.

As described, the posture is the state of equilibrium in which the net torque and force generated by gravity and muscles are zero, and only minimal sway exists around the quasi-stable inverted pendulum position. Walking occurs once the equilibrium ceases to exist because of the change of internal forces caused by muscle activity. The change of internal forces will cause the center of gravity to move out of the stability zone, and the body will start falling. Human walking starts, therefore, after the redistribution of internal forces allowing gravity to take over. The falling is prevented by bringing the contralateral leg in front of the body, hence, providing new support position. Once the contralateral leg supports the body weight and the ipsilateral leg pushes the body up and forward due to the momentum, the body will move in the direction of progression, and ultimately come directly above the supporting leg. This new inverted pendulum position is transitional; momentum and gravity will again bring the body into the falling pattern. Cyclic repetition of the described events is defined as bipedal locomotion or walking.

The major requirements for successful locomotion are (1) production of a locomotor rhythm to ensure support to the body against gravity; (2) production of muscle forces that will result with the friction force required for propelling it to the intended direction; (3) dynamic equilibrium of the moving body; and (4) adaptation of these movements to meet the environmental demands and the tasks selected by the individual.

Control of goal-directed movement: Goal-directed movement is a planned change of arm and hand segments positions, ultimately leading to a task. This movement depends on a balance of initial programming and subsequent correction. Initial programming is based partly on visual perception of objects, and partly on proprioception (e.g., a visual cue is used to decide whether to pick up the object with one or two hands, and what type of grasp to use). The accuracy of visual perception determines the initial programming.

The visual information is used to identify a target and its location in space, and also for corrections of ongoing movement. Goal-directed movement for a seen object usually benefits from visual feedback. This observation raises the question of how visual guidance is used in the control of reaches and grasps. There are at least three aspects of this problem (1) visual localization of the target in extra-personal space and suitable coding of that information for use by the arm motor system; (2) visual monitoring of the hand before and during its movement through space; and (3) visual adjustment of the final position of the hand to touch, grasp, or retrieve successfully the object of interest [7].

It has been shown unequivocally that reaching is more accurate in the presence than in the absence of vision of the arm just before [8] and during the movement [8–10]. Since this improvement was observed even for movements that were completed within 200 msec, it was proposed [11] that visual cues from arm motion are being processed at higher speeds than the timing assumed necessary (190 to 260 msec) to utilize external visual feedback [12].

The nervous system can learn to achieve desired levels of accuracy by adjusting control signals to accommodate factors such as changing musculoskeletal geometry, and dynamics. For example, when an object is grasped and lifted with fingers, the grip force varies directly in an anticipation of the load force as determined by mass and acceleration of the object [13–16].

Although the results of Morasso [17] are usually taken as strong evidence for spatial planning, several investigators have pointed out that end-point trajectories are not completely straight but instead gently curved in many parts of workspace, particularly in the sagittal plane [18]. This might be evidence for joint space trajectory planning, but the curvature seen in this movement is insufficient to support simple joint space interpolation, which would lead to much larger curvature. To account for this Hollerbach et al. [18] proposed a modification to joint space interpolation, which they termed "staggered joint interpolation," in which different joints begin moving at different times in order to produce straighter trajectories. However, this model cannot account for the reversals seen in the study of Morasso [17]. Hollerbach and Atkeson [19] proposed a way to directly control joint, which also yields straight-line hand paths. The method is to vary the onset times for the motions of the joints. Another experiment, which tried to prove that movement is joint space planned [20], was a simple act of pointing to a target.

Redundancy and motor equivalence: Bernstein [21] postulated the main problem of control of voluntary movement as the elimination of redundant degrees of freedom. The method used by nature to resolve the problem of redundancy and increase the efficiency of movement comes from the dependencies between components of the motor system. These dependencies could be understood as constraints and they ultimately decrease the number of variables to be controlled.

Motor equivalent behavior can be understood as the ability to use redundant degrees of freedom to compensate for temporary constraints on the effectors while producing movement trajectories to targets. There are some advantages of having the ability to perform a task in many ways (e.g., such as avoiding obstacles). The essence of motor equivalence is the ability to transform one type of sensory information into another. This is not present at birth. Transformations must be adapted (calibrated) in different circumstances like growth or handicap.

An important element to understand is the role and organization of the highly redundant muscles. The best way to do so is to analyze electrical activity of muscles, that is, the electromyography (EMG). The first detailed EMG analysis [22] of agonist and antagonist muscle activity in humans during flexion-extension movements of the arm showed a so-called triphasic pattern. The triphasic pattern is a strict alteration between agonist and antagonist EMG activity: the initiation of a distinct burst of activity in the agonist is followed by a distinct burst of activity in the antagonist. After a brief silent period in the agonist, activity returns in the form of a second burst. The existence of a consistent relationship between muscle activation patterns and the kinematic (or kinetic) variables of movement indicates which of these variables are important in planning appropriate motor output [23].

Grasping: Grasping is a part of the prehension, a process of orienting the hand, opening it so that the object fits comfortably, contacting the object, and forming a firm grip.

The selection of the grasp depends on both the function that has to be achieved and the physical constraints of the object and the hand. A fundamental functional constraint is that once the object is grasped it is not to be dropped. The posture used by the hand during the task must be capable of overcoming perturbations and include anticipated forces that may act at the object. There are different prehensile classifications, methods to classify hand postures, developed by researchers from different prospectives (e.g., medical, robotics) [24]. Schlesinger [25] suggested a taxotomy that was developed to capture the versatility of human hands for designing functionally effective prosthetic hands. The simplest taxotomy includes set of five grasp postures. For practical reasons this classification can be further reduced to only three grasps: lateral, palmar, and pinch grasps. Analyzing grasping in typical daily activities shows that these three grasps are responsible for almost 95% of all functions.

The task for the motor system of the hand is to build an "opposition space," which would take into account both the shape of the object and the biomechanics of the hand [26,27]. Experimental data suggest that there are preferred orientations for the hand opposition space. The hand posture selected during the preshape defines the optimal opposition space for applying the required forces to the object [28]. Using the term opposition authors described three basic directions along which the human hand can apply forces (1) pad opposition occurring between hand surfaces along a direction parallel to the palm. The surfaces are typically the volar surface of the fingers and thumb near or on the pads (pinch grasp); (2) palm opposition occurring between hand surfaces along a direction perpendicular to the palm (palmar grasp); and (3) side opposition occurring in the direction generally transverse to the palm (lateral grasp). Paulignan et al. [29] showed that the same orientation of the hand was retained during prehension of the same object placed at different positions in the working space, which implies different degrees of rotation of the wrist or the elbow.

15.3 Modeling of Human Extremities

Modeling of a human body with the emphasis to the extremities is the prerequisite for the synthesis of analytic control [30–33]. Human extremities are unlike any other plant encountered in control engineering especially in terms of joints, actuators, and sensors. This fact must be kept in mind when applying the general equations of mechanics to model the dynamics of functional motions. A simple extension of analytical tools used for the modeling of mechanical plants to the modeling of biomechanical systems may easily produce results in sharp discrepancy to reality.

A basic problem in motor control of human extremities is in *planning* of motions to solve a previously specified task, and, then, *controlling* the extremity as it implements the commands. In terms of mechanics, extremities could be adopted as the rigid mechanical segments connected by joints and surrounded by muscles, tendons, ligaments, and soft tissue that can set the joint angle, joint angular velocity, and acceleration to any value within its range. Muscles and tendons can also control the joint stiffness. The motions of extremities are called *trajectories* and consist of a sequence of positions, velocities, and accelerations of any part of the system (e.g., hand, fingertip, foot, etc.). It is anticipated that by using laws of mechanics one can determine necessary muscle forces to follow the given trajectory.

A body segment, when exposed to physiological loading, can be modeled as a **rigid body**, even though it contains somewhat flexible bones and soft tissue (e.g., muscles, tendons, ligaments, skin, etc). Inertial properties of a rigid body are its mass and the inertia tensor. The inertia tensor for a rigid body provides information on inertial properties of the body when rotating. The mass for a rigid body describes its inertia for translation type of movements. In reality the inertial properties change: the center of mass is shifting because the masses relatively move during contractions and passive stretching of muscles, relative movements of bones and other soft tissue modify the geometry, and polycentric joints virtually change the length of a body segment.

The second issue in the modeling relates to joint structures. A joint is modeled as a **kinematic pair**. The theory of mechanisms defines connection of neighboring segments as kinematic pairs having up to five degrees of freedom (DOF). Most common human joints are rotational kinematic pairs having three DOF (ball joint), or only one DOF (pin joint). However, many movements cannot be simplified to a pin or a ball joint. Some human joints must be represented with double mechanical joints (e.g., ankle joint consists of one joint for internal–external rotation, and inversion–eversion, and the other joint for movements in sagittal plane [flexion–extension]). Sometime the body segment rotation results from more complex structures such as two parallel bones connected between two neighboring joints (e.g., supination–pronation). Human joints are spatial and polycentric, and the displacement of the center of rotation results in the virtual change of the geometric and inertial properties of the body segment.

Speaking of mechanics one needs to distinguish the *forward kinematics* from the *inverse kinematics*. The direct kinematics is concerned with the determination of the position of body parts in the absolute reference frame given joint angles, whereas the inverse kinematics computes joint angles for a given position of the body part. Of these two, the direct **kinematic analysis** is the simplest by far, with a straightforward solution for the unique end point of the body part corresponding to the given joint angles. On the other hand, the feasibility of an inverse kinematics solution depends on the redundancy of the structure, as well as the offsets and constraints.

The redundancy is an important feature in biological systems. The concept of *redundancy* requires a distinction between a **degree of freedom** and a permissible motion (e.g., rotation). The term DOF pertains exclusively to that permissible motion which is independent from other motions. A free rigid body has a maximum of six DOF, and a rigid body connected to another rigid body by a ball joint can have a maximum of three DOF; thus, any body segment has less or maximum three DOF. Speaking of a structure as a whole, the total number of permissible rotations is termed system DOF. Some permissible rotations are not independent and they should not be called DOF (e.g., two parallel hinge joints). It is difficult to determine which permissible rotations should be controlled, and which will be constrained by themselves due to anatomical and physiological limitations.

Decomposing the linked structure into a set of single links is essential for numerical simulation. Internal forces within the body generated by muscle activities become external forces and torques when the dynamics of a single link is considered. The muscle is a linear actuator, with a very complex behavior depending on its length, velocity of shortening, firing rate, recruitment, and type. *Muscle models* [34] can be grouped to three classes (1) Crossbridge models including sarcomere — microscopic, conventional crossbridge, and unconventional crossbridge models; (2) Fiber models; and (3) Whole muscle — macroscopic models (viscoelastic and black box models). The distinctions between these classes are not absolute (e.g., micro–macro).

The modeling and control of movements in this chapter relates to external control of muscles via so-called functional electrical stimulation. Macroscopic viscoelastic models started from the observation that the process of electrical stimulation transforms the viscoelastic material from a compliant, fluent state into the stiff, viscous state. Levin and Wyman [35] proposed a three-element model — damped and undamped elastic element in series. Hill's work [36] demonstrated that the heat transfer depends upon the type of contraction (isometric, slow contracting, etc). The model includes the force generator, damping and elastic elements. Winters [37] generalized Hill's model in a simple enhancement of the original, which makes no claim to be based on the microstructure. Winters's model deals with joint moments:

$$M = M_0 - B\dot{\Theta}, \quad M_0 = AM_{0m}f(\Theta)$$

M is the muscle moment exerted about the joint, M_0 is the isometric moment (active state) with a maximum possible value M_{0m}, Θ is the joint angle corresponding to the current contractile element length, A is a normalized activation variable ($A = 0$ for relaxed muscle, $A = 1$ for a tetanized muscle), $f(\Theta)$ is the normalized tetanic length–tension relation, and B is a variable damping coefficient. For shortening muscle

$$B = M_0(1 + \alpha)/(\dot{\Theta} + \gamma\dot{\Theta}_0), \quad \dot{\Theta} < 0$$

whereas for lengthening muscle

$$B = M_0(1 - \beta)/(\dot{\Theta} + \gamma\dot{\Theta}_0), \quad \dot{\Theta} > 0$$

where α, β, and γ are constants.

Zajac [38] proposed an appealing new version of the Hill model designed primarily for use in studies of mechanical interactions in multiple muscle systems. Muscles are connected to a skeleton with tendons, and they have spring-like behavior when stretched. A variety of different nonrigid structures are included in the musculoskeletal system (e.g., ligaments) adding different elastic and damping effects. Nonlinear models of electrically stimulated muscle have been reviewed by Durfee [68]. Block models are only one of several possible structures, which can be used in biological system identification. Where there are only two blocks, one of that is nonlinear, may be placed before or after the dynamic block, in so-called Hammerstein or Wiener forms. Techniques for identifying the parameters for these models were investigated in details by Kearney and Hunter [40].

Dynamic analysis deals with two problems: determination of forces and torques when desired laws of motion are known (*forward dynamics*), and determination of trajectories and laws of motion when torques and forces are prescribed (*inverse dynamics*). Forward dynamics is a simple problem, and the only difficulty comes from error generated through numerical derivation on noisy input data. Using laws of mechanics (D'Alembert principle [41,42], Newton–Euler method [38,43–47], Lagrange equations [48–51], Basic theorems of mechanics [52], etc.) in inverse dynamics works only for open-chain structures such as an arm when reaching, or a leg during the swinging, but it is neither applicable for closed-chain structures such as legs during the double-support phase in walking, or the arm when contacting an immobile object, nor in redundant systems. Every closed, chained structure is dynamically undetermined and the only possibility to determine forces and torques is to use the theory of elasticity. The theory of elasticity assumes that the elements of the structure are solid (not rigid), and it is inappropriate for control design because of its extreme complexity. Approximate solution of the dynamics of a closed-chain mechanism assumes how forces and torques are distributed in the structure. In the case of locomotion, it is necessary to introduce at least three equations in order to be able to determine the dynamics of the process. In most cases the chain is limited to a small number of admissible rotations. The reason for simplification is twofold: the problem can be solved and the simulation results can be interpreted.

The complexity of a body segment dynamical model depends on the number and types of body segments, the joints connecting the segments, and the interaction among the segments and the environment. How complex is a model required for dynamic analysis of externally controlled walking, standing, manipulation, and grasping? Some decisions on how complex the model should be are simple, others are not. For instance, lower limb can be assumed rigid during standing and walking. More controversial is the decision on how many segments should be assumed, and how many DOFs should be assumed for each joint.

Several studies deal with strategies for prolonged standing [53–58] and functional electrical stimulation-aided gait [59–64].

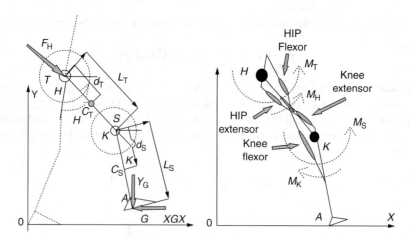

FIGURE 15.2 A sketch of a human body used for modeling of locomotion. Rigid body segments (left) are driven with two pairs of muscles (right). See the text for details.

Recent studies are concerned with estimating parameters required for modeling and simulation [65–74]. Many of the results are very useful; however, the presentations are incomplete and difficult to reproduce.

15.4 Analytic Models for Control of Movements

Attempts to analyze multijoint structures are often characterized by reducing the number of DOF to a manageable level. Locomotion is often decomposed into a component in the sagittal plane, and smaller components in the frontal and horizontal planes. Using smaller number of links is essential for simulation of gait.

A double, planar, pendulum with a moving hanging point, representing a human leg, is included here to illustrate the modeling. The remaining part of the body is represented as a single force acting to the moving hanging point (hip joint), hip joint torque (Figure 15.2). Two pairs of muscles acting around the hip and knee joints actuate the leg. Both monoarticular and biarticular muscles add to the joint torques. Estimating the relative contribution of monoarticular and biarticular muscles is very difficult but possible [75].

The model does not include ankle and phalangeal joints. The following system of differential equations describes the dynamics:

$$A_1\ddot{\phi}_S + A_2\ddot{\phi}_T \cos(\phi_T - \phi_S) + A_3\dot{\phi}_T^2 \sin(\phi_T - \phi_S) - A_4\ddot{x}_H \sin\phi_S$$
$$- A_5(\ddot{y}_H + g)\cos\phi_S - X_G L_S \sin\phi_S + Y_G L_S \cos\phi_S = M_S \qquad (15.1)$$

$$B_1\ddot{\phi}_T + B_2\ddot{\phi}_S \cos(\phi_T - \phi_S) + B_3\dot{\phi}_S^2 \sin(\phi_T - \phi_S)$$
$$- B_4\ddot{x}_H \sin\phi_T - B_5(\ddot{y}_H + g)\cos\phi_T - X_G L_T \sin\phi_T + Y_G L_T \cos\phi_T = M_T \qquad (15.2)$$

$$A_1 = J_{CS} + m_S d_S^2, \qquad B_1 = J_{CT} + m_S L_T^2 + m_T d_T^2$$
$$A_2 = m_S d_S L_T, \qquad B_2 = A_2, \qquad A_3 = -A_2, \qquad B_3 = B_2$$
$$A_4 = m_S d_S, \qquad B_4 = m_S L_T + m_T d_T, \qquad A_5 = -A_4, \qquad B_5 = -B_4$$

There are several torques contributing to the total torques acting at the links

$$M_S = -M_K, \qquad M_T = M_K + M_H$$
$$M_K = M_K^f - M_K^e - M_K^r, \qquad M_H = M_H^f - M_H^e - M_H^r \qquad (15.3)$$

The following notations are used: S — the shank segment (including the foot); T — the thigh segment; C_S, C_T — the center of the mass of the shank and thigh segments; H — the hip joint; K — the knee joint; G — the point of ground contact; d_S, d_T — distances of the proximal joint to the centers of the masses; L_S, L_T — lengths of the shank and thigh; m_S, m_T — masses of the shank and thigh; J_{CS}, J_{CT} — moments of inertia of the shank and thigh about the central axes perpendicular to xOy plane; g — gravitational acceleration; F_H — force acting at the hip joint; X_G, Y_G — horizontal and vertical components of the ground reaction force; M_S, M_T — total torques acting at the shank and thigh segments; M_K, M_H — joint torques at the knee and hip joints; $\ddot{x}_H$, $\ddot{y}_H$ — horizontal and vertical components of the hip acceleration; ϕ_S, ϕ_T — angles of the shank and thigh vs. the horizontal axis (Ox); ϕ_K, ϕ_H — angles of the knee and hip joint; ϕ_{TR} — angle of the trunk vs. the horizontal axis (Ox).

Flexion of a joint is defined to be the positive direction for angular changes; hence, the flexor torque is assumed to be positive. Index f is for the equivalent flexor muscle, and index e for the equivalent extensor muscle. The contribution of passive tissue crossing the joints is included by a "resistive" torque (index r), which will be described below.

A three-multiplicative-factor model used is a modified version of the Hill model (Figure 15.3). Active muscle force depends on the neural activation, muscle length, and velocity of shortening or lengthening [41,42]. The model is formulated as a function of joint angle and angular velocity, rather than muscle length and velocity. The three-factor model is given by:

$$M_a = A(u)f(\phi)g(\dot{\phi}) \qquad (15.4)$$

where M_a is the active torque generated by a muscle contraction; $A(u)$ is the dependence of a torque on the level of muscle activity u depending on the stimulus amplitude, pulse width, and stimulus frequency; $f(\phi)$ is the dependence on the angle ϕ; and $g(\dot{\phi})$ is the dependence on the angular velocity $\dot{\phi}$. The parameter u is normalized to the range $0 \leq u \leq 1$. According to the literature [76], the muscle model described by Equation 15.1 can predict the muscle torque with 85 to 90% accuracy during simultaneous, independent, pseudorandom variations of recruitment, angle, and angular velocity.

Activation $A(u)$: In accordance with the literature [76–79] the muscle response to electrical stimulation was approximated by a second-order, critically damped [76,77], low-pass filter with a delay. Thus, the

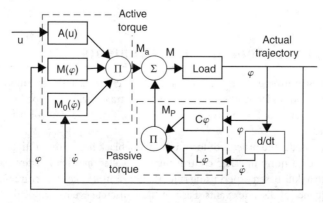

FIGURE 15.3 A three factor multiplicative model of a muscle (active torque). The model includes antagonist muscle (passive torque).

activation dynamics were assumed to be expressed by the following equation:

$$\frac{A(j\omega)}{U(j\omega)} = \frac{\omega_p^2}{\omega^2 + 2j\omega\omega_p + \omega_p^2} e^{-j\omega t_d} \tag{15.5}$$

where $A(j\omega)$ is the Fourier transform of the muscles' contractile activity, $U(j\omega)$ is the Fourier transform of the muscle's electrical activity, ω_p is muscle's natural frequency (typically in the range of 1 to 3 Hz), t_d is the excitation-contraction and other delays in the muscle.

Joint torque ($f(\phi)$) dependence on a joint angle: The nonlinear function relating torque and joint angle is simulated by a quadratic curve, $F = a_0 + a_1\phi + a_2\phi^2$. The torque generated can not be negative for any angle, so

$$f(\phi) = \begin{cases} F & \text{if } F \geq 0 \\ 0 & \text{if } F < 0 \end{cases} \tag{15.6}$$

Coefficients a_i define the shape of the torque-angle curve and they are determined as the best fit through the experimental data recorded. The quadratic polynomial was selected as the simplest adequate fitting curve as described elsewhere [73,80]. Note that each of the quantities is nonnegative.

Normalized joint torque ($g(\dot{\phi})$) dependence on the angular velocity: The normalized joint torques vs. joint angular velocities can be modelled piecewise linear:

$$g(\dot{\phi}) = \begin{cases} c_{ij}, & \dot{\phi} < (1 - c_{ij})/c_{ij} \\ 1 - c_{ij}\dot{\phi}, & (1 - c_{ij})/c_{ij} \leq \dot{\phi} < 1/c_{ij} \\ 0, & 1/c_{ij} \leq \dot{\phi} \end{cases} \tag{15.7}$$

The coefficients c_{ij} determine the slope and saturation level of the linearized torque vs. velocity of the muscle shortening. These coefficients can be determined using the method described in Reference 81.

Resistive joint torque: Soft tissue, passive stretching of antagonistic muscles, and ligaments introduce nonlinearities, which can be modeled as:

$$M^r = d_{11}(\phi - \phi_0) + d_{12}\dot{\phi} + d_{13}\, e^{d_{14}\phi} - d_{15}\, e^{d_{16}\phi} \tag{15.8}$$

The presented form was developed heuristically, and it shows that the resistive torques depend on both the joint angle and its angular velocity. The two first terms are the contributions of passive tissues crossing the joints (dissipative properties of joints) reduced to first-order functions. The other terms are the nonlinear components of the resistive torques around the terminal positions, and are modeled as double exponential curve [73].

15.5 Nonanalytic Modeling of Movements

As said, the control of movements in humans is a highly complex task, the model of the body and extremities is complicated and not observable per se, the trajectories are not known in advance, the driving resources are user specific and time variable; thus, real-time control using analytical tools is probably not feasible.

An alternative is to model the process of locomotion as a black box with multiple inputs and outputs. Tomović [82] proposed a nonnumerical control method, called **artificial reflex control** (ARC). ARC (Figure 15.4) refers to a skill-based expert using rules that have an *If–Then* structure [83]. The locomotion is presented as a sequence of discrete events. Each of these discrete events can be described in terms of a sensory pattern and a motor activity. A sensory pattern occurring during particular motor activity can be recognized with the use of human-made (artificial or natural) sensors. The specific discrete event is called

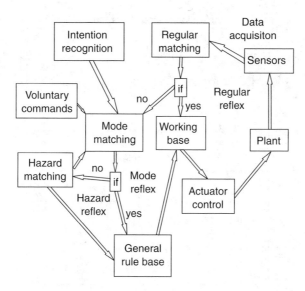

FIGURE 15.4 A scheme of the organization of a skill-based multilevel control for locomotion. Regular reflexes are sequences of system states connected with conditional If–Then expressions within a single mode of the gait, mode reflexes relate to the change of the mode of the gait (level, slope, stairs, etc.), and hazard reflexes are for situations where software or hardware cannot drive the system upon the preferred sequence of system states.

the state of the system by analogy to the state of finite-state automata [82,84]. This skill-based expert system is of the *On–Off* type and does not consider explicitly the system dynamics.

A rule-based control system has a hierarchical structure. The highest level is under volitional control of the user. Automatic adaptation to environmental changes and modes of gait is realized using artificial reflex control. The execution of the artificial reflex has to be tuned for smooth functional movements. Advantages of this **hierarchical control** method are the following (1) adaptivity, (2) modularity, (3) ease of application, and (4) possibility of integration into a man–machine system. Rule-based control was tested in hybrid assistive systems [85,86] and artificial legs [83].

Nonanalytic control can be described as cloning the biological control [87,88]. The basic mechanisms for implementation of such algorithms are rule-based controllers (RBCs) [89]. RBC were applied for assistive systems to restore locomotion with handcrafted [82,85,90,91], and lately automatically determined knowledge base [92–97] with limited success. An RBC is a system implementing "If–Then" **production rules**, where "If" part describes the sensory and motor state of the system, while "Then" part of a rule defines the corresponding motor activity to follow.

It was hypothesized that machine learning (ML) can acquire the needed knowledge for RBC (see Chapter 14 of Abbas, this book). Learning in general can be described as capturing and memorizing of connectivisms between facts (Figure 15.5). ML is a computerized capturing and memorizing process. The study [93] used simulation results of a fully customized biomechanical model as inputs and outputs required for an ML. The following MLs were compared (1) a multilayer perceptron (MLP) with the Levenberg–Marquardt improvement of backpropagation (BP) algorithm [98]; (2) an adaptive-network-based fuzzy inference system (ANFIS) [99]; and (3) combination of an entropy minimization type of inductive learning (IL) technique [92,97,100] and a radial basis function (RBF) type of artificial neural network (ANN) [101,102] with orthogonal least squares (OLS) learning algorithm [101].

A comparison of IL with adaptive logic networks (ALNs) using restriction rules [95,96] shows that ALNs have some advantages over IL. Heller et al. [92] compared an IL method based on an algorithm called "hierarchical mutual information classifier" [103] with an MLP with BP algorithm in reconstructing muscle activation from kinematic data during normal walking. The conclusion was that both techniques show comparable performance, although each technique has some advantages over the other. A comparison of IL method based on minimization of entropy and the RBF network in predicting muscle

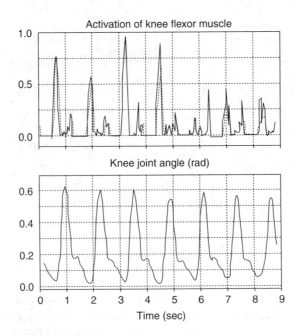

FIGURE 15.5 A mapping obtained as a result of radial basis function and artificial neural network (RBF ANN) learning algorithm. The knee joint angle sensory information for first four consecutive strides (full line, bottom panel), the ground reactions, and the hip accelerations were used as inputs for training. The activation of knee flexor muscles for the same four strides (full line, upper panel) was used for output during the training. The upper panel presents superimposed desired activation of muscles (full line) and a predicted activity of the muscle by a RBF ANN (dashed line) obtained from a trained network for seven consecutive steps. See text for details.

activation and sensory data from the history of sensory data for a human with spinal cord injury (SCI) [93] shows that the best generalization comes from combining both. The benefits of merging fuzzy logic and an ANN were explored extensively in the literature [99–104].

Investigations of MLPs have been intensified since the formulation of the BP learning algorithm [98]. An MLP is a feed-forward network, typically consisting of several layers of nonlinear processing nodes called hidden layers with a linear output layer. Processing nodes take as input only the outputs of the previous layer, which are combined as a weighted sum and then passed through a nonlinear processing function known as the "activation function." This activation function is typically sigmoidal in shape. An MLP with three hidden layers can form arbitrarily complex decision regions and can separate classes that are meshed together. It can form regions as complex as those formed using mixture distributions and nearest neighbor classifiers [105].

The BP learning algorithm is a generalization of a gradient descent algorithm. The BP algorithm may lead to a local, rather than a global error minimum. If the local minimum found is not satisfactory, use of several different sets of initial conditions or a network with more neurons can be tried. A simple BP algorithm is very slow because it must use low learning rates for stable learning. There are ways to improve the speed and general performance of a BP algorithm. It can be improved in two different ways: by heuristics and by using more powerful methods of optimization. Speed and reliability of BP can be increased by techniques called momentum and adaptive learning rates (e.g., Levenberg–Marquardt modification of BP algorithm).

Fuzzy sets are a generalization of conventional set theory. They were introduced by Zadeh [106] as a mathematical way to represent vagueness in everyday life. A formal definition of fuzzy sets that has been presented by many researchers is following: a fuzzy set A is a subset of the universe of discourse X that admits partial membership. The fuzzy set A is defined as the ordered pair $A = \{x, m_A(x)\}$, where $x \in X$ and $0 \le m_A(x) \le 1$. The membership function $m_A(x)$ describes the degree to which the object

x belongs to the set A, where $m_A(x) = 0$ represents no membership, and $m_A(x) = 1$ represents full membership.

One of the biggest differences between conventional (crisp) and fuzzy sets is that every crisp set always has a unique membership function, whereas every fuzzy set has an infinite number of membership functions that may represent it. This is at once both a drawback and advantage; uniqueness is sacrificed, but this gives a concomitant gain in terms of flexibility, enabling fuzzy models to be "adjusted" for maximum utility in a given situation.

The typical steps of a "fuzzy reasoning" consist of (1) Fuzzification, that is, comparing the input variables with the membership functions of the premise (IF) parts in order to obtain the membership values between 0 and 1; (2) Weighing, that is, applying specific fuzzy logic operators (e.g., AND operator, OR operator, etc.) on the premise parts membership values to get a single number between 0 and 1; (3) Generation, that is, creating the consequent (THEN) part of the rule; and (4) Defuzzification, that is, aggregating the consequent to produce the output.

There are several kinds of fuzzy rules used to construct fuzzy models. These fuzzy rules can be classified into the following three types according to their consequent form [107]:

1. Crisply defined constant in the consequent:

$$R_i : \text{IF } x_1 \text{ is } A_{i1} \text{ and } \cdots \text{ and } x_m \text{ is } A_{im} \text{ THEN } y \text{ is } c_i$$

2. A linear combination of the system's input variables in the consequent:

$$R_i: \text{IF } x_1 \text{ is } A_{i1} \text{ and } \cdots \text{ and } x_m \text{ is } A_{im} \text{ THEN } y \text{ is } g_i(x_1, \ldots, x_m) = b_0 + b_1 x_1 + \cdots + b_m x_m$$

3. Fuzzy set in the consequent:

$$R_i: \text{IF } x_1 \text{ is } A_{i1} \text{ and } \cdots \text{ and } x_m \text{ is } A_{im} \text{ THEN } y \text{ is } B_i$$

where R_i is the ith rule of the fuzzy system, x_j $(j = 1, 2, \ldots, m)$ are the inputs to the fuzzy system, and y is the output from the fuzzy system. The linguistic terms A_{ij} and B_i are fuzzy sets, c_i and b_j denote crisp constants.

The so-called zero-order Sugeno, or Takagi–Sugeno–Kang fuzzy model [108] has rules of the first type, whereas the first-order Sugeno fuzzy model has rules of the second type. The easiest way to visualize the first-order Sugeno fuzzy model is to think of each rule as defining the location of a "moving singleton" (a single spike from the consequent) depending on what the input is. Sugeno models are similar to the Mamdani model [109] which has rules of the third type, and which is more intuitive, but computationally less efficient. Fuzzification and weighing are exactly the same, but generation and defuzzification are different [107].

For the type of fuzzy rules used in Mamdani model various methods are available for defuzzification: the centroid of area, bisector of area, middle of maximum, largest of maximum, and so forth [110], but all of these methods are based on the calculation of the two-dimensional-shape surface, that is on the integration. The Sugeno style enhances the efficiency of the defuzzification process because it greatly simplifies the computation; that is, it has to find just the weighted average of a few data points. The implication method (generation) is simply multiplication and the aggregation operator just includes all of the singletons.

Membership functions are subjective and context-dependent, so there is no general method to determine them. Currently, when fuzzy set theory is applied in control systems, the system designers are given enough freedom to choose membership functions and operators, usually in a trial and error way. After a hand-tuning process, the system can function effectively. However, the same methodology is hardly applicable when the system is a general purpose one, or when the context changes dynamically. This suggests an explanation why the most successful applications of fuzzy logic happen in control systems, rather than in natural language processing, knowledge base management, and general purposes reasoning.

The IL is a symbolic technique, which uses supervised learning and generates a set of "if-then-else" decision rules. A method [97] is based on an algorithm called "hierarchical mutual information classifier" [92,103]. This algorithm produces a decision tree by maximizing the average mutual information at each partitioning step. It uses Shannon's entropy as a measure of information. Mutual information is a measure of the amount of information that one random variable contains about another random variable. It is a reduction of the uncertainty of one random variable due to the knowledge of the other. An effective method of integrating results of a mutual information algorithm into a production rule formalism, following the original work of Watanabe [100] and Pitas [111], was done by Nikolić [112]. While generating the decision tree, the algorithm performs a hierarchical partitioning of the domain multidimensional space. Each new node of the decision tree contains a rule based on a threshold of one of the input signals. Each new rule further subdivides the example set. The training is finished when each terminal node contains members of only one class. An excellent feature of this algorithm is that it determines threshold automatically based on the minimum entropy. This minimum entropy method is equivalent to determination of the maximum probability of recognizing a desired event (output) based on the information from input.

Radial basis function (RBF) network is a feed-forward network. The RBF has a single output node and a single hidden layer which contains as many neurons as are required to fit the function within the specifications of error goal. The transformation from the input space to the hidden-unit space is nonlinear, whereas the transformation from the hidden-unit space to the output space is linear. A common learning algorithm for RBF networks is based on first choosing randomly some data points as radial basis function centers and then using singular value decomposition to solve for the weights of the network. An arbitrary selection of centers may not satisfy the requirement that centers should suitably sample the input domain. Furthermore, in order to achieve a given performance, an unnecessarily large RBF network may be required. Since a performance of an RBF network critically depends upon the chosen centers, we used an alternative learning procedure based on the OLS learning algorithm [101]. By providing a set of inputs and corresponding outputs, the values of weights and bias, and RBF centers (parameters for RBF network) can be determined using the OLS algorithm in one pass of the learning data so that a network of an adequate size can be constructed.

When an input vector is presented to such a network, each neuron in the hidden layer will output a value according to how close the input vector is to the centers vector of each neuron. The result is that neurons with centers vector are very different from the input vector will have outputs near zero. These small outputs will have a negligible effect on the linear output neurons. In contrast, any neuron whose centers vector is very close to the input vector will output a value near 1. If a neuron has an output of 1, its output weights in the second layer pass their values to the neuron in the second layer. The width of an area in the input space to which each radial basis neuron responds can be set by defining a spread constant for each neuron. This constant should be big enough to enable neurons to respond strongly to overlapping regions of the input space. The same spread constant is usually selected for each neuron.

15.6 Hybrid Modeling of Controllers

Feedback error learning (FEL) is a hybrid technique [113] using the mapping to replace the estimation of parameters within the feedback loop in a closed-loop control scheme. FEL is a feed-forward neural network structure, under training, learning the inverse dynamics of the controlled object. This method is based on contemporary physiological studies of the human cortex [114], and is shown in Figure 15.6.

The total control effort u applied to the plant is the sum of the feedback control output and network control output. The ideal configuration of the neural network would correspond to the inverse mathematical model of the system's plant. The network is given information of the desired position and its derivatives, and it will calculate the control effort necessary to make the output of the system follow the desired trajectory. If there are no disturbances the system error will be zero.

The configuration of the neural network should represent the inverse dynamics of the system when training is completed. It was prudent to use a total energy approach as basis for the neural network, because

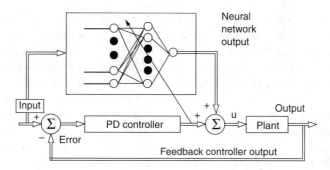

FIGURE 15.6 Model for the hybrid modeling of controllers using feedback error learning algorithm. The inclined arrow represents the learning.

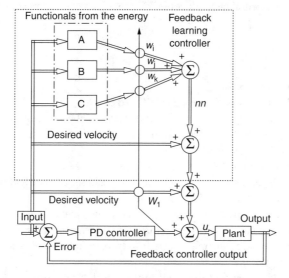

FIGURE 15.7 Scheme of the feedback error learning controller used for the one degree of freedom system. See text for details.

only the commanded input and its first derivative is required for the FEL controller. By comparison, if the FEL were based on the mathematical model, the second derivative would be needed for the neural network to operate [115].

Figure 15.7 depicts a more in-depth explanation of the FEL strategy. The system input and output are labeled θ_d and θ. The proportional-plus-derivative (PD) feedback controller is included to provide stability during training of the neural network [114,116–118]. Enclosed in the dashed rectangle is an FEL controller, which outputs the necessary control signal, based on the desired inputs. The total energy of the system (nn) is calculated through parallel processing within the neural network, consisting of the functionals (A,B,C, ...) obtained from the total energy expression, the synaptic weights w_i, w_j, and w_k. In addition to the above-mentioned synaptic weights, w_l is associated with damping losses. The training of the FEL controller is facilitated by changing the synaptic weights based on the output from a PD controller. The learning rule used, was proposed by Kawato et al. [119] and it is given as follows:

$$w_{i\text{new}} = w_{i\text{old}} + u_{\text{PD}} A \eta \Delta t$$

where $w_{i\text{new}}$ is the new value of the synaptic weight, $w_{i\text{old}}$ is the old value, u_{PD} is the output from the PD controller, A is the network functional associated with weight w_i, η is the learning rate, and Δt is the integration step used in the computer simulation. A learning rate is included to control the rate of growth of the synaptic weights. The learning rule, as proposed by Kawato et al. [113], is based on the assumption of slow growth of the synaptic weights. The weights are initialized at zero, and the learning rates adjusted so the growths of the weights are uniform. This causes the weights to reach their final value at the same point in time, causing the error to approach zero. Subsequently, the learning as a function of error will level off, and the training of the neural network will be completed. However, if the growth of the weights is not homogeneous, it will result in an unbounded growth of the weights. The vertical line in Figure 15.7 pointing upward through w_i, w_j, w_k, and w_l symbolizes the learning. After the total energy is calculated, the time derivative is taken and divided by the desired velocity. The losses are calculated by multiplying the desired velocity by the weight w_l, and are then added to the control signal. Finally, the control effort from the FEL controller is added to the PD control effort.

In essence, the output of the feedback controller is an indication of the mismatch between the dynamics of the plant and the inverse-dynamics model obtained by the neural network. If the true inverse-dynamic model has been learned, the neural network alone will provide the necessary control signal to achieve the desired trajectory [118,120].

Defining Terms

Actuator: Device that power a system.

Artificial reflex control: Expert system using rule-based control.

Closed-loop system: Control system which uses information about the output to correct the control parameters to minimize the error between the desired and actual trajectory.

Controls: The signals driving the actuators.

Controller: Process by which the controls are generated.

Degree of freedom: Independent variable defining the position. A free rigid body has six degrees of freedom, a ball joint three, and a hinge joint one.

Dynamic analysis: Analytic simulation of movements of the system considering forces, torques, and kinematics. Forward dynamics uses the geometry and kinematics as input, and provides forces and torques as outputs; inverse dynamics starts from forces and torques and determines kinematics and geometry of the system.

Hierarchical control: Multilevel control allowing the vertical decomposition of the system.

Kinematic analysis: Analytic simulation of movements of the system considering positions, velocities, and accelerations.

Kinematic pair: Connection of two neighboring segments.

Nonanalytic control: Mappings between inputs and outputs to be used for control.

Open-loop control: Control method that uses a prestored trajectory and the model of the system to control the plant.

Plant: The mechanical system being controlled.

Production rule: "If–Then" conditional expression used in experts systems.

Reference-based open-loop control: Control which precomputes and stores control signals, and execute the desired motor task in real-time.

Rigid body: Set of material points with the distances between points being fixed.

State: The configuration of the system at any instant in time.

Trajectory: The time histories of the plant states in response to the control signals.

References

[1] Latash, M.L., *Control of Human Movement*. Human Kinetics Publishers, Champaign, IL, 1993.

[2] Sherrington, C.S., *The Integrative Action of the Nervous System*. Yale University Press, New Haven, CT, 1906 (reprinted 1961).

[3] Magnus, R., *Der Körperstellung*. Springer-Verlag, Berlin, 1924.

[4] Kuypers, H.G., Anatomy of the descending pathways. In Brook, V.B. (Ed.), *Handbook of Physiology: The Nervous System* (Vol. II). American Physiological Society, Bethesda, pp. 597–666, 1981.

[5] Bouisset, S., Do, M.C., and Zattara, M. Posturo-kinetic capacity assessed in paraplegics and Parkinsonians. In Woollacott, M. and Horak, F. (Eds.), *Posture and Gait: Control Mechanisms*. University Oregon Books, Portland, OR, pp. 19–22, 1992.

[6] Massion, J., Postural control systems in developmental perspective. *Neurosci. Behav. Rev.* 22: 465–472, 1998.

[7] Georgopoulos, A.P., On reaching. *Ann. Rev. Neurosci.* 9: 147–170, 1986.

[8] Prablanc, C., Echallier, J.F., Komilis, E., and Jeannerod, M., Optimal response of eye and hand motor systems in pointing at visual target. II. Static and dynamic visual cues in the control of hand movements. *Biol. Cybern.* 35: 183–187, 1979.

[9] Conti, P. and Beaubaton, D., Utilisation des informations visuelles dans le controle du mouvement: etude de la precision des pointages chez l'homme. *Le Trav. Hum.* 39: 19–32, 1976.

[10] Prablanc, C., Echallier, J.F., Komilis, E., and Jeannerod, M., Optimal response of eye and hand motor systems in pointing at visual target. I. Spatio-temporal characteristics of eye and hand movements and their relationships when varying the amount of visual information. *Biol. Cybern.* 35: 113–124, 1979.

[11] Paillard, J., The contribution of peripheral and central vision to visually guided reaching. In Ingle, D.J., Goodale, M.A., and Mansfield, R.J.W. (Eds.), *Visually Oriented Behavior*. MIT Press, Cambridge, MA, pp. 367–385, 1982.

[12] Keele, S.W. and Posner, M.I., Processing of visual feedback in rapid movements. *J. Exp. Physiol.* 77: 155–158, 1968.

[13] Flanagan, J.R. and Wing, A.M., Modulation of grip force with load force during point-to-point arm movements. *Exp. Brain Res.* 95: 131–143, 1993.

[14] Flanagan, J.R. and Wing, A.M., Effects of surface texture and grip force on the discrimination of hand-held loads. *Percept. Psychophys.* 59: 111–118, 1997.

[15] Flanagan, J.R. and Wing, A.M., The role of internal models in motion planning and control: evidence from grip force adjustments during movements of hand-held loads. *J. Neurosci.* 17: 1519–1528, 1997.

[16] Ghilardi, M., Gordon, J., and Ghez, C., Learning a visuomotor transformation in a local area of work space produces directional biases in other areas. *J. Neurophysiol.* 73: 2535–2539, 1995.

[17] Morasso, P., Spatial control of arm movements. *Exp. Brain Res.* 42: 223–227, 1981.

[18] Hollerbach, J.M., Moore, S.P., and Atkeson, C.G., Workspace effect in arm movement kinematics derived by joint interpolation. In Ganchev, G., Dimitrov, B., and Patev, P. (Eds.), *Motor Control*, Plenum, 1986.

[19] Hollerbach, J.M. and Atkeson, C.G., Deducing planning variables from experimental arm trajectories: pitfalls and possibilities. *Biol. Cybern.* 56: 279–292, 1987.

[20] Soechting, J.F. and Lacquaniti, F., Invariant characteristics of a pointing movement in man. *J. Neurosci.* 1: 710–720, 1981.

[21] Bernstein, N.A., *The Coordination and Regulation of Movements*. Pergamon Press, London (original work in 1926–1935), 1967.

[22] Wachholder, K. and Altenburger, H., Beitrage zur Physiologie der willkurlichen Bewegung. X Mitteilung. Einzelbewegungen. *Pflügers Arch. Ges. Physiol.* 214: 642–661, 1926.

[23] Soechting, J.F., Elements of coordinated arm movements in three-dimensional space. In Wallace, S.A. (Ed.), *Perspectives on the Coordination of Movement*. North-Holland, Amsterdam, pp. 47–83, 1989.

[24] MacKenzie, C.L. and Iberall, T., *The Grasping Hand*. North-Holland, 1994.

[25] Schlesinger, G., Der Mechanisce Aufbau der kunstlischen Glieder. In Borchardt, M. (Ed.), *Ersatzglieder und Arbeitshilfen für Kriegsbeshadigte und Unfallverletzte*. Springer, Berlin, pp. 21–600, 1919.

[26] Arbib, M.A., Schemas for the temporal control of behavior. *Hum. Neurobiol.* 4: 63–72, 1985.

[27] Iberall, T. and MacKenzie, C.L., Opposition space and human prehension. In Venkataraman, S.T. and Iberall, T. (Eds.), *Dexterous Robot Hands.* Springer-Verlag, New York, pp. 32–54, 1990.

[28] Iberall, T., Bingham, G., and Arbib, M.A., Opposition space as a structuring concept for the analysis of skilled hand movements. In Heuer, H. and Fromm, C. (Eds.), *Generation and Modulation of Action Pattern.* Plenum, New York, 1986.

[29] Paulignan, Y., MacKenzie, C.L., Marteniuk, R.G., and Jeannerod, M., Selective perturbation of visual input during prehension movements. I. The effects of changing object position. *Exp. Brain Res.* 83: 502–512, 1991.

[30] Winter, D.A., *Biomechanics and Motor Control of Human Movement*, 2nd ed. Wiley-Interscience, New York, 1990.

[31] Popović, D.B. and Sinkjær, T., *Control of Movement for the Physically Disabled*, Springer-Verlag, London, 2000.

[32] Winters, J.M. and Crago, E.P. (Eds.), *Biomechanics and Neural Control of Posture and Movement.* Springer-Verlag, New York, 2000.

[33] Zajac, F.E. and Gordon, M.E., Determining muscles's force and action in multi-articular movement. In Pandoff, K. (Ed.), *Exercise Sport Science Review*, Vol. 17. Williams and Wilkins, Baltimore, pp. 187–230, 1989.

[34] Zahalak, G.I., Modeling muscle mechanics (and energetics). In Winters, J.M. and Woo, S.L.-Y. (Eds.), *Multiple Muscle Systems: Biomechanics and Movement Organization*, Springer-Verlag, New York, pp. 1–23, 1990.

[35] Levin, A. and Wyman, J., The viscous elastic properties of muscle, *Proc. R. Soc. Lond. Biol.* 101: 218–243, 1927.

[36] Hill, T.L., The heat of shortening and the dynamic constants of muscle, *Proc. R. Soc. Lond. Biol.* 126: 135–195, 1938.

[37] Winters, J.M., Hill-based muscle models: a systems engineering prospective. In Winters, J.M. and Woo, S.L.-Y. (Eds.), *Multiple Muscle Systems: Biomechanics and Movement Organization.* Springer-Verlag, New York, pp. 66–93, 1990.

[38] Zajac, F.E., Muscle and tendon: properties: models, scaling, and application to biomechanics and motor control, *CRC Crit. Rev. Biomed. Eng.* 17: 359–411, 1989.

[39] Shue, G., Crago, P.E., and Chizeck, H.J., Muscle-joint models incorporating activation dynamics, moment-angle and moment-velocity properties, *IEEE Trans. Biomed. Eng.* BME-42: 212–223, 1995.

[40] Kearney, R.E. and Hunter, I.W., System identification of human joint dynamics, *CRC Crit. Rev. Biomed. Eng.* 18: 55–87, 1990.

[41] Huston, R.L., Passerello, C.E., and Harlow, M.W., On human body dynamics, *Ann. Biomed. Eng.* 4: 25–43, 1976.

[42] Huston, R.L., Passerello, C.E., and Harlow, M.W., Dynamics of multirigid-body systems, *J. Appl. Mech.* 45: 889–894, 1978.

[43] Stepanenko, Y. and Vukobratoviæ M., Dynamics of articulated open-chain active mechanisms, *Math. Biosci.* 28: 137–170, 1976.

[44] Orin, D.E., McGhee, R.B., Vukobratović, M., and Hartoch, G., Kinematic and kinetic analysis of open-chain linkages utilizing Newton–Euler methods, *Math. Biosci.* 43: 107–130, 1979.

[45] Marshall, R.N., Jensen, R.K., and Wood, G.A., A general Newtonian simulation of an n-segment open chain model, *J. Biomech.* 18: 359–367, 1985.

[46] Khang, G. and Zajac, F.E., Paraplegic standing controlled by functional electrical stimulation: part I — computer model and control-system design; part II —computer simulation studies, *IEEE Trans. Biomed. Eng.* BME-36: 873–893, 1989.

[47] Yamaguchi, G.T. and Zajac, F.E., Restoring unassisted natural gait to paraplegics via functional neuromuscular stimulation: a computer simulation study, *IEEE Trans. Biomed. Eng.* BME-37: 886–902, 1990.

[48] Onyshko, S. and Winter, D.A., A mathematical model for the dynamics of human locomotion, *J. Biomech.* 13: 361–368, 1980.

[49] Hatze, H., A complete set of control equations for the human musculo-skeletal system, *J. Biomech.* 10: 799–805, 1977.

[50] Hatze, H., Neuromusculoskeletal control systems modeling — a critical survey of recent developments, *IEEE Trans. Automat. Control* AC-25: 375–385, 1980.

[51] Zheng, Y.F. and Shen, J.S., Gait synthesis for the SD-2 biped robot to climb sloping surfaces, *IEEE Trans. Robot. Automat.* RA-6: 86–96, 1990.

[52] Koozekanani, S.H., Barin, K., McGhee, R.B., and Chang, H.T., A recursive free body approach to computer simulation of human postural dynamics, *IEEE Trans. Biomed. Eng.* BME-30: 787–792, 1983.

[53] Davoodi, R. and Andrews, B.J., Computer simulation of FES standing up in paraplegia: a self-adaptive fuzzy controller with reinforcement learning, *IEEE Trans. Rehabil. Eng.* TRE-6: 151–161, 1998.

[54] Donaldson, N. and Yu, C., A strategy used by paraplegics to stand up using FES, *IEEE Trans. Rehabil. Eng.* TRE-6: 162–166, 1998.

[55] Hunt, K.J., Munih, M., and Donaldson, N., Feedback control of unsupported standing in paraplegia — part I: optimal control approach and part II: experimental results, *IEEE Trans. Rehabil. Eng.* TRE-5: 331–352, 1997.

[56] Matjačić, Z. and Bajd, T., Arm-free paraplegic standing — part I: control model synthesis and simulation and part II: experimental results, *IEEE Trans. Rehabil. Eng.* TRE-6: 125–150, 1998.

[57] Riener, R. and Fuhr, T., Patient-driven control of FES supported standing up: a simulation study, *IEEE Trans. Rehabil. Eng.* TRE-6: 113–124, 1998.

[58] Veltink, P.H. and Donaldson, N., A perspective on the controlled FES-supported standing, *IEEE Trans. Rehabil. Eng.* TRE-6: 109–112, 1996.

[59] Abbas, J.J. and Chizeck, H.J., Neural network control of functional neuromuscular stimulation systems: computer simulation studies, *IEEE Trans. Biomed. Eng.* BME-42: 1117–1127, 1995.

[60] Abbas, J.J. and Triolo, R.J., Experimental evaluation of an adaptive feedforward controller for use in functional neuromuscular stimulation systems, *IEEE Trans. Rehabil. Eng.* TRE-5: 12–22, 1997.

[61] Gilchrist, L.A. and Winter, D.A., A multisegment computer simulation of normal human gait, *IEEE Trans. Rehabil. Eng.* TRE-5: 290–299, 1997.

[62] Graupe, D. and Kordylewaki, H., Artificial neural network control of FES in paraplegics for patient responsive ambulation, *IEEE Trans. Biomed. Eng.* BME-42: 699–707, 1995.

[63] Kobetic, R. and Marsolais, E.B., Synthesis of paraplegic gait with multichannel functional electrical stimulation, *IEEE Trans. Rehabil. Eng.* TRE-2: 66–79, 1994.

[64] Kobetic, R., Triolo, R.J., and Marsolais, E.B., Muscle selection and walking performance of multichannel FES systems for ambulation in paraplegia, *IEEE Trans. Rehabil. Eng.* TRE-5: 23–29, 1997.

[65] Crago, P.E., Muscle input–output model: the static dependence of force on length, recruitment and firing period, *IEEE Trans. Biomed. Eng.* BME-39: 871–874, 1992.

[66] Durfee, W.K. and Mac Lean, K.E., Methods of estimating the isometric recruitment curve of electrically stimulated muscle, *IEEE Trans. Biomed. Eng.* BME-36: 654–667, 1989.

[67] Durfee, W.K., Model identification in neural prostheses system, In Stein, R.B., Pechkam, P.H., and Popović, D. (Eds.), *Neural Prostheses: Replacing Motor Function After Disease or Disability.* Oxford University Press, New York, pp. 58–87, 1992.

[68] Durfee, W.K. and Palmer, K.I. Estimation of force activation, force–length, and force–velocity properties in isolated electrically stimulated muscle, *IEEE Trans. Biomed. Eng.* BME-41: 205–216, 1994.

[69] Franken, H.M., Veltink, P.H. et al. Identification of passive knee joint and shank dynamics in paraplegics using quadriceps stimulation, *IEEE Trans. Rehabil. Eng.* TRE-1: 154–164, 1993.

[70] Franken, H.M., Veltink, P.H. et al., Identification of quadriceps-shank dynamics using randomized interpulse interval stimulation, *IEEE Trans. Rehabil. Eng.* TRE-4: 182–192, 1995.

[71] Hunter, I. and Korenburg, M., The identification of nonlinear biological systems: Wiener and Hammersteiin cascade models, *Biol. Cybern.* 55: 135–144, 1986.

[72] Kearney, R.E., Stein, R.B., and Parameswaran, L., Identification of intrinsic and reflex contribution of human ankle stiffness dynamics, *IEEE Trans. Biomed. Eng.* BME-44: 493–504, 1997.

[73] Stein, R.B., Zehr, E.P. et al., Estimating mechanical parameters of leg segments in individuals with and without physical disabilities, *IEEE Trans. Rehabil. Eng.* TRE-4: 201–212, 1996.

[74] Xu, Y. and Hollerbach, J.M., Identification of human joint mechanical properties from single trial data, *IEEE Trans. Biomed. Eng.* BME-45: 1051–1060, 1998.

[75] Herzog, W. and derKeurs, H.E.D.J., Force–length relation of *in vivo* human rectus femoris muscles, *P. Flügens Arch.* 411: 643–647, 1988.

[76] Veltink, P.H., Chizeck, H.J., Crago, P.E., and El-Bialy, A., Nonlinear joint angle control for artificially stimulated muscle, *IEEE Trans. Biomed. Eng.* BME-39: 368–380, 1992.

[77] Bajzek, T.J. and Jaeger, R.J., Characterization and control of muscle response to electrical stimulation, *Ann. Biomed. Eng.* 15: 485–501, 1987.

[78] Baratta, R. and Solomonow, M., The dynamic response model of nine different skeletal muscles, *IEEE Trans. Biomed. Eng.* BME-36: 243–251, 1989.

[79] Chizeck, H.J., Lan, N., Sreeter-Palmiere, L., and Crago, P.E., Feedback control of electrically stimulated muscle using simultaneous pulse width and stimulus period variation, *IEEE Trans. Biomed. Eng.* BME-38: 1224–1234, 1991.

[80] Scheiner, A., Stein, R.B., Ferencz, D., and Chizeck, H.J., Improved models for the lower leg in paraplegics, *Proceedings of the IEEE Annual Conference on EMBS*, San Diego, pp. 1151–1152, 1993.

[81] Popović, D., Stein, R.B., et al., Optimal control of walking with functional electrical stimulation: a computer simulation study, *IEEE Trans. Rehabil. Eng.* TRE-7(1): 69–79, 1999.

[82] Tomović, R., Control of assistive systems by external reflex arcs. In Popović, D. (Ed.), *Advances in External Control of Human Extremities VIII*. Belgrade, Yugoslav Committee for ETAN, pp. 7–21, 1984.

[83] Popović, D., Tomović, R., Schwirtlich, L., and Tepavac, D., Control aspects on active A/K prosthesis, *Int. J. Man Mach. Stud.* 35: 750–767, 1991.

[84] Tomović, R., Popović, D., and Tepavac, D., Adaptive reflex control of assistive systems. In Popović D. (Ed.), *Advances in External Control of Human Extremities IX*. Belgrade, Yugoslav Committee for ETAN, pp. 207–214, 1987.

[85] Andrews, B.J., Barnett, R.W. et al., Rule-based control of a hybrid FES orthosis for assisting paraplegic locomotion, *Automedica* 11: 175–199, 1989.

[86] Popović, D., Schwirtlich, L., and Radosavljević, S., Powered hybrid assistive system, In Popović, D. (Ed.), *Advances in External Control of Human Extremities X*, Belgrade, Nauka, pp. 177–187, 1990.

[87] Popović, D., Finite state model of locomotion for functional electrical stimulation systems, *Progr. Brain Res.* 97: 397–407, 1993.

[88] Popović, D., Stein, R.B. et al., Sensory nerve recording for closed-loop control to restore motor functions, *IEEE Trans. Biomed. Eng.* BME-40: 1024–1031, 1993.

[89] Tomović, R., Popović, D., and Stein, R.B., *Nonanalytical Methods for Motor Control*. World Scientific Publication, Singapore, 1995.

[90] Aeyels, B., Peeraer, L., Van der Sloten, J., and Van der Perre, G., Development of an above-knee prosthesis equipped with a microprocessor-controlled knee joint: first test results, *J. Biomed. Eng.* 14: 199–202, 1992.

[91] Bar, A., Ishai, P., Meretsky, P., and Koren, Y., Adaptive microcomputer control of an artificial knee in level walking, *J. Biomech. Eng.* 5: 145–150, 1983.

[92] Heller, B., Veltink, P.H. et al., Reconstructing muscle activation during normal walking: a comparison of symbolic and connectionist machine learning techniques, *Biol. Cybern.* 69: 327–335, 1993.

[93] Jonić, S., Janković, T., Gajić, V., and Popović D., Three machine learning techniques for automatic determination of rules to control locomotion, *IEEE Trans. Biomed. Eng.* BME-46: 300–311, 1999.

[94] Kirkwood, C.A., Andrews, B.J., and Mowforth, P., Automatic detection of gait events: a case study using inductive learning techniques, *J. Biomed. Eng.* 11: 511–516, 1989.

[95] Kostov, A., Stein, R.B., Popović, D.B., and Armstrong, W.W., Improved methods for control of FES for locomotion, *Proceedings of IFAC Symposium Biomedical Model*, Galveston, Texas, pp. 422–428, 1994.

[96] Kostov, A., Andrews, B.J., Popović, D. et al., Machine learning in control of functional electrical stimulation (FES) for locomotion, *IEEE Trans. Biomed. Eng.* BME-42: 541–552, 1995.

[97] Nikolić, Z. and Popović, D., Automatic rule determination for finite state model of locomotion, *IEEE Trans. Biomed. Eng.* BME-45: 1081–1085, 1998.

[98] Rumelhart, D.E., Hinton, G.E., and Williams, R.J., Learning interval representation by error propagation, In *Parallel Distributed Processing*, MIT Press, Cambridge, MA, Chap. 8, pp. 318–361, 1986.

[99] Jang, J.S.R., ANFIS: Adaptive-network-based fuzzy inference systems, *IEEE Trans. Syst. Man Cybern.* SMC-23: 665–685, 1993.

[100] Watanabe, S., *Pattern Recognition.* Wiley Interscience, New York, 1985.

[101] Chen, S., Cowan, C.F.N., and Grant, P.M., Orthogonal least squares learning algorithm for radial basis function networks, *IEEE Trans. Neural Network* NN-2: 302–309, 1991.

[102] Nikolić, Z., Automatic rule determination for finite state model of locomotion. Ph.D. thesis, University of Miami, Miami, FL, 1995.

[103] Sethi, I.K. and Sarvarayudu, G.P.R., Hierarchical classifier design using mutual information, *IEEE Trans. Pattern Anal. Mach. Intel.* PAM-4: 441–445, 1992.

[104] Lin, C.T. and Lee, C.S.G., Neural-network-based fuzzy logic control and decision system, *IEEE Trans. Comput.* C-40: 1320–1336, 1991.

[105] Lippmann, R.P., An introduction to computing with neural nets, *IEEE ASSP Mag.* 3: 4–22, 1987.

[106] Zadeh, L.A., Fuzzy sets. *Information Control* 8: 338–352, 1965.

[107] Lee, K.M., Kwak, D.K., and Lee-Kwang, H., Fuzzy inference neural network for fuzzy model tuning, *IEEE Trans. Syst. Man Cybern.* SMC-26: 637–645, 1996.

[108] Sugeno, M., *Industrial Applications of Fuzzy Control.* Elsevier Science, New York, 1985.

[109] Mamdani, E.H. and Assilian, S., An experiment in linguistic synthesis with a fuzzy logic controller, *Int. J. Man-Mach. Stud.* 7: 1–13, 1975.

[110] Hellendoorn, H. and Thomas, C., Defuzzification in fuzzy controllers, *J. Intel. Fuzzy Syst.* 1: 109–123, 1993.

[111] Pitas, I., Milios, E., and Venetsanopoulos, A.N., Minimum entropy approach to rule learning from examples, *IEEE Trans. Syst. Man Cybern.* SMC-22: 621–635, 1992.

[112] Nikolić, Z. and Popović, D., Automatic detection of production rules for locomotion, *J. Autom. Control* 6: 81–94, 1996.

[113] Kawato, M., Computational schemes and neural network models for formation and control of multi-joint arm trajectory, In Miller, W.T., Sutton, R.T., and Werbos, P.J. (Eds.), *Neural Network for Control.* MIT Press, Cambridge, MA, 1990.

[114] Kawato, M., Feedback-error-learning neural network for supervised motor learning, *Adv. Neural Comput.* 365–372, 1990.

[115] Kalanović, V.D. and Tseng, W.H., Back propagation in feedback error learning, *Proc. Neural, Parallel Sci. Comput.* 1: 239–242, 1995.

[116] Miyamoto, H., Kawato, M., Setoyama, T., and Suzuki, R., Feedback-error-learning neural network for trajectory control of a robotic manipulator. *Neural Network* 1: 251–265, 1988.

[117] Nordgren, R.E. and Meckl, P.M., An analytical comparison of a neural network and a model-based adaptive controller, *IEEE Trans. Neural Network* NN-4: 595–601, 1993.

[118] Roa, D.H., Bitner, D., and Gupta, M.M., Feedback-error learning scheme using recurrent neural networks for nonlinear dynamic systems, *Proc. IEEE* 21–38, 1994.

[119] Kawato, M., Furukawa, K., and Suzuki, R., A hierarchical neural-network model for control and learning of voluntary movement, *Biol. Cybern.* 57: 169–185, 1987.

[120] Szabo, P. and Pandya, A.S., Neural network as robot arm manipulator controller, *Proc. IEEE* 321–328, 1996.

Further Reading

Popović, D.B. and Sinkjær, T. *Control of Movement for the Physically Disabled*, 2nd ed., Aalborg University, Aalborg, 2003.

Latash, M., *Control of Human Movements*, Human Kinetics Publication, Urbana, IL, 1993.

Tomović, R., Popović, D., and Stein, R.B., *Nonanalytical Methods for Motor Control*, World Scientific Publication, Singapore, 1995.

Winters, J.M. and Woo, S.L.-Y. (Eds.), *Multiple Muscle Systems: Biomechanics and Movement Organization*, Springer-Verlag, New York, 1990.

Periodicals

IEEE Transactions on Robotics and Automation, IEEE Press.
IEEE Transactions on Biomedical Engineering, IEEE Press.
IEEE Transactions on Neural Engineering and Rehabilitation Engineering, IEEE Press.
IEEE Transactions on Neural Networks, IEEE Press.
IEEE Transactions on System, Man and Cybernetics, IEEE Press.
Medical Engineering and Physics, Elsevier.
Journal of Biomechanics, Elsevier.
Gait and Posture, Elsevier.

16

The Fast Eye Movement Control System

John D. Enderle
University of Connecticut

16.1 Introduction

In this section, a broad overview of the fast eye movement control system is presented. A fast eye movement is usually referred to as a **saccade**, and involves quickly moving the eye from one image to another image. This type of eye movement is very common and is observed most easily while reading — when the end of a line is reached the eyes are moved quickly to the beginning of the next line. A qualitative description of the fast eye movement system is given first in the introduction and then followed by a brief description of saccade characteristics. Next, the earliest quantitative saccade model is presented and then followed by more complex and physiologically accurate models. Finally, the saccade generator, or saccade controller is then discussed on the basis of anatomical pathways and control theory. The purpose of this review is focused on mathematical models of the fast eye movement system and its control strategy, rather than on how visual information is processed. The literature on the fast eye movement system is vast, and thus this review is not exhaustive, but rather a representative sample from the field.

The **oculomotor system** responds to visual, auditory, and vestibular stimuli, which results in one of five types of eye movements: fast eye movements, smooth pursuit eye movements, vestibular ocular movements, vergence eye movements, and optokinetic eye movements. Each of these movements is controlled by a different neuronal system and all of these controllers share the same final common pathway to the muscles of the eye. In addition to the five types of eye movements, these stimuli also cause head and body movements. Thus, the visual system is part of a multiple input–multiple output system.

Regardless of the input, the oculomotor system is responsible for movement of the eyes so that images are focused on the central $\frac{1}{2}°$ region of the retina known as the fovea. Lining the retina are photoreceptive cells that translate images into neural impulses. These impulses are then transmitted along the optic nerve to the central nervous system (CNS) via parallel pathways to the superior colliculus (SC) and the cerebral cortex. The fovea is more densely packed with photoreceptive cells than the retinal periphery; thus a higher resolution image (or higher visual acuity) is generated in the fovea than the retinal periphery. The purpose of the fovea is to allow us to *clearly* see an object and the purpose of the retinal periphery is to allow us to *detect* a new object of interest. Once a new object of interest is detected in the periphery, the saccade system redirects the eyes, as fast as possible, to the new object. This type of saccade is typically called a goal-directed saccade.

During a saccade, the oculomotor system operates in an open-loop mode. After the saccade, the system operates in a closed-loop mode to ensure that the eyes reached the correct destination. The reason that the saccade system operates without feedback during a fast eye movement is simple; information from the retina and muscle proprioceptors is not transmitted quickly enough during the eye movement for use in altering the control signal.

The oculomotor plant and saccade generator are the basic elements of the saccadic system. The oculomotor plant consists of three muscle pairs and the eyeball. These three muscle pairs contract and lengthen to move the eye in horizontal, vertical, and torsional directions. Each pair of muscles acts in an antagonistic fashion due to reciprocal innervation by the saccade generator. For simplicity, the models described here involve only horizontal eye movements and one pair of muscles, the lateral and medial rectus muscle.

16.2 Saccade Characteristics

Saccadic eye movements, among the fastest voluntary muscle movements the human is capable of producing, are characterized by a rapid shift of gaze from one point of fixation to another. The usual experiment for recording saccades is for a subject to be made to sit before a horizontal target display of small light emitting diodes (LEDs), and instructed to maintain their eyes on the lit LED by moving their eyes as fast as possible to avoid errors. A saccade is made by the subject when the active LED is switched off, and another LED is switched on. Saccadic eye movements are conjugate and ballistic, with a typical duration of 20–100 msec and a latency of 150–300 msec. The **latent period** is thought to be the time interval during which the CNS determines whether to make a saccade, and if so, calculates the distance the eyeball is to be moved, transforming retinal error into transient muscle activity.

Generally, saccades are extremely variable, with wide variations in the latent period, time to peak velocity, peak velocity, and saccade duration. Furthermore, variability is well coordinated for saccades of the same size; saccades with lower peak velocity are matched with longer saccade durations, and saccades with higher peak velocity are matched with shorter saccade durations. Thus, saccades driven to the same destination usually have different trajectories.

To appreciate differences in saccade dynamics, it is often helpful to describe them with saccade **main sequence diagrams** [Bahill, 1975]. The main sequence diagrams plot saccade peak velocity–saccade magnitude, saccade duration–saccade magnitude, and saccade latent period–saccade magnitude. Shown in Figure 16.1 are the main sequence characteristics for a subject executing 54 saccades. Notice that the peak velocity–saccade magnitude is basically a linear function until approximately 15° after which it levels off to a constant for larger saccades. Many researchers have fit this relationship to an exponential function. The solid lines in Figure 16.1a include an exponential fit to the data for positive and negative eye movements. The lines in the first graph are fitted to the equation

$$V = \alpha_i (1 - e^{-x/\beta_i}) \tag{16.1}$$

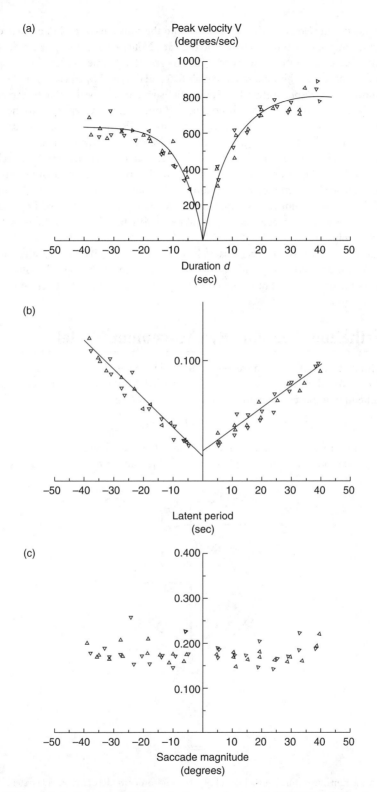

FIGURE 16.1 Main sequence diagrams. (a) peak velocity–saccade magnitude, (b) saccade duration–saccade magnitude, and (c) latent period–saccade magnitude for 54 saccadic eye movement by a single subject. (From Enderle, J.D. 1988. *Aviation, Space, Environ. Med.* 59:309–313. With permission.)

where V is the maximum velocity, x the saccade size, and the constants α_i and β_i evaluated to minimize the summed error squared between the model and the data. Note that α_i is to represent the steady state of the peak velocity–saccade magnitude curve and β_i is to represent the "time constant" for the peak velocity–saccade magnitude curve. For this data set, α_i equals 825 and 637, and β_i equals 9.3 and 6.9, for positive and negative movements, respectively. The exponential shape of the peak velocity–saccade amplitude relationship might suggest that the system is nonlinear, if one assumes a step input to the system. A step input would provide a linear peak velocity–saccade amplitude relationship. In fact, the saccade system is not driven by a step input, but rather a more complex pulse-step waveform. Thus, one cannot conclude that the saccade system is nonlinear solely based on the peak velocity–saccade amplitude relationship.

Shown in Figure 16.1b is data depicting a linear relationship between saccade duration–saccade magnitude. The dependence between saccade duration and saccade magnitude also might suggest that the system is nonlinear, if one assumes a step input. Since the input is not characterized by a step waveform, one cannot conclude that the saccade system is nonlinear solely based on the saccade duration–saccade magnitude relationship.

Shown in Figure 16.1c is the latent period–saccade magnitude data. It is quite clear that the latent period does not show any linear relationship with saccade size, that is, the latent period's value is independent of saccade size. In the development of the oculomotor plant models, the latent period will be implicitly assumed within the model.

16.3   Westheimer Saccadic Eye Movement Model

The first quantitative saccadic eye movement model, illustrated in Figure 16.2, was published by Westheimer [1954]. Based on visual inspection of a recorded 20° saccade, and the assumption of a step controller, Westheimer proposed the following second order model:

$$J\ddot{\theta} + B\dot{\theta} + K\theta = \tau(t) \tag{16.2}$$

To analyze the characteristics of this model and compare it to data, it is convenient to solve Equation 16.2 for peak velocity and duration through Laplace analysis. The transfer function of Equation 16.2, written

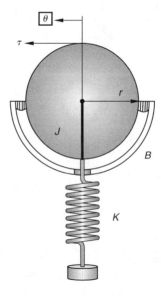

FIGURE 16.2   A diagram illustrating Westheimer's [1954] second-order model of the saccade system. The parameters J, B, and K are rotational elements for moment of inertia, friction, and stiffness, respectively, and represent the eyeball and its associated viscoelasticity. The torque applied to the eyeball by the lateral and medial rectus muscles is given by $\tau(t)$, and θ is the angular eye position. (Reprinted from Enderle, J.D., Blanchard, S., and Bronzino, J. 2005, *Introduction to Biomedical Engineering, Second Edition*, p. 729, Figure 12.12. With permission from Elsevier.)

in standard form, is given by:

$$H(s) = \frac{\theta(s)}{\tau(s)} = \frac{\omega_n^2/K}{s^2 + 2\zeta\omega_n s + \omega_n^2} \tag{16.3}$$

where $\omega_n = \sqrt{(K/J)}$ and $\zeta = B/(2\sqrt{KJ})$. Based on the saccade trajectory for a 20° saccade, Westheimer estimated $\omega_n = 120$ rad/sec, and $\zeta = 0.7$. With the input $\tau(s) = \gamma/s$, $\theta(t)$ is determined as:

$$\theta(t) = \frac{\gamma}{K}\left[1 + \frac{e^{-\zeta\omega_n t}}{\sqrt{1-\zeta^2}}\cos(\omega_d t + \phi)\right] \tag{16.4}$$

where

$$\omega_d = \omega_n\sqrt{1-\zeta^2} \quad \text{and} \quad \phi = \pi + \tan^{-1}\frac{-\zeta}{\sqrt{1-\zeta^2}}$$

Duration, T_p, is found by first calculating

$$\frac{\partial\theta}{\partial t} = \frac{\gamma e^{-\zeta\omega_n t}}{K\sqrt{1-\zeta^2}}[-\zeta\omega_n\cos(\omega_d t + \phi) - \omega_d\sin(\omega_d t + \phi)] \tag{16.5}$$

then determining T_p from $(\partial\theta/\partial t)|_{t=T_p} = 0$, yielding

$$T_p = \frac{\pi}{\omega_n\sqrt{1-\zeta^2}} \tag{16.6}$$

With Westheimer's parameter values, $T_p = 37$ msec for saccades of all sizes, which is independent of saccade magnitude and not in agreement with the experimental data that has a duration which increases as a function of saccade magnitude.

Predicted saccade peak velocity, $\dot\theta(t_{mv})$, is found by first calculating

$$\frac{\partial^2\theta}{\partial t^2} = \frac{-\gamma e^{-\zeta\omega_n t}}{K\sqrt{1-\zeta^2}}(-\zeta\omega_n(\zeta\omega_n\cos(\omega_d t + \phi) + \omega_d\sin(\omega_d t + \phi))$$

$$+ (-\zeta\omega_n\omega_d\sin(\omega_d t + \phi) + \omega_d^2\cos(\omega_d t + \phi))) \tag{16.7}$$

and then determining time at peak velocity, t_{mv}, from $(\partial^2\theta/\partial t^2)|_{t=t_{mv}} = 0$, yielding

$$t_{mv} = \frac{1}{\omega_d}\tan^{-1}\left(\frac{\sqrt{1-\zeta^2}}{\zeta}\right) \tag{16.8}$$

Substituting t_{mv} into Equation 16.7 gives the peak velocity $\dot\theta(t_{mv})$. Using Westheimer's parameter values and with the saccade magnitude given by $\Delta\theta = \gamma/K$ based on the steady state value from Equation 16.3, we have from Equation 16.5

$$\dot\theta(t_{mv}) = 55.02\Delta\theta \tag{16.9}$$

that is, peak velocity is directly proportional to saccade magnitude. As illustrated in the main sequence diagram shown in Figure 16.1a, experimental peak velocity data has an exponential form, and not a linear function as predicted by the Westheimer model.

Westheimer noted the differences between saccade duration–saccade magnitude and peak velocity–saccade magnitude in the model and the experimental data and inferred that the saccade system was not linear because the peak velocity–saccade magnitude plot was nonlinear, and the input was not an abrupt step function. Overall, this model provided a satisfactory fit to the eye position data for a saccade of 20°, but not for saccades of other magnitudes. Interestingly, Westheimer's second-order model proves to be an adequate model for saccades of all sizes, if one assumes a different input function as described in the next section. Due to its simplicity, the Westheimer model of the oculomotor plant is still popular today.

16.4   Robinson's Model of the Saccade Controller

In 1964, Robinson performed an experiment to measure the input to the eyeballs during a saccade. To record the input, one eye was held fixed using a suction contact lens, while the other eye performed a saccade from target to target. Since the same innervation signal is sent to both eyes during a saccade, Robinson inferred that the input, recorded through the transducer attached to the fixed eyeball, was the same input driving the other eyeball. He estimated that the neural commands controlling the eyeballs during a saccade are a pulse plus a step, or simply, a pulse-step input.

It is important to distinguish between the tension or force generated by a muscle, called muscle tension, and the force generator within the muscle, called the **active state tension generator**. The active state tension generator creates a force within the muscle that is transformed through the internal elements of the muscle into the muscle tension. Muscle tension is external and measurable, and the active state tension is internal and unmeasurable. Moreover, Robinson [1981] reports that the active state tensions are not identical to the neural controllers, but described by low-pass filtered pulse-step waveforms. The neural control and the active state tension signals are illustrated in Figure 16.3. The agonist pulse input is required to get the eye to the target as soon as possible, and the step is required to keep the eye at that location.

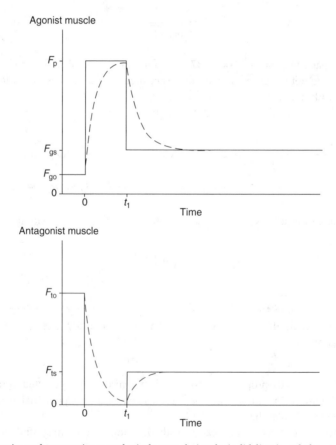

FIGURE 16.3   Agonist and antagonist neurological control signals (solid lines) and the agonist and antagonist active state tensions (dashed lines). Note that the time constant for activation is different than the time constant for deactivation. (From Enderle, J.D. and Wolfe, J.W. 1987. *IEEE Trans. Biomed. Eng.* 34:43–55. With permission.)

Robinson [1964] also described a model for fast eye movements (constructed from empirical consid-erations), which simulated saccades over a range of 5 to 40° by changing the amplitude of the pulse-step input. Simulation results were adequate for the position–time relationship, but the velocity–time relation-ship was inconsistent with physiological evidence. To correct this deficiency of the model, physiological studies of the oculomotor plant were carried out during the 1960s through the 1970s that allowed the development of a more **homeomorphic** oculomotor plant. Essential to this work was the construction of oculomotor muscle models.

16.5   A Linear Homeomorphic Saccadic Eye Movement Model

In 1980, Bahill and coworkers presented a linear fourth order model of the oculomotor plant, based on physiological evidence, that provides an excellent match between model predictions and eye movement data. This model eliminates the differences seen between velocity predictions of the model and the data, and also the acceleration predictions of the model and the data. For ease in presentation, the modification of this model by Enderle and coworkers [1984] will be used.

Figure 16.4 illustrates the mechanical components of the oculomotor plant for horizontal eye move-ments, the lateral and medial rectus muscle, and the eyeball. The agonist muscle is modeled as a parallel combination of an active state tension generator F_{AG}, viscosity element B_{AG}, and elastic element K_{LT}, con-nected to a series elastic element K_{SE}. The antagonist muscle is similarly modeled as a parallel combination of an active state tension generator F_{ANT}, viscosity element B_{ANT}, and elastic element K_{LT}, connected to a series elastic element K_{SE}. The eyeball is modeled as a sphere with moment of inertia J_P, connected to viscosity element B_P and elastic element K_P. The passive elasticity of each muscle is included in spring K_P for ease in analysis. Each of the elements defined in the oculomotor plant is ideal and linear.

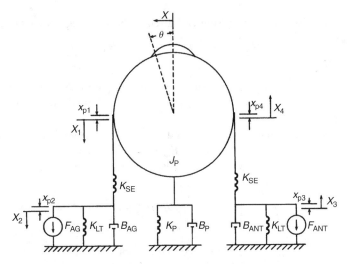

FIGURE 16.4   This diagram illustrates the mechanical components of the oculomotor plant. The muscles are shown to be extended from equilibrium, a position of rest, at the primary position (looking straight ahead), consistent with physiological evidence. The average length of the rectus muscle at the primary position is approximately 40 mm, and at the equilibrium position is approximately 37 mm. θ is the angle the eyeball is deviated from the primary position, and variable x is the length of arc traversed. When the eye is at the primary position, both θ and x are equal to zero. Variables x_1 through x_4 are the displacements from equilibrium for the stiffness elements in each muscle. Values x_{p1} through x_{p4} are the displacements from equilibrium for each of the variables x_1 through x_4 at the primary position. The total extension of the muscle from equilibrium at the primary position is x_{p1} plus x_{p2} or x_{p3} plus x_{p4}, which equals approximately 3 mm. It is assumed that the lateral and medial rectus muscles are identical, such that x_{p1} equals x_{p4} and x_{p3} equals x_{p2}. The radius of the eyeball is r. (From Enderle, J.D., Wolfe, J.W., and Yates, J.T. 1984. *IEEE Trans. Biomed. Eng.* 31:717–720. With permission.)

Physiological support for this model is based on the muscle model by Wilkie [1968], and estimates for the **extraocular muscle** elasticities and the passive tissues of the eyeball are based on experiments by Robinson et al. [1969, 1981] and Collins [1975] and studies of extraocular muscle viscosity by Bahill et al. [1980].

By summing the forces at junctions 2 and 3 (the equilibrium positions for x_2 and x_3) and the torques acting on the eyeball, using Laplace variable analysis about the operating point, the linear homeomorphic model, as shown in Figure 16.4, is derived as

$$\delta(K_{SE}(K_{ST}(F_{AG} - F_{ANT}) + B_{ANT}\dot{F}_{AG} - B_{AG}\dot{F}_{ANT})) = \dddot{\theta} + P_3\ddot{\theta} + P_2\ddot{\theta}P_1\dot{\theta} + P_0\theta \tag{16.10}$$

where

$$K_{ST} = K_{SE} + K_{LT}, \quad J = \frac{57.296 J_P}{r^2}, \quad B = \frac{57.296 B_P}{r^2}, \quad K = \frac{57.296 K_P}{r^2}, \quad \delta = \frac{57.296}{rJB_{ANT}B_{AG}}$$

$$C_3 = \frac{JK_{ST}(B_{AG} + B_{ANT}) + BB_{ANT}B_{AG}}{JB_{ANT}B_{AG}}$$

$$C_2 = \frac{JK_{ST}^2 + BK_{ST}(B_{AG} + B_{ANT}) + B_{ANT}B_{AG}(K + 2K_{SE})}{JB_{ANT}B_{AG}}$$

$$C_1 = \frac{BK_{ST}^2 + (B_{AG} + B_{ANT})(KK_{ST} + 2K_{SE}K_{ST} - K_{SE}^2)}{JB_{ANT}B_{AG}}$$

$$C_0 = \frac{KK_{ST}^2 + 2K_{SE}K_{ST}K_{LT}}{JB_{ANT}B_{AG}}$$

The agonist and antagonist active state tensions, are given by the following low-pass filtered waveforms:

$$\dot{F}_{AG} = \frac{N_{AG} - F_{AG}}{\tau_{AG}} \quad \text{and} \quad \dot{F}_{ANT} = \frac{N_{ANT} - F_{ANT}}{\tau_{ANT}} \tag{16.11}$$

where N_{AG} and N_{ANT} are the pulse-step waveforms shown in Figure 16.3, and $\tau_{ag} = \tau_{ac}(u(t) - u(t - t_1)) + \tau_{de}u(t - t_1)$ and $\tau_{ant} = \tau_{de}(u(t) - u(t - t_1)) + \tau_{ac}u(t - t_1)$ are the time-varying time constants [Bahill et al., 1980].

Based on an analysis of experimental evidence, Enderle and Wolfe [1988] determined parameter estimates for the oculomotor plant as: $K_{SE} = 125\,\text{Nm}^{-1}$, $K_{LT} = 32\,\text{Nm}^{-1}$, $K = 66.4\,\text{Nm}^{-1}$, $B = 3.1\,\text{Nsec m}^{-1}$, $J = 2.2 \times 10^{-3}\,\text{Nsec}^2\,\text{m}^{-1}$, $B_{AG} = 3.4\,\text{Nsec m}^{-1}$, $B_{ANT} = 1.2\,\text{Nsec m}^{-1}$ and $\delta = 72.536 \times 10^6$, and the steady state active state tensions as:

$$F_{AG} = \begin{cases} 0.14 + 0.01850\theta\ N & \text{for } \theta < 14.23° \\ 0.02830\theta\ N & \text{for } \theta \geq 14.23° \end{cases} \tag{16.12}$$

$$F_{ANT} = \begin{cases} 0.14 - 0.009800\theta\ N & \text{for } \theta < 14.23° \\ 0\ N & \text{for } \theta \geq 14.23° \end{cases} \tag{16.13}$$

Since saccades are highly variable, estimates of the dynamic active state tensions are carried out on a saccade-by-saccade basis. One method to estimate the active state tensions is using the system identification technique, a conjugate gradient search program carried out in the frequency domain [Enderle and Wolfe, 1988]. Figure 16.5 to Figure 16.7 show the system identification technique results for an eye movement response to a 15° target movement. A close fit between the data and model prediction is seen in Figure 16.5. Figure 16.6 and Figure 16.7 further illustrate the accuracy of the final parameter estimates for velocity and acceleration. Estimates for agonist pulse magnitude are highly variable for saccade to saccade, even for the same size (see Figure 9 of Enderle and Wolfe [1988]). Agonist pulse duration is closely coupled with pulse amplitude; as the pulse amplitude increases, the pulse duration decreases for saccades of the same

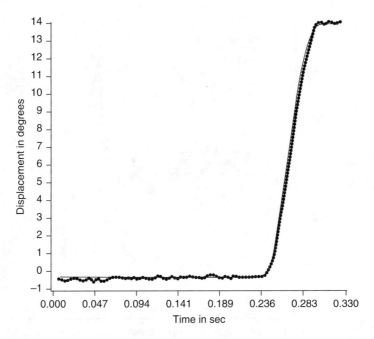

FIGURE 16.5 Saccadic eye movement in response to a 15° target movement. Solid line is the prediction of the saccadic eye movement model with the final parameter estimates computed using the system identification techniques. Dots are the data. (From Enderle, J.D. and Wolfe, J.W. 1987. *IEEE Trans. Biomed. Eng.* 34:43–55. With permission.)

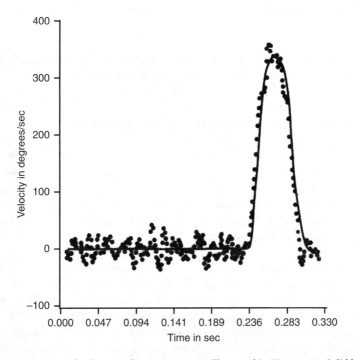

FIGURE 16.6 Velocity estimates for the saccadic eye movement illustrated in Figure 16.5. Solid line is the saccadic eye movement model velocity prediction with the final parameter estimates computed using the system identification techniques. The dots are the two-point central difference estimates of velocity computed with a step size of 3 and a sampling interval of 1 msec. (From Enderle, J.D. and Wolfe, J.W. 1987. *IEEE Trans. Biomed. Eng.* 34:43–55. With permission.)

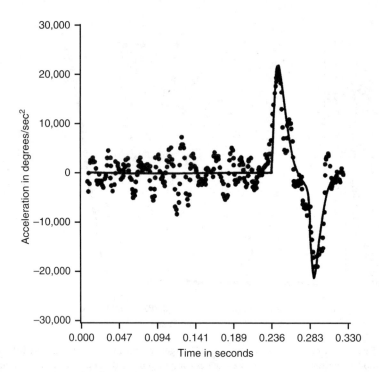

FIGURE 16.7 Acceleration estimates for the saccadic eye movement illustrated in Figure 16.6. Solid line is the saccadic eye movement model acceleration prediction with the final parameter estimates computed using the system identification techniques. The dots are the two-point central difference estimates of velocity computed with a step size of 4 and a sampling interval of 1 msec. (From Enderle, J.D. and Wolfe, J.W. 1987. *IEEE Trans. Biomed. Eng.* 34:43–55. With permission.)

magnitude. Reasonable values for the pulse amplitude for this model range from about 0.6 to 1.4 N. The larger the magnitude of the pulse the larger the peak velocity of the eye movement.

16.6 Another Linear Homeomorphic Saccadic Eye Movement Model

The previous linear model of the oculomotor plant is derived from a nonlinear oculomotor plant model by Hsu et al. [1976], and based on a linearization of the force–velocity curve [Bahill et al., 1980]. Muscle viscosity traditionally has been modeled with a hyperbolic force–velocity relationship. Using the linear model of muscle reported by Enderle and coworkers [1991], it is possible to avoid the linearization, and derive an updated linear homeomorphic saccadic eye movement model.

The linear muscle model has the static and dynamic properties of rectus eye muscle, a model without any nonlinear elements. The model has a nonlinear force–velocity relationship that matches muscle data using linear viscous elements; and the length tension characteristics are also in good agreement with muscle data within the operating range of the muscle. Some additional advantages of the linear muscle model are that a passive elasticity is not necessary if the equilibrium point $x_e = -19.3°$, rather than 15°, and muscle viscosity is constant that does not depend on the innervation stimulus level.

Figure 16.8 illustrates the mechanical components of the updated oculomotor plant for horizontal eye movements, the lateral and medial rectus muscle, and the eyeball. The agonist muscle is modeled as a parallel combination of viscosity B_2 and series elasticity K_{SE}, connected to the parallel combination of active state tension generator F_{AG}, viscosity element B_1, and length tension elastic element K_{LT}. Since viscosity does not change with innervation level, agonist viscosity is set equal to antagonist viscosity. The

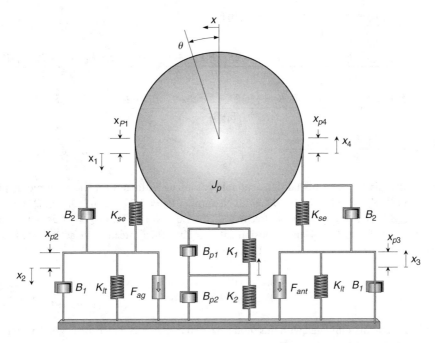

FIGURE 16.8 This diagram illustrates the mechanical components of the updated oculomotor plant. The muscles are shown to be extended from equilibrium, a position of rest, at the primary position (looking straight ahead), consistent with physiological evidence. The average length of the rectus muscle at the primary position is approximately 40 mm, and at the equilibrium position is approximately 37 mm. θ is the angle the eyeball is deviated from the primary position, and variable x is the length of arc traversed. When the eye is at the primary position, both θ and x are equal to zero. Variables x_1 through x_4 are the displacements from equilibrium for the stiffness elements in each muscle, and θ_5 is the rotational displacement for passive orbital tissues. Values x_{p1} through x_{p4} are the displacements from equilibrium for each of the variables x_1 through x_4 at the primary position. The total extension of the muscle from equilibrium at the primary position is x_{p1} plus x_{p2} or x_{p3} plus x_{p4}, which equals approximately 3 mm. It is assumed that the lateral and medial rectus muscles are identical, such that x_{p1} equals x_{p4} and x_{p3} equals x_{p2}. The radius of the eyeball is r. (Reprinted from Enderle, J.D., Blanchard, S., and Bronzino, J. 2005, *Introduction to Biomedical Engineering, Second Edition*, p. 764, Figure 12.33. With permission from Elsevier.)

antagonist muscle is similarly modeled with a suitable change in active state tension to F_{ANT}. The eyeball is modeled as a sphere with moment of inertia J_P, connected to a pair of viscoelastic elements connected in series; the update of the eyeball model is based on observations by Robinson [1981]. Each of the elements defined in the oculomotor plant is ideal and linear.

The differential equation describing oculomotor plant model shown in Figure 16.8 is derived by summing the forces acting at junctions 2 and 3, and the torques acting on the eyeball and junction 5, and using Laplace variable analysis about the operating point, is given by

$$\delta(K_{\text{SE}}K_{12}(F_{\text{AG}} - F_{\text{ANT}}) + (K_{\text{SE}}B_{34} + B_2 K_{12})(\dot{F}_{\text{AG}} - \dot{F}_{\text{ANT}}) + B_2 B_{34}(\ddot{F}_{\text{AG}} - \ddot{F}_{\text{ANT}}))$$
$$= \dddot{\theta} + P_3 \dddot{\theta} + P_2 \ddot{\theta} + P_1 \dot{\theta} + P_0 \theta \tag{16.14}$$

where

$$J = \frac{57.296 J_{\text{p}}}{r^2}, \quad B_3 = \frac{57.296 B_{\text{p1}}}{r^2}, \quad B_4 = \frac{57.296 B_{\text{p2}}}{r^2}, \quad K_1 = \frac{57.296 K_{\text{p1}}}{r^2}, \quad K_2 = \frac{57.296 K_{\text{p2}}}{r^2},$$

$$B_{12} = B_1 + B_2, \quad B_{34} = B_3 + B_4, \quad K_{12} = K_1 + K_2, \quad \delta = \frac{57.296}{rJ B_{12} B_{34}}$$

$$C_3 = \frac{B_{12}(JK_2 + B_3B_4) + JB_4K_{ST} + 2B_1B_2B_{34}}{JB_{12}B_4}$$

$$C_2 = \frac{JK_{ST}K_2 + B_3B_4K_{ST} + B_{12}B_3K_2 + 2K_{SE}B_{34}B_1 + K_1B_{12}B_4 + 2B_2K_{LT}B_{34} + 2B_1K_{12}B_2}{JB_{12}B_4}$$

$$C_1 = \frac{K_{ST}(B_3K_2 + K_1B_4) + K_1K_2B_{12} + 2K_{LT}K_{SE}B_{34} + 2B_1K_{12}K_{SE} + 2B_2K_{LT}K_{12}}{JB_{12}B_4}$$

$$C_0 = \frac{2K_{LT}K_{SE}K_{12} + K_1K_{ST}K_2}{JB_{12}B_4}$$

Based on an analysis of experimental data, suitable parameter estimates for the oculomotor plant are: $K_{SE} = 125$ Nm^{-1}, $K_{LT} = 60.7$ Nm^{-1}, $B_1 = 2.0$ Nsec m^{-1}, $B_2 = 0.5$ Nsec m^{-1}, $J = 2.2 \times 10^{-3}$ Nsec^2 m^{-1}, $B_3 = 0.538$ Nsec m^{-1}, $B_4 = 41.54$ Nsec m^{-1}, $K_1 = 26.9$ Nm^{-1}, and $K_2 = 41.54$ Nm^{-1}. Based on the updated model of muscle and length tension data [Collins, 1975], steady state active state tensions are determined (as described in Enderle et al. [1991]) as:

$$F = \begin{cases} 0.4 + 0.0175\theta \ N & \text{for } \theta \geq 0° \\ 0.4 + 0.0125\theta \ N & \text{for } \theta < 0° \end{cases} \tag{16.15}$$

Saccadic eye movements simulated with this model have characteristics which are in good agreement with the data, including position, velocity and acceleration, and the main sequence diagrams.

16.7   Saccade Pathways

Clinical evidence, lesion, and stimulation studies all point toward the participation of vitally important neural sites in the control of saccades, including the cerebellum, superior colliculus (SC), thalamus, cortex, and other nuclei in the brain stem, and that saccades are driven by two parallel neural networks [Enderle, 1994, 2002]. From each eye, the axons of retinal ganglion cells exit and join other neurons to form the optic nerve. The optic nerves from each eye then join at the optic chiasm, where fibers from the nasal half of each retina cross to the opposite side. Axons in the optic tract synapse in the lateral geniculate nucleus (a thalamic relay), and continue to the visual cortex. This portion of the saccade neural network is concerned with the recognition of visual stimuli. Axons in the optic tract also synapse in the SC. This second portion of the saccade neural network is concerned with the location of visual targets and is primarily responsible for goal-directed saccades.

Saccadic neural activities of the SC and cerebellum, in particular, have been identified as the saccade initiator and terminator, respectively, for a goal-directed saccade. The impact of the frontal eye field and the thalamus, while very important, has less important roles in the generation of goal-directed saccades to visual stimuli. The frontal eye fields are primarily concerned with voluntary saccades, and the thalamus appears to be involved with corrective saccades. Shown in Figure 16.9 is a diagram illustrating important sites for the generation of a conjugate goal-directed horizontal saccade in both eyes [Enderle, 1994, 2002]. Each of the sites and connections detailed in Figure 16.9 are fully supported by physiological evidence. Some of these neural sites are briefly described herein.

The SC contains two major functional divisions: a superficial division and an intermediate or deep. Inputs to the superficial division are almost exclusively visual and originate from the retina and the visual cortex. The deep layers provide a site of convergence for sensory signals from several modalities and a source of efferent commands for initiating saccades. The SC is the initiator of the saccade and thought to translate visual information into motor commands.

The deep layers of the SC initiate a saccade based on the distance between the current position of the eye and the desired target. The neural activity in the SC is organized into movement fields that are associated with the direction and saccade amplitude, and does not involve the initial position of

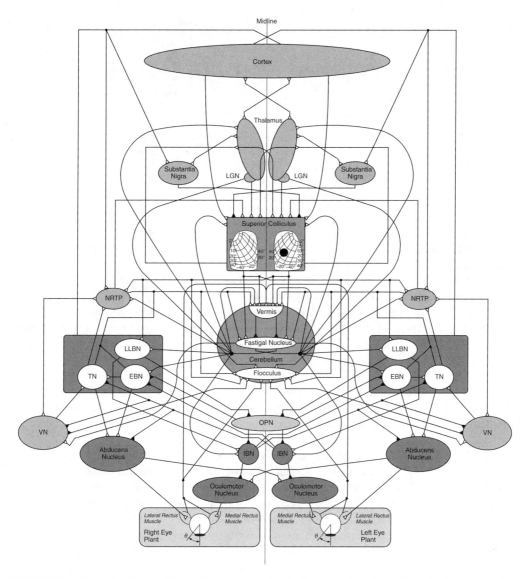

FIGURE 16.9 Shown is a diagram illustrating important sites for the generation of a conjugate horizontal saccade in both eyes. It consists of the familiar premotor excitatory burst neurons (EBN), inhibitory burst neurons (IBN), long-lead burst neurons (LLBN), omnipause neurons (OPN), tonic neurons (TN), and the vestibular nucleus, abducens nucleus, oculomotor nucleus, cerebellum, substantia nigra, nucleus reticularis tegmenti pontis (NRTP), the thalamus, the deep layers of the superior colliculus (SC), and the oculomotor plant for each eye. Excitatory inputs are shown with Δ, inhibitory inputs are shown with a ▲. Consistent with current knowledge, the left and right structures of the neural circuit model are maintained. This circuit diagram was constructed after a careful review of the current literature. Each of the sites and connections is supported by firm physiological evidence. Since interest is in goal-directed visual saccades, the cortex has not been partitioned into the frontal eye field and posterior eye field (striate, prestriate, and inferior parietal cortices).

the eyeball whatsoever. The movement field is shown in Figure 16.10 for a 20° saccade. Neurons active during a particular saccade are shown as the dark circle, representing a desired 20° eye movement. Active neurons in the deep layers of the SC generate a high frequency burst of activity beginning 18–20 msec before a saccade and end sometime toward the end of the saccade; the exact timing for the end of the burst firing is quite random and can occur slightly before or slightly after the saccade ends. Each active bursting

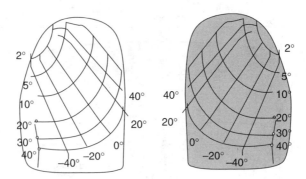

FIGURE 16.10   Movement fields of the superior colliculus.

neuron discharges maximally, regardless of the initial position of the eye. Neurons discharging for small saccades have smaller movement fields, and those for larger saccades have larger movement fields. All of the movement fields are connected to the same set of long-lead burst neurons (LLBN).

The cerebellum is responsible for the coordination of movement, and is composed of a cortex of gray matter, internal white matter, and three pairs of deep nuclei: fastigial nucleus (FN), the interposed and globose nucleus, and dentate nucleus. The deep cerebellar nuclei and the vestibular nuclei transmit the entire output of the cerebellum. Output of the cerebellar cortex is carried through Purkinje cells. Purkinje cells send their axons to the deep cerebellar nuclei and have an inhibitory effect on these nuclei. The cerebellum is involved with both eye and head movements, and both tonic and phasic activities are reported in the cerebellum. The cerebellum is not directly responsible for the initiation or execution of a saccade, but contributes to saccade precision. Sites within the cerebellum important for the control of eye movements include the oculomotor vermis, FN and the flocculus. Consistent with the operation of the cerebellum for other movement activities, the cerebellum is postulated here to act as the coordinator for a saccade, and act as a precise gating mechanism.

The cerebellum is included in the saccade generator as a time-optimal gating element using three active sites during a saccade: the vermis, FN and flocculus. The vermis is concerned with the absolute starting position of a saccade in the movement field and corrects control signals for initial eye position. Using proprioceptors in the oculomotor muscles and an internal eye position reference, the vermis is aware of the current position of the eye. The vermis is also aware of the signals (dynamic motor error) used to generate the saccade via the connection with the nucleus reticularis tegmenti pontis (NRTP) and the SC.

With regard to the oculomotor system, the cerebellum has inputs from SC, lateral geniculate nucleus (LGN), oculomotor muscle proprioceptors, and striate cortex via NRTP. The cerebellum sends inputs to the NRTP, LLBN, excitatory burst neurons (EBN), VN, thalamus, and SC. The oculomotor vermis and FN are important in the control of saccade amplitude, and the flocculus, perihypoglossal nuclei of the rostral medulla, and possibly the pontine and mesencephalic reticular formation are thought to form the integrator within the cerebellum. One important function of the flocculus may be to increase the time constant of the neural integrator for saccades starting at locations different from primary position.

The FN receives input from the SC, as well as other sites. The output of the FN is excitatory and projects ipsilaterally and contralaterally as shown in Figure 16.9. During fixation, the FN nucleus fires tonically at low rates. Twenty msec prior to a saccade, the contralateral FN bursts, and the ipsilateral FN pauses and then is discharged with a burst. The pause in ipsilateral firing is due to Purkinje cell input to the FN. The sequential organization of Purkinje cells along beams of parallel fibers suggests that the cerebellar cortex might function as a delay, producing a set of timed pulses that could be used to program the duration of the saccade. If one considers nonprimary position saccades, different temporal and spatial schemes, via cerebellar control, are necessary to produce the same size saccade. It is postulated here that the cerebellum acts as a gating device, which precisely terminates a saccade based on the initial position of the eye in the orbit.

The PPRF (paramedian pontine reticular formation) has neurons that burst at frequencies up to 1000 Hz during saccades and are silent during periods of fixation, and neurons that fire tonically during periods of fixation. Neurons that fire at steady rates during fixation are called tonic neurons (TN) and are responsible for holding the eye steady. The TN firing rate depends on the position of the eye (presumably through a local integrator type network). The TN are thought to provide the step component to the motoneuron. There are two types of burst neurons in the PPRF called the long-lead burst neuron (LLBN) and a medium-lead burst neuron (MLBN); during periods of fixation, these neurons are silent. The LLBN burst at least 12 msec before a saccade and the MLBN burst <12 msec (typically 6 to 8 msec) before the saccade. The MLBN are connected monosynaptically with the Abducens Nucleus.

There are two types of neurons within the MLBN, the EBN and the inhibitory burst neurons (IBN). The EBN and IBN label describe the synaptic activity upon the motoneurons; the EBN excite and are responsible for the burst firing, and the IBN inhibit and are responsible for the pause. A mirror image of these neurons exists on both sides of the midline. The IBN inhibit the EBN on the contralateral side.

Also within the brain stem is another type of saccade neuron called the omnipause neuron (OPN). The OPN fires tonically at approximately 200 Hz during periods of fixation, and is silent during saccades. The OPN stops firing approximately 10 to 12 msec before a saccade and resumes tonic firing approximately 10 msec before the end of the saccade. The OPN are known to inhibit the MLBN, and are inhibited by the LLBN. The OPN activity is responsible for the precise timing between groups of neurons that causes a saccade.

To execute a saccade, a sequence of complex activities takes place within the brain, beginning from the detection of an error on the retina, to the actual movement of the eyes. A saccade is directly caused by a burst discharge (pulse) from motoneurons stimulating the agonist muscle and a pause in firing from motoneurons stimulating the antagonist muscle. During periods of fixation, the motoneurons fire at a rate necessary to keep the eye stable (step). The pulse discharge in the motoneurons is caused by the EBN and the step discharge is caused by the TN in the PPRF.

Consider the saccade network in Figure 16.9 that is programmed to move the eyes 20° [Enderle, 2002]. The contralateral SC begins firing within an appropriate locus of neurons for a 20° saccade due to a LGN retinal error. The contralateral SC then stimulates the ipsilateral LLBN and contralateral FN. The contralateral FN also stimulates the ipsilateral LLBN, and the LLBN then inhibits the tonic firing of the OPN. When the OPN cease firing, the MLBN is released from inhibition and begins firing. The ipsilateral IBN is stimulated by the ipsilateral LLBN and the contralateral FN of the cerebellum. When released from inhibition, it has been proposed that the ipsilateral EBN fire spontaneously [Enderle, 2002]. The EBN are also stimulated by the contralateral FN of the cerebellum; however, FN stimulation is not required for a saccade to be generated. The burst firing in the ipsilateral IBN inhibits the contralateral EBN, TN, and Abducens Nucleus, and the ipsilateral Oculomotor Nucleus. The burst firing in the ipsilateral EBN cause the burst in the ipsilateral Abducens Nucleus, which stimulates the ipsilateral lateral rectus muscle and the contralateral Oculomotor Nucleus. With the stimulation of the ipsilateral lateral rectus muscle by the ipsilateral Abducens Nucleus and the inhibition of the ipsilateral medial rectus muscle via the Oculomotor Nucleus, a saccade occurs in the right eye.

Simultaneously, the contralateral medial rectus muscle is stimulated by the contralateral Oculomotor Nucleus, and with the inhibition of the contralateral lateral rectus muscle via the Abducens Nucleus, a saccade occurs in the left eye. Thus the eyes move conjugately under the control of a single drive center.

The end of the saccade is normally terminated by the cerebellum. In most saccades, the SC continues to fire even though the saccade has ended. At the termination time, the cerebellar vermis, operating through the Purkinje cells, inhibits the contralateral FN and stimulates the ipsilateral FN. Some of the stimulation of the ipsilateral LLBN and IBN is lost because of the inhibition of the contralateral FN.

The ipsilateral FN stimulates the contralateral LLBN, EBN, and IBN. The contralateral EBN then stimulates the contralateral Abducens Nucleus. Further simulation of the contralateral IBN occurs from the contralateral LLBN. The contralateral IBN then inhibits the ipsilateral EBN, TN, and Abducens Nucleus, and contralateral Oculomotor Nucleus. With this inhibition, the stimulus to the agonist muscles ceases.

The ipsilateral FN stimulation of the contralateral EBN allows for modest bursting in the contralateral EBN, which stimulates the contralateral Abducens Nucleus and Ipsilateral Oculomotor Nucleus. With the stimulation from the contralateral EBN through the contralateral Abducens Nucleus and Ipsilateral Oculomotor Nucleus, the antagonist muscles fire, causing a dynamic break. Once the SC cease firing, the stimulus to the LLBN ends allowing the resumption of OPN firing that inhibits the MLBN.

16.8   Saccade Control Mechanism

Although the purpose for a saccadic eye movement is clear, that is, to quickly redirect the eyeball to the destination, the neural control mechanism is not. Until quite recently, saccade generator models involved a ballistic or preprogrammed control to the desired eye position based on retinal error alone. Today, an increasing number of investigators are putting forth the idea that visual goal-directed saccades are controlled by a local feedback loop that continuously drives the eye to the desired eye position. This hypothesis first gained acceptance in 1975 when Robinson suggested that saccades originate from neural commands that specify the desired position of the eye rather than the preprogrammed distance the eye must be moved. The value of the actual eye position is subtracted from the desired position to create an error signal that completes the local feedback loop that drives a high-gain burst element to generate the neural pulse. This neural pulse continuously drives the eye until the error signal is zero.

Subsequently, a number of other investigators have modified the local feedback mechanism proposed by Robinson [1975] to better describe the neural connections and firing patterns of brainstem neurons in the control of horizontal saccadic eye. In addition to the Robinson model, two other models describe a saccade generator [Scudder, 1988; Scudder et al., 2002; Enderle, 1994, 2002]. All of the models involve three types of premotor neurons: burst, tonic, and pause cells, as previously described, and involve a pulse-step change in firing rate at the motoneuron during a saccadic eye movement.

While the general pattern of motoneuron activity is qualitatively accepted during a saccadic eye movement, there is little agreement on a quantitative discharge description. The saccade generator models by Robinson and Scudder are structured to provide a control signal that is proportionally weighted (or dependent) to the desired saccade size, as opposed to the saccade generator model structured to provide a control signal that is independent of saccade amplitude. Using time-optimal control theory and the system identification technique, Enderle and Wolfe [1988] investigated the control of saccades and reported that the system operates under a first-order time-optimal control. The concepts underlying this hypothesis are that each muscle's active state tension is described by a low-pass filtered pulse-step waveform in which the magnitude of the agonist pulse is a maximum regardless of the amplitude of the saccade, and that only the duration of the agonist pulse affects the size of the saccade. The antagonist muscle is completely inhibited during the period of maximum agonist stimulation. The saccade generator illustrated in Figure 16.9 operates under these principles, and provides simulations that match the data very well.

Saccadic eye movements were simulated using TUTSIM, a continuous time simulation program for the saccade generator model presented in Figure 16.9, and compared with experimental data. Neural sites (nucleus) are described via a *functional* block diagram description of the horizontal saccade generator model as shown in Figure 16.11 and Figure 16.12. Table 16.1 summarizes additional firing characteristics for the neural sites. The output of each block represents the firing pattern at each neural site observed during the saccade; time zero indicates the start of the saccade and T represent the end of the saccade. Naturally, the firing pattern observed for each block represents the firing pattern for a single neuron, as recorded in the literature, but the block represents the cumulative effect of all of the neurons within that site. Consistent with a time optimal control theory, neural activity is represented within each of the blocks as pulses and steps to reflect their operation as timing gates. The SC fires maximally, as long as the dynamic motor error is greater than zero, which is in agreement with the first-order time optimal controller and physiological evidence. Notice that the LLBN's are driven by the SC as long as there is a feedback error maintained by the cerebellar vermis. In all likelihood, the maximal firing rate by the SC is stochastic, depending on a variety of physiological factors such as the interest in tracking the target, anxiety, frustration, stress, and other factors. The actual firing patterns in the SC, the burst neurons in the PPRF (LLBN, EBN, and IBN) and abducens nucleus are simulated with filtered pulse signals, consistent

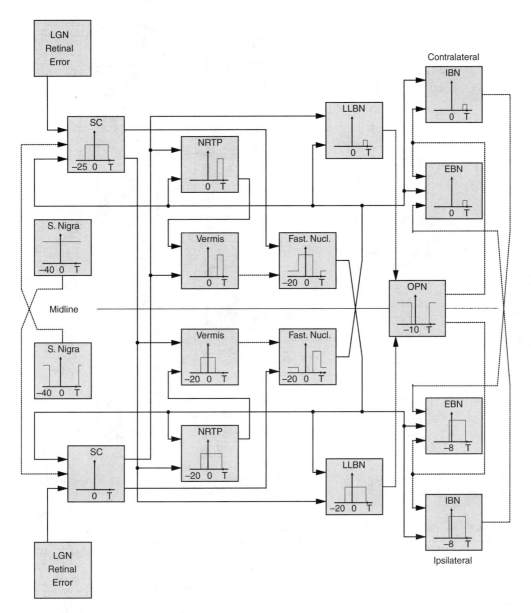

FIGURE 16.11 Part A: a functional block diagram of the saccade generator model. Solid lines are excitatory and dashed lines are inhibitory.

with the physical limitations of neurons. For the SC and the LLBN, this involves a single pulse, but for the EBN and IBN, this involves two pulses with different filters (the first pulse describes the brief rise and subsequent fall within the first 10 msec during a saccade, and the second pulse describes the steady state pulse during the saccade) and match the electrophysiological data.

Illustrated in Figure 16.13 is an extracellular single unit recording for the EBN, eye position data and a simulation for a 20° saccade. Details of the experiment are given in Enderle [1994]. A 20° saccade was simulated by using EBN data as input and the oculomotor plant in Figure 16.8. Little difference between the data and the simulation results are observed for this movement, as well as other eye movements. The saccade generator model in Figure 16.9 also provides an excellent description of the saccade system, and matches the data very well for all naturally occurring saccades, including saccades with dynamic overshoot and glissadic behavior, without parametric changes [Enderle, 1994].

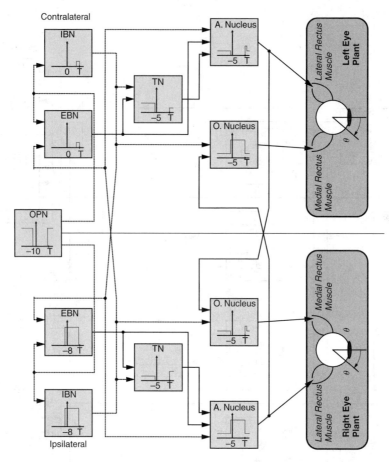

FIGURE 16.12   Part B: a functional block diagram of the saccade generator model. Solid lines are excitatory and dashed lines are inhibitory.

TABLE 16.1   Activity of Neural Sites during a Saccade

Neural site	Onset before saccade (msec)	Peak firing rate (Hz)	End time
Abducens nucleus	5	400–800	Ends approx. 5 msec before saccade ends
Contralateral FN	20	200	Pulse ends with pause approx. 10 msec before saccade ends, resumes tonic firing approx. 10 msec after saccade ends
Contralateral SC	20–25	800–1000	Ends approx. when saccade ends
Ipsilateral cerebellar vermis	20–25	600–800	Ends approx. 25 msec before saccade ends
Ipsilateral EBN	6–8	600–800	Ends approx. 10 msec before saccade ends
Ipsilateral FN	20	Pause during saccade, and a burst of 200 Hz toward the end of the saccade	Pause ends with burst approx. 10 msec before saccade ends, resumes tonic firing approx. 10 msec after saccade ends
Ipsilateral FEF	>30	600–800	Ends approx. when saccade ends
Ipsilateral IBN	6–8	600–800	Ends approx. 10 msec before saccade ends
Ipsilateral LLBN	20	800–1000	Ends approx. when saccade ends
Ipsilateral NRTP	20–25	800–1000	Ends approx. when saccade ends
Ipsilateral substantia nigra	40	40–100	Resumes firing approx. 40–150 msec after saccade ends
OPN	6–8	150–200 (before and after)	Ends approx. when saccade ends

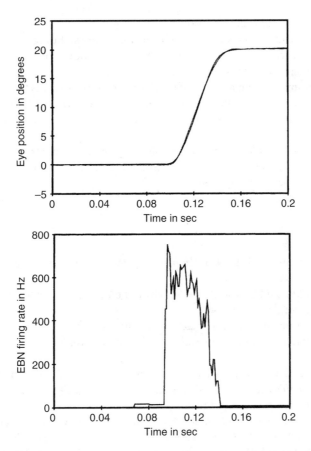

FIGURE 16.13 Simulated eye position in solid line shown in top graph, generated with EBN saccade data (shown in lower graph) and the oculomotor plant in Figure 16.8. Actual eye movement data recorded with the EBN data during a saccadic eye movement. (Data provided by Dr. David Sparks from his laboratory while at the University of Alabama.)

16.9 Conclusion

This section has focused on quantitative models and control of the fast eye movement system. Each of the oculomotor plant models described here are linear. Beginning with the most simple quantitative model of saccades by Westhiemer [1954], important characteristics of saccades were determined as a means of evaluating the quality of saccade models. Next, models of increasing complexity were presented with the end goal of constructing a homeomorphic saccade model of the oculomotor plant. These plant models were driven by improved models of muscle that ultimately provided an excellent match of the static and dynamic properties of rectus eye muscle. Finally, the control of saccades was considered from the basis of systems control theory and anatomical considerations. Many nonlinear models of the oculomotor plant exist and readers interested in learning about them should consult [Robinson, 1981].

Defining Terms

Active state tension generator: The active state tension generator describes the element within the muscle which creates a force. This force is different than muscle tension, which is the force due to the active state tension generator and all of the other elements within the muscle.

Extraocular muscles: The six muscles attached directly to the outside of the eyeball, and consists of the medial, lateral, superior, inferior recti, and the superior and inferior oblique muscles.

Homeomorphic: As close to reality as possible.
Latent period: The latent period is thought to be the time interval during which the CNS determines whether to make a saccade, and if so, calculates the distance the eyeball is to be moved, transforming retinal error into transient muscle activity.
Main-sequence diagrams: Summary plots of the characteristics of saccades that allows one to compare inter- and intrassubject variations. Commonly used characteristics include (1) peak velocity–saccade magnitude, (2) saccade duration–saccade magnitude, and (3) latent period–saccade magnitude.
Oculomotor system: The oculomotor system consists of the eyeball and extraocular muscles (also called the oculomotor plant), and the neural sites responsible for the eye movement.
Saccade: A saccade is a fast eye movement.

References

Bahill, A.T., Clark, M.R., and Stark, L. 1975. The main sequence, a tool for studying human eye movements. *Math. Biosci.* 24: 194–204.

Bahill, A.T., Latimer, J.R., and Troost, B.T. 1980. Linear homeomorphic model for human movement. *IEEE Trans. Biomed. Eng.* 27: 631–639.

Collins, C.C. 1975. The human oculomotor control system. In G. Lennerstrand and P. Bach-y-Rita (Eds.), *Basic Mechanisms of Ocular Motility and Their Clinical Implications*, pp. 145–180. Pergamon Press, Inc., Oxford.

Enderle, J.D. 2002. Neural control of saccades. In J. Hyönä, D. Munoz, W. Heide, and R. Radach (Eds.), *The Brain's Eyes: Neurobiological and Clinical Aspects to Oculomotor Research, Progress in Brain Research*, Vol. 140, pp. 21–50. Elsevier, Amsterdam.

Enderle, J.D. 1994. A physiological neural network for saccadic eye movement control. *Armstrong Laboratory/AO-TR-1994-0023*. Air Force Material Command, Brooks Air Force Base, Texas.

Enderle, J.D., Blanchard, S., and Bronzino, J. 2005, *Introduction to Biomedical Engineering, Second Edition*, p. 729, Figure 12.12.

Enderle, J.D., Blanchard, S., and Bronzino, J. 2005, *Introduction to Biomedical Engineering, Second Edition*, p. 764, Figure 12.33.

Enderle, J.D., Engelken, E.J., and Stiles, R.N. 1991. A comparison of static and dynamic characteristics between rectus eye muscle and linear muscle model predictions. *IEEE Trans. Biomed. Eng.* 38: 1235–1245.

Enderle, J.D. and Wolfe, J.W. 1988. Frequency response analysis of human saccadic eye movements. *Comput. Biol. Med.* 18: 195–219.

Enderle, J.D. 1988. Observations on pilot neurosensory control performance during saccadic eye movements. *Aviation, Space Environ. Med.* 59: 309–313.

Enderle, J.D. and Wolfe, J.W. 1987. Time-optimal control of saccadic eye movements. *IEEE Trans. Biomed. Eng.* BME-34: 43–55.

Enderle, J.D., Wolfe, J.W., and Yates, J.T. 1984. The linear homeomorphic saccadic eye movement model — a modification. *IEEE Trans. Biomed. Eng.* 31: 717–720.

Hsu, F.K., Bahill, A.T., and Stark, L. 1976. Parametric sensitivity of a homeomorphic model for saccadic and vergence eye movements. *Comput. Prog. Biomed.* 6: 108–116.

Robinson, D.A. 1981. Models of mechanics of eye movements. In B.L. Zuber (Ed.), *Models of Oculomotor Behavior and Control*, pp. 21–41. CRC Press, Boca Raton, FL.

Robinson, D.A. 1975. Oculomotor control signals. In G. Lennerstrand and P. Bach-y-Rita (Eds.), *Basic Mechanisms of Ocular Motility and their Clinical Implication*, pp. 337–374. Pergamon Press, Oxford.

Robinson, D.A., O'Meara, D.M., Scott, A.B., and Collins, C.C. 1969. Mechanical components of human eye movements. *J. Appl. Physiol.* 26: 548–553.

Robinson, D.A. 1964. The mechanics of human saccadic eye movement. *J. Physiol. (Lond.)* 174: 245–264.

Scudder, C.A., Kaneko, C.R.S., and Fuchs, A.F. 2002. The brainstem burst generator for saccadic eye movements — a modern synthesis. *Exp. Brain Res.* 142: 439–462.

Scudder, C. A. 1988. A new local feedback model of the saccadic burst generator. *J. Neurophysiol.* 59: 1454–1475.

Westheimer, G. 1954. Mechanism of saccadic eye movements. *AMA Archiv. Ophthalmol.* 52: 710–724.

Wilkie, D.R. 1968. *Muscle: Studies in Biology*, Vol. 11. Edward Arnold Ltd., London, United Kingdom.

Further Information

Readers interested in additional information on the subject of fast eye movements should consult the following books. There are many journals that publish articles on saccadic eye movements — for a sample of these journals, see the references listed within the following books as well.

Bahill, A.T. 1981. *Bioengineering, Biomedical, Medical and Clinical Engineering.* Englewood Cliffs, NJ, Prentice-Hall.

Carpenter, R.H.S. 1988. *Movements of the Eyes*, 2nd revised ed. London, Pion Ltd.

Enderle, J.D., Blanchard, S.M., and Bronzino, J.D. 2000. *Introduction to Biomedical Engineering.* San Diego, CA, Academic Press, p. 1062.

Leigh, R.J. and Zee, D.S. 1999. *The Neurology of Eye Movements*, 3rd ed. New York, Oxford University Press.

Wurtz, R.H. and Goldberg, M.E. 1989. *The Neurobiology of Saccadic Eye Movements.* Elsevier, New York.

17

A Comparative Approach to Analysis and Modeling of Cardiovascular Function

John K-J. Li
Rutgers University

Ying Zhu
Adow Innovation

Abraham Noordergraaf
University of Pennsylvania

17.1 Introduction

Although the cardiovascular system and its parts do not always work as simple linear systems, they frequently work, similarly, and in some cases, optimally. One can only marvel at the amazing similarities that exist, structurally and dynamically, across a large number of mammalian species. These similarities occur in spite of grossly different body weights and social–ecological environments of the many different species. The constant biological transformations that occurred did not seem to alter these similarities significantly.

Using physical principles and applying engineering techniques, we can model the cardiovascular systems of different mammals. However, the complexity of the beat-to-beat dynamic performance of the heart and its interaction with the vascular systems makes this a major challenge. This complexity can be substantially reduced when we first impose appropriate biological scaling laws and identify relevant invariant features that appear across species in the mammalian class.

In terms of structure and function, there are a number of characteristics that must vary with size, and they are consequently scaled with respect to body weight. Examples include: size of the heart, volume of blood, length of the aorta, and cardiac output. Other characteristics however, are invariant. Examples are: blood pressure, ejection fraction, heart beats per life time, capillary, and red blood cell sizes.

It was not until the 17th century that Harvey [1628], in his now famous "De Motu Cordis," rejected Gaelenus' theory, and proposed the closed circulation. This allowed him to explain the intermittent pumping function of the heart as a consequence of systolic ejection and diastolic filling. He also made comparisons of circulatory function from his many "Anatomical Exercises Concerning the Motion of the Heart and Blood in Living Creatures," performed on several mammalian species, avians, and amphibians. The quantification of blood pressure amplitudes and cardiac output in mammalian species, however, was first introduced by Hales [1733] a century later. Until this day, blood pressure and cardiac output are still regarded as the most pertinent clinical variables that govern the function of the cardiovascular system.

D'Arcy Thompson's [1917] "On Growth and Form" paved yet another path to modern comparative biological studies. This is followed by Huxley's [1932] work on the "Problems of Relative Growth" in which he based many of his biological interpretations on allometric relations.

Allometry is defined as the change of proportions with increase of size both within a single species and between adults of related groups. The allometric formula relates any measured physical quantity Y to body mass M, with a and b as derived or measured empirical constants. This resulted in the now familiar power law,

$$Y = aM^b \tag{17.1}$$

This formula expresses simple allometry. In the special case when the exponent is 0, Y is independent of body mass M: the physical variable is said to be invariant with body mass. When b is 1/3, the variable is said to be dependent on body length; when b is 2/3, Y is dependent on body surface area, and when $b = 1$, Y is simply proportional to body mass. This provided what is known as the basis of the "one-third power law" or geometric scaling [Lambert and Teissier, 1927]. It has recently been challenged by the "one-fourth power law" as the basis of biological allometric formulation [West et al., 1997].

The allometric equation has proven to be powerful for characterization of similarities among species. It is effective in relating a physiological phenomenon, either structural or functional, among mammals of grossly different body mass. A similarity criterion is established when Y, formulated in terms of either product(s) or ratio(s) of physically measurable variables, remains constant despite changes in body mass, and is dimensionless. Thus, the exponent b must necessarily be zero. In other words, similarity is present whenever any two, dimensionally identical, measurements occur in a constant ratio to each other. If such a ratio exists among different species, then a similarity criterion is established as the scaling law. This approach of establishing biological similarity criteria has been very useful [Stahl, 1963a, b, 1965; Gunther and DeLa Barra, 1966a, b; Gunther, 1975; Li, 1987, 1996, 2000].

17.2 Dimensional Analysis of Physiological Function

The theorem of dimensional analysis was introduced by Buckingham in 1915. It states that if a physical system can be properly described by a certain set of dimensional variables, it may also be described by a lesser number of dimensionless parameters which incorporate all the variables.

We shall now illustrate the use of dimensional analysis with the application of Laplace's law to mammalian hearts. The beat-to-beat pumping ability of the mammalian heart is determined by its force-generating capability and the lengths of its constituent muscle fibers, as governed by the Starling's experimental observations on the heart. The formula for calculating force or tension, however, has been based on the law of Laplace

$$T = pr \tag{17.2}$$

which states that the pressure difference, p, across a curved membrane in a state of tension is equal to the tension in the membrane, T, divided by its radius of curvature, r [Woods, 1892]. This law has been applied to both blood vessels [Burton, 1954] and the heart [Li, 1986a]. To apply this formula, a certain geometric shape of the heart has to be assumed in order to arrive at the radius or radii of curvature. The ventricle has therefore been described geometrically as either a thin-walled or thick-walled sphere or ellipsoid. The myocardium, which encloses the ventricular chamber, actually, has finite wall thickness. Also, the long-axis diameter that is, the base-to-apex distance is greater than the short-axis diameter. When the left ventricle is considered as thin-walled ellipsoid, there are two principle radii of curvature, r_1 and r_2. Laplace's law dictates:

$$p = T(1/r_1 + 1/r_2) \tag{17.3}$$

For the ventricle as a sphere, $r_1 = r_2$ so that

$$p = 2T/r \tag{17.4}$$

In a cylinder such as the blood vessel, one radius is infinite, so that

$$p = T/r \tag{17.5}$$

which indicates that a greater tension in the wall is needed to balance the same distending pressure. Both arterial pressure and ventricular pressure have been found to be similar in many mammalian species.

The larger the size of the mammalian heart, the greater the tension exerted on the myocardium. To sustain this greater amount of tension, the wall of the larger mammal must thicken proportionally with increasing radius of curvature. This results in a larger heart weight. The Lame relation that accounts for wall thickness, h, therefore substitutes Laplace's law:

$$T = pr/h \tag{17.6}$$

A dimensional matrix can be readily formed by first expressing T, r, p, and h in the mass (M), length (L), and time (T) system, that is, $4T = M^1 T^{-2}$, $r = L^1$, $p = M^1 L^{-1} T^{-2}$, and $h = L^1$:

$$
\begin{array}{c|cccc}
 & T & r & p & h \\
\hline
M & 1 & 0 & 1 & 0 \\
L & 0 & 1 & -1 & 1 \\
T & -2 & 0 & -2 & 0 \\
\end{array}
\tag{17.7}
$$

To derive dimensionless parameters (π_i), Buckingham's pi-theorem needs to be utilized. To reiterate, the number of pi-numbers (j) is equal to the number of physical quantity considered ($n = 4$) minus the rank ($r = 2$) of the matrix (Li, 1983, 1986a). Thus, there will be two pi-numbers, denoted π_1 and π_2.

$$\pi_1 = T/ph \quad \text{and} \quad \pi_2 = h/r \tag{17.8}$$

They provide a description of the geometric and mechanical relations of the mammalian hearts and Laplace's Law is implicit in the ratio of the two,

$$I = \pi_1/\pi_2 = T/pr \tag{17.9}$$

17.3   Invariant Numbers and Their Physiological Applications

In general, both π_1 and π_2 and their ratio, I, are not only dimensionless, they are also independent of mammalian body mass. That is, π_2 indicates that ratio of ventricular wall thickness to its radius, h/r, is invariant among mammals. This also establishes a scaling factor. They are thus considered invariant numbers, that is, of the form $[M]^0[L]^0[T]^0$ = a dimensionless constant. This invariance implies that Laplace's law applies to all mammalian hearts [Martin and Haines, 1970; Li, 1986a].

Clinical implications of some of this finding can be easily appreciated. For instance, in the case of pathological cardiac hypertrophy, the h/r ratio is significantly altered as a consequence of increased wall thickness [Li et al., 1997]. This latter increase has been suggested as the result of an adaptation process by which the wall tension is normalized Equation 17.6. While in an enlarged and failing heart, the greater tension due to a larger radius of curvature results in excess myocardial oxygen demand.

Another example of scaling invariance can be found in blood flow in arteries. A dimensional matrix is first formed by incorporating parameters that are thought of as pertinent. These are the density (ρ) and viscosity (η) of the fluid, diameter (D) of the blood vessel, and velocities of the flowing blood (v) and of the pulse wave (c).

$$
\begin{array}{c|ccccc}
 & \begin{array}{c}\rho \\ (\text{g/cm}^3)\end{array} & \begin{array}{c}c \\ (\text{cm/sec})\end{array} & \begin{array}{c}D \\ (\text{cm})\end{array} & \begin{array}{c}\eta \\ (\text{poise})\end{array} & \begin{array}{c}v \\ (\text{cm/sec})\end{array} \\
\hline
M & 1 & 0 & 0 & 1 & 0 \\
L & -3 & 1 & 1 & -1 & 1 \\
T & 0 & -1 & 0 & -1 & -1 \\
\hline
 & k_1 & k_2 & k_3 & k_4 & k_5
\end{array}
\tag{17.10}
$$

where k_ns are Rayleigh indices referring to the exponents of the parameters. The pi-numbers can readily be obtained. Two of these are the well-known Reynold's number (Re), essential for identifying viscous similitude and laminar to turbulent flow transitions [Li, 1988], Re = $\rho v D/\eta$, and the Mach number, Ma = v/c, or the ratio of blood velocity to pulse wave velocity. Allometric relation gives

$$
\text{Ma} = 0.04\, M^{0.0}
\tag{17.11}
$$

which is nondimensional and invariant with respect to mammalian body mass. Although the Reynold's number is also dimensionless, it is not an invariant function of mammalian body mass,

$$
\text{Re} = 260.76\, M^{0.42}
\tag{17.12}
$$

Thus, dimensionless pi-numbers do not necessarily expose similarity principles, that is, scaling factors are not necessarily invariant numbers.

17.4   Comparative Analysis of the Mammalian Circulatory System

Allometric relations of anatomic structures and physiological functions are useful for identifying similarities of the circulatory function of different mammalian species [Li, 1996, 1998]. Obvious factors that are important in determining function are heart rate and size, cardiac efficiency and contractility, stroke volume, and blood pressure. Some examples of circulatory allometry are given in Table 17.1, and can be found in other sources [Stahl, 1963a, b, 1965; Juznic and Klensch, 1964; Holt et al., 1968, 1981; Calder III, 1981, 1996; Dawson, 1991; Li, 1987, 1996, 1998].

TABLE 17.1   Allometric Relations of Some Hemodynamic Parameters, $Y = aM^b$
(M in kg)

Parameter	Y	a	b	Reference
Heart rate (sec^{-1})	f_h	3.60	−0.27	Adolph [1949]
Stroke volume (ml)	V_s	0.66	1.05	Holt et al. [1968]
Pulse velocity (cm/sec)	c	446.0	0.0	Li [1987, 1996]
Arterial pressure (dyn/cm^2)	p	1.17×10^5	0.033	Gunther and Guerra [1955]
Radius of aorta (cm)	r	0.205	0.36	Holt et al. [1981]
Length of aorta (cm)	L	17.5	0.31	Li [1987, 1996]
Metabolic rate (ergs/sec)	MR	3.41×10^7	0.734	Kleiber [1947]
Heart weight (kg)	M_h	0.0066	0.98	Adolph [1949]

In mammals, the ratio of heart weight to body mass is an invariant with the heart accounting for about 0.6% of body mass. In allometric form [Adolph, 1949; Gunther and DeLa Barra, 1966a], this is

$$M_h = 6.6 \times 10^{-3} M^{0.98} \tag{17.13}$$

where the heart weight M_h and body weight M are both in grams. With M_h in g and M in kg, this has been given [Holt et al., 1968] as

$$M_h = 2.61 M^{1.10} \tag{17.14}$$

It should be readily apparent that experimental conditions and ecological factors can influence the empirical constants a and b. The above exponents for the heart weight (M_h), however, do not differ significantly from the theoretical exponent of 1.0 ($M^{1.0}$). The deviations arise from statistical fits of regressions to experimental data. It is also readily apparent that if a variable scales as $M^{1.0}$, then the allometric equation can be made invariant by taking a ratio with M in denominator, that is, normalizing with body mass.

The stroke volume (V_s) is also an invariant when normalized to heart weight or to body mass,

$$V_s = 0.66 M^{1.05} \text{ ml} \quad \text{or} \quad 0.74 M^{1.03} \text{ ml} \tag{17.15}$$

Stroke volume has long been considered a critical hemodynamic quantity in assessing ventricular function. Its product with mean blood pressure, bears a direct relation to the energy expenditure of the heart, or the external work, EW,

$$\text{EW} = pV_s \tag{17.16}$$

This is the work performed by the heart in order to perfuse the vasculature during each contraction, or in other words, the work necessary to overcome the arterial load during each ejection. Blood pressures are generally invariant with respect to body mass in mammals. Of course, there are exceptions due to unusual body size and shape [McMahon, 1973, 1983], such as the giraffe [Goetz et al., 1960] for identifiable reasons. This also indicates that the heart is basically a pressure source; maintaining an average constant blood pressure is of utmost importance. The process of blood pressure control is complex, and important roles are played by baroreceptors, the renin–angiotensin system and the autonomic nervous system, just to name a few subsystems. Allometrically, the mean arterial pressure is expressed as

$$p = 1.17 \times 10^5 M^{0.033} \text{ dynes/cm}^2 = 87.8 M^{0.033} \text{ mm Hg} \tag{17.17}$$

The exponent is slightly, though statistically it is not significantly different from 0 ($p = aM^0$). Thus, the external work is given by

$$\text{EW} = 0.87 \times 10^5 M^{0.063} \text{ ergs} = 0.0087 M^{1.06} \text{ J} \tag{17.18}$$

A larger ventricle generates a greater amount of external work. The quantity of blood that is ejected per beat (stroke volume), however, is a constant fraction of the amount contained in the heart as end-diastolic volume. Thus, ejection fraction, as it is termed, is thus an invariant among mammals,

$$F_{ej} = V_s/V_{ed} = 0.6\text{--}0.7 \qquad (17.19)$$

In a failing heart, the ejection fraction can decrease substantially (to 0.2 say), as a result of a reduced stroke volume and an enlarged heart size.

The smaller the mammal, the smaller is its heart weight, but the faster its heart rate (f_h;7):

$$tf_h = 4.02\ M^{-0.25}\ \text{sec}^{-1} \qquad (17.20)$$

Smaller mammals have shorter life spans, since the total number of heart beats in a mammal's lifetime is invariant. Within an individual mammal, rapid (and random) heart rhythms beyond normal often result in cardiac arrhythmias, such as ventricular tachycardia. On the other hand, it is interesting to note here that "cardiac slowing," which reduces heart rate, can actually have the beneficial consèquence of increasing longitivity.

Cardiac output, deemed by Hales [1733] as a valuable quantity describing ventricular function is given as the product of stroke volume and heart rate, or the amount of blood pumped out of the ventricle per minute,

$$CO = V_s f_h = (0.74\ M^{1.03})(4.02\ M^{-0.25})60/1000 = 0.178\ M^{0.78}\ \text{l/min} \qquad (17.21)$$

Cardiac output is closely related to metabolic rate, since the heart supplies oxygen and nutrients for metabolism. Table 17.2 gives a comparison of cardiac output in several species. Deviations from this equation have been found in very small mammals [White et al., 1968]. Since blood pressure is invariant, cardiac output is limited by the total peripheral resistance to blood flow of the mammalian systemic arterial tree, which is obtained as

$$R_s = p/CO = 2.8 \times 10^6 M^{-0.747}\ \text{dyn sec cm}^{-5} \qquad (17.22)$$

Thus, the peripheral resistance follows the $-3/4$ power of mass [West et al., 1997], and is inversely proportional to the metabolic rate ($+3/4$). This relation can be strongly altered under local conditions, such as vasoconstriction or vasodilation. This derived allometric equation can be compared to that reported by Gunther and Guerra [1955] who gave an equation conforming more closely to the 2/3 power:

$$R_s = 3.35 \times 10^6\ M^{-0.68}\ \text{dyn sec cm}^{-5} \qquad (17.23)$$

TABLE 17.2   Cardiac Output of Some Mammalian Hearts Based on the Allometric Equation $CO = 0.178\ M^{0.78}$ l/min

Species	Body weight (kg)	Cardiac output (l/min)
Elephant	2000	67
Horse	400	19
Man	70	5
Dog	20	1.8
Rabbit	3.5	0.5
Mouse	0.25	0.06
Tree Shrew	0.005	0.003

17.5   Metabolic Turn-Over Rate and Cardiac Work

The energy requirement of cardiac muscle fibers and the useful work they can generate are of considerable interest [Starling and Visscher, 1926; Robard et al., 1959; Li, 1983; Liao et al., 2003]. They define the mechanical efficiency of the cardiac pump. In hemodynamic terms, the efficiency of the heart is defined as the ratio of external mechanical work (EW) to myocardial oxygen consumption (MVO_2):

$$e = \text{EW}/\text{MVO}_2 \tag{17.24}$$

The efficiency of the heart is an invariant among mammalian species [Li, 1983a, b].

EW is also termed stroke work and is represented as the area encircled by the left ventricular pressure–volume (P–V) diagram during each heart beat. The external mechanical work generated by the heart per unit body or heart weight is constant for mammalian species [Li, 1983a, b], that is,

$$\text{EW}/M = \text{constant} = (pV_s)/M \tag{17.25}$$

This result is also of considerable physiological importance, since it states that the cardiac external work intensity, is invariant among mammals. Species differences in cardiac energetics, however, have been reported [Loiselle and Gibbs, 1979]. For man, taking $V = 75$ ml, $p = 100$ mm Hg, $M = 70$ kg, and $M_h = 370$ g, the external work is about 1 J and the coefficient is about 2.7 J/kg. In terms of heart weight, this is

$$\text{EW} = 2.7 \text{ J/kg} \quad \text{or} \quad \text{EW} = 1/70 \text{ J/kg} \tag{17.26}$$

in terms of body mass. For a 2100-kg elephant, its left ventricle is estimated to generate about 30 J for each heart beat. Examination of the dimensions gives:

$$\text{EW}/M = [M]^0[L]^2[T]^{-2} \tag{17.27}$$

Although this ratio is constant among mammalian species, it is not dimensionless. Therefore, it is not an invariant number.

17.6   Comparative Pulse Transmission Characteristics

Mammalian arterial system exhibits geometric and elastic nonuniformities. Geometric taper of the aorta alone is associated with an increased elastic modulus away from the heart. Vascular branching occurs where target organ perfusion is necessary, increasing the total vascular cross-sectional area. Arterial wall-thickness-to-lumen-radius ratios are invariant at corresponding anatomic sites in mammalian species. The ratio of aortic length to its diameter is also an invariant [Holt et al., 1981; Li, 1987]. In addition, the sizes of terminal arterioles and capillaries, as well as of red blood cells are also virtually invariant among mammalian species regardless of their body size. These represent structural invariants, giving rise to global vascular perfusion characteristics that are amazingly similar.

Similar pressure and flow waveforms are recorded in aortas of different mammalian species [Kenner, 1972; Noordergraaf et al., 1979; Li, 1987, 2000; Figure 17.1]. This suggests that corresponding pulse transmission characteristics may also be similar. Nonuniformities in geometry and elasticity, as well as viscous damping, could give rise to varying impedances to blood flow along the arterial tree. Pressure and flow pulses could therefore be modified as they travel away from the heart as they encounter mismatches of these impedances. Impedance to pulsatile flow is like resistance to steady flow and can be viewed as complex resistances that vary with frequency. Impedance is calculated as the complex ratio of pressure to flow for each harmonic, or multiples of heart rate. When the impedance is determined at the ascending aorta, or the entrance to the arterial tree, it is termed input impedance. Vascular input impedance (Z_{in}) can be used to characterize the global properties of the arterial system.

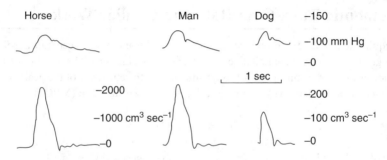

FIGURE 17.1 Simultaneously measured ascending aortic pressure and flow waveforms in three mammalian species, namely the horse, man, and dog, with grossly different body weights. Similarities in waveforms are obvious. Blood pressure magnitudes are similar.

TABLE 17.3 Data for Different Mammals for Analysis of Arterial Pulse Transmission Characteristics

| | Body mass M (kg) | Heart rate f_h (beats/min) | Phase velocity c (cm/sec) | System length l (cm) | Reflection coefficient | | Propagation constant $\times l$ γl |
					Γ (experimental)	Γ (non-dimensional)	
Horse	400	36	400	110	0.36	0.42	1.13
Man	70	70	500	65	0.38	0.45	1.06
Dog	20	90	400	45	0.39	0.42	1.01
Rabbit	3	210	450	25	0.41	0.48	0.93

$Z_0/R_s = 0.1$ is used in the calculation of Γ and γ.

When the characteristic impedance of the proximal aorta (Z_0) is matched to the input impedance of the arterial tree, that is, $Z_{in} = Z_0$, maximum transmission is present and reflection of the propagating pulse does not occur. Under this "matched impedances" condition, the pulsatile energy is totally transmitted to organ vascular beds. In normal physiological conditions, however, there is some mismatching of the impedances close to the peripheral organs. This causes the reflection of the propagating pressure and flow pulses. The fraction of the propagating pulse that is reflected is given by the reflection coefficient [Li, 1986, 2004], related to the impedances as

$$\Gamma = (Z_{in} - Z_0)/(Z_{in} + Z_0) \tag{17.28}$$

The magnitude of the reflection coefficient at normal resting heart rate is about 0.4, similar for many mammalian species (Table 17.3). The resolution of pressure and flow waveforms into their respective forward and reflected components [Li, 2000, 2004] are shown in Figure 17.2.

Pulse propagation characteristics [Li et al., 1981] can be quantified with a propagation constant,

$$\gamma = \alpha + j\beta \tag{17.29}$$

where α is the attenuation coefficient, describing pulse damping due to viscous losses and β, the phase constant, denoting the relative amount of phase shift or pulse transmission time delay due to finite pulse propagation velocity, c. In the mammalian aorta, the pulse wave velocity is invariant, as seen from the allometric relation

$$c = \omega/\beta = 446\, M^0 \text{ cm sec}^{-1} \tag{17.30}$$

where $\omega = 2\pi f_h$, $f_h =$ heart rate (sec^{-1}).

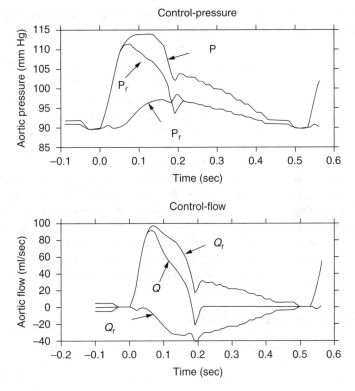

FIGURE 17.2 Simultaneously measured canine aortic pressure and flow in the aorta when resolved into its forward (P_f, Q_f) and reflected (P_r, Q_r) components.

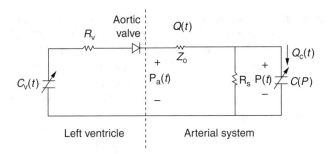

FIGURE 17.3 The coupled model of the left ventricle (LV) and the arterial system (AS). The LV is represented here by a time-varying compliance and a resistance. The AS is represented by the modified windkessel model with characteristic impedance, Z_o, peripheral resistance, R_s, and compliance of the arterial system, C. $C(P)$ denotes the case when compliance is allowed to change with blood pressure levels.

To compare gross features of the arterial trees of different mammals, modeling approach can be particularly useful. The modified windkessel model of the systemic arterial system that is coupled to the heart (Figure 17.3) has been shown to represent well the features of the input impedance of the systemic arterial tree. For this representation, the input impedance is

$$Z_{\text{in}} = Z_o + R_s/(1 + j\omega CR_s) \qquad (17.31)$$

dominated by Z_0, R_s, the systemic peripheral resistance as shown before, and C, the total systemic arterial compliance, representing the elastic storage properties of the arteries:

$$C = 0.18 \times 10^{-4} \, M^{0.95} \, \text{g cm}^4 \, \text{sec}^2 \qquad (17.32)$$

It is clear that the peripheral resistance decreases, while compliance increases with mammalian body size. Thus, the dynamic features of blood pressure and flow pulse transmission can be scaled through this kind of modeling. The ratio of Z_0/R_s corresponds to the ratio of pulsatile energy loss due to oscillatory flow to the energy dissipated due to steady flow (to overcome R_s) and has been reported to be between 5 and 10% and is an invariant for the mammalian arterial circulation [Li, 1996, 2004].

Some of the pulse transmission characteristics for horse, man, dog and rabbit are summarized in Table 17.3. The ratio of pulse propagation wavelength, λ, for the fundamental harmonic, to the length of the aorta, l, equals about 6, independent of the body mass of the mammal. The product of γl is about 1, again independent of the mammalian body mass and confirming that the propagation characteristics along mammalian aortas are similar. The global reflection coefficient is also practically invariant. This occurs in spite of vast differences in heart rate, systemic peripheral resistance, total systemic arterial compliance, and aortic characteristic impedance that are associated with different body sizes.

17.7   Optimal Design Features

These observed phenomena concerning pulse transmission, pulse wave velocity, and input impedance as discussed above must all be attributed to a common mechanism [Li and Noordergraaf, 1991]. The architecture of the branching arterial junctions is such that only a portion of the pulse wave generated by the ventricle reaches the capillaries. Another part is reflected in the periphery, principally in the arteriolar beds. Reflected waves encounter mismatched branching sites on their return trip to the ventricle. As a result, a negligible fraction of the reflected pulse wave actually reaches the heart, with the exception of the lowest frequency component for which the wavelength is comparable to the effective length of the vascular system.

Another important feature of the optimal design of the mammalian arterial tree network is that there is minimal loss of pulsatile energy due to vascular branching [Li et al., 1984]. The vascular junctions are practically impedance matched. In other words, the characteristic impedance of the mother vessel is closely matched to the branching daughter vessels. This implies that the geometric and elastic properties of the daughter vessels match that of the mother vessel. As such, pulse transmission at a vascular branching junction is met with minimal local reflection. This results in the facilitation of vascular perfusion with minimal energy loss en route to organ vascular beds.

References

Adolph, E.F. Quantitative relations in the physiological constitutions of mammals. *Science* 109: 579, 1949.

Buckingham, E. On physically similar systems; illustrations of the use of dimensional equations. *Phys. Rev.* 4: 345, 1915.

Burton, A.C. Relation of structure to function of the tissues of walls of blood vessels. *Physiol. Rev.* 34: 619–642, 1954.

Calder, W.A., III. Scaling of physiological processes in homeothermic animals. *Ann. Rev. Physiol.* 43: 301, 1981.

Calder, W.A. III. *Size, Function and Life History.* Dover, New York, 1996.

Dawson, T.H. *Engineering Design of the Cardiovascular System of Mammals.* Prentice-Hall, Englewood Cliffs, NJ, 1991.

Goetz, R.H., J.V. Warren, O.H. Gauer, J.L. Patterson Jr., J.T. Doyle, E.N. Keen, and M. McGregor. Circulation of the giraffe. *Circ. Res.* 8: 1049–1058, 1960.

Gunther, B. Allometric ratios, invariant numbers and the theory of biological similarity. *Physiol. Rev.* 55: 659, 1975.

Gunther, B. and L. DeLa Barra. Physiometry of the mammalian circulatory system. *Acta Physiol. Lat.-Am.* 16: 32, 1966a.

Gunther, B. and L. DeLaBarra. Theories of biological similarities, non-dimensional parameters and invariant numbers. *Bull. Math. Biophys.* 28: 9–102, 1966b.

Gunther, B. and B. Guerra. Biological similarities. *Acta Physiol. Lat.-Am.* 5: 169, 1955.

Hales, S. *Statical Essays Containing Haemostaticks.* London, 1733.

Harvey, W. *De Motu Cordis.* London, 1628. Dover edition, New York, 1995.

Holt, J.P., E.A Rhode, and H. Kines. Ventricular volumes and body weights in mammals. *Am. J. Physiol.* 215: 704, 1968.

Holt, J.P., E.A. Rhode, W.W. Holt, and H. Kines. Geometric similarity of aorta, venae cavae, and certain of their branches in mammals. *Am. J. Physiol.* 241: R100, 1981.

Huxley, J.S. *Problems of Relative Growth.* Methuen, London, 1932.

Juznic, G. and H. Klensch. Vergleichende physiologische untersuchunger uber das verhalten der indices fur energieaufwand und leistung des herzens. *Arch. ges Physiol.* 280: 3845, 1964.

Kenner, T. Flow and pressure in arteries. In *Biomechanics*, Y.C. Fung, N. Perroue, and M. Anliker (Eds.). Prentice-Hall, NJ, 1972.

Kleiber, M. Body size and metabolic rate. *Physiol. Rev.* 27: 511–541, 1947.

Lambert, R. and G. Teissier. Theorie de la similitude biologique. *Ann. Physiol. Physiocochem. Biol.* 3: 212, 1927.

Li, J.K.-J. A new similarity principle for cardiac energetics. *Bull. Math. Biol.* 45: 1005–1011, 1983a.

Li, J.K.-J. Hemodynamic significance of metabolic turnover rate. *J. Theor. Biol.* 103: 333–338, 1983b.

Li, J.K.-J. Comparative cardiac mechanics: Laplace's law, *J. Theor. Biol.* 118: 339–343, 1986a.

Li, J.K.-J. Time domain resolution of forward and reflected waves in the aorta. *IEEE Trans. Biomed. Eng.* BME-33: 783–785, 1986b.

Li, J.K.-J. *Arterial System Dynamics.* New York University Press, New York, 1987.

Li, J.K.-J. Laminar and turbulent flow in the mammalian aorta: Reynolds number. *J. Theor. Biol.* 135: 409–414, 1988.

Li, J.K.-J. *Comparative Cardiovascular Dynamics of Mammals.* CRC Press, Boca Raton, FL, 1996.

Li, J.K.-J. A new approach to the analysis of cardiovascular function: allometry. In *Analysis and Assessment of Cardiovascular Function*, G. Drzewiecki and J.K.-J. Li (Eds.). Springer-Verlag, New York, 1998, pp. 13–29.

Li, J.K.-J. *The Arterial Circulation: Physical Principles and Clinical Application.* Humana Press, Totowa, NJ, 2000.

Li, J.K.-J. *Dynamics of the Vascular System.* World Scientific, Singapore, New York, 2004.

Li, J.K.-J., J. Melbin, R.A. Riffle, and A. Noordergraaf. Pulse wave propagation. *Circulation Res.* 49: 442–452, 1981.

Li, J.K.-J., J. Melbin, and A. Noordergraaf. Directional disparity of pulse wave reflections in dog arteries. *Am. J. Physiol.* 247: H95–H99, 1984.

Li, J.K.-J. and A. Noordergraaf. Similar pressure pulse propagation and reflection characteristics in aortas of mammals. *Am. J. Physiol.* 261: R519–R521, 1991.

Li, J.K.-J., Y. Zhu, and M. Nanna. Computer modeling of the effects of aortic valve stenosis and arterial system afterload on left ventricular hypertrophy. *Comput. Biol. Med.* 27: 477–485, 1997.

Liao, J., J.K.-J. Li, and D. Metaxas. Characterization of time-varying properties and regional strains in myocardial ischemia. *Cardiovasc. Eng. Int. J.* 3: 109–116, 2003.

Loiselle, D.S. and C.L. Gibbs. Species differences in cardiac energies. *Am. J. Physiol.* 490–498, 1979.

Martin, R.R. and H. Haines. Application of Laplace's law to mammalian hearts. *Comp. Biochem. Physiol.* 34: 959, 1970.

McMahon, T.A. Size and shape in biology. *Science* 179: 1201–1204, 1973.

McMahon, T.A. and J.T. Bonner. *On Size and Life.* Scientific American Library, New York, 1983.

Noordergraaf, A., J.K.-J. Li, and K.B. Campbell. Mammalian hemodynamics: a new similarity principle. *J. Theor. Biol.* 79: 485, 1979.

Robard, S., F. Williams, and C. Williams. The spherical dynamics of the heart. *Am. Heart J.* 57: 348–360, 1959.

Stahl, W.R. Similarity analysis of biological systems. *Persp. Biol. Med.* 6: 291, 1963a.

Stahl, W.R. The analysis of biological similarity. *Adv. Biol. Med. Phys.* 9: 356, 1963b.

Stahl, W.R. Organ weights in primates and other mammals. *Science* 150: 1039–1042, 1965.

Starling, E.H. and M.B. Visscher. The regulation of the energy output of the heart. *J. Physiol.* 62: 243–261, 1926.

Thompson, D.W. *On Growth and Form.* Cambridge University Press, 1917.

West, G.B., J.H. Brown, and B.J. Enquist. A general model for the origin of allometric scaling laws in biology. *Science* 276: 122–126, 1997.

White, L., H. Haines, and T. Adams. Cardiac output related to body weights in small mammals. *Comp. Biochem. Physiol.* 27: 559–565, 1968.

Woods, R.H. A few applications of a physical theorem to membranes in the human body in a state of tension. *J. Anat. Physiol.* 26: 362–370, 1892.

18

Cardiopulmonary Resuscitation: Biomedical and Biophysical Analyses

Gerrit J. Noordergraaf
St. Elisabeth Hospital

Johnny T. Ottesen
University of Roskilde

Gert J. Scheffer
University Medical Center

Wil H.A Schilders
Technical University

Abraham Noordergraaf
University of Pennsylvania

18.1 Introduction

The evolution of the human in caring for others is reflected in the development of cardiopulmonary resuscitation (CPR). Superstition, divine intervention, and, finally, science have contributed to the development of a technique which may allow any person to save another's life. Fully 50% of the first presentation of coronary artery disease is sudden death, typically in (western) men [1]. However, achieving a clear understanding of why CPR saves some lives remains shrouded in mist; mist made even thicker by contradictory reports, different schools of thought, and persistently low-survival rates.

Despite the suggestion that much remains unclear, CPR is not new. Initially known as closed-chest cardiac resuscitation (CCCR), an early report of CPR as performed today, in an 18-year-old woman, dates from 1858 [2]. Following airway obstruction and hypoxia, cardiac arrest occurred. Artificial respiration and compressions on the anterior chest wall for 6 min resolved the incident successfully. Surprisingly little seems to have changed in CCCR since that early report.

Even though CPR has been researched extensively, the number of survivors remains disappointingly small. Survival rates as low as a few percent and extending upward to 30% (most frequently around 10%) survival for "out-of-hospital" resuscitation have been reported, without a clear understanding of why some patients do and others do not survive when given the same care. CPR is a technique taught to tens of thousands each year.

This chapter addresses functional aspects of CPR required for a working understanding of the biomedical aspects of CPR. It does not purport to be a CPR course, although practical aspects relevant to understanding will be addressed, though not exhaustively. The development in CPR and the contributions of science to this development is presented, with emphasis on the cardiovascular system and only on the artificial respiratory aspects when needed. Schools of thought, chronologically organized, with the effects of physical and experimental models on their development and validity will allow the reader to analyze strengths and weaknesses.

18.2 Basic Models and Methods in CPR: Fundamental Characteristics

Cardiopulmonary resuscitation, as a generally known and accepted technique, typically addresses the combination of some form of artificial respiration and artificial mechanical support for the circulation. The most clear-cut case for application of CPR is that of a heart attack: electromechanical dysfunction of the heart, leading to uncoordinated movement of the ventricles and loss of cardiac output. As the brain is starved for oxygen, loss of consciousness follows within seconds and breathing ceases shortly thereafter. If no support is given, death will follow in minutes.

Initially, resuscitation focused on what is now known as opening the airway and artificial respiration and was performed when breathing had stopped (a clearly visible aspect), or after drowning. Recognition of the separate entity of the circulation and of the appearance of arrhythmias did not occur until the 1900s.

18.2.1 Open-Chest Cardiac Resuscitation

Early CPR was associated with specific illnesses and often a perioperative occurrence. Interest surged with the advent of large-scale use of inhalation anesthesia during the late 1840s [3]. The first report of an unsuccessful human attempt is attributed to Niehaus in 1880, and the first successful case is attributed to Igelsrud in 1904 [4,5].

The technique for open-chest cardiac resuscitation (OCCR) was simple and based on experimental work done in the 1870s by Schiff on laboratory animals [6]. Ventilation was provided by opening the airway and blowing in air. The chest could be opened between two ribs (fourth and fifth) on the left side so that the heart could be stimulated and compressed by enveloping the ventricles with one hand and squeezing rhythmically and pressing against an inside wall of the chest. Care was taken to compress the heart below the annulus (the border between ventricles and the atria) in order to avoid interference with coronary arterial or venous flow. During abdominal surgery the heart could be approached sub- or transdiaphragmatically, in which the subdiaphragmatical approach was most common. In 1953, Stephenson et al. [7] published a manuscript describing an international accumulation of 1200 cases, reporting a 28% long-term survival rate. It should be noted that 21% of these patients was less than 10 years old and that while ventricular fibrillation was recognized, electric defibrillation may have been utilized. This contrasted with a retrospective report with by Briggs et al. [8] of 58% survival, using data from the Massachusetts General Hospital.

Using open-chest cardiac compression a cardiac output approaching 90% of normal could be achieved and maintained for long periods of time. Mortality due to infection was low (ca. 4.7%) even by modern standards, undermining suggestions that a "second killer" exists in the use of OCCR [9]. In this series of 43 patients a definitive survival rate of 74% was described.

Pike et al. [3] compared OCCR with CCCR and reported, "where we have been sure that the heart has stopped entirely, although for the briefest period, extra-thoracic massage alone has proved useless."

Open-chest cardiac resuscitation, mainly an in-hospital procedure, remained the method of choice until the beginning of the 1960s, when it was quickly replaced by the CCCR technique. The change from OCCR to CCCR occurred rapidly, despite scientific evidence strongly holding that this transition was controversial. Regular, resurgent efforts to reintroduce OCCR have found only a minor toehold in medicine, despite recent insights and many contemporary reports [10]. (See Section 18.3.1.13 on minimally invasive direct cardiac massage.)

18.2.2   The Transition to Closed-Chest Cardiac Resuscitation

Creating movement of blood without opening the chest and enclosing the heart by the hand and directly compressing it, was first described in a series of human case reports by Koenig in 1885 [11]. In 1960, Kouwenhoven et al. [12] published what later became known as a landmark article, describing CCCR in general terms and claiming a 70% permanent success rate. The mechanism underlying their technique mimicked that of OCCR, based on the assumption that artificial CPR or compression systole caused direct compression of the heart between the sternum and the thoracic vertebral column at about Th_7–Th_8. During CPR systole the pressure in the (left) ventricle was assumed to be higher than the pressure in the atria, closing the atrioventricular valves, allowing for (right) atrial inflow, and creating a systemic and pulmonary arterial to venous pressure gradient [13]. This was thought to cause forward flow of sufficient magnitude to support life for up to several hours.

A clinical follow-up paper was published by Jude et al. [14]. While return of spontaneous circulation (ROSC) was achieved in 78%, only 24% survived to leave the hospital. If further subdivision is made for the patients with recognizable sudden cardiac death (24 patients), then the intervention length was 2 to 120 min, with 20% reaching ROSC and only 13% of this group to leave the hospital alive.

Further studies, in humans, comparing OCCR and CCCR were not performed [15], and OCCR gradually was reduced to a specialized technique, performed by a few physicians under a limited number of conditions.

18.2.3   Application of Closed-Chest Cardiac Resuscitation

Closed-chest cardiac resuscitation quickly gained popularity as a procedure that lay people could perform, and a number of psychomotor aspects became important. The term CCCR gradually transformed to CPR, in order to emphasize the cardiac and pulmonary aspects in resuscitation, while de-emphasizing the suggestion that the heart was being pumped. The psychomotor skills, often synonymous with basic life support (BLS), became central issues on how CPR is performed, and it has been suggested that they are core issues in survival.

The key psychomotor aspects include compression depth, compression frequency, duty cycle, and interruption of chest compression (for ventilation), and were defined in the early papers, although in some cases the motivation for the specific choice was unclear.

Compression depth is reported as the distance that the sternum is moved from its neutral position in the direction of the vertebral column. It is performed by applying significant external force on the lower half of the sternum, typically with one hand overlying the other. Compression frequency refers to the number of compression–relaxation cycles per minute, and is typically reported as the frequency without subtraction of noncompression time (i.e., for ventilation). The duty cycle refers to the fractions of time,

TABLE 18.1   Summary of the Values Given for Essential Aspects of CCCR (External Cardiac Massage), with Emphasis on the Circulatory Aspects

Year	Hand placement on the sternum	Impression depth	C : R ratio	Frequency (frequency during compressions)	Other aspects
1960	Lower half	1.5–2 in.	n.a.	60 min^{-1}	5 : 1 compression : ventilation
1974	Lower half (1.5 in. above xyphoid)	1.5–2 in.	1 : 1	60 min^{-1} (2 caregivers) 80 min^{-1} (1 caregiver)	No pause for ventilation (5 : 1) 5 sec pause allowed
1980	Lower half	1.5–2 in.	1 : 1	60 min^{-1} (2 caregivers) 80 min^{-1} (1 caregiver)	No pause for ventilation 5 sec pause allowed
1992	Lower half	1.5–2 in.	1 : 1	80–100 min^{-1} (both)	6 sec ventilation pause
2000	Lower half	1.5–2 in.	1 : 1	100 min^{-1}	2 sec per ventilation (15 : 2)

Note that the table is adapted from the American Heart Association "Standards and Guidelines." For explanation of abbreviations, see text. Abbreviations: C : R = compression to relaxation ratio. See Section 18.2.2 for a detailed explanation. (5 : 1) = 5 compressions followed by 1 ventilation. No pause implies that the chest compression will continue, that is, the time available for ventilation is 0.5 sec.

expressed as percentages, for compression as opposed to relaxation, and may also incorporate maintenance of compression or relaxation state. For example: a 40% duty cycle refers to (a) 40% compression, (b) 40% relaxation, and (c) 20% maintenance of relaxation. During one-rescuer CCCR, interruption of the compressions is required to clear the airway, ventilate the patient, and reposition the hands on the sternum. It may also include time needed to evaluate the electrocardiogram, check for respiration or pulsations, defibrillation, etc.

Other aspects such as hand position, use of a noncompressible underlying surface, opening the airway, and ventilation volumes have been discussed and adapted over time but have remained less central to the survival question. In Table 18.1 a summary is presented showing the consistency of the values over time.

Clinical realism requires that several additional concepts be understood. These are:

- *Oxygen delivery*: The purpose of CPR is to create sufficient circulation of oxygenated blood to maintain cellular metabolism and integrity.
- *Pressure*: Not arterial systolic or diastolic, but mean pressure is related to perfusion. Flow may be extrapolated by (mean) pressure differences at two different points in the vasculature. Direct measurement of flow in CPR conditions remains difficult.
- *Flow*: This is extrapolated from pressure differences. Coronary perfusion pressure (CPP) or myocardial perfusion pressure (MPP) is mean diastolic arterial pressure minus mean diastolic right atrial pressure. CPP is also used to denote cerebral perfusion pressure, equal to mean arterial minus mean intracranial pressures. In the former at least 15 mmHg [16] and in the latter 60 mmHg have been suggested as being required to sustain oxygenation of the myocardium and neuronal integrity [17]. Coronary perfusion occurs during diastole and remains dependant on myocardial wall tension, intrapericardial pressure.
- *Critical coronary perfusion pressure*: As stated above, flow is related to the pressure gradient. However, in stenotic vessels, flow will remain disproportionally low, as autoregulation cannot cause the maximal vasodilation in the healthier vessels. This may exacerbate regional hypoxia, the build up of low energy phosphates and acidosis.

18.2.4 The "Cardiac" and the "Thoracic" Pump Theories

Gradually, divergent opinions appeared as to the mechanism by which blood was actually pumped. Two schools of thought developed. The "cardiac" pump theory [12] suggested that pumping was achieved by direct compression of the heart, despite doubts expressed about the ability of the heart to function as a unidirectional pump under CCCR conditions as early as 1961 [18]. Weale, in his "letter to the

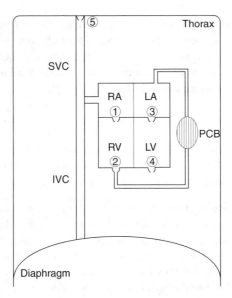

FIGURE 18.1 Schematics of the heart and the relevant structures for CPR. Valves listed as numbers. (1) Right atrioventricular valve or tricuspid valve; (2) right ventricular valve or pulmonary valve; (3) left atrioventricular valve or mitral valve (4–6 cm^2); (4) left ventricular valve or aortic valve (2.6–3.5 cm^2); (5) Niemann's valve, a nonanatomical valve in the cerebral-to-thoracic venous circulation. SVC = superior vena cava; IVC = inferior vena cava; RA = right atrium (pressure −1 to +7 mmHg); LA = left atrium; RV = right ventricle (pressure 15–25/0–8 mmHg), ejection fraction 40–60% with end-diastolic volume of 100–160 ml; LV = left ventricle (ejection fraction 40–75%). PA = pulmonary artery (15–25/8–15 mmHg); PCB = pulmonary capillary bed.

editor," proposed an alternative theory. It became popularized as the "thoracic" pump theory, but was not functionally reported until 1976 [19].

Central to the theoretical models of cardiac or thoracic pumping are two biomedical aspects. These are the actions of valves and the source of the blood volume that is being displaced. In Figure 18.1, a much-simplified representation of the relevant structures in CPR is given, to support and lend clarity to the modeling strategies described later.

The cardiac pump theory advocates that there is (direct) pressure on the ventricles. This is supported by indications that compression depth is related to output, that cardiac (or more specifically ventricular) deformation is related to stroke volume, that the duration of compression has no effect, and that an increased compression rate will increase flow [17]. In the original manuscripts, as well as over time, 1.5 to 2 in. (4 to 5 cm) has been maintained as standard. Forward flow of blood is assumed to be caused by competent atrioventricular valves and sufficient competence of the aortic and pulmonary valves to avoid regurgitation during CPR diastole. Implicitly, ventricular filling is essential and artificial systole must be sufficiently frequent to generate acceptable flow, as stroke volumes may be relatively small compared to the normal 60 to 100 ml per beat at ejection fractions of 40 to 75%. Mitral valve closure during CPR systole is deemed essential for the "cardiac" pump theory to work.

The "thoracic" pump theory [19] was suggested when patients with proven ventricular fibrillation on the EKG remained conscious for up to 90 sec, if they coughed forcefully, and kept coughing. Both fibrillation and cough had been triggered by the coronary catheterization procedure which prompted this clinical observation. The thoracic pump theory suggests that it is not the heart which is forced to pump by compression during CCCR or which supplies the volume to be displaced, but the blood volume in the thoracic cavity (i.e., the pulmonary circulation), with forward flow being generated by the arteriovenous pressure gradient, and (functional) valves at the thoracic outlet. The pressure chamber has been suggested to be the right ventricle, the pulmonary vasculature, and the complete left heart all connected in series. Transmitral flow during compression systole is considered characteristic of "thoracic" pump thinking.

This controversy remains active, although there is increasing evidence that in any one clinical case both theories may pertain. In both cases optimal performance of the technique seems to produce no more than 30% of normal cardiac output. It is recognized that many factors may be involved, for example, chest diameter, which confuse study outcomes [20]. Duration of circulatory failure, pH in tissue and in blood, underlying disease, and other causes, may also be factors.

18.2.5 Animal Models

When looking at the literature, the reader will note that animal models have long been used in the absence of the opportunity to study CPR in humans carefully and in an organized fashion. The choice of animal model may influence the outcome. Aspects to consider are:

- The anterior to posterior dimensions of the chest in relationship to the heart. This may be reported as anterior–posterior to lateral sizing. Increasingly small animals have been seen as models for humans with highly compliant, relatively oblong chests, as in children.
- The support/position of the animal. Many animals are unstable in a pure dorsal decubitus (lying on their back). A lateral decubitus, or a dorsal position, but supported by a "V" shaped cradle may be used to overcome this, but the former influences the distances between compression surfaces and the latter may limit lateral movement of the chest wall.
- The force, velocity, or distance used during CPR. Moving the sternum 2 in. in a small animal (chest diameter of 5 in.) may not translate to movement of 2 in. in a human (chest diameter upward of 10 in. or 24 cm).
- The method of inducing anesthesia, inducing ventricular fibrillation for CPR [21].
- The length of time between steps/series/controls. In series of experiments animals may be used as their own controls, with a few minutes between one technique followed by another. Return to baseline conditions is often impossible.
- The type of monitoring used for data acquisition.

The current standard (animal) model for CPR is the pig. However, care should be taken in extrapolating this data to humans for the same reasons [22].

18.2.6 Summary of This Section

Two distinct conceptual theories have been purported to explain why blood moves during CPR. Animal models may provide increased insights, but may also give rise to confusion. Although the "cardiac" pump theory (Kouwenhoven) and the "thoracic" pump theory (Criley) have been promoted as one-or-the-other mechanism, it has gradually become accepted over time that depending on the physiology of the patient the blood flow may be caused by either or both, perhaps alternating or time sensitive.

18.3 Variations in CPR Technique Based on Physiological Expectations and Modeling

The poor results, in terms of cardiac output, as well as in terms of survivors, found when larger-scale studies were published, initiated the development of what has become known as "adjuvants" to standard CPR or alternative CPR techniques. These techniques, all based on the application of CPR as CCCR, described by Kouwenhoven et al. [12] in 1960, attempt to improve survival using a variation of the baseline technique. The main line of adjuvants is presented in the order of their initial publication. Their underlying conceptual models are explained. Where possible, human data is referenced.

Standard CPR (S CPR), or basic life support (BLS) anno 2000 consists of a device-free, one- or two-caregiver technique, involving external chest compression on the lower half of the sternum, with a compression depth of 4 to 5 cm, at a frequency of 100 compression per minute with a duty cycle of 50%.

Compressions are supplemented by ventilations in a ratio of 15 compression to 2 ventilations of about 800 ml (one caregiver), and this respiratory pause should be shorter than 6 sec.

18.3.1 Adjuvant Techniques in CPR

18.3.1.1 Simultaneous Ventilation and Chest Compression (SVC) CPR

As an early variation of CCCR [23], this adjuvant, functionally a model supportive of the "thoracic" pump theory, suggests that insufflating the lungs, with simultaneous compression on the chest, should create optimal flow of blood out of the thoracic cavity by the (high) intrathoracic pressures generated. The technique, known as SVC-CPR, requires a formal airway to avoid excessive gastric insufflation, as high airway pressures are used to add to intrathoracic pressure change caused by the external compression. This mechanism was not supported by Harris et al. [24], due to other considerations and remained a dormant technique until the 1980s when Chandra et al. [25] revitalized it. This group, noting airway pressures of 60 to 110 cm H_2O, found more than a 100% improvement over baseline values for carotid flow, while working in humans. However, a large study (994 enrolled) in humans found a significantly detrimental effect in outcome [26], and it is currently not advocated for general use by the ILCOR 2000 guidelines [1]. The cause of the detrimental effect may be that open alveoli become severely overdistended, and that the pulmonary capillary bed becomes underperfused.

18.3.1.2 Static (Manual) Abdominal Binding

Having noted the limited cardiac output under CCCR conditions, experiments were performed with the use of epinephrine, volume loading, and static abdominal binding over the whole abdomen [27]. While demonstrating improvement in cerebral blood flow, at unspecified pressures, by improving the arterial to venous pressure gradient, as well as improving cardiac filling, the technique was not deemed useful due to extensive abdominal trauma. Not until the 1980s did further human data support static binding. The improvements were suggested to (a) increase intrathoracic pressure (decrease in pressure loss due to movement of the flaccid diaphragm and abdominal wall), (b) increase functional arterial resistance, and (c) redistribute blood volume to compartments above the diaphragm out of the abdominal compartment due to the flaccid nature of the diaphragm [28]. In a laboratory study in dogs, Niemann et al. [29] could not support the premises, finding that venous return is dependent on venous capacitance more than on the peripheral-to-central venous pressure gradient. Static abdominal binding is not in clinical use. No original research papers have appeared on this specific topic in more than 10 years. While listed separately, MAST-CPR is a specific form of static abdominal binding (see Section 18.3.1.6).

18.3.1.3 Cough CPR

Cough CPR [19,30], and its external variant, vest CPR, have been mentioned as the prototype for CPR without (direct) cardiac compression and is a "pure" application of the "thoracic" pump theory. The mechanism for coughing is clear: the diaphragm contracts strongly after a deep breath. With the upper airway partially obstructed forceful contraction will compress the air in the lungs and create equal pressure change on all intrathoracic structures. The intrathoracic pressure can reach 100 to 140 mmHg during the 0.2 to 0.5 sec of glottic closure and exhalation. Blood, not compressible, will move out of the high-pressure area to low-pressure areas. To achieve effective forward flow some (at least one) anatomical or functional valves and resistance differences are required. Reflux into the cerebral venous system is avoided by Niemann's valves, a functional set of valves at the thoracic outlets [31]. A similar functional valvular obstruction at the level of the diaphragm is unproven, with retrograde flow being limited by the peripheral capillary beds and arteriolar resistance. Cough CPR is considered a proven and useful clinical entity within specific settings, such as the coronary catheterization laboratory. Some hospitals routinely describe it in patient information folders and have the nursing staff issue instructions on the technique prior to procedures.

18.3.1.4 Altered Compression Duration

Birch et al. [33,35] suggested that the duration of compression might be an important factor in effective CCCR. In a prospective human study, increasing the duration of standard CPR systole to 60% of cycle time, in the range of 40 to 80 compressions per minute, improved the arterial flow index to 185% of control value. A 50% compression duration (compression : relaxation ratio of 1), was introduced as standard and still is advocated. Caregiver skills evaluation has demonstrated that at higher frequencies, that is, compression rates greater than 120 cpm, the compression : relaxation ratios almost always approach 1.

Later, other studies, typically in conjunction with much higher compression rates or increased force of compression (see Section 18.3.1.9), suggested that the rate in which compressions are performed may be more important than the duty cycle (duration of the compression as little as 20%). In addition, it became clear that only CPR performed mechanically (i.e., the Thumper®) is able to effectively perform short duty cycles at higher compression rates. Duty cycle alteration might be expected to effect output during CPR only from a "thoracic" pump approach [17].

18.3.1.5 Negative Airway Pressure

The use of negative airway pressure [34] in a noncardiac pump and nonthoracic pump model promised potential improvement in CPR. The concept rests on basic physiological principles directly relating to intrathoracic pressure changes influencing venous return. Cardiac output is dependent on venous return. With intermittent positive-pressure ventilation (mouth-to-mouth or using a respirator), intrathoracic pressure is predominantly positive, reducing venous return by interfering with the pressure gradient. The negative airway pressure creates an artificially normal negative segment in the pressure curve, in theory recreating a pressure cycle similar to that seen under spontaneous breathing. The technique has fallen into disuse due to extensive ventilation to perfusion mismatch (shunting) in the lung and severe atelectasis. However, a variation on this concept, in the form of a transient occlusion of the airway during decompression of the chest is currently under clinical investigation (see Section 18.3.1.15).

18.3.1.6 MAST-Augmented CPR

This technique uses pneumatically inflated "military antishock trousers" with an abdominal compartment and two-leg compartments [35]. Conceptually, it will decrease the arterial inflow into the lower extremities by increasing the peripheral resistance and decrease the venous pool in the legs by compression of the superficial and deep veins. This should generate a small, one-time, fluid challenge to the central circulation, known as autotransfusion and decrease the systemic vascular bed size. The autotransfusion has been suggested to be in the order of 8 to 12 ml/kg body weight. Since low peripheral vascular resistance during CPR is a major concern, with the MAP generally lower than 40 mmHg, improvements are theoretically possible. Studies in humans have not been able to demonstrate improved outcome, perhaps due to the involved nature of application. As opposed to static abdominal binding (Section 18.3.1.2), the MAST does not explicitly cause diaphragmatic splinting.

18.3.1.7 Synchronized Ventilation and Abdominal Compression

As a byproduct of work on cough CPR (Section 18.3.1.3 and Section 18.3.1.10), Rosborough found that using ventilation to increase intrathoracic pressure with simultaneous compression of the abdominal compartment maintained carotid artery flows similar to flows from standard CPR in dog experiments [36]. This model, based on a pure "thoracic" pump concept, has not been demonstrated to improve outcome in humans, and has been associated with pulmonary complications attributed to high airway pressures.

18.3.1.8 Interposed Abdominal Compression (IAC) CPR

Compression of the (central) abdomen [37], with 120 to 150 mmHg, between compressions of the chest (IAC-CPR), also known as abdominal counterpulsation CPR, or phased thoracic–abdominal compression (PTAC-CPR), was shown by Ralston, in a carefully documented analysis in a small- and large-dog series, to systematically improve systolic and diastolic arterial pressure as well as the central diastolic arteriovenous pressure gradient which is also known as CPP. The mechanism for improvement has been thought to be counterpulsation in the aorta and increased venous loading of the thoracic cavity, as demonstrated by increased antegrade flow in the vena cava inferior [38], and typically involves at least three well-trained caregivers. The Lifestick® may simplify the use of the technology, and incorporates active decompression (PTACD-CPR). Babbs [39] recently published a comprehensive review supporting IAB-CPR, which is one of the most extensively modeled and investigated concepts in CPR, presenting both the mathematical, animal, and clinical support for this technique. The safety of IAC-CPR has been investigated, without demonstrating increased aspiration or emesis, perhaps due to an increase in intra-abdominal pressure during artificial ventilation. The lifestick is in limited clinical use and has been accepted by the ILCOR guidelines for in-hospital use.

18.3.1.9   High Impact or Impulse CPR

This theory [16,40], uses high force/velocity for the external cardiac compressions. As a by-product, this technique uses a shorter-compression duration (i.e., as little as 20% instead of the usual 50%), without having the active intention of changing the compression depth. Rates of up to 150 compression per minute (100 compressions per minute is currently advised, see Table 18.1), have been proposed. When modeling from the cardiac pump theory, as long as the compression allows the mitral valve to close, and allows for sufficient filling time, artificial cardiac output will be determined by left ventricular end-diastolic volume. Higher compression rates will create more output. Modeled from the thoracic pump theory, the benefit may be due to the overall increase in the percentage of time actually allotted to compression.

18.3.1.10   Vest CPR

An external variant of cough CPR, vest CPR [41], has been mentioned as the prototype for CPR without (direct) cardiac compression and is conceptually pure "thoracic" pump theory. Halperin [17], working in dogs, compared standard CPR with high-frequency CPR and OCCR. Using a mechanical compression device, exact massage depths could be reproduced at any given frequency or compression duration. Vest CPR was demonstrated to displace the sternum by 0.5 ± 0.1 cm as opposed to 4.6 ± 0.1 cm in the external series. For the OCCR series the heart itself was compressed the same 4.6 ± 0.1 cm distance. Halperin notes that the rate and force (400 N) dependence as well as the outputs generated by the vest CPR, support its use and the thoracic pump model. In 1993, this was followed up by a report of 17 clinical cases [42]. This preliminary study demonstrated a small improvement in initial outcome, with better perfusion gradients. However, time needed to apply the vest, as well as its bulkiness have limited its general use. An interesting, but unsupported, anecdotal suggestion is that Vest CPR should be the principle technique used for research purposes. This is due to its independence from changes in thoracic compliance, myocardial stiffness, and ventilation parameters.

18.3.1.11   Simultaneous Chest and Abdominal Compressions (SCAC) CPR

This technique (SCAC-CPR) [43] is a variation on the model suggested by interposed abdominal compression CPR (Section 18.3.1.8). Conceptually, the simultaneous compression of chest and abdomen should create an improvement in the pressure rise, due to coupling of the thoracic and abdominal cavities (thoracic pump theory). Initial investigations seem to support improved pressure gradients, but as improved outcome has not been demonstrated, little recent work has been presented.

18.3.1.12   Active Compression–Decompression (ACD) CPR

After an anecdotal report of CPR performed successfully with a "plumbers helper," interest was stimulated in active decompression of the chest, allowing for negative intrathoracic pressure and increased venous return [44,45]. This technique became known as active compression – decompression (ACD-CPR), and has achieved routine clinical use in some countries, such as France. While discussion continues as to whether definitive survival is increased, studies have shown that flow, filling pressure, and valve movement (as "thoracic" pump) is improved with respect to standard CPR. Initial reports of significant improvement of outcome have been challenged by others who were unable to find improvements [46]. ACD-CPR is performed as a clinical tool in many settings. Steen et al. [47], have developed a mechanical, pressure-driven device, which can combine compression with active decompression (LUCAS®) addressing the issue that ACD-CPR is caregiver unfriendly. Use of ACD-CPR, in conjunction with an inspiratory impedance valve (Section 18.3.1.15) has also been advocated recently and the preliminary results are promising.

18.3.1.13 Minimal Invasive Direct Cardiac Massage Device (MID-CM) CPR

The use of minimally invasive direct cardiac massage [48], performed by inserting a plunger-like device through a 7.5 cm incision, makes direct compression of the ventricles through the intact pericardium possible. It was introduced as part of a resurgence of OCCR in a well-defined number of situations, and is a technique similar to insertion of a chest drain. Insertion time is less than 30 sec, and as little as 10 sec may be required in trained hands. Early human work, in the prehospital setting, in patients with failed basic and advanced life support, demonstrated good clinical parameters, although one cardiac rupture was noted [49]. The conceptual model is OCCR.

18.3.1.14   pGz-CPR

A highly technical and experimental procedure, it involves horizontal head-to-foot oscillations at frequency of about 2 Hz, over small, horizontal distances. The name, pGz, refers to a periodic fractional part of the acceleration of gravity, applied along the head to foot or "Z"-axis. It has been demonstrated to produce blood flow and ventilation proportional to the amplitude and frequency of the force applied. At 2 Hz and approximately 0.6 G, 20% of baseline cardiac output, at a very low peripheral and pulmonary vascular resistance, can be achieved in a fibrillating swine model with 100% of animals achieving ROSC or initial success. Using radiolabeled microspheres injected into the circulation, preferential flow to vital organs, including the splanchic microcirculation, could be detected. Separate mechanical ventilation was not used, as pGz-CPR [50] has been shown to generate adequate ventilation and oxygenation if some positive pressure is supplied. This concept is unrelated to classic CPR models.

18.3.1.15   Inspiratory Impedance Valve (ITV or ITD) CPR

Improvement in venous return can be expected if negative intrathoracic pressure is created by "closing" the airway during the decompression phase of the external CPR cycle [51]. This induces extra priming of the pump as a mechanism to improve cardiac output, similar to the concept underlying the active compression–decompression technique. Conceptually, this model is independent of the "cardiac" or "thoracic" pump theories, although the "thoracic" (volume) aspect does play a role. This procedure involves utilizing a valvular device in combination with a facemask or attached to the endotracheal tube. It harnesses the kinetic energy stored in the compressed chest wall, creating down to -40 cmH$_2$O (current model: -6 to -12 cmH$_2$O) when used in combination with active decompression (Section 18.3.1.12), and with most other CPR techniques, including standard CPR. It has been FDA-approved. Early clinical studies suggest interesting possibilities, with 40% improvement in cerebral blood flow noted. Improvement in outcome is attributed to the increased venous return, as well as improvements in CPR technique due to feedback mechanisms included in the valve. The valve must be removed when a spontaneous circulation is reinstituted or if spontaneous ventilation returns. Clinical data has been presented, showing promise, when used in conjunction with active decompression CPR [52].

18.3.1.16   Prone CPR

Alteration of the position of the whole patient (prone vs. the standard recumbent position, in both cases on a hard surface) is an anecdotal technique, which may have its roots in the classic Schafer [53] technique of artificial ventilation. This technique has the suggested advantage of no mouth-to-mouth contact and cleared airway, with ventilation caused by the chest compressions, which are bilateral on the lower ribs. By implication, prone CPR may be included in the "thoracic" pump school. Recently, the use of the prone CPR position has been reported due to dictation by positioning for a surgical procedure [54], as well as on potential psychological merits [55].

No current human or animal series, or modeling of this technique is known. Suggestions that the technique might be "thoracic" pump dependent are based solely on the noncentral hand placements [55]. It is interesting to note that one of the figures supplied earlier by Jude et al. [14] depicts the prone position.

Despite all the above mentioned CPR techniques and variations, a recent meta-analysis demonstrated that the survival of prehospital arrest is no greater than 6.4%, even when the best of the U.S. situations (Cook County, Seattle Washington) is factored in [30]. This rate has not only not improved but has decreased over earlier reports.

18.3.2 Summary of This Section

A plethora of functional and conceptual models for external support of the collapsed circulation are available. It remains disturbing that definitive survival in the majority of these applications continues to be poor. Devices, used in ACD-CPR (Section 18.3.1.12) and the ITD-CPR (Section 18.3.1.15) offer windows of opportunity, but have — as yet — not lived up to expectations, although the sum of knowledge is increasing. Additions to the basis laid down in the 1960s, plus the polarization offered by the "cardiac" or "thoracic" pump conceptual models, clearly fail to fully explain the behavior of the circulation in arrest. The commitment to simplicity in CPR teaching is a refreshing balm in the face of all the theoretical, modeling, and device options. However, it should not become its own goal.

18.4 From Clinical Experiments to Biomedical and Biophysical Understanding

Animal, and even more so human, experiments are handicapped by restrictions that nature and moral attitude impose. For example, it is difficult to direct changes in intrathoracic pressure, generated by compression of the thorax, to particular organs while excluding others. Similar difficulties apply to alterations in air pressure caused by the respiratory system. These examples may be supplemented by any number of other experiments, which should be performed using current technology in view of their presumed instructive value. Some of the confusing results from both animal and clinical research may be caused by limitations in experimental techniques. An example of this was the use of labeled microspheres to document myocardial perfusion.

Progress in understanding of the complex phenomena related to CPR suffered seriously during the entire period in which experiments were performed without the benefit of analytical studies.

18.4.1 Earlier Mathematical, Mechanical, and Animal Models in CPR

In Section 18.3, a wide variety of variations on the principle of external cardiac massage, as suggested by Kouwenhoven et al. [12] were summarized. Mathematical models with distributed properties have found extensive application for the purpose of supporting the experimental observations related to these variations, especially by Babbs et al. and by Beyar et al., both teams starting in 1984, later joined by other teams (see Reference 56, for an extensive review). Mathematical modeling addressing fundamental aspects in this area is of recent vintage [57].

18.4.1.1 Mechanical and Animal Models

Central to CPR is displacement of the sternum in order to either compress the heart directly or to achieve an increase in intrathoracic pressure. In most cases, the thoracic rib cage, responsible for most of the viscoelastic stiffness, will be relatively rigid (i.e., most patients requiring resuscitation are elderly), and a careful balance is required between applying enough force to depress the sternum, without causing undue damage. A consensus exists about the complexity of the psychomotor skills needed to sustain life, and the need to train and retrain these skills in order to achieve adequate life support. The most frequently used mechanical model in CPR remains the training manikin, of which a wide scale of models is available.

An analysis of force deemed adequate for chest compressions demonstrates a surprising range in human experiments, when standardized to Newtons based on area of compression. The range is 245–769 N, with compliances of 0.1 to 2.9×10^{-2} cm N^{-1}. In a review of forces used in mathematical modeling experiments, the range is 59–400 N [56].

Investigation directed at modeling the compliance of the human thoracic cavity in the elderly, has been performed. As early as 1976 the Emergency Care Research Institute suggested that 30 kg should produce a sternal depression of 3.8 to 5 cm [58]. Little work has been done to validate mechanical models in use [59], while work by Gruben et al. [60] on dogs, and Bankman et al. [61] on humans is not reflected in the mechanics modeled in CPR manikins. Force needed to compress the sternum in different manikins varied up to 140% at compression depth of 4 to 5 cm. Within one type of commonly used manikin, differing only in length of time in use, differences in pressure needed to reach 5 cm were found to vary from 37 to 46.5 kPs.

Recently, devices have been introduced to improve compression pressure. These devices, placed between the hands and the anterior chest wall, offer a visual reference to the force being applied. One such device, the CPREzy is being subjected to extensive clinical and bench testing, and seems to improve the consistency of the compression pressure. However, the "correct" depth of an individual patient remains a matter of individual caregiver interpretation.

For many years, small animal models have been utilized for modeling CPR in humans. Small animals, such as cats, pigs, and dogs, weighing from 5 to 20 kg have been used. Regrettably, small-animal experiments are dissimilar to the (elderly) human, but may be carefully applied for neonatal or small pediatric models. More recently, swine, weighing at least 20 kg have become the standard for experiments. This is not only due to improved similarity between the position of the heart and availability of the model, but is mostly due to improved estimation of the cardiac to thoracic cavity size ratio, and the similar ventrodorsal and lateral ratios to humans.

18.4.2 Recent Biomedical Insights: Compression Depth

Much of the research and development in CPR has followed the line of thinking set out by Kouwenhoven in 1960. In the following section the emphasis is shifted to evaluation of a widely accepted aspect, which was not properly scrutinized before, namely the sternum depression depth, discussed in Section 18.2.3, earlier. Additional information is needed to verify whether depression depth may or may not be a factor in the poor outcome after sudden cardiac death. This threshold, conceptually, applies to the "cardiac" pump theory.

There have been suggestions that a threshold depression depth must be observed before cardiac compression becomes effective [62]. Of principal interest would be whether the current recommendations could, in fact, directly cause cardiac compression in the general population (i.e., when the Kouwenhoven et al. recommendations are actually followed with 1.5 to 2 in. depression depth). Noordergraaf et al. [56] measured the transverse distances from the internal border of the sternum to the most ventral aspect of the curved, underlying, vertebral body using CT-scans in 50 cases. Each structure (cardiac, vascular, and esophagus) in these planes was listed, with the diameters of cardiac and vascular cavities described at T_1 and T_2. The cranial transverse slice, T_1, was taken to be the lowest visible border of the pulmonary valve, effectively the upper edge of the hand position on a standard sternum as well as the upper edge of the heart. The T_2 position was taken to be the lowest border of the tricuspid valve, that is, the mid position of the hand.

In this study, representative data was sought, with regard to age, gender, and weight. The distance, at the upper measuring plane, from the inside border of the sternum to the ventral aspect of the underlying vertebral body was 12.6 ± 2.4 cm. In this transverse plane the following structures were identified: the outflow tracts in all patients, which were in 80% of cases central veins, in 35% of cases the descending thoracic aorta, and incidentally the esophagus.

The internal distance T_2 was 13.4 ± 2.3 cm, with a difference of 11.1 ± 1.2 cm between outside and inside diameters. The structures found in the plane between the sternum and the vertebral body were predominantly the right atrium, the esophagus, which was in a majority of cases part of the right ventricle, and in some cases the left atrium with only an edge of the left ventricle. The descending thoracic aorta lay, in most cases, lateral of the vertebral column. The cardiac structures in this line being 8.6 ± 1.6 cm. The "noncardiac" distance available was 4.6 ± 1.6 cm (with a range of 1.8 to 7.3 cm).

These results do not contradict Kouwenhoven et al. [12] in suggesting that part of the heart may not be directly compressed between bony structures when moving the sternum dorsally for up to 5.1 cm to cover the mean value of 4.2 cm between bony and cardiac structures. Initially noted in clinical instructions adjusting the compression depth to the individual characteristics of the patient has recently resurfaced as a brief aside [1]. With part of the cardiac structure subject to direct compression, notably the right atrium and to a lesser degree the right ventricle, it remains difficult to explain significant size reduction of the left ventricle reported in clinical and animal echocardiographic studies, even when supposed restrictive aspects of the pericardium are incorporated [63,64].

These experimental observations lead to the conclusion that CCCR is not, in general, imitation of OCCR, because the heart, as a whole, and in particular the left ventricle, is not in the line of compression and the space to be bridged is too large.

18.4.3 Description of a Model to Assist Analysis

Careful formulation and development of mathematical expressions offer a way to resolve some of the difficulties mentioned above between the differing conceptual models in CPR. Figure 18.2 shows a schematic of the cardiovascular closed loop, consisting of eight blocks, anatomically identified in the figure. Cardiovascular events within each block are specified by algebraic and differential equations, as needed. The equations contain the unknown blood pressure and blood flow variables as they relate to parameters covering effects of the viscous and inertial properties of blood, elastic properties of heart and vessels, controls, such as ventricular stimulation and relaxation, and valves. The blocks are interconnected as dictated by anatomical and physiological requirements. These equations permit inclusion of local, regional, or global respiratory influences at the discretion of the user. By defining terms with the circulation, that is, the peripheral resistance, and keeping this constant without the use of drugs, the effect of compression force on the heart can be measured as a single variable.

The results of a long-ranging effort to restrict the size of models to their dominant features by elimination of small effects or details no longer popular were incorporated throughout [65]. This action had a significant effect on the number of equations, currently standing at around 50, replacing several hundreds originally [66]. Such reduction must be carried out judiciously; arbitrary reduction of the size may have ruinous effects on the behavior of the model, pointed out as early as 1943 by Landes [67]. In addition

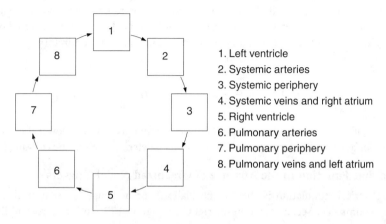

1. Left ventricle
2. Systemic arteries
3. Systemic periphery
4. Systemic veins and right atrium
5. Right ventricle
6. Pulmonary arteries
7. Pulmonary periphery
8. Pulmonary veins and left atrium

FIGURE 18.2 Schematic of the circulatory model. Each of the eight blocks represents one section in the model. The two ventricles (blocks 1 and 5) feature both inlet and outlet valves.

careful use of physiologic data for each parameter is required. Inasmuch as the heart plays a central role in this chapter, its model will be described in more detail in this section.

It will be recalled that the Frank mechanism [68] deals with isovolumetric contraction, while Patterson and Starling's observations [69] focus on the ejecting ventricle. Both phenomena can be integrated into a single analytical expression describing ventricular pressure, p_v, as a function of ventricular volume, V_v, and time, t, formally written as $p_v(V_v, t)$. From experiments on isolated dog hearts, it was found

$$p_v(V_v, t) = \pm a(V_v - b)^2 + (cV_v - d)f(t) \tag{18.1}$$

The first term on the right, applying to the relaxed ventricle, is complemented by the second term, which covers systolic augmentation of pressure. The parameter a relates to diastolic compliance, and b denotes the diastolic volume for which the pressure equals zero. The negative sign applies only to the first term on the right and only when $V_v < b$, manifesting a suction effect at small volumes. In the second term on the right the parameters c and d determine the volume related and volume unrelated components of developed pressure. The normalized function $f(t)$ describes crossbridge formation and detachment [70,71].

Comparison between predicted (Equation 18.1) and measured pressure curves exposed the so-called ejection effect: early into ejection the predicted pressure is higher, later in ejection it is lower than the measured one (akin to Hill's 1938 force–velocity relation). To include the ejection effect quantitatively, the function $f(t)$ must be modified and Equation 18.1 becomes

$$p_v(V_v, t, Q_{ej}) = \pm a(V_v - b)^2 + (cV_v - d)F(t, Q_{ej}) \tag{18.2}$$

with

$$F(t, Q_{ej}) = f(t) - k_1 Q_{ej}(t) + k_2 Q_{ej}^2(t - k_3 t) \tag{18.3}$$

in which Q_{ej} denotes ejection flow, while k_1, k_2, and k_3 are parameters [72].

Equation 18.2 may be further generalized by inclusion of the pericardium and by taking into account the detrimental effect of ventricular overfilling [73].

Much of the criticism of the interpretation of Starling's original measured input–output relations was resolved by the introduction of a family of cardiac function curves [74], which accommodated neural and metabolic stimulation of the heart. Such influences manifest themselves in graphs of input (preload)–output (stroke volume, stroke work, etc.) as counter clockwise rotation (steeper) and stretch along the output (vertical) axis. Alteration in parameter c in Equation 18.1 and Equation 18.2 carries major responsibility for these modifications. In addition, it has recently been found that the cardiac function curve can be shifted along the horizontal (preload) axis [75]. This shift is effected by changes in air pressure, p_e, external to the cardiac chambers, such as caused by the respiratory system, or by CPR, and modifies Equation 18.2 by approximation to

$$p_v(V_v, t, Q_{ej}) - p_e = \pm a(V_v - b)^2 + (cV_v - d)F(t, Q_{ej}) \tag{18.4}$$

The new term, p_e, if negative as during inhalation, shifts the function curve to lower preloads, if positive to higher ones. For additional information about the model, Reference 76 may be consulted.

18.4.3.1 Cardiac Function in the Absence of Organized Nodal Triggers

If the heart's electrical stimulation is chaotic (fibrillation), or no longer present at all (asystole), its chambers fail to pump. The second term on the right in Equation 18.1 tends to zero, and Equation 18.1 degenerates to

$$p_v = a(V_v - b)^2 + p_e \tag{18.5}$$

Returning to CPR, the second term on the right in Equation 18.5 is now the application of external pressure, either directly as in the "cardiac" pump theory, or via general intrathoracic pressure increase as in the "thoracic" pump theory.

With positive p_e, as occurs in chest compression, ventricular blood pressure is raised by an amount p_e and ejection is promoted. There is reason to believe, however, that venous return will be impeded by the presence of this same p_e, resulting in the possibility of ejecting less blood at a higher rate of flow.

18.4.4   Impedance-Defined Flow

William Harvey [77] taught that the heart is the only pump that propels blood around the closed circulatory loop. Liebau [78], on the other hand, based on experiments with fluid mechanical models of his own design, concluded that blood could be propelled around the loop without the benefit of cardiac and venous valves. Liebau demonstrated with his simplest model, consisting of two tubes with different elastic properties, free of valves, making a closed water-filled loop, that periodic compression at an appropriate, fixed site caused steady net fluid flow around the loop, but could not explain the reason why this occurred. The explanation, developed in 1998 [57], was that Liebau worked with an asymmetric loop to which he provided energy by periodic compression at some site. This was termed impedance defined flow, in view of the nonuniform distribution of impedances around the loop. (Compression at a symmetric point, if any, generates no steady net flow, either experimentally or theoretically.)

There is, therefore no doubt whether flow can be generated in a closed loop, free of valves. Thus, it becomes of interest to determine whether the far more complex closed cardiovascular loop qualifies. Two conditions make it a candidate in principle. The first is in the human embryo, which by the end of the third week has a coordinated heart beat, that is, local compression, prior to the formation of cardiac valves about a week later [79]. The second can reportedly occur in total circulatory and respiratory collapse during the application of CPR [80].

In the postembryonic normal circulation at least two cardiac valves are always closed. This makes inapplicable the valveless closed loop, though the impedance-defined flow principle remains intact, but now at the local or regional level. This can easily be appreciated without looking in detail at the corresponding mathematical analysis. The presence of ventricular exit valves, in conjunction with high peripheral resistances results in two high-pressure reservoirs, one in the systemic, the other in the pulmonary arteries. From the peripheral resistances onward to the corresponding ventricles, impedances become smaller and pressures drop, together promoting return flow to the heart in the presence of local compression. Local compression, or contraction, occurs at many sites, including in the venules (venomotion) at the terminations of the microvasculature.

However, this set of conditions cannot remain satisfied indefinitely around a closed loop. At some point, a transformation of impedance levels must necessarily take place. Nature has solved this problem by the insertion of two sets of valves in the heart, three sets not being required [66].

If, for any reason, the heart continues to contract and relax without functional valves (open conduit), conditions revert to those visualized by Liebau, but net cardiac output reduces to a negligible level. Noordergraaf et al. [71] measured less than 60 ml/min on the model referred to earlier without valves and around 5000 ml/min with valves. This invalidates Liebau's suggestion that the cardiac valves might be superfluous.

18.4.5   Summary of This Section

Previous research in CPR appears to have focused on variations of the standard method and their validation, on the design of mechanical models, on experiments in animals in which the chest has a different shape as well as different mechanical properties, rather than on the basic features fundamental to CPR.

New research suggests that the *key function of CPR is reestablishment of cardiac valvular function* in a patient who presents with the same low blood pressure all around the cardiovascular loop.

18.5 Expectations and Current Developments

Thinking in cardiopulmonary resuscitation has, over the last decennium, seen a return to fundamentals. This restored interest in why CPR may or may not lead to survival has surpassed the tendency to expect improvements based solely on adaptation of techniques as well as simplification of techniques and is focusing more and more on understanding the circulation.

Looking forward to the "consensus in science on CPR," representing a new international standard for care in cardiopulmonary resuscitation, with both European and American (ILCOR) collaboration and expected in 2005, laboratory and clinical investigations may be focusing on a number of issues:

Modeling, using up-to-date computing and mathematical opportunities and based on valid physiological and pathophysiological data may become a leading resource in increasing understanding by allowing greater control over variables involved in CPR, while avoiding limitations created by animal and laboratory conditions. The selection and careful use of one animal substrate including correlation to human chest diameters should contribute less equivocal data [81].

Recent clinical insights may also further understanding, such as the effect of the changing compliance of the myocardium (stone heart) over time following circulatory collapse [82], and sufficient decrease in intrathoracic pressure to allow for venous return (i.e., decrease of ventilation frequency and volume), decrease in adrenergic medication, reduction in the amount of time to commencement of cardiac compressions, overfilling of the right heart, and a realistic analysis of clinical technique during CPR. These can all lay groundwork for fundamental improvements.

18.6 Summary

Open-chest cardiac resuscitation was introduced in the 19th century as a surgical procedure to force the ventricles to expel their volumes. It was replaced through Kouwenhoven's influence, by the noninvasive CCCR procedure that gained popularity after 1960. Kouwenhoven's instructions on how to apply CCCR are taught today virtually intact, though it quickly had become apparent that survival rates left much to be desired.

There has been no lack of efforts to improve outcome. In an attempt to achieve better understanding [83], literal Kouwenhoven adherents believe in what became known as the "cardiac" pump theory, while other investigators prefer the "thoracic" pump theory, since they believe that alterations in intrathoracic pressure prevail. A wide variety in "adjuvant" techniques — most but not all of them paralleling either of the two theories — was conceived and developed. Thus far, little of this effort has borne fruit convincingly.

The new century gave rise to a more basic approach. Fundamental models, using computers were introduced. As known, but not applied, it was found, with the aid of CT scans, that the ventricles are not compressed by impression of the sternum for two reasons: impression may often be too shallow and at least the left ventricle is outside the main line of compression; hence CCCR is not a straight imitation of OCCR as had been assumed.

In addition, investigators of impedance-defined flow found that when all cardiac valves are open (open conduit [80]) flow around a closed loop reduces to negligible values even when ventricular contraction is normal. Hence, CPR as a technique, should attempt to reestablish (at least part of) valvular operation in order to allow for survival of a heart too good to die.

References

[1] Guidelines 2000 for cardiopulmonary resuscitation and emergency cardiovascular care. *JAMA*, 102, I-1–384, 2000.

[2] Husveti, S. and Ellis, H. Janos Balassa, pioneer of cardiac resuscitation. *Anaesthesia*, 24, 113–115, 1969.

[3] Pike, F.H., Gurthie, C.C., and Steward, G.N. Studies in resuscitation: 1. The general considerations affecting resuscitation of the blood and the heart. *J. Exp. Med.*, 10, 371–418, 1908.

[4] Zesas D.G., Über Massage des freigelegten Herzens beim Chloroformkollaps. *Zentralblatt für Chirurgie.* 30, 588, 1903.

[5] Keen, W.W. Case of total laryngectomy (unsuccessful) and a case of abdominal hysterectomy (successful) in both of which massage of the heart for chloroform collapse was employed, with notes of 25 other cases of cardiac massage. *Ther. Gaz.*, 28, 217, 1904.

[6] Hake, T. Studies on ether and chloroform from Prof. Schiff's physiological laboratory. *Practitioner*, 12, 241, 1874.

[7] Stephenson, H.E. Jr., Read, L.C., and Hinton, J.W. Some common denominators in 1200 cases of cardiac arrest. *Ann. Surg.*, 137, 731–744, 1953.

[8] Briggs, B.D., Sheldon, D.B., and Beecher, H.K. Cardiac arrest: study in a 30 year period of operating room deaths at Massachusett General Hospital (1925–1954). *JAMA*, 160, 1439–1444, 1956.

[9] Altemeier, W.A. and Todd, J. Studies on the incidence of infection following open-chest cardiac massage for cardiac arrest. *Ann. Surg.*, 158, 596–607, 1963.

[10] Geehr, E.C. Failure of open-heart massage to improve survival after prehospital cardiac arrests. *N. Engl. J. Med.*, 314, 1189–1190, 1986.

[11] Koenig, F. *Lehrbuch der Allgemeinen Chirurgie.* Göttingen, pp. 60–61, 1883.

[12] Kouwenhoven, W.B., Jude, J.R., and Knickerbocker, G.G. Closed chest cardiac massage. *JAMA*, 173, 1064–1067, 1960.

[13] Kouwenhoven, W.B., Jude, J.R., and Knickerbocker, G.G. Closed-chest cardiac massage. *Circulation*, 173, 94–97, 1960.

[14] Jude, J.R., Kouwenhoven, W.B., and Knickerbocker, G.G. Cardiac arrest. Report of application of external cardiac massage on 118 patients. *JAMA*, 178, 1063–1071, 1961.

[15] Redding, J.S. and Cozine, R.A. A comparison of open chest and closed chest cardiac massage in dogs. *Anesthesia*, 22, 280–285, 1961.

[16] Redberg, R.F., Tucker, K.J., Cohen, T.J., Dutton, J.P., Callahan, M.L., and Schiller, N.B. Physiology of blood flow during cardiopulmonary resuscitation: a transesophageal echocardiographic study. *Circulation*, 88, 534–542, 1993.

[17] Halperin, H.R., Tsitlik, J.E., Geurci, A.D., Mellits, E.D., Levin, H.R., Shi, A.Y., Chandra, N., and Weisfeldt, M.L. Determinants of blood flow to vital organs during cardiopulmonary resuscitation in dogs. *Circulation*, 73, 539–550, 1986.

[18] Weale, F.E. External cardiac massage (letter to the editor). *Lancet*, I, 172, 1961.

[19] Criley, M., Blaufuss, A.H., and Kissel, G.L. Cough-induced cardiac compression: self administrated form of cardiopulmonary resuscitation. *JAMA*, 236, 1246–1250, 1976.

[20] Babbs, C.F. New versus old theories of blood flow during cardiopulmonary resuscitation. *Crit. Care Med.*, 8, 191–195, 1980.

[21] Wenzel,V., Padosch, S.A., Voelckel, W.G., Idris, A.H., Krismer, A.C., Bettsch, A., Wolfensberger, R., and Linder, K.H. Survey of effects of anesthesia protocols on hemodynamic variables in porcine cardiopulmonary resuscitation laboratory models before induction of cardiac arrest. *Comp. Med.*, 50, 644–648, 2000.

[22] Hannon, J.P., Bossone, C.A., and Wade, C.E. Normal physiological values for conscious pigs used in biomedical research. *Lab. Animal Sci.*, 40, 293–298, 1990.

[23] Wilder, R.J., Weir, D., Rush, B.F., and Ravitch, M.M. Methods of coordinating ventilation and closed chest cardiac massage in the dog. *Surgery*, 53, 186–194, 1963.

[24] Harris, L.C., Kirimli, B., and Safar, P. Ventilation — cardiac compression rates and ratios in cardiopulmonary resuscitation. *Anesthesia*, 28, 806–813, 1967.

[25] Chandra, N.C., Rudikoff, M., and Weisfeldt, M.L. Simultaneous chest compression and ventilation at high airway pressure during cardiopulmonary resuscitation. *Lancet*, I, 175–178, 1980.

[26] Krischer, J.P., Fine, E.G., Weisfeldt, M.L., Geurci, A.D., Nagel, E., and Chandra, N.C. Comparison of prehospital conventional and simultaneous compression ventilation cardiopulmonary resuscitation. *Crit. Care Med.*, 17, 1263–1269, 1989.

[27] Harris, L.C., Kirimli, B., and Safar, P. Augmentation of artificial circulation during cardiopulmonary resuscitation. *Anesthesia*, 28, 730–734, 1967.

[28] Chandra, N.C., Snyder, L.D., and Weisfeldt, M.L. Abdominal binding during cardiopulmonary resuscitation. *JAMA*, 246, 351–353, 1981.

[29] Niemann, J.T., Rosborough, J.P., Hausknecht, M., Garner, D., and Criley, J.M. Pressure-synchronized cineangiography during experimental cardiopulmonary resuscitation. *Circulation*, 64, 985–991, 1981.

[30] Nicol, G., Stiel, I.G., Laupais, A., De Mario, V.J., and Wells, G.A. A cumulative meta-analysis of the effectivity of defibrillator capable emergency medical services for victims of out-of-hospital cardiac arrest. *Ann. Emerg. Med.*, 34, 517–525, 1999.

[31] Niemann, J.T., Rosborough, J., Hausknecht, M., Brown, D., and Criley, J.M. Cough-CPR: documentation of systemic perfusion in man and in an experimental model: a "window" to the mechanism of blood flow in external CPR. *Crit. Care Med.*, 8, 141–146, 1980.

[32] Birch, L.H., Kenny, L.J., Doornbos, F., Kosht, D.W., and Barkalow, C.E. A study of external compression. *J. Mich. State Med. Soc.*, 61, 1346–1352, 1962.

[33] Taylor, G.J., Tucker, W.M., Greene, H.L., Rudikoff, M.T., and Weisfeldt, M.L. Importance of prolonged compression during cardiopulmonary resuscitation in man. *N. Engl. J. Med.*, 296, 1515–1517, 1977.

[34] Chandra, N.C., Cohen, J.M., Tsitlik, J., and Weisfeldt, M.L. Negative airway pressure between compressions augments flow during CPR. *Circulation*, 60, 46–46, 1979.

[35] Bircher, N., Safar, P., and Steward, R. A comparison of standard, "MAST" augmented, and open-chest CPR in dogs. *Crit. Care Med.*, 8, 147–152, 1980.

[36] Rosborough, J.P., Niemann, J.T., and Criley, J.M. Lower abdominal compression with synchronized ventilation — a CPR modality. *Circulation*, 64, 303–309, 1981.

[37] Plaisance, P., Lurie, K.G., Vicaut, E., Martin, D., Gueugniaud, P.Y., Petit, J.L., and Payen, D. Evaluation of an impedance threshold device in patients receiving active compression–decompression cardiopulmonary resuscitation for out of hospital cardiac arrest. *Resuscitation*, 61, 265–271, 2004.

[38] Voorhees, W.D., Niebauer, M.J., and Babbs, C.F. Improved oxygen delivery during cardiopulmonary resuscitation with interposed abdominal compressions. *Ann. Emerg. Med.*, 12, 128–135, 1983.

[39] Babbs, C.F. Interposed abdominal compression CPR: a comprehensive evidence based review. *Resuscitation*, 59, 71–82, 2003.

[40] Maier, G.W., Tyson, G.S., Olsen, C.O., Kernstein, K.H., Davis, J.W., Conn, E.H., Sabiston, D.C., and Rankin, J.S. The physiology of external cardiac massage: high-impulse cardiopulmonary resuscitation. *Circulation*, 70, 86–101, 1984.

[41] Halperin, H.R., Guerci, A.D., Chandra, N., Herskowitz, A., Tsitlik, J.E., Niskanen, R.A., Wurmb, E., and Weisfeldt, M.L. Vest inflation without simultaneous ventilation during cardiac arrest in dogs: improved survival from prolonged cardiopulmonary resuscitation. *Circulation*, 74, 1407–1415, 1986.

[42] Halperin, H.R., Tsitlik, J.E., Gelfand, M., Myron, M.S., Weisfeldt, M.L., Gruben, K.G., Levin, H.R., Raybun, B.K., Chandra, N.C., Scott, C.J., Kreps, B.J., Siu, C.O., and Guerci, A.D. A preliminary study of cardiopulmonary resuscitation by circumferential compression of the chest with the use of a pneumatic vest. *N. Engl. J. Med.*, 329, 762–768, 1993.

[43] Barranco, F., Lesmes, A., Irles, J.A., Blasco, J., Leal, J., Rodriquez, J., and Leon, C. Cardiopulmonary resuscitation with simultaneous chest and abdominal compression: comparative study in humans. *Resuscitation*, 20, 67–77, 1990.

[44] Cohen, T.J., Tucker, K.J., Lurie, K.G., Redberg, R.F., Dutton, J.P., Dwyer, K.A., Scwab, T.M., Chin, M.C., Gelb, A.M., Scheinman, M.M., Schiller, N.B., and Callaham, M.L. Active compression–decompression: a new method of cardiopulmonary resuscitation. *JAMA*, 267, 2916–2923, 1992.

[45] Patterson, S.W. and Starling, E.H. On the mechanical factors which determine the output of the ventricles. *J. Physiol.*, 48, 357–379, 1914.

[46] Lafeunte-Lafuente, C. and Melero-Bascones, M. Active chest compression–decompression for cardiopulmonary resuscitation. *Cochrane Database Syst. Rev.*, 2, CD002751, 2004.

[47] Steen, S., Liao, Q., Pierre, L., Paskevicius, A., and Sjoberg, T. Evaluation of LUCAS, a new device for automatic mechanical compression and active decompression resuscitation. *Resuscitation*, 55, 285–299, 2002.

[48] Buckman, R.F. Jr., Badellino, M.M., Mauro, L.H., Aldridge, S.C., Milner, R.E., Malaspina, P.J., Merchant, N.B., and Buckman, R.F. III. Direct cardiac massage without major thoracotomy feasibility and systemic blood flow. *Resuscitation*, 29, 237–248, 1995.

[49] Rozenberg, A., Incagnoli, P., Delpech, P., Spaulding, C., Vivien, B., Kern, K., and Carli, P. Prehospital use of minimally invasive direct cardiac massage (MID-CM): a pilot study. *Resuscitation*, 50, 257–262, 2001.

[50] Adams, J.A., Mangino, M.J., Bassuk, J., Kurlansky, P., and Sackner, M.A. Novel CPR with periodic Gz acceleration. *Resuscitation*, 51, 55–62, 2001.

[51] Lurie, K.G., Coffen, P., Shultz, J., McKnite, S., Detloff, B., and Mulligan, K. Improving active compression–decompression cardiopulmonary resuscitation with an inspiratory impedance valve. *Circulation*, 92, 1629–1632, 1995.

[52] Plaisance, P., Adnet, F., Vicaut, E., Hennquin, B., Magne, P., Prudhomme, C., Lambert, Y., Cantineau, J.P., Leopold, C., Ferracci, C., Gizzi, M., and Payen, D. Benefit of active compression–decompression cardiopulmonary resuscitation as a prehospital advanced cardiac life support. *Circulation*, 95, 955–961, 1997.

[53] Schafer, E.A. Artificial respiration in its physiologic aspects. *JAMA*, LI, 801–803, 1908.

[54] Brown, J., Rogers, J., and Soar, J. Cardiac arrest during surgery and ventilation in the prone position: a case report and systematic review. *Resuscitation*, 50, 233–238, 2001.

[55] Steward, J.A. Resuscitating an idea: prone CPR. *Resuscitation*, 54, 231–236, 2002.

[56] Noordergraaf, G.J., Van Tilborg, G.F.A.J.B., Schoonen, J.A.P., Ottesen, J.T., and Noordergraaf, A. 2004. Thoracic CT-scans and cardiovascular models: the effect of external force in CPR. *Int. J. Cardiov. Med. Sci.*, 5(1), 1–7, 2005.

[57] Moser, M., Huang, J.W., Schwarz, G.S., Kenner, T., and Noordergraaf, A. Impedance defined flow. Generalisation of William Harvey's concept of the circulation — 370 years later. *Int. J. Cardiov. Med. Sci.*, 1, 205–211, 1998.

[58] Knickerbocker, G.G. Evaluation of CPR manikins. *Health Dev.*, 10, 228–246, 1981.

[59] Baubin, M.A., Gilly, H., Posch, A., Schinnerl, A., and Kroesen, G.A. Compression characteristics of CPR manikins. *Resuscitation*, 30, 117–126, 1995.

[60] Gruben, K.G., Halperin, H.R., Popel, A.S., and Tsitlik, J.E. Canine sternal force–displacement relationship during cardiopulmonary resuscitation. *IEEE Trans. Biomed. Eng.*, 46, 788–796, 1999.

[61] Bankman, I.N., Gruben, K.G., Halperin, H.R., Popel, A.S., Geurci, A.D., and Tsitlik, J.E. Identification of dynamic mechanical parameters of the human chest during manual CPR. *IEEE Trans. Biomed. Eng.*, 37, 211–217, 1990.

[62] Babbs, C.F., Voorhees, W.D., Fitzgerald, K.R., Holmes, E.R., and Geddes L.A. Relationship of blood pressure and flow during CPR to chest compression amplitude: evidence for an effective compression threshold. *Ann. Emerg. Med.*, 12, 527–532, 1983.

[63] Ralston, S.H., Babbs, C.F., and Niebauer, M.J. Cardiopulmonary resuscitation with interposed abdominal compression in dogs. *Anesth. Analg.*, 61, 645–651, 1982.

[64] Klouche, K., Weil, M.H., Sun, S., Tang, W., Provoas, H., and Bisera, J. Stroke volumes generated by precordial compressions during cardiac resuscitation. *Crit. Care Med.*, 30, 2626–2631, 2002.

[65] Noordergraaf, G.J., Dijkema, T.J., Kortsmit, W.J.P.M., Schilders, W.H.A., Scheffer, G.J., and Noordergraaf, A. Modeling in cardiopulmonary resuscitation: pumping the heart. *Cardiovascular Engineering*, 5(3), 105–118, 2005.

[66] Noordergraaf, A. *Circulatory System Dynamics*. Academic Press, New York, 1978.

[67] Landes, G. Einige Untersuchungen an electrischen Analogieschaltungen zum Kreislaufsystem. *Z. Biol.*, 101, 418–429, 1943.

[68] Frank, O. Die Grundform des arteriellen Pulsus. *Z. Biol.*, 37, 483–526, 1899.

[69] Palladino, J.L., Drzewiecki, G.M., and Noordergraaf, A. *Modeling Strategies in Physiology*. CRC Handbook, 3rd ed., Chap. 8.

[70] Mulier, J.P. Ventricular pressure as a function of volume and flow. Ph.D. dissertation, Catholic University of Leuven, 1994.

[71] Noordergraaf, G.J., Schilders, W.H.A., Scheffer, G.J., and Noordergraaf, A. Essential factors in CPR? Modeling and clinical aspects. (Abstract) Annual meeting Dutch Society of Anesthesiology. Amsterdam, NL, Sept 30, 2005.

[72] Danielsen, M., Palladino, J.L., and Noordergraaf, A. The left ventricular ejection effect. In *Mathematical Modelling in Medicine*. Ottesen. J.T. and Danielsen, M. (Eds.), IOS Press, Amsterdam, 2000, pp. 3–11.

[73] Niemann, J.T., Rosborough, J.P., and Pelikan, P.C. Hemodynamic determinants of subdiaphragmatic venous return during closed-chest CPR in a canine cardiac arrest model. *Ann. Emerg. Med.*, 19, 1232–1237, 1990.

[74] Sarnoff, S.J. and Berglund, E. Ventricular function I. Starling's law of the heart studied by means of simultaneous right and left ventricular function curves in the dog. *Circulation*, IX, 706–719, 1954.

[75] Noordergraaf, A. *Blood in Motion*. Springer-Verlag, New York, N.Y., 2006.

[76] Palladino, J.L. and Noordergraaf, A., Muscle contraction mechanics from ultrastructural dynamics. In *Analysis and Assessment of Cardiovascular Function*. Drzewiecki, G.M. and Li, J.K-J. (Eds.), Chap. 3, Springer, New York, 1998.

[77] Harvey, G. *Exercitatio Anatomica, de motu Cordis Et Sanguinis in Animalibus*, Frankford, 1628.

[78] Liebau, G. Möglichkeit der Förderung des Blutes im Herz- und Gefäszsystem ohne Herz- und Venenklappenfunktion. *Verh. Deutschen Ges. Kreislauff.*, 22. Tagung. Seite 354–359, 1956.

[79] Moore, K.L. *Embryology*. Schattauer, Stuttgart, 2nd ed., pp. 340–358, 1985.

[80] Swenson, R.D., Weaver, W.D., Niskanen, R.A., Martin, J., and Dahlberg, S. Hemodynamics in humans during conventional and experimental methods of cardiopulmonary resuscitation. *Circulation*, 78, 630–663, 1988.

[81] Steen, S., Liao, Q., Pierre, L., Paskevicius, A., and Sjöberg, T. The critical importance of minimal delay between chest compressions and subsequent defibrillation: a hemodynamic explanation. *Resuscitation*, 58, 249–258, 2003.

[82] Takino, M. and Okada, Y. Firm myocardium in cardiopulmonary resuscitation. *Resuscitation*, 33, 101–106, 1996.

[83] Rudikoff, M.T., Maughan, W.L., Effron, M., Freund, P., and Weisfeldt, M.L. Mechanism of blood flow during cardiopulmonary resuscitation. *Circulation*, 61, 345–352, 1980.

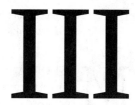

III

Bioelectric Phenomena

William M. Smith

University of Alabama at Birmingham

MOST ORGANS DEPEND IN SOME WAY on electrical currents for proper function. Disruptions in normal electrophysiology can lead to serious, sometimes fatal, pathology. The currents, composed of moving ions, are the culmination of complex cellular and subcellular processes that have been and continue to be the subjects of intense investigation. In some cases, notably the brain, the currents are the immediate mediators of the ultimate role of the organ. In others, for example the heart, the currents control other processes, in this case mechanical activity, that lead to the fulfillment of the role of the organ. In either case, appropriate bioelectric activity is a necessary condition for normal physiology. Because of the centrality of bioelectricity and biomagnetics to the maintenance of health and homeostasis, many experimental and theoretical techniques have been developed to study them. This section of *The Biomedical Engineering Handbook* explores many of them and some important results that have been attained by their use.

Chapter 19 introduces the basic concepts of bioelectricity. These include the cellular level currents and voltages that initiate electrical events; the manner by which electrical currents are propagated through excitable tissue; the mechanism by which microscopic phenomena give rise to macroscopic, measurable variables; and the relationship between bioelectricity and biomagnetism. Much of what we measure in medicine and physiology are biopotentials at a distance from the source, seen through conducting but inexcitable tissue. Chapter 20 provides a mathematical basis for understanding the effects of these volume conductors. Chapter 21 provides a valuable discussion of the electrical conductivities of tissue. An understanding of basic substrate characteristics is necessary for carrying out effective experiments and formulating accurate and relevant mathematical models. For many years, investigators have sought a complete understanding of the activity of the cell membrane in excitable tissue. Chapter 22 is a description of the functional role of the membrane in a wide variety of cell types in regulation of the biochemical and electrophysiological environments of tissue. Chapter 23 provides a description of how rigorous, verified numerical techniques have been adapted and extended to accommodate models of electrophysiological phenomena. One of the first investigations into bioelectricity and its clinical and physiological importance was the development of the electrocardiogram. Chapter 24 recounts the history, physiological basis, instrumentation, and applications of the ECG. Another, less well studied, clinical application is electromyography, the study of the electrophysiological phenomena associated with skeletal muscle, described in Chapter 25. Of course, a major application of bioelectric recording and analysis is in the brain, where the electroencephalogram (EEG) reveals important information concerning physiology and pathology. Chapter 26 is a complete account of the use of the EEG. The electrical currents in tissue give rise to magnetic fields. In some applications, the acquisition and analysis of these fields using magnetocardiography and magnetoencephalography yield complementary information about the underlying processes, as described in Chapter 27. Most excitable cells require an external stimulus for activation. The stimulus can be either biochemical or electrical. Chapter 28 presents the theory and practice of stimulating tissue.

Thus, this section contains a quite broad presentation of the topic of bioelectric phenomena. At the same time, there is sufficient depth to allow an appreciation of the complexity and subtlety of the beautiful processes involved. These chapters should provide the reader with enough basic information to allow him or her to select more focused reading as necessary.

19

Basic Electrophysiology

Roger C. Barr
Duke University

19.1 Membranes

Bioelectricity has its origin in the voltage differences present between the inside and outside of cells. These potentials arise from the specialized properties of the cell membrane, which separates the intracellular from the extracellular volume. From the perspective of electrophysiology, cell membranes are not just containers separating intracellular from extracellular volumes, rather, membranes are the site of the electrically active elements — pumps, channels, and connexons joining cells — that create the voltages and currents that cause electrical events to occur. (In contrast, both intracellular and extracellular volumes serve largely as passive conductors of current, though differences in ionic concentrations between inside and outside are large and electrically significant.) Much of the membrane surface is made of a phospholipid bilayer, an electrically inert material [Byrne and Schultz, 1988]. Because the membrane is thin (about 75 Å), it has a high capacitance, about 1 uF/cm^2. (Membrane capacitance is less in nerve, except at nodes, because most of the membrane is myelinated, which makes it much thicker.)

Electrically active membrane also includes a number of integral proteins of different kinds, with genetic origins that are increasingly well understood [Marban, 1999]. Integral proteins are compact but complex structures extending across the membrane. Each integral protein is composed of a large number of amino acids, often in a single long polypeptide chain, which folds into multiple domains. Each domain may span the membrane several times. The multiple crossings may build the functional structure, for example, a channel, through which electrically charged ions may flow. The structure of integral proteins is loosely analogous to that of a length of thread passing back and forth across a fabric to form a buttonhole. As a buttonhole allows movement of a button from one side of the fabric to the other, an integral protein may allow passage of ions from the exterior of a cell to the interior, or vice versa. In contrast to a buttonhole, an integral protein has active properties, for example, the ability to open or close. Excellent drawings of channel structure and function are given by Watson et al. [1992].

Cell membrane possesses a number of active characteristics of marked importance to its bioelectric behavior, including these (1) Some integral proteins function as pumps. These pumps use energy to transport ions across membrane, working against a concentration gradient, a voltage gradient, or both. The most important pump moves sodium ions out of the intracellular volume and potassium ions in. (2) Other integral proteins function as channels, that is, openings through the membrane that open and close over time. These channels can function selectively so that, for a particular kind of channel, only sodium ions may pass through. Another kind of channel may allow only potassium ions or calcium ions. (3) The activity of the membrane's integral proteins is modulated by signals specific to its particular function. For example, some channels open or close in response to photons or to odorants; thus they function as sensors for light or smell. Pumps respond to the concentrations of the ions they move. Rapid electrical impulse transmission in nerve and muscle is made possible by changes that respond to the **transmembrane potential** itself, forming a feedback mechanism. These active mechanisms provide ion-selective means of current crossing the membrane, both against the concentration or voltage gradients (pumps) or in response to them (channels). While the pumps build up the concentration differences (and thereby the potential energy) that allow events to occur, channels utilize this energy actively to create the fast changes in voltage and small intense current loops that constitute nerve signal transmission, initiate muscle contraction, and participate in other essential bioelectric phenomena.

19.2   Bioelectric Current Loops

Because of the electrical conductivity of tissues, voltages generated across cell membranes are associated with currents that flow across the membrane in the surrounding tissues. Bioelectricity normally flows in current loops, as illustrated in Figure 19.1. A loop includes four segments: an outward traversal of the cell membrane (current I_m^1 at position $z = z_1$), an extracellular segment (current I_e, along a path outside a cell or cells), an inward traversal of the cell membrane (current I_m^2 at $z = z_2$), and an intracellular segment (current I_i, along a segment inside the cell membrane). Each of the segments has aspects that give it a unique importance to the current loop. Intense current loops often are contained within a millimeter or less, although loops of weaker intensity may extend throughout the whole body volume. The energy that supports the current flow arises from one or both of the segments of the loop that cross the membrane. Current loops involve potential differences of about 100 mV between extremes. The charge carriers are mobile ions. Especially important are ions of sodium, potassium, calcium, and chloride because some membranes allow one or more of these ion species to move across when others cannot. Such current loops not only exist within tissue but in electrically active tissue often modify the electrical state of surrounding tissue in such a way that the loop propagates along a nerve or muscle.

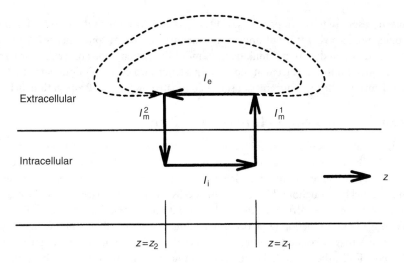

FIGURE 19.1 Bioelectric current loop, concept drawing. Current enters the membrane at $z = z_1$, flows intracellularly and emerges at z_2. Flow in the extracellular volume may be along the membrane (solid) or throughout the surrounding volume conductor (dashed).

19.2.1 Membrane Currents

Total membrane current I_m may be given mathematically as

$$I_m = I_c + I_{ion} \qquad (19.1)$$

where each of these currents often is given per unit area, for example, milliamperes per square centimeter.

The first component, I_c, corresponds to the charging or discharging of the membrane capacitance. Thus

$$I_c = C_m \frac{\partial V_m}{\partial t} \qquad (19.2)$$

where C_m is the membrane capacitance per unit area, V_m is the transmembrane voltage, and t is time.

The second component, I_{ion}, corresponds to the current through the membrane carried by ions such as those of sodium, potassium, or calcium. It normally is found by summing each of the individual components, for example,

$$I_{ion} = I_K + I_{Na} + I_{Ca} \qquad (19.3)$$

In turn, each of the component currents is often written in a form such as

$$I_K = g_K (V_m - E_K) \qquad (19.4)$$

where E_K is the equilibrium potential for K (see below), a function of K concentrations, and g_K is the conductivity of the membrane to K ions. The conductivity g_K is not constant but rather varies markedly as a function of transmembrane voltage and time. More positive transmembrane voltages normally are associated with higher conductivities, at least transiently.

When a more detailed knowledge of channel structure is included, as in the DiFrancesco–Noble model for cardiac membrane, each of the individual ionic components, for example, I_K is found in turn as a sum of the currents through each kind of channel or pump through which that ion moves.

The total transmembrane current I_m contains the summed contributions from Ic and I_{ion}, as given by Equation 19.1 This equations holds at each site on the membrane at each time, that is, all three currents are functions of both space and time. Under most circumstances, when thinking of cause and effect, it is better for one to think of I_m as a value imposed on the cell by its environment, and I_c and I_{ion} as currents which change in response to the imposed I_m. (Often I_c is initially dominant, but subsides in magnitude as I_{ion} responds more slowly.) It is not unusual for membrane current components I_c and I_{ion} to differ both in magnitude and in direction. Thinking in terms of the current loops that exist during membrane **excitation**, one often finds that current at the site of peak outward current is dominated by I_c. At the site of peak inward current, the total current I_m usually dominated by I_{ion} (see **Propagation**, below).

19.2.2 Conduction along an Intracellular Path

Flow of electricity along a nerve or within a muscle occurs passively through the conducting medium inside the cell. The nature of the intracellular current path is closely related to the function of the current within that kind of cell. Nerve cells may have lengths of a meter or more, so intracellular currents can flow unimpeded and quickly throughout this length. Other cells, such as the muscle cells of the heart, are much smaller (about 100 mm in length). In cardiac cells, current flows intracellularly from cell to cell through specialized passages, called junctions, that occur in regions where the cell membranes fuse together. Thus intracellular regions may be connected over lengths of centimeters or more, even though each cell is much smaller. Mathematically, the intracellular current in a one-dimensional cable may be given as [Plonsey and Barr, 2000]

$$I_i = -\frac{1}{r_i}\frac{\partial \phi_i}{\partial z} \tag{19.5}$$

where, ϕ is the intracellular potential, z is the axial coordinate, r_i is the intracellular resistance per unit length, and I_i is the longitudinal axial current per unit cross-sectional area.

19.2.3 Conduction along an Extracellular Path

When current flows outside of cells, it is not constrained to a particular path but rather flows throughout the whole surrounding conducting volume, which may be the whole body. The study of these extracellular currents, and the effects of interfaces among structures, boundaries, and changes in conductivity is called **volume conductor** theory. Current intensity is highest near the places where current enters or leaves cells through the membrane. (These sites are called sinks and sources, respectively, in view of their relation to the extracellular volume.) Current flow from bioelectric sources through the volume conductor generates small potential differences, usually with a magnitude of a millivolt or less, between different sites within the volume or on the body surface. (Current flow from artificial sources, such as stimulators or defibrillators, may generate much higher voltages.) The naturally occurring potential differences between points in the volume conductor, for example, between the arms or across the head, are those commonly measured in the study of the heart (electrocardiography), the nerves and muscles (electromyography), and the brain (electroencephalography).

Mathematically, the extracellular current is easy to specify only in the special case where the extracellular current is confined to a small space surrounding a single fiber or nerve, as shown diagramatically by the solid I_e line in Figure 19.1. In this special case, the extracellular current is equal in magnitude (but opposite in direction) to the intracellular current, that is, $I_e = -I_i$.

In most living systems, however, extracellular currents extend throughout a more extensive volume conductor, as suggested by the dashed lines for I_e in Figure 19.1. Their direction and magnitude must be found as a solution to Poisson's equation in the extracellular medium, with the sources and sinks around the active medium used as boundary conditions. In this context, Poisson's equation becomes [Plonsey and Barr, 2000]

$$\nabla^2 \phi_e = -\frac{I_v}{\sigma_e} = -\frac{\nabla \cdot \vec{J}}{\sigma_e} \tag{19.6}$$

where I_v is the volume density of the sources (sinks being negative sources), σ_e is the conductivity of the extracellular medium, and J is the current density. The fact that, $\nabla \cdot \vec{J}$ takes on nonzero values appears at first to be physically unrealistic because it seems to violate the principle of conservation of charge. In fact, it only reflects the practice of solving for potentials and currents in the extracellular volume separately from those in the intracellular volume. Thus the nonzero divergence represents the movement of currents from the intracellular volume across the membrane and into the extracellular volume, where they appear from sources or disappear into sinks.

19.2.4 Duality

Note the duality Equation 19.6 and the form of Poisson's equation commonly used in problems in electrostatics. There, $\nabla^2/(-\rho/\varepsilon)$, where ρ is the charge density, and ε is the permittivity. Recognition of this duality is useful not only in locating solution methods for bioelectric problems, since the mathematics is the same, but also in avoiding confusion between electrostatics and problems of extracellular current flow through a volume conductor. The problems obviously are physically quite different (e.g., permittivity ε is not conductivity σ_e).

19.3 Membrane Polarization

Ionic pumps within membranes operate, over time, to produce markedly different concentrations of ions in the intracellular and extracellular volumes around cells. In cardiac cells, the sodium–potassium pump produces concentrations (millimoles per liter) for Purkinje cells as shown in Table 19.1.

A transmembrane voltage, or polarization, develops across the membrane because of the differences in concentrations across the membrane. In the steady state, the transmembrane potential for a two-ion system is, according to Goldman's equation [Plonsey and Barr, 2000],

$$V_m = \frac{RT}{F} \ln\left(\frac{P_K[K]_e + P_{Na}[Na]_e}{P_K[K]_i + P_{Na}[Na]_i}\right) \tag{19.7}$$

where R is the gas content, T is the temperature, and F is Faraday's constant ($RT/F \approx 25$ mV). P_K and P_{Na} are the permeabilities to potassium and sodium ions, respectively. [K] and [Na] are the concentrations of these ions, and the subscripts i and e indicate intracellular and extracellular, respectively. V_m is the transmembrane voltage at steady state.

19.3.1 Polarized State

At rest, P_{Na} is much smaller than P_K. Using Equation 19.6, approximating $P_{Na} = P_K/100$, and using the concentrations in Table 19.1,

$$V_m \approx 25 \text{ mV} \times \ln\left[\frac{4 + (0.01 \times 140)}{140 + (0.01 \times 8)}\right] \approx -82 \text{ mV} \tag{19.8}$$

Cardiac Purkinje cells show a polarization at rest of about this amount. The negative sign indicates that the interior of the cell is negative with respect to the exterior.

One way to think about why this voltage exists at the steady state is as follows: In the steady state, diffusion tends to move K^+ from inside because of the much higher concentration of K^+ intracellularly. This flow is offset, however, by a flow from outside to inside due to the potential gradient, with a higher potential outside, since K^+ is a positively charged ion. With the concentrations of Table 19.1, the effects of the

TABLE 19.1 Ionic Concentrations (mmol/l)

	Na^+	K^+
Intracellular	8	140
Extracellular	140	4

diffusion gradient and potential gradient are almost equal and opposite when the potential intracellularly is about -82 mV with respect to the **extracellular potential**. The result is a steady state. Rather than a true equilibrium, this state has a small but nonzero flow of sodium ions, offset electrically by a sustained flow of potassium ions. Thus the **membrane potential** would run down over time were there no $Na^+ - K^+$ pumps maintaining the transmembrane concentrations. (In the absence of such pumps, concentration differences diminish over a period of hours.)

19.3.2 Depolarized State

Suppose the permeabilities to sodium and potassium of Equation 19.7 are changed from the values used for Equation 19.8, which approximated membrane at rest (polarized). Instead, to approximate excited membrane, suppose that P_{Na} rises in comparison with P_K so that $P_K = P_{Na}/2$. Now,

$$V_m = 25 \text{ mV} \times \ln\left[\frac{4 + (2 \times 140)}{140 + (2 \times 8)}\right] \approx 15 \text{ mV} \qquad (19.9)$$

Here the positive sign for V_m indicates that the interior of the membrane is positive with respect to the exterior. Because V_m is here more nearly zero in magnitude, this excited state is called depolarized.

19.4 Action Potentials

Membranes create action potentials by actively changing their permeabilities to ions such as sodium and potassium. A comparison of the results of Equation 19.8 and Equation 19.9 shows a swing of about 100 mV between the resting and excited states (polarized to depolarized). The change of permeability from resting to excited values and then back again allows the membrane to generate an **action potential**.

Among the most important developments of the past 50 years has been the creation of a series of mathematical and numerical models of the time course and voltage dependence of the change in membrane permeabilities. These "membrane models" originally described the behavior of nerve membrane and has now been extended to many other tissues, such as skeletal muscle and cardiac muscle.

19.4.1 Cardiac Action Potentials

Action potentials that characterize actual tissue have the roughly rectangular shape that is suggested by the preceding calculation, but only as an approximation. An action potential for the cardiac conduction system simulated with the DiFrancesco–Noble model is shown in Figure 19.2. Initially, V_m has a baseline voltage (B) near -80 mV. During excitation (E), the membrane permeabilities change, and V_m rises abruptly. After the peak overshoot at about $+20$ mV, the potential maintains a plateau voltage (P) near -20 mV for nearly 300 msec and then recovers (R) rapidly to a baseline phase. The overall action potential duration is about 400 msec.

19.4.2 Nerve Action Potentials

For comparison, an action potential simulated with the Hodgkin–Huxley model for nerve is shown in Figure 19.3. Corresponding baseline, excitation, plateau, and recovery phases may be identified, and the voltage change between resting and excited states is again about 100 mV. The plateau phase is so short as to be virtually nonexistent, and the overall action potential duration is much shorter than that of Figure 19.2, only about 4 msec.

19.4.3 Wave Shape and Function

All excitable membranes are characterized by their ability to change membrane permeabilities and to do so selectively. Both the cardiac action potential of Figure 19.2 and the nerve action potential of Figure 19.3

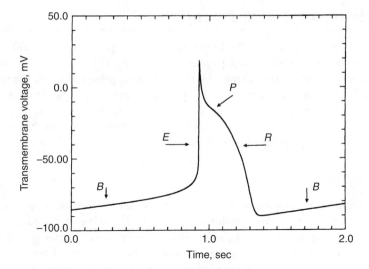

FIGURE 19.2   Cardiac action potential. Computed with the DiFrancesco–Noble membrane model for the cardiac conduction system (membrane patch). *B*, baseline; *E*, excitation; *R*, recovery (repolarization).

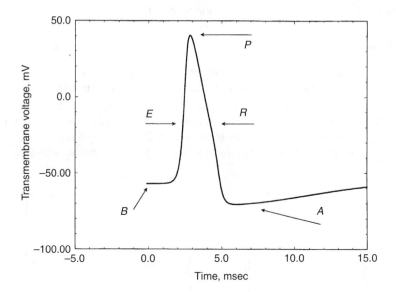

FIGURE 19.3   Nerve action potential. Computed with the Hodgkin–Huxley model for nerve membrane (membrane patch). *B*, baseline; *E*, excitation; *P*, plateau; *R*, recovery; *A*, afterpotential.

demonstrated rapid depolarization and a subsequent slower repolarization associated with membrane permeability changes and changes of about 100 mV in V_m amplitude. Conversely, the differences also have marked importance. Cardiac action potentials have a long duration that limits the shortest interval between heartbeats. This interval must be several hundred milliseconds long to allow time for movement of blood. The extended plateau of the cardiac action potential is associated with the movement of calcium ions, which is associated with muscle contraction. In contrast, nerve action potentials perform a signaling function. This function is supported by a shorter action potential duration, which allows more variability in the number of action potentials propagated per second, an important signaling variable. Conversely, nerves had no need for contraction and no need for a plateau period for calcium ion movement.

19.5   Initiation of Action Potentials

Action potentials of tissue with a specialized sensing function (e.g., for sight or smell) have membrane channels linked to receptors for the initiating agent [Watson et al., 1992]. In contrast, a large number of membrane channels are controlled by changes in transmembrane voltage. In particular, when the potential rises from its baseline value to a threshold level, the membrane initiates the sequence of permeability changes that create an action potential. The change of transmembrane voltage initiating the action potential normally comes from currents originating in adjacent tissue (see Propagation, below). Such currents also may come from artificial sources, such as stimulators.

19.5.1   Examples

Responses of a DiFrancesco–Noble membrane to transmembrane stimuli of three magnitudes are shown in Figure 19.4. All three stimuli were 1 msec in duration. Stimulus $S1$, the largest, caused the transmembrane potential to rise from its baseline value to about -65 mV and initiated an action potential (ap1), which followed a few milliseconds after the stimulus. Stimulus $S2$ had only 80% of the intensity of $S1$, and the stimulus itself caused a transmembrane voltage change that was proportionally smaller. As did $S1$, stimulus $S2$ initiated an action potential (ap2), although there was a delay of about 200 msec before excitation occurred, and the action potential itself was somewhat diminished in amplitude. Stimulus $S3$ had 80% of the magnitude of $S2$ and caused a transmembrane voltage change that again was proportionally smaller. $S3$, however, produced no subsequent action potential.

19.5.2   Threshold

An important general result demonstrated in Figure 19.4 is that action potential initiation has a threshold behavior. That is, stimuli producing transmembrane voltages above a threshold value initiate action potentials, while those below do not. This response is called "all or none," although (as Figure 19.4 shows) there is a variation in response for near-threshold stimuli. Threshold values are not constant. The threshold value for a particular stimulus varies depending on factors such as the location of the electrodes relative to the tissue that is excited, the stimulus duration, and the amount of membrane affected.

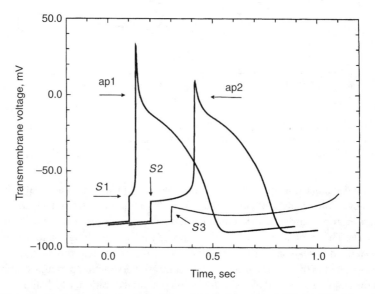

FIGURE 19.4   Variation in stimulus magnitude. In different trials, three stimuli ($S1$, $S2$, $S3$) of decreasing magnitude were applied. Action potentials followed the first two, but not the third.

19.6   Propagation

Initiation of excitation at one end of a excitable fiber leads to an action potential there. Subsequently, action potentials may be observed at sites progressively further away. Propagating current loops are of fundamental importance to nerve or muscle function, as they allow for the transmission of information in nerves or initiation of contraction through the release of calcium, in muscle. The deterioration of propagation with disease may be in the form of a failure to propagate, or propagation with an abnormally slow velocity. In the heart, propagation along a closed path ("re-entrant propagation") is one source of cardiac disrhythmias and even death. The theory of the electric telegraph as put forward by Kelvin was perhaps the origin of the core-conductor model, which forms much of the analytical basis for the present understanding of propagation.

19.6.1   Numerical Model

Numerical models of propagation were introduced by Hodgkin and Huxley [1952] in the 1950s to demon-strate quantitatively how the events of propagation arise from the elemental flow of ionic currents in nerves. While experimentally based, such models have become increasingly precise, increasingly specialized, and much more detailed so as to reflect accurately the properties of particular tissues [e.g., Spach et al., 2004]. Such numerical models allow a consistent picture to be obtained of action potentials at different sites along a nerve or muscle structure. They are based on analyzing the interaction of spatially distributed events at one time, so as to see the consequences at a short time later.

Such a model is used here. Consider the cylindrical fiber shown in Figure 19.5, having radius $a = 75\ \mu m$ and a length of 10 μm. The fiber is surrounded by an extracellular volume extending $3a$ beyond the membrane. To establish a symmetric reference potential, the outside edge of the extracellular region was connected via resistances to a junction where $\phi_e = 0$. Intracellular specific resistance R_i was 250 Ω cm, and R_e was one-third of R_i. Solutions for intracellular, extracellular, and transmembrane potentials were obtained through a process of numerical simulation. The structure of this example follows that of Spach et al. [1973], where cardiac Purkinje fibers were studied. Most of the examples below use the DiFrancesco–Noble model for Purkinje membrane [Noble et al., 1994].

19.6.2   Sequence of Action Potentials

Action potentials simulated for the cylindrical fiber are shown in Figure 19.6. Waveforms are shown following a transmembrane stimulus at $z = 0$, where the first action potential originates, and also for sites

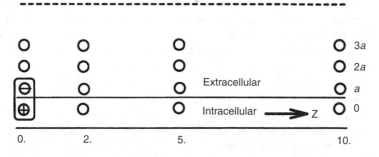

FIGURE 19.5   Geometry for numerical model. The model represented a fiber 10 mm in length. The cross section was a series of concentric bands. Nodes were spaced along the axial (z) dimension every 100 μm. These nodes are portrayed by the columns of circles drawn at four axial positions, although actually there were 101 columns. The innermost (lower) row of nodes, row 0, were sites where intracellular potentials were determined; four surrounding rows (rows 1 to 4), at increasing distances, were sites for extracellular potentials. The outermost boundary (dashed line) was assigned $\phi_c = 0$. Separation between all rows was the same as the fiber radius, $a = 75\ \mu m$. Transmembrane stimuli were applied across the membrane at $z = 0$ (nodes enclosed).

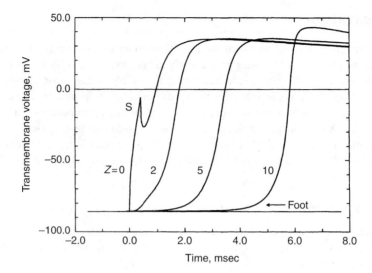

FIGURE 19.6   Action potentials for a 10-mm fiber. Transmembrane potentials $V_m(t)$ arising at z positions of 0, 2, 5, and 10 mm. The waveform at $z = 0$ shows a stimulus artefact S. $V_m(t)$ at $z = 10$ has a larger peak-to-peak rise because excitation terminates there, at the end of the fiber.

2, 5, and 10 mm away. All the action potentials have similar wave shapes, differing mainly in their timing. Although these are cardiac waveforms simulated with the DiFrancesco–Nobel model, note the markedly different impression of the wave shape seen in this figure as compared with Figure 19.2. Note also that the waveform at $z = 0$ has progressed through excitation, but not into the plateau phase, by the time of excitation at $z = 1$ cm. Secondary changes of action potential wave shape as a function of z, other than the stimulus artefact, can be discerned mainly in the baseline as it rises into the upstroke, a region called the foot. Differences in the duration of the foot reflect the time that other tissue has been excited, prior to the start of excitation at a particular site; that is, the foot is longer at sites further down the fiber.

19.6.3   Biophysical Basis

Although propagation in nerves and muscles often is compared to wave propagation of sound or light, to waves in the ocean, or to electrical waves in cables, bioelectric propagation does not have an analogous physical basis. In the former categories, energy used at the source creates a disturbance that propagates to the observer through an intervening passive medium. Propagation velocity depends on the properties of that medium. In bioelectric propagation, what is meant is that the source itself is moving down an excitable medium, the membrane, in a process more similar to setting off a chain of firecrackers. The velocities associated with bioelectric propagation relate to the magnitudes of transmembrane current passing through one site on the membrane and flowing to another and how fast the active responses of the membrane occur at the downstream sites. Although short intervals are required for passive propagation of the consequences of the active events through the surrounding tissue, these intervals are minuscule in comparison with the times required for the active changes. Consequently, most bioelectric events are analyzed as a sequence of "quasi-static" stages.

19.6.4   Velocity of Propagation

It is difficult to predict the velocity of propagation for a particular tissue structure prior to its measurement. Reported experimental velocities of propagation range from less than 0.01 m/sec to more than 10 m/sec, depending on the particular membrane and structure involved and its environment. Within a particular nerve or muscle, however, velocities vary little under normal conditions. Changes in the velocity of propagation θ as a result of changes in fiber diameter a or specific resistivity R_i can be approximated by the equation

$$\theta = \frac{Ka}{2R_i} \tag{19.10}$$

Here K is a constant determined by the membrane properties, a is the fiber radius, and R_i is the specific resistance of the intracellular medium [Plonsey and Barr, 2000], and the equation assumes relatively low extracellular resistance.

An important relationship shown by Equation 19.10 is the proportionality of the velocity to the square root of the fiber's radius. Living systems take advantage of this relationship by having larger-diameter fibers where higher velocity is essential. For example, the giant axon of the squid carries the signal by which the squid responds to predators.

19.6.5 Transmembrane Current

The mathematical analysis of propagation is greatly aided by using the principle of conservation of charge to develop an equation for membrane current I_m that depends on the local distribution of intracellular potential rather than on currents through the membrane, as in Equation 19.1. Conservation of current requires that current through the membrane at an axial position z be the difference between current coming to that site and current leaving that site (on one side, e.g., intracellularly). Because intracellular currents follow the first derivative of ϕ_i (Equation 19.5), then for one-dimensional flow [Plonsey and Barr, 2000],

$$I_m = \frac{1}{2\pi \, a r_i} \frac{\partial^2 \phi_i}{\partial z^2} \tag{19.11}$$

Here r_i is the axial resistance per unit length, a is the fiber radius, and ϕ_i is the intracellular potential. This result is used below, as well as in many mathematical analyses of propagation, because it provides a means (sometimes the sole means) of linking the membrane current at one site to electrical events at neighboring sites.

19.6.6 Movement of the Local Current Loop

Propagation occurs when a local current loop initiates an action potential in an adjacent region. The concept of how this occurs is illustrated in Figure 19.7. At time t_1, a local current loop exists, as shown in Figure 19.7a. This local loop produces outward current at site $z = z_1$. That there must be outward current at z_1 is shown by Figure 19.7b, which plots $f(z)$ for time t_1. The gradient of ϕ_i between z_2 and z_1 is shown in Figure 19.7b. This gradient produces intracellular current into z_1 from the left but not current out on the right (because the gradient is zero to the right). Current must therefore leave through the membrane at z_1. This positive membrane current is indicated by the upward arrow at z_1 in Figure 19.7b. The positive membrane current at z_1 discharges the membrane capacitance there, so the potential at z_1 rises, producing a new voltage distribution. The change in the intracellular voltage distribution produces a shift in the site of the current loop; that is, the loop propages to the right, as shown in Figure 19.7c.

More mathematically, at z_1 at time t_1 the value of $\partial^2 \phi_i / \partial_z^2$ is markedly positive, because ϕ_i changes slope there from negative to zero. Therefore, by Equation 19.11, I_m is large and positive at $z = z_1$. Additionally, I_{ion} is relatively small at z_1 because the intracellular voltage is at its resting value, so (by Equation 19.1) I_c must be large. By Equation 19.2, if I_c is large and positive, then $\partial V_m / \partial t$ is large and positive. Thus the transmembrane potential at z_1 rises rapidly, and soon the current loop shown in Figure 19.7c is achieved.

For comparison with the schematic drawings in Figure 19.7, the distribution of voltages and currents in the 1-cm simulated fiber is shown in Figure 19.8. The figure shows the transmembrane potential V_m and the total membrane current I_m. Both are shown as a function of axial distance z along the strand at time $t = 3$ msec after the stimulus. (This spatial plot came from the same simulation as the set of waveforms

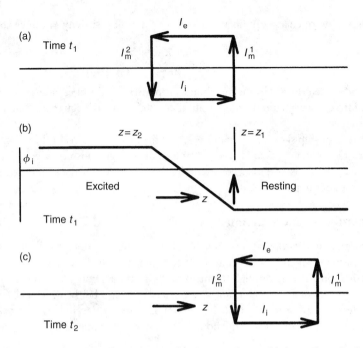

FIGURE 19.7 Propagation of a current loop, concept drawing. Panels a and b draw a hypothetical current loop as it might exist at time t_1. At this time, outward current is causing the potential to rise at $z = z_1$, as indicated by the upward arrow there, in panel b. The result is a shift in the distribution of intracellular potential θ_i. Thus the current loop moves to the position shown in panel c.

vs. time shown in Figure 19.6.) Because $V_m = \phi_i - \phi_e$, and because in this example the extracellular potentials ϕ_e are relatively small in magnitude (see below), V_m in Figure 19.8 is a close approximation to ϕ_i in Figure 19.7.

In Figure 19.8, the total membrane current I_m is biphasic, with the outward current on the leading edge of the propagating waveform. Propagation is to the right, consistent with the direction of downward slope of V_m and consistent with the direction of movement of Figure 19.7. The inward and outward currents of the distributed pattern in Figure 19.8 are consistent with the concept of Figure 19.7, where the distribution is lumped. (One might place $z_1 \approx 4.8$ mm in Figure 19.8 and $z_2 \approx 4.0$ mm.) Figure 19.8 shows that the local current loop is more accurately described as a local current distribution, extending over a distance of a few millimeters (about 0.8 mm between the maximum and minimum of the I_m curve).

The composition of $I_m(z)$ can be evaluated by comparing I_m with its components, the ionic current I_{ion} and the membrane capacitative current I_c. At the outward current peak (the maximum of I_m), the magnitude of the capacitive component I_c is greater than the magnitude of the ionic component I_{ion}. At the inward peak (the minimum of I_m), $|I_{ion}| > |I_c|$, although both magnitudes are significant. That is, the dominant components of I_m in Figure 19.8 are consistent with the drawings in Figure 19.7. In contrast to Figure 19.7, however, the peak outward current occurs near where $V_m \approx -40$ mV rather than near the baseline value (≈ -85 mV). Consistent with Figure 19.7, Figure 19.8 shows that I_m is dominated by I_c at the peak outward I_m and increasingly more so as one moves forward on the leading edge.

19.7 Extracellular Waveforms

An understanding of the origin of extracellular waveforms is important because most electrophysiologic recordings, including those of most clinical studies, are observations of extracellular events rather than underlying transmembrane or intracellular events.

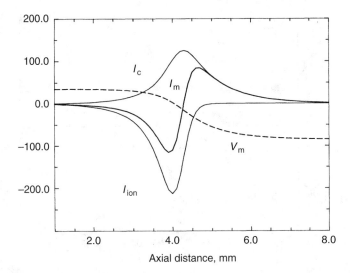

FIGURE 19.8   Potential and current distribution in a 10-mm fiber at $t = 3$ msec following a transmembrane stimulus applied at $z = 0$. The vertical scale is in millivolts for the V_m plot and in microamperes per square centimeter for the current plots. Results are from a numerical simulation using the geometry of Figure 19.6. Transmembrane potential V_m at this moment is shown by the dashed line. Note the inward and outward peaks of the transmembrane current I_m near $z = 4$ and 4.8 mm. Plots for I_c and I_{ion}, the components of I_m, also are shown. They demonstrate that on the leading edge of the waveform (higher values of z), current I_c dominates. Compare the results with the concept drawing of Figure 19.7.

Historically, extracellular waveforms were observed and their correspondence with many diseases established empirically well before their sources were known. In recent years, extracellular fields have been mapped in detail, both in time and space [Taccardi, 2002]. Though extracellular waveforms arise from membrane sources and corresponding intracellular action potentials, the extracellular–intracellular relationship is not a simple one, because it involves distance from the membrane sources, and because a given extracellular site usually is affected by currents from many different excitable fibers. Numerical models for bioelectric field problems [Gulrajani, 1998] prove extremely helpful in understanding extracellular waveforms and extracellular potential distributions ("potential maps") as they can take into account a complex pattern of current sources and the geometrical irregularities of the volume conductor, including the body surface itself.

Although extracellular waveforms $\phi_e(t)$ reflect the same current loops as the intracellular or transmembrane waveforms, their magnitude, wave shape, and timing usually are entirely different. (The greatest similarity occurs with a highly restricted extracellular volume.) With an extensive extracellular volume, the normal situation, waveforms such as those in Figure 19.9 are seen. The three waveforms come from "electrodes" just outside the fiber at $z = 0$, $z = 5$, and $z = 10$ mm, or in other words at the site of the stimulus, the middle of the strand, and the end where excitation terminates. (For reference, the intracellular potential from the middle of the fiber also is shown, reduced to 2% of its true magnitude.) All three extracellular waveforms shown are small in comparison with transmembrane waveforms, less than 1 mV peak to peak. Their wave shapes differ: Near the stimulus (0), the wave shape has a negative deflection from the stimulus and continues to be negative thereafter. In the middle, the wave shape is biphasic. A positive deflection occurs as excitation approaches, and a negative deflection occurs once it goes past (compare the timing of the extracellular and intracellular waveforms, which are from the same axial position). At the terminating end (10), the extracellular wave shape is predominantly positive, showing also a long initial rise as excitation approaches.

It is interesting that these extracellular waveforms show such large changes in wave shape as a function of position, whereas their underlying transmembrane waveforms, at the same z values, show no such

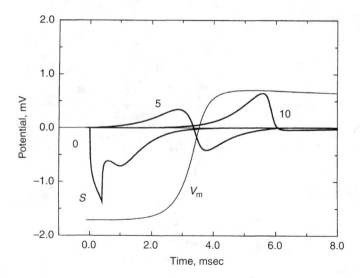

FIGURE 19.9 Extracellular waveforms from a 10-mm fiber. Extracellular potentials $\phi_e(t)$ are plotted for positions just outside the membrane at $z = 0, 5$, and 10 mm. The transmembrane stimulus at $z = 0$ affected the waveform there, as seen by stimulus artefact S. For reference, $V_m(t)$ at $z = 5$ mm also is drawn, reduced to 2% of its true amplitude.

changes, as can be seen by comparison with the transmembrane waveforms shown in Figure 19.6. The relative timing of the extracellular as compared with the transmembrane waveforms also is noteworthy: Close to the membrane, most of the major deflections of the extracellular waveforms are confined to the short time period when the transmembrane potential is undergoing excitation. During the hundreds of milliseconds thereafter, the intracellular potential is large but changing slowly (e.g., Figure 19.2), so the transmembrane currents are small. These smaller currents are distributed and produce proportionally small deflections. As the recording site moves away from the membrane, however, the distributed recovery currents do not decline as rapidly with distance, so the potentials they produce become larger in relation to potentials produced by the currents of excitation. On the body surface, the voltages produced during recovery may have similar magnitudes and play a large role in waveform interpretation (e.g., the T wave of the electrocardiogram).

Biphasic waveforms are observed at most extracellular sites, because most sites are neither the origin or termination of excitation. Further, most real extracellular waveforms are more complicated and last longer than those shown in Figure 19.9, because they show the composite effect from many different fibers rather than a single one in isolation.

19.7.1 Spatial Relation to Intracellular

Extracellular waveforms are created by the flow of current through the volume conductor surrounding the active membrane. An expression for the extracellular potential ϕ_e, outside a cylindrical fiber with a large conducting volume was given by Spach et al. [1973] as

$$\phi_e(t_o, z) = \frac{a\sigma}{4\sigma} \int_{-\infty}^{\infty} \frac{(\partial^2 \phi_i / \partial z'^2)_{to}}{\left(\frac{d+a}{a}\right)^2 + \left[\frac{(z'-z)}{a}\right]^2} dz' \qquad (19.12)$$

where z is the axial coordinate of the fiber, t_o is the time when the spatial distribution was obtained, ϕ_i is the intracellular potential, a is the fiber radius, and d is the perpendicular distance from the fiber membrane to the electrode. Conductivities σ_i and σ_e apply to the intracellular and extracellular conducting media, respectively. The integration limits of $\pm\infty$ recognize that the integration should be over the entire fiber.

Note that t_o must be chosen in a succession of values to generate a temporal waveform at position z and that the right-hand side of Equation 19.12 has t_o be evaluated separately for each to choice.

A number of examples of extracellular waveforms, as compared with their underlying intracellular ones, are given by Spach et al. [1973], together with an evaluation of the accuracy of Equation 19.12. A central feature of the equation is that the extracellular waveform is a weighted summation of the second spatial derivative of the intracellular potential. This relationship holds, to a good approximation, for all the extracellular waveforms shown in Figure 19.9. The different weighting for different waveforms (variation in $z' - z$ for different choices of z) produces the varying shapes of the extracellular waveforms at different sites.

19.7.2 Temporal Relation to Intracellular

If an action potential is assumed to be propagating with constant velocity θ on a long fiber, then the spatial derivative in the preceding equation can be converted to a temporal derivative using $z = \theta t$ so that

$$\phi_e(t_o, z) = \frac{a\sigma}{4\sigma} \int_{-\infty}^{\infty} \frac{(\partial^2 \phi_i/\partial z'^2)_{z0}}{\left(\frac{d+a}{a}\right)^2 + \left[\frac{\theta(t'-t)}{a}\right]^2} \, dt' \tag{19.13}$$

where t is time, z_0 is the axial coordinate of the position where the intracellular and extracellular "electrodes" are located, and θ is the velocity with which the action potential is moving along the z-axis. The integration limits of $\pm\infty$ recognize that only in long fibers does the velocity remain approximately constant over a significant period of time.

Some of the limitations of Equation 19.13 are apparent when considering the waveforms of Figure 19.9. The equation would be suitable only for the extracellular waveform in the middle of the fiber ($z = 5$ mm). At either end, the equation would be unsuitable, because velocity is not constant through initiation or through termination of propagation.

While the general principles given above apply to virtually all extracellular waveforms, many specific features characterize the extracellular waveforms observed from individual organs. In view of their clinical importance, extensive study has thus been given to the principles of electrocardiography (heart), principles of electromyography (skeletal muscle), and principles of electroencephalography (brain).

19.8 Stimulation

Natural **stimulation** of nerves and muscle occurs in sensory sites, and artificial electrical stimulation can initiate action potentials can initiate action potentials and control propagation in much the same way.

Most stimulation for clinical purposes and most experimental studies use extracellular electrodes because positioning the electrodes outside the active tissue can be done, usually, with little or no tissue damage. Such electrical stimulation of excitable tissue has become a subject of great practical import-ance, particularly so now that technology allows small stimulators to be implanted and to function well over periods of many years. An analytical understanding of stimulation has been markedly advanced by the introduction by Rattay [1990] of the "activating function," a mathematical expression that identifies regions along a membrane of excitable cells where stimulation introduces currents either entering or leaving the extracellular volume. The effect of a stimulus then may be understood as a convolution of the activating function with the membrane response, e.g., the analysis by Barr and Plonsey [2003] for a tissue sheet.

As an example of some of the principles of artificial stimulation, suppose two stimulating electrodes are placed just outside the 1-cm fiber, as identified in Figure 19.10. Note that the anode is placed at $z = 10$ mm (encircled +), and the cathode is placed at $z = 0$ (encircled −). Both electrodes are extracellular. When current is injected through these electrodes, most of the current will flow along the extracellular path (thick flow line). Some current also will cross the resistive barrier formed by the membrane and flow

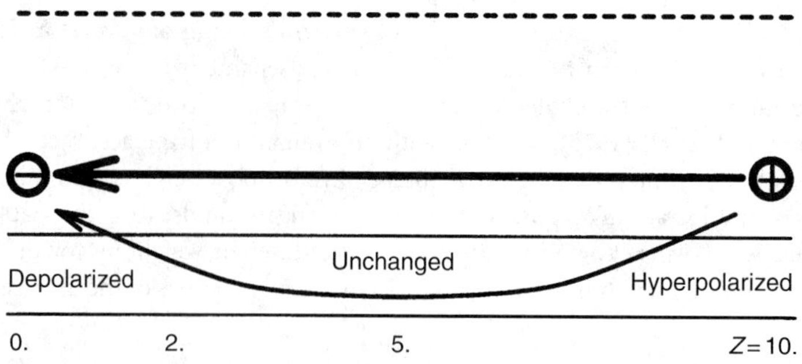

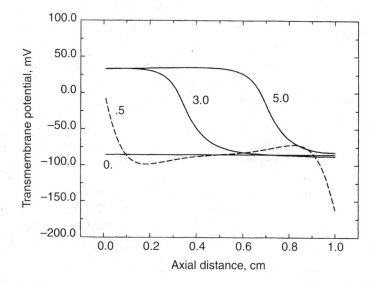

FIGURE 19.10 Extracellular stimulus currents, concept drawing. A stimulus is applied between and extracellular anode, at $z = 10$, and an extracellular cathode, at $z = 0$. Most current will flow in the extracellular volume (thick line). Some current will enter the intracellular volume (thin line). Current entering or leaving the membrane causes that portion of the membrane to become hyperpolarized (high z region) or depolarized (low z region).

FIGURE 19.11 Transmembrane potentials following an extracellular stimulus. The simulation used the geometry of Figure 19.5, except that the stimulus was applied to the row 2 nodes at $z = 0$ and $z = 10$ (similar to Figure 19.10). Successive plots show the transmembrane potentials as a function of z at time 0 (just before the stimulus), 0.5 msec (end of the stimulus), 3.0 msec (propagation underway), and 5.0 msec. The potential distribution at 0.5 msec is consistent in its major features with the concept drawing of Figure 19.10.

intracellularly (thin flow line). Where the intracellular current emerges from the membrane, it will tend to depolarize the membrane. (Note the effects of the stimulus on potential differences: The region depolarized is the region where the intracellular potential becomes higher as compared with the extracellular potential directly across the membrane. In contrast, the region depolarized has a lower potential near the cathode as compared with the potential at the other end of the fiber, near the anode, in both the intracellular and extracellular volumes.) If the magnitude of the depolarization is large enough in relation to the size of the depolarized region, then the stimulus will initiate action potentials and propagation.

Transmembrane potential distributions following the extracellular stimulus are shown in Figure 19.11. At time $t = 0$, the transmembrane potential (as a function of z) is flat, indicating that the membrane is uniformly in the resting state. Then a stimulus of 0.05 mA amplitude and 0.5 msec duration is applied to the stimulus electrodes, with the source–sink positioning that of Figure 19.10. Figure 19.11 shows the distribution of transmembrane potentials at $t = 0.5$ msec, the time of the end of the stimulus.

At $t = 0.5$ msec, the membrane is depolarized near the cathode (near $z = 0$) and is hyperpolarized near the anode (near $z = 10$). Interestingly, there is a small region of hyperpolarization beside the depolarized end (near $z = 2$ mm) and depolarization near the hyperpolarized end (near $z = 8$ mm), a predictable effect [Plonsey and Barr, 2000]. The transmembrane potentials along the central part of the fiber are much less affected by the stimulus than are the ends, even though the same magnitude of stimulus current flows along the entire length. This stimulus was large enough to produce action potentials, as can be seen by inspecting the transmembrane potentials for 3 msec. Figure 19.11 shows that the excitation wave that began near $z = 0$ has, by 3 msec, progressed about a third of the way down the fiber. Propagation to a further point is seen at 5.0 msec.

Many devices for medical stimulation have now come into routine use over long periods of time, for example, cardiac pacemakers. Large currents ("shocks") of artificial origin also are used to terminate action potentials in some cases, for example, cardiac defibrillators. The transmembrane potential changes induced by such shocks now have been measured in considerable detail [e.g., Zhou et al., 1996; Ideker et al., 2000].

19.9 Biomagnetism

Panofsky and Phillips [1962] show the connection between the electric field E to the magnetic field B and current j_{true} by giving two (of the four) Maxwell's equations as

$$\nabla \times H = -j_{\text{true}} + \frac{\partial D}{\partial t} \tag{19.14}$$

and

$$\nabla \times E = -\frac{\partial B}{\partial t} \tag{19.15}$$

together with the constituitive relations $H = B/\mu$ and $D = k\varepsilon_0 E$, where μ, k, and ε_0 are constants for a given medium.

Both currents j_{true} and changing electric fields (E and thereby D) are present naturally in and around excitable membranes, so Equation 19.14 shows that corresponding magnetic fields are to be expected. These magnetic fields are small, however, even in comparison with the earth's magnetic field. They can nonetheless be precisely measured if careful attention is paid to the design of equipment and the surroundings, as demonstrated by Wikswo and Egeraat [1991]. At present, magnetic fields are not routinely measured for clinical purposes, largely because the required equipment is more cumbersome and more expensive. Nonetheless, in principle, biomagnetic recordings offer some important advantages, including the absence of required electrode contact.

In a complementary way, rapidly changing magnetic fields induce electric fields (and thereby currents) in living tissue, as indicated by Equation 19.15. Stimulation of nerves or muscles is thereby possible, either by design (see, e.g., Roth and Basser 1990) or as a side effect of magnetic resonance imaging (MRI). Extensive consideration of biomagnetism has been presented by Malmivuo and Plonsey [1994], and Gulrajani [1998].

Defining Terms

Action potential: The cycle of changes of transmembrane potential, negative to positive to negative again, that characterizes excitable tissue. This cycle also is described as resting to excited and returning to rest.

Excitation: The change of the membrane from resting to excited states, characterized by the movement of the transmembrane potential across a threshold.

Extracellular potentials: Potentials generated between two sites outside the membrane (external to active cells), for example, between two sites on the skin, due to current flow in the volume conductor.

Intracellular (extracellular):   Inside (outside) cells.

Membrane polarization: The sustained (and approximately constant) transmembrane potential of a cell at rest that arises due to different intracellular and extracellular ionic concentrations.

Propagation: Excitation of one region of tissue as a result of an action potential in an adjacent region.

Stimulation: Change in the transmembrane potential at a site due to an influence from another site. The term is used most frequently when current is applied through wires from an artificial current source.

Transmembrane potential: The potential inside a cell membrane minus the potential just outside the membrane.

Volume conductor: The electrically conductive interior region of the body surrounding electrically active membrane.

References

Barr R.C. and Plonsey R. 2003. Field stimulation of 2-D sheets of excitable tissue. *IEEE Trans. Biomed. Eng.* 51: 539–540.

Byrne J.H. and Schultz S.G. 1988. *An Introduction to Membrane Transport and Bioelectricity*. New York, Raven Press.

Cabo C. and Barr R.C. 1992. Propagation model using the DiFrancesco–Nobel equations. *Med. Biol. Eng. Comput.* 30: 292.

Gulrajani R. 1998. *Bioelectricity and Biomagnetism*. New York, John Wiley and Sons, pp. 525–610.

Hodgkin A.L. and Huxley A.F. 1952. A quantitative description of membrane current and its application to conduction and excitation in nerve. *J. Physiol.* 117: 500–544.

Ideker R.E., Chattipakorn T.N., and Gray R.A. 2000. Defibrillation mechanisms: the parable of the blind men and the elephant. *J. Cardiovasc. Electrophysiol.* 11: 1008–1013.

Malmivuo J. and Plonsey R. 1995. *Bioelectromagnetism: Principles and Applications of Bioelectric and Biomagnetic Fields*. New York, Oxford University Press.

Marban E. 1999. Molecular approaches to arrhythmogenesis. In *Molecular Basis of Cardiovascular Disease* (K.R. Chien, Ed.), Philadelphia, W.B. Saunders, Chapter 14, pp. 313–328.

Noble D., DiFrancesco D., Noble S. et al. 1994. *Oxsoft Heart Program Manual*. Wellesley Hills, MA, NB Datyner.

Panofsky W.K.H. and Phillips M. 1962. *Classical Electricity and Magnetism*, 2nd ed. New York, Addison-Wesley.

Plonsey R. and Barr R.C. 2000. *Bioelectricity: A Quantitative Approach*. 2nd ed. New York, Kluwer Acedemic/Plenum Publishers.

Rattay F. 1990. *Electrical Nerve Stimulation*. Wien, New York, Springer-Verlag.

Roth B.J. and Passer P.J. 1990. A model of the stimulation of a nerve fiber by electromagnetic stimulating. *IEEE Trans. BME* 37: 588–597.

Spach M.S., Barr R.C., Johnson E.A., and Kootsey J.M. 1973. Cardiac extracellular potentials: analysis of complex waveforms about the Purkinje network in dogs. *Circ. Res.* 31: 465.

Watson J.D., Gilman M., Witkowski J., and Zoller M. 1992. *Recombinant DNA*, 2nd ed. New York, Scientific American Books.

Spach M.S., Heidlage F., Barr R.C., and Dolber P. 2004. Cell size and communication: role in structural and electrical development and remodeling of the heart. *Heart Rhythm* 1: 235–251.

Taccardi B. and Punske B.B. 2002. Body surface and epicardial mapping: state of the art and future perspectives. *IJBEM* 4: 91–94.

Wikswo J.P. Jr and van Egeraat J.M. 1991. Cellular magnetic fields: fundamental and applied measurements on nerve axons, peripheral nerve bundles, and skeletal muscle. *J. Clin. Neurophysiol.* 8: 170.

Zhou X.H., Smith W.M., Rollins D.L., and Ideker R.E. 1996. Transmembrane potential changes caused by shocks in guinea pig papillary muscle. *Am. J. Physiol.* 271: H2536–H2546.

20

Volume Conductor Theory

Robert Plonsey
Duke University

This chapter considers the properties of the volume conductor as it pertains to the evaluation of electric and magnetic fields arising therein. The sources of the aforementioned fields are described by $\vec{J}^i$, a function of position and time, which has the dimensions of current per unit area *or* dipole moment per unit volume. Such sources may arise from active endogenous electrophysiologic processes such as propagating action potentials, generator potentials, synaptic potentials, etc. Sources also may be established exogenously, as exemplified by electric or magnetic field stimulation. Details on how one may quantitatively evaluate a source function from an electrophysiologic process are found in other chapters. For our purposes here, we assume that such a source function $\vec{J}^i$ is known and, furthermore, that it has well-behaved mathematical properties. Given such a source, we focus attention here on a description of the volume conductor as it affects the electric and magnetic fields that are established in it. As a loose definition, we consider the *volume conductor* to be the contiguous passive conducting medium that surrounds the region occupied by the source $\vec{J}^i$. (This may include a portion of the excitable tissue itself that is sufficiently far from $\vec{J}^i$ to be described passively.)

20.1 Basic Relations in the Idealized Homogeneous Volume Conductor

Excitable tissue, when activated, will be found to generate currents both within itself and also in all surrounding conducting media. The latter passive region is characterized as a *volume conductor*. The adjective *volume* emphasizes that current flow is three-dimensional, in contrast to the confined one-dimensional flow within insulated wires. The volume conductor is usually assumed to be a monodomain (whose meaning will be amplified later), isotropic, resistive, and (frequently) homogeneous. These are simply assumptions, as will be discussed subsequently. The permeability of biologic tissues is important when examining magnetic fields and is usually assumed to be that of free space. The permittivity is a more complicated property, but outside cell membranes (which have a high lipid content) it is also usually considered to be that of free space.

A general, mathematical description of a current source is specified by a function $\vec{J}^i\,(x, y, z, t)$, namely, a vector field of current density in say milliamperes per square centimeter that varies both in space and time. A study of sources of physiologic origin shows that their temporal behavior lies in a low-frequency range. For example, currents generated by the heart have a power density spectrum that lies mainly under 1 kHz (in fact, clinical ECG instruments have upper frequency limits of 100 Hz), while most other electrophysiologic sources of interest (i.e., those underlying the EEG, EMG, EOG, etc.) are of even lower frequency. Examination of electromagnetic fields in regions with typical physiologic conductivities, with dimensions of under 1 m and frequencies less than 1 kHz, shows that *quasi-static* conditions apply. That is, at a given instant in time, source–field relationships correspond to those found under static conditions.[1] Thus, in effect, we are examining direct current (dc) flow in physiologic volume conductors, and these can be maintained only by the presence of a supply of energy (a "battery"). In fact, we may expect that wherever a physiologic current source $\vec{J}^i$ arises, we also can identify a (normally nonelectrical) energy source that generates this current. In electrophysiologic processes, the immediate repository of energy is the potential energy associated with the varying chemical compositions encountered (extracellular ionic concentrations that differ greatly from intracellular concentrations), but the long-term energy source is the adenosine triphosphate (ATP) that drives various pumps that create and maintain the aforementioned concentration gradients.

Based on the aforementioned assumptions, we consider a uniformly conducting medium of conductivity σ and of infinite extent within which a current source $\vec{J}^i$ lies. This, in turn, establishes an electric field $\vec{E}$ and, based on Ohm's law, a conduction current density $\sigma\vec{E}$. The total current density $\vec{J}$ is the sum of the aforementioned currents, namely,

$$\vec{J} = \sigma\vec{E} + \vec{J}^i \tag{20.1}$$

Now, by virtue of the quasi-static conditions, the electric field may be derived from a scalar potential Φ [Plonsey and Heppner, 1967] so that

$$\vec{E} = -\nabla\Phi \tag{20.2}$$

Since quasi-steady-state conditions apply, $\vec{J}$ must be solenoidal, and consequently, substituting Equation 20.2 into Equation 20.1 and then setting the divergence of Equation 20.1 to zero show that Φ must satisfy Poisson's equation, namely,

$$\nabla^2\Phi = \left(\frac{1}{\sigma}\right)\nabla\cdot\vec{J}^i \tag{20.3}$$

An integral solution to Equation 20.3 is [Plonsey and Collin, 1961]

$$\Phi_p(x', y', z') = -\frac{1}{4\pi\sigma}\int_v \frac{\nabla,\vec{J}^i}{r}\,dv \tag{20.4}$$

where r in Equation 20.4 is the distance from a field point $P(x', y', z')$ to an element of source at $dv(x, y, z)$, that is,

$$r = \sqrt{(x - x')^2 + (y - y')^2 + (z - z')^2} \tag{20.5}$$

---

[1]Note that while, in effect, we consider relationships arising when $\partial/\partial t = 0$, all fields are actually assumed to vary in time synchronously with $\vec{J}^i$. Furthermore for the special case of magnetic field stimulation, the source of the primary electric field, $\partial\vec{A}/\partial t$, where $\vec{A}$ is the magnetic vector potential, must be retained.

Equation 20.4 may be transformed to an alternate form by employing the vector identity

$$\nabla \cdot \left[\left(\frac{1}{r} \right) \vec{J}^i \right] \equiv \left(\frac{1}{r} \right) \nabla \cdot \vec{J}^i + \nabla \left(\frac{1}{r} \right) \cdot \vec{J}^i \tag{20.6}$$

Based on Equation 20.6, we may substitute for the integrand in Equation 20.4 the sum $\nabla \cdot [(1/r)\vec{J}^i] - \nabla(1/r) \cdot \vec{J}^i$, giving the following:

$$\Phi_p(x', y', z') = -\frac{1}{4\pi\sigma} \left\{ \int_v \nabla \cdot \left[\left(\frac{1}{r} \right) \vec{J}^i \right] dv - \int_v \nabla \left(\frac{1}{r} \right) \vec{J}^i dv \right\} \tag{20.7}$$

The first term on the right-hand side may be transformed using the divergence theorem as follows:

$$\int_v \nabla \cdot \left[\left(\frac{1}{r} \right) \vec{J}^i \right] dv = \int_s \left(\frac{1}{r} \right) \vec{J}^i \cdot d\vec{S} = 0 \tag{20.8}$$

The volume integral in Equation 20.4 and Equation 20.8 is defined simply to include all sources. Consequently, in Equation 20.8, the surface S, which bounds V, necessarily lies away from $\vec{J}^i$. Since $\vec{J}^i$ thus is equal to zero on S, the expression in Equation 20.8 must likewise equal zero. The result is that Equation 20.4 also may be written as

$$\Phi_p(x', y', z') = -\frac{1}{4\pi\sigma} \int_v \frac{\nabla \cdot \vec{J}^i}{r} dv = \frac{1}{4\pi\sigma} \int_v \vec{J}^i \cdot \nabla \left(\frac{1}{r} \right) dv \tag{20.9}$$

We will derive the mathematical expressions for monopole and dipole fields in the next section, but based on those results, we can give a physical interpretation of the source terms in each of the integrals on the right-hand side of Equation 20.9. In the first, we note that $-\nabla \cdot \vec{J}^i$ is a volume source density, akin to charge density in electrostatics. In the second integral of Equation 20.9, $\vec{J}^i$ behaves with the dimensions of dipole moment per unit volume. This confirms an assertion, above, that $\vec{J}^i$ has a dual interpretation as a current density, as originally defined in Equation 20.1, or a volume dipole density, as can be inferred from Equation 20.9; in either case, its dimension are $mA/cm^2 = mA \cdot cm/cm^3$.

20.2 Monopole and Dipole Fields in the Uniform Volume of Infinite Extent

The monopole and dipole constitute the basic source elements in electrophysiology. We examine the fields produced by each in this section.

If one imagines an infinitely thin wire insulated over its extent except at its tip to be introducing a current into a uniform volume conductor of infinite extent, then we illustrate an idealized point source. Assuming the total applied current to be I_0 and located at the coordinate origin, then by symmetry the current density at a radius r must be given by the total current I_0 divided by the area of the spherical surface, or

$$\vec{J} = \frac{I_0}{4\pi r^2} \vec{a}_r \tag{20.10}$$

and $\vec{a}_r$ is a unit vector in the radial direction. This current source can be described by the nomenclature of the previous section as

$$\nabla \cdot \vec{J}^i = -I_0 \delta(r) \tag{20.11}$$

where δ denotes a volume delta function.

One can apply Ohm's law to Equation 20.10 and obtain an expression for the electric field, and if Equation 20.2 is also applied, we get

$$\vec{E} = -\nabla\Phi = \frac{I_0}{4\pi\sigma r^2}\vec{a}_r \tag{20.12}$$

where σ is the conductivity of the volume conductor. Since the right-hand side of Equation 20.12 is a function of r only, we can integrate to find Φ, which comes out

$$\Phi = \frac{I_0}{4\pi\sigma r} \tag{20.13}$$

In obtaining Equation 20.13, the constant of integration was set equal to zero so that the point at infinity has the usually chosen zero potential.

The dipole source consists of two monopoles of equal magnitude and opposite sign whose spacing approaches zero and whose magnitude during the limiting process increases such that the product of spacing and magnitude is constant. If we start out with both component monopoles at the origin, then the total source and field are zero. However, if we now displace the positive source in an arbitrary direction $\vec{d}$, then cancellation is no longer complete, and at a field point P we see simply the change in monopole field resulting from the displacement. For a very small displacement, this amounts to (i.e., we retain only the linear term in a Taylor series expansion)

$$\Phi_P = \frac{\partial}{\partial d}\left(\frac{I_0}{4\pi\sigma r}\right)d \tag{20.14}$$

The partial derivative in Equation 20.14 is called the *directional derivative*, and this can be evaluated by taking the dot product of the gradient of the expression enclosed in parentheses with the direction of d (i.e., $\nabla() \cdot \vec{a}_d$, where $\vec{a}_d$ is a unit vector in the $\vec{d}$ direction). The result is

$$\Phi_P = \frac{I_0 d}{4\pi\sigma}\vec{a}_d \cdot \nabla\left(\frac{1}{r}\right) \tag{20.15}$$

By definition, the dipole moment $\vec{m} = I_0\vec{d}$ in the limits as $d \to 0$; as noted, m remains finite. Thus, finally, the dipole field is given by [Plonsey, 1969]

$$\Phi_P = \frac{1}{4\pi\sigma}\vec{m} \cdot \nabla\left(\frac{1}{r}\right). \tag{20.16}$$

20.3 Volume Conductor Properties of Passive Tissue

If one were considering an active single isolated fiber lying in an extensive volume conductor (e.g., an *in vitro* preparation in a Ringer's bath), then there is a clear separation between the excitable tissue and the surrounding volume conductor. However, consider in contrast activation proceeding in the *in vivo* heart. In this case, the source currents lie in only a portion of the heart (nominally where $\nabla V_m \neq 0$). The volume conductor now includes the remaining (passive) cardiac fibers along with an inhomogeneous torso containing a number of contiguous organs (internal to the heart are blood-filled cavities, while external are pericardium, lungs, skeletal muscle, bone, fat, skin, air, etc.).

The treatment of the surrounding multicellular cardiac tissue poses certain difficulties. A recently used and reasonable approximation is that the intracellular space, in view of the many intercellular junctions, can be represented as a continuum. A similar treatment can be extended to the interstitial space. This results in two domains that can be regarded as occupying the same physical space; each domain is separated from the other by the membrane. This view underlies the *bidomain* model [Plonsey, 1989]. To reflect the

TABLE 20.1 Conductivity Values
for Cardiac Bidomain

S/mm	Clerc [1976]	Roberts [1982]
g_{ix}	1.74×10^4	3.44×10^{-4}
g_{iy}	1.93×10^{-5}	5.96×10^{-5}
g_{ax}	6.25×10^{-4}	1.17×10^{-4}
g_{ay}	2.36×10^{-4}	8.02×10^{-5}

underlying fiber geometry, each domain is necessarily anisotropic, with the high conductivity axes defined by the fiber direction and with an approximate cross-fiber isotropy. A further simplification may be possible in a uniform tissue region that is sufficiently far from the sources, since beyond a few space constants transmembrane currents may become quite small and the tissue would therefore behave as a single domain (a *monodomain*). Such a tissue also would be substantially resistive. On the other hand, if the membranes behave passively and there is some degree of transmembrane current flow, then the tissue may still be approximated as a uniform monodomain, but it may be necessary to include some of the reactive properties introduced via the highly capacitive cell membranes. A classic study by Schwan and Kay [1957] of the macroscopic (averaged) properties of many tissues showed that the displacement current was normally negligible compared with the conduction current.

It is not always clear whether a bidomain model is appropriate to a particular tissue, and experimental measurements found in the literature are not always able to resolve this question. The problem is that if the experimenter believes the tissue under consideration to be, say, an isotropic monodomain, measurements are set up and interpreted that are consistent with this idea; the inherent inconsistencies may never come to light [Plonsey and Barr, 1986]. Thus one may find impedance data tabulated in the literature for a number of organs, but if the tissue is truly, say, an anisotropic bidomain, then the impedance tensor requires six numbers, and anything less is necessarily inadequate to some degree. For cardiac tissue, it is usually assumed that the impedance in the direction transverse to the fiber axis is isotropic. Consequently, only four numbers are needed. These values are given in Table 20.1 as obtained from, essentially, the only two experiments for which bidomain values were sought.

20.4 Effects of Volume Conductor Inhomogeneities: Secondary Sources and Images

In the preceding we have assumed that the volume conductor is homogeneous, and the evaluation of fields from the current sources given in Equation 20.9 is based on this assumption. Consider what would happen if the volume conductor in which $\vec{J}^i$ lies is bounded by air, and the source is suddenly introduced. Equation 20.9 predicts an initial current flow into the boundary, but no current can escape into the nonconducting surrounding region. We must, consequently, have a transient during which charge piles up at the boundary, a process that continues until the field from the accumulating charges brings the net normal component of electric field to zero at the boundary. To characterize a steady-state condition with no further increase in charge requires satisfaction of the boundary condition that $\partial\Phi/\partial n = 0$ at the surface (within the tissue). The source that develops at the bounding surface is secondary to the initiation of the primary field; it is referred to as a *secondary source*. While the secondary source is essential for satisfaction of boundary conditions, it contributes to the total field everywhere else.

The preceding illustration is for a region bounded by air, but the same phenomena would arise if the region were simply bounded by one of different conductivity. In this case, when the source is first "turned on," since the primary electric field $\vec{E}_a$ is continuous across the interface between regions of different conductivity, the current flowing into such a boundary (e.g., $\sigma_1\vec{E}_a$) is unequal to the current flowing away from that boundary (e.g., $\sigma_2\vec{E}_a$). Again, this necessarily results in an accumulation of charge, and a secondary source will grow until the applied plus secondary field satisfies the required continuity of current density, namely,

$$-\sigma_1 \partial \frac{\Phi_1}{\partial_n} = -\sigma_2 \partial \frac{\Phi_2}{\partial_n} = J_n \tag{20.17}$$

where the surface normal n is directed from region 1 to region 2. The accumulated single source density can be shown to be equal to the discontinuity of $\partial \Phi / \partial_n$ in Equation 20.17 [Plonsey, 1974], in particular,

$$K_s = J_n \left(\frac{1}{\sigma_1} - \frac{1}{\sigma_2} \right) \sigma$$

The magnitude of the steady-state secondary source also can be described as an *equivalent double layer*, the magnitude of which is [Plonsey, 1974]

$$\vec{K}_k^i = \Phi_k (\sigma_k'' - \sigma_k') \vec{n} \tag{20.18}$$

where the condition at the kth interface is described. In Equation 20.18, the two abutting regions are designated with prime and double-prime superscripts, and $\vec{n}$ is directed from the primed to the double-primed region. Actually, Equation 20.18 evaluates the double-layer source for the scalar function $\Psi = \Phi \sigma$, its strength being given by the discontinuity in Ψ at the interface [Plonsey, 1974] (the potential is necessarily continuous at the interface with the value Φ_k called for in Equation 20.18). The (secondary) potential field generated by $\vec{K}_k^i$, since it constitutes a source for Ψ with respect to which the medium is uniform and infinite in extent, can be found from Equation 20.9 as

$$\Psi_P^S = \sigma_P \Phi_P^S = \frac{1}{4\pi} \sum_k \int_k \Phi_k (\sigma_k'' - \sigma_k') \vec{n} \cdot \nabla \left(\frac{1}{r} \right) ds \tag{20.19}$$

where the superscript S denotes the secondary source/field component (alone). Solving Equation 20.19 for Φ, we get

$$\Phi_P^S = \frac{1}{4\pi \sigma_P} \sum_k \int_k \Phi_k (\sigma_k'' - \sigma_k') \vec{n} \cdot \nabla \left(\frac{1}{r} \right) ds \tag{20.20}$$

where σ_P in Equation 20.19 and Equation 20.20 takes on the conductivity at the field point. The total field is obtained from Equation 20.20 by adding the primary field. Assuming that all applied currents lie in a region with conductivity σ_a, then we have

$$\Phi_P^S = \frac{1}{4\pi \sigma_a} \int \vec{J}^i \cdot \nabla \left(\frac{1}{r} \right) dv + \frac{1}{4\pi \sigma_P} \sum_k \int_k \Phi_k (\sigma_k'' - \sigma_k') \vec{n} \cdot \nabla \left(\frac{1}{r} \right) ds \tag{20.21}$$

(If the primary currents lie in several conductivity compartments, then each will yield a term similar to the first integral in Equation 20.21.) Note that in Equation 20.20 and Equation 20.21 the secondary source field is similar in form to the field in a homogeneous medium of infinite extent, except that σ_P is piecewise constant and consequently introduces interfacial discontinuities. With regard to the potential, these just cancel the discontinuity introduced by the double layer itself so that Φ_k is appropriately continuous across each passive interface.

The primary and secondary source currents that generate the electrical potential in Equation 20.21 also set up a magnetic field. The primary source, for example, is the forcing function in the Poisson equation for the vector potential $\vec{A}$ [Plonsey, 1981], namely,

$$\nabla^2 \vec{A} = -\vec{J}^i \tag{20.22}$$

From this it is not difficult to show that, due to Equation 20.21 for Φ, we have the following expression for the magnetic field $\vec{H}$ [Plonsey, 1981]:

$$\vec{H} = \frac{1}{4\pi} \int \vec{J}^i \times \nabla \left(\frac{1}{r}\right) dv + \frac{1}{4\pi} \sum_k \int \Phi_k (\sigma_k'' - \sigma_k') \vec{n} \times \nabla \left(\frac{1}{r}\right) dS \qquad (20.23)$$

A simple illustration of these ideas is found in the case of two semi-infinite regions of different conductivity, 1 and 2, with a unit point current source located in region 1 a distance h from the interface. Region 1, which we may think of as on the "left," has the conductivity σ_1, while region 2, on the "right," is at conductivity σ_2. The field in region 1 is that which arises from the actual point current source plus an image point source of magnitude $(\rho_2 - \rho_1)/(\rho_2 + \rho_1)$ located in region 2 at the mirror-image point [Schwan and Kay, 1957]. The field in region 2 arises from an equivalent point source located at the actual source point but of strength $[1 + (\rho_2 - \rho_1)/(\rho_2 + \rho_1)]$. One can confirm this by noting that all fields satisfy Poisson's equation and that at the interface Φ is continuous while the normal component of current density is also continuous (i.e., $\sigma_1 \partial \Phi_1 / \partial n = \sigma_2 \partial \Phi_2 / \partial n$).

The potential on the interface is constant along a circular path whose origin is the foot of the perpendicular from the point source. Calling this radius r and applying Equation 20.13, we have for the surface potential Φ_S

$$\Phi_S = \frac{\rho_1}{4\pi \sqrt{h^2 + r^2}} \left(1 + \frac{\rho_2 - \rho_1}{\rho_2 + \rho_1}\right) \qquad (20.24)$$

and consequently a secondary double-layer source $\vec{K}_S$ equals, according to Equation 20.18,

$$\vec{K}_S = \frac{\rho_1}{4\pi \sqrt{h^2 + r^2}} \left(1 + \frac{\rho_2 - \rho_1}{\rho_2 + \rho_1}\right) (\sigma_2 - \sigma_1) \vec{n} \qquad (20.25)$$

where $\vec{n}$ is directed from region 1 to region 2. The field from $\vec{K}_S$ in region 1 is exactly equal to that from a point source of strength $(\rho_2 - \rho_1)/(\rho_2 + \rho_1)$ at the mirror-image point, which can be verified by evaluating and showing the equality of the following:

$$\Phi_P = \frac{1}{4\pi \sigma_1} \int \vec{K}_S \cdot \nabla \left(\frac{1}{r}\right) ds = \frac{(\rho_2 - \rho_1)/(\rho_2 - \rho_1)}{4\pi \sigma_1 R} \qquad (20.26)$$

where R in Equation 20.26 is the distance from the mirror-image point to the field point P, and r in Equation 20.26 is the distance from the surface integration point to the field point.

References

Clerc, L. 1976. Directional differences of impulse spread in trabecular muscle from mammalian heart. *J. Physiol. (Lond.)* 255: 335.

Plonsey, R. 1969. *Bioelectric Phenomena*. New York, McGraw-Hill.

Plonsey, R. 1974. The formulation of bioelectric source–field relationship in terms of surface discontinuities. *J. Frank Inst.* 297: 317.

Plonsey, R. 1981. Generation of magnetic fields by the human body (theory). In S.-N. Erné, H.-D. Hahlbohm, and H. Lübbig (Eds.), *Biomagnetism*, pp. 177–205. Berlin, W de Gruyter.

Plonsey, R. 1989. The use of the bidomain model for the study of excitable media. *Lect. Math. Life Sci.* 21: 123.

Plonsey, R. and Barr, R.C. 1986. A critique of impedance measurements in cardiac tissue. *Ann. Biomed. Eng.* 14: 307.

Plonsey, R. and Collin, R.E. 1961. *Principles and Applications of Electromagnetic Fields*. New York, McGraw-Hill.

Plonsey, R. and Heppner, D. 1967. Consideration of quasi-stationarity in electrophysiological systems. *Bull. Math. Biophys.* 29: 657.

Roberts, D. and Scher, A.M. 1982. Effect of tissue anisotropy on extracellular potential fields in canine myocardium *in situ*. *Circ. Res.* 50: 342.

Schwan, H.P. and Kay, C.F. 1957. The conductivity of living tissues. *NY Acad. Sci.* 65: 1007.

21

The Electrical Conductivity of Tissues

Bradley J. Roth
Oakland University

21.1 Introduction

One of the most important problems in bioelectric theory is the calculation of the electrical potential, Φ (V), throughout a **volume conductor**. The calculation of Φ is important in impedance imaging, cardiac pacing and defibrillation, electrocardiogram and electroencephalogram analysis, and functional electrical stimulation. In bioelectric problems, Φ often changes slowly enough that we can assume it is **quasistatic** [Plonsey, 1969]; we ignore capacitive and inductive effects and the finite speed of propagation of electromagnetic radiation. (Usually for bioelectric phenomena, this assumption is valid for frequencies below about 100 kHz.) Under the quasistatic approximation, the continuity equation states that the divergence, $\nabla \cdot$, of the current density, J (A/m^2), is equal to the applied or endogenous source of electrical current, S (A/m^3):

$$\nabla \cdot J = S. \tag{21.1}$$

In regions of tissue where there are no sources, S is zero. In these cases, the divergenceless of J is equivalent to the law of **conservation of current** that is often invoked when analyzing electrical circuits. Another property of a volume conductor is that the current density and the electric field, E (V/m), are related linearly by **Ohm's Law**,

$$J = gE, \tag{21.2}$$

where g is the electrical **conductivity** (S/m). Finally, the relationship between the electric field and the gradient, ∇, of the potential is

$$E = -\nabla \Phi. \tag{21.3}$$

The purpose of this chapter is to characterize the electrical conductivity. This task is not easy, because g is generally a macroscopic parameter (an "effective conductivity") that represents the electrical properties of the tissue averaged over many cells. The effective conductivity can vary with direction, can be complex (contain real and imaginary parts), and can depend on the temporal and spatial frequencies.

Before discussing the conductivity of tissue, consider one of the simplest and most easily understood volume conductors: saline. The electrical conductivity of saline arises from the motion of free ions in response to a steady electric field, and is on the order of 1 S/m. Besides conductivity, another property of saline is its electrical **permittivity**, ε (S sec/m). This property is related to the dielectric constant, κ (dimensionless), by $\varepsilon = \kappa \varepsilon_0$, where ε_0 is the permittivity of free space, 8.854×10^{-12} S sec/m. Dielectric properties arise from bound charge that is displaced by the electric field, creating a dipole. They can also arise if the applied electric field aligns molecular dipoles (such as the dipole moments of water molecules) that are normally oriented randomly. The DC dielectric constant of saline is similar to that of water (about $\kappa = 80$).

The movement of free charge produces conductivity, whereas stationary dipoles produce permittivity. In steady state, the distinction between the two is clear, but at higher frequencies the concepts merge. In such a case, we can combine the electrical properties into a complex conductivity, g':

$$g' = g + i\omega\varepsilon, \tag{21.4}$$

where ω (rad/sec) is the angular frequency ($\omega = 2\pi f$, where f is the frequency in Hz) and i is $\sqrt{-1}$. The real part of g' accounts for the movement of charge in phase with the electric field; the imaginary part accounts for out-of-phase motion. Both the real and the imaginary parts of the complex conductivity may depend on the frequency. For many bioelectric phenomena, the first term in Equation 21.4 is much larger than the second, so the tissue can be represented as purely conductive [Plonsey, 1969]. (The imaginary part of the complex conductivity represents a capacitive effect, and therefore technically violates our assumption of quasistationarity. This violation is the only exception we will make to our general rule of a quasistatic potential.)

21.2 Cell Suspensions

The earliest and simplest model describing the electrical conductivity of a biological tissue is a suspension of cells in a saline solution [Cole, 1968; Peters et al., 2001]. Let us consider a suspension of spherical cells, each of radius a (Figure 21.1a). The saline surrounding the cells constitutes the **interstitial space** (conductivity σ_e), while the conducting fluid inside the cells constitutes the intracellular space (conductivity σ_i). (We shall follow Henriquez [1993] in denoting macroscopic effective conductivities by g and microscopic conductivities by σ.) The cell membrane separates the two spaces; a thin layer having conductivity per unit area G_m (S/m^2) and capacitance per unit area C_m (F/m^2). One additional parameter — the intracellular volume fraction, f (dimensionless) — indicates how tightly the cells are packed together. The volume fraction can range from nearly zero (a dilute solution) to almost 1. (Spherical cells cannot approach a volume fraction of 1, but tightly packed, nonspherical cells can). For irregularly shaped cells, the "radius" is difficult to define. In these cases, it is easier to specify the surface-to-volume ratio of the tissue (the ratio of the membrane surface area to tissue volume). For spherical cells, the surface-to-volume ratio is $3f/a$.

We can define operationally the effective conductivity, g, of a cell suspension by the following process (Figure 21.1a): Place the suspension in a cylindrical tube of length L and cross-sectional area A (be sure L and A are large enough so the volume contains many cells). Apply a DC potential difference V across

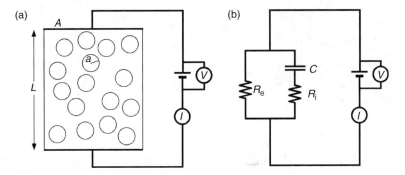

FIGURE 21.1 (a) A schematic diagram of a suspension of spherical cells; the effective conductivity of this suspension is *IL/VA*. (b) An electric circuit equivalent of the effective conductivity of this suspension.

the two ends of the cylinder (so that the electric field has strength V/L) and measure the total current, I, passing through the suspension. The effective conductivity is *IL/VA*.

Deriving an expression for the effective conductivity of a suspension of spheres in terms of microscopic parameters is an old and interesting problem in electromagnetic theory [Cole, 1968]. For DC fields, the effective conductivity, g, of a suspension of insulating spheres placed in a solution of conductivity σ_e is

$$g = \frac{2(1-f)}{2+f}\sigma_e. \tag{21.5}$$

For most cells, G_m is small enough so that the membrane behaves as an insulator, and hence the assumption of insulating spheres is applicable. The net effect of the cells is to decrease the conductivity of the solution (the decrease can be substantial for tightly packed cells).

The cell membrane has a capacitance of about 0.01 F/m² (or, in traditional units, 1 μF/cm²), which causes the electrical conductivity to depend on frequency. The electrical circuit in Figure 21.1b represents the suspension of cells: R_e is the effective resistance to current passing entirely through the interstitial space; R_i is the effective resistance to current passing into the intracellular space; and C is the effective membrane capacitance. (The membrane conductance is usually small enough so that it has little effect, regardless of the frequency.) At low frequencies all of the current is restricted to the interstitial space, and the electrical conductivity is given approximately by Equation 21.5 above. At high frequencies, C shunts current across the membrane, so that the effective conductivity of the tissue is:

$$g = \frac{2(1-f)\sigma_e + (1+2f)\sigma_i}{(2+f)\sigma_e + (1-f)\sigma_i}\sigma_e. \tag{21.6}$$

At intermediate frequencies, the effective conductivity has both real and imaginary parts, because the membrane capacitance contributes significantly to the effective conductivity. In these cases, Equation 21.6 still holds if σ_i is replaced by σ_i^*, where

$$\sigma_i^* = \frac{\sigma_i Y_m a}{\sigma_i + Y_m a} \quad \text{with } Y_m = G_m + i\omega C_m. \tag{21.7}$$

Figure 21.2 shows the effective conductivity (magnitude and phase) as a function of frequency for a typical tissue. The increase in the phase at about 300 kHz is sometimes called the "beta dispersion."

21.3 Fiber Suspensions

Many of the most interesting electrically active tissues, such as nerve and skeletal muscle, are better approximated as a suspension of cylinders rather than a suspension of spheres. This difference has profound

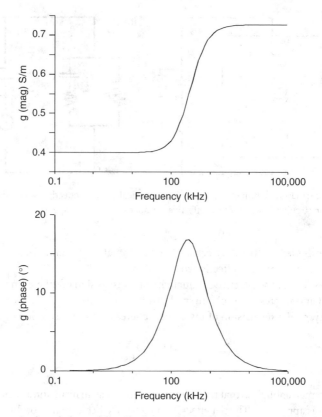

FIGURE 21.2 The magnitude and phase of the effective conductivity as a function of frequency, for a suspension of spherical cells: $f = 0.5$; $a = 20\ \mu\text{m}$; $\sigma_e = 1$ S/m; $\sigma_i = 0.5$ S/m; $G_m = 0$; and $C_m = 0.01$ F/m^2.

implications because it introduces **anisotropy**. The effective electrical conductivity depends on direction. Henceforth, we must speak of the longitudinal effective conductivity parallel to the cylindrical fibers, g_L, and the transverse effective conductivity perpendicular to the fibers, g_T. (In theory, the conductivity could be different in three directions; however, often the electrical properties in the two directions perpendicular to the fibers are the same.) In general, the conductivity is no longer a scalar quantity, but is a tensor instead, and must be represented by a 3×3 symmetric matrix. If our coordinate axes lie along the principle directions of this matrix (invariably, the directions parallel to and perpendicular to the fibers), then the off-diagonal terms of the matrix are zero. If, however, we choose our coordinate axes differently, or if the fibers curve so that the direction parallel to the fibers varies over space, we have to deal with tensor properties, including off-diagonal components.

When the electric field is applied perpendicular to the fiber direction, a suspension of fibers is similar to the suspension of cells described above (in Figure 21.1a, we must now imagine that the circles represent cross sections of cylindrical fibers, rather than spherical cells). The expression for the effective transverse conductivity of a suspension of cylindrical cells, of radius a and intracellular conductivity σ_i, placed in a solution of conductivity σ_e, with intracellular volume fraction f, is [Cole, 1968]

$$g_T = \frac{(1-f)\sigma_e + (1+f)\sigma_i^*}{(1+f)\sigma_e + (1-f)\sigma_i^*}\sigma_e, \qquad (21.8)$$

where Equation 21.7 defines σ_i^*. At DC, and for $G_m = 0$, Equation 21.8 reduces to

$$g_T = \frac{1-f}{1+f}\sigma_e. \qquad (21.9)$$

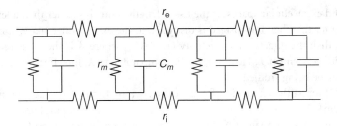

FIGURE 21.3 An electrical circuit representing a one-dimensional nerve or muscle fiber: r_i and r_e are the intracellular and extracellular resistances per unit length (Ω/m); r_m is the membrane resistance times unit length (Ω m); and c_m is the membrane capacitance per unit length (F/m).

When an electric field is applied parallel to the fiber direction, a new behavior arises that is fundamentally different from that observed for a suspension of spherical cells. Return for a moment to our operational definition of the effective conductivity. Surprisingly, the effective longitudinal conductivity of a suspension of fibers depends on the length L of the tissue sample used for the measurement. To understand this dependence, we must consider one-dimensional **cable theory** [Plonsey, 1969]. The circuit in Figure 21.3a approximates a single nerve or muscle fiber. Adopting the traditional electrophysiology nomenclature, we denote the intracellular and extracellular resistances per unit length along the fiber by r_i and r_e (Ω/m), the membrane resistance times unit length by r_m(Ω m), and the capacitance per unit length by c_m (F/m). The cable equation governs the transmembrane potential, V_m:

$$\lambda^2 \frac{\partial^2 V_m}{\partial x^2} = \tau \frac{\partial V_m}{\partial t} + V_m, \tag{21.10}$$

where τ is the time constant, $r_m c_m$, and λ is the length constant, $\sqrt{r_m/(r_i + r_e)}$. For a truncated fiber of length L (m) with sealed ends, and with a steady-state current I (A) injected into the extracellular space at one end and removed at the other, the solution to the cable equation is

$$V_m = I r_e \lambda \frac{\sinh(x/\lambda)}{\cosh(L/2\lambda)}, \tag{21.11}$$

where the origin of the x-axis is at the midpoint between electrodes. The extracellular potential, V_e, consists of two terms: One is proportional to x, and the other is $r_e/(r_i + r_e)$ times V_m. We can evaluate V_e at the two ends of the fiber to obtain the voltage drop between the electrodes, ΔV_e

$$\Delta V_e = \frac{r_i r_e}{r_i + r_e} I \left[L + \frac{r_e}{r_i} 2\lambda \tanh\left(\frac{L}{2\lambda}\right) \right]. \tag{21.12}$$

If L is very large compared to λ, the extracellular voltage drop reduces to

$$\Delta V_e = \frac{r_i r_e}{r_i + r_e} LI \quad L \gg \lambda. \tag{21.13}$$

The leading factor is the parallel combination of the intracellular and extracellular resistances. If, on the other hand, L is very small compared to λ, the extracellular voltage drop becomes

$$\Delta V_e = r_e LI \quad L \ll \lambda. \tag{21.14}$$

In this case, the leading factor is simply the extracellular resistance alone. Physically, there is a redistribution of current into the intracellular space that occurs over a distance on the order of a length constant. If the tissue length is much longer than a length constant, the current is redistributed completely between the intracellular and extracellular spaces. If the tissue length is much smaller than a length constant, the current does not enter the fiber, but instead is restricted to the extracellular space. If either of these two conditions is met, then the effective conductivity ($IL/A\Delta V_e$, where A is the cross-sectional area of the tissue strand) is independent of L. However, if L is comparable to λ, the effective conductivity depends on the size of the tissue being studied.

Roth et al. [1988] recast the expression for the effective longitudinal conductivity in terms of **spatial frequency**, k (rad/m). This approach has two advantages. First, the temporal and spatial behaviors are both described using frequency analysis. Second, a parameter describing the size of a specific piece of tissue is not necessary: the spatial frequency dependence becomes a property of the tissue, not the measurement. The expression for the DC effective longitudinal conductivity is

$$g_L = \frac{(1-f)\sigma_e + f\sigma_i}{1 + \dfrac{f\sigma_i}{(1-f)\sigma_e}\dfrac{1}{1 + \left(\dfrac{1}{\lambda k}\right)^2}} \tag{21.15}$$

To relate the effective longitudinal conductivity to Equation 21.13 and Equation 21.14 above, note that $1/k$ plays the same role as L. If $k\lambda \ll 1$, g_L reduces to $(1-f)\sigma_e + f\sigma_i$, which is equivalent to the parallel combination of resistances in Equation 21.13. If $k\lambda \gg 1$, g_L becomes $(1-f)\sigma_e$, implying that the current is restricted to the interstitial space, as in Equation 21.14. Equation 21.15 can be generalized to all temporal frequencies by defining λ in terms of Y_m instead of G_m [Roth et al., 1988]. Figure 21.4 shows the magnitude and phase of the longitudinal and transverse effective conductivities as functions of the temporal and spatial frequencies.

The measurement of effective conductivities is complicated by the traditionally used electrode geometry. Typically, one uses a four-electrode technique [Steendijk et al., 1993], in which two electrodes inject current and two others measure the potential (Figure 21.5). Gielen et al. [1984] used this method to measure the electrical properties of skeletal muscle and found that the effective conductivity depended on the interelectrode distance. Roth [1989] reanalyzed Gielen et al.'s data using the spatial frequency dependent model and found agreement with some of the more unexpected features or their data (Figure 21.6). Table 21.1 contains typical values of skeletal muscle effective conductivities and microscopic tissue parameters. Table 21.2 lists nerve effective conductivities.

21.4 Syncytia

Cardiac tissue is different from the other tissues we have discussed in that it is an electrical **syncytium**: the cells are coupled through intercellular junctions. The **bidomain** model describes the electrical properties of cardiac muscle [Henriquez, 1993]. It is essentially a two- or three-dimensional cable model that takes into account the resistance of both the intracellular and the interstitial spaces (Figure 21.7). Thus, the concept of current redistribution, discussed earlier in the context of the longitudinal effective conductivity of a suspension of fibers, now applies in all directions. Furthermore, cardiac muscle is markedly anisotropic. These properties make impedance measurements of cardiac muscle difficult to interpret [Plonsey and Barr, 1986; Le Guyader et al., 2001]. The situation is complicated further because the intracellular space is more anisotropic than is the interstitial space (in the jargon of bidomain modeling, this condition is known as "unequal anisotropy ratios") [Roth, 1997]. Consequently, an expression for a single effective conductivity for cardiac muscle is difficult, if not impossible, to derive. In general, one must solve a pair of coupled partial differential equations simultaneously for the intracellular and interstitial potentials.

The bidomain model characterizes the electrical properties of the tissue by four effective conductivities: g_{iL}, g_{iT}, g_{eL}, and g_{eT}, where i and e denote the intracellular and interstitial spaces, and L and T denote the

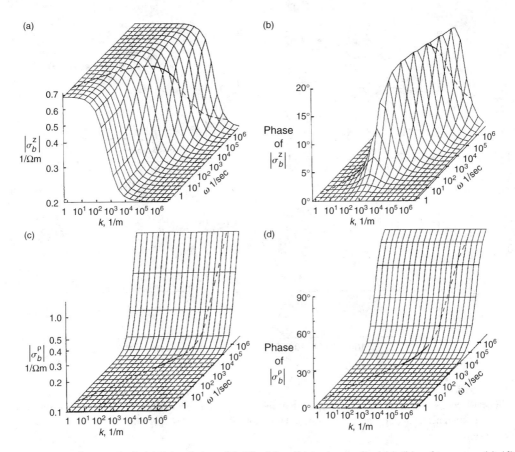

FIGURE 21.4 The magnitude (a), (c) and phase (b), (d) of the effective longitudinal (a), (b) and transverse (c), (d) effective conductivities, calculated using the spatial, k, and temporal, ω, frequency model. The parameters used in this calculation are $G_m = 1$ S/m^2; $C_m = 0.01$ F/m^2; $f = 0.9$; $a = 20$ μm; $\sigma_i = 0.55$ S/m; and $\sigma_e = 2$ S/m. (From Roth, B.J., Gielen, F.L.H., and Wikswo, J.P., Jr. 1988. *Math. Biosci.* 88: 159–189. With permission.)

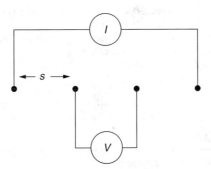

FIGURE 21.5 A schematic diagram of the four-electrode technique for measuring tissue conductivities. Current, I, is passed through the outer two electrodes, and the potential, V, is measured between the inner two. The interelectrode distance is s.

directions parallel to and perpendicular to the myocardial fibers. We can relate these parameters to the microscopic tissue properties by using an operational definition of an effective bidomain conductivity, similar to the operational definition given earlier. To determine the interstitial conductivity, first dissect a cylindrical tube of tissue of length L and cross-sectional area A (one must be sure that L and A are large

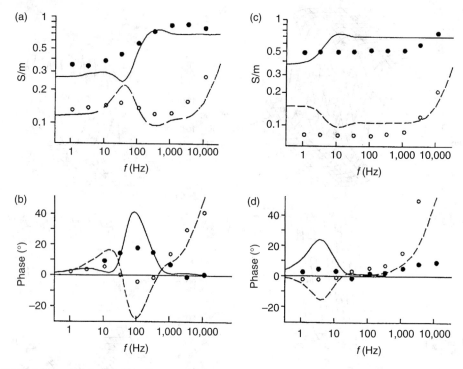

FIGURE 21.6   The calculated (a) amplitude and (b) phase of g_L (solid) and g_T (dashed) as a function of frequency, for an interelectrode distance of 0.5 mm; (c) and (d) show the quantities for an interelectrode distance of 3.0 mm. Circles represent experimental data; g_L (filled), g_T (open). (From Roth, B.J. 1989. *Med. Biol. Eng. Comput.*, 27: 491–495. With permission.)

TABLE 21.1   Skeletal Muscle

Macroscopic effective conductivities (S/m)			
g_L	g_T	Note	Reference
0.35	0.086	10 Hz, IED = 3 mm	Gielen et al. [1984]
0.20	0.092	10 Hz, IED = 0.5 mm	
0.52	0.076	20 Hz, IED = 17 mm	Epstein and Foster [1983]
0.70	0.32	100 kHz, IED = 17 mm	
0.67	0.040	0.1 sec pulse	Rush et al. [1963]

Microscopic tissue parameters					
σ_i (S/m)	σ_e (S/m)	f	C_m (F/m^2)	G_m (S/m^2)	References
0.55	2.4	0.9	0.01	1.0	Gielen et al. [1986]

Note: IED = interelectrode distance.

enough so the volume contains many cells, and that the dissection does not damage the tissue). Next, apply a drug to the tissue that makes the membrane essentially insulating (i.e., the length constant is much longer than L). Finally, apply a DC potential difference, V, across the two ends of the cylinder and measure the total current, I. The effective interstitial conductivity is IL/VA. This procedure must be performed twice, once with the fibers parallel to the axis of the cylinder, and once with the fibers perpendicular to it. To determine the effective intracellular conductivities, follow the above procedure but apply the voltage difference to the intracellular space instead of the interstitial space. Although the procedure would be

TABLE 21.2 Nerve

Macroscopic effective conductivities (S/m)			
g_L	g_T	Note	Reference
0.41	0.01	Toad sciatic nerve	Tasaki [1964]
0.57	0.083	Cat dorsal column, 10 Hz	Ranck and BeMent [1965]

Microscopic tissue parameters					
σ_i (S/m)	σ_e (S/m)	f	C_m (F/m^2)	G_m (S/m^2)	Reference
0.64	1.54	0.35	1	0.44	Roth and Altman [1992]

Note: Volume fraction of myelin = 0.27, G_m is proportional to axon diameter; the above value is for an axon with outer diameter of 6.5 μm.

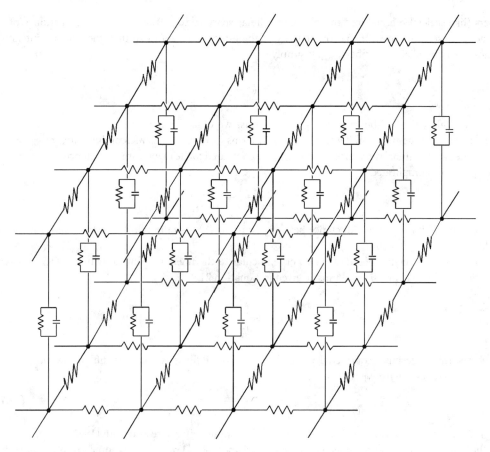

FIGURE 21.7 A circuit representing a two-dimensional syncytium (i.e., a bidomain). The lower array of resistors represents the intracellular space, the upper array represents the extracellular space, and the parallel resistors and capacitors represent the membrane.

extraordinarily difficult in practice, we can imagine two arrays of microelectrodes that impale the cells at both ends of the cylinder and maintain a constant potential at each end.

Expressions have been derived for the effective bidomain conductivities in terms of the microscopic tissue parameters [Roth, 1988; Henriquez, 1993; Neu and Krassowska, 1993]. The effective conductivities in the direction parallel to the fibers are simplest. Imagine that the tissue is composed of long, straight

TABLE 21.3   Cardiac Muscle

Macroscopic effective conductivities (ventricular muscle) (S/m)				
g_{iL}	g_{iT}	g_{eL}	g_{eT}	Reference
0.17	0.019	0.62	0.24	Clerc
0.28	0.026	0.22	0.13	Roberts et al.
0.34	0.060	0.12	0.080	Roberts and Scher

Microscopic tissue parameters						
σ_i (S/m)	σ_e (S/m)	f	a (μm)	b (μm)	G (μS)	Reference
1	1	0.7	100	10	3	Roth [1988]
0.4	2	0.85	100	7.5	0.05	Neu and Krassowska [1993]

fibers (like skeletal muscle) and that the intracellular space of these fibers occupies a fraction f of the tissue cross-sectional area. If the conductivity of the interstitial fluid is σ_e, then the effective interstitial conductivity parallel to the fibers, g_{eL}, is simply

$$g_{eL} = \left(1 - f\right)\sigma_e. \tag{21.16}$$

If we neglect the resistance of the gap junctions, we obtain a similar expression for the effective intracellular conductivity parallel to the fibers in terms of the myoplasmic conductivity, σ_i: $g_{iL} = f\sigma_i$. When the gap junctional resistance is not negligible compared to the myoplasmic resistance, the expression for g_{iL} is more complicated:

$$g_{iL} = \frac{1}{1 + (\pi a^2 \sigma_i)/(bG)} f\sigma_i, \tag{21.17}$$

where G is the junctional conductance between two cells (S), b is the cell length (m), and a is the cell radius (m).

The effective interstitial conductivity perpendicular to the fibers is identical with the DC transverse effective conductivity for skeletal muscle given in Equation 21.9

$$g_{eT} = \frac{1 - f}{1 + f}\sigma_e. \tag{21.18}$$

The effective intracellular conductivity perpendicular to the fibers is the most difficult to model, but a reasonable expression for g_{iT} is

$$g_{iT} = \frac{1}{1 + (b\sigma_i)/G}\sigma_i. \tag{21.19}$$

Table 21.3 contains measured values of the bidomain conductivities (see also Roth [1997]). Typical values of the microscopic tissue parameters are also given in Table 21.3, although some are quite uncertain (particularly G).

If the intercellular junctions contribute significantly to the intracellular resistance, the bidomain model only approximates the tissue behavior [Neu and Krassowska, 1993]. For sufficiently large junctional resistance, the discrete cellular properties become important, and a continuum model no longer represents the tissue well. Interestingly, as the junctional resistance increases, cardiac tissue behaves less like a syncytium and more like a suspension of cells. Thus we have come a full circle. We started by considering a suspension of cells, then examined suspensions of fibers, and finally generalized to syncytia. Yet, when the intercellular junctions in a syncytium are disrupted, we find ourselves again thinking of the tissue as a suspension of cells.

Defining Terms

Anisotropy: Having different properties in different directions.

Bidomain: A two- or three-dimensional cable model that takes into account the resistance of both the intracellular and the extracellular spaces.

Cable theory: Representation of a cylindrical fiber as two parallel rows of resistors (one each for the intracellular and extracellular spaces) connected in a ladder network by a parallel combination of resistors and capacitors (the cell membrane).

Conservation of current: A fundamental law of electrostatics, stating that there is no net current entering or leaving at any point in a volume conductor.

Conductivity: A parameter (g) that measures how well a substance conducts electricity. The coefficient of proportionality between the electric field and the current density. The units of conductivity are siemens per meter (S/m). A siemens is an inverse ohm, sometimes called a "mho" in the older literature.

Interstitial space: The extracellular space between cells in a tissue.

Ohm's law: A linear relation between the electric field and current density vectors.

Permittivity: A parameter (ε) that measures the size of the dipole moment induced in a substance by an electric field. The units of permittivity are siemens second per meter (S sec/m), or farads per meter (F/m).

Quasistatic: A potential distribution that changes slowly enough that we can accurately describe it by the equations of electrostatics (capacitive, inductive, and propagation effects are ignored).

Spatial frequency: A parameter governing how rapidly a function changes in space; $k = 1/(2\pi/s)$, where s is the wavelength of a sinusoidally varying function.

Syncytium (pl., syncytia): A tissue in which the intracellular spaces of adjacent cells are coupled through intercellular channels, so that current can pass between any two intracellular points without crossing the cell membrane.

Volume conductor: A three-dimensional region of space containing a material that passively conducts electrical current.

Acknowledgments

I thank Dr. Craig Henriquez for several suggestions and corrections, and Barry Bowman for carefully editing the manuscript.

References

Clerc, L. 1976. Directional differences of impulse spread in trabecular muscle from mammalian heart. *J. Physiol.* 255: 335–346.

Cole, K.S. 1968. *Membranes, Ions, and Impulses,* University of California Press, Berkeley, CA.

Epstein, B. R. and Foster, K. R. 1983. Anisotropy in the dielectric properties of skeletal muscle. *Med. Biol. Eng. Comput.* 21: 51–55.

Gielen F. L. H., Cruts, H. E., Albers, B. A., Boon, K. L., Wallinga-de Jonge, W., and Boom, H. B. 1986. Model of electrical conductivity of skeletal muscle based on tissue structure. *Med. Biol. Eng. Comput.* 24: 34–40.

Gielen, F.L.H., Wallinga-de Jonge, W., and Boon, K.L. 1984. Electrical conductivity of skeletal muscle tissue: experimental results from different muscles *in vivo. Med. Biol. Eng. Comput.* 22: 569–577.

Henriquez, C.S. 1993. Simulating the electrical behavior of cardiac tissue using the bidomain model. *Crit. Rev. Biomed. Eng.* 21: 1–77.

Le Guyader, P., Trelles, F., and Savard, P. 2001. Extracellular measurement of anisotropic bidomain myocardial conductivities. I. Theoretical analysis. *Ann. Biomed. Eng.* 29: 862–877.

Neu, J.C. and Krassowska, W. 1993. Homogenization of syncytial tissues. *Crit. Rev. Biomed. Eng.* 21: 137–199.

Peters, M.J., Hendriks, M., and Stinstra, J.G. 2001. The passive DC conductivity of human tissues described by cells in solution. *Bioelectrochemistry* 53: 155–160.

Plonsey, R. 1969. *Bioelectric Phenomena*, McGraw-Hill, New York.

Plonsey, R. and Barr, R.C. 1986. A critique of impedance measurements in cardiac tissue. *Ann. Biomed. Eng.* 14: 307–322.

Ranck, J.B. Jr. and BeMent, S. L. 1965. Specific impedance of the dorsal columns of cat: an anisotropic medium. *Exp. Neurol.* 11: 451–463.

Roberts, D.E., Hersh, L.T. and Scher, A.M. 1979. Influence of cardiac fiber orientation on wavefront voltage, conduction velocity, and tissue resistivity in the dog. *Circ. Res.* 44: 701–712.

Roberts, D.E. and Scher, A.M. 1982. Effect of tissue anisotropy on extracellular potential fields in canine myocardium in situ. *Circ. Res.* 50: 342–351.

Roth, B.J. and Altman, K.W. 1992. Steady-state point-source stimulation of a nerve containing axons with an arbitrary distribution of diameters. *Med. Biol. Eng. Comput.* 30: 103–108.

Roth, B.J. 1988. The electrical potential produced by a strand of cardiac muscle: a bidomain analysis. *Ann. Biomed. Eng.* 16: 609–637.

Roth, B.J. 1989. Interpretation of skeletal muscle four-electrode impedance measurements using spatial and temporal frequency-dependent conductivities. *Med. Biol. Eng. Comput.* 27: 491–495.

Roth, B.J. 1997. Electrical conductivity values used with the bidomain model of cardiac tissue. *IEEE Trans. Biomed. Eng.* 44: 326–328.

Roth, B.J., Gielen, F.L.H., and Wikswo, J.P., Jr. 1988. Spatial and temporal frequency-dependent conductivities in volume-conduction for skeletal muscle. *Math. Biosci.* 88: 159–189.

Rush, S., Abildskov, J. A., and McFee, R. 1963. Resistivity of body tissues at low frequencies. *Circ. Res.* 12: 40–50.

Steendijk, P., Mur, G., van der Velde, E.T., and Baan, J. 1993. The four-electrode resistivity technique in anisotropic media: theoretical analysis and application on myocardial tissue *in vivo*. *IEEE Trans. Biomed. Eng.* 40: 1138–1148.

Tasaki, I. 1964. A new measurement of action currents developed by single nodes of Ranvier. *J. Neurophysiol.* 27: 1199–1206.

Further Information

Mathematics and Physics

Jackson, J.D. *Classical Electrodynamics*, 3rd ed., John Wiley & Sons, New York, 1999. *(The classic graduate level physics text.)*

Purcell, E.M. *Electricity and Magnetism*, Berkeley Physics Course, Vol. 2, McGraw-Hill Book Co., New York, 1963. *(A wonderfully written undergraduate physics text full of physical insight.)*

Schey, H.M. *Div, Grad, Curl and All That*, 3rd ed., Norton, New York, 1997. *(An accessible and useful introduction to vector calculus.)*

Bioelectric Phenomena and Tissue Models

The texts by Cole and Plonsey, cited above, are classics in the field.

Gabriel, C., Gabriel, S., and Corthout, E. 1996. The dielectric properties of biological tissues: I. Literature survey. *Phys. Med. Biol.* 41: 2231–2249.

Geddes, L.A. and Baker, L.E. 1967. The specific resistance of biologic material — a compendium of data for the biomedical engineer and physiologist. *Med. Biol. Eng. Comput.* 5: 271–293. *(Measured conductivity values for a wide variety of tissues.)*

Plonsey, R. and Barr, R.C. *Bioelectricity, A Quantitative Approach*, 2nd ed., Plenum Press, New York, 2000. *(An updated version of Plonsey's "Bioelectric Phenomena," and a standard textbook for bioelectricity courses.)*

Polk, C. and Postow, E. (Eds.) *CRC Handbook of Biological Effects of Electromagnetic Fields*, CRC Press, Boca Raton, FL, 1986.

Journals: IEEE Transactions on Biomedical Engineering, Medical and Biological Engineering and Computing, Annals of Biomedical Engineering.

22

Membrane Models

Anthony Varghese
University of Minnesota

The models discussed in this chapter involve the time behavior of electrochemical activity in excitable cells. These models are systems of ordinary differential equations where the independent variable is time. While a good understanding of linear circuit theory is useful in order to understand the models presented in this chapter, most of the phenomena of interest involve nonlinear circuits with time-varying components.

Electrical activity in plant and animal cells are caused by two main factors: first, there are differences in the concentrations of ions inside and outside the cell; and second, there are molecules embedded in the cell membrane that allow these ions to be transported across the membrane. The ion concentration differences and the presence of large membrane-impermeant anions inside the cell result in the existence of a polarity: the potential inside a cell is typically 30 to 100 mV lower than that in the external solution. It is important to note that almost all of this potential difference occurs across the membrane itself. The bulk solutions both inside and outside the cell are, for the most part, at a uniform potential. This **transmembrane potential difference** is in turn sensed by molecules in the membrane that control the flow of ions.

The lipid bilayer, which constitutes the majority of the cell membrane, acts as a capacitor with a specific capacitance that is typically $1 \, \mu F/cm^2$. The rest of the membrane comprises large protein molecules that act

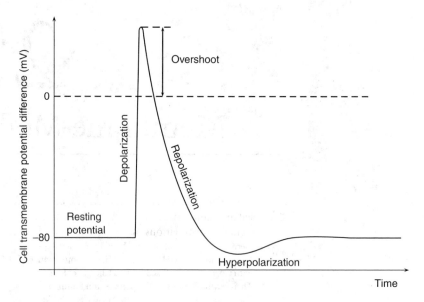

FIGURE 22.1 Schematic representation of an action potential in an excitable cell. The abscissa represents time and the ordinate represents the transmembrane potential.

as (1) **ion channels**, (2) **ion pumps**, or (3) **ion exchangers**. The flow of ions across the membrane causes changes in the transmembrane potential, which is typically the main observable quantity in experiments.

22.1 The Action Potential

The main behavior that will be examined in this chapter is the **action potential**. This is a term used to denote a temporal phenomenon exhibited by every electrically excitable cell. A schematic representation of an action potential is shown in Figure 22.1. The transmembrane potential difference of most excitable cells usually stays at some negative potential called the *resting potential*. External current or voltage inputs can cause the potential of the cell to deviate in the positive direction and if the input is large enough the result is an action potential. An action potential is characterized by a **depolarization**, which typically results in an *overshoot*, beyond the 0 mV level (see Figure 22.1) followed by **repolarization**. Some cells may actually *hyperpolarize* before returning to the resting potential.

A key concept in the modeling of excitable cells is the idea of *ion channel selectivity*. A particular type of ion channel will only allow certain ionic species to pass through; most types of ion channels are modeled as being permeant to a single ionic species. In most excitable cells at rest, the membrane is most permeable to potassium. This is because only potassium channels (i.e., channels selective to potassium) are open at the resting potential. For a given stimulus to result in action potential the cell has to be brought to **threshold**, it, that is, the stimulus has to be larger than some critical size; smaller subthreshold stimuli will result in an exponential decay to the resting potential. The upstroke, or fast initial depolarization, of the action potential is caused by a large influx of sodium ions as sodium channels open (in some cells, entry of calcium ions through calcium channels is responsible for the upstroke) in response to a stimulus. This is followed by repolarization as potassium ions starts flowing out of the cell in reponse to the new potential gradient. While responses of most cells to subthreshold inputs are usually linear and passive, the suprathreshold response — the action potential — is a nonlinear phenomenon. Unlike linear circuits where the principle of superposition holds, the nonlinear processes in cell membranes do not allow responses of two stimuli to be added. If an initial stimulus results in an action potential a subsequent stimulus administered at the peak voltage will not produce an even larger action potential; instead it may have no effect at all. Following an action potential most cells have a **refractory period**, during which they are unable to respond to stimuli. Nonlinear features such as these make modeling of excitable cells a nontrivial task. In addition, the molecular behavior of ion channels includes a stochastic component and is not completely understood, and therefore, it is not feasible to construct membrane models from first principles. The models in this chapter were all constructed using empirical data.

In 1952, Alan Hodgkin and Andrew Huxley published a paper showing how a nonlinear empirical model of the membrane processes could be constructed [Hodgkin and Huxley, 1952]. In the five decades since their work, the Hodgkin–Huxley (abbreviated *HH*) paradigm of modeling cell membranes has been enormously successful. While the concept of ion channels was not established when they performed their work, one of their main contributions was the idea that ion-selective processes existed in the membrane. It is now known that most of the passive transport of ions across cell membranes is accomplished by ion-selective channels. In addition to constructing a nonlinear model, they also established a method to incorporate experimental data into a nonlinear mathematical membrane model.

22.2 Patch Clamp Data

The main source of experimental data used to construct models of cell electrophysiology is the *patch clamp* method [Hamill et al., 1981]. In the *whole-cell* patch clamp configuration, a glass pipette with a very fine tip, typically 1 μm in diameter, containing a solution that is close in ionic composition to the intracellular fluid is brought to the external surface of the cell. A small amount of suction is applied to form at tight seal between the tip of the glass pipette and the membrane and by applying additional suction, the cell membrane under the tip can be ruptured and fluid in the electrode is allowed to come in physical contact with the internal fluid of the cell. With electrical contact thus established between the fluid of the glass pipette and the interior of the cell, it becomes possible to monitor as well as control cell electrical activity using electronic instruments.

The components of cellular electrophysiology can be summarized schematically in Figure 22.2a. Cell membranes may contain ion channels that allow ions to flow down their electrochemical gradient and ion pumps that move ions against their gradients. The various cell membrane channel, pump, and exchanger currents are summed in $I_{ion} = I_{ion}(V_m, \vec{y})$, which is a nonlinear function of V_m and $\vec{y}$, a vector representing the kinetics of the various channels, and so forth. The capacitance of the membrane, C_m, responds to changes in the cell transmembrane potential difference, V_m, with a capacitative current, $I_C = C_m \frac{dV_m}{dt}$. Using Kirchoff's Current Law from electrical circuit theory,

$$I_C + I_{ion} = 0 \tag{22.1}$$

which yields the basic differential equation for the cell transmembrane potential difference, V_m:

$$C_m \frac{dV_m}{dt} = -I_{ion}(V_m \cdot \vec{y}) \tag{22.2}$$

The kinetics of $\vec{y}$ is usually defined by a system of equations of the form:

$$\frac{d\vec{y}}{dt} = F(V_m, \vec{y}) \tag{22.3}$$

Cell patch-clamping allows experimenters to either inject a current while observing the response in V_m, (*current-clamp mode*, Figure 22.2b) or impose a waveform, $V_{clamp}(t)$, on the cell transmembrane potential and observe membrane current, I_m (*voltage-clamp mode*, Figure 22.2). By choosing appropriate voltage-clamp waveforms, $V_{clamp}(t)$, experimenters can make deductions about the structure of the nonlinear function $F(V_m, \vec{y})$ in Equation 22.3. The membrane current measured during voltage-clamp experiments, $I_m(t) = C_m \frac{dV_{clamp}}{dt} + I_{ion}(V_{clamp}, \vec{y})$ is then painstakingly dissected into its essential components due to the various ion channels, pumps, and exchangers by established protocols as well as by trial and error.

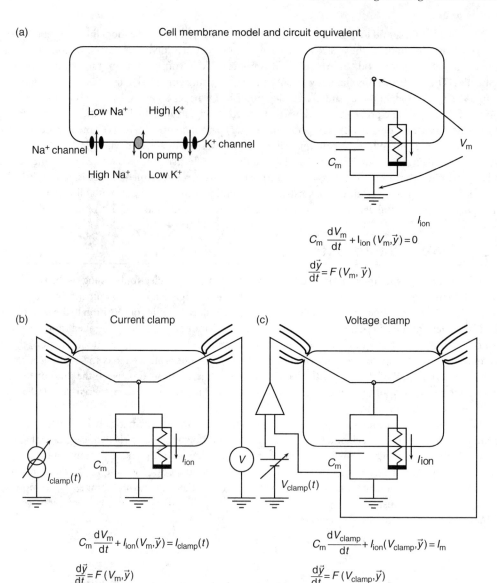

(a) Cell membrane model and circuit equivalent

$$C_m \frac{dV_m}{dt} + I_{ion}(V_m, \vec{y}) = 0$$

$$\frac{d\vec{y}}{dt} = F(V_m, \vec{y})$$

(b) Current clamp

$$C_m \frac{dV_m}{dt} + I_{ion}(V_m, \vec{y}) = I_{clamp}(t)$$

$$\frac{d\vec{y}}{dt} = F(V_m, \vec{y})$$

(c) Voltage clamp

$$C_m \frac{dV_{clamp}}{dt} + I_{ion}(V_{clamp}, \vec{y}) = I_m$$

$$\frac{d\vec{y}}{dt} = F(V_{clamp}, \vec{y})$$

FIGURE 22.2 Schematic view of membrane currents and patch clamp techniques. Most cells have a low internal concentration of sodium (Na^+) and a high internal concentration of potassium (K^+) ions while the external concentrations are reversed. Sodium and potassium channels allow these ions to run down their electrochemical gradients while ion pumps can pump these ions against their respective electrochemical gradients. This electrical activity can be represented by an equivalent circuit shown to the left. The cell membrane capacitance is represented by the capacitor C_m and the various ionic currents are added together into a single nonlinear element through which the current I_{ion} passes. Thus the equation of circuit equivalent is: $C_m \frac{dV_m}{dt} + I_{ion}(V_m, \vec{y}) = 0$ and the time-dependent properties of the nonlinearities of I_{ion} are described by the vector equation $\frac{d\vec{y}}{dt} = F(V_m, \vec{y})$. In the *current-clamp* mode of the whole-cell patch clamp configuration, one electrode is used to inject a known current $I_{clamp}(t)$ while the other electrode is used to sense the potential inside the cell. In **voltage-clamp** mode the potential inside the cell is compared to a known voltage supplied by the experimenter and an amplifier is used to supply whatever current is required to keep the cell potential at the specified voltage $V_{clamp}(t)$. The resulting circuit equations are indicated below the circuit diagrams.

Using cloned channels overexpressed in cultured cells or *Xenopus* oocytes, a relatively pure current can be studied in isolation.

22.3 General Formulations of Membrane Currents

In this section we examine the various components common to membrane models. We start with the Nernst–Planck formulation of ion flow across a membrane. Although it is seldom used now, this equation is needed to derive other, more practical models such as the resistor-battery model or the Goldman–Hodgkin–Katz (GHK) current model. Some preliminary remarks are in order before examining these models. At dilute concentrations, ions in aqueous solutions behave like gas molecules. This is why the *gas constant*, R, is ubiquitous in models of ion flow in cells. Similarly, the phenomenon of chemisorption of gas molecules is used as an analog to study the binding of ions (and drug molecules) to receptors in the cell membrane. In chemisorption under equilibrium conditions, the fraction of gas molecules bound to fixed reaction sites is given by an expression of the form: $[C]^n/(k + [C]^n)$ where $[C]$ is the concentration of gas, k is a constant, and n is typically a small positive number. This expression is also derived from Michaelis–Menten type kinetic schemes. Similar terms arise in many membrane models cited in this chapter and they indicate that some fraction of an ionic species, C, is binding to receptor molecules on the cell surface.

22.3.1 Nernst–Planck Equations

One of the most general description of ion flow across a membrane is given by the Nernst–Planck equations. This is a partial differential equation where the independent variables represent space (x) and time (t). The main dependent variable is the concentration of the ion ($c(x, t)$). The potential ($u(x, t)$) is usually a fixed function but can be made a dependent variable in which case an additional equation is required. The Nernst-Planck equations can be written as:

$$\frac{\partial c(x, t)}{\partial t} = \frac{\partial}{\partial x} \frac{\mu(x, t)}{|z|} \left[\frac{RT}{F} \frac{\partial c(x, t)}{\partial x} + zc(x, t) \frac{\partial u}{\partial x}(x, t) \right] \quad (22.4)$$

where the symbols are defined thus:

Variable	Description	Dimensions
R	Gas constant	8314.41 mJ/(mole°K)
T	Temperature	310°K
F	Faraday's constant	96485 C/mole
u	potential	mV
c	ion concentration	$\mathrm{mol}\,\mathrm{l}^{-1}$
z	valence of the ion	
E	electric field force	$\mathrm{mV}\,\mathrm{m}^{-1}$
μ	ion mobility	$\mathrm{m}^2\mathrm{mV}^{-1}\mathrm{sec}^{-1}$

Note that that μ can vary with both space and time depending on the type of ion channel or pump and its gating properties. Due to the complexity of this formulation, it is of limited use when examining behavior at the cellular level but it can be used to derive simpler formulations under certain assumptions as shown in the following section.

22.3.2 Hodgkin–Huxley Resistor Battery Model

This is the model that is most frequently employed to look at ions flowing through channels and is shown in terms of its circuit equivalent in Figure 22.3. This models the passive flow of ions due to a transmembrane

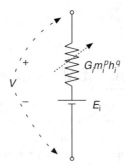

FIGURE 22.3 Circuit representation of membrane current. The conductance can be nonlinear as indicated by the powers p and q on the state variables m_i and h_i, respectively. These state variables are typically time-varying functions of the transmembrane potential difference, V. The battery, E_i represents the electrochemical gradient of the ionic species responsible for the current.

potential gradient, V_m, and a concentration gradient (represented in the battery, E_i) through a nonlinear membrane conductance. From the structure of the circuit, we see that the equation for the current for ionic species i has the form:

$$I_i = G_i m_i^p h_i^q (V_m - E_i) \tag{22.5}$$

where G_i represents the maximum value of the conductance of the membrane, and m_i and h_i are gating variables that vary in time and take values between 0 and 1. p and q are integers that depend on the kinetic characteristics of the membrane channel. For example, in the formulation of the sodium current in the Hodgkin and Huxley (HH, see below) equations, the conductance is $G_{Na} m^3 h$, that is, p is 3 and q is 1, and these values were found to result in the best fit with experimental data.

The above expression can be derived from the Nernst–Planck equations with the assumption that concentration does not vary with time. In addition the space dimension of Equation 22.4 is reduced to a two-compartment — cell interior and exterior — model. Thus the steady-state of Equation 22.4 tells us that when there is no net current flow, the transmembrane potential will equal a quantity called the "Nernst" potential: $E_i = (RT/z_i F) \ln([C]_o/[C]_i) \cdot z_i$ is the valence of the ion, $[C_i]_o$ is the concentration of the ion on the outside, and $[C_i]_i$ is the concentration on the inside. Quantities such as ion mobility are effectively lumped into a nonlinear time-varying conductance ($G_i m_i^p h_i^q$).

First order differential equations are used to model the time behavior of m_i and h_i. For example the equation for m_i will have the form:

$$\frac{dm_i}{dt} = \alpha_m (1 - m_i) - \beta_m m_i \tag{22.6}$$

where the α_m and β_m are empirically determined functions of the membrane potential. This equation is also written as: $dm_i/dt = (m_{i\infty} - m_i)/\tau_i$ where $m_{i\infty} = \alpha_m/(\alpha_m + \beta_m)$ and $\tau_i = 1/(\alpha_m + \beta_m)$. Voltage-clamp protocols are used by experiments to characterize $m_{i\infty}$ and τ_i empirically as functions of V_m for a given cell. As a result there is no unique derivation for the differential equations describing the time behavior of the gating variables. $m_{i\infty}$ and τ_i are usually nonlinear functions of voltage. This nonlinear dependence on V_m makes the coupled system of Equation 22.2 and Equation 22.3 a nonlinear system of ordinary differential equations. **Selectivity** is implicitly modeled by assuming that only one ionic species flows though a current branch. A number of current branches, one for each type of ion channel, are connected in parallel to model the interaction of the various ion currents.

Gating variables, ion channel kinetics, and Markov-state models   Gating variables such as m_i and h_i earlier model the kinetic behavior of ion channels. For example, in the HH equations (see below), the variable "m" is used to model the process of *activation* of the sodium current. At polarized potentials, the sodium current is turned off: m is close to 0 and therefore the sodium current conductance, $G_{Na}m^3h$, is close to 0. As the cell depolarizes (V_m increases, see Figure 22.1), the sodium current turns on (activates) and this is modeled as an increase in the value of m until it approaches 1. Concomitant with this activation is a process that desensitizes (inactivates) the sodium current thus guaranteeing that the sodium current is transient. This is modeled using the inactivation variable h, which goes from a resting value of 1 to a value closer to 0 as V_m increases. This decrease in h causes the sodium conductance, $G_{Na}m^3h$, to decrease even though m may be close to 1. In an excitable cell such as a nerve, skeletal, or cardiac cell, activation of the sodium current causes inward flow of sodium ions resulting in depolarization of the cell; this depolarization further activates the sodium current and a regenerative activation process continues until inactivation desensitizes the current. In the absence of other currents, the cell will stay depolarized but most excitable cells will have an outward potassium current that activates much more slowly than the fast inward sodium current. This outward potassium current causes potassium ions to leave the cell and repolarizes the cell, that is, it brings the transmembrane potential closer to the reversal potential for potassium. The sodium current is affected by repolarization in two ways: it turns off (deactivates) and it becomes resensitized (recovers from inactivation). The deactivation is modeled as a return of the m variable to values close to 0 and the recovery from inactivation is modeled as a return of h to a value closer to 1. These four processes: activation, inactivation, deactivation, and recovery from inactivation are present in many ion channels. Investigations of these processes in squid axons, native mammalian cells, and in cloned channels revealed that the *HH* formulation of these four processes were deficient in at least three ways. First, inactivation was often found to be coupled to activation rather than being independently voltage dependent as in the Hodgkin–Huxley model. Second, multiple steps were involved each of the four processes and these steps could not be adequately modeled using different values for the exponents (p and q above). Third, unlike the HH model, the speed of activation, for instance, is in some cases decoupled from the speed of deactivation. These observations resulted in the need for a more general framework for kinetics and the most commonly used one is Markov-state models [see Hille, 2001].

22.3.3 GHK Constant Field Formulation

From Equation 22.4, assuming that potential varies linearly across the membrane and that the ion flux is constant, we obtain an expression for current flow of the form [Goldman, 1943]:

$$I_i = P_i d_i^p f_i^q \frac{\frac{V_m}{RT/zF}}{1 - e^{-\frac{V_m}{RT/zF}}} \left[[C_i]_i - [C_i]_o e^{-\frac{V_m}{RT/zF}} \right] \tag{22.7}$$

where P_i is the maximum permeability of the membrane and d and f are gating variables such as m and h in Equation 22.5. This equation is frequently used when large concentration gradients are present.

22.3.4 GHK with Correction for Fixed Surface Charge

When surface charge is present on the inside or outside of the cell membrane, the effective potential gradient sensed by the channel is modified by a correction factor, $V_{surface}$, and the current then has the form [Frankenhaeuser, 1960]:

$$I_i = P_i d_i^p f_i^q \frac{\frac{V_m - V_{surface}}{RT/zF}}{1 - e^{-\frac{V_m - V_{surface}}{RT/zF}}} \left[[C_i]_i - [C_i]_o e^{-\frac{V_m - V_{surface}}{RT/zF}} \right] \tag{22.8}$$

22.3.5 Eyring Rate Theory Models of Ionic Currents

An alternative to the Nernst–Planck models of charge diffusion is the rate theory model, which views ion permeation through a channel or pump from a statistical thermodynamics perspective. In this approach, one or more energy barriers are assumed to exist at fixed points in the channel and ions permeate

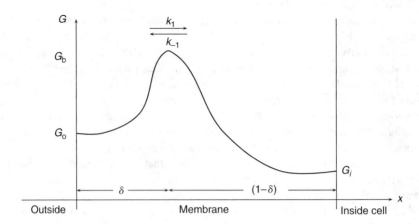

FIGURE 22.4 Schematic representation of energy barrier in a rate theory model of ionic current. A single energy barrier of height G_b located at a fraction δ of the membrane thickness is assumed in this example.

the channel when the energy of the ions overcomes the energy barrier. The case of one barrier is shown schematically in Figure 22.4. The forward and backward ion flux rates can be described using Boltzmann equations as shown below.

$$k_1 = \nu e^{-(G_b - G_o) - z\delta \frac{V_m}{RT/F}} \tag{22.9}$$

$$k_{-1} = \nu e^{-(G_b - G_i) - z(1-\delta) \frac{V_m}{RT/F}} \tag{22.10}$$

where k_1 is the forward flux rate from the outside to the inside, and k_{-1} is the flux rate in the other direction; ν is some nominal flux; G_o and G_i are the the energies at the external and internal surfaces of the cell membrane; G_b is the height of the energy barrier; z is the valence of the permeating ion; δ is the location of the membrane barrier as measured from the external side of the membrane; V_m is the transmembrane potential difference and is implicitly assumed to vary linearly through the thickness of the membrane; and R, T, and F are as defined earlier. Given these flux rates, we can write the flux equations as

$$\text{influx} = [C]_o k_1 \tag{22.11}$$

$$\text{efflux} = [C]_i k_{-1} \tag{22.12}$$

If the net current is then assumed to be the difference between the efflux and the influx, it can be written as:

$$I_i = \nu \left([C]_i e^{-(G_b - G_i) + z(1-\delta) \frac{V_m}{RT/F}} - [C]_o e^{-(G_b - G_o) - z\delta \frac{V_m}{RT/F}} \right) \tag{22.13}$$

The equations for the case of multiple barriers can be derived in a similar way but are much more tedious to work through.

22.3.6 Ion Pump

Ion pumps are membrane molecules that unlike channels, require energy to function. While the workings of ion pumps can get quite complex especially if the source of energy for these pumps need to be modeled, most models in use assume a simplied form using Michaelis–Menten terms such as:

$$I_p = I_{p\,max} \frac{[X]_i}{[X]_i + k_x} \frac{[Y]_o}{[Y]_o + k_y} \tag{22.14}$$

In the above equation, $I_{p\,max}$ is the maximum pump current, $[X]_i$ is the concentration of the ionic species on the inside being pumped out and $[Y]_o$ is the concentration of the ionic species on the outside being pumped in. k_x and k_y represent sensitivities of the pump to these ion concentrations.

22.3.7 Ion Exchangers

Ion exchangers are similar to ion pumps but do not require energy directly. Instead exchangers use the energy stored in a concentration gradient of ion X to transport ion Y in the opposite direction. An example of an exchanger current is the cardiac Na–Ca exhanger, which uses the concentration gradient of sodium (high outside, low inside) to pump one calcium ion out of the cell for every three sodium ions allowed into the cell. An additional difference between exchangers and pumps is that exchangers are more voltage-sensitive and are thus more readily operated in the reverse direction under physiological conditions.

22.3.8 Synapses

Yamada and Zucker [1992] have tested various kinetic mechanisms to model calcium control of presynaptic release of transmitters. The classic model of postsynaptic response to a synaptic input is the so-called *alpha* function due to Rall [1967] and has the form:

$$G(t) = \frac{t - t_0}{t_{peak}} e^{\frac{t - t_0}{t_{peak}}} \tag{22.15}$$

where G is usually a conductance in a resistor–battery type branch circuit. Although the alpha function is the one that is most commonly used, more detailed schemes have been constructed using kinetic models [Destexhe et al., 1994].

22.3.9 Calcium as a Second Messenger

Calcium entry into a cell frequently has a number of secondary effects such as initiation of contraction, release of neurotransmitters, and modulation of membrane ion channels. This is usually accomplished by the binding of calcium ions to calcium receptors inside the cell. Michaelis–Menten kinetic schemes with steady-state assumptions are used to model this binding and therefore expressions of the form $f = [Ca^{++}]_i^n / ([Ca^{++}]_i^n + K)$ are frequently employed. Here f is the fraction of calcium that is bound to the receptor and K is the dissociation constant for the reaction, and n is the number of calcium ions that bind to each receptor molecule.

22.4 Nerve Cells

Nerve cells typically have complex geometries with axons, branching dendrites, spines, and synapses. While it was thought for a long time that dendrites could be modeled using linear resistor–capacitor circuits, it is becoming increasingly clear that nonlinear ionic currents are present in many dendritic trees. Due to technical difficulties in measuring currents in dendrites and synapses directly, most neuronal models in this chapter describe ionic currents of cell soma or axons. Since the Hodgkin–Huxley equations constitutes the basis for membrane modeling, the reader should be familiar with this model before examining the others.

Squid axon: Hodgkin and Huxley Most models of excitable cells are descendents of this model. The basic circuit equivalent of this model comprises a linear capacitance in parallel with three resistor-battery subcircuits (one each for sodium, potassium, and a nonspecific leakage channel). The *HH* equations in their original form were:

$$C_m \frac{dV}{dt} = -G_{Na} m^3 h(V - E_{Na}) - G_K n^4 (V - E_K) - G_l(V - E_l)$$

$$\frac{dm}{dt} = \alpha_m(1 - m) - \beta_m m$$

$$\frac{dh}{dt} = \alpha_h(1 - h) - \beta_h h \tag{22.16}$$

$$\frac{dn}{dt} = \alpha_n(1 - n) - \beta_n n$$

The rate constants were given originally as:

$$\alpha_m = \frac{(V + 25)/10}{e^{(V+25)/10} - 1} \tag{22.17}$$

$$\beta_m = 4e^{V/18} \tag{22.18}$$

$$\alpha_h = 0.07 e^{V/20} \tag{22.19}$$

$$\beta_h = \frac{1}{e^{(V+30)/10} + 1} \tag{22.20}$$

$$\alpha_n = \frac{1}{10} \frac{(V + 10)/10}{e^{(V+10)/10} - 1} \tag{22.21}$$

$$\beta_n = \frac{e(V/80)}{8} \tag{22.22}$$

The physical constants used in these equations are: $G_{Na} = 120$ mS/cm^2, $G_K = 36$ mS/cm^2, $G_l = 0.3$ mS/cm^2, $C_m = 1$ μF/cm^2, $E_{Na} = -115$ mV, $E_K = 12$ mV, and $E_l = -10.613$. The original equations as listed by Hodgkin and Huxley [1952] unfortunately used a sign convention that has not been followed since. Using the sign convention of today for the transmembrane potential, the rate constants can be rewritten by replacing all occurences of V with $-(V_m + 60)$.

The successes of this model include the ability to predict the velocity of action potential propagation when the spatial aspect is included, the continuous nature of the threshold of the nerve, and the repetitive firing behavior seen under the influence of a constant current. A number of remarks should be made regarding this model that hold for other models as well. First, L'Hopital's Rule allows us to compute the value of expressions of the form x/e^{x-1} as in Equation 22.17 at the point $x = 0$. Second, for temperatures other than 6.3°C an acceptable correction is the Q_{10} scaling: multiply each α and β by $\phi = 3^{(T-6.3)/10}$ where the 3 indicates that for each 10°C change in temperature, the speed of the reaction increases threefold (T is in degree Celsius). It has been found that the ratio of 3.33 for $G_{Na} : G_K$ in this model achieves a balance between a quick repolarization and continued excitability.

Toad myelinated neuron Frankenhaeuser and Huxley [1964] modified the *HH* model to describe the fast sodium and delayed rectifier potassium currents with the GHK model rather than the resistor-battery formulation used by Hodgkin and Huxley. In addition they added a small non-specific current to account for inward currents late in action potentials of myelinated neurons of the toad *Xenopus laevis*.

Gastropod neuron The model of Connor and Stevens [1971] used a *HH*-type system of differential equations to model repetitive firing in isolated gastropod neurons. This was the first model to include an inactivating potassium current (the A-type current) that has since been used in a number of other cells.

Aplysia abdominal ganglion R15 cell The bursting behavior of *Aplysia* neurons have been extensively studied. The first model was that of Plant [1976] who extended the *HH* equations to include an inactivating potassium current, a slow potassium current, and a constant hyperpolarizing current due to the Na/K pump. Bertram [1993] modeled bursting in these cells by augmenting an *HH* model with a calcium current, a second delayed rectifier type potassium current, and serotonin-activated inward-rectifying potassium current and a negative slope region calcium current. A detailed model including a fast inward sodium current, fast and slow calcium currents, a delayed rectifier and an inward rectifier potassium currents, a sodium–potassium pump, a sodium–calcium exchanger, a calcium pump, and a leakage current was described in Butera et al. [1995].

CA3 hippocampal pyramidal neurons Traub et al. [1991] have constructed a multicompartment — soma and dendrites — model of hippocampal neurons with upto six membrane currents in each compartment (i) a fast sodium current, (ii) a calcium current, (iii) a delayed rectifier potassium current, (iv) an inactivating (A-type) potassium current, (v) a long-duration calcium-activated potassium current, and (vi) a short-duration calcium-activated potassium current. Furthermore, calcium concentration changes in a restricted space beneath the membrane is modeled using a simplified linear buffering scheme. Good and Murphy [1996] modified this model to include N-, L-, and T-type calcium currents along with an AMPA-activated current and the effects of β-amyloid block of the A-type current. A branching dendritic version of the Traub et al. [1991] model with synaptic input is described in Traub and Miles [1995].

CA1 hippocampal pyramidal neurons A model that accurately predicts accomodation in CA1 neurons was constructed by Warman et al. [1994]. Using the previous work of Traub et al. [1991] and taking experimental data into consideration, they constructed a 16-compartment model with the following membrane currents (i) a fast sodium current, (ii) a calcium current, (iii) a delayed rectifier potassium current, (iv) an inactivating (A-type) potassium current, (v) a long-duration calcium-dependent potassium current, (vi) a short-duration calcium- and voltage-activated potassium current, (vii) a persistent muscarinic potassium current, and (viii) a leakage current. Unlike the Traub model separate pools of calcium were used to modulate the potassium currents. A linear buffering scheme was assumed for both internal calcium pools but the decay times were assumed to be different in each pool.

Stomatogastric ganglion neurons Epstein and Marder [1990] constructed a *HH*-type model of the lobster stomatogastric ganglion neuron with a fast sodium current, a delayed rectifier potassium current a voltage-dependent calcium current, a calcium-dependent potassium current, and a linear leakage current in order to study the mechanism of bursting oscillations in these cells.

Chopper units in the anteroventral cochlear nucleus Banks and Sachs [1991] constructed an equivalent cylinder model of chopper units in the anteroventral cochlear nucleus. The model of the soma membrane included a fast sodium current, a delayed rectifier current, a linear leakage current, and inhibitory and excitatory synaptic currents using the Rall α-wave model.

Lamprey CNS neurons The model of Brodin et al. [1991] consisted of voltage-gated sodium, potassium and calcium currents, a calcium-activated potassium current, and an NMDA receptor channel. The voltage-dependent block by magnesium of the NMDA was also modeled in this paper. Two compartments were used to model calcium concentration changes inside the cells.

Thalamocortical cells Neurons in the thalamocortical systems show various kinds of oscillatory behavior during sleep and wake cycles. It has been shown in the last decade that these neurons interact to produce a wide range of oscillatory activity. Huguenard and McCormick [1992] constructed a model of thalamic relay neurons with (i) a low-threshold transient calcium current, (ii) an inactivating (A-type) potassium current, (iii) a slowly inactivating potassium current, and (iv) a **hyperpolarization**-activated nonspecific current. McCormick and Huguenard [1992] extended the above model to simulate the behavior of thalamocortical relay neurons by adding (i) a fast sodium current, (ii) a persistent sodium current, (iii) a high-threshold calcium current, (iv) a calcium-activated potassium current, and (v) linear leakage currents. Destexhe et al. [1993a,b] have examined similar models as well.

Human node of Ranvier Schwartz et al. [1995] measured action potentials and separated membrane currents in nodes of Ranvier in human nerve trunks. Their model comprises a fast sodium current, fast and slow potassium currents, and a leakage current.

Dopaminergic neurons A minimal model of the soma with a fast sodium current and a delayed rectifier potassium current and a dendritic compartment with a sodium–potassium pump, NMDA-activated current, and leakage current was augmented with an L-type calcium current in the dendritic compartment and an A-type potassium current, T-type calcium current and a calcium-sensitive potassium current in the soma by Li et al. [1996]. An improved model with an additional N-type calcium current and another high-voltage-activated calcium current, a sodium–calcium exchanger, a calcium pump, a hyperpolarization-activated cation current, and cytosolic calcium buffering was constructed by Aminis et al. [1999] and a model focusing on the GABA- and NMDA-mediated currents was published by Komendantov et al. [2004].

Cerebellar granule cells A model of the soma with three sodium currents (a fast, a persistent, and a resurgent current), a high-threshold calcium current, and five potassium currents (fast and slow delayed rectifier currents, an A-type, an inward rectifier, and a calcium-activated potassium current) was constructed by DAngelo et al. [2001].

22.4.1 Sensory Neurons

Rabbit sciatic nerve axons A fast sodium current and a leak current was found to be sufficient to model single action potentials in the nodes of Ranvier of axons from rabbit sciatic nerve by Chiu et al. [1979]. It is likely that this model should be augmented to include potassium currents in order to model trains of action potentials accurately.

Myelinated auditory nerve neuron A detailed model of the morphology of myelination and ion channel distribution was formulated by Colombo and Parkins [1987] using the Frankenhaeuser–Huxley model as a base: it includes a fast sodium current, fast potassium current, a leakage current, and a slow sodium current.

Retinal ganglion cells Fohlmeister et al. [1990] modeled the retinal ganglion cells using a fast inactivating sodium current, a calcium current, a noninactivating (delayed-rectifier) potassium current, an inactiavating potassium current, and a calcium-activated potassium current. An important feature in this model is that it models the calcium concentration inside the cell using a simplified buffering scheme and in this way they are able to model the modulation of potassium currents by calcium. A model with separate L-type and N-type calcium currents was constructed by Benison et al. [2001].

Retinal horizontal cells The model of Winslow and Knapp [1991] consisted of a fast sodium current, an inactivating (A-type) potassium current, a noninactivating potssium current, an anomalous rectifier potassium current, a calcium-inactivated calcium current, and a linear leakage current. In addition calcium concentration changes in a restricted region beneath the membrane was also modeled.

Rat Nodose neurons Schild et al. [1994] built a model comprising fast and slow sodium currents, an A-type potassium current, a delayed rectifier potassium current, T- and L-type calcium currents, a calcium-activated potassium current, a slowly inactivating potassium current, a sodium–calcium exchanger, a sodium–potassium pump, a calcium pump current, and background currents. This model was enhanced with descriptions of vesicular storage and release in Schild et al. [1995] and further tuned to fit myelinated and nonmyelinated neurons in Schild and Kunze [1997].

Muscle spindle primary endings Otten et al. [1995] extended the Frankenhaeuser–Huxley model with modifications to reproduce repetitive firing in sensory endings: in addition to the fast sodium current, fast potassium current and leakage currents of the FH model a slowly activating delayed rectifier current was required.

Vertebrate retinal cone photoreceptors A model of vertebrate photoreceptor cells that includes a light-sensitive current, an L-type calcium current, a delayed rectifier potassium current, calcium-sensitive potassium and chloride currents, a hyperpolarization-activated current, a sodium–potassium pump, and a leak current in addition to the response of the cell to a channel blocker was published by Usui et al. [1996].

Primary and secondary sensory neurons of the enteric nervous system A model of primary and secondary afferents with a fast sodium current, an N-type calcium current, a delayed rectifier potassium current, a calcium-sensitive potassium current, and a chloride current was set up by Miftakhov and Wingate [1996].

Invertebrate photoreceptor neurons The membrane properties of nerve terminals, axons, soma, and microvilli of Type-B photoreceptors of the invertebrate *Hermissenda* were modeled using a fast sodium current, an A-type potassium current, a calcium-dependent potassium current, a delayed rectifier potassium current, a noninactivating calcium current, light-induced sodium and calcium currents, and a leakage current by Fost and Clark [1996].

Fly optic lobe tangential cells Three families of tangential cells of the blowfly were modeled by Haag et al. [1997]. The centrifugal–horizontal cell has an inward calcium current and outward potassium currents. The other cells have a fast sodium current, a delayed rectifier potassium current, and a sodium-dependent potassium current.

Rat mesencephalic trigeminal neurons Negro and Chandler [1997] have constructed a model of sensory neurons involved in brain stem control of jaw musculature. This model of the trigeminal neurons includes a fast sodium current, N- and T-type calcium currents, two A-type potassium currents, a sustained potassium current, a delayed rectifier potassium current, a calcium-dependent potassium current, a hyperpolarization-activated current, and a leakage current.

Primary afferents and related efferents A model comprising a fast sodium current, a delayed rectifier potassium current, a calcium current, and a calcium-dependent potassium current was used to model primary afferents as well as interneurons and efferent neurons connected to the afferents by Saxena et al. [1997]. A modification of the *HH* model was used in Amir et al. [2002] to model A-type dorsal root ganglion neuron cell bodies.

Myelinated Ia primary afferent neurons The intraspinal collateral of a myelinated primary afferent neuron was modeled with a myelination morphology by D'Incamps et al. [1998] and included a fast sodium current, a delayed rectifier potassium current, and a Rall synaptic current at a particular node of Ranvier in the network.

22.4.2 Efferent Neurons

Sympathetic neurons of the superior cervical ganglia Superior cervical ganglion neurons were modeled by Belluzzi and Sacchi [1991] using the following membrane currents (i) sodium currents with fast and slow components, (ii) a GHK-type calcium current, (iii) a delayed rectifier potassium current, (iv) an inactivating (A-type) potassium current, and (v) a calcium-activated potassium current. One drawback of this model is that the calcium activation of the potassium channels was modeled using a fixed time delay rather than by allowing the internal calcium concentration to change.

Small intestine cholinergic and adrenergic neurons Miftakhov and Wingate [1994a] used the *HH* equations (fast sodium current, delayed rectifier potassium current, and a leakage current attributed to chloride channels) and added a system of equations to model the release of the neurotransmitter acetylcholine by the presynaptic terminal. Similarly release of noradrenaline was modeled in Miftakhov and Wingate [1994b].

Pyloric constrictor neurons of the lobster Models of the crab lateral pyloric neuron were modified to include a fast sodium current, an A-type potassium current, a delayed rectifier potassium current, a calcium current, a calcium-dependent potassium current, and a leak current by Harris-Warrick et al. [1995] to examine the effect of the neurotransmitter dopamine on the A-type current. This model was augmented by Harris-Warrick et al. [1995] to include a hyperpolarization-activated current.

Mammalian Spinal Motoneuron Halter et al. [1995] set up a detailed model of myelinated motoneurons with myelination morphology and ionic currents including: a fast sodium current, fast and slow delayed rectifier potassium currents, and a leak current.

Leech heartbeat oscillator Interneuron Interneurons controlling the leech heartbeat were modeled using: a fast sodium current, an A-type potassium current, an inward rectifier current, fast and slowly inactivating calcium currents, a persistent sodium current, a hyperpolarization-activated current, slowly inactivating and persistent potassium currents, and synaptic chloride currents [Nadim et al., 1995].

Snail RPa1 bursting neuron A model including a fast sodium current, a delayed rectifier potassium current, a voltage-dependent calcium current, a voltage- and calcium-dependent calcium current, and a leak current was constructed by Berezetskaya et al. [1996] to investigate the bursting behavior of pacemaker cells of the *Helix pomatia.*

Vertebrate motoneuron Data from motoneurons from various species were put together to construct a generic model of vertebrate motoneurons by Booth et al. [1997]. This model contains a fast sodium current, a delayed rectifier potassium current, L- and N-type calcium currents, and a calcium-dependent potassium current.

Xenopus central pattern generator neuron A model of *Xenopus* embryo swimming central pattern generator neurons with *HH* currents was modified by Tabak and Moore [1998] to include a voltage- and magnesium-sensitive NMDA channel current and a Rall alpha-wave mechanism for non-NMDA postsynaptic currents.

22.5   Skeletal Muscle Cells

Frog Sartorius muscle cell Skeletal muscle cells have a significant amount of current flowing through the cell membrane in the T-tubules of the cells. For this reason, it becomes imperative to model the currents in the T-tubules along with the rest of the cell membrane. The Adrian and Peachey [1973] equations are a system of coupled *HH*-type circuits and thus have a significant spatial component. The equations describing the velocity field have the same structure as the Hodgkin–Huxley equations. Two models were suggested in the paper: if sodium and potassium channels are assumed to exist in the T-tubules, the usual *HH* formulation of the corresponding currents are used; otherwise, only a linear leakage current appears in the voltage equation.

Barnacle muscle Morris and Lecar [1981] sought to model the oscillatory activity in current-clamped barnacle muscle fibers using just two noninactivating currents: a fast calcium current and a potassium current. It should be kept in mind that their model does not take into account the presence of a calcium chelator (EGTA) inside the cells used to obtain experimental results. Their equations have the same general structure as the *HH* equations:

$$C_m \frac{dV}{dt} = -G_L(V - E_L) - G_{Ca}m(V - E_{Ca}) - G_K n(V - E_K) \tag{22.23}$$

$$\frac{dm}{dt} = \lambda_m(m_\infty - m) \tag{22.24}$$

$$\frac{dn}{dt} = \lambda_n(m_\infty - n) \tag{22.25}$$

where:

$$m_\infty = \frac{1}{2}\left(1 + \tan h \frac{V - v_1}{v_2}\right) \tag{22.26}$$

$$\lambda_m = \overline{\lambda_m} \cos h \frac{V - v_1}{2v_2} \tag{22.27}$$

$$n_\infty = \frac{1}{2}\left(1 + \tan h \frac{V - v_3}{v_4}\right) \tag{22.28}$$

$$\lambda_n = \overline{\lambda_n} \cos h \frac{V - v_3}{2v_4} \tag{22.29}$$

Typical values of the parameters are: $C_m = 20 \ \mu F/cm^2$, $G_L = 2 \ mS/cm^2$, $G_K = 8 \ mS/cm^2$, $G_{Ca} = 4 \ mS/cm^2$, $E_L = -50 \ mV$, $E_K = -70 \ mV$, $E_{Ca} = 100 \ mV$, $v_1 = 10 \ mV$, $v_2 = 15 \ mV$, $v_3 = 10 \ mV$, $v_4 = 14.5 \ mV$, $\overline{\lambda_m} = 0.1$, and $\overline{\lambda_n} = 0.06667$. An alternative model of the calcium current was also proposed. Instead of the *HH* resistor-battery type formulation, a GHK formulation was suggested:

$$I_{Ca} = G_{Ca} m \frac{V/12.5}{1 - e^{V/12.5}} \left[1 - \frac{[Ca^{++}]_i}{[Ca^{++}]_o} e^{V/1.25} \right] \tag{22.30}$$

where typical values of $[Ca^{++}]_i$ and $[Ca^{++}]_o$ were 0.001 and 100 mM, respectively.

22.6   Endocrine Cells

Pancreatic β-cells An interesting electrophysiological phenomena occurs in the Islet of Langerhans of the pancreas: the release of insulin is controlled in these islets by trains of action potentials occuring in rapid bursts followed by periods of quiescence. This "bursting" behavior occurs only in intact islets: single cells do not display such bursting activity. Chay and Keizer [1983] was the first attempt to model this phenomenon quantitatively. Sherman et al. [1988] sought to explain the absence of bursting β-cells using the idea of "channel-sharing." Keizer [1988] modified this model by substituting an ATP- and ADP-dependent K channel instead of the Ca-dependent K channel. This model was then further improved by Keizer and Magnus [1989]. Sherman et al. [1990] constructed a domain model to examine the effect of Ca on Ca channel inactivation. Further refinements have been made by Keizer and Young [1993]. A new slowly activating calcium-dependent potassium current and a calcium subspace model was added in Goforth et al. [2002] and Zhang et al. [2003]. A recent model [Fridlyand et al., 2003] incorporates a detailed model of calcium uptake and release and sodium, IP3, and ATP signaling.

Pituitary Gonadotrophs and Corticotrophs Li et al. [1995] have constructed a model of membrane fluxes and calcium release from the endoplasmic reticulum of rat pituitary gonadotrophs. The membrane currents modeled include an L- and T-type calcium currents, delayed rectifier and calcium-sensitive potassium currents and a leak current. A modification of this model was used by LeBeau et al. [1997] to model pituitary corticotroph cells.

22.7   Cardiac Cells

Purkinje fiber Older models of the Purkinje fiber [Noble, 1960, 1962; Noble and Tsien, 1969; McAllister et al., 1975] failed to model the pacemaking currents correctly. Also, external and internal concentration changes were not modeled until the work of DiFrancesco and Noble [1985]. (The original paper contained a number of errors and a corrected listing of the model equations can be found in Varghese and Winslow [1993]). Despite the fact that the magnitude of the changes in calcium concentrations is at odds with recent experimental observations, this model has been very influential in directing modeling efforts. Most cardiac models being constructed now use the DiFrancesco–Noble structure.

Sinoatrial node As was the case with Purkinje fibers, the pacemaking mechanism was not modeled correctly in older models [Yanagihara et al., 1980; Bristow and Clark, 1982] and it was only after the Purkinje fiber model of DiFrancesco and Noble [1985] that accurate models of the sinoatrial node models could be constructed. An excellent summary of these modeling efforts can be found in Wilders et al. [1991] complete with listings of the equations. The most detailed model of sinoatrial node cells to-date is that of Demir et al. [1994]; this model includes a biophysically accurate description of internal calcium buffering and varying extracellular concentrations. A model similar to ones in Wilders et al. [1991] was augmented to model the effects of acetylcholine changes outside sinoatrial node cells by Dokos et al. [1996].

Atrial muscle The first detailed model of the excitation–contraction coupling mechanism in heart cells was constructed by Hilgemann and Noble [1987] and a single cell model was completed by Earm and Noble [1990]. A similarly detailed model of rabbit atrial cells was constructed by Lindblad et al. [1996] and modified to fit data from human atrial cells by Nygren et al. [1998]. Another model of human atrial cells based on the ventricular cell model of Luo and Rudy [1994] but with improved calcium handling equations was formulated by Courtemanche et al. [1998]. The main differences between the Nygren and

Courtemanche models are that the latter uses a steady-state approximation for the calcium buffers and that the relative sizes of the rapid and slow components of the delayed rectifier are reversed.

Ventricular muscle The first model of ventricular cells [Beeler and Reuter, 1977] consisted of (i) a fast inward sodium current, (ii) a slow inward calcium current, (iii) an inward-rectifying potassium current, and (iv) a voltage-dependent potassium current. A simple linear model of calcium buffering was also included. Drouhard and Roberge [1987] improved the Beeler–Reuter model by varying parameters and the equations for the rate constants for sodium activation and inactivation in order to match experimental results. Noble et al. [1991] constructed a model of the guinea-pig ventricular cell by varying parameters in equations for the atrial cell model of Earm and Noble [1990]. Further refinements including better handling of the fast and slow components of the delayed rectifier current and feedback of length and tension changes on the electrophysiology was incorporated in Noble et al. [1998]. Nordin [1993] modified the DiFrancesco and Noble [1985] equations to model ventricular cells. His model included membrane calcium and potassium pumps and subcompartments inside the cell for sodium and calcium concentrations. Luo and Rudy [1991] brought further improvements by including a plateau potassium current and updating all the current characteristics to match data from whole-cell and patch-clamp experiments. A more detailed model with more accurate descriptions of internal calcium concentration changes has also been constructed [Luo and Rudy, 1994]. The main disadvantage of this effort is the formulation of the calcium release current: it depends on the time of the maximum rate of depolarization and activates with a time delay. This was remedied by the model of Jafri et al. [1998] and also by Priebe and Beuckelmann [1998] for human ventricular cells. A model incorporating a Markov-state model of the transient outward current along with the other ionic currents in Jafri et al. [1998] was described in Greenstein et al. [2000] and a significantly more detailed model comprising a number of stochastically activated calcium release units and a Markov-state model formulation of L-type calcium currents was constructed by Greenstein and Winslow [2002].

Amphibian sinus venosus and atrial cells Rasmusson et al. [1990] have constructed a detailed model of the bullfrog sinus venosus pacemaker cells that includes (i) a delayed rectifier potassium current, (ii) a GHK-type calcium current, linear background, (iii) sodium current (iv) calcium current, (v) a Na/K pump current, (vi) a Na/Ca exchanger current, and (vii) a calcium pump current. Calcium binding to troponin, troponin-Mg, and calmodulin was also included in the model. Furthermore, internal and external sodium, calcium, and potassium were also modeled as time-varying quantities. In addition to the features of the sinus venosus cell, the bullfrog atrial cell [Rasmusson et al., 1990] includes a fast sodium current and an inward-rectifying potassium current.

22.8 Epithelial Cells

A detailed model of the slow processes in principal cells of the cortical collecting tubule of the mammalian kidney was built by Tang and Othmer [1996] and includes: sodium, potassium, and chloride channels; a sodium–potassium pump; a calcium pump; a sodium–potassium–chloride cotransporter; and a sodium–calcium exchanger.

22.9 Smooth Muscle

Smooth muscle cells like many other kinds of cells have significant currents carried by pumps and exchangers. A simple model of smooth muscle cell membrane electrical activity was constructed by Gonzalez-Fernandez and Ermentrout [1994]. This model has the same structure as the Morris–Lecar model of barnacle muscle fibers. Besides model parameter differences, the gating variable m was set to its steady-state value of m_∞ and internal calcium was modeled as a time-varying quantity with a simple linear model of internal buffering. A detailed model of electrical activity in smooth muscle of the small bowel with L- and T-type calcium currents, a calcium-dependent potassium current, a delayed rectifier potassium current, and a background chloride current has been published by Miftakhov et al. [1996].

22.10 Plant Cells

The electrophysiology of a number of plant cells have been studied and characterized. A plasmalemmal proton pump, a hydrogen–chloride symporter, inward- and outward-rectifying K^+ currents, and a chloride channel were modeled in the equations representing electrical activity in *Egeria densa* Planchon by Buschmann et al. [1996].

22.11 Simplified Models

There is a large number of papers investigating the dynamics of cell electrophysiology using simplifications of models listed above. A good reason to use simplified models is that mathematical analysis of such models is tractable.

Hill The model constructed by Hill [1936] was one of the earliest differential equation models of nerve electrical activity. While the behavior of this model was compared with experimental observations in animal preparations, the model is a phenomenological one that only reproduced subthreshold responses. Hill's main focus was the modeling of accomodation and he modeled this using a time-varying "threshold," U.

The basic model is a linear differential equation with time being the independent variable and voltage, V, and threshold voltage, U, being the dependent variables:

$$\dot{V} = \frac{-1}{k}(V - V_o) + I(t)$$
$$\dot{U} = \frac{-1}{\lambda}(U - U_o) + \frac{1}{\beta}(V - V_o)$$

(22.31)

where V_o and U_o are some steady-state values of voltage and the threshold function; k, λ, and β are relaxation time-constants (k is a few milliseconds and λ and β are a few hundred milliseconds); and $I(t)$ is some time-varying current source. The above equations can be solved using the variation of constants method and Hill documented the responses of the model to various functions, $I(t)$, and various parameter values. Such a model is only of use if one is not interested in suprathreshold behavior.

FitzHugh–Nagumo The FitzHugh–Nagumo equations are also called the Bonhoeffer–Van der Pol equations and have been used as a generic system that shows excitability and oscillatory activity. FitzHugh [1969] showed that much of the behavior of the Hodgkin–Huxley equations can be reproduced by a system of two differential equations:

$$\dot{V} = V - \frac{V^3}{3} - U + I(t)$$
$$\dot{U} = \phi(V - bU + a)$$

(22.32)

where a, b, and ϕ are positive constants (typical values are: $a = 0.7$, $b = 0.8$, and $\phi = 0.08$). With no input current ($I = 0$) the system has a stable resting state and at $I = 0.4$ the system exhibits oscillatory activity. This model reproduces excitability, threshold phenomena, and repetitive firing.

Hindmarsh–Rose models The first model of Hindmarsh and Rose [1982a] was an attempt to improve on the FitzHugh–Nagumo model without increasing the number of state variables. In most neurons undergoing repetitive firing, the time between action potentials is usually much greater than the duration of action potentials; however, the FHN model has an action potential duration that is roughly the same order of magnitude as the inter-spike interval. In addition, FHN does not yield a linear current–frequency relationship. These inadequacies were addressed by Hindmarsh and Rose and in their model the action potential duration and the inter-spike interval are closer to experimental recordings. Their model can be written as:

$$\dot{V} = -a(f(V) - y - I)$$
$$\dot{y} = b(g(V) - y) \tag{22.33}$$

where the nonlinearities are defined to be: $f(V) = cV^3 + dV^2 + eV + h$ and $g(V) = f(V) - ge^{rV} + s$. The constants used to model action potentials in snail visceral ganglion neurons were: $a = 5400$ MΩ/sec, $b = 30$ sec^{-1}, $c = 0.00017$, $d = 0.001$, $e = 0.01$, $h = 0.1$, $q = 0.022$, $r = 0.088$, and $s = 0.046$.

A second model [Hindmarsh and Rose, 1982b] sought to include the phenomenon of bursting by adding a third variable. The model had the following form:

$$\dot{V} = -aV^3 + bV^2 + y - z + I$$
$$\dot{y} = c - dV^2 - y \tag{22.34}$$
$$\dot{z} = r(s(V - V_1) - z)$$

where $a = 1$, $b = 3$, $c = 1$, $d = 5$, $r = 0.001$, $s = 1$, and setting $I = 1$ for a short period triggers the bursting response.

Defining Terms

Action potential: A phenomenon involving temporal changes in the transmembrane potential. An action potential is typically characterized by a fast depolarization follwed by a slower repolarization and sometimes hyperpolarization as well.

Depolarization: Depolarization is a process that is said to occur whenever the transmembrane potential becomes more positive than some "resting" potential.

Hyperpolarization: A deviation of the transmembrane potential in the negative direction from a "resting" state is called hyperpolarization.

Ion Channel: An ion channel is a protein molecule embedded in the cell membrane. It is thought to have the structure of a pipe with obstructions that gate the flow of ions into and out of the cell.

Ion Exchanger: An ion exchanger molecule uses the potential energy in the electrochemical gradients to pump one ionic species into the cell and another species out.

Ion Pump: An ion pump molecule uses energy (in the form of ATP molecules) to pump ions against their electrochemical gradients.

Refractory period: A period of time after an action potential during which the cell is unable to undergo another action potential in response to a second stimulus.

Repolarization: Repolarization is a process that usually follows depolarization and causes the transmembrane potential to return to a polarized state.

Selectivity: This is a property of ion channels where a certain type of channel only allows a specific ionic species to pass through it. Some channels are less specific than others and may allow more than one ionic species to pass through it.

Threshold: There is no satisfactory definition or quantitative description of threshold that will work for all conditions. A working definition of threshold would be the state the cell has to reach in order to produce an action potential. It is usually characterized by the strength of an external stimulus required to bring the cell from some initial state to the threshold state. The problem with this definition is that the threshold stimulus will vary considerably depending on the initial state of the cell: the cell may be in a resting state or it may be undergoing repolarization or depolarization.

Transmembrane potential difference: The potential difference between the inside and the outside of a cell manifests itself very close to membrane. In many cases the potential of the external fluid is taken to be the reference or ground potential and the transmembrane potential difference is the same as the cell potential otherwise also called the membrane potential.

Voltage clamp: This refers to the experimental procedure of using active electronic circuits to hold the transmembrane potential difference at a fixed value by pumping current into the cell.

References

Adrian, R.H. and L.D. Peachey (1973). Reconstruction of the action potential of frog sartorius muscle. *J. Physiol. (Lond.)* 235, 103–131.

Amini, B., J.W. Clark, and C.C. Canavier (1999). Calcium dynamics underlying pacemaker-like and burst firing oscillations in midbrain dopaminergic neurons: a computational study. *J. Neurophysiol.* 82, 2249–2261.

Amir, R., M. Michaelis, and M. Devor (2002). Burst discharge in primary sensory neurons: triggered by subthreshold oscillations, maintained by depolarizing afterpotentials. *J. Neurosci.* 22, 1187–1198.

Banks, M.I. and M.B. Sachs (1991). Regularity analysis in a compartmental model of chopper units in the anteroventral cochlear nucleus. *J. Neurophysiol.* 65, 606–629.

Beeler, G.W. and H. Reuter (1977). Reconstruction of the action potential of ventricular myocardial fibres. *J. Physiol. (Lond.)* 268, 177–210.

Belluzzi, O. and O. Sacchi (1991). A five-conductance model of the action potential in the rat sympathetic neurone. *Prog. Biophys. Mol. Biol.* 55, 1–30.

Benison, G., J. Keizer, L.M. Chalupa, and D.W. Robinson (2001). Modeling temporal behavior of postnatal cat retinal ganglion cells. *J. Theor. Biol.* 210, 187–199.

Berezetskaya, N.M., V.N. Kharkyanen, and N.I. Kononenko (1996). Mathematical model of pacemaker activity in bursting neurons of snail, *Helix pomatia. J. Theor. Biol.* 183, 207–218.

Bertram, R. (1993). A computational study of the effects of serotonin on a molluscan burster neuron. *Biol. Cybern.* 69, 257–267.

Bertram, R., M.J. Butte, T. Kiemel, and A. Sherman (1995). Topological and phenomenological classification of bursting oscillations. *Bull. Math. Biol.* 57, 413–439.

Booth, V., J. Rinzel, and O. Kiehn (1997). Compartmental model of vertebrate motoneurons for Ca^{2+}-dependent spiking and plateau potentials under pharmacological treatment. *J. Neurophysiol.* 78, 3371–3385.

Bristow, D.G. and J.W. Clark (1982). A mathematical model of primary pacemaking cell in sa node of the heart. *Am. J. Physiol.* 243, H207–H218.

Brodin, L., H.G.C. Traven, A. Lansner, P. Wallen, O. Ekeberg, and S. Grillner (1991). Computer simulations of n-methyl-d-aspartate receptor-induced membrane properties in a neuron model. *J. Neurophysiol.* 66, 473–484.

Buschmann, P., H. Sack, A.E. Kohler, and I. Dahnse (1996). Modeling plasmalemmal ion transport of the aquatic plant egeriadensa. *J. Membr. Biol.* 154, 109–118.

Butera, R.J., J.W. Clark, C.C. Canavier, D.A. Baxter, and J.H. Byrne (1995). Analysis of the effects of modulatory agents on a modeled bursting neuron: dynamic interactions between voltage and calcium dependent stores. *J. Comput. Neurosci.* 2, 19–44.

Chay, T.R. and J. Keizer (1983). Minimal model for membrane oscillations in the pancreatic β-cell. *Biophys. J.* 42, 181–190.

Chiu, S.Y., J.M. Ritchie, R.B. Rogart, and D. Stagg (1979). A quantitative description of membrane currents in rabbit myelinated nerve. *J. Physiol. (Lond.)* 292, 149–166.

Colombo, J. and C.W. Parkins (1987). A model of electrical excitation of the mammalian auditory-nerve neuron. *Heart Res.* 31, 287–312.

Connor, J.A. and C.F. Stevens (1971). Prediction of repetitive firing behaviour from voltage clamp data on an isolated neurone soma. *J. Physiol. (Lond.)* 213, 31–53.

Courtemanche, M., R.J. Ramirez, and S. Nattel (1998). Ionic mechanisms underlying human atrial action potential properties: insights from a mathematical model. *Am. J. Physiol.* 275, H301–H321.

DAngelo, E., T. Nieus, A. Maffei, S.A.P. Rossi, V. Taglietti, A. Fontana, and G. Naldi (2001). Theta-frequency bursting and resonance in cerebellar granule cells: experimental evidence and modeling of a slow K^+-dependent mechanism. *J. Neurosci.* 21, 759–770.

Demir, S.S., J.W. Clark, C.R. Murphey, and W.R. Giles (1994). A mathematical model of a rabbit sinoatrial node cell. *Am. J. Physiol.* 266, C832–C852.

Destexhe, A., A. Babloyantz, and T.J. Sejnowski (1993a). Ionic mechanisms for intrinsic slow oscillations in thalamic relay neurons. *Biophys. J.* 65, 1538–1552.

Destexhe, A., D.A. McCormick, and T.J. Sejnowski (1993b). A model for 8–10 hz spindling in interconnected thalamic relay and reticularis neurons. *Biophys. J.* 65, 2473–2477.

Destexhe, A., Z.F. Mainen, and T.J. Sejnowski (1994). An efficient method for computing synaptic conductances based on a kinetic model of receptor binding. *Neural Comput.* 6, 14–18.

DiFrancesco, D. and D. Noble (1985). A model of cardiac electrical activity incorporating ionic pumps and concentration changes. *Phil. Trans. R. Soc. Lond. B* 307, 353–398.

D'Incamps, B.L., C. Meunier, M.-L. Monnet, L. Jami, and D. Zytnicki (1998). Reduction of presynaptic action potentials by pad: model and experimental study. *J. Comput. Neurosci.* 5, 141–156.

Dokos, S., B.G. Celler, and N.H. Lovell (1996). Vagal control of sinoatrial node rhythm: a mathematical model. *J. Theor. Biol.* 182, 21–44.

Drouhard, J.-P. and F.A. Roberge (1987). Revised formulation of the Hodgkin–Huxley representation of the sodium current in cardiac cells. *Comput. Biomed. Res.* 20, 333–350.

Earm, Y.E. and D. Noble (1990). A model of the single atrial cell: relation between calcium current and calcium release. *Proc. R. Soc. Lond. Series B* 240, 83–96.

Epstein, I.R. and E. Marder (1990). Multiple modes of a conditional neural oscillator. *Biol. Cybern.* 63, 25–34.

FitzHugh, R. (1969). Mathematical models of excitation and propagation in nerve. In H.P. Schwan (Ed.), *Biological Engineering*, Chapter 1, pp. 1–85. New York: McGraw-Hill Book Co. Inc.

Fohlmeister, J.F., P.A. Coleman, and R.F. Miller (1990). Modeling the repetitive firing of retinal ganglion cells. *Brain Res.* 510, 343–345.

Fost, J.W. and G.A. Clark (1996). Modeling *hermissenda*: I. Differential contributions of ia and ic to type-b cell plasticity. *J. Comput. Neurosci.* 3, 137–153.

Frankenhaeuser, B. (1960). Sodium permeability in toad nerve and in squid nerve. *J. Physiol. (Lond.)* 152, 159–166.

Frankenhaeuser, B. and A.F. Huxley (1964). The action potential in the myelinated nerve fibre of *Xenopus laevis* as computed on the basis of voltage clamp data. *J. Physiol. (Lond.)* 171, 302–315.

Fridlyand, L.E., N. Tamarina, and L.H. Philipson (2003). Modeling of Ca^{2+} flux in pancreatic β-cells: role of the plasma membrane and intracellular stores. *Am. J. Physiol.* 285, E138–E154.

Goforth, P.B., R. Bertram, F.A. Khan, M. Zhang, A. Sherman, and L.S. Satin (2002). Calcium-activated K^+ channels of mouse β-cells are controlled by both store and cytoplasmic Ca^{2+}: experimental and theoretical studies. *J. Gen. Physiol.* 120, 307–322.

Goldman, D.E. (1943). Potential, impedence, and rectification in membranes. *J. Gen. Physiol.* 27, 37–60.

Gonzalez-Fernandez, J.M. and B. Ermentrout (1994). On the origin and dynamics of the vasomotion of small arteries. *Math. Biosci.* 119, 127–167.

Good, T.A. and R.M. Murphy (1996). Effect of β-amyloid block of the fast-inactivating K^+ channel on intracellular Ca^{2+} and excitability in a modeled neuron. *Proc. Natl Acad. Sci. USA* 93, 15130–15135.

Greenstein, J.L. and R.L. Winslow (2002). An integrative model of the cardiac ventricular myocyte incorporating local control of Ca^{2+} release. *Biophys. J.* 83, 2918–2945.

Greenstein, J.L., R. Wu, S. Po, G.F. Tomaselli, and R.L. Winslow (2000). Role of the calcium-independent transient outward current i_{to1} n shaping action potential morphology and duration. *Circ. Res.* 87, 1026–1033.

Guckenheimer, J., R. Harris-Warrick, J. Peck, and A. Willms (1997). Bifurcation, bursting, and spike frequency adaptation. *J. Comput. Neurosci.* 4, 257–277.

Haag, J., F. Theunissen, and A. Borst (1997). The intrinsic electrophysiological characteristics of fly lobula plate tangential cells: I. Active membrane properties. *J. Comput. Neurosci.* 4, 349–369.

Halter, J.A., J.S. Carp, and J.R. Wolpaw (1995). Operantly conditioned motoneuron plasticity: possible role of sodium channels. *J. Neurophysiol.* 73, 867–871.

Hamill, O.P., A. Marty, E. Neher, B. Sakmann, and F.J. Sigworth (1981). Improved patch-clamp techniques for high resolution current recording from cells and cell-free membrane patches. *Pflugers Arch. ges. Physiol.* 391, 85–100.

Harris-Warrick, R.M., L. Coniglio, N. Barazangi, J. Guckenheimer, and S. Gueron (1995a). Dopamine modulation of transient potassium current evokes phase shifts in a central pattern generator network. *J. Neurosci.* 15, 342–358.

Harris-Warrick, R.M., L. Coniglio, R.M. Levini, S. Gueron, and J. Guckenheimer (1995b). Dopamine modulation of two subthreshold currents produces phase shifts in activity of an identified motoneuron. *J. Neurophysiol.* 74, 1404–1420.

Hilgemann, D.W. and D. Noble (1987). Excitation–contraction coupling and extracellular calcium transients in rabbit atrium: reconstruction of basic cellular mechanisms. *Proc. R. Soc., Lond., Ser. B* 230, 163–205.

Hill, A.V. (1936). Excitation and accomodation in nerve. *Proc. R. Soc., Ser. B* 119, 305–355.

Hille, B. (2001). *Ion Channels of Excitable Membranes* (3rd ed.). Sunderland, MA: Sinauer Associates.

Hindmarsh, J.L. and R.M. Rose (1982a). A model of the nerve impulse using two first-order differential equations. *Nature* 296, 162–164.

Hindmarsh, J.L. and R.M. Rose (1982b). A model of the neuronal bursting using three coupled first order differential equations. *Proc. R. Soc., Ser. B* 221, 87–102.

Hodgkin, A.L. and A.F. Huxley (1952). A quantitative description of membrane current and its application to conduction and excitation in nerve. *J. Physiol. (Lond.)* 117, 500–544.

Huguenard, J.R. and D.A. McCormick (1992). Simulation of the currents involved in rhythmic oscillations in thalamic relay neurons. *J. Neurophysiol.* 68, 1373–1383.

Hunter, P., P. Robbins, and D. Noble (2002). The IUPS human physiome project. *Pflugers Arch.* 445, 1–9.

Jafri, M.S., J.J. Rice, and R.L. Winslow (1998). Cardiac Ca^{2+} dynamics: the roles of ryanodine receptor adaptation and sarcoplasmic reticulum load. *Biophys. J.* 74, 1149–1168.

Keizer, J. (1988). Electrical activity and insulin release in pancreatic beta cells. *Math. Biosci.* 90, 127–138.

Keizer, J. and G. Magnus (1989). ATP-sensitive potassium channel and bursting in the pancreatic beta cell. A theoretical study. *Biophys. J.* 89, 229–242.

Keizer, J. and G.W.D. Young (1993). Effect of voltage-gated plasma membrane Ca^{2+} fluxes on IP_3-linked Ca^{2+} oscillations. *Cell Calcium* 14, 397–410.

Koch, C., O. Bernander, and R.J. Douglas (1995). Do neurons have a voltage or a current threshold for action potential initiation? *J. Comput. Neurosci.* 2, 63–82.

Komendantov, A.O., O.G. Komendantova, S.W. Johnson, and C.C. Canavier (2004). A modeling study suggests complementary roles for $gaba_a$ and nmda receptors and the sk channel in regulating the firing pattern in midbrain dopamine neurons. *J. Neurophysiol.* 91, 346–357.

LeBeau, A.P., A.B. Robson, A.E. McKinnon, R.A. Donald, and J. Sneyd (1997). Generation of action potentials in a mathematical model of corticotrophs. *Biophys. J.* 73, 1263–1275.

Li, Y.-X., R. Bertram, and J. Rinzel (1996). Modeling n-methyl-d-aspartate-induced bursting in dopamine neurons. *Neuroscience* 71, 397–410.

Li, Y.-X., J. Rinzel, L. Vergara, and S.S. Stojilkovic (1995). Spontaneous electrical and calcium oscillations in unstimulated pituitary gonadotrophs. *Biophys. J.* 69, 785–795.

Lindblad, D.S., C.R. Murphey, J.W. Clark, and W.R. Giles (1996). A model of the action potential and underlying membrane currents in a rabbit atrial cell. *Am. J. Physiol.* 271, H1666–H1696.

Luo, C. and Y. Rudy (1991). A model of the ventricular cardiac action potential. *Circ. Res.* 68, 1501–1526.

Luo, C. and Y. Rudy (1994). A dynamic model of the cardiac ventricular action potential: I. Simulations of ionic currents and concentration changes. *Circ. Res.* 74, 1071–1096.

McAllister, R.E., D. Noble, and R.W. Tsien (1975). Reconstruction of the electrical activity of cardiac Purkinje fibres. *J. Physiol. (Lond.)* 251, 1–59.

McCormick, D.A. and J.R. Huguenard (1992). A model of the electrophysiological properties of thalamocortical relay neurons. *J. Neurophysiol.* 68, 1373–1383.

Miftakhov, R.N., G.R. Abdusheva, and D.L. Wingate (1996). Model predictions of myoelectrical activity of the small bowel. *Biol. Cybern.* 74, 167–179.

Miftakhov, R.N. and D.L. Wingate (1994a). Mathematical modelling of the enteric nervous network 1: cholinergic neuron. *Med. Eng. Phys.* 16, 67–73.

Miftakhov, R.N. and D.L. Wingate (1994b). Mathematical modelling of the enteric nervous network 3: adrenergic neuron. *Med. Eng. Phys.* 16, 451–457.

Miftakhov, R.N. and D.L. Wingate (1996). Electrical activity of the sensory afferent pathway in the enteric nervous system. *Biol. Cybern.* 75, 471–483.

Morris, C. and H. Lecar (1981). Voltage oscillations in the barnacle giant muscle fiber. *Biophys. J.* 35, 193–213.

Nadim, F., O.H. Olsen, E. DeSchutter, and R.L. Calabrese (1995). Modeling the leech heartbeat elemental oscillator i. Interactions of intrinsic and synaptic currents. *J. Comput. Neurosci.* 2, 215–235.

Negro, C.A.D. and S.H. Chandler (1997). Physiological and theoretical analysis of K^+ currents controlling discharge in neonatal rat mesencephalic trigeminal neurons. *J. Neurophysiol.* 77, 537–553.

Noble, D. (1960). A description of cardiac pacemaker potentials based on the Hodgkin–Huxley equations. *J. Physiol. (Lond.)* 154, 64P–65P.

Noble, D. (1962). A modification of the Hodgkin–Huxley equations applicable to Purkinje fibre action and pace-maker potentials. *J. Physiol. (Lond.)* 160, 317–352.

Noble, D. and R.W. Tsien (1969). Reconstruction of the repolarization process in cardiac Purkinje fibres based on voltage clamp measurements of membrane current. *J. Physiol. (Lond.)* 200, 205–231.

Noble, D., S.J. Noble, G.C.L. Bett, Y.E. Earm, W.K. Ho, and I.K. So (1991). The role of sodium–calcium exchange during the cardiac action potential. *Ann. N.Y. Acad. Sci.* 639, 334–353; Sodium–Calcium Exchange: *Proceedings of the 2nd International Conference*, April 1991, Baltimore, MD.

Noble, D., A. Varghese, P. Kohl, and P. Noble (1998). Improved guinea-pig ventricular cell model incorporating a diadic space, i_{Kr} and i_{Ks}, and length- and tension-dependent processes. *Can. J. Cardiol.* 14, 123–134.

Nordin, C. (1993). Computer model of membrane current and intracellular Ca^{2+} flux in the isolated guinea-pig ventricular myocyte. *Am. J. Physiol.* 265, H2117–H2136.

Nygren, A., C. Fiset, L. Firek, J.W. Clark, D.S.L.R.B. Clark, and W.R. Giles (1998). Mathematical model of an adult human atrial cell. The role of K^+ currents in repolarization. *Circ. Res.* 82, 63–81.

Otten, E., M. Hulliger, and K.A. Scheepstra (1995). A model study on the influence of a slowly activating potassium conductance on repetitive firing patterns of muscle spindle primary endings. *J. Theor. Biol.* 173, 67–78.

Plant, R.E. (1976). Mathematical description of a bursting pacemaker neuron by a modification of the Hodgkin–Huxley equations. *Biophys. J.* 16, 227–244.

Priebe, L. and D.J. Beuckelmann (1998). Simulation study of cellular electric properties in heart failure. *Circ. Res.* 82, 1206–1223.

Rall, W. (1967). Distinguishing theoretical synaptic potentials computed for different soma-dendritic distributions of synaptic input. *J. Neurophysiol.* 30, 1138–1168.

Rasmusson, R.L., J.W. Clark, W.R. Giles, K. Robinson, R.B. Clark, E.F. Shibata, and D.L. Campbell (1990). A mathematical model of electrophysiological activity in a bullfrog atrial cell. *Am. J. Physiol.* 259, H370–H389.

Rasmusson, R.L., J.W. Clark, W.R. Giles, E.F. Shibata, and D.L. Campbell (1990). A mathematical model of a bullfrog cardiac pacemaker cell. *Am. J. Physiol.* 259, H352–H369.

Saxena, P., R. Goldstein, and L. Isaac (1997). Computer simulation of neuronal toxicity in the spinal cord. *Neurol. Res.* 19, 340–349.

Schild, J.H. and D.L. Kunze (1997). Experimental and modeling study of Na^+ current heterogeneity in rat nodose neurons and it impact on neuronal discharge. *J. Neurophysiol.* 78, 3198–3209.

Schild, J.H., J.W. Clark, C.C. Canavier, D.L. Kunze, and M.C. Andresen (1995). Afferent synaptic drive of rat medial nucleus tractus solitarius neurons: dynamic simulation of graded vesicular mobilization, release, and non-NMDA receptor kinetics. *J. Neurophysiol.* 74, 1529–1548.

Schild, J.H., J.W. Clark, M. Hay, D. Mendelowitz, M.C. Andresen, and D.L. Kunze (1994). A- and c-type rat nodose sensory neurons: model interpretations of dynamic discharge characteristics. *J. Neurophysiol.* 71, 2338–2358.

Schwartz, J.R., G. Reid, and H. Bostock (1995). Action potentials and membrane currents in the human node of ranvier. *Pflugers Arch.* 430, 283–292.

Sherman, A., J. Keizer, and J. Rinzel (1990). Domain model for Ca^{2+}-inactivation of Ca^{2+} channels at low channel density. *Biophys. J.* 58, 985–995.

Sherman, A., J. Rinzel, and J. Keizer (1988). Emergence of organized bursting in clusters of pancreatic β-cells by channel sharing. *Biophys. J.* 54, 411–425.

Tabak, J. and L.E. Moore (1998). Simulation and parameter estimation study of a simple neuronal model of rhythm generation: role of NMDA and non-NMDA receptors. *J. Comput. Neurosci.* 5, 209–235.

Tang, Y. and H.G. Othmer (1996). Calcium dynamics and homeostasis in a mathematical model of the principal cell of the cortical collecting tubule. *J. Gen. Physiol.* 107, 207–230.

Traub, R.D. and R. Miles (1995). Pyramidal cell-to-inhibitory cell spike transduction explicable by active dendritic conductances in inhibitory cell. *J. Comput. Neurosci.* 2, 291–298.

Traub, R.D., R.K.S. Wong, R. Miles, and H. Michelson (1991). A model of a ca3 hippocampal pyramidal neuron incorporating voltage-clamp data on intrinsic conductances. *J. Neurophysiol.* 66, 635–650.

Usui, S., Y. Kamiyama, T. Ogura, I. Kodama, and J. Toyama (1996). Effects of zatebradine (ul-fs 49) on the vertebrate retina. In J. Toyama, M. Hiraoka, and I. Kodama (Eds.), *Recent Progress in Electropharmacology of the Heart*, Chapter 4, pp. 37–46. Boca Raton, FL: CRC Press.

Varghese, A. and R.L. Winslow (1993). Dynamics of the calcium subsystem in cardiac Purkinje fibers. *Physica D: Nonlinear Phenomena* 68, 364–386.

Warman, E.N., D.M. Durand, and G.L.F. Yuen (1994). Reconstruction of hippocampal ca1 pyramidal cell electrophysiology by computer simulation. *J. Neurophysiol.* 71, 2033–2045.

Wilders, R., H.J. Jongsma, and A.C.G. van Ginneken (1991). Pacemaker activity of the rabbit sinoatrial node: a comparison of mathematical models. *Biophys. J.* 60, 1202–1216.

Winslow, R.L. and A.G. Knapp (1991). Dynamic models of the retinal horizontal cell network. *Prog. Biophys. Mol. Biol.* 56, 107–133.

Yamada, W.M. and R.S. Zucker (1992). Time course of transmitter release calculated from simulations of a calcium diffusion model. *Biophys. J.* 61, 671–682.

Yanagihara, K., A. Noma, and H. Irisawa (1980). Reconstruction of sino-atrial node pacemaker potential based on the voltage clamp experiments. *Japan. J. Physiol.* 30, 841–857.

Zhang, M., P. Goforth, R. Bertram, A. Sherman, and L. Satin (2003). The Ca^{2+} dynamics of isolated mouse β-cells and islets: implications for mathematical models. *Biophys. J.* 84, 2852–2870.

Further Information

The best introduction to ion channels and excitable behavior in cells can be found in *Ion Channels of Excitable Membranes*, 3rd ed. by Bertil Hille (Sunderland, MA: Sinauer Associates; 2001).

In the case of neurons, *Principles of Neural Science* by Kandel, Schwartz, and Jessell (New York: Elsevier; 1991) is the bible. Detailed discussions of cardiovascular cell membrane phenomena can be found in *The Heart and Cardiovascular System* edited by Fozzard et al. (New York: Raven Press; 1992).

Mathematical analysis of cell models can be found in Guckenheimer et al. (1997); Bertram et al. (1995); and Koch et al. (1995).

Numerical methods: Most of the models presented in this chapter are systems of first-order nonlinear ordinary differential equations. While the solution of linear ordinary differential equations can be written down explicitly, this is usually impossible for nonlinear systems. The only option to investigate the behavior of these solutions is to compute approximate solutions using numerical time-integration. There are a number of numerical methods with varying degrees of accuracy and they fall into two main classes: explicit and implicit methods. The advantage of explicit methods is that they are simpler to implement whereas implicit methods require the use of a nonlinear solver, which can be extremely complicated. The disadvantage of explicit methods is that the errors of these methods are very sensitive to the time-step used and generally very small time-steps are required to ensure accuracy; implicit methods generally allow much larger time-steps. A general guideline would be to try a variable-step explicit method such as a Runge-Kutta method with tight tolerances to control the error; if this proves to be too slow, an implicit method such as the backward difference formula can be used. A good source of integration packages is http://www.netlib.org.

Databases: A number of databases of membrane models are being constructed. The IUPS Physiome project (Hunter et al., 2002) is an attempt to make mathematical models freely available on the internet although tools to translate the stored models (in XML) into machine executable form are not freely available at the time of this writing.

23

Computational Methods and Software for Bioelectric Field Problems

Christopher R. Johnson
University of Utah

23.1 Introduction

Computer modeling and simulation continue to grow more important to the field of Bioengineering. The reasons for this growing importance are manyfold. First, mathematical modeling has shown to be a substantial tool for the investigation of complex biophysical phenomena. Second, since the level of complexity one can model parallels existing hardware configurations, advances in computer architecture have made it feasible to apply the computational paradigm to complex biophysical systems. Hence, while biological complexity continues to outstrip the capabilities of even the largest computational systems, the computational methodology has taken hold in bioengineering and has been used successfully to suggest physiologically and clinically important scenarios and results.

This section provides an overview of numerical techniques which can be applied to a class of bioelectric field problems. Bioelectric field problems are found in a wide variety of biomedical applications which range from single cells [1], to organs [2], up to models which incorporate partial to full human structures [3–5]. We describe some general modeling techniques which will be applicable, in part, to all the aforementioned applications. We focus our study on a class of bioelectric volume conductor problems which arise in electrocardiography (ECG) and electroencephalography (EEG).

We begin by stating the mathematical formulation for a bioelectric volume conductor, continue by describing the model construction process, and follow with sections on numerical solutions and computational considerations. We conclude with a section on error analysis coupled with a brief introduction to adaptive methods.

23.2   Problem Formulation

As noted in the chapter on Volume Conductor Theory, most bioelectric field problems can be formulated in terms of either the Poisson or the Laplace equation for electrical conduction. Since Laplace's equation is the homogeneous counterpart of the Poisson equation, we will develop the treatment for a general three-dimensional Poisson problem and discuss simplifications and special cases when necessary.

A *typical* bioelectric volume conductor can be posed as the following boundary value problem:

$$\nabla \cdot \sigma \nabla \Phi = -I_V \quad \text{in } \Omega \tag{23.1}$$

where Φ is the electrostatic potential, σ is the electrical conductivity tensor, and I_V is the current per unit volume defined within the solution domain, Ω. The associated boundary conditions depend on what type of problem one wishes to solve. There are generally considered to be two different types of direct and inverse volume conductor problems.

One type of problem deals with the interplay between the description of the bioelectric volume source currents and the resulting volume currents and volume and surface voltages. Here, the problem statement would be to solve Equation 23.1 for Φ with a known description of I_V and the Neumann boundary condition:

$$\sigma \nabla \Phi \cdot \mathbf{n} = 0 \quad \text{on } \Gamma_T \tag{23.2}$$

which says that the normal component of the electric field is zero on the surface interfacing with air (here denoted by Γ_T). This problem can be used to solve two well-known problems in medicine, the direct EEG and ECG volume conductor problems. In the direct EEG problem, one usually discretizes the brain and surrounding tissue and skull. One then assumes a description of the bioelectric current source within the brain (this usually takes the form of dipoles or multipoles) and calculates the field within the brain and on the surface of the scalp. Similarly, in one version of the direct ECG problem, one utilizes descriptions of the current sources in the heart (either dipoles or membrane current source models such as the FitzHugh Nagumo and Beeler Reuter, among others) and calculates the currents and voltages within the volume conductor of the chest and voltages on the surface of the torso. The inverse problems associated with these direct problems involve estimating the current sources I_V within the volume conductor from measurements of voltages on the surface of either the head or body. Thus, one would solve Equation 23.1 with the boundary conditions:

$$\Phi = \Phi_0 \quad \text{on } \Sigma \subseteq \Gamma_T \tag{23.3}$$

$$\sigma \nabla \Phi \cdot \mathbf{n} = 0 \quad \text{on } \Gamma_T \tag{23.4}$$

The first is the Dirichlet condition, which says that one has a set of discrete measurements of the voltage of a subset of the outer surface. The second is the natural Neumann condition. While it does not look much different from the formulation of the direct problem, the inverse formulations are ill-posed. The bioelectric inverse problem in terms of primary current sources does not have a unique solution, and the solution does not depend continuously on the data. Thus, to obtain *useful* solutions, one must try to restrict the solution domain (i.e., number of physiologically plausible solutions) [6] for the former case, and apply so-called *regularization* techniques to attempt to restore the continuity of the solution on the data in the latter case.

Another bioelectric direct/inverse formulation poses both the problems in terms of scalar values at the surfaces. For the EEG problem, one would take the surface of the brain (cortex) as one bounded surface and the surface of the scalp as the other surface. The direct problem would involve making measurements of voltage of the surface of the cortex at discrete locations and then calculating the voltages on the surface of the scalp. Similarly, for the ECG problem, voltages could be measured on the surface of the heart and used to calculate the voltages at the surface of the torso, as well as within the volume conductor of the thorax. To formulate the inverse problems one uses measurements on the surface of the scalp (torso) to calculate the voltages on the surface of the cortex (heart). Here we solve Laplace's equation instead of Poisson's equation, because we are interested in the distributions of voltages on a surface instead of current sources within a volume. This leads to the following boundary value problem:

$$\nabla \cdot \sigma \nabla \Phi = 0 \quad \text{in } \Omega \tag{23.5}$$

$$\Phi = \Phi_0 \quad \text{on } \Sigma \subseteq \Gamma_T \tag{23.6}$$

$$\sigma \nabla \Phi \cdot \mathbf{n} = 0 \quad \text{on } \Gamma_T \tag{23.7}$$

For this formulation, the solution to the inverse problem is unique [7]; however, there still exists the problem of continuity of the solution on the data. The linear algebraic counterpart to the elliptic boundary value problem is often useful in discussing this problem of noncontinuity. The numerical solution to all elliptic boundary value problems (such as the Poisson and Laplace problems) can be formulated in terms of a set of linear equations, $A\Phi = \mathbf{b}$. For the solution of Laplace's equation, the system can be reformulated as:

$$A\Phi_{\text{in}} = \Phi_{\text{out}} \tag{23.8}$$

where Φ_{in} is the vector of data on the inner surface bounding the solution domain (the electrostatic potentials on the scalp or heart, for example), Φ_{out} is the vector of data which bounds the outer surface (the subset of voltage values on the surface of the cortex or torso, for example), and A is the *transfer matrix* between Φ_{out} and Φ_{in}, which usually contains the geometry and physical properties (conductivities, dielectric constants, etc.) of the volume conductor. The direct problem is then simply (well) posed as solving Equation 23.8 for Φ_{out} given Φ_{in}. Likewise, the inverse problem is to determine Φ_{in} given Φ_{out}.

A characteristic of A for ill-posed problems is that it has a very large condition number. In other words, the ill-conditioned matrix A is very near to being singular. Briefly, the condition number is defined as $\kappa(A) = \|A\| \cdot \|A^{-1}\|$ or the ratio of maximum to minimum singular values measured in the L_2 norm. The ideal problem conditioning occurs for orthogonal matrices which have $\kappa(A) \approx 1$, while an ill-conditioned matrix will have $\kappa(A) \gg 1$. When one inverts a matrix which has a very large condition number, the inversion process is unstable and is highly susceptible to errors. The condition of a matrix is relative. It is related to the precision level of computations and is a function of the size of the problem. For example, if the condition number exceeds a linear growth rate with respect to the size of the problem, the problem will become increasingly ill-conditioned. See Reference 58 for more about the condition number of matrices.

A number of techniques have arisen to deal with ill-posed inverse problems. These techniques include truncated singular value decompostion (TSVD), generalized singular value decompostion (GSVD), maximum entropy, and a number of generalized least squares schemes, including Twomey and Tikhonov regularization methods. Since this section is concerned more with the numerical techniques for approximating bioelectric field problems, the reader is referred to Reference 8 to Reference 11 to further investigate the regularization of ill-posed problems. A particularly useful reference for discrete ill-posed problems is the Matlab package developed by Per Christian Hansen, which is available via netlib [12].

23.3   Model Construction and Mesh Generation

Once we have stated or derived the mathematical equations which define the physics of the system, we must figure out how to solve these equations for the particular domain we are interested in. Most numerical methods for solving boundary value problems require that the continuous domain be broken up into discrete elements, the so-called *mesh* or *grid*, which one can use to approximate the governing equation(s) using the particular numerical technique (finite element, boundary element, finite difference, or multigrid) best suited to the problem.

Because of the complex geometries often associated with bioelectric field problems, construction of the polygonal mesh can become one of the most time-consuming aspects of the modeling process. After deciding upon the particular approximation method to use (and the most appropriate type of element), we need to construct a mesh of the solution domain which matches the number of degrees of freedom of our fundamental element. For the sake of simplicity, we will assume that we will use linear elements, either tetrahedrons, which are usually used for modeling irregular three-dimensional domains, or hexahedrons used for modeling regular, uniform domains.

There are several different strategies for discretizing the geometry into fundamental elements. For bioelectric field problems, two approaches to mesh generation have become standard: the *divide and conquer* (or subsequent subdivision) strategy; and the so-called *Delaunay triangulation* strategy.

In using the divide and conquer strategy one starts with a set of points which define the bounding surface(s) in three dimensions (contours in two dimensions). The volume (surface) is repeatedly divided into smaller regions until a satisfactory discretization level has been achieved. Usually, the domain is broken up into eight-node cubic elements, which can then be subdivided into five (minimally) or six tetrahedral elements if so desired. This methodology has the advantage of being fairly easy to program; furthermore, commercial mesh generators exist for the divide and conquer method. For use in solving bioelectric field problems, its main disadvantage is that it allows elements to overlap interior boundaries. A single element may span two different conductive regions, for example, when part of an element represents muscle tissue (which could be anisotropic) and the other part of the element falls into a region representing fat tissue. It then becomes very difficult to assign unique conductivity parameters to each element and at the same time accurately represent the geometry.

A second method of mesh generation is the Delaunay triangulation strategy. Given a three-dimensional set of points which define the boundaries and interior regions of the domain to be modeled, one tessellates the point cloud into an optimal mesh of tetrahedra. For bioelectric field problems, the advantages and disadvantages tend to be exactly contrary to those arising from the divide and conquer strategy. The primary advantage is that one can create the mesh to fit any predefined geometry, including subsurfaces, by starting with points which define all the necessary surfaces and subsurfaces and then adding additional interior points to minimize the aspect ratio. For tetrahedra, the aspect ratio can be defined as $4\sqrt{(3/2)}(\rho_k/h_k)$, where ρ_k denotes the diameter of the sphere circumscribed about the tetrahedron, and h_k is the maximum distance between two vertices. These formulations yield a value of 1 for an equilateral tetrahedron and a value of 0 for a degenerate (flat) element [13]. The closer to the value of 1, the better. The Delaunay criterion is a method for minimizing the occurrence of obtuse angles in the mesh, yielding elements which have aspect ratios as close as possible to 1, given the available point set. While the ideas behind Delaunay triangulation are straightforward, the programming is nontrivial and is the primary drawback to this method. Fortunately, there exist several public domain, two-dimensional (2D) versions, including one from netlib called sweep2.c from the directory Voronoi, as well as at least one three-dimensional (3D) package [14]. For more information on mesh generation and various aspects of biomedical modeling, see References 15 to 23.

23.4 Numerical Methods

Because of the geometrical complexity of, and numerous inhomogeneities inherent in, anatomical structures in physiological models, solutions of bioelectric field problems are usually tractable (except in the most simplified of models) only when one employs a numerical approximation method such as the finite difference (FD), the finite element (FE), boundary element (BE), or the multigrid (MG) method to solve the governing field equation(s).

23.4.1 Approximation Techniques — The Galerkin Method

The problem posed in Equation 23.1 can be solved using any of the aforementioned approximation schemes. One technique which addresses three of the previously mentioned techniques (FD, FE, and BE) can be derived by the Galerkin method. The Galerkin method is one of the most widely used methods for discretizing elliptic boundary value problems such as Equation 23.1 and for treating the spatial portion of time-dependent parabolic problems, which are common in models of cardiac wave propagation. While the Galerkin technique is not essential to the application of any of the techniques, it provides for a unifying bridge between the various numerical methods. To express our problem in a Galerkin form, we begin by rewriting Equation 23.1 as:

$$A\Phi = -I_v \tag{23.9}$$

where A is the differential operator, $A = \nabla \cdot (\sigma \nabla)$. An equivalent statement of Equation 23.9 is, find Φ such that $(A\Phi + I_v, \overline{\Phi}) = 0$. Here, $\overline{\Phi}$ is an arbitrary *test function*, which can be thought of physically as a virtual potential field, and the notation $(\phi_1, \phi_2) \equiv \int_\Omega \phi_1 \phi_2 \, d\Omega$ denotes the inner product in $L_2(\Omega)$. Applying Green's theorem, we can equivalently write,

$$(\sigma \nabla \Phi, \nabla \overline{\Phi}) - \left\langle \frac{\partial \Phi}{\partial n}, \overline{\Phi} \right\rangle = -(I_v, \overline{\Phi}) \tag{23.10}$$

where the notation $\langle \phi_1, \phi_2 \rangle \equiv \int_S \phi_1 \phi_2 \, dS$ denotes the inner product on the boundary S. When the Dirichlet, $\Phi = \Phi_0$, and Neumann, $\sigma \nabla \Phi \cdot \mathbf{n} = 0$, boundary conditions are specified on S, we obtain the *weak form* of Equation 23.1:

$$(\sigma \nabla \Phi, \nabla \overline{\Phi}) = -(I_v, \overline{\Phi}) \tag{23.11}$$

It is understood that this equation must hold for all test functions, $\overline{\Phi}$, which must vanish at the boundaries where $\Phi = \Phi_0$. The Galerkin approximation ϕ to the weak form solution Φ in Equation 23.11 can be expressed as:

$$\phi(\mathbf{x}) = \sum_{i=0}^{N} \phi_i \psi_i(\mathbf{x}) \tag{23.12}$$

The trial functions $\psi_i, i = 0, 1, \ldots, N$ form a basis for an $N + 1$ dimensional space $\mathcal{S}$. We define the *Galerkin approximation* to be that element $\phi \in \mathcal{S}$ which satisfies

$$(\sigma \nabla \phi, \nabla \psi_j) = -(I_v, \psi_j) \quad (\forall \psi_j \in \mathcal{S}) \tag{23.13}$$

Since our differential operator A is positive definite and self adjoint (i.e., $(A\Phi, \Phi) \geq \alpha(\Phi, \Phi) > 0$ for some nonzero positive constant α and $(A\Phi, \overline{\Phi}) = (\Phi, A\overline{\Phi})$, respectively), then we can define a space E with an inner product defined as $(\Phi, \overline{\Phi})_E = (A\Phi, \overline{\Phi}) \equiv a(\Phi, \overline{\Phi})$ and norm (the so-called energy norm) equal to:

$$\|\Phi\|_E = \left\{ \int_\Omega (\nabla \Phi)^2 \, d\Omega \right\}^{1/2} = (\Phi, \Phi)_E^{1/2} \tag{23.14}$$

The solution Φ of Equation 23.9 satisfies

$$(A\Phi, \psi_i) = -(I_v, \psi_i) \quad (\forall \psi_i \in S) \tag{23.15}$$

and the approximate Galerkin solution obtained by solving (23.13) satisfies

$$(A\phi, \psi_i) = -(I_v, \psi_i) \quad (\forall \psi_i \in S) \tag{23.16}$$

Subtracting Equation 23.15 from Equation 23.16 yields

$$(A(\phi - \Phi), \psi_i) = (\phi - \Phi, \psi_i)_E = 0 \quad (\forall \psi_i \in S) \tag{23.17}$$

The difference $\phi - \Phi$ denotes the error between the solution in the infinite dimensional space V and the $N+1$ dimensional space S. Equation 23.17 states that the error is orthogonal to all basis functions spanning the space of possible Galerkin solutions. Consequently, the error is orthogonal to all elements in S and must therefore be the minimum error. Thus the Galerkin approximation is an orthogonal projection of the true solution Φ onto the given finite dimensional space of possible approximate solutions. Therefore, the Galerkin approximation is the best approximation in the energy space E. Since the operator is positive definite, the approximate solution is unique. Assume for a moment there are two solutions, ϕ_1 and ϕ_2, satisfying

$$(A\phi_1, \psi_i) = -(I_v, \psi_i) \quad (A\phi_2, \psi_i) = -(I_v, \psi_i) \quad (\forall \psi_i \in S) \tag{23.18}$$

respectively. Then, the difference yields

$$(A(\phi_1 - \phi_2), \psi_i) = 0 \quad (\forall \psi_i \in S). \tag{23.19}$$

The function arising from subtracting one member from another member in S also belongs in S; hence, the difference function can be expressed by the set of A orthogonal basis functions spanning S:

$$\sum_{j=0}^{N} \Delta\phi_j(A(\psi_j, \psi_i)) = 0 \quad (\forall \psi_i \in) \tag{23.20}$$

When $i \neq j$, the terms vanish due to the basis functions being orthogonal with respect to A. Since A is positive definite:

$$(A\Phi_i, \Phi_i) > 0 \quad i = 0, \dots, N \tag{23.21}$$

Thus, $\Delta\phi_i = 0$, $i = 0, \dots, N$, and by virtue of Equation 23.20, $\delta\phi = 0$, such that $\phi_1 = \phi_2$. The identity contradicts the assumption of two distinct Galerkin solutions. This proves the solution is unique [24].

23.4.2 The Finite Difference Method

Perhaps the most traditional way to solve Equation 23.1 utilizes the FD approach by discretizing the solution domain Ω using a grid of uniform hexahedral elements. The coordinates of a typical grid point are $x = lh$, $y = mh$, $z = nh$ ($l, m, n =$ integers), and the value of $\Phi(x, y, z)$ at a grid point is denoted by $\Phi_{l,m,n}$. Taylor's theorem can then be utilized to provide the difference equations. For example:

$$\Phi_{l+1,m,n} = \left(\Phi + h\frac{\partial \Phi}{\partial x} + \frac{1}{2}h^2\frac{\partial^2 \Phi}{\partial x^2} + \frac{1}{6}h^3\frac{\partial^3 \Phi}{\partial x^3} + \cdots \right)_{l,m,n} \tag{23.22}$$

with similar equations for $\Phi_{l-1,m,n}, \Phi_{l,m+1,n}, \Phi_{l,m-1,n},...$. The finite difference representation of Equation 23.1 is

$$\frac{\Phi_{l+1,m,n} - 2\Phi_{l,m,n} + \Phi_{l-1,m,n}}{h^2} + \frac{\Phi_{l,m+1,n} - 2\Phi_{l,m,n} + \Phi_{l,m-1,n}}{h^2}$$

$$+ \frac{\Phi_{l,m,n+1} - 2\Phi_{l,m,n} + \Phi_{l,m,n-1}}{h^2} = -I_{l,m,n}(v) \tag{23.23}$$

or, equivalently,

$$\Phi_{l+1,m,n} + \Phi_{l-1,m,n} + \Phi_{l,m+1,n} + \Phi_{l,m-1,n} + \Phi_{l,m,n+1} + \Phi_{l,m,n-1} - 6\Phi_{l,m,n} = -h^2 I_{l,m,n}(v) \tag{23.24}$$

If we define the vector $\boldsymbol{\Phi}$ to be $[\Phi_{1,1,1} \cdots \Phi_{1,1,N-1}; \cdots \Phi_{1,N-1,1} \cdots \Phi_{N-1,N-1,N-1}]^T$ to designate the $(N-1)^3$ unknown grid values, and pull out all the known information from Equation 23.24, we can reformulate Equation 23.1 by its finite difference approximation in the form of the matrix equation $A\boldsymbol{\Phi} = \mathbf{b}$, where $\mathbf{b}$ is a vector which contains the sources and modifications due to the Dirichlet boundary condition.

Unlike the traditional Taylor's series expansion method, the Galerkin approach utilizes basis functions, such as linear piecewise polynomials, to approximate the true solution. For example, the Galerkin approximation to the sample problem Equation 23.1 would require evaluating Equation 23.13 for the specific grid formation and specific choice of basis function:

$$\int_\Omega \left(\sigma_x \frac{\partial \phi}{\partial x} \frac{\partial \psi_i}{\partial x} + \sigma_y \frac{\partial \phi}{\partial y} \frac{\partial \psi_i}{\partial y} + \sigma_z \frac{\partial \phi}{\partial z} \frac{\partial \psi_i}{\partial z} \right) d\Omega = - \int_\Omega I_v \psi_i d\Omega \tag{23.25}$$

Difference quotients are then used to approximate the derivatives in Equation 23.25. We note that if linear basis functions are utilized in Reference 23.25, one obtains a formulation which corresponds exactly with the standard finite difference operator. Regardless of the difference scheme or order of basis function, the approximation results in a linear system of equations of the form $A\boldsymbol{\Phi} = \mathbf{b}$, subject to the appropriate boundary conditions.

23.4.3 The Finite Element Method

As we have seen above, in the classical numerical treatment for partial differential equations — the FD difference method — the solution domain is approximated by a grid of uniformly spaced nodes. At each node, the governing differential equation is approximated by an algebraic expression which references adjacent grid points. A system of equations is obtained by evaluating the previous algebraic approximations for each node in the domain. Finally, the system is solved for each value of the dependent variable at each node. In the FE method, the solution domain can be discretized into a number of uniform or nonuniform finite elements that are connected via nodes. The change of the dependent variable with regard to location is approximated within each element by an interpolation function. The interpolation function is defined relative to the values of the variable at the nodes associated with each element. The original boundary value problem is then replaced with an equivalent integral formulation (such as Equation 23.13). The interpolation functions are then substituted into the integral equation, integrated, and combined with the results from all other elements in the solution domain. The results of this procedure can be reformulated into a matrix equation of the form $A\boldsymbol{\Phi} = \mathbf{b}$, which is subsequently solved for the unknown variable [16,25].

The formulation of the finite element approximation starts with the Galerkin approximation, $(\sigma \nabla \Phi, \nabla \overline{\Phi}) = -(I_v, \overline{\Phi})$, where $\overline{\Phi}$ is our test function. We now use the finite element method to turn the continuous problems into a discrete formulation. First we discretize the solution domain, $\Omega = \cup_{e=1}^E \Omega_e$, and define a finite dimensional subspace, $V_h \subset V = \{\overline{\Phi} : \overline{\Phi} \text{ is continuous on } \Omega, \nabla \overline{\Phi} \text{ is piecewise continuous on } \Omega\}$. One usually defines parameters of the function $\overline{\Phi} \in V_h$ at node points $\alpha_i = \overline{\Phi}(x_i)$, $i = 0, 1, \ldots, N$. If we now define the basis functions, $\psi_i \in V_h$, as linear continuous piecewise functions that take the value 1 at node points and zero at other node points, then we can represent the function $\overline{\Phi} \in V_h$ as

$$\overline{\Phi}(x) = \sum_{i=0}^{N} \alpha_i \Psi_i(x) \tag{23.26}$$

such that each $\overline{\Phi} \in V_h$ can be written in a unique way as a linear combination of the basis functions $\Psi_i \in V_h$. Now the finite element approximation of the original boundary value problem can be stated as

$$\text{Find } \Phi_h \in V_h \text{ such that } (\sigma \nabla \Phi_h, \nabla \overline{\Phi}) = -(I_v, \overline{\Phi}) \tag{23.27}$$

Furthermore, if $\Phi_h \in V_h$ satisfies Equation 23.27, then we have $(\sigma \nabla \Phi_h, \nabla \Psi_i) = -(I_v, \Psi_i)$ [26]. Finally, since Φ_h itself can be expressed as the linear combination

$$\Phi_h = \sum_{i=0}^{N} \xi_i \Psi_i(x) \quad \xi_i = \Phi_h(x_i) \tag{23.28}$$

we can then write Equation 23.27 as

$$\sum_{i=0}^{N} \xi_i (\sigma_{ij} \nabla \Psi_i, \nabla \Psi_j) = -(I_v, \Psi_j) \quad j = 0, \ldots, N \tag{23.29}$$

subject to the Dirichlet boundary condition. Then the finite element approximation of Equation 23.1 can equivalently be expressed as a system of N equations with N unknowns $\xi_i, \ldots, \xi_N$ (e.g., the electrostatic potentials). In matrix form, the above system can be written as $A\xi = b$, where $A = (a_{ij})$ is called the global stiffness matrix and has elements $(a_{ij}) = (\sigma_{ij} \nabla \Psi_i, \nabla \Psi_j)$, while $b_i = -(I_v, \Psi_i)$ and is usually termed the load vector.

For volume conductor problems, A contains all of the geometry and conductivity information of the model. The matrix A is symmetric and positive definite; thus, it is nonsingular and has a unique solution. Because the basis function differs from zero for only a few intervals, A is sparse (only a few of its entries are nonzero).

23.4.3.1   Application of the FE Method for 3D Domains

We now illustrate the concepts of the FE method by considering the solution of Equation 23.1 using linear 3D elements. We start with a 3D domain Ω which represents the geometry of our volume conductor and break it up into discrete elements to form a finite dimensional subspace, Ω_h. For 3D domains we have the choice of representing our function as either tetrahedra,

$$\tilde{\Phi} = \alpha_1 + \alpha_2 x + \alpha_3 y + \alpha_4 z \tag{23.30}$$

or hexahedra,

$$\tilde{\Phi} = \alpha_1 + \alpha_2 x + \alpha_3 y + \alpha_4 z + \alpha_5 xy + \alpha_6 yz + \alpha_7 xz + \alpha_8 xyz \tag{23.31}$$

Because of space limitations we restrict our development to tetrahera, knowing that it is easy to modify our formulae for hexahedra. We take out a specific tetrahedra from our finite dimensional subspace and apply the previous formulations for the four vertices,

$$\begin{pmatrix} \tilde{\Phi}_1 \\ \tilde{\Phi}_2 \\ \tilde{\Phi}_3 \\ \tilde{\Phi}_4 \end{pmatrix} = \begin{pmatrix} 1 & x_1 & y_1 & z_1 \\ 1 & x_2 & y_2 & z_2 \\ 1 & x_3 & y_3 & z_3 \\ 1 & x_4 & y_4 & z_4 \end{pmatrix} \begin{pmatrix} \alpha_1 \\ \alpha_2 \\ \alpha_3 \\ \alpha_4 \end{pmatrix} \tag{23.32}$$

or

$$\tilde{\mathbf{\Phi}}_i = \mathbf{C}\alpha \tag{23.33}$$

which define the coordinate vertices, and

$$\alpha = \mathbf{C}^{-1}\tilde{\mathbf{\Phi}}_i \tag{23.34}$$

which defines the coefficients. From Equation 23.30 and Equation 23.34 we can express $\tilde{\Phi}$ at any point within the tetrahedra,

$$\tilde{\Phi} = [1, x, y, z]\alpha = \mathbf{S}\alpha = \mathbf{S}\mathbf{C}^{-1}\tilde{\mathbf{\Phi}}_i \tag{23.35}$$

or, most succinctly,

$$\tilde{\Phi} = \sum_i N_i \tilde{\Phi}_i \tag{23.36}$$

$\tilde{\Phi}_i$ is the solution value at node i, and $\mathbf{N} = \mathbf{S}\mathbf{C}^{-1}$ is the local *shape function* or *basis function*. This can be expressed in a variety of ways in the literature (depending, usually, on whether you are reading engineering or mathematical treatments of finite element analysis):

$$\Phi_j(N_i) = N_i(x, y, z) = f_i(x, y, z) \equiv \frac{a_i + b_i x + c_i y + d_i z}{6V} \tag{23.37}$$

where

$$6V = \begin{vmatrix} 1 & x_1 & y_1 & z_1 \\ 1 & x_2 & y_2 & z_2 \\ 1 & x_3 & y_3 & z_3 \\ 1 & x_4 & y_4 & z_4 \end{vmatrix} \tag{23.38}$$

defines the volume of the tetrahedra, V.

Now that we have a suitable set of basis functions, we can find the finite element approximation to our 3D problem. Our orginal problem can be formulated as

$$a(u, v) = (I_v, v) \quad \forall v \in \Omega \tag{23.39}$$

where

$$a(u, v) = \int_{\Omega} \nabla u \cdot \nabla v \, d\Omega \tag{23.40}$$

and

$$(I_v, v) = \int_{\Omega} I_v \cdot v \, d\Omega \tag{23.41}$$

The finite element approximation to the original boundary value problem is

$$a(u_h, v) = (I_v, v) \quad \forall v \in \Omega_h \tag{23.42}$$

which has the equivalent form

$$\sum_{i=1}^{N} \xi_i a(\Phi_i, \Phi_j) = (I_v, \Phi_j) \tag{23.43}$$

where

$$a(\Phi_i, \Phi_j) = a(\Phi_i(N_j), \Phi_j(N_i)) \tag{23.44}$$

which can be expressed by the matrix and vector elements

$$(a_{ij}) = \int_{\Omega_E} \left(\frac{\partial N_i}{\partial x} \frac{\partial N_j}{\partial x} + \frac{\partial N_i}{\partial y} \frac{\partial N_j}{\partial y} + \frac{\partial N_i}{\partial z} \frac{\partial N_j}{\partial z} \right) d\Omega \tag{23.45}$$

and

$$I_i = \int_{\Omega_E} N_i I_v \, d\Omega \tag{23.46}$$

Fortunately, the above quantities are easy to evaluate for linear tetrahedra. As a matter of fact, there are closed form solutions for the matrix elements (a_{ij}):

$$\int_{\Omega_h} N_1^a N_2^b N_3^c N_4^d \, d\Omega = 6V \frac{a!b!c!d!}{(a+b+c+d+3)!} \tag{23.47}$$

Therefore,

$$(a_{ij}) = \int_{\Omega_E} \frac{b_i b_j + c_i c_j + d_i d_j}{6V^2} \, d\Omega = \frac{b_i b_j + c_i c_j + d_i d_j}{6V} \tag{23.48}$$

and, for the right-hand side (RHS), we have, assuming constant sources,

$$I_i = \int_{\Omega_E} \frac{a_i + b_i x + c_i y + d_i z}{6V} I_v \, d\Omega = \frac{V I_v}{4} \tag{23.49}$$

which have the compact forms

$$a_{ij}^{(n)} = \frac{1}{6V} \left(b_i^{(n)} b_j^{(n)} + c_i^{(n)} c_j^{(n)} + d_i^{(n)} d_j^{(n)} \right) \tag{23.50}$$

and

$$I_i^{(n)} = \frac{V I_v}{4} \quad \text{for constant sources} \tag{23.51}$$

Now we add up all the contributions from each element into a global matrix and global vector.

$$\sum_{n=1}^{\text{Nel}} \left(a_{ij}^{(n)} \right) (\xi_i) = \left(I_i^{(n)} \right) \tag{23.52}$$

where Nel is equal to the total number of elements in the discretized solution domain and i represents the node numbers (vertices). This yields a linear sytem of equations of the form $\mathbf{A\Phi} = \mathbf{b}$, where $\mathbf{\Phi}$ is our solution vector of voltages, $\mathbf{A}$ represents the geometry and conductivity of our volume conductor, and $\mathbf{b}$ represents the contributions from the current sources and boundary conditions.

For the FD method, it turns out that the Dirichlet boundary condition is easy to apply while the Neumann condition takes a little extra effort. For the FE method it is just the opposite. The Neumann boundary condition

$$\nabla\Phi \cdot \mathbf{n} = 0 \tag{23.53}$$

is satisfied automatically within the Galerkin and variational formulations. This can be seen by using Green's divergence theorem,

$$\int_{\Omega} \nabla \cdot \mathbf{A} \, dx = \int_{\Gamma} \mathbf{A} \cdot \mathbf{n} \, dS \tag{23.54}$$

and applying it to the left-hand side (LHS) of the Galerkin finite element formulation:

$$
\begin{aligned}
\int_{\Omega} \nabla v \cdot \nabla w \, d\Omega &\equiv \int_{\Omega} \left[\frac{\partial v}{\partial x_1} \frac{\partial w}{\partial x_1} + \frac{\partial v}{\partial x_2} \frac{\partial w}{\partial x_2} \right] d\Omega \\
&= \int_{\Gamma} \left[v \frac{\partial w}{\partial x_1} n_1 + v \frac{\partial w}{\partial x_2} n_2 \right] dS - \int_{\Omega} v \left[\frac{\partial^2 w}{\partial x_1^2} + \frac{\partial^2 w}{\partial x_2^2} \right] d\Omega \\
&= \int_{\Gamma} v \frac{\partial w}{\partial n} \, dS - \int_{\Omega} v \nabla^2 w \, d\Omega
\end{aligned}
\tag{23.55}
$$

If we multiply our original differential equation, $\nabla^2 \Phi = -I_v$, by an arbitrary test function and integrate, we obtain

$$
(I_v, v) = -\int_{\Omega} (\nabla^2 \Phi) v \, d\Omega = -\int_{\Gamma} \frac{\partial \Phi}{\partial n} v \, dS + \int_{\Omega} \nabla \Phi \cdot \nabla v \, d\Omega = a(\Phi, v)
\tag{23.56}
$$

where the boundary integral term, $\partial \Phi / \partial n$ vanishes and we obtain the standard Galerkin finite element formulation.

To apply the Dirichlet condition, we have to work a bit harder. To apply the Dirichlet boundary condition directly, one usually modifies the (a_{ij}) matrix and b_i vector such that one can use standard linear system solvers. This is accomplished by implementing the following steps:

Assuming we know the ith value of u_i:

1. Subtract from the ith member of the RHS the product of a_{ij} and the known value of Φ_i (call it $\bar{\Phi}_i$) this yields the new RHS, $\hat{b}_i = b_i - a_{ij} \bar{\Phi}_j$
2. Zero the ith row and column of A: $\hat{a}_{ij} = \hat{a}_{ji} = 0$
3. Assign $\hat{a}_{ii} = 1$
4. Set the jth member of the RHS equal to $\bar{\Phi}_i$
5. Continue for each Dirichlet condition
6. Solve the augmented system, $\hat{A}\Phi = \hat{b}_v$

23.4.4 The Boundary Element Method

For bioelectric field problems with isotropic domains (and few inhomogeneities), another technique, called the BE method, may be utilized. This technique utilizes information only upon the boundaries of interest, and thus reduces the dimension of any field problem by one. For differential operators, the response at any given point to sources and boundary conditions depends only on the response at neighboring points. The FD and FE methods approximate differential operators defined on subregions (volume elements) in the domain; hence, direct mutual influence (connectivity) exists only between neighboring elements, and the coefficient matrices generated by these methods have relatively few nonzero coefficients in any given matrix row. As is demonstrated by Maxwell's laws [27], equations in differential forms can often be replaced by equations in integral forms; for example, the potential distribution in a domain is uniquely defined by the volume sources and the potential and current density on the boundary. The BE method utilizes this fact by transforming the differential operator defined in the domain to integral operators defined on the boundary. In the boundary element method [28–30], only the boundary is discretized; hence, the mesh generation is considerably simpler for this method than for the volume methods. Boundary solutions are obtained directly by solving the set of linear equations; however, potentials and gradients in the domain can be evaluated only after the boundary solutions have been obtained. As this method has a rich history in bioelectric field problems, the reader is referred to some of the classic references for further information regarding the application of the BE method to bioelectric field problems [31–34].

23.4.5   Solution Methods and Computational Considerations

Application of each of the previous approximation methods to Equation 23.1 yields a system of linear equations of the form $\mathbf{A\Phi} = \mathbf{b}$, which must be solved to obtain the final solution. There are a plethora of available techniques for the solutions of such systems. The solution techniques can be broadly catagorized as *direct* and *iterative* solvers. Direct solvers include Gaussian elimination and LU decomposition, while iterative methods include Jacobi, Gauss-Seidel, successive overrelaxation (SOR),and conjugate gradient (CG) methods, among others. The choice of the particular solution method is highly dependent upon the approximation technique employed to obtain the linear system, upon the size of the resulting system, and upon accessible computational resources. For example, the linear system resulting from the application of the FD or FE method will yield a matrix $\mathbf{A}$ that is symmetric, positive definite, and sparse. The matrix resulting from the FD method will have a specific band-diagonal structure which is dependent on the order of difference equations one uses to approximate the governing equation. The matrix resulting from the FE method will be exceedingly sparse that only a few of the off-diagonal elements will be nonzero. The application of the BE method, on the other hand, will yield a matrix $\mathbf{A}$ that is dense and nonsymmetric and thus requires a different choice of solver.

The choice of the optimal solver is further complicated by the size of the system vs. access to computational resources. Sequential direct methods are usually confined to single workstations and thus the size of the system should fit in memory for optimal performance. Sequential iterative methods can be employed when the size of the system exceeds the memory of the machine; however, one pays a price in terms of performance as direct methods are usually much faster than iterative methods. In many cases, the size of the system exceeds the computational capability of a single workstation and one must resort to the use of clusters of workstations or parallel computers.

While new and improved methods continue to appear in the numerical analysis literature, the author's studies comparing various solution techniques for direct and inverse bioelectric field problems have resulted in the conclusion that the preconditioned CG methods and MG methods are the best overall performers for volume conductor problems computed on single workstations. Specifically, the incomplete Choleski conjugate gradient (ICCG) method works well for the FE method[1] and the preconditioned biconjugate gradient (BCG) methods are often utilized for BE methods. When clusters of workstations and parallel architectures are considered, the choice is less clear. For use with some high-performance architectures that contain large amounts of memory, parallel direct methods such as LU decomposition become attractive; however, preconditioned CG methods still perform well.

A discussion of parallel computing methods for the solution of biomedical field problems could fill an entire text. Thus, the reader is directed to the following references on parallel scientific computing [35–37].

23.4.6   Comparison of Methods

Since we do not have space to give a detailed, quantitative description of each of the aforementioned methods, we give an abbreviated summary of the applicability of each method in solving different types of bioelectric field problems.

As outlined above, the FD, FE, and BE methods can all be used to approximate the boundary value problems which arise in biomedical research problems. The choice depends on the nature of the problem. The FE and FD methods are similar in that the entire solution domain must be discretized, while with the BE method only the bounding surfaces must be discretized. For regular domains, the FD method is generally the easiest method to code and implement, but the FD method usually requires special modifications to define irregular boundaries, abrupt changes in material properties, and complex boundary conditions. While typically more difficult to implement, the BE and FE methods are preferred for problems with irregular, inhomogeneous domains, and mixed boundary conditions. The FE method is superior to the

---

[1] This is specifically for the FE method applied to elliptic problems. Such problems yield a matrix which is symmetric and positive definite. The Choleski decomposition only exists for symmetric, positive definite matrices.

BE method for representing nonlinearity and true anisotropy, while the BE method is superior to FE method for problems where only the boundary solution is of interest or where solutions are wanted in a set of highly irregularly spaced points in the domain. Because the computational mesh is simpler for the BE method than for the FE method, the BE program requires less book-keeping than a FE program. For this reason BE programs are often considered easier to develop than FE programs; however, the difficulties associated with singular integrals in the BE method are often highly underestimated. In general, the FE method is preferred for problems where the domain is highly heterogeneous, whereas the BE method is preferred for highly homogeneous domains.

23.5 Adaptive Methods

Thus far we have discussed how one formulates the problem, discretizes the geometry, and finds an approximate solution. We are now faced with answering the difficult question pertaining to the accuracy of our solution. Without reference to experimental data, how can we judge the validity of our solutions? To give yourself an intuitive feel for the problem (and possible solution), consider the approximation of a 2D region discretized into triangular elements. We will apply the FE method to solve Laplace's equation in the region.

First, consider the approximation of the potential field $\Phi(x, y)$ by a 2D Taylor's series expansion about a point (x, y):

$$\Phi(x + h, y + k) = \Phi(x, y) + \left[h \frac{\partial \Phi(x, y)}{\partial x} + k \frac{\partial \Phi(x, y)}{\partial y} \right]$$
$$+ \frac{1}{2!} \left[h^2 \frac{\partial^2 \Phi(x, y)}{\partial^2 x} + 2hk \frac{\partial^2 \Phi(x, y)}{\partial x \partial y} + k^2 \frac{\partial^2 \Phi(x, y)}{\partial^2 y} \right] + \cdots \qquad (23.57)$$

where h and k are the maximum x and y distances within an element. Using the first two terms (up to first-order terms) in the above Taylor's expansion, we can obtain the standard linear interpolation function for a triangle:

$$\frac{\partial \Phi(x_i, y_i)}{\partial x} = \frac{1}{2A} [\Phi_i(y_j - y_m) + \Phi_m(y_i - y_j) + \Phi_j(y_m - y_i)] \qquad (23.58)$$

where A is the area of the triangle. Likewise, one could calculate the interpolant for the other two nodes and discover that

$$\frac{\partial \Phi(x_i, y_i)}{\partial x} = \frac{\partial \Phi(x_j, y_j)}{\partial x} = \frac{\partial \Phi(x_m, y_m)}{\partial x} \qquad (23.59)$$

is constant over the triangle (and thus so is the gradient in y as well). Thus, we can derive the standard linear interpolation formulas on a triangle which represent the first two terms of the Taylor's series expansion. This means that the error due to discretization (from using linear elements) is proportional to the third term of the Taylor's expansion:

$$\epsilon \approx \frac{1}{2!} \left[h^2 \frac{\partial^2 \Phi(x, y)}{\partial^2 x} + 2hk \frac{\partial^2 \Phi(x, y)}{\partial x \partial y} + k^2 \frac{\partial^2 \Phi(x, y)}{\partial^2 y} \right] \qquad (23.60)$$

where Φ is the exact solution. We can conjecture, then, that the error due to discretization for first-order linear elements is proportional to the second derivative. If Φ is a linear function over the element, then the first derivative is a constant and the second derivative is zero and there is no error due to discretization. This implies that the gradient must be constant over each element. If the function is not linear, or the gradient is not constant over an element, the second derivative will not be zero and is proportional to the error incurred due to "improper" discretization. Examining Equation 23.60 we can easily see that one way to decrease the error is to decrease the size of h and k. As h and k go to zero, the error tends to zero as well. Thus, decreasing the mesh size in places of high errors due to high gradients decreases the error. Besides, we note that if one divides Equation 23.9 by h/k, one can also express the error in terms of the elemental aspect ratio h/k, which is a measure of the relative shape of the element. It is easy to see that one must be careful to maintain an aspect ratio as close as possible to unity.

The problem with the preceding heuristic argument is that one has to know the exact solution a priori before one can estimate the error. This is certainly a drawback considering the fact that we are trying to accurately approximate Φ.

23.5.1 Convergence of a Sequence of Approximate Solutions

Let us try to quantitfy our error a bit further. When we consider the preceding example, it seems to make sense that if we increase the number of degrees of freedom (DOF) we used to approximate our function, the accuracy must approach the true solution. That is, we would hope that the sequence of approximate solutions will *converge* to the exact solution as the number of DOF increases indefinitely:

$$\|\Phi(x) - \tilde{\Phi}_n(x)\| \to 0 \quad \text{as } N \to \infty \tag{23.61}$$

This is a statement of *pointwise convergence*. It describes the approximate solution as approaching arbitrarily close to the exact solution at each point in the domain as the number of DOF increases.

Measures of convergence often depend on how the *closeness* of measuring the distance between functions is defined. Another common description of measuring convergence is *uniform convergence*, which requires that the maximum value of $\|\Phi(x) - \tilde{\Phi}_n(x)\|$ in the domain vanish as $N \to \infty$. This is stronger than pointwise convergence as it requires a uniform rate of convergence at every point in the domain. Two other commonly used measures are *convergence in energy* and *convergence in mean*, which involve measuring an *average* of a function of the pointwise error over the domain [38].

In general, proving pointwise convergence is very difficult except in the simplest cases, while proving the convergence of an averged value, such as energy, is often easier. Of course, scientists and engineers are often much more interested in assuring that their answers are accurate in a pointwise sense than in an energy sense because they typically want to know values of the solution $\Phi(x)$ and gradients, $\nabla\Phi(x)$ at specific places.

One intermediate form of convergence is called the *Cauchy convergence*. Here, we require the sequences of two different approximate solutions to approach arbitrarily close to each other:

$$\|\Phi_m(x) - \tilde{\Phi}_n(x)\| \to 0 \quad \text{as } M, N \to \infty \tag{23.62}$$

While the pointwise convergence expression would imply the previous equation, it is important to note that the Cauchy convergence does not imply pointwise convergence, as the functions could converge to an answer other than the true solution.

While we cannot be assured pointwise convergence of these functions for all but the simplest cases, there do exist theorems that ensure that a sequence of approximate solutions must converge to the exact solution (assuming no computational errors) if the basis functions satisfy certain conditions. The theorems can only ensure convergence in an average sense over the entire domain, but it is usually the case that if the solution converges in an averge sense (energy, etc.), then it will converge in the pointwise sense as well.

23.5.1.1 Energy Norms

The error in energy, measured by the *energy norm*, is defined in general as [39–41]

$$\|e\| = \left(\int_\Omega e^T L e \, d\Omega \right)^{1/2} \tag{23.63}$$

where $e = \Phi(x) - \tilde{\Phi}_n(x)$ and L is the differential operator for the governing differential equation (i.e., it contains the derivatives operating on $\Phi(x)$ and any function multiplying $\Phi(x)$). For physical problems this is often associated with the energy density.

Another common measure of convergence utilizes the L_2 norm. This can be termed the average error and can be associated with errors in any quantity. The L_2 norm is defined as

$$\|e\|_{L_2} = \left(\int_{\Omega} e^T e \, d\Omega \right)^{1/2} \tag{23.64}$$

While the norms given above are defined on the whole domain, one can note that the square of each can be obtained by summing element contributions,

$$\|e\|^2 = \sum_{i=1}^{M} \|e\|_i^2 \tag{23.65}$$

where i represents an element contribution and m the total element number. Often for an *optimal* finite element mesh, one tries to make the contributions to this square of the norm equal for all elements.

While the absolute values given by the energy or L_2 norms have little value, one can construct a relative percentage error that can be more readily interpreted:

$$\eta = \frac{\|e\|}{\|\Phi\|} \times 100 \tag{23.66}$$

This quantity, in effect, represents a weighted RMS error. The analysis can be determined for the whole domain or for element subdomains. One can use it in an adaptive algorithm by checking element errors against some predefined tolerance, η_0, and increasing the DOF only of those areas above the predefined tolerance.

Two other methods, the p and the hp methods, have been found, in most cases, to converge faster than the h method. The p method of refinement requires that one increase the order of the basis function that was used to represent the interpolation (i.e., linear to quadratic to cubic, etc.). The hp method is a combination of the h and p methods and has recently been shown to converge the fastest of the three methods (but, as you might imagine, it is the hardest to implement). To find out more about adaptive refinement methods, see References 23, 26, 37, 38, and 41–43.

23.6 Software for Bioelectric Field Problems

23.6.1 SCIRun

In the past few years, there have been a number of research software systems that have been created for the computational study of biomedical problems, including bioelectric field problems. These include ECGSIM [45], EEGLAB [46], BrainStorm [47], CardioWave[48], SCIRun [49], and BioPSE [50].

In this section, I give a brief overview of the SCIRun and BioPSE problem-solving environments and give examples of their use for the solution of bioelectric field problems.

The SCIRun[2] software system is an integrated, extensible, visualization-driven, open source, problem solving environment that has been developed at the University of Utah's Scientific Computing and Imaging Institute [51].

---

[2] SCIRun is pronounced "ski-run" and derives its name from the Scientific Computing and Imaging (SCI) Institute, which is pronounced "ski" as in "Ski Utah."

For an application developer, SCIRun provides a software platform, upon which other applications can be rapidly constructed. SCIRun provides native support for interprocess communication, resource management (e.g., thread migration, memory management), and parallel computing. These operating system type services enable the dataflow aspects of the system. In addition to these low-level services, SCIRun also provides a number of built-in libraries and data structures that developers can use and can build upon. And at the highest level, SCIRun provides a rich set of algorithms for modeling, simulation, and visualization. All of these levels of functionality can be leveraged by the developer when constructing new algorithms or applications in SCIRun [49].

The application program interface (API) to SCIRun is the visual dataflow environment called the network editor. Within the network editor, programs can be visually assembled from the library of available algorithms. The dataflow network for a sample bioelectric field simulation is shown in Figure 23.1.

The boxes in the network are called *modules*, and the lines connecting them are called *datapipes*. The point of attachment, where a datapipe attaches to a module, is called a *dataport*; the dataports on the tops of the modules are input ports, and the ports on the bottoms of the modules are output ports. In SCIRun, the dataports are color-coded to indicate the type of the data. For example, the blue datapipes are for Matrices, and the yellow datapipes are for Fields. Fields are used to represent 3D geometry, as well as the data values that are defined over that geometry. Taken as a whole, the collection of modules and datapipes in a dataflow application is called a *network*, or *net*. Each module can have an optional user-interface (UI) button on its module; if the user presses the UI button, a separate window appears, with controls for viewing and modifying the state of the module's parameters.

23.6.2 BioPSE

SCIRun comes with a set of general purpose modules that are not specific to any particular application. Modules can also be generated for a specific application, or for adding a set of optional functionality (such as raster data processing), in which case they are organized into a *package*. The package that has been primarily used and extended in this work is called BioPSE [50]. BioPSE stands for biomedical problem solving environment, and contains all of the functionality that is specific to bioelectric field problems.

The example network in Figure 23.1, is solving a bioelectric field problem for a dipolar source in a volume conductor model of a head. The domain is discretized with linear tetrahedral finite elements, with five different conductivity types assigned through the volume. The problem is numerically approximated with a linear system, and is solved using the CG method. A set of virtual electrode points are rendered as pseudocolored spheres, to visualize the potentials at those locations on the scalp, and an iso-potential surface and several pseudocolored electric field streamlines are also shown.

The BioPSE network implements this simulation and visualization with a collection of interconnected modules. The tetrahedral finite element mesh with conductivity values is read in with one of the FieldReaders. That Field is then passed into the SetupFEMatrix module, which produces a stiffness matrix, $\mathbf{A}$, as output. The RHS of the linear system, $\mathbf{b}$, is generated by the ApplyFEMCurrentSource module, which applies the dipole source as a boundary condition. The linear system $\mathbf{A\Phi} = \mathbf{b}$ is then solved by the SolveMatrix module to recover the potentials at all of the nodes in the domain. This solution is then attached to the geometry with the ManageFieldData module, and the results are visualized. A complete description of this application is available in the tutorial section of the SCIRun User's Guide, and can be downloaded from the SCI Institute's website [52].

In addition to the BioPSE modules that appear in the above net, BioPSE also contains modules for generating and using finite element lead fields, for constructing separating surfaces from segmented volumes or planar contours, for running BEM simulations, and for visualizing lead potentials over time.

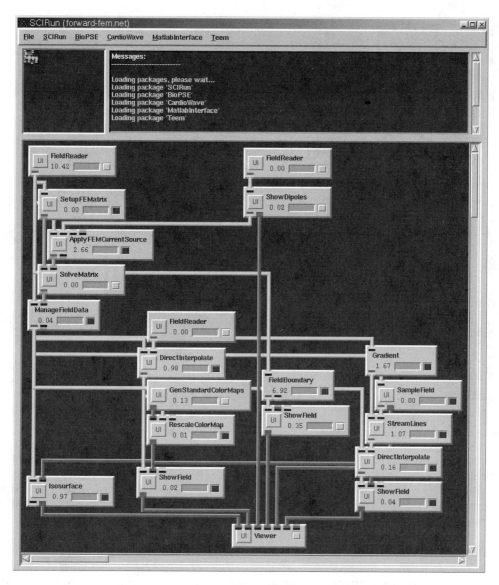

FIGURE 23.1   (See color insert following page **32**-14.) BioPSE dataflow network for modeling, simulating, and visualizing the bioelectric field generated in a realistic head model, due to a single dipole source.

23.6.3   PowerApps

Historically, one of the major hurdles to SCIRun becoming a tool for the scientist as well as the engineer has been SCIRun's dataflow interface. While visual programming is natural for computer scientists and engineers, who are accustomed to writing software and building algorithmic pipelines, it is overly cumbersome for application scientists. Even when a dataflow network implements a specific application (such as the forward bioelectric field simulation network provided with BioPSE and detailed in the BioPSE Tutorial), the UI components of the network are presented to the user in separate UI windows, without any semantic context for their settings. For example, SCIRun provides file browser UIs for reading in data. However, on the dataflow network all of the file browsers have the same generic presentation. Historically, there has not been a way to present the filename entries in their semantic context, for example to indicate that one entry should identify the electrodes input file and another should identify the finite element mesh file.

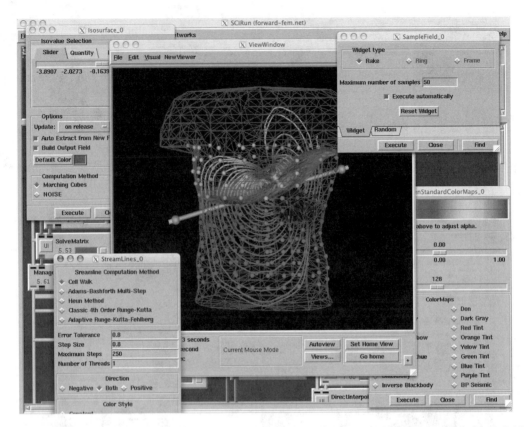

FIGURE 23.2   (See color insert following page **32**-14.) BioPSE dataflow interface to the forward bioelectric field application. The underlying dataflow network implements the application with modular interconnected components called modules. Data are passed between the modules as input and output parameters to the algorithms. While this is a useful interface for prototyping, it is nonintuitive for end-users; it is confusing to have a separate UI window to control the settings for each module. Moreover, the entries in the UI windows fail to provide semantic context for their settings. For example, the text-entry field on the SampleField UI that is labeled "Maximum number of samples" is controlling the number of electric field streamlines that are produced for the visualization.

While this interface shortcoming has long been identified, it has only recently been addressed. With the 1.20 release of BioPSE/SCIRun (in October 2003), we introduced *PowerApps*. A PowerApp is a customized interface built atop a dataflow application network. The dataflow network controls the execution and synchronization of the modules that comprise the application, but the generic UI windows are replaced with entries that are placed in the context of a single application-specific interface window.

With the 1.20 release of BioPSE, we released a PowerApp called BioFEM. BioFEM has been built atop the dataflow network shown in Figure 23.1, and provides a useful example for demonstrating the differences between the dataflow and PowerApp views of the same functionality. In Figure 23.2, the dataflow version of the application is shown: the user has separate interface windows for controlling different aspects of the simulation and visualization. In contrast, the PowerApp version is shown in Figure 23.3: here, the application has been wrapped up into a single interface window, with logically arranged and semantically labeled UI elements composed within panels and notetabs.

In addition to bioelectric field problems, the BioPSE system can also be used to investigate other biomedical applications. For example, we have wrapped the tensor and raster data processing functionality of the Teem toolkit into the Teem package of BioPSE, and we have used that increased functionality to develop the BioTensor PowerApp, as seen in Figure 23.4. BioTensor presents a customized interface to a 140-module dataflow network. With BioTensor the user can visualize diffusion weighted imaging (DWI) datasets in order to investigate the anisotropic structure of biological tissues. The application supports

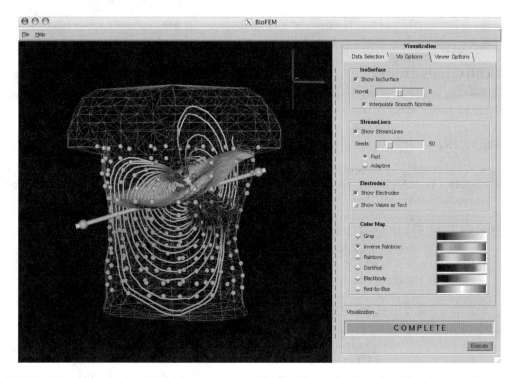

FIGURE 23.3 (See color insert following page **32**-14.) The BioFEM custom interface. Though the application is functionality equivalent to the dataflow version shown in Figure 23.1 and Figure 23.2, this PowerApp version provides an easier-to-use custom interface. Everything is contained within a single window; the user is lead through the steps of loading and visualizing the data with the tabs on the right; and generic control settings have been replaced with contextually appropriate labels; and application-specific tooltips (not shown) appear when the user places the cursor over any UI element.

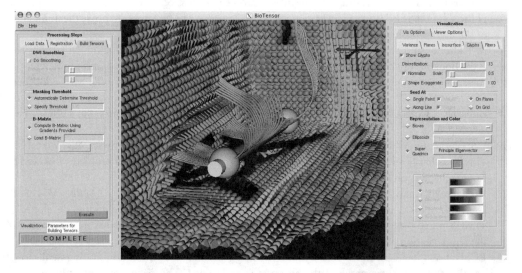

FIGURE 23.4 (See color insert following page **32**-14.) The BioTensor PowerApp. Just as with BioFEM, we have wrapped up a complicated dataflow network into a custom application. In the left panel, the user is guided through the stages of loading the data, co-registering the diffusion weighted images, and constructing diffusion tensors. On the right panel, the user has controls for setting the visualization options. In the rendering window in the middle, the user can render and interact with the dataset.

the import of DICOM and Analyze datasets, and implements the latest diffusion tensor visualization techniques, including superquadric glyphs [53] and tensorlines [54] (both shown).

Acknowledgments

This work was supported in part by awards from the NIH NCRR. I would like to thank David Weinstein for his contribution of the section on SCIRun and BioPSE.

References

[1] C.E. Miller and C.S. Henriquez. Finite element analysis of bioelectric phenomena. *Crit. Rev. Biomed. Eng.*, 18: 181–205, 1990. This represents the first review paper on the use of the finite element method as applied to biomedical problems. As the authors note, bioengineers came to these methods only fairly recently, as compared to other engineers. It contains a good survey of applications.

[2] J. Nenonen, H.M. Rajala, and T. Katilia. *Biomagnetic Localization and 3D Modelling*. Helsinki University of Technology, Espoo, Finland, 1992. Report TKK-F-A689.

[3] C.R. Johnson, R.S. MacLeod, and P.R. Ershler. A computer model for the study of electrical current flow in the human thorax. *Comp. Biol. Med.*, 22(3): 305–323, 1992. This paper details the construction of a three-dimensional thorax model.

[4] C.R. Johnson, R.S. MacLeod, and M.A. Matheson. Computer simulations reveal complexity of electrical activity in the human thorax. *Comp. Phys.*, 6(3): 230–237, May/June 1992. This paper deals with the computational and visualization aspects of the forward ECG problem.

[5] Y. Kim, J.B. Fahy, and B.J. Tupper. Optimal electrode designs for electrosurgery. *IEEE Trans. Biomed. Eng.*, 33:845–853, 1986. This paper discusses an example of the modeling of bioelectric fields for applications in surgery.

[6] F. Greensite, G. Huiskamp, and A. van Oosterom. New quantitative and qualitative approaches to the inverse problem of electrocardiology: their theoretical relationship and experimental consistency. *Med. Phys.*, 17(3): 369–379, 1990. This paper describes methods for constraining the inverse problem of electrocardiology in terms of sources. Methods are developed which put bounds on the space of acceptable solutions.

[7] Y. Yamashita. Theoretical studies on the inverse problem in electrocardiography and the uniqueness of the solution. *IEEE Trans. Biomed. Eng.*, 29: 719–725, 1982. The first paper to prove the uniqueness of the inverse problem in electrocardiography.

[8] A. Tikhonov and V. Arsenin. *Solution of Ill-Posed Problems*. Winston, Washington, DC, 1977. This is the book in which Tikhonov describes his method of regularization for ill-posed problems.

[9] A.N. Tikhonov and A.V. Goncharsky. *Ill-Posed Problems in the Natural Sciences*. MIR Publishers, Moscow, 1987. This is a collection of research papers from physics, geophysics, optics, medicine, etc., which describe ill-posed problems and the solution techniques the authors have developed.

[10] V.B. Glasko. *Inverse Problems of Mathematical Physics*. American Institute of Physics, New York, 1984. This book has several introductory chapters on the mathematics of ill-posed problems followed by several chapters on specific applications.

[11] P.C. Hansen. Analysis of discrete ill-posed problems by means of the L-curve. *SIAM Rev.*, 34(4):561–580, 1992. This is an excellent review paper which describes the various techniques developed to solve ill-posed problems. Special attention is paid to the selection of the a priori approximation of the regularization parameter.

[12] P.C. Hansen. Regularization tools: a matlab package for analysis and solution of discrete ill-posed problems. Available via netlib in the library numeralgo/no4. This is an excellent set of tools for experimenting with and analyzing discrete ill-posed problems. The netlib library contains several Matlab routines as well as a postscript version of the accompanying technical report/manual.

[13] O. Bertrand. 3d finite element method in brain electrical activity studies. In J. Nenonen, H.M. Rajala, and T. Katila (Eds.), *Biomagnetic Localization and 3D Modeling*, pp. 154–171. Helsinki University of

Technology, Helsinki, 1991. This paper describes the inverse MEG problem using the finite element method.

[14] C.B. Barber, D.P. Dobkin, and H. Huhdanpaa. The quickhull algorithm for convex hull. Geometry Center Technical Report GCG53. A public domain two- and three-dimensional Delaunay mesh generation code. Available via anonymous ftp from: geom.umn.edu:/pub/software/qhull.tar.Z. There is also a geometry viewer available from geom.umn.edu:/pub/software/geomview/geomview-sgi.tar.Z.

[15] A. Bowyer. Computing Dirichlet tesselations. *Comp. J.*, 24: 162–166, 1981. One of the first papers on the Delaunay triangulation in 3-space.

[16] S.R.H. Hoole. *Computer-Aided Analysis and Design of Electromagnetic Devices.* Elsevier, New York, 1989. While the title wouldn't make you think so, this is an excellent introductory text on the use of numerical techniques to solve boundary value problems in electrodynamics. The text also contains sections on mesh generation and solution methods. Furthermore, it provides pseudocode for most of the algorithms discussed throughout the text.

[17] R.S. MacLeod, C.R. Johnson, and M.A. Matheson. Visualization tools for computational electrocardiography. In Richard Robb (Ed.), *Visualization in Biomedical Computing*, pp. 433–444, 1992. This paper, and the paper which follows, concern the modeling and visualization aspects of bioelectric field problems.

[18] R.S. MacLeod, C.R. Johnson, and M.A. Matheson. Visualization of cardiac bioelectricity — a case study. In Arie E. Kaufman and Gregory M. Nielson (Eds.), *IEEE Visualization 92*, pp. 411–418, 1992. See previous comment.

[19] T.C. Pilkington, B. Loftis, J.F. Thompson, S.L-Y. Woo, T.C. Palmer, and T.F. Budinger. *High-Performance Computing in Biomedical Research.* CRC Press, Boca Raton, FL, 1993. This edited collection of papers gives an overview of the state of the art in high performance computing (as of 1993) as it pertains to biomedical research. While certainly not comprehensive, the text does showcase several interesting applications and methods.

[20] J. Thompson and N.P. Weatherill. Structed and unstructed grid generation. In T.C. Pilkington, B. Loftis, J.F. Thompson, S.L-Y. Woo, T.C. Palmer, and T.F. Budinger (Eds.), *High-Performance Computing in Biomedical Research*, pp. 63–112. CRC Press, Boca Raton, FL, 1993. This paper contains some extensions of Thompson's classic textbook on numerical grid generation.

[21] P.L. George. *Automatic Mesh Generation.* Wiley, New York, 1991. This is an excellent introduction to mesh generation. It contains a survey of all the major mesh generation schemes.

[22] J.F. Thompson, Z.U.A. Warsi, and C.W. Mastin. *Numerical Grid Generation.* North-Holland, New York, 1985. This is the classic on mesh generation. The mathematical level is higher than that of George's book, and most of the applications are directed toward computational fluid dynamics.

[23] J.A. Schmidt, C.R. Johnson, J.A. Eason, and R.S. MacLeod. Applications of automatic mesh generation and adaptive methods in computational medicine. In I. Babuska, J. Flaherty, J. Hopcroft, W. Henshaw, J. Olinger, and T. Tezduyar (Eds.), *Modeling, Mesh Generation, and Adaptive Methods for Partial Differential Equations.* Springer-Verlag, pp. 367–394, 1995.

[24] C.S. Henriquez, C.R. Johnson, K.A. Henneberg, L.J. Leon, and A.E. Pollard. Large scale biomedical modeling and simulation: from concept to results. Scientific computing and imaging technical report, Number UUSCI-1995-001, pp. 1–42, University of Utah, 1995. Available from the SCI Institute, web site: www.sci.utah.edu/publications.

[25] J.E. Akin. *Finite Element Analysis for Undergraduates.* Academic Press, New York, 1986. This is an easy to read, self contained text on the finite element method aimed at undergraduate engineering students.

[26] C. Johnson. *Numerical solution of Partial Differential Equations by the Finite Element Method.* Cambridge University Press, Cambridge, 1990. An excellent introductory book on the finite element method. The text assumes mathematical background of first year graduate students in applied mathematics and computer science. An excellent introduction to the theory of adaptive methods.

[27] J.D. Jackson. Classical Electrodynamics. John Wiley, New York, 1973.

[28] C.A. Brebbia and J. Dominguez. *Boundary Elements: An Introductory Course.* McGraw-Hill, Boston, MA, 1989. This is an introductory book on the boundary element method by one of the foremost experts on the subject (C.A.B.).

[29] M.A. Jawson and G.T. Symm. *Integral Equation Methods in Potential Theory and Elastostatics.* Academic Press, London, 1977. An introduction to the boundary integral method as applied to potential theory and elastostatics.

[30] G. Beer and J.O. Watson. *Introduction to Finite and Boundary Element Methods for Engineers.* Wiley, New York, 1992. This is an excellent first book for those wishing to learn about the practical aspects of the numerical solution of boundary value problems. The book covers not only finite and boundary element methods, but also sections on mesh generation and the solution of large systems.

[31] R.C. Barr, T.C. Pilkington, J.P. Boineau, and M.S. Spach. Determining surface potentials from current dipoles, with application to electrocardiography. *IEEE Trans. Biomed. Eng.*, 13: 88–92, 1966. This is the first paper on the application of the boundary element method to problems in electrocardiography.

[32] R. Plonsey. *Bioelectric Phenomena.* McGraw-Hill, New York, 1969. This is the first text using physics, mathematics, and engineering principles to quantify bioelectric phenomena.

[33] Y. Rudy and B.J. Messinger-Rapport. The inverse solution in electrocardiography: solutions in terms of epicardial potentials. *CRC Crit. Rev. Biomed. Eng.*, 16: 215–268, 1988. An excellent overview on the inverse problem in electrocardiography as well as a section on the application of the boundary element method to bioelectric field problems.

[34] R.M Gulrajani, F.A. Roberge, and G.E. Mailloux. The forward problem of electrocardiography. In P.W. Macfarlane and T.D. Lawrie (Eds.), *Comprehensive Electrocardiology*, pp. 197–236. Pergamon Press, Oxford, England, 1989. This contains a nice overview of the application of the boundary element method to the direct ECG problem.

[35] G. Golub and J.M. Ortega. *Scientific Computing: An Introduction with Parallel Computing.* Academic Press, New York, 1993. An excellent introduction to scientific computing with sections on sequential and parallel direct and iterative solvers, inlcuding a short section on the multigrid method.

[36] T.L. Freeman and C. Phillips. *Parallel Numerical Algorithms.* Prentice Hall, New York, 1992. A good introduction to parallel algorithms with emphasis on the use of BLAS subroutines.

[37] E.F. Van de Velde. *Concurrent Scientific Computing.* Springer-Verlag, New York, 1994. This text contains an excellent introduction to parallel numerical algorithms including sections on the finite difference and finite element methods.

[38] D.S. Burnett. *Finite Element Method.* Addison Wesley, Reading, MA, 1988. This is an excellent introduction to the finite element method. It covers all the basics and introduces more advanced concepts in a readily understandable context.

[39] O.C. Zienkiewicz. *The Finite Element Method in Engineering Science.* McGraw-Hill, New York, 1971. This is a classic text on the finite element method. It is now in its fourth edition, 1991.

[40] O.C. Zienkiewicz and J.Z. Zhu. A simple error estimate and adaptive procedure for practical engineering analysis. *Int. J. Num. Meth. Eng.*, 24: 337–357, 1987. This is a classic paper which describes the use of the energy norm to globally refine the mesh based upon a priori error estimates.

[41] O.C. Zienkiewicz and J.Z. Zhu. Adaptivity and mesh generation. *Int. J. Num. Meth. Eng.*, 32: 783–810, 1991. This is another good paper on adaptive methods which describes some more advanced methods than their 1987 paper.

[42] C.R. Johnson and R.S. MacLeod. Nonuniform spatial mesh adaption using a posteriori error estimates: applications to forward and inverse problems. *Appl. Numer. Math.*, 14: 331–326, 1994. This is a paper by the author which describes the application of the h-method of mesh refinement for large scale two- and three-dimensional bioelectric field problems.

[43] J.E. Flaherty. *Adaptive Methods for Partial Differential Equations.* SIAM, Philadelphia, PA, 1989. This is a collection of papers on adaptive methods, many by the founders in the field. Most of the

papers are applied to adaptive methods for finite element methods and deal with both theory and applications.

[44] M. Ainsworth. *A Posteriori Error Estimation in Finite Element Analysis*. Wiley-Interscience, 2000.

[45] A. van Oosterom and T. Oostendorp. ECGSIM; an interactive tool for studying the genesis of QRST waveforms. *Heart*, 90: 165–168, 2004.

[46] A. Delorme and S. Makeig. EEGLAB: an open source toolbox for analysis of single-trial dynamics including independent component analysis. *J. Neurosci. Meth.*, 134: 9–21, 2004.

[47] S. Baillet, J.C. Mosher, R.M. Leahy, and D.W. Shattuck. BrainStorm: a Matlab toolbox for the processing of MEG and EEG signals. *Proceedings of the 5th International Conference on Human Brain Mapping, NeuroImage*, 9(6): S246, June 1999.

[48] John B. Pormann. A modular simulation system for the bidomain equations. PhD Thesis, Duke University, January 1999.

[49] S.G. Parker, D.M. Weinstein, and C.R. Johnson. The SCIRun computational steering software system. In E. Arge, A.M. Bruaset, and H.P. Langtangen (Eds.), *Modern Software Tools in Scientific Computing*, pp. 1–40. Birkhäuser Press, Boston, 1997.

[50] BioPSE: Biomedical Problem Solving Environment for modeling, simulation, and visualization. Scientific Computing and Imaging Institute (SCI), http://software.sci.utah.edu/biopse.html, 2002.

[51] S.G. Parker. The SCIRun Problem Solving Environment and Computational Steering Software System, University of Utah, 1999.

[52] Scientific Computing and Imaging Institute, University of Utah, http://www.sci.utah.edu.

[53] G. Kindlmann. Superquadric tensor glyphs. In *Proceedings of IEEE TVCG/EG Symposium on Visualization*, pp. 147–154, 2004.

[54] D.M. Weinstein, G. Kindlmann, and E. Lundberg. Tensorlines: advection-diffusion based propagation through diffusion tensor fields. In *Proceedings of IEEE Visualization*, pp. 249–253, IEEE Press, New York, 1999.

[55] C.S. Henriquez and R. Plonsey. Simulation of propagation along a bundle of cardiac tissue. I. Mathematical formulation. *IEEE Trans. Biomed. Eng.*, 37: 850–860, 1990. This paper and the companion paper below, describe the bidomain approach to the propagation of electrical signals through active cardiac tissue.

[56] C.S. Henriquez and R. Plonsey. Simulation of propagation along a bundle of cardiac tissue. II. Results of simulation. *IEEE Trans. Biomed. Eng.*, 37: 861–887, 1990.

[57] J.P. Keener. Waves in excitable media. *SIAM J. Appl. Math.*, 46: 1039–1056, 1980. This paper describes mathematical models for wave propagation in various excitable media. Both chemical and physiological systems are addressed.

[58] J. Hadamard. Sur les problemes aux derivees parielies et leur signification physique. *Bull. Univ. Princeton*, 49–52, 1902. This is Hadamard's original paper describing the concepts of well- and ill-posedness. In French.

[59] G.H. Golub and C.F. Van Loan. *Matrix Computations*. Johns Hopkins, Baltimore, MD, 1989. This is a classic reference for matrix computations and is highly recommended.

24

Principles of Electrocardiography

Edward J. Berbari
Indiana University-Purdue University

24.1 Introduction

The electrocardiogram (ECG) is the recording on the body surface of the electrical activity generated by the heart. It was originally observed by Waller in 1889 [1] using his pet bulldog as the signal source and the capillary electrometer as the recording device. In 1903 Einthoven [2] enhanced the technology by using the string galvanometer as the recording device and using human subjects with a variety of cardiac abnormalities. Einthoven is chiefly responsible for introducing some concepts still in use today including the labeling of the various waves, defining some of the standard recording sites using the arms and legs, and developing the first theoretical construct whereby the heart is modeled as a single time-varying dipole. We also owe the "EKG" acronym to Einthoven's native Dutch language where the root word "cardio" is spelled with a "k."

In order to record an ECG waveform, a differential recording between two points on the body are made. Traditionally each differential recording is referred to as a lead. Einthoven defined three leads numbered with the Roman numerals I, II, and III. They are defined as:

$$I = V_{\text{LA}} - V_{\text{RA}}$$

$$II = V_{\text{LL}} - V_{\text{RA}}$$

$$III = V_{\text{LL}} - V_{LA}$$

where RA = right arm, LA = left arm, LL = left leg. Because the body is assumed to be purely resistive, at ECG frequencies, the four limbs can be thought of as wires attached to the torso. Hence, lead I could be recorded from the respective shoulders without a loss of cardiac information. Note that these are not independent and the following relationship II = I + III holds.

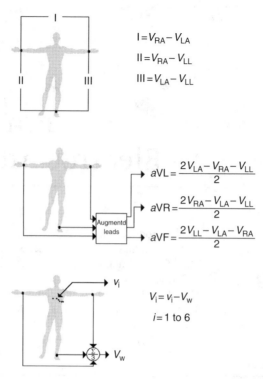

$$I = V_{RA} - V_{LA}$$
$$II = V_{RA} - V_{LL}$$
$$III = V_{LA} - V_{LL}$$

$$aVL = \frac{2V_{LA} - V_{RA} - V_{LL}}{2}$$
$$aVR = \frac{2V_{RA} - V_{LA} - V_{LL}}{2}$$
$$aVF = \frac{2V_{LL} - V_{LA} - V_{RA}}{2}$$

$$V_i = v_i - V_w$$
$$i = 1 \text{ to } 6$$

FIGURE 24.1   The 12-lead ECG is formed by the three bipolar surface leads: I, II, and III; the augmented Wilson terminal referenced limb leads: aVR, aVL, aVF; and the Wilson terminal referenced chest leads: V_1, V_2, V_3, V_4, V_5, and V_6.

For 30 years the evolution of the ECG proceeded when F.N. Wilson [3] added concepts of a "unipolar" recording. He created a reference point by tying the three limbs together and averaging their potentials so that individual recording sites on the limbs or chest surface would be differentially recorded with the same reference point. Wilson extended the biophysical models to include the concept of the cardiac source enclosed within the volume conductor of the body. He erroneously thought that the central terminal was a true zero potential. However, from the mid-1930s until today the 12 leads composed of the 3 limb leads, 3 leads in which the limb potentials are referenced to a modified Wilson terminal (the augmented leads [4]), and 6 leads placed across the front of the chest and referenced to the Wilson terminal form the basis of the standard 12-lead ECG. Figure 24.1 summarizes the 12-lead set. These sites are historically based, have a built in redundancy, and are not optimal for all cardiac events. The voltage difference from any two sites will record an ECG, but it is these standardized sites with the massive 90-year collection of empirical observations that has firmly established their role as the standard. Figure 24.2 is a typical or stylized ECG recording from lead II. Einthoven chose the letters of the alphabet from P–U to label the waves and to avoid conflict with other physiologic waves being studied at the turn of the century. The ECG signals are typically in the range of ∀2 mV and require a recording bandwidth of 0.05 to 150 Hz. Full technical specification for ECG equipment has been proposed by both the American Heart Association [5] and the Association for the Advancement of Medical Instrumentation [6].

There have been several attempts to change the approach for recording the ECG. The vectorcardiogram used a weighted set of recording sites to form an orthogonal *XYZ* lead set. The advantage here was minimum lead set but in practice it gained only a moderate degree of enthusiasm among physicians. Body surface mapping refers to the use of many recording sites (>64) arranged on the body so that isopotential surfaces could be computed and analyzed over time. This approach still has a role in research investigations. Other subsets of the 12-lead ECG are used in limited mode recording situations such as the tape-recorded ambulatory ECG (usually 2 leads) or in intensive care monitoring at the bedside

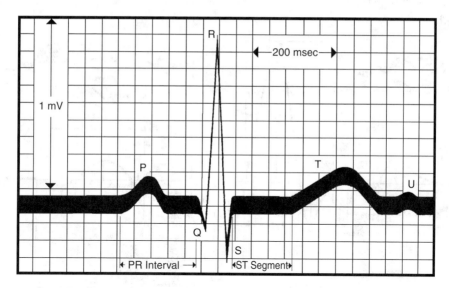

FIGURE 24.2 This is a stylized version of a normal lead II recording showing the P wave, QRS complex, and the T and U waves. The PR interval and the ST segment are significant time windows. The peak amplitude of the QRS is about 1 mV. The vertical scale is usually 1 mV/cm. The time scale is usually based on millimeter per second scales with 25 mm/sec being the standard form. The small boxes of the ECG are 1×1 mm^2.

(usually 1 or 2 leads) or telemetered within regions of the hospital from patients who are not confined to bed (1 lead). The recording electronics of these ECG systems have followed the typical evolution of modern instrumentation, for example, vacuum tubes, transistors, ICs, and microprocessors.

Application of computers to the ECG for machine interpretation was one of the earliest uses of computers in medicine [7]. Of primary interest in the computer-based systems was the replacement of the human reader and the elucidation of the standard waves and intervals. Originally this was performed by linking the ECG machine to a centralized computer via phone lines. The modern ECG machine is completely integrated with an analog front end, a 12–16 bit A/D converter, a computational microprocessor, and dedicated I/O processors. These systems compute a measurement matrix derived from the 12-lead signals and analyze this matrix with a set of rules to obtain the final set of interpretive statements [8]. Figure 24.3 shows the ECG of a heartbeat and the types of measurements that might be made on each of the component waves of the ECG and used for classifying each beat type and the subsequent cardiac rhythm. The depiction of the 12 analog signals and this set of interpretive statements form the final output with an example shown in Figure 24.4. The physician will over-read each ECG and modify or correct those statements that are deemed inappropriate. The larger hospital-based system will record these corrections and maintain a large database of all ECGs accessible by any combination of parameters, for example, all males, older than 50, with an inferior myocardial infarction.

There are hundreds of interpretive statements from which a specific diagnosis is made for each ECG, but there are only about five or six major classification groups for which the ECG is used. The first step in analyzing an ECG requires the determination of the rate and rhythm for the atria and ventricles. Included here would be any conduction disturbances either in the relationship between the various chambers or within the chambers themselves. Then one would proceed to identify features that would relate to the presence or absence of scarring due to a myocardial infarction. There may also be evidence of acute events occurring that would occur with ischemia or an evolving myocardial infarction. The ECG has been a primary tool for evaluating chamber size or enlargement, but one might argue that more accurate information in this area would be supplied by noninvasive imaging technologies.

More recently the high resolution ECG has been developed whereby the digitized ECG is signal averaged to reduce random noise [9,10]. This approach, coupled with postaveraging high-pass filtering, is used to

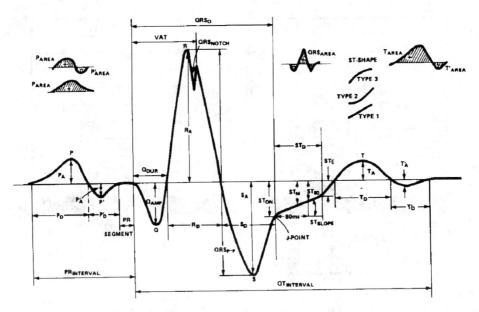

FIGURE 24.3 The ECG depicts numerous measurements that can be made with computer-based algorithms. These are primarily durations, amplitudes, and areas. (This figure is courtesy of the Hewlett Packard Co., Palo Alto, CA.)

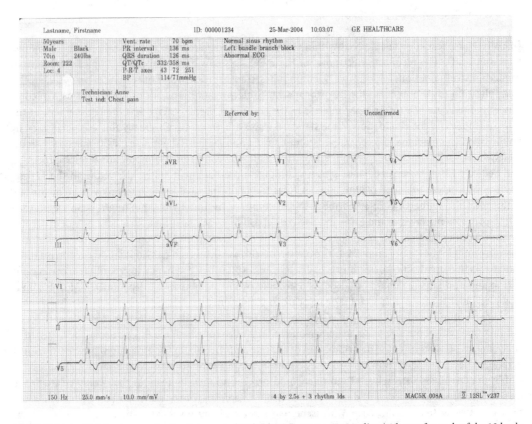

FIGURE 24.4 This is an example of an interpreted 12 lead ECG. A 2.5 sec recording is shown for each of the 12 leads. The bottom trace is a continuous 10 sec rhythm strip of lead II. Patient information is given in the top area, below which is printed the computerized interpretive statements. (Diagram is courtesy of GE Healthcare Technologies, Waukesha, WI.)

detect and quantify low-level signals (1.0 μV) not detectable with standard approaches. This computer-based approach has enabled the recording of events which are predictive of future life-threatening cardiac events [11,12].

24.2 Physiology

The heart has four chambers, the upper two chambers are called the atria and the lower two chambers are called the ventricles. The atria are thin-walled, low-pressure pumps that receive blood from venous circulation. Located in the top right atrium are a group of cells which act as the primary pacemaker of the heart. Through a complex change of ionic concentration across the cell membranes (the current source) an extracellular potential field is established which then excites neighboring cells and a cell-to-cell propagation of electrical events occur. Because the body acts as a purely resistive medium these potential fields extend to the body surface [13]. The character of the body surface waves depends upon the amount of tissue activating at one time and the relative speed and direction of the activation wave front. Therefore the pacemaker potentials which are generated by a small tissue mass are not seen on the ECG. As the activation wave front encounters the increased mass of atrial muscle, the initiation of electrical activity is observed on the body surface and the first ECG wave of the cardiac cycle is seen. This is the P wave and it represents activation of the atria. Conduction of the cardiac impulse proceeds from the atria through a series of specialized cardiac cells (the A–V node and the His–Purkinje system), which again are too small in total mass to generate a signal large enough to be seen on the standard ECG. There is a short relatively isoelectric segment following the P wave. Once the large muscle mass of the ventricles is excited, a rapid and large deflection is seen on the body surface. The excitation of the ventricles causes them to contract and provides the main force for circulating blood to the organs of the body. This large wave appears to have several components. The initial downward deflection is called the Q wave, the initial upward deflection is the R wave, and the terminal downward deflection is the S wave. The polarity and actual presence of these three components depends upon the position of the leads on the body as well as a multitude of abnormalities that may exist. In general the large ventricular waveform is generically called the QRS complex regardless of its makeup. Following the QRS complex is another relatively short isoelectric segment. After this short segment the ventricles return to their electrical resting state and a wave of repolarization is seen as a low-frequency signal called the T wave. In some individuals a small peak occurs at the end or after the T wave and is called the U wave. Its origin has never been fully established but is believed to be a repolarization potential.

24.3 Instrumentation

The general instrumentation requirements for the ECG have been addressed by professional societies through the years [5,6]. Briefly they recommend a system bandwidth between 0.05 and 150 Hz. Of great importance in ECG diagnosis is the low-frequency response of the system because shifts in some of the low-frequency regions, for example, the ST segment, have critical diagnostic value. While the heart rate may only have a 1 Hz fundamental frequency, the phase response of typical analog high-pass filters are such that the system corner frequency must be much smaller than the 3 db corner frequency where only the amplitude response is considered. The system gain depends upon the total system design. The typical ECG amplitude is ± 2 mV and if A/D conversion is used in a digital system, then enough gain to span the only 20% of the A/D converter's dynamic range is needed. This margin allows for recording abnormally large signals as well as accommodating base line drift if present and not corrected.

To first obtain an ECG the patient must be physically connected to the amplifier front end. The patient/amplifier interface is formed by a special bioelectrode that converts the ionic current flow of the body to the electron flow of the metallic wire. These electrodes typically rely on a chemical paste or gel with a high ionic concentration. This acts as the transducer at the tissue–electrode interface. For short-term applications the use of silver-coated suction electrodes or "sticky" metallic foil electrodes are used. Long-term recordings, such as the case for the monitored patient, require a stable electrode/tissue interface and special adhesive tape material surrounds the gel and an Ag^+/Ag^+Cl electrode.

At any given time, the patient may be connected to a variety of devices, for example, respirator, blood pressure monitor, temporary pacemaker, etc., some of which will invade the body and provide a low resistance pathway to the heart. It is essential that the device not act as a current source and inject the patient with enough current to stimulate the heart and cause it to fibrillate. Some bias currents are unavoidable for the system input stage and recommendations are that these leakage currents be less than 10 μA per device. In recent years, there has been some controversy regarding the level of allowable leakage current. The Association for the Advancement of Medical Instrumentation [5] has written its standards to allow leakage currents as high as 50 μA. Recent studies [14,15] have shown that there may be complex and lethal physiological response to 60 Hz currents as low as 32 μA. In light of the reduced standards these research results were commented on by members of the American Heart Association Committee on Electrocardiography [16].

There is also 10 μA maximum current limitation due to a fault condition if a patient comes in contact with the high voltage side of the AC power lines. In this case the isolation must be adequate to prevent 10 μA of fault current as well. This mandates that the ECG reference ground not be connected physically to the low side of the AC power line or its third ground wire. For ECG machines the solution has typically been to AM modulate a medium-frequency carrier signal (400 kHz) and use an isolation transformer with subsequent demodulation. Other methods of signal isolation can be used but the primary reason for the isolation is to keep the patient from being part of the AC circuit in the case of a patient to power line fault. In addition, with many devices connected in a patient-monitoring situation it is possible that ground loop currents will be generated. To obviate this potential hazard a low-impedance ground buss is often installed in these rooms and each device chassis will have an external ground wire connected to the buss. Another unique feature of these amplifiers is that they must be able to withstand the high-energy discharge of a cardiac defibrillator.

Older-style ECG machines recorded one lead at a time, then evolved to three simultaneous leads. This necessitated the use of switching circuits as well as analog weighting circuits to generate the various 12 leads. This is usually eliminated in modern digital systems by using an individual single-ended amplifier for each electrode on the body. Each potential signal is then digitally converted and all of the ECG leads can be formed mathematically in software. This would necessitate a 9-amplifier system. By performing some of the lead calculations with the analog differential amplifiers this can be reduced to an 8-channel system. Thus only the individual chest leads V_1 through V_6 and any two of the limb leads, for example, I and III, are needed to calculate the full 12-lead ECG. Figure 24.5 is a block diagram of a modern digital-based ECG system. This system uses an amplifier per lead wire and a 16 bit A/D converter, all within a small lead wire manifold or amplifier lead stage. The digital signals are sent via a high-speed link to the main ECG instrument. Here the embedded microprocessors perform all of the calculations and a hard copy report is generated (Figure 24.4). Note that each functional block has its own controller and the system requires a sophisticated real-time operating system to coordinate all system functions. Concomitant with the data acquisition is the automatic interpretation of the ECG. These programs are quite sophisticated and are continually evolving. It is still a medical/legal requirement that these ECGs be over-read by the physician.

24.3.1 Applications

Besides the standard 12-lead ECG, there are several other uses of ECG recording technology which rely on only a few leads. These applications have had a significant clinical and commercial impact. Following are brief descriptions of several ECG applications that are aimed at introducing the reader to some of the many uses of the ECG.

24.3.1.1 The Ambulatory ECG

The evolution of the ambulatory or Holter ECG has an interesting history and its evolution closely followed both technical and clinical progress. The original, analog tape-based, portable ECG resembled

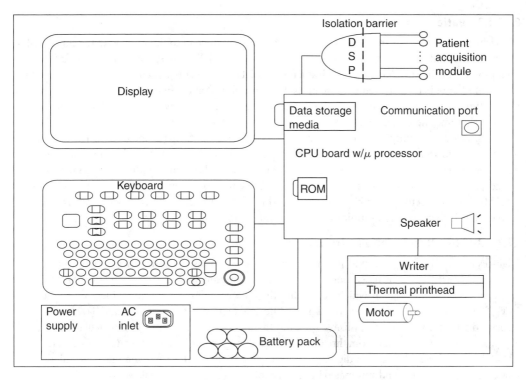

FIGURE 24.5 This is a block diagram of microprocessor-based ECG system. (Diagram is courtesy of GE Healthcare Technologies, Waukesha, WI.)

a fully loaded backpack and was developed by Dr. Holter in the early 1960s [17], but was soon followed by more compact devices that could be worn on the belt. The original large-scale clinical use of this technology was to identify patients who developed heart block transiently and could be treated by implanting a cardiac pacemaker. This required the secondary development of a device which could rapidly play back the 24 h of tape-recorded ECG signals and present to the technician or physician a means of identifying periods of time where the patient's heart rate became abnormally low. The scanners had the circuitry to not only playback the ECG at speeds 30 to 60 times real time, but to detect the beats and display them in a superimposed mode on a cathode ray tube (CRT) screen. In addition, an audible tachometer could be used to identify the periods of low heart rate. With this playback capability came numerous other observations such the identification of premature ventricular beats (PVBs) which lead to the development of techniques to identify and quantify their number. Together with the development of antiarrhythmic drugs a marriage was formed between pharmaceutical therapy and the diagnostic tool for quantifying PVBs. ECG tapes were recorded before and after drug administration and drug efficacy was measured by the reduction of the number of PVBs. The scanner technology for detecting and quantifying these arrhythmias was originally implemented with analog hardware but soon advanced to computer technology as it became economically feasible. Very sophisticated algorithms were developed based on pattern recognition techniques and were sometimes implemented with high-speed specialized numerical processors as the tape playback speeds became several hundred times real time [18]. Unfortunately this approach using the ambulatory ECG for identifying and treating cardiac arrhythmias has been on the decline as the rationale of PVC suppression was found to be unsuccessful for improving cardiac mortality. However, the ambulatory ECG is still a widely used diagnostic tool and modern units often have built-in microprocessors with considerable amounts (1.0 Gbyte) of random access memory. Here the data can be analyzed on line with large segments of data selected for storage and later analysis with personal computer-based programs.

24.3.1.2 Patient Monitoring

The techniques for monitoring the ECG in real time were developed in conjunction with the concept of the coronary care unit or CCU. Patients were placed in these specialized hospital units to carefully observe their progress during an acute illness such as a myocardial infarction or after complex surgical procedures. As the number of beds increased in these units it became clear that the highly trained medical staff could not continually watch a monitor screen and computerized techniques were added which monitored the patient's rhythm. These programs were not unlike those developed for the ambulatory ECG and the high-speed numerical capability of the computer was not taxed by monitoring a single ECG. The typical CCU would have 8 to 16 beds and hence the computing power was taken to its limit by monitoring multiple beds. The modern units have the central processing unit (CPU) distributed within the ECG module at the bedside, along with modules for measuring many other physiological parameters. Each bedside monitor would be interconnected with a high-speed digital line, for example, Ethernet, to a centralized computer used primarily to control communications and maintain a patient database.

24.3.1.3 High Resolution Electrocardiography

High-resolution (HR) capability is now a standard feature on most digitally based ECG systems, or as a stand-alone microprocessor based unit [19]. The most common application of the HRECG is to record very low level (1.0 μV) signals which occur after the QRS complex but are not evident on the standard ECG. These "late potentials" are generated from abnormal regions of the ventricles and have been strongly associated with the substrate responsible for a life-threatening rapid heart rate (ventricular tachycardia). The typical HRECG is derived from three bipolar leads configured in an anatomic XYZ coordinate system. These three ECG signals are then digitized at a rate of 1000 to 2000 Hz per channel, time aligned via a real-time QRS correlator, and summated in the form of a signal average. Signal averaging will theoretically improve the signal to noise ratio by the square root of the number of beats averaged. The underlying assumptions are that the signals of interest do not vary, on a beat-to-beat basis, and that the noise is random. Figure 24.6 has four panels depicting the most common sequence for processing the HRECG to measure the late potentials. Panel A depicts a 3 sec recording of the XYZ leads close to normal resolution. Panel B was obtained after averaging 200 beats and with a sampling frequency of ten times that shown in panel A. The gain is also five times greater. Panel C is the high-pass filtered signal using a partially time-reversed digital filter having a second order Butterworth response and a 3 db corner frequency of 40 Hz [12]. Note the appearance of the signals at the terminal portion of the QRS complex. A common method of analysis, but necessarily optimal, is to combine the filters XYZ leads into a vector magnitude, $(X^2 + Y^2 + Z^2)^{1/2}$. This waveform is shown in panel D. From this waveform several parameters have been derived such as total QRS duration, including late potentials, the RMS voltage value of the terminal 40 msec, and the low-amplitude signal (LAS) duration from the 40 μV level to the end of the late potentials. Abnormal values for these parameters are used to identify patients at high risk of ventricular tachycardia following a heart attack.

24.3.1.4 His Bundle Electrocardiography

The electrocardiogram can be directly recorded from the heart's surface as in a modern electrophysiology (EP) study where the evaluation of the heart relies on both the body surface ECG and direct recordings obtained from within the heart using electrode catheters. Such catheters are introduced into a leg or arm vein or artery and advanced, under fluoroscopic control, into the interior of one of the four chambers of the heart. An electrode catheter is an insulated set of wires bundled within a polyurethane sheath. The diameters of these catheters range from about 1.0 to 2.5 mm. As many as 16 wires may be in the total assembly with ring electrodes, exposed on the outer surface of the catheter, attached to each internal wire. In addition, there are usually structural internal wires used to stiffen the catheter. With a proper controller at the rear of the catheter a trained operator can flex the catheter in a loop of almost 180 degrees. Together with the torsional properties of the catheter almost every point within the heart can be probed for electrical events. Direct contact recordings are called electrograms to distinguish then from body surface electrocardiograms.

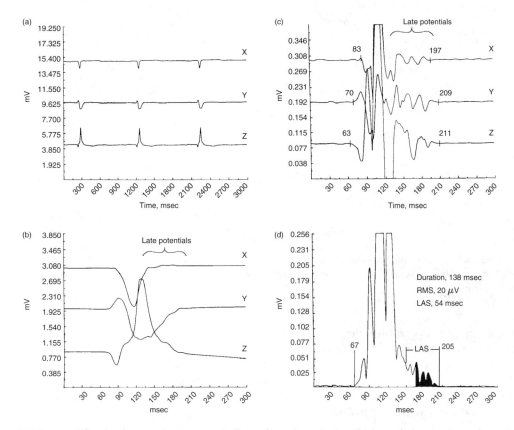

FIGURE 24.6 The signal processing steps typically performed to obtain a high resolution ECG are shown in panels A to D. See text for a full description.

Figure 24.7 shows an example of a His bundle recording. The top two traces are leads II and V_6 of the ECG and the bottom trace is the voltage difference from two electrodes on the indwelling electrode catheter. This internal view of cardiac activation combined with the His bundle electrogram has been referred to as His bundle electrocardiography [20]. Atrial activation on the catheter recording is called the "A" deflection and ventricular activation called the "V" deflection. The His bundle potential is the central "H" deflection. Since the catheter is located very close to the His bundle and AV node, it is assumed that the A deflection arises from atrial muscle tissue close to the AV node. When combined with the surface lead information a number of new intervals can be obtained. These are the PA, AH, and HV intervals. The PA interval is a measure of atrial muscle activation time, the AH interval is a measure of AV nodal activation time, and the HV interval is a measure of the ventricular conduction system activation time.

The modern electrophysiological evaluation, or EP study, may involve as many as 64 individual recordings within the heart. In addition, current can be passed through these electrodes to stimulate the heart. A variety of atrial and ventricular stimulation protocols can be used, which then allows the cardiac electrophysiologist to identify pathways and mechanisms involved in most forms of arrhythmias. Besides this diagnostic function, it is now possible to locate abnormal structures or regions of the heart that are critical to arrhythmogenesis. By passing high-energy radio frequency waves through one or more of the internal electrodes it is possible to cauterize or ablate the suspect tissue without causing any widespread injury to the rest of the heart. In many forms of arrhythmias this ablation therapy can produce a cure for the patient.

In addition to the EP study and ablation therapy internal electrodes are the primary form of signal recording for both the cardiac pacemaker and implantable defibrillator. These devices both sense cardiac activation from permanent indwelling catheters and deliver energy to the heart through them. In the

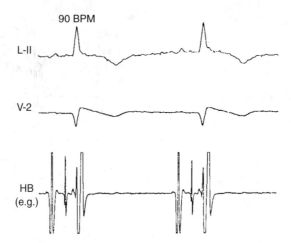

FIGURE 24.7 The top two traces are ECG leads II and V-2 and the bottom trace is a bipolar catheter recording, properly positioned inside the heart, showing the His Bundle deflection (HB), and intracardiac atrial (A) and ventricular (V) activity.

case of the cardiac pacemaker these are low-level shocks which maintain the patient's heart rhythm. In the case of the implantable defibrillator the device will monitor the patient's rhythm until a serious or life-threatening arrhythmia occurs and then a high-energy pulse will be delivered in order to convert the rhythm back to normal. Both devices rely heavily on continuous monitoring of the cardiac signals obtained from internal catheter recordings using sophisticated implanted microprocessors and accurate means of signal detection and analysis.

24.4 Conclusions

The ECG is one of the oldest, instrument-bound measurements in medicine. It has faithfully followed the progression of instrumentation technology. Its most recent evolutionary step, to the microprocessor-based system, has allowed patients to wear their computer monitor or provided an enhanced, high-resolution ECG which has opened new vistas of ECG analysis and interpretation. The intracardiac ECG also forms the basis of modern diagnostic EP studies and therapeutic devices, such as the pacemaker and implantable defibrillator.

References

[1] Waller A.D. One the electromotive changes connected with the beat of the mammalian heart, and the human heart in particular. *Phil. Trans. B*, 180: 169, 1889.

[2] Einthoven W. Die galvanometrische Registrirung des menschlichen Elektrokardiogramms, zugleich eine Beurtheilung der Anwendung des Capillar-Elecktrometers in der Physiologie. *Pflugers Arch. ges. Physiol.* 99: 472, 1903.

[3] Wilson F.N., Johnston F.S., and Hill I.G.W. The interpretation of the falvanometric curves obtained when one electrode is distant from the heart and the other near or in contact with the ventricular surface. *Am. Heart J.* 10: 176, 1934.

[4] Goldberger E. A simple, indifferent, electrocardiographic electrode of zero potential and a technique of obtaining augmented, unipolar, extremity leads. *Am. Heart J.* 23: 483, 1942.

[5] Bailey J.J., Berson A.S., Garson A., Horan L.G., Macfarlane P.W., Mortara D.W., and Zywietz C. Recommendations for standardization and specifications in automated electrocardiography: bandwidth and digital signal processing: a report for health professionals by an ad hoc writing group

of the committee on electrocardiography and cardiac electrophysiology of the Council on Clinical Cardiology, American Heart Association. *Circulation* 81: 2, 730–739, 1990.

[6] *Safe Current Limits for Electromedical Apparatus: American National Standard, ANSI/AAMI ES1–1993.* Arlington, VA: Association for the Advancement of Medical Instrumentation; 1993.

[7] Jenkins J.M. Computerized electrocardiography. *CRC Crit. Rev. Bioeng.* 6: 307, 1981.

[8] Pryor T.A., Drazen E., and Laks M. (Eds.), *Computer Systems for the Processing of Diagnostic Electrocardiograms.* IEEE Computer Society Press, Los Alamitos, CA, 1980.

[9] Berbari E.J., Lazzara R., Samet P., and Scherlag B.J. Noninvasive technique for detection of electrical activity during the PR segment. *Circulation* 48: 1006, 1973.

[10] Berbari E.J., Lazzara R., and Scherlag B.J. A computerized technique to record new components of the electrocardiogram. *Proc. IEEE* 65: 799, 1977.

[11] Berbari E.J., Scherlag B.J., Hope R.R., and Lazzara R. Recording from the body surface of arrhythmogenic ventricular activity during the ST segment. *Am. J. Cardiol.* 41: 697, 1978.

[12] Simson M.B. Use of signals in the terminal QRS complex to identify patients with ventricular tachycardia after myocardial infarction. *Circulation* 64: 235, 1981.

[13] Geselowitz D.B. On the theory of the electrocardiogram. *Proc. IEEE* 77: 857, 1989.

[14] Swerdlow C.D., Olson W.H., O'Connor M.E. et al. Cardiovascular collapse caused by electrocardiographically silent 60 Hz intracardiac leakage current: implications for electrical safety. *Circulation* 99: 2559–2564, 1999.

[15] Malkin R.A. and Hoffmeister B.K. Mechanisms by which AC leakage currents cause complete hemodynamic collapse without inducing fibrillation. [see comment]. *J. Cardiovasc. Electrophysiol.* 12: 1154–1161, 2001.

[16] Laks M.M., Arzbaecher R., Geselowitz D., Bailey J.J., and Berson A. Revisiting the question: will relaxing safe current limits for electromedical equipment increase hazards to patients? *Circulation* 102: 823–825, 2000.

[17] Holter N.J. New method for heart studies: continuous electrocardiography of active subjects over long periods is now practical. *Science* 134: 1214–1220, 1961.

[18] Ripley K.L. and Murray A. (Eds.), *Introduction to Automated Arrhythmia Detection*, IEEE Computer Society Press, Los Alamitos, CA, 1980.

[19] Berbari E.J. Berbari and Steinberg J.S. *A Practical Guide to High Resolution Electrocardiography.* Futura Publishers, Armonk, NY, 2000.

[20] Scherlag B.J., Samet P., and Helfant R.H. His bundle electrogram: a critical appraisal of its uses and limitations. *Circulation* 46: 601–613, 1972.

Further Information

Comprehensive Electrocardiology: Theory and Practice in Health and Disease, Vol. 1–3, P.W. Macfarlane and T.D. Veitch Lawrie, Eds., England: Pergamon Press, 1989.

A Practical Guide to the Use of the High-Resolution Electrocardiogram, Edward J. Berbari and Jonathan S. Steinberg, Eds., Armonk, NY: Futura Publishers, 2000.

Medical Instrumentation: Application and Design, 3rd ed., J.G. Webster, Ed., Boston: Houghton Mifflin, 1998.

Cardiac Electrophysiology: From Cell to Bedside, 4th ed., D.P. Zipes and J. Jalife, Eds., Philadelphia: W.B. Saunders & Co., 2004.

25

Principles of Electromyography

Kaj-Åge Henneberg
University of Montreal

Movement and position of limbs are controlled by electrical signals traveling back and forth between the muscles and the peripheral and central nervous system. When pathologic conditions arise in the motor system, whether in the spinal cord, the motor neurons, the muscle, or the neuromuscular junctions, the characteristics of the electrical signals in the muscle change. Careful registration and study of electrical signals in muscle (**electromyograms**) can thus be a valuable aid in discovering and diagnosing abnormalities not only in the muscles but also in the motor system as a whole. Electromyography (EMG) is the registration and interpretation of these muscle action potentials. Until recently, electromyograms were recorded primarily for exploratory or diagnostic purposes; however, with the advancement of bioelectric technology, electromyograms also have become a fundamental tool in achieving artificial control of limb movement, that is, functional electrical stimulation (FES) and rehabilitation. This chapter will focus on the diagnostic application of electromyograms, while FES will be discussed in Chapter 30.

Since the rise of modern clinical EMG, the technical procedures used in recording and analyzing electromyograms have been dictated by the available technology. The concentric needle electrode introduced by Adrian and Bronk in 1929 provided an easy-to-use electrode with high mechanical qualities and stable, reproducible measurements. Replacement of galvanometers with high-gain amplifiers allowed smaller electrodes with higher impedances to be used and potentials of smaller amplitudes to be recorded. With these technical achievements, clinical EMG soon evolved into a highly specialized field where electromyographists with many years of experience read and interpreted long paper EMG records based on the visual appearance of the electromyograms. Slowly, a more quantitative approach emerged, where features such as potential duration, peak-to-peak amplitude, and number of phases were measured on the paper records and compared with a set of normal data gathered from healthy subjects of all ages. In the last decade, the general-purpose rack-mounted equipment of the past have been replaced by ergonomically designed EMG units with integrated computers. Electromyograms are digitized, processed, stored on

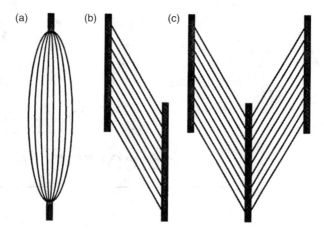

FIGURE 25.1   Schematic illustration of different types of muscles: (a) fusiform, (b) unipennate, and (c) bipennate.

removable media, and displayed on computer monitors with screen layouts that change in accordance with the type of recording and analysis chosen by the investigator.

With this in mind, this chapter provides an introduction to the basic concepts of clinical EMG, a review of basic anatomy, the origin of the electromyogram, and some of the main recording procedures and signal-analysis techniques in use.

25.1   The Structure and Function of Muscle

Muscles account for about 40% of the human mass, ranging from the small extraocular muscles that turn the eyeball in its socket to the large limb muscles that produce locomotion and control posture. The design of muscles varies depending on the range of motion and the force exerted (Figure 25.1). In the most simple arrangement (*fusiform*), parallel fibers extend the full length of the muscle and attach to tendons at both ends. Muscles producing a large force have a more complicated structure in which many short muscle fibers attach to a flat tendon that extends over a large fraction of the muscle. This arrangement (*unipennate*) increases the cross-sectional area and thus the contractile force of the muscle. When muscle fibers fan out from both sides of the tendon, the muscle structure is referred to as *bipennate*.

A lipid bilayer (sarcolemma) encloses the muscle fiber and separates the intracellular myoplasma from the interstitial fluid. Between neighboring fibers runs a layer of connective tissue, the endomysium, composed mainly of collagen and elastin. Bundles of fibers, fascicles, are held together by a thicker layer of connective-tissue called the perimysium. The whole muscle is wrapped in a layer of connective tissue called the epimysium. The connective tissue is continuous with the tendons attaching the muscle to the skeleton.

In the myoplasma, thin and thick filaments interdigitate and form short, serially connected identical units called sarcomeres. Numerous sarcomeres connect end to end, thereby forming longitudinal strands of myofibrils that extend the entire length of the muscle fiber. The total shortening of a muscle during contraction is the net effect of all sarcomeres shortening in series simultaneously. The individual sarcomeres shorten by forming cross-bridges between the thick and thin filaments. The cross-bridges pull the filaments toward each other, thereby increasing the amount of longitudinal overlap between the thick and thin filaments. The dense matrix of myofibrils is held in place by a structural framework of intermediate filaments composed of desmin, vimetin, and synemin [Squire, 1986].

At the site of the neuromuscular junction, each motor neuron forms collateral sprouts (Figure 25.2) and innervates several muscle fibers distributed almost evenly within an elliptical or circular region ranging from 2 to 10 mm in diameter. The motor neuron and the muscle fibers it innervates constitute a functional unit, the **motor unit**. The cross section of muscle occupied by a motor unit is called the

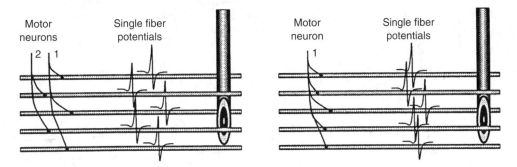

FIGURE 25.2 Innervation of muscle fibers. (a) Two normal motor units with intermingled muscle fibers. (b) Reinnervation of muscle fibers. The second and fourth muscle fibers have lost their motor neuron (2) and subsequently have become reinnervated by newly formed sprouts from the motor neuron (1) innervating adjacent muscle fibers. Not drawn to scale.

motor unit territory (MUT). A typical muscle fiber is only innervated at a single point, located within a cross-sectional band referred to as the end-plate zone. While the width of the end-plate zone is only a few millimeters, the zone itself may extend over a significant part of the muscle. The number of muscle fibers per motor neuron (i.e., the innervation ratio) ranges from 3 : 1 in extrinsic eye muscles where fine-graded contraction is required to 120 : 1 in some limb muscles with coarse movement [Kimura, 1981]. The fibers of one motor unit are intermingled with fibers of other motor units; thus several motor units reside within a given cross section. The fibers of the same motor unit are thought to be randomly or evenly distributed within the motor unit territory; however, reinnervation of denervated fibers often results in the formation of fiber clusters (see Figure 25.2).

25.2   The Origin of Electromyograms

Unlike the myocardium, skeletal muscles do not contain pacemaker cells from which excitations arise and spread. Electrical excitation of skeletal muscle is initiated and regulated by the central and peripheral nervous systems. Motor neurons carry nerve impulses from the anterior horn cells of the spinal cord to the nerve endings, where the axonal action potential triggers the release of the neurotransmitter acetylcholine (Ach) into the narrow clefts separating the sarcolemma from the axon terminals. As Ach binds to the sarcolemma, Ach-sensitive sodium channels open, and miniature end-plate potentials arise in the sarcolemma. If sufficient Ach is released, the summation of miniature end-plate potentials, that is, the end-plate potential, reaches the excitation threshold, and sarcolemma action potentials propagate in opposite directions toward the tendons. As excitation propagates down the fiber, it spreads into a highly branched transverse network of tubules (T system) which interpenetrate the myofibrils. The effective radial conduction velocity ($\sim$4 cm/sec) is about two orders of magnitude slower than the longitudinal conduction velocity (2 to 5 m/sec). This is due to the fact that the main portion of the total membrane capacitance is located in the T system and that the lumen of the T system constitutes a higher electrical resistance than the myoplasma.

The slower tubular conduction velocity implies an increasingly delayed onset of tubular action potentials toward the center of the fiber relative to that of the sarcolemmal action potential (Figure 25.3a). However, compared with the time course of the subsequent contraction, the spread of excitation along and within the muscle fiber is essentially instantaneous, thereby ensuring simultaneous release of calcium from the sarcoplasmic reticulum throughout the entire volume of the muscle. If calcium release were restricted to a small longitudinal section of the muscle fiber, only sarcomeres in this region would contract, and sarcomeres in the rest of the fiber would stretch accordingly. Similarly, experiments in detubulated muscle fibers, that is, fibers in which the continuation between the sarcolemmal and the tubular membrane has

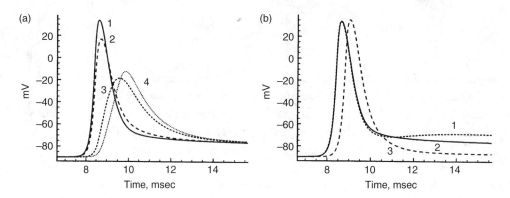

FIGURE 25.3 Simulated sarcolemmal and tubular action potentials of frog sartorius muscle fiber. (a) Temporal membrane action potentials calculated in a transverse plane 5 mm from the end-plate zone of a fiber with radius $a = 50$ μm. Curve 1: Sarcolemmal action potential; curves 2 to 4: action potentials in tubular membrane patches at $r = a$ (2), $r = a/2$ (3), and $r = a/20$ (4). (b) Sarcolemmal action potentials for fibers with radius 70 (1), 50 (2), and 30 (3) μm. The time axes have been expanded and truncated.

been disrupted, have demonstrated that only a thin layer of superficial myofibrils contracts when tubular action potentials fail to trigger calcium release deep in the muscle fiber.

It is well known that the shape of the skeletal muscle action potential differs from that of nerve action potentials with regard to the repolarization phase. In skeletal muscle, the falling phase of the action potential is interrupted by a long, slowly decaying potential known as the afterpotential. This late potential is caused by two opposing forces, the repolarization force due to the efflux of potassium through the sarcolemma and a depolarization force due to an influx of current from the interstitial space into the tubular lumen. The latter current is drawn in through the tubular openings by the repolarizing tubular membrane. Large muscle fibers have a higher tubular-sarcolemma area ratio; hence the inward surge of tubular current increases with fiber size. Figure 25.3b illustrates this by comparing sarcolemmal action potentials for fibers of increasing diameter. The small fiber has only a small amount of tubular membrane; hence the sarcolemmal potassium current has sufficient strength to rapidly repolarize the membrane. For the large fiber, inward tubular current actually depolarizes the sarcolemma slightly during repolarization of the tubular membrane system, thereby producing a small hump on the afterpotential. Since the hump on the *afterpotential* is influenced primarily by fiber size, this feature is more typical for large frog fibers than for smaller human fibers. Experiments have demonstrated that the sarcolemma action potential of detubulated fibers hyperpolarizes in a manner similar to that of a nerve action potential.

In Figure 25.4a, the time course of the sarcolemmal current density is compared with that of the current passing through the tubular mouth during the time course of the sarcolemmal action potential. The positive (outward) peak of the tubular current overlaps in time with the small capacitive sarcolemmal displacement current (initial positive peak) and the negative peak (inward sarcolemmal sodium current). As a result, the net current has a much larger positive peak than that of the sarcolemma alone, and the negative peak of the net current is only about half that of the sarcolemmal current. The outward sarcolemmal potassium current (late positive phase) is almost completely opposed by an antisymmetric inward tubular current, that is, the current drawn into the tubular lumen by the repolarizing T system. The combined effect of the sarcolemmal and tubular interaction is a net current with an almost biphasic waveform and with similar amplitudes of the positive and negative peaks.

As the net current source propagates toward the tendon, an extracellular potential field arises and follows the action potential complex. At a given field point, this phenomenon is observed as a temporal potential waveform (Figure 25.4b); however, a more complete picture of the phenomenon is obtained by considering the spatial distribution of potentials in the cross section of the motor unit. Figure 25.5 shows schematically how the concentric isopotential lines of individual fibers overlap with those of other fibers in the same motor unit. In a typical healthy motor unit (Figure 14.5a), the mean interfiber distance

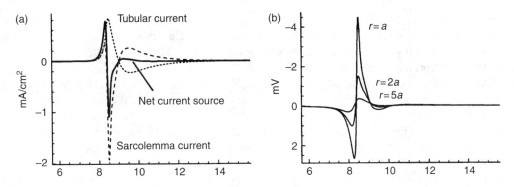

FIGURE 25.4 Simulated currents and extracellular potentials of frog sartorius muscle fiber (radius $a = 50\ \mu m$). (a) The net fiber current density is the summation of the current density through the sarcolemma and that passing the tubular mouth. (b) Extracellular action potentials calculated at increasing radial distances (in units of fiber radius) using a bidomain volume conductor model and the net current source in panel (a). The time axes have been expanded and truncated.

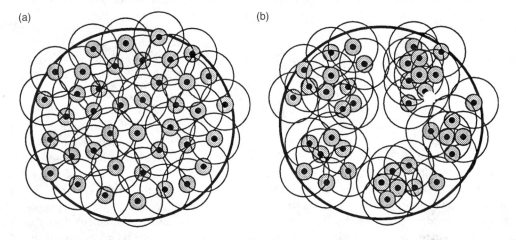

FIGURE 25.5 Schematic cross-sectional view of overlapping single-fiber action potential distributions in a normal (a) and reinnervated (b) motor unit. Muscle fibers are represented by filled black circles. Concentric rings represent axisymmetric isopotential lines of the individual single-fiber potentials at 2 (gray) and 5 radii from the fiber center, respectively. Compare with radial decline of extracellular potentials in Figure 25.4. See text for discussion of simplifying assumptions.

is on the order of a few hundred microns. Taking into account the steep radial decline of the potential amplitudes illustrated in Figure 25.4b, it is evident that **single-fiber action potential (SFAP)** overlapping occurs between low-magnitude isopotential lines. Figure 25.5b illustrates how spatial overlapping between SFAPs might look like in a motor unit with extensive fiber grouping. In this case, higher-level isopotential lines overlap within the clusters, while regions with no fibers would appear as electrically silent.

Several factors ignored in Figure 25.5 need further discussion. All fibers are assumed to be of the same size and with identical, perfectly axisymmetric potential distributions. The net single-fiber current source is an increasing function of fiber size; thus the magnitude of the potential distribution will vary with varying fiber size. Fibers can to a good approximation be considered as constant current sources; hence if the resistivity of the muscle tissue increases, for example, due to increased fiber packing density, the potential difference between an observation point and a reference point also will increase. It follows that local variations in fiber packing density in the region of an active fiber will destroy the axisymmetric appearance of its potential distribution. Muscle fibers are not perfect cylinders, and angular variation in the shape of the sarcolemma must be expected to create angular variations in the potential distribution. However, due to the relatively high conductivity of the volume conductor, it is plausible that such variations become increasingly insignificant as the distance to the fiber is increased.

A very important factor not considered in Figure 25.5 concerns the degree of longitudinal alignment of SFAPs in the motor unit. As illustrated in Figure 25.2, SFAPs are usually dispersed along the motor unit axis, and their potential distributions do not sum up in a simple manner. SFAPs can be misaligned for several reasons. The end plates are not aligned; hence some SFAPs originate ahead of others. Variations in fiber size and packing density cause variations in conduction velocity; thus the dispersion of SFAPs may actually increase with increasing distance from the end-plate zone. Neuropathologic conditions can affect the alignment of SFAPs. Complete or partial failure of collateral nerve sprouts to conduct nerve action potentials can abolish or delay the onset of action potentials, and immature sprouts formed during reinnervation may cause significant variability (**jitter**) in the onset of muscle action potentials. Denervated muscle fibers shrink; hence a newly reinnervated muscle fiber is likely to have a slower conduction velocity. An increased dispersion of SFAPs creates a very complex and irregular spatial potential distribution. The superimposed temporal potential waveform in a fixed observation point, that is, the **motor unit potential** (**MUP**), is therefore comprised of several peaks rather than a simple bi- or triphasic waveform. MUPs with five or more peaks are classified as polyphasic. A **satellite potential** is an SFAP that is so misaligned from the main potential complex that its waveform is completely separated from the MUP.

25.3   Electromyographic Recordings

A considerable amount of information regarding the bioelectrical state of a muscle is hidden in the time-varying spatial distribution of potentials in the muscle. Unfortunately, it is not clinically feasible to obtain high-resolution three-dimensional samples of the spatial potential distribution, since this would require the insertion of hundreds of electrodes into the muscles. In order to minimize the discomfort of the patient, routine EMG procedures usually employ only a single electrode that is inserted into different regions of the muscle. As the SFAPs of an active motor unit pass by the electrode, only their summation, that is, the MUP, will be registered by the electrode. The electrode is effectively integrating out the spatial information hidden in the passing potential complex, leaving only a time-variant potential waveform to be recorded and interpreted. It goes without saying that such a constraint on the recording procedure puts the electromyographist at a considerable disadvantage. To partially circumvent this setback, technical innovations and new procedures have continued to refine EMG examinations to such a level that some of the spatial information originally obscured by the electrode can be extracted intuitively from the temporal waveforms by an experienced electromyographist. With a detailed understanding of the bioelectric principles involved, for example, the bioelectric sources, the volume conductor, and the recording properties of the electrode, the electromyographist can quickly recognize and explain the waveform characteristics associated with various neuromuscular abnormalities.

To increase the amount of diagnostic information, several sets of EMG investigations may be performed using electrodes with different recording characteristics. Figure 25.6 illustrates three of the most popular EMG needle electrodes. The concentric and monopolar electrodes have an intermediate pickup range and are used in conventional recordings. The single-fiber electrode is a more recent innovation. It has a very small pickup range and is used to obtain recordings from only one or two muscle fibers. The macro electrode, which is the cannula of either the concentric or single-fiber electrode in combination with a remote reference electrode, picks up potentials throughout the motor unit territory. This section will review these EMG electrodes, the waveforms they produce, and the signal analysis performed in each case.

25.3.1   Concentric Electrode EMG

Adrian and Bronk developed the concentric electrode (see Figure 25.6) in order to obtain a pickup range that is smaller than that of wire electrodes. The modern version of the concentric electrode consists of a

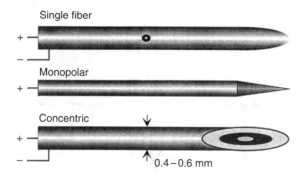

FIGURE 25.6   Needle electrodes for subcutaneous EMG recordings. For the single-fiber and concentric electrodes, the cannula of the hypodermic needle acts as reference electrode. The monopolar electrode is used with a remote reference electrode.

platinum or stainless steel wire located inside the lumen of a stainless steel cannula with an outer diameter of about 0.5 mm. The tip is beveled at 15 to 20 degrees, thereby exposing the central wire as an oblique elliptical surface of about $150 \times 580\ \mu$m. The central wire is insulated from the cannula with araldite or epoxy.

The concentric electrode is connected to a differential amplifier; thus common-mode signals are effectively rejected, and a relatively stable baseline is achieved. The cannula cannot be regarded as an indifferent reference electrode because it is located within the potential distribution and thus will pick up potentials from active fibers. Simulation studies [Henneberg and Plonsey, 1993] have shown that the cannula shields the central wire from picking up potentials from fibers located behind the tip. The sensitivity of the concentric electrode is therefore largest in the hemisphere facing the oblique elliptical surface. Due to the asymmetric sensitivity function, the waveshape of the recorded potentials will vary if the electrode is rotated about its axis. This problem is not observed with the axisymmetric monopolar electrode; however, this electrode has a more unstable baseline due to the remote location of the reference electrode. Both the concentric and monopolar electrodes (see Figure 25.6) are used in conventional EMG. Because of the differences in recording characteristics, however, concentric and monopolar recordings cannot be compared easily. A particular EMG laboratory therefore tends to use the one and not the other.

During the concentric needle examination, the investigator searches for abnormal insertional activity, spontaneous activity in relaxed muscles, and motor unit potentials with abnormal appearance. The waveshape of motor unit potentials is assessed on the basis of the quantitative waveform features defined in Figure 25.7:

- *Amplitude* is determined by the presence of active fibers within the immediate vicinity of the electrode tip. Low-pass filtering by the volume conductor attenuates the high-frequency spikes of remote SFAPs; hence the MUP amplitude does not increase for a larger motor unit. However, MUP amplitude will increase if the tip of the electrode is located near a cluster of reinnervated fibers. Large MUP amplitudes are frequently observed in neurogenic diseases.
- *Rise time* is an increasing function of the distance between the electrode and the closest active muscle fiber. A short rise time in combination with a small MUP amplitude might therefore indicate that the amplitude is reduced due to fiber atrophy rather than to a large distance between the electrode and the closest fiber.
- *Number of phases* indicates the complexity of the MUP and the degree of misalignment between SFAPs. In neurogenic diseases, polyphasic MUPs arise due to slow conduction velocity in immature nerve sprouts or slow conduction velocity in reinnervated but still atrophied muscle fibers. Variation in muscle fiber size also causes polyphasic MUPs in myopathic diseases. To prevent noisy baseline fluctuations from affecting the count of MUP phases, a valid baseline crossing must exceed a minimum absolute amplitude criterion.

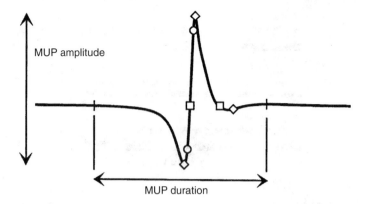

FIGURE 25.7 Definition of quantitative waveform features of MUPs recorded with a **concentric EMG electrode**. MUP area is defined as the rectified area under the curve in the interval between the onset and end. The number of MUP phases is defined as the number of baseline crossings (□) plus one. MUP turns are marked by a ◇. MUP rise time is the time interval between the 10% and 90% deflection (○) of the main negative-going slope. As by convention, negative voltage is displayed upward.

- *Duration* is the time interval between the first and last occurrence of the waveform exceeding a predefined amplitude threshold, for example, 5 μV. The MUP onset and end are the summation of low-frequency components of SFAPs scattered over the entire pickup range of the electrode. As a result, the MUP duration provides information about the number of active fibers within the pickup range. However, since the motor unit territory can be larger than the pickup range of the electrode, MUP duration does not provide information about the total size of a large motor unit. MUP duration will increase if a motor unit has an increased number of fibers due to reinnervation. MUP duration is affected to a lesser degree by SFAP misalignment.
- *Area* indicates the number of fibers adjacent to the electrode; however, unlike MUP amplitude, MUP area depends on MUP duration and is therefore influenced by fibers in a larger region compared with that of MUP amplitude.
- *Turns* is a measure of the complexity of the MUP, much like the number of phases; however, since a valid turn does not require a baseline crossing like a valid phase, the number of turns is more sensitive to changes in the MUP waveshape. In order to distinguish valid turns from signal noise, successive turns must be offset by a minimum amplitude difference.

Based on the complimentary information contained in the MUP features defined above, it is possible to infer about the number and density of fibers in a motor unit as well as the synchronicity of the SFAPs. However, the concentric electrode is not sufficiently selective to study individual fibers, nor is it sufficiently sensitive to measure the total size of a motor unit. The following two techniques were designed with these objectives in mind.

25.3.2 Single-Fiber EMG

The positive lead of the **single-fiber** electrode (see Figure 25.6) is the end cap of a 25-μm wire exposed through a side port on the cannula of a steel needle. Due to the small size of the positive lead, bioelectric sources, which are located more than about 300 μm from the side port, will appear as common-mode signals and be suppressed by the differential amplifier. To further enhance the selectivity, the recorded signal is high-pass filtered at 500 Hz to remove low-frequency background activity from distant fibers.

Due to its very small pickup range, the single-fiber electrode rarely records potentials from more than one or two fibers from the same motor unit. Because of the close proximity of the fibers, potentials are of large amplitudes and with small rise times. When two potentials from the same motor unit are picked up, the slight variation in their *interpotential interval* (IPI) can be measured (Figure 25.8). The mean IPI

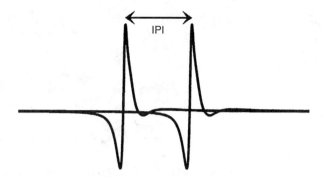

FIGURE 25.8   Measurement of interpotential interval (IPI) between single-fiber potentials recorded simultaneously from two fibers of the same motor unit.

(jitter) is normally 5 to 50 μsec but increases when neuromuscular transmission is disturbed. When the single-fiber electrode records potentials from an increased number of fibers, it usually indicates that the side port is close to either a cluster of fibers (reinnervation) or that the positive lead is close to fibers in the process of splitting.

25.3.3   Macro EMG

For this electrode, the cannula of a single-fiber or concentric electrode is used as the positive lead, while the reference electrode can be either a remote subcutaneous or remote surface electrode. Due to the large lead surface, this electrode picks up both near- and far-field activity. However, the signal has very small amplitude, and the macro electrode must therefore be coupled to an electronic averager. To ensure that only one and the same MUP is being averaged, the averager is triggered by a SFAP picked up from that motor unit by the side port wire of the single-fiber electrode or by the central wire of the concentric electrode. Since other MUPs are not time-locked to the triggering SFAP, they will appear as random background activity and become suppressed in the averaging procedure. Quantitative features of the macro MUP include the peak-to-peak amplitude, the rectified area under the curve, and the number of phases.

Defining Terms

Concentric electrode EMG: Registration and interpretation of motor unit potentials recorded with a concentric needle electrode.

Electromyograms (EMGs):   Bioelectric potentials recorded in muscles.

Jitter: Mean variation in interpotential interval between single-fiber action potentials of the same motor unit.

Macro EMG: The registration of motor unit potentials from the entire motor unit using the cannula of the single-fiber or concentric electrode.

Motor unit: The functional unit of an anterior horn cell, its axon, the neuromuscular junctions, and the muscle fibers innervated by the motor neuron.

Motor unit potential (MUP):   Spatial and temporal summation of all single-fiber potentials innervated by the same motor neuron. Also referred to as the *motor unit action potential* (MUAP).

Motor unit territory (MUT):   Cross-sectional region of muscle containing all fibers innervated by a single motor neuron.

Satellite potential: An isolated single-fiber action potential that is time-locked with the main MUP.

Single-fiber action potential (SFAP):   Extracellular potential generated by the extracellular current flow associated with the action potential of a single muscle fiber.

Single-fiber EMG (SFEMG):   Recording and analysis of single-fiber potentials with the single-fiber electrode.

References

Henneberg, K. and Plonsey, R. 1993. Boundary element analysis of the directional sensitivity of the concentric EMG electrode. *IEEE Trans. Biomed. Eng.* 40: 621.

Kimura, J. 1981. *Electrodiagnosis in Diseases of Nerve and Muscle: Principles and Practice.* Philadelphia, FA Davis.

Squire, J. 1986. *Muscle: Design, Diversity and Disease.* Menlo Park, CA, Benjamin/Cummings.

Further Information

Barry, D.T. 1991. AAEM minimonograph no. 36: basic concepts of electricity and electronics in clinical electromyography. *Muscle Nerve* 14: 937.

Buchthal, F. 1973. Electromyography. In *Handbook of Electroencephalography and Clinical Neurophysiology,* Vol. 16. Amsterdam, Elsevier Scientific.

Daube, J.R. 1991. AAEM minimonograph no. 11: needle examination in clinical electromyography. *Muscle Nerve* 14: 685.

Dumitru, D. and DeLisa, J.A. 1991. AAEM minimonograph no. 10: volume conduction. *Muscle Nerve* 14: 605.

Stålberg, E. 1986. Single fiber EMG, macro EMG, and scanning EMG: new ways of looking at the motor unit. *CRC Crit. Rev. Clin. Neurobiol.* 2: 125.

26

Principles of Electroencephalography

Joseph D. Bronzino
Trinity College

Electroencephalograms (EEGs) are recordings of the minute (generally less that 300 μV) electrical potentials produced by the brain. Since 1924, when Hans Berger reported the recording of rhythmic electrical activity from the human scalp, analysis of EEG activity has been conducted primarily in clinical settings to detect gross pathologies and epilepsies and in research facilities to quantify the central effects of new pharmacologic agents. As a result of these efforts, cortical EEG patterns have shown to be modified by a wide range of variables, including biochemical, metabolic, circulatory, hormonal, neuroelectric, and behavioral factors. In the past, interpretation of the EEG was limited to visual inspection by an electro-encephalographer, an individual trained to qualitatively distinguish normal EEG activity from localized or generalized abnormalities contained within relatively long EEG records. This approach left clinicians and researchers alike buried in a sea of EEG paper records. The advent of computers and the technologies associated with them has made it possible to effectively apply a host of methods to quantify EEG changes. With this in mind, this chapter provides a brief historical perspective followed by some insights regarding EEG recording procedures and an in-depth discussion of the quantitative techniques used to analyze alterations in the EEG.

26.1 Historical Perspective

In 1875, Richard Caton published the first account documenting the recording of spontaneous brain electrical activity from the cerebral cortex of an experimental animal. The amplitude of these electrical oscillations was so low (i.e., in the microvolt range) that Caton's discovery is all the more amazing because it was made 50 years before suitable electronic amplifiers became available.

In 1924, Hans Berger of the University of Jena in Austria, carried out the first human EEG recordings using metal strips pasted to the scalps of his subjects as electrodes and a sensitive galvanometer as the recording instrument. Berger was able to measure the irregular, relatively small electrical potentials (i.e., 50 to 100 μV) coming from the brain. By studying the successive positions of the moving element of the galvanometer recorded on a continuous roll of paper, he was able to observe the resultant patterns in these brain waves as they varied with time. From 1924 to 1938, Berger laid the foundation for many of the present applications of electroencephalography. He was the first to use the word **electroencephalogram** in describing these brain potentials in humans. Berger also noted that these brain waves were not entirely random but instead displayed certain periodicities and regularities. For example, he observed that although these brain waves were slow (i.e., exhibited a synchronized pattern of high amplitude and low frequency, <3 Hz) during sleep, they were faster (i.e., exhibited a desynchronized pattern of low amplitude and higher frequency, 15 to 25 Hz) during waking behaviors. He suggested, quite correctly, that the brain's activity changed in a consistent and recognizable fashion when the general status of the subject changed, as from relaxation to alertness. Berger also concluded that these brain waves could be greatly affected by certain pathologic conditions after noting a marked increase in the amplitude of these brain waves recorded during convulsive seizures. However, despite the insights provided by these studies, Berger's original paper, published in 1929, did not excite much attention. In essence, the efforts of this remarkable pioneer were largely ignored until similar investigations were carried out and verified by British investigators.

It was not until 1934, however, when Adrian and Matthews published their classic paper verifying Berger's findings that the concept of "human brain waves" was truly accepted and the study of EEG activity was placed on a firm foundation. One of their primary contributions was the identification of certain rhythms in the EEG, for example, a regular oscillation at approximately 10 to 12 Hz recorded from the occipital lobes of the cerebral cortex, which they termed the "alpha rhythm." This alpha rhythm was found to disappear when a subject displayed any type of attention or alertness or focused on objects in the visual field. The physiologic basis for these results, the "arousing influence" of external stimuli on the cortex, was not formulated until 1949, when Moruzzi and Magoun demonstrated the existence of pathways widely distributed through the central reticular core of the brainstem that were capable of exerting a diffuse-activating influence on the cerebral cortex. This "reticular activating system" has been called the brain's response selector because it alerts the cortex to focus on certain pieces of incoming information, while ignoring others. It is for this reason that a sleeping mother will immediately be awakened by her crying baby or the smell of smoke and yet, ignores the traffic outside her window or the television playing in the next room. (*Note:* For the interested reader, an excellent historical review of this early era in brain research is provided in a fascinating text by Brazier [1968].)

26.2   EEG Recording Techniques

Scalp recordings of spontaneous neuronal activity in the brain, identified as the EEG, allow measurement of potential changes over time between a signal electrode and a reference electrode. Compared with other biopotentials, such as the electrocardiogram, the EEG is extremely difficult for an untrained observer to interpret, partially as a result of the spatial mapping of functions onto different regions of the brain and electrode placement. Recognizing that some standardization was necessary, the International Federation in Electroencephalography and Clinical Neurophysiology adopted the 10–20 electrode placement system. In addition to the standard 10–20 scalp array, electrodes to monitor eye movement, ECG, and muscle activity are essential for discrimination of different vigilance or behavioral states [Kondraski, 1986; Smith, 1986; Bronzino, 1995, 2000].

Any EEG system consists of electrodes, amplifiers (with appropriate filters), and a recording device. Instrumentation required for recording EEG activity can be simple or elaborate. (*Note:* Although the discussion presented in this section is for a single-channel system, it can be extended to simultaneous multichannel recordings simply by multiplying the hardware by the number of channels required. In cases that do not require true simultaneous recordings, special electrode selector panels can minimize hardware requirements.)

Commonly used scale electrodes consist of Ag–AgCl disks, 1 to 3 mm in diameter, with long flexible leads that can be plugged into an amplifier. Although a low-impedance contact is desirable at the electrode–skin interface ($<10 \text{ k}\Omega$), this objective is confounded by hair and the difficulty of mechanically stabilizing the electrode. Conductive electrode paste helps obtain low impedance and keep the electrodes in place. Often a contact cement (collodion) is used to fix small patches of gauze over the electrodes for mechanical stability, and leads are usually taped to the subject to provide some strain relief. Slight abrasion of the skin is sometimes used to obtain lower electrode impedance, but this can cause slight irritation and sometimes infection (as well as pain in sensitive subjects).

For long-term recordings, as in seizure monitoring, electrodes present major problems. Needle electrodes, which must be inserted into the tissue between the surface of the scalp and the skull, are sometimes useful. However, the danger of infection increases significantly. Electrodes with self-contained miniature amplifiers are somewhat more tolerant because they provide a low-impedance source to interconnecting leads, but they are expensive. Despite numerous attempts to simplify the electrode application process and to guarantee long-term stability, no single method has been widely accepted.

Instruments are available for measuring impedance between electrode pairs. The procedure is recommended strongly as a good practice, since high impedance leads to distortions that may be difficult to separate from actual EEG signals. In fact, electrode impedance monitors are built into some commercially available EEG devices. Note that standard DC ohmmeters should not be used, since they apply a polarizing current that can result in a buildup of noise at the skin–electrode interface.

From carefully applied electrodes, signal amplitudes of 1 to 10 μV can be obtained. Considerable amplification (gain = 10^6) is required to bring signal strength up to an acceptable level for input to recording devices. Because of the length of electrode leads and the electrically noisy environment where recordings commonly take place, differential amplifiers with inherently high input impedance and high common-mode rejection ratios are essential for high-quality EEG recordings.

In some facilities, special electrically shielded rooms minimize environmental electrical noise, particularly 60 Hz alternating current (AC) line noise. Since much of the information of interest in the EEG lies in frequency bands below 40 Hz, low-pass filters in the amplifier can be used to greatly reduce 60 Hz noise. For attenuating AC noise when the low-pass cutoff is above 60 Hz, many EEG amplifiers employ a notch filter specific only for frequencies in a narrow band centered around 60 Hz.

When trying to eliminate or minimize the effect of 60-Hz sources, it is sometimes useful to use a dummy source, such as a fixed 100-kΩ resistor attached to the electrodes. By employing a dummy source as one of the input signals, the output of the differential amplifier represents only contributions from interfering sources. If noise can be reduced to an acceptable level (at least by a factor of 10 less than EEG signals), it is likely that uncontaminated EEG records can be obtained.

Different types of recording instruments obtain a temporary or permanent record of the EEG. The most common recording device is a pen or chart recorder (usually multichannel), which is an integral part of most commercially available EEG instruments. Recordings are on a long sheet of continuous paper (from a folded stack) fed past the moving pen at one of several selectable constant speeds. Paper speed is selected according to the monitoring situation at hand: slow speed (10 mm/sec) for observing the spiking characteristically associated with seizure activity and faster speeds (up to 120 mm/sec) to identify the presence of individual frequency bands in the EEG.

In addition to (or instead of) a pen recorder, the EEG may be recorded on a multichannel frequency-modulated (FM) analog tape recorder. During such recordings, a visual output device such as an oscilloscope or video display is often used to allow visual monitoring of signals.

Sophisticated FM tape recording and playback systems allow clinicians to review long EEG recordings over a greatly reduced time compared with that required to flip through stacks of paper or to observe recordings in real time. Such systems take advantage of time-compensation schemes, whereby a signal recorded at one speed can be played back at a faster speed. The ratio of playback to recording speed is known, so appropriate correction factor can be applied to played-back data generating a properly scaled video display. A standard ratio of 60 : 1 is often used. Thus a trained clinician can review each minute of real-time EEG in 1 sec. The display is scrolled at a high rate horizontally across the display screen. Features of such instruments allow the clinician to freeze a segment of EEG on the display and to slow down or accelerate tape speed from the standard playback as needed. A vertical "tick" mark is usually displayed at periodic intervals by one channel as a time mark to provide a convenient timing reference. Computers also can be used as recording devices. In such systems, one or more channels of analog EEG signal are repeatedly sampled at a fixed time interval (sampling interval), and each sample is converted into a digital representation by an analog-to-digital (A/D) converter. The A/D converter is interfaced to a computer system so that each sample can be saved in the computer's memory. The resolution of the A/D converter is determined by the smallest amplitude that can be sampled. This is determined by dividing the voltage range of the A/D converter by 2 raised to the power of the number of bits of the A/D converter. For example, an A/D converter with a range of ± 5 V and 12-bit resolution can resolve sample amplitudes as small as ± 2.4 mV. Appropriate matching of amplification and A/D converter sensitivity permits resolution of the smallest signal while preventing clipping of the largest signal amplitudes.

A set of such samples, acquired at a sufficient sampling rate (at least twice the highest frequency component of interest in the sampled signal), is sufficient to represent all the information in the waveform. To ensure that the signal is band-limited, a low-pass filter with a cutoff frequency equal to the highest frequency of interest is used. Since physically realizable filters do not have ideal characteristics, the sampling rate is usually set to twice the cutoff frequency of the filter or more. Furthermore, once converted to digital format, digital filtering techniques can be used.

Online computer recordings are only practical for short-term recordings or for situations in which the EEG is immediately processed. This limitation is primarily due to storage requirements. For example, a typical sampling rate of 128 Hz yields 128 new points per second that require storage. For an 8-sec sample, 1024 points are acquired per channel recorded. A 10-min recording period yields 76,800 data points per channel. Assuming 12-bit resolution per sample, one can see that available computer memory quickly becomes a significant factor in determining the length (in terms of time) as well as the number of channels of EEG activity to be acquired in real time by the computer.

Further data processing can consist of compression for more efficient storage (with associated loss of total information content), as in the use of compressed spectral arrays, determination of a reduced features set including only data needed for quantification, as in evoked response recordings, or feature extraction and subsequent pattern recognition, as in automated spike detection during monitoring for epileptic seizure activity.

In addition to the information available from spontaneous EEG activity, the brain's electrical response to sensory stimulation is also important. Due to the relatively small amplitude of a stimulus-evoked potential compared with that of spontaneous EEG potentials, the technique of signal averaging is often used to enhance the characteristics of stimulus-evoked responses. Stimulus averaging takes advantage of the fact that the brain's electrical response is time locked to the onset of the stimulus, while nonevoked, background potential changes are randomly distributed in time. Consequently, the averaging of multiple stimulus-evoked responses results in the enhancement of the time-locked activity, while average random background activity approaches zero. The result is an evoked response that consists of a number of discrete and replicable peaks that occur, depending on the stimulus and recording parameters, at predictable latencies associated with the onset of stimulation.

26.3   Use of Amplitude Histographs to Quantify the EEG

In general, the EEG contains information regarding changes in the electrical potential of the brain obtained from a given set of recording electrodes. These data include the characteristic waveforms with accompanying variations in amplitude, frequency, phase, and so on, as well as the brief occurrence of electrical patterns, such as spindles. *Any analysis procedure cannot simultaneously provide information regarding all these variables.* Consequently, the selection of any analytical technique will emphasize changes in one particular variable at the expense of the others. This observation is extremely important if one is to properly interpret the results obtained using a given technique.

In the computation of amplitude distributions of the EEG, for example, successive EEG amplitudes must be measured and ordered into specific amplitude classes, or *bins*. The amplitude histogram that results from this process is often a symmetrical, essentially Gaussian distribution. The primary characteristics of the Gaussian distribution are summarized simply by specifying its mean and standard deviation, since the higher control moments of the distribution, such as skewness and kurtosis, are equal to zero. However, in non-Gaussian distributions, the measures of skewness and kurtosis assume nonzero values and can be used to characterize that particular amplitude distribution. The four primary statistical measures used to characterize an EEG amplitude histogram include the mean, standard amplitude, skewness, and kurtosis.

26.3.1 Mean

Since the sum of (positive and negative) EEG potential is usually on the order of a few microvolts when the analysis time is not too short, the mean is essentially a constant, although of small value. Any shifts in values of the mean, therefore, are indicative of changes in potential that are of technical origin, such as amplifier drifts, and the like.

26.3.2 Standard Amplitude

The variance of the EEG amplitude distribution is directly related to the total power of the EEG. For example, a flat EEG will provide low variance values, while a widely oscillating EEG will yield high variance values. To avoid confusion and use units that are more familiar to electroencephalographers, the term *standard amplitude* is often used.

26.3.3 Skewness

The degree of deviation from the symmetry of a normal or Gaussian distribution is measured by skewness. This third central moment of the amplitude histogram has a value of zero when the distribution is completely symmetrical and assumes some nonzero value when the EEG waveforms are asymmetrical with respect to the baseline (as is the case in some characteristic sleep patterns, murhythms, morphine spindles, barbiturate spiking, etc.). In general, a nonzero value of the skewness index reflects the presence of monophasic events in the waveform. The following methods can be used to obtain the measure of skewness:

Moment coefficient of skewness:

$$S_{K\mathrm{mc}} = \frac{\sum_{i=1}^{N}(x_i - \bar{x})^3/N}{\left[\sum_{i=1}^{N}(x_i - \bar{x})^2/N\right]^{3/2}} \tag{26.1}$$

Pearson's second coefficient of skewness:

$$S_{K_{2c}} = \frac{3(\bar{x}\ \mathrm{median})}{\mathrm{SD}} \tag{26.2}$$

Centile index of skewness:

$$S_{K_{\mathrm{cent}}} = \frac{(\text{number of points} > \bar{x})}{N} \tag{26.3}$$

26.3.4 Kurtosis

The *kurtosis* measure reveals the peakedness or flatness of a distribution. A kurtosis value greater than that of a normal distribution means that the distribution is leptokurtic, or simply more peaked than

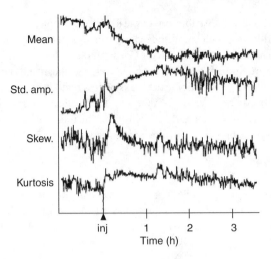

FIGURE 26.1 Plot of the indices of the amplitude distribution, that is, the mean, standard amplitude, skewness, and kurtosis, of the EEG recorded from a rat prior to and for 3 h following intraperitoneal injection of morphine sulfate (30 mg/kg). *Arrow (inj)* indicates time of injection.

the normal curve. A value less than that of a normal distribution indicates a flatter distribution. In clinical electroencephalography, when analyzing EEGs with little frequency and amplitude modulation, one observes negative values of kurtosis. High positive values of kurtosis are present when the EEG contains transient spikes, isolated high-voltage wave groups, and so on. The following methods can be used to obtain the measure of kurtosis.

Moment coefficient of kurtosis:

$$K_{mc} = \frac{\sum_{i=1}^{N}(x_i - \bar{x})^4 / N}{\left[\sum_{i=1}^{N}(x_i - \bar{x})^2 / N\right]^2} - 3 \tag{26.4}$$

Centile index of lurtosis:

$$K_{cent} \frac{\text{number of patients such that } |x_i - \bar{x}| > \text{ standard amplitude}}{N} \tag{26.5}$$

A normal distribution will have a value of 0.5 for this measure.

Figure 26.1 illustrates the sensitivity of these measures in analyzing the effect of systemic (IP) administration of morphine sulfate (30 mg/kg) on the cortical EEC. It will be noted that the skewness measure changes abruptly only immediately after the morphine injection, when the EEG was dominated by the appearance of spindles. However, the index of kurtosis characterizes the entire extent of the drug effect from onset to its return to baseline.

The central moments of the EEC amplitude histogram, therefore, are capable of (1) characterizing the amplitude distributions of the EEG and (2) quantifying alterations in these electrical processes brought about by pharmacologic manipulations. In addition, use of the centile index for skewness and kurtosis provides a computer-efficient method for obtaining these measures in real time.

26.4 Frequency Analysis of the EEG

In early attempts to correlate the EEG with behavior, analog frequency analyzers were used to examine single channels of EEG data. Although disappointing, these initial efforts did introduce the use of frequency

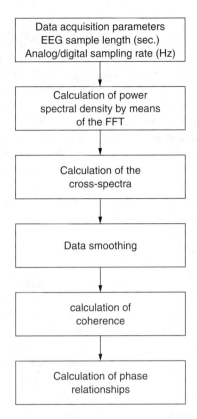

FIGURE 26.2   Block diagram illustrating the steps involved in conventional (linear) spectral analysis of EEG activity.

analysis to the study of gross brain wave activity. Although **power spectral analysis**, that is, the magnitude square of the Fourier transform, provides a quantitative measure of the frequency distribution of the EEG, it does so, as mentioned above, at the expense of other details in the EEG such as the amplitude distribution and information concerning the presence of specific EEG patterns.

The first systematic application of power spectral analysis by general-purpose computers was reported in 1963 by Walter; however, it was not until the introduction of the **fast Fourier transform (FFT)** by Cooley and Tukey in 1965 that machine computation of the EEG became commonplace. Although an individual FFT is ordinarily calculated for a short section of EEG data (e.g., from 1 to 8 sec), such signal segmentation with subsequent averaging of individual modified periodograms has been shown to provide a consistent estimator of the power spectrum. An extension of this technique, the compressed spectral array, has been particularly useful for evaluating EEG spectra over long periods of time. A detailed review of the development and use of various methods to analyze the EEG is provided by Bronzino et al. [1995, 2000] and others [Barlow, 1993; Dempster, 1993]. Figure 26.2 provides an overview of the computational processes involved in performing spectral analysis of the EEG, that is, including computation of auto- and **cross-spectra**. It is to be noted that the power spectrum is the *autocorrelellogram*, that is, the correlation of the signal with itself. As a result, the power spectrum provides only magnitude information in the frequency domain; it does not provide any data regarding phase. The power spectrum is computed by Equation 26.6, where $X(f)$ is the Fourier transform of the EEG signal.

$$P(f) = R_e^2[X(f)] + I_m^2[X(f)] \qquad (26.6)$$

Power spectral analysis not only provides a summary of the EEG in a convenient graphic form but also facilitates statistical analysis of EEG changes that may not be evident on simple inspection of the records.

In addition to absolute power derived directly from the power spectrum, other measures calculated from absolute power have been demonstrated to be of value in quantifying various aspects of the EEG. Relative power expresses the percentage contribution of each frequency band to the total power and is calculated by dividing the power within a band by the total power across all bands. Relative power has the benefit of reducing the intersubject variance associated with absolute power that arises from subject differences in skull and scalp conductance. The disadvantage of relative power is that an increase in one frequency band will be reflected in the calculation by a decrease in other bands; for example, it has been reported that directional shifts between high and low frequencies are associated with changes in cerebral blood flow and metabolism. Power ratios between low (0 to 7 Hz) and high (10 to 20 Hz) frequency bands have been demonstrated to be an accurate estimator of changes in cerebral activity during these metabolic changes.

Although the power spectrum quantifies activity at each electrode, other variables derivable from the FFT offer a means of quantifying the relationships between signals recorded from multiple electrodes or sites. Coherence (which is a complex number), calculated from the cross-spectrum analysis of two signals, is similar to cross-correlation in the time domain.

The cross-spectrum is computed by

$$\text{Cross-spectrum} = X(f)Y^*(f) \tag{26.7}$$

where $X(f)$ and $Y(f)$ are Fourier transforms, and $*$ indicates the complex conjugate.

Coherence is calculated by

$$\text{Coherence} = \frac{\text{cross-spectrum}}{\sqrt{PX(f) - PY(f)}} \tag{26.8}$$

The **magnitude squared coherence (MSC)** values range from 1 to 0, indicating maximum and no synchrony, respectively. The temporal relationship between two signals is expressed by the phase angle, which is a measure of the lag between two signals of common frequency components or bands.

Since coherence is a complex number, the phase is simply the angle associated with the polar expression of that number. MSC and phase then represent measures that can be employed to investigate interactions of cerebral activity recorded from separate brain sites. For example, short (intracortical) and long (corti-cocortical) pathways have been proposed as the anatomic substrates underlying the spatial frequency and patterns of coherence. Therefore, discrete cortical regions linked by such fiber systems should demonstrate a relatively high degree of synchrony, while the temporal difference between signals, represented by the phase measure, quantifies the extent to which one signal leads another.

26.5   Nonlinear Analysis of the EEG

As mentioned earlier, the EEG has been studied extensively using signal-processing schemes, most of which are based on the assumption that the EEG is a linear, Gaussian process. Although linear analysis schemes are computationally efficient and useful, they only utilize information retained in the autocorrelation function (i.e., the second-order cumulant). Additional information stored in higher-order cumulants is therefore ignored by linear analysis of the EEG. Thus, while the power spectrum provides the energy distribution of a stationary process in the frequency domain, it cannot distinguish nonlinearly coupled frequency from spontaneously generated signals with the same resonance.

There is evidence showing that the amplitude distribution of the EEG often deviates from Gaussian behavior. It has been reported, for example, that the EEG of humans involved in the performance of mental arithmetic tasks exhibits significant non-Gaussian behavior. In addition, the degree of deviation from gaussian behavior of the EEG has been shown to depend on the behavioral state, with the state of slow-wave sleep showing less Gaussian behavioral than quiet waking, which is less Gaussian than rapid eye movement (REM) sleep [Ning and Bronzino, 1989a,b]. Nonlinear signal-processing algorithms such as bispectral analysis are therefore necessary to address non-Gaussian and nonlinear behavior of the EEG in order to better describe it in the frequency domain.

But what exactly is the bispectrum? For a zero-mean, stationary process $\{X(k)\}$, the bispectrum, by definition, is the Fourier transform of its third-order cumulant (TOG) sequence:

$$B(\omega_1, \omega_2) = \sum_{m=-\alpha}^{\alpha} \sum_{m=-\alpha}^{\alpha} C(m, n) e^{-j(w_1 m + w_2 n)} \tag{26.9}$$

The TOG sequence $[C(m, n)]$ is defined as the expected value of the triple product

$$C(m, n) = E\{X(k)X(k + m)X(k + n)\} \tag{26.10}$$

If process $X(k)$ is purely Gaussian, then its third-order cumulant $C(m, n)$ is zero for each (m, n), and consequently, its Fourier transform, the bispectrum, $B(\omega_1, \omega_2)$ is also zero. This property makes the estimated bispectrum an immediate measure describing the degree of deviation from gaussian behavior. In our studies [Ning and Bronzino, 1989a,b], the sum of magnitude of the estimated bispectrum was used as a measure to describe the EEG's deviation from Gaussian behavior, that is,

$$D = \sum_{(\omega_1 \omega_2)} |B(\omega_1, \omega_2)| \tag{26.11}$$

Using bispectral analysis, the existence of significant **quadratic phase coupling** (QPC) in the hippocampal EEG obtained during REM sleep in the adult rat was demonstrated [Ning and Bronzino, 1989a,b, 1990]. The result of this nonlinear coupling is the appearance, in the frequency spectrum, of a small peak centered at approximately 13 to 14 Hz (beta range) that reflects the summation of the two theta frequency (i.e., in the 6- to 7-Hz range) waves (Figure 26.3). Conventional power spectral (linear) approaches are incapable of distinguishing the fact that this peak results from the interaction of these two generators and is not intrinsic to either.

To examine the phase relationship between nonlinear signals collected at different sites, the cross-bispectrum is also a useful tool. For example, given three zero-mean, stationary processes $\{x_j(n)_j = 1, 2, 3\}$, there are two conventional methods for determining the cross-bispectral relationship, direct and indirect. Both methods first divide these three processes into M segments of shorter but equal length. The direct method computes the Fourier transform of each segment for all three processes and then estimates the cross-bispectrum by taking the average of triple products of Fourier coefficients over M segments, that is,

$$B_{x_1 x_2 x_3}(\omega_1, \omega_2) = \frac{1}{M} \sum_{m=1}^{M} X_1^m(\omega_1) X_2^m(\omega_2) X_3^{m*}(\omega_1 + \omega_2) \tag{26.12}$$

where $X_j^m(\omega)$ is the Fourier transform of the mth segment of $\{x_j(n)\}$, and $*$ indicates the complex conjugate.

The indirect method computes the third-order cross-cumulant sequence for all segments:

$$C_{x_1 x_2 x_3}(k, l) = \sum_{n \in \tau} x_1^m(n) x_2^m(n + k) x_3^m(n + l) \tag{26.13}$$

where τ is the admissible set for argument n. The cross-cumulant sequences of all segments will be averaged to give a resultant estimate:

$$Cx_1 x_2 x_3(k, l) = \frac{1}{M} \sum_{m=1}^{M} C_{x_1 x_2 x_3}^m(k, l) \tag{26.14}$$

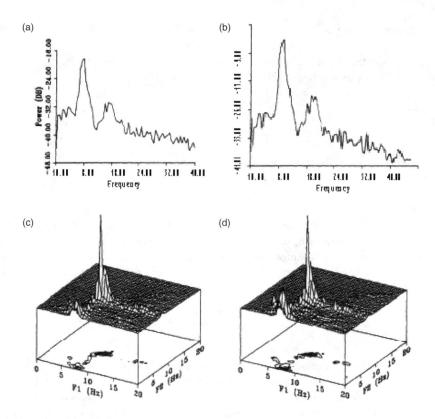

FIGURE 26.3 Plots (a) and (b) represent the averaged power spectra of sixteen 8-sec epochs of REM sleep (digital sampling rate = 128 Hz) obtained from hippocampal subfields CA1 and the dentate gyrus, respectively. Note that both spectra exhibit clear power peaks at approximately 8 Hz (theta rhythm) and 16 Hz (beta activity). Plots (c) and (d) represent the **bispectra** of these same epochs, respectively. Computation of the bicoherence index at $f(1) = 8$ Hz, $f(2) = 8$ Hz showed significant quadratic phase coupling (QPC), indicating that the 16-Hz peak seen in the power spectra is not spontaneously generated but rather results from the summation of activity between the two recording sites.

The cross-bispectrum is then estimated by taking the Fourier transform of the third-order cross-cumulant sequence:

$$B x_1 x_2 x_3(\omega_1, \omega_2) = \sum_{k=-\alpha}^{\alpha} \sum_{l=-\alpha}^{\alpha} C x_1 x_2 x_3(k, l) e^{-j(\omega_1 k + \omega_2 l)} \tag{26.15}$$

Since the variance of the estimated cross-bispectrum is inversely proportional to the length of each segment, computation of the cross-bispectrum for processes of finite data length requires careful consideration of both the length of individual segments and the total number of segments to be used.

The cross-bispectrum can be applied to determine the level of cross-QPC occurring between $\{x_1(n)\}$ and $\{x_2(n)\}$ and its effects on $\{x_3(n)\}$. For example, a peak at $B x_1 x_2 x_3(\omega_1, \omega_2)$ suggests that the energy component at frequency $\omega_1 + \omega_2$ of $\{x_3(n)\}$ is generated due to the QPC between frequency ω_1 of $\{x_1(n)\}$, and frequency ω_2 of $\{x_2(n)\}$. In theory, the absence of QPC will generate a flat cross-bispectrum. However due to the finite data length encountered in practice, peaks may appear in the cross-bispectrum at locations where there is no significant cross-QPC. To avoid improper interpretation, the cross-bicoherence index, which indicates the significance level of cross-QPC, can be computed as follows:

$$bic_{x_1 x_2 x_3}(\omega_1, \omega_2) = \frac{B x_1 x_2 x_3(\omega_1, \omega_2)}{\sqrt{P_{x_1}(\omega_1) P_{x_2}(\omega_2) P_{x_3}(\omega_1 + \omega_2)}} \tag{26.16}$$

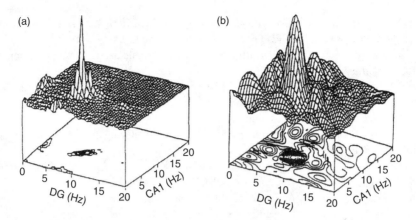

FIGURE 26.4 Cross-bispectral plots of $B_{CA1-DG-CA1}(\omega_1, \omega_2)$ computed using (a) the direct method and (b) the indirect method.

where $P_{xj}(w)$ is the power spectrum of process $\{x(n)\}$. The theoretical value of the bicoherence index ranges between 0 and 1, that is, from nonsignificant to highly significant.

In situations where the interest is the presence of QPC and its effects on $\{x(n)\}$, the cross-bispectrum equations can be modified by replacing $\{x_1(n)\}$ and $\{x_3(n)\}$ with $\{x(n)\}$ and $\{x_2(n)\}$ with $\{y(n)\}$, that is,

$$B_{xyz}(\omega_1, \omega_2) = \frac{1}{M} \sum_{m=1}^{M} X^m(\omega_1) Y^m(\omega_2) X^{m*}(\omega_1 + \omega_2) \tag{26.17}$$

In theory, both methods will lead to the same cross-bispectrum when data length is infinite. However, with finite data records, direct and indirect methods generally lead to cross-bispectrum estimates with different shapes (Figure 26.4). Therefore, like power spectrum estimation, users have to choose an appropriate method to extract the information desired.

Defining Terms

Bispectra: Computation of the frequency distribution of the EEG exhibiting nonlinear behavior.

Cross-spectra: Computation of the energy in the frequency distribution of two different electrical signals.

Electroencephalogram (EEG): Recordings of the electrical potentials produced by the brain.

Fast Fourier transform (FFT): Algorithms that permit rapid computation of the Fourier transform of an electrical signal, thereby representing it in the frequency domain.

Magnitude squared coherence (MSC): A measure of the degree of synchrony between two electrical signals at specified frequencies.

Power spectral analysis: Computation of the energy in the frequency distribution of an electrical signal.

Quadratic phase coupling (QPC): A measure of the degree to which specific frequencies interact to produce a third frequency.

References

Barlow J.S. 1993. *The Electroencephalogram.* Cambridge, MA: MIT Press.

Brazier M. 1968. *Electrical Activity of the Nervous System*, 3rd ed. Baltimore, Williams & Wilkins.

Bronzino J.D. 1984. Quantitative analysis of the EEG: general concepts and animal studies. *IEEE Trans. Biomed. Eng.* 31: 850.

Bronzino J.D. 2000. *Principles of Electroencephalography. The Biomedical Engineering Handbook*, Vol. 1, pp. 15.1–12. Boca Raton, FL, CRC Press, 1st ed., 1995; 2nd ed., 2000.

Cooley J.W. and Tukey J.S. 1965. An algorithm for the machine calculation of complex Fourier series. *Math. Comput.* 19: 267.

Dempster J. 1993. *Computer Analysis of Electrophysiological Signals.* New York, NY: Academic Press.

Kondraske G.V. 1986. *Neurophysiological Measurements. Biomedical Engineering and Instrumentation*, pp. 138–179. Boston, PWS Publishing.

Ning T. and Bronzino J.D. 1989a. Bispectral analysis of the rat EEG during different vigilance states. *IEEE Trans. Biomed. Eng.* 36: 497.

Ning T. and Bronzino J.D. 1989b. Bispectral analysis of the EEG in developing rats. In *Proceedings of the Workshop Higher-Order Spectral Analysis*, Vail, CO, pp. 235–238.

Ning T. and Bronzino J.D. 1990. Autoregressive and bispectral analysis techniques: EEG applications. Special Issue on Biomedical Signal Processing. *IEEE Eng. Med. Biol. Mag.* 9: 47.

Smith J.R. 1986. Automated analysis of sleep EEG data. In *Clinical Applications of Computer Analysis of EEG and Other Neurophysiological Signals, EEG Handbook*, revised series, Vol. 2, pp. 93–130. Amsterdam, Elsevier.

Further Information

See the journals, *IEEE Transactions in Biomedical Engineering* and *Electroencephalography* and *Clinical Neurophysiology*.

27

Biomagnetism

Jaakko Malmivuo
Tampere University of Technology

Since the first detection of the magnetocardiogram (MCG) in 1963 by Baule and McFee [Baule and McFee, 1963], new diagnostic information from biomagnetic signals has been widely anticipated. The first recording of the magnetoencephalogram (MEG) was made in 1968 by David Cohen [Cohen, 1968], but it was not possible to record biomagnetic signals with good signal quality before the invention of the superconducting quantum interference device (SQUID) in 1970 [Zimmerman et al., 1970].

27.1 Theoretical Background

27.1.1 Origin of Bioelectric and Biomagnetic Signals

In 1819, Hans Christian Örsted demonstrated that when an electric current flows in a conductor, it generates a magnetic field around it [Örsted, 1820]. This fundamental connection between electricity and magnetism was expressed in exact form by James Clerk Maxwell in 1864 [Maxwell, 1865]. In bioelectromagnetism, this means that when electrically active tissue produces a bioelectric field, it simultaneously produces a biomagnetic field as well. Thus the origin of both the bioelectric and the biomagnetic signals is the bioelectric activity of the tissue.

The following equations describe the electric potential field and the magnetic field of a volume source distribution $\bar{J}^i$ in an inhomogeneous volume conductor. The inhomogeneous volume conductor is represented by a piecewise homogeneous conductor where the regions of different conductivity σ are separated by surfaces S.

$$4\pi\sigma\Phi(r) = \int_v \bar{J}^i \cdot \nabla\left(\frac{1}{r}\right) dv + \sum_j \int_{S_j} (\sigma_j'' - \sigma_j')\Phi\nabla\left(\frac{1}{r}\right) dS_j \tag{27.1}$$

$$4\pi\bar{H}(r) = \int_v \bar{J}^i \cdot \nabla\left(\frac{1}{r}\right) dv + \sum_j \int_{S_j} (\sigma_j'' - \sigma_j')\Phi\nabla\left(\frac{1}{r}\right) dS_j \tag{27.2}$$

The first term on the right-hand side of Equation 27.1 and Equation 27.2 describes the *contribution of the volume source*, and the second term describes the contribution of boundaries separating regions of different conductivity, that is, the *contribution of the inhomogeneities* within the volume conductor. These equations were developed by David Geselowitz [Geselowitz, 1967, 1970].

27.1.2 Measurement of the Biomagnetic Signals

The amplitude of the biomagnetic signals is very low. The strongest of them is the MCG, having an amplitude on the order of 50 pT. This is roughly one-millionth of the static magnetic field of the earth. The amplitude of the MEG is roughly 1% of that of the MCG. This means that, in practice, the MEG can only be measured with the SQUID and that the measurements must be done in a magnetically shielded room. The MCG, instead, can be measured in the clinical environment without magnetic shielding.

27.1.3 Independence of Bioelectric and Biomagnetic Signals

The source of the biomagnetic signal is the electric activity of the tissue. Therefore, the most interesting and most important question in biomagnetism is whether the biomagnetic signals contain new information that cannot be obtained from bioelectric signals; in other words, whether the bioelectric and biomagnetic signals are fully independent or whether there is some interdependence. If the signals were fully independent, the biomagnetic measurement would possibly give about the same amount of new information as the bioelectric method. If there were some interdependence, the amount of new information would be reduced.

Helmholtz's theorem states that "A general vector field, that vanishes at infinity, can be completely represented as the sum of two independent vector fields, one that is irrotational (zero curl) and another that is solenoidal (zero divergence)" [Morse and Feshbach, 1953; Plonsey and Collin, 1961]. The impressed current density $\bar{J}^i$ is a vector field that vanishes at infinity and, according to the theorem, may be expressed as the sum of two components:

$$\bar{J}^i = \bar{J}^i_F + \bar{J}^i_V \tag{27.3}$$

where the subscripts F and V denote *flow* and *vortex*, respectively. By definition, these vector fields satisfy $\nabla \times \bar{J}^i_F = 0$ and $\nabla \times \bar{J}^i_V = 0$. We first examine the independence of the electric and magnetic signals in the infinite homogeneous case, when the second term on the right-hand side of Equation 27.1 and Equation 27.2, caused by inhomogeneities, is zero. The equation for the electric potential may be rewritten as

$$4\pi\sigma\Phi = \int_v \nabla\left(\frac{1}{r}\right)\cdot \bar{J}^i \mathrm{d}v = \int_v \frac{\nabla\cdot\bar{J}^i}{r}\mathrm{d}v \tag{27.4}$$

and that for the magnetic field may be rewritten as

$$4\pi\bar{H} = -\int_v \nabla\left(\frac{1}{r}\right)\times \bar{J}^i \mathrm{d}v = -\int_v \frac{\nabla\times\bar{J}^i}{r}\mathrm{d}v \tag{27.5}$$

Substituting Equation 27.3 into Equation 27.4 and Equation 27.5 shows that under homogeneous and unbounded conditions, the bioelectric field arises from $\nabla\cdot\bar{J}^i_F$, which is the *flow source*, and the biomagnetic field arises from $\nabla\times\bar{J}^i_V$, which is the *vortex source*. For this reason, in the early days of biomagnetic research it was generally believed that the bioelectric and biomagnetic signals were fully independent. However, it was soon recognized that this could not be the case. For example, when the heart beats, it produces an electric field recorded as the P, QRS, and T waves of the ECG, and it simultaneously produces the corresponding magnetic waves recorded as the MCG. Thus the ECG and MCG signals are not fully independent.

There have been several attempts to explain the independence/interdependence of bioelectric and biomagnetic signals. Usually these attempts discuss different detailed experiments and fail to give a satisfying general explanation. This important issue may be easily explained by considering the sensitivity distributions of the ECG and MCG lead systems, and this will be discussed in the next section.

27.2 Sensitivity Distribution of Dipolar Electric and Magnetic Leads

27.2.1 Concepts of Lead Vector and Lead Field

27.2.1.1 Lead Vector

Let us assume that two electrodes (or sets of electrodes) are placed on a volume conductor to form a lead. Let us further assume that inside the volume conductor in a certain location Q there is placed a unit dipole consecutively in the x, y, and z directions (Figure 27.1a). Due to the sources, we measure from the lead the signals c_x, c_y, and c_z, respectively. Due to *linearity*, if instead of the unit dipoles we place in the source location dipoles that are p_x, p_y, and p_z times the unit vectors, we measure signals that are $c_x p_x$, $c_y p_y$, and $c_z p_z$, respectively.

If these dipoles are placed simultaneously to the source location, due to the principle of *superposition*, we measure from the lead a voltage, that is,

$$V = c_x p_x + c_y p_y + c_z p_z \tag{27.6}$$

These dipoles can be considered to be components of a dipole $\bar{p}$, that is, $\bar{p} = p_x\bar{i} + p_y\bar{j} + p_z\bar{k}$. We may understand the coefficients c_x, c_y, and c_z to be components of a vector $\bar{c}$, that is, $\bar{c} = c_x\bar{i} + c_y\bar{j} + c_z\bar{k}$. Now we may express the lead voltage Equation 27.6 as the scalar product of the vector $\bar{c}$ and the dipole $\bar{p}$ as

$$V = \bar{c}\cdot\bar{p} \tag{27.7}$$

The vector $\bar{c}$ is a three-dimensional transfer coefficient that describes how a dipole source $\bar{p}$ at a fixed point Q inside a volume conductor influences the voltage measured from the lead and is called the *lead vector*.

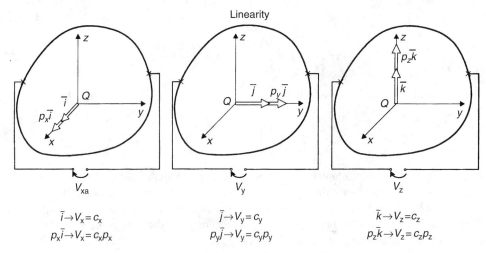

Because of linearity, in each case V is linearly proportional to the dipole magnitude.

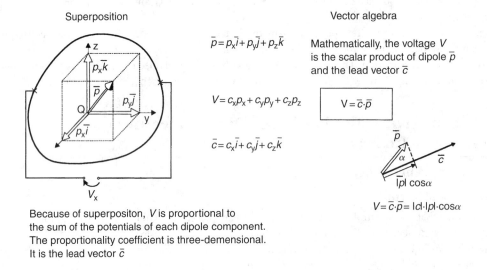

Because of superpositon, V is proportional to
the sum of the potentials of each dipole component.
The proportionality coefficient is three-demensional.
It is the lead vector $\bar{c}$

FIGURE 27.1   The concepts of (a) lead vector and (b) lead field. (See the text for more details.)

The lead vector $\bar{c}$ describes what is the sensitivity of the lead to a source locating at the source location. It is self-evident that for another source location the sensitivity may have another value. Thus the sensitivity, that is, the lead vector, varies as a function of the location, and we may say that it has a certain distribution in the volume conductor. This is called the *sensitivity distribution*.

27.2.1.2 Lead Field

We may define the value of the lead vector at every point in the volume conductor. If we then place the lead vectors to the points for which they are defined, we have a field of lead vectors throughout the volume conductor. This field of lead vectors is called the *lead field* J_L. The lead field illustrates the behavior of the sensitivity in the volume conductor and is a very powerful tool in analyzing the properties of electric and magnetic leads (see Figure 27.1b).

It follows from the *principle of reciprocity*, described by Hermann von Helmholtz in 1853 [Helmholtz, 1853], that the lead field is identical to the electric current field that arises in the volume conductor if a unit current, called reciprocal current I_R, is fed to the lead.

Field of lead vectors

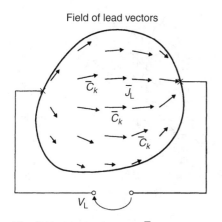

The field of the lead vectors $\bar{c}_k$ is the lead field $\bar{J}_L$

Lead voltage

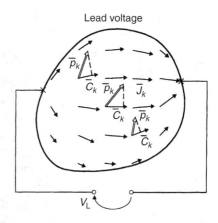

Each dipole element p_k con-
tributes to the lead voltage by $V_k = \bar{c}_k \cdot \bar{p}_k$
The toal lead voltage is the sum
of the lead voltage elements $V_L = \sum_k \bar{c}_k \cdot \bar{p}_k$

Reciprocity

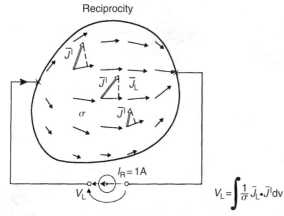

$$V_L = \int \frac{1}{\sigma} \bar{J}_L \cdot \bar{J}^i dv$$

Because of reciprocity, the field of lead vectors $\bar{J}_L$
is the same as the current field $\bar{J}_L$ raised by
feeding a reciprocal current of 1A to the lead.

Alternative illustration

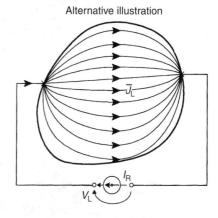

The lead field may also be illustrated
with lead field current flow lines.

FIGURE 27.1   Continued.

When we know the lead field $\bar{J}_L$, we can determine the signal V_L in the lead due to the volume source distribution $\bar{J}^i$. For each source element the signal is, of course, proportional to the dot product of the source element and the lead field at the source location, as shown in Equation 27.7. The contributions of the whole volume source is obtained by integrating this throughout the volume source. Thus the signal the volume source generates to the lead is

$$V_L = \int \frac{1}{\sigma} \bar{J}_L \cdot \bar{J}^i dv \qquad (27.8)$$

The lead field may be illustrated either with lead vectors in certain locations in the volume conductor or as the flow lines of the distribution of the reciprocal current in the volume conductor. This is called the *lead current field*. In the latter presentation, the lead field current flow lines are oriented in the direction of the sensitivity, and their density is proportional to the magnitude of the sensitivity.

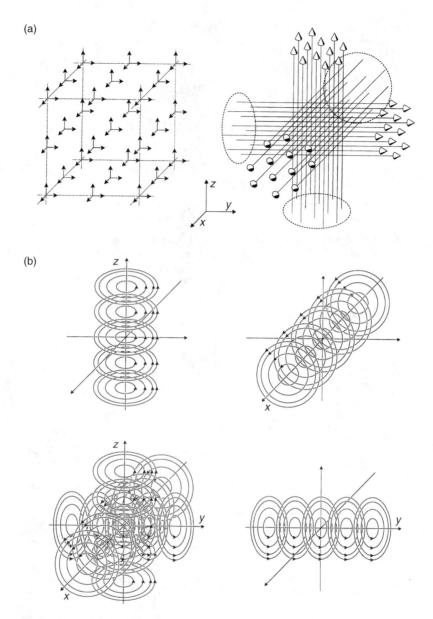

FIGURE 27.2 Sensitivity distributions, that is, lead fields of lead systems detecting (a) electric and (b) magnetic dipole moments of a volume source. The lead field of the electric lead is shown both with vectors representing the magnitude and direction of the lead field (on the left) and with lead field current flow lines (on the right).

27.2.2 Lead Fields of Leads Detecting the Electric and Magnetic Dipole Moments of a Volume Source

27.2.2.1 Electric Lead

The sensitivity of a lead system that detects the electric dipole moment of a volume source consists of three orthogonal components (Figure 27.2a). Each of these is linear and homogeneous. In other words, one component of the electric dipole moment is detected when the corresponding component of all elements of the impressed current density $\bar{J}^i$ are detected with the same sensitivity throughout the source area.

27.2.2.2 Magnetic Lead

The sensitivity distribution of a lead system that detects the magnetic dipole moment of a volume source also consists of three orthogonal components (Figure 27.2b). Each of these has such a form that the sensitivity is always tangentially oriented around the symmetry axis (the coordinate axis). The magnitude of the sensitivity is proportional to the radial distance from the symmetry axis and is zero on the symmetry axis.

27.2.3 Independence of Dipolar Electric and Magnetic Leads

27.2.3.1 Electric Lead

The sensitivity distributions of the three components of the lead system detecting the electric dipole moment of a volume source are orthogonal. This means that none of them can be obtained as a linear combination of the two other ones. (Note that any fourth measurement having a similar linear sensitivity distribution would always be a linear combination of the three previous ones.) Thus the sensitivity distributions, that is, the leads, are orthogonal and thus independent. However, because the three electric signals are only different aspects of the same volume source, they are not (fully) independent.

27.2.3.2 Magnetic Lead

The sensitivity distributions of the three components of the lead system detecting the magnetic dipole moment of a volume source are also orthogonal, meaning that no one of them can be obtained as a linear combination of the two other ones. Thus, similarly, as in measurement of the electric dipole moment, the sensitivity distributions, that is, the leads, are orthogonal and thus independent. However, because the three magnetic signals are only different aspects of the same volume source, they are not (fully) independent.

On the basis of the sensitivity distributions, we also can similarly explain the independence between the electric and magnetic signals. According to Helmholtz's theorem, the electric leads are orthogonal to the three magnetic leads. This means that none of these six leads can be obtained as a linear combination of the other five. However, the six signals, which they measure, are not independent because they arise from the same electrically active volume source.

27.3 Magnetocardiography

27.3.1 Selection of the Source Model for MCG

In ECG and MCG it is the clinical problem to solve the inverse problem, that is, to solve the source of the detected signal in order to get information about the anatomy and physiology of the source. Although the actual clinical diagnostic procedure is based on measuring certain parameters, such as time intervals and amplitudes, from the detected signal and actually not to display the components of the source, the selection of the source model is very important from the point of view of available information.

In clinical ECG, the source model is a dipole. This is the model for both the 12-lead ECG and vectorcardiography (VCG). In 12-lead ECG, the volume conductor (thorax) model is not considered, which causes considerable distortion of the leads. In VCG, only the form of the volume conductor is modeled. This decreases the distortion in the lead fields but does not eliminate it completely. Note that today the display systems used in these ECG and VCG systems do not play any role in the diagnostic procedure because the computerized diagnosis is always based on the signals, not on the display.

In selection of the source model for MCG, it is logical, at least initially, to select the magnetic source model to be on the same theoretical level with the ECG. Only in this way is it possible to compare the diagnostic performance of these methods. It is clear, of course, that if the source model is more accurate, that is, has more independent variables, the diagnostic performance is better, but when comparing ECG and MCG, the comparison is relevant only if their complexity is similar [Malmivuo and Plonsey, 1995].

(a)   (b)

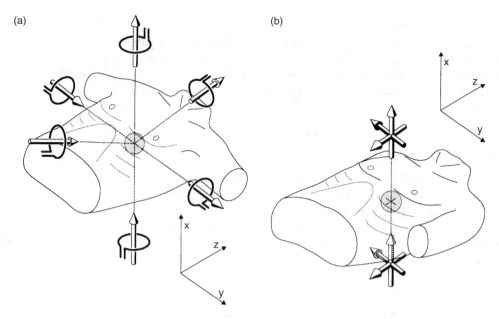

FIGURE 27.3   Measurement of the three orthogonal components of the magnetic dipole moment of the heart (a) on the coordinate axis (*xyz* lead system) and (b) at a single location over and under the chest (unipositional lead system).

27.3.2   Detection of the Equivalent Magnetic Dipole of the Heart

The basic detection method of the equivalent magnetic dipole moment of a volume source is to measure the magnetic field on each coordinate axis in the direction of that axis. To idealize the sensitivity distribution throughout the volume source, the measurements must be made at a distance that is large compared with the source dimensions. This, of course, decreases the signal amplitude. The quality of the measurement may be increased considerably if bipolar measurements are used; that is, measurements are made on both sides of the source. Measurement of the magnetic field on each coordinate axis is, however, difficult to perform in MCG due to the geometry of the human body. It would require either six sequential measurements with one magnetometer (dewar) or six simultaneous measurements using six dewars (Figure 27.3).

It has been shown [Malmivuo, 1976] that all three components of the magnetic dipole also can be measured from a single location. Applying this unipositional method symmetrically so that measurements are made on both the anterior and posterior sides of the thorax at the same distance from the heart, only two dewars are needed and a very high quality of lead fields is obtained. Figure 27.4 illustrates the sensitivity distributions in nonsymmetrical and symmetrical measurements [Malmivuo and Plonsey, 1995].

27.3.3   Diagnostic Performance of ECG and MCG

The diagnostic performances of ECG and MCG were compared in an extensive study made at the Ragnar Granit Institute [Oja, 1993]. The study was made using the asymmetrical unipositional lead system, that is, making measurements only on the anterior side of the thorax. The patient material was selected, however, so that myocardial changes were located dominantly on the anterior side.

This study consisted of 290 normal subjects and 259 patients with different myocardial disorders. It was found that the diagnostic performance of ECG and MCG is about the same (83%). Diagnostic parameters were then selected from both ECG and MCG. With this combined method, called *electromagnetocardiogram* (EMCG), a diagnostic performance of 90% was obtained. This improvement in diagnostic

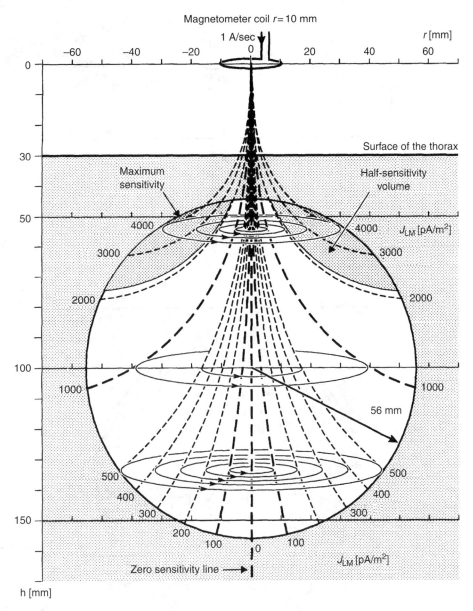

FIGURE 27.4   Sensitivity distributions in the measurement of the magnetic dipole moment of the heart. (a) Non-symmetrical and (b) symmetrical measurements of the x component. (c) Symmetrical measurement of the y and z components.

performance was obtained without increasing the number of parameters used in the diagnostic procedure. Moreover, this improvement is significant because it means that the number of incorrectly diagnosed patients was reduced by approximately 50%.

This important result may be explained as follows: The lead system recording the electric dipole moment of the volume source has three independent leads. (This is also the case in the 12-lead ECG system.) Similarly, the lead system detecting the magnetic dipole moment of the volume source has three independent leads. Therefore, the diagnostic performances of these methods are about the same. However, because the sensitivity distributions of electric and magnetic leads are different, the patient groups diagnosed correctly with both methods are not identical.

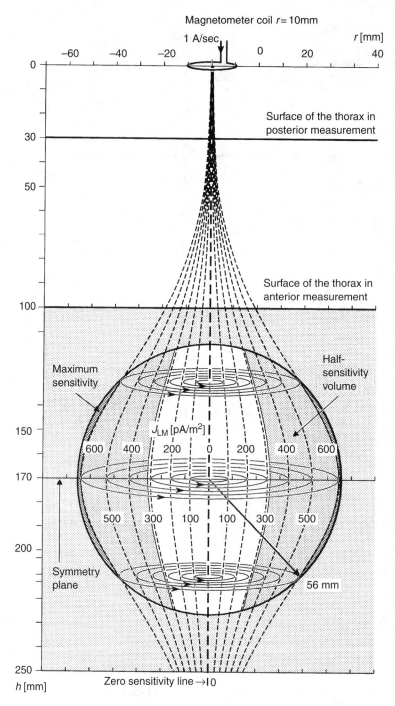

FIGURE 27.4 Continued.

As stated before, the electric leads are independent of the magnetic leads. If the diagnostic procedure simultaneously uses both the ECG and the MCG leads, we obtain $3 + 3 = 6$ independent leads, and the correctly diagnosed patient groups may be combined. Thus the diagnostic performance of the combined method is better than that of either method alone. This is the first large-scale statistically relevant study of the clinical diagnostic performance of biomagnetism.

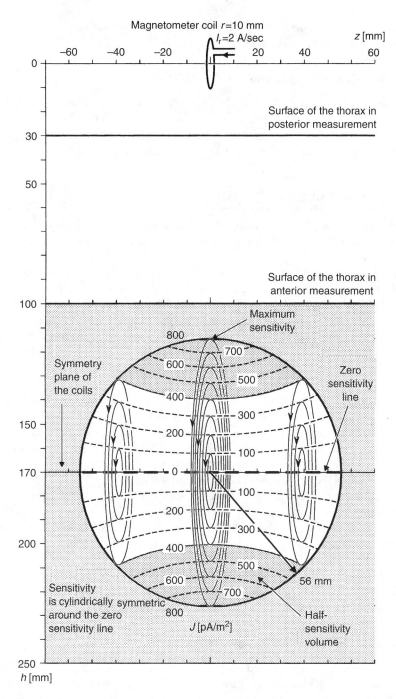

FIGURE 27.4 Continued.

27.3.4 Technical Reasons to Use the MCG

The technical differences between ECG and MCG include the MCG's far better ability to record static sources, sources on the posterior side of the heart, monitor the fetal heart, and perform electrodeless recording. As a technical drawback, it should be mentioned that the MCG instrument costs 2 to 3 times more. An important feature of MCG is that, unlike the MEG instrument, it does not need a magnetically shielded room. This is very important because the shielded room is not only very expensive but also limits application of the technique to a certain laboratory space.

27.3.5 Theoretical Reasons to Use the MCG

It has been shown that MCG has clinical value and that it can be used either alone or in combination with ECG as a new technique called the *electromagnetocardiogram* (EMCG). The diagnostic performance of the combined method is better than that of either ECG or MCG alone. With the combined method, the number of incorrectly diagnosed patients may be reduced by approximately 50%.

27.4 Magnetoencephalography

Similarly as in the cardiac applications, in the magnetic measurement of the electric activity of the brain, the benefits and drawbacks of the MEG can be divided into theoretical and technical ones. First, the theoretical aspects are discussed.

The two main theoretical aspects in favor of MEG are that it is believed that because the skull is transparent for magnetic fields, the MEG should be able to concentrate its measurement sensitivity in a smaller region than the EEG, and that the sensitivity distribution of these methods are fundamentally different. These questions are discussed in the following: The analysis is made using the classic spherical head model introduced by Rush and Driscoll [1969]. In this model, the head is represented with three concentric spheres, where the outer radii of the scalp, skull, and brain are 92, 85, and 80 mm, respectively. The resistivities of the scalp and the brain are 2.22 Ω cm, and that of the skull is 80 times higher, being 177 Ω cm.

The two basic magnetometer constructions in use in MEG are axial and planar gradiometers. In the former, both coils are coaxial, and in the latter, they are coplanar. The minimum distance of the coil from the scalp in a superconducting magnetometer is about 20 mm. The coil radius is usually about 10 mm. It has been shown [Malmivuo and Plonsey, 1995] that with this measurement distance, decreasing the coil radius does not change the distribution of the sensitivity in the brain region. In the following the sensitivity distribution of these gradiometer constructions is discussed.

To indicate the magnetometer's ability to concentrate its sensitivity to a small region, the concept of *half-sensitivity volume* has been defined. This concept means the region in the source area (brain) where the detector sensitivity is one-half or more from the maximum sensitivity. The smaller the half-sensitivity volume, the better is the detector's ability to focus its sensitivity to a small region.

In magnetocardiography, it is relevant to detect the magnetic dipole moment of the volume source of the heart and to make the sensitivity distribution within the heart region as independent of the position in the axial direction as possible. In magnetoencephalography, however, the primary purpose is to detect the electric activity of the cortex and to localize the regions of certain activity.

27.4.1 Sensitivity Distribution of the Axial Magnetometer

In a cylindrically symmetrical volume conductor model, the lead field flow lines are concentric circles and do not cut the discontinuity boundaries. Therefore, the sensitivity distribution in the brain area of the spherical model equals that in an infinite, homogeneous volume conductor.

Figure 27.5 illustrates the sensitivity distribution of an axial magnetometer. The thin solid lines illustrates the lead field flow lines. The dashed lines join the points where the sensitivity has the same value, being thus so-called isosensitivity lines. The half-sensitivity volume is represented by the shaded region.

27.4.2 Sensitivity Distribution of the Planar Gradiometer

Figure 27.6 illustrates the sensitivity distribution of a planar gradiometer. Again, the thin solid lines illustrate the lead field flow lines, and the dashed lines represent the isosensitivity lines. The half-sensitivity

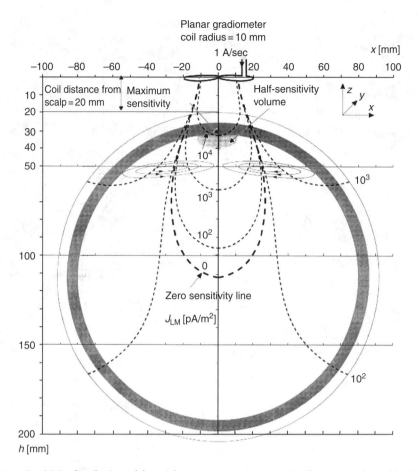

FIGURE 27.5 Sensitivity distribution of the axial magnetometer in measuring the MEG (spherical lead model).

volume is represented by the shaded region. The sensitivity of the planar gradiometer is concentrated under the center of the two coils and is mainly linearly oriented. Further, there exist two zero-sensitivity lines.

27.4.3 Half-Sensitivity Volumes of Electro- and Magnetoencephalography Leads

The half-sensitivity volumes for different EEG and MEG leads as a function of electrode distance and gradiometer baselines are shown in Figure 27.7. The minimum half-sensitivity volume is, of course, achieved with the shortest distance/baseline. For three- and two-electrode EEG leads, the half-sensitivity volumes at 1 degree of electrode distance are 0.2 and 1.2 cm^3, respectively. For 10-mm-radius planar and axial gradiometer MEG leads, these volumes at 1 degree of coil separation (i.e., 1.6-mm baseline for axial gradiometer) are 3.4 and 21.8 cm^3, respectively.

The 20-mm coil distance from scalp and 10-mm coil radii are realistic for the helmet-like whole-head MEG detector. There exist, however, MEG devices for recording at a limited region where the coil distance and the coil radii are on the order of 1 mm. Therefore, the half-sensitivity volumes for planar gradiometers with 1-mm coil radius at 0- to 20-mm recording distances are also illustrated in Figure 27.7. These curves show that when the recording distance is about 12 mm and the distance/baseline is 1 mm, such a planar gradiometer has about the same half-sensitivity volume as the two-electrode EEG.

Short separation will, of course, also decrease the signal amplitude. An optimal value is about 10 degrees of separation. Increasing the separation to 10 degrees increases the EEG and MEG signal amplitudes to

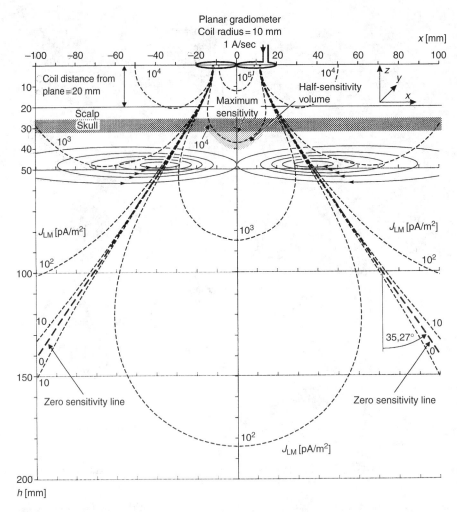

FIGURE 27.6 Sensitivity distribution of the planar gradiometer (half-space model).

approximately 70 to 80% of their maximum value, but the half-sensitivity volumes do not increase considerably from their values at 1 degree of separation.

Thus, contrary to general belief, the EEG has a better ability to focus its sensitivity to a small region in the brain than the whole-head MEG. At about 20 to 30 degrees of separation, the two-electrode EEG lead needs slightly smaller separation to achieve the same half-sensitivity volume as the planar gradiometer. The sensitivity distributions of these leads are, however, very similar. Note that if the sensitivity distributions of two different lead systems, whether they are electric or magnetic, are the same, they detect exactly the same source and produce exactly the same signal. Therefore, the planar gradiometer and two-electrode EEG lead detect very similar source distributions.

27.4.4 Sensitivity of EEG and MEG to Radial and Tangential Sources

The three-electrode EEG has its maximum sensitivity under that electrode which forms the terminal alone. This sensitivity is mainly directed radially to the spherical head model. With short electrode distances, the sensitivity of the two-electrode EEG is directed mainly tangentially to the spherical head model. Thus with the EEG it is possible to detect sources in all three orthogonal directions, that is, in the radial and in the two tangential directions, in relation to the spherical head model.

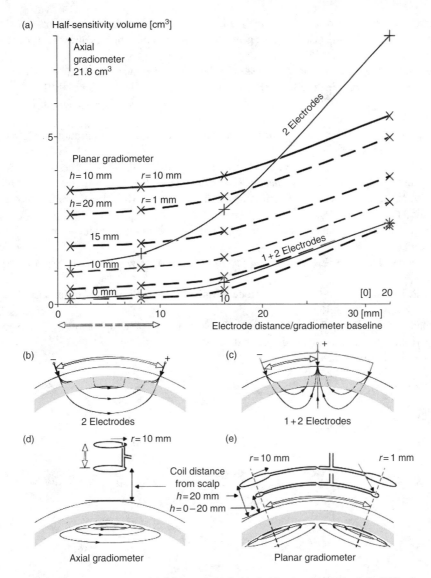

FIGURE 27.7 Half-sensitivity volumes of different EEG leads (*dashed lines*) and MEG leads (*solid lines*) as a function of electrode distance and gradiometer baseline, respectively.

In the axial gradiometer MEG lead, the sensitivity is directed tangentially to the gradiometer symmetry axis and thus also tangentially to the spherical head model. In the planar gradiometer, the sensitivity has its maximum under the center of the coils and is directed mainly linearly and tangentially to the spherical head model. The MEG lead fields are oriented tangentially to the spherical head model everywhere. This may be easily understood by recognizing that the lead field current does not flow through the surface of the head because no electrodes are used. Therefore, the MEG can only detect sources oriented in the two tangential directions in relation to the spherical head model.

References

Baule, G.M. and McFee, R. 1963. Detection of the magnetic field of the heart. *Am. Heart J.* 55: 95.
Cohen, D. 1968. Magnetoencephalography: evidence of magnetic fields produced by alpha-rhythm currents. *Science* 161: 784.

Geselowitz, D.B. 1967. On bioelectric potentials in an inhomogeneous volume conductor. *Biophys. J.* 7: 1.

Geselowitz, D.B. 1970. On the magnetic field generated outside an inhomogeneous volume conductor by internal current sources. *IEEE Trans. Magn. MAG*-6: 346.

Helmholtz, H.L.F. 1853. Ueber einige Gesetze der Vertheilung elektrischer Ströme in körperlichen Leitern mit Anwendung auf die thierisch-elektrischen Versuche. *Ann. Physik. Chem.* 89: 211.

Malmivuo, J. and Plonsey, R. 1995. *Bioelectromagnetism: Principles and Applications of Bioelectric and Biomagnetic Fields.* New York, Oxford University Press.

Malmivuo, J.A. 1976. On the detection of the magnetic heart vector: An application of the reciprocity theorem. *Acta Polytechnol. Scand.* 39: 112.

Maxwell, J. 1865. A dynamical theory of the electromagnetic field. *Phil. Trans. R. Soc. (Lond.)* 155: 459.

More, P.M. and Feshbach, H. 1953. *Methods of Theoretical Physics, Part I.* New York, McGraw-Hill.

Oja, O.S. 1993. Vector magnetocardiogram in myocardial disorders, M.D. thesis, University of Tampere, Medical Faculty.

Örsted, H.C. 1820. Experimenta circa effectum conflictus electrici in acum magneticam. *J. F. Chem. Phys.* 29: 275.

Plonsey, R. and Collin, R. 1961. *Principles and Applications of Electromagnetic Fields.* New York, McGraw-Hill.

Rush, S. and Driscoll, D.A. 1969. EEG-electrode sensitivity: An application of reciprocity. *IEEE Trans. Biomed. Eng. BME*-16: 15.

Zimmerman, J.E., Thiene, P., and Hardings, J. 1970. Design and operation of stable rf biased superconducting point-contact quantum devices. *J. Appl. Phys.* 41: 1572.

28

Electrical Stimulation of Excitable Systems

Dominique M. Durand
Case Western Reserve University

28.1 Introduction

Functional electrical stimulation (FES) of neural tissue provides a method to restore normal function to neurologically impaired individuals. By inserting electrode inside or near nerves, it is possible to activate pathways to the brain or to muscles. Functional nerve stimulation (FNS) is often used to describe applications of electrical stimulation in the peripheral nervous system. Neural prostheses refer to applications for which electrical stimulation is used to replace a function previously lost or damaged.

Electrical stimulation has been used to treat several types of neurological dysfunction with varying amount of success [see Hambrecht, 1979]. For example, electrical stimulation of the auditory nerves to restore hearing in deaf patients has proved to be not only feasible but also clinically useful [Clark, 1990]. Similarly, the phrenic nerve of patients with high-level spinal cord injury can be stimulated to produce diaphragm contractions and restore ventilation [Glenn, 1984]. Electrical stimulation of the visual cortex produces visual sensations called phosphenes [Brindley, 1968] and a visual prosthesis for the blind is currently being tested. Electrical stimulation in the peripheral nerves of paralyzed patients can restore partial function of both the upper extremities for hand function [Peckham and Mortimer, 1977] and lower extremities for gait [Marsolais and Kobetic, 1988]. Several other attempts were not so successful. Electrical stimulation of the cerebellum cortex for controlling epileptic seizures has been tried but was not reliable. However, a new method involving the stimulation of the vagus nerve looks promising [Rutecki, 1990]. There are many other applications of electrical stimulation of the nervous system and many problems associated with each one but it is now clear that the potential and the limits of the technique have not yet been realized.

Stimulation of the nervous system can also be achieved with magnetic field [Chokroverty, 1990]. A coil is placed near the excitable tissue and a capacitor is rapidly discharged into the coil. Large magnetic fluxes are generated and the induced electrical fields can generate excitation. Magnetic stimulation has several advantages over electrical stimulation. Magnetic fields can easily penetrate low-conductivity tissues such as bone and the stimulation it is completely noninvasive. However, magnetic stimulation requires a large amount of energy and the magnetic field is difficult to localize. Magnetic stimulation of excitable tissue shares many aspects with electrical stimulation since the electrical field is, in both cases, the source of the stimulus [Roth and Basser, 1990]. However, there are several important differences [Durand et al., 1989; Nagarajan and Durand, 1993] that are not reviewed below.

What is the basis for the effect of electric stimulation of the nervous system? Clearly, it comes from the fact that a propagated action potential can be triggered by applying a rapidly changing electric field near excitable tissue. This fact was demonstrated early in this century and clinical experimental applications resulted in the 1950s with the highly successful cardiac pacemaker. Other clinical applications have been slow in coming for several reasons that are to be discussed in later sections of this chapter. One of the difficulties is that the fundamental principles of the interaction of electrical fields and neurons is not completely understood. In order to understand how applied currents can generate excitation, it will be necessary to describe the mechanisms underlying excitation (Section 28.1), the distribution of currents inside the volume conductor (Section 28.2), and the interaction between the axon and applied electric fields (Section 28.3).

Another difficulty lies at the interface between electrodes applying the current and neural tissue to be stimulated. Electrons carry current in the wires to the electrodes whereas current in the volume conductor is carried by ions. Chemical reactions at the interface will take place and these reactions are still poorly understood. The waveforms used to apply the current can significantly affect the threshold, the electrochemistry at the electrode site, and tissue damage. These issues are reviewed in Section 28.4.

28.2 Physiology of Excitation

Electrical stimulation of excitable tissue is mediated by artificially depolarizing membrane containing channels capable of producing action potentials. Action potentials are normally elicited by synaptic currents, which in turn produce depolarization of the somatic membrane. The sodium channels are responsible for the generation of the depolarizing phase of the action potential and are sensitive to membrane voltage [Ferreira and Marschall, 1985]. Once initiated in the soma, the action potential is carried unattenuated along the axon to its intended target such as another neuron or neuromuscular junction for muscle contraction (see Figure 28.1). Unmyelinated axons have ionic channels distributed throughout their membrane and the action potential is carried smoothly along their length. The membrane of the axons containing the channels behaves as resistive and capacitive elements limiting the conduction velocity. Myelinated axons are surrounded by an insulation sheath of myelin, which significantly decreases the membrane capacitance, thereby increasing the speed of propagation. Conduction of the action potential is no longer smooth but takes place in discrete steps (saltatory conduction). The myelin sheath is broken at regularly spaced intervals (nodes of Ranvier) to allow the current to flow through the membrane [Aidley, 1978].

Action potential can be artificially generated by placing electrodes directly inside a cell. Current flowing from the inside to the outside will produce depolarization followed by excitation provided that the current amplitude is large enough. This technique cannot be used for functional stimulation since we do not yet have the technology to interface electrodes with large numbers of single axons. Therefore electrodes must be placed in the extracellular space near the tissue to be excited. It is then possible to activate simultaneously many cells. However, stimulation must be selective. Selectivity is defined as the ability of a stimulation system to activate any chosen set of axons. For example, the nervous system chooses to recruit small fibers connected to small motor units followed by large fibers connected to large motor units for smooth motor

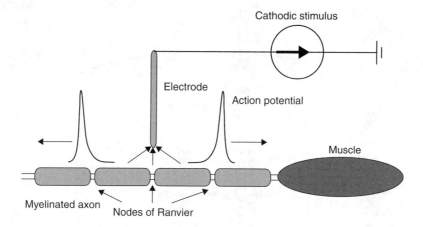

FIGURE 28.1 Electrical stimulation of a myelinated fiber. An electrode is located near the axon and a cathodic stimulus is applied to the electrode. The current flow in and around the axon is described in this chapter and causes depolarization of the membrane at the sites closest to the electrodes. Action potentials are generated underneath the electrode and propagate orthodromically and antidromically.

control. Applied current pulses activate first large fibers and then small fibers with increasing current (reverse recruitment) for reasons described in Section 28.4. The reverse recruitment order as well as our inability to recruit a chosen set of axons within a nerve bundle makes electrical stimulation a powerful but difficult-to-control tool for the activation of the nervous system.

28.3   Electric Fields in Volume Conductors

The excitable tissue to be stimulated (peripheral nerves, motor neurons, CNS neurons, etc.) are in all cases surrounded by an extracellular fluid with a relatively high conductivity (80 to 300 Ω cm). The electrodes used for electrical stimulation are always placed in this "volume conductor" and it is essential to understand how the currents and the electric fields are distributed [Heringa et al., 1982]. The calculation of the current density and electric fields can be easily done in simple cases such as a homogenous conductivity (the same everywhere) and isotropic conductivity (the same in all directions).

Quasi-static formulation: The calculation of the electric fields generated by an electrode located in a conducting volume conductor can be done by solving Maxwell equations. The frequencies used for electric stimulation are generally under 10 kHz, and therefore a simplified set of equations known as the quasi-static formulation can be used [Plonsey, 1969]:

$$\text{Conservation of charge:}\quad \nabla \cdot J = 0 \tag{28.1}$$

$$\text{Gauss' law:}\quad \nabla \cdot E = \frac{\rho}{\varepsilon} \tag{28.2}$$

$$\text{Ohm's law for conductors:}\quad J = \sigma E \tag{28.3}$$

$$\text{Electric field:}\quad E = -\nabla \phi \tag{28.4}$$

where E is the electric field (V/m) defined as gradient of the scalar potential ϕ, J the current density (defined as the current crossing a given surface in A/m^2), σ the conductivity (inverse of resistivity) in S/m, ρ the charge density in C/m^3, ε the permittivity of the medium, and $\nabla \cdot \mathbf{A}$ the divergence of vector $\mathbf{A}$.

Equivalence between dielectric and conductive media: Assuming an infinite homogeneous conducting medium with conductivity σ with a single point source as shown in Figure 28.2a, the current density

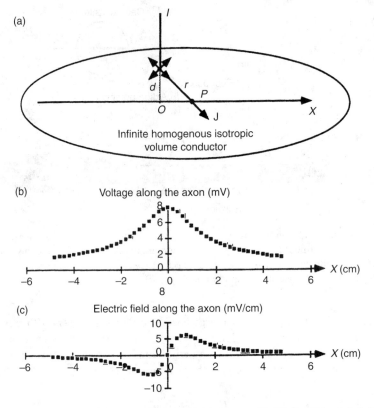

FIGURE 28.2 Voltage and electric field along an axon. (a) The current density J within an infinite, homogenous, and isotropic volume conductor is radial and is inversely proportional to the square of the distance. (b) Voltage along an axon located 1 cm from an anode with 1 mA of current. (c) Electric field along the same axon.

J at any point is the sum of a source term J_s and an ohmic term σE.

$$J = \sigma E + J_s \qquad (28.5)$$

Using Equation 28.1:

$$\nabla \cdot J = \nabla \cdot \sigma E + \nabla \cdot J_s = 0 \qquad (28.6)$$

Since the volume conductor is homogeneous, $\nabla \cdot (\sigma E) = \sigma \nabla \cdot E$ and we then have:

$$\sigma \nabla \cdot E = -\nabla \cdot J_s \qquad (28.7)$$

Since $E = -\nabla \phi$ and $\nabla \cdot (\nabla \mathbf{A})$ is by definition the Laplacian of $\mathbf{A}$, $\nabla^2 \mathbf{A}$, we then have

$$\nabla^2 \phi = \nabla \cdot \frac{J_s}{\sigma} = -\frac{I_v}{\sigma} \qquad (28.8)$$

where I_v is a source term in A/m^3. The source term I_v is zero everywhere except where the sources are located. This equation is nearly identical to the Poisson equation derived from Equation 28.2

[Kraus and Carver, 1973]:

$$\nabla^2 \phi = -\frac{\rho}{\varepsilon} \tag{28.9}$$

derived for dielectric media. Using the following equivalence:

$$\rho \rightarrow I_v$$

$$\varepsilon \rightarrow \sigma$$

the solution of the Poisson equation for dielectric problems can then be used for the solution of the current in volume conductors.

Potential from a monopole source: Given a point source (monopolar) in an infinite homogeneous and isotropic volume conductor connected to a current source I, the potential and currents anywhere can be easily derived. Using spherical symmetry, the current density J at a point P located at a distance r from the source is equal to the total current crossing a spherical surface with radius r (see Figure 28.2).

$$J = \frac{I}{4\pi r^2} \mathbf{u_r} \tag{28.10}$$

where $\mathbf{u_r}$ is the unit radial vector, r the distance between the electrode and the measurement point. The electric field is then obtained from Equation 28.3:

$$E = \frac{I}{4\pi \sigma r^2} \mathbf{u_r} \tag{28.11}$$

The electrical field is the gradient of the potential. In spherical coordinates:

$$E = -\frac{d\phi}{dr} \mathbf{u_r} \tag{28.12}$$

Therefore the potential at point P is obtained by integration:

$$\phi = \frac{I}{4\pi \sigma r} \tag{28.13}$$

It can be easily shown that this solution satisfies the Poisson equation. For a monopolar electrode, the current distribution is radial and is inversely proportional to the conductance of the medium and the distance to the source. The potential decays to zero far away from the electrode and goes to infinity on the electrode. The singularity at $r = 0$ can be eliminated by assuming that the electrode is spherical with finite radius a. Equation 28.13 is then valid on the surface of the electrode $r = a$ and for $r > a$ [Nunez, 1981].

Equation 28.13 can be generalized to several monopolar electrodes. Assuming n electrodes with a current I_i located at a distance r_i from the recording point, the voltage is then given by:

$$\phi = \frac{1}{4\pi \sigma} \sum_n \frac{I_i}{r_i} \tag{28.14}$$

For an axon located in the volume conductor as shown in Figure 28.2, the voltage along the axon located 1 cm away from an anode with a 1-mA current source is given by the following equation and is plotted in

Figure 28.2b:

$$\phi = \frac{I}{4\pi\sigma\sqrt{d^2 + x^2}} \qquad (28.15)$$

The electric field along the axon can be obtained by taking the spatial derivative of Equation 28.15 and is plotted in Figure 28.2b.

Potential from bipolar electrodes and dipoles: In the derivation of the potential generated by a monopolar electrode, the current enters the volume conductor at the tip of the electrode and exits at infinity. However, in the following example (salt water tank), a current is applied through two monopolar electrodes separated by a distance d as shown in Figure 28.3a. The potential generated by this bipolar configuration can be calculated at point P (assuming that the voltage reference is at infinity) as follows:

$$\phi = \frac{I}{4\pi\sigma}\left(\frac{1}{r_1} - \frac{1}{r_2}\right) \qquad (28.16)$$

When the distance d between the two electrodes is small compared to the distance r, the equation for the potential is given by the following dipole equation valid for $r \gg d$:

$$\phi = \frac{Id\cos\theta}{4\pi\sigma r^2} \qquad (28.17)$$

where the angle θ is defined in Figure 28.3. The current distribution for a current dipole is no longer radial and is shown in Figure 28.3b. The voltage along the line perpendicular to the axis of the dipole and passing through a point equidistant from the electrodes is zero. Therefore an axon located in that region would not be excited regardless of the current amplitude. The potential generated by a dipole is inversely proportional to the square of the distance and therefore decays faster than the monopole. Therefore,

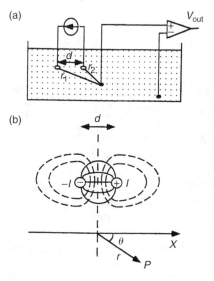

FIGURE 28.3 Voltage generated by bipolar electrodes. (a) Salt water tank. Two electrodes are located within a large tank filled with a conduction solution. The voltage generated by the bipolar arrangement can be measured as shown provided that the reference electrode is located far away from the stimulation electrode. The effect of the stimulation electrode on the reference potential can also be taken into account. (b) Current lines and equipotential voltage distributions (dashed lines) for a dipole. The distance r between the observation P and the electrodes is much greater than the distance d between the electrodes.

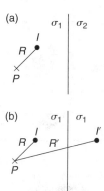

FIGURE 28.4 Method of images. The method of images can be used to calculate the voltage generated by an electrode in a homogenous volume conductor. The two semi-infinite volume conductors with conductivities σ_1 and σ_2 (a) are replaced by a single infinite volume conductor with conductivity σ_1 and an additional image electrode (b).

the dipole configuration will have a more localized excitation region. However, the excitation thresholds are higher since most of the current flows around the electrode. For an observation point located at a distance r from a dipole or monopole with the same current, the ratio of the monopole voltage to that of the dipole voltage is proportional to r/d. Since r is assumed to be much larger than d, then the monopole voltage is much larger than the voltage generated by the dipole.

Inhomogenous volume conductors: For practical applications of electrical stimulation, electrodes are placed in various parts of the body. The volume conductors are clearly not homogenous since we must consider the presence of bone with a conductivity significantly higher than that of extracellular space or even air above the skin with a conductivity of zero. How do those conductivities affect the potentials generated by the electrode? This question can usually only be answered numerically by computer models, which take into account these various compartments such as finite differences, finite elements, or boundary elements methods. A simple solution, however, can be obtained in the case of a semi-infinite homogeneous volume conductor using the method of images. Consider two volume conductors with conductivities σ_1 and σ_2 separated by an infinite plane as shown in Figure 28.4. A monopolar stimulating electrode is placed in region 1. Potential recordings are made in that same region. It can be easily shown that the inhomogenous volume conductor can be replaced by a homogenous volume by adding another current located on the other side of the plane (see Figure 28.4) with an amplitude equal to [Nunez, 1981]:

$$I' = \frac{\sigma_1 - \sigma_2}{\sigma_1 + \sigma_2} I \tag{28.18}$$

The voltage at point P is then given by Equation 28.13. The mirror image theory is only applicable in simple cases but can be useful to obtain approximations when the distance between the recording electrode and the surface of discontinuity is small, thereby approximating an infinite surface [Durand et al., 1992].

28.4 Electric Field Interactions with Excitable Tissue

When axons are placed inside a volume conductor with a stimulation electrode, current flows according to equations derived in the previous section. Some of the current lines enter and exit the axon at different locations and will produce excitation or inhibition. An example of this current distribution is shown in Figure 28.5a for a monopolar anodic electrode. A length Δx of the axonal membrane can be modeled at rest by a capacitance C_m in parallel with a series combination of a battery (E_r) for the resting potential and a resistance R_m simulating the combined resistance at rest of all the membrane channels (see Figure 28.5b).

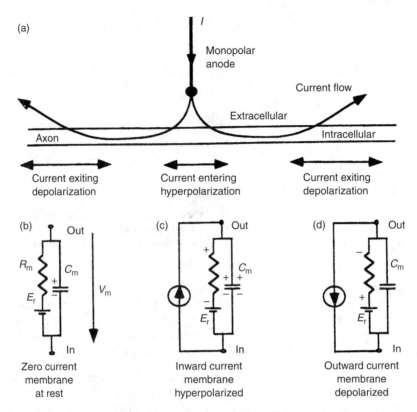

FIGURE 28.5 Effect of extracellular current on axon membrane polarization. (a) A monopolar anode is located near an axon and current enters and exits the membrane. (b) At rest the membrane can be modeled by a simple RC network. (c) When current enters the membrane, charge is added to the membrane capacitance and additive membrane polarization is generated. Therefore the membrane is hyperpolarized. (d) When current exits the axon, the membrane is depolarized.

Nonlinear ionic channels conductances can be added in parallel with the membrane resistance and capacitance. Their contribution at rest is small and becomes significant only around threshold. Since we are interested mainly how to drive the membrane potential toward threshold from resting values, their contribution is ignored. When current enters the membrane flowing from the outside to the inside, the membrane is hyperpolarized (moved closer to threshold) as illustrated in Figure 28.5c. Similarly, when the current exits the membrane, depolarization is generated (the membrane voltage is moved closer to the threshold). In the case of an anodic electrode illustrated in Figure 28.5, stimulation should not take place directly underneath the electrode but further along the axon where the membrane is depolarized.

A more quantitative approach to this problem can be obtained by modeling the interaction of the model with the applied current. The applied current I generates a voltage distribution in the extracellular space, which can be calculated using Equation 28.15 assuming a homogeneous and isotropic medium. An unmyelinated fiber is modeled as a one-dimensional network by linking together electrical models of the membrane with a resistance R_a to account for the internal resistance of the axon as shown in Figure 28.6a. The circuit can be simulated using numerical methods [Koch and Segev, 1989] or by using already available general software packages such as Pspice or neuronal simulation packages such as Neuron [Hines, 1984]. The variable of interest is the transmembrane potential V_m since the sodium channels are sensitive to the voltage across the membrane. V_m is defined as the difference between the intracellular voltage V_i and the extracellular voltage V_e minus the resting potential E_r in order the reflect the change from resting values. Stimulation of the fiber can occur when the extracellular voltage difference between two nodes is large enough to generate transmembrane voltage greater than the firing threshold. Applying Kirchoff's law at

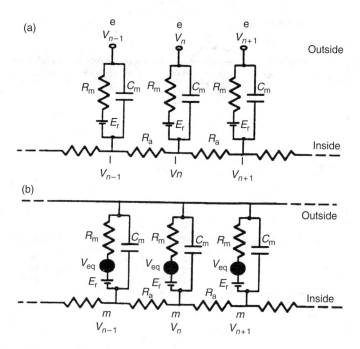

FIGURE 28.6 Model of extracellular voltage and axon interactions. (a) The effect of the extracellular voltage generated by the stimulating electrode on the axon can be modeled by connecting directly the membrane compartment to the extracellular source. The effect of the ion channels can be taken into account by adding nonlinear conductances and an equilibrium battery (not shown). (b) The axon with an extracellular voltage in (a) is equivalent to an axon inside an infinite conductance medium (zero voltage) and an equivalent voltage source inside the membrane.

each node and taking the limit when the length of membrane Δx goes to zero, one obtains the following inhomogenous cable equation [Clark and Plonsey, 1966; Rall, 1979; Altman, 1988; Ratty, 1989]:

$$\lambda^2 \frac{\partial^2 V_m}{\partial x^2} - \tau_m \frac{\partial V_m}{\partial t} - V_m = -\lambda^2 \frac{\partial^2 V_e}{\partial x^2} \tag{28.19}$$

V_m and V_e are the transmembrane and extracellular voltage, respectively. λ is the space constant of the fiber and depends only on the geometric and electric properties of the axon:

$$\lambda = \frac{1}{2} \sqrt{\frac{R_m^s d}{R_a^s}} \tag{28.20}$$

where R_m^s is the specific membrane resistance, R_a^s the axoplasmic specific resistance, and d the diameter of the axon. τ_m is the time constant of the axon and is given by:

$$\tau_m = R_m C_m \tag{28.21}$$

The term on the right side of Equation 28.21 is called the source term or forcing function and is the product of the square of the space constant with the second spatial derivative of the extracellular voltage. In order to explain the significance of this term, it can be easily shown that the model in Figure 28.6a is equivalent to a model in which the extracellular space with its electrode and voltage has been replaced by

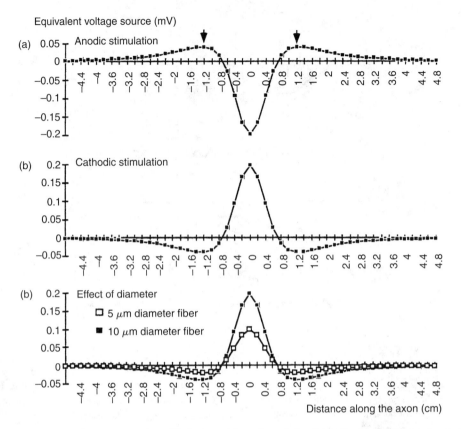

FIGURE 28.7 Equivalent source voltage (V_{eq}). A positive value of the V_{eq} indicates membrane depolarization and a negative value indicates membrane hyperpolarization. (a) Equivalent source voltage plotted along the axon for an anodic stimulus. The peak value is negative and therefore the membrane is hyperpolarized underneath the electrode. Depolarization occurs at the sites of maximum value of V_{eq} (arrows). (b) Cathodic stimulation generates depolarization underneath the electrode and the amplitude of V_{eq} is larger than that for anodic stimulation. Therefore, a cathodic stimulus has a lower threshold than an anodic stimulus. (c) V_{eq} is larger for fibers with larger diameter; therefore large diameter fibers are recruited first.

a set of equivalent voltage sources inside the nerve given by:

$$V_{eq} = \lambda^2 \frac{\Delta^2 V_e}{\Delta x^2} = \lambda^2 \frac{d^2 V_e}{dx^2}\bigg|_{\Delta x \to 0} \tag{28.22}$$

The amplitude of the equivalent voltage sources is plotted in Figure 28.7a for a 10-μm axon stimulated by a 1-mA anodic current located 1 cm away from the axon. A positive value for the equivalent indicates membrane depolarization while negative value indicates hyperpolarization. The peak value of the depolarization indicates the excitation site. Therefore, one would predict that for anodic stimulation, excitation would take place at the peak of the two depolarized regions and two action potentials would propagate toward the ends of the axon away from the electrode. Note that the shape of V_{eq} calculated is similar to that predicted by simply examining the current flow and out of the axon in Figure 28.5. This analysis is valid only at the onset of the pulse, since during the pulse, currents will be distributed throughout the cable and will affect the transmembrane potential [Warman et al., 1993]. However, it has been shown that for short pulses, these effects are small and the shape of the transmembrane voltage can be predicted using the source term of the cable equation.

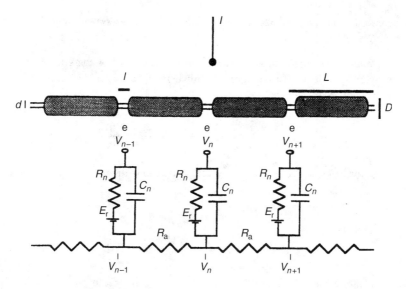

FIGURE 28.8 Discrete model for myelinated fibers. The resistance R_n and capacitance C_n of the node of Ranvier is modeled with an additional internodal resistance R_a. The resistance of the myelin is assumed to be infinite in this model. Extracellular voltages are calculated or measured at each node and the transmembrane voltage can be estimated.

Discrete cable equation for myelinated axons: Electrical stimulation of myelinated fibers is significantly different from unmyelinated fibers since the presence of myelin sheath around the axon forces the current to flow in and out of the membrane only at the nodes (see Figure 28.1). The action potential propagates from one node to the next (saltatory conduction). The effect of an applied electrical field on a myelinated fiber can be described using a discrete model of the axon and extracellular voltage [McNeal, 1976; Rattay, 1989]. Such a model is shown in Figure 28.8 in which voltages are applied at each node. The resistance R_n represents the membrane resistance at the node of Ranvier only since the myelin resistance is considered very high for this model and is neglected. C_n is the capacitance at the node of Ranvier. R_a represents the resistance between two nodes. The battery for the resting potential is removed for simplification by shifting the resting potential to zero. R_n, C_n, and R_a are given by:

$$R_n = \frac{R_n^s}{\pi \, dl} \tag{28.23}$$

$$R_a = \frac{4 R_a^s L}{\pi \, d^2} \tag{28.24}$$

$$C_n = C_n^s \pi \, dl \tag{28.25}$$

where d is the inner fiber diameter, l the width of the node, and L the internodal distance R_n^s and R_a^s are the specific membrane and axosplasmic resistance at the node respectively (Figure 28.8). The cable equation for this model can be derived using Kirchoff's law:

$$\frac{R_n}{R_a} \Delta^2 V_m - R_n C_n \frac{\partial V_m}{\partial t} - V_m = -\frac{R_n}{R_a} \Delta^2 V_e \tag{28.26}$$

Δ^2 is the second difference operator: $\Delta^2 V = V_{n-1} - 2V_n + V_{n+1}$. Using Equation 28.23 to Equation 28.25 one can show that $R_n C_n$ and R_n/R_a is independent of the diameter since $L/D = 100$ and $d/D = 0.7$ and l is constant. Therefore, the left part of Equation 28.26 is independent of the diameter. The source term, however, does depend on the diameter but only implicitly. As the distance between the node increases with the diameter of the fiber, the voltage across the nodes also increases suggesting that fiber with larger diameters are more easily excitable since they "see" larger potentials along the nodes.

Equivalent cable equation for myelinated fibers: The fiber dependence of these fibers can be expressed explicitly by using an equivalent cable equation recently derived [Basser, 1993] and adapted here to take into effect the extracellular voltage:

$$\lambda_{\text{my}}^2 \frac{\partial^2 V_m}{\partial x^2} - \tau_{\text{my}} \frac{\partial V_m}{\partial t} - V_m = -\lambda_{\text{my}}^2 \frac{\partial^2 V_e}{\partial x^2} \tag{28.27}$$

where λ_{my} is the equivalent space constant for the case of an axon with myelin sheath of infinite resistance and is defined as:

$$\lambda_{\text{my}} = \frac{1}{2} \sqrt{\frac{R_n^s \, dL}{R_a^s l}} \tag{28.28}$$

Unmyelinated/myelinated fibers: The equivalent cable equation for the myelinated fibers is similar to Equation 28.20 derived for unmyelinated axons. The forcing function is also proportional to the first derivative of the extracellular electrical field along the nerve. The dependence on the diameter can directly be observed by expressing the equivalent voltage source for myelinated fibers (V_{eqmy}) as a function of the inner diameter d:

$$V_{\text{eqmy}} = 35.7 \frac{R_n^s}{R_a^s} \frac{d^2}{e} \frac{d^2 V_e}{dx^2} \tag{28.29}$$

Equation 28.29 shows that V_{eqmy} is proportional to the square of the diameter of the fiber d while the equivalent voltage source for unmyelinated fiber is proportional to its diameter (Equation 28.22).

Anodic/cathodic stimulation: It has been demonstrated experimentally that in the case of electrical stimulation of peripheral nerves, cathodic stimulation has a lower threshold (less current required) than anodic stimulation. This experimental result can be directly explained by plotting V_{eq} for a cathodic and anodic electrode (1 mA) located 1 cm away from an 10-μm unmyelinated fiber (Figure 28.7). The maximum value of V_{eq} for anodic stimulation is 0.05 mV at the two sites indicated by the arrow. However, the maximum depolarization for the cathodic electrode is significantly larger at 0.2 mV with the site of excitation located directly underneath the electrode. In special cases, such as an electrode located on the surface of a cortex, cathodic stimulation can have a higher threshold [Ranck, 1975].

Large/small diameter axons: The equivalent voltage source of the cable equation is proportional to the square of the space constant λ. λ^2 is proportional to the diameter of the fiber (Equation 28.20) for myelinated fibers and to the square of the diameter (Equation 28.29) for myelinated fibers. Therefore, in both cases, V_{eq} is higher for fibers with larger diameter (see Figure 28.7c) and large diameter fibers have a lower threshold. Since the physiological recruitment order by the central nervous system (CNS) is to first recruit the small fibers followed by large ones, electrical stimulation produces a reverse recruitment order. However, techniques have been developed to recruit small fiber before large fibers by using a different stimulation waveform [Fang and Mortimer, 1991 and Lertmanorat and Durand, 2004a, b]. Since λ^2 is also dependent on the electrical properties of the axons, it is then possible to predict that fibers with a larger membrane resistance or lower axoplasmic resistance will also have lower thresholds.

Spatial derivative of the electrical field: The first spatial derivative (or the second spatial derivative of the voltage along the nerve) is responsible for electrical excitation of the nerve. Therefore, an electrical field with a nonzero second spatial derivative is required for excitation. An axon with a linearly decreasing voltage distribution would not be excited despite the presence of a large voltage difference along the axon.

This is due to the fact that a linear voltage distribution gives a constant electrical field and therefore the spatial derivative of the field is zero.

Activating function: The second spatial derivative term of the equivalent voltage source is also known as the activation function [Rattay, 1990]:

$$f_{unmy} = \frac{d^2 V_e}{dx^2} \tag{28.30}$$

This function can be evaluated from knowledge of the extracellular voltage alone and can be used to predict the location of excitation. For unmyelinated fibers, the activation function does not contain any information about the axon to be stimulated. In the case of myelinated fibers where the voltage is evaluated at the nodes of Ranvier, the activating function becomes:

$$f_{my} = \frac{\Delta^2 V_e}{\Delta x^2} \tag{28.31}$$

The new function contains implicit information about the fiber diameter since the distance L between the nodes of Ranvier is directly proportional to fiber diameter D ($L = 100 \times D$). The diameter dependence can be made explicit in Equation 28.29.

Net driving function: The equivalent voltage source or the activating function represent only the source term in the electrical model of the axon (Figure 28.6). However, the transmembrane voltage is determined by a weighted sum of the currents flowing at all the nodes. A net driving function which takes into account both the source term at each node and the passive redistribution from sources at other nodes has been defined and found useful for accurate prediction of the excitation threshold for any applied field [Warman et al., 1992].

Current–distance relationship: The amount of current required to activate a fiber with a given diameter depends of its geometry but also on its distance from the electrode. The farther away the fiber, the lower the voltage along the fiber (Equation 28.15); therefore larger current will be required to reach threshold. This effect is illustrated in Figure 28.9 for myelinated fibers. The distance as a function of current amplitude at threshold is plotted for several experiments [Ranck, 1975]. With a current of 1 mA, all fibers within 2 mm are activated. The calculated current–distance relationship for a 10-μm fiber has been shown to approximate well the experimental data (see dashed line in Figure 28.9) [Rattay, 1989]. The current–distance relationship is linear only for small distances. For distances above 1 mm, doubling the distance will require four times the current amplitude.

Longitudinal/transverse field: The equivalent voltage source is also proportional to the second spatial derivative of the potential present at each point along the axon. It is important to note that it is the longitudinal component of the electrical field, which is responsible for exciting the nerve. Therefore, electrodes placed longitudinally generate the most efficient stimulus since this placement would produce a large longitudinal electric field component. Conversely, electrodes placed transversely (on each side of the axon) require a much higher current since the largest component of the field does not contribute to the excitation of the nerve (Figure 28.10a).

Anodal surround block: As shown by the current–distance relation, the current amplitudes required for excitation decrease with distance. This is not entirely true for cathodic stimulation. Cathodic stimulation produces membrane depolarization underneath the electrode and membrane hyperpolarization on both sides of the electrodes (Figure 28.7b). As the current amplitude is increased, the hyperpolarization also increases and can block the propagation of the action potential along the axon. This effect is known as anodal surround block and is shown in Figure 28.10b. It is possible to identify three regions around the electrode each giving different responses. There is a spherical region close to the electrode (I) in which no

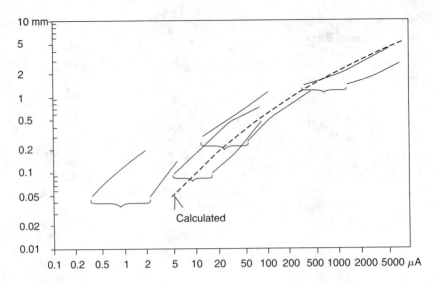

FIGURE 28.9 Current–distance relationship for monopolar cathodic stimulation of myelinated axons. The distance between the axon and the electrode is plotted as a function of current threshold amplitude for many experiments from several authors. The dashed line shows the current–distance relation calculated for 10-μm fiber stimulated with a 200-μsec pulse. (From Rattay F. *IEEE Trans. Biomed. Eng.* 36:676–681, 1989. With permission.)

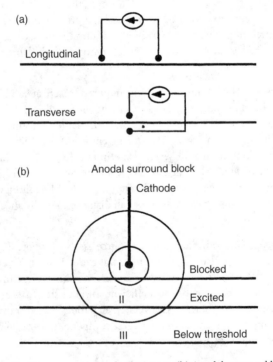

FIGURE 28.10   (a) Longitudinal/transverse electrode placement. (b) Anodal surround block.

excitation will take place due to the surround block. Fibers located in the region (II) are excited and fibers still further away (III) from the electrode are below threshold and are not excited.

Unidirectionally propagated action potentials: Electrical stimulation of nerves with electrodes normally depolarizes the membrane to threshold producing two action potentials propagating in opposite directions as shown in Figure 28.1. Stimulation techniques have been developed to generate action potential propagating in one direction only [Sweeney and Mortimer, 1981]. The techniques rely on the fact that bipolar stimulation generates depolarization under the cathode and hyperpolarization under the anode. By increasing the amount of hyperpolarization relative to the depolarization, the action potential generated underneath the cathode and traveling toward the anode can be blocked while the action potential traveling in the other direction can escape.

28.5   Electrode–Tissue Interface

At the interface between the electrode and the tissue, the shape of the waveform can influence the threshold for activation as well as the corrosion of the electrode and the tissue damage generated.

28.5.1   Effect of Stimulation Waveform on Threshold

Strength–duration curve: It has been known for a long time that it is the time-change in the applied current and not the continuous application of the external stimulus which can excite. DC currents cannot excite and even in small amplitudes can cause significant tissue damage. It has also been observed experimentally that the relationship between the pulse width and the amplitude suggests that it is the total charge injected which is the important parameter. This relationship between the amplitude and the width of a pulse required to bring an excitable tissue to threshold is shown in Figure 28.11a. The amplitude of the current threshold stimulus (I_{th}) decreases with increasing pulse width (W) and can be modeled by the following relationship derived experimentally [Lapicque, 1907]:

$$I_{th} = \frac{I_{rh}}{1 - \exp(-W/T)} \tag{28.32}$$

The smallest current amplitude required to cause excitation is known as the rheobase current (I_{rh}). T is the membrane time constant of the axon if the axon is stimulated intracellularly. For extracellular stimulation, T is a time constant which takes into account the extracellular space resistance. The relationship between current amplitude and pulse width can also be derived theoretically using the cable equation by assuming that total charge on the cable for excitation is constant [Jack et al., 1983].

Charge duration curve: The threshold charge injected $Q_{th} = I_{th} \times W$ is plotted in Figure 28.11b and increases as the pulse width increases.

$$Q_{th} = \frac{I_{rh}W}{1 - \exp(-W/T)} \tag{28.33}$$

The increase in the amount of charge required to fire the axon with increasing pulse width is due to the fact that for long pulse duration, the charge is distributed along the cable and does not participate directly to raising the membrane voltage at the excitation site. The minimum amount of charge Q_{min} required for stimulation is obtained by taking the limit of Q_{th} (Equation 28.33) when W goes to zero is equal to $I_{rh} \times T$. In practice, this minimum charge can be nearly achieved by using narrow current pulses.

Anodic break: Excitation generated by cathodic current threshold normally takes place at the onset of the pulse. However, long-duration, subthreshold cathodic or anodic current pulses have been observed experimentally to generate excitation at the end of the pulse. This effect has been attributed to the voltage sensitivity of the sodium channel. The sodium channel is normally partially inactivated at rest. However, when the membrane is hyperpolarized during the long-duration pulse, the inactivation of the sodium channel is completely removed. Upon termination of the pulse, an action potential is generated since the inactivation gate has a slow time constant relative to the activation time constant and cannot recover fast enough [Mortimer, Chapter 3 in Agnew and McCreery, 1990]. This effect can be observed with an anodic

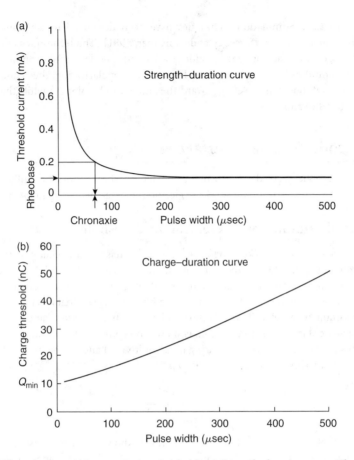

FIGURE 28.11 Effect of pulse width on excitation threshold. (a) Strength–duration curve. The amplitude of the current required to reach threshold decreases with the width of the pulse. This effect can be derived theoretically by assuming that the charge on the cable at threshold is constant. (b) The threshold charge (amplitude × pulsewidth) injected into the tissue increases with the pulse width. Narrow pulse are recommended to minimize charge injection.

or cathodic pulse since both can generate hyperpolarization. Anodic break can be prevented by avoiding abrupt termination of the current. Pulse shapes with slow decay phases such as exponential or trapezoidal decay shapes have been successfully used [Fang and Mortimer, 1991].

Electrochemistry of stimulation: Conduction in the metal is carried by electrons; while in the tissue, current is carried by ions. Although capacitive mechanisms have been tested, electrodes have not yet been developed which can store enough charge for stimulation. Therefore most electrical stimulation electrodes rely on Faradaic mechanisms at the interface between the metal and the tissue. Faradaic mechanisms require that oxidation and reduction takes place at the interface [Roblee and Rose, chapter 2 in Agnew and McCreery, 1990]. Faradaic stimulation mechanisms can be divided into reversible and nonreversible mechanisms. Reversible mechanisms occur at or near the electrode potential and include oxide formation and reduction, hydrogen plating. Irreversible mechanisms occur when the membrane is driven far away from its equilibrium potential and include corrosion, hydrogen, or oxygen evolution. Those irreversible processes can cause damage to both the electrode and the tissue since they alter the composition of the electrode surface and can generate toxic products with pH changes in the surrounding tissue. During charge injection, the electrode potential is modified by an amount related to the charge density (total charge divided by the surface area). In order to maintain the electrode potential within regions producing only minimal irreversible changes, this charge density must be kept below some values. The maximum charge density allowed depends on the metal used for the electrode [Merrill et al., 2005], the stimulation waveform, the type of electrode used, and the location of the electrode within the body.

Stimulation of brain tissue: Electrodes can be placed on the surface of the brain and directly into the brain to activate CNS pathways. Experiments with stimulation of electrodes arrays made of platinum and placed on the surface of the brain indicate that damage was produced for charge density between 50 and 300 $\mu C/cm^2$, but that the total charge/phase was also an important factor and should be kept below 3 μC [Pudenz, 1975a, b]. Intracortical electrodes with small surface area can tolerate a charge density as high as 1600 $\mu C/cm^2$ provided that the charge/phase remains below 0.0032 μC [Agnew, 1986]. More recently, studies have shown that prolonged stimulation by electrode cortical arrays can significantly decrease the excitability of the neural tissue [McCreery et al., 2002].

Stimulation of the peripheral nerve: The electrodes used in the peripheral nerves are varied and include extraneural designs such as the spiral cuffs or helix electrode [Naples et al., 1991] with electrode contacts directly on the surface of the nerve or intraneural designs placing electrodes' contacts directly inside the nerve [Nannini et al., 1991; Rutten et al., 1991]. Intraneural electrodes can cause significant damage since electrodes are inserted directly into the nerve through the perineurium. However, these electrodes can display good selectivity. Extraneural electrodes are relatively safe since the newer designs such as those at the spiral or helix are self-sizing and allow swelling without compression but display poor selectivity. Damage in peripheral nerve stimulation can be caused by the constriction of the nerve as well as neuronal hyperactivity and irreversible reactions at the electrode [McCreery et al., 1992]. New electrode designs aimed at producing selective stimulation by recruiting only small portions of the nerve have been proposed [Veraart et al., 1993; Tyler and Durand, 1994]. An electrode array has been designed to place electrodes directly into the nerve through the epineurium and the perinerium [Branner et al., 2001]. Another design takes advantage of the plasticity of the nerve and reshapes the nerve cross section into a flatter configuration. With this flat interface nerve electrode (FINE) design, electrodes can be placed close to the fascicles without damaging the perineurium [Tyler and Durand, 2002, 2003].

Stimulation of muscle tissue: Muscle tissue can be best excited by electrodes located on the nerve supplying the muscle [Popovic, 1991]. However, for some applications, electrodes can be placed directly on the surface of the skin (surface stimulation, Myklebust et al., 1985), directly into the muscle (intramuscular electrode, Caldwell and Reswick, 1975), or on the surface of the muscle (epimysial electrode, Grandjean and Mortimer, 1986). The current thresholds are higher when compared to nerve stimulation unless the electrode is carefully placed near the point of entry of the nerve [Mortimer, 1981]. Stainless steel is often used for these electrodes and is safe below 40 $\mu C/cm^2$ for coiled wire intramuscular electrodes [Mortimer, 1980].

Corrosion: Corrosion of the electrode is a major concern since it can cause electrode damage, metal dissolution, and tissue damage. However, corrosion occurs only during the anodic phase of the stimulation. Therefore, by using monophasic waveform as shown in Figure 28.12b, corrosion can be avoided. Conversely, the monophasic anodic waveform (Figure 28.12a) must be avoided since it will cause corrosion. (This not true, however for capacitive electrode metals such as tantalum for which a dielectric layer of tantalum pentoxide is formed during the anodic phase and reduced during the cathodic phase.) For most applications, cathodic stimulation has a lower threshold than that of anodic stimulation. It appears, therefore, that monophasic cathodic waveforms (Figure 28.11a) would be a preferred stimulation waveform since it minimizes both the current to be injected and the corrosion. However, since the current only flows in one direction, the chemical reactions at the interface are not reversed and the electrode is driven in the irreversible region.

Tissue damage: Electrodes operating in the irreversible region can cause significant tissue damage since irreversible process can modify the pH of the surrounding tissue and generate toxic products. Balanced biphasic waveforms are preferred since the second phase can completely reverse the charge injected into the tissue. Provided that the amplitude of the current is small, the electrode voltage can then be maintained within the reversible region. Waveforms that have the most unrecoverable charge are the most likely to induce tissue damage. Tissue damage can also be caused by generating high rate of neural activity

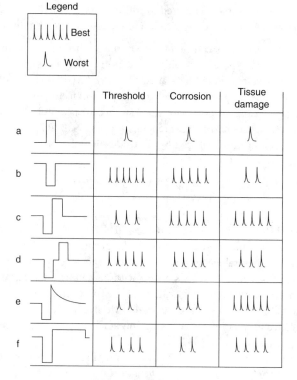

FIGURE 28.12 Comparison of stimulation waveforms. The waveforms are ranked for their ability to generate low threshold stimulation, low corrosion, and low tissue damage.

[Agnew et al., chapter 6 in Agnew and McCreery, 1990]. The mechanisms underlying this effect are still unclear but could include damage to the blood–nerve barrier, ischemia, or a large metabolic demand on the tissue leading to changes in ionic concentration both intra- and extracellularly.

Biphasic waveforms: Common biphasic waveforms for stainless steel or platinum use a cathodic pulse followed by anodic phase. An example of a square-balanced biphasic waveform is shown in Figure 28.12c. Another commonly used biphasic waveform easily implemented with capacitor and switches is shown in Figure 28.12e. This waveform ensures that the charge is exactly balanced since a capacitor is inserted in series with the tissue to be stimulated and the charge injected is then reversed by discharging the capacitor [Mortimer, 1981]. Biphasic cathodic-first waveforms have a higher threshold than monophasic waveforms since the maximum depolarization induced by the cathodic pulse is decreased by the following anodic pulse [Mortimer, chapter 3 in Agnew and McCreery, 1990]. A delay can then be inserted between the cathodic and anodic phase as shown in Figure 28.12d. However, the time delay can also prevent adequate charge reversal and can be dangerous to the electrode and the tissue. An alternative method is to decrease the maximum amplitude of the anodic phase but increase its length as shown in Figure 28.12f. However, this can also be damaging to the electrode since the charge is not reversed fast enough following the cathodic pulse. The various waveforms shown in Figure 28.12 are ranked for their effect on tissue damage, corrosion, and threshold of activation [See also Merrill et al, 2005].

28.6   Conclusion

Electrical stimulation of excitable tissue has been used for over a century and important discoveries have been made concerning the mechanisms underlying the interactions between the applied fields with the tissue and the electrochemistry at the electrode–tissue interface. It is now clear that electrical stimulation is a powerful technique, which could potentially activate any excitable tissue in the body and replace damaged functions. It is also clear, however, that if our goal is to provide intimate interfacing between excitable tissue and electrodes in order to reproduce the normal function of the nervous system, present technology is not adequate. The electrodes are too large relative to the size of the axons and can only access either a few elements separately or a large number of elements simultaneously. Moreover, it is also clear that our understanding of the electrochemistry at the interface between the electrode and tissue is limited as well as the mechanisms underlying tissue damage. However, the substantial gains to be made are worth the efforts required to solve these problems.

Acknowledgments

I am grateful to Srikantan Nagarajan for critically reviewing this manuscript. Supported by NIH grant RO1 NS 32845-09.

References

Agnew W.F. and McCreery D.B. *Neural Prostheses: Fundamental Studies*, Prentice Hall, 1990.

Agnew W.F., Yuen T.G.H., McCreery D.B., and Bullara L.A. Histopathologic evaluation of prolonged intracortical electrical stimulation. *Exp. Neurol.* 92: 162–185, 1986.

Aidley D.J. *The Physiology of Excitable Cells*, Cambridge University Press, 1978.

Altman K.W. and Plonsey R. Development of a model for point source electrical fibre bundle stimulation. *Med. Biol. Eng. Comput.* 26: 466–475, 1988.

Basser P.J. Cable equation for a myelinated axon derived from its microstructure. *Med. Biol. Eng. Comput.* 31: S87–S92, 1993.

Branner A., Stein R.B., and Normann R.A. Selective stimulation of cat sciatic nerve using an array of varying-length microelectrodes. *J. Neurophysiol.* 85: 1585–1594, 2001.

Brindley G.S. and Lewin W.S. The sensations produced by electrical stimulation of the visual cortex. *J. Physiol.* 106: 479–493, 1968.

Caldwell C.W. and Reswick J.B. A percutaneous wire electrode for chronic research use. *IEEE Trans. Biomed. Eng.* 22: 429–432, 1975.

Chokroverty S. *Magnetic Stimulation in Clinical Neurophysiology*, Butterworths, 1990.

Clark G.M., Tong Y.C., and Patrick J.F. *Cochlear Prostheses*, Churchill Linvinston, NY, 1990.

Clark J. and Plonsey R. A mathematical evaluation of the core conductor model. *Biophys. J.* 6: 95–112, 1966.

Durand D., Ferguson A.S.F., and Dalbasti T. Effects of surface boundary on neuronal magnetic stimulation. *IEEE Trans. Biomed. Eng.* 37: 588–597, 1992.

Fang Z.P. and Mortimer J.T. A method to effect physiological recruitment order in electrically activated muscle. *IEEE Trans. BME* 38: 175–179, 1991.

Ferreira H.G. and Marshal M.W. *The Biophysical Basis of Excitibility*, Cambridge, 1985.

Lertmanorat Z. and Durand D.M. Extracellular voltage profile for reversing the recruitment order of peripheral nerve stimulation: a stimulation study. *J. Neurol. Engineering*, 4: 202–211, 2004.

Lertmanorat Z. and Durand D.M. A novel electrode array for diameter dependent control of axonal excitability: a simulation study IEEE transactions on BME. 7, 1242–1250, 2004.

Glenn W.W.L., Hogan J.F., Loke J.S.O., Ciesielski T.E., Phelps M.L., and Rowedder R. Ventilatory support by pacing of the conditioned diaphragm in quadraplegia. *New Engl. J. Med.* 310: 1150–1155, 1984.

Grandjean P.A. and Mortimer J.T. Recruitment properties of monopolar and bipolar epimysial electrodes. *Ann. Biomed. Eng.* 14: 429–432, 1985.

Hambrecht F.T. Neural prostheses. *Ann. Rev. Biophys. Bioeng.* 8: 239–267, 1979.

Heringa A., Stegeman D.F., Uijen G.J.H., and deWeerd J.P.C. Solution methods of electrical field in physiology. *IEEE Trans. Biomed. Eng.* 29: 34–42, 1982.

Hines M. Efficient computation of branched nerve equations. *Int. J. Bio. Med. Comp.* 15: 69–76, 1984.

Jack J.J.B., Noble D., and Tsien R.W. *Electrical Current Flow in Excitable Cells*, Clarendon Press, Oxford, 1983.

Koch C. and Segev I. *Methods in Neural Modelling*, MIT Press, 1989.

Kraus J.D. and Carver K.R. *Electromagnetics*, McGraw Hill, 1973.

Lapicque L. Recherches quantitatives sure l'excitation electrique des nerfs traites comme une polarization. *J. Physiol. (Paris)* 9: 622–635, 1907.

Marsolais E.B. and Kobetic R. Development of a practical electrical stimulation system for restoring gait in the paralyzed patient. *Clin. Ortho. Relat. Res.* 233: 64–74, 1988.

McCreery D.B., Agnew W.F., and Bullara L.A. The effects of prolonged intracortical microstimulation on the excitability of pyramidal tract neurons in the cat. *Ann. Biomed. Eng.* 30: 107–119, 2002.

McCreery D.B., Agnew W.F., Yuen T.G.H., and Bullara L.A. Damage in peripheral nerve from continuous electrical stimulation: comparison of two stimulus waveforms. *Med. Biol. Eng. Comp.* 30: 109–1124, 1992.

McNeal D.R. Analysis of a model for excitation of myelinated nerve. *IEEE Trans. BME* 23: 329–337, 1976.

Mortimer J.T., Kaufman D., and Roessmann U. Coiled wire electrode intramuscular electrode: tissue damage. *Ann. Biomed. Eng.* 8: 235–244, 1980.

Mortimer J.T. Motor prostheses, In *Handbook of Physiology — The Nervous System III*, Ed. V.B. Brooks, American Physiological Society, pp. 155–187, 1981.

Myklebust J., Cusick B., Sances A., and Larson S.L.J. *Neural Stimulation*, CRC Press Inc, Boca Raton, FL, 1985.

Nagarajan S.S., Durand D., and Warman E.N. Effects of induced electric fields on finite neuronal structures: a simulation study. *IEEE Trans. Biomed. Eng.* 40: 1175–1188, 1993.

Nannini N. and Horch K. Muscle recruitment with intrafascicular electrodes. *IEEE Trans. Biomed. Eng.* 38: 769–776, 1991.

Nunez P.L. *Electric Fields in the Brain, The Neurophysics of EEG*, Oxford University Press, 1981.

Plonsey R. *Bioelectric Phenomena*, McGraw-Hill Series in Bioengineering, 1969.

Pudenz R.H.L., Bullara A., Dru D., and Tallala A. Electrical stimulation of the brain:II. Effects on the blood–brain barrier. *Surg. Neurol.* 4: 265–270, 1975a.

Pudenz R.H., Bullara L.A., Jacques P., and Hambrecht F.T. Electrical stimulation of the brain:III. The neural damage model. *Surg. Neurol.* 4: 389–400, 1975b.

Rall W. Core conductor theory and cable properties of neurons. In *Handbook of Physiology — The Nervous System I*. Bethesda, Maryland, Chap. 3, pp. 39–96, 1979.

Ranck J.B. Which elements are excited in electrical stimulation of mammalian central nervous system: a review. *Brain Res.* 98: 417–440, 1975.

Rattay F. Analysis of models for extracellular fiber stimulation. *IEEE Trans. Biomed. Eng.* 36: 676–681, 1989.

Rattay F. *Electrical Nerve Stimulation, Theory, Experiments and Applications*, Springer-Verlag, Wien, New York, 1990.

Roth B.J. and Basser P.J. A model for stimulation of a nerve fiber by electromagnetic induction. *IEEE Trans. Biomed. Eng.* 37: 588–597, 1990.

Rutecki P. Anatomical, physiological and theoretical basis for the antiepileptic effect of vagus nerve stimulation. *Epilepsia* 31: S1–S6, 1990.

Merrill D.R., Bikson M., and Jefferys J.G. Electrical stimulational of excitable tissue: design of efficacious and safe protocols. *J. Neuroscience methods*, 141: 171–198, 2005.

Rutten W.L.C., vanWier H.J., and Put J.J.M. Sensitivity and selectivity of intraneural stimulation using a silicon electrode array. *IEEE Trans. Biomed. Eng.* 38: 192–198, 1991.

Sweeney J.D. and Mortimer J.T. An asymetric two electrode cuff for generation of unidirectionally propagated action potentials. *IEEE Trans. Biomed. Eng.* 33: 541–549, 1986.

Tyler D.J. and Durand D.M. Functionally selective peripheral nerve stimulation with a flat interface nerve electrode. *IEEE Trans. Neural Syst. Rehabil. Eng.* 10: 294–303, 2002.

Tyler D.J. and Durand D.M. Chronic response of the rat sciatic nerve to the flat interface nerve electrode. *Ann. Biomed. Eng.* 31: 633–642, 2003.

Veraart C., Grill W.M., and Mortimer J.T. Selective control of muscle activation with a multipolar nerve cuff electrode. *IEEE Trans. Biomed. Eng.* 37: 688–698, 1990.

Warman N.R., Durand D.M., and Yuen G. Reconstruction of hippocampal CA1 pyramidal cell electrophysiology by computer simulation. *IEEE Trans. Biomed. Eng.* 39: 1244–1254, 1994.

Further Information

Neural Engineering Center: http://nec.cwru.edu/

Functional Electrical Stimulation Center: http://feswww.fes.cwru.edu/

Articles concerning the latest research can be found mainly in the following journals:

IEEE Transactions in Biomedical Engineering

IEEE Transactions on Neural Systems and Rehabilitation Engineering

Annuals of Biomedical Engineering

Medical and Biological Engineering and Computing

Journal of Neural Engineering

IV

Neuroengineering

Daniel J. DiLorenzo
BioNeuronics Corporation

Cedric F. Walker
Tulane University

Ross Davis
Neural Engineering Clinic and Alfred Mann Foundation for Scientific Research

WE ARE AT THE CUSP OF A TECHNOLOGICAL REVOLUTION that holds promise to have more of an impact on human health, disease, and quality of life than any other development in history. Based on a foundation of fundamental science and empirical observation, engineering research and design has brought us into an era where it is no longer boastful to expect that the blind will see and the paralyzed will walk. We have seen how the development of implantable pacemakers and defibrillators over the last half century has redefined life for patients with heart disease. We are about to witness a far more dramatic revolution. The convergence of decades of neuroscience research and technology development has now reached critical mass and is propelling the neural engineering field into the commercialization phase. First-generation pacemakers, *surface stimulators* and *single-channel* neural prosthetic implants were essentially miniaturized benchtop pulse generators, and the engineering challenges involved in their production were encapsulation, battery life, and component reliability. Now we are conceiving and implanting multichannel implants with closed-loop feedback and autonomous control systems, and the engineering challenges push the limits of medical knowledge and human creativity. We are developing a depth knowledge of neural function never before dreamed of ... as we must, if we are to be successful in our charge to augment and ultimately to replace neural function. *The payoff is huge: improved quality-of-life and functional restoration following stroke, spinal cord injury, and traumatic brain injury, with extension into deafness, blindness, paralysis, and movement disorders, and even some mental illness and seizure disorders.*

Neural Engineering has taken longer to reach the cusp of commercialization than many other medical device fields, such as that of pacemakers, largely because of the number and complexity of the multiple fields of knowledge in neuroscience, biomaterials, and engineering required to achieve acceptable efficacy. But Neural Engineering has the potential for impact on many disease states that are far from the realm of the neurologist or neurosurgeon, because excitable and hence stimulatable, tissue is implicated in the functioning of virtually every organ system in the body.

This volume represents contributions from a sampling of thought leaders in industry, academia, and clinical medicine and provides an understanding of the history, physiology, and some of the most promising engineering technologies in the industry. An exhaustive compilation is beyond the scope of this volume and is the subject of a planned separate text. DiLorenzo and Gross relate the extraordinary breadth and duration of investigation and discovery that has led up to the current flood of innovation. *Grill, an early leader in functional electrical stimulation (FES), describes the theoretical foundation for stimulation of cells of the nervous system. Graupe, an early pioneer in the research and clinical application of noninvasive FES for gait restoration discusses the research and commercialization efforts behind ParaStep. Davis et al. have outlined the development, success, and difficulties of a multichannel wired-linked stimulating system for functional restoration in paraplegia.* Kennedy, a pioneer in neural interfacing and the first to chronically record neural signals from a human, describes and compares various neural recording technologies. Schulman, a cofounder of Pacesetter systems and now president of The Alfred Mann Foundation, and colleagues describe the BION, a broadly applicable platform technology for minimally invasive neural stimulation and sensing. Greenberg, president of Second Sight, provides insight into the development of a breathtaking technology which offers hope to the blind. Velasco et al., leaders in the field of neurostimulation for the treatment of epilepsy, describe their experiences with seizure control. Roth and Zangen describe promising innovations in the noninvasive transcranial magnetic stimulation technology, which is being commercialized for a number of promising indications.

The convergence of disciplines described herein is becoming apparent to researchers, engineers, clinicians, established medical device companies, early stage venture capital investors, and a wave of startup companies. We are witnessing the transition of Neural Engineering from basic research to intense commercialization and widespread clinical application and acceptance. The impact of this industry on medicine and on society promises to be as dramatic as that of the development of antibiotics. We are entering an era in which the nervous system is replaceable and augmentable . . . the Neurological Age. The future is upon us.

29

History and Overview of Neural Engineering

Daniel J. DiLorenzo
BioNeuronics Corporation

Robert E. Gross
Emory University

29.1   Background

Recent years have witnessed remarkable advances in the development of technology and its practical applications in the amelioration of neurological dysfunction. This encompasses a wide variety of disorders and their treatment has been the purview of different, partially overlapping, medical and scientific specialties and societies. As a result of these advances, three somewhat independent and long-standing fields with unique origins — stereotactic and functional neurosurgery, neuromodulation, and functional electrical stimulation — are experiencing increasing convergence and overlap and the distinctions separating them are beginning to blur.

Stereotactic and functional neurosurgery — which takes its origins at the beginning of neurosurgery in the late 19th century, but which as a society dates to the 1940s — has mainly concerned itself with the surgical treatment of nervous system conditions that manifest as disordered function, including movement disorders (Parkinson's disease [PD], tremor, dystonia), pain, epilepsy, and psychiatric illnesses. In the first part of the last century, the surgical treatment of these disorders usually involved ablation of nervous tissue but this has almost completely been supplanted by the advent of electrical neurostimulation. Other modalities within the purview of stereotactic and functional neurosurgery include pharmacological and biological therapies that are delivered via surgical techniques.

Neuromodulation broadly involves alteration of the function of the nervous system. The International Neuromodulation Society was established in the 1990s and dedicated itself to the treatment of nervous system disorders — mostly pain and spasticity — with implantable devices, including pumps and stimulators. However, with the advances in the field, this society has broadened its scope to include implantable devices used to treat disorders of sensory and motor functions of the body. This society has been driven by both anesthesiologists and neurosurgeons, but has mainly been clinical in its purview.

Functional electrical stimulation has pertained mostly to the restoration of upper and lower limb function (after injury and ischemia), bowel, bladder and sexual function, and respiratory function. This field, represented by the International Functional Electrical Stimulation Society, also is interested in auditory and visual prostheses, and has — in contrast to the two other societies — a distinctly engineering bias, limited as it has been to electrical stimulation.

It is quite clear that each of these areas has strong overlap, both clinically as well as technologically. While one or the other may have been more clinical or basic in its scientific approach, with the progress in both technology development and its translation into the clinic, these distinctions are becoming increasingly blurred. Advances in functional neurosurgery have been driven by clinical empiricism and advances in pathophysiological understanding of the target disorders, but also by technological advancement (e.g., the development of the stereotactic frame and then frameless image guidance stereotactic technology and the development of implantable neurostimulation systems). Neuromodulation — based as it is on the use of implantable devices — has been driven by technical and pharmacological innovation coupled to increased understanding of neurophysiology and the pathophysiological manifestations in states of disease. Finally, functional electrical stimulation (FES) has mostly been an undertaking driven by engineering technology, since from the outset the goals have been restoration of motor function using controlled electrical stimulation. Clinical application has always been the long-term objective and with the current synergy of technological innovation and increasing clinical experimentalism (e.g., motor prosthesis trials for spinal cord injury) the field is making great strides.

The technology that is a main driver behind each of these overlapping disciplines can be coined "neural engineering." Although this domain might seem like a relatively recent innovation, a view into the historical underpinnings of neuromodulation in the 18th century reveals that in fact from the start, technological innovation and neuromodulation developed hand in hand, and some of this pioneering foundation building of the last several centuries might reasonably be called neural engineering.

29.1.1 The Early History of Electrical Stimulation of the Nervous System

The use of electricity for therapeutic purposes can arguably be said to date back even to the use of amber and magnetite in jewelry around 9000 BC [1]. The use of the torpedo fish or electric eel was advocated by Scribonius Largus — one of the first Roman physicians in the first millennium — for the treatment of headache and gout [2]. The patient would apply the fish to the painful region until numb (but not too long) [3]. Its use continued into the 16th century by which time the indications were broadened to include melancholy, migraine, and epilepsy.

By the 17th century electricity was identified as a form of energy and primitive devices to induce electric current were developed. The first electrostatic generator was constructed in 1672, but electrical sparks from a modified electrostatic generator were first used therapeutically to treat paralysis in 1744 [3] (the first example of neural engineering?). In 1745 in Leyden, the capacity of an electrified glass jar and tin foil — the Leyden jar — to store electrical charge was inadvertently discovered when its discharge caused a physiological effect so severe that the experimenter took two days to recover [4]. Electricity and the nervous system were intricately associated early on because the most sensitive electrical detector at the time was in fact the nervous system. The new phenomenon was quickly embraced by the medical field, and "cures" of paralysis and other ailments rapidly proliferated, yielding many fantastic books from "electrotherapists" such as John Wesley the divine [3,4]. By 1752, even Benjamin Franklin was using it, to treat a 24-year-old woman with convulsions [5], and various palsies, but he at least was not convinced of any persistent benefits from the electrical treatments [4].

Albrecht von Haller felt that nerves and muscles were sensitive to the effects of electrical current, but he and others did not believe that electricity played a role in normal functioning [6]. In 1791, Galvani published his famous experiments in which he induced muscular contractions in frog leg muscle using a metallic device constructed of dissimilar metals [7]. He reasoned that the electrical current was being "discharged" from the muscle, a view which was countered by Volta who felt that the electrical current flowed from the dissimilar metals [8] and which led him to develop the voltaic bimetallic pile — the first battery — based on this insight [9]. Electrophysiological experiments using voltaic piles to generate "Galvanic current" rapidly proliferated, including important experiments by Aldini, Galvani's nephew, who was interested in, among other things, the therapeutic applications of galvanism [6] (more examples of neural engineering). His particular interest was in "reanimation" especially following near-drowning, and this work included electrically stimulating both animals and men — the latter following the not infrequent hangings and decapitations [10]. He was successful at provoking muscular contractions of the somatic musculature, but was disappointed that he could not get similar results with the heart [6]. In fact, Aldini was likely the first to induce facial muscle contractions with direct brain electrical stimulation in both oxen and human cadavers, predating Fritsch and Hitzig's influential work by many years [11]. A particularly dramatic demonstration on a hanged criminal in England garnered widespread lay coverage, possibly contributing to the inspiration behind the *Frankenstein* myth [6]. He also used the voltaic piles to treat "mental disorders" including depression — a precursor to electroconvulsive therapy — after first applying the pile safely to his own head [10].

The next major advance arose from Faraday's invention of the first electric generator in 1831, which induced alternating or "Faradic current" by rotating wires inside a magnetic field. Dubois-Reymond in 1848 demonstrated that the time-varying nature of Faradic current was important in efficient stimulation, and he formulated an early expression of the strength–duration curve relating the threshold for activating the neuromuscular system to the intensity and duration of the current pulse [3]. G.B. Duchenne — regarded as the father of "electrotherapy" — established it as a separate discipline ("De l'Electrisation localisee," 1855) [3]. He used Faradic current applied through moistened electrode pads, preferring it to Galvanic current because of its warming properties. In 1852 he stimulated the facial nerve for palsy [12]. With Duchenne's influence and the proliferation of induction coils and batteries, therapeutic electrical stimulation spread widely. By 1900, according to McNeal, most physicians in the United States had an "electrical machine" for the treatment of a plethora of ailments — many neurological, including pain. Many different and interesting devices were constructed, for use in every part of the body (literally), including the "hydroelectric bath" (not recommended!) [3]. Called the "Golden Age of Medical Electricity," the close of the 19th century would only be eclipsed by the close of the following century in the proliferation of the use of electricity in medical therapeutics.

Fritsch and Hitzig [11] are said to have been the first to stimulate the cortex in living animals and systematic mapping of cerebrocortical function was described in animals by Ferrier [13]. The first time the human brain was directly stimulated in a conscious patient was in 1878 by Barthlow, who introduced a stimulating needle into a patient's brain through an eroding scalp and skull tumor [14]. Low amplitude Faradic current elicited contralateral muscle contractions and an unpleasant tingling feeling, initiating the field of cerebral localization using electrical stimulation. Cushing observed the effects of intraoperative faradic stimulation in 1909 [15], and Forester's intraoperative work in the 1930s influenced Wilder Penfield [16], culminating in Penfield and Jasper's seminal publication of *Functional Anatomy of the Human Brain* in 1954.

29.2 Neural Augmentation — Neural Prostheses

29.2.1 Origins of the Field of Neural Prostheses

The field of neural prostheses encompasses the set of technologies relevant to the restoration of neurological and neuromuscular function and this includes both motor prostheses and sensory prostheses. The early motor work focused on technologies for restoration of limb motor function, these having clinical relevance to the treatment of both paralyzed and amputee patients. In the last several decades, as microelectronic and microfabrication technologies have progressed, sensory prostheses have reached the state of practicality and cochlear implants have become a standard of care in the treatment of sensorineural deafness. Research and commercialization efforts continue in remaining areas, including restoration of the motor and sensory functions of the limbs, motor functions of the bladder, bowel, and diaphragm, and sensory functions including tactile, visual, and vestibular.

In the 1950s, a human study showing sound perception arising from electrode implantation inspired researchers across the world to investigate the possibility of a cochlear prosthesis, which, after several decades of development in academia and industry, became the first FDA approved neural prosthesis [17].

The Neural Prosthesis Program, launched in 1972 and spearheaded by F. Terry Hambrecht, MD, brought funding, focus, and coordination to the multidisciplinary effort to develop technologies to restore motor function in paralyzed individuals. The initial efforts were in electrode–tissue interaction, biomaterials and neural interface development, cochlear and visual prosthesis development and control of motor function using implanted and nonimplanted electrodes.

In his 1980 UC Davis Ph.D. thesis, David Edell [18,19] demonstrated chronic recording from peripheral nerve using a multichannel micromachined silicon regeneration electrode array . This was a major achievement, as it proved that chronic recording from the nervous system was possible. Furthermore, his silicon-based implant was proof of concept that biocompatible recording interfaces could be made from silicon using existing etching and microfabrication technology and could therefore be made to incorporate electrodes, preamplifiers, processing, memory, and telemetry elements on the same silicon substrate implanted in the nervous system.

29.2.2   Neural Augmentation — Motor Prostheses

29.2.2.1   Neuromuscular Stimulation for Control of Limb Movement

Liberson and coworkers [20] are credited as being the first to utilize FES to restore functional control of movement to a paralyzed limb. They treated over 100 hemiplegic patients with foot-drop using a transistorized stimulator and conductive rubber electrodes placed on the skin overlying the peroneal nerve. A switch under the sole triggered stimulation during the swing phase of gait causing contraction of the tibialis anterior and dorsiflexion of the foot [21]. All patients were reported to have received some benefit but acceptance was limited due to skin irritation from the electrode, need for precise electrode placement, hassle in applying the device compared to functional benefit, and electrode lead breakage. Liberson termed this "functional electrotherapy." However, this term did not gain widespread acceptance; rather, "functional electrical stimulation," coined by Moe and Post did [22].

Long and Masciarelli [23], intrigued by Liberson's lower extremity work, devised a system for upper extremity functional restoration in high cervical quadriplegic patients. Using FES controlled finger extension, via extensor digitorum stimulation, coupled with spring loaded thumb and finger flexion, the device enabled control of grasp in the paralyzed limb. Though patients tolerated it very well it did not gain widespread clinical acceptance.

Peckham and colleagues [24] at Case Western Reserve University used chronic percutaneous stimulation of forearm muscles to provide hand grasp, including both palmar and lateral prehension and release, in C5 quadriplegic patients.

Restoration of some form of assisted gait in spinal cord injured patients has been the focus of several research groups. In 1960, Kantrowitz [25] reported the use of surface stimulation of quadriceps and gluteal muscles to effect rising and standing for several minutes from a sitting position in a paraplegic patient. In 1973, Cooper [26] reported bilateral implantation of the femoral and sciatic nerves in a T11-12 paraplegic and claimed ambulation of up to 40 feet using a walker for balance assistance.

Using implanted stimulators and electrodes on the femoral nerves bilaterally, Brindley [27] was able to achieve in a paraplegic the movement of rising from a sitting position and limited gait assisted

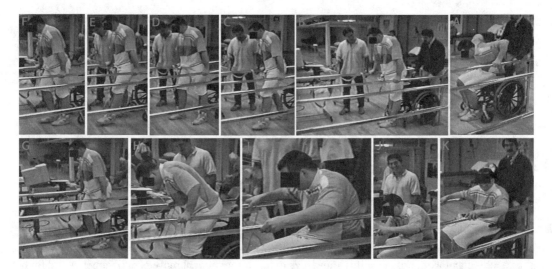

FIGURE 29.1 Series of still images from 4-channel FES gait sequence performed by author (DJD) at MIT in 1990. (A) Subject bracing to stand, (B) Standing under FES control with computer controlled stimulator on the far left (L to R: author DJD, subject, Allen Wiegner, PhD), (C) First step, (D) Second step, (E) Third step, (F) Fourth step, (G) Preparing to sit, (H) Sitting down, (I) Seated in wheelchair after walking, (J) Repositioning feet, (K) Smiling.

with elbow crutches but not requiring a walker, braces, or other support. Several more sophisticated devices followed. Kralj et al. [28,29] described a 4- to 6-channel skin surface electrode FES systems in which patients ambulated with the assistance of parallel bars or a roller walker. At MIT in 1990, DiLorenzo and Durfee [30] implemented a computer-controlled 4-channel skin surface electrode FES system with bilateral quadricep stimulation and peroneal nerve withdrawal reflex stimulation and achieved 60 feet of handrail balance-assisted gait in a thoracic spinal cord injured patient and developed adaptive closed-loop controllers which compensated for time-varying muscle performance, including gaint changes due to muscle fatigue [31,32]. Figure 29.1 shows a sequence of still frames from a gait sequence using this 4-channel surface FES configuration [30]. Convinced of the greater potential for clinical efficacy and market success with implanted technologies, DiLorenzo [30,33–36] pursued related implanted FES work, and Goldfarb and Durfee [37] continued this line of surface FES work to include a long-legged brace with a computer-controlled friction brake for improved energy efficiency and control.

Marsolais [38] reported improved motor function in patients with intramuscular stainless steel electrodes implanted in the quadriceps, hip flexors, extensors, and abductors. Though significant motor torque improvement was achieved in some of these patients, all of whom had some motor function preimplantation, patients required supervision for ambulation.

Dan Graupe [39,40] extended the surface FES technology developed by Lieberson and Kralj to include a patient borne and controlled system. Graupe then commercialized this technology for clinical use as the ParaStep system. The history of the field of FES for ambulation and the commercialization of ParaStep is described in more detail in the chapter by Graupe in this volume.

The first generation of implanted FES systems for upper extremity functional restoration were developed at Case Western Reserve University and Cleveland Veterans Affairs Medical Center for the restoration of hand grasp to patient with cervical spinal cord injury [41]. This system allowed the paraplegic patient to control hand grasp on an otherwise paralyzed limb by generating movement commands using contralateral shoulder movements. This technology was commercialized by NeuroControl Corporation, which was founded by Hunter Peckham, Ph.D., Ronald Podraza, and colleagues at Case Western Reserve University in Cleveland, Ohio. NeuroControl received FDA approval in 1997 to market the grasp restoration device, known as the FreeHand System.

29.2.2.2 Chronically Implanted Neuroelectric Interfaces (Recording Arrays)

29.2.2.2.1 Basic Neuroscience

Separate but concurrent research efforts by many investigators in basic neurophysiology were making significant advancements in developing an understanding of how cortical and spinal neural systems control motor function. Extensive research on control of movement by hundreds of neuroscientists has revealed correlations between parameters of limb movement and neural activity in many motor centers, including the primary motor cortex, premotor and supplementary motor cortex, cerebellum, and spinal cord.

The motor cortex was the first area to undergo detailed quantitative study of neuronal activity during whole-arm reaching movements in an awake behaving primate [42]. Georgopoulos et al. [42] first demonstrated a relation between neural cell activity and movement direction. They found that cell firing rates are directionally sensitive in a graded manner, that is, the firing rate is maximal in a so-called preferred direction and the firing rate tapers off gradually as the direction of movement deviates form this preferred direction. In 1984, Georgopoulos et al. [43] demonstrated the presence of cells in both primary motor cortex and in area 5, the firing rates of which correlate linearly with position of the hand in two-dimensional space. Subsequent work expanded this knowledge to include additional movement parameters and limb movement in three-dimensional space [44–48].

Later research, beginning in the 1990s focused on control using neural signals, in both nonhuman primate and human subjects, lending credence to the notion that sufficient information may be extracted from neural signals to be used as a control signal for a prosthetic system. Schwartz extended this work and characterized neural firing patterns associated with limb movement in three-dimensional space [46] and with Talyor and Tillary developed a real-time adaptive prediction algorithm with which a primate was able to control robot arm movement [49]. Donoghue et al. [50] pursued similar lines of research and characterized patterns of behavior from large populations of cells. DiLorenzo [51] showed evidence for the presence of real-time motor feedback error signals in the primate motor cortex, suggesting the presence of feedforward and feedback signals in primary motor cortex. Using the 100 channel intracortical array developed by Richard Normann, Donoghue characterized additional information content in correlations between neuronal activity [52]. Using wire electrode arrays, Nicolelis also characterized real-time prediction of limb trajectory using neural ensembles and in collaboration with Srinivasan showed remote control of robot movement by a nonhuman primate [53].

29.2.2.2.2 Initial Application to Humans

Kennedy and Bakay [54–56] demonstrated human 2-D control of cursor movement by a paralyzed human patient using the cone neurotrophic electrode. This novel electrode facilitates regeneration of neural processes into an insulating glass cone where a stable electrical and mechanical interface forms, providing a long-term high signal to noise ratio. In 1987, Kennedy founded Neural Signals to develop the cone electrode for clinical use; however, the company has refocused its direction on the commercialization of a less invasive EMG driven system for locked-in patients.

A spinout from Donoghue's and Normann's research efforts, Cyberkinetics Neurotechnology Systems, Inc., has demonstrated in pilot studies human control of cursor movement using a 4×4 mm 96-channel intracortical microelectrode array chronically implanted into the primary motor cortex [57]. As of this writing, they have demonstrated the ability to record over 6 months postimplantation.

29.2.3 Neural Augmentation — Sensory Prostheses

29.2.3.1 Sensory Stimulation — Auditory (Cochlear Implant)

Auditory prostheses, which provide patterned stimulation of the eighth cranial nerve, were the first commercially available sensory neural prosthesis. As of this writing, it is the only approved sensory prosthesis; however, visual prostheses are already in clinical trials and are likely to be available in the not too distant future.

An experiment published in 1957 by Djourno and Eyries [17] is credited with inspiring the development of the cochlear implant. Paris otologist C. Eyries, and neurophysiologist A. Djourno implanted wires in the inner ear of a deaf patient and were able to elicit sensations of sound with electrical stimulation. This experiment was reproduced in 1964 by Doyle et al. [58] in Los Angeles.

Inspired by this 1957 Djourno article, William House, MD, joined with Jack Urban, president of an electronics company, in Los Angeles to develop a cochlear implant and they published results on their first patients in 1973 [59]. Working with investigators at the House Ear Institute, founded by his brother Howard House [60], MD, also an otolaryngologist, William House pioneered the development of the single-channel cochlear implant and achieved its approval by the FDA.

Blair Simmons of Stanford University first evaluated multichannel cochlear stimulation, placing four wires into the auditory nerve [61]. Several years later, Dr. Robin Michelson, an otolaryngologist at the University of California San Francisco (UCSF), implanted a multichannel cochlear implant placed in the scala tympani [62]. Michael Merzenich, also of UCSF, lead the research and development of this and subsequent multichannel cochlear implants [63]. Al Mann founded Advanced Bionics® Corporation in 1993, licensed the UCSF cochlear implant technology, and recruited Joe Schulman, Ph.D. and Tom Santogrossi to develop this technology into the CLARION cochlear implant [64–67].

In parallel with developments in the United States, in Melbourne, Australia, Graeme Clark initiated a large and extremely productive clinical and research program at the University of Melbourne in Australia [68–71]. The implants developed under Clark are manufactured by Cochlear Ltd., a subsidiary of Nucleus Pty. Ltd. in Sydney and Cochlear has the largest worldwide population of implanted patients, with over 65,000 patients having been implanted with the Nucleus worldwide [72].

In 1975, Ingeborg and Erwin Hochmair began development of a multichannel cochlear implant, which was implanted in Vienna 2 years later [73,74]. They continued development of the device for nearly a decade and in 1989 founded MED-EL, which has since become the third major manufacturer of cochlear implants.

There are several factors that have contributed to the success of the cochlear implant. (1) Well-developed foundation of basic science, particularly in the area of auditory neurophysiology. (2) Focused and coordinated research programs and funding including that of the NIH Neural Prosthesis Program. (3) Clinician champions who were active in the research and facilitated its clinical acceptance as early adopters themselves and as thought leaders. (4) Cochlear anatomy, including the tonotopic arrangement of sensory receptors and their protection by a bony encasement, facilitating stable chronic neuroelectric interfacing. Because of this surgically accessible anatomy, an electrode array may be placed and press chronically against a rigid surface while being in close proximity to neural cells, without the risk of damage to or migration through soft neural tissues. This neural interfacing problem is a major hurdle in the development of visual, somatosensory, and motor prostheses, which generally must interface directly with soft neural tissues, which are subject to perpetually changing forces and displacements.

29.2.3.2 Sensory Stimulation — Visual

The restoration of vision has captivated the imagination of man since biblical times. Now, after 4 decades of modern research, beginning with the stimulation of the visual cortex by Giles Brindley in 1966 [75], visual prostheses are making the transition from basic science research to commercialization. William Dobelle, Ph.D. achieved similar results using cortical stimulation to evoke phospheses in 1974 [76,77], and he was a pioneer in the drive to commercialize the visual cortex prosthesis. In 1983, he acquired Avery Labs, a manufacturer of electrodes for brain stimulation. From this and other ventures he derived funds to advance his vision prosthesis research and developments efforts at the Dobelle Institute, located in Portugal. An excellent historical review is provided in this volume by Greenberg.

Retinal Implant: Microelectrode array for retinal activation fabricated on flexible
substrate for adherence to retinal curvature: Schematic implanted eye (left), photomicrograph of 1 of 10 bipolar gold electrode pairs with 25 mm inner electrode (right)

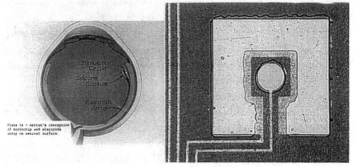

FIGURE 29.2   Example of an early microfabricated Pt–Ir bipolar electrode for acute preclinical experimentation in retinal stimulation built in 1991 by author (DID) [78].

29.2.3.3   Sensory Stimulation — Tactile

Electrocutaneous nerve stimulation was discovered in 1745 by von Kleist who described a shock from an electrostatically charged capacitor [79]. Studies published by von Frey in 1915 [80] and Adrian in 1919 [81] demonstrated the spectrum of sensations elicited by electrocutaneous stimulation, ranging from vibration to prickling pain and stinging pain. In 1966, Beeker [82] described an artificial hand with electrocutaneous feedback of thumb contact pressure. Initial results, although qualitative, were positive. In 1977, Schmidl [83] reported that electrocutaneous sensory feedback of grip strength improved control of an experimental hand. He found electrocutaneous feedback to be less susceptible to adaptation than vibrotactile feedback. In 1979, Shannon showed that electrocutaneous feedback on the skin above the median nerve is used to encode gripping force in a myoelectrically controlled prosthesis and patients reported an improved level of confidence when using the prosthesis [84].

In 1974 at Duke University, Clippinger implanted a sensory feedback system incorporating an electrode pair to stimulate the median nerve. He provided a frequency-modulated signal that transmitted gripping force at the terminal hook. Patients were able to perceive grip force as well as object consistency [85]. In 1977, Clippinger [86] reported a system using implanted electrodes to provide afferent sensory feedback for upper extremity amputees. The same year, he reported that postoperative stimulation of the sciatic nerve by a lower-extremity prosthesis offered the additional benefit of postoperative pain reduction, and in 1982, he reported 6 year success in a lower-extremity amputee using sciatic nerve stimulation to transmit heel strike force and leg structure bending movement on a single channel [87]. No further work on implanted sensory feedback prostheses is published by Clippinger.

In 1995 at MIT, DiLorenzo and Edell demonstrated functionality of a chronically implanted multichannel intrafascicular peripheral electrode array in an animal model using behavioral and neurophysiological recording, including eye blink reflexes and somatosensory evoked potentials. These studies demonstrated the functionality of sensory afferent fibers following transaction as well as the functionality of a chronically implanted intrafascicular stimulating neuroelectric interface [33–35,78] (Figure 29.2). Horch et al. [88–90] have developed percutaneous flexible microwires for intrafascicular stimulation of neural tissue.

29.3   Neuromodulation

29.3.1   Chronic Electrical Stimulation of the Nervous System for Functional Disorders

The early history of the use of electrical stimulation of the nervous system was limited to the acute setting because of the lack of availability of implantable stimulators for chronic use. The first progress in this regard was in the area of cardiac pacing, which only recently has come to be viewed, rightfully, as neuromodulation. Although Aldini was motivated to "reanimate" the heart with Galvanic stimulation [6], the first successes were by Albert Hyman who used faradic stimulation to resuscitate the heart in animals and apparently some patients as well after cardiac arrest [3]. It was not until 1952 that an artificial pacemaker was successfully used by Paul Zoll, and in 1958, a chronic pacemaker was used for 96 days (although it had to be wheeled around on a table!) [91]. An implantable device that had to be charged through the skin was implanted the next year in Sweden [92], followed by a radio-frequency coupled pacemaker [93,94], and the first fully implantable, self-powered device was implanted in 1960 [95].

29.3.2 Early Development of Deep Brain Stimulation for Psychiatric Disorders and Pain

The availability of implantable pacemakers paved the way for their use in treating nervous system disorders of "function," including movement disorders (tremor, PD, dystonia), pain, epilepsy, and psychiatric disorders. Until this time, a common procedure in the 1950s was subfrontal leucotomy for various psychiatric indications and in fact Spiegel and Wycis developed their stereotactic frame mainly for use in this surgery. J. Lawrence Pool at the Neurological Institute at Columbia University was the first to reason that electrical stimulation might provide a nondestructive, reversible alternative to ablative procedures; in this case for psychiatric indications. He had previously — in 1945 — implanted the first patient with an induction coil for stimulating the femoral nerve for paraparesis (the first example of true functional electrical stimulation) [96] and in 1948 he placed a silver electrode in the caudate nucleus of a patient with PD afflicted with intractable depression, coupled to a permanent mini induction coil placed in the skull. His intent was to activate the caudate with electrical stimulation (although his reasoning is not made clear) and indeed he reported that the patient had some benefits from daily stimulation (with an external primary coil?) for 8 weeks, but a wire broke and therapy was discontinued. Pool also implanted a psychotic patient in 1948 with a cingulate gyrus stimulator.

Neural ablation within the pain-mediating pathways of the brain and spinal cord was the standard treatment for deafferentation (neuropathic) or cancer-related (nociceptive) pain, which was refractory to medical treatment. Thus the nonablative treatment of pain was advanced when in 1954, R.G. Heath at Tulane reported pain relief in schizophrenic patients following electrical stimulation of the septal nuclei via a stereotactic approach (first done in 1950) [97], and similar results were reported by Pool using Heath's technique in a patient treated exclusively for pain (with an externalized electrode wire) [98]. In his 1954 monograph, Pool reported that "focal electrical stimulation of deep midline frontal lobe structures is a new technique that is now being used more and more frequently" [98], which apparently included both himself and Heath in patients with psychiatric disease and pain. By this time, Spiegel and Wycis [99] were also implanting chronic electrodes for stimulation through a stereotactic approach. However, there were as yet no reports of the use of chronic stimulation for the treatment of movement disorders. In the 1960s, levo-dopa for the treatment of PD arrived, and virtually eliminated — for the next several decades — the surgical treatment of PD, except for severe tremor. Moreover, by this time, public outcry eliminated the surgical treatment of psychiatric disorders, which, although mainly directed against leucotomy and lobotomy, also included electrical brain stimulation. Thus, the next advances occurred exclusively in the treatment of pain.

By 1960 Heath and colleagues were stimulating the septal nuclei for pain (without concurrent psychiatric disorder) and in 1961 Mazars and colleagues [100,101] introduced the sensory thalamus as a target with the idea that stimulation of the deafferented neurons in the thalamus following amputation or stroke, for example, would relieve neuropathic pain. In these and other reports of brain stimulation for pain (septal region [102]; caudate [103]), only acute stimulation through externalized wires was used. However, Glenn pioneered the use of his RF-coupled device — first introduced for cardiac pacing in 1959 [94] — to pace the phrenic nerve in a paralyzed patient in 1963 [104]. Shortly thereafter, Sweet and Wepsic [105] implanted an RF stimulator to suppress pain in the peripheral nervous system, and it was used in the first dorsal column stimulator implantation in 1967 by Shealy [106], based on the Melzack and Wall "gate control" theory of pain transmission in the spinal cord [107]. In 1982 at Duke, Nashold et al. [108] demonstrated a technique for intraoperatively mapping peripheral nerve bundles in order to accurately place electrodes on individual fasciculi to relieve chronic limb pain.

Pursuing an anatomically more central approach, Hosobuchi and colleagues [109] reported successful chronic stimulation of the sensory thalamus for facial pain in 1973 and this was followed by chronic stimulation of sensory thalamus by Mazars [110] and of other regions as well. Notable amongst these is the periventricular gray region which — based on the findings of analgesia induced by electrical stimulation in the rat by Reynolds [111] — was chronically stimulated in patients in 1973 by Hosobuchi and colleagues [112] and Richardson and Akil [113,114]. Ultimately, the fully implantable battery-powered stimulator was developed for cardiac pacing [95] and then adapted for use in the treatment of pain [14].

29.3.3 The Dawn of Deep Brain Stimulation for Movement Disorders

The earliest use of chronic therapeutic stimulation for movement disorders appears to be that of Bechtereva and colleagues in the erstwhile U.S.S.R. They implanted 24 to 40 electrodes in 4 to 6 bundles into the "thalamic — striopallidal nuclei" for patients with hyperkinesias as a result of PD, torsion dystonia, and other causes [115,116]. Benefits of intermittent stimulation were seen for as long as 3 years, although no implantable stimulator was used. Other early results were from electrical stimulation of sensory thalamus [110,117] or centromedian-parafascicular complex (CM/Pf) [118] for thalamic deafferentation pain, when improvements in the often associated dyskinesia were noted. Another avenue was that of Cooper and colleagues in the 1970s [119] who stimulated the anterior lobe of the cerebellum to treat various movement disorders, including spasticity and dystonia. Davis and colleagues performed cerebellar stimulation on 316 patients between 1974 and 1981 for spastic motor disorders with good success [120].

By the 1970s, when PD was mostly being treated pharmacologically, the usual indication for stereotactic surgery in movement disorders was tremor and hyperkinesias (e.g., in dystonia) and the preferred operation was thalamotomy of the ventral intermediate (Vim) nucleus. It had long been appreciated that acute high-frequency, but not low-frequency electrical stimulation of Vim led to immediate tremor arrest, which was used as a final check prior to radio-frequency ablation [121,122]. The first chronic stimulator implantations directed at movement disorders per se were by Mundinger in 1975 [123]. Brice and McLellan [124] implanted deep brain stimulator (DBS) leads in the subthalamic region (a common site for subthalamotomy at the time) in 3 patients for severe intention tremor resulting from multiple sclerosis. The latter paper is of special interest in that it anticipates by decades the idea of a contingent, on-demand system. Andy [125] implanted 9 patients with stimulating electrodes in the thalamus but concluded that the likely target was CM/Pf.

At about the same time in 1987, Benabid [126,127] and Seigfried [128] began implanting DBSs into Vim of the thalamus for tremor from PD and essential tremor. Benabid's report of his large series of Vim stimulators in 1996 [129], followed shortly thereafter by the North American series [130] brought international attention to the field of electrical brain stimulation. The field came full circle as a result of other important trends. The limitations and complications of levo-dopa treatment for PD began to become apparent by the 1980s and as a result Laitinen — a student of Leksell, a leader in functional neurosurgery in the 1950s during which time pallidotomies were performed — began to revisit ablative surgery for PD. His influential report in 1992 of the results of pallidotomy refocused attention on the surgical treatment of PD [131]. With a large experience by then in DBS, Siegfried performed the first implantation of a stimulator electrode into the posteroventral internal globus pallidus for PD in 1992 [132]. The next advance resulted from new insights into the pathophysiology of PD: the report of DeLong and colleagues of the amelioration of experimental PD in nonhuman primates by the ablation of the subthalamic nucleus, whose glutamatergic driving actions on the globus pallidus interna was elucidated [133]. Benabid then targeted this novel region for deep brain stimulation in 1993 (the subthalamic region, including white matter projections, had been the target for "subthalamotomies," but never before had the subthalamic nucleus per se been targeted because of concerns over the development of hemiballism) [134].

29.3.4   The Efforts toward Neurostimulation for Epilepsy

In the 1950s Cooke [135] and Dow [136] described their work in rats and primates showing that stimulation of the cerebellum had effects on the electroencephalogram and the frequency of seizures. On this basis, in 1973 Cooper and colleagues reported the use of chronic cerebellar stimulation in patients with epilepsy. They also reported benefits for spasticity [119]. Unfortunately, several subsequent clinical series were unable to replicate Cooper's results with epilepsy [137]. Also in the 1970s, Chkhenkeli reported preliminary results of stimulating the caudate nucleus for epilepsy (followed in 1997 by a larger series) (Chkhenkeli and Chkhenkeli, 1997).

Based on the idea that anterior nucleus of the thalamus (ANT) has widespread connections with and therefore possible modulatory effects on the cortex, Cooper also investigated and reported the results of stimulation of the anterior nucleus of the thalamus for epilepsy [138]. Also around that time Mirski and Fisher began providing experimental evidence for a role of the anterior nucleus in epilepsy [139,140] and that electrical stimulation can mitigate seizure activity [141]. This has provided the impetus to revisit this target for epilepsy [142,143] and current trials are underway. Meanwhile, Velasco reported that DBS of the centromedian nucleus (CM) — an intralaminar nucleus with widespread connections to the striatum and cortex — reduced seizure frequency in medically refractory patients [144]. Although not replicated in a limited clinical trial [145], results continue to be good for generalized epilepsy [12].

Also during the 1980s, the groups of Gale [146] and Moshe [147] independently began to report a role for the basal ganglia in regulating seizures. These and other lines of investigation paved the way for two small clinical series involving electrical stimulation of the subthalamic nucleus [148,149] which, although providing mixed results, have led to a larger clinical trial currently underway.

As early as the 1960s, the role of electrical stimulation of vagal nerve afferents on the electroencephalogram was appreciated [150]. This observation led Jacob Zabara, a physiologist at Temple University, to investigate the effect of vagal afferent stimulation on seizures in animal models [151,152]. These pre-clinical findings were the basis for launching Cyberonics, founded by Jacob Zabara and Reese S. Terry Jr. in 1987, which developed an implantable vagus nerve stimulator (VNS). Cyberonics conducted trials of vagal nerve stimulation for epilepsy in human patients beginning in 1988 [153,154] and achieved clinical approval for its use as an adjuvant therapy in 1997.

In the 1990s, Lesser [155] discovered the phenomenon of afterdischarges in the cortex, following electrical stimulation and he found that subsequent electrical stimulation can terminate these afterdischarges.

In 1997, Robert Fishell founded NeuroPace to develop an implant that applies the principle of afterdischarge termination to the treatment of seizures. In 2001, NeuroPace licensed seizure detection technology developed by Brian Litt, Ph.D. Frank Fisher and Ben Pless were recruited as CEO and CTO of NeuroPace and as of this writing, the company is in clinical trials for its Responsive Neurostimulator (RNS) device.

In the 1990s, DiLorenzo designed a closed-loop Neuromodulation technology, and in 2002 he founded NeuroBionics Corporation. In 2004, he recruited John Harris and Kent Leyde to join the company which was renamed BioNeuronics Corporation and as of this writing they are in development of a proprietary technology addressing this market.

Several trials of deep brain stimulation are currently underway. In addition, direct electrical stimulation of the epileptic focus in the cortex or hippocampus, in some cases coupled to contingent and others to closed-loop stimulation algorithms are being examined by a number of investigators.

29.3.5   Current State of the Art of Neurostimulation

Electrical stimulation of the central, peripheral, and autonomic nervous systems has reached the point of standard clinical practice for an expanding list of indications (see table). New indications are under active investigation, such as Tourette's syndrome [156] and cluster headache [157]. Vagal nerve stimulation is routinely performed for epilepsy but deep brain stimulation and cortical stimulation are actively being studied. As a nondestructive alternative, electrical stimulation is spurring a judicious resurgence of psychosurgery for obsessive compulsive disorder (OCD) (internal capsule, nucleus accumbens) and depression (same targets as for OCD, plus vagus nerve, and area 25 [158]) which disable a large number of patients and are treatment-resistant. The treatment of pain continues to lag behind even though it was one of the earliest indications for DBS studies. Spinal cord stimulation is frequently performed for various types of peripheral pain as is peripheral nerve stimulation. Motor cortex stimulation is under active investigation for neuropathic deafferentation pain (as well as for movement disorders [159] and for rehabilitation after stroke [160]).

In addition to advancing the field through expanding indications, technological and scientific advances are promising to increase effectiveness in certain settings. Most promising is the development of closed-loop strategies for the treatment of the epilepsies, and perhaps other disorders (recall the early work of Brice and McClellan [124] with tremor, discussed earlier). The ability to detect and predict [161] seizures is being capitalized on to tailor stimulation or other neuromodulatory interventions. This promises to increase effectiveness and decrease cellular injury, adaptation, or habituation, and to decrease battery drain as well. Other advances may include new electrode designs and stimulation strategies aimed at optimizing activation (or inhibition) of selected neural elements, such as axons over cell bodies. This work will be advanced by increasing understanding of the mechanisms of neurostimulation, which has lagged behind empirical, clinically based progress. Of course, progress in battery technology, including rechargeability and miniaturization, will increase long-term ease-of-use and tolerability of neurostimulation devices. With the more sophisticated neurostimulators on the drawing board and in development at several companies, the battery lifetime becomes an even more important issue than in first generation devices.

At the turn of the 20th century, the remarkable results seen with deep brain stimulation in movement disorders (historically, the last indication for which it was tried) have led to the great resurgence in the use of electrical stimulation for the treatment of a wide variety of neurological disorders. Not since the turn of the 19th century has interest in this therapy been so widespread. The difference, hopefully, is that we are now also in the age of evidence-based medicine so that the seemingly striking benefits of electrical neuromodulation have been and will continue to be subjected to objective standards of evaluation and that the enormous potential neural engineering holds will be responsibly harnessed for the patient's best interest.

References

[1] Velasco, F., Neuromodulation: an overview. *Arch. Med. Res.* 2000, **31**: 232–236.

[2] Largus, S., *Compositiones medicae. Joannes Rhodius recensuit, notis illustrauit, lexicon scriboniaum adiecit.* 1655, P. Frambotti: Patavii.

[3] McNeal, D.R., 2000 years of electrical stimulation, in *Funtional Electrical Stimulation*, F.T. Hambrecht and J.B. Reswick, Eds. 1977, Marcel Dekker: New York, pp. 3–33.

[4] Chaffe, E. and R. Light, A method for remote control of electrical stimulation of the nervous system. *Yale J. Biol. Med.*, 1934, **7**: 83.

[5] Evans, C., Medical observations and inquiries by a society of physicians in London. 1757, **I**: 83–86.

[6] Parent, A., Giovanni Aldini: From animal electricity to human brain stimulation. *Can. J. Neurol. Sci.*, 2004, **31**: 576–584.

[7] Galvani, L., De viribus electricitatis in motu musculari, commentarus. *De Bononiensi Scientiarum et Artium Inst. atque Acad.*, 1791, **7**: 363–418.

[8] Volta, A., Account of some discoveries made by Mr. Galvani from Mr. Alexander Volta to Mr. Tiberius Cavallo. *Phil. Trans. R. Soc.*, 1793, **83**: 10–44.

[9] Volta, A., On the electricity excited by the mere contact of conducting substances of different kinds. *Phil. Trans.*, 1800, **90**: 403.

[10] Aldini, J., *Essai theìorique et expeìrimental sur le galvanisme, avec une seìrie d'expeìriences faites devant des commissaires de l'Institut national de France, et en divers amphithéatres anatomiques de Londres.* 1804, Paris: Fornier Fils.

[11] Fritsch, G. and E. Hitzig, Ü"ber die elektrische Erregbarkeit des Grosshirns. *Arch. Anat. Physiol. wissenschaftl Med.*, 1870, **37**: 300–322.

[12] Velasco, M., et al., Acute and chronic electrical stimulation of the centromedian thalamic nucleus: modulation of reticulo-cortical systems and predictor factors for generalized seizure control. *Arch. Med. Res.*, 2000, **31**: 304–315.

[13] Ferrier, D., The localization of function in the brain. *Proc. R. Soc. Lond.*, 1873, **22**: 229.

[14] Davis, R., Chronic stimulation of the central nervous system, in *Textbook of Stereotactic and Functional Neurosurgery*, P.L. Gildenberg and R.R. Tasker, Eds. 1998, McGraw-Hill: New York, p. 963.

[15] Cushing, H., Faradic stimulation of postcentral gyrus in conscious patients. *Brain*, 1909, **32**: 44–53.

[16] Penfield, W. and H.H. Jasper, *Epilepsy and the Functional Anatomy of the Human Brain.* 1954, Boston: Little, Brown and Co.

[17] Djourno, A. and C.H. Eyries, Prothese auditive par excitation electrique a distance du nerf sensoriel a l'aide d'un bobinage inclus a demeure. *La Presse Medicale*, 1957. **65**: 1417.

[18] Edell, D., A peripheral nerve information transducer for amputees: long-term multichannel recordings from rabbit peripheral nerves. *IEEE Trans. Biomed. Eng.*, 1986. **33**: 203–214.

[19] Edell, D.J., Development of a chronic neuroelectronic interface, 1980, Ph.D. thesis, U.C. Davis, Davis, CA,

[20] Liberson, W.T., et al., Functional electrotherapy: Stimulation of the peroneal nerve synchronized with the swing phase of the gait of hemiplegic patients. *Arch. Phys. Med. Rehabil.*, 1961, **42**: 101–105.

[21] Liberson, W.T., Functional neuromuscular stimulation: historical background and personal experience, in *Functional Neuromuscular Stimulation: Report of a Workshop. April 27–28, 1972*, M.A. LeBlanc, Ed. 1972, Washington, DC, pp. 147–156.

[22] Moe, J.H. and H.W. Post, Functional electrical stimulation for ambulation in hemiplegia. *Lancet*, 1962, **82**: 285–288.

[23] Long, C. and V. Masciarelli, An electrophysiological splint for the hand. *Arch. Phys. Med. Rehabil.*, 1963, **44**: 449–503.

[24] Peckham, P.H., J.T. Mortimer, and E.B. Marsolais, Controlled prehension and release in the C5 quadriplegic elicited by functional electrical stimulation of the paralyzed forearm musculature. *Ann. Biomed. Eng.*, 1980, **8**: 369–388.

[25] Kantrowitz, A., *Electronic Physiologic Aids: A Report of the Maimonides Hospital.* 1960, New York: Brooklyn, pp. 4–5.

[26] Cooper, E.B., W.H. Bunch, and J.H. Campa, Effects of chronic human neuromuscular stimulation. *Surg. Forum.*, 1973. **24**: 477–479.

[27] Brindley, G.S., C.E. Polkey, and D.N. Ruston, Electrical splinting of the knee in paraplegia. *Paraplegia*, 1978, **16**: 434–441.

[28] Bajd, T. et al., The use of a four-channel electrical stimulator as an ambulatory aid for paraplegic patients. *Phys. Ther.*, 1983, **63**: 1116–1120.

[29] Kralj, A. et al., Gait restoration in paraplegic patients: a feasibility demonstration using multichannel surface electrode FES. *J. Rehabil.*, 1983, **20**: 3–20.

[30] DiLorenzo, D.J. and W.K. Durfee, *Unpublished Data on 4-Channel Surface FES for Gait Restoration*, 1990, Massachusetts Institute of Technology.

[31] Durfee, W.K. and D.J. DiLorenzo. Linear and nonlinear approaches to control of single joint motion by functional electrical stimulation, in *Proceedings of the 1990 American Control Conference*, 1990.

[32] Durfee, W.K. and D.J. DiLorenzo, Sliding mode control of FNS knee joint motion. *Abstr. First World Cong. Biomech.*, 1990, **2**: 329.

[33] DiLorenzo, D.J. et al. Chronic intraneural electrical stimulation for prosthetic sensory feedback, in *IEEE EMBS 1st International Conference on Neural Engineering*, 2003. Capri Island, Italy: IEEE.

[34] DiLorenzo, D.J. et al. Multichannel intraneural electrical stimulation for prosthetic sensory feedback, in *Society for Neuroscience Annual Meeting*. 1997, New Orleans, LA.

[35] DiLorenzo, D.J. et al. Multichannel intraneural electrical stimulation for prosthetic sensory feedback, in *Congress of Neurological Surgeons Annual Meeting*. 1997, New Orleans, LA.

[36] DiLorenzo, D.J., Cortical technologies: innovative solutions for neurological disease, 1999, Masters thesis, Massachusetts Institute of Technology, MIT Sloan School of Management: Management of Technology (MOT) Program, Cambridge, MA, p.72.

[37] Goldfarb, M. and W.K. Durfee, Design of a controlled-brake orthosis for FES-aided gait. *IEEE Trans. Rehabil. Eng.*, 1996, **4**: 13–24.

[38] Marsolais, E.B. and R. Kobetic, Functional walking in paralyzed patients by means of electrical stimulation. *Clin. Orthop. Relat. Res.*, 1983, 30–36.

[39] Graupe, D. et al. *EMG-controlled electrical stimulation*, in *Proceedings of the IEEE Frontiers of Engineering and Computer in Health Care*. 1983, Columbus, OH.

[40] Graupe, D. and K.H. Kohn, *Functional Electrical Stimulation for Ambulation by Paraplegics*. 1994, Malabar, FL: Krieger Publishing Co.

[41] Keith, M.W. et al., Implantable functional neuromuscular stimulation in the tetraplegic hand. *J. Hand Surg.*, 1989, **14A**: 524–530.

[42] Georgopoulos, A.P. et al., On the relations between the direction of two-dimensional arm movements and cell discharge in primate motor cortex. *J. Neurosci.*, 1982, **2**: 1527–1537.

[43] Georgopoulos, A.P., R. Caminiti, and J.F. Kalaska, Static spatial effects in motor cortex and area 5: quantitative relations in a two-dimensional space. *Exp. Brain Res.*, 1984, **54**: 446–454.

[44] Caminiti, R. et al., Shift of preferred directions of premotor cortical cells with arm movements performed across the workspace. *Exp. Brain Res.*, 1990, **83**: 228–232.

[45] Kalaska, J.F. et al., A comparison of movement direction-related versus load direction-related activity in primate motor cortex, using a two-dimensional reaching task. *J. Neurosci.*, 1989, **9**: 2080–2102.

[46] Schwartz, A.B., R.E. Kettner, and A.P. Georgopoulos, Primate motor cortex and free arm movements to visual targets in three-dimensional space. I. Relations between single cell discharge and direction of movement. *J. Neurosci.*, 1988, **8**: 2913–2927.

[47] Georgopoulos, A.P., R.E. Kettner, and A.B. Schwartz, Primate motor cortex and free arm movements to visual targets in three-dimensional space. II. Coding of the direction of movement by a neuronal population. *J. Neurosci.*, 1988, **8**: 2928–2937.

[48] Kettner, R.E., A.B. Schwartz, and A.P. Georgopoulos, Primate motor cortex and free arm movements to visual targets in three-dimensional space. III. Positional gradients and population coding of movement direction from various movement origins. *J. Neurosci.*, 1988, **8**: 2938–2947.

[49] Taylor, D.M., S.I. Tillary, and A.B. Schwartz, Direct cortical control of 3D neuroprosthetic devices. *Science*, 2002, **296**: 1828–1832.

[50] Hatsopoulos, N.G. et al., Information about movement direction obtained from synchronous activity of motor cortical neurons. *Proc. Natl Acad. Sci. USA*, 1998, **95**: 15706–15711.

[51] DiLorenzo, D.J., Neural correlates of motor performance in primary motor cortex, 1999, Ph.D. thesis, Massachusetts Institute of Technology, Department of Mechanical Engineering, Cambridge, MA, p. 104.

[52] Maynard, E.M. et al., Neuronal interactions improve cortical population coding of movement direction. *J. Neurosci.*, 1999, **19**: 8083–8093.

[53] Wessberg, J. et al., Real-time prediction of hand trajectory by ensembles of cortical neurons in primates. *Lett. Nature*, 2000, **408**: 361–365.

[54] Kennedy, P.R., The cone electrode: a long-term electrode that records from neurites grown onto its recording surface. *J. Neurosci. Meth.*, 1989, **29**: 181–193.

[55] Kennedy, P.R. and R.A. Bakay, Restoration of neural output from a paralyzed patient by a direct brain connection. *Neuroreport*, 1998, **9**: 1707–1711.

[56] Kennedy, P.R. et al., Direct control of a computer from the human central nervous system. *IEEE Trans. Rehabil. Eng.*, 2000, **8**: 198–202.

[57] Saleh, M. et al. Case study: reliability of multi-electrode array in the knob area of human motor cortex intended for a neuromotor prosthesis application. in *ICORR — 9th International Conference On Rehabilitation Robotics*. 2005, Chicago, IL.

[58] Doyle, J.H., J.B. Doyle, and F.M. Turnbull, Electrical stimulation of eighth cranial nerve. *Arch. Otolaryngol. Head Neck Surg.*, 1964, **80**: 388.

[59] House, W.F. and J. Urban, Long term results of electrode implantation and electronic stimulation of the cochlea in man. *Ann. Otol. Rhinol. Laryngol.*, 1973, **82**: 504.

[60] House, W.F. and K.I. Berliner, Safety and efficacy of the House/3M cochlear implant in profoundly deaf adults. *Otolaryngol. Clin. North Am.*, 1986, **19**: 275.

[61] Simmons, F.B. et al., Auditory nerve: electrical stimulation in man. *Science*, 1965, **148**: 104.

[62] Michelson, R.P., Electrical stimulation of the human cochlea: a preliminary report. *Arch. Otolaryngol. Head Neck Surg.*, 1971, **93**: 317.

[63] Merzenich, M.M., D.N. Schindler, and M.W. White, Feasibility of multichannel scala tympani stimulation. *Laryngoscope*, 1974, **84**: 1887.

[64] Kessler, D.K., The CLARION multi-strategy cochlear implant. *Ann. Otol. Rhinol. Laryngol.*, 1999, **177**(Suppl.): 8–16.

[65] Schindler, R.A. and D.K. Kessler, The UCSF/Storz cochlear implant: patient performance. *Am. J. Otol.*, 1987. **8**: 247–255.

[66] Schindler, R.A., D.K. Kessler, and H.S. Haggerty, Clarion cochlear implant: phase I investigational results [see comment] [erratum appears in *Am. J. Otol.* 1993; **14**: 627]. *Am. J. Otol.*, 1993. **14**: 263–272.

[67] Schindler, R.A. et al., The UCSF/Storz multichannel cochlear implant: patient results. *Laryngoscope*, 1986, **96**: 597–603.

[68] Clark, G.M., A surgical approach for a cochlear implant: an anatomical study. *J. Laryngol. Otol.*, 1975, **89**: 9–15.

[69] Clark, G.M. et al., The University of Melbourne — nucleus multi-electrode cochlear implant. *Adv. Oto-Rhino-Laryngol.*, 1987, **38**: V–IX.

[70] Clark, G.M. and R.J. Hallworth, A multiple-electrode array for a cochlear implant. *J. Laryngol. Otol.*, 1976, **90**: 623–627.

[71] Clark, G.M., R.J. Hallworth, and K. Zdanius, A cochlear implant electrode. *J. Laryngol. Otol.*, 1975, **89**: 787–792.

[72] Cochlear Limited. Cochlear limited corporate website. [Corporate Website] 2005 [cited 2005 July 18, 2005]; Available from: http://www.cochlear.com/.

[73] Burian, K. et al., Designing of and experience with multichannel cochlear implants. *Acta Oto-Laryngol.*, 1979, **87**: 190–195.

[74] Burian, K. et al., Electrical stimulation with multichannel electrodes in deaf patients. *Audiology*, 1980, **19**: 128–136.

[75] Brindley, G.S. and W.S. Lewin, The sensations produced by electrical stimulation of the visual cortex. *J. Physiol.*, 1968, **196**: 479–493.

[76] Dobelle, W.H. and M.G. Mladejovsky, Phosphenes produced by electrical stimulation of human occipital cortex, and their application to the development of a prosthesis for the blind. *J. Physiol.*, 1974, **243**: 553–576.

[77] Dobelle, W.H. et al., "Braille" reading by a blind volunteer by visual cortex stimulation. *Nature*, 1976, **259**: 111–112.

[78] DiLorenzo, D.J., Unpublished Data on Microfabricated Multichannel Electrode Array for Retinal Stimulation, 1991, Massachusetts Institute of Technology.

[79] Canby, E.T., *A History of Electricity*. New York: Hawthorne Books, 1962, p. 21.

[80] Frey, V.M., Physiological experiments on the vibratory sensation [German]. *Z. Biol.*, 1915. **65**: 417–427.

[81] Adrian, E.D., The response of human sensory nerves to currents of short duration. *J. Physiol. (Lond.)*, 1919. **53**: 70–85.

[82] Beeker, T.W., J. During, and A. Den Hertog, Technical note: artificial touch in a hand prosthesis. *Med. Biol. Eng.*, 1967. **5**: 47–49.

[83] Schmidl, H., The importance of information feedback in prostheses for the upper limbs. *Prosthet. Orthot. Int.*, 1977. **1**: 21–24.

[84] Shannon, G.F., A myoelectrically-controlled prosthesis with sensory feedback. *Med. Biol. Eng. Comput.*, 1979. **17**: 73–80.

[85] Clippinger, F.W., A sensory feedback system for an upper-limb amputation prosthesis. *Bull. Prosthet. Res.*, 1974. **BPR 10-22**: 247–258.

[86] Clippinger, F.W., *Textbook of Surgery: The Biological Basis of Modern Surgical Practice*, D.C.e. Sabiston, Ed. 1977, W.B. Saunders: Philadelphia. pp. 1582–1594.

[87] Clippinger, F.W., Afferent sensory feedback for lower extremity prosthesis. *Clin. Orthop.*, 1982, **169**: 202–206.

[88] Malmstrom, J.A., T.G. McNaughton, and K.W. Horch, Recording properties and biocompatibility of chronically implanted polymer-based intrafascicular electrodes. *Ann. Biomed. Eng.*, 1998, **26**: 1055–1064.

[89] McNaughton, T.G. and K.W. Horch, Metallized polymer fibers as leadwires and intrafascicular microelectrodes. *J. Neurosci. Meth.*, 1996, **70**: 103–110.

[90] Lawrence, S.M. et al., Long-term biocompatibility of implanted polymer-based intrafascicular electrodes. *J. Biomed. Mater. Res.*, 2002, **63**: 501–506.

[91] Furman, S. and J.B. Schwedel, *N. Engl. J. Med.*, 1959, **261**: 943–948.

[92] Senning, A., *Mal. Cardiovasc.*, 1963, **4**: 503–512.

[93] Glenn, W.W. et al., Total ventilatory support in a quadriplegic patient with radiofrequency electrophrenic respiration. *N. Engl. J. Med.*, 1972, **286**: 513–516.

[94] Glenn, W.W. et al., *N. Engl. J. Med.*, 1959, **261**: 948–951.

[95] Chardack, W.M., A.A. Gage, and W. Greatbatch, *Surgery*, 1960, **48**.

[96] Pool, J.L., Nerve stimulation in paraplegic patients by means of buried induction coil. Preliminary report. *J. Neurosurg.*, 1946, **3**: 192.

[97] Heath, R.G., *Studies in Schizophrenia: A Multidisciplinary Approach to Mid Brain Relationships.* 1954, Cambridge, MA: Harvard University Press.

[98] Pool, J.L., Psychosurgery in older people. *J. Am. Geriatr. Soc.*, 1954, **2**: 456–466.

[99] Spiegel, E.A. and H.T. Wycis, Chronic implantation of intracerebral electrodes in humans, in *Electrical Stimulation of the Brain*, D.E. Sheer, Ed. 1961, University of Texas Press: Austin, TX, pp. 37–44.

[100] Mazars, G., L. Merienne, and C. Ciolocca, [Intermittent analgesic thalamic stimulation. Preliminary note]. *Rev. Neurol.* (Paris), 1973, **128**: 273–279.

[101] Mazars, G.J., Intermittent stimulation of nucleus ventralis posterolateralis for intractable pain. *Surg. Neurol.*, 1975, **4**: 93–95.

[102] Gol, H., Relief of pain by electrical stimulation of the septal area. *J. Neurol. Sci.*, 1967, **5**: 115–120.

[103] Ervin, F.R., C.E. Brown, and V.H. Mark, Striatal influence on facial pain. *Conf. Neurol.*, 1966, **27**: 75–86.

[104] Glenn, W.W. et al., Diaphragm pacing by radiofrequency transmission in the treatment of chronic ventilatory insufficiency. Present status. *J. Thorac Cardiovasc. Surg.*, 1973, **66**: 505–520.

[105] Sweet, W. and J. Wepsic, Control of pain by focal electrical stimulation for suppression. *Arizona Med.*, 1969, **26**: 1042–1045.

[106] Shealy, C.N., J.T. Mortimer, and J.B. Reswick, Electrical inhibition of pain by stimulation of the dorsal columns: preliminary clinical report. *Anesth. Analg.*, 1967, **46**: 489–491.

[107] Melzack, R. and P.D. Wall, Pain mechanisms: a new theory. *Science*, 1965, **150**: 971–979.

[108] Mullen, J.B., C.F. Walker, and B.S. Nashold, Jr., An electrophysiological approach to neural augmentation implantation for the control of pain. *J. Bioeng.*, 1978, **2**: 65–67.

[109] Hosobuchi, Y., J.E. Adams, and B. Rutkin, Chronic thalamic stimulation for the control of facial anesthesia dolorosa. *Arch. Neurol.*, 1973, **29**: 158–161.

[110] Mazars, G., L. Merienne, and C. Cioloca, [Use of thalamic stimulators in the treatment of various types of pain]. *Ann. Med. Int. (Paris)*, 1975, **126**: 869–871.

[111] Reynolds, D.V., Surgery in the rat during electrical analgesia induced by focal brain stimulation. *Science*, 1969, **164**: 444–445.

[112] Hosobuchi, Y., J.E. Adams, and R. Linchitz, Pain relief by electrical stimulation of the central gray matter in humans and its reversal by naloxone. *Science*, 1977, **197**: 183–186.

[113] Richardson, D.E. and H. Akil, Pain reduction by electrical brain stimulation in man. Part 2: Chronic self-administration in the periventricular gray matter. *J. Neurosurg.*, 1977, **47**: 184–194.

[114] Richardson, D.E. and H. Akil, Pain reduction by electrical brain stimulation in man. Part 1: Acute administration in periaqueductal and periventricular sites. *J. Neurosurg.*, 1977, **47**: 178–183.

[115] Bechtereva, N.P. et al., Therapeutic electrostimulation of deep brain structures. *Vopr. Neirokhir.*, 1972, **1**: 7–12.

[116] Bechtereva, N.P. et al., Method of electrostimulation of the deep brain structures in treatment of some chronic diseases. *Confin. Neurol.*, 1975, **37**: 136–140.

[117] Mazars, G., L. Merienne, and C. Cioloca, Control of dyskinesias due to sensory deafferentation by means of thalamic stimulation. *Acta Neurochir. Suppl. (Wien.)*, 1980, **30**: 239–243.

[118] Andy, O.J., Parafascicular-center median nuclei stimulation for intractable pain and dyskinesia (painful-dyskinesia). *Appl. Neurophysiol.*, 1980, **43**: 133–144.

[119] Cooper, I.S. et al., Chronic cerebellar stimulation in cerebral palsy. *Neurology*, 1976, **26**: 744–753.

[120] Davis, R. et al., Update of chronic cerebellar stimulation for spasticity and epilepsy. *Appl. Neurophysiol.*, 1982, **45**: 44–50.

[121] Hassler, R. et al., Physiological observations in stereotaxic operations in extrapyramidal motor disturbances. *Brain*, 1960, **83**: 337–350.

[122] Jurko, M.F., O.J. Andy, and D.P. Foshee, Diencephalic influence on tremor mechanisms. *Arch. Neurol.*, 1963, **9**: 358–362.

[123] Mundinger, F. and H. Neumuller, Programmed stimulation for control of chronic pain and motor diseases. *Appl. Neurophysiol.*, 1982, **45**: 102–111.

[124] Brice, J. and L. McLellan, Suppression of intention tremor by contingent deep-brain stimulation. *Lancet*, 1980, **1**: 1221–1222.

[125] Andy, O.J., Thalamic stimulation for control of movement disorders. *Appl. Neurophysiol.*, 1983, **46**: 107–111.

[126] Benabid, A.L. et al., Combined (thalamotomy and stimulation) stereotactic surgery of the VIM thalamic nucleus for bilateral Parkinson disease. *Appl. Neurophysiol.*, 1987, **50**: 344–346.

[127] Benabid, A.L. et al., Long-term suppression of tremor by chronic stimulation of the ventral intermediate thalamic nucleus. *Lancet*, 1991, **337**: 403–406.

[128] Siegfried, J., Therapeutical neurostimulation — indications reconsidered. *Acta Neurochir. Suppl. (Wien)*, 1991, **52**: 112–117.

[129] Benabid, A.L. et al., Chronic electrical stimulation of the ventralis intermedius nucleus of the thalamus as a treatment of movement disorders. *J. Neurosurg.*, 1996, **84**: 203–214.

[130] Koller, W. et al., High-frequency unilateral thalamic stimulation in the treatment of essential and Parkinsonian tremor. *Ann. Neurol.*, 1997, **42**: 292–299.

[131] Laitinen, L.V., A.T. Bergenheim, and M.I. Hariz, Leksell's posteroventral pallidotomy in the treatment of Parkinson's disease. *J. Neurosurg.*, 1992, **76**: 53–61.

[132] Siegfried, J. and B. Lippitz, Bilateral chronic electrostimulation of ventroposterolateral pallidum: a new therapeutic approach for alleviating all parkinsonian symptoms. *Neurosurgery*, 1994, **35**: 1126–1129; discussion 1129–1130.

[133] Bergman, H., T. Wichmann, and M.R. DeLong, Reversal of experimental parkinsonism by lesions of the subthalamic nucleus. *Science*, 1990, **249**: 1436–1438.

[134] Benabid, A.L. et al., Acute and long-term effects of subthalamic nucleus stimulation in Parkinson's disease. *Stereotact Funct. Neurosurg.*, 1994, **62**: 76–84.

[135] Cooke, P.M. and R.S. Snider, Some cerebellar influences on electrically-induced cerebral seizures. *Epilepsia*, 1955, **4**: 19–28.

[136] Dow, R.S., A. Fernandez-Guardiola, and E. Manni, The influence of the cerebellum on experimental epilepsy. *Electroencephalogr. Clin. Neurophysiol.*, 1962, **14**: 383–398.

[137] Krauss, G.L. and R.S. Fisher, Cerebellar and thalamic stimulation for epilepsy. *Adv. Neurol.*, 1993, **63**: 231–245.

[138] Upton, A.R. et al., Suppression of seizures and psychosis of limbic system origin by chronic stimulation of anterior nucleus of the thalamus. *Int. J. Neurol.*, 1985, **19–20**: 223–230.

[139] Mirski, M.A. and J.A. Ferrendelli, Interruption of the mammillothalamic tract prevents seizures in guinea pigs. *Science*, 1984, **226**: 72–74.

[140] Mirski, M.A. and J.A. Ferrendelli, Anterior thalamic mediation of generalized pentylenetetrazol seizures. *Brain Res.*, 1986, **399**: 212–223.

[141] Mirski, M.A. et al., Anticonvulsant effect of anterior thalamic high frequency electrical stimulation in the rat. *Epilepsy Res.*, 1997, **28**: 89–100.

[142] Hodaie, M. et al., Chronic anterior thalamus stimulation for intractable epilepsy. *Epilepsia*, 2002, **43**: 603–608.

[143] Kerrigan, J.F. et al., Electrical stimulation of the anterior nucleus of the thalamus for the treatment of intractable epilepsy. *Epilepsia*, 2004, **45**: 346–354.

[144] Velasco, F. et al., Electrical stimulation of the centromedian thalamic nucleus in the treatment of convulsive seizures: a preliminary report. *Epilepsia*, 1987, **28**: 421–430.

[145] Fisher, R.S. et al., Placebo-controlled pilot study of centromedian thalamic stimulation in treatment of intractable seizures. *Epilepsia*, 1992, **33**: 841–851.

[146] Gale, K., Mechanisms of seizure control mediated by gamma-aminobutyric acid: role of the substantia nigra. *Fed. Proc.*, 1985, **44**: 2414–2424.

[147] Moshe, S.L. and B.J. Albala, Nigral muscimol infusions facilitate the development of seizures in immature rats. *Brain Res.*, 1984, **315**: 305–308.

[148] Benabid, A.L. et al., Deep brain stimulation of the corpus luysi (subthalamic nucleus) and other targets in Parkinson's disease. Extension to new indications such as dystonia and epilepsy. *J. Neurol.*, 2001, **248 (Suppl 3)**: III37–III47.

[149] Loddenkemper, T. et al., Deep brain stimulation in epilepsy. *J. Clin. Neurophysiol.*, 2001, **18**: 514–532.

[150] Chase, M.H., M.B. Sterman, and C.D. Clemente, Cortical and subcortical patterns of response to afferent vagal stimulation. *Exp. Neurol.*, 1966, **16**: 36–49.

[151] Zabara, J., Time course of seizure control to brief, repetitive stimuli. *Epilepsia*, 1985, **28**: 604.

[152] Zabara, J., Control of hypersynchronous discharge in peilepsy. *Electroencephalogr. Clin. Neurophysiol.*, 1985, **61**: 162.

[153] Penry, J.K. and J.C. Dean, Prevention of intractable partial seizures by intermittent vagal stimulation in humans: preliminary results. *Epilepsia*, 1990, **31 (Suppl 2)**: S40–S43.

[154] Uthman, B.M. et al., Treatment of epilepsy by stimulation of the vagus nerve. *Neurology*, 1993, **43**: 1338–1345.

[155] Lesser, R.P. et al., Brief bursts of pulse stimulation terminate afterdischarges caused by cortical stimulation. *Neurology*, 1999, **53**: 2073–2081.

[156] Visser-Vandewalle, V. et al., Chronic bilateral thalamic stimulation: a new therapeutic approach in intractable Tourette syndrome. Report of three cases. *J. Neurosurg.*, 2003, **99**: 1094–1100.

[157] Franzini, A. et al., Stimulation of the posterior hypothalamus for treatment of chronic intract-able cluster headaches: first reported series. *Neurosurgery,* 2003, **52**: 1095–1099; discussion 1099–1101.

[158] Mayberg, H.S. et al., Deep brain stimulation for treatment-resistant depression. *Neuron,* 2005, **45**: 651–660.

[159] Pagni, C.A., S. Zeme, and F. Zenga, Further experience with extradural motor cortex stimulation for treatment of advanced Parkinson's disease. Report of 3 new cases. *J. Neurosurg. Sci.,* 2003, **47**: 189–193.

[160] Brown, J.A. et al., Motor cortex stimulation for enhancement of recovery after stroke: case report. *Neurol. Res.,* 2003, **25**: 815–818.

[161] Litt, B. and J. Echauz, Prediction of epileptic seizures. *Lancet Neurol.,* 2002, **1**: 22–30.

30

Electrical Stimulation of the Central Nervous System

Warren M. Grill
Duke University

30.1 Introduction

Electrical stimulation is a widespread method to study the form and function of the nervous system and a technique to restore function following disease or injury. The central nervous system (CNS) includes the brain and spinal cord (Figure 30.1). Both the spinal cord and brain include regions primarily populated by cell bodies (somas) of neurons, and termed gray matter for its color, and regions primarily populated by axons of neurons, and termed white matter. The diversity of neuronal elements and complexity of the volume conductor make understanding the effects of stimulation more challenging in the case of CNS stimulation than in the case of peripheral stimulation. Specifically, it is unclear, in many cases, what neuronal elements (axons, cell bodies, presynaptic terminals; Figure 30.1) are activated by stimulation [Ranck, 1975]. Further, it is unclear how targeted neural elements can be stimulated selectively without coactivation of other surrounding elements. This chapter presents a review of the properties of CNS stimulation as required for rational design and interpretation of therapies employing electrical stimulation.

Electrical stimulation has been used to determine the structure of axonal branching [Jankowska and Roberts, 1972], examine strength of connections between neurons, and determine the projection patterns of neurons [Lipski, 1981; Tehovnik, 1996]. Examples of application of CNS stimulation from treatment

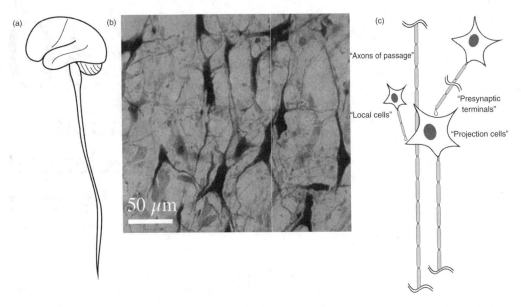

FIGURE 30.1 Structure of the central nervous system (CNS). (a) The CNS includes the brain and the spinal cord. (b) The gray matter of the CNS contains the cell bodies of neurons as well as dendritic and axonal processes. (c) When an electrode is placed within the heterogeneous cellular environment of the CNS it is unclear which neuronal elements are effected by stimulation.

of neurological disorders include the treatment of pain by stimulation of the brain [Coffey, 2001] and spinal cord [Cameron, 2004], treatment of tremor and the motor system symptoms of Parkinson's disease [Gross and Lozano, 2000], as an experimental treatment for epilepsy [Velasco et al., 2001; Hodaie et al., 2002], as well as a host of other neurological disorders [Gross, 2004]. In addition CNS stimulation is being developed for restoration of hearing by electrical stimulation of the cochlear nucleus [Otto et al., 2002] and for restoration of vision [Brindley and Lewin, 1968; Schmidt et al., 1996; Troyk et al., 2003].

A nerve cell or a nerve fiber can be artificially stimulated by depolarization of the cell's membrane. The resulting action potential propagates to the terminal of the neuron leading to release of neurotransmitter that can impact the postsynaptic cell. Passage of current through extracellular electrodes positioned near neurons creates extracellular potentials in the tissue. The resulting potential distribution can result in an outward flowing transmembrane current and depolarization. Alternately, extracellular potentials may modulate or block ongoing neuronal firing depending on the magnitude, distribution, and polarity of the potentials.

The objective of this chapter is to present the biophysical basis for electrical stimulation of neurons in the CNSs. The focus is on using fundamental understanding of both the electric field and its effects on neurons to determine the site of neuronal excitation or modulation in the CNS where electrodes are placed among heterogeneous populations of neuronal elements including cells, axons, and dendrites.

30.2 Generation of Potentials in CNS Tissues

Passage of current through tissue generates potentials in the tissue (recall Ohm's Law: $V = IR$). The potentials are dependent on the electrode geometry, the stimulus parameters (current magnitude), and the electrical properties of the tissue. For example, the potential generated by a monopolar point source can be determined analytically using the relationship $V_e(r) = I/4\pi\sigma r$ where I is the stimulating current, σ is the conductivity of the tissue medium (Table 30.1), and r is the distance between the electrode and the measurement point. The point source model is a valid approximation for sharp electrodes with small

TABLE 30.1 Electrical Conductivity of CNS Tissues

Tissue type	Electrical conductivity (S/m)	Reference
Dura	0.030	Holsheimer et al., 1995
Cerebrospinal fluid	1.5; 1.8	Crile et al., 1922; Baumann et al., 1997
Gray matter	0.20	Ranck, 1963; Li et al., 1968; Sances and Larson, 1975
White matter		Anisotropic
Transverse		
	0.6	Ranck and BeMent, 1965 (cat dorsal columns)
	1.1	Nicholson, 1965 (cat internal capsule)
Longitudinal		
	0.083	Ranck and BeMent, 1965
	0.13	Nicholson, 1965
Encapsulation tissue	0.16	Grill and Mortimer, 1994

tips [McIntyre and Grill, 2001]. Larger electrodes are typically used for chronic stimulation of the CNS, and the spatial distribution of the potentials in the tissue differs from those produced by a point source electrode (Figure 30.2). Examples of the spectrum of electrode types used for CNS stimulation (and recording) are shown in Figure 30.3.

The extracellular potentials generated by the passage of current are dependent on the electrical properties of the tissue. The electrical properties of the CNS are both inhomogeneous and anisotropic (Table 30.1), and the distribution of potentials within the tissue will depend strongly on the tissue and electrode geometries. In general, biological conductivities have a small reactive component [Ackman and Seitz, 1984; Eisenberg and Mathias, 1980], and thus a relatively small increase in conductivity at higher frequencies [Ranck, 1963; Nicholson, 1965; Ranck and BeMent, 1965].

Spatial variations in the electrical properties of the tissue can cause changes in the patterns of activation [Grill, 1999]. In most cases, to calculate accurately the extracellular potentials generated by extracellular stimulation requires a numerical solution using a discretized model, for example with the finite element method [e.g., Veltink et al., 1989; McIntyre and Grill, 2002].

30.3 Response of Neurons to Imposed Extracellular Potentials

As described in the previous section, the distribution of extracellular potentials is dependent on the electrode geometry, the electrical properties of the extracellular tissue, and the stimulation amplitude. The effect of the potentials on neurons is dependent on the nerve cell type, its size and geometry, as well as the temporal characteristics of the stimulus. During stimulation of peripheral nerves it is clear that it is the axons in the vicinity of the electrodes that are activated. However, the CNS contains a heterogeneous population of neuronal elements including local cells projecting locally around the electrode as well as those projecting away from the region of stimulation, axons passing by the electrode, and presynaptic terminals projecting onto neurons in the region of the electrode (Figure 30.1c). Effects of stimulation can be mediated by activation of any or all of these elements and include both direct effects of stimulation of postsynaptic elements, as well as indirect effects mediated by electrical stimulation of presynaptic terminals that mediate the effects of stimulation via synaptic transmission.

From this complexity arise two principal questions during stimulation of the CNS [Grill and McIntyre, 2001]: what neuronal elements are activated by extracellular stimulation? and how can targeted elements be stimulated selectively? Computational modeling provides a powerful tool to study extracellular excitation of CNS neurons. The volume of tissue stimulated, both for fibers and cells, and how this changes with electrode geometry, stimulus parameters, and the geometry of the neuronal elements is quite challenging to determine experimentally. Using a computer model enables these parameters to be examined under controlled conditions and enables determination of the effects of stimulation on all the different neural

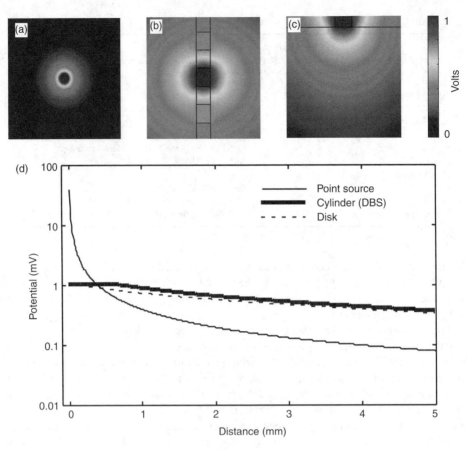

FIGURE 30.2 (See color insert following page **32**-14.) Electric fields generated by passage of current in CNS tissue. The first step in determining the response of CNS neurons to extracellular stimulation is to calculate the electric potentials generated in the tissue by passage of current through the electrode. Potentials produced by passage of current into a homogenous region of the CNS ($\sigma = 0.2$ S/m) using a point source electrode (a), a cylindrical electrode (b), as used for deep brain stimulation, and a disk electrode (c), as used for epidural or cortical surface stimulation. (d) Although a simple analytical solution exists for the potentials generated by a point source electrode, they differ substantially from the potentials generated by larger cylindrical or disk electrodes.

elements around the electrode simultaneously. Computational modeling of the effects of extracellular stimulation on neurons involves a two-step approach. The first step is to calculate the electric potentials generated in the tissue by passage of current through the electrode. The second step is to determine the effect of those potentials on the surrounding neurons.

30.4   From Cell to Circuit — Construction of Models of CNS Neurons

Electrical circuits are used to model the electrical behavior of neurons. These electrical-equivalent circuits, often referred to as cable models, represent the neuron as a series of cylindrical elements. Each cylinder is in turn replaced by a "compartment," representing the neuronal membrane, and a resistor representing the intracellular space. Thus the model becomes a series of membrane compartments, connected by resistors. Each compartment is itself an electrical circuit that includes a capacitor representing the membrane capacitance of the lipid bilayer, resistors representing the ionic conductances of the transmembrane

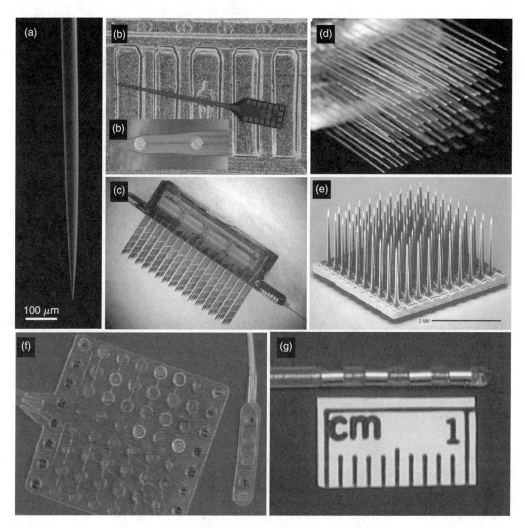

FIGURE 30.3 (See color insert following page **32**-14.) Electrodes for central nervous system stimulation. (a) Single iridium microwire electrode developed at Huntington Medical Research Institutes that can be used for extracellular recording from single units or extracellular microstimulation of small populations of neurons [McCreery et al., 1997]. (b) Multisite silicon microprobe developed at the University of Michigan. Inset shows higher magnification view of two electrode sites near the tip (Images courtesy of J.F. Hetke, University of Michigan). (c) Three-dimensional assembly of multisite silicon microprobes [Bai et al., 2000]. The array is four probes, 256 sites on 400 μm centers in 3D. There are 16 parallel stimulating channels (16 sites active at any time) with off-chip current generation. The array is fed by a 7-lead ribbon cable at a data rate of up to 10 Mbps. It operates from $\pm$5V supplies. (Image courtesy of K.D. Wise, University of Michigan). (d) Arrays of up to 128 microwires enable simultaneous extracellular recording from multiple single neurons. Each wire is 50 μm diameter stainless steel, insulated with Teflon [Nicolelis et al., 2003]. (e) Multielectrode silicone array developed at the University of Utah [Normann et al., 1999]. (f) Subdural grid and strip electrode arrays used for cortical stimulation and recording (PMT Corporation, Chanhassen, MN). (g) Quadrapolar electrode used for deep brain stimulation (Medtronic Inc., Minneapolis, MN).

proteins (ion channels), and batteries representing the differences in potential (Nernst potential) arising from ionic concentration differences across the membrane. The process of constructing an equivalent electric-circuit model of a CNS neuron is illustrated in Figure 30.4.

The values of circuit elements can be readily calculated from the geometry of the neurons and the specific values of neuron electrical properties. Consider a cylindrical representation of a segment of

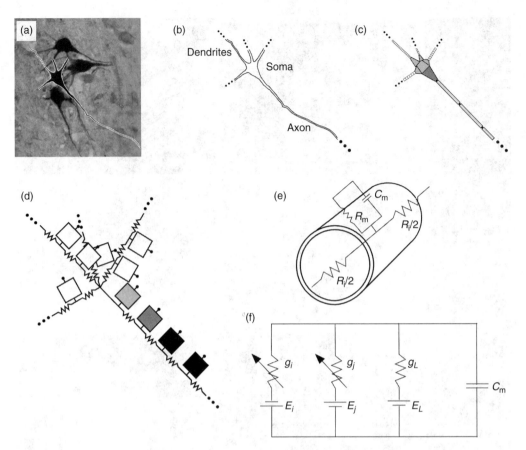

FIGURE 30.4 Construction of models of central nervous system (CNS) neurons. (a) Examples of stained neurons in the CNS. (b) The morphology of stained neurons can be reconstructed in three dimensions. (c) The morphology is then converted into a series of equivalent cylindrical elements. (d) The cylindrical elements are subsequently replaced by electrical equivalent circuits with resistive elements representing the intracellular space and compartmental models representing the membrane. (e) Each cylindrical segment includes a representation of the membrane and the intracellular space and the values of the equivalent circuit elements can be calculated from the geometry of the cylinder and specific parameter values. (f) Each compartment model of the membrane may contain several nonlinear ionic conductances (g_i, g_j) and linear ionic conductance (g_L) representing various ionic channels in the membrane, batteries representing the Nernst potential arising from the difference in concentration of ions on the inside and outside of the membrane (E_i, E_j, E_L), and a capacitor (C_m) representing the capacitance arising from the lipid bilayer of the cell.

neuronal element, with diameter d and length l (Figure 30.4e). If we cut and "unroll" the cylinder then the membrane resistance, R_m, can be calculated as: R_m = specific membrane resistance/area of segment = $r_m / \pi \times l \times d$, where typical values for the specific membrane resistance are from 1000 to 5000 Ω-cm^2. The membrane resistance is nonlinear, where the value of the membrane resistance depends on the voltage across the membrane (transmembrane potential). Further, separate elements (typically calculated as conductances) are used to represent the transmembrane paths for different ionic species, and the model of a patch of membrane includes several of these in parallel (Figure 30.4e). Similarly, the membrane capacitance, C_m, can be calculated as: C_m = specific membrane capacitance × area of segment = $c_m / \pi \times l \times d$, where typical values of the specific membrane capacitance are from 1 to 2 μF/cm^2. The intracellular resistance, R_i, can be calculated as: R_i = intracellular resistivity × segment length/cross sectional area of segment = $\rho_i \times l / (\pi \times (d/2)^2)$, where typical values of the intracellular resistivity are from 50 to 400 Ω-cm.

(a)   (b)   (c)

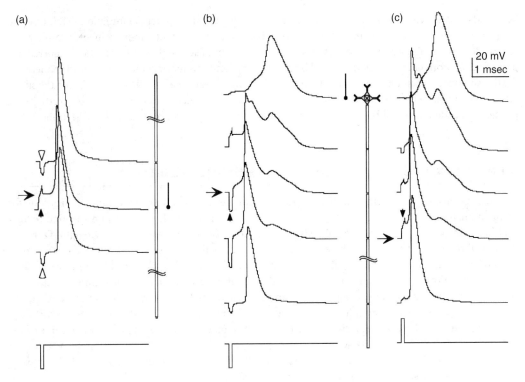

20 mV
1 msec

FIGURE 30.5   Action potential initiation by extracellular stimulation of CNS neurons by cathodic and anodic stimuli. Each trace shows transmembrane voltage as a function of time for different sections of the neuron. (a) Stimulation with a monophasic cathodic stimulus pulse from an electrode positioned 1 mm over a node of Ranvier of the axon. Depolarization occurs in the node directly beneath the electrode (solid arrowhead) and hyperpolarization occurs in the adjacent nodes of Ranvier (open arrowhead). Action potential initiation occurs in the node of Ranvier directly under the electrode (arrow) and the action potential propagates in both directions. (b) During threshold stimulation with an electrode positioned 1 mm over the cell body, action potential initiation occurs at a node of Ranvier of the axon. With cathodic stimuli (duration 0.1 msec) action potential initiation occurred at the second node of Ranvier from the cell body (arrow). (c) With anodic stimuli (duration 0.1 msec) action potential initiation occurred in the third node of Ranvier from the cell body (arrow).

30.5   Sites of Action Potential Initiation in CNS Neurons

The response of a cable model, representing a CNS neuron, to extracellular electrical stimulation is shown in Figure 30.5. The transmembrane potential as a function of time, in different segments of the neuron, is shown for a cathodic electrode positioned over the axon (Figure 30.5a), for a cathodic electrode positioned over the cell body (Figure 30.5b), and for an anodic electrode positioned over the cell body (Figure 30.5c).

During stimulation over the axon with a cathodic current the axon is depolarized immediately beneath the electrode, and hyperpolarized in regions lateral to the electrode (arrowheads Figure 30.5a). Action potential initiation occurs in the most depolarized node of Ranvier, immediately beneath the electrode (arrow) and then propagates in both directions.

The response of a CNS neuron is more complex. With both cathodic and anodic stimuli delivered through an electrode placed 1 mm above the cell body, action potential initiation occurred in the axon, even though the electrode is positioned directly over the soma. With 0.1 msec duration cathodic stimuli action potential initiation occurred at the second node of Ranvier from the cell body (arrow), and with 0.1 msec duration anodic stimuli action potential initiation occurred in the third node of Ranvier from the cell body (arrow). During the cathodic stimulus pulse, the node of Ranvier where action potential initiation occurred was hyperpolarized by the stimulus (arrowhead). Following termination of the stimulus, the cell body and dendritic tree discharged through the axon, leading to action potential initiation [McIntyre and Grill, 1999]. This finding in a computational model is consistent with contemporary in vitro results from cortex [Nowak and Bullier, 1998a, b]. Thus, with cathodic stimuli action potential initiation occurred in a part of the neuron that was hyperpolarized by the stimulus, and this indirect mode of activation increases the threshold for activation of local cells with cathodic stimuli. Conversely, with anodic stimuli, the site of action potential initiation was at the node that was most depolarized by the stimulus (arrowhead). These position dependent thresholds are reflected in exciting populations of neurons, as well (see Section 30.6.3).

30.6 Excitation Properties of CNS Stimulation

The finding that action potential initiation occurs in the axon has several important implications for CNS stimulation. First, since excitation occurs in the axon there is little difference in the extracellular chronaxie times for excitation of local cells and excitation of passing axons (see "Strength–Duration Relationship," in Section 30.6.1). Therefore, chronaxie time is not a sensitive indicator of the neuronal element that is activated by extracellular stimulation [Miocinovic and Grill, 2004]. Second, since action potential initiation occurs at some distance from the site of integration of synaptic inputs, the effects of coactivation of presynaptic fibers may be less than expected and the axon may still fire even when the cell body is hyperpolarized, for example by inhibitory synaptic inputs (see "Indirect Effects," Section 30.6.4). Therefore, extracellular unit recordings of cell body firing may not accurately reflect the output of the neuron [Grill and McIntyre, 2001; McIntyre et al., 2004]. Finally, the difference in the mode of activation of local cells by cathodic stimuli and anodic stimuli is the basis for the difference in threshold between cathodic and anodic stimuli (see "Effect of Stimulus Polarity," Section 30.6.3).

30.6.1 Strength–Duration Relationship

The stimulus amplitude necessary for excitation, I_{th}, increases as the duration of the stimulus is decreased. The strength–duration relationship describes this phenomena and is given by

$$I_{th} = I_{rh} \left[1 + \frac{T_{ch}}{PW} \right]$$

where the parameter I_{rh} is the rheobase current, and is defined as the current amplitude necessary to excite the neuron with a pulse of infinite duration, and the parameter T_{ch} is the chronaxie and is defined as the pulse duration necessary to excite the neuron with pulse amplitude equal to twice the rheobase current.

Measurements with intracellular stimulation have demonstrated that the temporal excitation characteristics, including chronaxie (T_{ch}) and refractory period, of cells and axons differ (Figure 30.6a). However, during extracellular stimulation of neurons, action potential initiation occurs in the axon, even with the stimulating electrode positioned over the cell body or dendrites (see above). Although with intracellular activation the chronaxies of many cell bodies exceed 1 msec, with extracellular activation they are below 1 msec [Stoney et al., 1968; Ranck, 1975; Asanuma, 1976; Swadlow, 1992] and lie within the ranges determined for extracellular activation of axons [Ranck, 1975; Li and Bak, 1976; West and Wolstencroft, 1983]. For stimulation of cortical gray matter, the mean T_{ch} for *intracellular* stimulation of cells (15 msec) was substantially longer than T_{ch} for *extracellular* stimulation of axons (0.27 msec), but the mean T_{ch} for *extracellular* stimulation of local cells (0.38 msec) was comparable to that for extracellular stimulation of axons [Nowak and Bullier, 1998a]. Further, the chronaxies measured with extracellular stimulation were dependent on a number of factors other than the neuronal element that was stimulated [Miocinovic and Grill, 2004]. The chronaxies of different neuronal elements determined with extracellular stimulation overlap and do not enable unique determination of the neuronal element stimulated.

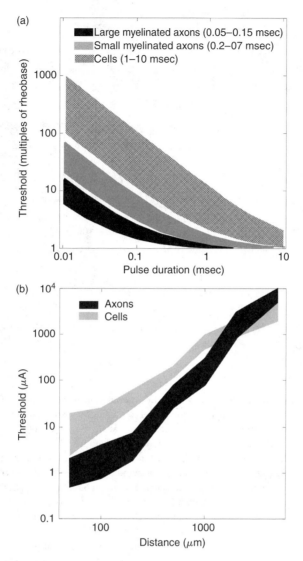

FIGURE 30.6 Properties of central nervous system stimulation. (a) The strength–duration relationship describes the amplitude required for stimulation as a function of the stimulation pulse duration. Strength–duration curves for intracellular stimulation of different neural elements were constructed from data summarized in Ranck, 1976. (b) The current–distance relationship describes the threshold intensity required for stimulation as a function of the distance between the electrode and the neuron. Current–distance curves for axons and cells were constructed from data summarized in Ranck, 1976.

30.6.2 Current–Distance Relationship

The threshold current required for extracellular stimulation of neurons, I_{th}, increases as the distance between the electrode and the neuron, r, increases. This is described by the current–distance relationship [Stoney et al., 1968]:

$$I_{th} = I_R + k \cdot r^2$$

where the offset, I_R, determines the absolute threshold and the slope, k, determines the threshold difference between neurons at different distances from the electrode. Current–distance relationship for excitation of

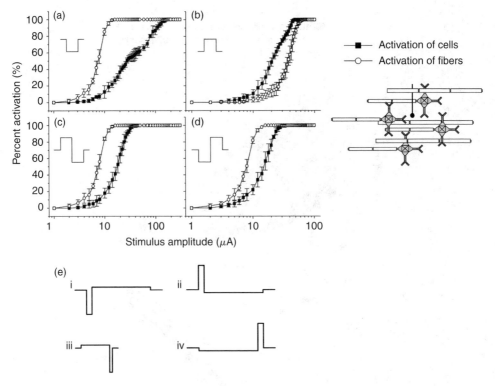

FIGURE 30.7 Effect of stimulus polarity and waveform on excitation of populations of local cells and passing axons. (a)–(d) Input–output curves from a population model containing 50 passing axons and 50 local cells randomly positioned around a point source stimulating electrode. The curves are the percent of neurons (passing axons, local cells) activated as a function of the stimulation amplitude for excitation with (a) 0.2 msec duration monophasic cathodic pulses, (b) 0.2 msec duration monophasic anodic pulses, (c) anodic-phase-first biphasic symmetric pulses (0.2 msec per phase), and (d) cathodic-phase-first biphasic symmetric pulses (0.2 msec per phase) [modified from McIntyre and Grill, 2000]. (e) Examples of asymmetric charge-balanced biphasic pulses. Cathodic-phase-first (i) and anodic-phase-first psuedomonophasic pulses have a low-amplitude second phases and exhibit excitation properties similar to monophasic cathodic and anodic stimuli, respectively. Novel asymmetric pulses manipulate neuronal excitability via a subthreshold first that also balances the charge. The anodic prepulse (0.2 msec) followed by a cathodic stimulus phase (0.02 msec) enables preferential excitation of passing axons, while a cathodic prepulse (1.0 msec) followed by an anodic stimulus pulse (0.1 msec) enables preferential excitation of local cells [McIntyre and Grill, 2000].

axons and cells in the CNS have been measured in a large number of preparations, and current–distance curves for these two populations are summarized in Figure 30.6b.

30.6.3 Effect of Stimulus Polarity and Stimulus Waveform on CNS Stimulation

During excitation of axons in the peripheral nervous system different stimulus polarities produce changes in the threshold as well as changes in the site of action potential initiation, and similar, but more pronounced effects occur during CNS stimulation. In Figure 30.7 are shown the results of a computational study to determine which neuronal elements are activated by extracellular stimulation in the CNS. A model including populations of local cells and axons of passage, randomly positioned around a point source stimulating electrode, was used to compare activation of local cells to activation of passing fibers with different stimulation waveforms [McIntyre and Grill, 2000]. Using cathodic pulses the threshold for activation of passing axons was less than the threshold for activation of local neurons, and when 70%

of the axons were activated approximately 10% of the local cells were also activated. When using anodic pulses, the threshold for activation of local cells is less than the threshold for activation of passing axons, and the stimulus amplitude that activated 70% of the local cells also activated 25% of the passing axons. The basis for this effect can be understood by comparing action potential initiation in local cells using cathodic and anodic stimuli described earlier.

To prevent possible degradation of the stimulating electrodes or damage to the tissue, chronic stimulation is conducted with biphasic stimulus pulses [Lilly et al., 1955; Robblee and Rose, 1990]. The response of passing axons and local cells to symmetric biphasic pulses is shown in Figure 30.7c and Figure 30.7d. Using either anodic-phase-first or cathodic-phase-first pulses, the threshold for activation of passing axons was less than the threshold for activation of local neurons, and the relative selectivity for axons was lower with either pulse than with monophasic cathodic pulses.

These results and previous experimental evidence demonstrate that different neuronal elements have similar thresholds for extracellular stimulation [Roberts and Smith, 1973; Gustafsson and Jankowska, 1976] and illustrates the need for design of methods that enable selective stimulation. Stimulus waveforms can be designed explicitly to take advantage of the nonlinear conductance properties of neurons and thereby increase the selectivity between activation of different neuronal elements. Biphasic asymmetrical stimulus waveforms capable of selectively activating either local cells or axonal elements consist of a long-duration low-amplitude prepulse followed by a short-duration high-amplitude stimulation phase. The long-duration prepulse phase of the stimulus is designed to create a subthreshold depolarizing prepulse in the nontarget neurons and a hyperpolarizing prepulse in the target neurons [Grill and Mortimer, 1995; McIntyre and Grill, 2000]. Recall that during cathodic stimulation, the site of excitation in axons is the depolarized node of Ranvier, while the site of excitation in local cells is a node of Ranvier that is hyperpolarized by the stimulus (Figure 30.5). Conversely, with anodic stimuli, the site of excitation in local cells is a depolarized node of Ranvier, and the most polarized node of passing axons is hyperpolarized by the stimulus. Thus, the same polarity prepulse will produce opposite polarization at the sites of excitation in local cells and passing axons. The effect of this subthreshold polarization is to decrease the excitability of the nontarget population and increase the excitability of the target population via alterations in the degree of sodium channel inactivation [Grill and Mortimer, 1995]. Therefore, when the stimulating phase of the waveform is applied, the neuronal population targeted for stimulation will be activated with greater selectively [McIntyre and Grill, 2000]. Asymmetrical charge-balanced biphasic cathodic-phase-first stimulus waveforms result in selective activation of local cells, while asymmetrical charge-balanced biphasic anodic-phase-first stimulus waveforms result in selective activation of fibers of passage. Further, charge balancing is achieved as required to reduce the probability of tissue damage and electrode corrosion. Note that these prepulse waveforms differ from the pseudomonophasic waveforms used in some stimulators in that the low-amplitude long-duration phase of the waveform precedes rather than follows the high-amplitude short-duration phase of the waveform (Figure 30.7e).

30.6.4 Indirect Effects of Extracellular Stimulation

The thresholds for excitation of presynaptic terminals and subsequent indirect effects on local neurons (mediated by synaptic transmission) are similar to thresholds for direct effects (mediated by stimulus current) during extracellular stimulation (Figure 30.8a) of spinal cord motoneurons [Gustafsson and Jankowska, 1976], rubrospinal neurons [Baldissera et al., 1972], and corticospinal neurons [Jankowska et al., 1975]. Further, the chronaxie of presynaptic terminals (~0.14 msec in frog spinal cord, Tkacs and Wurster, 1991; 0.06 to 0.54 msec in rat subthalamic nucleus, Hutchison et al., 2002) is comparable to that of passing axons, and thus effects may be attributed to activation of passing axons when in fact they arise from activation of presynaptic elements. These "indirect" effects of stimulation must be considered when electrodes are placed within the heterogeneous environment of the CNS. During extracellular stimulation, release of inhibitory and excitatory neurotransmitters from presynaptic terminals can result in complex polyphasic changes in the firing rate of postsynaptic neurons (Figure 30.8b) [Butovas and Schwarz, 2003] and modulate the threshold for excitation of the postsynaptic neuron

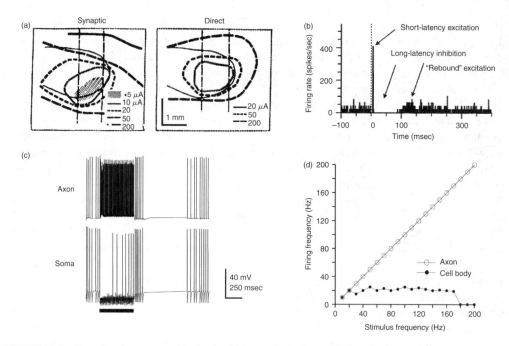

FIGURE 30.8 Central nervous system (CNS) stimulation results in direct effects and indirect effects on CNS neurons. (a) Two-dimensional maps of thresholds for indirect (synaptic) and direct activation of neurons in the red nucleus [from Baldissera et al., 1972]. (b) Complex polyphasic changes in the firing rate of a cortical neuron in response to extracellular stimulation [from Butovas and Schwarz, 2003]. (c) Transmembrane potential in the axon (top trace) and cell body (bottom trace) of a model thalamocortical neuron before, during (black bar at bottom), and after extracellular stimulation [from McIntyre et al., 2004]. Extracellular stimulation results in simultaneous inhibition of the cell body, as a result of activation of presynaptic terminals and subsequent indirect effects, and excitation of the axon, as a result of direct action potential initiation in a node of Ranvier. (d) Firing rate in the cell body and axon during extracellular stimulation of a model thalamocortical neuron [modified from McIntyre et al., 2004]. The firing rate in the cell body is lower than that in the axon, as a result of simultaneous indirect synaptic effects on the soma, and direct excitation of the axon.

[Swadlow, 1992; McIntyre and Grill, 2002]. Thus, indirect effects mediated by synaptic transmission may alter the direct effects of stimulation on the postsynaptic cell. Further, antidromic propagation of action potentials originating from activation of axon terminals can lead to widespread activation or inhibition of targets distant from the site of stimulation through axon collaterals. However, recall that action potential initiation occurs at some distance from the soma, where integration of synaptic inputs occurs, and thus the axon may be excited even when the cell body is hyperpolarized (Figure 30.8c). Therefore, extracellular unit recordings of firing in the soma may not accurately reflect the output of the neuron (Figure 30.8d) [Grill and McIntyre, 2001; McIntyre et al., 2004].

30.7   Summary

This chapter described electrical activation of neurons within the CNS. Electrical stimulation is used to study the form and function of the nervous system and a technique to restore function following disease or injury. Successful application of electrical stimulation to treat nervous system disorders as well as interpretation of the results of stimulation requires understanding of the cellular level effects of stimulation. Quantitative models provide a means to understand the response of neurons to extracellular stimulation. Further, accurate quantitative models provide powerful design tools that can be used to engineer stimuli that produce a desired response.

The fundamental properties of excitation of CNS neurons were presented with a focus on what neural elements around the electrode are activated under different conditions. During CNS stimulation action potentials are initiated in the axons of local cells, even for electrodes positioned over the cell body. The threshold difference between cathodic and anodic stimuli arises due to differences in the mode of activation. Anodic stimuli cause depolarization of the axon and excitation via a "virtual cathode," while cathodic stimuli cause hyperpolarization at the site of excitation and the action potential is initiated during repolarization. The threshold for activation of presynaptic terminals projecting into the region of stimulation is often less than or equal to the threshold for direct excitation of local cells, and indirect effects mediated by synaptic transmission may alter the direct effects of stimulation on the postsynaptic cell. The fundamental understanding provided by this analysis enables rational design and interpretation of studies and devices employing electrical stimulation of the brain or spinal cord.

Acknowledgments

Research in Dr. Grill's laboratory and preparation of this chapter were supported by NIH Grant R01 NS-40894.

References

Ackman, J.J. and Seitz, M.A. Methods of complex impedance measurement in biologic tissue. *CRC Crit. Rev. Biomed. Eng.* 1984; 11: 281–311.

Asanuma, H., Arnold, A., and Zarezecki, P. Further study on the excitation of pyramidal tract cells by intracortical microstimulation. *Exp. Brain Res.* 1976; 26: 443–461.

Bai, Q., Wise, K.D., and Anderson, D.J. A high-yield microassembly structure for three-dimensional microelectrode arrays. *IEEE Trans. Biomed. Eng.* 2000; 47: 281–289.

Baldissera, F., Lundberg, A., and Udo, M. Stimulation of pre- and postsynaptic elements in the red nucleus. *Exp. Brain. Res.* 1972; 15: 151–167.

Baumann, S.B., Wozny, D.R., Kelly, S.K., and Meno, F.M. The electrical conductivity of human cerebrospinal fluid at body temperature. *IEEE Trans. Biomed. Eng.* 1997; 44: 220–223.

Brindley, G.S. and Lewin, W.S. The sensations produced by electrical stimulation of the visual cortex. *J. Physiol.* 1968; 196: 479–493.

Butovas, S. and Schwarz, C. Spatiotemporal effects of microstimulation in rat neocortex: a parametric study using multielectrode recordings. *J. Neurophysiol.* 2003; 90: 3024–3039.

Cameron, T. Safety and efficacy of spinal cord stimulation for the treatment of chronic pain: a 20-year literature review. *J. Neurosurg.* 2004; 100: 254–267.

Coffey, R.J. Deep brain stimulation for chronic pain: results of two multicenter trials and a structured review. *Pain Med.* 2001; 2: 183–192.

Crile, G.W., Hosmer, H.R., and Rowland, A.F. The electrical conductivity of animal tissues under normal and pathological conditions. *Am. J. Physiol.* 1922; 60: 59–106.

Eisenberg, R.S. and Mathias, R.T. Structural analysis of electrical properties of cells and tissues. *CRC Crit. Rev. Biomed. Eng.* 1980; 4: 203–232.

Grill, W.M. and McIntyre, C.C. Extracellular excitation of central neurons: implications for the mechanisms of deep brain stimulation. *Thalamus Relat. Syst.* 2001; 1: 269–277.

Grill, W.M. and Mortimer, J.T. Electrical properties of implant encapsulation tissue. *Ann. Biomed. Eng.* 1994; 22: 23–33.

Grill, W.M. and Mortimer, J.T. Stimulus waveforms for selective neural stimulation. *IEEE Eng. Med. Biol.* 1995; 14: 375–385.

Grill, W.M. Modeling the effects of electric fields on nerve fibers: influence of tissue electrical properties. *IEEE Trans. Biomed. Eng.* 1999; 46: 918–928.

Gross, R.E. and Lozano, A.M. Advances in neurostimulation for movement disorders. *Neurol. Res.* 2000; 22: 247–258.

Gross, R.E. Deep brain stimulation in the treatment of neurological and psychiatric disease. *Expert Rev. Neurother.* 2004; 4: 465–478.

Gustafsson, B. and Jankowska, E. Direct and indirect activation of nerve cells by electrical pulses applied extracellularly. *J. Physiol.* 1976; 258: 33–61.

Hodaie, M., Wennberg, R.A., Dostrovsky, J.O., and Lozano, A.M. Chronic anterior thalamus stimulation for intractable epilepsy. *Epilepsia* 2002; 43: 603–608.

Holsheimer, J., Struijk, J.J., and Tas, N.R. Effects of electrode geometry and combination on nerve fibre selectivity in spinal cord stimulation. *Med. Biol. Eng. Comput.* 1995; 33: 676–682.

Hutchison, W.D., Chung, A.G., and Goldsmidt, A. Chronaxie and refractory period of neuronal inhibition by extracellular stimulation in the region of rat STN. Program No. 416.3. 2002 Abstract Viewer/Itinerary Planner CD-ROM, Society for Neuroscience, Washington, DC.

Jankowska, E., Padel, Y., and Tanaka, R. The mode of activation of pyramidal tract cells by intracortical stimuli. *J. Physiol.* 1975; 249: 617–636.

Jankowska, E. and Roberts, W.J. An electrophysiological demonstration of the axonal projections of single spinal interneurones in the cat. *J. Physiol.* 1972; 222: 597–622.

Li, C.-H., Bak, A.F., and Parker, L.O. Specific resistivity of the cerebral cortex and white matter. *Exp. Neurol.* 1968; 20: 544–557.

Li, C.L. and Bak, A. Excitability characteristics of the A- and C-fibers in a peripheral nerve. *Exp. Neurol.* 1976; 50: 67–79.

Lilly, J.C., Hughes, J.R., Alvord, E.C. Jr, and Galkin, T.A. Brief noninjurious electric waveform for stimulation of the brain. *Science*, 1955; 121: 468–469.

Lipski, J. Antidromic activation of neurons as an analytic tool in the study of the central nervous system. *J. Neurosci. Meth.* 1981; 4: 1–32.

McCreery, D.B., Yuen, T.G., Agnew, W.F., and Bullara, L.A. A characterization of the effects on neuronal excitability due to prolonged microstimulation with chronically implanted microelectrodes. *IEEE Trans. Biomed. Eng.* 1997; 44: 931–939.

McIntyre, C.C. and Grill, W.M. Excitation of central nervous system neurons by nonuniform electric fields. *Biophys. J.* 1999; 76: 878–888.

McIntyre, C.C. and Grill, W.M. Selective microstimulation of central nervous system neurons. *Ann. Biomed. Eng.* 2000; 28: 219–233.

McIntyre, C.C. and Grill, W.M. Finite element analysis of the current-density and electric field generated by metal microelectrodes. *Ann. Biomed. Eng.* 2001; 29: 227–235.

McIntyre, C.C. and Grill, W.M. Extracellular stimulation of central neurons: influence of stimulus waveform and frequency on neuronal output. *J. Neurophysiol.* 2002; 88: 1592–1604.

McIntyre, C.C., Grill, W.M., Sherman, D.L., and Thakor, N.V. Cellular effects of deep brain stimulation: model-based analysis of activation and inhibition. *J. Neurophysiol.* 2004; 91: 1457–1469.

Miocinovic, S. and Grill, W.M. Sensitivity of temporal excitation properties to the neuronal element activated by extracellular stimulation. *J. Neurosci. Meth.* 2004; 132: 91–99.

Nicholson, P.W. Specific impedance of cerebral white matter. *Exp. Neurol.* 1965; 13: 386–401.

Nicolelis, M.A.L., Dimitrov, D., Carmena, J.M., Crist, R., Lehew, G., Kralik, J.D., and Wise, S.P. Chronic, multisite, multielecrode recording in macaque monkeys. *Proc. Nat. Acad. Sci. USA*, 2003, 100: 11041–11046.

Normann, R.A., Maynard, E.M., Rousche, P.J., and Warren, D.J. A neural interface for a cortical vision prosthesis. *Vision Res.* 1999; 39: 2577–2587.

Nowak, L.G. and Bullier, J. Axons, but not cell bodies, are activated by electrical stimulation in cortical gray matter. I. Evidence from chronaxie measurements. *Exp. Brain. Res.* 1998a; 118: 477–488.

Nowak, L.G. and Bullier, J. Axons, but not cell bodies, are activated by electrical stimulation in cortical gray matter. II. Evidence from selective inactivation of cell bodies and axon initial segments. *Exp. Brain. Res.* 1998b; 118: 489–500.

Otto, S.R., Brackmann, D.E., Hitselberger, W.E., Shannon, R.V., and Kuchta, J. Multichannel auditory brainstem implant: update on performance in 61 patients. *J. Neurosurg.* 2002; 96: 1063–1071.

Ranck, J.B. Jr. Which elements are excited in electrical stimulation of mammalian central nervous system: a review. *Brain Res.* 1975; 98: 417–440.

Ranck, J.B., Jr. Analysis of specific impedance of rabbit cerebral cortex. *Exp. Neurol.* 1963; 7: 153–174.

Ranck, J.B., Jr. and BeMent, S.L. The specific impedance of the dorsal columns of the cat: an anisotropic medium. *Exp. Neurol.* 1965; 11: 451–463.

Robblee, L.S. and Rose, T.L. Electrochemical guidelines for selection of protocols and electrode materials for neural stimulation. In Agnew, W.F. and McCreery, D.B. Eds., *Neural Prostheses: Fundamental Studies*, Prentice-Hall, Englewood Cliffs, NJ, pp. 25–66, 1990.

Roberts, W.J. and Smith, D.O. Analysis of threshold currents during microstimulation of fibers in the spinal cord. *Acta Physiol. Scand.* 1973; 89: 384–394.

Sances A., Jr. and Larson, S.J. Impedance and current density studies. In Sances, A. and Larson, S.J. Eds., *Electroanesthesia: Biomedical and Biophysical Studies*, Academic Press, NY, 1975, pp. 114–124.

Schmidt, E.M., Bak, M.J., Hambrecht, F.T., Kufta, C.V., O'Rourke, D.K., and Vallabhanath, P. Feasibility of a visual prosthesis for the blind based on intracortical microstimulation of the visual cortex. *Brain* 1996; 119: 507–522.

Stoney, S.D. Jr, Thompson, W.D., and Asanuma, H. Excitation of pyramidal tract cells by intracortical microstimulation: effective extent of stimulating current. *J. Neurophys.* 1968; 31: 659–669.

Swadlow, H.A. Monitoring the excitability of neocortical efferent neurons to direct activation by extracellular current pulses. *J. Neurophysiol.* 1992; 68: 605–619.

Tehovnik, E.J. Electrical stimulation of neural tissue to evoke behavioral responses. *J. Neursci. Meth.* 1996; 65: 1–17.

Tkacs, N.C. and Wurster, R.D. Strength–duration and activity-dependent excitability properties of frog afferent axons and their intraspinal projections. *J. Neurophysiol.* 1991; 65: 468–476.

Troyk, P., Bak, M., Berg, J., Bradley, D., Cogan, S., Erickson, R., Kufta, C., McCreery, D., Schmidt, E., and Towle, V. A model for intracortical visual prosthesis research. *Artif. Organs* 2003; 27: 1005–1015.

Velasco, F., Velasco, M., Jimenez, F., Velasco, A.L., and Marquez, I. Stimulation of the central median thalamic nucleus for epilepsy. *Stereotact. Funct. Neurosurg.* 2001; 77: 228–232.

West, D.C. and Wolstencroft, J.H. Strength–duration characteristics of myelinated and non-myelinated bulbospinal axons in the cat spinal cord. *J. Physiol.* 1983; 337: 37–50.

31

Transcutaneous FES for Ambulation: The Parastep System

Daniel Graupe
University of Illinois

31.1 Introduction and Background

31.1.1 Historical Background

Functional electrical (neuromuscular) stimulation, denoted as FES (or FNS) has its origins in Luigi Galvani's experiment on electrically exciting a frog's leg in the 1780s as described by him in "De Viribus Electricitatis in Motu Muscular" (1791), which despite some faults due to the state of scientific knowledge at its time, can be shown to lay the foundation to two great disciplines, electrical engineering and neurophysiology [l].

The first demonstrated modern application of FNS to a human patient for functional movements of extremities was reported by Lieberson in 1960 [2] in the case of a hemiplegic patient, whereas the first application to a paraplegic patient is that by Kantrowitz [3].

Unbraced short-distance ambulation by transcutaneous FNS of a complete paraplegic was first described in 1980 by Kralj et al. [4].

In early 1982, the first patient-controlled ambulation for a complete paraplegic as necessary for independent ambulation was achieved by Graupe et al. [5–7] employing EMG (electromyograph) control. A manually controlled system, known as the Parastep FNS system was tested from 1982 and received FDA approval in 1994 to become the first FNS ambulation system to be so approved and to be commercially available for use by individuals beyond research environments.

The systems of Graupe et al. [5,7] employ a walker for balancing support. It was commercialized by Sigmedics, Inc. (founded for this purpose in 1987) as the Parastep System (Parastep-I System) and was the first (and still is the only) FES ambulation system to have received FDA approval in 1994 [8] and approval by Medicare/Medicid for reimbursement 2003 [9,10].

In parallel, work was carried out since the early 1980s on percutaneous FNS, especially at Case Western Reserve University [11,12] in Vienna, Austria [13], and in Augusta, Maine [14].

FNS as above is applicable for traumatic complete (or near-complete as far as sensation, leg extension, and hip flexion are concerned) upper-motor-neuron thoracic level paraplegics. To date, approximately 1000 such patients are or have been able to ambulate over short distances with the FDA-approved Parastep system. They have been trained in over 20 hospitals or rehabilitation centers in the USA and in Europe, with no known detrimental effects. These patients can ambulate independently between 20 and several hundred meters (some up to one mile) without sitting down. The number of complete paraplegic patients who ambulate with implanted (percutaneous) electrodes is very small — about a dozen. The latter patients must undergo surgery (often of several hours) and they require occasional repeat surgery to correct electrode breakage or slippage, which are still unresolved problems. They also experience infections at the sites of electrode penetration through the skin. Consequently, at the present state of implantation, and noting the performance of the transcutaneous Parastep FNS users, it appears that for some time to come, the transcutaneous approach will be the more common one, and not just due to it being the only one available outside the research lab. It is for these reasons and since it is the only system for which there exists a body of independent source published material on clinical experience and data collection that this chapter concentrates on the Parastep ambulation system. Still, for completeness of this chapter, a very brief discussion on the major other ambulation systems is discussed.

31.1.2 Brief Review of FES Systems for Ambulation by Paraplegics

A very brief discussion on the major other FES ambulation systems is discussed here, for completeness.

1. *Noninvasive (Transcutaneous) FES systems:* The only other transcutaneous FES system (but for the PARASTEP) or both standing and ambulation that has been used outside their inventors' laboratory is the *Ljubljana FES system*, which is based on the work of Kralj et al. [15,16] and which emanated from that group's earlier pioneering work [4] on FES (related to the still earlier work of Lieberson et al. [2] concerning hemiplegia). The bench-model of the Ljubljana system was the first to achieve ambulation via FES by a complete thoracic-level paraplegic [4]. Its principles are similar to those of the Parastep system in their purpose and in their general function, which can, in part, already be found in the principles of the earlier Ljubljana work on hemiplegia and in Lieberson's work. It differs from the Parastep system in that it was not designed to maximize walking distance and it also differs in its control and in its channel coordination (to result in a bulkier system than the Parastep system). Its patient-borne version is usually a four-channel system. Its signal generation is essentially a two-channel signal generator, such that the four-channel system is a double two-channel system. The Ljubljana system is not yet commercially available (at least, not outside the use in research programs, mainly in Europe) and is presently not FDA-approved. No independent multi-patient ambulation-performance studies and statistics and no multi-patient medical evaluations or psychological evaluations were published on that system.

Other noninvasive (transcutaneous) FES systems for standing and ambulation, apart from the Ljubljana system and the Parastep system, are essentially all *bench-devices*, as developed in various research laboratories for the purpose of their own research (see D. Popovic et al. [17], Mayagoitia et al. [18], and the Stanmore system of Phillips et al. [19]). Whereas all FES ambulation systems can be and are used for *standing*, there are several transcutaneous FES systems for standing alone (see Jaeger [20]; Kralj and Bajd [21];

the Odstock standing system of Taylor et al. [22]). These are obviously limited in scope and are not within the main theme of this review. None is commercially available.

2. *Hybrid FES-Long-Leg Brace Ambulation Systems:* Hybrid FES-Long-Leg-Brace or FES-Body-Brace systems, which combine trascutaneous FES with a long-leg brace or with a body brace for standing and ambulation by paraplegics, have been developed since the 1970s ([8,23,24], Solomonow et al. [the LSU system] [25]). These systems are also intended for upper-motor-neuron (thoracic level) LSI. They represent a regression from FES, since they give up one of the major goals of FES ambulation, namely, patient's independence. Since hybrid systems use a body brace or long-leg braces, they are far heavier and far more cumbersome than, say, the 10.5 ounce Parastep. They require 30 min to don and a long time to doff, requiring help from an able-bodied person in donning and in doffing the system. This also affects patient compliance and regular use of the system, while the system's weight reduces ambulation distances [25].

3. *Implanted FES Ambulation Systems:* As stated earlier in this section, research on implanted FES for standing and ambulation has been carried out in parallel with the work on transcutaneous noninvasive FES, the latter being the subject of the present review. It is however important for the completeness of this review to comment briefly on implanted FES.

Work on both invasive FES and noninvasive FES started in the late 1970s and early 1980s. Also, the first applications to thoracic-level complete traumatic paraplegic were reported for both approaches in the early 1980s [4–6,11,13]. Also, both approaches are based on the fundamental user by Lieberson et al. [2]. However, invasive methods, both *percutaneous* [11,13] and fully implanted systems [26] always involve major surgery in contrast to the noninvasive transcutaneous methods on which this review concentrates. It is not just the surgery (and its cost). Furthermore, so far all noninvasive methods encounter loss of contact of electrodes, wire breakage, and sometimes even tearing of nerve fibers. Such occurrences then require resurgery. Fully implanted FES [27] does not encounter infections at locations where wires penetrate the skin as it happens with percutaneous methods. (In fully implanted systems, a radio-frequency [RF] receiver is implanted that receives RF signals through the skin, from a transmitter attached above the skin and the received RF is rectified to provide electric power.) All invasive systems require some kind of patient control from a nonimplanted device, as do noninvasive systems. Also all invasive systems require similar patient training and muscle strengthening. Of course, an implanted device requires no electrode placement each morning and removal each evening. However, with the Parastep system, donning time is 5–8 min for a trained user and doffing time is 3–4 min. Connection and disconnection of the FES control device and, in percutaneous systems, connection of wires to the implanted electrodes from outside, also takes a few minutes. It is therefore not surprising that the Parastep system was the first and is still the only FES system for standing and ambulation that has received (1994) FDA approval and is commercially available. We note that there are presently some 600 users of the Parastep and it is used both at home and at workplace. In contrast, there are presently only a few (in the order of a dozen) users of even the most advanced percutaneous system (based on Marsolais work and that of his colleagues in Cleveland, as mentioned above), whereas the fully implanted system is not yet complete to allow out-of-clinic ambulation.

We comment that the work on implanted FES has resulted in great advances in implantation techniques and materials that are of value in situations where there is no alternative to implantation (unlike the case of FES for standing and ambulation). However, the difficulties in implanted systems are still with us and they will always require surgery.

31.2 The Parastep System

31.2.1 System's Electric Charge and Charge Density Parameters

The FNS consists of sequences (trains) of electrical impulses that are applied transcutaneously so that stimulation reaches peripheral motor neurons at selected sites. Stimulation serves only to trigger action

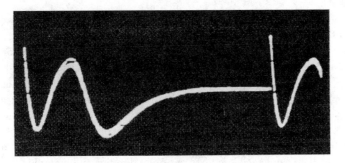

FIGURE 31.1   Action potential in response to stimulation at a quadriceps stimulated site.

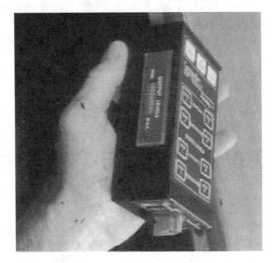

FIGURE 31.2   The parastep unit.

potentials at these motor units. The resultant action potentials produced in the motor neurons concerned, in response to these triggers (stimulation impulses), subsequently cause contraction of muscle fibers that are associated with these motor neuron [27,28], see Figure 31.1.

Comment: This action potential (AP) is a summation of many synchronous action potentials produced in response to a stimulation signal. It is recoded by surface electrodes at the stimulation site. The sharp peak at the beginning of each AP is an artifact of the stimulus.

31.2.1.1 Parameters of Stimulation Signals and safety Standard Constraints

The stimulation trains that are employed are trains of impulses of 120–150 μsec in duration (width) and their rate is of 20–25 pulses/sec. The pulse duration above is selected to be as low as possible while still allowing full contractions [27,29]. This is necessitated by considerations of minimizing the electrical charge density applied to the stimulation site for the patient's safety: it, therefore, also minimizes battery power, to result in a compact light-weight portable system (Figure 31.2). The system is powered by a 9.6 VDC battery pack consisting of 8 AA or AAA Ni-Cad rechargeable batteries, to power the stimulator and its computer.

The maximal current per pulse is limited [27] in our system to 0.3 A = Io. As per the 1985 ANSI standard, Section 3.2.2.2 of the Association for Advancement of Medical Instrumentation and the American National Standard Institute [30], stimulation should be limited to below 10 mA average current. Hence, stimuli of

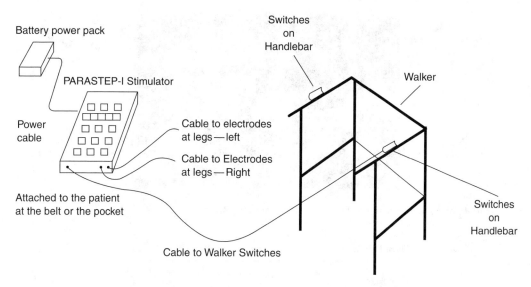

FIGURE 31.3   Parastep system with battery pack and walker.

$T = 150 \ \mu$sec duration (pulse-width) at $f = 24$ pulses/sec, result in average current I_{ave} of

$$I_{ave} = Io \times T \times f \tag{31.1}$$

namely $0.3 \times 24 \times 0.00015 = 0.00108$ A or 1.08 mA, as is well below the ANSI limit. Another critical ANSI parameter is that of maximal electrical charge per pulse of 75 μC/pulse. The Parastep system's maximal output electrical charge value is given by

$$Q = IoT \tag{31.2}$$

or 0.3×0.00015 C $= 45 \ \mu$C $=$ Q. Thus the current density I_{ave}/S is for electrodes of 1.75×3.75 in.^{2} (namely $S = 40$ cm$^2 = 4000$ mm^2). The current density in the case of the Parastep system is therefore:

$$I_{ave}/S = 0.00108/4000 \ \text{A/mm}^2 = 0.25 \ \mu\text{C/mm}^2 \tag{31.3}$$

which is well below the ANSI limit of 10 μC/sq.mm.

31.2.2   System Parameters and Design

The Parastep system is based on a single microprocessor [27,29] which is its main component and where the stimulation signals of all channels are shaped and controlled and where synchronization between channels is performed for the four different stimulation operational menus. The microprocessor generates and shapes trains of stimulation pulses that are multiplexed and directed by the algorithm imbedded in that microcomputer to 6 output channels, which are individually controlled by the microcomputer, in response to menu selection by the patient to avoid robot-like movements. Channel separation is performed by a timing program, which is passed from the microcomputer to an array of microcomputer-controlled opto-isolators and then appropriately amplified, thus providing the system's outputs to 12 surface electrodes that are attached to the skin at appropriate placements. These skin electrodes are self-adhesive and are reusable for 14 days. They are to be attached by the patient himself in the morning and removed each evening or as desired at locations that the patient has been taught to remember. The stimulator unit weighs 7.6 ounces (Figure 31.2), excluding a battery pack of six AA 1.5 V rechargeable alkaline (or 8 rechargeable NiMH) batteries to allow at least 60 min of standing or walking [27]. The system is shown in Figure 31.3 and Figure 31.4.

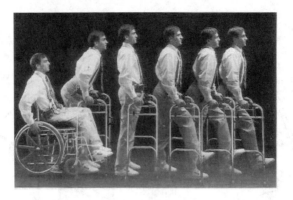

FIGURE 31.4 Parastep system in use during walk by paraplegic patient.

TABLE 31.1 Stimulation Frequency vs. Rate of Muscle Fatigue

Stimulation frequency (Hz)	% Drop in isometric moment at ankle joint		
	After 10 min	After 20 min	After 30 min
20	<2	<2	3
30	4	14	40
50	17	53	71

Pulse duration: 300 μsec throughout.

The same microchip also controls optic isolation chips to allow using a single power amplifier for all channels. This allows the Parastep to employ six stimulation channels (12 electrodes) rather than the usual four stimulation channels and to integrate them to reduce system's weight, while facilitating full patient control of all channels. Furthermore, it facilitates considerable battery power savings. The additional two stimulation channels (at the paraspinals for trunk stability) play a major role in enhancing standing time, ambulation distances, and speeds as compared with four channel systems.

31.2.2.1 Pulse Width and Pulse Repetition-Rate (Frequency)

Pulse durations (widths) are set to be of 120 to 150 μsec [27]. Higher durations are undesirable and unnecessary. Higher pulse width speeds up the rate of muscle fatigue and therefore reduces the maximal ambulation distance (see Table 31.1) and the maximal time a patient can stand or walk via FES. It also sends into the body more electrical charge than is needed and requires higher battery power and hence higher battery weight.

The inter-pulse repetition rate (frequency) is set higher than the average pulse rate in the able-bodied individual, but is still kept as low as possible (22 to 24 pulses/sec) to reduce rate of fatigue (see Table 31.1). It is determined by considerations of fatigue, tetanization, and force (note that while standing or walking, the body weight dampens vibrations considerably). At even lower frequencies, muscle vibrations are observed that are no more dampened and that may affect the patient's balance when standing or walking. Higher frequencies also imply that a higher electrical charge enters the body and requires higher battery power and heavier batteries. Furthermore higher pulse rates speed up the rate of muscle fatigue to reduce duration and range of ambulation. Both pulse widths and rates, while constant, can be adjusted if necessary (see Figure 31.5).

Therefore, a combination of a short pulse duration, low stimulation levels, and low pulse rate is essential to reduce muscle fatigue, thus extending walking distance (walking time) per walk [5]. The consequences of lower battery power needs, of lower system weight, and of the resultant effect on compactness are of course also significant for a patient-borne system and for user friendliness, especially, in a body-borne system.

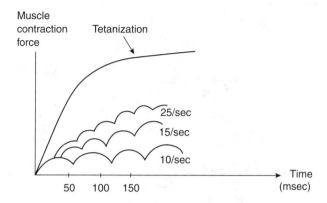

FIGURE 31.5 Muscle contraction force vs. stimulation rate and time.

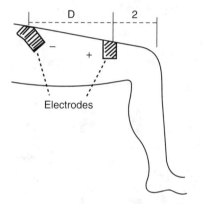

FIGURE 31.6 Placement of quadriceps stimulation electrodes (right leg, lateral side view).

31.2.2.2 Menus for Pulse Shaping and Synchronization

Pulse amplitude shaping is a major aspect of the pulse shaping algorithm and it is the subject of four different menus within that algorithm. The menus are patient selectable, through touch of finger-touch switches located on the Parastep's walker or on the Parastep's elbow-support canes. The menus are those for standing up, for right step, for left step, and for sitting down (see Figure 31.6). Pulse-amplitude shaping is dynamic and varies for each of the six stimulation channels and as per each menu, as does the distribution of output signal to each output channel [5,11]. The time variation of the pulse amplitudes in each menu and per each channel, as in Figure 31.6, is therefore unique and is based on considerations of the executions of the given menu's function (say, taking a right step) and of doing so safely, efficiently, and smoothly.

31.2.2.3 Stimulation Sites

The stimulation electrodes are self-adhesive electrodes (12 in total), placed at six stimulation sites [27], two electrodes per site, as follows: two over the right quadriceps and two over the left quadriceps, to stimulate knee extension; two over the common peroneal nerve right and left (to activate dorsi-flexion and to elicit a hip flexion reflex via sensory neural feedback). Finally, two electrodes are placed over the right paraspinals at right and two at left, for upper trunk stability in patients with lesions at T7 or higher (to be placed approximately 1 in. below the level of start of sensation, but not too close to the heart). Patients with SCI lesions at lower levels will have electrodes placed over the gluteus medius and maximus for improved stability, whereas patients with lesions at T-1 0 or lower usually do not require paraspinal stimulation at all (Figure 31.6 to Figure 31.8). We comment that improved trunk stability affects not

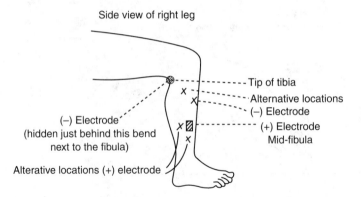

FIGURE 31.7 Placement of peroneal nerve electrodes (to elicit step via hip flexion reflex).

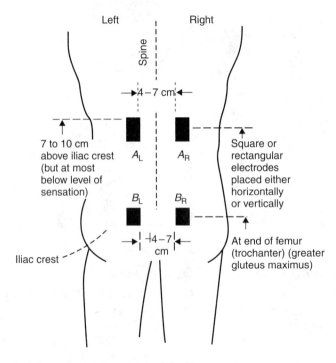

FIGURE 31.8 Paraspinal electrodes placement (patient's back).

just patient safety, but helps to reduce fatigue, thus improving ambulation performance and appearance (which is not just an esthetic aspect but also a psychological one).

As shown in Figure 31.8, alternatives to the peroneal nerve placements are possible in some cases (see Chapter 7 of Reference 5). These alternatives involve other branches of the sciatic nerve, which trigger the hip flexion reflex.

The number of channels (of electrode pairs) to be used is a matter of trade-off. Obviously, with more channels more muscle groups (at below the SCI lesion) can contract. However, when increasing the number of channels, say from six to eight, the patient must place (every morning) 16 electrodes instead of 12 and for a paraplegic patient this involves a lot of additional effort and time. Furthermore, the six channels that are stimulated by the Parastep system, as discussed above are the ones that are the easiest to be reached by the user and the ones where there is the greatest tolerance in terms of error in placement's localization, while additional sites will require more care in exact placement. It is our experience that with

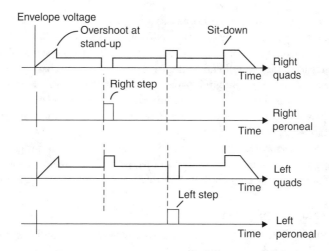

FIGURE 31.9 Synchronization scheme of envelopes of stimulation signals at various channels. (*Note:* Broken vertical lines divide between the four Parastep menus. Paraspinal signal envelopes correspond in shape to quadriceps channels except for peaks.)

more than 6 channels, most patients will soon stop using the system. Hence, human factor considerations imply to limit the system to the most important functions (channels) as far as performance is concerned. The resulting performance, as discussed later in this review (Section 31.5) appears to justify this choice and to result in a rather smooth walk that can be viewed in a 15-min movie of a walk of a complete thoracic-level paraplegic using the Parastep system (see http://www.ece.uic.edu/~graupe).

31.2.2.4 Sequencing-Control Menus for the Stimulation Signals

Pulse-amplitude shaping is a major aspect of the pulse-shaping algorithm and it is the subject of four different menus within that algorithm. The menus are patient selectable, through touch of finger-touch switches located on the Parastep's walker or on the Parastep's elbow-support canes. The menus are those for standing up, for right step, for left step, and for sitting down (see Figure 31.9). Pulse-amplitude shaping is dynamic and varies for each of the six stimulation channels and per each menu, as does the distribution of output signal to each output channel [6,27]. The time variation of the pulse amplitudes in each menu and per each channel, as in Figure 31.9, is therefore unique and is based on considerations of the executions of the given menu's function (say, taking a right step), and of doing so safely, efficiently, and smoothly.

The stimulation signals are sequenced at the system's microcomputer chip as in Figure 31.9, where the envelope patterns of the stimulation impulses (and not the individual pulses) are illustrated. This pattern is automatically sequenced by the stimulator's computer to give a ramp increase of impulse levels for stand-up to be followed by a lower constant level while the patient is standing, both being applied to the right and left quadriceps electrodes and to the right and left paraspinal/gluteal electrodes. When a left step menu is selected, either manually or through above-lesion (chest-level) EMG (as described later), then stimulation is stopped at the left quadriceps and paraspinals/gluteus while at the same time the common peroneal nerve is being stimulated to elicit a step. This lasts for a fixed duration of $T = 0.4$ to 1.0 sec, as is preselected for the convenience of the patient. At the end of this period T, stimulation to the left common peroneal stops and the left quadriceps and left paraspinals/gluteus are stimulated. However, during the step period, the level of stimulation at the right quadriceps is automatically increased by the sequencing program to compensate for the fact that full body weight is borne by the right leg over that period. If a right step is selected, then the same menu is employed, with a reversal of roles of right and left. When a sit-down menu is selected, then the sequencing program first triggers an audible and a visual warning to allow the patient to abort the sit-down if he is not ready to sit and to allow for time to reach a chair and to comfortably sit down. Also, at that time, stimulation to the quadriceps is increased to compensate for possible weakening of the quadriceps that may have caused the patient to decide to sit.

The microchip also controls optic isolation chips to allow using a single power amplifier for all channels. This allows the Parastep to employ six rather than the usual four stimulation channels and to integrate them to reduce system weight, while facilitating full patient control of all channels. Furthermore, it facilitates considerable further battery power savings. The additional two stimulation channels (at the paraspinals, for trunk stability) play a major role in enhancing standing time, ambulation distances, and speeds as compared to four channel systems.

Control of the FES is performed by the stimulation signal's sequencing program of the Parastep's microcomputer, while selection of menus of that program is performed either manually (as in the Parastep commercial system) or via an above-lesion EMG control algorithm for menu selections [5,7,29].

31.2.2.5 Finger-Touch Menu Selection

Menu-selection finger-touch switches [27,29] are located on the walker's handlebars for easy finger reach while normally holding the walker (or cane). They require only a light single and quick (short) finger touch without changing hand position on the bars. Adaptation and learning of balancing and of menu selection (only two menus during walking; of right and of left step, activated at right or left handlebar), is very easy and fast. Only finger-touch selection is available in the commercial Parastep system.

31.2.2.6 Above-Lesion EMG-Controlled Menu Selection

While the commercial PARASTEP system employs only manual touch buttons for menu selection, the laboratory Parastep system, that was tested on 14 patients at Michael Reese Hospital, Chicago, IL, allowed for above-lesion surface-EMG (electromyographic) menu selection too with good results [7,27,29]. However, menu-selection EMG-control was not incorporated in the commercial system (and is not covered by its FDA approval), since training is far lengthier and requires the donning of four more electrodes (for EMG pickup). This was felt to greatly limit the number of users. We comment that EMG electrode placement is much more critical than that of placing the stimulation electrodes themselves.

The above-lesion EMG-based menu selections employ surface-EMG signals from electrodes placed at above-lesion locations on the patient's chest. The thus obtained EMG signal (see Figure 31.8) serves to map a pattern of upper-trunk posture that has been shown [5,7,27], to predict intended body function, corresponding to the four menus above (stand, left step, right step, and sit menus), with an accuracy of better than 99.8%. In this case, no finger controls are needed.

We emphasize that the relevant information from the above-lesion EMG signal is NOT based on the EMG level (power), but on the whole stochastic time-series pattern of that signal [27,29]. Therefore, the patient does not have to produce a specific produce upper-body above-lesion (shoulder) movement to select a particular menu. The patient's natural walk and the natural changes in the above-lesion muscles as are needed to move the walker and to otherwise balance when intending a particular step (or to stand up or to sit down) causes dynamic changes in the whole EMG stochastic pattern. These pattern changes are then recognized in the microchip's algorithm as a command to select a particular menu (from the menus above). In this way, the above-lesion EMG control differs from others that require unnatural pulling of shoulders or of arms to produce an EMG-based command. Such intentional and unnatural movements divert patient's concentration and yield an unnatural walk.

The mapping of the upper-trunk posture considers the above-lesion EMG signal, dented as $y(k)$, to satisfy a pure autoregressive (AR) time-series model [7,29]:

$$y(k) = a(1)y(k-1) + a(2)y(k-2) + \cdots + a(n)y(k-n) + w(k) \qquad (31.4)$$

where k is discrete time, such that $k = n+1, n+2, n+3, \ldots$, and $w(k)$ denotes a discrete white-noise process.

We comment that both under finger-touch control (menu selection) and under EMG menu selection, the direction of step (and hence, of a walk) is determined by the shoulder movement of the patient as naturally performed when intuitively moving the walker to any desired direction.

31.2.2.7 Stimulation Signal's Level Control

The stimulation level is adjusted at the Paraestep's microcomputer chip, in accordance to either the patient's single finger-touch menu switching command or t in response to an above-lesion EMG signal from the patent's chest that is interpreted in the same microchip.

31.2.2.8 Finger-Touch Force Level Control

The degree of recruitment of motor neurons determines the contraction force exerted by the muscle fibers that are associated with these neurons [27,29]. The degree of recruitment is, in turn, dependent on the level of the stimulation signal when the motor neurons are triggered by FES stimuli. In the commercial Parastep, the stimulation level is controlled by the touch buttons at the left and right hand side of the walker. Each finger touch raises the level by a single increment. Out of 10 possible level increments that are color marked most patients use one of the 3 lowest levels to start their walk, in order to minimize rate of fatigue. During a half-hour walk a patient will usually have to adjust FES level only 2 to 3 times by a single discrete increment. The range of levels can be factory-set to suit special needs (patients).

31.2.2.9 Below-Lesion Response-EMG FES Level Control

Alternatively, in the Parastep lab system tried at Michael Reese Hospital, a below-lesion surface-EMG Stimulation-Level Control, denoted as Response-EMG Level Control, was successfully tested on some patients [27,29].

Obviously, in complete upper-motor neuron paraplegics (thoracic level SCI patients), no EMG occurs below the level of the lesion, since the lower-extremity neurons do not fire. However, under FES, action potentials arise at the stimulated motor neurons. These produce action potentials similar to those in nonimpaired situations. Furthermore, since any stimulation electrode-pair activates many hundreds of motor neurons simultaneously, all resultant action potentials are fully synchronized and appear as one very strong action potential due to this combined and synchronized firing (see Figure 31.1). This is in contrast to the surface-EMG above the lesion, which results from unsynchronized firing of hundreds of neurons. Furthermore, the resulting response-EMG increases with the degree of recruitment. It can thus serve to detect progression of fatigue and serve to adjust stimulation levels accordingly. The commercial system uses only finger-touch level control, since the reliability in calibration of relations between response-EMG level (and shape) against desired FES stimuli strength (to counter the fatigue) is still not sufficiently reliable. It is also not covered by the Parastep's FDA approval. However, when using opto-isolators, the stimulation electrodes can simultaneously serve as response-EMG electrodes. This is due to the very short duration of the Parastep's stimulus in relation to the duration of a single action potential (which is given by the stimulation of low pulse-rate used by the Parastep system).

31.2.2.10 Peripheral Equipment

The Parastep FES system uses a walker (see Figure 31.3 and Figure 31.4), or in a few cases, a pair of elbow-support (Canadian) canes [27,29]. Walkers are employed in all other FES ambulation systems, invasive or not. Walkers (or elbow-support canes) serve mainly for balance. Walkers carry (in the Parastep system) only 5% or less of body weight in trained FES users during standing and are crucial during the standing-up mode. Their balancing role is due to the fact that complete SCI paraplegics have no sensation (in addition to having no motor functions below their lesion). Hence, indirect sensation coming through their arms and hands, while holding the walker's handlebars, lets the users sense the ground to provide a certain psychological security. It thus allows the users to balance their body by slight shoulder and arm movements to better balance during standing and walking. The users are able to easily and rather naturally change direction of walking, at will, through shoulder positioning by which they turn their steps. One major function of the walker is during the stand-up phase from a seated position. The patient then gets up with the arms leaning on the walker. All these reasons indicate the crucial role of walkers toward achieving independent standing and walking.

The Parastep system is described in further detail in Graupe and Kohn [27,28].

31.3   Patient Admissibility, Contraindications, and Training

31.3.1   Patient Admissibility Criteria

The cardiovascular status of the patients must be good. Hence, the criteria for a patient to be admitted to train and to use the Parastep standing/ambulation system are as follows [7,27,29]:

1. The patient must be in good general health and with a complete traumatic spinal cord lesion at levels no higher than C-7 and no lower than T-12.
2. Intact lower motor units (lumbar level L-1 and below).
3. Must have a complete/near-complete SCI lesion that do not allow the patient to stretch his/her knees for standing up and where the patient has no substantial sensation (pain) of the stimuli.
4. Surgery/wound following SCI must have healed, or as determined by the surgeon.
5. Stable ortho-neuro-metabolic systems.
6. No recent history of long bone stress fractures, osteoporosis, or severe hip or knee joint disease. A bone density test is advisable in case of women over 40 or patients who are many years (10 or more) beyond date of injury. The author had a patient 40 years postinjury who had no problem and was accepted to the FES ambulation program.
7. No history of cardiac or respiratory problems.
8. Adequate trunk stability so that once quadriceps are stimulated, the patient can hold his upper trunk upright while supporting himself with a walker.
9. The patient demonstrates appropriate muscle contractions in response to stimulation (absence of such response usually implies some lesions below T-12).
10. Standing tolerance: The patient has adequate fatigue tolerance to practice and perform standing and walking functions after initial training.
11. Balance and trunk control (at least when paraspinals are stimulated).
12. The patient must have adequate hand and finger control or VOICE control to manipulate the system controls. Future systems may circumvent the need for finger control via speech recognition to allow patients lacking hand/finger control to use the system.
13. Sufficient upper body and arm strength to lift oneself up to the walker for a second or two without stimulation and to grasp chair when stimulation is stopped for any reason.
14. No severe scoliosis.
15. No irreversible contractures.
16. No morbid obesity.
17. Patient is not pregnant.
18. Motivation: The patient demonstrates and expresses appropriate desire and commitment to the training program.

Also, interference of stimulation signal with an electronic cardiac pacemaker must be avoided.

31.3.2   Contraindications

Once the admission criteria of Section 31.3.1 are followed, no contraindications are known to the author from his personal observations or training experience with approximately 100 patients. Also, none are known to have been reported in the literature.

31.3.3 Patient Training

The author's experience of over 23 years of working with patients and of observing Parastep training programs outside his own training program in the use of the Parastep FES system for standing indicates that once the patient satisfies the criteria as above the patient is able to stand and to ambulate, if trained properly. Distances and speed vary widely and even distances (and speeds) well below the averages mentioned in this chapter may be a major achievement for some patients, depending on their general health, level of lesion, age, and any other limitations they may have. The author had trained a 62-year-old T-3/T-4 complete paraplegic patient (gunshot wounds) who was in the wheelchair for 40 years and never been stimulated. This patient stood up in his first session and took 12 steps in his third one-hour session. Motivation is the definite key factor and this also implies family/friends' and (and physician's) encouragement and support. Family/friends' support is crucial. This should not just be verbal, but also in terms of helping the candidate stand/walk at home after or between training sessions by walking next to him/her to be able to prevent the patient from a possible fall, and moving (sharp) obstacles from the way. The patient should have at least one strong armchair (possibly a metal chair) with arm rests at an adequate height for the patient to be able to get up and sit down independently of the walker. Some patients do initially need help in placing the lower paraspinal or gluteus electrodes on the skin. It is very advisable that a family member or friend should observe at least part of one training session. The skin electrodes need be replaced once every 2 weeks (or less, if contact to skin is inadequate). Bad electrodes or broken electrode connectors are the main reasons for stimulation failure.

Training programs vary widely and so do their respective results. This author is familiar with Parastep training programs that involve 5 to 6 h a day of supervised training for 5 or 10 consecutive days, of Parastep programs of one hourly session every week or every 2 weeks for over 1 year, of Parastep programs of three 1-h sessions a week for 11 weeks (Klose et al. [31], the University of Miami program), and of Parastep programs of 2 h per day, 5 days a week for over 4 months (Cerrel-Bazo et al. [32], the Vicenza program, Italy). Since all these programs use the same FES system (the Parastep system) only the performance results shed a light on their efficiency. However, they differ widely in cost and in the required commitment of time by the patient. Therefore, the decision on which kind of program to attend is usually not a matter of choice.

Regardless of the training program, it is of utmost importance that the patient complements each supervised training session with after-hour home exercise of at least 15 min (many programs require much more).

In almost all training programs, training starts with reconditioning and strengthening of the muscles involved and also of arm muscles. First, the quadriceps muscles, which are those that are the most involved in stand-up and in standing require strengthening. Treadmill exercises in walking are often used. In many programs, monitoring of heart rate and of blood pressure is done during treadmill training. Parallel-bar standing and walking are sometimes used at the initial stages, during a muscle-strengthening phase. But parallel-bar exercise does not help in learning to rely on and to balance oneself with the walker and may therefore be counter productive. Muscle strengthening while seated is a very major part of the home exercise throughout training, but takes place only in the first or second supervised sessions. It is psychologically most important to stand a patient up, even for 20 to 30 sec (as long as is safe) even in the first session. This and taking of the first few steps (even 2 or 3) early on are great motivators. Hence, the first step should be taken after the patient can stand safely (with a walker) for about 3 min. Eventually, training and muscle strengthening should aim at standing for 10 min or more and walking for as long as is possible. These sessions should start with treadmill standing and walking. At the last stages of training, patients should be taught to fall, by sudden power shutdown (they will learn to avoid an actual fall through proper use of walker). They will also learn to lift themselves up from the ground with no help, to walk on rough ground, and on reasonable slopes. They will train in getting in and out of a car unaided. The most advanced T-9 to T-12 patients can then train on using elbow-support cane.

Continuous walking after end of training on a near-daily basis, for at least 45 min a day (not necessarily in one session per day) is essential for progress and for improved performance.

The first training session must involve getting sufficient quadriceps contraction to have each leg lift while the patient is in a seated position. Psychologically and motivationally, it is desired that the patient gets up (to a walker, not to parallel bars) in the first or second session. However, this should not defer rigorous muscle strengthening in future sessions (actually, until end of the training program). For best results, daily (5 days/week) training of 1–2 h/day, followed by home exercises, yields far better outcomes at end of training than a 3 h/week program and even more, if the whole training program is condensed over only 1–2 weeks. Still, whatever the training program, if after completion of training, the patient continues to walk daily for 30–45 min he will continue improving and his performance will equal the best program (of course, considering his individual status, lesion level, age, and general health).

Home exercising while undergoing training should be done when the patient stimulates while seated — except when, later in training (and with trainer's explicit permission) the patient is permitted to take a walker home and stands/takes steps WHILE an able-bodied person is close at hand.

31.4   Walking Performance, and Medical and Psychological Benefits Evaluation Results

31.4.1   Walking Performance Data

Walking distances covered by Parastep users vary with the individual user's level of injury, training, learned skills, and physical condition. Distance walked will vary and increase with practice and training. Individual goals are established for each user by the physical therapist. Studies conducted in different clinical settings reported distances walked by individual users ranging from a few feet to over a mile at a time, with the average distance being around 1450 ft (450 m/walk) for fully trained patients in certain training programs [32,33].

Performance is influenced by the training program, but mostly by how rigorously the patient continues to actively stand and walk with the FES system after end of training. Improvements in performance will be very noticeable 1 or 2 years after end of formal training. Approximately 5% of the Parastep users known to the author (from several U.S. training programs) can ambulate one mile per walk on occasions (usually one year or more after end of formal training). The author expects this to be the case too for the Vicenza (Italy) training program.

The Miami Project to Cure Paralysis of the University of Miami reports average ambulation distances for Parastep users of 115 m/walk at a mean pace of 5 m/min, at the end of the training program of 33 sessions over 11 weeks [31]. For the Parastep training program of daily sessions over 4 months at the Centro di Rehabilitazione di Villa Margherita in Argugnano, Vicenza, Italy, an average distance of 444 m per walk was reported, at a mean speed of 14.5 m/min and with mean daily walk time of 90 min [32]. See also Chaplin [33]. These performance differences are very significant.

Still, there is no reason to assume that persistent FES users in the 11-week program cannot do as well as those in the 4-month program at 1 year after end of training. However, continuous use may be higher for patients whose performance at end of training is considerably higher. This is the author's experience in his own (once weekly over 1-year program). The Vicenza program reports zero dropout 14 to 39 months after end of training [32]. The author is not aware of other training programs with similar results.

We comment that the averages given are for patients whose SCI lesion levels are more or less evenly distributed between T-1 and T-12. Usually, performance is better if the LSI lesion is lower (toward T-12). However, motivation and persistence often makes up for level of lesion. Still, patients who for various medical or age reasons cannot walk more than 10 m (per walk) at end of training should still continue exercising, since benefits of FES exercise are more than just a matter of distance or speed, as is discussed later. Kralj et al. [15] give the general utilization statistics on the Ljubljana FES system for performance tests carried out by its developers.

However, these do not include performance data or medical or psychological patient evaluation on that system. The data given here on the Parastep system, are from independent centers (University of

TABLE 31.2 Ambulation Performance Results (Parastep Users)

Ave. speed	Ave. distance	
	m/walk	m/min
Approx 85 sessions daily over 4 months Vicenza [32]	444.3	14.5
32 sessions 3/week, 12 weeks University of Miami [31]	115	5.0

Miami Medical School, the Vicenza Rehabilitation Center, Italy) that are not connected with the system's manufacturers or its developers.

Table 31.2 gives further ambulation performance data.

A 14 min video of complete thoracic-level paraplegic patients, while walking with the Parastep system, is shown in www.ece.uic.edu/~graupe.

31.4.2 Evaluation Results on Medical Benefits for Walking with the Parastep System

The benefits in using the Parastep system go well beyond the benefits in the ability of walking, as discussed in Section 31.4.1. Medical and psychological evaluation that were published on Parastep users, show several medical and psychological benefits to walking with the Parastep. These are discussed in this and in the next section. Most important medically is the major improvement in circulation at below the level of the SCI lesion. We discuss the medical and physiological evaluation results here, while psychological evaluation outcomes are summarized in Section 31.4.3.

1. *Lower-Extremity Blood Flow:* A study performed as a part of the Miami Project, to Cure Paralysis of the Departments of Neurological Surgery and of Orthopedics and Rehabilitation of the University of Miami, authored by Nash et al. [34] and involving 12 Parastep users, reports an average increase of lower-extremity blood inflow volume f 56% (from 417 to 650 ml/min) after 12 weeks (32 sessions) of Parastep training. Dr. Cerrel-Bazo reported (verbally) to this author similar improvements (at the Vicenza program in Italy). It is noted that, after paralysis due to thoracic level SCI, blood flow to the lower extremities decreases considerably, with detrimental subsequent effects on kidney function and eventual cardiovascular effects. Hence, such improvement is of major significance.

2. *Other Cardiovascular Effects:* The above 12-patient study at the Miami Project of the University of Miami [34] has shown that the average resting heartbeat of Parastep users decreased from 70.1 (prior to FES training) to 63.2 (posttraining). Also, the Common Femoral Artery cross-sectional area increased by 50%, from 0.36 cm^2 (pretraining) to 0.48 cm^2 (post-FES training).

3. *Physiological Responses to Peak Arm Ergometry:* A study on physiological responses by 15 Parastep users [27] to peak-arm ergometry exercises have shown that average time to fatigue has improved from 15.3 min prestart of FES training to 19.2 min after 33 sessions of training. Also, the peak workload increased from 48.1 to 60 W. Oxygen uptake at peak-arm ergometry increased from 20.02 ml/kg/min pretraining to 23.01 ml/kg/min posttraining, while the respiratory exchange ratio dropped from 1.26 pretraining to 1.18 posttraining, to indicate improvement in all these parameters. The patients (12 men, 3 women) ranged in age from 21 to 45, in years from injury from 0.7 to 8.8, and in body weight from 53.6 to 83.5 kg.

4. *Muscle Mass:* A significant increase (10 to 22%) in high circumference was measured on Parastep users after 3 to 6 months of training at the University of Illinois/Michael Reese Hospital training program in Chicago [5].

5. *Spasticity:* Spasticity is common to all SCI patients with upper-motor lesions. In the authors experience in 19 years of observing well over 100 patients training with or using the Parastep system, almost all patients who complained of spasticity commented on either considerable or some improvement in spasticity. This improvement was usually observed after the first 2 to 3 training sessions. Usually,

TABLE 31.3 Medical and Physiological Evaluation Data (Parastep Users)

	Pre-FES-training (Ave.)	Post-FES-training (Ave.)	
Lower-extremity blood flow	417 ml/min	650 ml/min (improv.)	12 patient data/ U. of Miami [34]
Heart rate	70.1	63.2 (improv.)	12 patients/Miami [34]
Time to fatigue (at peak-arm ergometry test)	15.3 min	19.2 min (improv.)	15 patients/Miami [35]
Peak workload heart rate (pk arm ergom. test)	188.5	183.1 (improv.)	15 patients/Miami [35]
Oxygen uptake (pk arm ergom. test)	20 ml/kg/min	23 ml/kg/min (improv.)	15 patients/Miami [35]
Spasticity		Usually improvement, especially for very spastic pre-training Training, where no significant change was reported	Michael Reese Hospital, Chicago [6,27,29]

the higher the degree of spasticity, the greater was the improvement that was reported. This improvement was often reported as one of the reasons for participating in the FES program. The improvement in spasticity is important with regard to the detrimental effect of medications (Baclofen, Valium, Lioresal) on alertness and fatigue as medication doses can then be reduced in many cases [5].

6. *Bone Density:* Practically all paraplegics suffer from reduced bone density. This happens right after injury and may be aggravated when the patient does not put weight on the legs. One of the Parastep patients in the author's program recorded a 50% bone density prior to training (but no bone injuries) with no improvement after one year though he continued to walk and reached 1 mile/walk. The only study published till now (Needham-Shropshire et al. [36]) does not show any improvement in bone density due to FES ambulation. However, this study refers to the end of 11 weeks of training. No study exists on patients who have consistently walked via FES for several years.

7. *Pressure Ulcers (Decubitus Ulcers):* Almost all paraplegics suffer from decubitus ulcers. However, all but one patient at the author's FES program (at Michel Reese Hospital, Chicago), had no occurrence of a new ulcer while regularly using FES. Improved blood circulation at below the lesion is most likely the cause for this [27]. The exception was due to a cut from a sharp object.

The medical and physiological evaluation data are summarized in Table 31.3.

31.4.3 Psychological Outcome Evaluation Results

1. *Psychological Evaluation Results — Self-Concept Scores:* A study on 14 Parastep users after 11 weeks of training at the Miami program [37] concerning physical self-concept using the Tennessee Self-Concept Scale (TSCS), compares TSCS scores before the beginning of Parastep training against the score at the end of the 11-week program. It shows that the average TSCS score improved in a statistically significant manner from 44.3 to 52.0. Furthermore, all patients with a score below 50 prior to FES-training, have improved, whereas no patient with an initial score above 50 dropped to below 50.

2. *Psychological Observations – Depression scores:* The same study [37] as in Section 31.4.3 reports on comparing Beck Depression Inventory (BDI) scores for measuring depression before and after 11 weeks of Parastep training. BDI scores of below 9 refer to no depression and scores below 18 to mild depression, whereas scores from 18 to 29 point to moderate depression. The results of the study show that all five patients who were initially at the mild or moderate depression score levels (one was initially even beyond the moderate range) did improve significantly. The patient who was initially beyond the moderate depression range (31 DBI score) improved to 24 (mild depression range). One of the two patients, who were initially

TABLE 31.4   Psychological Evaluation Results — For Parastep Users

	Pre-FES-Training (Ave.)	Post-FES-Training (Ave.)	
Physical Self Concept (TSCS scores)	43.2 TSCS	52 TSCS (improv.)	15 patients/Miami [37]
Depression Scores (BDI scores)	8.8 BDI	5.4 BDI (improv.)	15 patient data [37]

in the moderate range, improved to the low-mild range and the other to the no-depression range. All patients who were initially in the low-depression range stayed in that range.

The psychological evaluation results, as in the present section, are summarized in Table 31.4.

31.5   Regulatory Status

The Parastep-I functional neuromuscular (electrical) system (referred to throughout this chapter as the Parastep system) for standing and for ambulation by thoracic-level paraplegics received FDA approval on April 20, 1994 [8]. It was the first and is still the only noninvasive FES ambulation system to have received FDA approval. Furthermore, effective April 1, 2003 the Centers for Medicare and Medicaid Services (CMS) made a National Coverage Determination extending coverage to the Parastep-I System for qualifying Medicare beneficiaries. Specific HCPCS codes have been assigned to cover costs associated with both the acquisition of the Parastep-I equipment [9] and for the physical therapy training services Parastep-I [10]. Medicare covers approximately 80% of equipment acquisition costs. Following the CMS example, most major medical insurers in the United States have already amended their policies to cover the Parastep system. The Parastep's manufacturer, Sigmedics, Inc. of Fairborn, Ohio, physical therapy training services has set up its own Patient Case Management Department for the purpose of facilitating insurance reimbursement process.

31.6   Concluding Comments

This chapter discusses the Parastep system, which is the first and still, the only FDA-approved transcutaneous (noninvasive) FES system for ambulation by complete or near-complete thoracic-level paraplegics. It describes what this system can already do for the thoracic-level (complete) paraplegic patient in noninvasive FES. It gives concrete data from many studies on how that system performs. It also discusses its design, operation, admission criteria, contraindications, and training.

We thus conclude that a totally noninvasive FES for independent standing and mobility is already a reality for complete upper-motor-neuron thoracic-level traumatic paraplegics. Furthermore, it is commercially available and it received (2003) approval for reimbursement by the Center for Medicare and Medicaid Services (CMS) that regulates Medicare and Medicaid reimbursements policies in the United States and subsequently, by practically all medical insurance companies in the United States. Training programs for that system exist in many hospitals and rehabilitation centers. As was discussed above, upon completion of 4 months of daily training, ambulation distances for the Parastep system were reported to average 444 [32] or 115 m/walk in a 33-session 11-week program [31]. Medical benefits have been documented, in terms of greatly increased blood flow to the lower extremities [34], reduced spasticity [29], reduced incidence of decubiti [27], increased thigh circumference [27], and of psychological benefits (improved self-concept and depression scores) [37].

However, even 10 years after FDA approval of such a noninvasive FES system and 2 years after reimbursement was approved by Medicare, Medicaid, and by most insurers, there is great ignorance in the paraplegics community about the availability of such a system and of its performance and benefits. In Reference [38], a statement by a patient is quoted (made in a recent symposium of prospective FES users, funded by the Whitaker Foundation), that "in 3 to 4 different rehabilitation facilities and (having) talked to over 200 patients...none of them ever mentioned FES." These indicate ignorance, regarding the role of FES in paraplegia, among physicians involved in caring for paraplegics, and among the (physical and occupational) therapists and other related staff.

The consensus of the Symposium above (and which agrees with what this author repeatedly hears from patients) was that desire to stand upright independently and to ambulate even short distances is the prime desire of paraplegics long-term compliance and long-term use of FES is also a problem. However, the circulatory benefits and the other medical and psychological befits should play an important role, for patients, for physicians, and for insurance companies involved.

All this does not detract in any way from the urgent need to repair the spinal cord through regeneration. Neither the Parastep nor any other FES approach can substitute for this, since FES does not heal. It is an aid, just like eyeglasses or a hearing aid. It is hoped that regeneration will be a reality for human SCI patients. In the meantime, a realistic aid does exists that is already FDA-approved and reimbursable. It can always be and will be improved, but its performance even now is usually pretty good.

References

[1] Galvani, L. (1791), *Commentary on the Effect of Electricity on Muscular Motion*, Translated by R.M. Green (1953), Elizabeth Licht Publishing Co., Cambridge, MA.

[2] Lieberson, W.T., Holmquest, H.J., Scott, D., and Dow, H. (1961), Functional electrotherapy stimulation of the swing phase of the gait in hemiplegic patients, *Arch. Phys. Med. Rehabil.*, 101.

[3] Kantrowitz, A. (1960), *A Report of the Maimonides Hospital*, Brooklyn, NY, pp. 4–5.

[4] Kralj, A., Bajd, T., and Turk, R. (1980), Electrical stimulation providing functional use of paraplegic patients muscles, *Med. Prog. Technol.*, 7: 3.

[5] Graupe, D., Kralj, A., and Kohn, K.H. (1982), Computerized signature discrimination of above-lesion EMG for stimulating peripheral nerves of complete paraplegics, *Proceedings of the IFAC Symposium Prosthetics Control*, Columbus, OH, March.

[6] Graupe, D., Kohn, K.H., Basseas, S., and Naccarato, E. (1983), EMG-controlled electrical stimulation, *Proc. IEEE Frontiers of Eng. & Comp. in Health Care*, Columbus, OH.

[7] Graupe, D., Kohn, K.H., Basseas, S., and Naccarato, E. (1984), Electromyographic control of functional electric stimulation in selected paraplegics, *Orthopedks*, 7: 1134–1138; Graupe, D. (1989), EMG pattern analysis for patient-responsive control of FES in paraplegics, *IEEE Trans. Biomed. Eng.*, **36**: 711–719.

[8] FDA approval P900038 (1994), http://www.fda.gov/cdrh/pma94.html, April 20.

[9] Centers for Medicare and Medicaid Services (CMS), Code K0600 (Parastep-I equipment acquisition), http://www.cms.hhs.gov/coverage, 2003.

[10] Centers for Medicare and Medicaid Centers (CMS), Code 97116 (physical training services with Parastep-I), http://www.cms.hhs.gov/coverage, 2003.

[11] Marsolais, E.B. and Kobetic, R. (1983), Functional walking in paralyzed patients by means of electrical stimulation, *Clin. Orthop.*, 175: 30–36.

[12] Marsolais, E.B. and Kobetic, R. (1986), Implantation techniques and experience with percutaneous intramuscular electrodes in the lower extremities, *J. Rehabil. Res. De.*, **23**.

[13] Holle, J., Frey, M., Gruber, H., Kern, H., Stoehr, H., and Thoma, H. (1984), Functional electrostimulation of paraplegics, experimental investigations and first — clinical experience — with an implantable stimulation device, *Orthopedks*, 7: 1145–1155.

[14] Davis, R., Kuzma, J., Patrick, J., Heller, J.W., McKendry, J., Eckhouse, R., and Emmons, S.E. (1992), Nucleus FES-22 stimulator for motor function in a paraplegic subject, *Proceedings of the RESNA International Conference*, June 6–11.

[15] Kralj, A. and Bajd, T. (1989), *Functional Electrical Stimulation: Standing and Walking After Spinal Cord Injury*, CRC Press, Boca Raton, FL.

[16] Kralj, A., Turk, R., Bajd, T., Stafancic, M., Sarvin, R., Benko, H., and Obreza, P. (1993), FES Utilization Statistics for 94 Patients, *Proceedings of the Ljubljana FES Conference*, Ljubljana, Slovenia, pp. 79–81.

[17] Popovic, D. (1986), Control methodology for gait restoration, *Proceedings of the 8th Annual Conference of IEEE Engineering in Medical and Biological Society*, Dallas-Ft. Worth, TX, pp. 675–678.

[18] Mayagoitia, R.E., Phillips, G.F., and Martinez, L.M. (1993), Mexican Programmable Eight Channel Surface Stimulator, *Proceedings of the Ljubljana FES Conference*, Ljubljana, Slovenia, pp. 169–170.

[19] Phillips, G.F., Adler, J.R., and Taylor, S.J.G. (1993), A portable stimulator for surface FES, *Proceedings of the Ljubljana FES Conference*, Ljubljana, Slovenia, pp. 166–168.

[20] Jaeger, R. (1986), Design and simulation of closed-loop electrical stimulation orthoses for restoration of quiet standing in paraplegia, *J. Biomech.*, p. 825.

[21] Kralj, A., Bajd, T., Turk, R., and Benko, H. (1989), Paraplegic patients standing by functional electrical stimulation, *Digest 12th International Conference of Medical Biology Engineering*, Jerusalem, Israel. Paper 59.3.

[22] Taylor, P.N., Ewins, D.J., and Swain, I.D. (1993), The odstock closed-loop FES standing system — experience in clinical use, *Proceedings of the Ljubljana FES Conference*, Ljubljana, Slovenia, pp. 97–100.

[23] Tomovic, R., Vukobratovic, M., and Vodovnik, L. (1973), Hybrid actuators for orthotic systems — hybrid assistive system, *Proceedings of the International Symposium on External Conference Human Extremities*, Dubrovnik, Yugoslavia, p. 73.

[24] Andrews, B.J. and Bajd, T. (1984), Hybrid orthoses for paraplegics, *Proceedings of the International Symposium on External Control Human Extremities*, Dubrovnik, Yugoslavia, p. 55.

[25] Solomonov, M., Best, R., Aguilar, E., Cetzee, T., D'Ambrosia, R., and Rarrata, R.V. (1997), Reciprocating gait orthosis powered with electrical muscle stimulation (RGO-2), *Orthopedics*, pp. 315–324 (Part 1); pp. 411–418 (Part 2).

[26] Davis, R., MacFarland, W., and Emmons, S. (1994), Initial results of the nucleus FES-22 stimulator implanted system for limb movement in paraplegia, *Stereotat. Funct. Neurosurg.*, **63**: 192–197.

[27] Graupe, D. and Kohn, K.H. (1994), *Functional Electrical Stimulation for Ambulation by Paraplegics*, Krieger Publishing Co., Malabar, FL.

[28] Graupe, D. and Kohn, K.H. (1998), Functional neuromuscular stimulator for short-distance ambulation by certain thoracic-level spinal-cord-injured paraplegics, *Surg. Neurol.*, **36**: 202–207.

[29] Graupe, D. and Kohn, K.H. (1997), Transcutaneous functional neuromuscular stimulation of certain traumatic complete thoracic paraplegics for independent short-distance ambulation, *Neurol. Res.*, **19**: 323–333.

[30] Assoc for Advancement of Med Instrumentation/Amer. Nat. Standard Inst.: American National Standard for Transcutaneous Nerve Stimulators, *AINSllAAMI NS4 0* 1985, Arlington, VA, Approved: May 20, 1986.

[31] Klose, K.J., Jacobs. P.L., Broton, J.G., Guest, R.S., Needham-Shopshire, B.M., Lebwohl, N., Nash, M.S., and Green. B.A. (1997), Evaluation of a training program for persons with SCI paraplegia using the Parastep-I ambulation system, Part 1: ambulation performance and anthropometric measures, *Arch. Phys. Med. Rehabil.*, **78**: 789–793.

[32] Cerrel-Bazo, H.A., Rizetto, A., Pauletto, D., Lucca, L., and Caldana, L. (1997), Assisting paraplegic individuals to walk by means of electrically induced muscle contraction: gait performance and patient compliance, Session 91, Paper 66, *Eighth World Congress of the International Rehabilitation Medicine Association*, Kyoto, Japan.

[33] Chaplin, E. (1995), Functional neuromuscular stimulation for mobility in people with spinal cord injuries. The Parastep I system, *J. Spinal Cord Med.*, **19**: 99–105.

[34] Nash, M.S., Jacobs, P.L., Montalvo, P.M., Klose, K.J., Guest, R.S., and Needham-Shropshire, B.M. (1997), Evaluation of a training program for persons with SCI paraplegia using the Parastep-I ambulation system, Part 5: lower extremity blood flow and hypermic responses to occlusion are augmented by ambulation training, *Arch. Phys. Med. Rehabil.*, **78**: 808–814.

[35] Jacobs, P.L., Nash, M.S., Klose, K.J., Guest, R.S., Needham-Shropshire, B.M., and Green, B.A. (1997), Evaluation of a training program for patients with SCI paraplegia using the parastep-I ambulation

system, Part 2: effects on physiological responses of peak arm ergometry, *Arch. Phys. Med. Rehabil.*, **78**: 794–798.

[36] Needham-Shropshire, B.M., Broton, G.J., Klose, K.J., Lebwohl, N., Guest, R.S., and Jacobs, P.L. (1997), Evaluation of a training program for persons with SCI paraplegia using the Parastep-I ambulation system, Part 3: lack of effect on bone mineral density, *Arch. Phys. Med. Rehabil.*, **78**: 799–803.

[37] Guest, R.L., Klose, K.J., Needham-Shropshire, B.M., and Jacobs, P.L. (1997), Evaluation of a training program for persons with SCI paraplegia using the Parastep-I ambulation system, Part 4: effects on physical self-concept and depression, *Arch. Phys. Med. Rehabil.*, **78**: 804–807.

[38] Kilgore, K.L., Scherer, M., Bobblit, R., Dettloff, J., Dombrowski, D.M., Goldbold, N., Jatich, J.W., Morris, R., Penko, J.S., Schremp, E.S., and Cash, L.A. (2001), Neuroprosthesis Consumers' Forum: consumer priorities for research directions, *Veterans Administration — J. Rehabil. Res. Develop.*, 655–660.

32

Comparing Electrodes for Use as Cortical Control Signals: Tiny Tines, Tiny Wires, or Tiny Cones on Wires: Which Is Best?

Philip R. Kennedy
Emory Uiversity

In the fields of neural prosthetics and neural engineering there are several viable contenders for the prize of best long-term electrode to access cortical control signals for restoration of communication and movement in humans. These contenders can be classified into three main groups. The first group includes those who have developed tiny tines that are driven into the cortex and provide signals for months and sometimes years [1–3]. The second group produces flexible wires that are inserted into the cortex and provide signals also for months and sometimes years [4]. The third type of electrode is also a wire configuration but allows for growth of the brain's neuropil into the hollow glass tip of the electrode. Robust signals have been recorded for years from this neurotrophic electrode (NE) [5]. Thus, these electrodes can be classified into (1) those that protrude toward neurons and (2) the NE that welcomes the neurites into its tip and thus fuses with the neuropil.

The holy grail of all these efforts is the restoration of movement to the paralyzed. For example, quadriplegics need to use their hands, and cortical control of functional neuromuscular stimulation devices would appear to be the answer to this need. These systems, though they will provide access to cortical control signals, may not alone restore movement to those with spinal cord injury; instead, I suspect these recording technologies will be hybridized with spinal cord regeneration efforts to restore movement to

TABLE 32.1   Characteristics of Electrodes

	Tines	Tines	Tines	Wires	Neurotrophic
Investigators	Anderson	Donoghue	Schwartz	Nicholelis	Kennedy
1 Longevity	1 + yrs	4 + yrs	1 + yrs	1 + yrs	4 + yrs human
2 Stability	No	No	No	No	Yes
3 Plasticity	Yes	Yes	Yes	Yes	Yes
4 Directionality	2D	2D	3D	2D	2D
5 Force	N/T	N/T	N/T	Yes	N/T
6 LFPs	Yes	N/T	N/T	N/T	Yes
7 Units/contact	1–2	1–2	1–2	1–2	19
8 Units/electrode	40	40	40	100++	19
9 EMG related	N/T	N/T	N/T	N/T	Yes
10 Stimulation	Yes	Yes	Yes	Yes	No

N/T = Not tested, yrs = years.

those paralyzed by spinal cord injuries. Similarly for amputees, robotic technologies will be wed with cortical control signal technologies for successful control of artificial limbs.

Herculean efforts have been expended by all workers in this field to provide single unit recordings in the belief that the precision needed for control of digits is found only in the firing patterns of cortical single units recorded from primates. While not doubting this conclusion, less precise control may be sufficient for some prosthetic applications. An example of less precision is found in local field potential recordings (LFPs), which are simply an aggregate of single unit recordings. These LFPs may prove very useful as prosthetic controllers [1,6–8]. Furthermore, this chapter will conclude with the surmise that not only precision, but plasticity too, may be the unique (and a very necessary) feature available from single unit recordings and not from LFPs. Yet LFPs may provide some degree of prosthetic control, which though less precise, may be useful.

First, let us look more closely at these three electrode categories and discuss the pros and cons. Conflict of Interest statement: yes, it is true that this author is the developer of the NE. Nevertheless, I will try to be as impartial as I can and assess the facts as published and known to me. Table 32.1 summarizes electrode similarities and differences. I apologize in advance if any worker in this field is underrepresented.

The first three investigators use tine type electrodes that are either the 100-pin array (devised by Dick Norman), and used by Donoghue and colleagues [2], or the Michigan probe used by Schwartz et al. [3]. Anderson and colleagues use their version of the array [1]. Nicholelis et al. use micro wires they have devised [4]. Let us take these characteristics point by point. Kennedy is the only one to use the NE so far [5,9,10].

1. Longevity is of prime importance in a chronic electrode that is to be implanted in a young adult human for a lifetime that can extend beyond 50 years. Clearly, the NE is ahead in this respect so far [5], though recent reports from Donoghue's lab show a few signals enduring for years [2]. In all animals and human subjects, the signals from the NE continued until the preparation was destroyed or the subject died. The NE has endured in two humans for over 4 years (in preparation).

2. Stability of signal is of great importance too. This is difficult to assess over long time periods especially if the subject is totally paralyzed because in that case there is no behavior or electromyographic (EMG) activity available for correlation. Stability has been shown in the NE [5,9–11] and to some extent in Donoghue's recordings [2]. One can argue, however, that stable single units may not be of great importance now with the advent of LFPs' recordings. Because the LFP signals are inherently more stable, the loss of a few single units may not matter to the overall quality of the LFP. Nevertheless, there is yet no firm evidence of that, so stability still remains important.

3. Plasticity is one important feature of single units that is probably not available from LFPs. It ought to be easier to train one unit, than an unruly classroom of poorly correlated units. The expectation is that perhaps any unit recorded from anywhere in the brain can be trained to control a specific output. If this plasticity expectation is to be fulfilled, however, there must be a priori stability of the unit. Without stability and longevity, repeated sessions of retraining would be required. So far, the NE is unique in achieving the goals of plasticity, stability, and longevity [5,10 in prep.].

4. Directionality has been tested by all investigators and found to be present. Schwartz and colleagues are the only ones to have shown directionality in three dimensions using a virtual reality environment [3]. In these trials the cursor was driven under the influence of the single units into all eight corners of the virtual cube space. There does not seem to be any overwhelming reason why other electrode configurations should be deficient in this task. Directionality with the NE was achieved without resort to the firing rate, but was deduced from the initial direction of depolarization of the action potentials [11].

5. Force has been tested by the Nicholelis group who found that force and direction can be controlled by the monkey [4]. This feature has not been tested by others. Again, there is no overwhelming reason why force relationships could not be found with other electrode configurations.

6. Local field potentials have been studied by Anderson et al. [1], Kennedy et al. [6,7] and Leuthardt [8] and found to be useful. Anderson's group found that LFPs indicate cognitive state of the monkey and has also indicated directionality. The Kennedy group also found directionality within the LFPs [5], and in addition used them to control a cursor and a cyber hand on the computer monitor. The subject was able to flex the cyber digits under control of the LFPs with reasonable speed [5]. Again, there is no overwhelming reason why other electrode configurations should be deficient in recording LFPs. In fact, it may minimize the impact of unit instability inherent in other electrodes and thus improve their functional longevity.

7 and 8. Units per contact and per electrode have been presented by all authors. Tines and wires usually have only a few units, but have many tines or wires, thus providing a large number of units overall. This makes processing of the signal outputs per electrode relatively straightforward, but implies that a large number of electrodes are needed to provide many signals. On the other hand, the NE has 5 to 10 signals per electrode and up to 19 in one subject (in preparation), which means that fewer electrodes are required. Processing of these signals using spike-sorting technologies is complicated but very achievable with today's systems [2, in prep.]. The NE advantage is that fewer electrodes, and hence implantable amplifiers, are needed.

9. Relatedness to EMG Activity. Electromyographic activity has been studied by the Kennedy group in one almost paralyzed subject. They found that EMG was related to movement onsets, and poorly related to single unit recording, though fairly well related to LFP onsets (in preparation). Though interesting, these results are not essential to the success of any of the electrodes. After all, the subjects to be implanted will be paralyzed a priori. Furthermore, there is no overwhelming reason why other electrode configurations should be deficient in this task.

10. Stimulation of the underlying cortex can be achieved by all electrodes except the NE. The NE is not designed for stimulation. Its design constraints do not preclude it from being used as a stimulation electrode. Tests cannot be carried out in the human for technical reasons (no implantable stimulating electronics, subjects are paralyzed) and ethical reasons (implants are allowed so as to provide communication with the external world). In animal studies, stimulation was attempted and no response, such as limb movement, was seen. It would have been surprising if a response was seen because the NE contains a limited number of axons within its tip (see below) and stimulation with conventional electrodes affects a large number of neurons (with or without passing fibers) to produce a measurable response. If it can never be shown to produce a response with stimulation, then it has the disadvantage of being used only for recording.

Let us now look more closely at the evidence for some functional advantages of the NE in humans. Disadvantages will be enumerated and discussed at the end of this section. Published data have

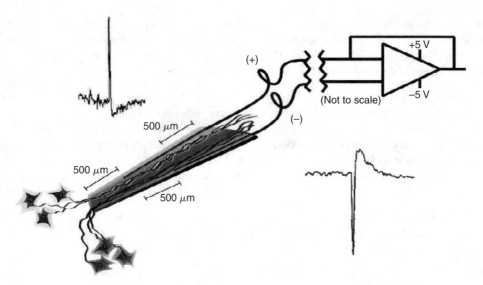

FIGURE 32.1   (See color insert following page **32**-14.) Neurotrophic electrode configuration.

shown the following:

1. Subjects drove a cursor in 2D for communication using single action potentials (APs) and LFPs [5,11]
2. Plasticity was demonstrated for single APs, but not attempted with LFPs [5,11]
3. Directionality was detected in single APs [5,11] and LFPs [6]
4. LFPs were used to drive simulated cyber digits [6]
5. Binary switch control was obtained from single APs [10] and LFPs [7]

32.1   A Brief Description of the NE

First, let us understand the unusual configuration of the NE. Figure 32.1 illustrates the salient features of the NE. The glass tip is 1 to 2 mm in length with a 50 μm diameter at the lower end where the neurites enter. The upper end is about 300 μm wide to allow at least two wires to enter. They are held in place by methylmethacrylate glue. The wire ends are usually 500 μm.

from each other and from the each end of the glass. The amplifier is connected to the wires. Because the ingrown neurites become myelinated, the neural signals recorded must be considered as APs (see histology discussion below). The APs shown have opposite initial depolarization directions. This is because the amplifier has fixed polarity with positive and negative wires. So axons close to one wire will have initial AP depolarizations opposite in direction to the AP depolarizations recorded at the other wire. This has important implications for directionality as discussed later.

A brief description of implantation techniques is required. Prior to surgery, localization of an active cortical site is essential and this is achieved using functional magnetic resonance imaging (MRI). An example of active areas is shown in red in Figure 32.2. The subject imagines movement of digits for example, and the scanner detects this as blood flow changes. We will describe this in detail in a further publication [in prep.]. All subjects undergo fMRI prior to implantation.

The implantation site is chosen based on stereotaxic 3D guidance using a system such as Stealth. Figure 32.3 shows the white pointer wand that is registered in 3D with the computer that contains the subject's MRI. The pointer indicates the active area by moving it over the active area of the fMRI.

Histological processing has shown that there are myelinated neurites inside the cone tip of the electrode as shown in this electron microscopic image. The tissue contains normal neuropil except for the lack

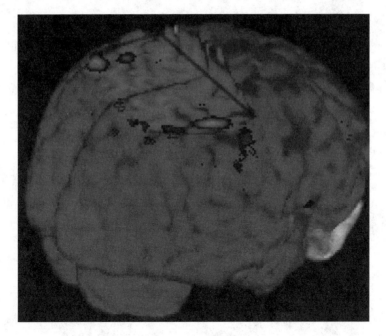

FIGURE 32.2   (See color insert following page **32**-14.) Three-dimensional reconstruction of implantation target site.

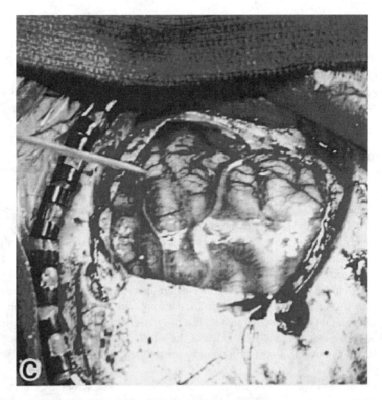

FIGURE 32.3   (See color insert following page **32**-14.) Surgical implantation site.

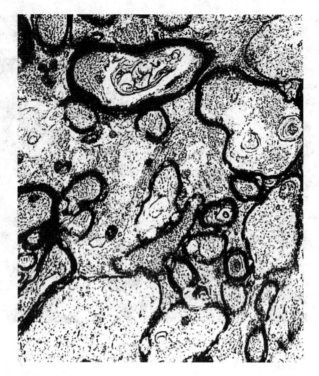

FIGURE 32.4   Electron microscopic histology.

of neurons [10]. There are myelinated neurites, axo-dendritic synapses, blood vessels, and dendroglial cells but no microglial scavenger cells, no gliosis, and no neurons. Our interpretation is that the neurons sprouted neurites that grew into the cone tip and became myelinated. Thus, the NE records APs from axons, and because there are usually many axons close together, we appear to be recording compound APs when the firing rates are high. *Long lasting (1) and stability (2)* signals have persisted in two subjects for over 4 years when the subjects died from their underlying diseases (Figure 32.4).

32.2   Functionality of the APs Recorded from the NE

32.2.1   Cursor Control

Subject JR was the world's first cyborg because he was the first to control a computer directly from his brain. Our first subject MH only provided binary signals and did not demonstrate control of a computer. JR was implanted on March 24th, 1998 and by mid-summer was controlling the cursor [10]. We thresholded his signals and separated them into large and small amplitude APs. One set drove the cursor in the horizontal and the large units drove the cursor in the vertical direction. The firing rate or the APs was directly proportional to the cursor movement above a user-determined threshold firing. Gain of firing rate to cursor velocity was also user determined but held fixed during trials. Results of testing on days 120, 121, and 122 after implantation demonstrated that within five trials he could control the cursor as shown in Figure 32.5. The cursor was placed at the top left of the screen and he had to move it across and down the screen as quickly as possible, thus forcing him to fire the large units that drove the cursor vertically downward.

When asked to drive the cursor to a particular icon about half way across the screen, he succeeded quite well as shown in Figure 32.6 for day 243. Target 4 (on the ordinate) was the requested target which he hit repeatedly after initial inaccurate hitting of target 3 for five trials. Gaps between bars indicate rest

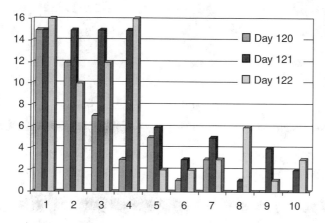

FIGURE 32.5   Learning curve for cursor control.

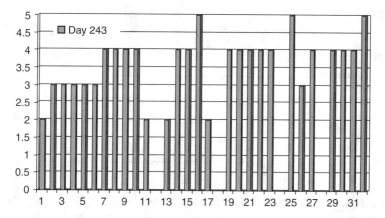

FIGURE 32.6   Learning curve for two-dimensional cursor control.

periods. Thus subject JR demonstrated cursor control in two dimensions even before it was demonstrated in monkeys [5].

3. Plasticity: In JR, we implanted area 4, hand representation, as determined by the functional MRI. We realized that he was moving facial muscles, specifically eyebrow movements, to produce neural activations. We preferred of course that he use neural activity that was not related to face or other residual movements. We asked JR not to use face movements of any kind during cursor driving. He appeared to comply with this request. To ensure that he did not move, we placed electrodes over his eyebrows to measure EMG activity. This activity would have driven the cursor in the vertical direction. This would have upset his performance in a task that required him to move horizontally to hit icons. Thus he had to maintain relaxation of his eyebrow muscles. The neural activity that drove the cursor is shown in Figure 32.7 with the target icon entry point on the right above, and the EMG activity shown below over a 10-sec timebase. Note the neural bursts that are not accompanied by the EMG activity.

His performance during this task is shown in Figure 32.8. When he tried to perform too quickly (less than 20 sec) he produced errors as shown by the grey bars. Trial 5 was error free with a time of 22 sec, whereas trials 3 and 4 performed in 11 or 12 sec produced errors. Thus he could perform without activating his face muscles.

When asked what he was thinking during these trials, he spelled out "nothing" [5]. However, the next day he admitted he was thinking of the cursor. He was focused on the cursor alone. He was driving the

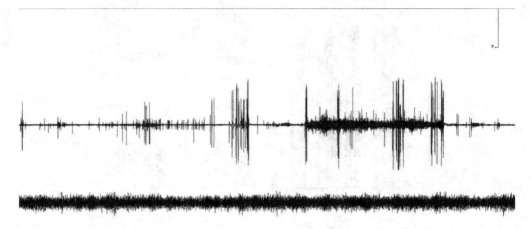

FIGURE 32.7 Neural signal activity during cursor movement with no EMG phasic activity.

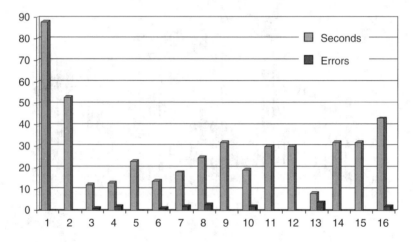

FIGURE 32.8 Learning curve while using neural signals alone.

cursor simply by thinking about it. Thus we concluded that what had once been hand-related cortex, was now cursor-related cortex. This is the first demonstration of plasticity in human cortical recording.

4. *Directionality*: In other electrode configurations, directionality is detected by the firing rate of a neuron in a specific direction [3]. With the NE however, fdirectionality is independent of firing rate. Instead, it is determined by the initial depolarization direction of the AP as shown in Figure 32.9. We noted that individual action potentials can be discrete depolarizations in positive or negative directions or can appear to be a single biphasic unit, which is in reality the overlying of positive and negative depolarizing directions.

Deflections in one direction are shown in the upper panel of Figure 32.10 where most APs have initial deflections in the negative or downward direction at rest. The subject JR was then requested to think of moving the cursor in the horizontal direction and all APs were thresholded as a group to drive the cursor. JR saw the cursor moving horizontally. The lower panel of Figure 32.10 shows the resultiing action potential directions, namely, upward or positive. Later recordings when all the action potentials were used to drive the cursor vertically downward, resulted in AP deflections in the opposite direction. Thus the initial direction of depolarization allows detection of directionality.

Directionality was also detected during LFP recordings as shown in Figure 32.11. In these recordings, LFPs were recorded separately from each wire inside the cone tip of the electrode. The wires are in the rows with 5 sec of recording in each panel. In the left column, the subject JR was moving the cursor

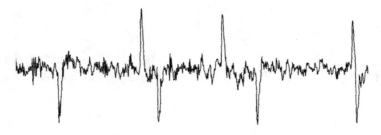

FIGURE 32.9 Action potentials.

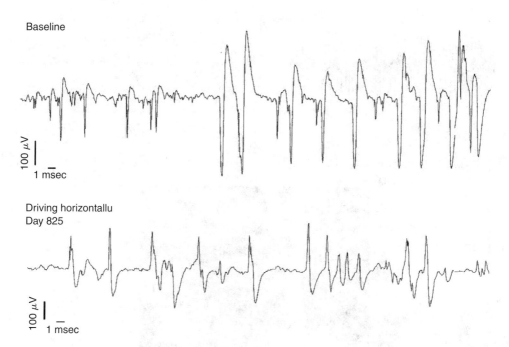

FIGURE 32.10 Directionality detected by phase relationships.

horizontally, and in the right column he was moving it vertically. Note the clearly distinct separation of activity for each wire that depended on the direction of cursor movement.

5. *Force.* Clearly, we cannot test force relationships in paralyzed people. Force relationships were not tested in animals.

6. *Local field potentials (LFPs).* Intracortical LFPs were tested in two subjects JR and TT as published [6]. Intracortical LFPs have large amplitudes as can be seen in the previous Figure 32.11. In one subject, JR, a cyber hand was developed with digits that moved with firing rate as shown in Figure 32.12. The subject received feedback visually, auditorially, and sensorially (with a finger tap) with each AP firing. He was instructed to move a digit on receiving a verbal "Go" signal. The latency between the "go" signal and movement onset is plotted in Figure 32.13. After 6 trials, he usually performed this task in under 5 sec. This performance improvement indicated that LFPs could be used in this crude manner for movement control.

Extracortical LFPs were recorded in two subjects, RR and GT [7]. The signal amplitudes were low in this mode and thus detection methods other than voltage thresholds were sought. Thus we analyzed the data using the frequency domain as shown in Figure 32.14. In this subject a stainless steel skull screw was implanted over the leg area of motor cortex. At rest, the dominant frequency was the resting 8 Hz (alpha waves) and a 16- to 20-Hz signal. During attempted (and very slight) foot movements, the 8-Hz

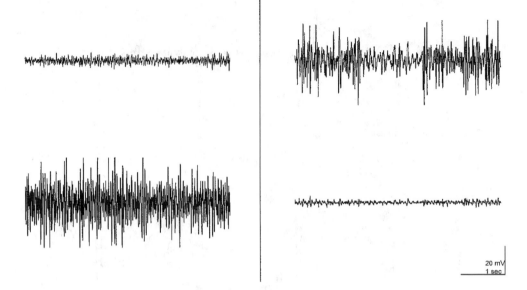

FIGURE 32.11   Directionality detected in LFPs.

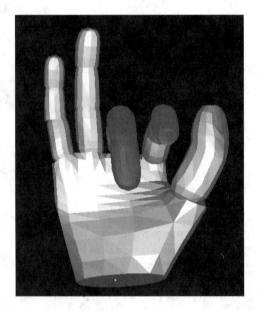

FIGURE 32.12   LFP control of cyber digit movements.

signal shifted lower and the lowest frequency increased in amplitude near 2 Hz. Changes such as these can provide a binary switch signal. In this subject, this binary output was used to operate a light switch as recently published [7].

Thus, LFPs can be used as binary outputs and for controlling crude movements.

7 and 8. Units per contact and per electrode. One of the misconceptions about the NE is that only one or two can be implanted and thus only one or two signals can be obtained. It is true that only a few can be implanted, and that is due to the bulk of the implanted electronics. Once the electronics can be further miniaturized, many electrodes can be implanted. Even with one electrode however, recent off-line analysis of human recorded data has revealed as many as 19 units from one electrode in subject JR as

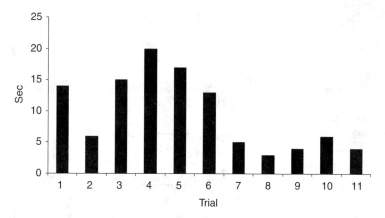

FIGURE 32.13   Learning curve for LFPs.

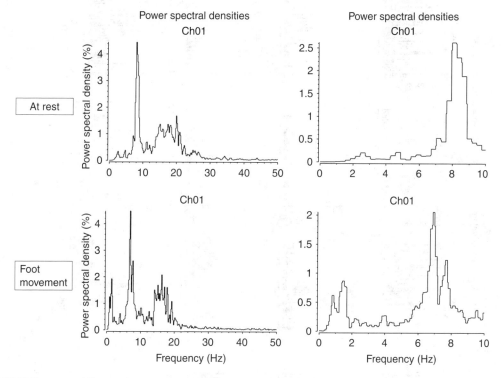

FIGURE 32.14   Differences in LFP spectrum during movement and rest.

shown in Figure 32.15. About half are not correlated and thus are expected to be independent channels of communication [in prep.]. Therefore it is not unrealistic to expect that each electrode will yield between 5 and 10 useful signals that the patient can control. Such control remains to be tested in subsequent subjects.

These large numbers of units per electrode are in sharp contrast to other electrodes where about one, maybe two, units are recorded at each electrode tip. With 100 tines on the Cyberkinetic's probe this is indeed impressive [2]. In fact, over time, this number drops to 40% or less of tines that continue to record unit activity. Furthermore, each unit varies due to micromovements, so the stability of units is questionable.

9. ElectroMyoGraphic (EMG) relatedness. In one subject, DJ, we were able to record EMG from the forearm as he made minute movements. The EMG was correlated with LFPs and APs recorded from

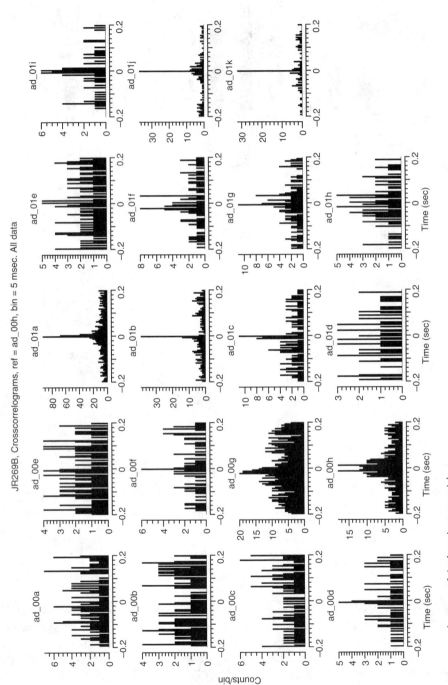

FIGURE 32.15   Cross correlograms of single action potentials.

the electrode implanted in the contralateral area 4 motor cortex [in prep.]. The LFPs were correlated and the APs had weak correlations as expected. Recording EMG in near paralyzed subjects is unique to our project but would be feasible with any of the electrodes.

10. Stimulation. Attempts at microstimulation in rats through the NE implanted in the leg area did not produce movement. Evoked movements would have been surprising because only a few tens of axons could have been stimulated and usually an observable movement of a leg in response to stimulation would be produced in response to a large area of stimulated neurons and passing axons. Increasing the stimulating current was not an option due to the danger of electrolytically destroying the axons inside the electrode tip. All other electrodes, whether wires or tines, have safely provided stimulation. Thus for stimulation, the other electrodes are preferred.

32.3 Conclusions

In nine of the 10 characteristics discussed earlier, the NE shines. The one exception is stimulation as discussed. Thus, it could be the outright winner in this race except that it has some unique problematic characteristics.

1. Accurate histological reconstruction of recorded units is not possible due to the destruction inherent in placing it in the cortex and the trophic changes that take place as the tissue grows into the cone tip. This is not, however, of importance in neural prosthetics where functionality is paramount.
2. Manufacture of the electrode at present is difficult and requires many months of practice.
3. Implantation of the electrode is also difficult and requires much practice by someone with microsurgical skills.
4. There is a delay of 3 or 4 months before the tissue has grown in and signals stabilize.
5. Replacement of the electrode in the exact same area would hardly produce the same signals unless many months passed to allow healing and reconstitution of the tissue.
6. Training time may be prolonged since plastic changes may be needed to produce useful function.

Thus for successful usage, skill in manufacture and implantation is required. The delay in signal acquisition of 3 months is surely tolerable for someone who requires a lifetime of use. Replacement is hardly going to be needed if it continues recording as studies strongly suggest. Training time again is hardly a problem when used for the lifetime of the subject.

We will allow the reader to judge for himself or herself as to who the winner will eventually be because I cannot be considered unbiased. The LFPs discussed earlier may allow other electrodes to produce useful signals even though they may not be able to retain single units over the required lifetime of the subject. LFPs may prove adequate when crude control is needed, but will hardly prove adequate for precise control. Only time and effort will tell which electrode and recording technique will be instrumental in providing cortical control of prosthetic devices.

Acknowledgments

Supported by the NIH, NINDS, Neural Prostheses Program, grant no. 2 R44 NS36913-02. Supported also by Neural Signals Inc. internal funds.

Financial Disclosure: The author PK may derive some financial gain from the sale of the Neurotrophic Electrode. USA patent number 4,852,573.

References

[1] Andersen R.A. and Buneo C.A. 2002. Intentional maps in posterior parietal cortex. *Ann. Rev. Neurosci.* 25: 189–220.

 [2] Serruya M.D., Hatsopoulos N.G., Paninski L., Fellows M.R., and Donoghue J.P. 2002. Instant neural control of a movement signal. *Nature* 416: 141.

 [3] Taylor D.M., Tillery S.I., and Schwartz A.B. 2002. Direct cortical control of 3D neuroprosthetic devices. *Science* 7: 1829–1832.

 [4] Carmena J.M., Lebedev M.A., Crist R.E., O'Doherty J.E., Santucci D.M., Dimitrov D.F., Patil P.G., Henriquez C.S., and Nicholelis M.A.L. 2003. Learning to control a brain–machine interface for reaching and grasping by primates. *PloS Biol.* 1: 2, 193.

 [5] Kennedy P.R., Bakay R.A., Moore M.M., Adams K., and Goldwaithe J. 2000. Direct control of a computer from the human central nervous system. *IEEE Trans. Rehab. Eng.* 8: 198.

 [6] Kennedy P.R., Kirby M.T., King B., Mallory A., Adams K., and Moore M.M. 2004. computer control using human cortical local field potentials. *IEEE Trans. Neural Syst. Rehab. Eng.* (accepted 2004).

 [7] Kennedy P., Andreasen D., Ehirim P., King B., Kirby T., Mao H., and Moore M.M. 2004. Using human extra-cortical local field potentials to control a switch. *J. Neural. Eng.* 1: 63–71. FDA approval number: G960032/S10, Brain to computer interfacing device.

 [8] Leuthardt E.C., Schalk G., Wolpaw J.R., Ojemann J.G., and Moran D.W. 2004. A brain–computer interface using electrocorticographic signals in humans. *J. Neural. Eng.* 1: 63–71.

 [9] Kennedy P.R., Mirra S., and Bakay R.A.E. 1992. The cone electrode: ultrastructural studies following long-term recording. *Neurosci. Lett.* 142: 89–94.

[10] Kennedy P. 1989. A long-term electrode that records from neurites grown onto its recording surface. *J. Neurosci. Meth.* 29: 181–193.

[11] Kennedy P.R. and King B. 2001. Dynamic interplay of neural signals during the emergence of cursor related cursor in a human implanted with the Neurotrophic electrode. In *Neural Prostheses for Restoration of Sensory and Motor Function.* Chapin J. and Moxon K. (Eds.). CRC Press, Boca Raton, FL, 2001.

[12] Plexon Inc. Dallas Tx; Neuralynx Inc., Denver CO.

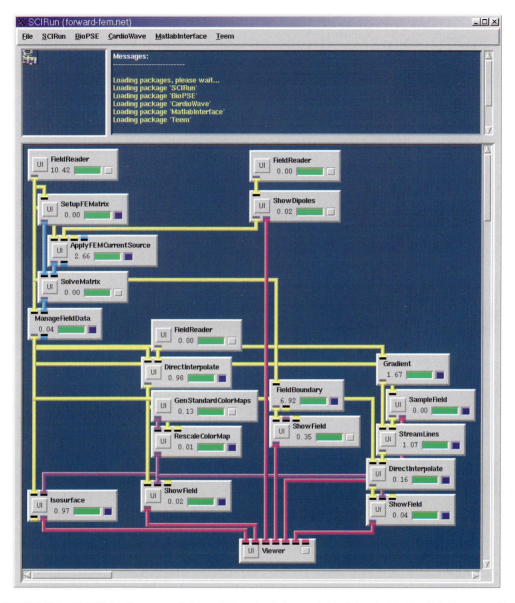

FIGURE 23.1 BioPSE dataflow network for modeling, simulating, and visualizing the bioelectric field generated in a realistic head model, due to a single dipole source.

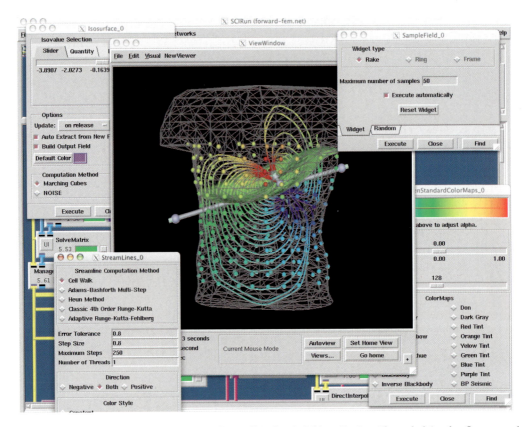

FIGURE 23.2 BioPSE dataflow interface to the forward bioelectric field application. The underlying dataflow network implements the application with modular interconnected components called modules. Data are passed between the modules as input and output parameters to the algorithms. While this is a useful interface for prototyping, it is nonintuitive for end-users; it is confusing to have a separate UI window to control the settings for each module. Moreover, the entries in the UI windows fail to provide semantic context for their settings. For example, the text-entry field on the SampleField UI that is labeled "Maximum number of samples" is controlling the number of electric field streamlines that are produced for the visualization.

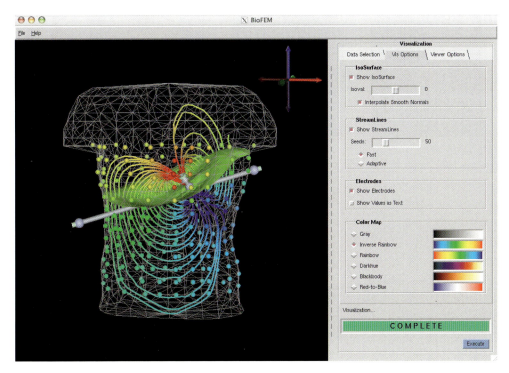

FIGURE 23.3 The BioFEM custom interface. Though the application is functionality equivalent to the dataflow version shown in Figures 23.1 and 23.2, this PowerApp version provides an easier-to-use custom interface. Everything is contained within a single window; the user is lead through the steps of loading and visualizing the data with the tabs on the right; and generic control settings have been replaced with contextually appropriate labels; and application-specific tooltips (not shown) appear when the user places the cursor over any UI element.

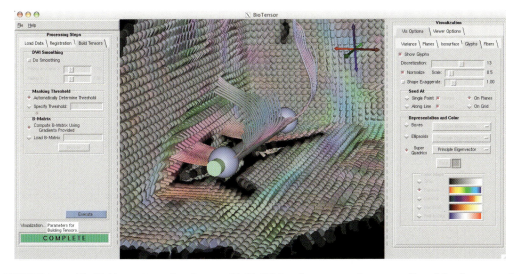

FIGURE 23.4 The BioTensor PowerApp. Just as with BioFEM, we have wrapped up a complicated dataflow network into a custom application. In the left panel, the user is guided through the stages of loading the data, co-registering the diffusion weighted images, and constructing diffusion tensors. On the right panel, the user has controls for setting the visualization options. In the rendering window in the middle, the user can render and interact with the dataset.

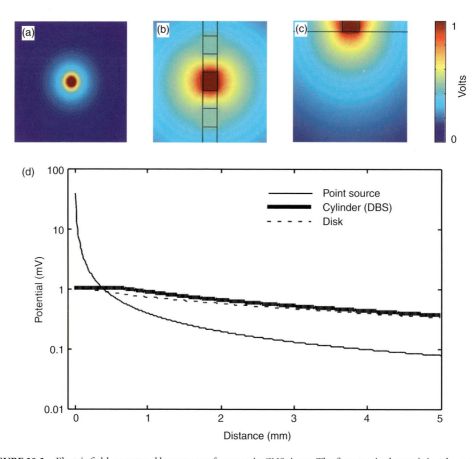

FIGURE 30.2 Electric fields generated by passage of current in CNS tissue. The first step in determining the response of CNS neurons to extracellular stimulation is to calculate the electric potentials generated in the tissue by passage of current through the electrode. Potentials produced by passage of current into a homogenous region of the CNS ($s = 0.2$ S/m) using a point source electrode (a), a cylindrical electrode (b), as used for deep brain stimulation, and a disk electrode (c), as used for epidural or cortical surface stimulation. (d) Although a simple analytical solution exists for the potentials generated by a point source electrode, they differ substantially from the potentials generated by larger cylindrical or disk electrodes.

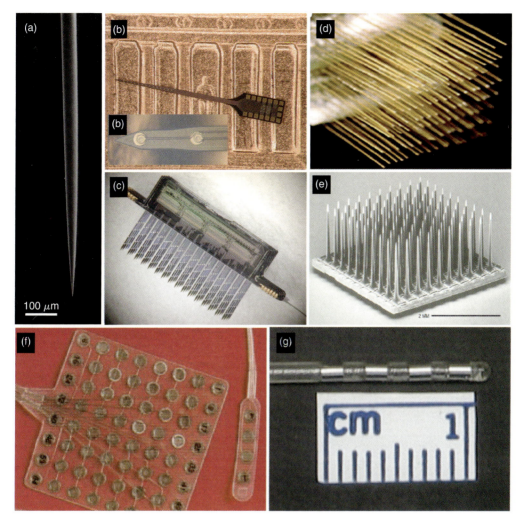

FIGURE 30.3 Electrodes for central nervous system stimulation. (a) Single iridium microwire electrode developed at Huntington Medical Research Institutes that can be used for extracellular recording from single units or extracellular microstimulation of small populations of neurons (McCreery et al., 1997). (b) Multisite silicon microprobe developed at the University of Michigan and higher magnification view (b) of two electrode sites near the tip (Images courtesy of J.F. Hetke, University of Michigan). (c) Three-dimensional assembly of multisite silicon microprobes (Bai et al., 2000). The array is four probes, 256 sites on 400 μm centers in 3D. There are 16 parallel stimulating channels (16 sites active at any time) with off-chip current generation. The array is fed by a 7-lead ribbon cable at a data rate of up to 10 Mbps. It operates from $\pm$5V supplies. (Image courtesy of K.D. Wise, University of Michigan). (d) Arrays of up to 128 microwires enable simultaneous extracellular recording from multiple single neurons. Each wire is 50 μm diameter stainless steel, insulated with Teflon (Nicolelis et al., 2003). (e) Multielectrode silicone array developed at the University of Utah (Normann et al., 1999). (f) Subdural grid and strip electrode arrays used for cortical stimulation and recording (PMT Corporation, Chanhassen, MN). (g) Quadrapolar electrode used for deep brain stimulation (Medtronic Inc., Minneapolis, MN).

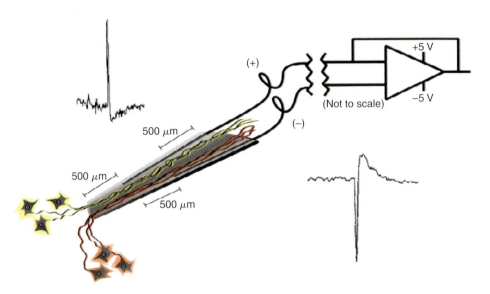

FIGURE 32.1   Neurotrophic electrode configuration.

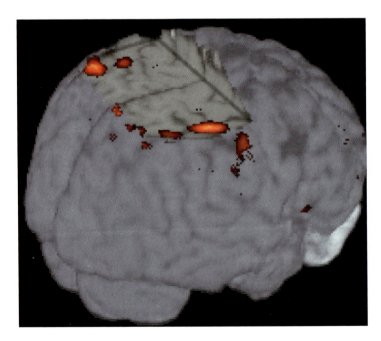

FIGURE 32.2   Three-dimensional reconstruction of implantation target site.

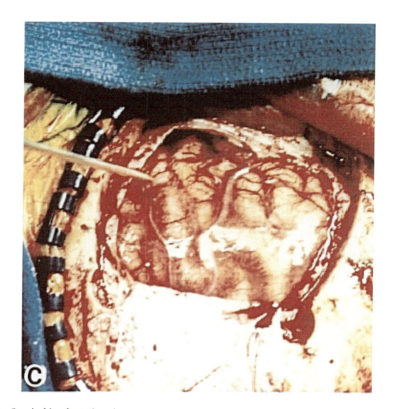

FIGURE 32.3 Surgical implantation site.

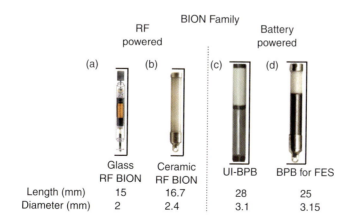

FIGURE 34.1 Evolution of the BION devices show 4 Bions to same scale.

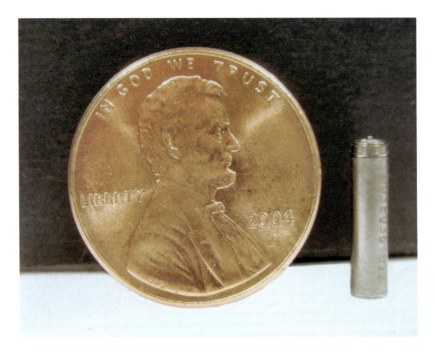

FIGURE 34.2 Quallion battery for the BPB.

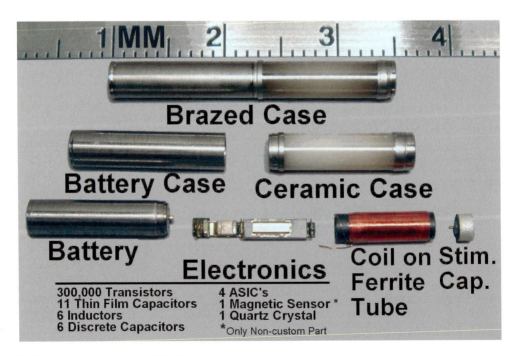

FIGURE 34.4 Battery-powered BION internal components.

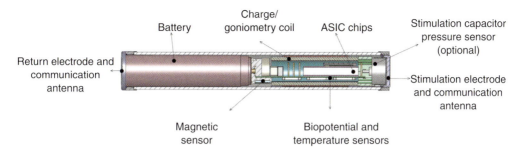

FIGURE 34.5   Battery-powered BION device cross section.

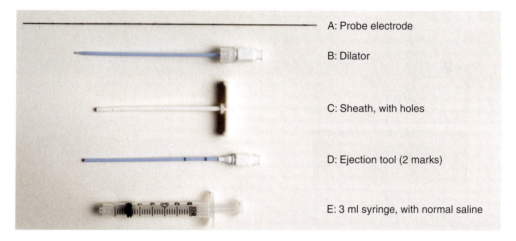

A: Probe electrode

B: Dilator

C: Sheath, with holes

D: Ejection tool (2 marks)

E: 3 ml syringe, with normal saline

FIGURE 34.10   BPB implantation tools.

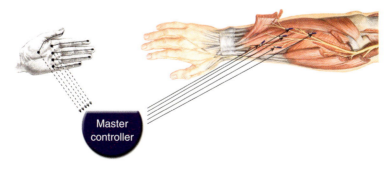

FIGURE 34.13   BPBs measuring pressure in fingers.

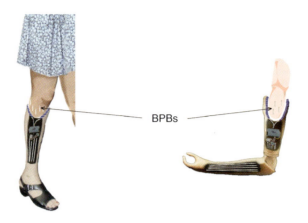

FIGURE 34.14 Use of BPBs in amputee patients.

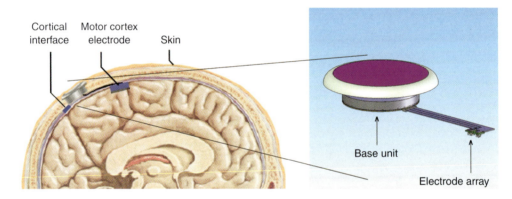

FIGURE 34.15 Cortical interface device.

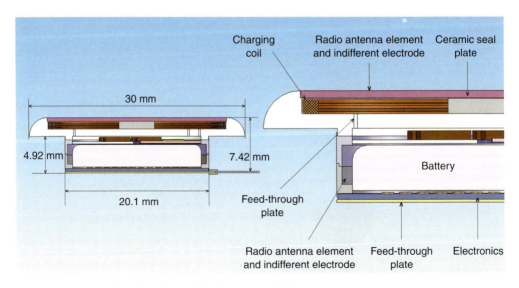

FIGURE 34.16 Cortical interface device (left) dimensions, (right) cross section.

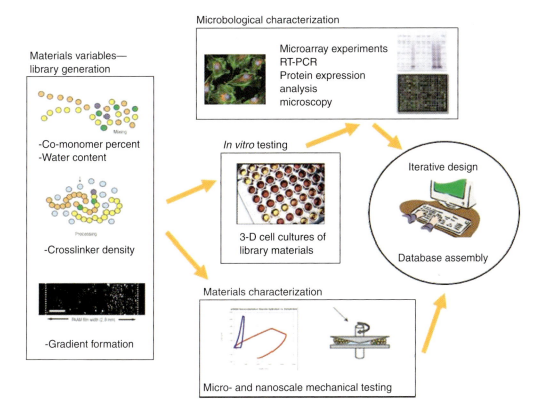

Materials variables—
library generation

-Co-monomer percent
-Water content

-Crosslinker density

-Gradient formation

Microbological characterization

Microarray experiments
RT-PCR
Protein expression
analysis
microscopy

In vitro testing

3-D cell cultures of
library materials

Materials characterization

Micro- and nanoscale mechanical testing

Iterative design

Database assembly

FIGURE 46.1 Schematic of the combinatorial approach using cell responses as variables in synthetic biomaterials design for tissue engineering applications. Libraries of chemically well-defined materials are generated combinatorially. The materials are characterized both chemically and mechanically at the nano- and microscale. *In vitro* cell-based assays are used to assess gene and protein expression. Cell–biomaterial interactions are visualized in 3-D culture using confocal microscopy. Finally, data is stored in an organized database for use in de novo materials design.

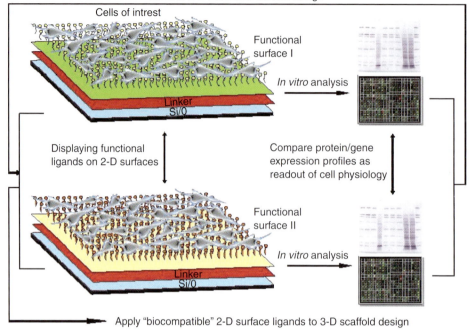

Iterative 2-D functional surface design

Cells of intrest

Functional
surface I

In vitro analysis

Linker
Si/O

Displaying functional
ligands on 2-D surfaces

Compare protein/gene
expression profiles as
readout of cell physiology

Functional
surface II

In vitro analysis

Linker
Si/O

Apply "biocompatible" 2-D surface ligands to 3-D scaffold design

FIGURE 46.2 A functional surface-based strategy to probe cell–ligand interactions — an iterative tissue engineering scaffold design approach. (Reproduced from Song, J. et al., *J. Mater. Chem.*, 2004, **14**: 2643–8. With permission.)

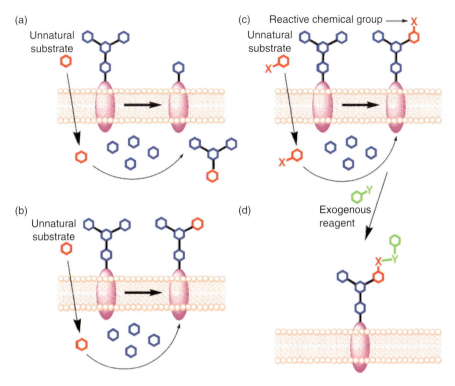

FIGURE 46.3 (Right) Modulating cell-surface glycosylation by metabolic interference. (a) Unnatural substrates fed to cells can divert oligosaccharide biosynthesis away from endogenous scaffolds, reducing the expression of specific carbohydrate structures. (b) Unnatural substrates can be used in biosynthetic pathways and incorporated into cell-surface glycoconjugates. (c) If the unnatural substrates possess unique functional groups, their metabolic products on the cell-surface can be chemically elaborated with exogenous reagents (d). (Reproduced from Bertozzi, C.R. and L.L. Kiessling, *Science*, 2001, **291**(5512): 2357–64. With permission.)

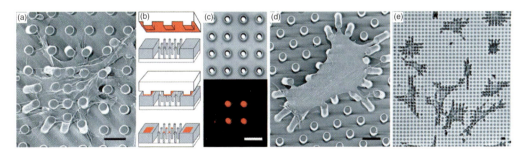

FIGURE 46.4 Cell culture on arrays of posts. (a) Scanning electron micrograph of a representative smooth muscle cell attached to an array of posts that was uniformly coated with fibronectin. Cells attached at multiple points along the posts as well as the base of the substrates. (b) Schematic of microcontact printing of protein (red), precoated on a PDMS stamp, onto the tips of the posts (gray). (c) Differential interference contrast (Upper) and immunofluorescence (Lower) micrographs of the same region of posts where a 2 × 2 array of posts has been printed with fibronectin. (d and e) Scanning electron micrograph (d) and phase-contrast micrograph (e) of representative smooth muscle cells attached to posts where only the tips of the posts have been printed with fibronectin by using a flat PDMS stamp. Cells deflected posts maximally during the 1 to 2-h period after plating, were fully spread after 2 h, and were fixed and critical point dried 4 h after plating. (Scale bars indicate 10 μm.) (Reproduced from Tan, J.L. et al., *Proc. Natl Acad. Sci. USA*, 2003, **100**(4): 1484–9. With permission.)

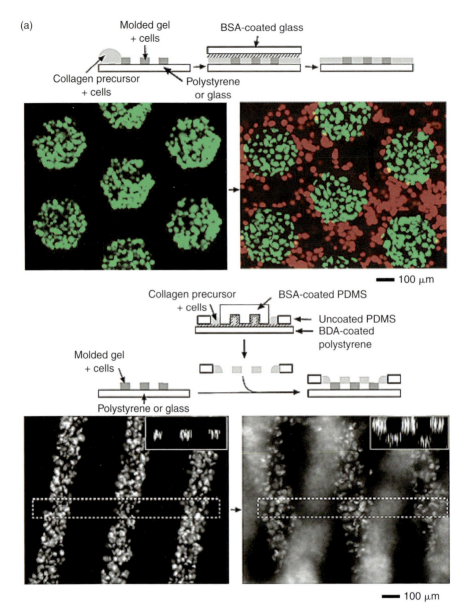

FIGURE 46.5 Schematic diagrams of the microfabrication of composite gels, and fluorescence images of cells in these gels. The shaded regions represent collagen gels in which fibroblasts are embedded. (a) (Left) An array of hexagonal gels (100 m on a side, 100 m thick) and cells on a glass coverslip. (Right) A composite structure that consists of an array of isolated hexagonal gels and a separate gel filling the spaces between the isolated gels on a glass coverslip. Fibroblasts in and between the hexagonal gels were prelabeled with green and red fluorescent dyes, respectively. (b) (Left) Lines (100 m wide, 100 m thick) of gel and cells formed by MIMIC on a glass coverslip. Nuclei of fibroblasts were labeled with the fluorescent dye Hoechst 33342 (1 g/ml; Molecular Probes). (Right) A bilayered structure that is composed of two layers of lines at a relative angle of ~30 on a glass coverslip. The top layer is in focus, and the layer below is out-of-focus. (Insets) Cross-sectional views (corresponding to the regions outlined by dashed boxes) of deconvolved images. (Reproduced from Tang, M.D., A.P. Golden, and J. Tien, *J. Am. Chem. Soc.*, 2003, **125**(43): 12988-9. With permission.)

33

Development of a Multi-Functional 22-Channel Functional Electrical Stimulator for Paraplegia

Ross Davis
T. Houdayer
Neural Engineering Clinic

T. Johnston
B. Smith
R. Betz
Shriners Hospital for Children

A. Barriskill
Neopraxis Pty. Ltd.

33.1 Introduction

The authors' aim has been to develop a generic functional electrical stimulation (FES) implant for the restoration of functions in spinal cord injured (SCI) paraplegic individuals, the functions or modes of which can be matched to an individual's requirements: upright functional mobility, pressure relief and lower extremity exercise, bladder and bowel control [1–6]. In addition, for bladder control, less invasive surgical procedures were proposed to avoid posterior conus rhizotomy, and sacral laminotomy in order to access the sacral nerve roots for stimulation [7,8]. It was hoped that this system would offer more functions and less surgery to patients with a cost–benefit ratio. This approach was termed "Multi-Functional."

Simple locomotor functions can complement the use of a wheelchair and be helpful in overcoming obstacles to wheelchair access specially doorsteps and unadapted bathroom facilities. In addition, being able to stand up to reach objects and perform prolonged manual tasks would be convenient for many workplace and home situations [3–5]. Five paraplegic volunteers (two at the Neural Engineering Clinic (NEC) in Augusta, ME and three at the Shriners Hospital for Children (SHC) in Philadelphia, PA) have participated in this device's evolution.

During 1983, R.D. (NEC) became aware of the possibilities of modifying and using the 22-channel cochlear implant technology (Cochlear Ltd., Lane Cove, N.S.W., Australia) as the basis for an implantable FES system for the restoration of multiple functions in SCI paraplegics.

The state of FES in paraplegia has been extensively reviewed [1–5]. These SCI individuals are unable to move their lower extremities or control bladder and bowel function. They must regularly self-catheterize (~3 to 6 times/day). Secondary medical problems are prone to occur, such as pressure sores, osteoporosis, muscular atrophy in the lower limbs, muscle spasticity, deep vein thrombosis, cardiovascular disease, and depression. Although considerable FES achievements have been made, there has yet to be developed a safe, practical FES system for these multiple functions that is completely independent of the laboratory and is an energy-efficient mobility aid for prolonged use at home and in the workplace. The reason lies in the fact that FES is addressing complex problems requiring not only interdisciplinary knowledge from muscle and nerve physiology and electrical stimulation technology, but also implementation of biomechanical and control principles [6].

Other reasons that limit clinical application may also be significant, for example cost-benefit considerations (especially for implanted systems). Although spinal injury results in loss of multiple physiological systems, neural implants to date have been developed to restore only specific functions. An approach was proposed to develop a generic FES implant the functions or modes of which can be matched to an individual patient's requirements. In addition, less invasive surgical procedures were proposed to avoid the posterior conus rhizotomies, and sacral laminectomy associated with existing implanted bladder implants [7,8].

Since 1984, three FES implant models have evolved from the Cochlear's technology and its subsidiary: Neopraxis Pty. Ltd. The initial Nucleus FES-22 Stimulator was implanted in 1991 after animal and human studies, and with the U.S. Food and Drug Administration's approval (IDE# G87014) and Institutional Review Board (IRB) approval in a 21 yr. Paraplegic Subject (ASIA: T10).

33.2   Historical Aspect

In 1984, the Veterans Administration (VA) funded the initial animal studies at the Togus VA Medical Center (Augusta, ME). These were aimed at determining what changes would be required to use a modified cochlear implant with a maximum pulse output of 4.3 mA and 0.4-msec pulse width, to be suitable for FES use in humans. An initial decision was taken to utilize epineurally placed electrodes (2.5-mm diameter platinum disks) in preference to epimysial or intramuscular electrodes because it was known that the stimulation currents would be lower and that there would be less movement of the electrodes. In order to determine exactly how low the stimulation currents would be and to determine the stimulation sites, initial anesthetized rabbits studies were conducted [9]. The threshold found for each branch of the split sciatic nerves was of 0.1 to 0.2 mA at 0.2 msec with 50 pps. Maximal stimulation was achieved usually between 0.5 and 1.0 mA. Simultaneous dorsiflexion of both paws as well as co-contraction in the anterior and posterior muscle groups could be achieved.

At the Togus VA Medical Center, with the approval of their IRB and volunteer patients undergoing lower extremity amputation, stimulation studies were carried out at 0.2-msec pulse duration with 20-pps frequency, with a portable, battery-operated, calibrated constant-current unit (Cordis Corp Miami, Fl.,

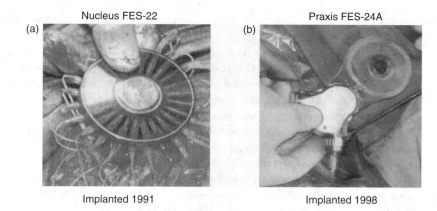

FIGURE 33.1   (a) The first 22-channel RF FES System (Nucleus FES-22) implanted in Subject A in 1991. (b) The second developed RF FES-24A Praxis System, implanted in Subject B in 1998.

Model 910 A). The pulse amplitudes for producing maximal stimulation and contraction in the largest of the nerves (medial sciatic) ranged from 0.6 to 2.5 mA, which falls well within the range of the Cochlear receiver-stimulating unit to be used [9,10]. Using the *Color Atlas of Human Anatomy*, First Edition edited by R.M.H. McMinn and R.T. Hutchings (Yearbook Medical Publishers, Inc., Chicago IL), whose dissections were reproduced as life-size photographs, allow measurements of the diameters to be made at different points along the nerves. These measurements were in relatively close agreement with the amputated nerve diameters of the nine volunteer patients [10].

33.3   Neural Engineering Clinic: 2 Male Subjects

33.3.1   Nucleus FES22 Stimulating System

As a first device, the FES22 stimulator was only intended to provide its recipient with enhanced mobility functions. During 1985, Roger Avery (Custom Med Laboratories, Durham, NH) started work on the design and manufacture for the implantable leads and electrodes. Because of the need for higher output currents it was also necessary to design a new transmitter coil capable of delivering the higher power. To make each of the 22 output channels individually available a circular epoxy housing was designed with 22 sockets around the perimeter (Figure 33.1a) with the diameter of the housing being determined by the diameter of the coil. During November/December 1991, the Nucleus FES-22 system was implanted in Subject A (21-year-old male paraplegic subject; ASIA: A T10) in 3 sessions at the Kennebec Valley Medical Center (now Maine General Medical Center), Augusta, ME. The receiver–stimulator was placed subcutaneously at the lower right anterior intercostal margin with 11 connecting leads subcutaneously tunneled to the right and another 11 to the left hip areas. Following this, 2.5-mm diameter platinum disc electrodes were placed epineurally on the individual branches of the right and left femoral nerves by suturing the silicone elastomer ring around each electrode to the connective tissues on each side of the nerve branches. In the second and third procedures, electrodes were attached over gluteal, posterior tibial, peroneal, and sciatic nerves bilaterally [11]. A total of 20 electrodes were implanted epineurally, with one electrode placed subcutaneously in a Teflon bag in each of the femoral triangles, as spare lead.

Six weeks following surgery (January 1992), the FES-22 system did produce threshold and maximal muscle contractions as tested in all 20 channels. At the second testing session in February 1992, the implanted system did not function properly owing to a suspected electrostatic damage in the implant resulting in the loss of 7 channels. Hardware and software changes were made allowing the remaining 15 channels to work. In December 1992, the 15 channels were retested for threshold and maximal muscle contractions; the multivariate analysis did not show any change with time or body side, but a significant effect was seen with the electrode locations [12].

Subject A exercised his lower extremity muscles at home using a PC computer to control the implanted stimulator. In January 1997, he was provided with a battery-operated external portable conditioning system ($19 \times 11 \times 6 \, cm^3$), which he uses at home and at work sitting in his wheelchair. The exercise protocol stimulates the right and left knee extensors and ankle plantar/dorsi flexors alternately 4 sec ON/4 sec OFF, for a total of 20 min. After the muscles have been conditioned, dynamometric testing (isometric mode) has shown that implanted FES stimulation produces bilateral knee extension torque of 45 to 55 Nm at $30°$ and 65 Nm at $60°$ of knee flexion. Subject A exercised at least 3 days a week, and found if he did not do so the spasticity in the lower extremities increased.

The laboratory PC-based FES-22 System implements a 10-msec duty-cycle state machine for open- and closed-loop control for use in prolonged standing mode. The controller is divided into three phases (1) open-loop "sit-to-stand"; (2) closed-loop stand; and (3) closed-loop "stand-to-sit." To initiate standing up and sitting down, the subject uses a remote switch on a hand glove. The sensors used for closed-loop control are electrogoniometers across both knees, which respond to a $10°$ knee buckle, and accelerometers attached to the back at T6 level.

Controlled Nucleus FES-22 stimulation to the motor nerves of the quadriceps and gluteal muscles has resulted in uninterrupted standing for over 60 min [12]. This has been achieved by use of the bilateral knee-angle goniometer sensors with the Andrews stabilizing anterior floor reaction orthosis (AFRO), which is an ankle–foot brace. With the knee goniometers sensing for a 10 degree, the stimulator would come "ON" to correct the buckle; usually this occurred between 3 and 8% of the standing time. On recovery, the automatic switch "OFF" occurs when knee flexion has returned to less than 5 degrees. Otherwise, lower extremity muscle activation is not required to maintain the upright posture [13].

33.4 Praxis FES24-A System

In 1998, Cochlear Ltd formed a subsidiary company: Neopraxis Pty. Ltd., which decided to build on the knowledge gained from the FES22 implant and to produce the Praxis FES24A System. This system was designed to provide multiple functions, bladder and bowel control, enhanced mobility, and seated pressure relief, in order to provide recipients with a cost-effective device that addresses their most important needs.

33.4.1 Bladder Control

The traditional bladder stimulator, Finetech–Brindley Stimulator, and now the "Vocare" (NeuroControl Corp., Cleveland, OH) operates by stimulating the sacral anterior roots [8]. This system has two primary drawbacks, which the Praxis system was designed to eliminate: (a) posterior sacral rhizotomies are done, via a laminectomy, in order to achieve an areflexive bladder with increased capacity; (b) a sacral laminectomy is done to access the anterior sacral roots for fitting cuff type electrodes. The rhizotomy procedure eliminates reflex erection in male recipients. Further, Creasey [8] states that "a patient who has the rhizotomies but does not use the implant (stimulator) would therefore be expected to become more constipated."

In August 1998, the Praxis FES24-A stimulator (Figure 33.1b) was developed by Neopraxis Pty. Ltd., and implanted in Subject B (35 year-old male paraplegic subject; ASIA: A, T10). Eighteen channels were used for stimulating individual nerves or branches for muscle contractions and limb movements, including exercise, pressure relief, and standing and stepping. The electrodes implanted for epineural stimulation were ten thin flexible platinum cuffs (Flexi-Cuff) that were sized, cut, and sutured closed with at least twice the diameter of encircled nerve. The other 8 electrodes were 3-mm-diameter, platinum buttons which were placed on the epineurium. Each button has an attached Dacron mesh surround that was sutured to the adjacent connective tissue on each side of the nerve.

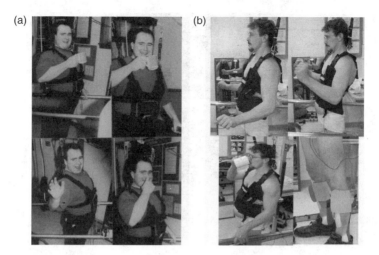

FIGURE 33.2 Prolonged standing (1 h): controlled FES + Andrews' AFO.

Three channels for bilateral sacral root stimulation (S2-4) for bladder control (bowel control and erection, if possible) were provided. Sacral root stimulation was achieved by three pairs of LPR electrodes (10-mm long, solid platinum tubing of 1.0-mm diameter) inserted into the external sacral foramina in a lateral direction to follow and to stimulate the nerve roots epidurally. One further channel was connected to an epidural spinal cord stimulating electrode (Pisces Quad: Medtronic Inc., Minneapolis, MN) for conus medullaris modulation of spastic bladder and bowel reflexes.

33.4.2 Praxis System Clinical Results

For the year prior to his implantation, Subject B was able to stand without knee bracing using a combination of the Andrews' AFRO and closed-loop skin surface FES applied directly over the femoral nerves, 2 to 3 cm below the inguinal ligament. With closed-loop control of stimulation, he would typically stand uninterrupted for 30 min, and up to 70 min. With training, Subject B did achieve the "C" posture and stood with the stimulation "OFF" for more than 50% of the standing time [14]. In December 1997, muscle strength tests done on the Biodex dynamometer (isometric mode) showed that surface stimulation of the right quadriceps (femoral nerve) was capable of eliciting 50 Nm of knee extension at 30° of knee flexion and 45 Nm at 45° [13–15].

After implantation of the Praxis FES 24-A system in August, 1998, Subject B carried out an FES exercise routine, which stimulated three separate sequences (quadriceps group, buttocks and posterior thigh group, and ankle group), each running initially for 5 min and extending to 15 min over a 2-week period. Each muscle in the sequence would be stimulated sequentially for 4 sec on and off. Subject B found that daily stimulation decreased his muscle spasms and spasticity level.

When standing with the implanted system, he was able to perform a variety of one-handed tasks including reaching for and holding a 2.2-kg object at arm's length. These tasks were achieved while in the "C" posture with closed-loop activation to the lower extremity muscles and balance maintained by the other upper extremity (Reference 15; Figure 33.2b).

33.4.3 Bladder Results

On September 4th 1998, in the Urodynamic Testing Laboratory, Subject 2 had his sacral roots (S3 and 4) bilaterally stimulated intermittently. This showed on three occasions the bladder contracted with recorded pressures of between 45 and 50 cm of water. On December 14th 1998, urodynamic testing again showed consistent results from S3 and 4 sacral root stimulation producing three sustained bladder contractions

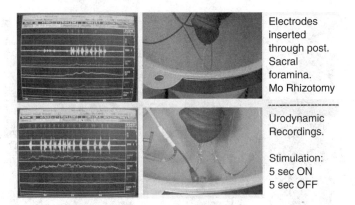

Electrodes
inserted
through post.
Sacral
foramina.
Mo Rhizotomy

Urodynamic
Recordings.

Stimulation:
5 sec ON
5 sec OFF

FIGURE 33.3   SCI: Bladder voiding: Bilateral S3 + 4 stimulation.

with pressures of 40 to 55 cm water and urination (Figure 33.3) with each stimulation pattern (5 sec on/5 sec off, 20 Hz, 8 bursts). On April 2nd 1999, urodynamic testing was repeated with two bladder reflex activations from each pattern of stimulation (5 sec on/5 sec off, 20 Hz, 8 to 14 bursts). Pressures of 50 to 70 cm of water were recorded.

In April 1999, the internal FES24-A unit's connecting wire between the internal antenna and the stimulator module broke as a result of subject B's repeated bending at the waist [15]. The Receiver/Stimulator unit was removed in 1999, as subject B complained of discomfort from the two connectors under the abdominal skin. The network of leads and electrodes were left for a possible replacement of the newly designed System.

33.5   Praxis FES24-B System

This third iteration system: FES24-B System (Figure 33.4), which eliminates this internal wire breakage possibility and consists of:

- A body-worn controller "Navigator" capable of executing a wide variety of software control Strategies.
- A skin surface stimulator "ExoStim" to mimic an implant and to provide simple exercise functions prior to implantation.
- Sensor packs incorporating accelerometers and a gyroscope to provide feedback information to control Strategies.
- A new implant receiver/stimulator was based on the latest cochlear implant control integrated circuit (IC), the "CIC3."
- A range of implantable electrode leads suitable for the system's multiple functions.

  The FES24-B System provides a maximum current output of 8 mA in a constant-current mode. Stimulation is achieved using biphasic (negative and positive phases, closely charge-matched) current pulses. Pulse widths can be varied from 25 to 500 μsec and a per channel pulse frequency of 0 to 400 Hz on each of the 22 channels can be obtained, which were designed as cathodes while the rear surface plate of the receiver/stimulator was connected to be the anode. The stimulator provides real time data telemetry functions including the ability to measure the impedance of the current path through each electrode and the ability to transmit voltage measurements from each electrode [16].

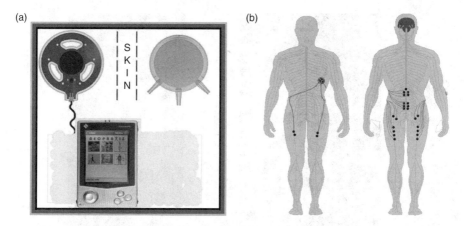

FIGURE 33.4 (a) The external parts of the Praxis FES24B System with the Control unit and surface applied antenna over the implanted Receiver-Stimulator. (b) The Radio-stimulator with the connecting 22 leads to the electrodes on nerves and spinal cord conus.

TABLE 33.1 Muscles Implanted Per Channel of Stimulation

Muscle(s)
Posterior adductor magnus
Biceps femoris — long head[a] or short head[b]
Gluteus maximus
Gluteus medius, minimus, and tensor fascia lata
Vastus lateralis and vastus intermedius
Vastus medialis and vastus lateralis
Tibialis anterior and extensor digitorum longus
Gastrocnemius, soleus, and flexor hallucis longus
Iliopsoas[c]

[a] Subjects 1 and 2.
[a] Subject 3.
[c] Subjects 2 and 3.

33.6 Experience at Shriners Hospitals for Children

Three males with paraplegia, ages 18, 21, and 21 years, underwent surgical implantation of the Praxis FES24-B System (Figure 33.4) between January 2002 and May 2003 at Shriners Hospital for Children, Philadelphia. Eighteen epineural electrodes (Table 33.1) were implanted for upright mobility in all three subjects, and three pairs of bifurcated linear pararadicular electrodes were placed extradurally on the bilateral S2, S3, and S4 mixed nerve roots for bladder and bowel function in the first 2 subjects.

33.6.1 Upright Mobility

Four weeks postimplantation, the subjects participated in 4 weeks of strengthening and conditioning of the implanted muscles followed by 17 to 22 weeks in which the focus was on programming of the upright mobility strategies and training for their functional use. Goals included achievement of the transitions between sitting and standing, swing through and reciprocal gait with a walker or crutches, and prolonged standing. For reciprocal gait, swing was achieved through stimulation to the iliopsoas, biceps femoris, and the tibialis anterior to create a flexor withdrawal response. Additional training goals

(a) 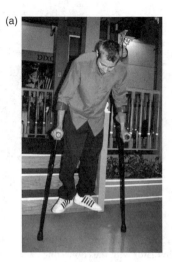   (b)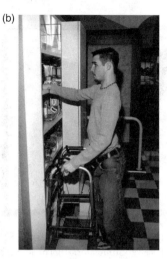

FIGURE 33.5   Two subjects using the Praxis System for functional activities (a) Subject 2 uses forearm crutches to descend stairs. (b) Subject 3 reaches for items on a shelf using a walker to support himself with one upper extremity.

include advanced activities, such as ascending and descending stairs (Figure 33.5a) and achievement of subject specific goals (Figure 33.5b). Bilateral ankle foot orthoses were worn for all upright mobility activities.

Following training, data were collected for a variety of mobility activities, including transitions between sitting and standing, a short (6 min) and a long (6 min) walk, ascending and descending stairs, and maneuvering in an inaccessible bathroom stall. All subjects chose to use a swing-through gait pattern for the tested activities, except Subject 2 who chose a reciprocal pattern for ascending stairs only. Subjects 1 and 3 each used a walker with wheels to perform the mobility activities and Subject 2 used forearm crutches. None of the subjects required physical assistance to complete the activities. Subjects 1 and 3 required supervision for all tested activities, and Subject 2 was independent for all activities except stairs where he required supervision. Data for ascending and descending stairs were not collected with Subject 1 as the activity was felt to be unsafe for him. Several activities could not be performed by Subject 3 secondary to complaints of shoulder pain related to poor scapular muscle control.

33.6.2 Sensors

Closed-loop standing using sensor packs incorporating accelerometers and a gyroscope was attempted with Subject 1. Sensor packs were attached externally on the thigh and the calf (Figure 33.6) to detect the position of the knee while standing. Stimulation would decrease until a change in the knee joint angle was detected, at which time stimulation would again increase to prevent a knee buckle.

Figure 33.7 demonstrates the use of the sensors for closed-loop feedback to the right quadriceps muscles during quiet standing. Using closed-loop control, the subject was able to stand with less stimulation to the quadriceps than what he had been using while standing with open-loop control. He was also able to stand for a longer period of time before the muscle fatigued, requiring him to sit. The algorithm for increasing and decreasing stimulation to the quadriceps did not create any balance disturbances for this subject.

33.6.3 Bladder and Bowel

Neuromodulation was attempted with Subject 1 and acute suppression of reflexive bladder contractions during bladder filling was observed. When using stimulation to both S3 nerve roots throughout the day, this subject maintained a catheterize schedule (every 6 h) comparable to that used when he took anti-cholenergic medication. This suggested that neuromodulation may have helped to suppress reflexive bladder activity on a daily basis during the control period (without the neuromodulation or medication) he catheterized more frequently, on an average of every 4 h. The ability to improve bowel evacuation was examined in Subject 2, using two different stimulation paradigms: low-frequency electrical stimulation (20 Hz, 350 μsec, 8 mA) and a combination of low frequency and high frequency (500 Hz, 350 μsec, 8 mA). The daily use of electrical stimulation appeared to cause a reduction in the time to complete defecation by 40% with the first stimulation strategy and by 60% with the second strategy.

Despite numerous attempts with varying stimulation parameters to the sacral nerve roots, neither subject could obtain detrusor pressures sufficient to provide voiding with stimulation. Both subjects continued to catheterize for bladder emptying.

33.6.4 Electrode Stability

Three of the 52 electrodes placed for lower extremity stimulation experienced changes in the responses of the muscles. One of these was due to a disconnection at the connector site between the implant and the electrode lead. This was repaired and the electrode continued to function without further problems. The remaining two electrodes (biceps femoris and tibial nerve) were not replaced, as they did not impact function for the subjects involved.

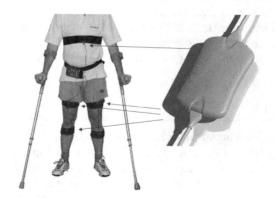

FIGURE 33.6 Sensor packs used for closed-loop standing.

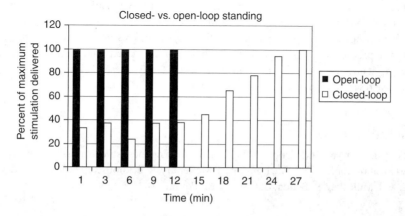

FIGURE 33.7 Using open-loop control, the stimulation remained at 100% for 12 min of standing after which the subject's muscles were too fatigued for him to remain upright. Using closed-loop control, stimulation could be maintained at a lower level, increasing over time as needed. With closed-loop control, standing time was more than doubled to 27 min.

33.7 Complications

Follow-up of the first two implanted at the NEC site, Subjects (A & B.): In 2002, Subject A accidentally cut his left foot, which was treated superficially. In 3 to 4 days, his left lower extremity was swollen with an infection, which immediately was treated with intravenous antibiotics for 2 weeks. The swelling resolved, but 6 weeks later the tissues around the Nucleus FES-22 system were swollen and inflamed. After 3 days of I.V. antibiotics, the implanted system was explanted taking as much time as when it was implanted. The most difficult part was finding and dissecting the small 2.5 mm platinum electrodes and their silastic backing. He recovered well without further complications.

In 2001, Subject B was experiencing intermittent severe pain in the T7-8 vertebra at the post-fractured site, after conservative treatment failed; the spine was fused in this area. By the time that he was ready for implanting the Praxis FES24-B stimulator in 2003, the Neopraxis Company was closed by Cochlear Ltd. However, he was offered the stimulator for implantation, but without further support by the Company, he decided not to continue and did have the leads and electrodes removed.

At the SHC site: During the training period Subject 2 sustained a stress fracture of the left proximal first metatarsal, which he believed happened when his left leg experienced greater impact at initial contact due to his poor control of swing for that step. The subject was immobilized for 6 weeks in a soft boot after which he was able to return to training without further problems. At the end of June 2002, Subject 1 sustained an abrasion near his ankle and antibiotics were started once this was reported. Then at the beginning of August 2002, he began experiencing high fever and complained of heat and inflammation around one of his surgical incisions. Despite treatment with intravenous antibiotics, this subject continued to experience problems with inflamed incisions, some of which resulted in open skin and fluid drainage. Antibiotic treatment appeared to temporarily suppress these reactions but problems continued. Due to this, the majority of the system has been removed with future surgeries planned to remove the remainder.

33.8 Conclusion

In the developing field of FES and implantable neural prosthetic devices, there has been a need for reliable and safe, multichannel implantable stimulating systems to restore multiple functions in neurologically impaired patients. In paraplegic individuals, the stimulating systems' functions should be designed to modulate spasticity and precisely activate individual muscles for joint movement and control of bladder and bowel functions. The more channels available, the more nerves can be activated and the more modes of functionality can be restored. Our contribution to this aim has been continuous since 1983, and the two Praxis FES Systems [11–16], have provided hope for a new rehabilitation aid for restoration of function in spinal cord injury paraplegia. Providing more functions with an FES system with a greater number of channels introduced new challenges to the subjects and research teams including the need for multiple surgical procedures, new surgical approaches to placing electrodes, increased risk of infection, and greater hospitalization and rehabilitation time. Importantly, these challenges are being addressed through multiple research efforts [17] at various centers.

Acknowledgments

Our thanks to Cochlear Ltd. and Neopraxis Ptv Ltd. for making these studies possible. Our sincere thanks to our many Collaborators at NEC: S.E. Emmons, J. McKendry, R. Eckhouse, A. Delehunty, W. MacFarland; and at SHC: M.J. Mulcahey, B. Benda, G. Creasey, M. Pontari.

References

[1] Kralj, A. and Bajd, T. *Functional Electrical Stimulation: Standing and Walking After Spinal Cord Injury.* CRC Press, Boca Raton, FL, 1989.

[2] Davis, R. International Functional Electrical Stimulation Society: the development of controlled neural prostheses for functional restoration. *Neuromod*, 2000; 3: 1–5.

[3] Agarwal, S., Triolo, R.J., Kobetic, R., Miller, M., Bieri, C., Kukke, S., Rohde, L., and Davis, J.A. Long-term user perceptions of an implanted neuroprosthesis for exercise, standing, and transfers after spinal cord injury. *J. Rehabil. Res. Dev.* 2003; 40: 241–252.

[4] Bonaroti, D., Akers, J., Smith, B.T., Betz, R.R., and Mulcahey, M.J. Comparison of functional electrical stimulation to long leg braces for upright mobility for children with complete thoracic level spinal injuries. *Arch. Phys. Med. Rehabil.* 80: 1047–1053, 1999.

[5] Johnston, T.E., Betz, R.R., Smith, B.T., and Mulcahey, M.J. Implanted functional electrical stimulation: an alternative for standing and walking in pediatric spinal cord injury. *Spinal Cord* 2003; 41: 144–152.

[6] Bajd, T. and Jaeger, R. FES for movement restoration. *BAM* 1994; 228–229.

[7] Brindley, G. The first 500 patients with sacral anterior root stimulator implants: general description. *Paraplegia* 1994; 32: 795–805.

[8] Creasey, G. Managing bladder, bowel and sexual function after spinal cord injury. In *Handbook of Neuro-Urology*, Rushton, D. (Ed.). Marcel Dekker, New York, 1994, pp. 233–251.

[9] Davis, R., Eckhouse, J., Patrick, J., and Delehunty, A. Computerized 22 channel stimulator for limb movement. *Appl. Neurophysiol.* 1987; 50: 444–448.

[10] Davis, R., Eckhouse, J., Patrick, J., and Delehunty, A. Computer-controlled 22-channel stimulator for limb movement. *Acta Neurochir.* 1987; 39: 117–120.

[11] Davis, R., Kuzma, J., Patrick, J., Heller, J., McKendry, J., Eckhouse, J., and Emmons, S. Nucleus FES-22 stimulator for motor function in a paraplegic subject. *RESNA Int.* 1992, 228–229.

[12] Davis, R., MacFarland, W., and Emmons, S. Initial results of the nucleus FES-22-implanted stimulator for limb movement in paraplegia. *Stereotact. Funct. Neurosurg.* 1994; 63: 192–197.

[13] Davis, R., Houdayer, T., Andrews, B., Emmons, S., and Patrick, P. Paraplegia: prolonged closed loop standing with implanted nucleus FES-22 stimulator and andrews foot-ankle orthosis. *Stereotact. Funct. Neurosurg.* 1997; 69: 281–287.

[14] Davis, R., Houdayer, T., Andrews, B., and Barriskill, A. Prolonged closed-loop functional electrical stimulation and andrews ankle-foot orthosis. *Artif. Organs* 1999; 23: 418–420.

[15] Davis, R., Houdayer, T., Andrews, B., Barriskill, A., and Parker, S. Paraplegia: implantable Praxis24-FES system and external sensors for multi-functional restoration. Proceedings of the 5th Annual Conference International Function Electrical Stimualtion Soc, Aalborg, Denmark, June 18–21, 2000; pp. 35–38.

[16] Davis, R., Patrick, J., and Barriskill, A. Development of functional electrical stimulators utilizing cochlear implant technology. *Med. Eng. Phys.* 2001; 23: 61–68.

[17] Schulman, J., Mobley, P., Wolfe, J., Voelkel, A., Davis, R., and Arcos, I. An implantable bionic network of injectable neural prosthetic devices: the future platform for functional electrical stimulation and sensing to restore movement and sensation. In *Biomedical Engineering Fundamentals*, Walker, C.F. and DiLorenzo, D.J. (eds). CRC Press, Boca Raton, FL, 2006, Chapter 34, pp. **34**-1–**34**-18.

34

An Implantable Bionic Network of Injectable Neural Prosthetic Devices: The Future Platform for Functional Electrical Stimulation and Sensing to Restore Movement and Sensation

Joe Schulman
Phil Mobley
Jamés Wolfe
Ross Davis
Isabel Arcos
*Alfred Mann Foundation for
Scientific Research*

34.1   Introduction

Functional electrical stimulation (FES) is a rehabilitation technique for the restoration of lost neurological function, resulting from conditions such as stroke, spinal cord injury, cerebral palsy, head injuries, and multiple sclerosis. FES utilizes low-level electrical current applied in programmed patterns to different nerves or reflex centers in the central nervous system to produce functional movements. The stimulation may be triggered by a single switch (open-loop) or from sensor(s) or neuronal activity (closed-loop).

While FES has been used successfully to pace the heart [1] and to restore hearing [2] in the past, it has not been widely adopted as a means of reanimating paralyzed limbs that result from stroke and spinal cord injury (SCI). It is estimated by the U.S. National Institutes of Health (NIH) that there are about 700,000 people who experience a stroke each year in the United States, with an associated comprehensive cost of $57.9 billion per year [3]. Of the more than 4 million stroke survivors alive today, many experience permanent impairments of their ability to move, think, understand and use language, or speak — losses that compromise their independence and quality of life. Furthermore, stroke risk increases with age, and as the American population is growing older, the number of persons at risk for experiencing a stroke is increasing. There is also an estimation of 250,000 Americans living with spinal cord injuries with 10,000 to 12,000 new spinal cord injuries reported every year in the United States. The cost of managing the care of SCI patients approaches $4 billion each year [4].

The potential of FES to restore function in these areas has been largely unfulfilled mostly due to the limitations of the FES devices currently available. FES could also be used in limb loss applications to reduce phantom pain and to restore functional movement of prosthetic limbs. In 2000/2001, about 130,000 lower-limb amputations were performed each year in the United States [5,6].

An optimal FES system should have the following fundamental characteristics. It should (1) provide both stimulating and sensing capabilities, (2) be fully implantable, (3) be minimally invasive, (4) have real-time communication capability, (5) allow a practically unlimited number of stimulation and sensing channels, and (6) function without external equipment or interconnected leads between components.

This chapter describes a network of wireless implantable microstimulators/microsensors, also known as Battery-Powered BION®[1] (BIOnic Neuron) devices for FES and Sensing (FES–BPB System). This new platform was designed to overcome the limitations of the current FES technology by providing:

1. Microdevices that can be programmed as either stimulators or sensors for use in closed-loop applications.
2. Minimally invasive implantation procedures to reduce labor intensive surgery and associated patient risks and to provide rapid recovery.
3. Wireless bidirectional communications and telemetry to all stimulators and sensors, which eliminates the use of both transcutaneous leads (which are susceptible to infection), and surface applied coils and stimulators.
4. Real-time communication between the stimulators, sensors, and control unit, to maintain continuous closed-loop control.
5. Flexibility and functional expandability since there are no leads and each implant has a full complement of programmable stimulators and sensors.
6. A large number of channels, which allows the same system to be used for a variety of applications without interference in the same patient.
7. Self-powered operation using rechargeable batteries to power the implantable devices. External equipment (e.g., power antennas) are only needed during battery recharging.
8. Wireless sensors capable of measuring biopotentials, angle, position, pressure, temperature, and permanent magnet fields.

---

[1] BION is a registered trademark of the Advanced Bionics Corporation, a Boston Scientific company.

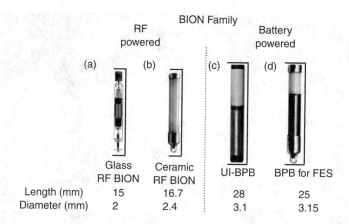

FIGURE 34.1   (See color insert following page 32-14.) Evolution of the BION devices show 4 Bions to same scale.

34.2   Evolution of the Implantable BION Devices

In 1988, G. Loeb proposed and W.J. Heetderks mathematically showed that the concept of a wireless network of injectable microstimulators powered by an external antenna/coil, was possible [7]. It was thought that these microstimulators would eliminate many of the problems associated with the use of percutaneous electrodes, since they do not incorporate leads. J.H. Schulman, G.E. Loeb, and P.R. Troyk, under support contracts from the U.S. NIH (contract N01-NS-9-2327), the Alfred Mann Foundation (AMF, Santa Clarita, CA), and the Canadian Network for Neural Regeneration and Functional Recovery, developed an injectable, glass-enclosed microstimulator (Figure 34.1a) that is powered and controlled by an external alternating magnetic field generated by a coil connected to a control unit. This first 255-channel stimulating system, later called the radio frequency (RF) BION device, allowed instantaneous control of stimulation pulse amplitude, frequency, pulse width, pulse position timing, and pulse charge-recovery current [8].

The AMF continued to develop and improve the wireless RF BION device. As a result of these efforts, a second-generation RF BION device, which incorporates a ceramic case, an output capacitor, and zener diodes to protect the device against electrostatic discharges was developed (Figure 34.1b) [9]. These RF BION devices are currently being used or have been used in several clinical studies being conducted by the AMF and its affiliated organizations, the Alfred Mann Institute (University of Southern California, Los Angeles, CA) and Advanced Bionics Corporation (Santa Clarita, CA). As of September, 2004, 33 patients have been implanted with RF BION devices for treatment of urinary incontinence, obstructive sleep apnea, pain associated with shoulder subluxation, knee osteoarthritis, forearm contracture, and foot drop applications [10–13].

While the wireless RF BION device eliminates the need for the leads associated with the percutaneous electrodes, it requires the patient to wear an external coil during use, to transmit power and data to the implanted device. Both to improve patient acceptance of this technology, and to increase the reliability of the system, it was necessary to eliminate the need to constantly use an external coil to power and control the device. Thus, the idea for a battery-powered BION device (hereinafter BPB) was conceived at the AMF.

The AMF, with guidance from Jet Propulsion Lab (JPL), developed a small cylindrical lithium ion rechargeable battery. A new company (Quallion, Inc.) was formed and financed by Alfred Mann to manufacture and improve these unique highly reliable batteries. Today, these batteries can be safely recharged if discharged to zero volts and are expected to operate for over 10 years. These batteries were designed specifically for the BPB (Figure 34.2).

The AMF licensed the BPB technology to Advanced Bionics Corp., which designed and implemented the first BPB (stimulator only) for urinary incontinence (referred to as the UI-BPB). This was the first BION to have a two-way telemetry (Figure 34.1c). The telemetry receiver in this UI-BPB turns on for a

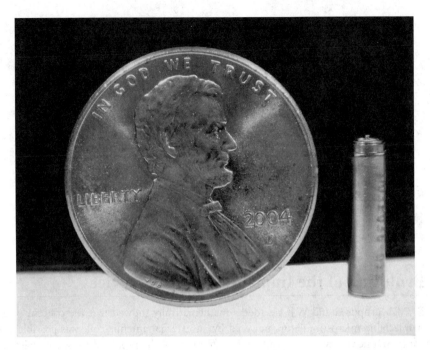

FIGURE 34.2   (See color insert following page **32**-14.) Quallion battery for the BPB.

very short time interval every 1.5 sec, to conserve battery power. Thus, rapid synchronization for limb control is not feasible with the UI-BPB. As of January 2006, over 100 patients have been implanted with the UI-BPB for the treatment of urinary incontinence, urinary frequency and migraine headaches [14]. Due to its lack of sensing capabilities, and slow communication response time, the UI-BPB is not well suited for FES applications.

The AMF is currently developing the next generation of the BPB. This BPB (Figure 34.1d) allows the creation of a wireless FES network including: both stimulation and sensing in each BPB for fully implantable closed-loop applications; data processing for sensed signals; high-speed bidirectional telemetry; wireless oscilloscope monitoring for fitting purposes, via back telemetry of voltage-sensed signals; a rechargeable battery (enabling prolonged operation without external power); and capability of communications with over 850 BPBs simultaneously (effectively 100 communications/sec/BPB) [15].

The ceramic BION devices (Figure 34.1b through Figure 34.1d) use an extremely strong Zirconia with 3% Ytrium ceramic case. The FDA pointed out that long-term immersion in water significantly weakens this ceramic [16]. Over a three-year period, the AMF came up with a process to improve the longevity of this ceramic. Today, accelerated life testing has shown that this ceramic will retain 80% of its strength after 40 years of soaking in saline solution [17–19].

34.3   Battery-Powered BION System for FES and Sensing

The FES–BPB System is a wireless, multichannel network of separately implantable battery-powered BION devices that can be used for both stimulation and sensing. The System is comprised of a master control unit (MCU), a Clinician's Programmer, a recharging subsystem (charger and coil), and BPBs. Additional equipment, dissolvable suture material, and surgical insertion tools (used only during the implantation procedure) are also part of the System. The FES–BPB System can be set up for use in two configurations: fitting mode and stand-alone mode. A block diagram of the FES–BPB System is shown in Figure 34.3.

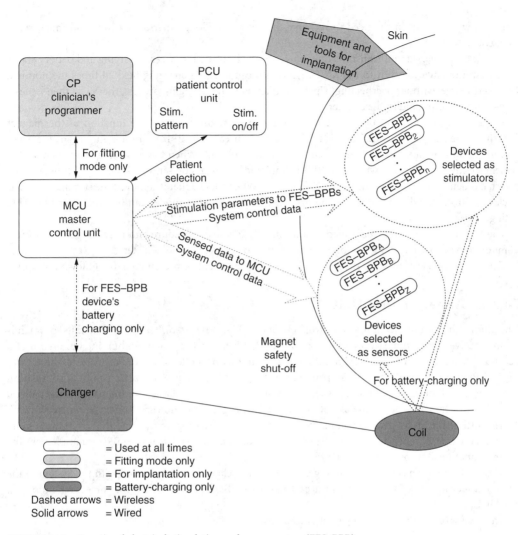

FIGURE 34.3 Functional electrical stimulation and sensor system (FES–BPB).

The MCU is the communication and control hub for the FES–BPB System. The MCU transmits commands to and receives data from all the BPBs and the recharging subsystem. There are two versions contemplated for the MCU packaging (1) an external MCU, which will be outside the body and have a few controls accessible to the patient; and (2) an implantable MCU, which will be implanted in a convenient location in the body. The implantable MCU version will have a small patient control unit (PCU).

The Clinician's Programmer consists of software loaded on a computer that allows the clinician to configure and test the FES–BPB System for each patient.

The recharging subsystem (charger and coil) is used when the rechargeable battery of the BPB needs to be recharged. The charging process requires the placement of the coil close to the area on the patient's body where the BPB is implanted. Recharging is mandatory when the battery of the BPB is low. Depending on the frequency of use and stimulation levels delivered by the BPB, the battery could potentially run down in 1–8 days. Under normal stimulation conditions (nerve stimulation of 1- to 2-mA pulse amplitude, 15- to 100-μsec pulse width, and 20 pulses/sec), charging for about 5–20 min/day is required to charge the battery. The BPB's maximum stimulation capability (20-mA pulse amplitude at 14 V compliance with 200-μsec pulse width and 125 pulses/sec) can rapidly discharge the battery in a very short time and would result in the need to recharge the battery for longer periods of time and much more frequently.

The external charger coil transmits only power to the implanted devices. Charging and battery status are transmitted by each BPB to the MCU. Each BPB can accept a charging field 20 times the nominal field to recharge, without overheating. Upon completion of the charging process, the MCU then issues a stop-charging command to the charger.

The BPB has a sensor to detect the field from a permanent magnet. The function of the magnet is to hold the stimulation off. This is a safety feature in case the BPB is stimulating in an undesired manner and the patient does not have access to his control unit. When the magnet is positioned on the patient's body over the area where the BPB is implanted, a magnetic sensor inside the BPB detects the external magnetic field and holds the stimulation off. When the magnet is removed the stimulation turns back on. This is the default mode of the magnetic detector. Other modes can be programmed during fitting.

The BPB implantation is performed in a minimally invasive procedure and is accomplished using a combination of specially designed insertion tools and commercially available items.

The functional description of the FES–BPB System components is presented in the following sections.

34.3.1 Master Control Unit

The MCU is the communication and control hub for the FES–BPB System. The MCU transmits commands to and receives data from each one up to a total of 850 BPBs in the system within one hundredth of a second. When the patient uses the FES–BPB System (stand-alone mode), the MCU coordinates the activity of the BPBs by receiving data from implanted devices programmed as sensors, transmitting stimulation commands, and monitoring overall System status. It also serves as the basic user interface for the patient, providing System ON/OFF control and alarms, as well as program selection and limited parameter control. During fitting, the MCU acts as a conduit between the Clinician's Programmer and the rest of the System, enabling the transparent setup of each BPB and the coordination needed among BPBs to implement the desired functional movement.

The MCU also manages the recharging subsystem. The charger communicates with the System in the same manner as that of the BPBs, and it can be turned ON/OFF or checked for correct operation via the MCU.

The MCU contains the following safety mechanisms:

- An emergency STOP button on the external MCU, which when depressed, immediately issues a "stop stimulation" command to all BPBs.
- During recharging, if any BPB overheats or overcharges and cannot protect itself, it would communicate this information to the MCU, which would issue a "stop charging" command to the charger and alert the patient. If an external MCU is being used, it would produce a sound to alert the patient. In the case where an implantable MCU is being used, the MCU would send a command to the BPBs to produce a specific stimulation pattern to alert the patient and would also communicate with the external PCU, if it is within communication range. The PCU would then generate an audible alert.

The MCU also stores patient usage data for the clinician. This data can be used to verify compliance and to analyze the stimulation and sensing parameters of each session. The approximate location of each BPB in the body is also maintained in this database.

34.3.2 Software and Firmware

The software for the FES–BPB System is divided into two components. One component is the Clinician's Programmer application, which runs on a laptop computer. The other component is the firmware running on the MCU. The PC with the Clinician's Programmer interfaces with the MCU via a serial

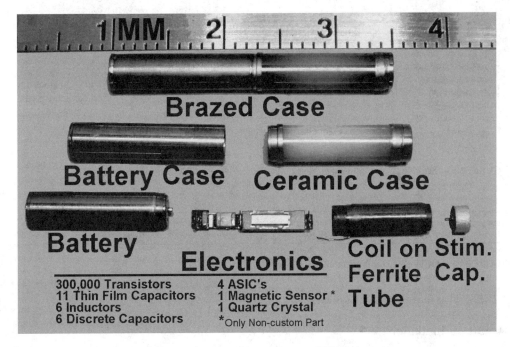

FIGURE 34.4 (See color insert following page **32**-14.) Battery-powered BION internal components.

communication link. During the fitting of the System to a particular patient, the two components work in concert to facilitate measurement and storage of the stimulation and sensor calibration parameters. Once these parameters have been gathered in a fitting session, the essential information can be stored in the MCU, so that the MCU can operate in stand-alone mode to facilitate the desired functional movement. Ultimately, the MCU will modulate the stimulation output in response to information it receives from the BPBs programmed as sensors.

The Clinician's Programmer uses a graphical interface, which contains screens to perform the following essential functions:

- Gather basic personal information for the patient, including information about the location in the body of his/her BPBs.
- Establish the stimulation range for each implanted BPB and allow selection of the stimulation parameters.
- Specify the details of the activity sequences that will be involved in the FES algorithm.
- Gather the trigger information that will be used to generate transitions between activity sequences in response to the sensor inputs.
- Compose the Finite State Machine functions that will drive a routine and download the complete program to the MCU for either immediate execution or later use.

34.3.3 Battery-Powered BION Device (BPB)

The BPB is a battery-powered microdevice that is capable of both delivering electrical stimulation and acting as a general-purpose sensor for recording biopotential signals, pressure, distance or angle between two BPBs, and temperature. The following sections describe the functional building blocks of the BPB, battery, and packaging. The specifications of the BPB are provided in Table 34.1. Figure 34.4 shows the internal components of the BPB and Figure 34.5 shows a cross section of an assembled BPB.

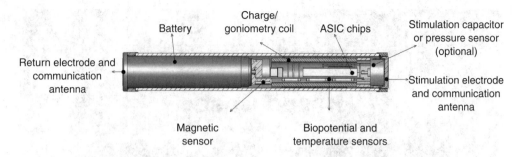

FIGURE 34.5   (See color insert following page **32**-14.) Battery-powered BION device cross section.

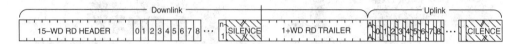

FIGURE 34.6   MCU–BPB communication protocol.

The BPB has the following subsystems:

34.3.3.1 Stimulation

The BPB is a single-channel, constant-current, charge-balanced stimulator. The stimulation output is capacitance-coupled, which also prevents direct connection between the battery or battery-generated DC voltages and the tissue. Stimulation pulse amplitude, width, and frequency can be independently adjusted. In addition, triggering events can cause the stimulation to be delivered continuously or in a pulse burst, which can be ramped up and down with a variety of Start/Stop times.

34.3.3.2 Communication

The bidirectional propagated wave RF communication between the MCU and the BPBs is established through a dipole antenna (Figure 34.5). This link operates at a frequency in the band 100 to 500 MHz, using quad phase modulation with a 5-MHz bandwidth. The BPB communication module includes a crystal-controlled transmitter, receiver, and digital processing unit that synchronizes with and processes the MCU transmissions. The digital processing unit in the BPB also corrects small numbers of errors in the received data, decodes the MCU commands, and generates the responses to the MCU including the reporting of higher numbers of communication errors that cannot be mathematically corrected. In this latter situation, the MCU would resend the message.

The communication protocol between the MCU and BPBs is shown in Figure 34.6. The timing of the frame is completely controlled by the MCU and every BPB will synchronize to its MCU's clock.

The header and trailer fields are used for frame synchronization and for carrying frame control data intended for all BPBs and for other MCUs. When an MCU detects another MCU, the one with the higher ID number shifts the time slots of all the BPBs it is controlling, to avoid communication interference. Once the MCU assigns the time slots for the downlink and uplink data packets to each one of the BPBs in the net, each BPB turns on its receiving or transmitting circuitry for only a few microseconds at the assigned times in each frame in order to save battery. The downlink data packets contain stimulation or sensing control data or both and forward error correction (FEC) bits to correct up to four or five bit errors. Bit errors beyond that number are reported to the MCU, which will then resend the message. If some messages are vital, the message would be sent twice or the value would be sent back to the MCU for the MCU to verify and authorize the command. Uplink data packets are transmitted by each of the BPBs and are used to carry information to the MCU (e.g., sensed data). The FEC in the uplink data packet only corrects one or two bit errors.

34.3.3.3   Power (Battery and Charging)

The main power source for the BPB is a 10-mW-Hr rechargeable lithium-ion battery that allows the implanted device to operate as a stand-alone stimulator/sensor. Its special nonflammable lithium ion chemistry provides long life and permits the voltage to go to zero and be recovered safely without damage to the battery. The recharge process is achieved via a low-frequency (127 kHz) magnetic link with an external coil worn or placed nearby when charging. Assuming continuous stimulation pulses at 20 pps with 100-μsec pulse width and 2-mA pulse amplitude into a 2-kΩ load, the battery of a BPB selected as a stimulator will provide 100 h of continuous operation. For a BPB selected as sensor, the battery will also provide 100 h of continuous operation.

The lithium ion battery is specified to have a cycle life of 2000 cycles for a standard charge/discharge cycle, which is a fairly deep discharge of the battery before recharge occurs. The nominal stimulation/sensing requirements in many applications are such that the battery would not be discharged to the standard low level (if recharged daily). Thus, the 2000 cycles represent a lifetime of over 10 years if the battery is recharged daily.

34.3.3.4   Safety

The BPB includes the following safety features:

- A miniature magnetic sensor that detects the magnetic field from an external magnet and holds off the stimulation if, for some reason, it needs to be turned off.
- A temperature sensor that communicates with the charger, via the MCU, to terminate charging, if appropriate and disconnects the battery when the temperature rises above a predetermined threshold.
- Battery safety circuitry that protects the battery from overvoltage, overdischarging, and overcharging.
- BPBs can protect themselves from magnetic fields in excess of 20 times the field necessary for maximum charging and, for a short time, for fields in excess of 50 times the field for maximum charging. This short time is more than sufficient for the BPB to send a message to the MCU to turn off the charger and to alert the patient of risk.

34.3.3.5   Biopotential Sensing, Data Display, and Data Analysis

The biopotential function is implemented to record neural or muscular electrical signals (EMG signals). Biopotential sensing is accomplished using a low-noise amplifier and band-pass filter circuit, followed by a digital postprocessing circuit. The amplifier is adjustable from a gain of 10 to a gain of 1000. The low-frequency setting of the band-pass filter is adjustable from below 1 to 300 Hz. The high-frequency setting is adjustable from 300 Hz to 10 kHz. Input referred noise is less than 5 μV rms (20 μV peak).

34.3.3.5.1   *Data Display: Oscilloscope Mode*

During fitting, the analog signal from the amplifier/filter section can be digitized and transmitted from the BPB to the MCU to the Clinician's Programmer screen at the rate of 40,000 samples per second. This "oscilloscope mode" (Figure 34.7) can be used when evaluating the placement of the BPB and during fitting, but it is not suitable for long-term use due to its high power demands.

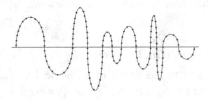

FIGURE 34.7   Biopotential sensing module, oscilloscope display mode.

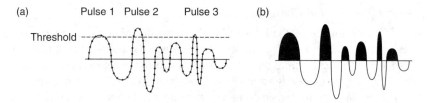

FIGURE 34.8 Data analysis with the BPB biopotential sensing module. (a) Counting pulses above threshold line. (b) Rectify and integrate neural signal.

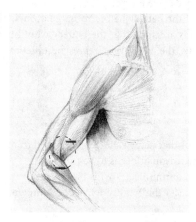

FIGURE 34.9 Use of BPBs for distance/angle measurements.

34.3.3.5.2 Data Analysis

The analog output of the biopotential sensor also passes to a programmable window detection circuitry that can be set by the clinician (1) count pulses that fall within (or above or below) the set thresholds (Figure 34.8a); or, (2) rectify and integrate the sensed signal (Figure 34.8b). (1) Counting pulses: The neuronal pulses that occur are accumulated every 10 msec and relayed to the MCU. (2) Rectify and integrate: Every 10 msec, if required, the circuit can rectify the amplitude of the biopotential sensor's analog output and sum up the average rectified signal. An output between 0 and 255 will be generated indicating the average energy occurring every 10 msec.

34.3.3.6 Pressure Sensing

Some BPBs will be fabricated with a pressure transducer mounted at one end. The initial version of this sensor is about 3 mm in diameter and is sensitive to pressures along the axial dimension of the BPB. Future versions will be sensitive to lateral pressure, and may be mounted remotely from the BPB. The present full-scale absolute pressure range is 400 to 900 mmHg. This signal can be read out either AC or DC coupled. When DC-coupled, it reads the absolute pressure. Since ambient pressure varies with altitude changes, this offset can be accounted for by placing a reference sensor of the same type in the MCU, then subtracting off this baseline.

34.3.3.7 Angle/Position Sensing (Goniometry)

The same internal coil that is used to receive the magnetic field to charge the BPB battery may also be programmed as a transmitter in any selected BPB or as a receiver in another selected BPB. The goniometry function is implemented using one BPB as a transmitter and the other BPB as a receiver. The BPB programmed as a receiver detects and measures the signal strength of the received signal (Figure 34.9).

The distance between two BPBs is derived from the intensity of the received magnetic field, which falls off approximately with the cube of the distance between the devices.

There are eight different programmable transmitter–receiver frequencies available for goniometry use. The eight frequencies are clustered around 127 kHz. This permits eight parallel goniometry systems consisting of one transmitter and any number of receivers. There is no limit on the number of BPB receivers that can process the signal strength to give distance measurements (from each of the transmitters). Each BPB receiver is able to send back a measurement 100 times/sec. A goniometry pair (transmitter–receiver) can be used to measure distances between 1 and 20 cm.

34.3.3.8 Temperature Sensing

An internal temperature sensor is incorporated as an additional safety mechanism to guard against overheating of the BPB and to provide temperature data to patients, such as certain quadriplegics, who do not sense temperature. The sensor is accurate to within one-third degree celsius and is operable over the range from 16 to 50°C. In the event a significant temperature rise is detected, the BPB can be shut down or communication with the MCU can be made to initiate appropriate external action (such as shutting down the charging field, if present). Readings are taken once per second and can be read by the MCU.

34.3.4 Recharging Subsystem (Charger and External Coil)

The charger produces a 127-kHz signal that generates a magnetic field in the charging coil. The MCU communicates with the charger to indicate when to turn on a charging field. The MCU interrogates each BPB to determine which BPB is going to be charged and when the BPB is fully charged. The MCU determines which BPBs are not being charged and indicates to the patient where the coil has to be moved to charge those BPBs. If the charger is coupled to several coils but can only power one coil at a time, the MCU can then cause the charger to switch coils so uncharged BPBs can be charged. The MCU can also determine the state of the charge in each BPB and can initially select the most discharged devices to be charged first.

The recharging subsystem includes a temperature sensor that stops the recharging process if the external coil temperature adjacent to the patient skin rises over 41°C.

34.3.5 Magnet

The patient can stop stimulation by placing an external magnet near the location of the implanted device(s). A Neodymium magnet is being used because it is small, lightweight and because it produces a very strong magnetic signal. The default mode of this magnet is to hold the stimulation off when the magnet is positioned on the patient's body, over the area where the BPB is implanted. When the magnet is removed, the stimulation turns back on. Other magnet control modes are available.

34.3.6 FES–BPB System Specifications

TABLE 34.1   Battery-Powered BION Device Specifications

1. Physical	
Implant weight	0.6 g
Implant length with eyelet[++] and diameter	25 mm_{max} length/3.15 mm_{max} diameter
Electrodes area	5.2 mm^2 (0.008 in.^{2}) stimulation electrode
	12.8 mm^2 (0.019 in.^{2}) return electrode
Case materials	Yttria stabilized Zirconia; Titanium 6Al4V alloy
Electrodes material	Iridium

Continued

TABLE 34.1   *Continued*

2. Stimulation parameters	
Pulse amplitude	5 μA–20 mA in 3.3% exponential steps (255 levels)
Pulse width	7.6–1953 μsec in 7.6 or 15.2 μsec steps
Pulse frequency	1–4096 pps
Stimulation control response time	10.6 msec maximum
Capacitor recharge current	10–500 μA
Compliance voltage	Up to 14 V automatically adjusted
Stimulation output capacitor	4 μF
Delay to start from a trigger	0–42.4 h in 15.6 μsec, 125 msec, 2 sec, 1 min, 10 min steps
Burst on/off time	Min Max Step
Range 1	0.031 sec 0.9996 sec 0.0156 sec
Range 2	0.25 sec 8.00 sec 0.125 sec
3. Sensors	
Temperature	16–50°C with 0.3% accuracy
Magnetic field to trigger shut off	10.0 Gauss threshold
Goniometry (number of frequency channels)	8
Range	1–20 cm
Repeatable accuracy error	Less than 1% for 1–10 cm
Pressure (range)	Readout = AC coupled. 300–900 mmHg absolute
Accuracy	±10 mmHg
Biopotential sensing (amplification)	10, 30, 100, 300, 1000
Low frequency roll-off	1, 10, 30, 100, 300 Hz
High frequency roll-off	300, 1 K, 3 K, 10 kHz
Notch filter	50 or 60 Hz
Input referred noise	5 μV rms
4. Communication	
Number of implants per patient	Up to 850 at 10 msec
ID, MCU/BPB	27/30 bits
Band width	5 MHz
Sense-to-stimulate delay	10.6 msec maximum
Frequency band	100–500 MHz
MCU to BPB data rate 15 bits/6 μsec	(15 bits data + 16 bits FEC[a])/6 μsec
BPB to MCU data rate 8 bits/5 μsec	(8 bits data + 8 bits FEC[a])/5 μsec
Data streaming (oscilloscope mode)	39.8 K samples/sec X 3 channels (8 bit resolution)
5. Charging	
Frequency of charging field	127 kHz
Excessive magnetic field permissible	20 times nominal
6. Battery: Lithium ion rechargeable, hermetically sealed	
Battery length and diameter	13 mm length, 2.5 mm diameter
Battery weight	0.21 g
Battery capacity	3.0 mA h, 10 mW h
Cell voltage range	3.0–4.0 V (3.6 V nom.)
Battery life	Nominally 10 year (usage dependent)

[a] FEC, forward error correction.

34.3.7   Minimally Invasive Procedure to Implant BPBs

To implant a BPB, a minimally invasive procedure is followed. The implantation procedure can be done in a clean Procedure Room, where the patient's implant sites can be surgically cleansed and draped with sterile towels and covered with adherent sterile plastic drapes. The implant physician scrubs his/her forearms and hands, is gowned and gloved, and wears a cap and mask.

The implantation (insertion) tools are shown in Figure 34.10. Under local anesthesia, a 5-mm skin incision is made. A sterile probe electrode (0.71 mm OD; insulated except at the tips, Figure 34.10)

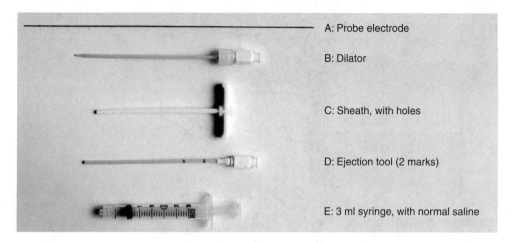

A: Probe electrode

B: Dilator

C: Sheath, with holes

D: Ejection tool (2 marks)

E: 3 ml syringe, with normal saline

FIGURE 34.10   (See color insert following page **32**-14.) BPB implantation tools.

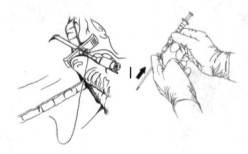

FIGURE 34.11   BPB implantation technique.

connected to an external stimulator is directed into the tissues to excite and find the target nerve/motor-point. With adjustments to the probe electrode, the optimal target muscle contraction is located. A customized introducer (dilator plus sheath) is then slid over the probe electrode. Stimulation with the probe electrode is repeated to ensure a similar optimal response and correct location. The probe electrode and dilator are then withdrawn, leaving the sheath in position.

The BPB has a dissolvable suture attached to the return electrode. The BPBs stimulation electrode end is inserted into the sheath and gently pushed by the ejection tool to the sheath tip, so that only the BPB stimulation electrode end protrudes. From the ejection tool tip, saline is infused into the sheath to allow the anodal end of the BPB to have electrical connection to the tissues through small holes in the distal sheath. The BPB is activated to test and confirm its optimal position relative to the target nerve/motor-point. By withdrawing the sheath over the ejection tool, the BPB is deposited into the tissues (Figure 34.11). The sheath and the ejection tool are then removed.

The BPB is retested to confirm that the optimal response is achieved. If this position is not satisfactory in regard to the responses to stimulation or recording, then the BPB can be retrieved by pulling on the suture attached to the BPB (Figure 34.12) and then reinserted. The emerging sutures are cut at the subcutaneous tissue level, and the wound is then closed.

The implanted BPB is tested one week after implantation to confirm that the responses are still adequate. If an inadequate response is observed, the wound could be reopened and the BPB retrieved by pulling on the sutures. A new BPB could then be reinserted to obtain proper response.

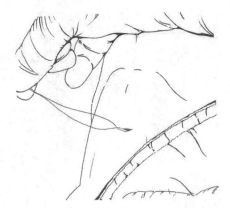

FIGURE 34.12 Retrieval of BPB.

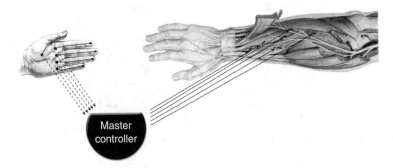

FIGURE 34.13 (See color insert following page 32-14.) BPBs measuring pressure in fingers.

34.4 Applications

The different functions of the BPB (as a stimulator, biopotential signal sensor, goniometry sensor, and pressure or temperature sensor) and the availability of multiple BPBs in one patient (up to 850 BPBs) gives the clinician many opportunities to restore neurological function, especially in poststroke syndrome, spinal cord injury, cerebral palsy, multiple sclerosis, traumatic brain injury, and for limb sensing in amputees to control fitted prostheses.

Take, for example, the case where a paralyzed upper extremity is implanted with multiple BPBs placed near motor-points or nerves of muscles in the arm, fore-arm, and hand. It will be possible to trigger sequential functional muscle actions to extend the arm and fore-arm, and open the hand to grasp an object. The limits of each functional action can be controlled from implanted BPBs working as goniometry sensors, measuring the angles of the elbow (see Figure 34.9) and wrist and implanted BPBs working as pressure sensors, measuring the pressure at the finger tip (Figure 34.13).

The reverse of this extension can be similarly achieved using this stimulating and sensing system to bring the grasped object, for example, to the mouth. Similar closed-loop controls of stimulation could be used in the lower extremities for standing and ambulation. For partially paralyzed extremities, sensing of the muscle activities using BPBs would act as triggers to other BPBs to stimulate the motor-points of these muscles, thus augmenting the total action. Goniometry sensors would add the closed-loop controls to reduce or stop the actions. This approach could be used to augment swallowing, bladder control, and respiration.

Where pressure points need to be monitored, for example, at the heel (as a trigger for improving walking on stroke patients) or buttock (to avoid pressure sores) or hand (to detect the grasping of an object), BPB

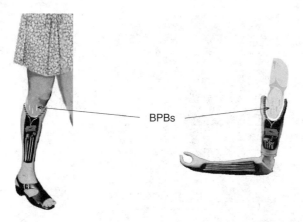

FIGURE 34.14   (See color insert following page **32**-14.) Use of BPBs in amputee patients.

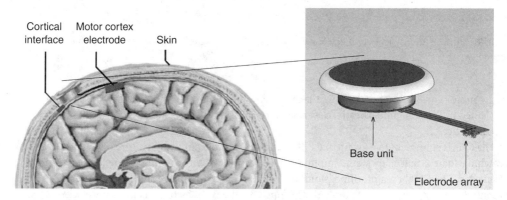

FIGURE 34.15   (See color insert following page **32**-14.) Cortical interface device.

devices placed in these sites can measure the pressure and either trigger motor-point functional stimulation to activate muscles or stop a functional stimulation sequence.

34.4.1 FES–BPB System in Amputee Patients: Controlling Artificial Limbs

For Amputee Patients (Figure 34.14) BPBs, working as biopotential sensors, would be inserted in the "stump to pick up motor nerve signals, which can be used to control movement of the artificial limb flexible components".

34.4.2 Cortical Interface Device: A Cortical Stimulator and Sensor Using the BPB System Technology

Individuals with spinal cord injury or disease that limits control over voluntary motion or sensing may be able to regain some of the ability of voluntary motion by monitoring the motor cortex and feeding back sensed response signals to the sensory cortex. Voluntary motion is expressed as neural activity in the motor cortex. The sensory cortex depends on muscle spindles and other sensors to help control the limb movement. By feeding back signals to the sensory cortex, the psychological use of the limb would be given back to the patient. The motor cortex signals can also be used to control wheel chairs and other assistive devices.

The miniaturized components developed for the BPB are used to create a cortical interface device (CID) with multiple stimulation and sensing electrodes within a single implantable package (Figure 34.15). The CID has the capability of monitoring up to several hundred electrodes that can be implanted or positioned

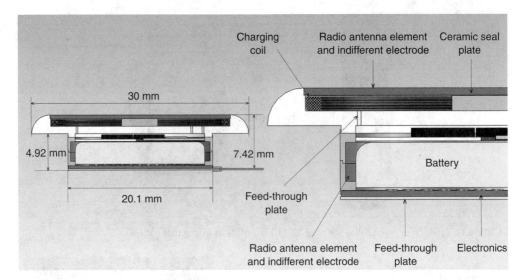

FIGURE 34.16 (See color insert following page **32**-14.) Cortical interface device (left) dimensions, (right) cross section.

in the motor cortex, sensory cortex, or a combination of both. The CID system consists of a base unit implanted in the skull, underneath the scalp and one or several electrode arrays placed on the sensory or motor cortices.

The CID is equivalent to a group of 64 BPBs in its communication ability. It also includes an additional switching matrix that allows any amplifier to sense voltages either unipolar or bipolar from any two electrodes. The CID base unit dimensions and internal components are shown in Figure 34.16. The CID is constructed with the same technology developed for the BPB. It contains the same electronics as those used in the BPB as far as the communication, charging, power management, biopotential sensing, and stimulation modules are concerned. A CID base unit contains 64 biopotential sensing modules attached to one or more electrode arrays. The battery used in the CID provides 50-mA-h at 3.6 V.

The electrode arrays could be configured for sensing or stimulating purposes. The sensing electrode array includes signal processing capabilities by using the same electronics as those in the biopotential sensing module in the BPB. The stimulating electrode array contains the same stimulation electronics as those in the BPB stimulation module. The CID contains a powerful microprocessor to analyze the signals from the motor cortex and to reduce the data to 64 eight-bit messages that the MCU can use to control up to 64 muscles.

References

[1] Heart Disease and Stroke Statistics — 2004 Update, American Heart Association.
[2] http://www.bionicear.com/support/clinical_papers/supp_research_demo2.html,
    http://www.bionicear.com/support/clinical_papers/supp_research_demo1.html,
    http://www.bionicear.com/printables/Bilateral.pdf;
    http://www.nidcd.nih.gov/health/hearing/coch_moreon.asp,
    http://www.cochlear.com/896.asp
[3] Heart Disease and Stroke Statistics — 2006 Update. A Report from the American Heart Association Statistics Committee and Stroke Statistics Subcommittee, January 11, 2006. http://circ.ahajournals.org
[4] Facts and Figures at a Glance. May 2001. National Spinal Cord Injury Statistical Center. Spinal Cord Injury: Hope Through Research. http://www.ninds.nih.gov/health_and_medical/pubs/sci.htm

[5] Complications of Diabetes in the United States. National Diabetes Statistics. http://www.diabetes.niddk.nih.gov/dm/pubs/statistics/

[6] Amputee Statistics (SAMPLE) from National Database. http://rehabtech.eng.monash.edu/techguide/als/Stats.htm

[7] Heetderks, W.J. RF powering of millimeter- and submillimeter-sized neural prosthetic implants. *IEEE Trans. Biomed. Eng.* 35, 323–327 (1988).

[8] Loeb, G.E., Zamin, C.J., Schulman, J.H., and Troyk, P.R. Injectable microstimulator for functional electrical stimulation. *Med. Biol. Eng. Comput.* 29, NS13–NS19 (1991).

[9] Arcos, I., Davis, R., Fey, K., Mishler, D., Sanderson, D., Tanacs, C., Vogel, M.J., Wolf, R., Zilberman, Y., and Schulman, J. Second-generation microstimulator. *Artif. Organs* 26, 228–231 (2002).

[10] Dupont, A.C., Bagg, S.D., Baker, L., Chun, S., Creasy, J.L., Romano, C., Romano, D., Waters, R.L., Wederich, C.L., Richmond, F.J.R., and Loeb, G.E. Therapeutic electrical stimulation with BIONS: clinical trial report. *Proceedings of the IEEE-EMBS Conference* (Houston, TX, 2002).

[11] Richmond, F.J.R., Dupont, A.C., Bagg, S.D., Chun, S., Creasy, J.L., Romano, C., Romano, D., Waters, R.L., Wederich, C.L., and Loeb, G.E. Therapeutic electrical stimulation with BIONs to rehabilitate shoulder and knee dysfunction. *Proceedings of the IFESS Conference* (Ljubljana, Slovenia, 2002).

[12] Buller, J.L., Cundiff, G.W., Noel, K.A., VanRooyen, J.A., Leffler, K.S., Ellerkman, R.M., Bent, A.E. RF BION™: An Injectable Microstimulator for the Treatment of Overactive Bladder Disorders in Adult Females. European Association of Urology (February 2002).

[13] Misawa, A., Shimada, Y., Matsunaga, T., Aizawa, T., Hatakeyama, K., Chida, S., Sato, M., Davis, R., Zilberman, Y., Cosendai, G., and Ripley, A.M. The use of the RF BION device to treat pain due to shoulder subluxation in chronic hemiplegic stroke patient — a case report. *Proceedings of the IFESS Conference* (United Kingdom, 2004).

[14] E-mail communication, Advanced Bionics Corporation, a Boston Scientific Company.

[15] J.H. Schulman, Mobley, J.P., Wolfe, J., Regev, E., Perron, C.Y., Ananth, R., Matei, E., Glukhovsky, A., and Davis, R. Battery Powered BION FES network. *Proceedings of the IEEE-EMBS Conference* (San Francisco, CA, 2004).

[16] Personal Communication, Joe Schulman.

[17] Jiang, G., Fay, K., and Schulman, J. *In-Vitro* and *In-Vivo* Aging Tests of BION® Micro-Stimulator. Biomedical Engineering Department, University of Southern California, Los Angeles, CA. Proceedings of the 7th Annual Fred S. Grodins Graduate Research Symposium, March 2003.

[18] Jiang, G., Purnell, K., and Schulman, J. Accelerated life tests and *in-vivo* tests of 3Y-TZP ceramics. Materials and Processes for Medical Devices Conference, *Proceedings* 2003.

[19] Jiang, G., Mishler, D., Davis, R., Mobley, P., and Schulman, J. Ceramic to Metal Seal for Implantable Medical Device. Biomedical Engineering Department, USC, Los Angeles, CA. *Proceedings of the 8th Annual F. Grodins Graduate Research Symposium*, pp. 92–92, March 2004.

35

Visual Prostheses

Robert J. Greenberg
Second Sight

The possibility of restoring vision to blind patients using electricity began with the discovery that an electric charge delivered to a blind eye produces a sensation of light. This discovery was made by LeRoy in 1755 [1]. However, it was not until 1966 that the first human experiments in this field began with Giles Brindley's experiments with electrical stimulation of the visual cortex [2]. He used 180 cortical surface electrodes on patients, who were then able to perceive spots of light called "phosphenes," but they were ill defined and could not be combined to make an image. This did fail to produce useful vision in these patients. Similar experiments by William Dobelle in 1974 produced essentially the same results [3,4].

Since these early experiments, efforts have been underway to produce penetrating arrays of electrodes that offer the possibility of more closely spaced electrodes and therefore higher resolution cortical devices [5–8]. Richard Normann (University of Utah) has micromachined 100 electrodes out of silicon, which was primarily used for recording in the sensory cortex of animals [5]. Another group at the University of Michigan led by Ken Wise has also produced micromachined penetrating electrodes for recording [6]. In the 1990s an effort at the NIH headed by Terry Hambrecht made an array of 38 penetrating microelectrodes, which were implanted in a patient and yielded separable phosphenes at electrode placements closer than had been produced with surface electrodes [7,8]. Electronics for an implantable cortical prosthesis are being developed (with 1024 channels) at the Illinois Institute of Technology by Philip Troyk (personal communication).

While the cortical stimulation approaches have made progress, it has been hampered by the physiology. The processing that has occurred by the time the neural signals have reached the cortex is greater than at the more distal sites such as the retina. This results in more complex phosphenes being perceived by the patient. The surgery and the implanted prosthesis do provide risks such as intracranial hemorrhage to a blind patient who has an otherwise normal brain. These factors and the lack of availability of implantable electronics have limited the clinical application of these devices.

The limitations of the cortical approach encouraged several groups in United States over the past 10 years to explore the possibility of producing vision in patients with an intact optic nerve with damaged photoreceptors by stimulating the retina [9–15]. Likely candidate diseases are retinitis pigmentosa (RP) or age-related macular degeneration (AMD). It is difficult to determine exactly how many patients are blinded by these diseases since patients often stop seeing their ophthalmologist after being told there is nothing that can be done. However, estimates of legal blindness in the West (developed world) run as high as 300,000 people with RP and 3,000,000 people with AMD. 1.2 million people are afflicted (but not yet blind) with retinitis pigmentosa worldwide and 10 million people are afflicted with AMD in the United States alone [16].

There have emerged two major approaches to retinal stimulation — epiretinal and subretinal. In the epiretinal approach, electrodes are placed on top of the retina to produce phosphenes. In the subretinal approach, photodiodes are implanted underneath the retina and used to generate currents, which stimulate the retina. The epiretinal approach has been pursued by a team at the Johns Hopkins University led by Eugene de Juan and Mark Humayun [9,15] and another at Harvard/MIT Centers led by Joseph Rizzo and John Wyatt [10]. Recently Rizzo and Wyatt have decided to pursue the subretinal approach. Second Sight, a privately held company in Sylmar, CA, is developing a permanently implantable epiretinal prosthesis. Six patients have been implanted with a first generation device containing 16 electrodes and a 60 electrode second generation device should be in patients soon. Patients with the first device have shown the ability to read large letters, locate objects and detect the direction of motion of objects and light. They have also shown the ability to discriminate multiple levels of gray. The second generation device is expected to work even better. The subretinal approach has been pursued by the Chow brothers in Chicago — one an ophthalmologist and the other an engineer — who have formed a company called Optobionics (Chicago, IL) [14]. They implanted ten patients in an initial feasibility study, which showed some temporary subjective improvements in vision that Optobionics believes was caused by a secondary neurotrophic effect and not direct stimulation by the implant. They have recently implanted 20 more patients at 3 centers with better vision than the first group in an attempt to demonstrate improvement in more than one center and to explore the effect in patients with better vision. Subretinal and epiretinal implants are also being pursued in Germany by large groups led by Eberhart Zrenner [11] and Rolf Eckmiller [12] respectively. Two companies have been formed in Germany by these individuals as well. There is also a group in Japan at Nagoya University led by Tohru Yagi. This group is focused primarily on cultured neuron preparations (personal communication).

Finally, there is a group at the Neural Rehabilitation Engineering Laboratory in Brussels, Belgium, led by Claude Veraart which has implanted a nerve cuff electrode with four electrodes around the optic nerve of a blind patient. That patient is able to identify in which quadrant she sees a phosphene [17]. Recently a second patient has been implanted with an eight-channel device. The new device was implanted inside the ocular orbit and has not performed as well as the first implant.

On February 19, 2000, the inaugural symposium of the Alfred Mann Institute-University of Southern California (AMI-USC) titled, "Can We Make the Blind See? — Prospects for Restoring Vision to the Blind" was held. The list of lecturers included Dean Baker Director of the AMI-USC; Gerald Loeb, a FES researcher at the AMI-USC; Dean Bok, a retinal physiologist from UCLA; Retinal prosthesis researchers — Robert Greenberg, Mark Humayun, Joseph Rizzo, John Wyatt, and Alan Chow; Cortical prosthesis researchers —Richard Normann and Philip Troyk; and Dana Ballard, a visual psychophysicist from the University of Rochester.

Dr. Baker provided the welcome and Dr. Loeb gave a brief history of neural prosthetics. Dr. Bok's talk highlighted biological approaches to inherited retinal degenerations, which result in photoreceptor loss. He chose to talk about two genes (rhodopsin and RDS) whose mutations cause a form of autosomal dominant inherited blindness — retinitis pigmentosa [18]. He discussed biological approaches to these diseases. Specifically, he described work by Matthew LaVail, William Hauswirth, and Al Lewin Laboratories where subretinal injections were performed in transgenic rats carrying one of the rhodopsin mutations (P23H). By injecting viral vectored ribozymes for the selective destruction of mutant mRNA produced by the P23H mutation, there was a dramatic arrest in the photoreceptor degeneration. Dr. Bok also spoke about his own work with Matthew LaVail and William Hauswirth laboratories where viral vectored secreted form of ciliary neurotrophic factor (CNTF) was injected subretinally (see Figure 35.1). When tested with transgenic rats containing an RDS mutation (peripherin P216L), the photoreceptor loss was again slowed.

After Dr. Greenberg gave a brief introduction to retinal prosthetics, Mark Humayun spoke about the epiretinal prosthesis efforts at the Johns Hopkins University [9,15]. He spoke about recent experiments of intraocular electrical stimulation in RP and AMD patients. Under local anesthesia, different stimulating

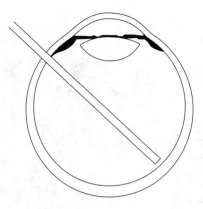

FIGURE 35.1   Experimental protocol for intraocular patient testing at the Johns Hopkins Medical Center.

electrodes were inserted through the eye-wall and positioned over the surface of the retina. Data from the ten most recently tested patients were reported. These awake patients reported simple forms in response to pattern electrical stimulation of the retina. A nonflickering perception was created with stimulating frequencies between 40 and 50 Hz. The stimulation threshold was also dependent on the targeted retinal area (higher in the extramacular region).

Next, Joseph Rizzo and John Wyatt spoke about the work at The Massachusetts Eye and Ear Infirmary and the Massachusetts Institute of Technology (MEEI-MIT) [10]. They reported tests on six humans tested intraocularly similar to the tests performed at the Johns Hopkins Medical Center. Using micro-fabricated electrode arrays placed in contact with the retina, five patients blind from retinitis pigmentosa and one volunteer with normal vision were tested. The normal volunteer was having their eye enucleated because of a cancer. Their most significant results included (1) safe contact of the retina with a microfabricated array (2) determination of strength-duration curves in two volunteers; and (3) creation of visual percepts with crude form. In the best cases, volunteers were able to distinguish two spots of light when two electrodes separated by roughly 2° of visual angle were driven. Thresholds reported exceed the accepted charge-density limits for chronic neural stimulation for the electrodes used. It was suggested that the quality of these results would improve with a chronically implantable prosthesis.

Alan Chow from Optobionics spoke about his Artificial Silicon Retina™ (ASR) [14]. ASRs are semiconductor-based silicon chip microphotodiode arrays (microscopic solar cells) designed to be surgically implanted into the subretinal space. The arrays are approximately 2 to 3 mm in diameter, 50 to 75 μm thick. Dr. Chow reported successful electrical stimulation of normal animal retinas.

Robert Greenberg spoke about "Second Sight" and its mission of producing a chronically implantable retinal prosthesis. "Second Sight" has chosen a retinal prosthesis approach over the cortical approach because of concerns of patient safety even though the cortical approach has the potential to treat the largest number of blind patients (since it does not require the patients to have an intact retina or optic nerve). Second Sight has also chosen the epiretinal approach (see Figure 35.2) over the subretinal approach because of the belief that the photodiodes used by Dr. Chow and Dr. Zrenner will not be able to produce enough electrical energy to stimulate abnormal human retinas.

Richard Normann from the University of Utah spoke about his electrode arrays, which have been used to record both acute and chronic electrophysiological recordings from various brain structures in monkeys, cats, and rats [5]. The standard array is a 4.2-mm square grid with 100 silicon microelectrodes, 1.0 mm long, and a spacing of 0.4 mm (see Figure 35.3). Dr. Normann also spoke about his new Utah Slant Array (USA) electrodes, which have been used to record signals from peripheral nerve.

Philip Troyk from the Illinois Institute of Technology spoke about the issues of implantable hardware. One issue raised was that the next-generation neuroprostheses would be five to ten times denser, electrically and physically than current neuroprosthetic devices. Dr. Troyk discussed the need for heat dissipation by

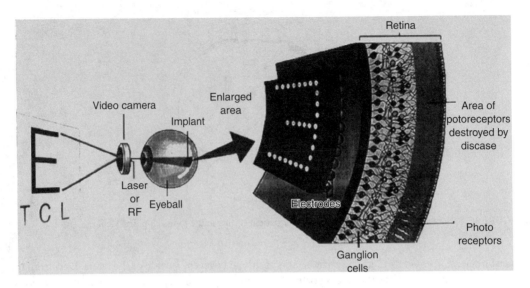

FIGURE 35.2   Concept for an epiretinal prosthesis.

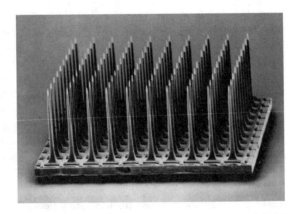

FIGURE 35.3   Penetrating cortical electrode array designed by Richard Normann's lab.

implanted prosthetics, particularly eye-mounted devices. Data was presented where a suspended-carrier closed-loop Class-E transcutaneous magnetic link was used to generate data transmission rates of over 1 M bit per second with a 5 MHz carrier [19]. Dr. Troyk also pointed out that the stimulation strategies to produce usable sight are still unknown. When reliable implantable hardware systems become available, testing can begin to devise efficacious image-to-stimulation transformations. It is important that the implantable hardware developed at this phase not restrict the nature of the stimulation sequences from the standpoint of amplitude, pulse width, frequency, and temporal modulation.

Then, Dana Ballard from the University of Rochester discussed the visual representations that affect sensory-motor task performance [20]. Volunteers were shown videos of a simulated driving environment and their eye movements, monitored. By tracking saccadic eye movements inferences can be drawn describing the underlying cortical processing [21].

Finally, a panel discussion was convened where the relative merits of the different approaches to visual prosthetics were debated. The session ended with a general consensus that visual prostheses are technically feasible and that chronically implanted devices and clinical testing are a necessary next step to assess efficacy.

Acknowledgments

This Review resulted from the Inaugural Symposium of the Alfred E. Mann Institute for Biomedical Engineering at University of Southern California, Los Angeles, California on February 19, 2000. The Alfred E. Mann Institute for Biomedical Engineering at the University of Southern California (AMI-USC) was established with a $150 million donation by Mr. Mann to the University and has as its goal the transfer of university research to the public sector for the benefit of patients.

References

[1] Clausen, J. Visual sensations (phosphenes) produced by ac sine wave stimulation. *Acta Physiol. Neurol. Scand. Suppl.* 94: 1–101, 1955.

[2] Brindley, G.and Lewin, W. The sensations produced by electrical stimulation of the visual cortex. *J. Physiol. (London)* 196: 479–493, 1968.

[3] Dobelle, W.H. and Mladwovsky, M.G. Phosphenes produced by electrical stimulation of human occipital cortex and their application to the development of a prosthesis for the blind. *J. Physiol.* 243: 553–576, 1974.

[4] Dobelle, W.H., Mladejovsky, M.G., Evans, J.K., Roberts, T.S., and Girvin, J.P. "Braille" reading by a blind volunteer by visual cortex stimulation. *Nature* 259: 111–112, 1976.

[5] Rousche, P.J. and Normann, R.A. Chronic recording capability of the Utah Intracortical Electrode Array in cat sensory cortex. *J. Neurosci. Meth.* 82: 1–15.

[6] Hoogerwerf, A.C. and Wise, K.D. A three-dimensional microelectrode array for chronic neural recording. *IEEE Trans. Biomed. Eng.* 41: 1136–1146.

[7] Bak, M., Girvin, J.P., Hambrecht, F.T., Kuftar, C.V., Loeb, G.E., and Schmidt, E.W. Visual sensations produced by intracortical microstimulation of the human occipital cortex. *Med. Biol. Eng. Comp.* 28: 257–259, 1990.

[8] Schmidt, E.M., Bak, M.J., Hambrecht, F.T., Kufta, C.V., O'Rourke, D.K., and Vallabhanath, P. Feasibility of a visual prosthesis for the blind based on intracortical microstimulation of the visual cortex. *Brain* 119: 507–522, 1996.

[9] Humayun, M.S., deJuan, E., Dagnelie, G., Greenberg, R.J., Propst, R., and Phillips, D.H. Visual perception elicited by electrical stimulation of retina in blind humans. *Arch. Ophthalmol.* 114: 40–46, 1996.

[10] Wyatt, J. and Rizzo, J. Ocular implants for the blind. *IEEE Spectrum* 47–53, 1996.

[11] Zrenner, E., Miliczek, K.D., Gabel, V.P., Graf, H.G., Guenther, E., Haemmerle, H. et al. The development of subretinal microphotodiodes for replacement of degenerated photoreceptors. *Ophthalm. Res.* 29: 269–80, 1997.

[12] Eckmiller, R. Learning retina implants with epiretinal contacts. *Ophthalmic Res.* 29: 281–289, 1997.

[13] Greenberg, R.J. Analysis of Electrical Stimulation of the Vertebrate Retina — Work Towards a Retinal Prosthesis (*thesis*) Johns Hopkins University, Baltimore, MD, 1998.

[14] Chow, A.Y. and Peachey, N.S. The subretinal microphotodiode array retinal prosthesis. *Ophthalmic Res.* 30: 195–198, 1998.

[15] Humayun, M.S., deJuan, E., Weiland, J.D., Dagnelie, G., Katona, S., Greenberg, R., and Suzuki, S. Pattern electrical stimulation of the human Retina. *Vision Res* 39: 2569–2576, 1999.

[16] Davis, R. Future possibilities for neural stimulation. In *Textbook of Stereotactic and Functional Neurosurgery.* Philip L. Gildenberg and Ronald R. Tasker (Eds.), McGraw-Hill, NY, Chapter 217, pp. 2064–2066, 1997.

[17] Veraart, C., Raftopoulos, C., Mortimer, J.T., Delbeke, J., Pins, D., Michaux, G. et. al. Visual sensations produced by optic nerve stimulation using an implanted self-sizing spiral cuff electrode. *Brain Res.* 813: 181–186, 1998.

[18] Kedzierski, W., Bok, D., and Travis, G.H. Transgenic analysis of rds/peripherin N-glycosylation: effect on dimerization, interaction with rom1, and rescue of the rds null phenotype. *J. Neurochem.* 72: 430–438, 1999.

[19] Troyk, P.R. and Schwan, M.A. Closed-loop class E transcutaneous power and data link for microimplants. *IEEE Trans. Biomed. Eng.* 39: 589–599, 1992.

[20] Smeets, J.B., Hayhoe, M.M., and Ballard, D.H. Goal-directed arm movements change eye-head coordination. *Exp. Brain Res.* 109: 434–440, 1996.

[21] Ballard, D.H., Hayhoe, M.M., Li, F., and Whitehead, S.D. Hand-eye coordination during sequential tasks. *Philos. Trans. R. Soc. Lond. B Biol. Sci.* 337: 331–339, 1992.

36

Interfering with the Genesis and Propagation of Epileptic Seizures by Neuromodulation

Ana Luisa Velasco
Francisco Velasco
Fiacro Jiménez
Marcos Velasco
Mexico City General Hospital

36.1 Introduction

Epilepsy is a medical condition that is very frequent around the world. It is estimated that 1% of the population suffers epilepsy. From these patients, only 70% are controlled with antiepileptic medication. The other 30% of patients may benefit from surgical intervention. The use of chronic stimulation of the brain, so called neuromodulation, has shown to be a reliable procedure in the control of epileptic seizures. In 1970, the first totally implantable stimulating systems were available [Rise, 2000]. Based on the work of Cooke and Snider [1955], Cooper et al. [1978] used cerebellar stimulation to control different varieties of epileptic seizures.

Our group has worked on two deep brain stimulation procedures according to the type of epileptic seizures (1) stimulation of the centromedian nucleus (CM) of the thalamus in the control of intractable generalized seizures and atypical absences of the Lennox–Gastaut syndrome (LGS) [Velasco et al., 1987,

1989, 1993a, b, 1995, 2000a, b, 2002] and (2) stimulation of the hippocampus for the control of mesial temporal lobe seizures [Velasco et al., 2000, 2001].

36.2 Electrical Stimulation of the Centromedian Thalamic Nuclei

Although electrical stimulation of the centromedian thalamic nuclei (ESCM) has been used in cases of difficult-to-control seizures with multifocal onset in the frontal and temporal lobes, as well as in cases of seizures with no evidence of focal onset such as LGS, it has proven to have its best result in the latter.

The role of midline and intralaminar thalamic nuclei in the genesis and propagation of epileptic attacks was proposed long ago on the basis of clinical observations [Penfield and Jasper, 1954]. Although the controversy on the anatomical initiation of the epileptic attacks remains, there seems to be an agreement that the thalamocortical interactions are essential in the development of most of them [Pollen et al., 1963; Gloor et al., 1977; Quesney et al., 1977; Avoli et al., 1983; Steriade, 1990; Velasco et al., 1991].

The decision to stimulate the CM was based on the idea to interfere with the thalamocortical interactions and thus stop either the genesis or propagation of the seizures. In 1984, our group performed the first ESCM trial on a 12-year-old male who had severe atypical absences refractory to high levels of antiepileptic medication. The CM was chosen as a target because of its relatively large size and close relationship to the conventional stereotaxic landmarks and because the CM is an intralaminar nucleus that forms part of the nonspecific reticular-thalamocortical system, which transmits and integrates the cerebral inputs of the generalized seizures [Jasper and Droogleever-Fortuyn, 1947; Hunter and Jasper, 1949; Gloor et al., 1979]. Since then, several types of seizures were included in the protocol of ESCM [Velasco et al., 1993a]. The best results were obtained in patients with generalized seizures of the LGS (associated with 2-Hz spike wave complexes and mental deterioration). Other forms of seizures particularly those with focal origins (as in temporal lobe seizures), are not significantly improved by ESCM to a lesser extent [Velasco et al., 2000b]. However secondary tonic–clonic generalization is relieved suggesting that ESCM interferes with the propagation mechanisms of focally initiated epileptic activity.

The ESCM procedure has been refined progressively by increasing the number of treated patients and lengthening the follow-up period. Our group has also better defined a number of predictor factors that must be taken into account to achieve a good outcome. There are three such main predictor factors (1) selection of responding patients, (2) verifying correct DBS implantation based on definition of the stereotaxic coordinates of the CM optimal effective areas and neurophysiologic characterization of the targeted area, and (3) performing periodic monitoring of the reliability of ESCM on a long-term follow-up [Velasco et al., 2000b, 2001].

36.2.1 Patient's Selection

In this chapter we analyze the last 13 patients with LGS selected from patients of the Epilepsy Surgery Clinic of the General Hospital of Mexico on the basis of having generalized difficult-to-control seizures of the LGS. They underwent ESCM with the idea to correlate seizure type, stereotaxic targeting, and neurophysiologic responses with the final outcome of the patient. The LGS is one of the most severe forms of childhood epilepsy. It is characterized by drug-resistant generalized seizures, the most characteristic being the tonic and atonic seizures, atypical absences, myoclonic attacks, episodes of nonconvulsive, and tonic *status epilepticus*. The peak onset is known to be between 1 and 7 years of age. It is usually preceded by other types of seizure disorders, especially infantile spasms. LGS is accompanied by severe mental deterioration as it progresses. From the electroencephalographic (EEG) standpoint, the diagnosis is based upon the presence of slow spike–wave complexes (<2.5 cps) and bursts of rapid (10 Hz) rhythms during slow sleep. The overall prognosis is very severe, 90% of the patients are mentally retarded and 80% continue to have seizures through adulthood [Aicardi, 1994]. The selected patients had either secondary LGS with stable or nonprogressive diseases (birth trauma, postencephalitic sequelae, cortical dysplasia, and stable tuberous sclerosis) or primary LGS with no demonstrable lesion in the magnetic resonance imaging (MRI).

36.2.2 Correct Targeting

To have the optimal results with ESCM, it is of extreme importance to have good patient selection combined with adequate target localization. The latter should be obtained from two points of view: stereotaxic (defined with ventriculography and MRI) and neurophysiologic definition.

36.2.2.1 Ventriculographic Definition of CM Target

Surgical technique: under general anesthesia, electrodes (Medtronic Model 3387 DBS lead Medtronic, Inc., Minneapolis, MN) are stereotactically placed in both left and right CM nuclei through a coronal incision and bifrontal burr holes made at a distance of 10 to 15 mm at each side of the midline at the level of the coronal suture. The CM localization is accomplished by air ventriculography. This method allows us to demonstrate the anterior commissure (AC) and posterior commissure (PC) of the third ventricle with remarkable precision. Two lines are drawn, the AC–PC line and the vertical line perpendicular to the PC (VPC). The target point for the electrode tip was a distance 10 mm from the midline and the intersection of the AC–PC line with the VPC [Velasco et al., 1989, 2000b].

Electrodes are fixed to burr holes using a plastic ring and silastic ring caps (Medtronic). The position of the contacts along the trajectory of the electrode is plotted on the sagittal and frontal sections of the Schaltenbrand and Bailey atlas [1959] according to the standardization technique described elsewhere [Velasco et al., 1975].

The optimal targets for seizure arrest are located in the basolateral portion of the CM, which corresponds to the parvocellular portion; this is an area of maximal neuronal population [Mehler, 1996] Figure 36.1. The best antiepileptic results are located as follows: LAT = 10.0 ± 2.0 mm from the midline, H = from 2.0 to 7.0 mm above the AC–PC line, and AP = from 3.0 to 5.0 mm in front or PC–VPC intersection. Since

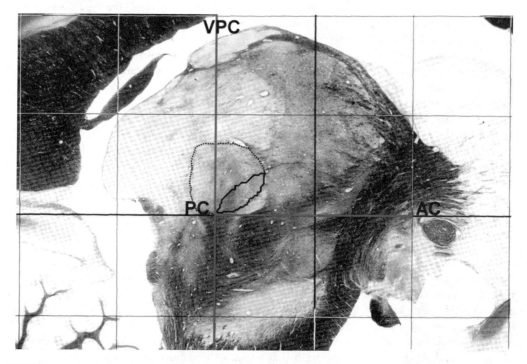

FIGURE 36.1 Optimal targets for seizure arrest located in the basolateral portion of the CM.

the CM is a large nucleus with several subdivisions, it is important to point out that the electrode contacts used for stimulation in patients with good outcome are positioned in the ventrolateral or parvocellular part of the CM considered by anatomists as the core of the CM nucleus of Luys, which is surrounded by denser fiber connections ascending from the brainstem to terminate in other nuclei of the thalamus [Mehler, 1996].

36.2.2.2 MRI Confirmation of the CM Target

Electrodes are left externalized to confirm their position by MRI. Scans are performed using 1.5 T Edge equipment software version 9.3 (Marconi Medical Systems, Cleveland, Ohio), using T2 weighted fast spin echo sequence (echo time 11 ms; repetition time 4070 msec; field of view 16.0 cm; 256×256 matrix). Sections are oriented parallel and perpendicular to the AC–PC line for axial and frontal views, and parallel to the midsagittal plane for sagittal sections [Velasco et al., 2000b, 2002].

36.2.2.3 Neurophysiologic Confirmation of the CM Target

Stimuli are delivered by a Grass S8 stimulator and isolation unit attached to the patient by means of a Tektronix CRU and a comparative 10 kΩ resistor in order to monitor the voltage (V), current flow (μA), and impedance (kΩ) of the stimulated contacts within the brain tissue [Velasco et al., 1993a].

The electrical incremental and desynchronizing responses are elicited by unilateral electrical stimulation through adjacent electrode contacts (where the cathode was always the lower contact). Stimuli consist of 5 to 30 sec trains of monophasic square pulses of 1.0 msec duration and 6- to 60-Hz frequency. Analysis of the scalp distribution of the incremental spike–wave and desynchronizing electrocortical responses is made from EEG recordings taken from frontopolar (FP2, FP1), frontal (F4, F3), central (C4, C3), parietal (P4, P3), occipital (O2, O1), frontotemporal (F8, F7), and anterior temporal (T4, T3) referred to ipsilateral ears (A2, A1) (Sensitivity = 10 μA/cm; time constant = 0.35 sec; paper speed = 15 mm/sec).

Low-frequency (6/sec), threshold (4–5 V = 320–400 μA) unilateral stimulation of CM elicits incremental responses with the typical waxing and waning profile. The incremental responses produced by this stimulation procedure along the CM or other structures are described elsewhere [Velasco et al., 1996]. Although there are three types of incremental responses that may be elicited, the Type A one points the best place to obtain the optimum antiepileptic effect. They are recruiting-like responses elicited by the stimulation of the caudal-basal portions of CM (parvocellular CM close to the nonspecific mesencephalic structures, such as the mesencephalic *tegmentum* tract). They consist of monophasic negative potentials with a latency of 20 msec and peak latency of 30–35 msec, see Figure 36.2a. Suprathreshold Type A responses show a bilateral regional scalp distribution with maximal amplitude at the frontal region ipsilateral to the stimulated side, see Figure 36.2b [Velasco et al., 1996].

Unilateral high-frequency (60/sec) threshold and suprathreshold stimulation of the caudal-basal and central CM elicits a regional EEG desynchronization consisting of an increased frequency of the EEG activity superimposed on a slow negative shift. It also shows a bilateral regional scalp distribution with maximal amplitude at the frontal region ipsilateral to the stimulated side, see Figure 36.2(c) [Velasco et al., 1996].

36.2.3 Periodic Monitoring of the Reliability of ESCM on a Long-Term Follow-Up

Incremental responses, EEG desynchronization, and slow negative shifts may be useful as biological responses for monitoring the efficiency of the ESCM, particularly when the stimulating electrodes are internalized subcutaneously and the physical characteristics of the electrical stimuli cannot be monitored any longer [Velasco et al., 1995]. In view of the patient's lack of subjective sensations and the long latency of the antiepileptic effects of ESCM, the reliability of ESCM is questionable. The use of 10 or 60/sec and 6 V (800 μA) transcutaneous activation of CM with the internalized pulse generator (IPG) by Medtronic, Inc., Minneapolis and the recording of scalp incremental responses, EEG desynchronization and slow negative shifts are advisable.

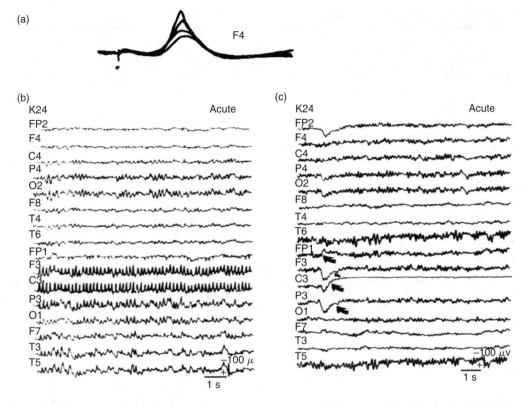

FIGURE 36.2 Neurophysiologic confirmation of the CM target. (a) Type A recruiting-like responses elicited by the stimulation of the caudal-basal portions of CM. They consist of monophasic negative potentials with a latency of 20 msec and peak latency of 30 to 35 msec. (b) Low-frequency (6/sec) stimulation elicits suprathreshold Type A responses showing a bilateral regional scalp distribution with maximal amplitude at the frontal region ipsilateral to the stimulated side. (c) Unilateral high-frequency (60/sec) threshold and suprathreshold stimulation of the caudal-basal and central CM elicits a regional EEG desynchronization consisting of an increased frequency of the EEG activity superimposed on a slow negative shift with a bilateral regional scalp distribution with maximal amplitude at the frontal region ipsilateral to the stimulated side.

36.2.3.1 Chronic Stimulation Parameters

The parameters recommended for ESCM are as follows: 2 h of daily stimulation sessions. Stimulus consists of 1-min trains of Lilly pulses with an interstimulus interval of 4 min, alternating right and left CM. Such trains consist in a 130-Hz frequency, with individual pulses of 450 μs in duration and amplitude of 400 to 600 μA.

36.2.4 Results

Electrical stimulation of the centromedian thalamic nuclei produces a significant reduction in the number of primary and secondary generalized tonic–clonic seizures (GTC) and atypical absences of the LGS, and also the number of interictal generalized slow spike–wave complexes.

As said above, the results depend on both the seizure type and correct target selection. Note that the patients with excellent result (i.e., 100% improvement) had generalized seizures and correct stereotaxic placement and electrophysiological responses. All patients who had less than 80% seizure improvement had either other seizure type (i.e., LC who had residual complex partial seizures [CXP]), or incorrect target selection according to either anatomic (stereotaxic) or physiologic parameters (Table 36.1).

TABLE 36.1 The Predictors of Seizure Relief Obtained after ESCM Are Shown

Initials	Seizure type			Stereotactic placement		Electro physiological		Final improvement (%)
	GTC	AA	CXP	RCM	LCM	RCM	LCM	
GA	Y	Y	N	C	C	C	C	100
MAM	Y	Y	N	C	C	C	C	100
AMP	Y	Y	N	C	I	C	C	95
MS	Y	Y	N	C	C	C	C	95
MAPR	Y	Y	N	C	I	C	C	95
JM	Y	Y	N	C	C	C	C	91
JS	Y	Y	N	C	C	C	C	89
IM	Y	Y	N	C	C	C	C	87
LC	Y	Y	Y	C	C	I	I	80
EGV	Y	Y	N	C	C	C	I	70
DC	N	Y	N	C	I	C	C	58
JR	Y	Y	N	C	I	I	I	53
LVAP	N	Y	N	C	C	I	I	30

Note all patients had generalized tonic–clonic seizures (GTC), atypical absences (AA) and only LC also had complex partial seizures (CXP). Correct (C) and Incorrect (I) stereotaxic and electrophysiological parameters are shown. Note that all patients with a seizure improvement 100% had generalized seizures and correct target localization parameters. (From Velasco et al., submitted for publication)

36.3 Electrical Stimulation of the Hippocampus (ESHC)

In the Epilepsy Surgery Clinic of the General Hospital of Mexico, 70% of patients referred for surgery have CXP arising from the hippocampal formation; other series have reported a similar referral number [Wieser et al., 1993; Williamson, 1993]. Resective surgery of the epileptic focus yields very good results [Engel, 1987; Velasco et al., 2000c], nevertheless there are cases that escape this surgical possibility, that is, patients with bilateral hippocampal foci or patients with epileptic foci located nearby eloquent areas for speech and memory (usually the left side). These latter patients cannot be operated on because it would mean having severe neurological impairment particularly related to short-term memory. These patients are candidates for neuromodulating procedures. Unfortunately, our experience with ESCM pointed out that CM is not the place to stimulate in patients with CXP originating in the temporal lobe. On the other hand, animal experiments showed that the application of an electrical stimulus to the amygdala or hippocampus following the kindling stimulus produces a significant and long-lasting suppressive effect on seizures [Weiss et al., 1995]. For these reasons we decided to perform a preliminary study in 10 patients with nonlesional temporal lobe epilepsy in whom intracranial electrodes were implanted (either subdural basotemporal grid or hippocampal electrodes) for the detection of the epileptic foci [Velasco et al., 2000c]. The study consisted in performing subacute hippocampal stimulation (SAHCS) trial for a duration of 2–3 weeks once the epileptic focus was located and before performing the temporal lobectomy. Two patients had bilateral hippocampal depth electrodes implanted to determine the lateralization of the epileptic focus and eight had unilateral subdural electrode grids on the pial surface of the basotemporal cortex to determine the precise site and extent of the focus (see Figure 36.3). In all patients, antiepileptic drugs were discontinued for 72 h before SAHCS initiation. Thereafter, SAHCS was applied for a minimum of 16 days. SAHCS was bipolar and between continuous electrode contacts (cathode attached to the most anterior contact) and consisted of continuous stimulation with biphasic Lilly pulses, 130-Hz frequency, 450 μsec in duration, and amplitude of 200–400 μA). The reliability of SAHCS was determined by daily measurement of voltage, impedance, and current flow at the intracerebral contacts by means of externalized electrode systems [Velasco et al., 1993a].

To evaluate the antiepileptic effects of SAHCS on temporal lobe epileptogenesis, the number and type of clinical seizures/day and the number of interictal negative EEG spikes at the epileptic focus/10 sec was

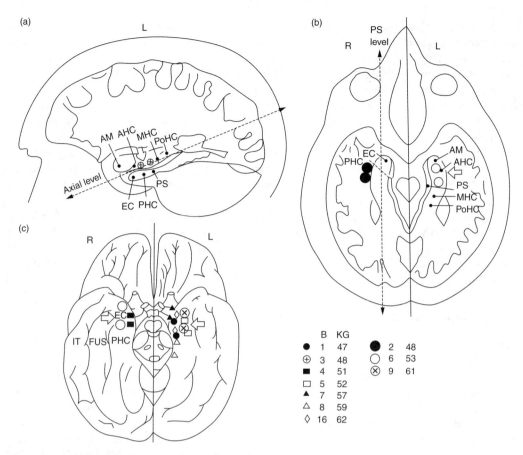

FIGURE 36.3 Diagrams showing the position of the depth and subdural electrode contacts for SAHCS. (a and b) show parasagittal and axial sections and (c) basotemporal cortex all of them showing the position of the stimulation contacts in different patients (indicated by different symbols at the right bottom corner). Arrows indicate sites where SAHCS produced evident and fast antiepileptic responses. Abbreviations: AHC, MHC, and PoHC: anterior, middle, and posterior hippocampus. AM: amygdala, PS presubiculum, PHC, EC, FUS, and IT: parahippocampal, entorhinal, fusiform, and inferior temporal gyri. (Reproduced from Velasco et al. *Arch. Med. Res.* 2000d, 31:316–328. With permission.)

evaluated. At completion of the clinical and EEG studies, SAHCS was discontinued, the electrodes were removed, and an anterior temporal lobectomy was performed ipsilateral to the epileptic focus and SAHCS. Biopsies of mesial and lateral temporal lobe were fixed in 10% formaldehyde buffer solution, embedded in paraffin, and cut in serial coronal sections of 10-μm thickness and perpendicular to the fascia dentata, taken every 1000 μm and stained with hematoxilin-eosin for perikarion and with Gomori's technique used for the collagen. Histopathological analysis of the temporal lobe tissue was performed under light microscope by comparing the contiguous hippocampal tissue at the stimulated vs. nonstimulated tissues.

In seven patients in whom stimulation sites were located within the hippocampal formation and gyrus, there was an evident antiepileptic response. Both CXP and secondary GTC seizures were abolished after 6 days of continuous stimulation and interictal EEG spikes were significantly reduced from days 4 to 11 of SAHCS. The most evident and fastest antiepileptic responses were found in five patients in whom the stimulation contacts were located at either the anterior pes hippocampus near the amygdala or at the anterior parahippocampal gyrus near the entorhinal cortex. Three patients did not respond, two of them when SAHCS was accidentally interrupted and the other patient when the stimulated contacts were located at the white matter lateral to the hippocampus.

Histopathological analysis of the hippocampal tissues revealed abnormalities due to depth electrode penetration or lesion due to the foreign body electrodes. However, no histopathological differences were found between stimulated and nonstimulated hippocampal tissues. Therefore, the SAHCS effect does not appear to depend on a lesional process but rather to a functional blockage of the hippocampus.

During this preliminary study we took advantage of this ethically permissible situation and studied some basic mechanisms underlying the beneficial therapeutic effect on seizures due to hippocampal stimulation [Velasco et al., 2000d, e, 2001a, b]. Such studies suggest that the antiepileptic effect of hippocampal stimulation is due to an inhibition mechanism, that is, increased threshold and decreased duration of the afterdischarges induced by acute hippocampal stimulation; depression of the paired pulse hippocampal recovery cycles; and single photon emission computed tomography (SPECT) hypoperfusion and autoradiographic increase of the benzodiazepine receptor binding in the stimulated hippocampal tissue [Cuéllar et al., 1994].

Based upon these results we decided to proceed with a long-term hippocampal stimulation protocol to demonstrate that chronic hippocampal stimulation (CHCS) may produce a sustained antiepileptic effect without undesirable effects on language and memory. So far, we have stimulated 8 patients on a long-term basis, but we will only take into consideration those 6 patients who have a follow-up period of at least 1 year (1 to 4 years).

36.3.1 Study Design

Candidates were selected from patients of the Epilepsy Surgery Clinic of the General Hospital of Mexico on the basis of having difficult-to-control temporal lobe seizures. All of them underwent a careful clinical history with special emphasis on the seizure type (CXP), adequate antiepileptic medication with adequate blood levels, four serial EEGs, magnetic resonance, SPECT, neuropsychological exam, and psychiatric evaluation. All of them had bilateral hippocampal transitory eight contact depth electrodes (SD 8P, Ad Tech Medical Instrument Co., Racine, WI, USA) implanted to be able to assess the epileptic foci. Two of them had bilateral independent hippocampal foci and the other four patients were selected on the basis of having their hippocampal focus on the dominant hemisphere, with neuropsychological evidence of verbal memory situated here.

Once the precise epileptic focus was defined, the transitory electrodes were replaced by four contact depth brain stimulation electrodes (3789 DBS and IPG by Medtronic, Inc., Minneapolis, MN) (Figure 36.4) and connected to an independent IPG system that were placed in a subcutaneous subclavicular pocket on each side. The target of the electrode contacts was the site of maximal interictal and ictal activities. All antiepileptic drugs were withdrawn to avoid any possible interference with the neuromodulation procedure [Velasco et al., 2000e] and were replaced with phenytoin.

36.3.1.1 Chronic Stimulation Parameters

The parameters recommended for ESHC are as follows: daily stimulation sessions with 1-min trains of Lilly pulses with an interstimulus interval of 4 min. Such trains consist in a 130-Hz frequency, with individual pulses of 450 μsec in duration and amplitude of 400 to 600 μA. In those patients with bilateral electrodes, the stimulation has the same characteristics but the stimulation alternates right and left hippocampus.

36.3.2 Results

In analyzing the antiepileptic effect of ESHC, the six patients were divided into two distinct groups: three patients had normal MRIs and the other three had ipsilateral hippocampal sclerosis. The best results were obtained in the first group with normal MRIs. The antiepileptic effect was evident since the stimulation started and the patients were seizure free after the first three to six months of stimulation. Our longest follow-up period is on patient KG67 who had bilateral hippocampal stimulation and has now been 4 years seizure free. Patient KG101 is under left hippocampal stimulation and has been seizure free for 15 months and the most recent patient KG109 also has left hippocampal stimulation and has been seizure

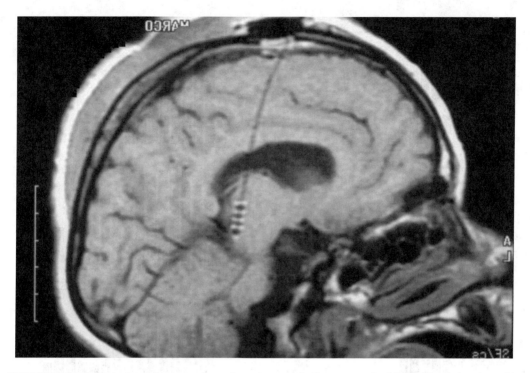

FIGURE 36.4   Illustrates the replacement of transitory electrodes by four contact depth brain stimulation electrodes.

free for a year. The neuropsychological tests in all of them became normal after 6 months of stimulation (Figure 36.5a).

The patients that constitute the second group have unilateral left mesial temporal sclerosis. Patient KG71 had bilateral epileptic foci. Even though he had a 75% seizure reduction, he persisted with auras during the 10-months follow-up. Unfortunately he had to undergo explantation because of skin erosion. Patient KG102 had 60% seizure improvement, which could be observed very slowly and took 9 months to reach its actual seizure number (follow-up of 20 months). KG106 has had only 50% seizure improvement after one year of stimulation (Figure 36.5b). In all the patients of this group there has only been a slight improvement in the neuropsychological tests. The three patients in this group improved only slightly in their memory tests after more than 6 months stimulation.

Even though these are preliminary results, we may say that stimulating the hippocampal epileptic focus is effective in the control of mesial temporal lobe seizures. The best cases are those who have normal MRI, in whom seizure control can be achieved up to 100%. This result is of extreme importance because these patients with intractable seizures and normal MRI are the ones that are excluded as candidates for temporal lobectomy and are left with no other alternative. Patients with mesial temporal lobe sclerosis do not do so well and their follow-up shows only 50 to 75% seizure reduction. If the patient has temporal sclerosis and the seizures are starting within the sclerotic hippocampus, lobectomy could be risked. Patients with bilateral hippocampal foci and unilateral sclerosis though should be considered for neuromodulation, since they could have better results and the risk of having residual seizures after unilateral lobectomy is high.

36.4   Conclusion

Neuromodulation constitutes an innovative neurosurgical technique in the treatment of difficult-to-control seizures. Stimulation should be targeted according to the seizure type: ESCM for generalized seizures and ESHC for mesial temporal lobe epilepsy. Neuromodulation is a method that has several

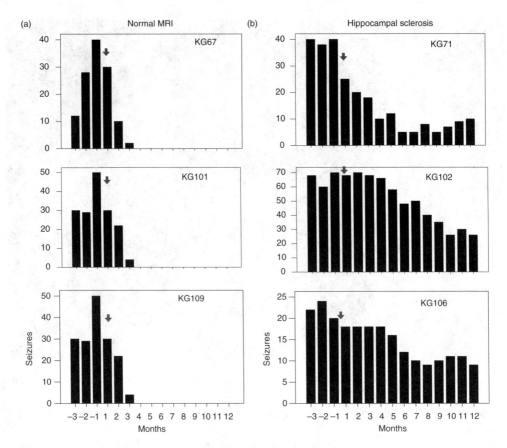

FIGURE 36.5 Seizure reduction per month in 6 patients with ESHC, graphs show 3-month baseline period, stimulation started at the fourth month (arrow) after that, 12-month stimulation follow-up. (a) Three patients with normal MRI. (b) Three patients with left hippocampal sclerosis.

advantages: it is nonlesional, with reversible effect when turned off, does not interfere with the functioning eloquent areas, and even improves neuropsychological performance. Unfortunately it has some disadvantages: neurostimulating systems are expensive, it needs periodic follow-up visits to verify whether it is functioning adequately, and the stimulators have to be exchanged when the batteries wear off, which implies a surgical procedure. Probably the most important disadvantage is the skin erosion due to the stimulating system that often leads to explantation mainly in young children.

Challenges remain. For the epileptologists there are a number of variables that are influencing the antiepileptic effect of neurostimulation that we are probably missing and there are as well other seizure types that are subject to be studied to know the antiepileptic effects of neuromodulation, that is, supplementary motor cortex epilepsy. For the engineers the need to improve neuromodulation systems so that they are less invasive (so that they are not rejected by the patients and can be implanted in small children), include rechargeable batteries, may even be remote controlled so the use of extension cables is discontinued. The systems have to be low cost so that they can be accessed by a larger number of epileptic patients. They also need to be more reliable and include user-friendly software so that the patient can check it by himself to avoid so many follow-up visits to guarantee reliable functioning.

References

Aicardi, J. Lennox–Gastaut Syndrome in *Epilepsy in Children*, 2nd ed. New York: Raven Press, 1994, pp. 44–66.

Avoli, M., Gloor, P., Kostopoulus, G., and Gutman, J. An analysis of penicillin-induced generalized spike and wave discharges using simultaneous recordings of cortical and thalamic single neurons. *J. Neurophysiol.* 1983, 50: 819–837.

Cooke, R.M. and Snider, R.S. Some cerebellar influences on electrically induced cerebral seizures. *Epilepsia* 1955, 4–19.

Cooper, I.S., Rickland, M., Amin, I., and Cullinan, T. A long term follow up study of cerebellar stimulation for the control of epilepsy. In Cooper, I. (Ed.), *Cerebellar Stimulation in Man*. New York: Raven Press, 1978, pp. 19–27.

Cuellar-Herrera, Velasco, M., Velasco, F., Velasco, A.L., Jiménez, F., Orozco, S., Briones, M., and Rocha, L. Evaluation of GABA system and cell damage in parahippocampus of patients with temporal lobe epilepsy showing antiepileptic effects alter subacute electrical stimulation. *Epilepsia* 2004, 45: 459–466.

Engel, J. Jr. (Ed.) Outcome with respect to epilepsy seizures. In *Surgical Treatment of the Epilepsies*. New York: Raven, 1987, pp. 553–569.

Gloor, P., Quesney, L.F., and Zumstein, H. Pathophysiology of generalized penicillin seizures in the cat. The role of cortical and subcortical structures. II. Topical application of penicillin to the cerebral cortex and to sucortical structures. *Electroencephalogr. Clin. Neurophysiol.* 1977, 48: 79–94.

Hunter, J. and Jasper, H.H. Effects of thalamic stimulation in unanesthetized animals. The arrest reaction and petit mal-like seizures activation patterns and generalized convulsions. *Electroenceph. Clin. Neurophysiol.* 1949, 11: 305–324.

Jasper, H.H. and Droogleever-Fortuyn, J. Experimental studies of the functional anatomy of petit mal epilepsy. *Res. Public Assoc. Nerv. Ment. Dis.* 1947, 26: 272–298.

Mehler, R.W. Further notes of the centromedian nucleus of Luys. In Purpura, D.P. and Yahr, M.D. (Eds.), *The Thalamus*. New York: Columbia University Press, 1996, pp. 102–111.

Penfield, W. and Jasper, H. *Epilepsy and the Functional Anatomy of the Human Brain*. Boston, MA: Little Brown, 1954, pp. 566–596.

Pollen, D.A., Perot, P., and Reid, K.H. Experimental bilateral spike and wave from thalamic stimulation in relation to the level of arousal. *Electroencephalogr. Clin. Neurophysiol.* 1963, 15: 459–473.

Quesney, L.F., Gloor, P., Kratzemberg, E., and Zumstein, H. Pathophysiology of generalized penicillin seizures in the cat. The role of cortical and subcortical structures. I. systemic application of penicillin. *Electroencephalogr. Clin. Neurophysiol.* 1977, 42: 640–655.

Rise, M.T. Instrumentation for neuromodulation. *Arch. Med. Res.* 2000, 34: 237–247.

Schaltebrand, G. and Bailey, P.: Stuttgart, Georg Thieme 1959, Vol IV.

Steriade, M. Spindling, incremental thalamo-cortical responses and spike-wave like epilepsy. In Avoli, M., Gloor, P., Kustopoulus, G., and Naquet, R. (Eds.), *Generalized Epilepsy: Neurobiological Approaches*. Boston, MA: Birkhouser, 1990, pp. 161–180.

Velasco, F., Velasco, M., and Machado, J.P. A statistical outline of the subthalamic target for the arrest of tremor. *Appl. Neurophysiol.* 1975, 38: 38–46.

Velasco, F., Velasco, M., Ogarrio, C., and Fanghänel, F. Electrical Stimulation of the centromedian thalamic nucleus in the treatment of convulsive seizures. A preliminary report. *Epilepsia* 1987, 28: 421–430.

Velasco, F., Velasco, M., and Alcalá, H. The electrical stimulation of the thalamus. In Kutt, H. and Resor, S.R. (Eds.), *Advances in Neurology. Medical treatment of Epilepsy*. New York: Marcel Decker, 1989, pp. 677–780.

Velasco, M., Velasco, F., Alcalá, H., Dávila, G., and Díaz de León, A.E. Epileptiform EEG activities in the centromedian thalamic nuclei in children with intractable generalizad seizures of the Lennox–Gastaut syndrome. *Epilepsia* 1991, 32: 310–321.

Velasco, F., Velasco, M., Velasco, A.L., and Jimenez, F. Effect of chronic electrical stimulation of the centromedian thalamic nuclei on various intractable seizure patterns: I. Clinical seizures and paroxysmal EEG activity. *Epilepsia* 1993a, 34: 1052–1064.

Velasco, M., Velasco, F., Velasco, A.L., Velasco, G., and Jimenez, F. Effect of chronic electrical stimula-tion of the centromedian thalamic nuclei on various intractable seizure patterns: II. Psychological performance and background activity. *Epilepsia* 1993b, 34: 1065–1074.

Velasco, F., Velasco, M., Velasco, A.L., Jimenez, F., and Rise, M. Electrical stimulation of the centromedian thalamic nucleus in control of seizures: long-term studies. *Epilepsia* 1995, 36: 63–71.

Velasco, M., Velasco, F., Velasco, A.L., Jimenez, F., Márquez, I., and Rojas, B. Electrocortical and behavioral responses produced by acute electrical stimulation of the human centromedian thalamic nucleus. *Electroenceph. Clin. Neurophysiol.* 1996, 102: 461–471.

Velasco, M., Velasco, F., Velasco, A.L., Jiménez, F., Brito, F., and Márquez, I. Acute and chronic electrical stimulation of the centromedian thalamic nucleus: modulation of reticulo-cortical systems and predictor factors for generalized seizure control. *Arch. Med. Res.* 2000a, 31: 304–315.

Velasco, F., Velasco, M., Jiménez, F., Velasco, A.L., Brito, F., Rise, M., and Carrillo-Ruiz, J.D. Predictors in the treatment of difficult to control seizures by electrical stimulation of the centromedian thalamic nucleus. *Neurosurgery* 2000b, 47: 295–305.

Velasco, A.L., Boleaga, B., Brito, F., Jiménez, F., Gordillo, J.L., Velasco, F., and Velasco, M. Absolute and relative predictor values of some non-invasive and invasive studies for the outcome of anterior temporal lobectomy. *Arch. Med. Res.* 2000c, 31: 62–74.

Velasco, A.L., Velasco, M., Velasco, F., Ménes, D., Gordon, F., Rocha, L., Briones, M., and Márquez, I. Subacute and chronic electrical stimulation of the hippocampus on intractable temporal lobe seizures. *Arch. Med. Res.* 2000d, 31: 316–328.

Velasco, M., Velasco, F., Velasco, A.L., Boleaga, B., Jiménez, F., Brito, F., and Márquez, I. Subacute electrical stimulation of the hippocampus blocks intractable temporal lobe seizures and paroxysmal EEG activities. *Epilepsia* 2000e, 41: 158–169.

Velasco, M., Velasco, F., and Velasco, A.L. Centromedian thalamic and hippocampal electrical stimulation for the control of intractable epileptic seizures. *Clin. Neurophysiol.* 2001a, 18: 1–15.

Velasco, F., Velasco, M., Velasco, A.L., Ménez, D., and Rocha, L. Electrical stimulation for epilepsy 1. Stimulation of hippocampal foci. *Stereotact. Funct. Neurosurg.* 2001b, 77: 223–227.

Velasco, F., Velasco, M., Jiménez, F., Velasco, A.L., Rojas, B., and Pérez, M.L. Centromedian nucleus stimulation for epilepsy: clinical, electroencephalographic and behavioral observations. *Thalamus Related Syst.* 2002, 34: 1–12.

Velasco, F., Velasco, A.L., Velasco, M., Rocha, L., and Ménes, D. Electrical stimulation of the epileptic focus in cases of temporal lobe seizures. In Lüders, H.O. (Ed.), *Electrical Stimulation for Epilepsy*. London: Taylor and Frances Health Sciences, 2003, pp. 287–300.

Weiss, S.B.R., Li, X.L., Rosen, J.B., Li, H., and Heynen, T. Post RM. Quenching: inhibition of development and expression of amygdale kindled seizures with low frequency stimulation. *Neuroreport* 1995, 4: 2171.

Wieser, H.G., Engel, J. Jr., Williamson, P.D., Babb, T.L., and Gloor, P. Surgically remediable temporal lobe syndromes. In Engel, J. Jr. (Ed.), *Surgical Treatment of the Epilepsies*. New York: Raven, 1993, pp. 49–63.

Williamson, P.D., French, J.A., and Thadani, V.M. Characteristics of medial temporal lobe epilepsy II. Inter-ictal and ictal scalp electroencephalography, neuropsychological testing, neuroimaging, surgical results and pathology. *Ann. Neurol.* 1993, 34: 781–787.

37

Transcranial Magnetic Stimulation of Deep Brain Regions

Yiftach Roth
Sheba Medical Center

Abraham Zangen
Weizmann Institute of Science

37.1 Introduction

Transcranial magnetic stimulation (TMS) is a noninvasive technique used to apply brief magnetic pulses to the brain. The pulses are administered by passing high currents through an electromagnetic coil placed upon the scalp that can induce electrical currents in the underlying cortical tissue, thereby producing a localized axonal depolarization. Neuronal stimulation by TMS was first demonstrated in 1985 [Barker et al., 1985], when a circular coil was placed over a normal subject vertex and evoked action potentials from the abductor digiti minimi. Since then this technique has been applied to studying nerve conduction, excitability, and conductivity in the brain and peripheral nerves, and to studying and treating various neurobehavioral disorders, primarily mood disorders [Kircaldie et al., 1997; Wassermann and Lisanby, 2001].

The ability of TMS technique to elicit neuronal response has until recently been limited to brain cortex. The coils used for TMS (such as round or a figure-of-eight coils) induce stimulation in cortical regions mainly just superficially under the windings of the coil. The intensity of the electric field drops dramatically deeper in the brain as a function of the distance from the coil [Maccabee et al., 1990; Tofts, 1990; Tofts et al., 1991; Eaton, 1992]. Therefore, to stimulate deep brain regions, a very high intensity would be needed. Such intensity cannot be reached by standard magnetic stimulators, using the regular figure-of-eight or circular coils. Stimulation of regions at depth of 3 to 4 cm, such as the leg motor area, may be achieved using coils such as the double cone coil [Terao et al., 1994, 2000; Stokic et al., 1997], which is a larger figure-of-eight with an angle of about 95° between the two wings. However, the intensity needed to stimulate deeper brain regions effectively would stimulate cortical regions and facial nerves over the level that might lead to facial pain, facial and cervical muscle contractions, and may cause epileptic seizures and other undesirable side effects.

This chapter describes principles and design of TMS coils for deep brain stimulation. The construction of such coils should meet simultaneously several goals:

1. High enough electric field intensity in the desired deep brain region that will surpass the threshold for neuronal activation
2. High percentage of electric field in the desired deep brain region relative to the maximal intensity in the cortex
3. Minimal aversive side effects during stimulation such as pain and activation of facial muscles

37.2   Basic Principles of TMS

The TMS stimulation circuit consists of a high-voltage power supply which charges a bank of capacitors, which are then rapidly discharged via an electronic switch into the TMS coil, to create the briefly changing magnetic field pulse. A typical circuit is shown in Figure 37.1, where low-voltage AC is transformed into high-voltage DC, which charges the capacitors. A crucial component is the thyristor switch, which has to traverse very high current at a very short time of 50 to 250 μsec. The cycle time depends on the capacitance (typically 10 to 250 μF) and on the coil inductance (typically 10 to 30 μH). Typical peak currents and voltages are 5000 A and 1500 V, respectively.

Most TMS stimulators produce a biphasic pulse of electric current. During the discharge cycle, the TMS circuit behaves like a RCL circuit, and the current I is given by:

$$I(t) = \frac{V}{wL}\exp(-\alpha t)\sin(wt) \tag{37.1}$$

where $\alpha = R/2L$, $w = \sqrt{((LC)^{-1} - \alpha^2)}$, and R, C, and L are the total values of the resistance, capacitance, and inductance, respectively, in the circuit. The inductance is mainly the coil inductance, but there is additional contribution from the cables, and the resistance includes contributions from the thyristor and the coil.

Biologically, the most relevant parameter for neuronal activation is the induced electric field, which is proportional to the rate of change of the current (dI/dt). The brief strong current generates a time-varying magnetic field B. An electric field E is generated in every point in space with direction perpendicular to the magnetic field, with amplitude proportional to the time-rate of change of the vector potential $A(r)$.

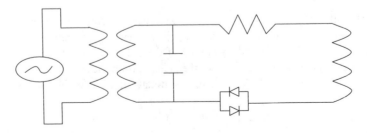

FIGURE 37.1   Typical magnetic stimulation circuit, including high-voltage transformer, capacitor, resistor, thyristor trigger, and stimulating coil.

The vector potential $A(r)$ in position r is related to the current in the coil I by the expression:

$$A(r) = \frac{\mu_0 I}{4\pi} \int \frac{dl'}{|r - r'|} \tag{37.2}$$

where $\mu_0 = 4\pi \times 10^{-7}$ Tm/A is the permeability of free space, the integral of dl' is over the wire path, and r' is a vector indicating the position of the wire element. The magnetic and electric fields are related to the vector potential through the expressions:

$$B_A = \nabla \times A \tag{37.3}$$

$$E_A = \frac{-\partial A}{\partial t} \tag{37.4}$$

The only quantity which is changing with time is the current I. Hence the electric field E_A can be written as:

$$E_A = \frac{-\mu_0}{4\pi} \frac{\partial I}{\partial t} \int \frac{dl'}{|r - r'|} \tag{37.5}$$

Since brain tissue has conducting properties, while the air and skull are almost complete insulators, the vector potential will induce accumulation of electric charge at the brain surface. This charge is another source for electric field, which can be expressed as:

$$E_\Phi = -\nabla \Phi \tag{37.6}$$

where Φ is the scalar potential produced by the surface electrostatic charge. The total field in the brain tissue E is the vectorial sum of these two fields:

$$E = E_A + E_\Phi \tag{37.7}$$

The influence of the electrostatic field E_Φ is in general to oppose the induced field E_A and consequently to reduce the total field E. The amount of surface charge produced and hence the magnitude of E_Φ depends strongly on coil configuration and orientation. This issue will be elaborated in the following sections.

Figure 37.2 demonstrates the electric field pulse produced by a figure-of-eight coil, as measured by a two-wire probe in a brain phantom filled with saline solution at physiologic concentration. In repetitive TMS (rTMS), several such pulses are administered in a train of between 1 and 20 Hz.

This electric field produces action potential in excitable neuronal cells, which might result in activation of neuronal circuits when applied above certain threshold. The neuronal response depends not only on the electric field strength, but also on the pulse duration through a strength–duration curve of the form:

$$E_{\text{th}} = b(1 + c/\tau) \tag{37.8}$$

where E_{th} is the threshold electric field required to induce neuronal response and τ is the duration the field was above this threshold. The biological parameters determining neural response are the threshold at infinite duration, termed the rheobase (b, measured in V/m), and the duration at which the threshold is twice the rheobase, termed the chronaxie (c, in μsec). Motor and sensory curves as reported by Bourland et al. [1996] are shown in Figure 37.3. These curves should be treated as illustrative only since the chronaxie and rheobase depend on many biological and experimental factors such as whether the nerves are myelinated or not (hence peripheral and cortical parameters should be different) and on train frequency in rTMS, which in general reduces the threshold for stimulation.

As shown by Heller and Van Hulstein [1992], the three-dimensional maximum of the electric field intensity will always be located at the brain surface for any configuration or superposition of TMS coils.

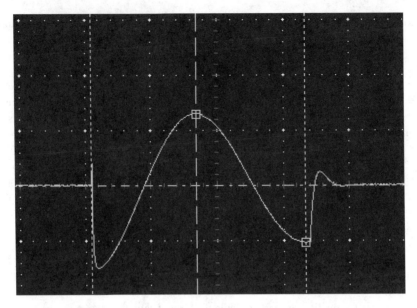

FIGURE 37.2 The induced electric field of a figure-of-eight coil vs. time over a TMS pulse cycle. The timescale is 100 μs.

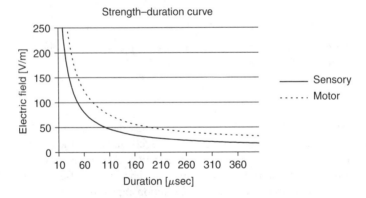

FIGURE 37.3 Neural strength–duration curve depicting stimulation threshold vs. duration.

It is possible, however, to increase considerably the depth penetration and the percentage of electric field intensity in deep brain regions, relative to the maximal field at the cortex. The next section outlines the construction principles for efficient deep brain stimulation, and the following sections demonstrates several examples of TMS coils designed to accomplish this goal.

37.3 Deep TMS Coils: Design Principles

While the activation of peripheral nerves depends mainly on the derivative of the electric field along the nerve fiber [Maccabee et al., 1993], the most relevant parameter for activation of brain structures seems to be the electric field intensity [Amassian et al., 1992; Thielscher and Kammer, 2002]. In both cases, however, Physiological studies indicate that optimal activation occurs when the field is oriented in the same direction as the nerve fiber [Durand et al., 1989; Roth and Basser 1990; Basser and Roth 1991; Brasil-Neto et al., 1992, Mills et al., 1992, Pascual-Leone et al., 1994, Niehaus et al., 2000, Kammer et al., 2001]. Hence, in order to stimulate deep brain regions, it is necessary to use coils in such an orientation that they will produce a significant field in the preferable direction to activate the neuronal structures or axons under consideration.

In light of these findings, the geometrical features of each specific design are mainly dependent on two goals:

1. The location and size of the deep brain region or regions intended to be activated
2. The preferred direction or directions we want to stimulate

The design of a specific coil is dictated by these goals. Nevertheless, all deep TMS coils have to share the following important features:

1. *Base complementary to the human head*: The part of the coil close to the head (the base) must be optimally complementary to the human skull at the desired region. In some coils the base may be flexible and be able to receive the shape of an individual patient, and in other coils it may be more robust, namely arcuated in a shape that fits the average human skull at the desired region. In the latter case there may be few similar models designed to fit smaller and larger heads.

2. *Proper orientation of stimulating coil elements*: Coils must be oriented such that they will produce a considerable field in a direction tangential to the surface, which should also be the preferable direction to activate the neurons under consideration. That is, wires of the coils are directed in one or more directions, which results in a preferred activation of neuronal structures orientated in these particular directions. In some cases, there is one preferred direction along the length or width axis, and in other cases, there are two preferred directions along both the length and width axes.

3. *Summation of electric impulses*: The induced electric field in the desired deep brain regions is obtained by optimal summation of electric fields, induced by several coil elements with common direction, located in different locations around the skull. The principle of summation may be applied either in time or in space or in a combination of both. The main kinds of summation are listed below:

(a) *One-point spatial summation*: In this kind of summation coil elements, carrying current in the desired direction, are placed in various locations around the head in such a configuration to create high electric field intensity in a specific deep brain region, which is simultaneously a high percent of the maximal electric field at the brain cortex.

(b) *Morphological line spatial summation*: The goal of this summation is to induce electric field at several points along a certain neuronal structure. This line should not be straight and may have a complex bent path. The application of diffusion tensor imaging (DTI) in magnetic resonance imaging (MRI) for fiber tracking is an evolving field, which may improve significantly the efficacy of TMS treatment. If, for example, we know the path of a certain axonal bundle, a coil shall be designed in a configuration that will produce significant electric field at several points along the bundle. This configuration may enable induction of an action potential in this bundle, while minimizing the activation of other brain regions. For example, the TMS coil may be activated in an intensity that will induce subthreshold electric field at most brain regions, which will not induce an action potential, while the induction of subthreshold field along the desired path may induce an action potential in this bundle, thus increasing the specificity of the TMS treatment.

(c) *Temporal summation*: The various coil elements may be stimulated consecutively and not simultaneously. As shown in Figure 37.3, the neuronal activation threshold depends on both electric field intensity and the stimulation duration. The TMS coil may be designed in such configuration that the various elements are scattered around the desired region or path, so that passing a current in each element will produce a significant field at the desired deep brain region. In such a case, the coil may be stimulated consecutively, so that at each time period only a certain element or a group of elements are activated. This way, in the desired deep brain region will be induced a significant electric field at all time periods while in more cortical regions a significant field will be induced mainly at certain periods when proximate coil elements are activated. This will enable stimulation of the deep brain structure while minimizing stimulation of other brain regions and specifically of cortical regions. A detailed study into the neural response to trains with inter-pulse intervals of milliseconds (instead of hundreds if milliseconds as in rTMS) will aid in refining this technique.

4. *Minimization of radial components*: Coil construction is meant to minimize wire elements carrying current components which are nontangential to the skull. Electrical field intensity in the tissue to be stimulated and the rate of decrease of electrical field as a function of distance from the coil depend on the orientation of the coil elements relative to the tissue surface. It has been shown that coil elements which are nontangential to the surface induce accumulation of surface charge, which leads to cancellation of the perpendicular component of the induced field at all points within the tissue, and reduction of the electrical field in all other directions. At each specific point, the produced electric field is affected by the lengths of the nontangential components, and their distances from this point. Thus, the length of coil elements which are not tangential to the brain tissue surface should be minimized. Furthermore, the nontangential coil elements should be as small as possible and placed as far as possible from the deep region to be activated.

5. *Remote location of return paths*: The wires leading currents in a direction opposite to the preferred direction (the return paths) should be located far from the base and the desired brain region. This enables higher absolute electric field in the desired brain region. In some cases the return paths may be in the air, namely, far from the head. In other cases part of the return paths may be adjacent to a different region in the head which is distant from the desired brain region.

6. *Shielding*: Feature 5 enables the possibility of screening. Since the return paths are far from the main base, it is possible to screen all, or part of their field, by inserting a shield around them or between them and the base. The shield is comprised of a material with high magnetic permeability, capable of inhibiting or diverting a magnetic field, such as mu metal, iron, or steel core. Alternatively the shield is comprised of a metal with high conductivity which can cause electric currents or charge accumulation that may oppose the effect produced by the return portions.

Specific deep TMS coils for stimulating different deep brain regions are described in the next sections.

37.4   A Coil for Stimulation of Deep Brain Regions Related to Mood Disorders: Simulations and Phantom Measurements

Accumulating evidence suggests that the nucleus accumbens plays a major role in mediating reward and motivation [Self and Nestler, 1995; Schultz et al., 1997; Breiter and Rosen, 1999; Ikemoto and Panksepp, 1999; Kalivas and Nakamura, 1999]. Functional MRI and positron emission tomographic studies showed that the nucleus accumbens is activated in cocaine addicts in response to cocaine administration [Lyons et al., 1996; Breiter et al., 1997]. Other brain regions are also associated with reward circuits, such as the ventral tegmental area, amygdala, and medial prefrontal, cingulate, and orbitofrontal cortices [Breiter and Rosen, 1999; Kalivas and Nakamura, 1999]. Moreover, neuronal fibers connecting the medial prefrontal, cingulate, or orbitofrontal cortex with the nucleus accumbens may have an important role in reward and motivation [Jentsch and Taylor, 1999; Volkow and Fowler, 2000]. The nucleus accumbens is also connected to the amygdala and the ventral tegmental area. Therefore, activation of these brain regions may affect neuronal circuits mediating reward and motivation. In rats and monkeys and even in humans, electrical stimulation of the median forebrain bundle is rewarding, and when a stimulating electrode is inserted into various parts of that bundle (including the ventral tegmental area, the median prefrontal cortex and the nucleus accumbens septi), compulsive self-stimulation can be obtained [Milner, 1991; Jacques, 1999]. The new coil (termed the *Hesed coil*) is designed to stimulate effectively deeper brain regions without increasing the electrical field intensity in the superficial cortical regions. Numeric simulations and phantom measurements of the total electrical field produced by the Hesed coil inside a homogeneous spherical volume conductor are presented and compared with results from a circular coil in different orientations and from the double-cone coil. The drop of the electrical field in the brain as a function of the distance from the new coil is much slower compared with previous coils. It is hoped that such a coil can stimulate deeper regions such as the nucleus accumbens and the fibers connecting the medial prefrontal or cingulate cortex with the nucleus accumbens. Activation of these fibers may induce reward, and chronic treatment may have antidepressant properties or serve as a new strategy against drug addiction.

37.4.1 Methods

37.4.1.1 Numerical Simulations

The simulations were conducted using a Mathematical program [Wolfram, 1999]. The head was modeled as a spherical homogeneous volume conductor with a radius of 7 cm. The induced and electrostatic field at a specific point inside the spherical volume were computed for several coil configurations, using the method presented by Eaton [1992], and the total electric fields in the x, y, and z directions were calculated.

The vector potential A and scalar potential Φ can be expanded in terms of spherical harmonic functions up to N order. After enforcing the boundary conditions at the sphere boundary, the final expressions for the total electric field in the three Cartesian directions are:

$$E_j = E_{Aj} + E_{\Phi j}, \quad j = x, y, z \tag{37.9}$$

where the induced field in each direction is given by:

$$E_{Aj} = -\mu_0 \frac{\partial I}{\partial t} \sum_{l=0}^{N} \sum_{m=-l}^{l} Y_{lm}(\theta, \varphi) C_{lm}^{j}, \quad j = x, y, z \tag{37.10}$$

where $Y_{lm}(\theta, \varphi)$ are spherical harmonic functions, r, θ, and φ are spherical coordinates of the point inside the conductive sphere where the electric field is calculated (see Figure 37.4), and C_{lm}^{j} are jth component of the integration over the coil path:

$$C_{lm}^{j} = \int_{coil} \frac{Y_{lm}^{*}(\theta', \varphi') dl j}{(2l+1) r'^{l+1}}, \quad j = x, y, z \tag{37.11}$$

where $*$ means complex conjugate, r', θ', and φ' are spherical coordinates of the coil element (Figure 37.4), and dlj is the jth component of the differential element of the coil.

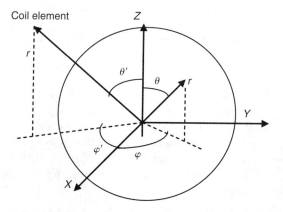

FIGURE 37.4 The relation between the spherical coordinate system and the Cartesian coordinate system in which the field components in every point were calculated. R is the radius vector to the point inside the sphere where the field is computed, and r' is the vector to the differential coil element on which the integration is performed.

The electrostatic fields in x, y, and z directions are given by:

$$E_{\Phi x} = -\sin(\theta)\cos(\varphi)\sum_{l=1}^{N+1}\sum_{m=-l}^{l} V_{lm} l r^{l-1} Y_{lm}(\theta,\varphi)$$

$$+ \cos(\varphi)\cos(\varphi)\sum_{l=1}^{N+1}\sum_{m=-l}^{l} V_{lm} r^{l-1}\tfrac{1}{2}[\exp(i\varphi)\sqrt{((l-m+1)(l+m))}Y_{l,m-1}(\theta,\varphi)$$

$$- \exp(-i\varphi)\sqrt{((l+m+1)(l-m))}Y_{l,m+1}(\theta,\varphi)]$$

$$+ \frac{\sin(\varphi)}{\sin(\theta)}\sum_{l=1}^{N+1}\sum_{m=-l}^{l} V_{lm} r^{l-1} im Y_{lm}(\theta,\varphi) \tag{37.12}$$

$$E_{\Phi y} = -\sin(\theta)\sin(\varphi)\sum_{l=1}^{N+1}\sum_{m=-l}^{l} V_{lm} l r^{l-1} Y_{lm}(\theta,\varphi)$$

$$+ \cos(\theta)\sin(\varphi)\sum_{l=1}^{N+1}\sum_{m=-l}^{l} V_{lm} r^{l-1}\tfrac{1}{2}[\exp(i\varphi)\sqrt{((l-m+1)(l+m))}Y_{l,m-1}(\theta,\varphi)$$

$$- \exp(-i\varphi)\sqrt{((l+m+1)(l-m))}Y_{l,m+1}(\theta,\varphi)]$$

$$+ \frac{\cos(\varphi)}{\sin(\theta)}\sum_{l=1}^{N+1}\sum_{m=-l}^{l} V_{lm} r^{l-1} im Y_{lm}(\theta,\varphi) \tag{37.13}$$

$$E_{\Phi z} = -\cos(\theta)\sum_{l=1}^{N+1}\sum_{m=-l}^{l} V_{lm} l r^{l-1} Y_{lm}(\theta,\varphi)$$

$$- \sin(\theta)\sum_{l=1}^{N+1}\sum_{m=-l}^{l} V_{lm} r^{l-1}\tfrac{1}{2}[\exp(i\varphi)\sqrt{((l-m+1)(l+m))}Y_{l,m-1}(\theta,\varphi)$$

$$- \exp(-i\varphi)\sqrt{((l+m+1)(l-m))}Y_{l,m+1}(\theta,\varphi)] \tag{37.14}$$

where $i = \sqrt{-1}$, and V_{lm} is a complex function of the integrals over coil path C_{lm}^{j}:

$$V_{lm} = -\frac{\mu_0}{l}\frac{\partial I}{\partial t}(\sqrt{[(l+m-1)(l+m)/(2l+1)(2l-1)]}0.5(C_{l-1,m-1}^{y} i - C_{l-1,m-1}^{x})$$

$$+ \sqrt{[(l-m-1)(l-m)/(2l+1)(2l-1)]}0.5(C_{l-1,m+1}^{y} i + C_{l-1,m+1}^{x})$$

$$+ \sqrt{[(l-m)(l+m)/(2l+1)(2l-1)]}C_{l-1,m}^{z}) \tag{37.15}$$

The simulations were performed using 10th order approximation. The summations in Equation 37.10 to Equation 37.15 were computed up to $N = 10$. The convergence rate depends on the distance from coil elements and on coil configuration, and in general, is faster for more remote points. For the new coil design, the convergence rate was faster than for the circular coil. For points close to the coils (up to 1.5 cm), the induced field was corrected by the exact formula (Equation 37.5). For more remote points the error was less than 1%. In all the calculations, the rate of current change was taken as 10,000 A/100 μsec. The field is given in volts per meter.

37.4.1.2 Measurements of the Electrical Field Induced in a Phantom Brain

The electrical field induced by the new coil and the double-cone coil (Magstim; Whitland, UK) was measured in a saline solution placed in a hollow glass model of the human head ($15 \times 17 \times 20$ cm^3; Cardinal

Industries, Inc., Milwaukee, WI, USA), using a two-wire probe. The distance between the noninsulated edges of the two wires of the probe was 14 mm. Voltage measured divided by the distance between the wire edges gives the induced electrical field figure. Stimulation was delivered using the Magstim Model 200 stimulator at 100% power level. The coils were placed on the glass surface and the electrical field was measured in numerous points within the saline solution.

37.4.2 Results

The simulations revealed that, in general, the presence of accumulating surface charge induced by coil configurations having a radial current component changes the total field in a nontrivial way. The presence of an electrostatic field not only reduces the total field at any point, but also leads to significant reduction in the percentage of the total field in depth, relative to total field at the surface. Moreover, both the total field and the percentage relative to the surface at any specific point depend on its distance from the nontangential coil elements.

The basic concept of the new coil design is to generate summation of the electrical field in depth by inducing electrical fields at different locations around the surface of the head, all of which have a common direction. Such an approach increased the percentage of electrical field induced in depth, relative to the field in the surface regions. In addition, because a radial component had a dramatic effect on the percentage of the electrical field in depth, an effort was made to minimize the overall length of nontangential coil elements, and to locate them as distant as possible from the deep region to be activated. This region simulated the location of the nucleus accumbens. Calculations for several coil configurations were made and the optimal configuration (termed the *Hesed coil*) was compared with standard circular coils and with the double-cone coil. We compare simulation results of field distribution of the Hesed coil design (Figure 37.5), of a double-cone coil, and of a circular coil oriented perpendicular (Figure 37.6[a]) and parallel (Figure 37.6b) to the head. Figure 37.5 shows the coil design when applied on the human head. The coil contains several strips (26 in the example of Figure 37.5) attached to the head, all connected serially, and having wires that induce stimulation in the desired direction. This desired direction is the anteroposterior direction in the example shown in Figure 37.5 (z direction). For each strip there is a return path wire having current component at the opposite direction (z direction), located 5 cm above the head. These return paths are located at the top edges of four fans to remove the currents flowing through them away from the deep regions of the head. The specific design of the fans is meant to reduce the inductance of the coil. The fans are connected to the frame near strips 7, 9, 18, and 20 (see Figure 37.5). These loci were chosen to remove the return paths as much as possible from the deep brain region to be activated most effectively. The only wires with currents that have radial components are those connecting the strips that are attached to the head with their return paths, along the sides of the fans. An optimized coil would have a flexible frame allowing all elements of the coil that are touching the head to be tangential to the head surface (see Figure 37.5).

In the calculations of the field produced by the Hesed coil design, we assumed that the only coil elements carrying current components that are not tangential to the surface are the wires connecting the return paths with the strips that are attached to the head (along the fans). This is a plausible assumption in the realistic case, where the coil is attached to the skull. In the human head, the cerebral spinal fluid is approximately parallel to the skull everywhere and it can be assumed that the conductive properties of the cerebral spinal fluid are similar to those of the brain. The electrostatic field resulting from the contribution of the nontangential elements was calculated for each point and subtracted from the induced field of the coil. To obtain maximal efficacy, given the limitations of the stimulator and the need for a specific range of the coil inductance (15 to 25 μH), the average lengths of the strips were taken as 8 cm. The simulations were made for strips of length of 9 cm over one hemisphere and of 7 cm over the other (to obtain a slight preference for one hemisphere stimulation and to have the opportunity to reach stimulation threshold in one hemisphere only). The wires connecting the head strips to their return paths (the nontangential elements) were taken as 5 cm long. The locations of the strips were determined to fit the human head, as in Figure 37.5. Hence, the distances of strips 13 and 14 from the sphere center were taken as approximately

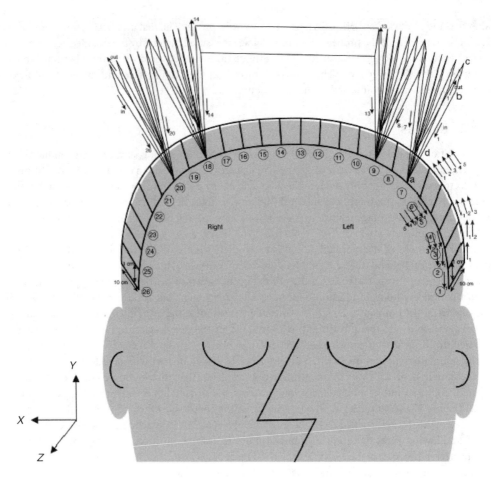

FIGURE 37.5   The Hesed coil shape when applied over the human head. The same coil can be placed around the forehead to stimulate nerve fibers in the superoinferior direction. The only elements that produce an electrical field in the z-direction are the 26 strips attached to the head (numbered 1 to 26), where the current is in the $+z$ direction, and the 26 return paths at the edges of the fans where the current is in the $-z$ direction.

6 cm; strips 3 and 24 were located approximately 7 cm from the sphere center. For the orientation shown in Figure 37.5, the maximal total field in the anteroposterior direction (z direction) was produced at the cortex near the center of strips 1 and 26 at the sides. The field at the top of the head was reduced considerably because of the influence of the return paths and of the nontangential wires along the sides of the fans.

Figure 37.7 shows the induced (Figure 37.7a) and total (Figure 37.7b) field in the z-direction (Ez, defined in Figure 37.6) of a one-turn 5.5-cm-diameter circular coil placed perpendicular and parallel to a 7-cm-radius spherical volume conductor, as a function of distance from the coil edge. The fields were calculated along the line connecting the sphere center to the coil point closest to the surface (line o–p in Figure 37.6). It is clear that the reduction in total field resulting from charge accumulation is much larger when the coil is oriented perpendicular to surface (Figure 37.7). In addition, a comparison was made with the induced and total fields of one winding from the new Hesed coil, including strip 1 with its connection to the return path and its return path itself (and taking strips length of 5.5 cm). The simulations show that although the induced field of the strip is slightly larger than that of a circular coil with similar dimensions (see Figure 37.7), the difference in the total field is much larger (see Figure 37.7). This results from the fact that the field reduction due to electrostatic charge accumulation in the case of the winding of strip 1 is very small, because the only elements carrying radial current components are the wires along paths

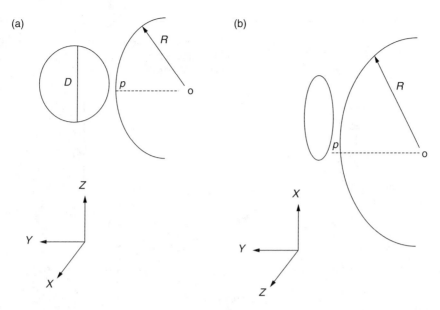

FIGURE 37.6 (a) A circular coil with diameter D placed perpendicular to the head surface. The head is modeled as a sphere with a radius $R = 7$ cm. The coil has current component in the y-direction, which is perpendicular to the head, and a component in the z-direction, which is completely parallel to the head surface only at the attachment point p. (b) A circular coil with diameter D placed tangential to the head surface. The coil has current components in the x- and z-directions, which are completely parallel to the head surface only at the attachment point p.

a–b and c–d (see Figure 37.5), which are a relatively small fraction of the winding length, and are distant from the points under consideration. The induced and total field in z-direction (Ez) resulting from the entire Hesed coil compared with the double-cone coil is shown in Figure 37.8. The field of the Hesed coil is computed along the line from strip 26 (where it is maximal) to the sphere center. The field of the double-cone coil is computed along the line from the junction at the coil center (where it is maximal) to the sphere center. Although the double-cone coil produces a much larger-induced field than the Hesed coil (see Figure 37.8a), the rate of decay of the effective total field with distance is much smaller for the Hesed coil (see Figure 37.8b). Hence, at depth of 6 cm, the total electrical field of the Hesed coil is already a little larger than that of the double-cone coil (see Figure 37.8b).

Figure 37.9 shows the z-component of the electrical field as a function of distance, relative to the field at a distance of 1 cm, for the Hesed coil, a double-cone coil with 14-cm diameter for each wing, and the 5.5-cm-diameter circular coil oriented tangential and perpendicular to the head surface. The field produced by the Hesed coil at a depth of 6 cm is approximately 35% of the field at a depth of 1 cm near the middle of strip 26 (where the field induced by the Hesed coil is highest throughout the brain). The field produced by the double-cone coil at a depth of 6 cm is only about 8% of the field 1 cm from the coil. The field produced by the 5.5-cm-diameter circular coil at this depth is less than 2% of the field 1 cm from the coil. For a larger circular coil, the percentage of field in depth is somewhat higher, but still smaller than that of the double-cone coil (data not shown).

Actual measurements of the electrical fields in a phantom brain using the first manufactured version of the Hesed coil and a double-cone coil basically confirmed our theoretical calculations. Both coils produced slightly lower fields at any point in the phantom brain compared with the theoretical calculations. However, this was more evident in the case of the Hesed coil, and the percentage of field in depth relative to the surface was slightly lower compared with our calculations. The results for the total field and the percentage in depth are presented in Figure 37.10.

It is clear that the total field induced by the double-cone coil, using the maximal output of the stimulator (10,000 A/100 μsec) produces a markedly greater electrical field up to 6-cm depth, compared with the

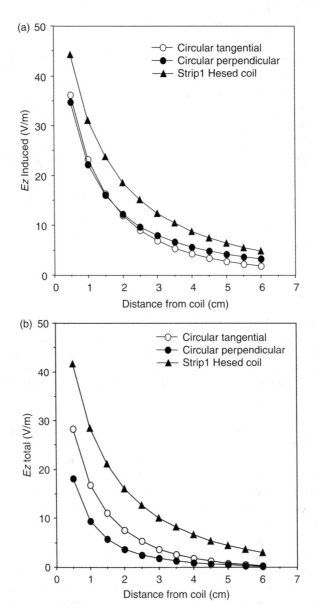

FIGURE 37.7   (a,b) Induced (a) and total (b) electrical field in the z-direction plotted as a function of distance from a one-turn circular coil of 5.5-cm diameter placed tangential or perpendicular to the head surface. In addition the induced and total fields of the winding of the Hesed coil connected to strip 1 (see Figure 37.2) is shown for the case of strip length of 5.5 cm.

Hesed coil (see Figure 37.10a), but the percentage in depth is markedly greater when the Hesed coil is used (see Figure 37.10b).

37.5   Transcranial Magnetic Stimulation of Deep Brain Regions: Evidence for Efficacy of the H-Coil

The biological efficacy of the H-coil was tested [Zangen et al., 2005] using the motor threshold as a measure of a biological effect. The rate of decrease of the electric field as a function of distance from the

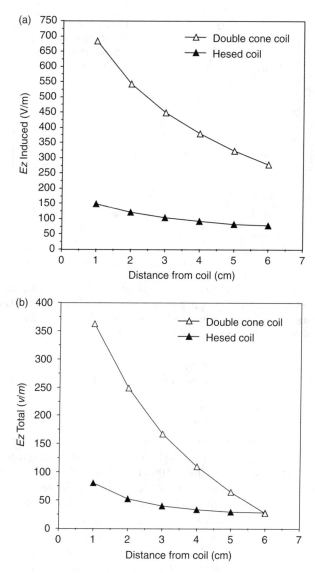

FIGURE 37.8 (a,b) Induced (a) and total (b) electrical field in the z-direction plotted as a function of distance for the double-cone coil and the Hesed coil. The electrical fields were calculated for a six-turn double-cone coil with a diameter of 14 cm for each wing, an opening angle of 95°, and a central linear section of 3 cm, and for the Hesed coil with strip lengths of 9 cm over the right hemisphere and 7 cm over the left hemisphere. The field of the Hesed coil is computed along the line from strip 26 (where Ez is maximal) to the sphere center. The field of the double-cone coil is computed along the line from the central linear section (where Ez is maximal) to the sphere center.

coil was measured by gradually increasing the distance of the coil from the skull and measuring the motor threshold at each distance. A comparison was made to the figure-8 coil.

37.5.1 Methods

37.5.1.1 Subject

Six healthy, right-handed volunteers (4 men and 2 women, mean age 36 yr, range 25 to 45 yr) gave written informed consent for the study, which was approved by the National Institute of Neurological Disorders

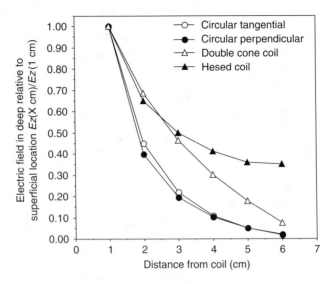

FIGURE 37.9 Electrical field in the z-direction relative to the field 1 cm from the coil as a function of distance. Data are presented for the Hesed coil, the double-cone coil, and the 5.5-cm-diameter circular coil oriented tangential and perpendicular to the head surface. The total electrical field in each point along the line from the point of maximal Ez to the sphere center was divided by the Ez value calculated at a 1-cm distance.

and Stroke Institutional Review Board. Subjects were interviewed and examined by a neurologist and found to be free of any significant medical illness or medications known to affect the CNS.

37.5.2 TMS Coils

The TMS coils used in this study were a specific version of the H-coil and a figure-of-eight coil. The H-coil version used in this study allows a comfortable placement above the hand motor cortex. The theoretical considerations and design principles of the H-coils are explained in our previous study [Roth et al., 2002]. In short, the coil is designed to generate summation of the electric field in a specific brain region by locating coil elements at different locations around this region, all of which have a common current component which induce electric field in the desired direction (termed $+z$ direction). In addition, since a radial component has a dramatic effect on electric field magnitude and on the rate of decay of the electric field with distance, the overall length of coil elements which are nontangential to the skull should be minimized, and these elements as well as coil elements having current component in the opposite direction ($-z$ direction) should be located as distant as possible from the brain region to be activated.

The H-coil version used in the present study is shown in Figure 37.11. The coil has 10 strips carrying a current in a common direction ($+z$ direction) and located around the desired motor cortex site (segments A–B and G–H in Figure 37.11). The average length of the strips is 11 cm. The only coil elements having radial current components are those connected to the return paths of five of the strips (segments C–I and J–F in Figure 37.1). The length of these wires is 8 cm. The return paths of the other five strips are placed on the head at the contralateral hemisphere (segment D–E in Figure 37.11). The wires connecting between the strips and the return paths (segments B–C and F–A in Figure 37.11) are on average 9-cm long. The H-coil was compared to a standard commercial Magstim figure-of-eight coil with internal loop diameters of 7 cm.

37.5.2.1 Experimental Setup

Subjects were seated with the right forearm and hand supported. Motor evoked potentials (MEPs) of the right APB muscle were recorded using silver–silver chloride surface electrodes. Subjects were instructed to maintain muscle relaxation throughout the study. Electromyogram (EMG) amplitude was amplified using a conventional EMG machine (Counterpoint, Dantec Electronics, Skovlunde, Denmark) with band-pass

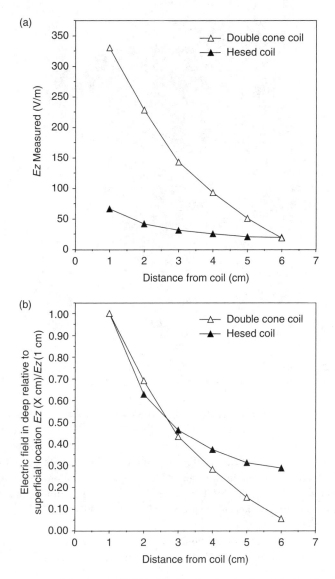

FIGURE 37.10 Measurements of the electrical field induced by the Hesed coil and the double-cone coil in a phantom brain. (a, b) The electrical field induced in the z-direction (a) and the electrical field in the z-direction *relative* to the field 1 cm from the coil (b) is plotted as a function of distance from the coil. For both coils, the data show the measurements along the line from the point where maximal Ez value is obtained (as described earlier) to the sphere center.

between 10 and 2,000 Hz. The signal was digitized at a frequency of 5 kHz and fed into a laboratory computer.

A magstim super rapid stimulator (The Magstim Company New York, NY), which produces a biphasic pulse, coupled with either the figure-8 coil or the H-coil, was used. Preliminary studies showed the H-coil to have a loudness when activated of 122 dB, similar to other coils used in our laboratory. As a standard laboratory practice, subjects were fitted with foam ear plugs to attenuate the sound.

The coil was placed on the scalp over the left motor cortex. The intersection of the figure-8 coil was placed tangentially to the scalp with the handle pointing backward and laterally at a 45° angle away from the midline. Thus the current induced in the neural tissue was directed approximately perpendicular to the line of the central sulcus and therefore optimal for activating the corticospinal pathways transsynaptically [Brasil-Neto et al. 1992; Kaneko et al. 1996]. Similarly, the H-coil was placed on the scalp with the handle

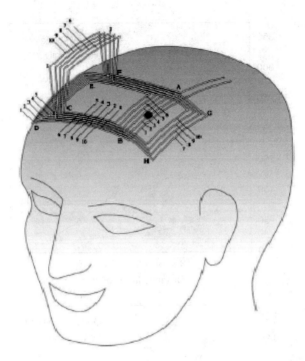

FIGURE 37.11   Sketch of the H-coil version used in this study placed on a human head. The coil orientation shown in the figure is designated for optimal stimulation of the left abductor pollicis brevis (APB) (indicated by a black spot).

pointing backward in such a way that the center of the strips cover the motor cortex and in such a direction that the current induced in the neural tissue would be perpendicular to the line of the central sulcus. With a slightly suprathreshold stimulus intensity, the stimulating coil was moved over the left hemisphere to determine the optimal position for eliciting MEPs of maximal amplitudes (the "hot spot"). The optimal position of the coil was then marked on the scalp to ensure coil placement throughout the experiment. Resting motor threshold was determined to the nearest 1% of the maximum stimulator output and was defined as the minimal stimulus intensity required to produce MEPs of >50 μV in document ≥ 5 of 10 consecutive trials at least 5 sec apart.

The coils were held in a stable coil holder, which could be adjusted at different heights above the "hot spot" on the scalp. The resting motor threshold was determined at different distances above the scalp, using increments of 0.5 cm.

37.5.2.2 Safety Measurements

Since the H-coil was not used in previous clinical TMS studies, we asked the subjects to report any side effects including pain, anxiety, or dizziness and we performed cognitive and hearing tests before and after the TMS session. For the cognitive testing we used the CalCap computer program to test immediate and delayed memory as described previously [Wassermann et al., 1996].

37.5.3 Results

None of the six subjects who participated in the study reported any significant side effects after the TMS session. We did not find any change in cognitive or hearing abilities in these six subjects. A slight and short-lasting headache was reported by one out of the six subjects. In a different experiment done subsequently, not reported in this book, we used the H-coil to deliver single or paired pulses at 1 Hz during 20 sec over five different locations on the scalp in three additional subjects. The third of these subjects experienced some hearing loss in his left ear, a 30-dB loss at 4000 Hz which has been stable for 10 months and appears permanent. The ear protection had fallen out transiently during the study.

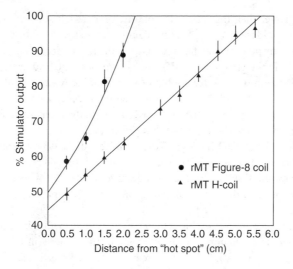

FIGURE 37.12   Intensity needed for APB stimulation at different heights above the scalp. Resting motor threshold of the APB was measured at different distances above the "hot spot" when using either the H-coil or the figure-8 coil. The percentage of stimulator power needed to reach the resting motor threshold vs. the distance of the coil from the "hot spot" on the skull is plotted. The points represent means and SDs of six healthy volunteers.

The percentage of stimulator output required for APB activation by each coil is plotted in Figure 37.12 as a function of distance from the "hot spot" on the scalp. It can be seen that the efficacy of the H-coil at large distances from the scalp was significantly greater as compared to the figure-8 coil. When using the maximal stimulation power output, the figure-8 coil can be effective (reach stimulation threshold) up to 2 cm away from the coil, while the H-coil can be effective at 5.5 cm away from the coil. Moreover, the rate of decay of effectiveness as a function of the distance from the coil is much slower in the H-coil relative to the figure-8 coil (Figure 37.12).

37.5.4   Discussion

The findings confirm our theoretical calculations and phantom brain measurements [Roth et al., 2002] indicating the ability of the H-coil to stimulate brain structures at a large distance from the coil. The comparison between the TMS coils demonstrated a significantly improved depth penetration, and a much slower rate of decay of effectiveness as a function of the distance from the coil, when using the H-coil relative to the regular figure-8 coil. This indicates that when stimulating deep brain regions by using the H-coil, the cortical stimulation is not much higher for the same activation in depth.

The H-coil produces a summation of the electric field from several coil elements carrying current in the same direction. In contrast, the electric field of the figure-8 coil is produced by a concentrated region in the center of the coil. In addition, the relative fraction of the figure-8 field that is produced by coil elements which are nontangential to skull surface is much larger then in the H-coil. These two reasons lead to the fact that although the figure 8 field is more focal, it has more significant reduction both in absolute field magnitude at any point and in the percentage of the deep region field relative to field at the surface.

According to our calculations and phantom brain measurements [Roth et al., 2002], the field induced in cortical regions by the H-coil is much lower than that of the double-cone coil. Therefore, it is likely that excitation threshold can be reached at 4 to 6 cm using the H-coil without inducing pain and other side effects.

It should be emphasized that although the structure stimulated in this study was in the motor cortex, and the medium between the coils and the "hot spot" was mainly air, the rate of decay within the brain itself should be very similar. This is a delicate point that should be elaborated. The electric conductivity of the brain is much greater then that of air. In conductive materials such as the brain, radial current components of the coil would lead to charge accumulation on the surface of the brain, which would cause a decrease of the field in any point inside the brain. Hence, the rate of decay of electric field with distance would be faster in the brain then that measured in air. Nevertheless, the field distribution inside the brain is *independent* of the location of the interface between the conductive and insulating media [Branston and Tofts 1990; Tofts 1990; Eaton 1992]. As a result, the rate of decay within the brain when attaching the coil to the skull would be similar to that measured in this study, where the coil was raised above the skull. Small changes are expected due to the fact that coil configuration relative to the skull is somewhat different when it is raised. The H-coil is designed to minimize radial current components when attached to the scalp; hence the amount of radial components may be slightly different and probably larger when the H-coil is raised above the scalp. Therefore, the advantage of the H-coil as compared to the figure-8 coil, in terms of the rate of decay of the field as a function of distance, may be even greater when the coils are attached to the scalp.

Although the H-coil has a remarkable ability to penetrate into deeper brain regions, due to the slower decay of the electric field as a function of distance, none of the subjects in the present study reported any side effects and cognitive or hearing abilities were not affected. Nevertheless, it should be emphasized that subjects in the present study experienced only 20 to 30 single pulses at intensities greater then those needed for minimal APB activation (when looking for the hot spot for APB activation) and that the rest of the pulses were given just at the minimal level for APB activation when the coil was placed either on the scalp or at different heights above the scalp. Future studies will address the safety and efficacy of the H-coil when used in higher doses. As we have reported, one subject has experienced some hearing loss in a subsequent experiment. Our past safety studies have not demonstrated that hearing loss is to be expected [Pascual-Leone et al., 1992]. As the loudness of the H-coil does not appear different from other coils, this result may be due in part to particularly sensitive hearing in this subject and lapse in the hearing protection. However, as we did caution before, the event does emphasize need in all TMS studies to take care to protect hearing.

37.6   Transcranial Magnetic Stimulation of Deep Prefrontal Regions

Medial prefrontal and orbitofrontal regions are known to be associated with reward circuits. The H1 and H2 coils are designed to stimulated deep prefrontal structures, with minimal undesired side effects such as pain, motor stimulation, and facial muscles activation. The coils are wounded with a double 14 AWG (American Wire Gauge) insulated cupper wire winded into several windings, connected in series. Detailed illustration of the wiring pattern of H1 is shown in Figure 37.13, and of H2 is shown in Figure 37.14.

The effective part of the H1 coil in contact with the patient scalp has a shape of half a donut, with 14 strips of 7–12-cm length (Figure 37.13). These strips produce the most effective field of the coil, and are oriented in an anterior–posterior axis. The 14 strips are distributed above the prefrontal cortex of the left hemisphere, with a separation of 1 cm between them. Three strips (8–10 in Figure 37.13) are elongated toward the forehead, and their continuations pass in the left–right direction along the orbitofrontal cortex (segments I–J 8–10 in Figure 37.13), with a separation of 1 cm between them. The return paths of strips 1–7 are attached to the head in the right hemisphere (segments D–E 1–7 in Figure 37.13), with a separation of 0.8 cm between them. The return paths of strips 8–14 are remote 7 cm from the head (segments M–G 8–14 in Figure 37.13), with a separation of 0.3 cm between them.

The frame of the inner rim of the half donut is flexible in order to fit the variability in human skull shape.

The paths of the 14 windings of the H1 coil are shown in Figure 37.13. The windings of strips 1–7 traverse the path A–B–C–D–E–F–G–H–A. The winding of strips 8–10 traverse the path A–I–J–K–L–M–G–H–A. The windings of strip 11–14 traverse the path A–N–L–M–G–H–A.

H1-Coil Specifications

Number of Windings	14 wire loops, including strips and return paths
Strips length	Strips 1–7, 11–14: 7 cm
	Strips 8–10: 10–12 cm
Main induced field direction	Anterior–posterior axis
Strips separation	1 cm (typical)
Connecting cable	2 ± 0.5 m
Coil inductance (including cable)	$30 \pm 1 \ \mu$H
Max. magnetic field strength	3.2 T
Max. electric field strength 0.5 cm from coil	200 V/m
Wire size (circular section copper)	Two 14 AWG Insulated Wires in Parallel
Wire length	750 cm

Figure 37.14 shows a diagram of the H2 coil, which is designed to stimulate deep brain regions and fit the human head. The effective part of the coil in contact with the patient scalp has a shape of half a donut, with 10 strips of 14–22 cm length (Figure 37.14). These strips produce the most effective field of the coil, and are oriented in a right–left direction (lateral–medial axis). Three strips pass in front of the forehead along the orbitofrontal cortex (1–3 in Figure 37.14), with a separation of 1 cm between them. Seven strips pass above the forehead along the prefrontal cortex (4–10 in Figure 37.14), with 0.8-cm separation.

The paths of the ten windings are shown in Figure 37.3. The windings of strips 1–3 traverse the path A–B–C–D–E–F–G–H–I–J–Q–R–S–T–K–L–A. The winding of strip four traverses the path A–B–G–H–I–J–Q–R–S–T–K–L–A. The winding of strip five traverses the path A–M–N–B–G–O–P–H–I–J–Q–R–S–T–K–L–A. The windings of strips 6–7 traverse the path A–M–N–B–G–O–P–H–I–J–K–L–A. The windings of strips 8–9 traverse the path A–B–G–H–I–J–K–L–A. The winding of strip ten traverses the path A–H–I–J–K–L–A.

H2-Coil Specifications

Number of windings	10 wire loops, including strips and return paths
Strips length	14–22 cm
Main induced field direction	Lateral–medial axis
Strips separation	0.8 cm (typical)
Connecting cable	2 ± 0.5 m
Coil inductance (including cable)	$25 \pm 1 \ \mu$H
Max. magnetic field strength	3.0 T
Max. electric field strength 0.5 cm from coil	190 V/m
Wire size (circular section copper)	Two 14 AWG insulated wires in parallel
Wire length	800 cm

37.6.1 Comparison of Electric Field Distributions

The electric field distribution produced by H1 and H2 coils, were measured in a brain phantom with general dimensions of $23 \times 19 \times 15$ cm^3, which was filled with 0.9% weight/volume saline. In order to determine output of the coil at depth, the induced electric field was measured using a two-wire probe. The distance between the ends of the two-wire of the probe was measured to be 12.7 ± 0.2 mm. Voltage measured divided by the distance between the wires gives the induced electric field value. The two coils were compared to a standard Magstim Figure-8 coil with internal loop diameter of 7 cm, and a Magstim double-cone coil. The double-cone coil is considered to be able to stimulate deeper brain regions compared to other coils [Terao et al., 1994, 2000; Stokic et al., 1997].

The depth penetration of the coils was tested by measuring the electric field along the up–down line (Z-axis) beneath the center of the most effective part of the coil, at 100% output of Magstim Rapid stimulator. In H1 the most effective part was under strip 8 (under third of A–I 8 segment in Figure 37.13 above), where the probe is oriented in an anterior–posterior direction (Y-axis). In H2 the most effective

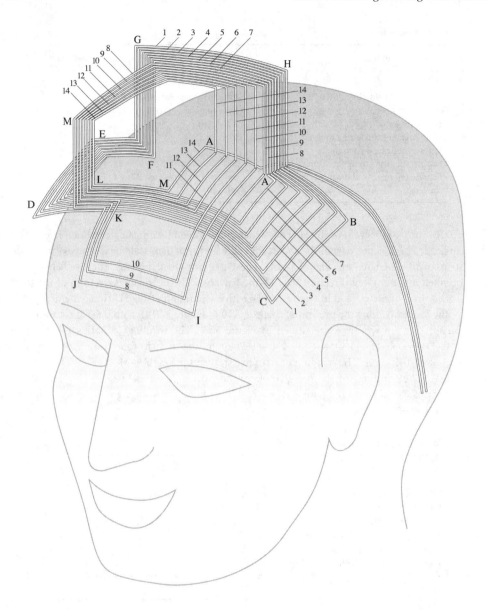

FIGURE 37.13   Sketch of the H1 coil near a human head. The coil orientation shown in the figure is designated for activation of structures in the prefrontal cortex, in the anterior–posterior direction.

part was the center of strip 5 (center of C–F 5 segment in Figure 37.14 above), where the probe is oriented in a lateral–medial direction (X-axis). In the double cone coil and the figure-8 coil, the most effective part was the junction at coil center, where the probe is oriented in an anterior–posterior direction (Y-axis). Plots of total electric field as a function of distance are shown in Figure 37.15.

Figure 37.16 shows the electric field as a function of distance, relative to the field at a distance of 1 cm, for the four coils.

It can be seen that the total electric field induced by the double-cone coil, and by the figure-8 coil, using the maximal output of the stimulator, is markedly greater than the field produced by the H1 and H2 at short distances of 1 to 2 cm. Yet, at distances of above 5 cm the fields of the H1 and H2 coils become greater, due to their much slower rate of decay. From Figure 37.16 it can be seen that the percentage in depth for the H coils is greater then the two other coils already at 2 cm distance, and this advantage of the

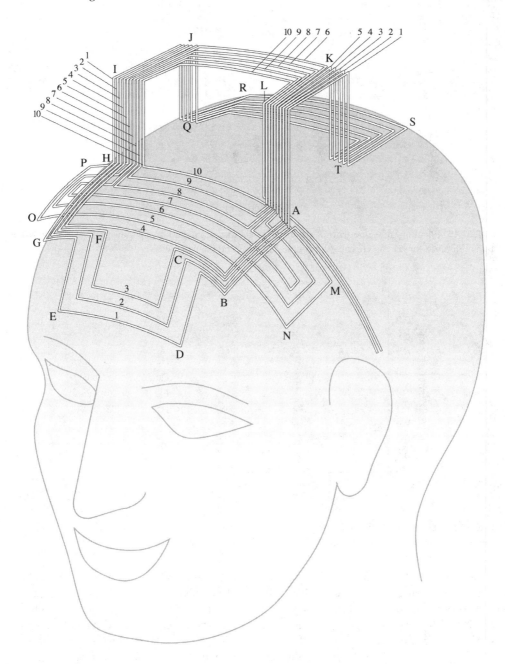

FIGURE 37.14 Sketch of the H2-coil near a human head. The coil orientation shown in the figure is designated for activation of structures in the prefrontal cortex, in the lateral–medial direction.

H coils becomes more prominent with increasing distance. Comparing between the two H coils it can be seen that H1 produces slightly smaller absolute field magnitude, but larger percentage in depth, relative to H2. The fields produced by the H1 and H2 at 6-cm depth are about 63 and 57% of the field 1 cm from the coil, respectively, while the fields of the double-cone coil and the figure-8 coil attenuate to 8 to 10% at this distance.

Stimulation of brain structures at 3–4 cm depth with the double-cone coil is painful since a much higher field is induced at superficial cortical areas and at the facial muscles. In order to reach stimulation

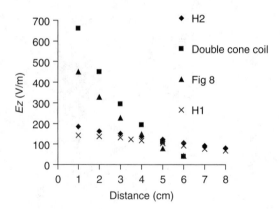

FIGURE 37.15 Phantom measurements of the electric field in the z-direction (up–down direction), plotted as a function of distance, for H1 and H2 coils, the double-cone coil, and the figure-8 coil.

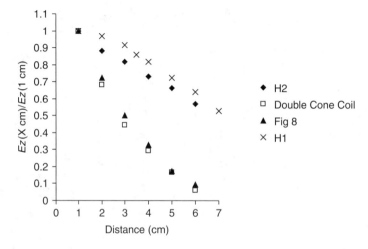

FIGURE 37.16 Electric field relative to the field 1 cm from coil, as a function of distance, for the H1 and H2 coils, the double-cone coil, and the figure-8 coil, according to the phantom brain measurements.

threshold at 5–8-cm depth, a much higher intensity would be needed which would increase pain and the risk for other side effects such as convulsions. The total field induced by the H1 and H2 coils, even at maximal power output, will be three to four times lower than the double cone in cortical regions. The H1 and H2 fields at 5–6-cm depth are not much smaller than their fields in the cortex and greater than the double-cone coil field at that depth. Therefore, it is likely that excitation threshold can be reached at 6–7 cm using the H coils, without the induction of pain and other side effects. The percentage of the electric field in depth produced by the standard figure-8 coils is similar to the double-cone coil, but the absolute field magnitude is much smaller. Therefore the figure-8 coil would not only cause greater side effects, but could not reach stimulation threshold in depth, even at maximal power output.

References

Amassian V.E., Eberle L., Maccabee P.J., and Cracco R.Q. Modeling magnetic coil excitation of human cerebral cortex with a peripheral nerve immersed in a brain-shaped volume conductor: the significance of fiber bending in excitation. *Electroenceph. Clin. Neurophysiol.* 1992; 85: 291–301.

Barker A.T., Jalinous R., and Freeston I.L. Non-invasive magnetic stimulation of the human motor cortex. *Lancet* 1985; 1: 1106–1107.

Barker A.T., Garnham C.W., and Freeston I.L. Magnetic nerve stimulation — the effect of waveform on efficiency, determination of neural membrane time constants and the measurement of stimulator output, in magnetic motor stimulation: basic principles and clinical experience. *Electroenceph. Clin. Neurophysiol.* 1991; 43: 227–237.

Basser P.J. and Roth B.J. Stimulation of a myelinated nerve axon by electromagnetic induction. *Med. Biol. Eng. Comput.* 1991; 29: 261–268.

Bohning D.H. Introduction and overview of TMS physics. In *Transcranial Magnetic Stimulation in Neuropsychiatry*, p. 13.

Bourland J.D., Nyenhuis J.A., Noe W.A., Schaefer J.D., Foster K.S., and Geddes L.A. Motor and sensory strength–duration curves for MRI gradient fields, in Proceedings of International Society Magnetic Resonance Medicine 4th *Scientific Meeting and Exhibit*, New York, 1996; p. 1724.

Branston N.M. and Tofts P.S. Magnetic stimulation of a volume conductor produces a negligible component of induced current perpendicular to the surface. *J. Physiol. (Lond.)* 1990; 423: 67.

Brasil-Neto J.P., Cohen L.G., Panizza M., Nilsson J., Roth B.J., and Hallett M. Optimal focal transcranial magnetic activation of the human motor cortex: effects of coil orientation, shape of the induced current pulse, and stimulus intensity. *J. Clin. Neurophysiol.* 1992; 9: 132–136.

Breiter H.C., Gollub R.L., Weisskoff R.M., et al. Acute effects of cocaine on human brain activity and emotion. *Neuron* 1997; 19: 591–611.

Breiter H.C. and Rosen B.R. Functional magnetic resonance imaging of brain reward circuitry in the human. *Ann. NY Acad. Sci.* 1999; 877: 523–547.

Cohen D. and Cuffin B.N. Developing a more focal magnetic stimulator. Part I: Some basic principles. *J. Clin. Neurophysiol.* 1991; 8: 102–111.

Cohen L.G., Roth B.J., Nilsson J., et al. Effects of coil design on delivery of focal magnetic stimulation. Technical considerations. *Electroencephal. Clin. Neurophysiol.* 1990; 75: 350–357.

Durand D., Ferguson A.S., and Dalbasti T. Induced electric fields by magnetic stimulation in non-homogeneous conducting media. *IEEE Eng. Med. Biol. Soc. 11th Annual International Conference*, Seatle, WA, 1989; 6: 1252–1253.

Eaton H. Electric field induced in a spherical volume conductor from arbitrary coils: application to magnetic stimulation and MEG. *Med. Biol. Eng. Comput.* 1992; 30: 433–440.

Heller L. and Van Hulstein D.B. Brain stimulation using electromagnetic sources: theoretical aspects. *Biophys. J.* 1992; 63: 129–138.

Ikemoto S. and Panksepp J. The role of nucleus accumbens dopamine in motivated behavior: a unifying interpretation with special reference to reward-seeking. *Brain. Res. Rev.* 1999; 31: 6–41.

Jacques S. Brain stimulation reward: "pleasure centers" after twenty five years. *Neurosurgery* 1999; 5: 277–283.

Jentsch J.D. and Taylor J.R. Impulsivity resulting from frontostriatal dysfunctionin drug abuse: implications for the control of behavior by reward-related behaviors. *Psychopharmacology* 1999; 146: 373–390.

Kalivas P.W. and Nakamura M. Neural systems for behavioral activation and reward. *Curr. Opin. Neurobiol.* 1999; 9: 223–227.

Kammer T., Beck S., Thielscher A., Laubis-Herrmann U., and Topka H. Motor thresholds in humans. Atranscranial magnetic stimulation study comparing different pulseforms, current directions and stimulator types. *Clin. Neurophysiol.* 2001; 112: 250–258.

Kaneko K., Kawai S., Fuchigami Y., Morita H., and Ofuji A. The effect of current direction induced by transcranial magnetic stimulation on the corticospinal excitability in human brain. *Electroenceph. Clin. Neurophysiol.* 1996; 101: 478–482.

Kirkcaldie M.T., Pridmore S.A., and Pascual-Leone A. Transcranial magnetic stimulation as therapy for depression and other disorders. *Aust. NZ J. Psychiat.* 1997; 31: 264–272.

Lyons D., Friedman D.P., Nader M.A., and Porrino L.J. Cocaine alters cerebral metabolism within the ventral striatum and limbic cortex of monkeys. *J. Neurosci.* 1996; 16: 1230–1238.

Maccabee P.J., Eberle L., Amassian V.E., Cracco R.Q., Rudell A., and Jayachandra M. Spatial distribution of the electric field induced in volume by round and figure "8" magnetic coils: relevance to activation of sensory nerve fibers. *Electroenceph. Clin. Neurophysiol.* 1990; 76: 131–141.

Maccabee P.J., Amassian V.E., Eberle V.E., and Cracco R.Q. Magnetic coil stimulation of straight and bent amphibian and mammalian peripheral nerve *in vitro*: Locus of excitation. *J. Physiol.* 1993; 460: 201–219.

Mills K.R., Boniface S.J., and Schubert M. Magnetic brain stimulation with a double coil: the importance of coil orientation. *Electroenceph. Clin. Neurophysiol.* 1992; 85: 17–21.

Milner P.M. Brain-stimulation reward: a review. *Can. J. Psychol.* 1991; 45: 1–36.

Niehaus L., Meyer B.U., and Weyh T. Influence of pulse configuration and direction of coil current on excitatory effects of magnetic motor cortex and nerve stimulation. *Clin. Neurophysiol.* 2000; 111: 75–80.

Pascual-Leone A., Cohen L.G., Shotland L.I., Dang N., Pikus A., Wassermann E.M., Brasil-Neto J.P., Valls-Sole J., and Hallett M. No evidence of hearing loss in humans due to transcranial magnetic stimulation. *Neurology* 1992; 42: 647–651.

Pascual-Leone A., Cohen L.G., Brasil-Neto J.P., and Hallett M. Non-invasive differentiation of motor cortical representation of hand muscles by mapping of optimal current directions. *Electroenceph. Clin. Neurophysiol.* 1994; 93: 42–48.

Ren C., Tarjan P.P., and Popovic D.B. A novel electric design for electromagnetic stimulation: the slinky coil. *IEEE Trans. Biomed. Eng.* 1995; 42: 918–925.

Roth B.J. and Basser P.J. A model of the stimulation of a nerve fiber by electromagnetic radiation. *IEEE Trans. Biomed. Eng.* 1990; 37: 588–597.

Roth B.J., Cohen L.G., Hallet M., Friauf W., and Basser P.J. A theoretical calculation of the electric field induced by magnetic stimulation of a peripheral nerve. *Muscle Nerve* 1990; 13: 734–741.

Roth Y., Zangen A., and Hallett M. A coil design for transcranial magnetic stimulation of deep brain regions. *J. Clin. Neurophysiol.* 2002; 19: 361–370.

Ruhonen J. and Ilmoniemi R.J. Focusing and targeting of magnetic brain stimulation using multiple coils. *Med. Biol. Eng. Comput.* 1998; 38: 297–301.

Schultz W., Dayan P., and Montague P.R. A neural substrate of prediction and reward. *Science* 1997; 275: 1593–1599.

Self D.W. and Nestler E.J. Molecular mechanisms of drug reinforcement and addiction. *Annu. Rev. Neurosci.* 1995; 18: 463–495.

Stokic D.S., McKay W.B., Scott L., Sherwood A.M., and Dimitrijevic M.R. Intracortical inhibition of lower limb motor-evoked potentials after paired transcranial magnetic stimulation. *Exp. Brain Res.* 1997;117: 437–443.

Terao Y., Ugawa Y., Sakai K., Uesaka Y., and Kanazawa I. Transcranial magnetic stimulation of the leg area of motor cortex in humans. *Acta. Neurol. Scand.* 1994; 89: 378–383.

Terao Y., Ugawa Y., Hanajima R., et al. Predominant activation of I1-waves from the leg motor area by transcranial magnetic stimulation. *Brain Res.* 2000; 859: 137–146.

Thielscher A. and Kammer T. Linking physics with physiology in TMS: A spherical field model to determine the cortical stimulation site in TMS. *Neuroimage* 2002; 17: 1117–1130.

Tofts P.S. The distribution of induced currents in magnetic stimulation of the brain. *Phys. Med. Biol.* 1990; 35: 1119–1128.

Tofts P.S. and Branston N.M. The measurement of electric field, and the influence of surface charge, in magnetic stimulation. *Electroenceph. Clin. Neurophysiol.* 1991; 81: 238–239.

Volkow N.D. and Fowler J.S. Addiction, a disease of compulsion and drive: involvement of the orbitofrontal cortex. *Cereb. Cortex* 2000; 10: 318–325.

Wassermann E.M., Grafman J., Berry C., Hollnagel C., Wild K., Clark K., and Hallett M. Use and safety of a new repetitive transcranial magnetic stimulator. *Electroenceph. Clin. Neurophysiol.* 1996; 10: 412–417.

Wassermann E.M. and Lisanby S.H. Therapeutic application of repetitive transcranial magnetic stimulation: a review. *Clin. Neurophysiol.* 2001; 112: 1367–1377.

Watson D., Clark L.A., and Tellegen A. Development and validation of brief measures of positive and negative affect: the PANAS scales. *J. Pers. Soc. Psychol.* 1988; 54: 1063–1070.

Zangen A., Roth Y., Voller B., and Hallett M. Transcranial magnetic stimulation of deep brain regions: evidence for efficacy of the H-coil. *Clin. Neurophysiol.* 2005; 116: 775–779.

Zimmermann K.P. and Simpson R.K. "Slinky" coils for neuromagnetic stimulation. *Electroenceph. Clin. Neurophysiol.* 1996; 101: 145–152.

V

Biomaterials

Joyce Y. Wong
Boston University

V.1   A Brief Note Regarding This Edition

Due to unforeseen circumstances, the bulk of this section is largely identical to the previous edition with the notable exception of the addition of a chapter relating to micro- and nanotechnologies in advanced **biomaterials**. The content remains current, and the following introduction is taken from the previous edition with minor changes describing the content of this Section. In addition, a number of relevant biomaterials journals have been added to the list.

Biomaterial is used to make devices to replace a part or a function of the body in a safe, reliable, economic, and physiologically acceptable manner [Hench and Erthridge, 1982]. A variety of devices and materials are used in the treatment of disease or injury. Commonplace examples include sutures, needles, catheters, plates, tooth fillings, etc. A biomaterial is a synthetic material used to replace part of a living system or to function in intimate contact with living tissue. The Clemson University Advisory Board for Biomaterials has formally defined a biomaterial to be "a systemically and pharmacologically inert substance designed for implantation within or incorporation with living systems." Black defined biomaterials as "a nonviable material used in a medical device, intended to interact with biological systems" [Black, 1992]. Others include "materials of synthetic as well as of natural origin in contact with tissue, blood, and biological fluids, and intended for use for prosthetic, diagnostic, therapeutic, and storage applications without adversely affecting the living organism and its components" [Bruck, 1980]. Still another definition of biomaterials is stated as "any substance (other than drugs) or combination of substances, synthetic or natural in origin, which can be used for any period of time, as a whole or as a part of a system which treats, augments, or replaces any tissue, organ, or function of the body" [Williams, 1987] and adds to the many ways of looking the same but expressing in different ways. By contrast, a **biological material** is a material such as skin or artery, produced by a biological system. Artificial materials that simply are in contact with the skin, such as hearing aids and wearable artificial limbs are not included in our definition of biomaterials since the skin acts as a barrier with the external world.

According to these definitions, one must have a vast field of knowledge or collaborate with different specialties in order to develop and use biomaterials in medicine and dentistry as Table V.1 indicates. The uses of biomaterials, as indicated in Table V.2, include replacement of a body part which has lost function due to disease or trauma, to assist in healing, to improve function, and to correct abnormalities. The role of biomaterials has been influenced considerably by advances in many areas of biotechnology and science. For example, with the advent of antibiotics, infectious disease is less of a threat than in former times so that degenerative disease assumes a greater importance. Moreover, advances in surgical technique and instruments have permitted materials to be used in ways which were not possible previously. This section of the handbook is intended to develop in the reader a familiarity with the uses of materials in medicine and dentistry and with some rational basis for these applications.

The performance of materials in the body can be classified in many ways. First, biomaterials may be considered from the point of view of the problem area which is to be solved, as in Table V.2. Second,

TABLE V.1   Fields of Knowledge to Develop Biomaterials

Discipline	Examples
Science and engineering	Materials sciences: structure–property relationship of synthetic and biological materials including metals, ceramics, polymers, composites, tissues (blood and connective tissues), etc.
Biology and physiology	Cell and molecular biology, anatomy, animal and human physiology, histopathology, experimental surgery, immunology, etc.
Clinical sciences	All the clinical specialties: dentistry, maxillofacial, neurosurgery, obstetrics and gynecology, ophthalmology, orthopedics, otolaryngology, plastic and reconstructive surgery, thoracic and cardiovascular surgery, veterinary medicine, and surgery, etc.

Source: Modified from von Recum, A.F. [1994] Boston, MA. Biomaterials Society.

TABLE V.2   Uses of Biomaterials

Problem area	Examples
Replacement of diseased or damaged part	Artificial hip joint, kidney dialysis machine
Assist in healing	Sutures, bone plates, and screws
Improve function	Cardiac pacemaker, intraocular lens
Correct functional abnormality	Cardiac pacemaker
Correct cosmetic problem	Augmentation mammoplasty, chin augmentation
Aid to diagnosis	Probes and catheters
Aid to treatment	Catheters, drains

TABLE V.3   Biomaterials in Organs

Organ	Examples
Heart	Cardiac pacemaker, artificial heart valve, total artificial heart
Lung	Oxygenator machine
Eye	Contact lens, intraocular lens
Ear	Artificial stapes, cochlea implant
Bone	Bone plate, intramedullary rod
Kidney	Kidney dialysis machine
Bladder	Catheter and stent

TABLE V.4   Biomaterials in Body Systems

System	Examples
Skeletal	Bone plate, total joint replacements
Muscular	Sutures, muscle stimulator
Circulatory	Artificial heart valves, blood vessels
Respiratory	Oxygenator machine
Integumentary	Sutures, burn dressings, artificial skin
Urinary	Catheters, stent, kidney dialysis machine
Nervous	Hydrocephalus drain, cardiac pacemaker, nerve stimulator
Endocrine	Microencapsulated pancreatic islet cells
Reproductive	Augmentation mammoplasty, other cosmetic replacements

we may consider the body on a tissue level, an organ level (Table V.3), or a system level (Table V.4). Third, we may consider the classification of materials as polymers, metals, ceramics, and composites as is done in Table V.5. In that vein, the role of such materials as biomaterials is governed by the interaction between the material and the body; specifically, the effect of the body environment on the material and the effect of the material on the body [Williams and Roaf, 1973; Bruck, 1980; Hench and Erthridge, 1982; von Recum, 1986; Black, 1992; Park and Lakes, 1992; and Greco, 1994].

It should be evident from any of these perspectives that most current applications of biomaterials involve structural functions, even in those organs and systems which are not primarily structural in their nature, or very simple chemical or electrical functions. Complex chemical functions such as those of the liver and complex electrical or electrochemical functions such as those of the brain and sense organs cannot be carried out by biomaterials at this time.

V.2   Historical Background

The use of biomaterials did not become practical until the advent of an aseptic surgical technique developed by Dr. J. Lister in the 1860s. Earlier surgical procedures, whether they involved biomaterials or not, were generally unsuccessful as a result of infection. Problems of infection tend to be exacerbated in the

TABLE V.5   Materials for Use in the Body

Materials	Advantages	Disadvantages	Examples
Polymers (nylon, silicone rubber, polyester, polytetrafuoroethylene, etc.)	Resilient Easy to fabricate	Not strong Deforms with time May degrade	Sutures, blood vessels, hip socket, ear, nose, other soft tissues, sutures
Metals (Ti and its alloys, Co–Cr alloys, stainless steels, Au, Ag, Pt, etc.)	Strong, tough, ductile	May corrode Dense Difficult to make	Joint replacements, bone plates and screws, dental root implants, pacer and suture wires
Ceramics (aluminum oxide, calcium phosphates including hydroxyapatite, carbon)	Very biocompatible, Inert Strong in compression	Brittle Not resilient Difficult to make	Dental; femoral head of hip replacement, coating of dental and orthopedic implants
Composites (carbon–carbon, wire or fiber reinforced bone cement)	Strong, tailor-made	Difficult to make	Joint implants, heart valves

presence of biomaterials, since the implant can provide a region inaccessible to the body's immunologically competent cells. The earliest successful implants, as well as a large fraction of modern ones, were in the skeletal system. Bone plates were introduced in the early 1900s to aid in the fixation of long-bone fractures. Many of these early plates broke as a result of unsophisticated mechanical design; they were too thin and had stress-concentrating corners. Also, materials such as vanadium steel that was chosen for its good mechanical properties corroded rapidly in the body and caused adverse effects on the healing processes. Better designs and materials soon followed. Following the introduction of stainless steels and cobalt chromium alloys in the 1930s, greater success was achieved in fracture fixation, and the first joint-replacement surgeries were performed. As for polymers, it was found that warplane pilots in World War II who were injured by fragments of plastic PMMA (polymethyl methacrylate) aircraft canopy, did not suffer adverse chronic reactions from the presence of the fragments in the body. PMMA became widely used after that time for corneal replacement and for replacements of sections of damaged skull bones. Following further advances in materials and in surgical technique, blood vessel replacements were tried in the 1950s and heart valve replacements and cemented joint replacements in the 1960s. Table V.6 lists notable developments relating to implants. Recent years have seen many further advances.

V.3 Performance of Biomaterials

The success of biomaterials in the body depends on factors such as the material properties, design, and **biocompatibility** of the material used, as well as other factors not under the control of the engineer, including the technique used by the surgeon, the health and condition of the patient, and the activities of the patient. If we can assign a numerical value f to the probability of failure of an implant, then the reliability can be expressed as

$$r = 1 - f \tag{V.1}$$

If, as is usually the case, there are multiple modes of failure, the total reliability r_t is given by the product of the individual reliabilities $r_1 = (1 - f_1)$, etc.

$$r_t = r_1 \cdot r_2 \cdots r_n \tag{V.2}$$

Consequently, even if one failure mode such as implant fracture is perfectly controlled so that the corresponding reliability is unity, other failure modes such as infection could severely limit the utility represented by the total reliability of the implant. One mode of failure which can occur in a biomaterial, but not in

TABLE V.6 Notable Developments Relating to Implants

Year	Investigators	Development
Late 18-19th century		Various metal devices to fix bone fractures; wires and pins from Fe, Au, Ag, and Pt
1860–1870	J. Lister	Aseptic surgical techniques
1886	H. Hansmann	Ni-plated steel bone fracture plate
1893–1912	W.A. Lane	Steel screws and plates (Lane fracture plate)
1912	W.D. Sherman	Vanadium steel plates, first developed for medical use; lesser stress concentration and corrosion (Sherman plate)
1924	A.A. Zierold	Introduced Stellites® (CoCrMo alloy)
1926	M.Z. Lange	Introduced 18-8sMo stainless steel, better than 18-8 stainless steel
1926	E.W. Hey-Groves	Used carpenter's screw for femoral neck fracture
1931	M.N. Smith-Petersen	First femoral neck fracture fixation device made of stainless steel
1936	C.S. Venable, W.G. Stuck	Introduced Vitallium® (19-9 stainless steel), later changed the material to CoCr alloys
1938	P. Wiles	First total hip replacement prosthesis
1939	J.C. Burch, H.M Carney	Introduced tantalum (Ta)
1946	J. and R. Judet	First biomechanically designed femoral head replacement prosthesis. First plastics (PMMA) used in joint replacements
1940s	M.J. Dorzee, A. Franceschetti	First used acrylics (PMMA) for corneal replacement
1947	J. Cotton	Introduced Ti and its alloys
1952	A.B. Voorhees, A. Jaretzta, A.B. Blackmore	First successful blood vessel replacement made of cloth for tissue ingrowth
1958	S. Furman, G. Robinson	First successful direct heart stimulation
1958	J. Charnley	First use of acrylic bone cement in total hip replacement on the advice of Dr. D. Smith
1960	A. Starr, M.L. Edwards	First commercial heart valves
1970s	W.J. Kolff	Total heart replacement

Source: Park, J.B. [1984] New York: Plenum Publishing Co.

engineering materials used in other contexts, is an attack by the body's immune system on the implant. Another such failure mode is an unwanted effect of the implant upon the body; for example, toxicity, inducing allergic reactions, or causing cancer. Consequently, biocompatibility is included as a material requirement in addition to those requirements associated directly with the function of the implant.

Biocompatibility involves the acceptance of an artificial implant by the surrounding tissues and by the body as a whole. Biocompatible materials do not irritate the surrounding structures, do not provoke an abnormal inflammatory response, do not incite allergic or immunologic reactions, and do not cause cancer. Other compatibility characteristics that may be important in the function of an implant device made of biomaterials include (1) adequate mechanical properties such as strength, stiffness, and fatigue properties; (2) appropriate optical properties if the material is to be used in the eye, skin, or tooth; and (3) appropriate density. Sterilizability, manufacturability, long-term storage, and appropriate engineering design are also to be considered.

The failure modes may differ in importance as time passes following the implant surgery. For example, consider the case of a total joint replacement in which infection is most likely soon after surgery, while loosening and implant fracture become progressively more important as time goes on. Failure modes also depend on the type of implant and its location and function in the body. For example, an artificial blood vessel is more likely to cause problems by inducing a clot or becoming clogged with thrombus than by breaking or tearing mechanically.

With these basic concepts in mind, the chapters in this book focus on biomaterials consisting of different materials such as metallic, ceramic, polymeric, and composite. The impact of recent advances in the area of nano- and microtechnology on biomaterial design is highlighted in Chapter 46.

Defining Terms

Biocompatibility: Acceptance of an artificial implant by the surrounding tissues and by the body as a whole.
Biological material: A material produced by a biological system.
Biomaterial: A synthetic material used to make devices to replace part of a living system or to function in intimate contact with living tissue.

References

Black, J. (1992) *Biological Performance of Materials*, 2nd ed. New York: M. Dekker, Inc.
Bruck, S.D. (1980) *Properties of Biomaterials in the Physiological Environment*. Boca Raton, FL: CRC Press.
Greco, R.S. (1994) *Implantation Biology*. Boca Raton, FL: CRC Press.
Hench, L.L. and Erthridge, E.C. (1982) *Biomaterials — An Interfacial Approach*, Vol. 4, A. Noordergraaf, Ed. New York: Academic Press.
Park, J.B. (1984) *Biomaterials Science and Engineering*. New York: Plenum Publishing Co.
Park, J.B. and Lakes, R.S. (1992) *Biomaterials: An Introduction*, 2nd ed. NY: Plenum Publishing Co.
von Recum, A.F. (1994) Biomaterials: educational goals. In: *Annual Biomaterials Society Meeting*. Boston, MA. Biomaterials Society.
von Recum, A.F. (1986) *Handbook of Biomaterials Evaluation*. New York: Macmillan Publishing Co., pp. 97–158 and 293–502.
Williams, D.F. (1987) Definition in biomaterials. In: *Progress in Biomedical Engineering*. Amsterdam: Elsevier, p. 67.
Williams, D.F. and Roaf, R. (1973) *Implants in Surgery*. London: W.B. Saunders.

Further Information

(Most important publications relating to the biomaterials area are given for further reference.)
Allgower, M., Matter, P., Perren, S.M., and Ruedi, T. 1973. *The Dynamic Compression Plate*, DCP, Springer-Verlag, New York.
Bechtol, C.O., Ferguson, A.B., and Laing, P.G. 1959. *Metals and Engineering in Bone and Joint Surgery*, Balliere, Tindall and Cox, London.
Black, J. 1992. *Biological Performance of Materials*, 2nd ed., Marcel Dekker, New York.
Bloch, B. and Hastings, G.W. 1972. *Plastic Materials in Surgery*, 2nd ed., C.C. Thomas, Springfield, IL.
Bokros, J.C., Arkins, R.J., Shim, H.S., Haubold, A.D., and Agarwal, N.K. 1976. Carbon in prosthestic devices. In: *Petroleum Derived Carbons*, M.L. Deviney and T.M. O'Grady, Eds. *Am. Chem. Soc. Symp.*, Series No. 21, American Chemical Society, Washington, D.C.
Boretos, J.W. 1973. *Concise Guide to Biomedical Polymers*, C.C. Thomas, Springfield, IL.
Boretos, J.W. and Eden, M. (Eds.) 1984. *Contemporary Biomaterials*, Noyes, Park Ridge, NJ.
Brown, P.W. and Constantz, B. 1994. *Hydroxyapatite and Related Materials*, CRC Press, Boca Raton, FL.
Bruck, S.D. 1974. *Blood Compatible Synthetic Polymers: An Introduction*, C.C. Thomas, Springfield, IL.
Bruck, S.D. 1980. *Properties of Biomaterials in the Physiological Environment*, CRC Press, Boca Raton, FL.
Chandran, K.B. 1992. *Cardiovascular Biomechanics*, New York University Press, New York.
Charnley, J. 1970. *Acrylic Cement in Orthopedic Surgery*, Livingstone, Edinborough and London.
Cooney, D.O. 1976. *Biomedical Engineering Principles*, Marcel Dekker, New York.
Cranin, A.N., Ed. 1970. *Oral Implantology*, C.C. Thomas, Springfield, IL.
Dardik, H., Ed. 1978. *Graft Materials in Vascular Surgery*, Year Book Medical Publishing, Chicago.
de Groot, K., Ed. 1983. *Bioceramics of Calcium Phosphate*, CRC Press, Boca Raton, FL.
Ducheyne, P., Van der Perre, G., and Aubert, A.E., Eds. 1984. *Biomaterials and Biomechanics*, Elsevier Science, Amsterdam.
Dumbleton, J.H. and Black, J. 1975. *An Introduction to Orthopedic Materials*, C.C. Thomas, Springfield, IL.

Edwards, W.S. 1965. *Plastic Arterial Grafts*, C.C. Thomas, Springfield, IL.

Edwards, W.S. 1965. *Plastic Arterial Grafts*, C.C. Thomas, Springfield, IL.

Eftekhar, N.S. 1978. *Principles of Total Hip Arthroplasty*, C.V. Mosby, St. Louis, MO.

Frost, H.M. 1973. *Orthopedic Biomechanics*, C.C. Thomas, Springfield, IL.

Fung, Y.C. 1993. *Biomechanics: Mechanical Properties of Living Tissues*, 2nd ed., Springer-Verlag, New York.

Ghista, D.N. and Roaf, R., Eds. 1978. *Orthopedic Mechanics: Procedures and Devices*, Academic Press, London.

Greco, R.S., Ed. 1994. *Implantation Biology*, CRC Press, Boca Raton, FL.

Guidelines for Blood–Material Interactions, Revised 1985. Report of the National Heart, Lung, and Blood Institute Working Group, Devices and Technology Branch, NHLBI, NIH Publication No. 80-2185.

Gyers, G.H. and Parsonet, V. 1969. *Engineering in the Heart and Blood Vessels*, J. Wiley & Sons, New York.

Hastings, G.W. and Williams, D.F., Eds. 1980. *Mechanical Properties of Biomaterials*, John Wiley & Sons, New York.

Hench, L.L. and Ethridge, E.C. 1982. *Biomaterials: An Interfacial Approach*, Academic Press, New York.

Hench, L.L. and Wilson, J., Eds. 1993. *An Introduction to Bioceramics*, World Scientific, Singapore.

Heppenstall, R.B., Ed. 1980. *Fracture Treatment and Healing*, W.B. Saunders, Philadelphia, PA.

Homsy, C.A. and Armeniades, C.D., Eds., 1972. Biomaterials for skeletal and cardiovascular applications, *J. Biomed. Mater. Symp.*, No. 3, John Wiley & Sons, New York.

Hulbert, S.F., Young, F.A., and Moyle, D.D., Eds. 1972. *J. Biomed. Mater. Res. Symp.*, No. 2.

Kawahara, H., Ed. 1989. *Oral Implantology and Biomaterials*, Elsevier Science, Armsterdam.

Kronenthal, R.L. and Oser, Z., Eds. 1975. *Polymers in Medicine and Surgery*, Plenum Press, New York.

Kuntscher, G. 1947. *The Practice of Intramedullary Nailing*, C.C. Thomas, Springfield, IL.

Lee, H. and Neville, K. 1971. *Handbook of Biomedical Plastics*, Pasadena Technology Press, Pasadena, CA.

Lee, S.M., Ed. *Advances in Biomaterials*, Technomic Pub. AG, Lancaster, PA, 1987.

Leinninger, R.I. 1972. Polymers as surgical implants, CRC *Crit. Rev. Bioeng.*, 2: 333–360.

Levine, S.N., Ed. 1968. Materials in Biomedical Engineering, *Ann. NY Acad. Sci.*, 146.

Levine, S.N., Ed. 1968. Polymers and Tissue Adhesives, *Ann. NY Acad. Sci.*, Part IV, 146.

Lynch, W. 1982. *Implants: Reconstructing Human Body*, Van Nostrand Reinhold, New York.

Martz, E.O., Goel, V.K., Pope, M.H., and Park, J.B., 1997 Materials and design of spinal implants — A review. *J. Biomed. Mat. Res. (App. Biomater.)*, 38: 267–288.

Mears, D.C. 1979. *Materials and Orthopedic Surgery*, Williams & Wilkins, Baltimore, MD.

Oonishi, H. Aoki, H. and Sawai, K., Eds. 1989. *Bioceramics*, Ishiyaku EuroAmerica, Tokyo.

Park, J.B. 1979. *Biomaterials: An Introduction*, Plenum Press, New York.

Park, J.B. 1984. *Biomaterials Science and Engineering*, Plenum Press, New York.

Park, J.B. and Lakes, R.S. 1992. *Biomaterials: An Introduction*, 2nd ed., Plenum Press, New York.

Park, K., Shalaby, W.S.W., and Park, H. 1993. *Biodegradable Hydrogels for Drug Delivery*, Technomic, Lancaster, PA.

Rubin, L.R., Ed. 1983. *Biomaterials in Reconstructive Surgery*, C.V. Mosby, St. Louis, MO.

Savastano, A.A., Ed. 1980. *Total Knee Replacement*, Appleton-Century-Crofts, New York.

Sawyer, P.N. and Kaplitt, M.H. 1978. *Vascular Grafts*, Appleton-Century-Crofts, New York.

Schaldach, M. and Hohmann, D., Eds. 1976. *Advances in Artificial Hip and Knee Joint Technology*, Springer-Verlag, Berlin.

Schnitman, P.A. and Schulman, L.B., Eds. 1980. Dental Implants: Benefits and Risk, A *NIH-Harvard Consensus Development Conference*, NIH Pub. No. 81-1531, U.S. Dept. Health and Human Services, Bethesda, MD.

Sharma, C.P. and Szycher, M., Eds. 1991. *Blood Compatible Materials and Devices*, Technomic, Lancaster, PA.

Stanley, J.C., Burkel, W.E., Lindenauer, S.M., Bartlett, R.H., and Turcotte, J.G., Eds. 1972. *Biologic and Synthetic Vascular Prostheses*, Grune & Stratton, New York.

Stark, L. and Agarwal, G., Eds. 1969. *Biomaterials*, Plenum Press, New York.

Swanson, S.A.V. and Freeman, M.A.R., Eds. 1977. *The Scientific Basis of Joint Replacement*, John Wiley & Sons, New York.

Syrett, B.C. and Acharya, A., Eds. 1979. *Corrosion and Degradation of Implant Materials*, ASTM STP 684, American Society for Testing and Materials, Philadelphia, PA.

Szycher, M. and Robinson, W.J., Eds. *Synthetic Biomedical Polymers, Concepts and Applications*, Technomic, Lancaster, PA.

Szycher, M., Ed. 1991. *High Performance Biomaterials*, Technomic, Lancaster, PA.

Taylor, A.R. 1970. *Endosseous Dental Implants*, Butterworths, London.

Uhthoff, H.K., Ed. 1980. *Current Concepts of Internal Fixation of Fractures*, Springer-Verlag, Berlin.

Venable, C.S. and Stuck, W.C. 1947 *The Internal Fixation of Fractures*, C.C. Thomas, Springfield, IL.

Webster, J.G., Ed. 1988. *Encyclopedia of Medical Devices and Instrumentation*, John Wiley & Sons, New York.

Williams, D.F. and Roaf, R. 1973. *Implants in Surgery*, W.B. Saunders, London.

Williams, D.F., Ed. 1976. *Compatibility of Implant Materials*, Sector Pub. Ltd., London, 1976.

Williams, D.F., Ed. 1981. *Fundamental Aspects of Biocompatibility*, vols I and II, CRC Press, Boca Raton, FL.

Williams, D.F., Ed. 1981. *Systemic Aspects of Blood Compatibility*, CRC Press, Boca Raton, FL.

Williams, D.F., Ed. 1982. *Biocompatibility in Clinical Practice*, vols I and II, CRC Press, Boca Raton, FL.

Wright, V., Ed. 1969. *Lubrication and Wear in Joints*, J.B. Lippincott, Philadelphia, PA.

Yamamuro, T., Hench, L.L., and Wilson J., Eds. 1990. *CRC Handbook of Bioactive Ceramics*, vols I and II, CRC Press, Boca Raton, FL.

Journals of Interest

Acta Biomaterialia
Annals of Biomedical Engineering
Bioconjugate Chemistry
Biomacromolecules
Biomaterials
Biomedical Materials and Engineering
CRC Critical Review in Bioengineering
Journal of Arthoplasty
Journal of Biomechanics
Journal of Biomedical Materials Research
Journal of Controlled Release
Journal of Applied Biomaterials
Journal of Medical Engineering and Technology
Journal of Orthopaedic Research
Journal of Biomaterials Science, Polymer Edition
Journal of Biomedical Engineering
Langmuir
Acta Orthopaedica Scandinavica
Clinical Orthopaedics and Related Research
Journal of Bone and Joint Surgery
International Orthopaedics
Medical Engineering and Physics
American Association of Artificial Internal Organs: Transactions
Tissue Engineering
Transactions of the Orthopaedic Research Society Meeting (annually held during February): Abstracts
Transactions of the Society for Biomaterials (annually held during April and May): Abstracts
Transactions of the American Society of Artificial Internal Organs (annually held in spring): Extended Abstracts
Society for Biomaterials: http://www.biomaterials.org/index.html

38

Metallic Biomaterials

Joon B. Park
University of Iowa

Young Kon Kim
Inje University

38.1 Introduction

Metals are used as biomaterials due to their excellent electrical and thermal conductivity and mechanical properties. Since some electrons are independent in metals, they can quickly transfer an electric charge and thermal energy. The mobile free electrons act as the binding force to hold the positive metal ions together. This attraction is strong, as evidenced by the closely packed atomic arrangement resulting in high specific gravity and high melting points of most metals. Since the metallic bond is essentially nondirectional, the position of the metal ions can be altered without destroying the crystal structure resulting in a plastically deformable solid.

Some metals are used as passive substitutes for hard tissue replacement such as total hip and knee joints, for fracture healing aids as bone plates and screws, spinal fixation devices, and dental implants because of their excellent mechanical properties and **corrosion** resistance. Some metallic alloys are used for more active roles in devices such as vascular stents, catheter guide wires, orthodontic archwires, and cochlea implants.

The first metal alloy developed specifically for human use was the "vanadium steel" which was used to manufacture bone fracture plates (Sherman plates) and screws. Most metals such as iron (Fe), chromium (Cr), cobalt (Co), nickel (Ni), titanium (Ti), tantalum (Ta), niobium (Nb), molybdenum (Mo), and tungsten (W), that were used to make alloys for manufacturing implants can only be tolerated by the body in minute amounts. Sometimes those metallic elements, in naturally occurring forms, are essential in red blood cell functions (Fe) or synthesis of a vitamin B_{12} (Co), but cannot be tolerated in large amounts in the body [Black, 1992]. The biocompatibility of the metallic implant is of considerable concern because these implants can corrode in an *in vivo* environment [Williams, 1982]. The consequences of corrosion are the disintegration of the implant material per se, which will weaken the implant, and the harmful effect of corrosion products on the surrounding tissues and organs.

38.2   Stainless Steels

The first stainless steel utilized for implant fabrication was the 18-8 (type 302 in modern classification), which is stronger and more resistant to corrosion than the vanadium steel. Vanadium steel is no longer used in implants since its corrosion resistance is inadequate *in vivo*. Later 18-8sMo stainless steel was introduced which contains a small percentage of molybdenum to improve the corrosion resistance in chloride solution (salt water). This alloy became known as *type 316 stainless steel*. In the 1950s the carbon content of 316 stainless steel was reduced from 0.08 to a maximum amount of 0.03% (all are weight percent unless specified) for better corrosion resistance to chloride solution and to minimize the sensitization and hence, became known as type *316L stainless steel*. The minimum effective concentration of chromium is 11% to impart corrosion resistance in stainless steels. The chromium is a reactive element, but it and its alloys can be *passivated* by 30% nitric acid to give excellent corrosion resistance.

The *austenitic stainless steels*, especially type 316 and 316L, are most widely used for implant fabrication. These cannot be hardened by heat treatment but can be hardened by cold-working. This group of stainless steels is nonmagnetic and possesses better corrosion resistance than any others. The inclusion of molybdenum enhances resistance to *pitting corrosion* in salt water. The American Society of Testing and Materials (ASTM) recommends type 316L rather than 316 for implant fabrication. The specifications for 316L stainless steel are given in Table 38.1. The only difference in composition between the 316L and 316 stainless steel is the maximum content of carbon, that is, 0.03 and 0.08%, respectively, as noted earlier.

The nickel stabilizes the austenitic phase [γ, face centered cubic crystal (fcc) structure], at room temperature and enhances corrosion resistance. The austenitic phase formation can be influenced by both the Ni and Cr contents as shown in Figure 38.1 for 0.10% carbon stainless steels. The minimum amount of Ni for maintaining austenitic phase is approximately 10%.

Table 38.2 gives the mechanical properties of 316L stainless steel. A wide range of properties exists depending on the heat treatment (annealing to obtain softer materials) or cold working (for greater strength and hardness). Figure 38.2 shows the effect of cold working on the yield and ultimate tensile strength of 18-8 stainless steels. The engineer must consequently be careful when selecting materials of this type. Even the 316L stainless steels may corrode inside the body under certain circumstances in a highly stressed and oxygen depleted region, such as the contacts under the screws of the bone fracture

TABLE 38.1   Compositions of
316L Stainless Steel (American
Society for Testing and Materials,
F139–86, p. 61, 1992)

Element	Composition (%)
Carbon	0.03 max.
Mangnese	2.00 max.
Phosphorus	0.03 max.
Sulfur	0.03 max.
Silicon	0.75 max.
Chromium	17.00–20.00
Nickel	12.00–14.00
Molybdenum	2.00–4.00

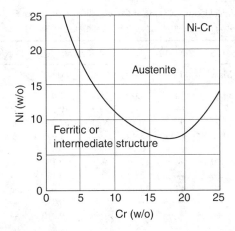

FIGURE 38.1 The effect of Ni and Cr contents on the austenitic phase of stainless steels containing 0.1% C [Keating, 1956].

TABLE 38.2 Mechanical Properties of 316L Stainless Steel for Implants
(American Society for Testing and Materials, F139–86, p. 61, 1992)

Condition	Ultimate tensile strength, min. (MPa)	Yield strength (0.2% offset), min. (MPa)	Elongation 2 in. (50.8 mm) min. %	Rockwell hardness
Annealed	485	172	40	95 HRB
Cold-worked	860	690	12	—

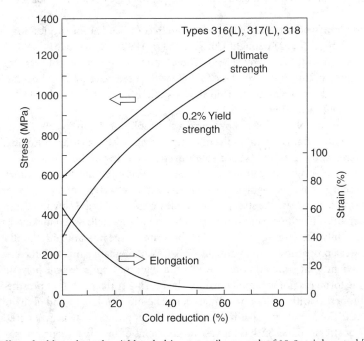

FIGURE 38.2 Effect of cold-work on the yield and ultimate tensile strength of 18-8 stainless steel [ASTM, 1980].

TABLE 38.3 Chemical Compositions of Co–Cr Alloys (American Society for Testing and Materials, F75–87, p. 42; F90–87, p. 47; F562–84, p. 150, 1992)

Element	CoCrMo (F75) Min.	Max.	CoCrWNi (F90) Min.	Max.	CoNiCrMo (F562) Min.	Max.	CoNiCrMoWFe (F563) Min.	Max.
Cr	27.0	30.0	19.0	21.0	19.0	21.0	18.00	22.00
Mo	5.0	7.0	—	—	9.0	10.5	3.00	4.00
Ni	—	2.5	9.0	11.0	33.0	37.0	15.00	25.00
Fe	—	0.75	—	3.0	—	1.0	4.00	6.00
C	—	0.35	0.05	0.15	—	0.025	—	0.05
Si	—	1.00	—	1.00	—	0.15	—	0.50
Mn	—	1.00	—	2.00	—	0.15	—	1.00
W	—	—	14.0	16.0	—	—	3.00	4.00
P	—	—	—	—	—	0.015	—	—
S	—	—	—	—	—	0.010	—	0.010
Ti	—	—	—	—	—	1.0	0.50	3.50
Co		Balance						

plate. Thus, these stainless steels are suitable to use only in temporary implant devices such as fracture plates, screws, and hip nails. Surface modification methods such as anodization, **passivation**, and glow-discharge nitrogen-implantation, are widely used in order to improve corrosion resistance, wear resistance, and fatigue strength of 316L stainless steel [Bordiji et al., 1996].

38.3   CoCr Alloys

There are basically two types of cobalt–chromium alloys (1) the castable CoCrMo alloy and (2) the CoNiCrMo alloy which is usually *wrought* by (hot) *forging*. The castable CoCrMo alloy has been used for many decades in dentistry and, relatively recently, in making artificial joints. The wrought CoNiCrMo alloy is relatively new, now used for making the stems of prostheses for heavily loaded joints such as the knee and hip.

The ASTM lists four types of CoCr alloys which are recommended for surgical implant applications (1) cast CoCrMo alloy (F75), (2) wrought CoCrWNi alloy (F90), (3) wrought CoNiCrMo alloy (F562), and (4) wrought CoNiCrMoWFe alloy (F563). The chemical compositions of each are summarized in Table 38.3. At the present time only two of the four alloys are used extensively in implant fabrications, the castable CoCrMo and the wrought CoNiCrMo alloy. As can be noticed from Table 38.3, the compositions are quite different from each other.

The two basic elements of the CoCr alloys form a solid solution of up to 65% Co. The molybdenum is added to produce finer grains which results in higher strengths after casting or forging. The chromium enhances corrosion resistance as well as solid solution strengthening of the alloy.

The CoNiCrMo alloy originally called MP35N (Standard Pressed Steel Co.) contains approximately 35% Co and Ni each. The alloy is highly corrosion resistant to seawater (containing chloride ions) under stress. Cold working can increase the strength of the alloy considerably as shown in Figure 38.3. However, there is a considerable difficulty of cold working on this alloy, especially when making large devices such as hip joint stems. Only hot-forging can be used to fabricate a large implant with the alloy.

The abrasive wear properties of the wrought CoNiCrMo alloy are similar to the cast CoCrMo alloy (about 0.14 mm/yr in joint simulation tests with ultra high molecular weight polyethylene acetabular cup); however, the former is not recommended for the bearing surfaces of joint prosthesis because of its poor frictional properties with itself or other materials. The superior fatigue and ultimate tensile strength of the wrought CoNiCrMo alloy make it suitable for the applications which require long service life without fracture or stress fatigue. Such is the case for the stems of the hip joint prostheses. This advantage is better appreciated when the implant has to be replaced, since it is quite difficult to remove the failed

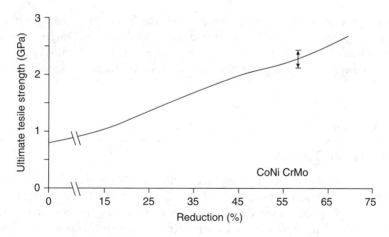

FIGURE 38.3 Relationship between ultimate tensile and the amount of cold-work for CoNiCrMo alloy [Devine and Wulff, 1975].

TABLE 38.4 Mechanical Property Requirements of Co-Cr Alloys (ASTM F76, F90, F562) (American Society for Testing and Materials, F75–87, p. 42; F90–87, p. 47; F562–84, p. 150, 1992)

Property	Cast CoCrMo (F75)	Wrought CoCrWNi (F90)	Wrought CoNiCrMo (F562) Solution annealed	Wrought CoNiCrMo (F562) Cold-worked and aged
Tensile strength (MPa)	655	860	793–1000	1793 min.
Yield strength (0.2% offset) (MPa)	450	310	240–655	1585
Elongation (%)	8	10	50.0	8.0
Reduction of area (%)	8	—	65.0	35.0
Fatigue strength (MPa)[a]	310	—	—	—

[a] From Semlitch, M. (1980). *Eng. Med.* 9, 201–207.

piece of implant embedded deep in the femoral medullary canal. Furthermore, the revision arthroplasty is usually inferior to the primary surgery in terms of its function due to poorer fixation of the implant.

The mechanical properties required for CoCr alloys are given in Table 38.4. As with the other alloys, the increased strength is accompanied by decreased ductility. Both the cast and wrought alloys have excellent corrosion resistance.

Experimental determination of the rate of nickel release from the CoNiCrMo alloy and 316L stainless steel in 37°C Ringer's solution showed an interesting result. Although the cobalt alloy has more initial release of nickel ions into the solution, the rate of release was about the same (3×10^{-10} g/cm^2/day) for both alloys [Richards-Mfg-Company, 1980]. This is rather surprising since the nickel content of the CoNiCrMo alloy is about three times that of 316L stainless steel.

The metallic products released from the prosthesis because of wear, corrosion, and fretting may impair organs and local tissues. *In vitro* studies have indicated that particulate Co is toxic to human osteoblast-like cell lines and inhibits synthesis of type-I collagen, osteocalcin and alkaline phosphatase in the culture medium. However, particulate Cr and CoCr alloy are well tolerated by cell lines with no significant toxicity. The toxicity of metal extracts *in vitro* have indicated that Co and Ni extracts at 50% concentration appear to be highly toxic since all viability parameters were altered after 24 h. However, Cr extract seems to be less toxic than Ni and Co [Granchi et al., 1996].

The modulus of elasticity for the CoCr alloys does not change with the changes in their ultimate tensile strength. The values range from 220 to 234 GPa which are higher than other materials such as stainless steels. This may have some implications of different load transfer modes to the bone in artificial joint replacements, although the effect of the increased modulus on the fixation and longevity of implants is not clear. Low wear (average linear wear on the MeKee-Farrar component was 4.2 μm/yr) has been recognized as an advantage of metal-on-metal hip articulations because of its hardness and toughness [Schmalzried et al., 1996].

38.4   Ti Alloys

38.4.1   Pure Ti and Ti6Al4V

Attempts to use titanium for implant fabrication dates to the late 1930s. It was found that titanium was tolerated in cat femurs, as was stainless steel and Vitallium® (CoCrMo alloy). Titanium's lightness (4.5 g/cm^3, see Table 38.5) and good mechanochemical properties are salient features for implant application.

There are four grades of unalloyed commercially pure (cp) titanium for surgical implant applications as given in Table 38.6. The impurity contents separate them; oxygen, iron, and nitrogen should be controlled carefully. Oxygen in particular has a great influence on the ductility and strength.

One titanium alloy (Ti6Al4V) is widely used to manufacture implants and its chemical requirements are given in Table 38.7. The main alloying elements of the alloy are aluminum (5.5–6.5%) and vanadium

TABLE 38.5   Specific Gravities of Some Metallic Implant Alloys

Alloys	Density (g/cm^3)
Ti and its allloys	4.5
316 Stainless steel	7.9
CoCrMo	8.3
CoNiCrMo	9.2
NiTi	6.7

TABLE 38.6   Chemical Compositions of Titanium and its Alloy (American Society for Testing and Materials, F67–89, p. 39; F136–84, p. 55, 1992)

Element	Grade 1	Grade 2	Grade 3	Grade 4	Ti6Al4V[a]
Nitrogen	0.03	0.03	0.05	0.05	0.05
Carbon	0.10	0.10	0.10	0.10	0.08
Hydrogen	0.015	0.015	0.015	0.015	0.0125
Iron	0.20	0.30	0.30	0.50	0.25
Oxygen	0.18	0.25	0.35	0.40	0.13
Titanium			Balance		

[a] Aluminum 6.00% (5.50–6.50), vanadium 4.00% (3.50–4.50), and other elements 0.1% maximum or 0.4% total.
All are maximum allowable weight percent.

TABLE 38.7   Mechanical Properties of Ti and its Alloys (ASTM F136) (American Society for Testing and Materials, F67–89, p. 39; F136–84, p. 55, 1992 and Davidson et al., 1994)

Properties	Grade 1	Grade 2	Grade 3	Grade 4	Ti6Al4V	Ti13Nb13Zr
Tensile strength (MPa)	240	345	450	550	860	1030
Yield strength (0.2% offset) (MPa)	170	275	380	485	795	900
Elongation (%)	24	20	18	15	10	15
Reduction of area (%)	30	30	30	25	25	45

(3.5∼4.5%). The Ti6Al4V alloy has approximately the same fatigue strength (550 MPa) of CoCr alloy after rotary bending fatigue tests [Imam et al., 1983]. Titanium is an allotropic material, which exists as a hexagonal close packed structure (hcp, α-Ti) up to 882°C and body-centered cubic structure (bcc, β-Ti) above that temperature. Titanium alloys can be strengthened and mechanical properties varied by controlled composition and thermomechanical processing techniques. The addition of alloying elements to titanium enables it to have a wide range of properties: (1) Aluminum tends to stabilize the α-phase, that is increase the transformation temperature from α- to β-phase (Figure 38.4). (2) Vanadium stabilizes the β-phase by lowering the temperature of the transformation from α to β.

The α-alloy has a single-phase microstructure (Figure 38.5a) which promotes good weldability. The stabilizing effect of the high aluminum content of these groups of alloys makes excellent strength

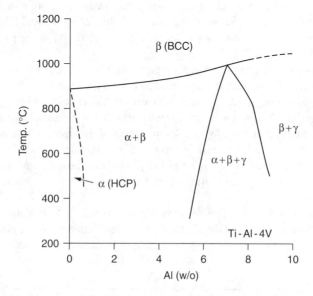

FIGURE 38.4 Part of Phase-diagram of Ti–Al–V at 4 w/o V [Smith and Hughes, 1966].

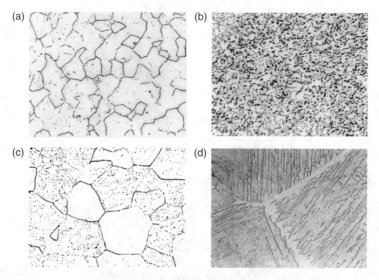

FIGURE 38.5 Microstructure of Ti alloys (all are 500X) [Hille, 1966]. (a) Annealed α-alloy. (b) Ti6Al4V, α–β alloy, annealed. (c) β-alloy, annealed. (d) Ti6Al4V, heat-treated at 1650°C and quenched [Imam et al., 1983].

characteristics and oxidation resistance at high temperature (300 to 600°C). These alloys cannot be heat-treated for precipitation hardening since they are single-phased.

The addition of controlled amounts of β-stabilizers causes the higher strength β-phase to persist below the transformation temperature which results in the two-phase system. The precipitates of β-phase will appear by heat treatment in the solid solution temperature and subsequent quenching, followed by aging at a somewhat lower temperature. The aging cycle causes the coherent precipitation of some fine α particles from the metastable β, imparting α structure may produce local strain field capable of absorbing deformation energy. Cracks are stopped or deterred at the α particles, so that the hardness is higher than for the solid solution (Figure 38.5b).

The higher percentage of β-stabilizing elements (13%V in Ti13V11Cr3Al alloy) results in a microstructure that is substantially β which can be strengthened by heat-treatment (Figure 38.5c). Another Ti alloy (Ti13Nb13Zr) with13%Nb and 13%Zr showed **martensite** structure after water quenched and aged, which showed high corrosion resistant with low modulus ($E = 79$ MPa) [Davidson et al., 1994]. Formation of plates of martensite induces considerable elastic distortion in the parent crystal structure and increases strength (Figure 38.5d).

The mechanical properties of the commercially pure titanium and its alloys are given in Table 38.7. The modulus of elasticity of these materials is about 110 GPa except 13Nb13Zr alloy. From Table 38.7 one can see that the higher impurity content of the cp-Ti leads to higher strength and reduced ductility. The strength of the material varies from a value much lower than that of 316 stainless steel or the CoCr alloys to a value about equal to that of annealed 316 stainless steel of the cast CoCrMo alloy. However, when compared by the specific strength (strength per density) the titanium alloys exceed any other implant materials as shown in Figure 38.6. Titanium, nevertheless, has poor shear strength making it less desirable for bone screws, plates, and similar applications. It also tends to gall or seize when in sliding contact with itself or another metal.

Titanium derives its resistance to corrosion by the formation of a solid oxide layer to a depth of 10 nm. Under *in vivo* conditions the oxide (TiO_2) is the only stable reaction product. However, micromotion at the cement-prosthesis and cement-bone are inevitable and consequently, titanium oxide and titanium

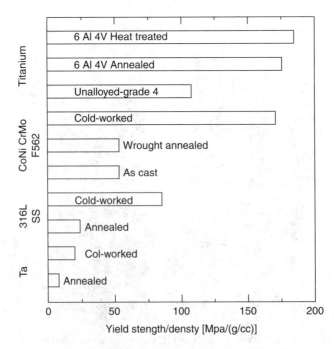

FIGURE 38.6   Yield strength to density ratio of some implant materials [Hille, 1966].

alloy particles are released in cemented joint prosthesis. Sometimes this wear debris accumulates as periprosthetic fluid collections and triggers giant cell response around the implants. This cystic collection continued to enlarge and aspiration revealed "dark" heavily stained fluid containing titanium wear particles and histiocytic cells. Histological examination of the stained soft tissue showed "fibrin necrotic debris" and collagenous, fibrous tissue containing a histiocytic and foreign body giant cell infiltrate. The metallosis, black staining of the periprosthetic tissues, has been implicated in knee implant [Breen and Stoker, 1993].

The titanium implant surface consists of a thin oxide layer and the biological fluid of water molecules, dissolved ions, and biomolecules (proteins with surrounding water shell) as shown in Figure 38.7. The microarchitecture (microgeometry, roughness, etc.) of the surface and its chemical compositions are important due to the following reasons:

1. Physical nature of the surface either at the atomic, molecular, or higher level relative to the dimensions of the biological units may cause different contact areas with biomolecules, cells, etc. The different contact areas, in turn, may produce different perturbations and types of bonding of the biological units, which may influence their conformation and function.
2. Chemical composition of the surface may produce different types of bonding to the biomolecules, which may then also affect their properties and function. Metals undergo chemical reactions at the surface depending on the environment which cause the difficulties of understanding the exact nature of the interactions.

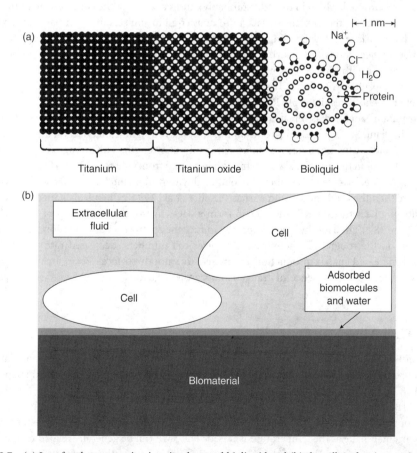

FIGURE 38.7 (a) Interface between a titanium implant and bioliquid and (b) the cell surface interaction [Kasemo and Lausma, 1988].

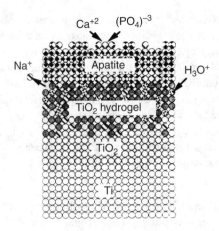

FIGURE 38.8   Chemical change of titanium implant surface of alkali following heat treatment [Kim et al., 1996].

The surface-tissue interaction is dynamic rather than static, i.e., it will develop into new stages as time passes, especially during the initial period after implantation. During the initial few seconds after implantation, there will be only water, dissolved ions, and free biomolecules in the closest proximity of the surface but no cells. The composition of biofluid will then change continuously as inflammatory and healing processes proceed, which in turn also probably causes changes in the composition of the adsorbed layer of biomolecules on the implant surface until quasiequilibrium sets in. Eventually, cells and tissues will approach the surface and, depending on the nature of the adsorbed layer, they will respond in specific ways that may further modify the adsorbed biomolecules. The type of cells closest to the surface and their activities will change with time. For example, depending on the type of initial interaction, the final results may be fibrous capsule formation or tissue integration [Kasemo and Lausma, 1988; Hazan et al., 1993; Takatsuka et al., 1995; Takeshita et al., 1997; Yan et al., 1997].

Osseointegration is defined as direct contact without intervening soft tissue between viable remodeled bone and an implant. Surface roughness of titanium alloys have a significant effect on the bone apposition to the implant and on the bone implant interfacial pull out strength. The average roughness increased from 0.5 to 5.9 μm and the interfacial shear strength increased from 0.48 to 3.5 MPa [Feighan et al., 1995]. Highest levels of osteoblast cell attachment are obtained with rough sand blast surfaces where cells differentiated more than those on the smooth surfaces [Keller et al., 1994]. Chemical changes of the titanium surface following heat treatment is thought to form a TiO_2 hydrogel layer on top of the TiO_2 layer as shown in Figure 38.8. The TiO_2 hydrogel layer may induce the apatite crystal formation [Kim et al., 1996].

In general, on the rougher surfaces there are lower cell numbers, decreased rate of cellular proliferation, and increased matrix production compared to smooth surface. Bone formation appears to be strongly related to the presence of transforming growth factor β_1 in the bone matrix [Kieswetter et al., 1996].

38.4.2   TiNi Alloys

The *titanium–nickel* alloys show unusual properties, that is, after it is deformed the material can snap back to its previous shape following heating of the material. This phenomenon is called **shape memory effect (SME)**. The SME of TiNi alloy was first observed by Buehler and Wiley at the U.S. Naval Ordnance Laboratory [Buehler et al., 1963]. The equiatomic TiNi or NiTi alloy (Nitinol) exhibits an exceptional SME near room temperature: if it is plastically deformed below the transformation temperature, it reverts back to its original shape as the temperature is raised. The SME can be generally related to a diffusionless martensitic phase transformation which is also thermoelastic in nature, the thermoelasticity being attributed to the ordering in the parent and martensitic phases [Wayman and Shimizu, 1972]. Another unusual

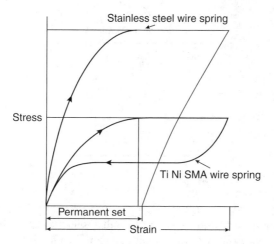

FIGURE 38.9 Schematic illustration of the stainless steel wire and TiNi SMA wire springs for orthodontic archwire behavior. (Modified from Wayman, C.M. and Duerig, T.W. (1990). London: Butterworth-Heinemann, pp. 3–20.)

property is the **superelasticity**, which is shown schematically in Figure 38.9. As can be seen, the stress does not increase with increased strain after the initial elastic stress region and upon release of the stress or strain the metal springs back to its original shape in contrast to other metals such as stainless steel. The superlastic property is utilized in orthodontic archwires since the conventional stainless steel wires are too stiff and harsh for the tooth. In addition, the shape memory effect can also be utilized.

Some possible applications of shape memory alloys are orthodontic dental archwire, intracranial aneurysm clip, *vena cava* filter, contractile artificial muscles for an artificial heart, vascular stent, catheter guide wire, and orthopedic staple [Duerig et al., 1990].

In order to develop such devices, it is necessary to understand fully the mechanical and thermal behavior associated with the martensitic phase transformation. A widely known NiTi alloy is 55-Nitinol (55 weight% or 50 atomic % Ni), which has a single phase and the mechanical memory plus other properties, for example, high acoustic damping, direct conversion of heat energy into mechanical energy, good fatigue properties, and low temperature ductility. Deviation from the 55-Nitinol (near stoichiometric NiTi) in the Ni-rich direction yields a second group of alloys which are also completely nonmagnetic but differ from 55-Nitinol in their ability to be thermally hardened to higher hardness levels. Shape recovery capability decreases and heat treatability increases rapidly as the Ni content approaches 60%. Both 55 and 60-Nitinols have relatively low modulus of elasticity and can be tougher and more resilient than stainless steel, NiCr, or CoCr alloys.

Efficiency of 55-Nitinol shape recovery can be controlled by changing the final annealing temperatures during preparation of the alloy device [Lee et al., 1988]. For the most efficient recovery, the shape is fixed by constraining the specimen in a desired configuration and heating to 482 to 510°C. If the annealed wire is deformed at a temperature below the shape recovery temperature, shape recovery will occur upon heating, provided the deformation has not exceeded crystallographic strain limits (~8% strain in tension). The NiTi alloys also exhibit good biocompatibility and corrosion resistance *in vivo*.

There is no significant difference between titanium and NiTi in the inhibition of mitosis in human fibroblasts. NiTi showed lower percentage bone and bone contact area than titanium and the Ti6Al4V alloy [Takeshita et al., 1997].

The mechanical properties of NiTi alloys are especially sensitive to the stoichiometry of composition (typical composition is given in Table 38.8) and the individual thermal and mechanical history. Although much is known about the processing, mechanical behavior, and properties relating to the shape memory effect, considerably less is known about the thermomechanical and physical metallurgy of the alloy.

TABLE 38.8   Chemical Composition of Ni–Ti Alloy Wire

Element	Composition (%)
Ni	54.01
Co	0.64
Cr	0.76
Mn	0.64
Fe	0.66
Ti	Balance

38.5 Dental Metals

Dental **amalgam** is an alloy made of liquid mercury and other solid metal particulate alloys made of silver, tin, copper, etc. The solid alloy is mixed with (liquid) mercury in a mechanical vibrating mixer and the resulting material is packed into the prepared cavity. One of the solid alloys is composed of at least 65% silver, and not more than 29% tin, 6% copper, 2% zinc, and 3% mercury. The reaction during setting is thought to be

$$\gamma + Hg \rightarrow \gamma + \gamma_1 + \gamma_2 \tag{38.1}$$

in which the γ phase is Ag_3Sn, the γ_1 phase is Ag_2Hg_3, and the γ_2 phase is Sn_7Hg. The phase diagram for the Ag-Sn-Hg system shows that over a wide compositional range all three phases are present. The final composition of dental amalgams typically contain 45% to 55% mercury, 35% to 45% silver, and about 15% tin after fully set in about one day.

Gold and gold alloys are useful metals in dentistry as a result of their durability, stability, and corrosion resistance [Nielsen, 1986]. Gold fillings are introduced by two methods: casting and malleting. *Cast* restorations are made by taking a wax impression of the prepared cavity, making a mold from this impression in a material such as gypsum silica, which tolerates high temperature, and casting molten gold in the mold. The patient is given a temporary filling for the intervening time. Gold *alloys* are used for cast restorations, since they have mechanical properties which are superior to those of pure gold. Corrosion resistance is retained in these alloys provided they contain 75% or more of gold and other **noble** metals. Copper, alloyed with gold, significantly increases its strength. Platinum also improves the strength, but no more than about 4% can be added, or the melting point of the alloy is elevated excessively. Silver compensates for the color of copper. A small amount of zinc may be added to lower the melting point and to scavenge oxides formed during melting. Gold alloys of different composition are available. Softer alloys containing more than 83% gold are used for inlays which are not subjected to much stress. Harder alloys containing less gold are chosen for crowns and cusps which are more heavily stressed.

Malleted restorations are built up in the cavity from layers of *pure* gold foil. The foils are welded together by pressure at ambient temperature. In this type of welding, the metal layers are joined by thermal diffusion of atoms from one layer to the other. Since intimate contact is required in this procedure, it is particularly important to avoid contamination. The pure gold is relatively soft, so this type of restoration is limited to areas not subjected to much stress.

38.6 Other Metals

Several other metals have been used for a variety of specialized implant applications. *Tantalum* has been subjected to animal implant studies and has been shown very biocompatible. Due to its poor mechanical properties (Table 38.9) and its high density (16.6 g/cm^3) it is restricted to few applications such as wire sutures for plastic surgeons and neurosurgeons and a radioisotope for bladder tumors.

TABLE 38.9 Mechanical Properties of Tantalum (American Society for Testing and Materials, F560–86, p. 143, 1992)

Properties	Annealed	Cold-worked
Tensile strength (MPa)	207	517
Yield strength (0.2% offset) (MPa)	138	345
Elongation (%)	20–30	2
Young's modulus (GPa)	—	190

Platinum group metals (PGM) such as Pt, Pd, Rh, Ir, Ru, and Os are extremely corrosion resistant but have poor mechanical properties [Wynblatt, 1986]. They are mainly used as alloys for electrodes such as pacemaker tips because of their high resistance to corrosion and low threshold potentials for electrical conductivity.

Thermoseeds made of 70% Ni and 30% Cu have been produced which possess Curie points in the therapeutic **hyperthermia** range, approximately 40 to 50°C [Ferguson et al., 1992]. Upon the application of an alternating magnetic field, eddy currents are induced, which will provide a continuous heat source through resistive heating of the material. As the temperature of a ferromagnetic substance nears its Curie point, however, there is a loss of ferromagnetic properties and a resulting loss of heat output. Thus, self-regulation of temperature is achieved and can be used to deliver a constant hyperthermic temperature extracorporeally at any time and duration.

Surface modifications of metal alloys such as coatings by plasma spray, physical or chemical vapor deposition, ion implantaion, and fluidized bed deposition have been used in industry [Smith, 1993]. Coating implants with tissue compatible materials such as hydroxyapatite, oxide ceramics, Bioglass®, and pyrolytic carbon are typical applications in implants. Such efforts have been largely ineffective if the implants are permanent and particularly if the implants are subjected to a large loading. The main problem is the delamination of the coating or eventual wear of the coating. The added cost of coating or ion implanting hinders the use of such techniques unless the technique shows unequivocal superiority compared to the non-treated implants.

38.7 Corrosion of Metallic Implants

Corrosion is the unwanted chemical reaction of a metal with its environment, resulting in its continued degradation to oxides, hydroxides, or other compounds. Tissue fluid in the human body contains water, dissolved oxygen, proteins, and various ions such as chloride and hydroxide. As a result, the human body presents a very aggressive environment for metals used for implantation. Corrosion resistance of a metallic implant material is consequently an important aspect of its biocompatibility.

38.7.1 Electrochemical Aspects

The lowest free energy state of many metals in an oxygenated and hydrated environment is that of the oxide. Corrosion occurs when metal atoms become ionized and go into solution, or combine with oxygen or other species in solution to form a compound which flakes off or dissolves. The body environment is very aggressive in terms of corrosion since it is not only aqueous but also contains chloride ions and proteins. A variety of chemical reactions occur when a metal is exposed to an aqueous environment, as shown in Figure 38.10. The electrolyte, which contains ions in solution, serves to complete the electric circuit. In the human body, the required ions are plentiful in the body fluids. Anions are negative ions which migrate toward the **anode**, and cations are positive ions which migrate toward the **cathode**. At the anode, or positive electrode, the metal oxidizes by losing valence electrons as in the following:

$$M \rightarrow M^{+n} + ne^{-}$$

(38.2)

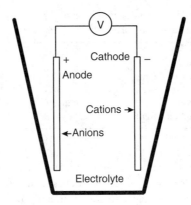

FIGURE 38.10   Electrochemical cell.

TABLE 38.10   Standard Electrochemical Series

Reaction	ΔE_0 [volts]
$Li \leftrightarrow Li^+$	−3.05
$Na \leftrightarrow Na^+$	−2.71
$Al \leftrightarrow Al^{+++}$	−1.66
$Ti \leftrightarrow Ti^{+++}$	−1.63
$Cr \leftrightarrow Cr^{++}$	−0.56
$Fe \leftrightarrow Fe^{++}$	−0.44
$Cu \leftrightarrow Cu^{++}$	−0.34
$Co \leftrightarrow Co^{++}$	−0.28
$Ni \leftrightarrow Ni^{++}$	−0.23
$H_2 \leftrightarrow 2H^+$	−0.00
$Ag \leftrightarrow Ag^+$	+0.80
$Au \leftrightarrow Au^+$	+1.68

At the cathode, or negative electrode, the following reduction reactions are important:

$$M^{+n} + ne^- \rightarrow M \tag{38.3}$$

$$M^{++} + OH^- + 2e^- \rightarrow MOH \tag{38.4}$$

$$2H_3O^+ + 2e^- \rightarrow H_2 \uparrow + 2H_2O \tag{38.5}$$

$$1/2 O_2 + H_2O + 2e^- \rightarrow 2OH^- \tag{38.6}$$

The tendency of metals to corrode is expressed most simply in the standard electrochemical series of **Nernst potentials**, shown in Table 38.10. These potentials are obtained in electrochemical measurements in which one electrode is a standard hydrogen electrode formed by bubbling hydrogen through a layer of finely divided platinum black. The potential of this reference electrode is defined to be zero. Noble metals are those which have a potential higher than that of a standard hydrogen electrode; base metals have lower potentials.

If two dissimilar metals are present in the same environment, the one which is most negative in the **galvanic series** will become the anode, and bimetallic (or galvanic) corrosion will occur. **Galvanic corrosion** can be much more rapid than the corrosion of a single metal. Consequently, implantation of dissimilar metals (mixed metals) is to be avoided. Galvanic action can also result in corrosion within a single metal, if there is inhomogeneity in the metal or in its environment, as shown in Figure 38.11.

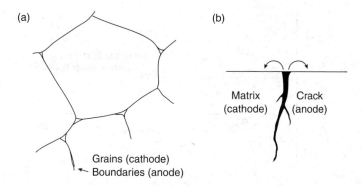

FIGURE 38.11   Micro-corrosion cells. (a) Grain boundaries are anodic with respect to the grain interior. (b) Crevice corrosion due to oxygen-deficient zone in metal's environment.

The potential difference, E, actually observed depends on the concentration of the metal ions in solution according to the Nernst equation,

$$E = E_o + (RT/nF) \ln[M^{+n}] \tag{38.7}$$

in which R is the gas constant, E_o is the standard electrochemical potential, T is the absolute temperature, F is Faraday's constant (96,487 C/mol), and n is the number of moles of ions.

The order of nobility observed in actual practice may differ from that predicted thermodynamically. The reasons are that some metals become covered with a *passivating* film of reaction products which protects the metal from further attack. The dissolution reaction may be strongly irreversible so that a potential barrier must be overcome. In this case, corrosion may be inhibited even though it remains energetically favorable. The kinetics of corrosion reactions are not determined by the thermodynamics alone.

38.7.2 Pourbaix Diagrams in Corrosion

The **Pourbaix diagram** is a plot of regions of *corrosion*, **passivity**, and **immunity** as they depend on electrode potential and pH [Pourbaix, 1974]. The Pourbaix diagrams are derived from the Nernst equation and from the solubility of the degradation products and the equilibrium constants of the reaction. For the sake of definition, the *corrosion region* is set arbitrarily at a concentration of greater than 10^{-6} g atom/l (molar) or more of metal in the solution at equilibrium. This corresponds to about 0.06 mg/l for metals such as iron and copper, and 0.03 mg/l for aluminum. *Immunity* is defined as equilibrium between metal and its ions at less than 10^{-6} M. In the region of immunity, the corrosion is energetically impossible. Immunity is also referred to as cathodic protection. In the passivation domain, the stable solid constituent is an oxide, hydroxide, hydride, or a salt of the metal. *Passivity* is defined as equilibrium between a metal and its reaction products (oxides, hydroxides, etc.) at a concentration of 10^{-6} M or less. This situation is useful if reaction products are adherent. In the biomaterials setting, passivity may or may not be adequate; disruption of a passive layer may cause an increase in corrosion. The equilibrium state may not occur if reaction products are removed by the tissue fluid. Materials differ in their propensity to re-establish a passive layer which has been damaged. This layer of material may protect the underlying metal if it is firmly adherent and nonporous; in that case further corrosion is prevented. Passivation can also result from a concentration polarization due to a buildup of ions near the electrodes. This is not likely to occur in the body since the ions are continually replenished. Cathodic depolarization reactions can aid in the passivation of a metal by virtue of an energy barrier which hinders the kinetics. Equation 38.5 and Equation 38.6 are examples.

There are two diagonal lines in the diagrams shown in Figure 38.12. The top oxygen line represents the upper limit of the stability of water and is associated with oxygen rich solutions or electrolytes near

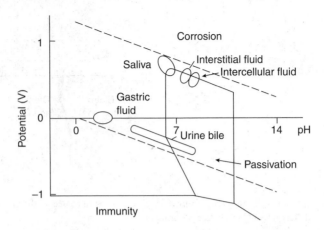

FIGURE 38.12   Pourbaix diagram for chromium, showing regions associated with various body fluids. (Modified from Black, J. (1992). *Biological Performance of Materials, 2nd ed.* New York: M. Dekker, Inc.)

oxidizing materials. In the region above this line, oxygen is evolved according to $2H_2O \rightarrow O_2 \uparrow + 4H^+ + 4e^-$. In the human body, saliva, intracellular fluid, and interstitial fluid occupy regions near the oxygen line, since they are saturated with oxygen. The lower hydrogen diagonal line represents the lower limit of the stability of water. Hydrogen gas is evolved according to Equation 38.5. Aqueous corrosion occurs in the region between these diagonal lines on the Pourbaix diagram. In the human body, urine, bile, the lower gastrointestinal tract, and secretions of ductless glands, occupy a region somewhat above the hydrogen line.

The significance of the Pourbaix diagram is as follows. Different parts of the body have different pH values and oxygen concentrations. Consequently, a metal which performs well (is immune or passive) in one part of the body may suffer an unacceptable amount of corrosion in another part. Moreover, pH can change dramatically in tissue that has been injured or infected. In particular, normal tissue fluid has a pH of about 7.4, but in a wound it can be as low as 3.5, and in an infected wound the pH can increase to 9.0.

Pourbaix diagrams are useful, but do not tell the whole story; there are some limitations. Diagrams are made considering equilibrium among metal, water, and reaction products. The presence of other ions, for example, chloride, may result in very much different behavior and large molecules in the body may also change the situation. Prediction of passivity may in some cases be optimistic, since reaction rates are not considered.

38.7.3   Rate of Corrosion and Polarization Curves

The regions in the Pourbaix diagram specify whether corrosion will take place, but they do not determine the rate. The rate, expressed as an electric current density (current per unit area), depends upon electrode potential as shown in the polarization curves shown in Figure 38.13. From such curves, it is possible to calculate the number of ions per unit time liberated into the tissue, as well as the depth of metal removed by corrosion in a given time. An alternative experiment is one in which the weight loss of a specimen of metal due to corrosion is measured as a function of time.

The rate of corrosion also depends on the presence of synergistic factors, such as those of mechanical origin (uneven distribution of mechanical stress). The stressed alloy failures occur due to the propagation of cracks in corrosive environments. For example, in corrosion fatigue (stress corrosion cracking), repetitive deformation of a metal in a corrosive environment results in acceleration of both the corrosion and the fatigue microdamage. Since the body environment involves both repeated mechanical loading and a chemically aggressive environment, fatigue testing of implant materials should always be performed under physiological environmental conditions; under Ringer's solution at body temperature. In *fretting corrosion*, rubbing of one part on another disrupts the passivation layer, resulting in accelerated corrosion. In

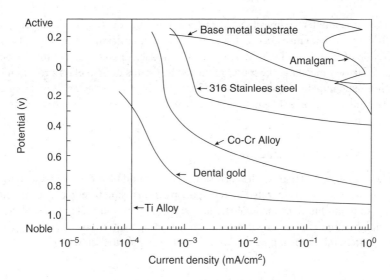

FIGURE 38.13   Potential-current density curves for some biomaterials [Greener et al., 1972].

pitting, the corrosion rate is accelerated in a local region. Stainless steel is vulnerable to pitting. Localized corrosion can occur if there is inhomogeneity in the metal or in the environment. *Grain boundaries* in the metal may be susceptible to the initiation of corrosion, as a result of their higher energy level. *Crevices* are also vulnerable to corrosion, since the chemical environment in the crevice may differ from that in the surrounding medium. The area of contact between a screw and a bone plate, for example, can suffer **crevice corrosion**.

38.7.4   Corrosion of Available Metals

Choosing a metal for implantation should take into account the corrosion properties discussed above. Metals which are in current use as biomaterials include gold, cobalt chromium alloys, type 316 stainless steel, cp-titanium, titanium alloys, nickel–titanium alloys, and silver-tin-mercury amalgam.

The noble metals are immune to corrosion and would be ideal materials if corrosion resistance were the only concern. Gold is widely used in dental restorations and in that setting it offers superior performance and longevity. Gold is not, however, used in orthopaedic applications as a result of its high density, insufficient strength, and high cost.

Titanium is a base metal in the context of the electrochemical series, however, it forms a robust passivating layer and remains passive under physiological conditions. Corrosion currents in normal saline are very low: 10^{-8} A/cm^2. Titanium implants remain virtually unchanged in appearance. Ti offers superior corrosion resistance but is not as stiff or strong as steel or Co–Cr alloys.

Cobalt–chromium alloys, like titanium, are passive in the human body. They are widely in use in orthopedic applications. They do not exhibit pitting corrosion.

Stainless steels contain enough chromium to confer corrosion resistance by passivity. The passive layer is not as robust as in the case of titanium or the cobalt chrome alloys. Only the most corrosion resistant of the stainless steels are suitable for implants. These are the austenitic types — 316, 316L, and 317, which contain molybdenum. Even these types of stainless steel are vulnerable to pitting and to crevice corrosion around screws.

The phases of dental amalgam are passive at neutral pH, the transpassive potential for the γ_2 phase is easily exceeded, due to interphase galvanic couples or potentials due to differential aeration under dental plaque. Amalgam, therefore, often corrodes and is the most active (corrosion prone) material used in dentistry.

Corrosion of an implant in the clinical setting can result in symptoms such as local pain and swelling in the region of the implant, with no evidence of infection; cracking or flaking of the implant as seen on x-ray films, and excretion of excess metal ions. At surgery, gray or black discoloration of the surrounding tissue may be seen and flakes of metal may be found in the tissue. Corrosion also plays a role in the mechanical failures of orthopaedic implants. Most of these failures are due to fatigue, and the presence of a saline environment certainly exacerbates fatigue. The extent to which corrosion influences fatigue in the body is not precisely known.

38.7.5 Stress Corrosion Cracking

When an implant is subjected to stress, the corrosion process could be accelerated due to the mechanical energy. If the mechanical stress is repeated then fatigue stress corrosion takes place such as in the femoral stem of the hip joint and hip nails made of stainless steels [Dobbs and Scales, 1979; Sloter and Piehler, 1979]. However, other mechanisms of corrosion such as fretting may also be involved at point of contact such as in the counter-sink of the hip nail or bone fracture plate for the screws.

38.8 Manufacturing of Implants

38.8.1 Stainless Steels

The austenitic stainless steels work-harden very rapidly as shown in Figure 38.2 and therefore, cannot be cold-worked without intermediate heat treatments. The heat treatments should not induce, however, the formation of chromium carbide (CCr_4) in the grain boundaries; this may cause corrosion. For the same reason, the austenitic stainless steel implants are not usually welded.

The distortion of components by the heat treatments can occur but this problem can be solved by controlling the uniformity of heating. Another undesirable effect of the heat treatment is the formation of surface oxide scales which have to be removed either chemically (acid) or mechanically (sand-blasting). After the scales are removed the surface of the component is polished to a mirror or mat finish. The surface is then cleaned, degreased, and passivated in nitric acid (ASTM Standard F86). The component is washed and cleaned again before packaging and sterilizing.

38.8.2 Co–Cr Alloys

The CoCrMo alloy is particularly susceptible to work-hardening so that the normal fabrication procedure used with other metals cannot be employed. Instead, the alloy is cast by a lost wax (or investment casting) method which involves making a wax pattern of the desired component. The pattern is coated with a refractory material, first by a thin coating with a slurry (suspension of silica in ethyl silicate solution) followed by complete investing after drying (1) the wax is then melted out in a furnace (100–150°C), (2) the mold is heated to a high temperature burning out any traces of wax or gas forming materials, (3) molten alloy is poured with gravitational or centrifugal force, and (4) the mold is broken after cooled. The mold temperature is about 800–1000°C and the alloy is at 1350–1400°C.

Controlling the mold temperature will have an effect on the grain size of the final cast; coarse ones are formed at higher temperatures which will decrease the strength. However, high processing temperature will result in larger carbide precipitates with greater distances between them resulting in a less brittle material. Again there is a complementary (trade off) relationship between strength and toughness.

38.8.3 Ti and Its Alloys

Titanium is very reactive at high temperature and burns readily in the presence of oxygen. Therefore, it requires an inert atmosphere for high temperature processing or is processed by vacuum melting. Oxygen diffuses readily in titanium and the dissolved oxygen embrittles the metal. As a result, any hot working or forging operation should be carried out below 925°C. Machining at room temperature is not the solution to all the problems since the material also tends to gall or seize the cutting tools. Very sharp tools with slow speeds and large feeds are used to minimize this effect. Electrochemical machining is an attractive means.

Defining Terms

Amalgam: An alloy obtained by mixing silver tin alloy with mercury.

Anode: Positive electrode in an electrochemical cell.

Cathode: Negative electrode in an electrochemical cell.

Corrosion: Unwanted reaction of metal with environment. In a Pourbaix diagram, it is the region in which the metal ions are present at a concentration of more than 10^{-6} M.

Crevice corrosion: A form of localized corrosion in which concentration gradients around pre-existing crevices in the material drive corrosion processes.

Curie temperature: Transition temperature of a material from ferromagnetic to paramagnetic.

Galvanic corrosion: Dissolution of metal driven by macroscopic differences in electrochemical potential, usually as a result of dissimilar metals in proximity.

Galvanic series: Table of electrochemical potentials (voltage) associated with the ionization of metal atoms. These are called Nernst potentials.

Hyperthermia: Application of high enough thermal energy (heat) to suppress the cancerous cell activities. Above 41.5°C (but below 60°C) is needed to have any effect.

Immunity: Resistance to corrosion by an energetic barrier. In a Pourbaix diagram, it is the region in which the metal is in equilibrium with its ions at a concentration of less than 10^{-6} M. Noble metals resist corrosion by immunity.

Martensite: A metastable structure formed by quenching of austenite (g) structure in alloys such as steel and Ti alloys. They are brittle and hard, and therefore, are further treated with heat to make tougher.

Nernst potential: Standard electrochemical potential measured with respect to a standard hydrogen electrode.

Noble: Type of metal with a positive standard electrochemical potential.

Passivation: Production of corrosion resistance by a surface layer of reaction products (Normally oxide layer which is impervious to gas and water.)

Passivity: Resistance to corrosion by a surface layer of reaction products. In a Pourbaix diagram, it is the region in which the metal is in equilibrium with its reaction products at a concentration of less than 10^{-6} molar.

Pitting: A form of localized corrosion in which pits form on the metal surface.

Pourbaix diagram: Plot of electrical potential vs. pH for a material in which the regions of corrosion, passivity, and immunity are identified.

Shape memory effect (SME):   Thermoelastic behavior of some alloys which can revert back to their original shape when the temperature is greater than the phase transformation temperature of the alloy.

Superelasticity: Minimal stress increase beyond the initial strain region resulting in very low modulus in the region for some shape memory alloys.

References

ASTM (1980). Annual Book of *ASTM Standards* (Philadelphia, PA).

Black, J. (1992). *Biological Performance of Materials*, 2nd ed. New York: M. Dekker, Inc.

Bordiji, K., Jouzeau, J., Mainard, D., Payan, E., Delagoutte, J., and Netter, P. (1996). Evaluation of the effect of three surface treatments on the biocompatibility of 316L stainless steel using human differentiated cells. *Biomaterials* 17, 491–500.

Breen, D.J. and Stoker, D.J. (1993). Titanium lines: a manifestation of metallosis and tissue response to titanium alloy megaprostheses at the knee. *Clin. Radiol.* 43, 274–277.

Buehler, W.J., Gilfrich, J.V., and Wiley, R.C. (1963). Effect of low-temperature phase changes on the mechanical properties of alloys near composition Ti–Ni. *J. Appl. Phys.* 34, 1475–1477.

Davidson, J.A., Mishra, A.K., Kovacs, P., and Poggie, R.A. (1994). New surface hardened, low-modulus, corrosion-resistant Ti–13Nb–13Zr alloy for total hip arthroplasty. *Biomed. Mater. Eng.* 4, 231–243.

Devine, T.M. and Wulff, J. (1975). Cast vs. wrought cobalt–chromium surgical implant alloys. *J. Biomed. Mater. Res.* 9, 151–167.

Dobbs, H.S. and Scales, J.T. (1979). Fracture and corrosion in stainless steel hip replacement stems. In *Corrosion and Degradation of Implant Materials*, Syrett, B.C. and Acharya, A. Eds. Philadelphia: American Society for Testing and Materials, pp. 245–258.

Duerig, T.W., Melton, K.N., Stockel, D., and Wayman, C.M. (1990). *Engineering Aspects of Shape Memory Alloys*. London: Butterworth-Heinemann.

Feighan, J.E., Goldberg, V.M., Davy, D., Parr, J.A., and Stevenson, S. (1995). The influence of surface-blasting on the incorporation of titanium–alloy implants in a rabbit intramedullary model. 77A, 1380–1395.

Ferguson, S.D., Paulus, J.A., Tucker, R.D., Loening, S.A., and Park, J.B. (1992). Effect of thermal treatment on heating characteristics of Ni–Cu Alloy for hyperthermie: preliminary studies. *J. Appl. Biomater.* 4, 55–60.

Granchi, D., Ciapetti, G., Savarino, L., Cavedagna, D., Donati, M.E., and Pizzoferrato, A. (1996). Assessment of metal extract toxicity on human lymphocytes cultured *in vitro*. *J. Biomed. Mater. Res.* 31, 183–191.

Greener, E.H., Harcourt, J.K., and Lautenschlager, E.P. (1972). *Materials Science in Dentistry*. Baltimore, MD: Williams and Wilkins.

Hazan, R., Brener, R., and Oron, U. (1993). Bone growth to metal implants is regulated by their surface chemical properties. *Biomaterials* 570–574.

Hille, G.H. (1966). Titanium for surgical implants. *J. Mater.* 1, 373–383.

Imam, M.A., Fraker, A.C., Harris, J.S., and Gilmore, C.M. (1983). Influence of heat treatment on the fatigue lives of Ti–6Al–4V and Ti–4.5Al–5Mo–1.5CR. In *Titanium Alloys in Surgical Implants*, Luckey, H.A. and Kubli, F.E. Eds. Philadelphia, PA: ASTM special technical publication 796, pp. 105–119.

Kasemo, B. and Lausma, J. (1988). Biomaterial and implant surface: A surface science approach. *Int. J. Oral Maxillofac Implant.* 3, 247–259.

Keating, F.H. (1956). *Chromium-Nickel Autentic Steels*. London: Butterworths.

Keller, J.C., Stanford, C.M., Wightman, J.P., Draughn, R.A., and Zaharias, R. (1994). Characterizations of titanium implant surfaces. III. *J. Biomed. Mater. Res.* 28, 939–946.

Kieswetter, K., Schwartz, Z., Hummert, T.W., Cochran, D.L., Simpson, J., and Boyan, B.D. (1996). Surface roughness modulates the local production of growth factors and cytokines by osteoblast-like MG-63 cells. *J. Biomed. Mater. Res.* 32, 55–63.

Kim, H., Miyaji, F., Kokubo, T., and Nakamura, T. (1996). Preparation of bioactive Ti and its alloys via simple chemical surface treatment. *J. Biomed. Mater. Res.* 32, 409–417.

Lee, J.H., Park, J.B., Andreasen, G.F., and Lakes, R.S. (1988). Thermomechanical study of Ni–Ti alloys. *J. Biomed. Mater. Res.* 22, 573–588.

Nielsen, J.P. (1986). Dental noble-metal casting alloys: composition and properties. In *Encyclopedia of Materials Science and Engineering*, Bever, M.B. Ed. Oxford, Cambridge: Pergamon Press, pp. 1093–1095.

Pourbaix, M. (1974). *Atlas of Electrochemical Equilibria in Aqueous Solutions*, 2nd ed. Houston/CEBELCOR, Brussels: NACE.

Richards-Mfg-Company. (1980). Biophase implant material, technical information publication 3846 Memphis, TN.

Schmalzried, T.P., Peters, P.C., Maurer, B.T., Bragdon, C.R., and Harris, W.H. (1996). Long-duration metal-on-metal total hip arthroplasties with low wear of the articulating surfaces. *J. Arthroplasty* 11, 322–331.

Semlitch, M. (1980). Properties of wrought CoNiCrMo alloy Protasul-10, a highly corrosion and fatigue resistant implant material for joint endoprostheses. *Eng. Med.* 9, 201–207.

Sloter, L.E. and Piehler, H.R. (1979). Corrosion-fatigue performance of stainless steel hip nails — Jewett type. In *Corrosion and Degradation of Implant Materials*, Syrett, B.C. and Acharya, A. Eds. Philadelphia, PA: American Society for Testing and Materials, pp. 173–195.

Smith, C.J.E. and Hughes, A.N. (1966). The corrosion-fatigue behavior of a titanium-6w/o aluminum-4w/o vanadium alloy. *Eng. Med.* 7, 158–171.

Smith, W.F. (1993). *Structure and Properties of Engineering Alloys*, 2nd ed. New York: McGraw-Hill.

Takatsuka, K., Yamamuro, T., Nakamura, T., and Kokubo, T. (1995). Bone-bonding behavior of titanium alloy evaluated mechanically with detaching failure load. *J. Biomed. Mater. Res.* 29, 157–163.

Takeshita, F., Ayukawa, Y., Iyama, S., Murai, K., and Suetsugu, T. (1997). Long-term evaluation of bone-titanium interface in rat tibiae using light microscopy, transmission electron microscopy, and image processing. *J. Biomed. Mater. Res.* 37, 235–242.

Wayman, C.M. and Duerig, T.W. (1990). An introduction of martensite and shape memory. In *Engineering Aspects of Shape Memory Alloys*, Duerig, T.W., Melton, K.N., Stockel, D., and Wayman, C.M. Eds. London: Butterworth-Heinemann, pp. 3–20.

Wayman, C.M. and Shimizu, K. (1972). The shape memory ('Marmem') effect in alloys. *Metal Sci. J.* 6, 175–183.

Williams, D.F. (1982). *Biocompatibility in Clinical Practice*. Boca Raton, FL: CRC Press.

Wynblatt, P. (1986). Platinum Group Metals and Alloys. In *Encyclopedia of Materials Science and Engineering*, Bever, M.B. Ed. Oxford, Cambridge: Pergamon Press, pp. 3576–3579.

Yan, W., Nakamura, T., Kobayashi, M., Kim, H., Miyaji, F., and Kokubo, T. (1997). Bonding of chemically treated titanium implants to bone. *J. Biomed. Mater. Res.* 37, 267–275.

Further Reading

American Society for Testing and Materials. 1992. *Annual Book of ASTM Standards*, vol. 13, *Medical Devices and Services*, American Society for Testing and Materials, Philadelphia, PA.

Bardos, D.I. 1977. Stainless steels in medical devices, in *Handbook of Stainless Steels*. Peckner, D. and Bernstein, I.M., Eds. pp. 1–10, McGraw-Hill, New York.

Bechtol, C.O., Ferguson, A.B., Jr., and Laing, P.G. 1959. *Metals and Engineering in Bone and Joint Surgery*, Williams and Wilkins, Baltimore, MD.

Comte, T.W. 1984. Metallurgical observations of biomaterials, in *Contemporary Biomaterials*, Boretos, J.W. and Eden, M., Eds., pp. 66–91, Noyes, Park Ridge, NJ.

Duerig, T.W., Melton, K.N., Stockel, D., and Wayman, C.M., Eds. 1990. *Engineering Aspects of Shape Memory Alloys*, Butterworth-Heinemann, London.

Dumbleton, J.H. and Black, J. 1975. *An Introduction to Orthopaedic Materials*, C. Thomas, Springfield, IL.

Fontana, M.G. and Greene, N.O. 1967. *Corrosion Engineering*, pp. 163–168, McGraw-Hill, New York.

Greener, E.H., Harcourt, J.K., and Lautenschlager, E.P. 1972. *Materials Science in Dentistry*, Williams and Wilkins, Baltimore, MD.

Hildebrand, H.F. and Champy, M., Eds. 1988. *Biocompatibility of Co–Cr–Ni Alloys*. Plenum Press, New York.

Levine, S.N., Ed. 1968. *Materials in Biomedical Engineering*, Annals of New York Academy of Science, vol. 146. New York.

Luckey H.A., Ed. 1983. *Titanium Alloys in Surgical Implants*, ASTM Special Technical Publication 796, Philadelphia, PA

Mears, D.C. 1979. *Materials and Orthopaedic Surgery*, Williams and Wilkins, Baltimore, MD.

Park, J.B. 1984. *Biomaterials Science and Engineering*, Plenum Pub., New York.

Perkins, J., Ed. 1975. *Shape Memory Effects in Alloys*, Plenum Press, New York.

Puckering, F.B., Ed. 1979. *The Metallurgical Evolution of Stainless Steels*, 1–42, American Society for Metals and the Metals Society, Metals Park, OH.

Smith, W.F. 1993. *Structure and Properties of Engineering Alloys*, 2nd ed., McGraw-Hill, New York.

Weinstein, A., Horowitz, E., and Ruff, A.W., Eds. 1977. *Retrieval and Analysis of Orthopaedic Implants*, NBS, U.S. Department of Commerce, Washington, D.C.

Williams, D.F. and Roaf, R. 1973. Implants in *Surgery*, W.B. Sauders Co., LTD, London.

39

Ceramic Biomaterials

W.C. Billotte
University of Dayton

39.1   Introduction

Ceramics are defined as the art and science of making and using solid articles that have as their essential component, inorganic nonmetallic materials [Kingery et al., 1976]. Ceramics are refractory, polycrystal line compounds, usually inorganic, including silicates, metallic oxides, carbides and various refractory hydrides, sulfides, and selenides. Oxides such as Al_2O_3, MgO, SiO_2, and ZrO_2 contain metallic and nonmetallic elements and ionic salts, such as $NaCl$, $CsCl$, and ZnS [Park and Lakes, 1992]. Exceptions to the preceding include covalently bonded ceramics such as diamond and carbonaceous structures like graphite and pyrolized carbons [Park and Lakes, 1992].

Ceramics in the form of pottery have been used by humans for thousands of years. Until recently, their use was somewhat limited because of their inherent brittleness, susceptibility to notches or micro-cracks, low tensile strength, and low impact strength. However, within the last 100 years, innovative techniques for fabricating ceramics have led to their use as "high tech" materials. In recent years, humans have realized that ceramics and their composites can also be used to augment or replace various parts of the body, particularly bone. Thus, the ceramics used for the latter purposes are classified as *bioceramics*. Their relative inertness to the body fluids, high compressive strength, and aesthetically pleasing appearance led to the use of ceramics in dentistry as dental crowns. Some carbons have found use as implants especially for blood interfacing applications such as heart valves. Due to their high specific strength as fibers and their biocompatibility, ceramics are also being used as reinforcing components of composite implant materials and for tensile loading applications such as artificial tendon and ligaments [Park and Lakes, 1992].

Unlike metals and polymers, ceramics are difficult to shear plastically due to the (ionic) nature of the bonding and minimum number of slip systems. These characteristics make the ceramics nonductile and are responsible for almost zero creep at room temperature [Park and Lakes, 1992]. Consequently, ceramics are very susceptible to notches or microcracks because instead of undergoing plastic deformation (or yield) they will fracture elastically on initiation of a crack. At the crack tip the stress could be many times higher than the stress in the material away from the tip, resulting in a *stress concentration* which weakens the material considerably. The latter makes it difficult to predict the tensile strength of the material (ceramic). This is also the reason ceramics have low tensile strength compared to compressive strength. If a ceramic is flawless, it is very strong even when subjected to tension. Flawless glass fibers have twice the tensile strengths of high strength steel ($\sim$7 GPa) [Park and Lakes, 1992].

Ceramics are generally hard; in fact, the measurement of hardness is calibrated against ceramic materials. Diamond is the hardest, with a hardness index of 10 on Moh's scale, and talc ($Mg_3Si_3O_{10}COH$) is the softest ceramic (Moh's hardness 1), while ceramics such as **alumina** (Al_2O_3; hardness 9), quartz (SiO_2; hardness 8), and apatite ($Ca_5P_3O_{12}F$; hardness 5) are in the middle range. Other characteristics of ceramic materials are (1) their high melting temperatures and (2) low conductivity of electricity and heat. These characteristics are due to the chemical bonding within ceramics.

In order to be classified as a bioceramic, the ceramic material must meet or exceed the properties listed in Table 39.1. The number of specific ceramics currently in use or under investigation cannot be accounted for in the space available for bioceramics in this book. Thus, this chapter will focus on a general overview of the relatively bioinert, bioactive or surface reactive ceramics, and biodegradable or resorbable bioceramics.

Ceramics used in fabricating implants can be classified as nonabsorbable (relatively inert), bioactive or surface reactive (semi-inert) [Hench, 1991, 1993] and biodegradable or resorbable (non-inert) [Hentrich et al., 1971; Graves et al., 1972]. Alumina, zirconia, silicone nitrides, and carbons are inert bioceramics. Certain **glass ceramics** and dense **hydroxyapatites** are semi-inert (bioactive) and **calcium phosphates** and calcium aluminates are resorbable ceramics [Park and Lakes, 1992].

39.2   Nonabsorbable or Relatively Bioinert Bioceramics

39.2.1   Relatively Bioinert Ceramics

Relatively bioinert ceramics maintain their physical and mechanical properties while in the host. They resist corrosion and wear and have all the properties listed for bioceramics in Table 39.1. Examples of relatively bioinert ceramics are dense and porous aluminum oxides, zirconia ceramics, and single phase calcium aluminates (Table 39.2). Relatively bioinert ceramics are typically used as structural-support

TABLE 39.1   Desired Properties of Implantable Bioceramics

1. Should be nontoxic
2. Should be noncarcinogenic
3. Should be nonallergic
4. Should be noninflammatory
5. Should be biocompatible
6. Should be biofunctional for its lifetime in the host

implants. Some of these are bone plates, bone screws, and femoral heads (Table 39.3). Examples of nonstructural support uses are ventilation tubes, sterilization devices [Feenstra and de Groot, 1983] and drug delivery devices (see Table 39.3).

39.2.2 Alumina (Al_2O_3)

The main source of high purity alumina (aluminum oxide, Al_2O_3) is bauxite and native corundum. The commonly available alumina (alpha, α) can be prepared by calcining alumina trihydrate. The chemical composition and density of commercially available "pure" calcined alumina are given in Table 39.4. The American Society for Testing and Materials (ASTM) specifies that alumina for implant use should contain 99.5% pure alumina and less than 0.1% combined SiO_2 and alkali oxides (mostly Na_2O) (F603-78).

Alpha alumina has a rhombohedral crystal structure ($a = 4.758$ Å and $c = 12.991$ Å). Natural alumina is known as sapphire or ruby, depending on the types of impurities which give rise to color. The single

TABLE 39.2 Examples of Relatively Bioinert Bioceramics

Bioinert Ceramics	References
1. Pyrolitic carbon coated devices	Adams and Williams, 1978
	Bokros et al., 1972
	Bokros, 1972
	Chandy and Sharma, 1991
	Dellsperger and Chandran, 1991
	Kaae, 1971
	More and Silver, 1990
	Shimm and Haubold, 1980
	Shobert, 1964
2. Dense and nonporous aluminum oxides	Hench, 1991
	Hentrich et al., 1971
	Krainess and Knapp, 1978
	Park, 1991
	Ritter et al., 1979
	Shackelford, 1988
3. Porous aluminum oxides	Hench, 1991
	Hentrich et al., 1971
	Park, 1991
	Ritter et al., 1979
	Shackelford, 1988
4. Zirconia ceramics	Barinov and Baschenko, 1992
	Drennan and Steele, 1991
	Hench, 1991
	Kumar et al., 1989
5. Dense hydroxyapatites	Bajpai, 1990
	Cotell et al., 1992
	Fulmer et al., 1992
	Huaxia et al., 1992
	Kijima and Tsutsumi, 1979
	Knowles et al., 1993
	Meenan et al., 1992
	Niwa et al., 1980
	Posner et al., 1958
	Schwartz et al., 1993
	Valiathan et al., 1993
	Whitehead et al., 1993
6. Calcium aluminates	Hammer et al., 1972
	Hentrich et al., 1971
	Hulbert and Klawitter, 1971

TABLE 39.3   Uses of Bioinert Bioceramics

Bioinert Ceramics	References
1. In reconstruction of acetabular cavities	Boutin, 1981
	Dorlot et al., 1986
2. As bone plates and screws	Zimmermann et al., 1991
3. In the form of ceramic–ceramic composites	Boutin, 1981
	Chignier et al., 1987
	Sedel et al.,1991
	Terry et al., 1989
4. In the form of ceramic–polymer composites	Hulbert, 1992
5. As drug delivery devices	Buykx et al., 1992
6. As femoral heads	Boutin, 1981
	Dörre, 1991
	Ohashi et al., 1988
	Oonishi, 1992
7. As middle ear ossicles	Grote, 1987
8. In the reconstruction of orbital rims	Heimke, 1992
9. As components of total and partial hips	Feenstra and de Groot, 1983
10. In the form of sterilization tubes	Feenstra and de Groot, 1983
11. As ventilation tubes	Feenstra and de Groot, 1983
12. In the repair of the cardiovascular area	Chignier et al., 1987
	Ely and Haubold, 1993

TABLE 39.4   Chemical Composition of Calcined Alumina

Chemicals	Composition (Weight %)
Al_2O_3	99.6
SiO_2	0.12
Fe_2O_3	0.03
Na_2O	0.04

Source: Park, J.B., and Lakes, R.S. 1992. *Ceramic Implant Materials.* In: *Biomaterials An Introduction,* 2nd ed., p. 121 Plenum Press, New York.

crystal form of alumina has been used successfully to make implants [Kawahara, 1989; Park 1991]. Single crystal alumina can be made by feeding fine alumina powders onto the surface of a seed crystal which is slowly withdrawn from an electric arc or oxy-hydrogen flame as the fused powder builds up. Single crystals of alumina up to 10 cm in diameter have been grown by this method [Park and Lakes, 1992].

The strength of polycrystalline alumina depends on its grain size and porosity. Generally, the smaller the grains, the lower the porosity and the higher the strength [Park and Lakes, 1992]. The ASTM standards (F603-78) requires a flexural strength greater than 400 MPa and elastic modulus of 380 GPa (Table 39.5).

Aluminum oxide has been used in the area of orthopaedics for more than 25 years [Hench, 1991]. Single crystal alumina has been used in orthopaedics and dental surgery for almost 20 years. Alumina is usually a quite hard material, its hardness varies from 20 to 30 GPa. This high hardness permits its use as an abrasive (emery) and as bearings for watch movements [Park and Lakes, 1992]. Both polycrystalline and single crystal alumina have been used clinically. The high hardness is accompanied by low friction and wear and inertness to the *in vivo* environment. These properties make alumina an ideal material for use in joint replacements [Park and Lakes, 1992]. Aluminum oxide implants in bones of rhesus monkeys have shown no signs of rejection or toxicity for 350 days [Graves et al., 1972; Hentrich et al., 1971]. One of the most popular uses for aluminum oxide is in total hip protheses. Aluminum oxide hip protheses

TABLE 39.5   Physical Property Requirements
of Alumina and Partially Stabilized Zirconia

Properties	Alumina	Zirconia
Elastic Modulus (GPa)	380	190
Flexural strength (GPa)	>0.4	1.0
Hardness, Mohs	9	6.5
Density (g/cm^3)	3.8–3.9	5.95
Grain size (μm)	4.0	0.6

Note: Both the ceramics contain 3 mole %Y_2O_3.
Source: Park, J.B. personal communication, 1993.

with an ultra-high molecular weight polyethylene (UHMWPE) socket have been claimed to be a better device than a metal prostheses with a UHMWPE socket [Oonishi, 1992]. However, the key for success of any implant, besides the correct surgical implantation, is the highest possible quality control during fabrication of the material and the production of the implant [Hench, 1991].

39.2.3   Zirconia (ZrO_2)

Pure zirconia can be obtained from chemical conversion of zircon ($ZrSiO_4$), which is an abundant mineral deposit [Park and Lakes, 1992]. Zirconia has a high melting temperature ($T_m = 2953$ K) and chemical stability with $a = 5.145$ Å, $b = 0.521$ Å, $c = 5.311$ Å, and $\beta = 99°14$ in [Park and Lakes, 1992]. It undergoes a large volume change during phase changes at high temperature in pure form; therefore, a dopant oxide such as Y_2O_3 is used to stabilize the high temperature (cubic) phase. We have used 6 mole% Y_2O_3 as dopant to make zirconia for implantation in bone [Hentrich et al., 1971]. Zirconia produced in this manner is referred to as *partially stabilized* zirconia [Drennan and Steele, 1991]. However, the physical properties of zirconia are somewhat inferior to that of alumina (Table 39.5).

High density zirconia oxide showed excellent compatibility with autogenous rhesus monkey bone and was completely nonreactive to the body environment for the duration of the 350 day study [Hentrich et al., 1971]. Zirconia has shown excellent biocompatibility and good wear and friction when combined with ultra-high molecular weight polyethylene [Kumar et al., 1989; Murakami and Ohtsuki, 1989].

39.2.4   Carbons

Carbons can be made in many allotropic forms: crystalline diamond, graphite, noncrystalline glassy carbon, and quasicrystalline pyrolitic carbon. Among these, only pyrolitic carbon is widely utilized for implant fabrication; it is normally used as a surface coating. It is also possible to coat surfaces with diamond. Although the techniques of coating with diamond have the potential to revolutionize medical device manufacturing, it is not yet commercially available [Park and Lakes, 1992].

The crystalline structure of carbon, as used in implants, is similar to the graphite structure shown in Figure 39.1. The planar hexagonal arrays are formed by strong covalent bonds in which one of the valence electrons or atoms is free to move, resulting in high but anisotropic electric conductivity. Since the bonding between the layers is stronger than the van der Waals force, it has been suggested that the layers are *cross-linked*. However, the remarkable lubricating property of graphite cannot be attained unless the cross-links are eliminated [Park and Lakes, 1992].

The poorly crystalline carbons are thought to contain unassociated or unoriented carbon atoms. The hexagonal layers are not perfectly arranged, as shown in Figure 39.2. Properties of individual crystallites seem to be highly anisotropic. However, if the crystallites are randomly dispersed, the aggregate becomes isotropic [Park and Lakes, 1992].

The mechanical properties of carbon, especially pyrolitic carbon, are largely dependent on its density, as shown in Figure 39.3 and Figure 39.4. The increased mechanical properties are directly related to increased

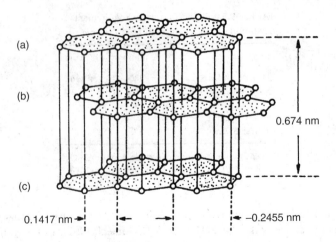

FIGURE 39.1 Crystal structure of graphite. (From Shobert, E.I. 1964. *Carbon and Graphite*. New York, Academic Press. With permission.)

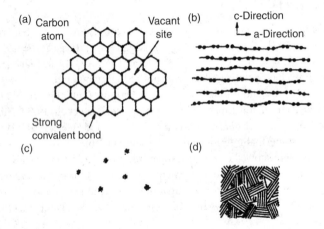

FIGURE 39.2 Schematic presentation of poorly crystalline carbon. (a) Single-layer plane, (b) parallel layers in a crystallite, (c) unassociated carbon, (d) an aggregate of crystallites, single layers and unassociated carbon. (From Bokros, J.C. 1972. *Chem. Phys. Carbon.* 5: 70–81, New York, Marcel Dekker. With permission.)

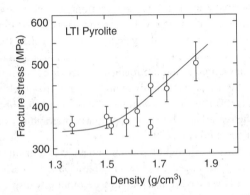

FIGURE 39.3 Fracture stress vs. density for unalloyed LTI pyrolite carbons. (From Kaae, J.L. 1971. *J. Nucl. Mater.* 38: 42–50. With permission.)

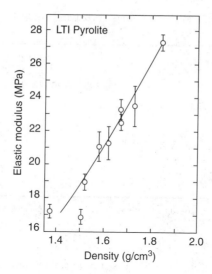

FIGURE 39.4   Elastic modulus vs. density for unalloyed LTI pyrolite carbons. (From Kaae, J.L. 1971. *J. Nucl. Mater.* 38:42–50. With permission.)

TABLE 39.6   Properties of Various Types of Carbon

Properties	Types of Carbon		
	Graphite	Glassy	Pyrolitica[a]
Density (g/cm3)	1.5–1.9	1.5	1.5–2.0
Elastic modulus (GPa)	24	24	28
Compressive strength (MPa)	138	172	517 (575[a])
Toughness (Mn/cm^3)[b]	6.3	0.6	4.8

[a] 1.0 w/o Si-alloyed pyrolitic carbon, Pyrolite ™(Carbomedics, Austin, TX).
[b] 1 m-N/cm^3 = 1.45 × 10^{-3} in.-lb/in.^{3}.
Source: Park, J.B., and Lakes, R.S. 1992. *Biomaterials An Introduction*, 2nd ed, p. 133. Plenum Press, New York.

density, which indicates that the properties of pyrolitic carbon depend mainly on the aggregate structure of the material [Park and Lakes, 1992].

Graphite and glassy carbon have a much lower mechanical strength than pyrolitic carbon (Table 39.6). However, the average modulus of elasticity is almost the same for all carbons. The strength of pyrolitic carbon is quite high compared to graphite and glassy carbon. Again, this is due to the fewer number of flaws and unassociated carbons in the aggregate.

A composite carbon which is reinforced with carbon fiber has been considered for making implants. However, the carbon–carbon composite is highly anisotropic, and its density is in the range of 1.4 to 1.45 g/cm^3 with a porosity of 35 to 38% (Table 39.7).

Carbons exhibit excellent compatibility with tissue. Compatibility of pyrolitic carbon-coated devices with blood have resulted in extensive use of these devices for repairing diseased heart valves and blood vessels [Park and Lakes, 1992].

Pyrolitic carbons can be deposited onto finished implants from hydrocarbon gas in a *fluidized bed* at a controlled temperature and pressure. The anisotropy, density, crystallite size and structure of the deposited carbon can be controlled by temperature, composition of the fluidized gas, the bed geometry, and the residence time (velocity) of the gas molecules in the bed. The microstructure of deposited carbon should be highly controlled, since the formation of growth features associated with uneven crystallization

TABLE 39.7   Mechanical Properties of Carbon Fiber-Reinforced Carbon

	Fiber lay-up	
Property	Unidirectional	0–90° Crossply
Flexural Modulus (GPa)		
Longitudinal	140	60
Transverse	7	60
Flexural Strength (MPa)		
Longitudinal	1,200	500
Transverse	15	500
Interlaminar shear strength (MPa)	18	18

Source: Adams, D. and Williams, D.F. 1978. *J. Biomed. Mater. Res.* 12: 38.

can result in a weaker material (Figure 39.5). It is also possible to introduce various elements into the fluidized gas and co-deposit them with carbon. Usually silicon (10 to 20 w/o) is co-deposited (or alloyed) to increase hardness for applications requiring resistance to abrasion, such as heart valve discs.

Recently, success was achieved in depositing pyrolitic carbon onto the surfaces of blood vessel implants made of polymers. This type of carbon is called ultra low temperature isotropic (ULTI) carbon instead of low temperature isotropic (**LTI**) **carbon**. The deposited carbon has excellent compatibility with blood and is thin enough not to interfere with the flexibility of the grafts [Park and Lakes, 1992].

The vitreous or glassy carbon is made by controlled pyrolysis of polymers such as phenolformaldehyde, Rayon (cellulose), and polyacrylnitrite at a high temperature in a controlled environment. This process is particularly useful for making carbon fibers and textiles which can be used alone or as components of composites.

39.3   Biodegradable or Resorbable Ceramics

Although Plaster of Paris was used in 1892 as a bone substitute [Peltier, 1961], the concept of using synthetic resorbable ceramics as bone substitutes was introduced in 1969 [Hentrich et al., 1969; Graves et al., 1972]. *Resorbable ceramics*, as the name implies, degrade upon implantation in the host. The resorbed material is replaced by endogenous tissues. The rate of degradation varies from material to material. Almost all bioresorbable ceramics except Biocoral and Plaster of Paris (calcium sulfate dihydrate) are variations of calcium phosphate (Table 39.8). Examples of resorbable ceramics are aluminum calcium phosphate, coralline, Plaster of Paris, hydroxyapatite, and tricalcium phosphate (Table 39.8).

39.3.1   Calcium Phosphate

Calcium phosphate has been used in the form of artificial bone. This material has been synthesized and used for manufacturing various forms of implants, as well as for solid or porous coatings on other implants (Table 39.9).

Calcium phosphate can be crystallized into salts such as hydroxyapatite and β-whitlockite depending on the Ca:P ratio, presence of water, impurities, and temperature. In a wet environment and at lower temperatures ($<900°C$), it is more likely that hydroxyl- or hydroxyapatite will form, while in a dry atmosphere and at a higher temperature, β-whitlockite will be formed [Park and Lakes 1992]. Both forms are very tissue compatible and are used as bone substitutes in a granular form or a solid block. The apatite form of calcium phosphate is considered to be closely related to the mineral phase of bone and teeth.

The mineral part of bone and teeth is made of a crystalline form of calcium phosphate similar to hydroxyapatite $[Ca_{10}(PO_4)_6(OH)_2]$. The apatite family of mineral $[A_{10}(BO_4)_6X_2]$ crystallizes into

TABLE 39.8 Examples of Biodegradable Bioceramics

Biodegradable or Resorbable Bioceramics	References
1. Aluminum–Calcium–Phosphorous Oxides	Bajpai et al., 1985 Mattie and Bajpai, 1988 Wyatt et al., 1976
2. Glass Fibers and their composites	Alexander et al., 1987 Zimmermann et al., 1991
3. Corals	Bajpai, 1983 Guillemin et al., 1989 Khavari and Bajpai, 1993 Sartoris et al., 1986 Wolford et al., 1987
4. Calcium Sulfates, including Plaster of Paris	Bajpai, 1983 Peltier, 1961 Scheidler and Bajpai, 1992
5. Ferric Calcium Phosphorous Oxides	Fuski et al., 1993 Larrabee et al., 1993 Stricker et al., 1992
6. Hydroxyapatites	Bajpai and Fuchs, 1985 Bajpai, 1983 Jenei et al., 1986 Ricci et al., 1986
7. Tricalcium Phosphate	Bajpai, 1983 Bajpai et al., 1988 Lemons et al., 1988 Morris and Bajpai, 1989
8. Zinc–Calcium–Phosphorous Oxides	Arar et al., 1989 Bajpai, US. Patent No. 4778471 Binzer and Bajpai, 1987 Gromofsky et al., 1988
9. Zinc-Sulfate–Calcium–Phosphorous Oxides	Scheidler and Bajpai, 1992

TABLE 39.9 Uses of Biodegradable Bioceramics

Biodegradable or resorbable ceramics	References
1. As drug delivery devices	Abrams and Bajpai, 1994 Bajpai, 1992 Bajpai, 1994 Benghuzzi et al., 1991 Moldovan and Bajpai, 1994 Nagy and Bajpai, 1994
2. For repairing damaged bone due to disease or trauma	Bajpai, 1990 Gromofsky et al., 1988 Khavari and Bajpai, 1993 Morris and Bajpai, 1987 Scheidler and Bajpai, 1992
3. For filling space vacated by bone screws, donor bone, excised tumors, and diseased bone loss	Bajpai and Fuchs, 1985 Ricci et al., 1986
4. For repairing and fusion of spinal and lumbo-sacral vertebrae	Bajpai et al., 1984 Yamamuro et al., 1988
5. For repairing herniated discs	Bajpai et al., 1984
6. For repairing maxillofacial and dental defects	Freeman et al., 1981
7. Hydroxyapatite Ocular Implants	De Potter et al., 1994 Shields et al., 1993

(a)

(b)

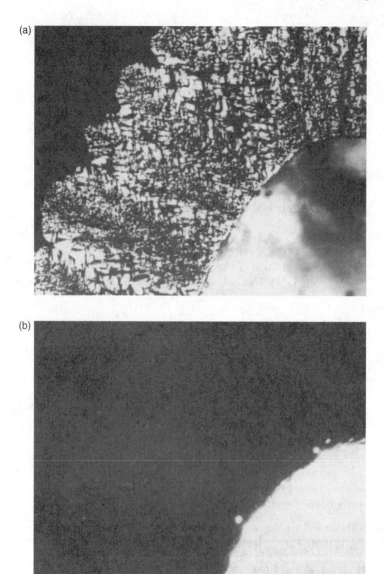

FIGURE 39.5   Microstructure of carbons deposited in a fluidized bed. (a) A granular carbon with distinct growth features. (b) An isotropic carbon without growth features. Both under polarized light. 240×. (From Bokros, J.C., LaGrange, L.D., and Schoen, G.J. 1972. *Chem. Phys. Carbon.* 9: 103–171. New York, Marcel Dekker. With permission,)

hexagonal rhombic prisms and has unit cell dimensions $a = 9.432$Å and $c = 6.881$ Å. The atomic structure of hydroxyapatite projected down the c-axis onto the basal plane is shown in Figure 39.6. Note that the hydroxyl ions lie on the corners of the projected basal plane and they occur at equidistant intervals (3.44 Å) along the columns perpendicular to the basal plane and parallel to the c-axis. Six of the ten calcium ions in the unit cell are associated with the hydroxyls in these columns, resulting in strong interactions among them [Park and Lakes, 1992].

The ideal Ca : P ratio of hydroxyapatite is 10 : 6 and the calculated density is 3.219 g/cm^3. Substitution of OH with fluoride gives the apatite greater chemical stability due to the closer coordination of fluoride (symmetric shape) as compared to the hydroxyl (asymmetric, two atoms) by the nearest calcium. This is why fluoridation of drinking water helps in resisting caries of the teeth [Park and Lakes, 1992].

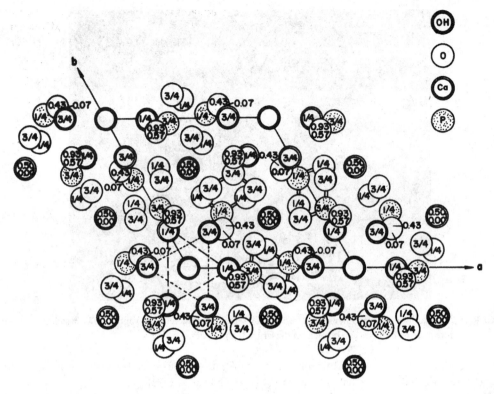

FIGURE 39.6 Hydroxyapatite structure projected down the *c*-axis onto the basal plane (From Posner A.S., Perloff A., and Diorio A.D. 1958. *Acta. Cryst.* 11: 308–309.)

TABLE 39.10 Physical Properties of Calcium Phosphate

Properties	Values
Elastic modulus (GPa)	4.0–117
Compressive strength (MPa)	294
Bending strength (MPa)	147
Hardness (Vickers, GPa)	3.43
Poisson's ratio	0.27
Density (theoretical, g/cm^3)	3.16

Source: Park J.B. and Lakes R.S. 1992. *Biomaterials: An Introduction*, 2nd ed., p. 125. Plenum Press, New York.

The mechanical properties of synthetic calcium phosphates vary considerably (Table 39.10). The wide variations in properties of polycrystalline calcium phosphates are due to the variations in the structure and manufacturing processes. Depending on the final firing conditions, the calcium phosphate can be calcium hydroxyapatite or β-whitlockite. In many instances, both types of structures exist in the same final product [Park and Lakes, 1992].

Polycrystalline hydroxyapatite has a high elastic modulus (40 to 117 GPa). Hard tissue such as bone, dentin, and dental enamel are natural composites which contain hydroxyapatite (or a similar mineral), as well as protein, other organic materials, and water. Enamel is the stiffest hard tissue, with an elastic modulus of 74 GPa, and contains the most mineral. Dentin ($E = 21$ GPa) and compact bone ($E = 12$ to

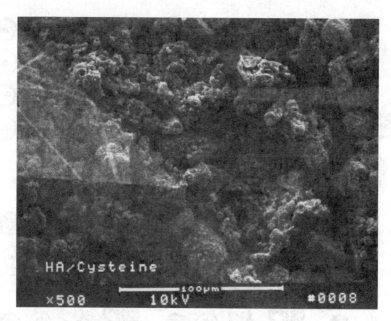

FIGURE 39.7   Scanning electron micrograph ($\times$500) of a set and hardened hydroxyaptite (HA)-cysteine composite. The small white cysteine particles can be seen on the larger HA particles.

18 GPa) contain comparatively less mineral. The Poisson's ratio for the mineral or synthetic hydroxyapatite is about 0.27 which is close to that of bone ($\approx$0.3) [Park and Lakes, 1992].

Hontsu et al. [1997] were able to deposit an amorphous HA film on Ti, α-Al_2O_3, SiO//Si(100), and $SrTiO_3$ using a pulsed ArF excimer laser. Upon heat treatment the amorphous film was converted to the crystalline form of HA. The HA film's electrical properties were measured for the first time (Table 39.14).

Among the most important properties of hydroxyapatite as a biomaterial is its excellent biocompatibility. Hydroxyapatite appears to form a direct chemical bond with hard tissues [Piattelli and Trisi, 1994]. On implantation of hydroxyapatite particles or porous blocks in bone, new lamellar cancellous bone forms within 4 to 8 weeks [Bajpai and Fuchs, 1985]. Scanning electron micrograph (500$\times$) of a set and hardened hydroxyapatite-cysteine composite is shown in Figure 39.7. The composite sets and hardens on addition of water.

Many different methods have been developed to make precipitates of hydroxyapatite from an aqueous solution of $Ca(NO_3)_2$ and NaH_2PO_4. There has been successful use of modifications to Jarcho and colleagues wet precipitation procedure for synthesizing hydroxyapatites for use as bone implants [Jarcho et al., 1979; Bajpai and Fuchs, 1985], and drug delivery devices [Bajpai, 1992, 1994; Parker and Bajpai, 1993; Abrams and Bajpai, 1994]. The dried, filtered precipitate is placed in a high-temperature furnace and calcined at 1150°C for 1 h. The calcined powder is then ground in a ball mill, and the particles are separated by an automatic sieve shaker and sieves. The sized particles are then pressed in a die and sintered at 1200°C for 36 h for making drug delivery devices [Bajpai, 1989, 1992; Abrams and Bajpai, 1994]. Above 1250°C, hydroxyapatite shows a second precipitation phase along the grain boundaries [Park and Lakes 1992].

39.3.2   Aluminum–Calcium–Phosphate (ALCAP) Ceramics

Initially we fabricated a calcium aluminate ceramic containing phosphorous pentoxide [Hentrich et al., 1969, 1971; Graves et al., 1972]. Aluminum–calcium–phosphorous oxide ceramic (ALCAP) was developed later [Bajpai and Graves, 1980]. ALCAP has insulating dielectric properties but no magnetic or piezoelectric properties [Allaire et al., 1989]. ALCAP ceramics are unique because they provide a multipurpose crystallographic system where one phase of the ceramic on implantation can be more rapidly resorbed than the others [Wyatt et al., 1976; Bajpai, 1983; Mattie and Bajpai, 1988]. ALCAP is prepared from stock powders of aluminum oxide, calcium oxide, and phosphorous pentoxide. A ratio of 50 : 34 : 16 by weight of $AlO_2 : CaO : P_2O_5$ is used to obtain the starting mixture for calcining at 1350°C in a high temperature furnace for 12 h. The calcined material is ground in a ball mill and sieved by an automatic siever to obtain particles of the desired size. The particulate powder is then pressed into solid blocks or hollow cylinders (green shape) and sintered at 1400°C for 36 h to increase the mechanical strength. ALCAP ceramic implants have given excellent results in terms of biocompatibility and gradual replacement of the ceramic material with endogenous bone [Bajpai, 1982; Mattie and Bajpai, 1988]. A scanning electron micrograph (1000×) of sintered porous ALCAP is shown in Figure 39.8.

39.3.3 Coralline

Coral is a natural substance made by marine invertebrates. According to Holmes et al. [1984], the marine invertebrates live in the limestone exostructure, or coral. The porous structure of the coral is unique for each species of marine invertebrate [Holmes et al., 1984]. Corals for use as bone implants are selected on the basis of structural similarity to bone [Holmes et al., 1984]. Coral provides an excellent structure for the ingrowth of bone, and the main component, calcium carbonate, is gradually resorbed by the body [Khavari and Bajpai, 1993]. Corals can also be converted to hydroxyapatite by a hydrothermal exchange process. Interpore 200, a coral hydroxyapatite, resembles cancellous bone [Sartoris et al., 1986]. Both pure coral (Biocoral) and coral transformed to hydroxyapatite are currently used to repair traumatized bone, replace diseased bone, and correct various bone defects.

Biocoral is composed of crystalline calcium carbonate or aragonite, the metastable form of calcium carbonate. The compressive strength of Biocoral varies from 26 (50% porous) to 395 MPa (dense) and depends on the porosity of the ceramic. Likewise, the modulus of elasticity (Young's Modulus) of Biocoral varies from 8 (50% porous) to 100 GPa (dense) [Biocoral, 1989].

39.3.4 Tricalcium Phosphate (TCP) Ceramics

A multicrystalline porous form of β-tricalcium phosphate [β-$Ca_3(PO_4)_2$] has been used successfully to correct periodontal defects and augment bony contours [Metsger et al., 1982]. X-ray diffraction

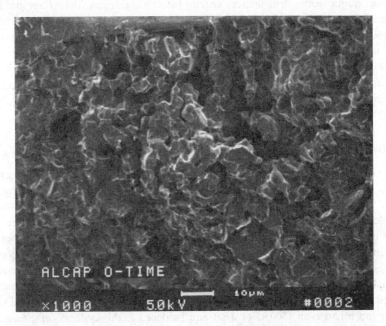

FIGURE 39.8 Scanning electron micrograph (×1000) of porous sintered ALCAP.

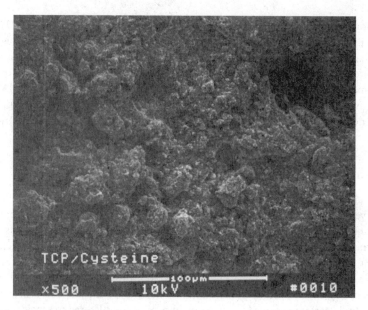

FIGURE 39.9   Scanning electron micrograph (×500) of a set and hardened TCP–cysteine composite. The small white cysteine particles can be seen on the larger TCP particles.

of β-tricalcium phosphate shows an average interconnected porosity of over 100 μm [Lemons et al., 1979]. Often tribasic calcium phosphate is mistaken for β-tricalcium phosphate. According to Metsger et al. [1982], tribasic calcium phosphate is a nonstoichiometric compound often bearing the formula of hydroxyapatite [$Ca_{10}(PO_4)_6(OH)_2$].

   β-Tricalcium phosphate is prepared by a wet precipitation procedure from an aqueous solution of $Ca(NO_3)_2$ and NaH_2PO_4 [Bajpai et al., 1988]. The precipitate is calcined at 1150°C for 1 h, ground, and sieved to obtain the desired size particles for use as bone substitutes [Bajpai et al., 1988; Bajpai, 1990] and for making ceramic matrix drug delivery systems [Morris and Bajpai, 1989; Nagy and Bajpai, 1994; Moldovan and Bajpai, 1994]. These particles are used as such or pressed into cylindrical shapes and sintered at 1150 to 1200°C for 36 h to achieve the appropriate mechanical strength for use as drug delivery devices [Bajpai, 1989, 1992, 1994; Benghuzzi et al., 1991]. A scanning electron micrograph (500×) of a set and hardened TCP-cysteine composite is shown in Figure 39.9. The composite sets and hardens on the addition of water. TCP is usually more soluble than synthetic hydroxyapatite and, on implantation, allows good bone ingrowth and eventually is replaced by endogenous bone.

39.3.5   Zinc–Calcium–Phosphorous Oxide (ZCAP) Ceramics

Zinc is essential for human metabolism and is a component of at least 30 metalloenzymes [Pories and Strain, 1970]. In addition, zinc may also be involved in the process of wound healing [Pories and Strain 1970]. Thus zinc–calcium–phosphorous oxide polyphasic ceramics (ZCAP) were synthesized to repair bone defects and deliver drugs [Binzer and Bajpai, 1987; Bajpai, 1988, 1993; Arar and Bajpai, 1992]. ZCAP is prepared by a thermal mixing of zinc oxide, calcium oxide, and phosphorous pentoxide powders [Bajpai, 1988]. ZCAP, like ALCAP, has insulating dielectric properties but no magnetic or piezoelectric properties [Allaire et al., 1989]. Various ratios of these powders have been used to produce the desired material [Bajpai, 1988]. The oxide powders are mixed in a ball mill and subsequently calcined at 800°C for 24 h. The calcined ceramic is then ground and sieved to obtain the desired size particles. Scanning electron micrograph (500×) of a set and hardened ZCAP–cysteine composite is shown in Figure 39.10. The composite sets and hardens on addition of water. To date, ZCAP ceramics have been

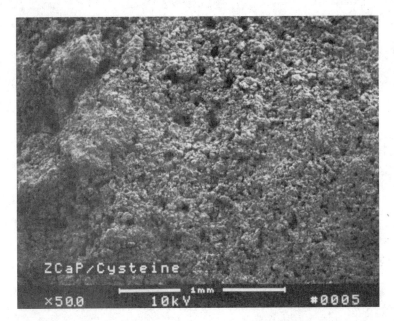

FIGURE 39.10 Scanning electron micrograph (×500) of a set and hardened ZCAP–cysteine composite. The small white cysteine particles have blended with the ZCAP particles.

used to repair experimentally induced defects in bone and for delivering drugs [Binzer and Bajpai, 1987; Bajpai, 1993].

39.3.6 Zinc–Sulfate–Calcium–Phosphate (ZSCAP) Ceramics

Zinc–sulfate–calcium–phosphate polyphasic ceramics (ZSCAP) are prepared from stock powders of zinc sulfate, zinc oxide, calcium oxide, and phosphorous pentoxide [Bajpai, 1988]. A ratio of $15:30:30:25$ by weight of $ZnSO_4:ZnO:CaO:P_2O_5$ is mixed in a crucible and allowed to cool for 30 min after the exothermal reaction has subsided. The cooled mixture is calcined in a crucible at 650°C for 24 h. The calcined ceramic is ground in a ball mill and the particles of the desired size are separated by sieving in an automatic siever. Scanning electron micrograph (2000×) of set and hardened ZSCAP particles (45 to 63 μm) is shown in Figure 39.11. ZSCAP sets and hardens on addition of water. ZSCAP particles, on implantation in bone, set and harden on contact with blood and have been used to repair experimentally induced defects in bone [Scheidler and Bajpai, 1992].

39.3.7 Ferric–Calcium–Phosphorous–Oxide (FECAP) Ceramics

Ferric–Calcium–Phosphorous–Oxide polyphasic ceramic (FECAP) is prepared from powders of ferric (III) oxide, calcium oxide, and phosphorous pentoxide [Stricker et al.,1992; Fuski et al., 1993; Larrabee et al., 1993]. The powders are combined in various ratios by weight and mixed in a blender. Blocks of the mixture are then pressed in a die by means of a hydraulic press and calcined at 1100°C for 12 h. The calcined ceramic blocks are crushed and ground in a ball mill. The calcined ceramic is ground in a ball mill and the particles of the desired size are separated by sieving in an automatic siever. A scanning electron micrograph (1000×) of a set and hardened FECAP-α ketoglutaric acid composite is shown in Figure 39.12. The composite sets and hardens on the addition of water. Studies conducted to date suggest complete resorption of FECAP particles implanted in bone within 60 days [Larrabee et al., 1993]. This particular ceramic could be used in patients suffering from anemia and similar diseases [Fuski et al., 1993].

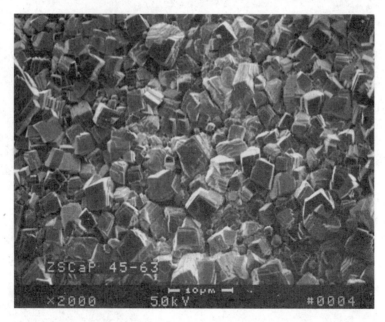

FIGURE 39.11   Scanning electron micrograph ($\times 2000$) of a set and hardened ZSCAP particles (45–63 μm). Sulfate is hardly visible between the cube-shaped ZCAP particles.

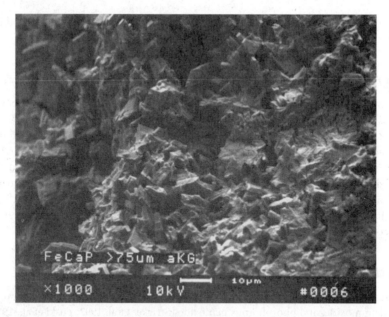

FIGURE 39.12   Scanning electron micrograph ($\times 1000$) of a set and hardened FECAP-α-ketoglutaric acid composite. Plate-shaped FECAP particles have been aggregated by the acid.

39.4   Bioactive or Surface-Reactive Ceramics

Upon implantation in the host, surface reactive ceramics form strong bonds with adjacent tissue. Examples of surface reactive ceramics are dense nonporous glasses, Bioglass and Ceravital, and hydroxyapatites (Table 39.11). One of their many uses is the coating of metal prostheses. This coating provides a stronger

TABLE 39.11   Examples of Surface Reactive Bioceramics

Surface reactive bioceramics	References
1. Bioglasses and Ceravital™	Ducheyne, 1985
	Gheyson et al., 1983
	Hench, 1991
	Hench, 1993
	Ogino et al., 1980
	Ritter et al., 1979
2. Dense and non-porous glasses	Andersson et al., 1992
	Blencke et al., 1978
	Li et al., 1991
	Ohtsuki et al., 1992
	Ohura et al., 1992
	Schepers et al., 1993
	Takatsuko et al., 1993
3. Hydroxyapatite	Bagambisa et al., 1993
	Bajpai, 1990
	Fredette et al., 1989
	Huaxia et al., 1992
	Knowles and Bonfield, 1993
	Niwa et al., 1980
	Park and Lakes, 1992
	Posner et al., 1958
	Schwartz et al., 1993
	Whitehead et al., 1993

bonding to the adjacent tissues, which is very important for protheses. A list of the uses of surface-reactive ceramics is shown in Table 39.12.

39.4.1   Glass Ceramics

Several variations of Bioglass and Ceravital glass ceramics have been used by various workers within the last decade. Glass ceramics used for implantation are silicon oxide based systems with or without phosphorous pentoxide.

Glass ceramics are polycrystalline ceramics made by controlled crystallization of glasses developed by S.D. Stookey of Corning Glass Works in the early 1960s [Park and Lakes, 1992]. Glass ceramics were first utilized in photosensitive glasses, in which small amounts of copper, silver, and gold are precipitated by ultraviolet light irradiation. These metallic precipitates help to nucleate and crystallize the glass into a fine grained ceramic which possesses excellent mechanical and thermal properties. Both Bioglass and Ceravital glass ceramics have been used as implants [Yamamuro et al., 1990].

The formation of glass ceramics is influenced by the nucleation and growth of small (<1 μm diameter) crystals as well as the size distribution of these crystals. It is estimated that about 10^{12} to 10^{15} nuclei/cm^3 are required to achieve such small crystals. In addition to the metallic agents already mentioned, Pt groups, TiO_2, ZrO_2, and P_2O_5 are widely used for nucleation and crystallization. The nucleation of glass is carried out at temperatures much lower than the melting temperature. During processing the melt viscosity is kept in the range of 10^{11} and 10^{12} Poise for 1 to 2 h. In order to obtain a larger fraction of the microcrystalline phase, the material is further heated to an appropriate temperature for maximum crystal growth. Deformation of the product, phase transformation within the crystalline phases, or redissolution of some of the phases should be avoided. The crystallization is usually more than 90% complete with grain sizes 0.1 to 1 μm. These grains are much smaller than those of conventional ceramics. Figure 39.13 shows a schematic representation of temperature–time cycle for a glass ceramic [Park and Lakes, 1992].

The glass ceramics developed for implantation are SiO_2–CaO–Na_2O–P_2O_5 and Li_2O–ZnO–SiO_2 systems. Two major groups are experimenting with the SiO_2–CaO–Na_2O–P_2O_5 glass ceramic. One group

TABLE 39.12   Uses of Surface Reactive Bioceramics

Surface Reactive Bioceramics	References
1. For coating of metal prostheses	Cotell et al., 1992
	Huaxia et al., 1992
	Ritter et al., 1979
	Takatsuko et al., 1993
	Whitehead et al., 1993
2. In reconstruction of dental defects	Hulbert et al., 1987
	Gheysen et al., 1983
	Schepers et al., 1988
	Schepers et al., 1989
3. For filling space vacated by bone screws, donor bone, excised tumors, and diseased bone loss	Hulbert et al., 1987
	Schepers et al., 1993
	Terry et al., 1989
4. As bone plates and screws	Doyle, 1990
	Ducheyne and McGuckin, 1990
	Yamamuro et al., 1988
5. As replacements of middle ear ossicles	Feenstra and de Groot, 1983
	Grote, 1987
	Hench, 1991
	Hench, 1993
	Reck et al., 1988
6. For lengthening of rami	Feenstra and de Groot, 1983
7. For correcting periodontal defects	Feenstra and de Groot, 1983
8. In replacing subperiosteal teeth	Hulbert, 1992

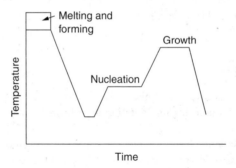

FIGURE 39.13   Temperature–time cycle for a glass-ceramic. (From Kingery W.D., Bowen H.K., and Uhlmann D.R. 1976. *Introduction to Ceramics*, 2nd ed., p. 368. New York, John Wiley & Sons, With permission.)

varied the compositions (except for P_2O_5) in order to obtain the best glass ceramic composition for inducing direct bonding with bone (Table 39.13). The bonding to bone is related to the simultaneous formation of a calcium phosphate and SiO_2-rich film layer on the surface, as exhibited by the 46S5.2 type Bioglass. If a SiO_2-rich layer forms first and a calcium phosphate film develops later (46 to 55 mol % SiO_2 samples) or no phosphate film is formed (60 mol % SiO_2) then direct bonding with bone does not occur [Park and Lakes, 1992]. The approximate region of the SiO_2–CaO–Na_2O system for the tissue–glass–ceramic reaction is shown in Figure 39.14. As can be seen, the best region (region A) for good tissue bonding is the composition given for 46S5.2 type Bioglass (see Table 39.13) [Park and Lakes, 1992].

39.4.2   Ceravital

The composition of Ceravital is similar to that of Bioglass in SiO_2 content but differs somewhat in other components (see Table 39.13). In order to control the dissolution rate, Al_2O_3, TiO_2, and Ta_2O_5 are added

TABLE 39.13   Compositions of Bioglass and Ceravital Glass Ceramics

Type	Code	SiO_2	CaO	Na_2O	P_2O_5	MgO	K_2O
Bioglass	42S5.6	42.1	29.0	26.3	2.6	—	—
	(45S5)46S5.2	46.1	26.9	24.4	2.6	—	—
	49S4.9	49.1	25.3	23.8	2.6	—	—
	52S4.6	52.1	23.8	21.5	2.6	—	—
	55S4.3	55.1	22.2	20.1	2.6	—	—
	60S3.8	60.1	19.6	17.7	2.6	—	—
Ceravital	Bioactive[a]	40–50	30–35	5–10	10–15	2.5–5	0.5–3
	Nonbioactive[b]	30–35	25–30	3.5–7.5	7.5–12	1–2.5	0.5–2

[a] The Ceravital® composition is in weight % while the Bioglass® compositions are in mol %.
[b] In addition Al_2O_3 (5.0–15.0), TiO_2 (1.0–5.0) and Ta_2O_5 (5–15) are added.
Source: Park J.B. and Lakes R.S. 1992. *Biomaterials: An Introduction*, 2nd ed., p. 127. Plenum Press, New York. With permission.)

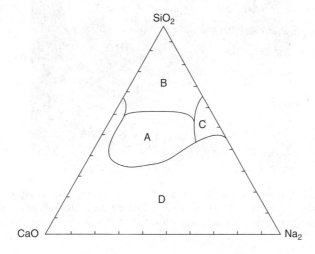

FIGURE 39.14   Approximate regions of the tissue-glass-ceramic bonding for the SiO_2–CaO–Na_2O system. A: Bonding within 30 days. B: Nonbonding; reactivity is too low. D: Bonding does not form glass. (From Hench L.L. and Ethridge E.C. 1982. *Biomaterials: An Interfacial Approach.* p. 147, New York, Academic Press. With permission.)

in Ceravital glass ceramic. The mixtures, after melting in a platinum crucible at 1500°C for three h, are annealed and cooled. The nucleation and crystallization temperatures are 680 and 750°C, respectively, each for 24 h. When the size of crystallites reaches approximately 4 Å and the characteristic needle structure is not formed, the process is stopped to obtain a fine grain structured glass ceramic [Park and Lakes, 1993].

Glass ceramics have several desirable properties compared to glasses and ceramics. The thermal coefficient of expansion is very low, typically 10^{-7} to 10^{-5}°C^{-1}, and in some cases it can even be made negative. Due to the controlled grain size and improved resistance to surface damage, the tensile strength of these materials can be increased by at least a factor of two, from about 100 to 200 MPa. The resistance to scratching and abrasion of glass ceramics is similar to that of sapphire [Park and Lakes, 1992].

A transmission electron micrograph of Bioglass glass ceramic implanted in the femur of rats for six weeks showed intimate contacts between the mineralized bone and the Bioglass (Figure 39.15). The mechanical strength of the interfacial bond between bone and Bioglass ceramic is on the same order of magnitude as the strength of the bulk glass ceramic (850 kg/cm^2 or 83.3 MPa), which is about three-fourths that of the host bone strength [Park and Lakes, 1992].

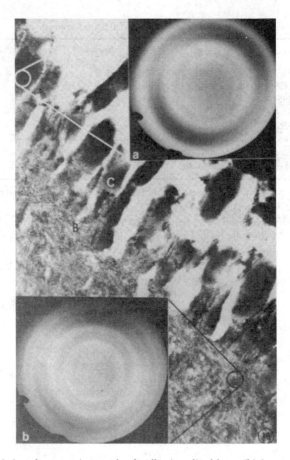

FIGURE 39.15 Transmission electron micrograph of well-mineralized bone (b) juxtaposed to the glass-ceramic (c) which fractured during sectioning. ×51,500. Insert a is the diffraction pattern from ceramic area and b is from bone area. (From Beckham C.A., Greenlee T.K. Jr, and Crebo A.R. 1971. *Calc. Tiss. Res.* 8: 165–171. With permission.)

A negative characteristic of the glass ceramic is its brittleness. In addition, limitations on the compositions used for producing a biocompatibile (or osteoconductive) glass ceramic hinders the production of a glass ceramic which has substantially higher mechanical strength. Thus glass ceramics cannot be used for making major load-bearing implants such as joint implants. However, they can be used as fillers for bone cement, dental restorative composites, and coating material (see Table 39.12). A glass ceramic containing 36 wt% of magnetite in a β-wollastonite- and $CaOSiO_2$-based glassy matrix has been synthesized for treating bone tumors by hyperthermia [Kokubo et al., 1992].

39.5 Deterioration of Ceramics

It is of great interest to know whether the inert ceramics such as alumina undergo significant static or dynamic fatigue. Even for the biodegradable ceramics, the rate of degradation *in vivo* is of paramount importance. Controlled degradation of an implant with time on implantation is desirable. Above a critical stress level, the fatigue strength of alumina is reduced by the presence of water. This is due to the delayed crack growth, which is accelerated by the water molecules [Park and Lakes, 1992]. Reduction in strength occurs if water penetrates the ceramic. Decrease in strength was not observed in samples which did not show water marks on the fractured surface (Figure 39.16). The presence of a small amount of silica in one sample lot may have contributed to the permeation of water molecules that is detrimental to the

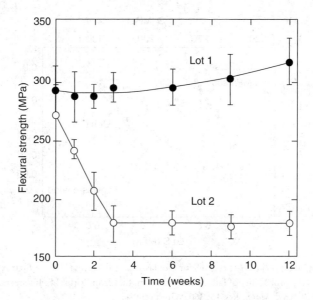

FIGURE 39.16   Flexural strength of dense alumina rods after aging under stress in Ringer's solution. Lot 1 and 2 are from different batches of production. (From Krainess F.E. and Knapp W.J. 1978. *J. Biomed. Mater. Res.* 12: 245. With permission.)

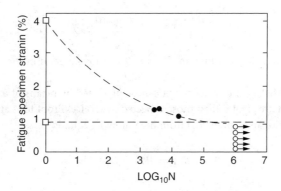

FIGURE 39.17   Strain vs. number of cycles to failure (○ = absence of fatigue cracks in carbon film; ● = fracture of carbon film due to fatigue failure of substrates; □ = data from substrate determined in single-cycle tensile test). (From Shimm H.S. and Haubold A.D. 1980. *Biomater. Med. Dev. Art. Org.* 8: 333–344. With permission.)

strength [Park and Lakes, 1992]. It is not clear whether the static fatigue mechanism operates in single crystal alumina. It is reasonable to assume, that static fatigue will occur if the ceramic contains flaws or impurities, because these will act as the source of crack initiation and growth under stress [Park and Lakes, 1992].

Studies of the fatigue behavior of vapor-deposited pyrolitic carbon fibers (4000 to 5000 Å thick) onto a stainless steel substrate showed that the film does not break unless the substrate undergoes plastic deformation at 1.3×10^{-2} strain and up to one million cycles of loading. Therefore, the fatigue is closely related to the substrate, as shown in Figure 39.17. Similar substrate-carbon adherence is the basis for the pyrolitic carbon deposited polymer arterial grafts [Park and Lakes, 1992].

The fatigue life of ceramics can be predicted by assuming that the fatigue fracture is due to the slow growth of preexisting flaws. Generally, the strength distribution, σ_i, of ceramics in an inert environment

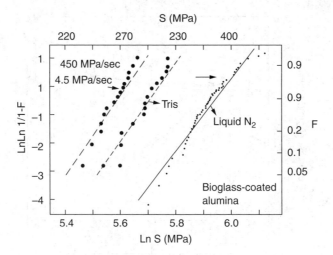

FIGURE 39.18 Plot of Ln Ln $[1/(1 - F)]$ vs. Ln S for Bioglass-coated alumina in a tris-hydroxyaminomethane buffer and liquid nitrogen. F is the probability of failure and S is strength. (From Ritter J.E. Jr, Greenspan D.C., Palmer R.A., and Hench L.L. 1979. *J. Biomed. Mater. Res.* 13: 260. With permission.)

can be correlated with the probability of failure F by the following equation:

$$\text{LnLn}\left(\frac{1}{1 - F}\right) = m\text{Ln}\left(\frac{s_i}{s_o}\right) \tag{39.1}$$

Both m and s_o are constants in the equation. Figure 39.18 shows a good fit for Bioglass coated alumina [Park and Lakes, 1992].

A minimum service life ($t_{\min}$) of a specimen can be predicted by means of a proof test wherein it is subjected to stresses that are greater than those expected in service. Proof tests also eliminate the weaker pieces. This minimum life can be predicted from the following equation:

$$t_{\min} = B\sigma_p^{N-2}\sigma_a^{-N} \tag{39.2}$$

Here σ_p is the proof test stress, σ_a is the applied stress, and B and N are constants.

Equation 39.2 after rearrangement, reads as follows:

$$t_{\min}\sigma_a^2 = B(\sigma_p/\sigma_a)^{N-2} \tag{39.3}$$

Figure 39.19 shows a plot of Equation 39.3 for alumina on a logarithmic scale [Park and Lakes, 1992].

39.6 Bioceramic Manufacturing Techniques

In order to fabricate bioceramics in more and more complex shapes, scientists are investigating the use of old and new manufacturing techniques. These techniques range from the adaptation of an age old pottery technique to the latest manufacturing methods for high temperature ceramic parts for airplane engines. No matter where the technique is perfected, the ultimate goal is the fabrication of bioceramic particles or devices in a desired shape in a consistent manner with the desired properties. The technique used to fabricate the bioceramic device will depend greatly on the ultimate application of the device, whether it is for hard tissue replacement or the integration of the device within the surrounding tissue.

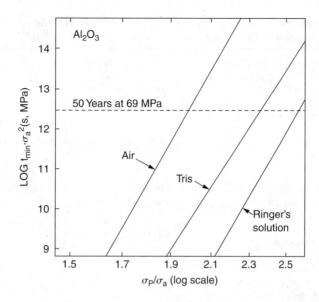

FIGURE 39.19 Plot of Equation 39.3 for alumina after proof testing. $N = 43.85$, $m = 13.21$, and $\sigma_o = 55728$ psi. (From Ritter J.E. Jr, Greenspan D.C., Palmer R.A., and Hench L.L. 1979. *J. Biomed. Mater. Res.* 13: 261. With permission.)

TABLE 39.14 Electrical properties of an HA Film

Dielectric constant (ε_r)	5.7 (25°C 1 MHz)
Loss tangent ($\tan \delta$)	<2%
Breakdown electric field	10^4 V cm^{-1}

Source: Hontsu S. et al. 1997. Electrical properties of hydroxyapatite thin films grown by pulsed laser deposition. *Thin Solid Films* 295: 214–217.

39.6.1 Hard Tissue Replacement

Hard tissue replacement implies that the bioceramic device will be used for load bearing applications. Although it is desirable to have a device with a sufficient porosity for the surrounding tissue to infiltrate and attach to the device, the most important and immediate property is the strength of the device. In order to accomplish this, one must manufacture a bioceramic implant with a density and strength sufficient to mimic that of bone. However, if the bioceramic part is significantly stronger than the surrounding bone, one runs into the common problem seen with metals called *stress shielding*. The density of the bioceramic greatly determines its overall strength. As the density increases so does the overall strength of the bioceramic. Some of the techniques used to manufacture dense bioceramics are injection molding, gel casting, bicontinuous microemulsion, inverse microemulsion, emulsion, and additives.

Injection molding is a common technique used to form plastic parts for many commercial applications such as automobile parts. Briefly, the process involves forcing a heated material into a die and then ejecting the formed piece from the die. Injection molding allows for making complex shapes. Cihlar and Trunec [1996] found that by calcining (1273 K, 3 h) and milling the hydroxyapatite (HA) prior to mixing with a binder, an ethylene vinyl acetate copolymer (EVA)/HA mixture of 63% HA, they achieved 98% relative density with only 16% shrinkage using injection molding. The maximum flexural strength was 60 MPa for HA products sintered at 1473 K. However, this is still not strong enough for load bearing applications.

TABLE 39.15 Bioceramic Manufacturing Techniques for Hard Tissue
Replacement or Tissue Integration

Manufacturing Technique	References
Hard Tissue Replacement	
Injection Molding	Cihlar and Trunec, 1996
Bicontinuous microemulsion	Lim et al., 1997
Inverse microemulsion	
Emulsion	
Additives	Fanovich et al., 1998; Kawashima et al., 1997;
	Suchanek et al., 1997
Tissue Integration	
Drip casting	Liu, 1996; Lyckfeldt and Ferreira, 1998
Starch consolidation	Lyckfeldt and Ferreira, 1998
Polymeric sponge method	
Foaming method	
Organic additives	
Gel casting	
Slip casting	
Direct coagulation consolidation	
Hydrolysis assisted solidification	
Freezing	

They also observed that HA decomposed to α-TCP at temperatures greater than 1573 K [Cihlar and Trunec, 1996].

In gel casting, HA is formed using the standard chemical precipitation. The calcium phosphate precipitant (30% w/v) is then mixed with glycerol and filtered. The "gel cake" is sintered at 1200°C for 2 h. This yielded a density of >99% and a highly uniform microstructure [Varma and Sivakumar, 1996].

Bicontinuous microemulsion, inverse microemulsion, and emulsion are all wet chemistry based methods to produce nanometer size HA powders. All three methods yield >97% relative density upon sintering at 1200°C for 2 h. The biocontinuous and inverse microemulsion resulted in the two smallest HA particle sizes, 22 and 24 nm respectively [Lim et al., 1997].

Another strategy to increase the density of ceramics is to use additives or impurities in small weight percents during sintering. The main disadvantages to this technique include (1) the possible decomposition of the original pure bioceramic and (2) results may end in all or portions of the bioceramic being nonbiocompatible.

Suchanek et al. [1997] studied the addition of several different additives to HA in 5 wt% amounts. The additives studied were K_2CO_3, Na_2CO_3, H_3BO_3, KF, $CaCl_2$, KCl, KH_2PO_4, $(KPO_3)_n$, $Na_2Si_2O_5$, $Na_2P_2O_7$, Na_3PO_4, $(NaPO_3)_n$, $Na_5P_3O_{10}$, and β-$NaCaPO_4$. HA has a fracture toughness of 1 MPa·m$^{1/2}$, whereas human bone has a fracture toughness of 2 to 12 MPa · m$^{1/2}$. One of the ways to improve the mechanical properties is to improve the densification of HA. Suchanek et al. [1997] found that the following additives (5 wt.%) did not improve the densification of HA: H_3BO_3, $CaCl_2$, KCl, KH_2PO_4, $(KPO_3)_n$, and $Na_2Si_2O_5$. The densification of HA was improved through the addition (5 wt.%) of K_2CO_3, Na_2CO_3, KF, $Na_2P_2O_7$, Na_3PO_4, $(NaPO_3)_n$, $Na_5P_3O_{10}$, and β-$NaCaPO_4$. However, H_3BO_3, $CaCl_2$, KH_2PO_4, $(KPO_3)_n$, $Na_2Si_2O_5$, K_2CO_3, Na_2CO_3, and KF produced the formation of β-TCP or CaO. The sodium phosphates used in this study were added to HA without the formation of β-TCP or CaO. The only compound that improved densification, did not cause formation of β-TCP or CaO, and provided a weak interface for HA was β-$NaCaPO_4$.

Another additive that has been investigated to improve the performance of HA is lithium (Li). The addition of lithium can increase the microhardness and produces a fine microstructure in HA. Fanovich et al. [1998] found that the addition of 0.2 wt% of Li to HA produced the maximum microhardness (5.9 GPa). However, the addition of high amounts of Li to HA results in abnormal grain growth and large pores. Furthermore, Li addition to HA results in the formation of β-TCP upon sintering.

Zirconia has been used as an additive to HA in order to improve its mechanical strength. Kawashima et al. [1997] found that addition of partially stabilized zirconia (PSZ) to HA can be used to increase the fracture toughness to 2.8 MPa · $m^{1/2}$. Bone has a fracture toughness of 2-12 MPa · $m^{1/2}$ [Suchanek et al., 1997]. PSZ was added to HA in different percentages (17, 33, 50 wt%) and it was found that 50 wt% PSZ had the highest fracture toughness. The surface energy of the PSZ-HA was not significantly different from HA alone. This suggests that the PSZ-HA composite could be biocompatible because of the similarity of the surface with HA [Kawashima et al., 1997].

39.6.2 Tissue Integration

The porosity is a critical factor for growth and integration of a tissue into the bioceramic implant. In particular the open porosity, that which is connected to the outside surface, is critical to the integration of tissue into the ceramic especially if the bioceramic is inert. Several methods have been developed to form porous ceramics, two of these are starch consolidation and drip casting.

In starch consolidation (Table 39.15), starch powders of a specific size are mixed with a bioceramic slurry at a predetermined weight percent. Upon heating, the starch will uptake water from the slurry mixture and swell. Upon sintering of the starch-bioceramic mixture, the starch is burned out and the pores are left in their place. Starch consolidation has been used to form complex shapes in alumina with ultimate porosities between 23 and 70 vol %. By controlling the starch content, one can control the ultimate porosity and resulting pore sizes. Large pores formed using starch consolidation in alumina were in the size range 10 to 80 μm whereas small pores varied between 0.5 and 9.5 μm [Lyckfeldt and Ferreira, 1998].

Liu [1996] used a drip casting technique (Table 39.15) to form porous HA granules with pore sizes from 95 to 400 μm. The granules had a total porosity from 24 to 76 vol %. The HA was made into a slurry using water and poly(vinyl butyral) powders. The slurry was then dripped onto a spherical mold surface. This technique is similar to that of drip casting by dripping an HA slurry into a liquid nitrogen bath. In both instances, calcining and sintering procedures are used to produce the final product [Liu, 1996].

39.6.3 Hydroxyapatite Synthesis Method

Prepare the following solutions:

Solution 1: Dissolve 157.6 g calcium nitrate tetrahydrate [$Ca(NO_3)_2 4H_2O$] in 500 ml DI water. Bring the solution to a pH of 11 by adding ≈70 ml ammonium hydroxide [NH_4OH]. Bring the solution to 800 ml with DI water.

Solution 2: Dissolve 52.8 g ammonium phosphate dibasic [$(NH_4)_2HPO_4$] in 500 ml DI water. Bring the solution to a pH of 11 by adding ≈150 ml ammonium hydroxide [NH_4OH]. Add DI water until the precipitate is completely dissolved, 250–350 ml.

39.6.3.1 Special Note

If you use calcium nitrate [$Ca(NO_3)_2 nH_2O$] instead of calcium nitrate tetrahydrate you need to recalculate the amount of calcium nitrate to add to make Solution 1 on the basis of the absence of the extra four waters. If you do not, you will have to add a large amount of ammonium hydroxide to pH the solution:

1. Add one-half of Solution 1 to a 2 l separatory funnel
2. Add one-half of Solution 2 to a 2 l separatory funnel
3. Titrate both solutions into a 4 l beaker with heat and constant stirring
4. Boil gently for 30 min
5. Repeat steps 1–4 for the rest of Solutions 1 and 2
6. Let cool completely allowing precipitate to settle to bottom of beaker
7. Pour contents of beaker into 250 ml polypropylene bottles
8. Centrifuge bottles for 10 min at (10,000 rpm) 16,000 g

9. Collect precipitate from the six bottles into two and resuspend with DI water
10. Fill the four empty bottles with the reaction mixture and centrifuge all six as before
11. Collect precipitant from the two bottles that were resuspended with DI water
12. Combine remaining four bottles into two bottles and resuspend with DI water
13. Repeat steps 10–12 as necessary
14. Dry precipitate for 24–48 h at 70°C
15. Calcine the precipitate for one hour at 1140°C
16. Grind and sieve product as desired

Defining Terms

Alumina: Aluminum oxide (Al_2O_3) which is very hard (Mohs hardness is 9) and strong. Single crystals are called sapphire or ruby depending on color. Alumina is used to fabricate hip joint socket components or dental root implants.

Calcium phosphate: A family of calcium phosphate ceramics including aluminum calcium phosphate, ferric calcium phosphate, hydroxyapatite and tricalcium phosphate (TCP), and zinc calcium phosphate which are used to substitute or augment bony structures and deliver drugs.

Glass-ceramics: A glass crystallized by heat treatment. Some of those have the ability to form chemical bonds with hard and soft tissues. Bioglass and Ceravital are well known examples.

Hydroxyapatite: A calcium phosphate ceramic with a calcium to phosphorus ratio of 5/3 and nominal composition $Ca_{1}0(PO_4)_6(OH)_2$. It has good mechanical properties and excellent biocompatibility. Hydroxyapatite is the mineral constituent of bone.

LTI carbon: A silicon alloyed pyrolitic carbon deposited onto a substrate at low temperature with isotropic crystal morphology. It is highly compatible with blood and used for cardiovascular implant fabrication such as artificial heart valve.

Maximum radius ratio: The ratio of atomic radii computed by assuming the largest atom or ion which can be placed in a crystal's unit cell structure without deforming the structure.

Mohs scale: A hardness scale in which 10 (diamond) is the hardest and 1 (talc) is the softest.

Acknowledgments

The author is grateful to Dr. Joon B. Park for inviting him to write this chapter and providing the basic shell from his book to expand upon. The author would like to thank his wife, Zoe, for her patience and understanding. The author would also like to thank Dr. M.C. Hofmann for her support and help.

In Memory Of

In memory of Dr. P.K. Bajpai who left us early in 1998, I would like to share our lab's recipe for hydroxyapatite. Dr. Bajpai's lab and research at the University of Dayton have ended after 30 plus years, but I felt it would be fitting to share this recipe as a way to encourage other scientists to continue exploring the possibilities of bioceramics.

References

Abrams L. and Bajpai P.K. 1994. Hydroxyapatite ceramics for continuous delivery of heparin. *Biomed. Sci. Instrum.* 30: 169–174.

Adams D. and Williams D.F. 1978. Carbon fiber-reinforced carbon as a potential implant material. *J. Biomed. Mater. Res.* 12: 35–42.

Alexander H., Parsons J.R., Ricci J.L., Bajpai P.K., and Weiss A.B. 1987. Calcium-based ceramics and composites in bone reconstruction. *Crit. Rev.* 4: 43–47.

Allaire M., Reynolds D., and Bajpai P.K. 1989. Electrical properties of biocompatible ALCAP and ZCAP ceramics. *Biomed. Sci. Instrum.* 25: 163–168.

Andersson O.H., Guizhi L., Kangasniemi K., and Juhanoja J. 1992. Evaluation of the acceptance of glass in bone. *J. Mat. Sci.: Mater. Med.* 3: 145–150.

Annual Book of ASTM Standards, part 46, F603-78, American Society for Testing and Materials, Philadelphia, 1980.

Arar H.A. and Bajpai P.K. 1992. Insulin delivery by zinc calcium phosphate (ZCAP) ceramics. *Biomed. Sci. Instrum.* 28: 172–178.

Bagambisa F.B., Joos U., and Schilli W. 1993. Mechanisms and structure of the bond between bone and hydroxyapatite ceramics. *J. Biomed. Mater. Res.* 27: 1047–1055.

Bajpai P.K., Fuchs C.M., and Strnat M.A.P. 1985. *Development of Alumino-Calcium Phosphorous Oxide (ALCAP) Ceramic Cements.* In: *Biomedical Engineering IV Recent Developments.* Proceedings of the Fourth Southern Biomedical Engineering Conference, Jackson, M.S. and B. Sauer (Ed.), pp. 22–25, Pergamon Press, New York, NY.

Bajpai P.K. 1994. Ceramic drug delivery systems. In: *Biomedical Materials Research in The Far East* (I). Xingdong Zhang and Yoshito Ikada (Eds.), pp. 41–42. Kobunshi Kankokai Inc., Kyoto, Japan.

Bajpai P.K. 1993. Zinc based ceramic cysteine composite for repairing vertebral defects. *J. Instrum. Sci.* 6: 346.

Bajpai P.K. 1992. Ceramics: a novel device for sustained long term delivery of drugs. In: *Bioceramics* Vol. 3, J.A. Hulbert and S.F. Hulbert (Eds.), pp. 87–99. Rose-Hulman Institute of Technology, Terra Haute, IN.

Bajpai P.K. 1990. Ceramic amino acid composites for repairing traumatized hard tissues. In: *Handbook of Bioactive Ceramics*, Vol. II: *Calcium Phosphate and Hydroxylapatite Ceramics.* T. Yamamuro, L.L. Hench, and J. Wilson-Hench (Eds.), pp. 255–270. CRC Press, Baton Raton, FL.

Bajpai P.K. 1989. Ceramic implantable drug delivery system. *T.I.B. & A.O.* 3: 203–211.

Bajpai P.K. 1988. ZCAP Ceramics. US. Patent No. 4778471.

Bajpai P.K. 1983. Biodegradable scaffolds in orthopedic, oral, and maxillo facial surgery. In: *Biomaterials in Reconstructive Surgery.* L.R. Rubin, Ed. pp. 312–328. C.V. Mosby Co., St. Louis, MO.

Bajpai P.K., Fuchs C.M., and McCullum D.E. 1988. *Development of tricalcium phosphate ceramic cements.* In: *Quantitative Characterization and Performance of Porous Implants for Hard Tissue Applications*, ASTM STP 953, J.E. Lemons (Ed.), pp. 377–388. American Society for Testing and Materials, Philadelphia, PA.

Bajpai P.K. and Fuchs C.M. 1985. Development of a hydroxyapatite bone grout. In: *Proceedings of the First Annual Scientific Session of the Academy of Surgical Research.* San Antonio, Texas. C.W. Hall, (Ed.), pp. 50–54. Pergamon Press, New York, NY.

Bajpai P.K., Graves G.A. Jr, Wilcox L.G., and Freeman M.J. 1984. Use of resorbable alumino-calcium-phosphorous-oxide ceramics (ALCAP) in health care. *Trans. Soc. Biomater.* 7: 353.

Bajpai P.K. and Graves G.A. Jr. 1980. Porous Ceramic Carriers for Controlled Release of Proteins, Polypeptide Hormones and other Substances within Human and/or Mammalian Species. US. Patent No. 4218255.

Barinov S.M. and Bashenko YuV. 1992. Application of ceramic composites as implants: result and problem. In: *Bioceramics and the Human Body.* A. Ravaglioli and A. Krajewski (Eds.), pp. 206–210. Elsevier Applied Science, London.

Beckham C.A., Greenlee T.K. Jr, and Crebo A.R. 1971. Bone formation at a ceramic implant interface. *Calc. Tiss. Res.* 8: 165–171.

Benghuzzi H.A., Giffin B.F., Bajpai P.K., and England B.G. 1991. Successful antidote of multiple lethal infections with sustained delivery of difluoromethylornithine by means of tricalcium phosphate drug delivery devices. *Trans. Soc. Biomater.* 24: 53.

Binzer T.J. and Bajpai P.K. 1987. The use of zinc–calcium-phosphorous oxide (ZCAP) ceramics in reconstructive bone surgery. *Digest of Papers, Sixth Southern Biomedical Engineering Conference.* Dallas, Texas. R.C. Eberhart (Ed.), pp. 182–185. McGregor and Werner, Washington, D.C.

Biocoral. 1989. From coral to biocoral, p. 46. *Innoteb*, Paris, France.

Blencke B.A., Bromer H., Deutscher K.K. 1978. Compatibility and long-term stability of glass-ceramic implants. *J. Biomed. Mater. Res.* 12: 307–318.

Bokros J.C. 1972. Deposition structure and properties of pyrolitic carbon. *Chem. Phys. Carbon.* 5: 70–81.

Bokros J.C., LaGrange L.D., and Schoen G.J. 1972. Control of structure of carbon for use in bioengineering. *Chem. Phys. Carbon.* 9: 103–171.

Boutin P. 1981. T.H.R. Using Alumina–Alumina Sliding and a Metallic Stem: 1330 Cases and an 11-Year Follow-up. In: *Orthopaedic Ceramic Implants*, Vol. 1. H. Oonishi and H.Y. Ooi (Eds.), Tokyo, Japanese Society of Orthopaedic Ceramic Implants.

Buykx W.J., Drabarek E., Reeve K.D., Anderson N., Mathivanar R., and Skalsky M. 1992. Development of porous ceramics for drug release and other applications. In: *Bioceramics*, Vol. 3. J.E. Hulbert and S.F. Hulbert (Eds.), pp. 349–354. Rose Hulman Institute of Technology, Terre Haute, Indiana.

Chandy T. and Sharma C.P. 1991. Biocomaptibility and toxicological screening of materials. In: *Blood Compatible Materials and Devices.* C.P. Sharma and M. Szycher (Eds.), pp. 153–166. Technomic Publishing Co., Lancaster, PA.

Chignier E., Monties J.R., Butazzoni B., Dureau G., and Eloy R. 1987. Haemocompatibility and biological course of carbonaceous composites for cardiovascular devices. *Biomaterials* 8: 18–23.

Cihlar J. and Trunec M. 1996. Injection moulded hydroxyapatite ceramics. *Biomaterials* 17: 1905–1911.

Cotell C.M., Chrisey D.B., Grabowski K.S., Sprague J.A., and Gossett C.R. 1992. Pulsed laser deposition of hydroxyapatite thin films on Ti–6Al–4V, *J. Appl. Biomater.* 3: 87–93.

de Groot K. 1983. *Bioceramics of Calcium Phosphate.* CRC Press, Boca Raton, FL.

De Potter P., Shields C.L., Shields J.L., and Singh A.D. 1994. Use of the hydroxyapatite ocular implant in the pediatric population. *Arch. Opthalmol.* 112: 208–212.

Dellsperger K.C. and Chandran K.B. 1991. Prosthetic heart valves. In: *Blood Compatible Materials and Devices.* C.P. Sharma and M. Szycher (Eds.), Technomic Publishing Co., Lancaster, PA.

Dorlot J.M., Christel P., and Meunier A. 1988. Alumina hip prostheses: long term behaviors. In: *Bioceramics. Proceedings of 1st International Symposium on Ceramics in Medicine.* H. Oonishi, H. Aoki, and K. Sawai (Eds.), pp. 236–301. Ishiyaku EuroAmerica, Inc. Tokyo.

Dörre E. 1991. Problems concerning the industrial production of alumina ceramic components for hip prosthesis. In: *Bioceramics and the Human Body.* A. Ravaglioli and A. Krajewski (Eds.), pp. 454–460. Elsevier Applied Science, London and New York.

Doyle C. 1990. Composite bioactive ceramic-metal materials. In: *Handbook of Bioactive Ceramics.* T. Yamamuro, L.L. Hench, and J. Wilson (Eds.), pp. 195–208. CRC Press, Boca Raton, FL.

Drennan J. and Steele B.C.H. 1991. Zirconia and hafnia, In: *Concise Encyclopedia of Advanced Ceramic Materials.* R.J. Brook (Ed.), pp. 525–528. Pergamon Press, Oxford, NY.

Ducheyne P. and McGuckin, J.F. Jr. 1990. Composite Bioactive Ceramic-Metal Materials. In: *Handbook of Bioactive Ceramics.* T. Yamamuro, L.L. Hench, and J. Wilson (Eds.), pp. 75–86. CRC Press, Boca Raton, FL.

Ducheyne P. 1985. Bioglass coatings and bioglass composites as implant materials. *J. Biomed. Mater. Res.* 19: 273–291.

Ely J.L. and Haubald A.O. 1993. Static fatigue and stress corrosion in pyrolitic carbon. In: *Bioceramics*, Vol. 6. P. Ducheyne and D. Christiansen (Eds.), pp. 199–204. Butterworth-Heinemann, Ltd. Boston. MA.

Fanovich M.A., Castro M.S., and Porto Lopez J.M. 1998. Improvement of the microstructure and microhardness of hydroxyapatite ceramics by addition of lithium. *Mat. Lett.* 33: 269–272.

Feenstra L and de Groot K. 1983. Medical use of calcium phosphate ceramics. In: *Bioceramics of calcium phosphate.* K. de Groot (Ed.), pp. 131–141, CRC Press, Boca Raton, FL.

Freeman M.J., McCullum D.E., and Bajpai P.K. 1981. Use of ALCAP ceramics for rebuilding maxillo-facial defects. *Trans. Soc. Biomater.* 4: 109.

Fredette S.A., Hanker J.S., Terry B.C., and Beverly L. 1989. Comparison of dense versus porous hydroxyapatite (HA) particles for rat mandibular defect repair. *Mat. Res. Soc. Symp. Proc.* 110: 233–238.

Fulmer M.T., Martin R.I., and Brown P.W. 1992. Formation of calcium deficient hydroxyapatite at near-physiological temperature. *J. Mat. Sci.: Mater. Med.* 3: 299–305.

Fuski M.P., Larrabee R.A., and Bajpai P.K. 1993. Effect of ferric calcium phosphorous oxide ceramic implant in bone on some parameters of blood. *T.I.B. & A.O.* 7: 16–19.

Gheysen G., Ducheyne P., Hench L.L., and de Meester P. 1983. Bioglass composites: a potential material for dental application. *Biomaterials* 4: 81–84.

Graves G.A. Jr, Hentrich R.L. Jr, Stein H.G., and Bajpai P.K. 1972. Resorbable Ceramic implants in bioceramics. In: *Engineering and Medicine (Part I).* C.W. Hall, S.F. Hulbert, S.N. Levine, and F.A. Young (Eds.), pp. 91–115. Interscience Publishers, New York, NY.

Grenoble D.E., Katz J.L., Dunn K.L., Gilmore R.S., and Murty K.L. 1972. The elastic properties of hard tissues and apatites. *J. Biomed. Mater. Res.* 6: 221–233.

Gromofsky J.R., Arar H., and Bajpai P.K. 1988. Development of zinc calcium phosphorous oxide ceramic–organic acid composites for repairing traumatized hard tissue. In: *Digest of Papers, Seventh Southern Biomedical Engineering Conference.* Greenville, S.C. and D.D. Moyle (Eds.), pp. 20–23. Mcgregor and Werner, Washington, D.C.

Grote J.J. 1987. Reconstruction of the ossicular chain with hydroxyapatite prostheses. *Am. J. Otol.* 8: 396–401.

Guillemin G., Meunier A., Dallant P., Christel P., Pouliquen J.C., and Sedel L. 1989. Comparison of coral resorption and bone apposition with two natural corals of different porosities. *J. Biomed. Mater. Res.* 23: 765–779.

Hammer J. III, Reed O., and Greulich R. 1972. Ceramic root implantation in baboons. *J. Biomed. Mater. Res.* 6: 1–13.

Heimke G. 1992. Use of alumina ceramics in medicine. In: *Bioceramics,* Vol. 3. J.E. Hulbert and S.F. Hulbert (Eds.), pp. 19–30. Rose Hulman Institute of Technology, Terre Haute, IN.

Hench L.L. 1991. Bioceramics: From concept to clinic. *J. Am. Ceram. Soc.* 74: 1487–1510.

Hench L.L. 1993. Bioceramics: From concept to clinic. *Am. Ceram. Soc. Bull.* 72: 93–98.

Hench L.L. and Ethridge E.C. 1982. *Biomaterials: An Interfacial Approach.* p.147, Academic Press, NY.

Hentrich R.L. Jr, Graves G.A. Jr, Stein H.G., and Bajpai P.K. 1971. An evaluation of inert and resorbable ceramics for future clinical applications. *J. Biomed. Mater. Res.* 5: 25–51.

Hentrich R.L. Jr, Graves G.A. Jr, Stein H.G., and Bajpai P.K. 1969. An evaluation of inert and resorbable ceramics for future clinical applications. Fall Meeting, Ceramics-Metals Systems, Division of the American Ceramic Society, Cleveland, Ohio.

Holmes R., Mooney V., Bucholz R., and Tencer A. 1984. A coralline hydroxyapatite bone graft substitute. *Clin. Orthopaed. Relat. Res.* 188: 252–262.

Hontsu S., Matsumoto T., Ishii J., Nakamori M., Tabata H., and Kawai T. 1997. Electrical properties of hydroxyapatite thin films grown by pulsed laser deposition. *Thin Solid Films* 295: 214–217.

Huaxia J.I., Ponton C.B., and Marquis P.M. 1992. Microstructural characterization of hydroxyapatite coating on titanium. *J. Mat. Sci.: Mater. Med.* 3: 283–287.

Hulbert S.F. 1992. Use of ceramics in medicine. In: *Bioceramics,* Vol. 3. J.E. Hulbert and S.F. Hulbert (Eds.), pp. 1–18. Rose Hulman Institute of Technology, Terre Haute, IN.

Hulbert S.F. and Klawitter J.J. 1971. Application of porous ceramics for the development of load-bearing internal orthopedic applications. *Biomed. Mater. Symp.* pp. 161–229.

Hulbert S.F., Bokros J.C., Hench L.L., Wilson J., and Heimke G. 1987. Ceramics in clinical applications: past, present, and future. In: *High Tech Ceramics.* P. Vincezini (Ed.), pp. 189–213. Elsevier, Amsterdam, Netherlands.

Jarcho M., Salsbury R.L., Thomas M.B., and Doremus R.H. 1979. Synthesis and fabrication of β-tricalcium phosphate (whitlockite) ceramics for potential prosthetic applications. *J. Mater. Sci.* 14: 142–150.

Jenei S.R., Bajpai P.K., and Salsbury R.L. Resorbability of commercial hydroxyapatite in lactate buffer. *Proceedings of the Second Annual Scientific Session of the Academy of Surgical Research.* S.C. Clemson and D.N. Powers (Ed.), pp. 13–16. Clemson University Press, Clemson, SC.

Kaae J.L. 1971. Structure and mechanical properties of isotropic pyrolitic carbon deposited below 1600°C. *J. Nucl. Mater.* 38: 42–50.

Kawahara H. Ed. 1989. *Oral Implantology and Biomaterials,* Elsevier, Amsterdam, Netherlands.

Kawashima N., Soetanto K., Watanabe K., Ono K., and Matsuno T. 1997. The surface characteristics of the sintered body of hydroxyapatite–zirconia composite particles. *Coll. Surf. B: Biointerf.* 10: 23–27.

Khavari F. and Bajpai P.K. 1993. Coralline-sulfate bone substitutes. *Biomed. Sci. Instrum.* 29: 65–69.

Kijima T. and Tsutsumi M. 1979. Preparation and thermal properties of dense polycrystalline oxyhydroxyapatite. *J. Am. Cer. Soc.* 62: 954–960.

Kingery W.D., Bowen H.K., and Uhlmann D.R. 1976. *Introduction to Ceramics,* 2nd ed., p. 368, John Wiley & New York.

Knowles J.C. and Bonfield W. 1993. Development of a glass reinforced hydroxyapatite with enhanced mechanical properties. the effect of glass composition on mechanical properties and its relationship to phase changes. *J. Biomed. Mater. Res.* 27: 1591–1598.

Kokubo T., Kushitani H., Ohtsuki C., Sakka S., and Yamamuro T. 1992. Chemical reaction of bioactive glass and glass-ceramics with a simulated body fluid. *J. Mat. Sci.: Mater. Med.* 3: 79–83.

Krainess F.E. and Knapp W.J. 1978. Strength of a dense alumina ceramic after aging *in vitro. J. Biomed. Mater. Res.* 12: 241–246.

Kumar P., Shimizu K., Oka M., Kotoura Y., Nakayama Y., Yamamuro T., Yanagida T., and Makinouchi K. 1989. Biological reaction of zirconia ceramics. In: *Bioceramics. Proceedings of 1st International Symposium on Ceramics in Medicine.* H. Oonishi, H. Aoki, and K. Sawai (Eds.), pp. 341–346, Ishiyaku Euroamerica, Inc., Tokyo.

Larrabee R.A., Fuski M.P., and Bajpai P.K. 1993. A ferric–calcium–phosphorous–oxide ceramic for rebuilding bone. *Biomed. Sci. Instrum.* 29: 59–64.

Lemons J.E., Bajpai P.K., Patka P., Bonel G., Starling L.B., Rosenstiel T., Muschler G, Kampnier S., and Timmermans T. 1988. Significance of the porosity and physical chemistry of calcium phosphate ceramics orthopaedic uses. In: *Bioceramics: Material Characteristics Versus In Vivo Behavior.* Annals of New York Academy of Sciences, Vol. 523, pp. 190–197.

Lemons J.E. and Niemann K.M.W. 1979. *Porous Tricalcium Phosphate Ceramic for Bone Replacement. 25th Annual O.R.S.,* Meetings, San Francisco, CA, February 20–22, p. 162.

Li R., Clark A.E., and Hench L.L. 1991. An investigation of bioactive glass powders by sol–gel processing, *J. Appl. Biomater.* 2: 231–239.

Lim G.K., Wang J., Ng S.C., Chew C.H., and Gan L.M. 1997. Processing of hydroxyapatite via microemulsion and emulsion routes. *Biomaterials* 18: 1433–1439.

Liu D. 1996. Fabrication and characterization of porous hydroxyapatite granules. *Biomaterials* 17: 1955–1957.

Lyckfeldt O. and Ferreira J.M.F. 1998. Processing of porous ceramics by starch consolidation. *J. Europ. Cer. Soc.* 18: 131–140.

Mattie D.R. and Bajpai P.K. 1988. Analysis of the biocompatibility of ALCAP ceramics in rat femurs. *J. Biomed. Mater. Res.,* 22: 1101–1126.

Meenen N.M., Osborn J.F., Dallek M., and Donath K. 1992. Hydroxyapatite-ceramic for juxta-articular implantation. *J. Mat. Sci.: Mater. Med.* 3: 345–351.

Metsger S., Driskell T.D., and Paulsrud J.R. 1982. Tricalcium phosphate ceramic — A resorbable bone implant: review and current status. *JADA* 105: 1035–1038.

Moldovan K. and Bajpai P.K. 1994. A ceramic system for continuous release of aspirin. *Biomed. Sci. Instrum.* 30: 175–180.

More R.B. and Silver M.D. 1990. Pyrolitic carbon prosthetic heart valve occluder wear: *in vitro* results for the Bjork–Shiley prosthesis. *J. Appl. Biomater.* 1: 267–278.

Morris L.M. and Bajpai P.K. 1989. Development of a resorbable tricalcium phosphate (TCP) amine antibiotic composite. *Mat. Res. Soc. Symp.* 110: 293–300.

Murakami T. and Ohtsuki N. 1989. Friction and wear characteristics of sliding pairs of bioceramics and polyethylene. In: *Bioceramics. Proceedings of 1st International Symposium on Ceramics in Medicine.* H. Oonishi, H. Aoki, and K. Sawai (Eds.), pp. 225–230. Ishiyaku Euroamerica, Inc., Tokyo.

Nagy E.A. and Bajpai P.K. 1994. Development of a ceramic matrix system for continuous delivery of azidothymidine. *Biomed. Sci. Instrum.* 30: 181–186.

Niwa S., Sawai K., Takahashie S., Tagai H., Ono M., and Fukuda Y. 1980. *Experimental Studies on the Implantation of Hydroxyapatite in the Medullary Canal of Rabbits, Trans. First World Biomaterials Congress*, Baden, Austria. p. 4.10.4.

Ogino M., Ohuchi F., and Hench L.L. 1980. Compositional dependence of the formation of calcium phosphate film on bioglass, *J. Biomed. Mater. Res.* 12: 55–64.

Ohashi T., Inoue S., Kajikawa K., Ibaragi K., Tada T., Oguchi M., Arai T., and Kondo K. 1988. The clinical wear rate of acetabular component accompanied with alumina ceramic head. In: *Bioceramics. Proceedings of 1st International Symposium on Ceramics in Medicine.* H. Oonishi, H. Aoki, and K. Sawai (Eds.), pp. 278–283. Ishiyaku EuroAmerica, Inc. Tokyo.

Ohtsuki C., Kokubo T., and Yamamuro T. 1992. Compositional dependence of bioactivity of glasses in the system $CaO–SiO_2–Al_2O_3$: its *in vitro* evaluation. *J. Mat. Sci.: Mater. Med.* 3: 119–125.

Ohura K., Nakamura T., Yamamuro T., Ebisawa Y., Kokubo T., Kotoura Y., and Oka M. 1992. Bioactivity of $Cao–SiO_2$ glasses added with various ions. *J. Mat. Sci.: Mater. Med.* 3: 95–100.

Oonishi H. 1992. Bioceramic in orthopaedic surgery — our clinical experiences. In: *Bioceramics*, Vol. 3. J.E. Hulbert and S.F. Hulbert (Eds.), pp. 31–42. Rose Hulman Institute of Technology, Terre Haute, IN.

Park J.B. and Lakes R.S. 1992. *Biomaterials — An Introduction*, 2nd ed., Plenum Press, New York.

Park J.B. 1991. Aluminum oxides: biomedical applications. In: *Concise Encyclopedia of Advanced Ceramic Materials*, R.J. Brook (Ed.), pp.13–16. Pergamon Press, Oxford.

Parker D.R. and Bajpai P.K. 1993. Effect of locally delivered testosterone on bone healing. *Trans. Soc. Biomater.* 26: 293.

Peltier L.F. 1961, The use of plaster of Paris to fill defects in bone. *Clin. Orthop.* 21: 1–29.

Piattelli A. and Trisi P. 1994. A light and laser scanning microscopy study of bone/hydroxyapatite-coated titanium implants interface: histochemical evidence of unmineralized material in humans. *J. Biomed. Mater. Res.* 28: 529–536.

Pories W.J. and Strain W.H. 1970. Zinc and wound healing. In: *Zinc Metabolism*, A.S. Prasad (Ed.), pp. 378–394. Thomas, Springfield, IL.

Posner A.S., Perloff A., and Diorio A.D. 1958. Refinement of hydroxyapatite structure. *Acta. Cryst.* 11: 308–309.

Reck R., Störkel S, and Meyer A. 1988. Bioactive glass-ceramics in middle ear surgery: an eight year review. In: *Bioceramics: Material Characteristics Versus In Vivo Behavior. Ann. NY Acad. Sci.* 253: 100–106.

Ricci J.L., Bajpai P.K., Berkman A., Alexander H., and Parsons J.R. 1986. Development of a fast-setting ceramic based grout material for filling bone defects. In: *Biomedical Engineering V Recent Developments. Proceedings of the Fifth Southern Biomedical Engineering Conference.* Shreveport L.A. and S. Saha (Eds.), pp. 475–481. Pergamon Press, New York.

Ritter J.E. Jr, Greenspan D.C., Palmer R.A., and Hench L.L. 1979. Use of fracture of an alumina and bioglass coated alumina, *J. Biomed. Mater. Res.* 13: 251–263.

Sartoris D.J., Gershuni D.H., Akeson W.H., Holmes R.E., and Resnick D. 1986. Coralline hydroxyapatite bone graft substitutes: Preliminary report of radiographic evaluation. *Radiology* 159: 133–137.

Scheidler P.A. and Bajpai P.K. 1992. Zinc sulfate calcium phosphate (ZSCAP) composite for repairing traumatized bone. *Biomed. Sci. Instrum.* 28: 183–188.

Schepers E., Ducheyne P., and De Clercq M. 1989. Interfacial analysis of fiber-reinforced bioactive dental root implants. *J. Biomed. Mater. Res.* 23: 735–752.

Schepers E., De Clercq M., and Ducheyne P. 1988. Interfacial behavior of bulk bioactive glass and fiber-reinforced bioactive glass dental root implants. *Ann. NY Acad. Sci.* 523: 178–189.

Schepers E.J.G, Ducheyne P., Barbier L., and Schepers S. 1993. Bioactive glass particles of narrow size range: A new material for the repair of bone defects. *Impl. Dent.* 2: 151–156.

Schwartz Z., Braun G., Kohave D., Brooks B., Amir D., Sela J., and Boyan B. 1993. Effects of hydroxyapatite implants on primary mineralization during rat tibial healing: Biochemical and morphometric analysis. *J. Biomed. Mater. Res.* 27: 1029–1038.

Sedel L., Meunier A., Nizard R.S., and Witvoet J. 1991. Ten year survivorship of cemented ceramic–ceramic total hip replacement. In: *Bioceramics* Volume 4. *Proceedings of the 4th International Symposium on Ceramics in Medicine.* W. Bonfield, G.W. Hastings, and K.E. Tanner (Eds.), pp.27–37. Butterworth-Heinemann Ltd., London, UK.

Shackelford J.F. 1988. *Introduction to Materials Science for Engineers*, 2nd ed., Macmillan Publishing Co., New York.

Shimm H.S. and Haubold A.D. 1980. The fatigue behavior of vapor deposited carbon films. *Biomater. Med. Dev. Art. Org.* 8: 333–344.

Shields J.A., Shields C.L., and De Potter P. 1993. Hydroxyapatite orbital implant after enucleation-experience with 200 cases. *Mayo Clinic Proc.* 68: 1191–1195.

Shobert E.I. II. 1964. *Carbon and Graphite*, Academic Press, N.Y.

Stricker N.J., Larrabee R.A., and Bajpai P.K. 1992. Biocompatibility of ferric calcium phosphorous oxide ceramics. *Biomed. Sci. Instrum.* 28: 123–128.

Suchanek W., Yashima M., Kakihana M., and Yoshimura M. 1997. Hydroxyapatite ceramics with selected sintering additives. *Biomaterials* 18: 923–933.

Sudanese A., Toni A., Cattaneo G.L., Ciaroni D., Greggi T., Dallart D., Galli G., and Giunti A. 1989. In *Bioceramics. Proceedings of 1st International Symposium on Ceramics in Medicine.* H. Oonishi, H. Aoki, and K. Sawai (Eds.), pp. 237–240, Ishiyaku Euroamerica, Inc., Tokyo.

Takatsuko K., Yamamuro T., Kitsugi T., Nakamura T., Shibuya T., and Goto T. 1993. A new bioactive glass-ceramic as a coating material on titanium alloy. *J. Appl. Biomater.* 4: 317–329.

Terry B.C., Baker R.D., Tucker M.R., and Hanker J.S. 1989. Alveolar ridge augmentation with composite implants of hydroxylapatite and plaster for correction of bony defects, deficiencies and related contour abnormalities. *Mat. Res. Soc. Symp.* 110: 187–198.

Valiathan A., Randhawa G.S., and Randhawa A. 1993. Biomaterial aspects of calcium hydroxyapatite, *T.I.B. & A.O.* 7: 1–7.

Varma H.K. and Sivakumar R. 1996. Dense hydroxyapatite ceramics through gel casting technique. *Mater. Lett.* 29: 57–61.

Whitehead R.Y., Lacefield W.R., and Lucas L.C. 1993. Structure and integrity of a plasma sprayed hydroxyapatite coating on titanium, *J. Biomed. Mater. Res.* 27: 1501–1507.

Wolford L.M., Wardrop R.W., and Hartog J.M. 1987. Coralline porous hydroxylapatite as a bone graft substitute in orthognathic surgery. *J. Oral. Maxillofacial. Surg.* 45: 1034–1042.

Wyatt D.F., Bajpai P.K., Graves G.A. Jr, and Stull P.A. 1976. Remodelling of calcium aluminate phosphorous pentoxide ceramic implants in bone. *IRCS. Med. Sci.* 4: 421.

Yamamuro T., Hench L.L., and Wilson J. 1990. *Handbook of Bioactive Ceramics I and II.* CRC Press, Boca Raton, FL.

Yamamuro T., Shikata J., Kakutani Y., Yoshii S., Kitsugi T., and Ono K. 1988. Novel methods for clinical applications of bioactive ceramics. In: *Bioceramics: Material Characteristics Versus In Vivo Behavior. Ann. NY Acad. Sci.* 523: 107–114.

Zimmerman M.C., Alexander H., Parsons J.R., and Bajpai P.K. 1991. The design and analysis of laminated degradable composite bone plates for fracture fixation. In: *High-Tech Textiles*, T.L. Vigo and A.F. Turbak (Eds.), pp. 132–148. ACS Symposium Series 457, American Chemical Society, Washington, D.C.

Further Information

Bajpai P.K. 1988. *ZCAP Ceramics.* US. Patent No. 4778471.

Bajpai P.K. 1987. *Surgical Cements.* US. Patent No. 4668295.

Bonfield W., Hastings G.W., and Tanner K.E. 1991. *Bioceramics, Vol. 4. Proceedings of the 4th International Symposium on Ceramics in Medicine.* Butterworth-Heinemann Ltd., London, UK.

Brook J. 1991. *Concise Encyclopedia of Advanced Ceramic Materials.* Pergamon Press, Oxford.

de Groot K. 1983. *Bioceramics of Calcium Phosphate.* CRC Press, Boca Raton, FL.

Ducheyne P. and Lemons J.E. 1988. Bioceramics: material characteristics versus *in vivo* behavior. *Ann. NY Acad. Sci.,* New York, NY.

Ducheyne P. and Christiansen D. 1993. *Bioceramics,* Vol. 6. Butterworth-Heinemann Ltd., Boston.

Filgueiras M.R.T., LaTorre G., and Hench L.L. 1993. Solution effects on the surface reactions of three bioactive glass compositions. *J. Biomed. Mater. Res.* 27: 1485–1493.

Frank R.M., Wiedemann P., Hemmerle J., and Freymann M. 1991. Pulp capping with synthetic hydroxyapatite in human premolars. *J. Appl. Biomater.* 2: 243–250.

Fulmer M.T. and Brown P.W. 1993. Effects of Na_2HPO_4 and NaH_2PO_4 on hydroxyapatite formation. *J. Biomed. Mater. Res.* 27: 1095–1102.

Garcia R. and Doremus R.H. 1992. Electron microscopy of the bone-hydroxyapatite interface from a human dental implant. *J. Mater. Sci.: Mater. Med.* 3: 154–156.

Hall C.W., Hulbert S.F., Levine S.N., and Young F.A. 1972. *Engineering and Medicine.* Interscience Publishers, New York.

Hench L.L. 1991. Bioceramics: From concept to clinic. *J. Am. Ceram. Soc.* 74: 1487–1510.

Hench L.L. and Ethridge E.C. 1982. *Biomaterials: An Interfacial Approach.* Academic Press, New York.

Hulbert J.A. and Hulbert S.F. 1992. *Bioceramics,* Vol. 3. *Proceedings of the 3rd International Symposium on Ceramics in Medicine,* Rose-Hulman Institute of Technology, Terra Haute, IN.

Kawahara H. Ed. 1989. *Oral Implantology and Biomaterials.* Elsevier, Amsterdam, Netherlands.

Kingery W.D., Bowen H.K., and Uhlmann D.R. 1976. *Introduction to Ceramics,* 2nd ed., p. 368, John Wiley & Sons, New York.

Lemons J.E. 1988. *Quantitative Characterization and Performance of Porous Implants for Hard Tissue Applications,* ASTM STP 953. American Society for Testing and Materials, Philadelphia, PA.

Mattie D.R. and Bajpai P.K. 1986. Biocompatibility testing of ALCAP ceramics. *IRCS. Med. Sci.* 14: 641–643.

Neo M., Nakamura T., Ohtsuki C., Kokubo T., and Yamamuro T. 1993. Apatite formation on three kinds of bioactive material at an early stage *in vivo*: A comparative study by transmission electron microscopy. *J. Biomed. Mater. Res.* 27: 999–1006.

Oonishi H., Aoki H., and Sawai K. 1988. *Bioceramics,* Vol. 1. *Proceedings of 1st International Symposium on Ceramics in Medicine.* Ishiyaku EuroAmerica, Inc. Tokyo.

Oonishi H. and Ooi Y. 1981. *Orthopaedic ceramic implants,* Vol. I. *Proceedings of Japanese Society of Orthopaedic Ceramic Implants.*

Park J.B. and Lakes R.S. 1992. *Biomaterials: An Introduction,* 2nd ed., Plenum Press, New York, NY.

Ravaglioli A. and Krajewski A. 1992. *Bioceramics and the Human Body.* Elsevier Applied Science, London and New York.

Rubin L.R. 1983. *Biomaterials in Reconstructive Surgery.* C.V. Mosby Co., St. Louis, MO.

Sharma C.P. and Szycher M. 1991. *Blood Compatible Materials and Devices: Perspectives Toward 21st Century.* Technomic Publishing Co., Lancaster, PA.

Signs S.A., Pantano C.G., Driskell T.D., and Bajpai P.K. 1979. In vitro dissolution of synthos ceramics in an acellular physiological environment. *Biomater. Med. Dev. Art. Org.* 7: 183–190.

Stea S., Tarabusi C., Ciapetti G., Pizzoferrato A., Toni A., and Sudanese A. 1992. Microhardness evaluations of the bone growing into porous implants. *J. Mater. Sci.: Mater. Med.* 3: 252–254.

van Blitterswijk C.A. and Grote J.J. 1989. Biological performance of ceramics during inflammation and infection. *Crit. Rev. Biocompatib.* 5: 13–43.

Wilson J. and Low S.B. 1992. Bioactive ceramics for periodontal treatment: Comparative studies in the patus monkey. *J. Appl. Biomater.* 3: 123–129.

Yamamuro T., Hench L.L., and Wilson J. 1990. *Handbook of Bioactive Ceramics.* CRC Press, Boca Raton, FL.

Zhang X. and Ikada Y. 1994. *Biomedical Materials Research in The Far East (I).* Kobunshi Kankokai Inc., Kyoto, Japan.

40

Polymeric Biomaterials

Hai Bang Lee
Korea Research Institute of
Chemical Technology

Gilson Khang
Chonbuk National University

Jin Ho Lee
Hannam University

40.1 Introduction

Synthetic polymeric materials have been widely used in medical disposable supply, prosthetic materials, dental materials, implants, dressings, extracorporeal devices, encapsulants, polymeric drug delivery systems, tissue engineered products, and orthodoses as that of metal and ceramics substituents [Lee, 1989]. The main advantages of the polymeric **biomaterials** compared to metal or ceramic materials are ease of manufacturability to produce various shapes (latex, film, sheet, fibers, etc.), ease of secondary processability, reasonable cost, and availability with desired mechanical and physical properties. The required properties of polymeric biomaterials are similar to other biomaterials, that is, **biocompatibility**, sterilizability, adequate mechanical and physical properties, and manufacturability as given in Table 40.1.

The objectives of this chapter are (1) the review of basic chemical and physical properties of the synthetic polymers, (2) the sterilization of the polymeric biomaterials, (3) the importance of the surface treatment for improving biocompatability, and (4) the application of the **chemogradient surface** for the study on cell to polymer interactions.

TABLE 40.1 Requirements for Biomedical Polymers

Properties	Description
Biocompatibility	Noncarcinogenesis, nonpyrogenicity, nontoxicity, and nonallergic response
Sterilizability	Autoclave, dry heating, ethylenoxide gas, and radiation
Physical property	Strength, elasticity, and durability
Manufacturability	Machining, molding, extruding, and fiber forming

Source: Modified from Ikada, Y. (Ed.) 1989. In: *High Technology Fiber*, Part B, Marcel Dekker, New York. With permission.

TABLE 40.2 Typical Condensation Polymers

Type	Interunit linkage
Polyester	$\begin{matrix} O \\ \| \\ -C-O- \end{matrix}$
Polyamide	$\begin{matrix} O\ \ H \\ \|\ \ \| \\ -C-N- \end{matrix}$
Polyurea	$\begin{matrix} H\ \ O\ \ H \\ \|\ \ \|\ \ \| \\ -N-C-N- \end{matrix}$
Polyurethane	$\begin{matrix} O\ \ H \\ \|\ \ \| \\ -O-C-N- \end{matrix}$
Polysiloxane	$\begin{matrix} R \\ \| \\ -Si-O- \\ \| \\ R \end{matrix}$
Protein	$\begin{matrix} O\ \ H \\ \|\ \ \| \\ -C-N- \end{matrix}$

40.2 Polymerization and Basic Structure

40.2.1 Polymerization

In order to link the small molecules one has to force them to lose their electrons by the chemical processes of condensation and addition. By controlling the reaction temperature, pressure, and time in the presence of catalyst(s), the degree to which **repeating units** are put together into chains can be manipulated.

40.2.1.1 Condensation or Step Reaction Polymerization

During **condensation polymerization** a small molecule such as water will be condensed out by the chemical reaction. For example

$$\underset{\text{(amine)}}{\text{R-NH}_2} + \underset{\text{(carboxylic acid)}}{\text{R}'\text{COOH}} \rightarrow \underset{\text{(amide)}}{\text{R}'\text{CONHR}} + \underset{\text{(condensed molecule)}}{\text{H}_2\text{O}} \tag{40.1}$$

This particular process is used to make polyamides (Nylons). Nylon was the first commercial polymer, made in the 1930s.

Some typical condensation polymers and their interunit linkages are given in Table 40.2. One major drawback of condensation polymerization is the tendency for the reaction to cease before the chains grow to a sufficient length. This is due to the decreased mobility of the chains and reactant chemical species as polymerization progresses. This results in short chains. However, in the case of Nylon the chains are polymerized to a sufficiently large extent before this occurs and the physical properties of the polymer are preserved.

Natural polymers, such as polysaccharides and proteins are also made by condensation polymerization. The condensing molecule is always water (H_2O).

40.2.1.2 Addition or Free Radical Polymerization

Addition polymerization can be achieved by rearranging the bonds within each monomer. Since each "mer" has to share at least two covalent electrons with other mers the monomer should have at least one double bond. For example, in the case of ethylene:

$$n \ \{ \overset{\overset{H}{|}}{\underset{\underset{H}{|}}{C}} = \overset{\overset{H}{|}}{\underset{\underset{H}{|}}{C}} \} \ \rightarrow \ -\overset{\overset{H}{|}}{\underset{\underset{H}{|}}{C}} \{ \overset{\overset{H}{|}}{\underset{\underset{H}{|}}{C}} - \overset{\overset{H}{|}}{\underset{\underset{H}{|}}{C}} \} \overset{\overset{H}{|}}{\underset{\underset{H}{|}}{C}} - \qquad (40.2)$$

The breaking of a double bond can be made with an **initiator**. This is usually a free radical such as benzoyl peroxide ($H_5C_6COO–OOCC_6H_5$). The initiation can be activated by heat, ultraviolet light, and other chemicals. The free radicals (initiators) can react with monomers and this free radical can react with another monomer and the process can continue on. This process is called propagation. The propagation process can be terminated by combining two free radicals, by transfer, or by disproportionate processes. Some of the free radical polymers are given in Table 40.3. There are three more types of initiating species for addition polymerization beside free-radicals; cations, anions, and coordination (stereospecific) catalysts. Some monomers can use two or more of the initiation processes but others can use only one process as given in Table 40.3.

TABLE 40.3 Monomers for Addition Polymerization and Suitable Process

Monomer names	Chemical structure	Polymerization mechanism			
		Radical	Cationic	Anionic	Coordination
Acrylonitrile	$CH_2=CH$ | $C≡N$	+	−	+	+
Ethylene	$CH_2=CH_2$	+	+	−	−
Methacrylate	$CH_2=CH$ | $COOCH_3$	+	−	+	+
Methylmethacrylate	$CH_2=CCH_3$ | $COOCH_3$	+	−	+	+
Propylene	$CH_2=CH$ | CH_3	−	−	−	+
Styrene	$CH_2=CH$ | C_6H_5	+	+	+	+
Vinylchloride	$CH_2=CH$ | Cl	+	−	−	+
Vinylidenechloride	$CH_2=C$ | Cl | Cl	+	−	+	−

+: high polymer formed.−: no reaction or oligomers only.
Source: Modified form Billmeyer, F.W.Jr. 1984. *Text Book of Polymer Scence*, 3rd ed. John Wiley & Sons; New York. With permission.

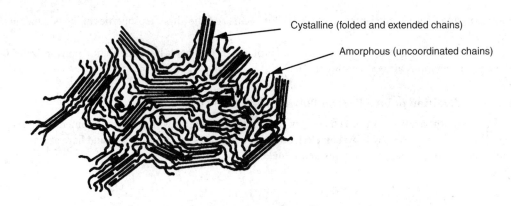

FIGURE 40.1   Fringed-micelle model of a linear polymer with semi-crystalline structure.

40.2.2 Basic Structure

Polymers have very long chain molecules which are formed by **covalent bonding** along the backbone chain. The long chains are held together either by secondary bonding forces such as van der Waals and hydrogen bonds or primary covalent bonding forces through crosslinks between chains. The long chains are very flexible and can be tangled easily. In addition, each chain can have **side groups**, branches and copolymeric chains or blocks which can also interfere with the long-range ordering of chains. For example, paraffin wax has the same chemical formula as polyethylene (PE) $[(CH_2CH_2)_n]$, but will crystallize almost completely because of its much shorter chain lengths. However, when the chains become extremely long {from 40 to 50 repeating units $[-CH_2CH_2-]$ to several thousands as in linear PE} they cannot be crystallized completely (up to 80 to 90% crystallization is possible). Also, branched PE in which side chains are attached to the main backbone chain at positions normally occupied by a hydrogen atom, will not crystallize easily due to the **steric hindrance** of side chains resulting in a more noncrystalline structure. The partially crystallized structure is called semicrystalline which is the most commonly occurring structure for linear polymers. The semicrystalline structure is represented by disordered noncrystalline (amorphous) regions and ordered crystalline regions which may contain folded chains as shown in Figure 40.1.

The degree of polymerization (DP) is defined as an average number of mers, or repeating units, per molecule, that is, chain. Each chain may have a different number of mers depending on the condition of polymerization. Also, the length of each chain may be different. Therefore, it is assumed there is an average degree of polymerization or average molecular weight (MW). The relationship between molecular weight and degree of polymerization can be expressed as:

$$\text{MW of polymer} = \text{DP} \times \text{MW of mer (or repeating unit)} \tag{40.3}$$

The two average molecular weights most commonly used are defined in terms of the numbers of molecules, Ni, having molecular weight, Mi; or wi, the weight of species with molecular weights Mi as follows:

1. The number-average molecular weight, Mn, is defined by

$$\text{Mn} = \frac{\Sigma NiMi}{\Sigma NiMi} = \Sigma niMi = \frac{\Sigma Wi}{\Sigma(Wi/Mi)} = \frac{1}{\Sigma(wi\ Mi)} \tag{40.4}$$

2. The weight average molecular weight, Mw, is defined by

$$\text{Mw} = \frac{\Sigma WiMi}{\Sigma Wi} = \Sigma wiMi = \frac{\Sigma NiMi^2}{\Sigma NiMi} \tag{40.5}$$

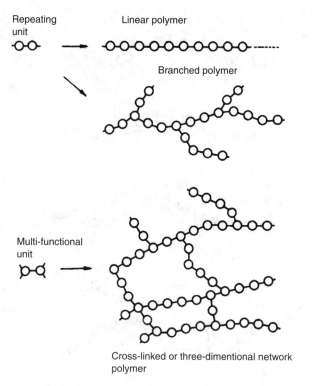

Repeating unit

Linear polymer

Branched polymer

Multi-functional unit

Cross-linked or three-dimentional network polymer

FIGURE 40.2 Arrangement of polymer chains into linear, branched, and network structure depending on the functionality of the repeating units.

An absolute method of measuring the molecular weight is one that depends on theoretical consider-ations, counting molecules and their weight directly. The relative methods require calibration based on an absolute method and include intrinsic viscosity and gel permeation chromatography (GPC). Absolute methods of determining the number-average molecular weight (Mn) include osmometry and other col-ligative methods, and end group analysis. Light-scattering yields an absolute weight-average molecular weight (Mw).

As the molecular chains become longer by the progress of polymerization, their relative mobility decreases. The chain mobility is also related to the physical properties of the final polymer. Generally, the higher the molecular weight, the less the mobility of chains which results in higher strength and greater thermal stability. The polymer chains can be arranged in three ways; linear, branched, and a cross-linked (or three-dimensional) network as shown in Figure 40.2. Linear polymers such as polyvinyls, polyamides, and polyesters are much easier to crystallize than the cross-linked or branched polymers. However, they cannot be crystallized 100% as with metals. Instead they become semicrystalline polymers. The arrangement of chains in crystalline regions is believed to be a combination of folded and extended chains. The chain folds, which are seemingly more difficult to form, are necessary to explain observed single crystal structures in which the crystal thickness is too small to accommodate the length of the chain as determined by electron and x-ray diffraction studies. The classical "fringed-micelle" model in which the amorphous and crystalline regions coexist has been modified to include chain folds in the crystalline regions. The cross-linked or three-dimensional network polymers such as polyphenolformaldehyde cannot be crystallized at all and they become noncrystalline, amorphous polymers.

Vinyl polymers have a repeating unit $-CH_2-CHX-$ where X is some monovalent side group. There are three possible arrangements of side groups (X) (1) atactic, (2) isotactic, and (3) syndiotactic. In atactic arrangements the side groups are randomly distributed while in syndiotactic and isotactic arrange-ments they are either in alternating positions or on one side of the main chain. If side groups are

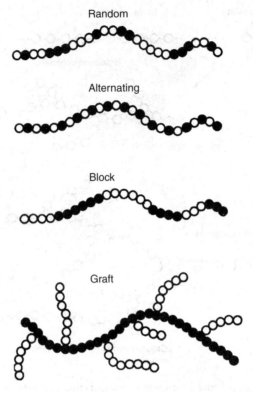

FIGURE 40.3   Possible arrangements of copolymers.

small like polyethylene (X = H) and the chains are linear, the polymer crystallizes easily. However, if the side groups are large as in polyvinyl chloride (X = Cl) and polystyrene (X = C_6H_5, benzene ring) and are randomly distributed along the chains (atactic), then a noncrystalline structure will be formed. The isotactic and syndiotactic polymers usually crystallize even when the side groups are large.

Copolymerization, in which two or more homopolymers (one type of repeating unit throughout its structure) are chemically combined, always disrupts the regularity of polymer chains thus promoting the formation of a noncrystalline structure. Possible arrangement of the different copolymerization is shown in Figure 40.3. The addition of **plasticizers** to prevent crystallization by keeping the chains separated from one another will result in more flexible polymers, a noncrystalline version of a polymer which normally crystallizes. An example is celluloid which is normally made of crystalline nitrocellulose plasticized with camphor. Plasticizers are also used to make rigid noncrystalline polymers like polyvinylchloride (PVC) into a more flexible solid (a good example is Tygon® tubing).

Elastomers, or rubbers, are polymers which exhibit large stretchability at room temperature and can snap back to their original dimensions when the load is released. The elastomers are non-crystalline polymers which have an intermediate structure consisting of long chain molecules in three-dimensional networks (see next section for more details). The chains also have "kinks" or "bends" in them which straighten when a load is applied. For example, the chains of *cis*-polyisoprene (natural rubber) are bent at the double bond due to the methyl group interfering with the neighboring hydrogen in the repeating unit [$-CH_2-C(CH_3)=CH-CH_2-$]. If the methyl group is on the opposite side of the hydrogen then it becomes *trans*-polyisoprene which will crystallize due to the absence of the steric hindrance present in the *cis* form. The resulting polymer is a very rigid solid called gutta percha which is not an elastomer. Below the **glass transition temperature** (T_g; second-order transition temperature between viscous liquid and solid) natural rubber loses its compliance and becomes a glass-like material. Therefore, to be flexible,

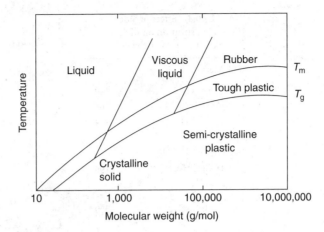

FIGURE 40.4 Approximate relations among molecular weight, T_g, T_m, and polymer properties.

all elastomers should have T_g well below room temperature. What makes the elastomers not behave like liquids above T_g is in fact due to the cross-links between chains which act as pinning points. Without cross-links the polymer would deform permanently. An example is latex which behaves as a viscous liquid. Latex can be cross-linked with sulfur (**vulcanization**) by breaking double bonds (C=C) and forming C–S–S–C bonds between the chains. The more cross-links are introduced the more rigid the structure becomes. If all the chains are cross-linked together, the material will become a three-dimensional rigid polymer.

40.2.3 Effect of Structural Modification on Properties

The physical properties of polymers can be affected in many ways. In particular, the chemical composition and arrangement of chains will have a great effect on the final properties. By such means the polymers can be tailored to meet the end use.

40.2.3.1 Effect of Molecular Weight and Composition

The molecular weight and its distribution have a great effect on the properties of a polymer since its rigidity is primarily due to the immobilization or entanglement of the chains. This is because the chains are arranged like cooked spaghetti strands in a bowl. By increasing the molecular weight the polymer chains become longer and less mobile and a more rigid material results as shown in Figure 40.4. Equally important is that all chains should be equal in length since if there are short chains they will act as plasticizers. Another obvious way of changing properties is to change the chemical composition of the backbone or side chains. Substituting the backbone carbon of a polyethylene with divalent oxygen or sulfur will decrease the melting and glass transition temperatures since the chain becomes more flexible due to the increased rotational freedom. On the other hand if the backbone chains can be made more rigid then a stiffer polymer will result.

40.2.3.2 Effect of Side Chain Substitution, Cross-Linking, and Branching

Increasing the size of side groups in linear polymers such as polyethylene will decrease the melting temperature due to the lesser perfection of molecular packing, that is, decreased crystallinity. This effect is seen until the side group itself becomes large enough to hinder the movement of the main chain as shown in Table 40.4. Very long side groups can be thought of as being branches.

  Cross-linking of the main chains is in effect similar to the side-chain substitution with a small molecule, that is, it lowers the melting temperature. This is due to the interference of the cross-linking which causes

TABLE 40.4   Effect of Side
Chain Substitution on Melting
Temperature in Polyethylene

Side chain	T_m (°C)
$-H$	140
$-CH_3$	165
$-CH_2CH_3$	124
$-CH_2CH_2CH_3$	75
$-CH_2CH_2CH_2CH_3$	−55
$-CH_2CHCH_2CH_3$ $\quad\quad CH_3$	196
$\quad\quad CH_3$ $\quad\quad\mid$ $-CH_2CCH_2CH_3$ $\quad\quad\mid$ $\quad\quad -CH_3$	350

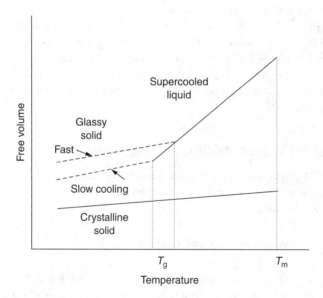

FIGURE 40.5   Change of volume vs. temperature of a solid. The glass transition temperature (T_g) depends on the rate of cooling and below (T_g) the material behaves as a solid like a window glass.

decreased mobility of the chains resulting in further retardation of the crystallization rate. In fact, a large degree of cross-linking can prevent crystallization completely. However, when the cross-linking density increases for a rubber, the material becomes harder and the glass transition temperature also increases.

40.2.3.3   Effect of Temperature on Properties

Amorphous polymers undergo a substantial change in their properties as a function of temperature. The glass transition temperature, T_g, is a boundary between the glassy region of behavior in which the polymer is relatively stiff and the rubbery region in which it is very compliant. T_g can also be defined as the temperature at which the slope of volume change versus temperature has a discontinuity in slope as shown in Figure 40.5. Since polymers are non-crystalline or at most semicrystalline, the value obtained in this measurement depends on how fast it is taken.

TABLE 40.5 Biomedical Application of Polymeric Biomaterials

Synthetic Polymers	Applications
Polyvinylchloride (PVC)	Blood and solution bag, surgical packaging, IV sets, dialysis devices, catheter bottles, connectors, and cannulae
Polyethylene (PE)	Pharmaceutical bottle, nonwoven fabric, catheter, pouch, flexible container, and orthopedic implants
Polypropylene (PP)	Disposable syringes, blood oxygenator membrane, suture, nonwoven fabric, and artificial vascular grafts
Polymethylmetacrylate (PMMA)	Blood pump and reservoirs, membrane for blood dialyzer, implantable ocular lens, and bone cement
Polystyrene (PS)	Tissue culture flasks, roller bottles, and filterwares
Polyethylenterephthalate (PET)	Implantable suture, mesh, artificial vascular grafts, and heart valve
Polytetrafluoroethylene (PTFE)	Catheter and artificial vascular grafts
Polyurethane (PU)	Film, tubing, and components
Polyamide (Nylon)	Packaging film, catheters, sutures, and mold parts

40.3 Polymers Used as Biomaterials

Although hundreds of polymers are easily synthesized and could be used as biomaterials only ten to twenty polymers are mainly used in medical device fabrications from disposable to long-term implants as given in Table 40.5. In this section, the general information of the characteristics, properties, and applications of the most commonly used polymers will be discussed [Billmeyer, 1984; Park, 1984; Leininger and Bigg, 1986; Shalaby, 1988; Brandrup and Immergut, 1989; Sharma and Szycher, 1991; Park and Lakes, 1992; Dumitriu, 1993; Lee and Lee, 1995; Ratner et al., 1996].

40.3.1 Polyvinylchloride (PVC)

The PVC is an amorphous, rigid polymer due to the large side group (Cl, chloride) with a T_g of 75 to 105°C. It has a high melt viscosity hence it is difficult to process. To prevent the thermal degradation of the polymer (HCl could be released), thermal stabilizers such as metallic soaps or salts are incorporated. Lubricants are formulated on PVC compounds to prevent adhesion to metal surfaces and facilitate the melt flow during processing. Plasticizers are used in the range of 10 to 100 parts per 100 parts of PVC resin to make it flexible. Di-2-ethylhexylphthalate (DEHP or DOP) is used in medical PVC formulation. However, the plasticizers of trioctyltrimellitate (TOTM), polyester, azelate, and phosphate ester are also used to prevent extraction by blood, aqueous solution, and hot water during autoclaving sterilization.

PVC sheets and films are used in blood and solution storage bags and surgical packaging. PVC tubing is commonly used in intravenous (IV) administration, dialysis devices, catheters, and cannulae.

40.3.2 Polyethylene (PE)

PE is available commercially in five major grades: (1) high density (HDPE), (2) low density (LDPE), (3) linear low density (LLDPE), (4) very low density (VLDPE), and (5) ultra high molecular weight (UHMWPE). HDPE is polymerized in a low temperature (60–80°C), and at a low pressure ($\sim$10 kg/cm^2) using metal catalysts. A highly crystalline, linear polymer with a density ranging from 0.94 to 0.965 g/cm^3 is obtained. LDPE is derived from a high temperature (150–300°C) and pressures (1000–3000 kg/cm^2) using free radical initiators. A highly branched polymer with lower crystallinity and densities ranging from 0.915 to 0.935 g/cm^3 is obtained. LLDPE (density: 0.91–0.94 g/cm^3) and VLDPE (density: 0.88–0.89 g/cm^3), which are linear polymers, are polymerized under low pressures and temperatures using metal catalysts with comonomers such as 1-butene, 1-hexene, or 1-octene to obtain the desired physical properties and density ranges.

HDPE is used in pharmaceutical bottles, nonwoven fabrics, and caps. LDPE is found in flexible container applications, nonwoven-disposable and laminated (or coextruded with paper) foil, and polymers for packaging. LLDPE is frequently employed in pouches and bags due to its excellent puncture resistance and VLDPE is used in extruded tubes. UHMWPE (MW $>2\times10^6$ g/mol) has been used for orthopedic implant fabrications, especially for load-bearing applications such as an acetabular cup of total hip and the tibial plateau and patellar surfaces of knee joints. Biocompatability tests for PE are given by ASTM standards in F981, F639, and F755.

40.3.3 Polypropylene (PP)

PP can be polymerized by a Ziegler-Natta stereospecific catalyst which controls the isotactic position of the methyl group. Thermal (T_g: $-12°$C, T_m: 125–167°C and density: 0.85–0.98 g/cm^3) and physical properties of PP are similar to PE. The average molecular weight of commercial PP ranges from 2.2 to 7.0×10^5 g/mol and has a wide molecular weight distribution (polydispersity) which is from 2.6 to 12. Additives for PP such as antioxidants, light stabilizer, nucleating agents, lubricants, mold release agents, antiblock, and slip agents are formulated to improve the physical properties and processability. PP has an exceptionally high flex life and excellent environment stress-cracking resistance, hence it had been tried for finger joint prostheses with an integrally molded hinge design [Park, 1984]. The gas and water vapor permeability of PP are in-between those of LDPE and HDPE. PP is used to make disposable hypothermic syringes, blood **oxygenator** membrane, packaging for devices, solutions, and drugs, **suture**, artificial vascular **grafts**, nonwoven fabrics, etc.

40.3.4 Polymethylmetacrylate (PMMA)

Commercial PMMA is an amorphous (T_g: 105°C and density: 1.15 to 1.195 g/cm^3) material with good resistance to dilute alkalis and other inorganic solutions. PMMA is best known for its exceptional light transparency (92% transmission), high **refractive index** (1.49), good weathering properties, and as one of the most biocompatible polymers. PMMA can be easily machined with conventional tools, molded, surface coated, and plasma etched with glow or corona discharge. PMMA is used broadly in medical applications such as a blood pump and reservoir, an IV system, membranes for blood dialyzer, and in *in vitro* diagnostics. It is also found in contact lenses and implantable ocular lenses due to excellent optical properties, dentures, and maxillofacial prostheses due to good physical and coloring properties, and **bone cement** for joint prostheses fixation (ASTM standard F451).

Another acrylic polymer such as polymethylacrylate (PMA), polyhydroxyethyl-methacrylate (PHEMA), and polyacrylamide (PAAm) are also used in medical applications. PHEMA and PAAm are **hydrogels**, lightly cross-linked by ethyleneglycoldimethylacrylate (EGDM) to increase their mechanical strength. The extended wear soft contact lenses are synthesized from PMMA and N-vinylpyrollidone or PHEMA which have high water content (above 70%) and a high oxygen permeability.

40.3.5 Polystyrene (PS) and Its Copolymers

The PS is polymerized by free radical polymerization and is usually atactic. Three grades are available; unmodified general purpose PS (GPPS, T_g: 100°C), high impact PS (HIPS), and PS foam. GPPS has good transparency, lack of color, ease of fabrication, thermal stability, low specific gravity (1.04–1.12 g/cm^3), and relatively high modulus. HIPS contains a rubbery modifier which forms chemical bonding with the growing PS chains. Hence the ductility and impact strength are increased and the resistance to environmental stress-cracking is also improved. PS is mainly processed by injection molding at 180–2?0°C. To improve processability additives such as stabilizers, lubricants, and mold releasing agents are ꞏulated. GPPS is commonly used in tissue culture flasks, roller bottles, vacuum canisters, and filterware. ꞏlonitrile–butadiene–styrene (ABS) **copolymers** are produced by three monomers; acrylonitrile, ꞏe, and styrene. The desired physical and chemical properties of ABS polymers with a wide range nal characteristics can be controlled by changing the ratio of these monomers. They are resistant to the common inorganic solutions, have good surface properties, and dimensional stability. ABS is used for IV sets, clamps, blood dialyzers, diagnostic test kits, and so on.

40.3.6 Polyesters

Polyesters such as polyethyleneterephthalate (PET) are frequently found in medical applications due to their unique chemical and physical properties. PET is so far the most important of this group of polymers in terms of biomedical applications such as artificial vascular graft, sutures, and meshes. It is highly crystalline with a high melting temperature (T_m: 265°C), hydrophobic and resistant to hydrolysis in dilute acids. In addition, PET can be converted by conventional techniques into molded articles such as luer filters, check valves, and catheter housings. Polycaprolactone is crystalline and has a low melting temperature (T_m: 64°C). Its use as a soft matrix or coating for conventional polyester fibers was proposed by recent investigation [Leininger and Bigg, 1986].

40.3.7 Polyamides (Nylons)

Polyamides are known as nylons and are designated by the number of carbon atoms in the repeating units. Nylons can be polymerized by step-reaction (or condensation) and ring-scission polymerization. They have excellent fiber-forming ability due to interchain **hydrogen bonding** and a high degree of crystallinity, which increases strength in the fiber direction.

The presence of –CONH– groups in polyamides attracts the chains strongly toward one another by hydrogen bonding. Since the hydrogen bond plays a major role in determining properties, the number and distribution of –CONH– groups are important factors. For example, T_g can be decreased by decreasing the number of –CONH– groups . On the other hand, an increase in the number of –CONH– groups improves physical properties such as strength as one can see that Nylon 66 is stronger than Nylon 610 and Nylon 6 is stronger than Nylon 11.

In addition to the higher Nylons (610 and 11) there are aromatic polyamides named aramids. One of them is poly (*p*-phenylene terephthalate) commonly known as **Kevlar®**, made by DuPont. This material can be made into fibers. The specific strength of such fibers is five times that of steel, therefore, it is most suitable for making composites.

Nylons are hygroscopic and lose their strength *in vivo* when implanted. The water molecules serve as plasticizers which attack the amorphous region. Proteolytic enzymes also aid in hydrolyzing by attacking the amide group. This is probably due to the fact that the proteins also contain the amide group along their molecular chains which the proteolytic enzymes could attack.

40.3.8 Fluorocarbon Polymers

The best known fluorocarbon polymer is polytetrafluoroethylene (PTFE), commonly known as **Teflon®** (DuPont). Other polymers containing fluorine are polytrifluorochloroethylene (PTFCE), polyvinylfluoride (PVF), and fluorinated ethylene propylene (FEP). Only PTFE will be discussed here since the others have rather inferior chemical and physical properties and are rarely used for implant fabrication.

PTFE is made from tetrafluoroethylene under pressure with a peroxide catalyst in the presence of excess water for removal of heat. The polymer is highly crystalline (over 94% crystallinity) with an average molecular weight of $0.5–5 \times 10^6$ g/mol. This polymer has a very high density (2.15–2.2 g/cm^3), low modulus of elasticity (0.5 GPa) and tensile strength (14 MPa). It also has a very low surface tension (18.5 erg/cm^2) and friction coefficient (0.1).

Standard specifications for the implantable PTFE are given by ASTM F754. PTFE also has an unusual property of being able to expand on a microscopic scale into a microporous material which is an excellent thermal insulator. PTFE cannot be injection molded or melt extruded because of its very high melt viscosity and it cannot be plasticized. Usually the powders are sintered to above 327°C under pressure to produce implants.

40.3.9   Rubbers

Silicone, natural, and synthetic rubbers have been used for the fabrication of implants. Natural rubber is made mostly from the latex of the Hevea brasiliensis tree and the chemical formula is the same as that of *cis*-1,4 polyisoprene. Natural rubber was found to be compatible with blood in its pure form. Also, cross-linking by x-ray and organic peroxides produces rubber with superior blood compatibility compared with rubbers made by the conventional sulfur vulcanization.

Synthetic rubbers were developed to substitute for natural rubber. The Ziegler-Natta types of stereospecific polymerization techniques have made this variety possible. The synthetic rubbers have rarely been used to make implants. The physical properties vary widely due to the wide variations in preparation recipes of these rubbers.

Silicone rubber, developed by Dow Corning company, is one of the few polymers developed for medical use. The repeating unit is dimethyl siloxane which is polymerized by a condensation polymerization. Low molecular weight polymers have low viscosity and can be cross-linked to make a higher molecular weight, rubber-like material. Medical grade silicone rubbers contain stannous octate as a catalyst and can be mixed with a base polymer at the time of implant fabrication.

40.3.10   Polyurethanes

Polyurethanes are usually thermosetting polymers: they are widely used to coat implants. Polyurethane rubbers are produced by reacting a prepared prepolymer chain with an aromatic di-isocyanate to make very long chains possessing active isocyanate groups for cross-linking. The polyurethane rubber is quite strong and has good resistance to oil and chemicals.

40.3.11   Polyacetal, Polysulfone, and Polycarbonate

These polymers have excellent mechanical, thermal, and chemical properties due to their stiffened main backbone chains. Polyacetals and polysulfones are being tested as implant materials, while polycarbonates have found their applications in the heart/lung assist devices, food packaging, etc.

Polyacetals are produced by reacting formaldehyde. These are also sometimes called polyoxymethylene (POM) and known widely as **Delrin®** (DuPont). These polymers have a reasonably high molecular weight ($>2 \times 10^4$ g/mol) and have excellent mechanical properties. More importantly, they display an excellent resistance to most chemicals and to water over wide temperature ranges.

Polysulfones were developed by Union Carbide in the 1960s. These polymers have a high thermal stability due to the bulky side groups (therefore, they are amorphous) and rigid main backbone chains. They are also highly stable to most chemicals but are not so stable in the presence of polar organic solvents such as ketones and chlorinated hydrocarbons.

Polycarbonates are tough, amorphous, and transparent polymers made by reacting bisphenol A and diphenyl carbonate. It is noted for its excellent mechanical and thermal properties (high T_g: 150°C), hydrophobicity, and antioxidative properties.

40.3.12   Biodegradable Polymers

Recently, several biodegradable polymers such as polylactide (PLA), polyglycolide (PGA), poly(glycolide-*co*-lactide) (PLGA), poly(dioxanone), poly(trimethylene carbonate), poly(carbonate), and so on are extensively used or tested on a wide range of medical applications due to their good biocompatibility, controllable biodegradability, and relatively good processability [Khang et al., 1997]. PLA, PGA, and PLGA are bioresorbable polyesters belonging to the group of poly α-hydroxy acids. These polymers degrade by nonspecific hydrolytic scission of their ester bonds. The hydrolysis of PLA yields lactic acid which is a normal byproduct of anaerobic metabolism in the human body and is incorporated in the tricarboxylic acid (TCA) cycle to be finally excreted by the body as carbon dioxide and water. PGA biodegrades by a combination of hydrolytic scission and enzymatic (esterase) action producing glycolic acid which can either enter the TCA cycle or is excreted in urine and can be eliminated as carbon dioxide and water. The degradation time of PLGA can be controlled from weeks to over a year by varying the ratio of monomers and the processing conditions. It might be a suitable biomaterial for use in tissue engineered repair systems in which cells are implanted within PLGA films or scaffolds and in drug delivery systems in which drugs are loaded within PLGA microspheres. PGA (T_m: 225–230°C, T_g: 35–40°C) can be melt spun into fibers which can be converted into bioresorbable sutures, meshes, and surgical products. PLA (T_m: 173–178°C, T_g: 60–65°C) exhibit high tensile strength and low elongation resulting in a high modulus suitable for load-bearing applications such as in bone fracture fixation. Poly-p-dioxanone (T_m: 107–112°C, T_g: ~10°C) is a bioabsorbable polymer which can be fabricated into flexible monofilament surgical sutures.

40.4 Sterilization

Sterilizability of biomedical polymers is an important aspect of the properties because polymers have lower thermal and chemical stability than other materials such as ceramics and metals, consequently, they are also more difficult to sterilize using conventional techniques. Commonly used sterilization techniques are dry heat, autoclaving, radiation, and ethylene oxide gas [Block, 1977].

In dry heat sterilization, the temperature varies between 160 and 190°C. This is above the melting and softening temperatures of many linear polymers like polyethylene and PMMA. In the case of polyamide (Nylon), oxidation will occur at the dry sterilization temperature although this is below its melting temperature. The only polymers which can safely be dry sterilized are PTFE and silicone rubber.

Steam sterilization (autoclaving) is performed under high steam pressure at relatively low temperature (125–130°C). However, if the polymer is subjected to attack by water vapor, this method cannot be employed. PVC, polyacetals, PE (low-density variety), and polyamides belong to this category.

Chemical agents such as ethylene and propylene oxide gases [Glaser, 1979], and phenolic and hypochloride solutions are widely used for sterilizing polymers since they can be used at low temperatures. Chemical agents sometimes cause polymer deterioration even when sterilization takes place at room temperature. However, the time of exposure is relatively short (overnight), and most polymeric implants can be sterilized with this method.

Radiation sterilization [Sato, 1983] using the isotopic ^{60}Co can also deteriorate polymers since at high dosage the polymer chains can be dissociated or cross-linked according to the characteristics of the chemical structures, as shown in Table 40.6. In the case of PE, at high dosage (above 10^6 Gy) it becomes a brittle and hard material. This is due to a combination of random chain scission cross-linking. PP articles will often discolor during irradiation giving the product an undesirable color tint but the more severe problem is the embrittlement resulting in flange breakage, luer cracking, and tip breakage. The physical properties continue to deteriorate with time, following irradiation. These problems of coloration and changing physical properties are best resolved by avoiding the use of any additives which discolor at the sterilizing dose of radiation [Khang, 1996c].

40.5 Surface Modifications for Improving Biocompatability

Prevention of **thrombus** formation is important in clinical applications where blood is in contact such as hemodialysis membranes and tubes, artificial heart and heart–lung machines, prosthetic valves, and artificial vascular grafts. In spite of the use of anticoagulants, considerable platelet deposition and thrombus formation take place on the artificial surfaces [Branger, 1990].

Heparin, one of the complex carbohydrates known as mucopolysaccharides or glycosaminoglycan is currently used to prevent formation of clots. In general, heparin is well tolerated and devoid of serious consequences. However, it allows platelet adhesion to foreign surfaces and may cause hemorrhagic complications such as subdural hematoma, retroperitoneal hematoma, gastrointestinal bleeding, hemorrage

TABLE 40.6 Effect of Gamma Irradiation on
Polymers Which Could be Cross-Linked or
Degraded

Cross-linking polymers	Degradable polymers
Polyethylene	Polyisobutylene
Polypropylene	Poly-α-methylstyrene
Polystyrene	Polymethylmetacrylate
Polyarylates	Polymethacrylamide
Polyacrylamide	Polyvinylidenechloride
Polyvinylchloride	Cellulose and derivatives
Polyamides	Polytetrafluoroethylene
Polyesters	Polytrifluorochloroethylene
Polyvinylpyrrolidone	
Polymethacrylamide	
Rubbers	
Polysiloxanes	
Polyvinylalcohol	
Polyacroleine	

into joints, ocular and retinal bleeding, and bleeding at surgical sites [Lazarus, 1980]. These difficulties give rise to an interest in developing new methods of hemocompatible materials.

Many different groups have studied immobilization of heparin [Kim and Feijen, 1985; Park et al., 1988] on the polymeric surfaces, heparin analogues and heparin-prostaglandin or heparin-fibrinolytic enzyme conjugates [Jozefowicz and Jozefowicz, 1985]. The major drawback of these surfaces is that they are not stable in the blood environment. It has not been firmly established that a slow leakage of heparin is needed for it to be effective as an immobilized antithrombogenic agent, if not its effectiveness could be hindered by being "coated over" with an adsorbed layer of more common proteins such as albumin and **fibrinogen**. Fibrinolytic enzymes, urokinase, and various prostaglandins have also been immobilized by themselves in order to take advantage of their unique fibrin dissolution or antiplatelet aggregation actions [Ohshiro, 1983].

Albumin-coated surfaces have been studied because surfaces that resisted platelet adhesion *in vitro* were noted to adsorb albumin preferentially [Keogh et al., 1992]. Fibronectin coatings have been used in *in vitro* endothelial cell seeding to prepare a surface similar to the natural blood vessel lumen [Lee et al., 1989]. Also, algin-coated surfaces have been studied due to their good biocompatibility and biodegradability [Lee et al., 1990b; 1997b].

Recently, plasma gas discharge [Khang et al., 1997a] and corona treatment [Khang et al., 1996d] with reactive groups introduced on the polymeric surfaces have emerged as other ways to modify biomaterial surfaces [Lee et al., 1991; 1992].

Hydrophobic coatings composed of silicon- and fluorine-containing polymeric materials as well as polyurethanes have been studied because of the relatively good clinical performances of Silastic®, Teflon®, and polyurethane polymers in cardiovascular implants and devices. Polymeric fluorocarbon coatings deposited from a tetrafluoroethylene gas discharge have been found to greatly enhance resistance to both acute thrombotic occlusion and embolization in small diameter **Dacron®** grafts.

Hydrophilic coatings have also been popular because of their low interfacial tension in biological environments [Hoffman, 1981]. Hydrogels as well as various combinations of hydrophilic and hydrophobic monomers have been studied on the premise that there will be an optimum polar-dispersion force ratio which could be matched on the surfaces of the most passivating proteins. The passive surface may induce less clot formation. Polyethylene oxide coated surfaces have been found to resist protein adsorption and cell adhesion and have therefore been proposed as potential "blood compatible" coatings [Lee et al., 1990a]. General physical and chemical methods to modify the surfaces of polymeric biomaterials are listed in Table 40.7 [Ratner et al., 1996].

TABLE 40.7 Physical and Chemical Surface Modification Methods for Polymeric
Biomaterials

To modify blood compatibility	Octadecyl group attachment to surface
	Silicon containing block copolymer additive
	Plasma fluoropolymer deposition
	Plasma siloxane polymer deposition
	Radiation-grafted hydrogels
	Chemically modified polystyrene for heparin-like activity
To influence cell adhesion and growth	Oxidized polystyrene surface
	Ammonia plasma-treated surface
	Plasma-deposited acetone or methanol film
	Plasma fluoropolymer deposition
To control protein adsorption	Surface with immobilized polyethyelenglycol
	Treated ELISA dish surface
	Affinity chromatography particulates
	Surface cross-linked contact lens
To improve lubricity	Plasma treatment
	Radiation-grafted hydrogels
	Interpenetrating polymeric networks
To improve wear resistance and corrosion resistance	Ion implantation
	Diamond deposition
	Anodization
To alter transport properties	Plasma deposition (methane, fluoropolymer, siloxane)
To modify electrical characteristics	Plasma deposition
	Solvent coatings
	Parylene coatings

Source: Ratner, B.D. et al. 1996. Academic Press, NY, p. 106.

Another way of making antithrombogenic surfaces is the saline perfusion method, which is designed to prevent direct contacts between blood and the surface of biomaterials by means of perfusing saline solution through the porous wall which is in contact with blood [Park and Kim, 1993; Khang et al., 1996a, b]. It has been demonstrated that the adhesion of the blood cells could be prevented by the saline perfusion through PE, alumina, sulfonated/nonsulfonated PS/SBR, ePTFE (expanded polytetrafluoroethylene), and polysulfone porous tubes.

40.6 Chemogradient Surfaces for Cell and Protein Interaction

The behavior of the adsorption and desorption of blood proteins or adhesion and proliferation of different types of mammalian cells on polymeric materials depends on the surface characteristics such as wettability, hydrophilicity/hydrophobicity ratio, bulk chemistry, surface charge and charge distribution, surface roughness, and rigidity.

Many research groups have studied the effect of the surface wettability on the interactions of biological species with polymeric materials. Some have studied the interactions of different types of cultured cells or blood proteins with various polymers with different wettabilities to correlate the surface wettability and blood- or tissue-compatibility [Baier et al., 1984]. One problem encountered from the study using different kinds of polymers is that the surfaces are heterogeneous, both chemically and physically (different surface chemistry, roughness, rigidity, crystallinity, etc.), which caused widely varying results. Some others have studied the interactions of different types of cells or proteins with a range of methacrylate copolymers with different wettabilities and have the same kind of chemistry but are still physically heterogeneous [van Wachem et al., 1987]. Another methodological problem is that such studies are often tedious, laborious, and time-consuming because a large number of samples must be prepared to characterize the complete range of the desired surface properties.

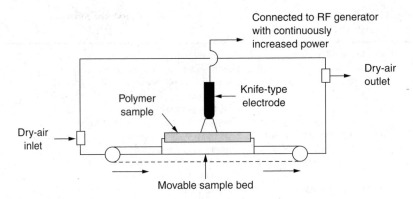

FIGURE 40.6   Schematic diagram showing corona discharge apparatus for the preparation of wettability chemo-gradient surfaces.

   Many studies have been focused on the preparation of surfaces whose properties are changed gradually along the material length. Such chemogradient surfaces are of particular interest in basic studies of the interactions between biological species and synthetic materials surfaces since the affect of a selected property can be examined in a single experiment on one surface preparation. A chemogradient of methyl groups was formed by diffusion of dimethyldichlorosilane through xylene on flat hydrophilic silicone-dioxide surfaces [Elwing et al., 1989]. The wettability chemogradient surfaces were made to investigate hydrophilicity-induced changes of adsorbed proteins.

   Recently, a method for preparing wettability chemogradients on various polymer surfaces was developed [Lee et al., 1989, 1990; Khang et al., 1997b]. The wettability chemogradients were produced via radio frequency (RF) and plasma discharge treatment by exposing the polymer sheets continuously to the plasma [Lee et al., 1991]. The polymer surfaces oxidized gradually along the sample length with increasing plasma exposure time and thus the wettability chemogradient was created. Another method for preparing a wettability chemogradient on polymer surfaces using corona discharge treatment has been developed as shown in Figure 40.6 [Lee et al., 1992]. The wettability chemogradient was produced by treating the polymer sheets with corona from a knife-type electrode whose power was gradually changed along the sample length. The polymer surface gradually oxidized with the increasing power and the wettability chemogradient was created. Chemogradient surfaces with different functional gruops such as –COOH, –CH$_2$OH, –CONH$_2$, and –CH$_2$NH$_2$ were produced on PE surfaces by the above corona treatment followed by vinyl monomer grafting and substitution reactions [Kim et al., 1993; Lee et al., 1994a, b]. We have also prepared chargeable functional groups [Lee et al., 1997c, d, 1998a], comb-like polyethyleneoxide (PEO) [Jeong et al., 1996; Lee et al., 1997a] and phospholipid polymer chemogradient surfaces [Iwasaki et al., 1997] by the corona discharge treatment, followed by the graft copolymerization with subsequent substitution reaction of functional vinyl monomers as acrylic acid, sodium p-sulfonic styrene and N, N-dimethyl aminopropyl acrylamide, poly(ethyleneglycol) mono-methacrylate, and ω-methacryloyloxyalkyl phosphorylcholine (MAPC), respectively.

   The water contact angles of the corona-treated PE surfaces gradually decrease along the sample length with increasing corona power (from about 95° to about 45°) as shown in Figure 40.7. The decrease in contact angles, that is, the increase in wettability along the sample length was due to the oxygen-based polar functionalities incorporated on the surface by the corona treatment. It was also confirmed also by fourier-transform infrared spectroscopy in the attenuated total reflectance mode and electron spectroscopy for chemical analysis (ESCA).

   In order to investigate the interaction of different types of cells in terms of the surface hydrophilicity/hydrophobicity of polymeric materials, Chinese hamster ovaries (CHO), fibroblasts, and bovine aortic endothelial cells (EC) were cultured for 1 and 2 days on the PE wettability chemogradient surfaces. The maximum adhesion and growth of the cells appeared around a water contact angle of 50 to 55°

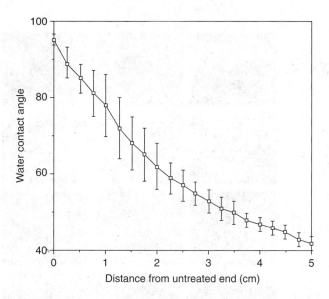

FIGURE 40.7 Changes in water contact angle of corona-treated PE surface along the sample length. Sample numbers, $n = 3$.

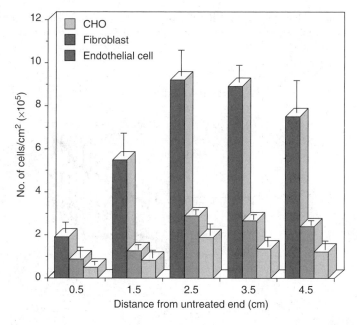

FIGURE 40.8 CHO, fibroblast, and endothelial cell growth on wettability chemogradient PE surfaces after 2 days culture (number of seeded cells, $4 \times 104/cm^2$). $n = 3$.

as shown in Figure 40.8. The observation of scanning electron microscopy (SEM) also verified that the cells are more adhered, spread, and grown onto the sections with moderate hydrophilicity as shown in Figure 40.9.

To determine the cell proliferation rates, the migration of fibroblasts on PE wettability chemogradient surfaces were observed [Khang et al., 1998b]. After the change of culture media at 24 h, cell growth morphology was recorded for 1 or 2 h intervals at the position of 0.5, 1.5, 2.5, and 4.5 cm for the counting

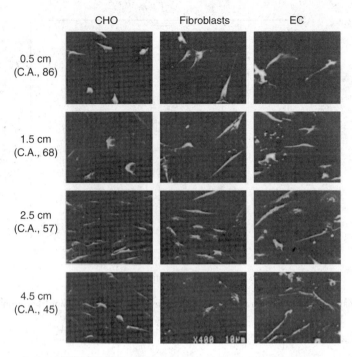

FIGURE 40.9 SEM microphotographs of CHO, fibroblast, and endothelial cells grown on PE wettability chemogradient surface along the sample length after 2 days culture (original magnification; ×400).

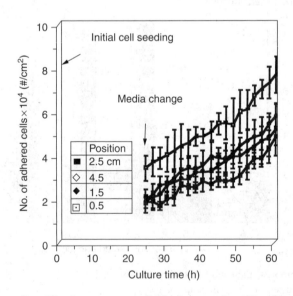

FIGURE 40.10 Fibroblast cell proliferation rates on wettability chemogradient PE surfaces (24 to 60 h culture).

of grown cells and the observation of cell morphology with a video tape recorder. The proliferation rates of fibroblast cells were calculated from the slopes of Figure 40.10 as given in Table 40.8. The proliferation rates on the PE surfaces with wettability chemogradient showed that as the surface wettability increased, it increased and then decreased. The maximum proliferation rate of the cells as 1111 cells/h · cm^2 appeared at around the position 2.5 cm.

TABLE 40.8 Proliferation Rates of Fibroblast Cells on Wettability Gradient PE Surfaces

Positions (cm)	Contact angle (°)	Cell proliferation rate (#cell/h cm^2)
2.5	55	1111
4.5	45	924
1.5	67	838
0.5	85	734

Note: 24 to 60 h culture.

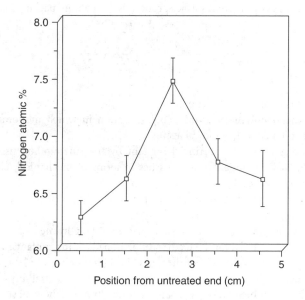

FIGURE 40.11 Serum protein adsorption on PE wettability chemogradient surface (1 h adsorption). $n = 3$.

To observe the effect of serum proteins on the cell adhesion and growth behaviors, fetal bovine serum (FBS), which contains more than 200 kinds of different proteins, was adsorbed onto the wettability gradient PE surfaces for 1 h at 37°C. Figure 40.11 shows the relative adsorbed amount of serum proteins on the wettability gradient surfaces determined by ESCA. The maximum adsorption of the proteins appeared at around the 2.5 cm position, which is the same trend as the cell adhesion, growth, and migration behaviors. It can be explained that preferential adsorption of some serum proteins, like fibronectin and vitronectin from culture medium, onto the moderately wettable surfaces may be a reason for better cell adhesion, spreading, and growth. Proteins like fibronectin and vitronectin are well known as cell-adhesive proteins. Cells attached on surfaces are spread only when they are compatible on the surfaces. It seems that surface wettability plays an important role for cell adhesion, spreading, and migration.

Also investigated were (1) platelet adhesion on wettability chemogradient [Lee and Lee, 1998b], (2) cell interaction on microgrooved PE surfaces (groove depth, 0.5 μm; groove width, 0.45 μm; and pitch, 0.9 μm) with wettability chemogradient [Khang et al., 1997c], (3) detachment of human endothelial under flow from wettability gradient surface with different functional groups [Ruardy et al., 1997], (4) cell interaction on microporous polycarbonate membrane with wettability chemogradient [Lee et al., 1998c], and (5) cell interaction on poly(lactide-*co*-glycolide) surface with wettability chemogradient [Khang et al., 1998a].

During the last several years, "chemogradient surfaces" have evolved into easier and more popular tools for the study of protein adsorption and platelet or cell interactions continuously which relate to the surface properties such as wettability, chemistry and charge, or dynamics of polymeric materials. In many studies, different kinds of polymeric materials with widely varying surface chemistries are used and the explanation of the results is often in controversy due to the surface heterogeneity. In addition, these studies are tedious, laborious, and time-consuming, and biological variations are more likely to occur. The application of chemogradient surfaces for these studies can reduce these discomforts and problems, and eventually save time and money. Also, chemogradient surfaces are valuable in investigating the basic mechanisms by which complicated systems such as proteins or cells interact with surfaces, since a continuum of selected and controlled physical–chemical properties can be studied in one experiment on the polymeric surface.

The possible applications of chemogradient surfaces in the near future are (1) separation devices of cells and/or biological species by different surface properties, (2) column packing materials for separation, (3) biosensing, etc.

Defining Terms

Acetabulum: The socket portion of the hip joint.

Addition (or free radical) polymerization: Polymerization in which monomers are added to the growing chains, initiated by free radical agents.

Biocompatibility: Acceptance of an artificial implant by the surrounding tissues and as a whole. The implant should be compatible with tissues in terms of mechanical, chemical, surface, and pharmacological properties.

Biomaterials: Synthetic materials used to replace part of a living system or to function in intimate contact with living tissue.

Bone cement: Mixture of polymethylmethacrylate powder and methylmethacrylate monomer liquid to be used as a grouting material for the fixation of orthopedic joint implants.

Branching: Chains grown from the sides of the main backbone chains.

Chemogradient surface: The surface whose properties such as wettability, surface charge, and hydrophilicity/hydrophobicity ratio are changed gradually along the material length.

Condensation (step reaction) polymerization: Polymerization in which two or more chemicals are reacted to form a polymer by condensing out small molecules such as water and alcohol.

Copolymers: Polymers made from two or more monomers which can be obtained by grafting, block, alternating, or random attachment of the other polymer segment.

Covalent bonding: Bonding of atoms or molecules by sharing valence electrons.

Dacron®: Polyethyleneterephthalate polyester that is made into fiber. If the same polymer is made into a film, it is called Mylar®.

Delrin®: Polyacetal made by Union Carbide.

Elastomers: Rubbery materials. The restoring force comes from uncoiling or unkinking of coiled or kinked molecular chains. They can be highly stretched.

Embolus: Any foreign matter, as a blood clot or air bubble, carried in the blood stream.

Fibrinogen: A plasma protein of high molecular weight that is converted to fibrin through the action of thrombin. This material is used to make (absorbable) tissue adhesives.

Filler: Materials added as a powder to a rubber to improve its mechanical properties.

Free volume: The difference in volume occupied by the crystalline state (minimum) and non-crystalline state of a material for a given temperature and a pressure.

Glass transition temperature: Temperature at which solidification without crystallization takes place from viscous liquid.

Grafts: A transplant.

Heparin: A substance found in various body tissues, especially in the liver, that prevents the clotting of blood.

Hydrogel: Polymer which can absorb 30% or more of its weight in water.

Hydrogen bonding: A secondary bonding through dipole interactions in which the hydrogen ion is one of the dipoles.

Hydroquinone: Chemical inhibitor added to the bone cement liquid monomer to prevent accidental polymerization during storage.

Initiator: Chemical used to initiate the addition polymerization by becoming a free radical which in turn reacts with a monomer.

Ionic bonding: Bonding of atoms or molecules through electrostatic interaction of positive and negative ions.

Kevlar®: Aromatic polyamides made by DuPont.

Lexan®: Polycarbonate made by General Electric.

Oxygenator: An apparatus by which oxygen is introduced into blood during circulation outside the body, as during open-heart surgery.

Plasticizer: Substance made of small molecules, mixed with (amorphous) polymers to make the chains slide more easily past each other, making the polymer less rigid.

Refractive index: Ratio of speed of light in vacuum to speed of light in a material. It is a measure of the ability of a material to refract (bend) a beam of light.

Repeating unit: Basic molecular unit which can represent a polymer backbone chain. The average number of repeating units is called the degree of polymerization.

Repeating unit: The smallest unit representing a polymer molecular chain.

Semi-crystalline solid: Solid which contains both crystalline and noncrystalline regions and usually occurs in polymers due to their long chain molecules.

Side group: Chemical group attached to the main backbone chain. It is usually shorter than the branches and exists before polymerization.

Steric hindrance: Geometrical interference which restrains movements of molecular groups such as side chains and main chains of a polymer.

Suture: Material used in closing a wound with stitches.

Tacticity: Arrangement of asymmetrical side groups along the backbone chain of polymers. Groups could be distributed at random (atactic), one side (isotactic), or alternating (syndiotactic).

Teflon®: Polytetrafluoroethylene made by DuPont.

Thrombus: The fibrinous clot attached at the site of thrombosis.

Udel®: Polysulfone made by General Electric.

Valence electrons: The outermost (shell) electrons of an atom.

van der Waals bonding: A secondary bonding arising through the fluctuating dipole-dipole interactions.

Vinyl polymers: Thermoplastic linear polymers synthesized by free radical polymerization of vinyl monomers having a common structure of $CH_2=CHR$.

Vulcanization: Cross-linking of a (natural) rubber by adding sulfur.

Ziegler–Natta catalyst: Organometallic compounds which have the remarkable capacity of polymerizing a wide variety of monomers to linear and stereoregular polymers.

Acknowledgments

This work was supported by grants from the Korea Ministry of Health and Welfare (grant Nos. HMP-95-G-2-33 and HMP-97-E-0016) and the Korea Ministry of Science and Technology (grant No. 97-N1-02-05-A-02).

References

Baier, R.E., Meyer, A.E., Natiella, J.R., Natiella, R.R., and Carter, J.M. 1984. Surface properties determine bioadhesive outcomes; methods and results, *J. Biomed. Mater. Res.*, 18: 337–355.

Billmeyer, F.W. Jr. 1984. *Textbook of Polymer Science*, 3rd ed. John Wiley & Sons, NY.

Block, S.S. (Ed.) 1977. *Disinfection, Sterilization, and Preservation*, 2nd ed. Rea and Febiger, Philadelphia, PA.

Bloch, B. and Hastings, G.W. 1972. *Plastic Materials in Surgery*, 2nd ed. C.C. Thomas, Springfield, IL.

Brandrup, J. and Immergut, E.H., Ed. 1989. Polymer Handbook, 3rd ed. Wiley-Interscience Pub., NY.

Branger, B., Garreau, M., Baudin, G., and Gris, J.C. 1990. Biocompatibility of blood tubings, *Int. J. Artif. Organs*, 13: 697–703.

Dumitriu, S. (Ed.) 1993. *Polymeric Biomaterials*, Marcell Dekker, Inc., NY.

Elwing, E., Askendal, A., and Lundstorm, I. 1989. Desorption of fibrinogen and γ-globulin from solid surfaces induced by a nonionic detergent, *J. Colloid Interface Sci.*, 128: 296–300.

Glaser, Z.R. 1979. Ethylene oxide: toxicology review and field study results of hospital use, *J. Environ. Pathol. Toxicol.*, 2: 173–208.

Hoffman, A.S. 1981. Radiation processing in biomaterials: A review, *Radiat. Phys. Chem.*, 18: 323–340.

Ikada, Y. (Ed.) 1989. Bioresorbable fibers for medical use. In: *High Technology Fiber*, Part B., Marcel Dekker, NY.

Iwasaki, Y., Ishihara, K., Nakabayashi, N., Khang, G., Jeon, J.H., Lee, J.W., and Lee, H.B. 1997. Preparation of gradient surfaces grafted with phospholipid polymers and evaluation of their blood compatibility. In: *Advances in Biomaterials Science*, Vol. 1, T. Akaike, T. Okano, M. Akashi, M. Terano, and N. Yui, Eds. pp. 91–100, CMC Co., LTD., Tokyo.

Jeong, B.J., Lee, J.H., and Lee, H.B. 1996. Preparation and characterization of comb-like PEO gradient surfaces. *J. Colloid Interface Sci.*, 178: 757–763.

Jozefowicz, M. and Jozefowicz, J. 1985. New approaches to anticoagulation: heparin-like biomaterials. *J. Am. Soc. Art. Intern. Org.* 8: 218–222.

Keogh, J.R., Valender, F.F., and Eaton, J.W. 1992. Albumin-binding surfaces for implantable devices, *J. Biomed. Mater. Res.*, 26: 357–372.

Khang, G., Park J.B., and Lee, H.B. 1996a. Prevention of platelet adhesion on the polysulfone porous catheter by saline perfusion, I. *In vitro* investigation, *Bio-Med. Mater. Eng.*, 6: 47–66.

Khang, G., Park, J.B., and Lee, H.B. 1996b. Prevention of platelet adhesion on the polysulfone porous catheter by saline perfusion, II. *Ex vivo* and *in vivo* investigation, *Bio-Med. Mater. Eng.*, 6: 123–134.

Khang, G., Lee, H.B., and Park, J.B. 1996c. Radiation effects on polypropylene for sterilization, *Bio-Med. Mater. Eng.*, 6: 323–334.

Khang, G., Kang, Y.H., Park, J.B., and Lee, H.B, 1996d. Improved bonding strength of poly-ethylene/polymethylmetacrylate bone cement — a preliminary study, *Bio-Med. Mater. Eng.*, 6: 335–344.

Khang, G., Jeon, J.H., Lee, J.W., Cho, S.C., and Lee, H.B. 1997a. Cell and platelet adhesion on plasma glow discharge-treated poly(lactide-*co*-glycolide), *Bio-Med. Mater. Eng.*, 7: 357–368.

Khang, G., Lee, J.H., and Lee, H.B. 1997b. Cell and platelet adhesion on gradient surfaces, In: *Advances in Biomaterials Science*. Vol. 1, T. Akaike, T. Okano, M. Akashi, Terano, and N. Yui, Eds. pp. 63–70, CMC Co., LTD., Tokyo.

Khang, G., Lee, J.W., Jeon, J.H., Lee, J.H., and Lee, H.B., 1997c. Interaction of fibroblasts on microgrooved polyethylene surfaces with wettabililty gradient, *Biomat. Res.*, 1: 1–6.

Khang, G., Cho, S.Y., Lee, J.H., Rhee, J.M. and Lee, H.B., 1998a. Interactions of fibroblast, osteo-blast, hepatoma, and endothelial cells on poly(lactide-*co*-glycolide) surface with chemogradient (to appear).

Khang, G., Jeon, J.H., and Lee, H.B., 1998b. Fibroblast cell migration on polyethylene wettability chemogradient surfaces, *to appear*.

Kim, H.G., Lee, J.H., Lee, H.B., and Jhon, M.S. 1993. Dissociation behavior of surface-grafted poly(acrylic acid): Effects of surface density and counterion size, *J. Colloid Interface Sci.*, 157: 82–87.

Kim, S.W. and Feijen, J. 1985. Surface modification of polymers for improved blood biocompatibility, *CRC Crit. Rev. Biocompat.*, 1: 229–260.

Lazarus, J.M. 1980. Complications in hemodialysis: An overview, *Kidney Int.*, 18: 783–796.

Lee, H.B. 1989. Application of synthetic polymers in implants. In: *Frontiers of Macromolecular Science*, T. Seagusa, T., Higashimura, and A. Abe, Eds. pp. 579–584, Blackwell Scientific Publications, Oxford.

Lee, H.B. and Lee, J.H. 1995. Biocompatibility of solid substrates based on surface wettability. In: *Encyclopedic Handbook of Biomaterials and Bioengineering: Materials*, Vol. 1., D.L. Wise, D.J. Trantolo, D.E. Altobelli, M.J. Yasemski, J.D. Gresser, and E.R. Schwartz, pp. 371–398, Marcel Dekker, New York.

Lee, J.H., Khang, G., Park, K.H., Lee, H.B., and Andrade, J.D. 1989. Polymer surfaces for cell adhesion: I. Surface modification of polymers and ESCA analysis. *J. Korea Soc. Med. Biol. Eng.*, 10: 43–51.

Lee, J.H., Khang, G., Park, J. W., and Lee, H. B. 1990a. Plasma protein adsorption on polyethyleneoxide gradient surfaces, *33rd IUPAC International Symposium on Macromolecules*, July 8–13, Montreal, Canada.

Lee, J.H., Shin, B.C., Khang, G., and Lee, H.B. 1990b. Algin impregnated vascular graft: I. *In vitro* investigation. *J. Korea Soc. Med. Biol. Eng.*, 11: 97–104.

Lee, J.H., Park, J.W., and Lee, H.B. 1991. Cell adhesion and growth on polymer surfaces with hydroxyl groups prepared by water vapor plasma treatment, *Biomaterials*, 12: 443–448.

Lee, J.H., Kim, H.G., Khang, G., Lee, H.B., and Jhon, M.S. 1992. Characterization of wettability gradient surfaces prepared by corona discharge treatment, *J. Colloid Interface Sci.*, 151: 563–570.

Lee, J.H., Kim, H.W., Pak, P.K., and Lee, H.B. 1994a. Preparation and characterization of functional group gradient surfaces, *J. Polym. Sci., Part A, Polym. Chem.*, 32: 1569–1579.

Lee, J.H., Jung, H.W., Kang, I.K., and Lee, H.B. 1994b. Cell behavior on polymer surfaces with different functional groups, *Biomaterials*, 15: 705–711.

Lee, J.H., Jeong, B.J., and Lee, H.B. 1997a. Plasma protein adsorption and platelet adhesion onto comb-like PEO gradient surface, *J. Biomed. Mater. Res.*, 34: 105–114.

Lee, J.H., Kim, W.G., Kim, S.S., Lee, J.H., and Lee, H.B., 1997b. Development and characterization of an alginate-impregnated polyester vascular graft, *J. Biomed. Mater. Res.*, 36: 200–208.

Lee, J.H., Khang, G., Lee, J.H., and Lee, H.B. 1997c. Interactions of protein and cells on functional group gradient surfaces, *Macromol. Symp.*, 118: 571–576.

Lee, J.H., Khang, G., Lee, J.H., and Lee, H.B. 1997d. Interactions of cells on chargeable functional group gradient surfaces, *Biomaterials*, 18: 351–358.

Lee, J.H., Khang, G., Lee, J.H., and Lee, H.B. 1998a. Platelet adhesion onto chargeable functional group gradient surfaces, *J. Biomed. Mater. Res.*, 40: 180–186.

Lee, J.H. and Lee, H.B. 1998b. Platelet adhesion onto wettability gradient surfaces in the absence and presence of plasma protein, *J. Biomed. Mater. Res.*, 41: 304–311.

Lee, J.H., Lee, S.J., Khang, G., and Lee, H.B. 1998c. Interactions of cells onto microporous polycarbonate membrane with wettability gradient surfaces, *J. Biomat. Sci., Polm. Edn.* (in press).

Leininger, R.I. and Bigg, D.M. 1986. Polymers. In: *Handbook of Biomaterials Evaluation*, pp. 24–37, Macmillian Publishing Co., NY.

Oshiro,T. 1983. Thrombosis, antithrombogenic characteristics of immobilized urokinase on synthetic polymers, In: *Biocompatible Polymers, Metals, and Composites*, M. Szycher, Ed. pp. 275–299. Technomic, Lancaster, PA.

Park, J.B. 1984. *Biomaterials Science and Engineering*, Plenum Publication, NY.

Park, J.B. and Lakes, R. 1992. *Biomaterials: An Introduction*, 2nd ed. pp. 141–168, Plenum Press, NY.

Park, J.B. and Kim S.S. 1993. Prevention of mural thrombus in porous inner tube of double-layered tube by saline perfusion. *Bio-Med. Mater. Eng.*, 3: 101–116.

Park, K.D., Okano, T., Nojiri, C., and Kim S.W. 1988. Heparin immobilized onto segmented polyurethane effect of hydrophillic spacers. *J. Biomed. Mater. Res.*, 22: 977–992.

Ratner, B.D., Hoffman, A.S., Schoen, F.J., and Lemons, J.E. 1996. *Biomaterials Science: An Introduction to Materials in Medicine*, Academic Press, NY.

Raurdy, T.G., Moorlag, H.E., Schkenraad, J.M., van der Mei, H.C., and Busscher, H.J. 1997. Detachment of human endothelial under flow from wettability gradient surface with different functional groups, *Cell Mat.*, 7: 123–133.

Sato, K. 1983. Radiation sterilization of medical products. *Radioisotopes*, 32: 431–439.

Shalaby, W.S. 1988. Polymeric materials. In: *Encyclopedia of Med. Dev. Instr.*, J.G. Webster, Ed. pp. 2324–2335, Wiley-Interscience Pub., NY.

Sharma, C.P. and Szycher, M. Eds., *Blood Compatible Materials and Devices: Perspective Toward the 21st Century*, Technomic Publishing Co. Inc., Lancaster, PA.

van Wachem, P.B., Beugeling. T., Feijen, J., Bantjes, A., Detmers, J.P., and van Aken, W.G. 1985. Interaction of cultured human endothelial cells with polymeric surfaces of different wettabilities, *Biomaterials*, 6: 403–408.

41

Composite Biomaterials

Roderic S. Lakes
University of Wisconsin-Madison

Composite materials are solids which contain two or more distinct constituent materials or phases, on a scale larger than the atomic. The term "composite" is usually reserved for those materials in which the distinct phases are separated on a scale larger than the atomic, and in which properties such as the elastic modulus are significantly altered in comparison with those of a homogeneous material. Accordingly, reinforced plastics such as fiberglass as well as natural materials such as bone are viewed as composite materials, but alloys such as brass are not. A foam is a composite in which one phase is empty space. Natural biological materials tend to be composites. Natural composites include bone, wood, dentin, cartilage, and skin. Natural foams include lung, cancellous bone, and wood. Natural composites often exhibit hierarchical structures in which particulate, porous, and fibrous structural features are seen on different micro-scales [Katz, 1980; Lakes, 1993]. In this segment, composite material fundamentals and applications in biomaterials [Park and Lakes, 1988] are explored. Composite materials offer a variety of advantages in comparison with homogeneous materials. These include the ability for the scientist or engineer to exercise considerable control over material properties. There is the potential for stiff, strong, lightweight materials as well as for highly resilient and compliant materials. In biomaterials, it is important that each constituent of the composite be biocompatible. Moreover, the interface between constituents should not be degraded by the body environment. Some applications of composites in biomaterial applications are (1) dental filling composites, (2) reinforced methyl methacrylate bone cement and ultra-high molecular weight polyethylene, and (3) orthopedic implants with porous surfaces.

41.1 Structure

The properties of composite materials depend very much upon *structure*. Composites differ from homogeneous materials in that considerable control can be exerted over the larger scale structure, and hence over the desired properties. In particular, the properties of a composite material depend upon the *shape* of the heterogeneities, upon the *volume fraction* occupied by them, and upon the *interface* among the constituents. The shape of the heterogeneities in a composite material is classified as follows. The principal inclusion shape categories are (1) the particle, with no long dimension, (2) the fiber, with one long dimension, and (3) the platelet or lamina, with two long dimensions, as shown in Figure 41.1. The inclusions may vary in size and shape within a category. For example, particulate inclusions may be spherical, ellipsoidal, polyhedral, or irregular. If one phase consists of voids, filled with air or liquid, the material is known as a cellular solid. If the cells are polygonal, the material is a honeycomb; if the cells are polyhedral, it is a foam. It is necessary in the context of biomaterials to distinguish the above structural cells from biological cells, which occur only in living organisms. In each composite structure, we may moreover make the distinction between random orientation and preferred orientation.

41.2 Bounds on Properties

Mechanical properties in many composite materials depend on structure in a complex way, however for some structures, the prediction of properties is relatively simple. The simplest composite structures are the idealized Voigt and Reuss models, shown in Figure 41.2. The dark and light areas in these diagrams represent the two constituent materials in the composite. In contrast to most composite structures, it is easy to calculate the stiffness of materials with the Voigt and Reuss structures, since in the Voigt structure the strain is the same in both constituents; in the Reuss structure the stress is the same. The Young's modulus, E, of the Voigt composite is:

$$E = E_i V_i + E_m [1 - V_i] \tag{41.1}$$

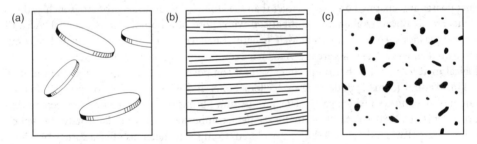

FIGURE 41.1   Morphology of basic composite inclusions. (a) Particle, (b) fiber, and (c) platelet.

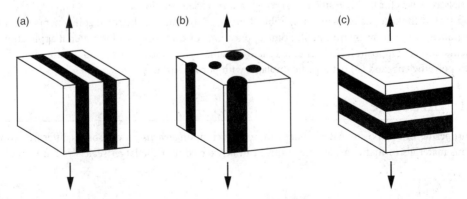

FIGURE 41.2   Voigt (a, laminar; b, fibrous) and Reuss (c) composite models, subjected to tension force indicated by arrows.

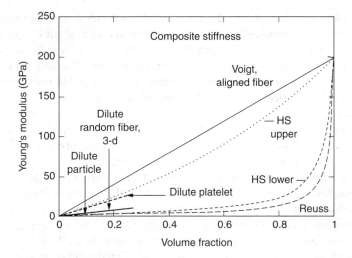

FIGURE 41.3   Stiffness vs. volume fraction for Voigt and Reuss models, as well as for dilute isotropic suspensions of platelets, fibers, and spherical particles embedded in a matrix. Phase moduli are 200 and 3 GPa.

in which E_i is the Young's modulus of the inclusions, and V_i is the volume fraction of inclusions, and E_m is the Young's modulus of the matrix. The Voigt relation for the stiffness is referred to as the rule of mixtures.

The Reuss stiffness E,

$$E = \left[\frac{V_i}{E_i} + \frac{1 - V_i}{E_m} \right]^{-1}$$ (41.2)

is less than that of the Voigt model. The Voigt and Reuss models provide upper and lower bounds respectively upon the stiffness of a composite of arbitrary phase geometry [Paul, 1960]. The bounds are far apart if, as is commonplace, the phase moduli differ a great deal, as shown in Figure 41.3. For composite materials which are isotropic, the more complex relations of Hashin and Shtrikman [1963] provide tighter bounds upon the moduli (Figure 41.3); both the Young's and shear moduli must be known for each constituent to calculate these bounds.

41.3   Anisotropy of Composites

Observe that the Reuss laminate is identical to the Voigt laminate, except for a rotation with respect to the direction of load. Therefore, the stiffness of the laminate is *anisotropic*, that is, dependent on direction [Lekhnitskii, 1963; Nye, 1976; Agarwal and Broutman, 1980]. Anisotropy is characteristic of composite materials. The relationship between stress σ_{ij} and strain ε_{kl} in anisotropic materials is given by the tensorial form of Hooke's law as follows:

$$\sigma_{ij} = \sum_{k=1}^{3} \sum_{l=1}^{3} C_{ijkl} \varepsilon_{kl}$$ (41.3)

Here C_{ijkl} is the elastic modulus tensor. It has $3^4 = 81$ elements, however since the stress and strain are represented by symmetric matrices with six independent elements each, the number of independent modulus tensor elements is reduced to 36. An additional reduction to 21 is achieved by considering elastic materials for which a strain energy function exists. Physically, C_{2323} represents a shear modulus since it couples a shear stress with a shear strain. C_{1111} couples axial stress and strain in the 1 or x direction, but it is not the same as Young's modulus. The reason is that Young's modulus is measured with the lateral strains free to occur via the Poisson effect, while C_{1111} is the ratio of axial stress to strain when there is only one nonzero strain value; there is no lateral strain. A modulus tensor with 21 independent elements describes a *triclinic* crystal, which is the least symmetric crystal form. The unit cell has three different oblique angles and three different side lengths. A triclinic composite could be made with groups of fibers of three different spacings, oriented in three different oblique directions. Triclinic modulus elements such as C_{2311}, known as cross-coupling constants, have the effect of producing a shear stress in response to a uniaxial strain; this is undesirable in many applications. An *orthorhombic* crystal or an *orthotropic* composite has a unit cell with orthogonal angles. There are nine independent elastic moduli. The associated engineering constants are three Young's moduli, three Poisson's ratios, and three shear moduli; the cross-coupling constants are zero when stresses are aligned to the symmetry directions. An example of such a composite is a unidirectional fibrous material with a rectangular pattern of fibers in the cross-section. Bovine bone, which has a laminated structure, exhibits orthotropic symmetry, as does wood. In a material with *hexagonal* symmetry, out of the nine C elements, there are five independent elastic constants. For directions in the transverse plane the elastic constants are the same, hence the alternate name transverse isotropy. A unidirectional fiber composite with a hexagonal or random fiber pattern has this symmetry, as does human Haversian bone. In *cubic* symmetry, there are three independent elastic constants, a Young's modulus, E, a shear modulus, G, and an independent Poisson's ratio, ν. Cross-weave fabrics have cubic symmetry. Finally, an *isotropic* material has the same material properties in any direction. There are only two independent elastic constants, hence E, G, ν, and also the bulk modulus B are related in an isotropic material. Isotropic materials include amorphous solids, polycrystalline metals in which the grains are randomly oriented, and composite materials in which the constituents are randomly oriented.

Anisotropic composites offer superior strength and stiffness in comparison with isotropic ones. Material properties in one direction are gained at the expense of properties in other directions. It is sensible, therefore, to use anisotropic composite materials only if the direction of application of the stress is known in advance.

41.4   Particulate Composites

It is often convenient to stiffen or harden a material, commonly a polymer, by the incorporation of particulate inclusions. The shape of the particles is important [see Christensen, 1979]. In isotropic systems, stiff platelet (or flake) inclusions are the most effective in creating a stiff composite, followed by fibers; and the least effective geometry for stiff inclusions is the spherical particle, as shown in Figure 41.3. A dilute concentration of spherical particulate inclusions of stiffness E_i and volume fraction V_i, in a matrix (with Poisson's ratio assumed to be 0.5) denoted by the subscript m, gives rise to a composite with a stiffness E:

$$E = \frac{5(E_i - E_m)V_i}{3 + 2(E_i/E_m)} + E_m \tag{41.4}$$

The stiffness of such a composite is close to the Hashin–Shtrikman lower bound for isotropic composites. Even if the spherical particles are perfectly rigid compared with the matrix, their stiffening effect at low concentrations is modest. Conversely, when the inclusions are more compliant than the matrix, spherical ones reduce the stiffness the least and platelet ones reduce it the most. Indeed, soft platelets are suggestive of crack-like defects. Soft platelets, therefore result not only in a compliant composite, but also a weak one. Soft spherical inclusions are used intentionally as crack stoppers to enhance the toughness of polymers such as polystyrene (high impact polystyrene), with a small sacrifice in stiffness.

Particle reinforcement has been used to improve the properties of bone cement. For example, inclusion of bone particles in PMMA cement somewhat improves the stiffness and improves the fatigue life considerably [Park et al., 1986]. Moreover, the bone particles at the interface with the patient's bone are

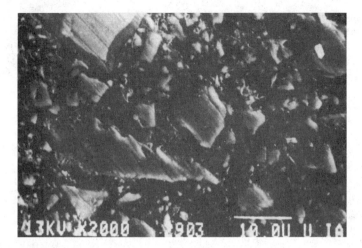

FIGURE 41.4   Microstructure of a dental composite. Miradapt® [Johnson & Johnson] 50% by volume filler: barium glass and colloidal silica [Park and Lakes, 1992].

ultimately resorbed and are replaced by ingrown new bone tissue. This approach is in the experimental stages.

Rubber used in catheters, rubber gloves, etc. is usually reinforced with very fine particles of silica (SiO_2) to make the rubber stronger and tougher.

Teeth with decayed regions have traditionally been restored with metals such as silver amalgam. Metallic restorations are not considered desirable for anterior teeth for cosmetic reasons. Acrylic resins and silicate cements had been used for anterior teeth, but their poor material properties led to short service life and clinical failures. Dental composite resins have virtually replaced these materials and are very commonly used to restore posterior teeth as well as anterior teeth [Cannon, 1988].

The dental composite resins consist of a polymer matrix and stiff inorganic inclusions [Craig, 1981]. A representative structure is shown in Figure 41.4. The particles are very angular in shape. The inorganic inclusions confer a relatively high stiffness and high wear resistance on the material. Moreover, since they are translucent and their index of refraction is similar to that of dental enamel, they are cosmetically acceptable. Available dental composite resins use quartz, barium glass, and colloidal silica as fillers. Fillers have particle size from 0.04 to 13 μm, and concentrations from 33 to 78% by weight. In view of the greater density of the inorganic filler phase, a 77% weight percent of filler corresponds to a volume percent of about 55%. The matrix consists of a polymer, typically BIS-GMA. In restoring a cavity, the dentist mixes several constituents, then places them in the prepared cavity to polymerize. For this procedure to be successful the viscosity of the mixed paste must be sufficiently low and the polymerization must be controllable. Low viscosity liquids such as triethylene glycol dimethacrylate are used to lower the viscosity and inhibitors such as BHT (butylated trioxytoluene) are used to prevent premature polymerization. Polymerization can be initiated by a thermochemical initiator such as benzoyl peroxide, or by a photochemical initiator (benzoin alkyl ether) which generates free radicals when subjected to ultraviolet light from a lamp used by the dentist.

Dental composites have a Young's modulus in the range 10 to 16 GPa, and the compressive strength from 170 to 260 MPa [Cannon, 1988]. As shown in Table 41.1, these composites are still considerably less stiff than dental enamel, which contains about 99% mineral. Similar high concentrations of mineral particles in synthetic composites cannot easily be achieved, in part because the particles do not pack densely. Moreover, an excessive concentration of particles raises the viscosity of the unpolymerized paste. An excessively high viscosity is problematical since it prevents the dentist from adequately packing the paste into the prepared cavity; the material will then fill in crevices less effectively.

The thermal expansion of dental composites, as with other dental materials, exceeds that of tooth structure. Moreover, there is a contraction during polymerization of 1.2 to 1.6%. These effects are thought

TABLE 41.1   Properties of Bone, Teeth, and Biomaterials

Material	Young's modulus E(GPa)	Density ρ (g/cm^3)	Strength (MPa)	References
Hard Tissue				
Tooth, bone, human compact bone, longitudinal direction	17	1.8	130 (tension)	Craig and Peyton, 1958; Reilly and Burstein, 1975: Peters et al., 1984; Park and Lakes, 1992
Tooth dentin	18	2.1	138 (compression)	
Tooth enamel	50	2.9		
Polymers				Park and Lakes, 1992
Polyethylene (UHMW)	1	0.94	30 (tension)	
Polymethyl methacrylate, PMMA	3	1.1	65 (tension)	
PMMA bone cement	2	1.18	30 (tension)	
Metals				Park and Lakes, 1992
316L Stainless steel (wrought)	200	7.9	1000 (tension)	
Co-Cr-Mo (cast)	230	8.3	660 (tension)	
Co Ni Cr Mo (wrought)	230	9.2	1800 (tension)	
Ti6A14V	110	4.5	900 (tension)	
Composites				
Graphite-epoxy (unidirectional fibrous, high modulus)	215	1.63	1240 (tension)	Schwartz, 1997
Graphite-epoxy (quasi-isotropic fibrous)	46	1.55	579 (tension)	Schwartz, 1997
Dental composite resins (particulate)	10–16		170–260 (compression)	Cannon, 1988
Foams				Gibson and Ashby, 1988
Polymer foams	10^{-4}–1	0.002–0.8	0.01–1 (tension)	

to contribute to leakage of saliva, bacteria, etc., at the interface margins. Such leakage in some cases can cause further decay of the tooth.

Use of colloidal silica in the so-called "microfilled" composites allows these resins to be polished, so that less wear occurs and less plaque accumulates. It is more difficult, however, to make these with a high fraction of filler. All the dental composites exhibit creep. The stiffness changes by a factor of 2.5 to 4 (depending on the particular material) over a time period from 10 sec to 3 h under steady load [Papadogianis et al., 1985]. This creep may result in indentation of the restoration, but wear seems to be a greater problem.

Dental composite resins have become established as restorative materials for both anterior and posterior teeth. The use of these materials is likely to increase as improved compositions are developed and in response to concern over long term toxicity of silver-mercury amalgam fillings.

41.5   Fibrous Composites

Fibers incorporated in a polymer matrix increase the stiffness, strength, fatigue life, and other properties [Agarwal and Broutman, 1980; Schwartz, 1992]. Fibers are mechanically more effective in achieving a stiff, strong composite than are particles. Materials can be prepared in fiber form with very few defects which concentrate stress. Fibers such as graphite are stiff (Young's modulus is 200–800 GPa) and strong (the tensile strength is 2.7–5.5 GPa). Composites made from them can be as strong as steel but much lighter, as shown in Table 41.1. The stiffness of a composite with aligned fibers, if it is loaded along the fibers, is equivalent to the Voigt upper bound, Equation 41.1. Unidirectional fibrous composites, when

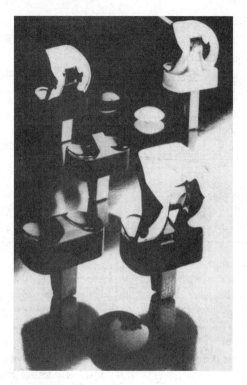

FIGURE 41.5   Knee prostheses with polyethylene tibial components reinforced with carbon fiber.

loaded along the fibers, can have strengths and stiffnesses comparable to that of steel, but with much less weight (Table 41.1). However if it is loaded transversly to the fibers, such a composite will be compliant, with a stiffness not much greater than that of the matrix alone. While unidirectional fiber composites can be made very strong in the longitudinal direction, they are weaker than the matrix alone when loaded transversely, as a result of stress concentration around the fibers. If stiffness and strength are needed in all directions, the fibers may be oriented randomly. For such a three-dimensional isotropic composite, for a low concentration of fibers,

$$E = \frac{E_i V_i}{6} + E_m \tag{41.5}$$

so the stiffness is reduced by about a factor of six in comparison with an aligned composite as illustrated in Figure 41.3. However if the fibers are aligned randomly in a plane, the reduction in stiffness is only a factor of three. The degree of anisotropy in fibrous composites can be very well controlled by forming laminates consisting of layers of fibers embedded in a matrix. Each layer can have fibers oriented in a different direction. One can achieve quasi-isotropic behavior in the laminate plane; such a laminate is not as strong or as stiff as a unidirectional one, as illustrated in Table 41.1. Strength of composites depends on such particulars as the brittleness or ductility of the inclusions and the matrix. In fibrous composites failure may occur by (1) fiber breakage, buckling, or pullout, (2) matrix cracking, or (3) debonding of fiber from matrix.

   Short fiber composites are used in many applications. They are not as stiff or as strong as composites with continuous fibers, but they can be formed economically by injection molding or by *in situ* polymerization. Choice of an optimal fiber length can result in improved toughness, due to the predominance of fiber pull-out as a fracture mechanism.

   Carbon fibers have been incorporated in the high density polyethylene used in total knee replacements (Figure 41.5). The standard ultra high molecular weight polyethylene (UHMWPE) used in these implants

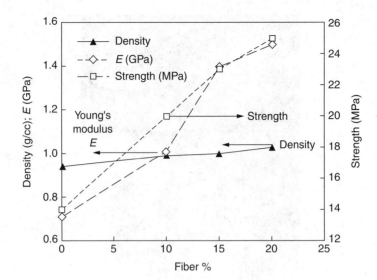

FIGURE 41.6   Properties of carbon fiber reinforced ultra high molecular weight polyethylene. (Replotted from Sclippa, E. and Piekarski, K. 1973. *J. Biomed. Mater. Res.*, **7**, 59–70. With permission.)

is considered adequate for most purposes for implantation in older patients. A longer wear-free implant lifetime is desirable for use in younger patients. It is considered desirable to improve the resistance to creep of the polymeric component, since excessive creep results in an indentation of that component after long term use. Representative properties of carbon reinforced ultra high molecular weight polyethylene are shown in Figure 41.6 [Sclippa and Piekarski, 1973]. Enhancements of various properties by a factor of two are feasible.

Polymethyl methacrylate (PMMA) used in bone cement is compliant and weak in comparison with bone. Therefore several reinforcement methods have been attempted. Metal wires have been used clinically as macroscopic "fibers" to reinforce PMMA cement used in spinal stabilization surgery [Fishbane and Pond, 1977]. The wires are made of a biocompatible alloy such as cobalt–chromium alloy or stainless steel. Such wires are not currently used in joint replacements owing to the limited space available. Graphite fibers have been incorporated in bone cement [Knoell et al., 1975] on an experimental basis. Significant improvements in the mechanical properties have been achieved. Moreover, the fibers have an added beneficial effect of reducing the rise in temperature which occurs during the polymerization of the PMMA in the body. Such high temperature can cause problems such as necrosis of a portion of the bone into which it is implanted. Thin, short titanium fibers have been embedded in PMMA cement [Topoleski et al., 1992]; a toughness increase of 51% was observed with a 5% volumetric fiber content. Fiber reinforcement of PMMA cement has not found much acceptance since the fibers also increase the viscosity of the unpolymerized material. It is consequently difficult for the surgeon to form and shape the polymerizing cement during the surgical procedure.

Metals are currently used in bone plates for immobilizing fractures and in the femoral component of total hip replacements. A problem with currently used implant metals is that they are much stiffer than bone, so they shield the nearby bone from mechanical stress. Stress-shielding results in a kind of disuse atrophy: the bone resorbs [Engh and Bobyn, 1988]. Therefore composite materials have been investigated as alternatives [Bradley et al., 1980; Skinner, 1988]. Fibrous composites can deform to higher strains (to about 0.01) than metals (0.001 for a mild steel) without damage. This resilience is an attractive characteristic for more flexible bone plates and femoral stems. Flexible composite bone plates are effective in promoting healing [Jockish, 1992]. Composite hip replacement prostheses have been made with carbon fibers in a matrix of polysulfone and polyetherether ketone (PEEK). These prostheses experience heavy load with a static component. Structural metals such as stainless steel and cobalt chromium alloys do not

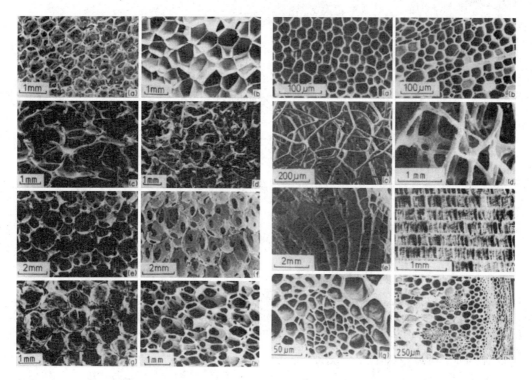

FIGURE 41.7 Cellular solids structures, after Gibson and Ashby [1988]. Left: synthetic cellular solids: (a) open-cell polyurethane, (b) closed-cell polyethylene, (c) foamed nickel, (d) foamed copper, (e) foamed zirconia, (f) foamed mullite, (g) foamed glass, (h) polyester foam with both open and closed cells. Right: natural cellular solids: (a) cork, (b) balsa wood, (c) sponge, (d) cancellous bone, (e) coral, (f) cuttlefish bone, (g) iris leaf, (h) plant stalk.

creep significantly at room or body temperature. In composites which contain a polymer constituent, creep behavior is a matter of concern. The carbon fibers exhibit negligible creep, but polymer constituents tend to creep. Prototype composite femoral components were found to exhibit fiber dominated creep of small magnitude and are not expected to limit the life of the implant [Maharaj and Jamison, 1993].

Fibrous composites have also been used in external medical devices such as knee braces [Yeaple, 1989], in which biocompatibility is not a concern but light weight is crucial.

41.6 Porous Materials

The presence of voids in porous or cellular solids will reduce the stiffness of the material. For some purposes, that is both acceptable and desirable. Porous solids are used for many purposes: flexible structures such as (1) seat cushions, (2) thermal insulation, (3) filters, (4) cores for stiff and lightweight sandwich panels, (5) flotation devices, and (6) to protect objects from mechanical shock and vibration; and in biomaterials, as coatings to encourage tissue ingrowth. Representative cellular solid structures are shown in Figure 41.7.

The stiffness of an open-cell foam is given by [Gibson and Ashby, 1988]

$$E = E_s[V_s]^2 \tag{41.6}$$

in which E_s is the Young's modulus and V_s is the volume fraction of the solid phase of the foam; V_s is also called the relative density.

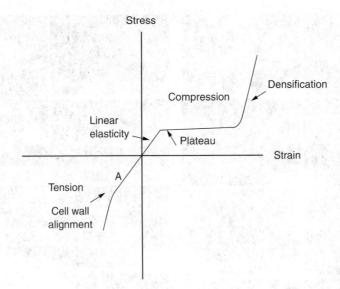

FIGURE 41.8   Representative stress-strain curve for a cellular solid. The plateau region for compression in the case of elastomeric foam (a rubbery polymer) represents elastic buckling; for an elastic-plastic foam (such as metallic foam), it represents plastic yield, and for an elastic-brittle foam (such as ceramic) it represents crushing. On the tension side, point 'A' represents the transition between cell wall bending and cell wall alignment. In elastomeric foam, the alignment occurs elastically, in elastic plastic foam it occurs plastically, and an elastic-brittle foam fractures at A.

The strength for crushing of a brittle foam and the elastic collapse of an elastomeric foam is given, respectively, by

$$\sigma_{\text{crush}} = 0.65\, \sigma_{\text{f,s}}[V_\text{s}]^{3/2} \tag{41.7}$$

$$\sigma_{\text{coll}} = 0.05\, E_\text{s}[V_\text{s}]^2 \tag{41.8}$$

Here $\sigma_{\text{f,s}}$ is the fracture strength of the solid phase. These strength relations are valid for relatively small density. Their derivation is based on the concept of *bending* of the cell ribs and is presented by Gibson and Ashby [1988]. Most man-made closed cell foams tend to have a concentration of material at the cell edges, so that they behave mechanically as open cell foams. The salient point in the relations for the mechanical properties of cellular solids is that the *relative density* dramatically influences the stiffness and the strength. As for the relationship between stress and strain, a representative stress strain curve is shown in Figure 41.8. The physical mechanism for the deformation mode beyond the elastic limit depends on the material from which the foam is made. Trabecular bone, for example, is a natural cellular solid, which tends to fail in compression by crushing. Many kinds of trabecular bone appear to behave mechanically as an open cell foam. For trabecular bone of unspecified orientation, the stiffness is proportional to the cube of the density and the strength as the square of the density [Gibson and Ashby, 1988], which indicates behavior dominated by bending of the trabeculae. For bone with oriented trabeculae, both stiffness and strength in the trabecular direction are proportional to the density, a fact which indicates behavior dominated by axial deformation of the trabeculae.

Porous materials have a high ratio of surface area to volume. When porous materials are used in biomaterial applications, the demands upon the inertness and biocompatibility are likely to be greater than for a homogeneous material.

Porous materials, when used in implants, allow tissue ingrowth [Spector et al., 1988a,b]. The ingrowth is considered desirable in many contexts, since it allows a relatively permanent anchorage of the implant to the surrounding tissues. There are actually two composites to be considered in porous implants (1) the implant prior to ingrowth, in which the pores are filled with tissue fluid which is ordinarily of no

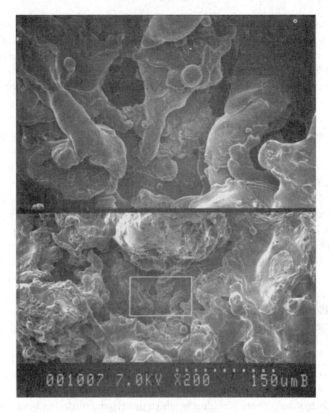

FIGURE 41.9 Irregular pore structure of porous coating in Ti5Al4V alloy for bony ingrowth. The top scanning electron microscopic picture is a 5× magnification of the rectangular region of the bottom picture (200×). (From Park, J.B. and Lakes, R.S. 1992. *Biomaterials*, Plenum, New York.)

mechanical consequence; and (2) the implant filled with tissue. In the case of the implant prior to ingrowth, it must be recognized that the stiffness and strength of the porous solid are much less than in the case of the solid from which it is derived.

Porous layers are used on bone compatible implants to encourage bony ingrowth [Galante et al., 1971; Ducheyne, 1984]. The pore size of a cellular solid has no influence on its stiffness or strength (though it does influence the toughness), however pore size can be of considerable biological importance. Specifically, in orthopedic implants with pores larger than about 150 μm, bony ingrowth into the pores occurs and this is useful to anchor the implant. This minimum pore size is on the order of the diameter of osteons in normal Haversian bone. It was found experimentally that pores <75 μm in size did not permit the ingrowth of bone tissue. Moreover, it was difficult to maintain fully viable osteons within pores in the 75 to 150 μm size range. Representative structure of such a porous surface layer is shown in Figure 41.9. Porous coatings are also under study for application in anchoring the artificial roots of dental implants to the underlying jawbone. Porous hydroxyapatite has been studied for use in repairing large defects in bone [Meffert et al., 1985; Holmes et al., 1986]. Hydroxyapatite is the mineral constituent of bone, and it has the nominal composition $Ca_{10}(PO_4)_6(OH)_2$. Implanted hydroxyapatite is slowly resorbed by the body over several years and replaced by bone. Tricalcium phosphate is resorbed more quickly and has been considered as an implant constituent to speed healing.

When a porous material is implanted in bone, the pores become filled first with blood which clots, then with osteoprogenitor mesenchymal cells, then, after about 4 weeks, bony trabeculae. The ingrown bone then becomes remodeled in response to mechanical stress. The bony ingrowth process depends on a degree of mechanical stability in the early stages of healing. If too much motion occurs, the ingrown tissue will be collagenous scar tissue, not bone.

Porous materials used in soft tissue applications include polyurethane, polyamide, and polyester velours used in percutaneous devices. Porous reconstituted collagen has been used in artificial skin, and braided polypropylene has been used in artificial ligaments. As in the case of bone implants, the porosity encourages tissue ingrowth which anchors the device.

Blood vessel replacements are made with porous materials which encourage soft tissue to grow in, eventually forming a new lining, or neointima. The new lining consists of the patient's own cells. It is a natural nonthrombogenic surface resembling the lining of the original blood vessel. This is a further example of the biological role of porous materials as contrasted with the mechanical role.

Ingrowth of tissue into implant pores is not always desirable. For example, sponge (polyvinyl alcohol) implants used in early mammary augmentation surgery underwent ingrowth of fibrous tissue, and contracture and calcification of that tissue, resulting in hardened, calcified breasts. Current mammary implants make use of a balloon-like nonporous silicone rubber layer enclosing silicone oil or gel, or perhaps a saline solution in water. A porous layer of polyester felt or velour attached to the balloon is provided at the back surface of the implant so that limited tissue ingrowth will anchor it to the chest wall and prevent it from migrating.

Foams are also used externally to protect the human body from injury. Examples include knee pads, elbow pads, wrestling mats, and wheelchair cushions. Since these foams are only in contact with skin rather than any internal organs, they are not subject to rigorous biocompatibility requirements. They are therefore designed based on mechanical considerations. Foam used in sports equipment must have the correct compliance to limit impact force without bottoming out. Foam used in wheelchair cushions is intended to prevent pressure sores in people who suffer limited mobility. The properties of cushions are crucial in reducing illness and suffering in people who are confined to wheelchairs or hospital beds for long periods. Prolonged pressure on body parts can obstruct circulation in the capillaries. If this lasts too long it may cause a sore or ulcer called a pressure sore, also called a bed sore. In its most severe manifestation, a pressure sore can form a deep crater-like ulcer in which underlying muscle or bone is exposed [Dinsdale, 1974]. A variety of flexible cushion materials have been tried to minimize the incidence and severity of pressure sores [Garber, 1985]. Viscoelastic foam allows the cushion to progressively conform to the body shape. However, progressive densification of the foam due to creep results in a stiffer cushion which must be periodically replaced.

Porous materials are produced in a variety of ways. For example, in the case of bone compatible surfaces they are formed by sintering of beads or wires. Vascular and soft tissue implants are produced by weaving or braiding fibers as well as by nonwoven "felting" methods. Protective foams for use outside the body are usually produced by use of a "blowing agent" which is a chemical which evolves gas during the polymerization of the foam. An interesting approach to producing micro-porous materials is the replication of structures found in biological materials: the *replamineform* process [White et al., 1976]. The rationale is that the unique structure of communicating pores is thought to offer advantages in the induction of tissue ingrowth. The skeletal structure of coral or echinoderms (such as sea urchins) is replicated by a casting process in metals and polymers; these have been tried in vascular and tracheal prostheses as well as in bone substitutes.

41.7 Biocompatibility

Carbon itself has been successfully used as a biomaterial. Carbon based fibers used in composites are known to be inert in aqueous (even seawater) environments, however they do not have a track record in the biomaterials setting. *In vitro* studies by Kovacs [1993] disclose substantial electrochemical activity of carbon fiber composites in an aqueous environment. If such composites are placed near a metallic implant, galvanic corrosion is a possibility. Composite materials with a polymer matrix absorb water when placed in a hydrated environment such as the body. Moisture acts as a plasticizer of the matrix and shifts the glass transition temperature towards lower values [DeIasi and Whiteside, 1978], hence a reduction in stiffness and an increase in mechanical damping. Water immersion of a graphite epoxy cross-ply composite [Gopalan et al., 1989] for 20 days reduced the strength by 13% and the stiffness by 9%. Moisture absorption by polymer constituents also causes swelling. Such swelling can be beneficial in dental composites since it offsets some of the shrinkage due to polymerization.

Flexible composite bone plates are effective in promoting healing [Jockish, 1992], but particulate debris from composite bone plates gives rise to a foreign body reaction similar to that caused by ultra high molecular weight polyethylene.

41.8 Summary

Composite materials are a relatively recent addition to the class of materials used in structural applications. In the biomaterials field, the ingress of composites has been even more recent. In view of their potential for high performance, composite materials are likely to find increasing use as biomaterials.

References

Agarwal, A.G. and Broutman, L.J. 1980. *Analysis and Performance of Fiber Composites*, John Wiley & Sons, New York.

Bradley, J.S., Hastings, G.W., and Johnson-Hurse, C. 1980. Carbon fiber reinforced epoxy as a high strength, low modulus material for internal fixation plates, *Biomaterials* 1, 38–40.

Cannon, M.L. 1988. Composite resins, in: *Encyclopedia of Medical Devices and Instrumentation*, J.G. Webster, Ed., John Wiley & Sons, New York.

Christensen, R.M. 1979. *Mechanics of Composite Materials*, John Wiley & Sons, New York.

Craig, R. 1981. Chemistry, composition, and properties of composite resins, In: *Dental Clinics of North America*, H. Horn, Ed., W.B. Saunders, Philadelphia, PA.

Craig, R.G. and Peyton, F.A. 1958. Elastic and mechanical properties of human dentin, *J. Dental Res.*, 37, 710–718.

DeIasi, R. and Whiteside, J.B. 1978. Effect of moisture on epoxy resins and composites: advanced composite materials — environmental effects, J.R. Vinson, Ed. *ASTM Publication STP 658*, Philadelphia, PA.

Dinsdale, S.M. 1974. Decubitus ulcers: role of pressure and friction in causation, *Arch. Phys. Med. Rehabil.*, 55, 147–152.

Ducheyne, P. 1984. Biological fixation of implants, in: *Functional Behavior of Orthopaedic Biomaterials*, G.W. Hastings and P. Ducheyne, Eds. CRC Press, Boca Raton, FL.

Engh, C.A. and Bobyn, J.D. 1988. Results of porous coated hip replacement using the AML prosthesis, In: *Non-Cemented Total Hip Arthroplasty*, Raven Press, New York.

Fishbane, B.M. and Pond, R.B. 1977. Stainless steel fiber reinforcement of polymethylmethacrylate, *Clin. Orthop.*, 128, 490–498.

Galante, J., Rostoker, W., Lueck, R., and Ray, R.D. 1971. Sintered fiber metal composites as a basis for attachment of implants to bone, *J. Bone Joint Surg.*, 53A, 101–114.

Garber, S.L. 1985. Wheelchair cushions: a historical review, *Am. J. Occup. Ther.*, 39, 453–459.

Gibson, L.J. and Ashby, M.F. 1988. *Cellular Solids*, Cambridge, England.

Gopalan, R., Somashekar, B.R., and Dattaguru, B. 1989. Environmental effects on fiber-polymer composites, *Polym. Degradat. Stabil.*, 24, 361–371.

Hashin, Z. and Shtrikman, S. 1963. A variational approach to the theory of the elastic behavior of multiphase materials, *J. Mech. Phys. Solids*, 11, 127–140.

Holmes, D.E., Bucholz, R.W., and Mooney, V. 1986. Porous hydroxyapatite as a bone graft substitute in metaphyseal defects, *J. Bone Jnt. Surg.*, 68, 904–911.

Katz, J.L. 1980. Anisotropy of Young's modulus of bone. *Nature*, 283, 106–107.

Kovacs, P. 1993. *In vitro* studies of the electrochemical behavior of carbon-fiber composites, in: *Composite Materials for Implant Applications in the Human Body: Characterization and Testing, ASTM STP 1178*. R.D. Jamison and L.N. Gilbertson, Eds. ASTM, Philadelphia, PA, pp. 41–52.

Jockish, K.A., Brown, S.A., Bauer, T.W., and Merritt, K. 1992. Biological response to chopped carbon reinforced PEEK, *J. Biomed. Mater. Res.*, 26, 133–146.

Knoell, A., Maxwell, H., and Bechtol, C. 1975. Graphite fiber reinforced bone cement, *Ann. Biomed. Eng.*, 3, 225–229.

Lakes, R.S. 1993. Materials with structural hierarchy, *Nature*, 361, 511–515.

Lekhniitski, 1963. Elasticity of an anisotropic elastic body, Holden Day.

Maharaj, G.R. and Jamison, R.D. 1993. Creep testing of a composite material human hip prosthesis, In: *Composite Materials for Implant Applications in the Human Body: Characterization and Testing*, ASTM STP 1178. R.D. Jamison and L.N. Gilbertson, Eds. Am. Soc. Testing, Materials, Philadelphia, PA, 86–97.

Meffert, R.M., Thomas, J.R., Hamilton, K.M., and Brownstein, C.N. 1985. Hydroxylapatite as allopathic graft in the treatment of periodontal osseous defects, *J. Periodontol.*, 56, 63–73.

Park, H.C., Liu, Y.K., and Lakes, R.S. 1986. The material properties of bone-particle impregnated PMMA, *J. Biomech. Eng.*, 108, 141–148.

Nye, J.F. 1976. *Physical Properties of Crystals*, Oxford University Press, Oxford.

Papadogianis, Y., Boyer, D.B., and Lakes, R.S. 1985. Creep of posterior dental composites, *J. Biomed. Mat. Res.*, 19, 85–95.

Park, J.B. and Lakes, R.S. 1992. *Biomaterials*, Plenum, New York.

Paul, B. 1960. Prediction of elastic constants of multiphase materials, *Trans. AIME*, 218, 36–41.

Peters, M.C., Poort, H.W., Farah, J.W., and Graig, R.G. 1983. Stress analysis of a tooth restored with a post and a core, *J. Dental Res.*, 62, 760–763.

Reilly, D.T. and Burstein, A.H. 1975. The elastic and ultimate properties of compact bone tissue, *J. Biomech.*, 8, 393–405.

Schwartz, M.M. 1992. *Composite Materials Handbook*, 2nd ed. McGraw-Hill, New York.

Sclippa, E. and Piekarski, K. 1973. Carbon fiber reinforced polyethylene for possible orthopaedic usage, *J. Biomed. Mater. Res.*, 7, 59–70.

Skinner, H.B. 1988. Composite technology for total hip arthroplasty. *Clin. Orthop. Rel. Res.*, 235, 224–236.

Spector, M., Miller, M., and Beals, N. 1988a. Porous materials, In: *Encyclopedia of Medical Devices and Instrumentation*, J.G. Webster, Ed. John Wiley & Sons, New York.

Spector, M., Heyligers, I., and Robertson, J.R. 1988b. Porous polymers for biological fixation, *Clin. Orthop. Rel. Res.*, 235, 207–219.

Topoleski, L.D.T., Ducheyne, P., and Cackler, J.M. 1992. The fracture toughness of titanium fiber reinforced bone cement, *J. Biomed. Mater. Res.*, 26, 1599–1617.

White, R.A., Weber, J.N., and White, E.W. 1976. Replamineform: a new process for preparing porous ceramic, metal, and polymer prosthetic materials, *Science*, 176, 922.

Yeaple, F. 1989. Composite knee brace returns stability to joint, *Design News*, 46, 116.

42

Biodegradable Polymeric Biomaterials: An Updated Overview

Chih-Chang Chu
Cornell University

42.1 Introduction

The term **biodegradation** is loosely associated with materials that could be broken down by nature either through hydrolytic mechanisms without the help of enzymes and/or enzymatic mechanism. Other terms like *absorbable, erodible, and resorbable* have also been used in the literature to indicate biodegradation.

TABLE 42.1 Properties of Commercially Important Synthetic Absorbable Polymers

Polymer	Crystallinity	T_m (°C)	T_g (°C)	T_{dec} (°C)	Fiber Strength MPa	Modulus GPa	Elongation (%)
PGA	High	230	36	260	890	8.4	30
PLLA	High	170	56	240	900	8.5	25
PLA	None	—	57	—	—	—	—
Polyglactin910[a]	High[c]	200	40	250	850	8.6	24
Polydioxanone	High	106	<20	190	490	2.1	35
Polyglyconate[b]	High[c]	213	<20	260	550	2.4	45
Poliglecaprone25[d]	—	<220	−36~15		91,100[e]	113,000[e]	39

[a] Glycolide per lactide = 9/1.
[b] Glycolide per trimethylene carbonate = 9/1.
[c] Depending on the copolymer composition.
[d] 2/0 size Monocryl (glycolide-ε-caprolactone copolymer).
[e] PSI unit.

Source: Kimura, Y., 1993. *Biomedical Applications of Polymeric Materials*, T. Tsuruta, T. Hayashi, K. Kataoka, K. Ishihara, and Y. Kimura, Eds. CRC Press, Boca Raton, FL and Chu, C.C., von Fraunhofer, J.A., and Greisler, H.P., 1996. *Wound Closure Biomaterials and Devices.* CRC Press, Boca Raton, FL.

The interests in biodegradable polymeric biomaterials for biomedical engineering use have increased dramatically during the past decade. This is because this class of biomaterials has two major advantages that non-biodegradable biomaterials do not have. First, they do not elicit permanent chronic foreign-body reactions due to the fact that they are gradually absorbed by the human body and do not permanently leave traces of residual in the implantation sites. Second, some of them have recently been found to be able to regenerate tissues, so called **tissue engineering**, through the interaction of their biodegradation with immunologic cells like macrophages. Hence, surgical implants made from biodegradable biomaterials could be used as a temporary scaffold for tissue regeneration. This approach toward the reconstruction of injured, diseased, or aged tissues is one of the most promising fields in the next century.

Although the earliest and most commercially significant biodegradable polymeric biomaterials were originated from linear aliphatic polyesters like polyglycolide and polylactide from poly(α-hydroxyacetic acids), recent introduction of several new synthetic and natural biodegradable polymeric biomaterials extends the domain beyond this family of simple polyesters. These new commercially significant biodegradable polymeric biomaterials include poly(orthoesters), polyanhydrides, polysaccharides, poly(ester-amides), tyrosine-based polyarylates or polyiminocarbonates or polycarbonates, poly(D,L-lactide-urethane), poly(β-hydroxybutyrate), poly(ε-caprolactone), poly[*bis*(carboxylatophenoxy) phosphazene], poly(amino acids), pseudo-poly(amino acids), and copolymers derived from amino acids and non-amino acids.

All the above biodegradable polymeric biomaterials could be generally divided into eight groups based on their chemical origin: (1) Biodegradable linear aliphatic polyesters (e.g., polyglycolide, polylactide, polycaprolactone, polyhydroxybutyrate) and their copolymers within the aliphatic polyester family like poly(glycolide-L-lactide) copolymer and poly(glycolide-ε-caprolactone) copolymer; (2) Biodegradable copolymers between linear aliphatic polyesters in (1) and monomers other than linear aliphatic polyesters like, poly(glycolide-trimethylene carbonate) copolymer, poly(L-lactic acid-L-lysine) copolymer, Tyrosine-based polyarylates or polyiminocarbonates or polycarbonates, poly(D,L-lactide-urethane), and poly(ester-amide); (3) Polyanhydrides; (4) Poly(orthoesters); (5) Poly(ester-ethers) like poly-p-dioxanone; (6) Biodegradable polysaccharides like hyaluronic acid, chitin, and chitson; (7) polyamino acids like poly-L-glutamic acid and poly-L-lysine; (8) Inorganic biodegradable polymers like polyphosphazene and poly[*bis*(carboxylatophenoxy)phosphazene] which have a nitrogen-phosphorus backbone instead of ester linkage. Recently, there is a new approach of making new biodegradable polymers through melt-blending of highly accepted biodegradable polymers like those of glycolide and lactide base [Shalaby, 1994].

The earliest, most successful, and frequent biomedical applications of biodegradable polymeric biomaterials have been in wound closure [Chu et al., 1996]. All biodegradable wound closure biomaterials are based upon the glycolide and lactide families. For example, polyglycolide (Dexon from American Cyanamid), poly(glycolide-L-lactide) random copolymer with 90 to 10 — ratio (Vicryl from Ethicon), poly(ester-ether) (PDS from Ethicon), poly(glycolide-trimethylene carbonate) random block copolymer (Maxon from American Cyanamid), and poly(glycolide-ε-caprolactone) copolymer (Monocryl from Ethicon). This class of biodegradable polymeric biomaterials is also the one most studied for their chemical, physical, mechanical, morphological, and biological properties and their changes with degradation time and environment. Some of the above materials like Vicryl have been commercially used as surgical meshes for repair of a hernia or the body wall.

The next largest biomedical application of biodegradable polymeric biomaterials that are commercially satisfactory is drug control/release devices. Some well-known examples in this application are polyanhydrides and poly(ortho-ester). Biodegradable polymeric biomaterials, particularly totally resorbable composites, have also been experimentally used in the field of orthopedics, mainly as components for internal bone fracture fixation like PDS pins. However, their wide acceptance in other parts of orthopaedic implants may be limited due to their inherent mechanical properties and their biodegradation rate. Besides the commercial uses described above, biodegradable polymeric biomaterials have been experimented with as (1) vascular grafts, (2) vascular stents, (3) vascular couplers for vessel anastomosis, (4) nerve growth conduits, (5) augmentation of defected bone, (6) ligament/tendon prostheses, (7) intramedullary plug during total hip replacement, (8) anastomosis ring for intestinal surgery, and (9) stents in ureteroureterostomies for accurate suture placement.

Due to space limitation, the emphasis of this chapter will be on the commercially most significant and successful biomedical biodegradable polymers based on (1) linear aliphatic polyesters, (2) some very recent research and development of important classes of synthetic biodegradable polymers, (3) a new theoretical approach to modeling the hydrolytic degradation of glycolide/lactide based biodegradable polymers, (4) the effects of some new extrinsic factors on the degradation of the most commercially significant biodegradable polymers, and (5) the new biomedical applications of this class of synthetic biodegradable polymers in tissue engineering and regeneration. The details of the applications of this family and other biodegradable polymeric biomaterials and their chemical, physical, mechanical, biological, and biodegradation properties can be found in other recent reviews [Barrows, 1986; Vert et al., 1992; Kimura, 1993; Park et al., 1993; Shalaby, 1994; Hollinger, 1995; Chu et al., 1996].

42.2 Glycolide/Lactide Based Biodegradable Linear Aliphatic Polyesters

This class of biodegradable polymers is the most successful, important, and commercially widely used biodegradable biomaterials in surgery. It is also the class of biodegradable biomaterials that were most extensively studied in terms of degradation mechanisms and structure–property relationships. Among them, polyglycolide or polyglycolic acid (PGA) is the most important one because most other biodegradable polymers are derived from PGA either through copolymerization, for example, poly(glycolide-L-lactide) copolymer or modified glycolide monomer, for example, poly-p-dioxanone.

42.2.1 Glycolide Based Biodegradable Homopolymers Polyesters

PGA can be polymerized either directly or indirectly from glycolic acid. The direct polycondensation produces a polymer of M_n less than 10,000 because of the requirement of a very high degree of dehydration (99.28% up) and the absence of monofunctional impurities. For PGA of molecular weight higher than 10,000 it is necessary to proceed through the ring-opening polymerization of the cyclic dimers

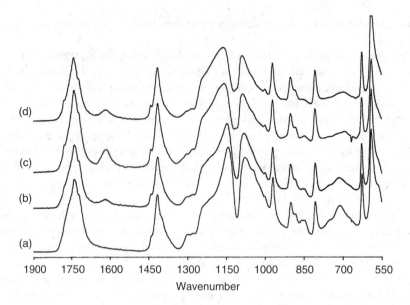

FIGURE 42.1   FTIR spectra of polyglycolic acid disks as a function of *in vitro* hydrolysis time in phosphate buffer of pH 7.44 at 37°C. (a) 0 day; (b) 55 h; (c) 7 days; (d) 21 days.

of glycolic acid. Numerous catalysts are available for this ring-opening polymerization. They include organometallic compounds and Lewis acids [Chujo et al., 1967; Wise et al., 1979]. For biomedical applications, stannous chloride dihydrate or trialkyl aluminum are preferred. PGA was found to exhibit an orthorhombic unit cell with dimensions $a = 5.22$ Å, $b = 6.19$ Å, and c(fiber axis) $= 7.02$ Å. The planar zigzag-chain molecules form a sheet structure parallel to the ac plane and do not have the polyethylene type arrangement [Chatani et al., 1968]. The molecules between two adjacent sheets orient in opposite directions. The tight molecular packing and the close approach of the ester groups might stabilize the crystal lattice and contribute to the high melting point, T_m, of PGA (224 to 230°C). The glass transition temperature, T_g, ranges from 36 to 40°C. The specific gravities of PGA are 1.707 for a perfect crystal and 1.50 in a completely amorphous state [Chujo et al., 1967a]. The heat of fusion of 100% crystallized PGA is reported to be 12 kJ/mol (45.7 cal/g) [Brandrup et al., 1975]. A recent study of injection molded PGA disks reveals their IR spectroscopic characteristics [Chu et al., 1995]. As shown in Figure 42.1, the four bands at 850, 753, 713, and 560 cm^{-1} are associated with the amorphous regions of the PGA disks and could be used to assess the extends of hydrolysis. Peaks associated with the crystalline phase included those at 972, 901, 806, 627, and 590 cm^{-1}. Two broad, intense peaks at 1142 and 1077 cm^{-1} can be assigned to C—O stretching modes in the ester and oxymethylene groups, respectively. These two peaks are associated mainly with ester and oxymethylene groups originating in the amorphous domains. Hydrolysis could cause both of these C—O stretching modes to substantially decrease in intensity.

42.2.2 Glycolide-Based Biodegradable Copolyesters Having Aliphatic Polyester Based Co-Monomers

Other commercially successful glycolide-based biodegradable polymeric biomaterials are the copolymers of glycolide with other monomers within linear aliphatic polyesters like lactides, carbonates, and ε-caprolactone. The glycolide-lactide random copolymers are the most studied and have a wide range of properties and applications, depending on the composition ratio of glycolide to lactide. Figure 42.2 illustrates the dependence of biodegradation rate on the composition of glycolide to lactide in the copolymer. For wound closure purposes, a high concentration of glycolide monomer is required for achieving proper mechanical and degradation properties. Vicryl sutures, sometime called polyglactin 910,

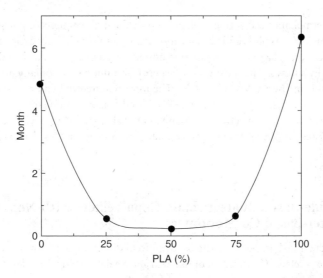

FIGURE 42.2 The effect of poly(L-lactide) composition in polyglycolide on the time required for 50% mass loss implanted under the dorsal skin of rat. (From Miller, R.A., Brady, J.M., and Cutright, D.E., 1977. *J. Biomed. Mater. Res.*, 11:711. With permission.)

contain a 90/10 molar ratio of glycolic to L-lactide and this molar ratio is important for the Vicryl suture to retain crystalline characteristics. For biomedical use, Lewis acid catalysts are preferred for the copolymers [Wise et al., 1979]. If D,L-instead of L-lactide is used as the co-monomer, the U-shape relationship between the level of crystallinity and glycolide composition disappears. This is because polylactide from 100% D,L-lactide composition is totally amorphous. IR bands associated with Vicryl molecules in the amorphous domains are 560, 710, 850, and 888 cm^{-1}, while 590, 626, 808, 900, and 972 cm^{-1} are associated with the crystalline domains [Frederick et al., 1984]. Like PGA, these IR bands could be used to assess the extent of hydrolysis.

A relatively new block copolymer of glycolide and carbonates, such as trimethylene carbonate, has been commercialized. Maxon is made from a block copolymer of glycolide and 1,3-dioxan-2-one (trimethylene carbonate or GTMC) and consists of 32.5% by weight (or 36 mol%) of trimethylene carbonate [Casey et al., 1984; Katz et al., 1985]. Maxon is a poly(ester-carbonate). The polymerization process of Maxon is divided into two stages. The first stage is the formation of a middle block which is a random copolymer of glycolide and 1,3-dioxan-2-one. Diethylene glycol is used as an initiator and stannous chloride dihydrate ($SnCl_2 \cdot 2H_2O$) serves as the catalyst. The polymerization is conducted at about 180°C. The weight ratio of glycolide to trimethylene carbonate in the middle block is 15:85. After the synthesis of the middle block, the temperature of the reactive bath is raised to about 220°C to prevent the crystallization of the copolymer and additional glycolide monomers as the end blocks are added into the reaction bath to form the final triblock copolymer.

The latest glycolide-based copolymer that has become commercially successful is Monocryl suture. It is a segmented block copolymer consisting of both soft and hard segments. The purpose of having soft segments in the copolymer is to provide good handling properties like pliability, while the hard segments are used to provide adequate strength. The generic copolymerization process between glycolic acid and ε-caprolactone was recently reported by Fukuzaki et al. in Japan [1989, 1991]. The resulting copolymers were low molecular weight biodegradable copolymers of glycolic acid and various lactones for potential drug delivery purposes. The composition of lactone ranged from as low as 15 to as high as 50 mol% and the weight average for molecular weight ranged from 4,510 to 16,500. The glass transition temperature ranged from 18 to −43°C, depending on the copolymer composition and molecular weight.

Monocryl is made from two stages of the polymerization process [Bezwada et al., 1995]. In the first stage, soft segments of prepolymer of glycolide and ε-caprolactone are made. This soft segmented prepolymer is further polymerized with glycolides to provide hard segments of polyglycolide. Monocryl has a composition of 75% glycolide and 25% ε-caprolactone and should have a higher molecular weight than those glycolide/ε-caprolactone copolymers reported by Fukuzaki et al., for adequate mechanical properties required by sutures. The most unique aspect of Monocryl monofilament suture is its pliability as claimed by Ethicon [Bezwada et al., 1995]. The force required to bend a 2/0 suture is only about 2.8×10^4 lb-in^2 for Monocryl, while the same size PDSII and Maxon monofilament sutures require about 3.9 and 11.6×10^4 lb-in^2 force, respectively. This inherent pliability of Monocryl is due to the presence of soft segments and T_g resulting from the ε-caprolactone co-monomer unit. Its T_g is expected to be between 15 and $-36°C$.

42.2.3   Glycolide-Based Biodegradable Copolyesters with Non-Aliphatic Polyester-Based Co-Monomers

In this category, the most important one is the glycolide copolymer consisting of poly(ethylene 1,4-phenylene-bis-oxyacetate) (PEPBO) (Jamiokowski and Shalaby, 1991). The development of this type of glycolide-based copolymer was initiated because of the adverse effect of γ irradiation on the mechanical properties of glycolide-based synthetic absorbable sutures. There is a great desire to develop γ-irradiation sterilizable, synthetic, absorbable polymers to take advantage of the highly convenient and reliable method of sterilization. Shalaby et al. recently reported that the incorporation of about 10 mol% of a polymeric radiostabilizer like PEPBO into PGA backbone chains would make the copolymer sterilizable by γ irradiation without a significant accelerated loss of mechanical properties upon hydrolysis when compared with the unirradiated copolymer control (MPG) [Jamiokowski et al., 1991]. The changes in tensile breaking force of both MPG and PGA sutures implanted intramuscularly and subcutaneously in rats for various periods show the great advantage of such copolymers. MPG fibers γ-irradiated at 2.89 Mrads did not show any loss in tensile breaking force during the first 14 days postimplantation when compared with unimplanted samples. On the contrary, PGA sutures γ-irradiated at 2.75 Mrads lost 62% of the tensile breaking force of their unimplanted samples. There was no tensile breaking force remaining for the irradiated PGA at the end of 21 days, while both 2.89 and 5 Mrads irradiated MPG retained 72 and 55% of their corresponding 0 day controls, respectively. The inherent more hydrolytic resistance of MPG must be attributed to the presence of an aromatic group in the backbone chains. This aromatic polyester component is also responsible for the observed γ-irradiation stability. It is not known at this time whether the new γ-irradiation-resistant MPG is biocompatible with biologic tissues due to the lack of published histologic data.

42.2.4   Glycolide-Derived Biodegradable Polymers Having Ether Linkage

Poly-p-dioxanone (PDS) is derived from the glycolide family with better flexibility. It is polymerized from ether-containing lactones, 1,4-dioxane-2,5-dione (i.e., p-dioxanone) monomers with a hydroxylic initiator and tin catalyst [Shalaby, 1994]. The resulting polymer is semi-crystalline with T_m about 106–115°C and T_g -10–0°C. The improved flexibility of PDS relative to PGA as evidenced in its lower T_g is due to the incorporation of an ether segment in the repeating unit which reduces the density of ester linkages for intermolecular hydrogen bonds. Because of the less dense ester linkages in PDS when compared with PGA or glycolide-L-lactide copolymers, PDS is expected and has been shown to degrade at a slower rate *in vitro* and *in vivo*. PDS having an inherent viscosity of 2.0 dl/g in hexafluoroisopropanol is adequate for making monofilament sutures. Recently, an advanced version of PDS, PDSII, was introduced. PDSII was achieved by subjecting the melt-spun fibers to a high temperature (128°C) for a short period of time. This additional treatment partially melts the outermost surface layer of PDS fibers and leads to a distinctive skin-core morphology. The heat employed also results in larger crystallites in the core of the fiber than the untreated PDS fiber. The tensile strength-loss profile of PDSII sutures is better than that of PDS sutures.

A variety of copolymers having high molar ratios of PDS compared to other monomers within the same linear aliphatic polyester family have been reported for the purpose of improving the mechanical and biodegradation properties [Shalaby, 1994]. For example, copolymer of PDS (80%) and PGA (up to 20%) has an absorption profile similar to Dexon and Vicryl sutures but it has compliance similar to PDS. Copolymer of PDS (85%) and PLLA (up to 15%) results in a more compliant (low modulus) suture than homopolymer PDS but with absorption profiles similar to PDS [Bezwada et al., 1990].

Copolymer fibers made from PDS and monomers other than linear aliphatic polyester like morpholine-2,5-dione (MD) exhibit rather interesting biodegradation properties. This copolymer fiber was absorbed 10 to 25% earlier than PDS. The copolymer, however, retained a tensile breaking strength profile similar to PDS with a slightly faster strength loss during the earlier stage, that is, the first 14 days [Shalaby, 1994]. This ability to break the inherent fiber structure–property relationship through copolymerization is a major improvement in biodegradation properties of absorbable sutures. It is interesting to recognize that a small % (3%) of MD in the copolymer suture is sufficient to result in a faster mass loss profile without the expense of its tensile strength-loss profile. The ability to achieve this ideal biodegradation property might be attributed to both an increasing hydrophilicity of the copolymer and the disruption of crystalline domains due to MD moiety. As described later, the loss of suture mass is mainly due to the destruction of crystalline domains, while the loss of tensile breaking strength is chiefly due to the scission of tie-chain segments located in the amorphous domains. The question is why MD–PDS copolymeric suture retains its strength-loss similar to PDS. The possible explanation is that the amide functional groups in MD could form stronger intermolecular hydrogen bonds than ester functional groups. This stronger hydrogen bond contributes to the strength retention of the copolymer of PDS and MD during *in vivo* biodegradation. The incorporation of MD moiety into PDS also lowers the unknot and knot strength of unhydrolyzed specimens, but increases elongation at break. This suggests that the copolymer of PDS and MD should have a lower level of crystallinity than PDS which is consistent with its observed faster mass loss *in vivo*.

To improve γ-irradiation stability of PDS, radiostabilizers like PEPBO have been copolymerized with PDS to form segmented copolymers the same way as PEPBO with glycolide described above [Koelmel et al., 1991; Shabaly, 1994]. The incorporation of 5 to 10% of such stabilizer in PDS has been shown not only to improve γ-irradiation resistance considerably but to also increase the compliance of the material. For example, PEPBO-PDS copolymer retained 79, 72, and 57% of its original tensile breaking strength at 2, 3, and 4 weeks in *in vivo* implantation, while PDS homopolymer retained only 43, 30, and 25% at the corresponding periods. It appears that an increasing (CH_2) group between the two ester functional groups of the radiation stabilizers improves the copolymer resistance toward γ-irradiation.

42.2.5 Lactide Biodegradable Homopolymers and Copolymers

Polylactides, particularly poly-L-lactide (PLLA), and copolymers having >50% L- or DL-lactide have been explored for medical use without much success mainly due to their much slower absorption and difficulty in melt processing. PLLAs are prepared in solid state through ring-opening polymerization due to their thermal instability and should be melt-processed at the lowest possible temperature [Shalaby, 1994]. Other methods like solution spinning, particularly for high molecular weight, and suspension polymerization have been reported as better alternatives. PLLA is a semi-crystalline polymer with $T_m = 170°C$ and $T_g = 56°C$. This high T_g is mainly responsible for the extremely slow biodegradation rate reported in the literature. The molecular weight of lactide-based biodegradable polymers suitable for medical use ranges from 1.5 to 5.0 dl/g inherent viscosity in chloroform. Ultra high molecular weight of polylactides have been reported [Tunc, 1983; Leenslag et al., 1984]. For example, an intrinsic viscosity as high as 13 dl/g was reported by Leenslag et al. High strength PLLA fibers from this ultra high molecular weight polylactide was made by hot-drawing fibers from solutions of good solvents. The resulting fibers had tensile breaking strength close to 1.2 GPa [Gogolewski et al., 1983]. Due to a dissymmetric nature of lactic acid, the polymer made from the optically inactive racemic mixture of D and L enantiomers, poly-DL-lactide, however, is an amorphous polymer.

Lactide-based copolymers having a high percentage of lactide have recently been reported, particularly those copolymerized with aliphatic polycarbonates like trimethylene carbonate (TMC) or 3,3-dimethyltrimethylene carbonate (DMTMC) [Shieh et al., 1990]. The major advantage of incorporating TMC or DMTMC units into lactide is that the degradation products from TMC or DMTMC are largely neutral pH and hence are considered to be advantageous. Both *in vitro* toxicity and *in vivo* non-specific foreign body reactions like sterile sinuses have been reported in orthopaedic implants made from PGA and/or PLLA [Eitenmuller et al., 1989; Bostman et al., 1990; Daniels et al., 1992; Hofmann, 1992; Winet et al., 1993]. Several investigators indicated that the glycolic or lactic-acid rich-degradation products have the potential to significantly lower the local pH in a closed and less body-fluid buffered regions surrounded by bone [Sugnuma et al., 1992]. This is particularly true if the degradation process proceeds with a burst mode (i.e., a sudden and rapid release of degradation products). This acidity tends to cause abnormal bone resorption and/or demineralization. The resulting environment may be cytotoxic [Daniels et al., 1992]. Indeed, inflammatory foreign body reactions with a discharging sinus and osteolytic foci visible on x-ray have been encountered in clinical studies [Eitenmuller et al., 1989]. Hollinger et al. recently confirmed the problem associated with PGA and/or PLLA orthopaedic implants [Winet et al., 1993]. A rapid degradation of a 50:50 ratio of glycolide-lactide copolymer in bone chambers of rabbit tibias has been found to inhibit bone regeneration. However, emphasis has been placed on the fact that extrapolation of *in vitro* toxicity to *in vivo* biocompatibility must consider microcirculatory capacity. The increase in the local acidity due to a faster accumulation of the highly acidic degradation products is also known to lead to an accelerated acid-catalyzed hydrolysis in the immediate vicinity of the biodegradable device. This acceleration in hydrolysis could lead to a faster loss of mechanical property of the device than we expect. This finding suggests the need to use components in totally biodegradable composites so that degradation products with less acidity would be released into the surrounding area. A controlled slow release rather than a burst release of degradation products at a level that the surrounding tissue could timely metabolize them would also be helpful in dealing with the acidity problem. Copolymers of composition ratio of 10DMTMC/90LLA or 10TMC/90LLA appear to be a promising absorbable orthopaedic device. Other applications of this type of copolymers include nerve growth conduits, tendon prostheses, and coating materials for biodegradable devices.

Another unique example of Llactide copolymer is the copolymer of L-lactide and 3-(S)[(alkyloxycarbonyl) methyl]-1,4-dioxane-2,5-dione, a cyclic diester [Kimura, 1993]. The most unique aspect of this new biodegradable copolymer is the carboxyl acid pendant group which obviously would make the new polymer not only more hydrophilic and hence faster biodegradation but also more reactive toward future chemical modification through the pendant carboxyl group. The availability of these carboxyl reactive pendant sites could be used to chemically bond antimicrobial agents or other biochemicals like growth factors for making future wound closure biomaterials having new and important biological functions. Unfortunately, there are no reported data to evaluate the performance of this new absorbable polymer for biomedical engineering use up to the present time.

Block copolymers of PLLA with poly(amino acids) have also been reported as a potential controlled drug delivery system [Nathan et al., 1994]. This new class of copolymers consists of both ester and amide linkages in the backbone molecules and is sometimes referred as poly(depsipeptides) or poly(esters-amides). Poly(depsipeptides) could also be synthesized from ring-opening polymerization of morpholine-2,5-dione and its derivatives [Helder et al., 1986]. Barrows has also made a series of poly(ester-amides) from polyesterification of diols that contain preformed amide linkages, such as amidediols [Barrows, 1994]. Katsarava and Chu et al. just reported the synthesis of high-molecular-weight poly(ester-amides) of M_w from 24,000 to 167,000 with narrow polydispersity ($M_w/M_n = 1.20-1.81$) via solution polycondensation of di-p-toluenesulfonic acid salts of *bis*-(α-amino acid) α, ω-alkylene diesters and di-p-nitrophenyl esters of diacids [Katsarava et al., In press]. These poly(ester-amide)s consisted of naturally occurring and non-toxic building blocks and had excellent film forming properties. These polymers were mostly amorphous materials with T_g from 11 to 59°C. The rationale for making poly(ester-amides) is to combine the well-known absorbability and biocompatibility of linear aliphatic polyesters with the high performance and the flexibility of potential chemical reactive sites of amide of polyamides. Poly(ester-amides) could be degraded either by enzyme and/or nonenzymatic mechanisms. There is no commercial use of this class of copolymers at the present time.

The introduction of poly(ethylene oxide) (PEO) into PLLA in order to modulate the hydrophilicity and degradability of PLLA for drug control/release biomaterials has been reported and an example is the triblock copolymer of PLA/PEO/PLA [Li et al., 1998a]. Biomaterials having an appropriate PLLA and PEO block length were found to have a hydrogel property that could deliver hydrophilic drugs as well as hydrophobic ones like steroids and hormones. Another unique biodegradable biomaterial consisting of a star-block copolymer of PLLA, PGA, and PEO was also reported for protein drug delivery devices [Li et al., 1998b]. This star-shaped copolymer has 4 or 8 arms made of PEO, PLLA, and PGA. The glass transition temperature and the crystallinity of this star-shaped block copolymer were significantly lower than the corresponding linear PLLA and PGA.

Because of the characteristic of very slow biodegradation rate of PLLA and the copolymers having a high composition ratio of PLLA, their biomedical applications have been mainly limited to (1) orthopaedic surgery, (2) drug control/release devices, (3) coating materials for suture, (4) vascular grafts, and (5) surgical meshes to facilitate wound healing after dental extraction.

42.3 Non-Glycolide/Lactide Based Linear Aliphatic Polyesters

All glycolide/lactide based linear aliphatic polyesters are based on poly(α-hydroxy acids). Recently, there are two unique groups of linear aliphatic polyesters based on poly(ω-hydroxy acids) and the most famous ones are poly(ε-caprolactone) [Kimura, 1993], poly(β-hydroxybutyrate) (PHB), poly(β-hydroxyvalerate) (PHV) and the copolymers of PHB/PHV (Gross, 1994). Poly(ε-caprolactone) has been used as a comonomer with a variety of glycolide/lactide based linear aliphatic polyesters described earlier. PHB and PHV belong to the family of poly(hydroxyalkanoates) and are mainly produced by prokaryotic types of microorganisms like *Pseudomonas olevorans* or *Alcaligenes eutrophus* through biotechnology. PHB and PHV are the principal energy and carbon storage compounds for these microorganisms and are produced when there are excessive nutrients in the environment. These naturally produced PHB and PHV are stereochemically pure and are isotactic. They could also be synthesized in labs, but the characteristics of steroregularity is lost.

This family of biodegradable polyesters is considered to be environmentally friendly because they are produced from propionic acid and glucose and could be completely degraded to water, biogas, biomass, and humic materials [Gross, 1994]. Their biodegradation requires enzymes. Hence, PHB, PHV, and their copolymers are probably the most important biodegradable polymers for environmental use. However, the biodegradability of this class of linear aliphatic polyesters in human or animal tissues has been questionable. For example, high molecular weight PHB or PHB/PHV fibers do not degrade in tissues or simulated environments over periods of up to six months [Williams, 1990]. The degradability of PHB could be accelerated by γ-irradiation or copolymerization with PHV.

An interesting derivative of PHB, poly(β-malic acid) (PMA), has been synthesized from β-benzyl malolactonate followed by catalytic hydrogenolysis. PMA differs from PHB in that the β-(CH_3) substituent is replaced by $-COOH$ [Kimura, 1993]. The introduction of pendant carboxylic acid group would make PMA more hydrophilic and easier to be absorbed.

42.4 Non-Aliphatic Polyesters Type Biodegradable Polymers

42.4.1 Aliphatic and Aromatic Polycarbonates

The most significant aliphatic polycarbonates are based upon DMTMC and TMC. They are made by the same ring-opening polymerization as glycolide-based biodegradable polyesters. The homopolymers are biocompatible with a controllable rate of biodegradation. Pellets of poly(ethylene carbonate) were absorbed completely in two weeks in the peritoneal cavity of rats. A slight variation of this polycarbonate, that is, poly(propylene carbonate), however, did not show any sign of absorption after two months [Barrows, 1986]. Copolymers of DMTMC/ε-caprolactone and DMTMC/TMC have been reported to have adequate properties for wound closure, tendon prostheses, and vascular grafts. The most important advantage of aliphatic polycarbonates is the neutral pH of the degradation products.

Poly(BPA-carbonates) made from bisphenol A (BPA) and phosgene is non-biodegradable, but an analog of poly(BPA-carbonate) like poly(iminocarbonates) have been shown to degrade in about 200 days [Barrows, 1986]. In general, this class of aromatic polycarbonates takes an undesirably long period to degrade, presumably due to the presence of an aromatic ring which could protect adjacent ester bonds to be hydrolyzed by water or enzymes. Different types of degradation products of this polymer under different pH environments are produced. At pH >7.0, the degradation products of this polymer are BPA, and ammonia and CO_2, while insoluble poly(BPA-carbonate) oligomers were produced with pH <7.0 [Barrows, 1986]. The polymer had good mechanical properties and acceptable tissue biocompatibility. Unfortunately, there is currently no commercial use of this class of polymer in surgery.

42.4.2 Poly(alkylene oxalates) and Copolymers

This class of high crystalline biodegradable polymers was initially developed [Shalaby, 1994] for absorbable sutures and their coating. They consist of $[-ROOC-COO-]_n$ repeating unit where R is $(CH_2)_x$ with x ranging from 4 to 12. R could also be cyclic (1,4-trans-cyclohexanedimethanol) or aromatic (1,4-benzene, 1,3-benzene dimethanol) for achieving higher melting temperature. The biodegradation properties depend on the number of (CH_2) group, x, and the type of R group (i.e., acyclic vs. cyclic or aromatic). In general, a higher number of methylene group and/or the incorporation of cyclic or aromatic R group would retard the biodegradation rate and hence make the polymer absorbed slower. For example, there was no mass of the polymer with $x = 4$ remaining in vivo (rats) after 28 days, while the polymer with $x = 6$ retained 80% of its mass after 42 days in vivo. An isomorphic copolyoxalate consisting of 80% cyclic R group like 1,4-trans-cyclohexanedimethanol and 20% with acyclic R group like 1,6-hexanediol retained 56% of its original mass after 180 days in vivo. By varying the ratio of cyclic to acyclic monomers, copolymers with a wide range of melting temperatures could be made, for example, copolymer of 95/5 ratio of cyclic (i.e., 1,4-trans-cyclohexanedimethanol)/acyclic (i.e., 1,6-hexanediol) monomers had a $T_m = 210°C$, while the copolymer with 5/95 ratio had a $T_m = 69°C$. Poly(alkylene oxalates) with $x = 3$ or 6 had been experimented with as drug control/release devices. The tissue reaction to this class of biodegradable polymers has been minimal.

42.5 Biodegradation Properties of Synthetic Biodegradable Polymers

The reported biodegradation studies of a variety of biodegradable polymeric biomaterials have mainly focused on their tissue biocompatibility, the rate of drug release, or loss of strength and mass. Recently, the degradation mechanisms and the effects of intrinsic and extrinsic factors, such as pH [Chu, 1981, 1982], enzymes [Williams et al., 1977, 1984; Williams, 1979; Chu et al., 1983], γ-irradiation [Campbell et al., 1981; Chu et al., 1982, 1983; Williams et al., 1984; Zhang et al., 1993], electrolytes [Pratt et al., 1993a], cell medium [Chu et al., 1992], annealing treatment [Chu et al., 1988], plasma surface treatment [Loh et al., 1992], external stress [Miller et al., 1984; Chu, 1985a], and polymer morphology [Chu et al., 1989] and on a chemical means to examine the degradation of PGA fibers [Chu et al., 1985] have been systemically examined and the subject has been recently reviewed [Chu, 1985b, 1991, 1995a, b; Hollinger, 1995; Chu et al., 1996]. Table 42.2 is an illustration of structural factors of polymers that could control their degradation [Kimura, 1993]. Besides these series of experimental studies of a variety of factors that could

TABLE 42.2   Structural Factors to Control the Polymer Degradability

Factors	Methods of control
Chemical structure of main chain and side groups	Selection of chemical bonds and functional groups
Aggregation state	Processing, copolymerization
Crystalline state	Polymer blend
Hydrophilic/hydrophobic balance	Copolymerization, introduction of functional groups
Surface area	Micropores
Shape and morphology	Fiber, film, composite

Source: Kimura, Y., 1993, in *Biomedical Applications of Polymeric Materials*, T. Tsuruta, T. Hayashi, K. Kataoka, K. Ishihara, and Y. Kimura, Eds. pp. 164–190. CRC Press, Boca Raton, FL.

affect the degradation of biodegradable polymeric biomaterials, there are two new areas that broaden the above traditional study of biodegradation properties of biodegradable polymers into the frontier of science. They are: theoretical modeling and the role of free radicals.

42.5.1   Theoretical Modeling of Degradation Properties

The most systematic theoretical modeling study of degradation properties of biodegradable biomaterials was reported by Pratt and Chu who used computational chemistry to theoretically model the effects of a variety of substituents which could exert either steric effect and/or inductive effect on the degradation properties of glycolide/lactide based biodegradable polymers [Pratt et al., 1993b, 1994a, b]. This new approach could provide scientists with a better understanding of the relationship between the chemical structure of biodegradable polymers and their degradation behavior at a molecular level. It also could help the future research and development of this class of polymers through the intelligent prediction of structure–property relationships. In those studies, Pratt and Chu examined the affect of various derivatives of linear aliphatic polyester (PGA) and a naturally occurring linear polysaccharide (hyaluronic acid) on their hydrolytic degradation phenomena and mechanisms.

The data showed a decrease in the rate of hydrolysis by about a factor of 106 with isopropyl α-substituents, but nearly a six-fold increase with *t*-butyl α-substituents [Pratt et al., 1993b]. The role of electron donating and electron withdrawing groups on the rate of hydrolytic degradation of linear aliphatic polyesters was also theoretically modeled by Pratt and Chu [Pratt et al., 1994a]. Electron withdrawing substituents a to the carbonyl group would be expected to stabilize the tetrahedral intermediate resulting from hydroxide attack, that is, favoring hydroxide attack but disfavoring alkoxide elimination. Electron releasing groups would be expected to show the opposite effect. Similarly, electronegative substituents on the alkyl portion of the ester would stabilize the forming alkoxide ion and favor the elimination step. Pratt and Chu found that the rate of ester hydrolysis is greatly affected by halogen substituents due primarily to charge delocalization. The data suggest that the magnitude of the inductive effect on the hydrolysis of glycolic esters decreases significantly as the location of the substituent is moved further away from the α-carbon because the inductive effect is very distance-sensitive. In all three locations of substitutions (α, β, and γ), Cl and Br substituents exhibited the largest inductive effect compared to other halogen elements.

Therefore, Pratt and Chu concluded that the rate of ester hydrolysis is greatly affected by both alkyl and halogen substituents due primarily to either steric hindrance or charge delocalization. In the steric effect, alkyl substituents on the glycolic esters cause an increase in activation enthalpies, and a corresponding decrease in reaction rate, up to about three carbon sizes, while bulkier alkyl substituents other than isopropyl make the rate-determining elimination step more facile. It appears that aliphatic polyesters containing a isopropyl groups, or slightly larger linear alkyl groups, such as n-butyl, n-pentyl, etc., would be expected to show a longer strength retention, given the same fiber morphology. In the inductive effect, α-substituents on the acyl portion of the ester favor the formation of the tetrahedral intermediate through charge delocalization, with the largest effect seen with Cl substitution, but retard the rate-determining alkoxide elimination step by stabilizing the tetrahedral intermediate. The largest degree of stabilization is caused by the very electronegative F substituent.

42.5.2 The Role of Free Radicals in Degradation Properties

Salthouse et al. had demonstrated that the biodegradation of synthetic absorbable sutures is closely related to macrophage activity through the close adhesion of macrophage onto the surface of the absorbable sutures [Matlaga et al., 1980]. It is also known that inflammatory cells, particularly leukocytes and macrophages are able to produce highly reactive oxygen species like superoxide ($\cdot O_2^-$) and hydrogen peroxide during inflammatory reactions toward foreign materials [Badwey et al., 1980; Devereux et al., 1991]. These highly reactive oxygen species participate in the biochemical reaction, frequently referred to as a respiratory burst, which is characterized by the one electron reduction of O_2 into superoxide via either NADPH or NADH oxidase as shown below. The reduction of O_2 results in an increase in O_2 uptake and the consumption of glucose.

$$2O_2 + \text{NADPH} \xrightarrow{\text{(NADPH Oxidase)}} 2\,\cdot O_2^- + \text{NADP}^+ + \text{H}^+ \tag{42.1}$$

The resulting superoxide radicals are then neutralized to H_2O_2 via cytoplasmic enzyme superoxide dismutase (SOD).

$$2\,\cdot O_2^- + 2\text{H}^+ \xrightarrow{\text{(SOD)}} \text{H}_2\text{O}_2 + \text{O}_2 \tag{42.2}$$

Very recently, Williams et al. suggested that these reactive oxygen species may be harmful to polymeric implant surfaces through their production of highly reactive, potent, and harmful hydroxyl radicals $\cdot$OH in the presence of metals like iron as shown in the following series of redox reactions [Williams et al., 1991; Ali et al., 1993; Zhong et al., 1994].

$$\cdot \text{O}_2 + \text{M}^{+n} \rightarrow \text{O}_2 + \text{M}^{+(n-1)} \tag{42.3}$$

$$\text{H}_2\text{O}_2 + \text{M}^{+(n-1)} \rightarrow \cdot\text{OH} + \text{HO}^- + \text{M}^{+n} \tag{42.4}$$

The net reaction will be:

$$\cdot \text{O}_2^- + \text{H}_2\text{O}_2 \rightarrow \cdot\text{OH} + \text{HO}^- + \text{O}_2 \tag{42.5}$$

and is often referred to as the metal-catalyzed Haber–Weiss reaction [Haber et al., 1934].

Although the role of free radicals in the hydrolytic degradation of synthetic biodegradable polymers is largely unknown, a very recent study using absorbable sutures like Vicryl in the presence of an aqueous free radical solution prepared from H_2O_2 and ferrous sulfate, $FeSO_4$, raised the possibility of the role of free radicals in the biodegradation of synthetic absorbable sutures [Williams et al., 1991; Zhong et al., 1994]. As shown below, both $\cdot$OH radicals and OH^- are formed in the process of oxidation of Fe^{+2} by H_2O_2 and could exert some influence on the subsequent hydrolytic degradation of Vicryl sutures.

$$\text{Fe}^{+2} + \text{H}_2\text{O}_2 \rightarrow \text{Fe}^{+3} + \cdot\text{OH} + \text{OH}^-$$

SEM results indicated that Vicryl sutures in the presence of free radical solutions exhibited many irregular surface cracks at both 7 and 14 days *in vitro*, while the same sutures in the two controls (H_2O_2 or $FeSO_4$ solutions) did not have these surface cracks. Surprisingly, the presence of surface cracks of Vicryl sutures treated in the free radical solutions did not accelerate the tensile breaking strength-loss as would be expected. Thermal properties of Vicryl sutures under the free radical and 3% H_2O_2 media showed the classical well-known maximum pattern of the change of the level of crystallinity with hydrolysis time. The level of crystallinity of Vicryl sutures peaked at 7 days in both media (free radical and 3% H_2O_2). The time for peak appearance in these two media was considerably earlier than Vicryl sutures in conventional physiological buffer media. Based on the Chu's suggestion of using the time of the appearance of the crystallinity peak as an indicator of degradation rate, it appears that these two media accelerated the degradation of Vicryl sutures when compared with regular physiological buffer solution. Based on their findings, Williams et al. proposed the possible routes of the role of $\cdot OH$ radicals in the hydrolytic degradation of Vicryl sutures [Zhong et al., 1994]. Unfortunately, the possible role of OH^-, one of the byproducts of Fenton reagents ($H_2O_2/FeSO_4$), was not considered in the interpretation of their findings. OH^- species could be more potent than OH toward hydrolytic degradation of synthetic absorbable sutures. This is because hydroxyl anions are the sole species which attack carbonyl carbon of the ester linkages during alkaline hydrolysis. Since an equal amount of $\cdot OH$ and OH^- are generated in Fenton reagents, the observed changes in morphological, mechanical, and thermal properties could be partially attributed to OH^- ions as well as $\cdot OH$ radicals.

Besides hydroxyl radicals, the production of superoxide ions and singlet oxygen during phagocytosis has been well documented [Babior et al., 1973]. Although the role of superoxide in simple organic ester hydrolysis has been known since the 1970s [Forrester et al., 1984, 1987; Johnson, 1976; Mango et al., 1976; San Fillipo et al., 1976], its role in the hydrolytic degradation of synthetic biodegradable polyester-based biomaterials has remained largely unknown. Such an understanding of the superoxide ion role during the biodegradation of foreign materials has become increasing desirable because of the advanced understanding of how the human immune system reacts to foreign materials and the increasing use of synthetic biomaterials for human body repair.

Lee and Chu very recently examined the reactivity of the superoxide ion towards biodegradable biomaterials having an aliphatic polyester structure at different reaction conditions such as temperature, time, and superoxide ion concentration [Lee et al., 1996a]. Due to the extreme reactivity of the superoxide ion, it has been observed that the effect of superoxide ion-induced hydrolytic degradation of PDLLA and PLLA was significant in terms of changes in molecular weights and thermal properties. The superoxide ion-induced fragmentation of PDLLA would result in a mixture of various species with different chain lengths. A combined GPC method with a chemical tagging method revealed that the structure of oligomer species formed during the superoxide-induced degradation of PDLLA and PLLA was linear. The significant reduction in molecular weight of PDLLA by superoxide ion was also evident in the change of thermal properties like T_g. The linear low molecular species (oligomer, trimers, and dimers) in the reaction mixture could act as an internal plasticizer to provide the synergetic effects of lowering T_g by increasing free volume. The effect of the superoxide ion-induced hydrolytic degradation on molecular weight of PLLA was similar to PDLLA but with a much smaller magnitude. The mechanism of simple hydrolysis of ester by superoxide ion proposed by Forrester et al. was subsequently modified to interpret the data obtained from the synthetic biodegradable polymers.

In addition to the PDLLA and PLLA, superoxide ions also have a significant adverse effect on the hydrolytic degradation of synthetic absorbable sutures [Lee et al., 1996c]. A significant reduction in molecular weight has been found along with mechanical and thermal properties of these sutures over a wide range of superoxide ion concentrations, particularly during the first few hours of contact with superoxide ions. For example, the PGA suture lost almost all of its mass at the end of 24 h contact with superoxide ions at 25°C, while the same suture would take at least 50 days in an *in vitro* buffer for a complete mass loss. The surface morphology of these sutures was also altered drastically. The exact mechanism, however, is not fully known yet; Lee et al. suggested the possibility of simultaneous occurrence of several main-chain scissions by three different nucleophilic species.

Lee and Chu also reported that the addition of Fenton agent or hydrogen peroxide to the degradation medium would retard the well-known adverse effect of the conventional γ-irradiation sterilization of synthetic absorbable sutures [Lee et al., 1996a]. They found that these γ-irradiated sutures retained better tensile breaking strength in the Fenton medium than in the regular buffer media. Chu et al. postulated that the γ-irradiation induced α-carbon radicals in these sutures react with the hydroxyl radicals from the Fenton agent medium and hence neutralize the adverse effect of α-carbon radicals on the backbone chain scission. This mechanism is supported by the observed gradual loss of ESR signal of the sutures in the presence of the Fenton agent in the medium.

Instead of the adverse effect of free radicals on the degradation properties of synthetic biodegradable polyesters, Lee and Chu described an innovative approach of covalent bonding nitroxyl radicals onto these biodegradable polymers so that the nitroxyl radical attached polymers would have biological functions similar to nitric oxide [Lee et al., 1996b, 1998]. A preliminary *in vitro* cell culture study of these new biologically active biodegradable polymers indicated that they could retard the proliferation of human smooth muscle cells as native nitric oxide. The full potential of this new class of biologically active biodegradable polymers is currently under investigation by Chu for a variety of therapeutic applications.

42.6   The Role of Linear Aliphatic Biodegradable Polyesters in Tissue Engineering and Regeneration

The use of biodegradable polymers as the temporary scaffolds either to grow cells/tissues *in vitro* for tissue engineering applications or to regenerate tissues *in vivo* has very recently become a highly important aspect of research and development that broadens this class of biodegradable polymers beyond their traditional use in wound closure and drug control/release biomaterials. The scaffolds used in either tissue engineering or regeneration are to provide support for cellular attachment and subsequent controlled proliferation into a predefined shape or form. Obviously, a biodegradable scaffold would be preferred because of the elimination of chronic foreign body reaction and the generation of additional volume for regenerated tissues.

Although many other biodegradable polymers of natural origin like alginate [Atala et al., 1994], hyaluronate [Benedetti et al., 1993; Larsen et al., 1993], collagen [Hirai et al., 1995] and laminin [Dixit, 1994] have been experimented with for such a purpose, synthetic biodegradable polymers of linear aliphatic polyesters like PGA, PLA, and their copolymers [Bowald et al., 1979, 1980; Greisler, 1982; Greisler et al., 1985, 1987a, b, 1988a, b, c, 1991a; Freed et al., 1993; Mikos et al., 1993; Yu et al., 1993, 1994; Mooney et al., 1994, 1995, 1996a, b, c; Kim et al., 1998a, b] have received more attention because of their consistent sources, reproducible properties, means to tailor their properties, and versatility in manufacturing processes.

Biodegradable polymers must be fabricated into stable textile structures before they can be used as the scaffold for tissue engineering or regeneration. The stability of the scaffold structure is important during tissue engineering and regeneration in order to maintain its proper size, shape, or form upon the shear force imposed by the circulating culture media in a bioreactor, the contractile force imposed by the growing cells on the scaffold surface, and other forces like the compression from surrounding tissues.

Kim et al. reported that, although ordinary non-woven PGA matrices have very good porosity (to facilitate diffusion of nutrients) with a high surface to volume ratio (to promote cell attachment and proliferation) and have been used to engineer dental pulp and smooth muscle tissues having comparable biological contents as the native tissues [Kim et al., 1998b; Mooney et al., 1996c], these non-woven PGA matrices could not maintain their original structure during tissue engineering due to the relatively weak non-woven textile structure and stronger contractile force exerted by the attached and proliferated cells/tissues [Kim et al., 1998a]. This led to deformed engineered tissues that may have undesirable properties; for example, the smooth muscle engineered on collagen gels exhibited significant contraction over time [Zeigler et al., 1994; Hirai et al., 1995].

Because of this shortcoming of the existing non-woven PGA matrices, Kim et al. very recently reported the use of PLLA to stabilize the PGA matrices [Kim et al., 1998a]. A 5% w/v PLLA solution in chloroform was sprayed onto PGA non-woven matrices (made of 12 μm diameter PGA fibers) of 97% porosity and either 3 mm or 0.5 mm thickness. The PLLA-impregnated PGA non-wovens could be subjected to additional heat treatment at 195°C to enhance their structural stability further. Figure 42.3 shows

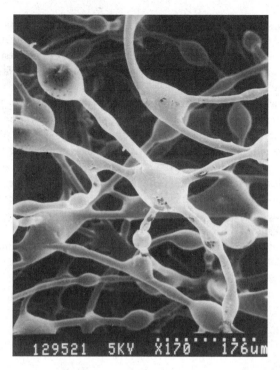

FIGURE 42.3 Scanning electron micrograph of the exterior of PLLA-impregnated and annealed PGA matrix. (From Kim, B.S. and Mooney, D.J., 1998a. *J. Biomed. Mater. Res.*, 41: 322–332. With permission).

the morphology of such a heat annealed PLLA-impregnated PGA non-woven matrix [Kim et al., 1998]. The PLLA was deposited mainly on the crosspoints of PGA fibers and hence interlocked the possible sliding of PGA fibers upon external force. Depending on the amount of PLLA used and subsequent heat treatment, the resulting PLLA-impregnated PGA non-woven matrices had an increase in compressive modulus of 10- to 35-fold when compared with the original PGA non-woven. The PLLA-impregnated PGA non-woven matrices also retained their initial volume (101 ± 4%) and about same shape as the original during the seven weeks in culture, while the untreated PGA non-woven exhibited severe distortion in shape and contracted about 5% of its original volume. Since PLLA is well-known to degrade at a much slower rate than PGA, its presence on the PGA fibers surface would be expected to make the treated PGA non-woven matrices degrade at a much slower rate than the untreated PGA non-woven. For example, the PLLA treated PGA non-woven retained about 80% of its initial mass, while the untreated PGA control had only 10% at the end of the seven week culture.

Linear aliphatic polyesters like PGA, its lactide copolymer, and poly-p-dioxanone have also been fabricated into both woven and knitted forms for the *in vivo* regeneration of blood vessels in animals [Bowald et al., 1979, 1980; Greisler, 1982; Greisler et al., 1985, 1987a, 1988c, 1991b; Yu et al., 1993, 1994]. The published results from a variety of animals like dogs and rabbits indicate that full-wall healing with pseudo-endothelial lining was observed. This class of synthetic biodegradable polymers are promising candidates for the regeneration of vascular tissue.

These encouraging findings were believed to be associated with the intense macrophage/biomaterial interactions. [Greisler, 1988a; Greisler et al., 1989]. This interaction leads to a differential activation of the macrophage which, in turn, yields different macrophage products being released into the microenvironment [Greisler et al., 1991b]. Greisler et al. [1988b] have documented active stimulatory or inhibitory effects of various bioresorbable and non-resorbable materials on myofibroblast, vascular smooth muscle cell, and endothelial cell regeneration, and has shown a transinterstitial migration to be their source when lactide/glycolide copolymeric prostheses are used. The rate of tissue ingrowth parallels the kinetics of macrophage mediated prosthetic resorption in all lactide/glycolides studied [Gresler, 1982; Greisler et al., 1985, 1987a, 1988a]. Macrophage phagocytosis of the prosthetic material is observed histologically as early as one week following implantation of a rapidly resorbed material, such as PGA or polyglactin 910 (PG910), and is followed by an extensive increase in the myofibroblast population and neovascularization of the inner capsules [Greisler, 1982; Greisler et al., 1985, 1986]. Autoradiographic analyses using tritiated thymidine demonstrated a significantly increased mitotic index within these inner capsular cells, that mitotic index paralleling the course of prosthetic resorption [Greisler et al., 1991a]. Polyglactin 910, for example, resulted in a mitotic index of $20.1 \pm 16.6\%$ three weeks following implantation, progressively decreasing to $1.2 \pm 1.3\%$ after 12 weeks. The more slowly resorbed polydioxanone prostheses demonstrated a persistently elevated mitotic index, $7.1 \pm 3.8\%$, 12 weeks after implantation, a time in which the prosthetic material was still being resorbed. By contrast Dacron never yielded greater than a $1.2 \pm 1.3\%$ mitotic index [Greisler et al., 1991a]. These mitotic indices correlated closely with the slopes of the inner capsule thickening curves suggesting that myofibroblast proliferation contributed heavily to this tissue deposition.

Therefore, the degradation property of synthetic biodegradable polymers somehow relates to macrophage activation which subsequently leads to the macrophage production of the required growth factors that initiate tissue regeneration. Different degradation properties of synthetic biodegradable polymers would thus be expected to result in different levels of macrophage activation, i.e., different degrees of tissue regeneration.

Defining Terms

Biodegradation: Materials that could be broken down by nature either through hydrolytic mechanisms without the help of enzymes and/or enzymatic mechanism. It is loosely associated with absorbable, erodable, resorbable.

Tissue Engineering: The ability to regenerate tissue through the help of artifical materials and devices.

References

Ali, S.A.M., Zhong, S.P., Doherty, P.J., and Williams, D.F., 1993. Mechanisms of polymer degradation in implantable devices. I. Poly(caprolactone). *Biomaterials*, 14: 648.

Atala, A., Kim, W., Paige, K.T., Vancanti, C.A., and Retil, A., 1994. Endoscopic treatment of vesicoureterall reflux with a chondrocye-alginate suspension. *J. Urol.*, 152: 641–643.

Babior, B.M., Kipnes R.S., and Cumutte, J.T., 1973. Biological defense mechanisms. The production by leukocytes of superoxide, A potential bactercidal agent. *J. Clin. Invest.*, 52: 741.

Badwey, J.A. and Kamovsky, M.L., 1980. Active oxygen species and the functions of phagocytic leucocytes. *Ann. Rev. Biochem.*, 49: 695.

Barrows, T.H., 1986, Degradable implant materials: a review of synthetic absorbable polymers and their applications. *Clin. Mater.*, 1: 233–257.

Barrows, T.H., 1994. Bioabsorbable poly(ester-amides). In: *Biomedical Polymers: Designed-to-Degrade Systems*, S.W. Shalaby, Ed., Hanser, New York, chap. 4.

Benedetti, L., Cortivo, R., Berti, T., Berti, A., and Pea, F., 1993. Biocompatibility and biodegradation of different hyaluronan derivatives (Hyaff) implanted in rats. *Biomaterials*, 14: 1154–1160.

Bezwada, R.S., Jamiolkowski, D.D., Lee, I.Y., Agarwal, V., Persivale, J., Trenka-Benthin, S., Erneta, M., Suryadevara, J., Yang, A., and Liu, S., 1995. Monocryl suture: a new ultra-pliable absorbable monofilament suture, *Biomaterials*, 16: 1141–1148.

Bezwada, R.S., Shalaby, S.W., Newman, H.D. Jr., and Kafrawy, A., 1990. Bioabsorbable copolymers of p-dioxanone and lactide for surgical devices. *Trans. Soc. for Biomater.* vol. XIII, p. 194.

Bostman, O., Hirvensalo, E., Vainionpaa, S. et al., 1990. Degradable polyglycolide rods for the internal fixation of displaced bimalleolar fractures. *Intern. Orthop. (Germany)*, 14: 1–8.

Bowald, S., Busch, C., and Eriksson, I., 1979. Arterial regeneration following polyglactin 910 suture mesh grafting, *Surgery*, 86: 722–729.

Bowald, S., Busch, C., and Eriksson, I., 1980. Absorbable material in vascular prosthesis. *Acta. Chir. Scand.*, 146: 391–395.

Brandrup, J., and Immergut, E.H., 1975. *Polymer Handbook*, 2nd ed., John Wiley & Sons, New York.

Campbell, N.D., and Chu, C.C., 1981. The effect of γ-irradiation on the biodegradation of polyglycolic acid synthetic sutures, the Tensile Strength Study. *27th International Symposium on Macromolecules*, Abstracts of Communications, Vol. II, pp. 1348–1352, Strasbourg, France, July 6–9, 1981.

Casey, D.J. and Roby, M.S., 1984. Synthetic copolymer surgical articles and method of manufacturing the same. US Patent 4,429,080, American Cyanamid.

Chatani, Y., Suehiro, K., Okita, Y., Tadokoro, H., and Chujo, K., 1968. Structural studies of polyesters, I. Crystal structure of polyglycolide. *Die Makromol. Chem.*, 113: 215–229.

Chu, C.C., 1981. The *In-vitro* degradation of poly(glycolic acid) sutures: effect of pH. *J. Biomed. Mater. Res.*, 15: 795–804.

Chu, C.C., 1982. The effect of pH on the *in vitro* degradation of poly(glycolide lactide) copolymer absorbable sutures. *J. Biomed. Mater. Res.*, 16: 117–124.

Chu, C.C., 1985a. Strain-accelerated hydrolytic degradation of synthetic absorbable sutures. In: *Surgical Research Recent Development*, C.W. Hall, Ed., Pergamon Press, San Antonio, Texas.

Chu, C.C., 1985b. The Degradation and biocompatibility of suture materials. In: *CRC Critical Reviews in Biocompat.*, D.F. Williams, Ed., Vol. 1 (3), CRC Press, Boca Raton, FL, pp. 261–322.

Chu, C.C., 1991. Recent advancements in suture fibers for wound closure. In: *High-Tech Fibrous Materials: Composites, Biomedical Materials, Protective Clothing, and Geotextiles*, T.L. Vigo and A.F. Turbak, Eds., ACS Symposium Series #457, American Chemical Society, Washington, D.C. pp. 167–213.

Chu, C.C., 1995a. Biodegradable suture materials: intrinsic and extrinsic factors affecting biodegradation phenomena. In: *Handbook of Biomaterials and Applications*, D.L. Wise, D.E. Altobelli, E.R. Schwartz, M. Yszemski, J.D. Gresser, and D.J. Trantolo, Eds., Marcel Dekker, New York.

Chu, C.C. 1995b. Biodegradable suture materials: intrinsic and extrinsic factors affecting biodegradation. In: *Encyclopedic Handbook of Biomaterials and Applications*, Part A: Materials, Vol. 1, D.L. Wise, Ed., Marcel Dekker, chap. 17, pp. 543–688.

Chu, C.C. and Browning, A., 1988. The study of thermal and gross morphologic properties of polyglycolic acid upon annealing and degradation treatments. *J. Biomed. Mater. Res.*, 22: 699–712.

Chu, C.C. and Campbell, N.D., 1982. Scanning electron microscope study of the hydrolytic degradation of poly(glycolic acid) suture. *J. Biomed. Mater. Res.*, 16: 417–430.

Chu, C.C., Hsu, A., Appel, M., and Beth, M. 1992. The effect of macrophage cell media on the *in vitro* hydrolytic degradation of synthetic absorbable sutures. *4th World Biomaterials Congress*, April 27–May 1, 1992, Berlin, Germany.

Chu, C.C. and Kizil, Z., 1989. The effect of polymer morphology on the hydrolytic degradation of synthetic absorbable sutures. *3rd International ITV Conference on Biomaterials — Medical Textiles*, Stuttgart, W. Germany, June 14–16, 1989.

Chu, C.C. and Louie, M., 1985. A chemical means to study the degradation phenomena of polyglycolic acid absorbable polymer. *J. Appl. Polym. Sci.*, 30: 3133–3141.

Chu, C.C., von Fraunhofer, J.A., and Greisler, H.P., 1996. *Wound Closure Biomaterials and Devices*. CRC Press, Boca Raton, FL.

Chu, C.C. and Williams, D.F., 1983. The effect of γ-irradiation on the enzymatic degradation of polyglycolic acid absorbable sutures. *J. Biomed. Mater. Res.*, 17: 1029.

Chu, C.C., Zhang, L., and Coyne, L., 1995. Effect of irradiation temperature on hydrolytic degradation properties of synthetic absorbable sutures and polymers. *J. Appl. Polym. Sci.* 56: 1275–1294.

Chujo, K., Kobayashi, H., Suzuki, J., Tokuhara, S., and Tanabe, M., 1967a. Ring-opening polymerization of glycolide. *Die Makromol. Chemi.*, 100: 262–266.

Chujo, K., Kobayashi, H., Suzuki, J., and Tokuhara, S., 1967b. Physical and chemical characteristics of polyglycolide. *Die Makromol. Chem.*, 100: 267–270.

Daniels, A.U., Taylor, M.S., Andriano, K.P., and Heller, J., 1992. Toxicity of absorbable polymers proposed for fracture fixation devices. *Trans. 38th Ann. Mtg. Orthop. Res. Soc.*, 17:88.

Devereux, D.F., O'Connell, S.M., Liesch, J.B., Weinstein, M., and Robertson, F.M., 1991. Induction of leukocyte activation by meshes surgically implanted in the peritoneal cavity. *Am. J. Surg.*, 162:243.

Dixit, V., 1994. Development of a bioartificial liver using isolated hepatocytes. *Artif. Organs*, 18:371–384.

Eitenmüller, K.L., Schmickal, G.T., and Muhr, G., 1989. Die versorgung von sprunggelenksfrakturen unter verwendung von platten und schrauben aus resorbierbarem polymer material. Presented at Jahrestagung der Deutschen Gesellschaft für Unfallheilkunde, Berlin, November 1989.

Forrester, A.R. and Purushotham, V., 1987. Reactions of carboxylic acid derivatives with superoxide. *J. Chem. Soc. Perkin Trans.* 1,945.

Forrester, A.R. and Purushotham, V., 1984. Mechnism of hydrolysis of esters by superoxide. *J. Chem. Soc., Chem. Commun.*, 1505.

Fredericks, R.J., Melveger, A.J., and Dolegiewitz, L.J., 1984. Morphological and structural changes in a copolymer of glycolide and lactide occurring as a result of hydrolysis. *J. Polym. Sci. Phy. Ed.* 22: 57–66.

Freed, L.E., Marquis, J.C., Nohia, A., Emmanual, J., Mikos, A.G., and Langer, R., 1993. Neocartilage formation *in vitro* and *in vivo* using cells cultured on synthetic biodegradable polymers. *J. Biomed. Mater. Res.*, 27: 11–23.

Fukuzaki, H., Yoshida, M., Asano, M., Aiba, Y., and Kumakura, M., 1989. Direct copolymerization of glycolic acid with lactones in the absence of catalysts. *Eur. Polym. J.*, 26: 457–461.

Fukuzaki, H., Yoshida, M., Asano, M., Kumakura, M., Mashimo, T., Yuasa, H., Imai, K., Yamandka, H., Kawaharada, U., and Suzuki, K., 1991. A new biodegradable copolymer of glycolic acid and lactones with relatively low molecular weight prepared by direct copolycondensation in the absence of catalysts. *J. Biomed. Mater. Res.*, 25: 315–328.

Gogolewski, S. and Pennings, A.J., 1983. Resorbable materials of poly(Llactide). II. Fibres spun from solutions of poly(Llactide) in good solvents. *J. Appl. Polym. Sci.*, 28: 1045–1061.

Greisler, H.P., 1982. Arterial regeneration over absorbable prostheses. *Arch. Surg.*, 117: 1425-1431.

Greisler, H.P., 1988a. Macrophage-biomaterial interactions with bioresorbable vascular prostheses. *Transactions of ASAIO*, 34: 1051–1059.

Greisler, H.P., 1991a. Macrophage activation in bioresorbable vascular grafts. In: *Vascular Endothelium: Physiological Basis of Clinical Problems*. J.D. Catravas, A.D. Callow, C.N. Gillis, and U. Ryan, Eds., Plenum Publishing, New York, NATO Advanced Study Institute. pp. 253–254.

Greisler, H.P., Dennis, J.W., Endean, E.D., Ellinger, J., Friesel, R., and Burgess, W., 1989. Macrophage/Biomaterial interactions: The stiulation of endotherlialization. *J. Vasc. Surg.*, 9: 588–593.

Greisler, H.P., Dennis, J.W., Endean, E.D., and Kim, D.U., 1988b. Derivation of neointima of vascular grafts. *Circ. Suppl. I*, 78: I6–I12.

Greisler, H.P., Ellinger, J., Schwarcz, T.H., Golan, J., Raymond, R.M., and Kim, D.U., 1987a. Arterial regeneration over polydioxanone prostheses in the rabbit. *Arch. Surg.*, 122: 715–721.

Greisler, H.P., Endean, E.D., Klosak, J.J., Ellinger, J., Dennis, J.W., Buttle, K., and Kim, D.U., 1988c. Polyglactin 910/polydioxanone bicomponent totally resorbable vascular prostheses. *J. Vasc. Surg.*, 7: 697–705.

Greisler, H.P., Kim, D.U., Dennis, J.W., Klosak, J.J., Widerborg, K.A., Endean, E.D., Raymond, R.M., and Ellinger, J., 1987b. Compound polyglactin 910/polypropylene small vessel prostheses. *J. Vasc. Surg.*, 5: 572–583.

Greisler, H.P., Kim, D.U., Price, J.B., and Voorhees, A.B., 1985. Arterial regenerative activity after prosthetic implantation. *Arch. Surg.*, 120: 315–323.

Greisler, H.P., Schwarcz, T.H., Ellinger, J., and Kim, D.U.,1986. Dacron inhibition of arterial regenerative activity. *J. Vasc. Surg.*, 747–756.

Greisler, H.P., Tattersall, C.W., Kloask, J.J. et al., 1991b. Partially bioresorbable vascular grafts in dogs. *Surgery*, 110: 645–655.

Gross, R.A., 1994. Bacterial polyesters: structural variability in microbial synthesis. In: *Biomedical Polymers: Designed-to-Degrade Systems*, S.W. Shalaby, Ed., chap. 7, Hanser, New York.

Haber, F. and Weiss, J., 1934. The catalytic decomposition of hydrogen peroxide by iron salts. *Proc. R. Soc. Lond.*, A, 147: 332.

Helder, J., Feijen, J., Lee, S.J., and Kim, W., 1986. Copolyemrs of DL-lactic acid and glycine. *Makromol. Chem. Rapid. Commun.*, 7: 193.

Hirai, J. and Matsuda, T., 1995. Self-organized, tubular hybrid vascular tissue composed of vascular cells and collagen for low pressure-loaded venous system, *Cell Transpl.*, 4: 597–608.

Hofmann, G.O., 1992. Biodegradable implants in orthopaedic surgery-A review of the state of the art. *Clin. Mater.*, 10: 75.

Hollinger, J.O., 1995. *Biomedical Applications of Synthetic Biodegradable Polymers*, CRC Press, Boca Raton, FL.

Jamiokowski, D.D. and Shalaby, S.W., 1991. A polymeric radiostabilizer for absorbable polyesters. In: Radiation Effect of Polymers, R.L. Clough and S.W. Shalaby, Eds., chap. 18, pp. 300–309. ACS Symposium Series # 475, ACS, Washington, D.C.

Johnson, R.A., 1976. *Tetrahedron Lett.*, 331.

Katsarava, R., Beridze, V., Arabuli, N. Kharadze, D., Chu, C.C., and Won, C.Y., Amino acid based bioanalogous polymers. Synthesis and study of regular poly(ester amide)s based on bis(α-amino acid) α, ω-alkylene diesters and aliphatic dicarboxylic acids. *J. Polym. Sci. Chem.* (in press).

Katz, A., Mukherjee, D.P., Kaganov, A.L., and Gordon, S., 1985. A new synthetic monofilament absorbable suture made from polytrimethylene carbonate. *Surg. Gynecol. Obstet.*, 161: 213–222.

Kim, B.S. and Mooney, D.J., 1998a. Engineering smooth muscle tissue with a predefined structure. *J. Biomed. Mater. Res.*, 41: 322.

Kim, B.S., Putman, A.J., Kulik, T.J., and Mooney, D.J., 1998b. Optimizing seeding and culture methods to engineer smooth muscle tissue on biodegradable polymer matrices. *Biotechnol. Bioeng.*, 57: 64–54.

Kimura, Y., 1993. Biodegradable polymers. In: *Biomedical Applications of Polymeric Materials*, T. Tsuruta, T. Hayashi, K. Kataoka, K. Ishihara, and Y. Kimura, Eds., pp. 164–190. CRC Press, Inc., Boca Raton, FL.

Koelmel, D.F., Jamiokowski, D.D., Shalaby, S.W., and Bezwada, R.S., 1991. Low modulus radiation sterilizable monofilament sutures. *Polym. Prepr.*, 32: 235–236.

Larsen, N.E., Pollak, C.T., Reiner, K., Leshchiner, E., and Balazs, E.A., 1993. Hylan gel biomaterial: Dermal and immunologic compatibility. *J. Biomed. Meter. Res.*, 27: 1129–1134.

Lee, K.H. and Chu, C.C., 1996a. The role of free radicals in hydrolytic degradation of absorable polymeric biomaterials. *5th World Biomaterials Congress*, Toronto, Canada, May 29–June 2.

Lee, K.H. and Chu, C.C., 1998. Molecular design of biologically active biodegradable polymers for biomedical applications. *Macromol. Symp.*, 130: 71.

Lee, K.H., Chu, C.C., and Fred, J., 1996b. Aminoxyl-containing radical spin in polymers and copolymers. U.S. Patent 5,516,881, May 16.

Lee, K.H., Won, C.Y., and Chu, C.C., 1996c. Hydrolysis of absorable polymeric biomaterials by superoxide. *5th World Biomaterials Congress*, Toronto, Canada, May 29–June 2.

Leenslag, J.W. and Pennings, A.J., 1984. Synthesis of high-molecular weight poly(L-lactide) initiated with tin 2-ethylhexanoate. *Makromol. Chem.*, 188: 1809–1814.

Li, S., Anjard, S., Tashkov, I., and Vert, M., 1998a. Hydrolytic degradation of PLA/PEO/PLA triblock copolymers prepared in the presence of Zn metal or CaH$_2$, *Polymer*, 39: 5421–5430.

Li, Y. and Kissel, T., 1998b. Synthesis, characteristics and *in vitro* degradation of star-block copolymers consisting of L-lactide, glycolide and branched multi-arm poly(ethylene oxide). *Polymer*, 39: 4421–4427.

Loh, I.H., Chu, C.C., and Lin, H.L., 1992. Plasma surface modification of synthetic absorbable fibers for wound closure. *J. Appl. Biomater.* 3: 131–146.

Magno, F. and Bontempelli, G., 1976. *J. Electroanal. Chem.*, 68: 337.

Matlaga, V.F. and Salthouse, T.N., 1980. Electron microscopic observations of polyglactin 910 suture sites, In *First World Biomaterials Congress*, Abstr., Baden, Austria, April 8–12, 2.

Mikos, A.G., Sarakinos, G., Leite, S.M., Vacanti, J.P., and Langer, R., 1993. Laminated three-dimensional biodegradable forms for use in tissue engineering. *Biomaterials*, 14: 323–330.

Miller, N.D. and Williams, D.F., 1984. The *in vivo* and *in vitro* degradation of poly(glycolic acid) suture material as a function of applied strain. *Biomaterials*, 5: 365–368.

Mooney, D.J., Baldwin, D.F., Vacanti, J.P., and Langer, R., 1996a. Novel approach to fabricate porous sponges of poly(D,L-lactic-co-glycolic acid) without the use of organic solvents. *Biomaterials*, 17: 1417–1422.

Mooney, D.J., Breuer, C., McNamara, K., Vacanti, J.P., and Langer, R., 1995. Fabricating tubular devices from polymers of lactic and glycolic acid for tissue engineering. *Tissue Eng.*, 1: 107–118.

Mooney, D.J., Mazzoni, C.L., Breuer, K., McNamara, J.P., Vacanti, J.P., and Langer, R., 1996b. Stabilized polyglycolic acid fibre-based tubes for tissue engineering. *Biomaterials*, 17: 115–124.

Mooney, D.J., Organ, G., Vacanti, J.P., and Langer, R., 1994. Design and fabrication of biodegradable polymer devices to engineer tubular tissue. *Cell Transplant*, 3: 203–210.

Mooney, D.J, Powell, C., Piana, J., and Rutherford, B., 1996c. Engineering dental pulp-like tissue *in vitro*. *Biotechnol. Prog.*, 12: 865–868.

Nathan, A. and Kohn, J., 1994. Amino acid derived polymers. In: *Biomedical Polymers: Designed-to-Degrade Systems*, S.W. Shalaby, chap. 5. Hanser Publishers, New York.

Park, K., Shalaby, W.S.W., and Park. H., 1993. *Biodegradable Hydrogels for Drug Delivery*, Technomic Publishing, Lancaster, PA.

Pratt, L., Chu, A., Kim, J., Hsu, A., and Chu, C.C., 1993a. The effect of electrolytes on the *in vitro* hydrolytic degradation of synthetic biodegradable polymers: mechanical properties, thermodynamics and molecular modeling. *J. Polym Sci. Chem. Ed.*, 31: 1759–1769.

Pratt, L. and Chu, C.C., 1993b. Hydrolytic degradation of α-substituted polyglycolic acid: a semi-empirical computational study. *J. Comput. Chem.*, 14: 809–817.

Pratt, L. and Chu, C.C., 1994a. The effect of electron donating and electron withdrawing substituents on the degradation rate of bioabsorbable polymers: a semi-empirical computational study. *J. Mol. Struct.*, 304: 213–226.

Pratt, L. and Chu, C.C., 1994b. A computational study of the hydrolysis of degradable polysaccharide biomaterials: substituent effects on the hydrolytic mechanism. *J. Comput. Chem.*, 15: 241–248.

Puelacher, W.C., Mooney, D., Langer, R., Upton, J., Vacanti, J.P., and Vananti, C.A., 1994. Design of nasoseptal cartilage replacements sunthesized from biodegradable polymers and chondrocytes. *Biomaterials*, 15: 774–778.

San Fillipo, Jr, J., Romano, L.J., Chem, C.I., and Valentine, J.S., 1976. Cleavage of esters by superoxide. *J. Org. Chem.*, 4: 586.

Shalaby, S.W., 1994. *Biomedical Polymers: Designed-to-Degrade Systems*, Hanser Publishers, New York.

Shieh, S.J., Zimmerman, M.C., and Parsons, J.R., 1990. Preliminary characterization of bioresorbable and nonresorbable synthetic fibers for the repair of soft tissue injuries. *J. Biomed. Mater. Res.*, 24: 789–808.

Sugnuma, J., Alexander, H., Traub, J., and Ricci, J.L., 1992. Biological response of intramedullary bone to poly-l-lactic acid. In: *Tissue-Inducing Biomater*, L.G. Cima and E.S. Ron, Eds., *Mater. Res. Soc. Sump. Proc.*, 252: 339–343.

Tunc, D.C., 1983. A high strength absorbable polymer for internal bone fixation. *Trans. Soc. Biomater.*, 6: 47.

Vert, M., Feijen, J., Albertsson, A., Scott, G., and Chiellini, E., 1992. *Biodegradable Polymers and Plastics*, Royal Society of Chemistry, Cambridge, England.

Williams, D.F., 1979. Some observations on the role of cellular enzymes in the In vivo degradation of polymers. *ASTM Spec. Tech. Publ.*, 684: 61–75.

Williams, D.F., 1990. Biodegradation of medical polymers. In: *Concise Encyclopedia of Medical and Dental Materials*, D.F. Williams, Ed., pp. 69–74. Pergamon Press, New York.

Williams, D.F. and Mort, E., 1977. Enzyme-accelerated hydrolysis of polyglycolic acid. *J. Bioeng.* 1: 231–238.

Williams, D.F. and Chu, C.C., 1984. The effects of enzymes and gamma irradiation on the tensile strength and morphology of poly(p-dioxanone) fibers. *J. Appl. Polym. Sci.*, 29: 1865–1877.

Williams, D.F. and Zhong, S.P., 1991. Are free radicals involved in the biodegradation of implanted polymers. *Advanced Materials*, 3: 623.

Winet, H. and Hollinger, J.O., 1993. Incorporation of polylactide–polyglycolide in a cortical defect: neoosteogenesis in a bone chamber. *J. Biomed. Mater. Res.*, 27: 667–676.

Wise, D.L., Fellmann, T.D., Sanderson, J.E., and Wentworth, R.L., 1979. Lactic/Glycolic acid polymers. In: *Drug Carriers in Biology and Medicine*, G. Gregoriadis, Ed., pp. 237–270. Academic Press, New York.

Yu, T.J. and Chu, C.C., 1993. Bicomponent vascular grafts consisting of synthetic biodegradable fibers. Part I. *In vitro* study. *J. Biomed. Mater. Res.*, 27: 1329–1339.

Yu, T.J., Ho, D.M., and Chu, C.C., 1994. Bicomponent vascular grafts consisting of synthetic biodegradable fibers. Part II. In vivo Healing Response. *J. Investigative Surg.* 7: 195–211.

Zhang, L., Loh, I.H., and Chu, C.C., 1993. A combined γ-irradiation and plasma deposition treatment to achieve the ideal degradation properties of synthetic absorbable polymers. *J. Biomed. Mater. Res.*, 27: 1425–1441.

Zhong, S.P., Doherty, P.J., and Williams, D.F., 1994. A preliminary study on the free radical degradation of glycolic acid/lactic acid copolymer. *Lastics, Rubber and Composites Processing and Application*, 21: 89.

Ziegler, T. and Nerem, R.M., 1994. Tissue engineering a blood vessel: Regulation of vascular biology by mechanical stress. *J. Cell. Biochem.*, 56: 204–209.

Further Information

Several recent books have very comprehensive descriptions of a variety of biodegradable polymeric biomaterials, their synthesis, physical, chemical, mechanical, biodegradable, and biological properties.

Barrows, T.H., 1986, Degradable implant materials: a review of synthetic absorbable polymers and their applications, *Clin. Mater.*, 1: 233–257.

Chu, C.C., Biodegradable suture materials: intrinsic and extrinsic factors affecting biodegradation phenomena, In: *Handbook of Biomaterials and Applications*, D.L. Wise, D.E. Altobelli, E.R. Schwartz, M. Yszemski, J.D. Gresser, and D.J. Trantolo, Eds., Marcel Dekker, New York (1995).

Chu, C.C., von Fraunhofer, J.A., and Greisler, H.P., 1996. *Wound Closure Biomaterials and Devices*. CRC Press, Boca Raton, FL.

Hollinger, J.O., Ed., 1995. *Biomedical Applications of Synthetic Biodegradable Polymers*, CRC Press, Boca Raton, FL.

Kimura, Y., 1993, Biodegradable polymers, In: *Biomedical Applications of Polymeric Materials*, T. Tsuruta, T. Hayashi, K. Kataoka, K. Ishihara, and Y. Kimura, Eds., pp. 164–190. CRC Press, Inc., Boca Raton, FL.

Park, K., Shalaby, W.S.W., and Park. H., 1993. *Biodegradable Hydrogels for Drug Delivery*, Technomic Publishing, Lancaster, PA.

Shalaby, S.W., 1994. *Biomedical Polymers: Designed-to-Degrade Systems*, Hanser Publishers, New York.

Vert, M., Feijen, J., Albertsson, A., Scott, G. and Chiellini, E., 1992. *Biodegradable Polymers and Plastics*, Royal Society of Chemistry, Cambridge, England.

The review by Barrows is brief with an emphasis on their applications with an extensive lists of patents. The book and chapter by Chu et al. focuses on the most successful use of biodegradable polymers in medicine, namely wound closure biomaterials like sutures. It is so far the most comprehensive review of all aspects of biodegradable wound closure biomaterials with very detailed chemical, physical, mechanical, biodegradable, and biological information. The chapter by Kimura is an overview of the subject with some interesting new polymers. The chapter includes both enzymatically degradable natural polymers and non-enzymatically degradable synthetic polymers. The biodegradable hydrogel book by Park et al. is the only book available that focuses on hydrogel. Probably the most broad coverage of biodegradable polymeric biomaterials is the very recent book edited by Shalaby. It has 8 chapters and covers almost all commercially and experimentally available biodegradable polymers. The book edited by Vert et al. is based on the *Proceedings of the 2nd International Scientific Workshop on Biodegradable Polymers and Plastics* held in Montpellier, France in November 1991. The book covers both medical and non-medical applications of biodegradable polymers. It has broader coverage of biodegradable polymers with far more chapters than Shalaby's book, but its chapters are shorter and less comprehensive than Shalaby's book which is far more focused on biomedical use.

Topics of biodegradable polymeric biomaterials can also be found in *Journal of Biomedical Materials Research, Journal of Applied Biomaterials, Biomaterials, Journal of Biomaterials Science: Polymer Ed., Journal of Applied Polymer Science, Journal of Materials Science,* and *Journal Polymer Science.*

43

Biologic Biomaterials: Tissue-Derived Biomaterials (Collagen)

Shu-Tung Li
Collagen Matrix, Inc.

43.1 Structure and Properties of Collagen and Collagen-Rich Tissues

43.1.1 Structure of Collagen

Collagen is a multifunctional family of proteins of unique structural characteristics. It is the most abundant and ubiquitous protein in the body, its functions ranging from serving crucial biomechanical functions in bone, skin, tendon, and ligament to controlling cellular gene expressions in development [Nimni and Harkness, 1988]. Collagen molecules like all proteins are formed *in vivo* by enzymatic regulated step-wise polymerization reaction between amino and carboxyl groups of amino acids, where R is a side group of an amino acid residue.

$$(\overset{\overset{\text{O}}{\|}}{-\text{C}} - \overset{\overset{\text{H}}{|}}{\text{N}} - \overset{\overset{\text{H}}{|}}{\underset{\underset{\text{R}}{|}}{\text{C}}} -)_n \tag{43.1}$$

The simplest amino acid is **glycine** (Gly) (R=H), where a hypothetical flat sheet organization of polyglycine molecules can form and be stabilized by intermolecular hydrogen bonds (Figure 43.1a). However, when R is a large group as in most other amino acids, the stereochemical constraints frequently force the **polypeptide** chain to adapt a less constraining conformation by rotating the bulky R groups away from the crowded interactions, forming a helix, where the large R groups are directed toward the surface of the helix (Figure 43.1b). The hydrogen bonds are allowed to form within a helix between the hydrogen attached to nitrogen in one amino acid residue and the oxygen attached to a second amino acid residue. Thus, the final conformation of a protein, which is directly related to its function, is governed primarily by the amino acid sequence of the particular protein.

Collagen is a protein comprised of three polypeptides (α chains), each having a general amino acid sequence of $(-\text{Gly}-X-Y-)_n$, where X is any other amino acid and is frequently **proline** (Pro) and Y is any other amino acid and is frequently *hydroxyproline* (Hyp). A typical amino acid composition of collagen is shown in Table 43.1. The application of helical diffraction theory to high-angle collagen x-ray

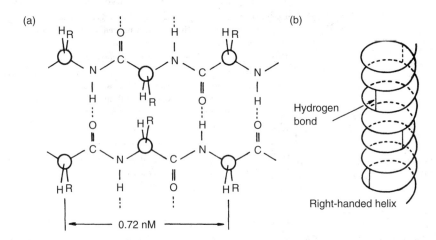

FIGURE 43.1   (a) Hypothetical flat sheet structure of a protein. (b) Helical arrangement of a protein chain.

TABLE 43.1   Amino Acid Content of Collagen

Amino Acids	Content, residues/1000 residues[a]
Gly	334
Pro	122
Hyp	96
Acid polar (Asp, Glu, Asn)	124
Basic polar (Lys, Arg, His)	91
Other	233

[a]Reported values are average values of 10 different determinations for tendon tissue.

Source: Eastoe,   J.E.   (1967).   *Treatise   on   Collagen*, G.N. Ramachandran (Ed.), pp. 1–72, Academic Press, New York. With permission.

diffraction pattern [Rich and Crick, 1961] and the stereochemical constraints from the unusual amino acid composition [Eastoe, 1967] led to the initial triple-helical model and subsequent modified triple helix of the collagen molecule. Thus, collagen can be broadly defined as a protein which has a typical triple helix extending over the major part of the molecule. Within the triple helix, glycine must be present as every third amino acid, and proline and hydroxyproline are required to form and stabilize the triple helix.

To date, 19 proteins can be classified as collagen [Fukai et al., 1994]. Among the various collagens, type I collagen is the most abundant and is the major constituent of bone, skin, ligament, and tendon. Due to the abundance and ready accessibility of these tissues, they have been frequently used as a source for the preparation of collagen. This chapter will not review the details of the structure of the different collagens. The readers are referred to recent reviews for a more in-depth discussion of this subject [Nimni, 1988; van der Rest et al., 1990; Fukai et al., 1994; Brodsky and Ramshaw, 1997]. It is, however, of particular relevance to review some salient structural features of the type I collagen in order to facilitate the subsequent discussions of properties and its relation to biomedical applications.

A type I collagen molecule (also referred to as *tropocollagen*) isolated from various tissues has a molecular weight of about 283,000 daltons. It is comprised of three left-handed helical polypeptide chains (Figure 43.2a) which are intertwined forming a right-handed helix around a central molecular axis (Figure 43.2b). Two of the polypeptide chains are identical (α_1) having 1056 amino acid residues, and the third polypeptide chain (α_2) has 1029 amino acid residues [Miller, 1984]. The triple-helical structure has a rise per residue of 0.286 nm and a unit twist of 108°, with 10 residues in three turns and a **helical pitch** (repeating distance within a single chain) of 30-residues or 8.68 nm [Fraser et al., 1983]. Over 95% of the amino acids have the sequence of Gly–X–Y. The remaining 5% of the molecule does not have the sequence of Gly–X–Y and is therefore not triple-helical. These nonhelical portions of the molecule are located at the N- and C-terminal ends and are referred to as **telopeptides** (9 to 26 residues) [Miller, 1984]. The whole molecule has a length of about 280 nm and a diameter of about 1.5 nm and has a conformation similar to a rigid rod (Figure 43.2c).

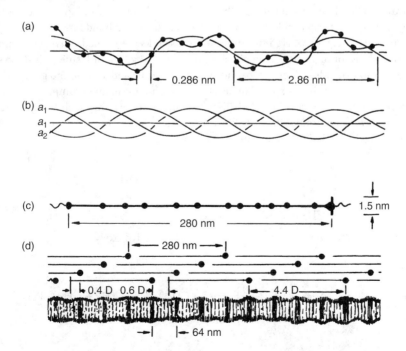

FIGURE 43.2 Diagram depicting the formation of collagen, which can be visualized as taking place in several steps: (a) single chain left-handed helix; (b) three single chains intertwined into a triple stranded helix; (c) a collagen (tropocollagen) molecule; (d) collagen molecules aligned in D staggered fashion in a fibril producing overlap and hole regions.

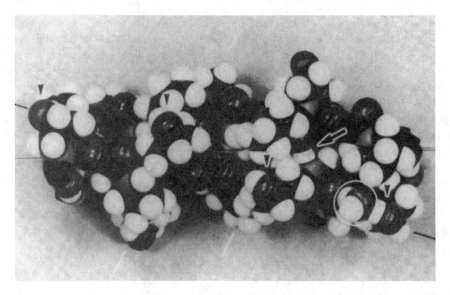

FIGURE 43.3 A space-filling model of the collagen triple helix, showing all the atoms in a ten-residue segment of repeating triplet sequence (Gly–Pro–Hyp)$_n$. The arrow shows an interchain hydrogen bond. The arrow heads identify the hydroxy groups of hydroxyproline in one chain. The circle shows a hydrogen-bonded water molecule. The short white lines identify the ridge of amino acid chains. The short black lines indicate the supercoil of one chain [Piez, 1984].

The triple-helical structure of a collagen molecule is stabilized by several factors (Figure 43.3): (1) a tight fit of the amino acids within the triple-helix — this geometrical stabilization factor can be appreciated from a space-filling model constructed from a triple helix with (Gly–Pro–Hyp) sequence (Figure 43.3); (2) the interchain hydrogen bond formation between the backbone carbonyl and amino hydrogen interactions; and (3) the contribution of water molecules to the interchain hydrogen bond formation.

The telopeptides are regions where **intermolecular crosslinks** are formed *in vivo*. A common inter-molecular crosslinks is formed between an **allysine** (the ε-amino group of **lysine** or hydroxy-lysine has been converted to an aldehyde) of one telopeptide of one molecule and an ε-amino group of a lysine or **hydroxylysine** in the triple helix or a second molecule (43.2). Thus the method commonly used to solubil-ize the collagen molecules from crosslinked **fibrils** with **proteolytic enzymes** such as **pepsin** removes the telopeptides (cleaves the intermolecular crosslinks) from the collagen molecule. The pepsin solubilized collagen is occasionally referred to as **atelocollagen** [Stenzl, 1974].

$$
\begin{array}{c}
\qquad\qquad\qquad\qquad\qquad\qquad\qquad\qquad OH \\
\qquad\qquad\qquad\qquad\qquad\qquad\qquad\qquad | \\
Pr - CH_2 - CH_2 - CH_2 - CHO \quad + \quad H_2N - CH_2 - CH - CH_2 - CH_2 - Pr \\
\text{Allysine} \qquad\qquad\qquad\qquad\qquad \text{Hydroxylysine} \\
\qquad\qquad\qquad\qquad\qquad\qquad\qquad OH \\
\qquad\qquad\qquad\qquad\qquad\qquad\qquad | \\
\rightarrow \ Pr - CH_2 - CH_2 - CH_2 - CH = N - CH_2 - CH - CH_2 - CH_2 - Pr \\
\qquad\qquad\qquad \text{Dehydrohydroxylysinonorleucine}
\end{array}
$$

(43.2)

Since the presence of hydroxyproline is unique in collagen **elastin** contains a small amount), the determ-ination of collagen content in a collagen-rich tissue is readily done by assaying the hydroxyproline content.

Collagen does not appear to exist as isolated molecules in the extracellular space in the body. Instead, collagen molecules aggregate into *fibrils*. Depending on the tissue and age, a collagen fibril varies from about 50 to 300 nm in diameter with indeterminate length and can be easily seen under electron microscopy (Figure 43.4). The fibrils are important structural building units for large **fibers** (Figure 43.5). Collagen molecules are arranged in specific orders both longitudinally and in cross-section, and the organization

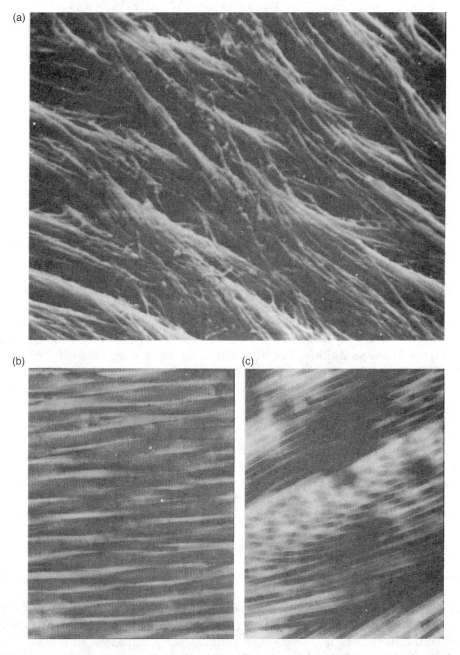

FIGURE 43.4 (a) Scanning electron micrograph of the surface of an adult rabbit bone matrix, showing how the collagen fibrils branch and interconnect in an intricate, woven pattern ($\times 4800$) (Tiffit, 1980). (b) Transmission electron micrographs of ($\times 24,000$) parallel collagen fibrils in tendon [Fung, 1992]. (c) Transmission electron micrographs of ($\times 24,000$) mesh work of fibrils in skin [Fung, 1993].

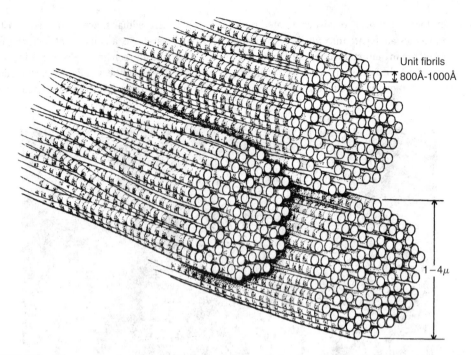

FIGURE 43.5 Diagram showing the collagen fibers of the connective tissue in general which are composed of unit collagen fibrils.

of collagen molecules in a fibril is tissue-specific [Katz and Li, 1972, 1973b]. The two-dimensional structure (the projection of a three-dimensional structure onto a two-dimensional plane) of a type I collagen fibril has been unequivocally defined both by an analysis of small-angle x-ray diffraction pattern along the meridian of a collagenous tissue [Bear, 1944] and by examination of the transmission electron micrographs of tissues stained with negative or positive stains [Hodge and Petruska, 1963]. In this structure (Figure 42.2d) the collagen molecules are staggered with respect to one another by a distance of D (64 to 67 nm) or multiple of D, where D is the fundamental repeat distance seen in the small-angle x-ray diffraction pattern, or the repeating distance seen in the electron micrographs. Since a collagen molecule has a length of about $4.4D$, this staggering of collagen molecules creates overlap regions of about $0.4D$ and hole or defect regions of about $0.6D$.

One interesting and important structural aspect of collagen is its approximate equal number of acidic (**aspartic** and **glutamic acids**) and basic (lysines and **arginines**) side groups. Since these groups are charged under physiological conditions, the collagen is essentially electrically neutral [Li and Katz, 1976]. The packing of collagen molecules with a D staggering results in clusters of regions where the charged groups are located [Hofmann and Kuhn, 1981]. These groups therefore are in close proximity to form intra- and intermolecular hydrogen-bonded **salt-linkages** of the form $(Pr - COO^{-+}H_3N - Pr)$ [Li et al., 1975]. In addition, the side groups of many amino acids are nonpolar [**alanine (Ala)**, **valine** (Val), **leucine** (Leu), **isoleucine** (Ile), *proline* (Pro), and *phenolalanine* (Phe)] in character and hence *hydrophobic*; therefore, chains with these amino acids avoid contact with water molecules and seek interactions with the nonpolar chains of amino acids. In fact, the result of molecular packing of collagen in a fibril is such that the nonpolar groups are also clustered, forming hydrophobic regions within collagen fibrils [Hofmann and Kuhn, 1981]. Indeed, the packing of the collagen molecules in various tissues is believed to be a result of intermolecular interactions involving both the electrostatic and hydrophobic interactions [Hofmann and Kuhn, 1981; Katz and Li, 1981; Li et al., 1975].

The three-dimensional organization of type I collagen molecules within a fibril has been the subject of extensive research over the past 40 years [Fraser et al., 1983; Katz and Li, 1972, 1973a, b, 1981; Miller, 1976; Ramachandran, 1967; Yamuchi et al., 1986]. Many structural models have been proposed based on an analysis of equatorial and off-equatorial x-ray diffraction patterns of rat-tail-tendon collagen [Miller, 1976; North et al., 1954], *intrafibrillar volume* determination of various collagenous tissues [Katz and Li, 1972, 1973a, b], intermolecular side chain interactions [Hofmann and Kuhn, 1981; Katz and Li, 1981; Li et al., 1981], and intermolecular crosslinking patterns studies [Yamuchi et al., 1986]. The general understanding of the three-dimensional molecular packing in type I collagen fibrils is that the collagen molecules are arranged in hexagonal or near hexagonal arrays [Katz and Li, 1972, 1981; Miller, 1976]. Depending on the tissue, the intermolecular distance varies from about 0.15 nm in rat tail tendon to as large as 0.18 nm in bone and dentin [Katz and Li, 1973b]. The axial staggering of the molecules by $1\sim 4D$ with respect to one another is tissue-specific and has not yet been fully elucidated.

There are very few interspecies differences in the structure of type I collagen molecule. The extensive homology of the structure of type I collagen may explain why this collagen obtained from animal species is acceptable as a material for human implantation.

43.1.2 Properties of Collagen-Rich Tissue

The function of collagenous tissue is related to its structure and properties. This section reviews some important properties of collagen-rich tissues.

43.1.2.1 Physical and Biomechanical Properties

The physical properties of tissues vary according to the amount and structural variations of the collagen fibers. In general, a collagen-rich tissue contains about 75 to 90% of collagen on a dry weight basis. Table 43.2 is a typical composition of a collagen-rich soft tissue such as skin. Collagen fibers (bundles of collagen fibrils) are arranged in different configurations in different tissues for their respective functions at specific anatomic sites. For example, collagen fibers are arranged in parallel in tendon (Figure 43.4b) and ligament for their high-tensile strength requirements, whereas collagen fibers in skin are arranged in random arrays (Figure 43.4c) to provide the resiliency of the tissue under stress. Other structure-supporting functions of collagen such as transparency for the lens of the eye and shaping of the ear or tip of the nose can also be provided by the collagen fiber. Thus, an important physical property of collagen is the three-dimensional organization of the collagen fibers.

The collagen-rich tissues can be thought of as a composite polymeric material in which the highly oriented crystalline collagen fibrils are embedded in the amorphous ground substance of noncollagenous **polysaccharides**, **glycoproteins**, and elastin. When the tissue is heated, its specific volume increases, exhibiting a glass transition at about 40°C and a melting of the crystalline collagen fibrils at about 56°C. The melting temperature of crystalline collagen fibrils is referred to as the *denaturation temperature* of collagenous tissues.

The stress–strain curves of a collagenous tissue such as tendon exhibit nonlinear behavior (Figure 43.6). This nonlinear behavior of stress–strain of tendon collagen is similar to that observed in synthetic fibers. The initial toe region represents alignment of fibers in the direction of stress. The steep rise in slope represents the majority of fibers stretched along their long axes. The decrease in slope following the steep rise may represent the breaking of individual fibers prior to the final catastrophic failure. Table 43.3 summarizes some mechanical properties of collagen and elastic fibers. The difference in biomechanical

TABLE 43.2 Composition of Collagen-Rich Soft Tissues

Component	Composition, %
Collagen	75 (dry), 30 (wet)
Proteoglycans and polysaccharides	20 (dry)
Elastin and glycoproteins	<5 (dry)
Water	60–70

Source: Park and Lakes (1992).

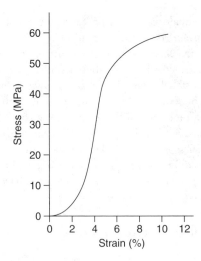

FIGURE 43.6   A typical stress-strain curve for tendon [Rigby et al., 1959].

TABLE 43.3   Elastic Properties of Collagen and Elastic Fibers

Fibers	Modulus of elasticity, MPa	Tensile strength, MPa	Ultimate elongation, %
Collagen	1000	50–100	10
Elastin	0.6	1	100

Source: Park, J.B. and Lakes, R.S. 1992. Structure-property relationships of biological materials. In *Biomaterials: An Introduction*, 2nd ed., pp. 185–222, Plenum Press, New York.

properties between collagen and elastin is a good example of the requirements for these proteins to serve their specific functions in the body.

Unlike tendon or ligament, skin consists of collagen fibers randomly arranged in layers or lamellae. Thus skin tissues show mechanics anisotropy (Figure 43.7). Another feature of the stress-strain curve of the skin is its extensibility under small load as compared to tendon. At small load the fibers are straightened and aligned rather than stretched. Upon further stretching the fibrous lamellae align with respect to each other and resist further extension. When the skin is highly stretched the modulus of elasticity approaches that of tendon as expected of the aligned collagen fibers.

Cartilage is another collagen-rich tissue which has two main physiological functions. One is the maintenance of shape (ear, tip of nose, and rings around the trachea), and the other is to provide bearing surfaces at joints. It contains very large and diffuse proteoglycan (protein-polysaccharide) molecules which form a gel in which the collagen-rich molecules entangled. They can affect the mechanical properties of the collagen by hindering the movements through the interstices of the collagenous matrix network.

The joint cartilage has a very low coefficient of friction (<0.01). This is largely attributed to the squeeze-film effect between cartilage and synovial fluid. The synovial fluid can be squeezed out through highly fenestrated cartilage upon compressive loading, and the reverse action will take place in tension. The lubricating function is carried out in conjunction with **glycosaminoglycans** (GAG), especially **chondroitin sulfates.** The modulus of elasticity (10.3 to 20.7 MPa) and tensile strength (3.4 MPa) are quite low. However, wherever high stress is required the cartilage is replaced by purely collagenous tissue. Mechanical properties of some collagen-rich tissues are given in Table 43.4 as a reference.

43.1.2.2   Physiochemical Properties

Electrostatic properties: A collagen molecule has a total of approximately 240 ε-amino and guanidino groups of lysines, hydroxylysines, and arginines and 230 carboxyl groups of aspartic and glutamic acids.

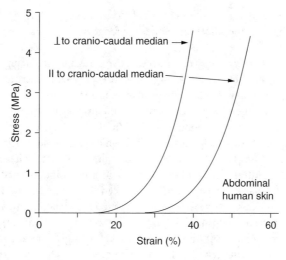

FIGURE 43.7   Stress–strain curves of human abdominal skin [Daly, 1966].

TABLE 43.4   Mechanical Properties of Some Nonmineralized Human Tissues

Tissues	Tensile strength, MPa	Ultimate elongation, %
Skin	7.6	78.0
Tendon	53.0	9.4
Elastic cartilage	3.0	30.0
Heart valves (aortic)		
Radial	0.45	15.3
Circumferential	2.6	10.0
Aorta		
Transverse	1.1	77.0
Longitudinal	0.07	81.0

Source: Park, J.B. and Lakes, R.S. 1992. Structure-property relationships of biological materials. In *Biomaterials: An Introduction*, 2nd ed., pp. 185–222, Plenum Press, New York.

These groups are charged under physiological conditions. In a native fibril, most of these groups interact either intra- or intermolecularly forming salt-linkages providing significant stabilization energy to the collagen fibril [Li et al., 1975]. Only a small number of charged groups are free. However, the electrostatic state within a collagen fibril can be altered by changing the pH of the environment. Since the pK for an amino group is about 10 and about 4 for a carboxyl group, the electrostatic interactions are significantly perturbed at a pH below 4 and above 10. The net result of the pH change is a weakening of the intra- and intermolecular electrostatic interactions, resulting in a swelling of the fibrils. The fibril swelling can be prevented by chemically introducing covalent intermolecular crosslinks. Any bifunctional reagent which reacts with amino, carboxyl, and hydroxyl groups can serve as a crosslinking agent. The introduction of covalent intermolecular crosslinks fixes the physical state of the fibrillar structure and balances the swelling pressures obtained from any pH changes.

Another way of altering the electrostatic state of a collagen fibril is by chemically modifying the electrostatic side groups. For example, the positively charged ε-amino groups of lysine and hydroxylysine can be chemically modified with acetic anhydride, which converts the ε-amino groups to a neutral acetyl group [Green et al., 1954]. The result of this modification increases the number of the net negative charges of the fibril. Conversely, the negatively charged carboxyl groups of aspartic and glutamic acid can be chemically modified to a neutral group by methylation [Fraenkel-Conrat, 1944]. Thus, by adjusting the pH of the solution and applying chemical modification methods, a range of electrostatic properties of collagen can be obtained.

Ion and macromolecular binding properties: In the native state and under physiological conditions, a collagen molecule has only about 60 free carboxyl groups [Li et al., 1975]. These groups have the capability of binding cations such as calcium with a free energy of formation for the protein-$COO-Ca^{++}$ of about 1.2 kcal/mol. This energy is not large enough to compete for the hydrogen bonded salt-linkage interactions, which have a free energy of formation of about -1.6 kcal/mol. The extent of ion binding, however, can be enhanced in the presence of lyotropic salts such as KCNS, which breaks the salt-linkages, or by shifting the pH away from the *isoelectric point* of collagen. Macromolecules can bind to collagen via covalent bonding, cooperative ionic binding, entrapment, entanglement, and a combination of the above. In addition, binding of charged ions and macromolecules can be significantly increased by modifying the charge profile of collagen as described previously. For example, a complete N-acetylation of collagen will eliminate all the positively charged ε-amino groups and, thus, will increase the free negatively charged groups. The resulting acetylated collagen enhances the binding of positively charged ions and macromolecules. On the other hand, the methylation of collagen will eliminate the negatively charged carboxyl groups and, thus, will increase the free positively charge moieties. The methylated collagen, therefore, enhances the binding of negatively charged ions and macromolecules [Li and Katz, 1976].

Fiber-forming properties: Native collagen molecules are organized in tissues in specific orders. *Polymorphic* forms of collagen can be reconstituted from the collagen molecules, obtained either from enzymatic digestion of collagenous tissues or by extracting the tissues with salt solutions. The formation of polymorphic aggregates of collagen depends on the environment for reconstitution [Piez, 1984]. Native arrangement of the collagen molecules is formed under physiological conditions. Various polymorphic molecular aggregates may be formed by changing the state of intermolecular interactions. For example, when collagen molecules are aggregated under high concentrations of a neutral salt or under nonaqueous conditions, the collagen molecules associate into random arrays having no specific regularities detectable by electron microscopy. The collagen molecules can be induced to aggregate into other polymorphic forms such as the **segment-long-spacing** (SLS) form where all heads are aligned in parallel and the **fibrous-long-spacing** (FLS) form where the molecules are randomly aligned in either a head-to-tail, tail-to-tail, or head-to-head orientation.

43.1.2.3 Biologic Properties

Hemostatic properties: Native collagen aggregates are intrinsically hemostatic. The mechanism of collagen-induced hemostasis has been the subject of numerous investigations [Wilner et al., 1968; Jaffe and Deykin, 1974; Wang et al., 1978]. The general conclusion from these studies is that **platelets** first adhere to a collagen surface. This induces the release of platelet contents, followed by platelet aggregation, leading to the eventual hemostatic plug. The hemostatic activity of collagen is dependent on the size of the collagen aggregate and the native organization of the molecules [Wang et al., 1978]. Denatured collagen (**gelatin**) is not effective in inducing hemostasis [Jonas et al., 1988].

Cell interaction properties: Collagen forms the essential framework of the tissues and organs. Many cells, such as epithelial and endothelial cells, are found resting on the collagenous surfaces or within a collagenous matrix such as that of many connective tissue cells. Collagen-cell interactions are essential features during the development stage and during wound healing and tissue remodeling in adults [Kleinman et al., 1981; Linbold and Kormos, 1991]. Studying collagen-cell interactions is useful in developing simulated tissue and organ structures and in investigating cell behavior in the *in vivo* simulated systems. Numerous studies have aimed at developing viable tissues and organs *in vitro* for transplantation applications [Bell et al., 1981; Montesano et al., 1983; Silbermann, 1990; Bellamkonda and Aebischer, 1994; Hubbel, 1995; Moghe et al., 1996; Sittinger et al., 1996].

Immunologic properties: **Soluble collagen** has long been known to be a poor immunogen [Timpl, 1982]. A significant level of antibodies cannot be raised without the use of Freund's complete adjuvant (a mixture of mineral oil and heat-killed *mycobacteria*) which augments antibody response. It is known that insoluble collagen is even less immunogenic [Stenzel et al., 1974]. Thus, xenogeneic collagenous tissue devices such as porcine and bovine pericardial heart valves are acceptable for long-term implantation in humans. The reasons for the low antibody response against collagen are not known. It may be related to the homology of the collagen structure from different species (low level of foreignness) or to certain structural features associated with collagen [Timpl, 1982].

43.2   Biotechnology of Collagen

43.2.1   Isolation and Purification of Collagen

There are two distinct ways of isolating and purifying collagen material. One is the molecular technology and the other is the fibrillar technology. These two technologies are briefly reviewed here.

43.2.1.1   Isolation and Purification of Soluble Collagen Molecules

The isolation and purification of soluble collagen molecules from a collagenous tissue is achieved by using a proteolytic enzyme such as pepsin to cleave the telopeptides [Miller and Rhodes, 1982]. Since telopeptides are the natural crosslinking sites of collagen, the removal of telopeptides renders the collagen molecules and small collagen aggregates soluble in an aqueous solution. The pepsin-solubilized collagen can be purified by repetitive precipitation with a neutral salt. Pepsin-solubilized collagen in monomeric form is generally soluble in a buffer solution at low temperature. The collagen molecules may be reconstituted into fibrils of various **polymorphisms**. However, the reconstitution of the pepsin-solubilized collagen into fibrils of native molecular packing is not as efficient as the intact molecules, since the telopeptides facilitate fibril formation [Comper and Veis, 1977].

43.2.1.2   Isolation and Purification of Fibrillar Collagen

The isolation and purification of collagen fibers relies on the removal of noncollagenous materials from the collagenous tissue. Salt extraction removes the newly synthesized collagen molecules that have not been covalently incorporated into the collagen fibrils. Salt also removes the noncollagenous materials that are soluble in aqueous conditions and are bound to collagen fibrils by nonspecific interactions. **Lipids** are removed by low-molecular-weight organic solvents such as low-molecular-weight ethers and alcohols. Acid extraction facilities the removal of acidic proteins and glycosaminoglycans due to weakening of the interactions between the acidic proteins and collagen fibrils. Alkaline extraction weakens the interaction between the basic proteins and collagen fibrils and thus facilitates the removal of basic proteins. In addition, various enzymes other than **collagenase** can be used to facilitate the removal of the small amounts of glycoproteins, proteoglycans, and elastins from the tissue. Purified collagen fibers can be obtained through these sequential extractions and enzymatic digestions from the collagen-rich tissues.

43.2.2   Matrix Fabrication Technology

The purified collagen materials obtained from either the molecular technology or from the fibrillar technology are subjected to additional processing to fabricate the materials into useful devices for specific medical applications. The different matrices and their medical applications are summarized in Table 43.5. The technology in fabricating these matrices are briefly outlined below.

43.2.2.1   Membranous Matrix

Collagen membranes can be produced by drying a collagen solution or a fibrillar collagen dispersion cast on a nonadhesive surface. The thickness of the membrane is governed by the concentration and the initial thickness of the cast solution or dispersion. In general, membrane thickness of up to 0.5 mm can be easily obtained by air drying a cast collagen material. Additional chemical crosslinking is required to stabilize the membrane from dissolution or dissociation. The membrane produced by casting and air drying does not permit manipulation of the pore structure. Generally, the structure of a cast membrane is dense and amorphous with minimal **permeability** to macromolecules [Li et al., 1991]. Porous membranes

TABLE 43.5   Summary of Different Collagen Matrices and Their Medical
Applications

Matrix form	Medical application
Membrane (film, sheet)	Oral tissue repair; wound dressings; dura repair; patches
Porous (sponge, felt, fibers)	Hemostats; wound dressings; cartilage repair; soft-tissue augmentation
Gel	Drug and biologically active macromolecule delivery; soft- and hard-tissue augmentation
Solution	Soft-tissue augmentation; drug delivery
Filament	Tendon and ligament repair; sutures
Tubular (membrane, sponge) Composite	Nerve repair; vascular repair
Collagen/synthetic polymer	Vascular repair; skin repair; wound dressings
Collagen/biological polymer	Soft-tissue augmentation; skin repair
Collagen/ceramic	Hard-tissue repair

may be obtained by freeze-drying a cast solution or dispersion of a predetermined density or by partially compressing a preformed porous matrix to a predetermined density and pore structure.

43.2.2.2   Porous Matrix

Porous collagen matrices are generally obtained by freeze-drying an aqueous volume of collagen solution or dispersion. The freeze-dried porous matrix requires chemical crosslinking to stabilize the structure. A convenient way to stabilize the porous matrix is to crosslink the matrix by vapor using a volatile crosslinking agent such as formaldehyde or glutaraldehyde. The pore structure of the matrix depends, to a large extent, on the concentration of the collagen in the solution or dispersion. Other factors that contribute to the pore structure include the rate of freezing, the size of fibers in the dispersion, and the presence and absence of other macromolecules. **Apparent densities** from 0.05 to 0.3 g matrix per cubic centimeter matrix volume can be obtained. These porous matrices generally have pores from about 50 μm to as large as 1500 μm.

43.2.2.3   Gel Matrix

A *gel matrix* may be defined as a homogeneous phase between a liquid and a solid. As such, a gel may vary from a simple viscous fluid to a highly concentrated putty-like material. Collagen gels may be formed by shifting the pH of a dispersion away from its isoelectric point. Alternatively, the collagen material may be subjected to a chemical modification procedure to change its charge profile to a net positively charged or a net negatively charged protein before hydrating the material to form a gel matrix. For example, native fibers dispersed in water at pH 7 will be in the form of two phases. The dispersed fibers become gel when the pH changes from 7 to 3. Succinylating the primary amino groups of collagen, which converts the positively charged amino groups to negatively charged carboxyl groups, changes the isoelectric point of collagen from about 7 to about 4.5. Such a collagen material swells to a gel at a pH of 7.

43.2.2.4   Solution Matrix

A collagen solution is obtained by dissolving the collagen molecules in an aqueous solution. Collagen molecules are obtained by digesting the insoluble tissue with pepsin to cleave the crosslinking sites of collagen (telopeptides) as previously described. The solubility of collagen depends on the pH, the temperature, the ionic strength of the solution, and the molecular weight. Generally, collagen is more soluble in the cold. Collagen molecules aggregate into fibrils when the temperature of the solution increases to the body temperature. pH plays an important role in solubilizing collagen. Collagen is more soluble at a pH away from the isoelectric point of the protein. Collagen is less soluble at higher ionic strength of a solution. The solubility of collagen decreases with increasing the size of molecular aggregates. Thus, collagen becomes increasingly less soluble with increasing the extent of crosslinking [Bailey et al., 1970].

43.2.2.5 Filamentous Matrix

Collagen filaments can be produced by extrusion techniques [Kemp et al., 1995; Li and Stone, 1993; Schimpf and Rodriquez, 1976]. A collagen solution or dispersion having a concentration in the range of 0.5 to 1.5% (w/v) is first prepared. Collagen is extruded into a coacervation bath containing a high concentration of a salt or into an aqueous solution at a pH of the isoelectric point of the collagen. Tensile strength of 30 MPa has been obtained for the reconstituted filaments.

43.2.2.6 Tubular Matrix

Tubular matrices may be formed by extrusion through a coaxial cylinder [Stenzl et al., 1974], or by coating collagen onto a mandrel [Li, 1990]. Different properties of the tubular membranes can be obtained by controlling the drying properties.

43.2.2.7 Composite Matrix

Collagen can form a variety of homogeneous composites with other water-soluble materials. Ions, peptides, proteins, and polysaccharides can all be uniformly incorporated into a collagen matrix. The methods of homogeneous composite formation include ionic and covalent bonding, entrapment, entanglement, and coprecipitation. A heterogeneous composite can be formed between collagen, ceramics, and synthetic polymers that have distinct properties for medical applications [Li, 1988].

43.3 Design of a Resorbable Collagen-Based Medical Implant

Designing a medical implant for tissue or organ repair requires a thorough understanding of the structure and function of the tissue and organ to be repaired, the structure and properties of the materials used for repair, and the design requirements. There are at present two schools of thought regarding the design of an implant, namely the permanent implant and the *resorbable implant*. The permanent implants are intended to permanently replace the damaged tissues or organs are fabricated from various materials including metals and natural or synthetic polymers. For example, most of the weight-bearing orthopedic and oral implants are made of metals or alloys. Non-weight-bearing tissues and organs are generally replaced with implants that are fabricated either from synthetic or natural materials. Implants for blood vessel, heart valve, and most soft tissue repair fall into this class. Permanent implants, particularly those made of synthetic and biological materials, frequently suffer from the long-term effects of material degradation. Material degradation can result from biological processes such as enzymatic degradation or environmentally induced degradation from mechanical, metal-catalyzed oxidation, and from the permeation of body fluids into the polymeric devices [Bruck, 1991]. The material degradation is particularly manifested in applications where there is repetitive stress-strain on the implant, such as artificial blood vessels and heart valves.

As a result of the lack of suitable materials for long-term implantation, the concept of using a resorbable template to guide host tissue regeneration (guided tissue regeneration) has received vigorous attention in recent years. This area of research can be categorized into synthetic and biological templates. **Polyglycolic acid** (PGA), **polylactic acid** (PLA), polyglycolic-polylactic acid copolymers, and **polydioxanone** are among the polymers most selected for resorbable medical implant development. Among the biological materials used for resorbable medical implant development, *collagen* has been one of the most popular materials in this category. Collagen-based templates have been developed for skin [Yannas and Burke, 1981], peripheral nerve [Li et al., 1990; Yannas et al., 1985], oral tissue [Altman and Li, 1990; Blumenthal, 1988], and meniscal regeneration [Li et al., 1994; Stone et al., 1997]. A variety of other collagen based templates are being developed for tissue repair and regeneration applications [Goldstein et al., 1989; Ma et al., 1990; Li, et al., 1997].

The following discussion is useful in designing a template for tissue repair and regeneration applications. By way of an example, the design parameters listed below are specifically applied to the development of a **resorbable collagen** based template for guiding meniscal tissue repair and regeneration in the knee joint.

Menisci are semilunar fibrocartilages that are anatomically located between the femoral condyles and tibial plateau, providing stability, weight bearing, shock absorption and assisting in lubrication of the knee joint. A major portion of the meniscal tissue is avascular except the peripheral rim, which comprises about 10 to 30% of the total width of the structure and which is nourished by the peripheral vasculature [Arnoczky and Warren, 1982]. Collagen is the major matrix material of the **meniscus**, and the fibers are oriented primarily in the circumferential direction in the line of stress for mechanical function. Repair of damaged meniscal tissue in the peripheral vascular rim can be accomplished with sutures. However, in cases where the injured site is in the avascular region, partial or total removal of the meniscal tissue is often indicated. This is primarily due to the inadequacy of the *fibrochondrocytes* alone to self-repair the damaged meniscal tissue. Studies in animals and humans have shown that removal of the meniscus is a prelude to degenerative knees manifested by the development of **osteoarthritis** [Hede and Sarberg, 1992; Shapiro and Glimcher, 1980]. At present there is no suitable permanent substitute for meniscal tissue.

43.3.1　Biocompatibility

Biocompatibility of the materials and their degraded products is a prerequisite for resorbable implant development. Purified collagen materials have been used either as implants or have been extensively tested in clinical studies as implants without adverse effects. The meniscus template can be fabricated from purified type I collagen fibers that are further crosslinked chemically to increase the stability and reduce the immunogenicity *in vivo*. In addition, small amounts of noncollagenous materials such as glycosaminoglycans and growth factors can be incorporated into the collagen matrix to improve the osmotic properties as well as the rate of tissue ingrowth.

Since the primary structure of a collagen molecule from bovine is homologous to human collagen [Miller, 1984], the *in vivo* degradation of bovine collagen implant should be similar to the normal host tissue remodeling process during wound healing. For a resorbable collagen template, the matrix is slowly degraded by the host over time. It is known that a number of cell types such as **polymorphonuclear leukocytes**, **fibroblasts**, and **macrophages**, during the wound healing period, are capable of secreting enzyme collagenases which cleave a collagen molecule at 1/4 position from the C-terminal end of the molecule [Woolley, 1984]. The enzyme first reduces a collagen molecule to two smaller triple helices which are not stable at body temperature and are subsequently denatured to random coiled polypeptides. These polypeptides are further degraded by proteases into amino acids and short peptides that are metabolized through normal metabolic pathways [Nimni and Harkness, 1988].

Despite the safety record of collagen materials for implantation, during the process of preparing the collagen template, small amounts of unwanted noncollagenous materials could be incorporated into the device such as salts and crosslinking agents. Therefore, a series of biocompatibility testing must be conducted to ensure the residuals of these materials do not cause any safety issues. The FDA has published a new guideline for biocompatibility testing of implantable devices (Biological Evaluation of Medical Devices, 1995).

43.3.2　Physical Dimension

The physical dimension of a template defines the boundary of regeneration. Thus, the size of the collagen template should match the tissue defect to be repaired. A properly sized meniscal substitute has been found to function better than a substitute which mismatches the physical dimension of the host meniscus [Rodkey et al., 1998; Sommerlath et al., 1991]. For a porous, elastic matrix such as the one designed from collagen for meniscal tissue repair, the shape of the meniscus is further defined *in vivo* by the space available between the femoral condyles and tibial plateau within the synovial joint.

43.3.3　Apparent Density

The apparent density as defined as the weight of the dry matrix in a unit volume of matrix. Thus, the apparent density is a direct measure of the empty space which is not occupied by the matrix material per se in the dry state. For example, for a collagen matrix of an apparent density 0.2 g/cm^3, the empty space would be 0.86 cm^3 for a 1 cm^3 total space occupied by the matrix, taking the density of collagen to be 1.41 g/cm^3 [Noda, 1992]. The apparent density is also directly related to the mechanical strength of a matrix. In weight-bearing applications, the apparent density has to be optimized such that the mechanical properties are not compromised for the intended function of the resorbable implant as described in the mechanical properties section.

43.3.4 Pore Structure

The dimension of a mammalian fibrogenic cell body is on the order of 10 to 50 μm, depending on the substrate to which the cell adheres [Folkman et al., 1978]. In order for cells to infiltrate into the interstitial space of a matrix, the majority of the pores must be significantly larger than the dimension of a cell such that both the cell and its cellular processes can easily enter the interstitial space. In a number of studies using collagen-based matrices for tissue regeneration, it has been found that pore size plays an important role in the effectiveness of the collagen matrix to induce host tissue regeneration [Chvapil, 1982; Dagalailis et al., 1980; Yannas, 1996]. It was suggested that pore size in the range of 100 to 400 μm was optimal for tissue regeneration. Similar observations were also found to be true for porous metal implants in total hip replacement [Cook et al., 1991]. The question of interconnecting pores may not be a critical issue in a collagen template as collagenases are synthesized by most **inflammatory cells** during wound healing and remodeling processes. The interporous membranes which exist in the noninterconnecting pores should be digested as part of resorption and wound healing processes.

43.3.5 Mechanical Property

In designing a resorbable collagen implant for weight-bearing applications, not only the initial mechanical strength is important, but the gradual strength reduction of the partially resorbed template has to be compensated by the strength increase from the regenerated tissue such that at any given time point, the total mechanical properties of the template are maintained. In order to accomplish this goal, one must first be certain that the initial mechanical properties are adequate for supporting the weight-bearing application. For example, compressing the implant with multiple body weights should not cause fraying of the collagen matrix material. It is also of particular importance to design an implant having an adequate and consistent suture pullout strength in order to reduce the incidence of detachment of the implant from the host tissue. The suture pullout strength is also important during surgical procedures as the lack of suture pull strength may result in retrieval and reimplantation of the template. In meniscal tissue repair the suture pullout strength of 1 kg has been found to be adequate for arthroscopically assisted surgery in simulated placement procedures in human cadaver knees, and this suture pullout strength should be maintained as the minimal strength required for this particular application.

43.3.6 Hydrophilicity

Hydration of an implant facilitates nutrient diffusion. The extent of hydration would also provide information on the space available for tissue ingrowth. The porous collagen matrix is highly hydrophilic and therefore facilitates cellular ingrowth. The biomechanical properties of the hydrophilic collagen matrix such as fluid outflow under stress, fluid inflow in the absence of stress, and the resiliency for shock absorption are the properties also found in the weight-bearing cartilagenous tissues.

43.3.7 Permeability

The permeability of ions and macromolecules is of primary importance in tissues that do not rely on vascular transport of nutrients to the end organs. The diffusion of nutrients into the interstitial space ensures the survival of the cells and their continued ability of growth and synthesis of tissue specific extracellular matrix. Generally, the permeability of a macromolecule the size of the bovine serum albumin

(MW 67,000) can be used as a guideline for probing accessibility of the interstitial space of a collagen template [Li et al., 1994].

43.3.7.1 *In Vivo* Stability

As stated above, the rate of template resorption and the rate of new tissue regeneration have to be balanced so that the adequate mechanical properties are maintained at all times. The rate of *in vivo* resorption of a collagen-based implant can be controlled by controlling the density of the implant and the extent of intermolecular crosslinking. The lower the density, the greater the interstitial space and generally the larger the pores for cell infiltration, leading to a higher rate of matrix degradation. The control of the extent of intermolecular crosslinking can be accomplished by using bifunctional crosslinking agents under conditions that do not denature the collagen. Glutaraldehyde, formaldehyde, adipyl chloride, hexamethylene diisocyanate, and carbodiimides are among the many agents used in crosslinking the collagen-based implants. Crosslinking can also be achieved through vapor phase of a crosslinking agent. The vapor phase crosslinking is effective using crosslinking agents of high vapor pressures such as formaldehyde and glutaraldehyde. The vapor crosslinking is particularly useful for thick implants of vapor permeable dense fibers where crosslinking in solution produces nonuniform crosslinking. In addition, intermolecular crosslinking can be achieved by heat treatment under high vacuum. This treatment causes the formation of an amide bond between an amino group of one molecule and the carboxyl group of an adjacent molecule and has often been referred to in the literature as dehydrothermal crosslinking.

The shrinkage temperature of the crosslinked matrix has been used as a guide for *in vivo* stability of a collagen implant [Li, 1988]. The temperature of shrinkage of collagen fibers measures the transition of the collagen molecules from the triple helix to a random coil conformation. This temperature depends on the number of intermolecular crosslinks formed by chemical means. Generally, the higher the number of intermolecular crosslinks, the higher the thermal shrinkage temperature and more stable the material *in vivo*.

A second method of assessing the *in vivo* stability is to determine the crosslinking density by applying the theory of rubber elasticity to denatured collagen [Wiederhorn and Beardon, 1952]. Thus, the *in vivo* stability can be directly correlated with the number of intermolecular crosslinks introduced by a given crosslinking agent.

Another method that has been frequently used in assessing the *in vivo* stability of a collagen-based implant is to conduct an *in vitro* collagenase digestion of a collagen implant. Bacterial collagenase is generally used in this application. The action of bacterial collagenase on collagen is different from that of mammalian collagenase [Woolley, 1984]. In addition, the enzymatic activity used in *in vitro* studies is arbitrarily defined. Thus, the data generated from the bacterial collagenase should be viewed with caution. The bacterial collagenase digestion studies, however, are useful in comparing a prototype with a collagen material of known rate of *in vivo* resorption.

Each of the above parameters should be considered in designing a resorbable implant. The interdependency of the parameters must also be balanced for maximal efficacy of the implant.

43.4 Tissue Engineering for Tissue and Organ Regeneration

Biomedical applications of collagen have entered a new era in the past decade. The potential use of collagen materials in medicine has increasingly been appreciated as the science and technology advances.

One major emerging field of biomedical research which has received rigorous attention in recent years is tissue engineering. Tissue engineering is an interdisciplinary science of biochemistry, cell and molecular biology, genetics, materials science, biomedical engineering, and medicine to produce innovative three-dimensional composites having structure/function properties that can be used either to replace or correct poorly functioning components in humans and animals or to introduce better functional components into these living systems. Thus, the field of tissue engineering requires a close collaboration among various disciplines for success.

TABLE 43.6　Survey of Collagen-Based Medical Products, and Research and Development Activities

Applications	Comments
Hemostasis	Commercial Products: Sponge, fiber, and felt forms are used in cardiovascular [Abbott and Austin, 1975]; neurosurgical [Rybock and Long, 1977]; dermatological [Larson, 1988]; ob/gyn [Cornell et al., 1985]; orthopaedic [Blanche and Chaux, 1988]; oral surgical applications [Stein et al., 1985]
Dermatology	Commercial Products: Injectable collagen for soft tissue augmentation [Webster et al., 1984]; collagen based artificial skins [Bell et al., 1981; Yannas and Burke, 1981]. Research and Development: Collagen based wound dressings [Armstrong et al., 1986]
Cardiovascular Surgery and Cardiology	Commercial Products: Collagen coated and gelatin coated vascular grafts [Jonas et al., 1988, Li, 1988]; chemically processed human vein graft [Dardik et al., 1974]; bovine arterial grafts [Sawyer et al., 1977]; porcine heart valves [Angell et al., 1982]; bovine pericardial heart valves [Walker et al., 1983]; vascular puncture hole seal device [Merino et al., 1992]
Neurosurgery	Research and Development: Guiding peripheral nerve regeneration [Archibald et al., 1991; Yannas et al., 1985]; dura replacement material [Collins et al., 1991]
Periodontal and Oral Surgery	Research and Development: Collagen membranes for periodontal ligament regeneration [Blumenthal, 1988]; resorbable oral tissue wound dressings [Ceravalo and Li, 1988]; collagen/hydroxyapatite for augmentation of alveolar ridge [Gongloff and Montgomery, 1985]
Ophthalmology	Commercial Products: Collagen corneal shield to facilitate epithelial healing [Ruffini et al., 1989]. Research and Development: Collagen shield for drug delivery to the eye [Reidy et al., 1990]
Orthopaedic Surgery	Commercial Products: Collagen with hydroxyapatite and autogenous bone marrow for bone repair [Hollinger et al., 1989]. Research and Development: Collagen matrix for meniscus regeneration [Li et al., 1994]; collagenous material for replacement and regeneration of Achilles tendon [Kato et al., 1991]; reconstituted collagen template for ACL reconstruction [Li et al., 1997]
Other Applications	Research and Development: Drug delivery support [Sorensen et al., 1990]; delivery vehicles for growth factors and bioactive macromolecules [Deatherage and Miller, 1987; Li et al., 1996]; collagenous matrix for delivery of cells for tissue and organ regeneration [Bell et al., 1981]

Tissue engineering consists primarily of three components: (1) extracellular matrix, (2) cells, and (3) regulatory signals (e.g., tissue specific growth factors). One of the key elements in tissue engineering is the extracellular matrix which either provides a scaffolding for cells or acts as a delivery vehicle for regulatory signals such as growth factors.

Type I collagen is the major component of the extracellular matrix and is intimately associated with development, wound healing, and regeneration. The development of the type I collagen based matrices described in this review article will greatly facilitate the future development of tissue engineering products for tissue and organ repair and regeneration applications.

To date, collagen-based implants have been attempted for many tissue and organ repair and regeneration applications. A complete historical survey of all potential medical applications of collagen is a formidable task but a selected survey of collagen-based medical products and the research and development activities are summarized in Table 43.6 as a reference.

Defining Terms

Alanine (Ala):　One of the amino acids in collagen molecules.

Allysine:　The ε-amino group of lysine has been enzymatically modified to an aldehyde group.

Apparent density:　Calculated as the weight of the dry collagen matrix per unit volume of matrix.

Arginine (Arg):　One of the amino acids in collagen molecules.

Aspartic acid (Asp):　One of the amino acids in collagen molecules.

Atelocollagen: A collagen molecule without the telopeptides.

Chondroitin sulfate: Sulfated polysaccharide commonly found in cartilages, bone, corea, tendon, and skin.

Collagen: A family fibrous insoluble proteins having a triple helical conformation extending over a major part of the molecule. Glycine is present at every third amino acid in the triple helix and proline and hydroxyproline are required in the triple helix.

Collagenase: A proteolytic enzyme that specifically catalyzes the degradation of collagen molecules.

Dehydrohydroxylysinonorleucine (deH-HLNL):   A covalently crosslinked product between an allysine and a hydroxylysine residues in collagen fibrils.

D spacing: The repeat distance observed in collagen fibrils by electron microscopic and x-ray diffraction methods.

Elastin: One of the proteins in connective tissue. It is highly stable at high temperatures and in chemicals. It also has rubberlike properties.

Fiber: A bundled group of collagen fibrils.

Fibril: A self-assembled group of collagen molecules.

Fibroblast: Any cell from which connective tissue is developed.

Fibrochondrocyte: Type of cells that are associated with special types of cartilage tissues such as meniscus of the knee and intervertebral disc of the spine.

Fibrous long spacing (FLS):   One of the polymorphic forms of collagen where the collagen molecules are randomly aligned in either head-to-tail, tail-to-tail, or head-to-head orientation.

Gelatin: A random coiled form (denatured form) of collagen molecules.

Glutamic acid (Glu):   One of the amino acids in collagen molecules.

Glycine (Gly):   One of the amino acids in collagen molecules having the simplest structure.

Glycoprotein: A compound consisting of a carbohydrate protein. The carbohydrate is generally hexosamine, an amino sugar.

Glycosaminoglycan (GAG):   A polymerized sugar (see polysaccharide) commonly found in various connective tissues.

Helical pitch: Repeating distance within a single polypeptide chain in a collagen molecule.

Hemostat: Device or medicine which arrests the flow of blood.

Hydrophilicity: The tendency to attract and hold water.

Hydrophobicity: The tendency to repel or avoid contact with water. Substances generally are nonpolar in character, such as lipids and nonpolar amino acids.

Hydroxylysine (Hyl):   One of the amino acids in collagen molecules.

Hydroxyproline (Hyp):   One of the amino acids uniquely present in collagen molecules.

Inflammatory cell: Cells associated with the succession of changes which occur in living tissue when it is injured. These include macrophages, polymorphonuclear leukocytes, and lymphocytes.

Intermolecular crosslink: Covalent bonds formed *in vivo* between a side group of one molecule and a side group of another molecule; covalent bonds formed between a side group of one molecule and one end of a bifunctional agent and between a side group of a second molecule and the other end of a bifunctional agent.

Intrafibrillar volume: The volume of a fibril excluding the volume occupied by the collagen molecule.

In vitro: In glass, as in a test tube. An *in vitro* test is one done in the laboratory, usually involving isolated tissues, organs, or cells.

In vivo: In the living body or organism. A test performed in a living organism.

Isoelectric point: Generally used to refer to a particular pH of a protein solution. At this pH, there is no net electric charge on the molecule.

Isoleucine (Ile):   One of the amino acids in collagen molecules.

Leucine (Leu):   One of the amino acids in collagen molecules.

Lipid: Any one of a group of fats or fat-like substances, characterized by their insolubility in water and solubility in fat solvents such as alcohol, ether, and chloroform.

Lysine (Lys):   One of the amino acids in collagen molecules.

Meniscus: A C-shaped fibrocartilage anatomically located between the femoral condyles and tibial plateau providing stability and shock absorption and assisting in lubrication of the knee joint.

Macrophage: Cells of the reticuloendothelial system having the ability to phagocytose particulate substances and to store vital dyes and other colloidal substances. They are found in loose connective tissues and various organs of the body.

Mycobacterium: A genus of acid-fast organisms belonging to the Mycobacteriaceae which includes the causative organisms of tuberculosis and leprosy. They are slender, nonmotile, gram-positive rods and do not produce spores or capsules.

Osteoarthritis: A chronic disease involving the joint, especially those bearing the weight, characterized by destruction of articular cartilage, overgrown of bone with impaired function.

Permeability: The space within a collagen matrix, excluding the space occupied by collagen molecules, which is accessible to a given size of molecule.

Pepsin: A proteolytic enzyme commonly found in the gastric juice. It is formed by the chief cells of gastric glands and produces maximum activity at a pH of 1.5 to 2.0.

Phenolalanine (Phe):   One of the amino acids in collagen molecules.

Platelet: A round or oval disk, 2 to 4 μm in diameter, found in the blood of vertebrates. Platelets contain no hemoglobin.

Polydioxanone: A synthetic polymer formed from dioxanone monomers which degrades by hydrolysis.

Polyglycolic acid (PGA):   A synthetic polymer formed from glycolic acid monomers which degrades by hydrolysis.

Polylactic acid (PLA):   A synthetic polymer formed from lactic acid monomers which degrades by hydrolysis.

Polymorphism: Different types of aggregated states of the collagen molecules.

Polymorphonuclear leukocyte: A white blood cell which possesses a nucleus composed of two or more lobes or parts; a granulocyte (neutrophil, eosinophil, basophil).

Polypeptide: Polymerized amino acid molecules formed by enzymatically regulated stepwise polymerization *in vivo* between the carboxyl group of one amino acid and the amino group of a second amino acid.

Polysaccharide: Polymerized sugar molecules found in tissues as lubricant (synovial fluid) or cement (between osteons, tooth root attachment) or complexed with proteins such as glycoproteins or proteoglycans.

Proline (Pro):   One of the amino acids commonly occurring in collagen molecules.

Proteolytic enzyme: Enzymes which catalyze the breakdown of native proteins.

Resorbable collagen: Collagen which can be biodegraded *in vivo*.

Salt-linkage: An electrostatic bond formed between a negative charge group and a positive charge group in collagen molecules and fibrils.

Segment-long-spacing (SLS):   One of the polymorphic forms of collagen where all heads of collagen molecules are aligned in parallel.

Soluble collagen: Collagen molecules that can be extracted with salts and dilute acids. Soluble collagen molecules contain the telopeptides.

Telopeptide: The two short nontriple helical peptide segments located at the ends of collagen molecules.

Valine (Val):   One of the amino acids in collagen molecules.

References

Abbott, W.M. and Austin, W.G. 1975. The effectiveness of mechanism of collagen-induced topical hemostasis. *Surgery* 78: 723–729.

Altman, R. and Li, S.T. 1990. Collagen matrix for oral surgical applications. *Int. J. Oral Implantol.* 7: 75.

Angell, W.W., Angell, J.D., and Kosek, J.C. 1982. Twelve year experience with gluteraldehyde preserved porcine xenografts. *J. Thorac Cardiovasc. Surg.* 83: 493–502.

Archibald, S.J., Krarup, C., Shefner, J., Li, S.T., and Madison, R. 1991. Collagen-based nerve conduits are as effective as nerve grafts to repair transected peripheral nerves in rodents and non-human primates. *J. Comp. Neurol.* 306: 685–696.

Armstrong, R.B., Nichols, J., and Pachance, J. 1986. Punch biopsy wounds treated with Monsel's solution or a collagen matrix.*Arch. Dermatol.* 122: 546–549.

Arnoczky, S.P. and Warren, R.F. 1982. Microvasculature of the human meniscus. *Am. J. Sport Med.* 10: 90–95.

Baily, A.J. and Rhodes, D.N. 1964. Irradiation-induced crosslinking of collagen. *Radiat. Res.* 22: 606–621.

Bear, R.S. 1952. The structure of collagen fibrils. *Adv. Prot. Chem.* 7: 69–160.

Bell, E., Ehrlich, H.P., Buttle, D.J., and Nakatsuji, T. 1981. Living tissue formed *in vitro* and accepted as skin equivalent tissue of full thickness. *Science* 211: 1042–1054.

Bellamkonda, R. and Aebischer, P. 1994. Review: tissue engineering in the nerve system. *Biotechnol. Bioeng.* 43: 543–554.

Biological evaluation and medical devices. Use of international standard ISO-10993. Blue Book memorandon G95-1, Rockville, MD, FDA, CDRH, Office of Device Evaluation, May 1, 1995.

Blanche, C. and Chaux, A. 1988. The use of absorbable microfibrillation collagen to control sternal bone marrow bleeding. *Int. Surg.* 73: 42–43.

Blumenthal, N.M. 1988. The use of collagen membranes to guide regeneration of new connective tissue attachment in dogs. *J. Periodontol* 59: 830–836.

Brodsky, B. and Ramshaw, J.A. 1997. The collagen triple-helix structure. *Matrix Biol.* 15: 545–554.

Bruck, S.D. 1991. Biostability of materials and implants. *J. Long-Term Effects Med. Implants* 1: 89–106.

Ceravolo, F. and Li, S.T. 1988. Alveolar ridge augmentation utilizing collagen wound dressing. *Int. J. Oral Implantol.* 4: 15–18.

Chvapil, M. 1982. Considerations on manufacturing principles of a synthetic burn dressing: a review. *J. Biomed. Mater. Res.* 16: 245–263.

Collins, R.L., Christiansen, D., Zazanis, G.A., and Silver, F.H. 1991. Use of collagen film as a dural substitute: Preliminary animal studies. *J. Biomed. Mater. Res.* 25: 267–276.

Comper, W.D. and Veis, A. 1977. Characterization of nuclei in vitro collagen fibril formation. *Biopolymers* 16: 2133–2142.

Cook, S.D., Thomas, K.A., Dalton, J.E., Volkman, T., and Kay, J.F. 1991. Enhancement of bone ingrowth and fixation strength by hydroxyapatite coating porous implants. *Trans. Orthop. Res. Soc.* 16: 550.

Correll, J.T., Prentice, H.R., and Wise, R.C. 1985. Biological investigations of a new absorbable sponge. *Surg. Gynecol. Obstet.* 81: 585–589.

Dagalailis, N., Flink, J., Stasikalis, P., Burke, J.F., and Yannas, I.V. 1980. Design of an artificial skin. III. Control of pore structure. *J. Biomed. Mater. Res.* 14: 511–528.

Daly, C.H. 1966. *The Biomechanical Characteristics of Human Skin.* Ph.D. thesis, University of Strathclyde, Scotland.

Dardik, H., Veith, F.J., Spreyregen, S., and Dardik I. 1974. Arterial reconstruction with a modified collagen tube. *Ann. Surg.* 180: 144–146.

Deatherage, J.R. and Miller, E.J. 1987. Packaging and delivery of bone induction factors in a collagen implant. *Collagen Rel. Res.* 7: 225–231.

Eastoe, J.E. 1967. Composition of collagen and allied proteins. In *Treatise on Collagen,* G.N. Ramachandran (Ed.), pp. 1–72, Academic Press, New York.

Ellis, D.L. and Yannas, I.V. 1996. Recent advances in tissue synthesis *in vivo* by use of collagen-glycosaminoglycans copolymers. *Biomaterials* 17: 291–299.

Folkman, J. and Moscona, A. 1978. Role of cell shape in growth control. *Nature* 273: 345–349.

Fraenkel-Conrat, H. and Olcott, H.S. 1945. Esterification of proteins with alcohols of low molecular weight. *J. Biol. Chem.* 161: 259–268.

Fraser, R.D.B., MacRae, T.P., Miller, A., and Suzuki, E. 1983. Molecular conformation and packing in collagen fibrils. *J. Mol. Biol.* 167: 497–510.

Fukai, N., Apte, S.S., and Olsen, B.R. 1994. Nonfibrillar collagens. *Meth. Enzymol.* 245: 3–28.

Fung, Y.C. 1993. Bioviscoelastic solids. In *Biomechanics, Mechanical Properties of Living Tissues*, 2nd ed., p. 255, Springer-Verlag, New York.

Goldstein, J.D., Tria, A.J., Zawadsky, J.P., Kato, Y.P., Christiansen, D., and Silver, F.H. 1989. Development of a reconstituted collagen tendon prosthesis. A preliminary implantation study. *J. Bone Joint Surg.* 71-A: 1183–1191.

Gongloff, R.K., Whitlow, W., and Montgomery, C.K. 1985. Use of collagen tubes for implantation of hydroxylapatite. *J. Oral Maxillofac. Surg.* 43: 570–573.

Green, R.W., Ang K.P., and Lam, L.C. 1953. Acetylation of collagen. *Biochem. J.* 54: 181–187.

Guidon, R., Marcean, D., Rao, T.J., Merhi, Y., Roy, P., Martin, L., and Duval, M. 1987. *In vitro* and *in vivo* characterization of an impervious polyester arterial prosthesis: the Gelseal Triaxial graft. *Biomaterials* 8: 433–441.

Hede, A., Larson, E., and Sanberg, H. 1992. The long term outcome of open total and partial meniscectomy related to the quantity and site of the meniscus removed. *Int. Orthop.* 16: 122–125.

Hodge, A.J. and Petruska, J.A. 1963. Recent studies with the electron microscope on the ordered aggregates of the tropocollagen molecule. In *Aspects of Proteins Structure*, G.N. Ramachandran (Ed.), pp. 289–300, Academic Press, New York.

Hofmann, H. and Kuhn, K. 1981. Statistical analysis of collagen sequences with regard to fibril assembly and evolution. In *Structural Aspects of Recognition and Assembly in Biological Macromolecules*, M. Balaban, J.L. Sussman, W. Traub, and A. Yonath (Eds.), pp. 403–425, Balabann ISS, Rehovot and Philadelphia.

Hollinger, J., Mark, D.E., Bach, D.E., Reddi, A.H., and Seyfer, A.E. 1989. Calvarial bone regeneration using osteogenin. *J. Oral Maxillofac. Surg.* 47: 1182–1186.

Hubbell, J.A. 1995. Biomaterials in tissue engineering. *Bio/technology* 13: 565–576.

Jaffe, R. and Deykin, D.J. 1974. Evidence for a structural requirement for the aggregation of platelet by collagen. *Clin. Invest.* 53: 875–883.

Kato, Y.P., Dunn, M.G., Zawadsky, J.P., Tria, A.J., and Silver, F.H. 1991. Regeneration of Achilles tendon with a collagen tendon prosthesis. *J. Bone Joint Surg.* 73-A: 561–574.

Katz, E.P. and Li, S.T. 1972. The molecular organization of collagen in mineralized and nonmineralized tissues. *Biochem. Biophys. Res. Commun.* 3: 1368–1373.

Katz, E.P. and Li, S.T. 1973a. The intermolecular space of reconstituted collagen fibrils. *J. Mol. Biol.* 73: 351–369.

Katz, E.P. and Li, S.T. 1973b. Structure and function of bone collagen fibrils. *J. Mol. Biol.* 80: 1–15.

Katz, E.P. and Li, S.T. 1981. The molecular packing of type I collagen fibrils. In *The Chemistry and Biology of Mineralized Connective Tissues*, A. Veis (Ed.), pp. 101–105, Elsevier, North Holland.

Kemp, P.D., Cavallaro, J.F., and Hastings, D.N. 1995. Effects of carbodiimide crosslinking and load environment on the remodeling of collagen scaffolds. *Tissue Eng.* 1: 71–79.

Kleinman, H.K., Klebe, R.J., and Martin, G.R. 1981. Role of collagenous matrices in the adhesion and growth of cells. *J. Cell Biol.* 88: 473–485.

Larson, P.O. 1988. Topical hemostatic agents for dermatologic surgery. *J. Dermatol. Surg. Oncol.* (14): 623–632.

Li, S.T. 1990. A multi-layered, semipermeable conduit for nerve regeneration comprised of type I collagen, its method of manufacture and a method of nerve regeneration using said conduit. U.S. Patent 4,963,146.

Li, S.T. and Stone, K.R. 1993. Prosthetic ligament. U.S. Patent 5,263,984.

Li, S.T. 1988. Collagen and vascular prosthesis. In *Collagen*, Vol. III., M.E. Nimni (Ed.), pp. 253–271, CRC Press, Boca Raton, FL.

Li, S.T. and Katz, E.P. 1976. An electrostatic model for collagen fibrils: the interaction of reconstituted collagen with Ca^{++}, Na^+, and Cl^-. *Biopolymers* 15: 1439–1460.

Li, S.T., Archibald, S.J., Krarup, C., and Madison, R.D. 1991. The development of collagen nerve guiding conduits that promote peripheral nerve regeneration. In *Biotechnology and Polymers*, C.G. Gebelein (Ed.), pp. 282–293, Plenum Press, New York.

Li, S.T., Archibald, S.J., Krarup, C., and Madison, R. 1990. Semipermeable collagen nerve conduits for peripheral nerve regeneration. *Polym. Mater. Sci. Eng.* 62: 575–582.

Li, S.T., Golub, E., and Katz, E.P. 1975. On electrostatic side chain complimentarity in collagen fibrils. *J. Mol. Biol.* 98: 835–839.

Li, S.T., Sullman, S., and Katz, E.P. 1981. Hydrogen bonded salt linkages in collagen. In *The Chemistry and Biology of Mineralized Tissues*, A. Veis (ed.), pp. 123–127, Elsevier, North Holland.

Li, S.T., Yuen, D., Li, P.C., Rodkey, W.G., and Stone, K.R. 1994. Collagen as a biomaterial: an application in knee meniscal fibrocartilage regeneration. *Mater. Res. Soc. Symp. Proc.* 331: 25–32.

Li, S.T., Yuen, D., Charoenkul, W., Ulreich, J.B., and Speer, D.P. 1997. A type I collagen ligament for ACL reconstruction. *Trans. Soc. Biomater.* 407.

Li, S.T., Bolton, W., Helm, G., Gillies, G., and Frenkel, S. 1996. Collagen as a delivery vehicle for bone morphogenetic protein (BMP). *Trans. Orthop. Res. Soc.* p 647.

Lindblad, W.J. and Kormos, A.I. 1991. Collagen: a multifunctional family of proteins. *J. Reconstruct. Microsurg.* 7: 37–43.

Ma, S., Chen, G., and Reddi, A.H. 1990. Collaboration between collagenous matrix and osteoginin is required for bone induction. *Ann. NY Acad. Sci.* 580: 524–525.

Merino, A., Faulkner, C., Corvalan, A., and Sanborn, T.A. 1992. Percutaneous vascular hemostasis device for interventional procedures. *Catheterizat. Cardiovasc. Diagn.* 26: 319–322.

Miller A. 1976. Molecular packing in collagen fibrils. In *Biochemistry of Collagen*, G.N. Ramachandran and H. Reddi (Eds.), pp. 85–136, Plenum Press, New York.

Miller, E.J. 1984. Chemistry of the collagens and their distribution. In *Extracellular Matrix Biochemistry*, K.A. Piez and A.H. Reddi (Eds.), pp. 41–82, Elsevier, New York.

Miller, E.J. and Rhodes, R.K. 1982. Preparation and characterization of the different types of collagen. *Meth. Enzymol.* 82: 33–63.

Moghe, P.V., Berthiaume, F., Ezzell, R.M., Toner, M., Tompkins, R.C., and Yarmush, M.L. 1996. Culture matrix configuration and composition in the maintenance of hepatocyte polarity and function. *Biomaterials* 17: 373–385.

Montesano, R., Mouron, P., Amherdt, M., and Orci, L. 1983. Collagen matrix promotes reorganization of pancreatic endocrine cell monolayers into islet-like organoids. *J. Cell Biol.* 97: 935–939.

Nimni M.E., (Ed.) 1988. *Collagen*, Vols. I, II, and III. CRC Press, Boca Raton, FL.

Nimni, M.E. and Harkness, R.D. 1988. Molecular structures and functions of collagen. In *Collagen*, Vol. I, M.E. Nimni (Ed.), pp. 1–78, CRC Press, Boca Raton, FL.

Noda, H. 1972. Partial specific volume of collagen. *J. Biochem.* 71: 699–703.

Park, J.B. and Lakes, R.S. 1992. Structure-property relationships of biological materials. In *Biomaterials: An Introduction*, 2nd ed., pp. 185–222, Plenum Press, New York.

Piez, K.A. 1984. Molecular and aggregate structures of the collagens. In *Extracellular Matrix Biochemistry*, K.A. Piez and A.H. Reddi (Eds.), p. 5, Elsevier, New York

Ramachandran, G.N. 1967. Structure of collagen at the molecular level. In *Treatise on Collagen*, Vol. I, G.N. Ramachandran (Ed.), pp. 103–183, Academic Press, New York, London.

Reidy, J.J., Limberg, M., and Kaufman, H.E. 1990. Delivery of fluorescein to the anterior chamber using the corneal collagen shield. *Ophthalmology* 97: 1201–1203.

Rich, A. and Crick, F.H.C. 1961. The molecular structure of collagen. *J. Mol. Biol.* 3: 483–505.

Rigby, B.J., Hiraci, N., Spikes, J.D., and Eyring H. 1959. The mechanical properties of rat tail tendon. *J. Gen. Physiol.* 43: 265–283.

Rodkey, W.G., Li, S.T., Arnoczky, S.P., McDevitt, C.A., Woo, SL-Y., and Steadman, J.R. 1998. Type I collagen based template for meniscal tissue regeneration: III. In vivo evaluations in humans. (In preparation.)

Ruffini, J.J., Aquavella, J.V., and LoCascio, J.A. 1989. Effect of collagen shields on corneal epithelialization following penetrating keratoplasty. *Ophthal. Surg.* 20: 21–25.

Rybock, J.D. and Long, D.M. 1977. Use of microfibrillar collagen as a topical hemostatic agent in brain tissue. *J. Neurosurg.* 46: 501–505.

Sawyer, P.N., Stanczewski, B., and Kirschenbaum, D. 1977. The development of polymeric cardiovascular collagen prosthesis. *Artif. Organs* 1: 83–91.

Schimpf, W.C. and Rodriquez F. 1976. Fibers from regenerated collagen. *Ind. Eng. Chem. Prod. Res. Rev.* 16: 90–92.

Shapiro, F. and Glimcher, M.J. 1980. Induction of osteoarthrosis in the rabbit knee joint: histologic changes following meniscectomy and meniscal lesions. *Clin. Orthop.* 147: 287–295.

Silbermann, M. 1990. *In vitro* systems for inducers of cartilage and bone development. *Biomaterials* 11: 47–49.

Sittinger, J.B., Bugia, J., Rotter, N., Reitzel, D., Minuth, W.W., and Burmester, G.R. 1996. Tissue engineering and autologous transplant formation: prectical approaches with resorbable biomaterials and new cell culture techniques. *Biomaterials* 17: 237–242.

Sommerlath, K., Gallino, M., and Gillquist, J. 1991. Biomechanical characteristics of different artificial substitutes for the rabbit medial meniscus and the effect of prosthesis size on cartilage. *Trans. Orthop. Res. Soc.* 16: 375.

Sorensen, T.S., Sorensen, A.I., and Merser, S. 1990. Rapid release of gentamicin from collagen sponge. *Acta Orthop. Scand.* 61: 353–356.

Stein, M.D., Salkin, L.M., Freedman, A.L., and Glushko, V. 1985. Collagen sponge as a topical hemostatic agent in mucogingival surgery. *J. Periodontol.* 56: 35–38.

Stenzl, K.H., Miyata, T., and Rubin, A.L. 1974. Collagen as a biomaterial. *Ann. Rev. Biophys. Bioeng.* 3: 231–253.

Stone, K.R., Steadman, J.R., Rodkey, W.R., and Li, S.T. 1997. Regeneration of meniscal cartilage with the use of a collagen scaffold. *J. Bone Joint Surg.* 79-A: 1770–1777.

Tiffit, J.T. 1980. The organic matrix of bone tissue. In *Fundamental and Clinical Bone Physiology*, M.R. Urist (Ed.), p. 51, JB Lippincott Co., PA.

Timpl, R. 1982. Antibodies to collagen and procollagen. *Meth. Enzymol.* 82: 472–498.

van der Rest, M., Dublet, B., and Champliaud, M.F. 1990. Fibril-associated collagens. *Biomaterials* 11: 28–31.

Walker, W.E., Duncan, J.M., Frazier, O.H., Liversay, J.J., Ott, D.A., Reul, G.J., and Cooly, D.A. 1983. Early experience with the Ionescu-Shiley pericardial xenograft valve. *J. Thorac Cardiovasc. Surg.* 86: 570–575.

Wang, C-L, Miyata, T., Weksler, B., Rubin, A., and Stenzel, K.H. 1978. Collagen-induced platelet aggregation and release: critical size and structural requirements of collagen. *Biochim. Biophys. Acta* 544: 568–577.

Webster, R.C., Kattner, M.D., and Smith, R.C. 1984. Injectable collagen for augmentation of facial areas. *Arch. Otolaryngol.* 110: 652–656.

Wiederhorn, N. and Beardon, G.V. 1952. Studies concerned with the structure of collagen: II. Stress-strain behavior of thermally controlled collagen. *J. Polym. Sci.* 9: 315–325.

Wilner, G.D., Nossel, H.L., and Leroy, E.C. 1968. Activation of Hageman factor by collagen. *J. Clin. Invest.* 47: 2608–2615.

Woolley, D.E. 1984. Mammalian Collagenases. In *Extracellular Matrix Biochemistry*, K.A. Piez and A.H. Reddi (Eds.), pp. 119–151, Elsevier, New York.

Yamuchi, M., Katz, E.P., and Mechanic, G.L. 1986. Intermolecular cross-linking and stereospecific molecular packing in type I collagen fibrils of the periodontal ligament. *Biochemistry* 25: 4907–4913.

Yannas, I.V. and Burke, J.F. 1981. Design of an artificial skin. I. Basic design principles. *J. Biomed. Mater. Res.* 14: 65–80.

Yannas, I.V., Orgill, D.P., Silver, J., Norregaad, T., Ervas, N.N., and Schoene, W.C. 1985. Polymeric template facilitates regeneration of sciatic nerve across a 15 mm gap. *Polym. Mater. Sci. Eng.* 53: 216–218.

44

Soft Tissue Replacements

K.B. Chandran
University of Iowa

K.J.L. Burg
Carolinas Medical Center

S.W. Shalaby
Poly-Med, Inc.

44.1 Blood Interfacing Implants

K.B. Chandran

44.1.1 Introduction

Blood comes in contact with foreign materials for a short term in extracorporeal devices such as **dialysers**, **blood oxygenators**, ventricular assist devices, and **catheters**. Long-term vascular implants include heart valve prostheses, **vascular grafts**, and **cardiac pacemakers** among others. In this section, we will be concerned with development of biomaterials for long-term implants, specifically for heart valve prostheses, total artificial heart (**TAH**), and vascular grafts. The primary requirements for biomaterials for long-term implants are biocompatibility, nontoxicity, and durability. Furthermore, the material should be nonirritating to the tissue, resistant to **platelet** and **thrombus** deposition, nondegradable in the physiological environment, and neither absorb blood constituents nor release foreign substances into the blood stream [Shim and Lenker, 1988]. In addition, design considerations include that the implant should mimic the function of the organ that it replaces without interfering with the surrounding anatomical structures and must be of suitable size and weight. The biomaterials chosen must be easily available, inexpensive, easily machinable, sterilizable, and have a long storage life. The selection of material will also be dictated by the strength requirement for the implant being made. As an example, an artificial heart valve prosthesis is required to open and close on an average once every second. The biomaterial chosen must be such that

TABLE 44.1   Heart Valve Prostheses Developed and Currently Available in the U.S.

Type	Name	Manufacturer
Caged ball	Starr-Edwards	Baxter Health Care, Irvine, CA
Tilting disc	Medtronic-Hall	Medtronic Blood Systems, Minneapolis, MN
	Lillehei-Kaster	Medical Inc., Inner Grove Heights, MN
	Omni-Science	
Bileaflet	St. Jude Medical	St. Jude Medical, Inc., St. Paul, MN
	Carbomedics	Carbomedics, Austin, TX
	ATS Valve[a]	ATS Medical, St. Paul, MN
	On-X Valve[a]	Medical Carbon Research Inst., Austin, TX
Porcine bioprostheses	Carpentier-Edwards Standard	Baxter Health Care, Irvine, CA
	Hancock Standard	Medtronic Blood Systems, Santa Ana, CA
	Hancock modified orifice	
	Hancock II	
Pericardial bioprostheses	Carpentier-Edwards	Edwards Laboratories, Santa Ana, CA

[a] FDA approval pending.

the valve is durable and will not fail under **fatigue stress** after implantation in a patient. As sophisticated measurement techniques and detailed computational analyses become available with the advent of super computers, our knowledge on the complex dynamics of the functioning of the implants is increasing. Improvements in design based on such knowledge and improvements in selection and manufacture of biomaterials will minimize problems associated with blood interfacing implants and significantly improve the quality of life for patients with implants. We will discuss the development of biomaterials for the blood interfacing implants, problems associated with the same, and future directions in the development of such implants.

44.1.2 Heart Valve Prostheses

Attempts at replacing diseased natural human valves with prostheses began about four decades ago. The details of the development of heart valve prostheses, design considerations, *in vitro* functional testing, and durability testing of valve prototypes can be found in several monographs [Shim and Lenker, 1988; Chandran, 1992]. The heart valve prostheses can be broadly classified into **mechanical prostheses** (made of non-biological material) and **bioprostheses** (made of biological tissue). Currently available mechanical and tissue heart valve prostheses in the United States are listed in Table 44.1.

44.1.2.1 Mechanical Heart Valves

Lefrak and Starr [1970] describe the early history of mechanical valve development. The initial designs of mechanical valves were of centrally occluding caged ball or caged disc type. The Starr–Edwards caged ball prostheses, commercially available at the present time, was successfully implanted in the mitral position in 1961. The caged ball prostheses is made of a polished Co–Cr alloy (**Stellite 21®**) cage and a silicone rubber ball (Silastic®) which contains 2% by weight barium sulfate for **radiopacity** (Figure 44.1). The valve **sewing rings** use a silicone rubber insert under a knitted composite polytetrafluorethylene (PTFE-**Teflon®**) and **polypropylene** cloth. Even though these valves have proven to be durable, the centrally occluding design of the valve results in a larger pressure drop in flow across the valve and higher **turbulent stresses** distal to the valve compared to other designs of mechanical valve prostheses [Yoganathan et al., 1979a, b; 1986; Chandran et al., 1983]. The relatively large profile design of caged ball or disc construction also increases the possibility of interference with anatomical structures after implantation. The **tilting disc valves**, with improved hemodynamic characteristics, were introduced in the late 1960s. The initial design consisted of a polyacetal (**Delrin®**) disc with a Teflon® sewing ring. Delrin acetal resins are thermoplastic

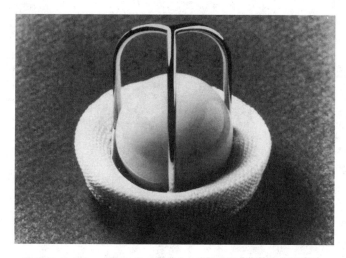

FIGURE 44.1   A caged-ball heart valve prosthesis. (Courtesy of Baxter Health Care, Irvine, CA.)

polymers manufactured by the polymerization of **formaldehyde** [Shim and Lenker, 1988]. Even though Delrin exhibited excellent wear resistance and mechanical strength with satisfactory performance after more than 20 years of implantation, it was also found to swell when exposed to humid environments such as **autoclaving** and blood contact. To avoid design and manufacturing difficulties due to the swelling phenomenon, the Delrin disc was soon replaced by the **pyrolytic carbon** disc and has become the preferred material for mechanical valve prostheses occluders to date. Pyrolytic carbons are formed in a fluidized bed by pyrolysis of a gaseous hydrocarbon in the range of 1000 to 2400°C. For biomedical applications, carbon is deposited onto a preformed polycrystalline graphite substrate at temperatures below 1500°C (low temperature isotropic pyrolytic carbon, **LTI** Pyrolite®). Increase in strength and wear resistance is obtained by codepositing silicone (up to 10% by weight) with carbon in applications for heart valve prostheses. The pyrolytic carbon discs exhibit excellent blood compatibility, as well as wear and fatigue resistance. The guiding **struts** of tilting disc valves are made of **titanium** or Co–Cr alloys (**Haynes 25®** and Stellite 21®). The Co–Cr based alloys, along with pure titanium and its alloy (Ti6A14V) exhibit excellent mechanical properties as well as resistance to corrosion and thrombus deposition. A typical commercially available tilting disc valve with a pyrolytic carbon disk is shown in Figure 44.2a. A tilting disc valve with the leaflet made of **ultra high molecular weight polyethylene** (Chitra valve — Figure 44.2b) is currently marketed in India. The advantages of **leaflets** with relatively more flexibility compared to pyrolytic carbon leaflets are discussed in Chandran et al. [1994a]. Another new concept in a tilting disc valve design introduced by Reul et al. [1995] has an S-shaped leaflet with leading and trailing edges being parallel to the direction of blood flow. The housing for the valve is nozzle-shaped to minimize flow separation at the inlet and energy loss in flow across the valve. Results from *in vitro* evaluation and animal implantation have been encouraging.

In the late 1970s, a bileaflet design was introduced for mechanical valve prostheses and several different bileaflet models are being introduced into the market today. The leaflets as well as the housing of the bileaflet valves are made of pyrolytic carbon and the bileaflet valves show improved hemodynamic characteristics especially in smaller sizes compared to tilting disc valves. A typical bileaflet valve is shown in Figure 44.3. Design features to improve the hydrodynamic characteristics of the mechanical valves include the opening angle of the leaflets [Baldwin et al., 1997] as well as having an open-pivot design in which the pivot area protrudes into the orifice and is exposed to the washing action of flowing blood [Drogue and Villafana, 1997]. Other design modifications to improve the mechanical valve function include: the use of double polyester (Dacron®) velour material for the suture ring to encourage rapid and controlled tissue ingrowth, and mounting the cuff on a rotation ring which surrounds the orifice ring to protect the cuff mounting mechanism from deeply placed annulus sutures. A PTFE (Teflon®) insert in the cuff provides pliability without excessive drag on the sutures. Tungsten (20% by weight) is incorporated into the leaflet substrate in order to visualize the leaflet motion *in vivo*.

(a)

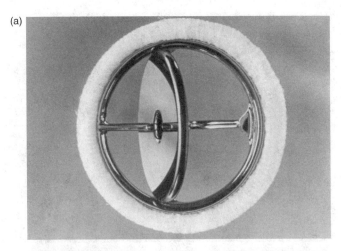

(b)

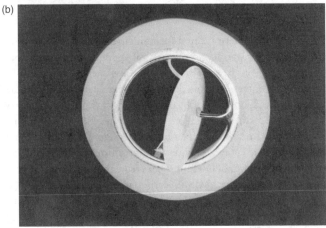

FIGURE 44.2   (a) Photograph of a typical tilting disc valve prosthesis. (Courtesy of Medtronic Heart Valves, Minneapolis, MN.) (b) Chitra tilting disc valve prosthesis with the occluder made of ultra high molecular weight polyethylene. (Courtesy of Sree Chitra Tirunal Institute for Medical Sciences and Technology, India.)

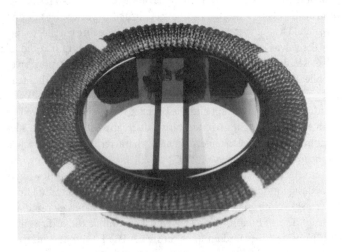

FIGURE 44.3   A CarboMedics bileaflet valve with pyrolytic carbon leaflets and housing. (Courtesy of Sulzer-CarboMedics, Austin, TX.)

(a)

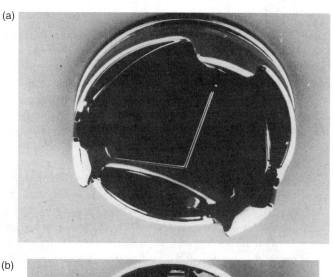

(b)

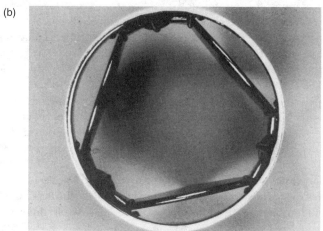

FIGURE 44.4 A tri-leaflet heart valve prosthesis under development. (Courtesy of Triflo Medical, Inc., Costa Mesa, CA.)

Another attempt to design a mechanical valve which mimics the geometry and function of the tri-leaflet aortic valve is that of Lapeyre et al. (1994) (Figure 44.4a, b). The geometry of the valve affords true central flow characteristics with reduced backflow. Accelerated fatigue tests have also shown good wear characteristics for this design and the valve is undergoing further evaluation including animal studies. Other improvements in the mechanical valves which augment performance include: machining of the valve housing to fit a disk so as to produce optimal washing and minimal regurgitation [McKenna, 1997]; a supra-annular design so that a larger-sized valve can be inserted in the aortic position in the case of patients with small aortic annulus [Bell, 1997]; and coating of a titanium alloy ring with a thin, uniform, and strongly adherent film of high-density turbostratic carbon (Carbofilm™) [Bona et al., 1997] in order to integrate the structural stability of the metal alloy to the non-thrombogenecity of pyrolytic carbon. Details of contemporary design efforts in mechanical valve design and potential future biomaterials such as Boralyn® (boron carbide) are discussed in Wieting [1997].

In spite of the desirable characteristics of the biomaterials used in the heart valve prostheses, problems with **thrombo-embolic complications** are significant with implanted valves and patients with mechanical valves are under long-term anticoagulant therapy. The mechanical stresses induced by the flow of blood across the valve prostheses have been linked to the lysis and activation of **formed elements of blood** (red blood cells, white blood cells, and platelets) resulting in the deposition of thrombi in regions with relative stasis in the vicinity of the prostheses. Numerous *in vitro* studies with mechanical valves in pulse duplicators simulating physiological flow have been reported in the literature and have been reviewed by Chandran [1988] and Dellsperger and Chandran [1991]. Such studies have included measurement of velocity profiles and turbulent stresses distal to the valve due to flow across the valve. The aim of these studies has been the correlation of regions prone to thrombus deposition and tissue overgrowth with explanted valves and the experimentally measured bulk turbulent shear stresses as well as regions of relative stasis. In spite of improvements in design of the prostheses to afford a centralized flow with minimal flow disturbances and fluid mechanical stresses, the problems with thrombus deposition remain significant.

Reports of strut failure, material **erosion** and leaflet escapes, as well as **pitting** and erosion of valve leaflets and housing, have resulted in numerous investigations of the **closing dynamics** of mechanical valves. The dynamics of the leaflet motion and its impact with the valve housing or seat stop is very complex and a number of experimental and numerical studies have appeared recently in the literature. As the leaflet impacts against the seat stop and comes to rest instantaneously, high positive and **negative pressure** transients are present on the outflow and inflow side of the occluder, respectively, at the instant when the leaflet impacts against the seat stop or the guiding strut [Leuer, 1986; Chandran et al., 1994a]. The *negative pressure transients* have been shown to reach magnitudes below the **liquid vapor pressure** and have been demonstrated to be a function of the loading rate on the leaflet inducing the valve closure. As the magnitudes of negative pressure transients go below the liquid vapor pressure, **cavitation bubbles** are initiated and the subsequent collapse of the cavitation bubbles may also be a factor in the lysis of red blood cells, platelets, and **valvular structures** [Chandran et al., 1994a; Lee et al., 1994]. Typical cavitation bubbles visualized in an *in vitro* study with tilting disc and bileaflet valves are shown in Figure 44.5. A correlation is also observed between the region where cavitation bubbles are present, even though for a period of time less than a millisecond after valve closure, and sites of pitting and erosion reported in the pyrolytic carbon material in the valve housing and on the leaflets with explanted valves [Kafesjian, 1994] as well as those used in total artificial hearts [Leuer, 1987]. An electron micrograph of pitting and erosion observed in the pyrolytic carbon valve housing of an explanted bileaflet mechanical valve is shown in Figure 44.6. The pressure transients at valve closure are substantially smaller in mechanical valves with a flexible occluder and leaflets made of ultra high molecular weight polyethylene (Figure 44.2b) may prove to be advantageous based on the closing dynamic analysis [Chandran et al., 1994a]. A correlation between the average velocity of the leaflet edge and the negative pressure transients in the same region at the instant of valve closure, as well as the presence of cavitation bubbles has been reported recently [Chandran et al., 1997]. This study demonstrated that for the valves of the same geometry (e.g., tilting disk) and size, the leaflet edge velocity as well as the negative pressure transients were similar. However, the presence of cavitation bubbles depended on the local interaction between the leaflet and the seat stop. Hence, it was pointed out that magnitudes of leaflet velocity or presence of pressure transients below the liquid vapor pressure might not necessarily indicate cavitation inception with mechanical valve closure. Chandran et al. [1998] have also demonstrated the presence of negative pressure transients in the atrial chamber with implanted mechanical valves in the mitral position in animals, demonstrating that potential for cavitation exists with implanted mechanical valves. Similar to the *in vitro* results, the transients were of smaller magnitudes with the Chitra valve made of flexible leaflets, and no pressure transients were observed with tissue valve implanted in the mitral position *in vivo*. The demonstration of the negative pressure transients with mechanical valve closure also shows that this phenomenon is localized and the flow chamber or valve holder rigidity with the *in vitro* experiments will not affect the valve closing dynamics.

The pressure distribution on the leaflets and impact forces between the leaflets and guiding struts have also been experimentally measured in order to understand the causes for strut failure [Chandran et al., 1994b]. The flow through the clearance between the leaflet and the housing at the instant of valve closure [Lee and Chandran, 1994a, b] and in the fully closed position [Reif, 1991] and the resulting wall shear stresses within the clearance are also being suggested as responsible for clinically significant hemolysis and thrombus initiation. Detailed analysis of the complex closing dynamics of the leaflets may also be exploited in improving the design of the mechanical valves to minimize problems with structural failure

(a)

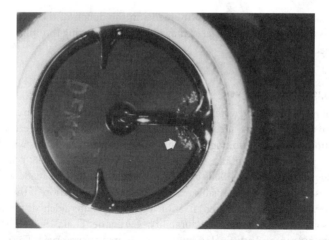

(b)

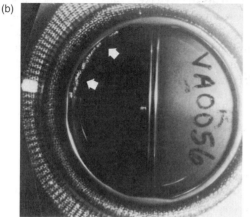

(c)

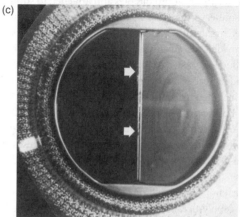

FIGURE 44.5 Cavitation bubbles visualized on the inflow side of the valves *in vitro* [Chandran et al., 1994a]: (a) Medtronic-Hall tilting disc valve; (b) Edwards-Duromedics bileaflet valve; (c) CarboMedics bileaflet valve.

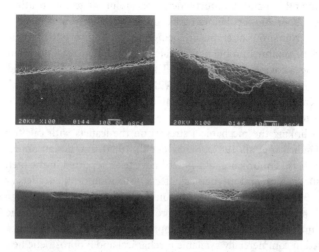

FIGURE 44.6 Photographs showing pitting on pyrolytic carbon surface of a mechanical heart valve. (Courtesy of Baxter Health Care, Irvine, CA.)

[Cheon and Chandran, 1994]. Further improvements in the design of the valves based on the closing dynamics as well as improvements in material may result in minimizing thrombo-embolic complications with implanted mechanical valves.

44.1.2.2 Biological Heart Valves

The first biological valves implanted were **homografts** with valves explanted from cadavers within 48 h after death. Preservation of the valves included various techniques of sterilization, freeze drying, and immersing in antibiotic solution. The use of homografts is not popular due to problems with long term durability and due to limited availability except in a few centers [Shim and Lenker, 1988; Lee and Boughner, 1991]. Attempts were also made in the early 1960s in the use of **xenografts** (valves made from animal tissue) and porcine bioprostheses became commercially available after the introduction of the gluteraldehyde (rather than formaldehyde which was initially used) fixation technique. Gluteraldehyde reacts with tissue proteins to form crosslinks and results in improved durability [Carpentier et al., 1969]. The valves are harvested from 7 to 12 month old pigs and attached to supporting **stents** and preserved. The stent provided support to preserve the valve in the natural shape and to achieve normal opening and closing. Initial supports were made of metal and subsequently flexible polypropylene stents were introduced. The flexible stents provided the advantage of ease of assembling the valve and **finite element analyses** have demonstrated reduction in stresses at the juncture between the stent and tissue leaflets resulting in increased durability and increased leaflet coaptation area [Reis et al., 1971; Hamid et al., 1985]. A typical porcine bioprosthesis is included in Figure 44.7a.

Fixed bovine pericardial tissue is also used to construct heart valves in which design characteristics such as orifice area, valve height, and degree of coaptation can be specified and controlled. Thus, the geometry and flow dynamics past **pericardial prostheses** mimic those of the natural human aortic valves more closely. Due to the low profile design of pericardial prostheses and increased orifice area, these valves are less stenotic compared to porcine bioprostheses, especially in smaller sizes [Chandran et al., 1984]. In the currently available bioprostheses, the stents are constructed from polypropylene, **Acetol®** homopolymer or copolymer, Elgiloy wire, or titanium. A stainless steel radiopaque marker is also introduced to visualize the valve *in vivo*. Other biomaterials, which have been employed in making the bioprostheses, include **fascia lata** tissue as well as human **duramater** tissue. The former was prone to deterioration and hence unsuitable for bioprosthetic application, while the latter lacked commercial availability.

The advantage with bioprostheses is the freedom from thrombo-embolism and hence not requiring long term anticoagulant therapy in general. These prostheses are preferable in patients who do not tolerate anticoagulants. On the other hand, bioprosthetic valves are prone to **calcification** and leaflet tear with an average lifetime of about 10 years before replacement is necessary, and is generally attributed to the tissue fixation process. Numerous attempts are being made to improve the design as well as fixation in bioprostheses in order to minimize problems with calcification and increase duration of the function of the implant. As an example, a bovine pericardial trileaflet valve (Figure 44.7[b]) treated with a non-aldehyde fixation resulting in collagen crosslink formation without a new "foreign" chemical process [Phillips and Printz, 1997] has been introduced in the European market. A non-aldehyde iodine-based sterilization process also sterilizes the valve.

Numerous studies linking the mechanical stresses on the leaflets with calcification, focal thinning, and leaflet failure [Thubrikar et al., 1982a; Sabbah et al., 1985], and design improvements to minimize the stresses on the leaflets [Thubrikar et al., 1982b] have been reported in the literature. Further details on the effects of tissue fixation and mechanical effects of fixation on the leaflets are reported elsewhere [Lee and Boughner, 1991]. Improvements in fixation techniques as well as in design of the bioprostheses are continually being made in order to minimize problems with calcification of the leaflets and improve the durability and functional characteristics of bioprosthetic heart valves [Piwnica and Westaby, 1998]. The biomaterials used in commercially available mechanical and bioprosthetic heart valves are included in Table 44.2. Table 44.3 includes a summary of the problems associated with implanted artificial heart valves.

(a)

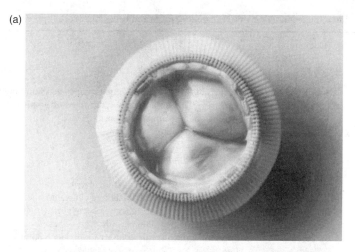

(b)

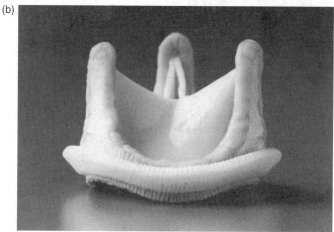

FIGURE 44.7 Typical bioprostheses: (a) Hancock porcine bioprosthesis (courtesy of Medtronic Heart Valves, Minneapolis, MN); (b) PhotoFix™ α pericardial prosthesis. (Courtesy of Sulzer-CarboMedics, Inc., Austin, TX.)

44.1.2.3 Synthetic Heart Valves

Concurrently, efforts have also been made in the development of valve prostheses made of synthetic material. Several attempts to make bileaflet [Braunwald et al., 1960] and trileaflet valves [Roe et al., 1958; Hufnagel, 1977; Gerring et al., 1974; Ghista and Reul, 1977] made of polyurethanes, polyester fabrics, and silicone rubber were not successful due to problems with durability of relatively thin leaflets made of synthetic material. With the advent of the total artificial hearts (TAH) and **left ventricular assist devices** (LVAD) in the 1980s, an additional impetus on the development of synthetic valves is present. Due to problems with thrombus deposition in the vicinity of the mechanical valves used in the TAH and subsequent stroke episodes in patients with permanent implants, the use of the device is currently restricted as a bridge to transplantation. In such temporary use before a donor heart becomes available (on an average of several weeks), the four mechanical prostheses used in the TAH results in substantial cost. Hence, efforts are being made to replace the mechanical valves with those made with synthetic material. With **vacuum forming** or **solution casting** techniques, synthetic valves can be made at a fraction of the cost of mechanical valves, provided their function in a TAH environment for several weeks will be satisfactory. Implantation of synthetic trileaflet valves [Russel et al., 1980; Harold et al., 1987], even more recently, have resulted in limited success due to leaflet failure and calcification. Hemodynamic comparison

TABLE 44.2 Biomaterial Used in Heart Valve Prostheses [Shim and Lenker, 1988; Dellsperger and Chandran, 1988]

Type	Component	Biomaterial
Caged ball	Ball/occluder	Silastic
	Cage	Stellite 21®/Titanium
	Suture ring	Silicone rubber insert under knitted composite Teflon®/polypropylene cloth
Tilting disc	Leaflet	Delrin®; Pyrolytic carbon (carbon deposited on graphite substrate); ultra high molecular polyethylene (UHMPE)
	Housing/strut	Haynes 25®/Titanium
	Suture ring	Teflon®/Dacron®
Bileaflet	Leaflets	Pyrolytic carbon
	Housing	Pyrolytic carbon
	Suture ring	Double velour Dacron® tricot knit polyester
Porcine bioprostheses	Leaflets	Porcine aortic valve fixed by stabilized gluteraldehyde
	Stents	Polypropylene stent covered with Dacron®; lightweight Elgiloy wire covered with porous knitted Teflon® cloth
	Suture ring	Dacron®; soft silicone rubber insert covered with porous, seamless Teflon® cloth
Pericardial bioprostheses	Leaflets	Porcine pericardial tissue fixed by stabilized gluteraldehyde before leaflets are sewn to the valve stents
	Stents	Polypropylene stent covered with Dacron®; Elgiloy wire and nylon support band covered with polyester and Teflon® cloth
	Suture ring	PTFE fabric over silicone rubber filter

TABLE 44.3 Common Problems with Implanted Prosthetic Heart Valves [Yoganathan et al., 1979a; Shim and Lenker, 1988; Chandran, 1992]

I. *Mechanical valves*
(a) Thromboembolism
(b) Structural failure
(c) Red blood cell and platelet destruction
(d) Tissue overgrowth
(e) Damage to endothelial lining
(f) Paravalvular/perivalvular leakage
(g) Tearing of sutures
(h) Infection

II. *Bioprosthetic valves*
(a) Tissue calcification
(b) Leaflet rupture
(c) Paravalvular/perivalvular leakage
(d) Infection

of vacuum formed and solution cast trileaflet valves to currently available bioprostheses have produced satisfactory results [Chandran et al., 1989a, b]. *Finite element analysis* of synthetic valves can be exploited in design improvements similar to those reported for bioprostheses [Chandran et al., 1991a].

44.1.3 Total Artificial Hearts (TAH) or Ventricular Assist Devices (VAD)

Artificial circulatory support can be broadly classified into two categories. The first category is for those patients who undergo open heart surgery to correct **valvular disorders**, ventricular *aneurysm*, or coronary **artery** disease. In several cases, the heart may not recover sufficiently after surgery to take over the pumping action. In such patients ventricular assist devices are used as extracorporeal devices to maintain circulation until the heart recovers. Other ventricular assist devices include **intra-aortic balloon pumps** as well as

cardiopulmonary bypass. Within several days or weeks, when the natural heart recovers, these devices will be removed. In the second category are patients with advanced stages of cardiomyopathy and are subjects for heart transplantation. Due to problems in the availability of suitable donor hearts, not all patients with a failed heart are candidates for heart transplantation. For those patients not selected for transplantation, the concept of replacing the natural heart with a total artificial heart has gained attention in recent years [Akutsu and Kolff, 1958; Jarvick, 1981; DeVries and Joyce, 1983; Unger, 1989; Kambic and Nose, 1991]. A number of attempts in the permanent implantation of TAH with pneumatically powered units were made in the 1980s. However, due to neurological complications as a result of thrombo-embolism, infection, and hematological and renal complications, permanent implantations are currently suspended. If a suitable donor heart is not readily available, TAHs can be used as "bridge to transplantation" for several weeks until a donor heart becomes available. Until recently, most of the circulatory assist devices were pneumatically driven and a typical pneumatic heart is shown in Figure 44.8a. It has two chambers for the left and right ventricle with inlet and outlet valves for each of the chambers. A line coming from the external pneumatic driver passes through the skin and is attached to the diaphragm housing through the connector shown in the photograph. Thus, the patient is tethered to an external pneumatic drive. He can move around for a short period of time by attaching the pneumatic line to a portable driver that he can carry.

Electrically driven blood pumps, which can afford tether-free operation within the body, unlike those of the pneumatically powered pumps, are currently at various stages of development for long-term use (of more than 2 years). The components of such devices include the blood pump in direct contact with blood, energy converter (from electrical to mechanical energy), variable column compensator, implantable batteries, transcutaneous energy transmission system, and external batteries. The blood pump configuration in these devices includes sac, diaphragm, and **pusher plate devices**. Materials used in blood contacting surfaces in these devices are synthetic polymers (polyurethanes, segmented polyurethanes, **Biomer**®, and others). Segmented polyurethane elastomer used in prosthetic ventricles with a thromboresistant additive modifying the polymeric surface have resulted in improved blood compatibility and reduced thrombo-embolic risk in animal trials [Farrar et al., 1988]. Design considerations include reduction of regions of stagnation of blood within the blood chamber and minimizing the mechanical stresses induced on the formed elements in blood. Apart from the characteristics of these materials to withstand repetitive high mechanical stresses and minimize failure due to fatigue, surface interaction with blood is also another crucial factor. An electrically powered total artificial heart intended for long term implantation is shown in Figure 44.8b. The details of the design considerations for the circulatory assist devices are included in Rosenberg [1995a] and details of the evaluation of the electrically powered heart is included in Rosenberg et al. [1995b].

Due to significant problems with thrombo-embolic complications and subsequent neurological problems with long-term implantation of TAH in humans, attention has been focused on minimizing factors responsible for thrombus deposition. In order to eliminate crevices formed with the quick connect system, valves sutured in place at the inflow and outflow orifices were offered as an alternative in the Philadelphia Heart [Wurzel et al., 1988]. An alternative quick connect system using precision machined components has been demonstrated to reduce valve- and connector-associated thrombus formation substantially [Holfert et al., 1987]. Several *in vitro* studies have been reported in the literature in order to assess the effect of fluid dynamic stresses on thrombus deposition [Phillips et al., 1979; Tarbell et al., 1986; Baldwin et al., 1990; Jarvis et al., 1991]. These have included flow visualization and **laser Doppler anemometry** velocity and turbulence measurements within the ventricular chamber as well as in the vicinity of the inflow and outflow orifices. The results of such studies indicate that the flow within the chamber generally has a smooth washout of blood in each pulsatile flow cycle with relatively large turbulent stresses and regions of stasis found near the valves. The thrombus deposition found with implanted TAH in the vicinity of the inflow valves also indicates that the major problem with the working of these devices are still with the flow dynamics across the mechanical valves. Computational flow dynamic analysis within the ventricular chamber may also be exploited to improve the design of the valve chambers and the mechanical valves in order to reduce the turbulent stresses near the vicinity of the inflow and outflow orifices [Kim et al., 1992]. Structural failure of the mechanical valves, initially reported with the TAH may have been the result of

(a)

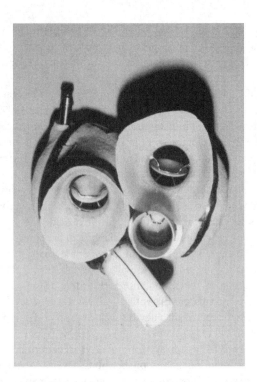

(b)

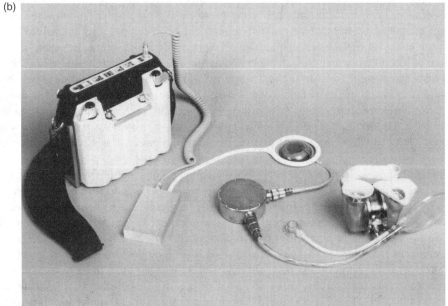

FIGURE 44.8 Typical prototype designs of total artificial hearts: (a) pneumatically powered TAH. The right and left ventricular chambers, inflow and outflow valves, as well as the connector for the pneumatic line are visible in the photograph; (b) electrically powered TAH. Shown are the external battery pack, transcutaneous energy transmission system (TETS) primary and secondary coils, implanted electronics, energy converter and the blood pumps, compliance chamber and the subcutaneous access port. (Courtesy of G. Rosenberg, Pennsylvania State University.)

TABLE 44.4 Classification of Vascular Prostheses

Prosthesis	Comments
Surgically-implanted biological grafts	
Autograft	Graft transplanted from part of a patient's body to another
	Example: saphenous vein graft for peripheral bypass
Allograft	Homograft. Transplanted vascular graft tissues derived from the
	same species as recipient. Example: glutaraldehyde treated umbilical cord vein graft
Xenograft	Heterograft. Surgical graft of vascular tissues derived from one
	species to a recipient of another species. Example: modified bovine heterograft
Surgically-implanted synthetic grafts	
Dacron (polyethylene terephthalate)	Woven, knitted
PTFE (polytetrafluoroethylene)	Expanded, knitted
Other	Nylon, polyurethane

increased load on the valves during closure due to the relatively large dp/dt (p is pressure, t is time) at which the TAH was operated. Attempts at reducing the dp/dt during closure of the inflow valves have also been reported with modified designs of the artificial heart driver [Wurzel et al., 1988]. Due to the relatively large dp/dt at which TAHs are operated, there is increased possibility of cavitation bubble initiation and subsequent collapse of the bubbles may also be another important reason for thrombus deposition near the mechanical valve at the inflow orifice. Introducing synthetic valves to replace the mechanical valves [Chandran et al., 1991b] may prove to be advantageous with respect to cavitation initiation and may minimize thrombus formation.

44.1.4 Vascular Prostheses

In advanced stages of vascular diseases such as obstructive **atherosclerosis** and aneurysmal dilatation, when other treatment modalities fail, replacement of diseased segments with vascular prostheses is a common practice. Vascular prostheses can be classified as given in Table 44.4.

44.1.4.1 Surgically Implanted Biological Grafts

Arterial homografts, even though initially used in large scale, resulted in aneurysm formation especially in the proximal suture line [Strandness and Sumner, 1975]. Still, a viable alternative is to use the saphenous vein graft from the same patient. Vein grafts have a failure rate of about 20% in one year and up to 30% in five years after implantation. Vein grafts from the same patients are also unavailable or unsuitable in about 10 to 30% of the patients [Abbott and Bouchier-Hayes, 1978]. Modified **bovine heterograft** and gluteraldehyde treated **umbilical cord vein grafts** have also been employed as vascular prostheses with less success compared to autologous vein grafts.

44.1.4.2 Surgically Implanted Synthetic Grafts

Prostheses made of synthetic material for vascular replacement have been used for over 40 years. Polymeric material currently used as implants include **nylon**, polyester, **polytetrafluoroethylene (PTFE)**, polypropylene, polyacrylonitrile, and silicone rubber [Park and Lakes, 1992]. However, Dacron® (polyethylene terephthalate) and PTFE are the more common vascular prostheses materials currently available. These materials exhibit the essential qualities for implants — they are biocompatible, resilient, flexible, durable, and resistant to sterilization and biodegradation. Detailed discussion on the properties, manufacturing techniques, and testing of Dacron® prostheses is included in Guidoin and Couture [1992]. Figure 44.9a depicts a Dacron vascular graft having a bifurcated configuration. Figure 44.9b shows expanded PTFE vascular grafts having a variety of configurations and sizes: straight, straight with external reinforcement rings (to resist external compression), and bifurcated.

(a)

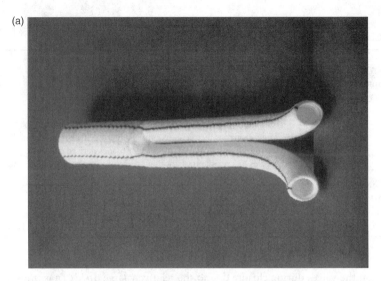

(b)

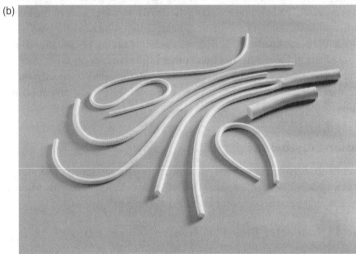

FIGURE 44.9   (a) Photograph of a Dacron vascular graft having a bifurcated configuration. (Courtesy of W.L. Gore and Associates, Inc., Flagstaff, AZ.) (b) Photographs of expanded PTFE vascular grafts with straight, straight with external reinforcement rings to resist compression, and bifurcated configurations. (Courtesy of W.L. Gore and Associates, Inc., Flagstaff, AZ.)

Synthetic vascular grafts implanted as large-vessel replacements have resulted in reasonable degrees of success. However, in medium- and small-diameter prostheses (less than 6 mm in diameter), loss of **patency** within several months after implantation is more acute. Graft failure due to thrombosis or intimal hyperplasia with thrombosis is primarily responsible in failures within 30 days after implantation, and intimal hyperplasia formation is the reason for failure within 6 months after surgery. Soon after implantation, a layer of **fibrin** and fibrous tissue covers the intimal and outer surface of the prosthesis, respectively. A layer of **fibroblasts** replaces the fibrin and is referred to as **neointima**. In the later stages, **neointimal hyperplasia** formation occurs and ultimately results in the occlusion of the vessels in small-diameter vascular grafts. Attempts are being made currently in suitably modifying the surface characteristics of the prostheses in order to reduce the problems with loss of patency. Studies are also being performed in order to understand the mechanical stresses induced at the anastomotic region, which may result in deposits on the intimal surface and occlusion of the vessels [Chandran and Kim, 1994]. The alterations in mechanical stresses with the implantation of vascular prostheses in the arterial circulation may include changes in the deformation and stress concentrations at the anastomotic site. Altered fluid shear stresses at the intimal surface in the vicinity of the anastomosis has also been suggested as important particularly since the loss of patency is present more often at the distal anastomosis. The vascular prostheses should have the same dynamic response after implantation as the host artery in order to reduce the effect of abnormal mechanical stresses at the junction. For a replacement graft of the same size as the host artery, mismatch in **compliance** may be the most important factor resulting in graft failure [Abbott and Bouchier-Hayes, 1978]. In implanting the prostheses, **end-to-end configuration** is common in the reconstruction of peripheral arteries. **End-to-side configuration** is common in coronary artery bypass where blood will flow from the host artery (aorta) to the prosthesis branching out at the anastomotic site. At the other end, the graft is attached distal to the occlusion in the host (coronary) vessel to enable perfusion of the vascular bed downstream from the occlusion. Numerous studies analyzing the abnormal flow dynamics within the anastomotic geometry and stress distribution within the vascular material at the junction to the prostheses have been reported in delineating the causes for intimal hyperplasia formation and loss of patency [Kim and Chandran, 1993; Kim et al., 1993; Ojha et al., 1990; Keynton et al., 1991; Chandran et al., 1992; Rodgers et al., 1987; Rhee and Tarbell, 1994] and a detailed discussion on the mechanical aspects of vascular prostheses can be found in Chandran and Kim [1994]. Improvements in the blood–surface interactions are also being attempted in order to improve the functioning capability of vascular grafts. Attempts at seeding the grafts with **endothelial cells** [Hunter et al., 1983], and modifying the graft material properties by removing the **crimping** and heat fusing a coil of bendable and dimensionally stable polypropylene at the outer surface to make it kink resistant [Guidoin et al., 1983], and employing a compliant and biodegradable graft which will promote regeneration of arterial wall in small caliber vessels [Van der Lei et al., 1985, 1986] are a few examples of such improvements.

44.1.4.3 Transluminally Placed Endovascular Prostheses (Stent-Grafts)

Endoluminal approaches to treating vascular disease involve the insertion of a prosthetic device into the vasculature through a small, often percutaneous, access site created in a remote vessel, followed by the intraluminal delivery and deployment of a prosthesis via transcatheter techniques [Veith et al., 1995]. In contrast to conventional surgical therapies for vascular disease, the use of transluminally placed endovascular prostheses are distinguished by their "minimally invasive" nature. Because these techniques do not require extensive surgical intervention, they have the potential to simplify the delivery of vascular therapy, improve procedural outcomes, decrease procedural costs, reduce morbidity, and broaden the patient population that may benefit from treatment. Not surprisingly, endoluminal therapies have generated intense interest within the vascular surgery, interventional radiology, and cardiology communities over recent years.

The feasibility of using transluminally placed endovascular prostheses, or stent-grafts, for the treatment of traumatic vascular injury [Marin et al., 1994], atherosclerotic obstructions [Cragg and Dake, 1993], and aneurysmal vascular disease [Parodi et al., 1991; Yusuf et al., 1994; Dake et al., 1994] has been demonstrated in human beings. Endoluminal stent-grafts continue to evolve to address a number of cardiovascular pathologies at all levels of the arterial tree. Figure 44.10a depicts endoluminal stent-grafts having a variety of configurations (straight, bifurcated) and functional diameters (peripheral, aortic) that are currently under clinical investigation.

Endoluminal stent-grafts are catheter-deliverable endoluminal prostheses comprised of an intravascular stent component and a biocompatible graft component. The function of these devices is to provide an intraluminal conduit that enables blood flow through pathologic vascular segments without the need for open surgery. The stent component functions as an arterial attachment mechanism and provides structural support to both the graft and the treated vascular segment. By design, stents are delivered to the vasculature in a low profile, small diameter delivery configuration, and can be elastically or plastically expanded to a secondary, large diameter configuration upon deployment. Vascular attachment is achieved by the interference fit created when a stent is deployed within the lumen of a vessel having a diameter smaller than that of the stent. The graft component, on the other hand, is generally constructed from a biocompatible material such as expanded polytetrafluoroethylene (ePTFE), woven polyester (Dacron), or polyurethane. The graft

(a)

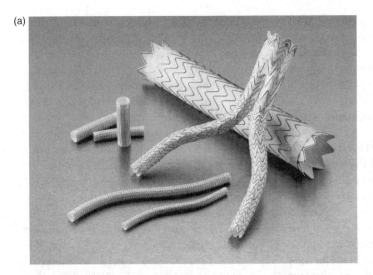

(b)

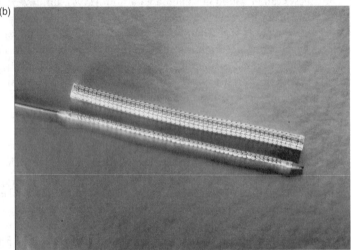

FIGURE 44.10   (a) Endoluminal stent-grafts of straight and bifurcated configurations and sizes currently under clinical investigation. (Courtesy of W.L. Gore and Associates, Inc., Flagstaff, AZ.) (b) A stent-graft implant consisting of an expanded PTFE graft that is externally supported by a self-expanding nitinol stent. (Courtesy of W.L. Gore and Associates, Inc., Flagstaff, AZ.)

component has a number of real and theoretical functions, including: segregating potential thromboemboli or atheroemboli from the bloodstream, presenting a physical barrier to mass transport between the bloodstream and arterial wall, and mitigating cellular infiltration and the host inflammatory response. Figure 44.10b shows a stent-graft implant consisting of an expanded polytetrafluoroethylene (ePTFE) graft that is externally supported along its entire length by a self-expanding nitinol stent. The implant is radially constrained and attached to the leading end of a dual lumen polyethylene delivery catheter that allows transluminal delivery and deployment. Following introduction into the vascular system, the implant is positioned fluoroscopically within the diseased segment and released from the delivery system.

Mechanical properties play an important role in determining the *in vivo* performance of an endoluminal stent-graft. Since the graft component typically lacks significant structural integrity, the mechanical behavior of the stent-graft predominantly depends upon the mechanical properties of its stent component. The type of mechanism required to induce dilatation from the delivery (small diameter) configuration, to the deployed (large diameter) configuration typically classifies stents. Self-expanding stents are designed to spontaneously dilate (i.e., elastically recover) from the delivery diameter up to a maximal, pre-determined deployed diameter; whereas balloon-expandable stents are designed to be plastically enlarged over a range of values with the use of appropriately sized and pressurized dilatation balloons. Consequently, self-expanding stents exert a continuous, radially outward directed force on periluminal tissues, while balloon-expandable stents assume a fixed diameter that resists recoil of the surrounding periluminal tissues. Both types of stents exhibit utilitarian features. For example, in comparison to balloon-expandable devices, self-expanding stents can be rapidly deployed without the use of dilatation balloons, are elastic and therefore less prone to external compression, can radially adapt to post-deployment vascular remodeling, and retain some of the natural compliance of the vascular tissues. In contrast, balloon-expandable stents are much more versatile when it comes to conforming to irregular vascular morphologies because their diameter can be radially adjusted via balloon dilatation. Since the luminal diameter of self-expanding stents cannot be adjusted (i.e., enlarged) to any appreciable degree, accurate sizing of the host vessel is critical. A sizing mismatch resulting in oversizing can cause overcompression of the self-expanding stent and obstructive invagination of the stent into the lumen. Undersizing, in turn, can result in a poor interference fit, inadequate anchoring, device migration, and/or leakage of blood into the abluminal compartment. In either case, the stent provides a scaffold that structurally supports the graft material. Ongoing work in the field of biomedical engineering is directed at optimizing the biomechanical and biological performance of these devices.

44.1.5 Conclusions

In the last four decades, we have observed significant advances in the development of biocompatible materials to be used in blood interfacing implants. In the case of mechanical heart valve prostheses, pyrolytic carbon has become the material of choice for the occluder and the housing. The pyrolytic carbon is chemically inert and exhibits very little wear even after more than 20 years of use. However, thrombo-embolic complications still remain significant with mechanical valve implantation. The complex dynamics of valve function and the resulting mechanical stresses on the formed elements of blood appear to be the main cause for initiation of thrombus. More recent reports of structural failure with implanted mechanical valves and pitting and erosion observed on the pyrolytic carbon surfaces have resulted in investigations on cavitation bubble formation during valve closure. Along with further improvements in biomaterials for heart valves, detailed analysis of the closing dynamics and design improvements to minimize the adverse effects of mechanical stresses may be the key to reducing thrombus deposition. Improvements on mechanical heart valves or further developments in durable synthetic leaflet valves may also be vital for the development of TAHs for long-term implantation without neurologic complications.

In the case of vascular grafts, the mismatch of material properties (compliance) between the host artery and the graft, as well as geometric considerations in end-to-side anastomoses, appear to be important for the loss of patency within several months after implantation particularly with medium and small diameter arterial replacement. Most of the vascular grafts are stiffer compared to the host artery and it has been suggested that the mechanical stresses resulting from the discontinuity at the junction is the major cause for neointimal hyperplasia formation and subsequent occlusion of the conduit. Developments with more compliant grafts and in modifying the surface interaction of the graft with blood (endothelialization or other treatment of the graft material) may result in reducing the problems with loss of patency. Recent advances in the use of minimally invasive stent-grafts also show promise in improving the quality of life of patients with vascular disease.

Defining Terms

Acetol: Product of the addition of two moles of alcohol to one of an aldehyde.
Aneurysms: Abnormal bulging or dilatation of a segment of a blood vessel or myocardium.
Artery: Blood vessel transporting blood in a direction away from the heart.
Atherosclerosis: Lipid deposits in the intima of arteries.

ATS valve: A bileaflet mechanical valve made by ATS (Advancing The Standard) Inc.

Autoclaving: Sterilizing by steam under pressure.

Biomer®:   Segmented polyurethane elastomer.

Bioprostheses: Prosthetic heart valves made of biological tissue.

Blood oxygenators: Extracorporeal devices to oxygenate blood during heart bypass surgery.

Bovine heterograft: Graft material (arterial) transplanted from bovine species.

Calcification: Deposition of insoluble salts of calcium.

Cardiac pacemakers: Prosthesis implanted to stimulate cardiac muscles to contract.

Cardiopulmonary bypass: Connectors bypassing circulation to the heart and the lungs.

Catheters: Hollow cylindrical tubing to be passed through the blood vessels or other canals.

Cavitation bubbles (vapor cavitation):   Formation of vapor bubbles due to transient reduction in pressure to below the liquid vapor pressure.

Closing dynamics: Dynamics during the closing phase of heart valves.

Compliance: A measure of ease with which a structure can be deformed; ratio of volumetric strain to increase in unit pressure.

Crimping: Creasing of the synthetic vascular grafts in the longitudinal direction to accommodate the large intermittent flow of blood.

Delrin®:   Polyacetal made by Union Carbide.

Dialysers: Devices to filter the blood of waste products taking over the function of the kidney.

dp/dt: Slope of the pressure vs. time curve of the ventricles.

Duramater: A tough fibrous membrane forming the outer cover of the brain and the spinal cord.

Electrohydraulic blood pump: Blood pumps energized by the conversion of electrical to hydraulic energy.

End-to-end configuration: End of the vascular graft anastamosed to the end of the host artery.

End-to-side configuration: End of the vascular graft anastamosed to the side of the host.

Endothelial cells: A layer of flat cells lining the intimal surface of blood vessels.

Erosion: A state of being worn away.

Fascia lata: A sheet of fibrous tissue enveloping the muscles of the thigh.

Fatigue stress: Level of stress below which the material would not undergo fatigue failure (107 cycles is used as the normal limit).

Fibrin: An elastic filamentous protein derived from fibrinogen in coagulation of the blood.

Fibroblasts: An elongated cell with cytoplasmic processes present in connective tissue capable of forming collagen fibers.

Finite element analysis: Structural analysis with the aid of a computer which divides the structure into finite elements and applies the laws of mechanics on each element.

Formaldehyde: Formic aldehyde, methyl aldehyde, a pungent gas used as antiseptic.

Formed elements in blood: Red blood cells, white blood cells, platelets, and other cells in whole blood.

Haynes 25®:   Co–Cr alloy.

Homografts: Transplants (heart valves, arterial segments, etc.) from the same species.

Intra-aortic balloon pumps: A balloon catheter inserted in the descending aorta and alternately inflated and deflated timed to the EKG in order to assist the ventricular pumping.

Laser Doppler anemometry: A velocity measurement device using the principle of Doppler shifted frequency of laser light by particles moving with the fluid.

Leaflets: Occluders on valves which open and close to aid blood flow in one direction.

Left ventricular assist devices: Prosthetic devices to assist the left ventricle in pumping blood.

Liquid vapor pressure: Pressure at which liquid vaporizes.

LTI: Low temperature (below 1500°C) isotropic pyrolytic carbon.

Mechanical prostheses: Prostheses made of non-biological material.

Negative pressure transients: Reduction in pressure for a short duration.

Neointima: Newly formed intimal surface.

Neointimal hyperplasia: Growth of new intimal surface formed by fibroblasts.

Nylon: Synthetic polymer with condensation polymerization.

Patency: State of being freely open.

Pericardial prostheses: Heart valve prosthesis made with fixed bovine pericardial tissue.

Pitting: Depression or indent on a surface.

Platelet: One of the formed elements of blood responsible for blood coagulation.

Polypropylene: One of the vinyl polymers with good flex life and good environmental stress crack resistance.

Polytetrafluoroethylene (PTFE):   A fluorocarbon polymer known as Teflon®.

Pusher plate devices: Artificial heart devices working with pusher plates moving the blood.

Pyrolytic carbon: Carbon deposited onto preformed polycrystalline graphite substrate.

Radiopacity: Being opaque to x-ray.

Sewing rings: Rings surrounding the housing of artificial heart valves used to sew the valve to the tissue orifice with suture.

Solution casting: Casting by pouring molten material on dyes to form a structure.

Stellite 21®:   Co–Cr alloy.

Stent: A device used to maintain the bodily orifice or cavity.

Strut: A projection in the structure such as guiding struts in heart valves used to guide the leaflets during opening and closing.

TAH: Total artificial heart replacing a failed natural heart.

Teflon®:   See PTFE.

Thrombo-embolic complications: Complications due to breaking away (emboli) of thrombus blocking the distal blood vessels.

Thrombus: A clot in the blood vessels or in the cavities of the heart formed from the constituents of blood.

Tilting disc valves: Valves with a single leaflet tilting open and shut.

Titanium: Highly reactive metal having low density, good mechanical properties, and biocompatibility due to tenacious oxide layer formation.

Turbulent stresses: Stresses generated in the fluid due to agitated random motion of particles.

Ultra high molecular weight polyethylene: Linear thermoplastics with very high molecular weight ($>2 \times 10^6$ g/mol) used for orthopedic devices such as acetabular cup for hip joint replacement.

Umbilical cord vein grafts: Vascular graft made from umbilical cord veins.

Vacuum forming: A manufacturing technique for thermoplastic polymer in which a sheet is heated and formed over a mold while a vacuum is present under the sheet.

Valvular disorders: Diseased states of valves such as stenosis.

Valvular structures: Components of valves such as leaflets, struts, etc.

Vascular grafts: Grafts to replace segments of diseased vessels.

Xenografts: Grafts obtained from species other than that of the recipient.

References

Abbott, W.M. and Bouchier-Hayes, D.J. 1978. The role of mechanical properties in graft design. In *Graft Materials in Vascular Surgery*, Dardick, H., Ed. Year Book Medical Publishers, Chicago, IL, pp. 59–78.

Akutsu, T. and Kolff, W.J. 1958. Permanent substitutes for valves and hearts. *Trans. Am. Soc. Art. Intern. Organs (ASAIO)* 4: 230–235.

Baldwin, J.T., Tarbell, J.M., Deutsch, S., Geselowitz, D.B., and Rosenberg, G. 1988. Hot-film wall shear probe measurements inside a ventricular assist device. *Am. Soc. Mech. Eng. (ASME) J. Biomech. Eng.* 110: 326–333.

Baldwin, J.T., Campbell, A., Luck, C., Ogilvie, W., and Sauter, J. 1997. Hydrodynamics of the CarboMedics® aortic kinetic™ prosthetic heart valve. In *Surgery for Acquired Aortic Valve Disease*. Piwnica, A. and Westaby, S., Eds., ISIS Medical Media, Oxford, pp. 365–370.

Bell, R.S. 1997. CarboMedics® supra-annular Top Hat™ aortic valve. In *Surgery for Acquired Aortic Valve Disease*. Piwnica, A. and Westaby, S., Eds., ISIS Medical Media, Oxford, pp. 371–375.

Bona, G., Rinaldi, S., and Vallana, F. 1997. Design characteristics of the BICARBON™ bileaflet heart valve prosthesis. In *Surgery for Acquired Aortic Valve Disease*. Piwnica, A. and Westaby, S. Eds., ISIS Medical Media, Oxford, pp. 392–396.

Braunwald, N.S., Cooper, T., and Morrow, A.G. 1960. Complete replacement of the mitral valve: successful application of a flexible polyurethane prosthesis. *J. Thorac. Cardiovasc. Surg.* 40: 1–11.

Carpentier, A., Lamaigre, C.G., Robert, L., Carpentier, S., and Dubost, C. 1969. Biological factors affecting long-term results of valvular heterografts. *J. Thorac. Cardiovasc. Surg.* 58: 467–483.

Chandran, K.B., Cabell, G.N., Khalighi, B., and Chen, C.J. 1983. Laser anemometry measurements of pulsatile flow past aortic valve prostheses. *J. Biomech.* 16: 865–873.

Chandran, K.B., Cabell, G.N., Khalighi, B., and Chen, C.J. 1984. Pulsatile flow past aortic valve bioprostheses in a model human aorta. *J. Biomech.* 17: 609–619.

Chandran, K.B. 1988. Heart valve prostheses: *in vitro* flow dynamics. In *Encyclopedia of Medical Devices and Instrumentation*, Vol. 3. Webster, J.G., Ed., Wiley Interscience, New York, pp. 1475–1483.

Chandran, K.B., Fatemi, R., Schoephoerster, R., Wurzel, D., Hansen, G., Pantalos, G., Yu, L.-S., and Kolff, W.J. 1989a. *In vitro* comparison of velocity profiles and turbulent shear distal to polyurethane trileaflet and pericardial prosthetic valves. *Artif. Organs* 13: 148–154.

Chandran, K.B., Schoephoerster, R.T., Wurzel, D., Hansen, G., Yu, L.-S., Pantalos, G., and Kolff, W.J. 1989b. Hemodynamic comparison of polyurethane trileaflet and bioprosthetic heart valves. *Trans. Am. Soc. Artif. Intern. Organs (ASAIO)* 35: 132–138.

Chandran, K.B., Kim, S.-H., and Han, G. 1991a. Stress distribution on the cusps of a polyurethane trileaflet heart valve prosthesis in the closed position. *J. Biomech.* 24: 385–395.

Chandran, K.B., Lee, C.S., Shipkowitz, T., Chen, L.D., Yu, L.S. and Wurzel, D. 1991b. *In vitro* hemodynamic analysis of flexible artificial ventricle. *Artif. Organs* 15: 420–426.

Chandran, K.B., Gao, D., Han, G., Baraniewski, H., and Corson, J.D. 1992. Finite element analysis of arterial anastomosis with vein, Dacron® and PTFE grafts. *Med. Biol. Eng. Comp.* 30: 413–418.

Chandran, K.B. 1992. *Cardiovascular Biomechanics*. New York University Press, New York.

Chandran, K.B., Lee, C.S., and Chen, L.D. 1994a. Pressure field in the vicinity of mechanical valve occluders at the instant of valve closure: correlation with cavitation initiation. *J. Heart Valve Dis.* 3 (Suppl. 1): S 65–S 76.

Chandran, K.B., Lee, C.S., Aluri, S., Dellsperger, K.C., Schreck, S., and Wieting, D.W. 1994b. Pressure distribution near the occluders and impact forces on the outlet struts of Björk–Shiley convexo-concave valves during closing. *J. Heart Valve Dis.* 5: 199–206.

Chandran, K.B. and Kim, Y.H. 1994. Mechanical aspects of vascular graft-host artery anastomoses. *IEEE Eng. Med. Biol. Mag.* 13: 517–524.

Chandran, K.B. and Aluri, S. 1997. Mechanical valve closing dynamics. Relationship between velocity of closing, pressure transients, and cavitation initiation. *Ann. Biomed. Eng.* 25: 926–938.

Chandran, K. B., Dexter, E. U., Aluri, S., and Richenbacher, W.E. 1998. Negative pressure transients with mechanical heart-valve closure: Correlation between *in vitro* and *in vivo* results. *Ann. Biomed. Eng.* 26: 546–556.

Cheon, G.J. and Chandran, K.B. 1994. Transient behavior analysis of a mechanical monoleaflet heart valve prosthesis in the closing phase. *Am. Soc. Mech. Eng. J. Biomech. Eng.* 116: 452–459.

Cragg A.H. and Dake M.D. 1993. Percutaneous femoropoliteal graft placement. *Radiology* 187: 643–648.

Dake M.D., Miller D.C., Semba C.P. et al. 1994. Transluminal placement of endovascular stent-grafts for the treatment of descending thoracic aortic aneurysms. *N. Engl. J. Med.* 331: 1729–34.

Dellsperger, K.C. and Chandran, K.B. 1991. Prosthetic heart valves. In *Blood Compatible Materials and Devices. Perspectives towards the 21st Century*. Sharma, C.P. and Szycher, M., Eds., Technomic Publishing Company Inc., Lancaster, PA, pp. 153–165.

DeVries, W.C. and Joyce, L.D. 1983. The artificial heart. *CIBA Clin. Symp.*, 35.

Drogue, J., and Villafana, M. 1997. ATS Medical open pivot™ valve. In *Surgery for Acquired Aortic Valve Disease.* Piwnica, A. and Westaby, S., Eds., ISIS Medical Media, Oxford, pp. 410–416.

Farrar, D.J., Litwak, P., Lawson, J.H., Ward, R.S., White, K.A., Robinson, A.J., Rodvein, R., and Hill, J.D. 1988. *In vivo* evaluations of a new thromboresistant polyurethane for artificial heart blood pumps. *J. Thorac. Cardiovasc. Surg.* 95: 191–200.

Gerring, E.L., Bellhouse, B.J., Bellhouse, F.H., and Haworth, F.H. 1974. Long term animal trials of the Oxford aortic/pulmonary valve prosthesis without anticoagulants. *Trans. ASAIO* 20: 703–708.

Ghista, D.N. and Reul, H. 1977. Optimal prosthetic aortic leaflet valve: design, parametric and longevity analysis: Development of the avcothane-51 leaflet valve based on the optimal design analysis. *J. Biomech.* 10: 313–324.

Guidoin, R., Gosselin, C., Martin, L., Marios, M., Laroche, F., King, M., Gunasekara, K., Domurado, D., and Sigot-Luizard, M.F. 1983. Polyester prostheses as substitutes in the thoracic aorta of dogs. I. Evaluation of commercial prostheses. *J. Biomed. Mater. Res.* 17: 1049–1077.

Guidoin, R. and Couture, J. 1991. Polyester prostheses: The outlook for the future. In *Blood Compatible Materials and Devices. Perspectives towards the 21st Century.* Sharma, C.P. and Szycher, M., Eds., Technomic Publishing Company Inc., Lancaster, PA, pp. 153–165.

Hamid, M.S., Sabbah, H.N., and Stein, P.D. 1985. Finite element evaluation of stresses on closed leaflets of bioprosthetic heart valves with flexible stents. *Finite Elem. Anal. Des.* 1: 213–225.

Harold, M., Lo, H.B., Reul, H., Muchter, H., Taguchi, K., Gierspien, M., Birkle, G., Hollweg, G., Rau, G., and Messmer, B.J. 1987. The Helmholtz Institute tri-leaflet polyurethane heart valve prosthesis: Design, manufacturing, and first *in vitro* and *in vivo* results. In *Polyurethanes in Biomedical Engineering II.* Planck, H., Syre, I., and Dauner, M., Eds., Elsevier Publishing Co., Amsterdam, pp. 321–356.

Holfert, J.W., Reibman, J.B., Dew, P.A., De Paulis, R., Burns, G.L., and Olsen, D.B. 1987. A new connector system for total artificial hearts: preliminary results. *Trans. ASAIO* 10: 151–156.

Hunter, G.C., Schmidt, S.P., Sharp, W.V., and Malindzak, G.S. 1983. Controlled flow studies in 4 mm endothelialized Dacron® grafts. *Trans. ASAIO* 29: 177–182.

Hufnagel, C.A. 1977. Reflections on the development of valvular prostheses. *Med. Instrum.* 11: 74–76.

Jarvick, R.K. 1981. The total artificial heart. *Sci. Am.* 244: 66–72.

Jarvis, P., Tarbell, J.M., and Frangos, J.A. 1991. An *in vitro* evaluation of an artificial heart. *Trans. ASAIO* 37: 27–32.

Kafesjian, R., Howanec, M., Ward, G.D., Diep, L., Wagstaff, L.S., and Rhee, R. 1994. Cavitation damage of pyrolytic carbon in mechanical heart valves. *J. Heart Valve Dis.* 3 (Suppl. 1): S 2–S 7.

Kambic, H.E. and Nose, Y. 1991. Biomaterials for blood pumps. In *Blood Compatible Materials and Devices. Perspectives Towards the 21st Century.* Sharma, C.P. and Szycher, M., Eds., Technomic Publishing Company Inc., Lancaster, PA, pp. 141–151.

Keynton, R.S., Rittgers, S.E., and Shu, M.C.S. 1991. The effect of angle and flow rate upon hemodynamics in distal vascular graft anastomoses: An *in vitro* model study. *ASME J. Biomech. Eng.* 113: 458–463.

Kim, S.H., Chandran, K.B., and Chen, C.J. 1992. Numerical simulation of steady flow in a two-dimensional total artificial heart model. *ASME J. Biomech. Eng.* 114: 497–503.

Kim, Y.H., Chandran, K.B., Bower, T.J., and Corson, J.D. 1993. Flow dynamics across end-to-end vascular bypass graft anastomoses. *Ann. Biomed. Eng.* 21: 311–320.

Kim, Y.H. and Chandran, K.B. 1993. Steady flow analysis in the vicinity of an end-to-end anastomosis. *Biorheol.* 30: 117–130.

Lapeyre, D.M., Frazier, O.H., and Conger, J.L. 1994. *In vivo* evaluation of a trileaflet mechanical heart valve. *ASAIO J.* 40: M707–M713.

Lee, C.S., Chandran, K.B., and Chen, L.D. 1994. Cavitation dynamics of mechanical heart valve prostheses. *Artif. Organs* 18: 758–767.

Lee, C.S. and Chandran, K.B. 1994. Instantaneous backflow through peripheral clearance of Medtronic Hall valve at the moment of closure. *Ann. Biomed. Eng.* 22: 371–380.

Lee, C.S. and Chandran, K.B. 1995. Numerical simulation of instantaneous backflow through central clearance of bileaflet mechanical heart valves at the moment of closure: shear stress and pressure fields within the clearance. *Med. Biol. Eng. Comp.* 33: 257–263.

Lee, J.M. and Boughner, D.R. 1991. Bioprosthetic heart valves: Tissue mechanics and implications for design. In *Blood Compatible Materials and Devices. Perspectives Towards the 21st Century.* Sharma, C.P. and Szycher, M., Eds., Technomic Publishing Company Inc., Lancaster, PA, pp. 167–188.

Lefrak, E.A. and Starr, A., Eds. 1970. *Cardiac Valve Prostheses.* Appleton-Century-Crofts, New York.

Leuer, L. 1987. Dynamics of mechanical valves in the artificial heart. *Proc. 40th Ann. Conf. Eng. Med. Biol. (ACEMB)*, p. 82.

Marin, M.L., Veith, F.J., Panetta, T.F. et al. 1994. Transluminally placed endovascular stented graft repair for arterial trauma. *J. Vasc. Surg.* 20: 466–73.

McKenna, J. 1997. The Ultracor™ prosthetic heart valve. In *Surgery for Acquired Aortic Valve Disease.* Piwnica, A. and Westaby, S., Eds., ISIS Medical Media, Oxford, pp. 337–340.

Ojha, M., Ethier, C.R., Johnston, K.W., and Cobbold, R.S.C. 1990. Steady and pulsatile flow fields in an end-to-side arterial anastomosis model. *J. Vasc. Surg.* 12: 747–753.

Park, J.B. and Lakes, R.S. 1992. *Biomaterials: An Introduction*, 2nd ed., Plenum Press, New York.

Parodi, J.C., Palmaz, J.C., and Barone, H.D. 1991. Transfemoral intraluminal graft implantation for abdominal aortic aneurysms. *Ann. Vasc. Surg.* 5: 491–9.

Phillips, W.M., Brighton, J.A., and Pierce, W.S. 1979. Laser Doppler anemometer studies in unsteady ventricular flows. *Trans. ASAIO* 25: 56–60.

Phillips, R.E., and Printz, L.K. 1997. PhotoFix™ α: a pericardial aortic prosthesis. In *Surgery for Acquired Aortic Valve Disease.* Piwnica, A. and Westaby, S., Eds., ISIS Medical Media, Oxford, pp. 376–381.

Piwnica, A. and Westaby, S., Eds. 1997. *Surgery for Acquired Aortic Valve Disease.* ISIS Medical Media, Oxford.

Reif, T.H. 1991. A numerical analysis of the back flow between the leaflets of a St. Jude Medical cardiac valve prosthesis. *J. Biomech.* 24: 733–741.

Reis, R.L., Hancock, W.D., Yarbrough, J.W., Glancy, D.L., and Morrow, A.G. 1971. The flexible stent. *J. Thorac. Cardiovasc. Surg.* 62: 683–691.

Reul, H., Steinseifer, U., Knoch, M., and Rau, G. 1995. Development, manufacturing and validation of a single leaflet mechanical heart valve prosthesis. *J. Heart Valve Dis.* 4: 513–519.

Rhee, K. and Tarbell, J.M. 1994. A study of wall shear rate distribution near the end-to-end anastomosis of a rigid graft and a compliant artery. *J. Biomech.* 27: 329–338.

Rodgers, V.G.J., Teodori, M.F., and Borovetz, H.S. 1987. Experimental determination of mechanical shear stress about an anastomotic junction. *J. Biomech.* 20: 795–803.

Roe, B.B., Owsley, J.W., and Boudoures, P.C. 1958. Experimental results with a prosthetic aortic valve. *J. Thorac. Cardiovasc. Surg.* 36: 563–570.

Rosenberg, G. 1995a. Artificial heart and circulatory assist devices. In *The Biomedical Engineering Handbook.* Bronzino, J.D., Ed., CRC Press, Boca Raton, FL, pp. 1839–1846.

Rosenberg, G., Snyder, A.J., Weiss, W.J., Sapirstein, J.S., and Pierce, W.S. 1995b. *In vivo* testing of a clinical-size totally implantable artificial heart. In *Assisted Circulation 4.* F. Unger, Ed., Springer-Verlag, Berlin, pp. 235–248.

Russel, F.B., Lederman, D.M., Singh, P.I., Cumming, R.D., Levine, F.H., Austen, W.G., and Buckley, M.J. 1980. Development of seamless trileaflet valves. *Trans. ASAIO* 26: 66–70.

Sabbah, H.N., Hamid, M.S., and Stein, P.D. 1985. Estimation of mechanical stresses on closed cusps of porcine bioprosthetic valves: effect of stiffening, focal calcium and focal thinning. *Am. J. Cardiol.* 55: 1091–1097.

Shim, H.S. and Lenker, J.A. 1988. Heart valve prostheses. In *Encyclopedia of Medical Devices and Instrumentation*, Vol. 3. Webster, J.G., Ed., Wiley Interscience, New York, pp. 1457–1474.

Strandness, D.E. and Sumner, D.S. 1975. Grafts and grafting. In *Hemodynamics for Surgeons*, Grune and Stratton, New York, pp. 342–395.

Tarbell, J.M., Gunishan, J.P., Geselowitz, D.B., Rosenberg, G., Shung, K.K., and Pierce, W.S. 1986. Pulsed ultrasonic Doppler velocity measurements inside a left ventricular assist device. *ASME J. Biomech. Eng.* 108: 232–238.

Thubrikar, M.J., Skinner, J.R., and Nolan, S.P. 1982a. Design and stress analysis of bioprosthetic valves *in vivo*. In *Cardiac Bioprostheses*. Cohn, L.H. and Gallucci, V., Eds., Yorke Medical Books, New York, pp. 445–455.

Thubrikar, M.J., Skinner, J.R., Eppink, T.R., and Nolan, S.P. 1982b. Stress analysis of porcine bioprosthetic heart valves *in vivo*. *J. Biomed. Mater. Res.* 16: 811–826.

Unger, F. 1989. *Assisted Circulation*, Vol. 3. Springer-Verlag, Berlin.

Van der Lei, B., Wildevuur, C.R.H., Niewenhuis, P., Blaauw, E.H., Dijk, F., Hulstaert, C.E., and Molenaar, I. 1985. Regeneration of the arterial wall in microporous, compliant, biodegradable vascular grafts after implantation into the rat abdominal aorta. *Cell Tissue Res.* 242: 569–578.

Van der Lei, B., Wildevuur, C.R.H., and Nieuwenhuis, P. 1986. Compliance and biodegradation of vascular grafts stimulate the regeneration of elastic laminae in neoarterial tissue: an experimental study in rats. *Surgery* 99: 45–51.

Veith, F.J., Abbott, W.M., Yao, J.S.T. et al. 1995. Guidelines for development and use of transluminally placed endovascular prosthetic grafts in the arterial system. *J. Vasc. Surg.* 21: 670–85.

Wieting, D.W. 1997. Prosthetic heart valves in the future. In *Surgery for Acquired Aortic Valve Disease*. Piwnica, A. and Westaby, S., Eds., ISIS Medical Media, Oxford, pp. 460–478.

Wurzel, D., Kolff, J., Missfeldt, W., Wildevuur, W., Hansen, G., Brownstein, L., Reibman, J., De Paulis, R., and Kolff, W.J. 1988. Development of the Philadelphia heart system. *Artif. Organs* 12: 410–422.

Yoganathan, A.P., Corcoran, W.H., and Harrison, E.C. 1979a. *In vitro* velocity measurements in the vicinity of aortic prostheses. *J. Biomech.* 12: 135–152.

Yoganathan, A.P., Corcoran, W.H., and Harrison, E.C. 1979b. Pressure drops across prosthetic aortic heart valves under steady and pulsatile flow — *in vitro* measurements. *J. Biomech.* 12: 153–164.

Yoganathan, A.P., Woo, Y.R., and Sung, H.W. 1986. Turbulent shear stress measurements in the vicinity of aortic heart valve prostheses. *J. Biomech.* 19: 433–442.

Yusef, S.W., Baker, D.M., Chuter, T.A.M. et al. 1994. Transfemoral endoluminal repair of abdominal aortic aneurysm with bifurcated graft. *Lancet* 344: 650–1.

44.2 Non-Blood-Interfacing Implants for Soft Tissues

K.J.L. Burg and S.W. Shalaby

Most tissues other than bone and cartilage are of the soft category. Implants do not generally interface directly with blood; the exceptions are located primarily in the cardiovascular systems. Non-blood-interfacing soft tissue implants are used to augment or replace natural tissues or to redirect specific biological functions. The implants can be transient; that is, of short-term function and thus made of absorbable materials, or they can be long-term implants which are expected to have prolonged functions and are made of nonabsorbable materials.

Toward the successful development of a new biomedical device or implant, including those used for soft tissues, the following milestones must be achieved: (1) acquire certain biologic and biomechanic data about the implant site and its function to aid in the selection of materials and engineering design of such an implant, to meet carefully developed product requirements; (2) construct a prototype and evaluate its physical and biologic properties both *in vitro* and *in vivo*, using the appropriate animal model; and (3) conduct a clinical study following a successful battery of animal safety studies depending on intended application and availability of historical safety and clinical data on the material or design. Extent of the studies associated with any specific milestone can vary considerably. Although different applications require different materials with specific properties, minimum requirements for soft-tissue implants should be met. The implant must (1) exhibit physical properties (e.g., flexibility and texture) which are equivalent or comparable to those called for in the product profile; (2) maintain the expected physical properties after implantation for a specific period; (3) elicit no adverse tissue reaction; (4) display no carcinogenic, toxic, allergenic, and/or immunogenic effect; and (5) achieve assured sterility without compromising the physicochemical properties. In addition to these criteria, a product of potentially broad applications is expected to (1) be easily mass produced at a reasonable cost; (2) have acceptable aesthetic quality; (3) be enclosed in durable, properly labeled, easy-access packaging; and (4) have adequate shelf stability.

The most common types of soft-tissue implants are (1) sutures and allied augmentation devices; (2) percutaneous and cutaneous systems; (3) maxillofacial devices; (4) ear and eye prostheses; (5) space-filling articles; and (6) fluid transfer devices.

44.2.1 Sutures and Allied Augmentation Devices

Sutures and staples are the most common types of augmentation devices. In recent years, interest in using tapes and adhesives has increased and may continue to do so, should new efficacious systems be developed.

44.2.1.1 Sutures and Suture Anchors

Sutures are usually packaged as a thread attached to a metallic needle. Although most needles are made of stainless steel alloys, the thread component can be made of various materials, and the type used determines the class of the entire suture. In fact, it is common to refer to the thread as the suture. Presently, most needles are drilled (mechanically or by laser) at one end for thread insertion. Securing the thread in the needle hole can be achieved by crimping or adhesive attachment. Among the critical physical properties of sutures are their diameter, *in vitro* knot strength, needle-holding strength, needle penetration force, ease of knotting, knot security, and *in vitro* strength retention profile.

Two types of threads are used in suture manufacturing and are distinguished according to the retention of their properties in the biologic environment, namely, absorbable and nonabsorbable. These may also be classified according to their source of raw materials, that is, natural (catgut, silk, and cotton), synthetic (nylon, polypropylene, polyethylene terephthalate, and polyglycolide and its copolymers), and metallic sutures (stainless steel and tantalum). Sutures may also be classified according to their physical form, that is, monofilament and twisted or braided multifilament (or simply braids).

The first known suture, the absorbable catgut, is made primarily of collagen derived from sheep intestinal submucosa. It is usually treated with a chromic salt to increase its *in vivo* strength retention and through imparted crosslinking that retards absorption. Such treatment extends the functional performance of catgut suture from 1 to 2 weeks up to about 3 weeks. The catgut sutures are packaged in a specially formulated fluid to prevent drying and maintain necessary compliance for surgical handling and knot formation.

The use of synthetic absorbable sutures exceeded that of catgut over the past two decades. This is attributed to many factors including (1) higher initial breaking strength and superior handling characteristics; (2) availability of sutures with a broad range of *in vivo* strength retention profiles; (3) considerably milder tissue reactions and no immunogenic response; and (4) reproducible properties and highly predictable *in vivo* performance. Polyglycolide (PG) was the first synthetic absorbable suture to be introduced, about three decades ago. Because of the high modulus of oriented fibers, PG is made mostly in the braided form. A typical PG suture braid absorbs in about 4 months and retains partial *in vivo* strength after 3 weeks. However, braids made of the 90/10 glycolide/l-lactide copolymer have a comparable or improved strength retention profile and faster absorption rate relative to PG. The copolymeric sutures absorb in about 3 months and have gained wide acceptance by the surgical community.

As with other types of braided sutures, an absorbable coating which improves suture handling and knot formation has been added to the absorbable braids. To minimize the risk of infection and tissue drag that are sometimes associated with braided sutures, four types of monofilament sutures have been commercialized. The absorbable monofilaments were designed specifically to approach the engineering compliance of braided sutures, by combining appropriate materials to achieve low moduli, for example, polydioxanone and copolymers of glycolide with caprolactone or trimethylene carbonate.

Members of the nonabsorbable family of sutures include braided silk (a natural protein), nylon, and polyethylene terephthalate (PET). These braids are used as coated sutures. Although silk sutures have retained wide acceptance by surgeons, nylon and particularly PET sutures are used for critical procedures where high strength and predictable long-term performance are required. Meanwhile, the use of cotton sutures is decreasing constantly because of their low strength and occasional tissue reactivity due to contaminants. Monofilaments are important forms of nonabsorbable sutures and are made primarily of polypropylene, nylon, and stainless steel. An interesting application of monofilament sutures is illustrated in the use of polypropylene loops (or haptics) for intraocular lenses. The polypropylene sutures exhibit not only the desirable properties of monofilaments but also the biologic inertness reflected in the minimal tissue reactions associated with their use in almost all surgical sites. With the exception of its natural tendency to undergo hydrolytic degradation and, hence, continued loss of mechanical strength postoperatively, nylon monofilament has similar attributes to those of polypropylene. Because of their exceptionally high modulus, stainless steel sutures are not used in soft-tissue repair because they can tear these tissues. All sutures can be sterilized by gamma radiation except those made of synthetic absorbable polymers, polypropylene, or cotton, which are sterilized by ethylene oxide.

Related to the suture is the tissue suture anchor, used to attach soft tissue to bone. The anchor is embedded into bone and the suture can be used to reattach the soft tissue. The most common anchor is polylactide-based and is used in shoulder repair.

44.2.1.2 Nonsuture Fibrous and Microporous Implants

Woven PET and polypropylene fabrics are commonly used as surgical meshes for abdominal wall repair and similar surgical procedures where surgical "patching" is required. Braid forms and similar construction made of multifilament PET yarns have been used for repairing tendons and ligaments. Microporous foams of polytetrafluoroethylene (PTFE) are used as pledgets (to aid in anchoring sutures to soft tissues) and in repair of tendons and ligaments. Microporous collagen-based foams are used in wound repair to accelerate healing.

44.2.1.3 Clips, Staples, and Pins

Ligating clips are most commonly used for temporary or long-term management of the flow in tubular tissues. Titanium clips are among the oldest and still-versatile types of clips. Thermoplastic polymers such as nylon can be injection-molded into different forms of ligating clips. These are normally designed to have a latch and living hinge. Absorbable polymers made of lactide/glycolide copolymers and polydioxanone have been successfully converted to ligating clips with different design features for a broad range of applications.

Metallic staples were introduced about three decades ago as strong competitors to sutures for wound augmentation; their use has grown considerably over the past 10 years for everything from skin closure procedures to a multiplicity of internal surgical applications. Major advantages associated with the use of staples are ease of application and minimized tissue trauma. Metallic staples can be made of tantalum, stainless steel, or titanium–nickel alloys. Staples are widely used to facilitate closure of large incisions produced in procedures such as Caesarean sections and intestinal surgery. Many interesting applications of small staples have been discovered for ophthalmic and endoscopic use, a fast-growing area of minimally invasive surgery.

Thermoplastic materials based on lactide/glycolide copolymers have been used to produce absorbable staples for skin and internal wound closures. These staples consist primarily of two interlocking components, a fastener and receiver. They are advantageous in that they provide a quick means of closure with comparable infection resistance. They are limited to locations which do not have large tensile loads and/or thicker or more sensitive tissue.

A new form of ligating device is the subcutaneous pin. This is designed with a unique applicator to introduce the pin parallel to the axis of the wound. During its application, the linear pin acquires a zig-zag-like configuration for stabilized tissue anchoring. The pins are made of lactide/glycolide polymers.

44.2.1.4 Surgical Tapes

Surgical tapes are intended to minimize necrosis, scar tissue formation, problems of stitch abscesses, and weakened tissues. The problems with surgical tapes are similar to those experienced with traditional skin tapes. These include (1) misaligned wound edges, (2) poor adhesion due to moisture or dirty wounds, and (3) late separation of tapes when hematoma or wound drainage occur.

Wound strength and scar formation in skin may depend on the type of incision made. If the subcutaneous muscles in the fatty tissue are cut and the overlying skin is closed with tape, then the muscles retract. This, in turn, increases the scar area, causing poor cosmetic appearance when compared to a suture closure. Tapes also have been used successfully for assembling scraps of donor skin for skin graft.

44.2.1.5 Tissue Adhesives

The constant call for tissue adhesives is particularly justified when dealing with the repair of exceptionally soft tissues. Such tissues cannot be easily approximated by sutures, because sutures inflict substantial mechanical damage following the traditional knotting scheme and associated shear stresses. However, the variable biological environments of soft tissues and their regenerative capacity make the development of an ideal tissue adhesive a difficult task. Experience indicates that an ideal tissue adhesive should (1) be able to wet and bond to tissues; (2) be capable of onsite formation by the rapid polymerization of a liquid monomer without producing excessive heat or toxic byproducts; (3) be absorbable; (4) not interfere with the normal healing process; and (5) be easily applied during surgery. The two common types of tissue adhesives currently used are based on alkyl-o-cyanoacrylates and fibrin. The latter is a natural adhesive derived from fibrinogen, which is one of the clotting components of blood. Although fibrin is used in Europe, its use in the United States has not been approved because of the risk of its contamination with hepatitis and/or immune disease viruses. Due to its limited mechanical strength (tensile strength and elastic modulus of 0.1 and 0.15 MPa, respectively), fibrin is used mostly as a sealant and for adjoining delicate tissues as in nerve anastomoses. Meanwhile, two members of the cyanoacrylate family of adhesives, n-butyl- and iso-butyl-cyano-acrylates, are used in a number of countries as sealants, adhesives, and blocking agents. They are yet to be approved for use in the United States because of the lack of sufficient safety data. Due to a fast rate of polymerization and some limited manageability in localizing the adhesive to the specific surgical site, the *in vivo* performance of cyanoacrylates can be unpredictable. Because of the low strength of the adhesive joints or sealant films produced on *in vivo* polymerization of these cyanoacrylates, their applications generally are limited to use in traumatized fragile tissues (such as spleen, liver, and kidney) and after extensive surgery on soft lung tissues. A major safety concern of these alkyl cyanoacrylates is related to their nonabsorbable nature. Hence, a number of investigators have directed their attention to certain alkoxy-alkyl cyanoacrylates which can be converted to polymeric adhesives with acceptable absorbable profiles and rheological properties. Methoxypropyl cyanoacrylate, for example, has demonstrated both the absorbability and high compliance that is advantageous to soft tissue repair.

44.2.2 Percutaneous and Skin Implants

The need for percutaneous (*trans* or through the skin) implants has been accelerated by the advent of artificial kidneys and hearts and the need for prolonged injection of drugs and nutrients. Artificial skin is urgently needed to maintain the body temperature and prevent infection in severely burned patients. Actual permanent replacement of skin by biomaterials is still a great clinical challenge.

44.2.2.1 Percutaneous Devices

The problem of obtaining a functional and viable interface between the tissue (skin) and an implant (percutaneous device) is primarily due to the following factors. First, although initial attachment of the tissue into the interstices of the implant surface occurs, attachment cannot be maintained for a sustained time since the dermal tissue cells turn over continuously. Downgrowth of epithelium around the implant or overgrowth on the implant leads to extrusion or invagination, respectively. Second, any opening near the implant that is large enough for bacteria to penetrate may result in infection, even though initially there may be a tight seal between skin and implant. Several factors are involved in the development of percutaneous devices:

1. Type of end use — this may deal with transmission of information (biopotentials, temperature, pressure, blood flow rate), energy (electrical stimulation, power for heart-assist devices), transfer of matter (cannula for blood), and load (attachment of a prosthesis);
2. Engineering factors — these may address materials selection (polymers, ceramics, metals, and composites), design variation (button, tube with and without skirt, porous or smooth surface), and mechanical stresses (soft and hard interface, porous or smooth interface);
3. Biologic factors — these are determined by the implant host (human, dog, hog, rabbit, sheep), and implant location (abdominal, dorsal, forearm);
4. Human factors — these can pertain to postsurgical care, implantation technique, and esthetic look.

No percutaneous devices are completely satisfactory. Nevertheless, some researchers believe that hydroxyapatite may be part of a successful approach. In one experimental trial, a hydroxyapatite-based percutaneous device was associated with less epidermal downgrowth (1 mm after 17 months vs. 4.6 mm after 3 months) when compared with a silicone rubber control specimen in the dorsal skin of canines. Researchers have also investigated coatings such as laminin-5 which has been shown to enhance epithelial attachment.

44.2.2.2 Artificial Skins

Artificial skin is another example of a percutaneous implant, and the problems are similar to those described above. Important for this application is a material which can adhere to a large (burned) surface and thus prevent the loss of fluids, electrolytes, and other biomolecules until the wound has healed.

In one study on wound-covering materials with controlled physicochemical properties, an artificial skin was designed with a crosslinked collagen-polysaccharide (chondroitin 6-sulfate) composite membrane. This was specifically chosen to have controlled porosity (5 to 150 μm in diameter), flexibility (by varying crosslink density), and moisture flux rate.

Several polymeric materials and reconstituted collagen have also been examined as burn dressings. Among the synthetic ones are the copolymers of vinyl chloride and vinyl acetate as well as polymethyl cyanoacrylate (applied as a fast-polymerizing monomer). The latter polymer and/or its monomer were found to be too brittle and histotoxic for use as a burn dressing. The ingrowth of tissue into the pores of polyvinyl alcohol sponges and woven fabric (nylon and silicone rubber velour) was also attempted without much success. Nylon mesh bonded to a silicone rubber membrane, another design attempt, prevented water evaporation but has not been found to induce fibrovascular growth.

Rapid epithelial layer growth by culturing cells *in vitro* from the skin of the burn patient for covering the wound area may offer a practical solution for less severely burned patients. Implantation of an allogenic fibroblast/polymer construct has proven useful for providing long-term skin replacement. Related to this, temporary tissue engineered replacements are possible alternatives for burns requiring larger area coverage. These can be similar to the synthetic dressing, a nylon mesh and silicone rubber component, but incorporates allogeneic fibroblasts. This temporary covering hopefully will stimulate or allow fibrovascular growth into the wound bed by providing the appropriate matrix proteins and growth factors.

44.2.3 Maxillofacial Implants

There are two types of maxillofacial implants: extraoral and intraoral. The former deals with the use of artificial substitutes for reconstructing defective regions in the maxilla, mandible, and face. Useful polymeric materials for extraoral implants require (1) match of color and texture with those of the patient; (2) mechanical and chemical stability (i.e., material should not creep or change color or irritate skin); and (3) ease of fabrication. Copolymers of vinyl chloride and vinyl acetate (with 5 to 20% acetate), polymethyl methacrylate, silicones, and polyurethane rubbers are currently used. Intraoral implants are used for repairing maxilla, mandibular, and facial bone defects. Material requirements for the intraoral implants are similar to those of the extraoral ones. For the latter group of implants, metallic materials such as tantalum, titanium, and CoCr alloys are commonly used. For soft tissues, such as gum and chin, polymers such as silicone rubber and polymethylmethacrylate are used for augmentation.

44.2.4 Ear and Eye Implants

Implants can be used to restore conductive hearing loss from otosclerosis (a hereditary defect which involves a change in the bony tissue of the ear) and chronic otitis media (the inflammation of the middle ear which can cause partial or complete impairment of the ossicular chain). A number of prostheses are available for correcting these defects. The porous polyethylene total ossicular implant is used to achieve a firm fixation by tissue ingrowth. The tilt-top implant is designed to retard tissue ingrowth into the section of the shaft which may diminish sound conduction. Materials used in fabricating these implants include polymethyl methacrylate, polytetrafluoroethylene, polyethylene, silicone rubber, stainless steel, and tantalum. More recently, polytetrafluoroethylene–carbon composites, porous polyethylene, and pyrolytic carbon have been described as suitable materials for cochlear (inner ear) implants.

Artificial ear implants capable of processing speech have been developed with electrodes to stimulate cochlear nerve cells. Cochlear implants also have a speech processor that transforms sound waves into electrical impulses that can be conducted through coupled external and internal coils. The electrical impulses can be transmitted directly by means of a percutaneous device.

Eye implants are used to restore the functionality of damaged or diseased corneas and lenses. Usually the cornea is transplanted from a suitable donor. In cataracts, eye lenses become cloudy and can be removed surgically. Intraocular lenses (IOL) are implanted surgically to replace the original eye lens and to restore function. IOL are made from transparent acrylics, particularly polymethyl methacrylate, which has excellent optical properties. Infection and fixation of the lens to the tissues are frequent concerns, and a number of measures are being used to address them. Transplantation of retinal pigmented epithelium can be used in the treatment of adult onset blindness; the challenge is developing readily detachable or absorbable materials on which to culture sheets of these cells.

44.2.5 Space-Filling Implants

Breast implants are common space-filling implants. At one time, the enlargement of breasts was done with various materials such as paraffin wax and silicone fluids, by direct injection or by enclosure in a rubber balloon. Several problems have been associated with directly injected implants, including progressive instability and ultimate loss of original shape and texture as well as infection and pain. One of the early efforts in breast augmentation was to implant a sponge made of polyvinyl alcohol. However, soft tissues grew into the pores and then calcified with time, and the so-called marble breast resulted. Although the enlargement or replacement of breasts for cosmetic reasons alone is not recommended, prostheses have been developed for patients who have undergone radical mastectomy or who have nonsymmetrical deformities. The development of the tissue-engineered breast is ongoing, where fat or normal breast tissue may be derived from the patient and combined with an absorbable scaffold for transplantation. A silicone rubber bag filled with silicone gel and backed with polyester mesh to permit tissue ingrowth for fixation is a widely used prosthesis, primarily for psychological reasons. The artificial penis, testicles, and vagina fall into the same category as breast implants, in that they make use of silicones and are implanted for psychological reasons rather than to improve physical health.

44.2.6 Fluid Transfer Implants

Fluid transfer implants are required for cases such as hydrocephalus, urinary incontinence, glaucoma-related elevated intraocular pressure, and chronic ear infection. Hydrocephalus, caused by abnormally high pressure of the cerebrospinal fluid in the brain, can be treated by draining the fluid (essentially an ultrafiltrate of blood) through a cannula. Earlier shunts had two one-way valves at either end. However, the more recent Ames shunt has simple slits at the discharging end, which opens when enough fluid pressure is exerted. The Ames shunt empties the fluid in the peritoneum while others drain into the blood stream through the right internal jugular vein or right atrium of the heart. The simpler peritoneal shunt shows less incidence of infection.

The use of implants for correcting the urinary system has not been successful because of the difficulty of adjoining a prosthesis to the living system for achieving fluid tightness. In addition, blockage of the passage by deposits from urine, salt for example, and constant danger of infection are major concerns. Several materials have been used for producing these implants, with limited long-term success; these include Dacron™, glass, polyvinyl alcohol, polyethylene, rubber, silver, tantalum, Teflon™, and Vitallium™. Tissue engineered devices also have application in urinary repair; for example, an alginate-chondrocyte system has been used clinically to treat vesicoureteral reflux. Preliminary results suggest that by transplanting the hydrogel system as a bulking agent below a refluxing ureter, neocartilage gradually develops to correct the reflux. Uroepithelial cells, combined with porous, absorbable polyester matrices show promise in the replacement of urologic tissues.

Drainage tubes, which are impermanent implants for chronic ear infection, can be made from polytetrafluoroethylene (Teflon™). Glaucoma-related elevated intraocular pressure may be relieved by implanting a tube connecting the anterior eye chamber to the external subconjunctival space in order to direct aqueous humor. Complications can arise with occlusion of the tube due to wound healing processes; however, researchers are investigating combining this device with an absorbable drug delivery plug to regulate flow and deliver drugs to regulate the wound healing process.

44.2.7 Technologies of Emerging Interest

A new process for uniaxial solid-state orientation, using a range of compressive forces and temperatures, has been developed to produce stock sheets of polyether-ether ketone (PEEK) for machining dental implants with substantially increased strength and modulus as compared to their unoriented counterparts.

Surface treatment of materials is another emerging interest, a process potentially influencing both surface charge, topography, and conductivity. The former has obvious effects on cell adhesion and integration of traditional implants with surrounding tissues, and it has a profound effect on the success or failure of a tissue-engineered device.

Pertinent to the effect of surface chemistry and texture on tissue regeneration/ingrowth, recent studies on surface-phosphonylation to create hydroxyapatite-like substrates show that (1) surface-microtextured polypropylene and polyethylene transcortical implants in goat tibia having phosphonate functionalities (with or without immobilized calcium ions) do induce bone ingrowth, and (2) microtexture and surface phosphonylated (with and without immobilized calcium ions) rods made of PEEK and similarly treated rods of carbon fiber-reinforced PEEK induce bone ingrowth when implanted in the toothless region of the lower jaw of goats. The use of surface-phosphonylated and post-treated (with a bridging agent) UHMW-PE fibers and fabric do produce high strength and modulus composites at exceptionally low filler loading. Among these composites are those based on methyl methacrylate matrices, similar to those used in bone cement.

Conductivity manipulation may be extremely useful in such areas as biosensor design. Surface-conducting phosphonylated, ultra-high molecular weight polyethylene may be formed by exposure to aqueous pyrole solution. Preliminary results suggest that this is a stable process, yielding no apparent cytotoxic effects due to the material or leachables. New surface treatments will be instrumental in the development of the two rapidly expanding areas of biosensor design and tissue engineering, both areas which encompass non-blood-interfacing soft tissue implants.

Further Reading

Allan, J. 1993. The molecular binding of inherently conducting polymers to thermoplastic substrates. M.S. thesis, Clemson University, Clemson, SC.

Allan, J.M., Wrana, J.S., Dooley, R.L., Budsberg, S., and Shalaby, S.W. 1999. Bone ingrowth into surface-phosphonylated polyethylene and polypropylene. *Trans. Soc. Biomat.* (submitted).

Allan, J.M., Wrana, J.S., Linden, D.E., Dooley, R.L., Farris, H., Budsberg, S., and Shalaby, S.W. 1999. Osseointegration of morphologically and chemically modified polymeric dental implants. *Trans. Soc. Biomater.* (submitted).

Allan, J.M., Kline, J.D., Wrana, J.S., Flagle, J.A., Corbett, J.T., and Shalaby, S.W. 1999. Absorbable gel-forming sealant/adhesives as a staple adjuvant in wound repair. *Trans. Soc. Biomater.* (submitted).

Chvapil, M. 1982. Considerations on manufacturing principles of a synthetic burn dressing: A review. *J. Biomed. Mater. Res.* 16:245.

Deng, M., Allan, J.M., Lake, R.A., Gerdes, G.A., and Shalaby, S.W. 1999. Effect of phosphonylation on UHMW-PE fabric-reinforced composites. *Trans. Soc. Biomater.* (submitted).

Deng, M., Wrana, J.S., Allan, J.M., and Shalaby, S.W. 1999. Tailoring mechanical properties of polyether-ether ketone for implants using solid-state orientation. *Trans. Soc. Biomater.* (submitted).

El-Ghannam, A., Starr, L., and Jones, J. 1998. Laminin-5 coating enhances epithelial cell attachment, spreading, and hemidesmosome assembly on Ti-6Al-4V implant material *in vitro. J. Biomed. Mater. Res.* 41:30.

Gantz, B.J. 1987. Cochlear implants: An overview. *Acta Otolaryng. Head Neck Surg.* 1:171.

Holder, W.D., Jr., Gruber, H.E., Moore, A.L., Culberson, C.R., Anderson, W., Burg, K.J.L., and Mooney, D.J. 1998. Cellular ingrowth and thickness changes in poly-L-lactide and polyglycolide matrices implanted subcutaneously in the rat. *J. Biomed. Mater. Res.* 41:412–421.

Kablitz, C., Kessler, T., Dew, P.A. et al. 1979. Subcutaneous peritoneal catheter: 1 1/2-years experience. *Artif. Organs* 3:210.

Lanza, R.P., Langer, R., and Chick, W.L., Eds. 1997. *Principles of Tissue Engineering*, Academic Press, San Diego, CA.

Lynch, W. 1982. *Implants: Reconstructing the Human Body*. Van Nostrand Reinhold, New York.

Park, J.B. and Lakes, R.S. 1992. *Biomaterials Science and Engineering*, 2nd ed., Plenum Press, New York.

Postlethwait, R.W., Schaube, J.F., and Dillan, M.L. et al. 1959. An evaluation of surgical suture material. *Surg. Gyn. Obstet.* 108:555.

Shalaby, S.W. 1985. Fibrous materials for biomedical applications. In *High Technology Fibers: Part A*. Lewin, M. and Preston, J., Eds., Dekker, New York.

Shalaby, S.W. 1988. Bioabsorbable polymers. In *Encyclopedia of Pharmaceutical Technology*, Vol. 1. Boylan, J.C. and Swarbrick, J., Eds., Dekker, New York.

Shalaby, S.W., Ed. 1994. *Biomedical Polymers Designed to Degrade Systems*, Hanser, New York.

Shall, L.M. and Cawley, P.W. 1994. Soft tissue reconstruction in the shoulder. Comparison of suture anchors, absorbable staples, and absorbable tacks. *Amer. J. Sports Med.* 22: 715.

VonRecum, A.G. and Park, J.B. 1979. Percutaneous devices. *Crit. Rev. Bioeng.* 5: 37.

Yannas, I.V. and Burke, I.F. 1980. Design of an artificial skin: 1. Basic design principles. *J. Biomed. Mater. Res.* 14: 107.

45

Hard Tissue Replacements

Sang-Hyun Park
Orthopedic Hospital

Adolfo Llinás
Pontificia Universidad Javeriana

Vijay K. Goel
J.C. Keller
University of Iowa

45.1 Bone Repair and Joint Implants

S.-H. Park, A. Llinás, and V.K. Goel

The use of biomaterials to restore the function of traumatized or degenerated connective tissues and thus improve the quality of life of a patient has become widespread. In the past, implants were designed with insufficient cognizance of biomechanics. Accordingly, the clinical results were not very encouraging. An upsurge of research activities into the mechanics of joints and biomaterials has resulted in better designs with better *in vivo* performance. The improving long-term success of total joint replacements for the lower limb is testimony to this. As a result, researchers and surgeons have developed and used fixation devices for the joints, including artificial spine discs. A large number of devices are also available for the repair of the bone tissue. This chapter provides an overview of the contemporary scientific work related to the use of biomaterials for the repair of bone (e.g., fracture) and joint replacements ranging from a hip joint to a spine.

45.1.1 Long Bone Repair

The principal functions of the skeleton are to provide a frame to support the organ-systems, and to determine the direction and range of body movements. Bone provides an anchoring point (insertion), for most skeletal muscles and ligaments. When the muscles contract, long bones act as levers, with the joints functioning as pivots, to cause body movement.

Bone is the only tissue able to undergo spontaneous regeneration and to remodel its micro- and macro-structure. This is accomplished through a delicate balance between an *osteogenic* (bone forming) and *osteoclastic* (bone removing) process [Brighton, 1984]. Bone can adapt to a new mechanical environment by changing the equilibrium between osteogenesis and osteoclasis. These processes will respond to changes in the static and dynamic stress applied to bone; that is, if more stress than the physiological is applied, the equilibrium tilts toward more osteogenic activity. Conversely, if less stress is applied the equilibrium tilts toward osteoclastic activity (this is known as **Wolff's Law** of bone remodeling) [Wolff, 1986].

Nature provides different types of mechanisms to repair fractures in order to be able to cope with different mechanical environments about a fracture [Hulth, 1989; Schenk, 1992]. For example, incomplete fractures (cracks), which only allow micromotion between the fracture fragments, heal with a small amount of fracture-line *callus*, known as **primary healing**. In contrast, complete fractures which are unstable, and therefore generate macromotion, heal with a voluminous callus stemming from the sides of the bone, known as **secondary healing** [Brighton, 1984; Hulth, 1989].

The goals of fracture treatment are obtaining rapid healing, restoring function, and preserving cosmesis without general or local complications. Implicit in the selection of the treatment method is the need to avoid potentially deleterious conditions, for example, the presence of excessive motion between bone fragments which may delay or prevent fracture healing [Brighton, 1984; Brand and Rubin, 1987].

Each fracture pattern and location results in a unique combination of characteristics ("fracture personality") that require specific treatment methods. The treatments can be non-surgical or surgical. Examples of non-surgical treatments are immobilization with casting (plaster or resin) and bracing with a plastic apparatus. The surgical treatments are divided into external fracture fixation, which does not require opening the fracture site, or internal fracture fixation, which requires opening the fracture.

With external fracture fixation, the bone fragments are held in alignment by pins placed through the skin onto the skeleton, structurally supported by external bars. With internal fracture fixation, the bone fragments are held by wires, screws, plates, and/or intramedullary devices. Figure 45.1a,b show radiographs of externally and internally fixed fractures.

All the internal fixation devices should meet the general requirement of biomaterials, that is, biocompatability, sufficient strength within dimensional constraints, and corrosion resistance. In addition, the device should also provide a suitable mechanical environment for fracture healing. From this perspective, stainless steel, cobalt–chrome alloys, and titanium alloys are most suitable for internal fixation. Detailed mechanical properties of the metallic alloys are discussed in the chapter on metallic biomaterials. Most internal fixation devices persist in the body after the fracture has healed, often causing discomfort and requiring removal. Recently, biodegradable polymers, for example, polylactic acid (PLA) and polyglycolic acid (PGA), have been used to treat minimally loaded fractures, thereby eliminating the need for a second surgery for implant removal. A summary of the basic application of biomaterials in internal fixation is presented in Table 45.1. A description of the principal failure modes of internal fixation devices is presented in Table 45.2.

45.1.1.1 Wires

Surgical wires are used to reattach large fragments of bone, like the greater trochanter, which is often detached during total hip replacement. They are also used to provide additional stability in long-oblique or spiral fractures of long bones which have already been stabilized by other means (Figure 45.1b). Similar approaches, based on the use of wires, have been employed to restore stability in the lower cervical spine region and in the lumbar segment as well (Figure 45.1c).

Twisting and knotting is unavoidable when fastening wires to bone; however, by doing so, the strength of the wire can be reduced by 25% or more due to stress concentration [Tencer et al., 1993]. This can be partially overcome by using a thicker wire, since its strength increases directly proportional to its diameter. The deformed regions of the wire are more prone to corrosion than the un-deformed because of the higher strain energy. To decrease this problem and ease handling, most wires are annealed to increase the ductility.

(a)

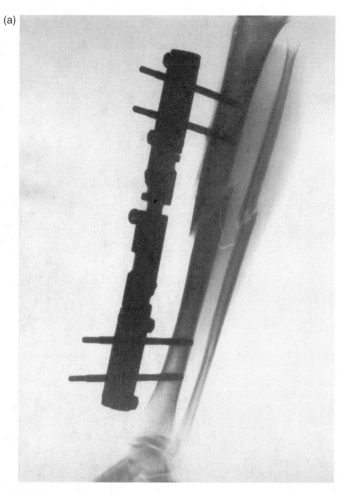

FIGURE 45.1 Radiographs of (a) tibial fracture fixed with four pins and an external bar; (b) a total hip joint replacement in a patient who sustained a femoral fracture and was treated with double bone plates, screws, and surgical wire (arrows); (c) application of wires, screws, and plates in the spine.

Braided multistrain (multifilament) wire is an attractive alternative because it has a similar tensile strength than a monofilament wire of equal diameter, but more flexibility and higher fatigue strength [Taitsman and Saha, 1977]. However, bone often grows into the grooves of the braided multistrain wire, making it exceedingly difficult to remove, since it prevents the wire from sliding when pulled. When a wire is used with other metallic implants, the metal alloys should be matched to prevent galvanic corrosion [Park and Lakes, 1992].

45.1.1.2 Pins

Straight wires are called Steinmann pins; however if the pin diameter is less than 2.38 mm, it is called Kirschner wire. They are widely used primarily to hold fragments of bones together provisionally or permanently and to guide large screws during insertion. To facilitate implantation, the pins have different tip designs which have been optimized for different types of bone (Figure 45.2). The trochar tip is the most efficient in cutting; hence, it is often used for cortical bone.

The holding power of the pin comes from elastic deformation of surrounding bone. In order to increase the holding power to bone, threaded pins are used. Most pins are made of 316L stainless steel; however, recently, biodegradable pins made of polylactic or polyglycolic acid have been employed for the treatment of minimally loaded fractures.

(b)

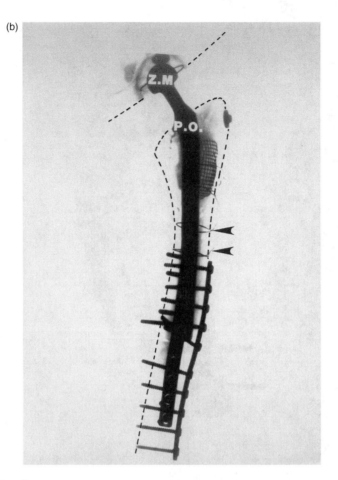

FIGURE 45.1   Continued.

The pins can be used as part of elaborate frames designed for external fracture fixation (Figure 45.1a). In this application, several pins are placed above and below the fracture, but away from it. After the fracture fragments are manually approximated (reduced) to resemble the intact bone, the pins are attached to various bars, which upon assembly will provide stability to the fracture.

45.1.1.3 Screws

Screws are the most widely used devices for fixation of bone fragments. There are two types of bone screws: (1) cortical bone screws, which have small threads, and (2) cancellous screws, which have large threads to get more thread-to-bone contact. They may have either V or buttress threads (Figure 45.3). The cortical screws are subclassified further according to their ability to penetrate, into self-tapping and non-self-tapping (Figure 45.3). The self-tapping screws have cutting flutes which thread the pilot drill-hole during insertion. In contrast, the non-self-tapping screws require a tapped pilot drill-hole for insertion.

The holding power of screws can be affected by the size of the pilot drill-hole, the depth of screw engagement, the outside diameter of the screw, and quality of the bone [Cochran, 1982; DeCoster et al., 1990]. Therefore, the selection of the screw type should be based on the assessment of the quality of the bone at the time of insertion. Under identical conditions, self-tapping screws provide a slightly greater holding power than non-self-tapping screws [Tencer et al., 1993].

Screw pullout strength varies with time after insertion *in vivo*, and it depends on the growth of bone into the screw threads and/or resorption of the surrounding bone [Schatzker et al., 1975]. The bone immediately adjacent to the screw often undergoes *necrosis* initially, but if the screw is firmly fixed, when

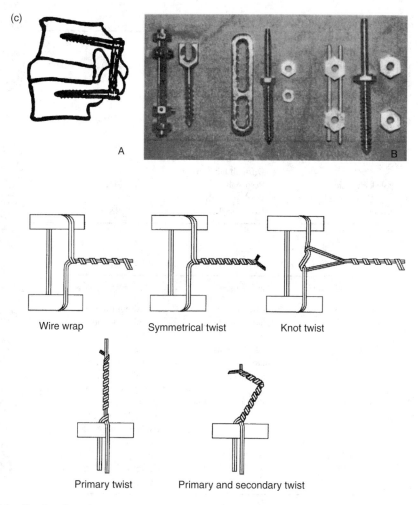

(c)

A   B

Wire wrap   Symmetrical twist   Knot twist

Primary twist   Primary and secondary twist

FIGURE 45.1 Continued.

the bone revascularizes, permanent secure fixation may be achieved. This is particularly true for titanium alloy screws or screws with a roughened thread surface, with which bone ongrowth results in an increase in removal torque [Hutzschenreuter and Brümmer, 1980]. When the screw is subject to micro- or macro-movement, the contacting bone is replaced by a membrane of fibrous tissue, the purchase is diminished, and the screw loosens.

The two principal applications of bone screws are (1) as interfragmentary fixation devices to "lag" or fasten bone fragments together, or (2) to attach a metallic plate to bone. Interfragmentary fixation is used in most fractures involving cancellous bone and in those oblique fractures in cortical bone. In order to lag the fracture fragments, the head of the screw must engage the cortex on the side of insertion without gripping the bone, while the threads engage cancellous bone and/or the cortex on the opposing side. When screws are employed for bone plate fixation, the bone screw threads must engage both cortices. Screws are also used for the fixation of spine fractures (for plate fixation or compression of bone fragment; Figure 45.1c).

45.1.1.4 Plates

Plates are available in a wide variety of shapes and are intended to facilitate fixation of bone fragments. They range from the very rigid, intended to produce primary bone healing, to the relatively flexible, intended to facilitate physiological loading of bone.

TABLE 45.1   Biomaterials Applications in Internal Fixation

Materials	Properties	Application
Stainless steel	Low cost, easy fabrication	Surgical wire (annealed)
		Pin, plate, screw
		IM nail
Ti alloy	High cost	Surgical wire
	Low density and modulus	Plate, screws, IM nails
	Excellent bony contact	
Co–Cr alloys (wrought)	High cost	Surgical wire
	High density and modulus	IM nails
	Difficult fabrication	
Poly lactic acid	Resorbable	Pin, screw
Poly glycolic acid	Weak strength	
Nylon	Non-resorbable plastic	Cerclage band

TABLE 45.2   Failure Modes of Internal Fixation Devices

Failure mode	Failure location	Reasons for failure
Overload	Bone fracture site	Small size implant
	Implant screw hole	Unstable reduction
	Screw thread	Early weight bearing
Fatigue	Bone fracture site	Early weight bearing
	Implant screw hole	Small size implant
	Screw thread	Unstable reduction
		Fracture non-union
Corrosion	Screw head-plate hole	Different alloy implants
	Bent area	Over-tightening screw
		Misalignment of screw
		Over-bent
Loosening	Screw	Motion
		Wrong choice of screw type
		Osteoporotic bone

The rigidity and strength of a plate in bending depend on the cross-sectional shape (mostly thickness) and material of which it is made. Consequently, the weakest region in the plate is the screw hole, especially if the screw hole is left empty, due to a reduction of the cross-sectional area in this region. The effect of the material on the rigidity of the plate is defined by the elastic modulus of the material for bending, and by the shear modulus for twisting [Cochran, 1982]. Thus, given the same dimensions, a titanium alloy plate will be less rigid than a stainless steel plate, since the elastic modulus of each alloy is 110 and 200 GPa, respectively.

Stiff plates often shield the underlying bone from the physiological loads necessary for its healthful existence [Perren et al., 1988; O'Slullivan et al., 1989]. Similarly, flat plates closely applied to the bone prevent blood vessels from nourishing the outer layers of the bone [Perren, 1988]. For these reasons, the current clinical trend is to use more flexible plates (titanium alloy) to allow micromotion, and low-contact plates (only a small surface of the plate contacts the bone, LCP), to allow restoration of vascularity to the bone [Uhthoff and Finnegan, 1984; Claes, 1989]. The underlying goals of this philosophical change are to increase the fracture healing rate, to decrease the loss of bone mass in the region shielded by the plate, and consequently, to decrease the incidence of re-fractures which occur following plate removal.

The interaction between bone and plate is extremely important since the two are combined into a composite structure. The stability of the plate-bone composite and the service life of the plate depends upon accurate fracture reduction. The plate is most resistant in tension; therefore, in fractures of long bones, the plate is placed along the side of the bone which is typically loaded in tension. Having excellent

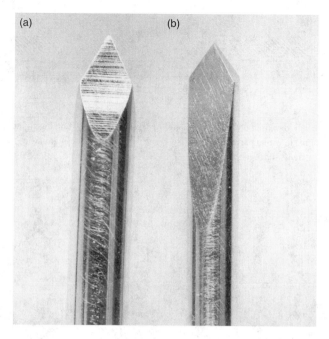

FIGURE 45.2   Types of metallic pin tip: (a) trochar end and (b) diamond end.

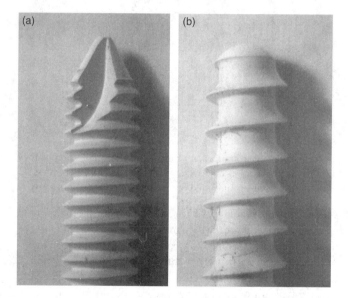

FIGURE 45.3   Bone screws: (a) a self-tapping V-threaded (has a cutting flute), and (b) a non-self-tapping, buttress threaded screw.

apposition of the bone fragments, as well as developing adequate compression between them, is critical in maintaining the stability of the fixation and preventing the plate from repetitive bending and fatigue failure. Interfragmentary compression also creates friction at the fracture surface, increasing resistance to torsional loads [Perren, 1991; Tencer et al., 1993]. On the contrary, too much compression causes micro fractures and necrosis of contacting bone due to the collapse of vesicular canals.

Compression between the fracture fragments can be achieved with a special type of plate called a *dynamic compression plate* (DCP). The dynamic compression plate has elliptic shape screw holes with its

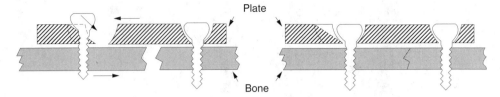

FIGURE 45.4 Principle of a dynamic compression plate for fracture fixation. During tightening a screw, the screw head slides down on a ramp in a plate screw hole which results in pushing the plate away from a fracture end and compressing the bone fragments together.

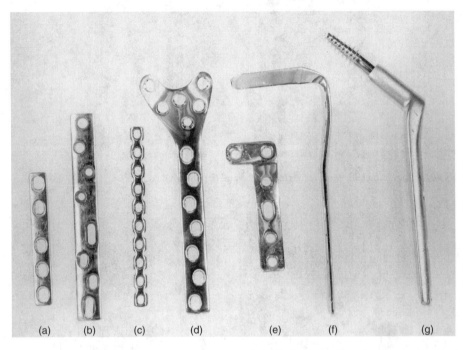

FIGURE 45.5 Bone plates: (a) dynamic compression plate, (b) hybrid compression plate (lower part has dynamic compression screw holes), (c) reconstruction bone plate (easy contouring), (d) buttress bone plate, (e) L shaped buttress plate, (f) nail plate (for condylar fracture), and (g) dynamic compression hip screw.

long axis oriented parallel to that of the plate. The screw hole has a sliding ramp to the long axis of the plate. Figure 45.4 explains the principle of the dynamic compression plate.

Bone plates are often contoured in the operating room in order to conform to an irregular bone shape to achieve maximum contact of the fracture fragments. However, excessive bending decreases the service life of the plate. The most common failure modes of a bone plate-screw fixation are screw loosening and plate failure. The latter typically occurs through a screw hole due to fatigue and/or crevice corrosion [Weinstein et al., 1979].

In the vicinity of the joints, where the diameter of long bones is wider, the cortex thinner, and cancellous bone abundant, plates are often used as a buttress or retaining wall. A buttress plate applies force to the bone perpendicular to the surface of the plate, and prevents shearing or sliding at the fracture site. Buttress plates are designed to fit specific anatomic locations and often incorporate other methods of fixation besides cortical or cancellous screws, for example, a large lag screw or an I-beam. For the fusion of vertebral bodies following diskectomy, spinal plates are used along with bone grafts. These plates are secured to the vertebral bodies using screws (Figure 45.1c). Similar approaches have been employed to restore stability in the thoracolumbar and cervical spine region as well. Figure 45.5 illustrates a variety of types of bone plates.

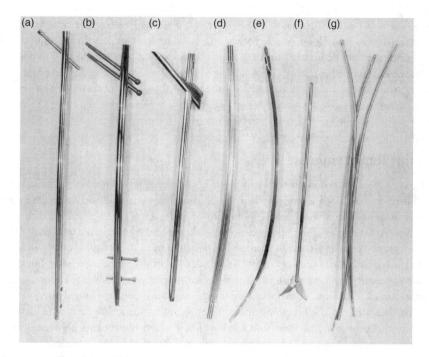

FIGURE 45.6   Intramedullary devices: (a) Gross-Kempf (slotted), (b) Uniflex (Ti alloy, slotted), (c) Kuntscher, (d) Samson, (e) Harris, (f) Brooker-Wills distal locking pin, and (g) Enders pins.

45.1.1.5   Intramedullary Nails

Intramedullary devices (IM nails) are used as internal struts to stabilize long bone fractures. IM nails are also used for fixation of femoral neck or intertrochanteric bone fractures; however, this application requires the addition of long screws. A gamut of designs are available, going from solid to cylindrical, with shapes such as cloverleaf, diamond, and "C" (slotted cylinders). Figure 45.6 shows a variety of intramedullary devices.

Compared to plates, IM nails are better positioned to resist multi-directional bending than a plate or an external fixator, since they are located in the center of the bone. However, their torsional resistance is less than that of the plate [Cochran, 1982]. Therefore, when designing or selecting an IM nail, a high polar moment of inertia is desirable to improve torsional rigidity and strength. The torsional rigidity is proportional to the elastic modulus and the moment of inertia. For nails with a circular cross-section, torsional stiffness is proportional to the fourth power of the nail's radius. The wall thickness of the nail also affects the stiffness. A slotted, open section nail is more flexible in torsion and bending, and it allows easy insertion into a curved medullary canal for example, that of the femur [Tencer, 1993]. However, in bending, a slot is asymmetrical with respect to rigidity and strength. For example, a slotted nail is strongest when bending is applied so that the slot is near the neutral plane; the nail is weakest when oriented so that the slot is under tension.

In addition to the need to resist bending and torsion, it is vital for an IM nail to have a large contact area with the internal cortex of the bone to permit torsional loads to be transmitted and resisted by shear stress. Two different concepts are used to develop shear stress: (1) a three-point, high pressure contact, achieved with the insertion of curved pins, and (2) a positive interlocking between the nail and intramedullary canal, to produce a unified structure. Positive interlocking can be enhanced by reaming the intramedullary canal. Reaming permits a larger, longer, nail-bone contact area and allows the use of a larger nail, with increased rigidity and strength [Kessler et al., 1986].

The addition of screws through the bone and nail, proximal and distal to the fracture, known as interlocking, increases torsional stability and prevents shortening of the bone, especially in unstable fractures

[Perren, 1989]. The IM nail which has not been interlocked allows interfragmentary compressive force due to its low resistance to axial load. Another advantage of IM nails is that they do not require opening the fracture site, since they can be inserted through a small skin incision, typically located in one extreme of the bone. The insertion of an intramedullary nail, especially those that require reaming of the medullary canal, destroys the intramedullary vessels which supply two thirds of the cortex. However, this is not of clinical significance because revascularization occurs rapidly [Kessler et al., 1986; O'Slullivan et al., 1989].

45.1.2 Joint Replacements

Our ability to replace damaged joints with prosthetic implants has brought relief to millions of patients who would otherwise have been severely limited in their most basic activities and doomed to a life in pain. It is estimated that about 16 million people in the United States are affected by osteoarthritis, one of the various conditions that may cause joint degeneration and may lead a patient to a total joint replacement.

Joint degeneration is the end-stage of a process of destruction of the articular cartilage, which results in severe pain, loss of motion, and occasionally, an angular deformity of the extremity [Buckwalter et al., 1993]. Unlike bone, cartilage has a very limited capacity for repair [Salter, 1989]. Therefore, when exposed to a severe mechanical, chemical, or metabolic injury, the damage is permanent and often progressive.

Under normal conditions, the functions of cartilage are to provide a congruent articulation between bones, to transmit load across the joint, and to allow low-friction movements between opposing joint surfaces. The sophisticated way in which these functions are performed becomes evident from some of the mechanical characteristics of normal cartilage. For example, due to the leverage geometry of the muscles and the dynamic nature of human activity, the cartilage of the hip is exposed to about eight times body weight during fast walking [Paul, 1976]. Over a period of 10 years, an active person may subject the cartilage of the hip to more than 17 million weight bearing cycles [Jeffery, 1994]. From the point of view of the optimal lubrication provided by synovial fluid, cartilage's extremely low frictional resistance makes it 15 times easier to move opposing joint surfaces than to move an ice-skate on ice [Mow and Hayes, 1991; Jeffery, 1994].

Cartilage functions as a unit with subchondral bone, which contributes to shock absorption by undergoing viscoelastic deformation of its fine trabecular structure. Although some joints, like the hip, are intrinsically stable by virtue of their shape, the majority require an elaborate combination of ligaments, meniscus, tendons, and muscles for stability. Because of the large multidirectional forces that pass through the joint, its stability is a dynamic process. Receptors within the ligaments fire when stretched during motion, producing an integrated muscular contraction that provides stability for that specific displacement. Therefore, the ligaments are not passive joint restraints as once believed. The extreme complexity and high level of performance of biologic joints determine the standard to be met by artificial implants.

Total joint replacements are permanent implants, unlike those used to treat fractures, and the extensive bone and cartilage removed during implantation makes this procedure irreversible. Therefore, when faced with prosthesis failure and the impossibility to reimplant, the patient will face severe shortening of the extremity, instability or total rigidity of the joint, difficulty in ambulation, and often will be confined to a wheel chair.

The design of an implant for joint replacement should be based on the kinematics and dynamic load transfer characteristic of the joint. The material properties, shape, and methods used for fixation of the implant to the patient determines the load transfer characteristics. This is one of the most important elements that determines long-term survival of the implant, since bone responds to changes in load transfer with a remodeling process, mentioned earlier as Wollff's law. Overloading the implant-bone interface or shielding it from load transfer may result in *bone resorption* and subsequent loosening of the implant [Sarmiento et al., 1990]. The articulating surfaces of the joint should function with minimum friction and produce the least amount of wear products [Charnley, 1973]. The implant should be securely fixed to the body as early as possible (ideally immediately after implantation); however, removal of the implant should not require destruction of a large amount of surrounding tissues. Loss of tissue, especially

TABLE 45.3 Biomaterials for Total Joint Replacements

Materials	Properties	Application
Co–Cr alloy	Stem, head (ball)	Heavy, hard, stiff
(casted or wrought)	Cup, porous coating	High wear resistance
	Metal backing	
Ti alloy	Stem, porous coating	Low stiffness
	Metal backing	Low wear resistance
Pure titanium	Porous coating	Excellent osseousintegration
Tantalum	Porous structure	Excellent osseousintegration
	Good mechanical strength	
Alumina	Ball, cup	Hard, brittle
		High wear resistance
Zirconia	Ball	Heavy and high toughness
		High wear resistance
UHMWPE	Cup	Low friction, wear debris
		Low creep resistance
PMMA	Bone cement fixation	Brittle, weak in tension
		Low fatigue strength

Note: Stem: femoral hip stem/chondylar knee stem; head: femoral head of the hip stem; cup: acetabular cup of the hip.

TABLE 45.4 Types of Total Joint Replacements

Joint	Types
Hip	Ball and socket
Knee	Hinged, semiconstrained, surface replacement
	Unicompartment or bicompartment
Shoulder	Ball and socket
Ankle	Surface replacement
Elbow	Hinged, semiconstrained, surface replacement
Wrist	Ball and socket, space filler
Finger	Hinged, space filler

of bone, makes re-implantation difficult and often shortens the life span of the second joint replacement [Dupont and Charnley, 1972].

Decades of basic and clinical experimentation have resulted in a vast number of prosthetic designs and material combinations (Table 45.3 and Table 45.4) [Griss, 1984]. In the following section, the most relevant achievements in fixation methods and prosthetic design for different joints will be discussed at a conceptual level. Most joints can undergo partial replacement (hemiarthroplasty), that is, reconstruction of only one side of the joint while retaining the other. This is indicated in selected conditions when global joint degeneration has not taken place. This section will focus on total joint replacement, since this allows for a broader discussion of the biomaterials used.

45.1.2.1 Implant Fixation Method

The development of a permanent fixation mechanism of implants to bone has been one of the most formidable challenges in the evolution of joint replacement. There are three types of methods of fixation: (1) mechanical interlock, which is achieved by press-fitting the implant [Cameron, 1994a], by using polymethylmethacrylate, which is called bone cement, as a grouting agent [Charnley, 1979], or by using threaded components [Albrektsson et al., 1994]; (2) biological fixation, which is achieved by using textured or porous surfaces, which allow bone to grow into the interstices [Cameron, 1994b]; and (3) direct chemical bonding between implant and bone, for example, by coating the implant with calcium hydroxyapatite, which has a similar mineral composition to bone [Morscher, 1992]. Recently, direct bonding with bone was observed with Bioglass, a glass-ceramic, through selective dissolution of the surface film [Hench, 1994]; however, the likelihood of its clinical application is still under investigation.

Each of the fixation mechanisms has an idiosyncratic behavior, and their load transfer characteristics as well as the failure mechanisms are different. Further complexity arises from prostheses which combine two or more of the fixation mechanisms in different regions of the implant. Multiple mechanisms of fixation are used in an effort to customize load transfer to requirements of different regions of bone in an effort to preserve bone mass. Loosening, unlocking, or de-bonding between implant and bone constitute some of the most important mechanisms of prosthetic failure.

45.1.2.2 Bone Cement Fixation

Fixation of implants with polymethylmethacrylate (PMMA, bone cement) provides immediate stability, allowing patients to bare all of their weight on the extremity at once. In contrast, implants which depend on bone ingrowth require the patient to wait about 12 weeks to bear full weight.

Bone cement functions as a grouting material; consequently, its anchoring power depends on its ability to penetrate between bone trabeculae during the insertion of the prosthesis [Charnley, 1979]. Being a viscoelastic polymer, it has the ability to function as a shock absorber. It allows loads to be transmitted uniformly between the implant and bone, reducing localized high-contact stress.

Fixation with bone cement creates bone-cement and cement-implant interfaces, and loosening may occur at either one. The mechanisms to enhance the stability of the metal-cement interface constitute an area of controversy in joint replacement. Some investigators have focused their efforts on increasing the bond between metal and cement by roughening the implant, or pre-coating it with PMMA to prevent sinking of the prosthesis within the cement mantle, and circulation of debris within the interface [Park et al., 1978; Barb et al., 1982; Harris, 1988]. In contrast, others polish the implant surfaces and favor wedge-shaped designs which encourage sinking of the prosthesis within the cement, to profit from the viscoelastic deformation of the mantle by loading the cement in compression [Ling, 1992].

The problems with bone-cement interface may arise from intrinsic factors, such as the properties of the PMMA and bone, as well as extrinsic factors such as the cementing technique. Refinements in the cementing technique, such as pulsatile lavage of the medullary canal, optimal hemostasis of the cancellous bone, as well as drying of the medullary canal and pressurized insertion of the prosthesis, can result in a cement-bone interface free of gaps, with maximal interdigitation with cancellous bone [Harris and Davies, 1988]. Despite optimal cementing technique, a thin *fibrous membrane* may appear in various regions of the interface, due to various factors such as the toxic effect of free methylmethacrylate monomer, necrosis of the bone resulting from high polymerization temperatures, or devascularization during preparation of the canal [Goldring et al., 1983]. Although a fibrous membrane in the bone cement interface may be present in a well-functioning implant, it may also increase in width over time (most probably as a result of the accumulation of polyethylene wear debris from the bearing couple), and may result in macromotion, bone loss, and eventual loosening [Ebramzadeh et al., 1994]. Finally, the cement strength itself may be improved by removing air bubbles by mixing monomer and polymer under vacuum and/or centrifuging it [Harris, 1988]. During implantation, various devices are used to guarantee uniform thickness of the mantle to minimize risk of fatigue failure of the cement [Oh et al., 1978].

45.1.2.3 Porous Ingrowth Fixation

Bone ingrowth can occur with inert implants which provide pores larger than 25 μm in diameter, which is the size required to accommodate an osteon. For the best ingrowth in clinical practice, pore size range should be 100 to 350 μm and pores should be interconnected with each other with similar size of opening [Cameron, 1994b]. Implant motion inhibits bony ingrowth and large bone-metal gaps prolong or prevent the **osseointegration** [Curtis et al., 1992]. Therefore, precise surgical implantation and prevention of post-operative weight bearing for about 12 weeks are required for implant fixation.

The porous coated implants require active participation of the bone in the fixation of the implant, in contrast to cementation where the bone has a passive role. Therefore, porous coated implants are best indicated in conditions where the bone mass is near-normal. The implant design should allow ingrown

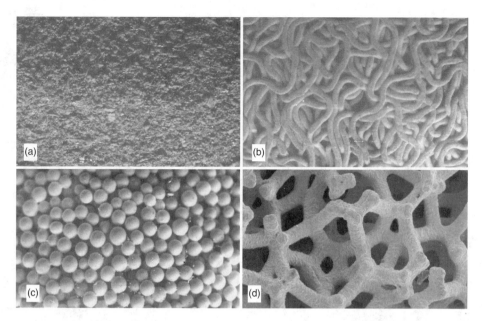

FIGURE 45.7   Scanning electron micrographs of four different types of porous structures: (a) plasma sprayed coating (7×), (b) sintered wire mesh coating (7×), (c) sintered beads coating (20×), and (d) Hedrocell porous tantalum (50×).

bone to be subjected to continuous loading within a physiologic range in order to prevent loss of bone mass due to **stress shielding**. Porous ingrowth prostheses are notoriously difficult to remove, and substantial bone damage often results from the removal process. For this reason, they should be optimized to provide predictable ingrowth with a minimal area of surgically accessible porous coated surface.

Commercially pure titanium, titanium alloy, tantalum, and calcium hydroxyapatite (HA) are currently used as porous coating materials. With pure titanium, three different types of porosity can be achieved: (1) plasma spray coating, (2) sintering of wire mesh, or (3) sintering of beads on an implant surface (Figure 45.7) [Morscher, 1992]. Thermal processing of the porous coating may weaken the underlying metal (implant). Additional problems may result from flaking of the porous coating materials, since loosened metal particles may cause severe wear when they migrate into the articulation (bearing couple) [Agins et al., 1988]. A thin calcium hydroxyapatite coating over the porous titanium surface has been used in an effort to enhance osseointegration; however, it improves only early-stage interfacial strength [Friedman, 1992; Capello and Bauer, 1994]. The long-term degradation and/or resorption of hydroxyapatite is still under investigation.

Recently, a cellular, structural biomaterial comprised of 15 to 25% tantalum (75 to 85% porous) has been developed. The average pore size is about 550 μm, and the pores are fully interconnected. The porous tantalum is a bulk material (i.e., not a coating) and is fabricated via a proprietary chemical vapor infiltration process in which pure tantalum is uniformly precipitated onto a reticulated vitreous carbon skeleton. The porous tantalum possesses sufficient compressive strength for most physiological loads, and tantalum exhibits excellent biocompatibility [Black, 1994]. This porous tantalum can be mechanically attached or diffusion bonded to substrate materials such as Ti alloy. Current commercial applications included polyethylene-porous tantalum acetabular components for total hip joint replacement and repair of defects in the acetabulum.

45.1.3   Total Joint Replacements

45.1.3.1   Hip Joint Replacement

The prosthesis for total hip replacement consists of a femoral component and an acetabular component (Figure 45.8a). The femoral stem is divided into head, neck, and shaft. The femoral stem is made of Ti (a)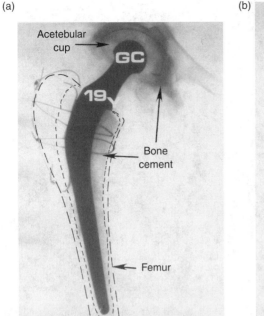

(b)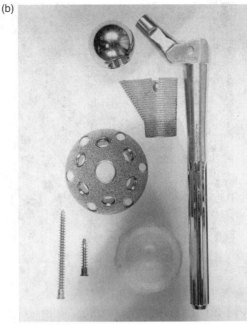

FIGURE 45.8   (a) Radiograph of bone cement fixed Charnley hip joint (monolithic femoral and acetabular component, 15-year follow-up). (b) Modular total hip system: head, femoral stem, porous coated proximal wedge, porous coated metal backing for cup, UHMWPE cup, and fixation screws.

alloy or CoCr alloy (316L stainless steel was used earlier) and is fixed into a reamed medullary canal by cementation or press fitting. The femoral head is made of CoCr alloy, alumina, or zirconia. Although Ti alloy heads function well under clean articulating conditions, they have fallen into disuse because of their low wear resistance to third bodies, for example, bone or cement particles. The acetabular component is generally made of ultra-high molecular weight polyethylene (UHMWPE).

The prostheses can be monolithic when they consist of one part, or modular when they consist of two or more parts and require assembly during surgery. Monolithic components are often less expensive, and less prone to corrosion or disassembly. However, modular components allow customizing of the implant intraoperatively, and during future revision surgeries, for example, modifying the length of an extremity by using a different femoral neck length after the stem has been cemented in place, or exchanging a worn polyethylene bearing surface for a new one without removing the well-functioning part of the prosthesis from the bone. In modular implants (Figure 45.8b), the femoral head is fitted to the femoral neck with a Morse taper, which allows changes in head material and size, and neck length. Table 45.5 illustrates the most frequently used combinations of material in total hip replacement.

When the acetabular component is monolithic, it is made of UHMWPE; when it is modular, it consists of a metallic shell and a UHMWPE insert. The metallic shell seeks to decrease the microdeformation of the UHMWPE and to provide a porous surface for fixation of the cup [Skinner, 1992]. The metallic shell allows worn polyethylene liners to be exchanged. In cases of repetitive dislocation of the hip after surgery, the metallic shell allows replacing the old liner with a more constrained one, to provide additional stability. Great effort has been placed on developing an effective retaining system for the insert, as well as on maximizing the congruity between insert and metallic shell (Figure 45.8[b]). Dislodgment of the insert results in dislocation of the hip and damage of the femoral head, since it contacts the metallic shell directly. Micromotion between insert and shell produces additional polyethylene debris which can eventually contribute to bone loss [Friedman, 1994].

The hip joint is a ball-and-socket joint, which derives its stability from congruity of the implants, pelvic muscles, and capsule. The prosthetic hip components are optimized to provide a wide range of motion

TABLE 45.5 Possible Combination of Total Hip Replacements

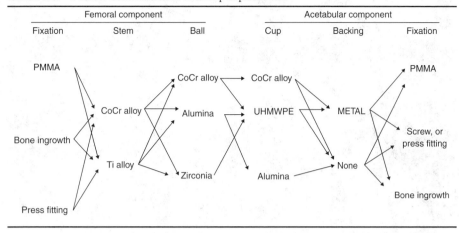

without impingement of the neck of the prosthesis on the rim of the acetabular cup to prevent dislocation. The design characteristics must enable implants to support loads that may reach more than eight times body weight [Paul, 1976]. Proper femoral neck length and correct restoration of the center of motion and femoral offset decrease the bending stress on the prosthesis–bone interface. High-stress concentration or stress shielding may result in bone resorption around the implant. For example, if the femoral stem is designed with sharp corners (diamond shaped in a cross-section), the bone in contact with the corners of the implant may necrose and resorb.

Load bearing and motion of the prosthesis produces wear debris from the articulating surface, and from the interfaces were there is micromotion, for example, stem–cement interface. Bone chip, cement chip, or broken porous coating are often entrapped in the articulating space and cause severe polyethylene wear (third-body wear). The principal source of wear under normal conditions is the UHMWPE bearing surface in the cup. Approximately 150,000 particles are generated with each step and a large proportion of these particles are smaller than 1 μm. Cells from the immune system of the host, for example, *macrophages*, are able to identify the polyethylene particles as foreign and initiate a complex inflammatory response. This response may lead to rapid focal bone loss (**osteolysis**), bone resorption, loosening, and/or fracture of the bone. Recently, low-wear UHMWPE has been developed using a cross-linking of polyethylene molecular chains. There are several effective methods of cross-linking polyethylene, including irradiation of cross-linking, peroxide cross-linking, and silane cross-linking [Shen et al., 1996]. However, none of the cross-linked polyethylene has been clinically tested yet. Numerous efforts are underway to modify the material properties of articulating materials to harden and improve the surface finish of the femoral head [Friedman, 1994]. There is growing interest in metal–metal and ceramic–ceramic hip prostheses as a potential solution to the problem of osteolysis induced by polyethylene wear debris.

45.1.3.2 Knee Joint Replacements

The prosthesis for total knee joint replacement consists of femoral, tibial, and patellar components. Compared to the hip joint, the knee joint has a more complicated geometry and movement biomechanics, and it is not intrinsically stable. In a normal knee, the center of movement is controlled by the geometry of the ligaments. As the knee moves, the ligaments rotate on their bony attachments and the center of movement also moves. The eccentric movement of the knee helps distribute the load throughout the entire joint surface [Burstein and Wright, 1993].

The prostheses for total knee replacement (Figure 45.9) can be divided according to the extent to which they rely on the ligaments for stability: (1) *Constrained*: these implants have a hinge articulation, with a fixed axis of rotation, and are indicated when all of the ligaments are absent, for example in reconstructive procedures for tumoral surgery. (2) *Semi-constrained*: these implants control posterior

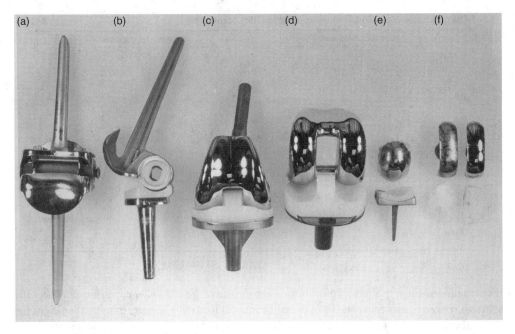

FIGURE 45.9 Various types of knee joints: (a) metal hinged, (b) hinged with plastic liner, (c) intramedullary fixed semiconstrained, (d) surface replacement, (e) uni-compartmental replacement, and (f) bi-compartmental replacement.

displacement of the tibia on the femur and medial-lateral angulation of the knee, but rely on the remaining ligaments and joint capsule to provide the rest of the constraint. Semi-constrained prostheses are often used in patients with severe angular deformities of the extremities, or in those that require revision surgery, when moderate ligamentous instability has developed. (3) *Non-constrained*: these implants provide minimal or no constraint. The prosthesis that provides minimal constraint requires resection of the posterior cruciate ligament during implantation, and the prosthetic constraint reproduces that normally provided by this ligament. The ones that provide no constraint spare the posterior cruciate ligament. These implants are indicated in patients who have joint degeneration with minimal or no ligamentous instability. As the degree of constraint increases with knee replacements, the need for the use of femoral and tibial intramedullary extensions of the prosthesis is greater, since the loads normally shared with the ligaments are then transferred to the prosthesis–bone interface.

Total knee replacements can be implanted with or without cement, the latter relying on porous coating for fixation. The femoral components are typically made of CoCr alloy and the monolithic tibial components are made of UHMWPE. In modular components, the tibial polyethylene component assembles onto a titanium alloy tibial tray. The patellar component is made of UHMWPE, and a titanium alloy back is added to components designed for uncemented use. The relatively small size of the patellar component compared to the forces that travel through the extensor mechanism, and the small area of bone available for anchorage of the prosthesis, make the patella vulnerable.

The wear characteristic of the surface of tibial polyethylene is different from that of acetabular components. The point contact stress and sliding motion of the components result in delamination and fatigue wear of the UHMWPE [Walker, 1993]. Presumably because of the relatively larger particle size of polyethylene debris, osteolysis around a total knee joint is less frequent than in a total hip replacement.

45.1.3.3 Ankle Joint Replacement

Total ankle replacements have not met with as much success as total hip and knee replacements, and typically loosen within a few years of service [Claridge et al., 1991]. This is mainly due to the high load

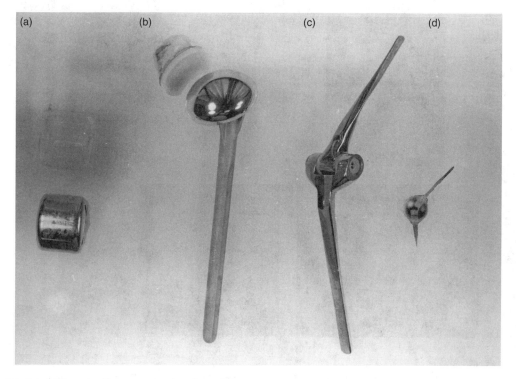

FIGURE 45.10   Miscellaneous examples of prostheses for total joint replacement: (a) ankle, (b) socket-ball shoulder joint, (c) hinged elbow joint, and (d) encapsulated finger joint.

transfer demand over the relatively small ankle surface area, and the need to replace three articulating surfaces (tibial, talar, and fibular). The joint configurations that have been used are cylindrical, reverse cylindrical, and spherical. The materials used to construct ankle joints are usually CoCr alloy and UHMWPE. Degeneration of the ankle joint is currently treated with fusion of the joint, since prostheses for total ankle replacement are still considered to be under initial development. Figure 45.10 shows ankle and other total joint replacements.

45.1.3.4   Shoulder Joint Replacements

The prostheses for total shoulder replacement consist of a humeral and a glenoid component. Like the femoral stem, the humeral component can be divided into head, neck, and shaft. Variations in the length of the neck result in changes in the length of the extremity. Even though the patient's perception of length of the upper extremity is not as accurate as that of the lower extremity, the various lengths of the neck are used to fine-tune the tension of the soft tissues to obtain maximal stability and range of motion.

The shoulder has the largest range of motion in the body, which results from a shallow ball and socket joint, which allows a combination of rotation and sliding motions between the joint surfaces. To compensate for the compromise in congruity, the shoulder has an elaborate capsular and ligamentous structure, which provides the basic stabilization. In addition, the muscle girdle of the shoulder provides additional dynamic stability. A decrease in the radius of curvature of the implant to compensate for soft tissue instability will result in a decrease in the range of motion [Neer, 1990].

45.1.3.5   Elbow Joint Replacements

The elbow joint is a hinge-type joint allowing mostly flexion and extension, but having a polycentric motion [Goel and Blair, 1985]. The elbow joint implants are either hinged, semi-constrained, or unconstrained. These implants, like those of the ankle, have a high failure rate and are not used commonly. The high loosening rate is the result of high rotational moments, limited bone stock for fixation, and minimal

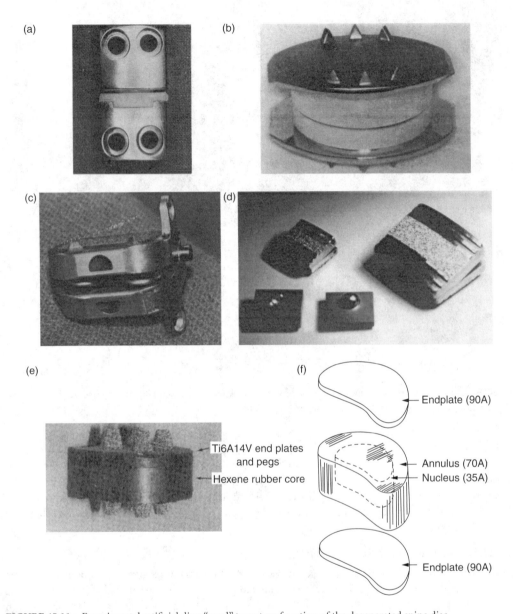

FIGURE 45.11   Experimental artificial discs "used" to restore function of the degenerated spine disc.

ligamentous support [Morrey, 1993]. In contrast to fusions of the ankle which function well, fusions of the elbow result in a moderate degree of incapacitation.

45.1.3.6   Finger Joint Replacements

Finger joint replacements are divided into three types: (1) hinge, (2) polycentric, and (c) space-filler. The most widely used are the space-filler type. These are made of high performance silicone rubber (polydimethylsiloxane) and are stabilized with a passive fixation method. This method depends on the development of a thin, fibrous membrane between implant and bone, which allows pistoning of the prosthesis. This fixation can provide only minimal rigidity of the joint [Swanson, 1973]. Implant wear and cold flow associated with erosive cystic changes of adjacent bone have been reported with silicone implants [Carter et al., 1986; Maistrelli, 1994].

45.1.3.7 Prosthetic Intervertebral Disk

Because of adjacent-level degeneration and other complications, such as non-fusion, alternatives to fusions have been proposed. One of the most recent developments for non-fusion treatment alternatives is replacement of the intervertebral discs [Hedman et al., 1991]. The goal of this treatment alternative is to restore the original mechanical function of the disc. One of the stipulations of artificial disc replacement is that remaining osseous spinal and paraspinal soft tissue components are not compromised by pathologic changes. Several artificial disk prostheses have been developed to achieve these goals (Figure 45.11).

45.1.3.8 Prostheses for Limb Salvage

Prosthetic implant technology has brought new lifestyles to thousands of patients who would lose their limbs due to bone cancer. In the past, the treatment for primary malignant bone cancer of the extremities was amputation. Significant advances in bone tumor treatment have taken place during the last two decades. The major treatment methods for limb reconstruction following bone tumor resection are resection arthrodesis (fusion of two bones), allograft-endoprosthetic composite, and endoprosthetic reconstruction. Endoprosthetic reconstruction is an extension of a total joint replacement(s) component to the resected bone area, and is the most popular option due to an advantage of fast postoperative recovery (Figure 45.12). Therefore, material and fixation methods for limb salvage endoprostheses are exactly the same as for total joint replacements. Femur, tibia, humerus, pelvis, and scapular are often resected and replaced endoprostheses. Similar to total joint replacements, disadvantages of the endoprosthetic

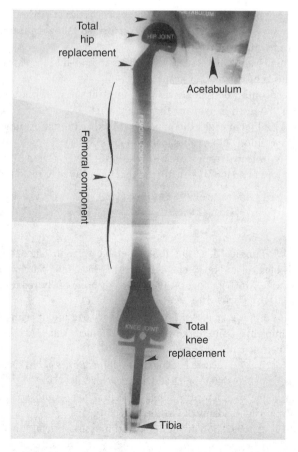

FIGURE 45.12 Radiographic appearance (montage) of a modular endoprosthetic replacement. Entire femur, hip joint, and knee joint of the bone tumor patient were replaced with prostheses for a limb salvage.

reconstruction are prosthesis loosening due to polyethylene wear and cement failure, and mechanical failure of the prostheses.

Most of the endoprostheses for limb salvage are of the expandable type [Ward et al., 1996]. Expandable endoprostheses are required for children who have a potential for skeletal growth. Several expandable prostheses require an open surgical procedure to be lengthened, whereas others have been developed that can be lengthened by servomechanisims within the endoprosthesis. The modular segmental system is a new option for expandable endoprosthesis. They can be revised easily to elongate modular components to gain length over time. The modular segmental system has several advantages over the mechanically expandable one. The use of the modular system allows intraoperative customization of the endoprosthesis during surgery. It minimizes discrepancies between custom implants and actual skeletal defects due to the radiographic magnification and uncertainty of margin of tumor resection. It allows the surgeon to assemble the prosthesis intraoperatively. The cost of the modular system is less than the cost of an expandable custom endoprosthesis. The modular system allows for simpler and less expensive revision when failures occur, obviating the need for an entirely new prosthesis when only one part needs to be replaced. On the other hand, the modular system has a high chance of corrosion failure at the Morse tapers and dislodgment at the Morse taper fittings. It can be lengthened only in certain increments. The modular component system has additional applications: metastatic bone disease, failure of internal fixation, severe acute fractures with poor bone quality, and failure of total joints with insufficient bone stock.

Defining Terms

Bone resorption: A type of bone loss due to the greater osteoclastic activity than the osteogenic activity.
Callus: Unorganized meshwork of woven bone which is formed following fracture of bone to achieve early stability of the fracture.
Fibrous membrane: Thin layer of soft tissue which covers an implant to isolate it from the body.
Necrosis: Cell death caused by enzymes or heat.
Osseointegration: Direct contact of bone tissues to an implant surface without fibrous membrane.
Osteolysis: Dissolution of bone mineral from the bone matrix.
Primary Healing: Bone healing in which union occurs directly without forming callus.
Secondary Healing: Bone union with a callus formation.
Stress shielding: Bone is protected from stress by the stiff implant.
Wolff's Law: Bone develops or adapts its structure to that most suited to resist the forces acting upon it.

References

Agins, H.J., Alcock, N.W., Bansal, M. et al., 1988. Metallic wear in failed Titanium-alloy total hip replacements. A istological and quantitative analysis. *J. Bone. Joint Surg.* 70-A: 347.

Albrektsson, T., Carlsson, L.V., Morberg, P. et al., 1994. Directly bone-anchored implants. In *Bone Implant Interface*, R. Hurley (Ed.), pp. 97–120, Mosby, St. Louis, MO.

Barb, W., Park, J.B., von Recum, A.F. et al., 1982. Intramedullary fixation of artificial hip joints with bone cement precoated implants: I. Interfacial strengths. *J. Biomed. Mater. Res.* 16: 447.

Black, J. 1994. Biological performance of tantalum. *Clin. Mater.* 16: 167.

Brand, R.A. and Rubin, C T. 1987. Fracture healing. In *Scientific Basics of Orthopaedics*, 2nd ed. J. Albert and R. Brand (Eds.), pp. 325–340, Appleton & Lange, Norwalk, CT.

Brighton, C.T. 1984. Principle of fracture healing, In *Instructional Course Lectures*, J. Murray (Ed.), pp. 60–106, The American Academy of Orthopaedic Surgeons.

Buckwalter, J.A., Woo, S. et al., 1993. Soft-tissue aging and musculoskeletal function. *J. Bone Joint Surg.* 75A: 1533.

Burstein, A.H. and Wright, T.H. 1993. Biomechanics. In *Surgery of the Knee*, 2nd ed., Vol. 7, J. Insall, R. Windsor, W. Scott et al. (Eds.), pp. 43–62, Churchill Livingstone, New York.

Cameron, H.U. 1994a. Smooth metal–bone interface. In *Bone Implant Interface*, R. Hurley (Ed.), pp. 121–144, Mosby, St. Louis, MO.

Cameron, H.U. 1994b. The implant–bone interface: porous metals. In *Bone Implant Interface*, R. Hurley (Ed.), pp. 145–168, Mosby, St. Louis, MO.

Capello, W.N. and Bauer, T.W. 1994. Hydroxyapatite in orthopaedic surgery. In *Bone Implant Interface*, R. Hurley (Ed.), pp. 191–202, Mosby, St. Louis, MO.

Carter, P., Benton, L., and Dysert, P. 1986. Silicone rubber carpal implants; A study of the incidence of late osseous complications, *J. Hand Surg.* 11A: 639.

Charnley, J. 1979. *Low Friction Arthroplasty of the Hip.* Springer-Verlag, Berlin.

Claes, L. 1989. The mechanical and morphological properties of bone beneath internal fixation plates of differing rigidity. *J. Orthop. Res.* 7: 170.

Claridge, R.J., Hart, M.B., Jones, R.A. et al., 1991. Replacement arthroplasties of the ankle and foot. In *Disorder of the Foot & Ankle*, 2nd ed. M. Jahss (Ed.), pp. 2647–2664, Saunders, Philedphia, PA.

Cochran, G.V.B. 1982. Biomechanics of orthopaedic structures. In *Primer in Orthopaedic Biomechanics*, pp. 143–215, Churchill Livingstone, New York.

Curtis, M.J., Jinnah, R.H., Wilson, V.D., and Hungerford, D.S. 1992. The initial stability of uncemented acetabular components. *J. Bone Joint Surg.* 74B: 372.

DeCoster, T.A., Heetderks, D.B. et al., 1990. Optimizing bone screw pullout force. *J. Orthop. Trauma* 4: 169.

Dupont, J.A. and Charnley, J. 1972. Low-friction arthroplasty of the hip for the failures of previous operations. *J. Bone Joint Surg.* 54B: 77.

Ebramzadeh, E., Sarmiento, A., McKellop, H.A. et al., 1994. The cement mantle in total hip arthroplasty. Analysis of long-term radiographic results. *J. Bone Joint Surg.* 76A: 77–87.

Friedman, R.F., Black, J., Galante, J.O. et al., 1994. Current concepts in orthopaedic biomaterials and implant fixation. In *Instructional Course Lectures*, J.M. Schafer (Ed.), pp. 233–255. The American Academy of Orthopaedic Surgeons.

Friedman, R.J. 1992. Advanced in biomaterials and factors affecting implant fixation. In *Instructional Course Lectures*, R.E. Eilert (Ed.), pp. 127–135, The American Academy of Orthopaedic Surgeons.

Goel, V.K. and Blair, W. 1985. Biomechanics of the elbow joint. *Automedica* 6: 119.

Goldring, S.R., Schiller, A.L., Roelke, M. et al., 1983. The synovial-like membrane at the bone–cement interface in loose total hip replacements and its proposed role in bone lysis. *J. Bone Joint Surg.* 65A: 575.

Griss, P. 1984. Assessment of clinical status of total joint replacement. In *Functional Behavior of Orthopaedic Biomaterials*, P. Ducheyne and G.W. Hastings (Eds.), pp. 21–48, CRC Press, Boca Raton, FL.

Harris, W.H. and Davies, J.P. 1988. Modern use of modern cement for total hip replacement. *Orthop. Clin. N. Am.* 19: 581.

Hedman, T.P., Kostuik, P.J., Fernie, G.R. et al., 1991. Design of an intervertebral disc prosthesis. *Spine* 16: 256.

Hench, L.L. 1994. Bioactive glasses, ceramics and composites. In *Bone Implant Interface*, R. Hurley (Ed.), pp. 181–190, Mosby, St. Louis, MO.

Hulth, A. 1989. Current concepts of fracture healing. *Clin. Orthop.* 249: 265.

Hutzschenreuter, P. and Brümmer, H. 1980. Screw design and stability. In *Current concepts of Internal Fixation*, H. Uhthoff (Ed.), pp. 244–250, Springer-Verlag, Berlin.

Jeffery, A.K. 1994. Articular cartilage and the orthopaedic surgeon. Part 1: structure and function. *Curr. Orthop.* 8: 38.

Kessler, S.B., Hallfeldt, K.K., Perren, S.M. et al., 1986. The effects of reaming and intramedullary nailing on fracture healing. *Clin. Orthop.* 212: 18.

Ling, R.S. 1992. The use of a collar and precoating on cemented femoral stems is unnecessary and detrimental. *Clin. Orthop.* 285: 73.

Maistrelli, G.L. 1994. Polymer in orthopaedic surgery. In *Bone Implant Interface*, R. Hurley (Ed.), pp. 169–190, Mosby, St. Louis, MO.

McKellop, H.A., Campbell, P., Park, S.H. et al., 1995 The origin of submicron polyethylene wear debris in total hip arthroplasty. *Clin. Orthop.* 311: 3.

Morrey, B.F. 1993. *The Elbow and its Disorders*, 2nd ed, Saunders, Philadelphia, PA.

Morscher, E.W. 1992. Current status of acetabular fixation in primary total hip arthroplasty. *Clin. Orthop.* 274: 172.

Mow, V.C. and Hayes, W.C. 1991. *Basic Orthopaedic Biomechanics*, Raven Press, New York.

Neer, C.S. 1990. *Shoulder Reconstruction*, Saunders, Philadelphia, PA.

Oh, I., Carlson, C.E., Tomford, W.W. et al., 1978. Improved fixation of the femoral component after total hip replacement using a methacrylate intramedullary plug. *J. Bone Joint Surg.* 60A: 608.

O'Slullivan, M.E., Chao, E.Y.S., and Kelly, P.J. 1989. Current concepts review. The effects of fixation on fracture healing. *J. Bone Joint Surg.* 71A: 306.

Park, J.B. and Lakes, R.S. 1992. *Biomaterials: An Introduction*, 2nd ed, Plenum, London.

Park, J.B., Malstrom, C.S., and von Recum, A.F. 1978 Intramedullary fixation of implants precoated with bone cement: A preliminary study. *Biomater. Med. Dev. Artif. Organs* 6: 361.

Paul, J.P. 1976. Loading on normal hip and knee joints and joint replacement., In *Advances in Hip and Knee Joint Technology*, M. Schaldach and D. Hohmann (Eds.), pp. 53–77, Springer-Verlag, Berlin.

Perren, S.M., 1989. The biomechnics and biology of internal fixation using plates and nails. *Orthopaedics* 12: 21.

Perren, S.M. 1991. Basic aspects of internal fixation. In *Manual of Internal Fixation*, 3rd ed., M. Müller, M. Allgöwer, R. Schneider, and H. Willenegger (Eds.), pp. 1–112, Springer-Verlag, Berlin.

Salter, R.B. 1988. The biologic concept of continuous passive motion of synovial joints. The first 18 years of basic research and its clinical application. *Clin. Orthop.* 242: 12.

Sarmiento, A., Ebramzadeh, E., Gogan, W.J. et al., 1990. Cup containment and orientation in cemented total hip arthroplasties. *J. Bone Joint Surg.* 72B: 996.

Schatzker, J., Sanderson, R., and Murnaghan, J.P. 1975. The holding power of orthopaedic screws *in vivo*. *Clin. Orthop.* 108: 115.

Schenk, R.K. 1992. Biology of fracture repair. In *Skeletal Trauma*, B. Browner, J. Jupitor, A. Levine, and P. Trafton (Eds.), pp. 31–75, W.B. Saunders, Philadephia, PA.

Shen, F.W., McKellop, H., and Salovey, R. 1996. Irradiation of chemically crosslinked ultrahigh molecular weight polyethylene. *J. Polym. Sci.: Part B: Polym. Phys.* 34: 1063.

Skinner, H.B. 1992. Current biomaterial problems in implants. In *Instructional Course Lectures*, R.E. Eilert (Ed.), pp. 137–144, The American Academy of Orthopaedic Surgeons.

Swanson, A.B. 1973. Concepts of flexible implant design. In *Flexible Implant Reconstruction Arthroplasty in the Hand and Extremity*, A. Swanson (Ed.), pp. 47–59, Mosby, St. Louis, MO.

Taitsman, J.P. and Saha, S. 1977. Tensile strength of wire-reinforced bone cement and twisted stainless-steel wire. *J. Bone Joint Surg.* 59A: 419.

Tencer, A.F., Johnson, K.D., Kely, R.F. et al., 1993. Biomechanics of fractures and fracture fixation. In *Instructional Course Lectures*, J.D. Heckman (Ed.), pp. 19–55, The American Academy of Orthopaedic Surgeons.

Uhthoff, H.K. and Finnegan, M.A. 1984. The role of rigidity in fracture fixation. *Arch. Orthop. Trauma Surg.* 102: 163.

Walker, P.S. 1993. Design of total knee arthroplasty. In *Surgery of the Knee*, 2nd ed., Vol. 7, J. Insall, R. Windsor, W. Scott et al. (Eds.), pp. 723–738, Churchill Livingstone, New York.

Ward, W.G., Yang, R.S., and Eckart, J.J. 1996. Endoprosthetic bone reconstruction following malignant tumor resection in skeletally immature patients. *Orthop. Clin. N. Am.* 27: 493.

Weinstein, A.M., Spires, W.P. Jr, Klawitter et al., 1979. Orthopaedic implant retrieval and analysis study. In *Corrosion and Degradation of Implant Materials*, B.C. Syrett and A. Acharya (Eds.), pp. 212–228, American Society for Testing and Materials Tech. Pub. No. 684, Philadelphia, PA.

Wolff, J. 1986. *The Law of Bone Remodeling*, R. Maquet and R. Furlong (trans.), Springer-Verlag, Berlin.

45.2 Dental Implants: The Relationship of Materials Characteristic to Biologic Properties

J.C. Keller

As dental implants have become an acceptable treatment modality for partially and fully edentulous patients, it has become increasingly apparent that the interaction of the host tissue with the underlying implant surface is of critical importance for long-term prognosis [Young, 1988; Smith, 1993]. From the anatomical viewpoint, it is generally accepted that dental implants must contact and become integrated with several types of host tissues. Due largely to the work of Branemark and his colleagues [Albrektsson et al., 1983; Branemark, 1983], the importance of developing and maintaining a substantial bone-implant interface for mechanical retention and transmission of occlusal forces was realized. Despite documented long-term success of dental implants, longer-term implant failures are noted due to poor integration of connective and epithelial tissues and subsequent failure to develop a permucosal seal akin to that with natural tooth structures. From a biologic point of view, the characteristics of the implant substrate which permit hard and soft tissue integration and prevent adhesion of bacteria and plaque need to be further understood. It is likely that as a more complete understanding of the basic biologic responses of host tissues becomes known, refinements in the currently employed materials as well as new and improved materials will become available for use in the dental implant field.

It is important to realize that the overall biologic response of host tissue to dental implants can be divided into two distinct but interrelated phases (as given in Table 45.6). Phase I consists of the tissue responses which occur during the clinical healing phase immediately following implantation of dental implants. During this healing phase, the initial biologic processes of protein and molecular deposition on the implant surface are followed by cellular attachment, migration, and differentiation [Stanford and Keller, 1991]. It is therefore important to understand the characteristics of the implant material which affect the initial formation of the host tissue–implant interface. The characteristics include materials selection and the physical and chemical properties of the implant surface. These initial tissue responses lead to the cellular expression and maturation of extracellular matrix and ultimately to the development of bony interfaces with the implant material. After the initial healing phase is complete, usually between 3 and 6 months according to the two-stage Branemark implant design, the bone interface remodels under the occlusal forces placed on the implant during the Phase II functional period [Skalak, 1985; Brunski, 1992]. The overall bioresponses including bone remodeling during the functional phase of implant service life are then strongly influenced by the characteristics of loading and distribution of stress at the interface [Brunski, 1992]. The ability of the maturing interface to "remodel" as stresses are placed on the implant thus depend in large part on the original degree of tissue–implant surface interaction.

TABLE 45.6 Correlation Between the Clinical Phases of Implant Service Life with Biologic Events and Important Implant Materials Characteristics

Clinical phase	Biological events	Influential materials characteristics
I (healing)	Protein deposition	Materials selection
	Cell attachment	Metals
	Cell migration	Ceramics
	Development of extracellular matrix	Chemical and physical characteristics
	Bone deposition	Topography
		Micro
		Macro
		Surface chemistry
		Inert
		Dissolution
II (functional)	Matrix and bone remodeling	

TABLE 45.7 Approximate Room Temperature Mechanical Properties of Selected Implant Materials Compared to Bone

	Elastic modulus ($MPa \times 10^3$)	Proportional limit (MPa)	Ultimate tensile strength (MPa)	Percent elongation
316L SS				
Annealed	200	240	550	50
Cold worked	200	790	965	20
CoCrMo(ASTM-F75)	240	500	700	10
Ti(ASTM-F67)	100	520	620	18
Ti-6A1-4V(ASTM-F136)	110	840	900	12
Cortical bone	18	130	140	1

Source: Keller, J.C. and Lautenschlager, E.P. 1986. Metals and alloys. In *Handbook of Biomaterials Evaluation*, A. Von Recon (Ed.), pp. 3–23, New York, Macmillan.

This chapter will focus on the factors concerning dental implants which affect biologic properties of currently available dental implant materials. As pertains to each major topic, the influence of the materials properties on biologic responses will be emphasized.

45.2.1 Effects of Materials Selection

45.2.1.1 Metals and Alloys

Previously, dental implants have been fabricated from several metallic systems, including stainless steel and cobalt–chrome alloys as well as from the titanium family of metals. Several studies have reported on the ability of host bone tissues to "integrate" with various metal implant surfaces [Albrektsson et al., 1983; Katsikeris et al., 1987; Johansson et al., 1989]. In current paradigms, the term osseointegration refers to the ability of host tissues to form a functional interface with implant surfaces without an intervening layer of connective tissue akin to a foreign body tissue capsule observable at the light microscopic level [Albrektsson et al., 1983; Branemark, 1983]. By this definition, it becomes apparent that several biomedical materials including Ti and Ti alloy fulfill this general criterion. Ultrastructural investigations using transmission electron microscopy (TEM) approaches have further refined descriptions of the tissue implant interface, and the early work by Albrektsson and colleagues [1983] has become the descriptive standard by which other materials interfaces are compared. When bone was allowed to grow on Ti, a partially calcified amorphous ground substance was deposited in immediate contact with the implant, followed by a collagenous fibril-based extracellular matrix, osteoblast cell processes, and a more highly calcified matrix generally 200 to 300 Å from the implant surface.

However, other metallic materials have fallen from favor for use as dental implants due to widely differing mechanical properties compared to bone (Table 45.7), which can result in a phenomenon termed stress shielding [Slalak, 1985; Brunski, 1992], and the propensity for formation of potentially toxic corrosion products due to insufficient corrosion resistance properties [Van Orden, 1985; Lucas et al., 1987]. Ultrastructurally, the interface between bone and 316L stainless steel was described as consisting of a multiple-cell layer separating the bone from metal. Inflammatory cells were prominent in this layer, and a thick proteoglycan noncollagenous coating was present. This histologic appearance resembled that of a typical foreign body reaction and typifies a nonosseointegration-type response. The poor biologic response to stainless steel alloys has been reconfirmed by recently conducted *in vitro* studies which related the inability of host tissue to attach to the metal surface to the toxicity associated with metal ion release [Vrouwenvelder et al., 1993].

Due in large measure to the introduction and overall clinical success of the Branemark system, the range of metallic materials utilized for dental implants has become limited largely to commercially pure titanium (cpTi > 99.5%) and its major alloy, Ti–6A1–4V [De Porter et al., 1986; Keller et al., 1987]. Controversy remains, largely due to commercial advertising interests, as to which material provides a more suitable

TABLE 45.8 Surface Characterizations of cpTi and Ti Alloy (means ± standard deviations)

	cpTi	Ti-6A1-4V
Surface roughness (Ra) (μm)		
Sandblasted	0.9 ± 0.2	0.7 ± 0.03
600 grit polish	0.2 ± 0.02	0.1 ± 0.02
Smooth, 1 μm polish	0.04 ± 0.01	0.03 ± 0.01
Atomic ratios to Ti		
C	1.5 ± 0.2	1.2 ± 0.1
O	2.8 ± 0.1	3.1 ± 0.2
N	0.08 ± 0.01	0.05 ± 0.01
Al	—	0.2 ± 0.04
V[a]	—	(0.02)[a]
Oxide thickness (Å)	32 ± 8	83 ± 12
Wetting angles (°)	52 ± 2	56 ± 4

[a] One specimen.

surface for tissue integration. Early work by Johansson and coworkers [1989] reported that sputtercoated Ti alloy surfaces resulted in wide (5000 Å) **amorphous zones** devoid of collagen filaments, compared to the thinner 200 to 400 Å collagen-free amorphous zone surrounding cpTi surfaces. Subsequent studies revealed differences in the oxide characteristics between these sputtercoated cpTi and Ti alloy surfaces used for histologic and ultrastructural interfacial analyses. Significant surface contamination and the presence of *V* was observed in the Ti alloy surface, which led to an overall woven bone interface compared to the cpTi surface which had a more compact bone interface. Orr and colleagues [1992] demonstrated a similar ultrastructural morphology for interfaces of bone to Ti and Ti alloy, respectively. In each case an afibrillar matrix with calcified globular accretions, similar in appearance to cement lines in haversian systems, were observed in intimate contact with the oxide surface. Any slight differences in morphology were attributed to minor differences in surface topography or microtexture rather than chemical differences between the two surface oxides.

This is an area that is still under investigation, although recent research indicates that the stable oxide of cpTi and Ti alloy provide suitable surfaces for biologic integration [Keller et al., 1994]. Studies involving comprehensive surface analyses of prepared bulk cpTi and Ti alloy indicated that although the oxide on Ti alloy is somewhat thicker following standard surface preparations (polishing, cleaning, and acid passivation), the overall topography, the chemical characteristics, including presence and concentration of contaminants, and surface energetics were virtually identical for both materials as given in Table 45.8. *In vitro* experiments confirmed that the inherently clean condition of these oxides supports significant osteoblast cell attachment and migration and provides a hospitable surface to allow *in vitro* mineralization processes to occur [Orr et al., 1992].

In vitro experiments designed to study the ultrastructural details of bone-implant interfaces made from cpTi and Ti alloy may provide additional clues as to the histologic and ultrastructural differences which have been observed with these materials. Since clinical implants made from both materials appear to be successful [Branemark, 1983; De Porter et al., 1986], it is possible that because of the difference in mechanical properties between unalloyed and Ti alloy material, the longer-term tissue interface results from differences in bone remodeling due to the local biomechanical environment surrounding these materials [Brunski, 1992]. This hypothesis requires continued investigation for more definitive answers.

45.2.1.2 Ceramics and Ceramic Coatings

The use of single crystal sapphire or Al_2O_3 ceramic implants has remained an important component in the dental implant field [Driskell et al., 1973]. Although this material demonstrates excellent biologic compatibility, implants fabricated from Al_2O_3 have not reached a high degree of popularity in the United

States. Morphologic analyses of the soft tissue interface with Al_2O_3 revealed a hemidesmosomal external lamina attachment adjacent to the **junctional epithelium** — implant interface [Steflik et al., 1984]. This ultrastructural description is often used for comparison purposes when determining the extent of soft-tissue interaction with dental implants. Similarly, *in vivo* studies of the bone — Al_2O_3 implant interface reveal high levels of bone-to-implant contact, with areas of intervening fibrous connective tissue. Although fibrous tissue was present at the interface, the implant remained immobile, and the interface was consistent with a dynamic support system. More recent ultrastructural studies have demonstrated a mineralized matrix in immediate apposition to the Al_2O_3 implants similar to that described for Ti implants [Steflik et al., 1993].

An approach to enhancing tissue responses at dental implant interfaces has been the introduction of ceramics like, *calcium-phosphate-containing (CP) materials* as implant devices. The use of calcium-phosphate materials, in bulk or particulate form or as coatings on metal substrates has taken a predominant position in the biomedical implant area and has been the focus of several recent reviews [Koeneman et al., 1990; Kay, 1992]. One of the most important uses of CP materials has been as a coating on metallic (cpTi and Ti alloy) substrates. This approach has taken advantage of thin-film-coating technology to apply thin coatings of hydroxyapatite (HA) and tricalcium phosphate (TCP) materials to the substrate in order to enhance bone responses at implant sites. The most popular method of coating has been the plasma spray process [Herman, 1988]; although this process has some advantages, there are reports of nonuniform coatings, interfacial porosity, and vaporization of elements in the powder [Cook et al., 1991; Kay, 1992].

The use of this class of materials is based on the premise that a more natural hydroxyapatite (HA-like) could act as a scaffold for enhanced bone response — osseointegration — and thereby minimize the long-term healing periods currently required for uncoated metal implants.

Numerous *in vivo* investigations have clearly demonstrated that HA-like coatings can enhance bone responses at implant interfaces [Cook et al., 1991; Jarcho et al., 1997], although the mechanisms responsible for the development of the interface between hard tissue and these ceramic coatings are not well understood [Jansen et al., 1993]. Histologically, the overall bone-coating interface is similar in appearance and chronologic development to that reported for uncoated implant surfaces. Initially, an immature, trabecular, woven bone interface is formed followed by more dense, compact lamellar supporting bone structure. Ultrastructurally, the interface is reported to consist of a globular, afibrillar matrix directly on the HA surface, an electron-dense, proteoglycan rich layer (20 to 60 nm thick) and the presence of a mineralized collagenous matrix [De Bruijn et al., 1993]. Although the morphologic descriptions of the HA and Ti interfaces are similar, numerous studies have shown that the bone response to HA coatings is more rapid than with uncoated Ti surfaces, requiring approximately one-third to one-half the time to establish a firm osseous bed as uncoated Ti. Likewise, the extent of the bone response to HA coatings is superior and, according to some studies, leads to a several-fold increase in interfacial strength compared to uncoated Ti [Cook et al., 1991].

The cellular events which take place and lead to the interfacial ultrastructure with bone tissue and ceramic surfaces are under current investigation. Based upon preliminary findings, the advantageous biologic properties of HA coatings do not appear to be related to recruitment of additional cells during the early attachment phase of healing. Although recent work indicated that bone cells and tissue form normal cellular focal contacts during attachment to HA coatings, the level of initial *in vitro* attachment generally only approximates that observed with Ti [Puleo et al., 1991; Keller et al., 1992]. Rather, the mechanisms for the enhanced *in vitro* cell responses appear to be related, to a certain degree, to the degradation properties and release of Ca^{+2} and PO_4^{-3} ions into the biologic milieu. This surface corrosion is associated with highly degradable amorphous components of the coating and leads to surface irregularities which may enhance the quality of cell adhesion to these roughened materials [Bowers et al., 1992; Chehroudi et al., 1992]. Cellular events which occur following attachment may be influenced by the nature of the ceramic surface. Emerging evidence from a number of laboratories suggests that cellular-mediated events, including proliferation, matrix expression, and bone formation are enhanced following attachment to HA coatings and appear to be related to the gene expression of osteoblasts when cultured on different ceramic materials. These early cellular events lead to histologic and ultrastructural descriptions of bone healing which take place on these surfaces and are very similar to those reported from *in vivo* studies [Orr et al., 1992; Steflik et al., 1993].

As determined from *in vitro* dissolution studies, there is general agreement that the biodegradation properties of the pertinent CP materials can be summarized as α-TCP $>$ β-TCP $>>>$ HA, whereas amorphous HA is more prone to biodegradation than crystalline HA [Koeneman et al., 1990]. Considerable attempts to investigate the effects of coating composition (relative percentages of HA, TCP) on bone integration have been undertaken. Using an orthopedic canine total hip model, Jasty and coworkers [1992] reported that by 3 weeks, a TCP/HA mixed coating resulted in significantly more woven bone apposition to the implants than uncoated implants. As determined by x-ray diffraction, the mixed coating consisted of 60% TCP, 20% crystalline HA, and 20% unknown Ca-PO$_4$ materials. Jansen and colleagues [1993] reported that, using HA-coated implants (90% HA, 10% amorphous CP), bony apposition was extensive in a rabbit tibia model by 12 weeks. However, significant loss of the coating occurred as early as 6 weeks after implantation. Most recently, Maxian and coworkers [1993] reported that poorly crystallized HA (60% crystalline) coatings demonstrated significant degradation and poor bone apposition *in vivo* compared to amorphous coatings. Both these reports suggest that although considerable bioresorption of the coating occurred in the cortical bone, there was significant bone apposition ($81 \pm 2\%$ for amorphous HA at 12 weeks, 77% for crystalline HA, respectively) which was not significantly affected by bioresorption.

From these *in vivo* reports, it is clear that HA coatings with relatively low levels of crystallinity are capable of significant bone apposition. However, as reported in a 1990 workshop report, the FDA is strongly urging commercial implant manufacturers to use techniques to increase the postdeposition crystallinity and to provide adequate adhesion of the coating to the implant substrate [Filiaggi et al., 1993]. Although the biologic responses to HA coatings are encouraging, other factors regarding HA coatings continue to lead to clinical questions regarding their efficacy. Although the overall bone response to HA-coated implants occurs more rapidly than with uncoated devices, with time an equivalent bone contact area is formed for both materials [Jasty et al., 1992]. These results have questioned the true need for HA-coated implants, especially when there are a number of disadvantages associated with the coating concept. Clinical difficulties have arisen due to failures within the coating itself and with continued dissolution of the coating, and to catastrophic failure at the coating–substrate interface [Koeneman et al., 1988].

Recent progress is reported in terms of the improvements in coating technology. Postdeposition heat treatments are often utilized to control the crystallinity (and therefore the dissolution characteristics) of the coatings, although there is still debate as to the relationship between compositional variations associated with differing crystallinity and optimization of biologic responses. Additional coating-related properties are also under investigation in regard to their effects on bone. These include coating thickness, level of acceptable porosity in the coating, and adherence of the coating to the underlying substrate. However, until answers concerning these variables have been more firmly established, HA coatings used for dental implants will remain an area of controversy and interest.

45.2.2 Effects of Surface Properties

45.2.2.1 Surface Topography

The effects of surface topography are different than the overall three-dimensional design or geometry of the implant, which is related to the interaction of the host tissues with the implant on a macroscopic scale as shown in Figure 45.13. This important consideration in overall biologic response to implants is discussed later in this chapter. In this discussion the concept of surface topography refers to the surface texture on a microlevel. It is on this microscopic level that the intimate cell and tissue interactions leading to osseointegration are based as shown in Figure 45.14.

The effects of surface topography on *in vitro* and *in vivo* cell and tissue responses have been a field of intense study in recent years. The overall goal of these studies is to identify surface topographies which

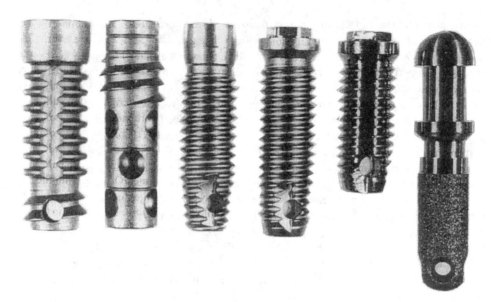

FIGURE 45.13 Examples of current dental implant designs, illustrating the variety of macroscopic topographies which are used to encourage tissue ingrowth. Left to right: Microvent, Corevent, Screw-vent, Swede-vent, Branemark, IMZ implant.

mimic the natural substrata in order to permit tissue integration and improve clinical performance of the implant. In terms of cell attachment, the *in vitro* work by Bowers and colleagues [1992] established that levels of short-term osteoblast cell attachment were higher on rough compared to smooth surfaces and cell morphology was directly related to the nature of the underlying substrate. After initial attachment, in many cases, cells of various origin often take on the morphology of the substrate as shown in Figure 45.15. Increased surface roughness, produced by such techniques as sand or grit blasting or by rough polishing, provided the rugosity necessary for optimum cell behavior.

Work in progress in several laboratories is attempting to relate the nature of the implant surface to cell morphology, intracellular cytoskeletal organization, and extracellular matrix development. Pioneering work by Chehroudi and coworkers [1992] suggests that microtextured surfaces (via micromachining or other techniques) could help orchestrate cellular activity and osteoblast mineralization by several mechanisms including proper orientation of collagen bundles and cell shape and polarity. This concept is related to the theory of **contact guidance** and the belief that cell shape will dictate cell differentiation through gene expression. In Chehroudi's work, both tapered pitted and grooved surfaces (with specific orientation and sequence patterns) supported mineralization with ultrastructural morphology similar in appearance to that observed by Davies and colleagues [1990]. However, mineralization was not observed on smooth surfaces in which osteoblastlike cells did not have a preferred growth orientation. Thus the control of surface microtopography by such procedures as micromachining may prove to be a valuable technology for the control and perhaps optimization of bone formation on implant surfaces.

It is apparent that macroscopic as well as microscopic topography may affect osteoblast differentiation and mineralization. In a recent study by Groessner-Schrieber and Tuan [1992], osteoblast growth, differentiation, and synthesis of matrix and mineralized nodules were observed on rough, textured, or porous coated titanium surfaces. It may be possible therefore, not only to optimize the interactions of host tissues with implant surfaces during the Phase I tissue responses but also to influence the overall bone responses to biomechanical forces during the remodeling phase (Phase II) of tissue responses.

Based on these concepts, current implant designs employ microtopographically roughened surfaces with macroscopic grooves, threads, or porous surfaces to provide sufficient bone ingrowth for mechanical

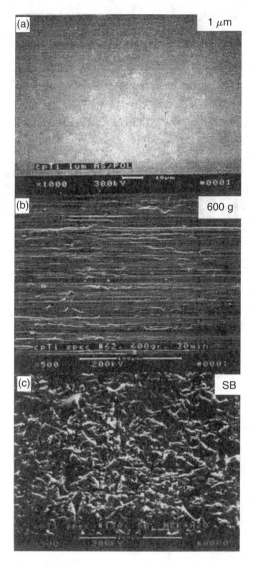

FIGURE 45.14 Laboratory-prepared cpTi surfaces with (a–c, top to bottom) smooth (1 μm polish), grooved (600 grit polish), and rough (sandblasted) surfaces.

stabilization and the prevention of detrimental micromotion as shown in Figure 45.16 and Figure 45.17 [De Porter et al., 1986; Keller et al., 1987; Pilliar et al., 1991; Brunski, 1992].

45.2.3 Surface Chemistry

Considerable attention has focused on the properties of the oxide found on titanium implant surfaces following surface preparation. Sterilization procedures are especially important and are known to affect not only the oxide condition but also the subsequent *in vitro* [Swart et al., 1992; Stanford et al., 1994] and *in vivo* [Hartman et al., 1989] biologic responses. Interfacial surface analyses and determinations of surface energetics strongly suggest that steam autoclaving is especially damaging to titanium oxide surfaces. Depending upon the purity of the autoclave water, contaminants have been observed on the metal oxide and are correlated with poor tissue responses on a cellular [Keller et al., 1990, 1994] and tissue [Meenaghan et al., 1979; Baier et al., 1984; Hartman et al., 1989] level.

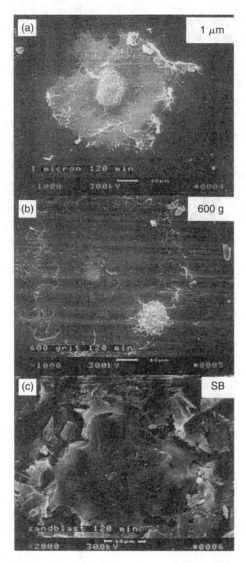

FIGURE 45.15   Osteoblastlike cell morphology after 2 h attachment on (a–c, top to bottom) smooth, grooved, and rough cpTi surfaces.

The role of multiple sterilization regimens on the practice of implant utilization is also under scrutiny. Many implants and especially bone plate systems are designed for repackaging if the kit is not exhausted. However, early evidence indicates that this practice is faulty and, depending on the method of sterilization, may affect the integrity of the metal oxide surface chemistry [Vezeau et al., 1991]. *In vitro* experiments have verified that multiple-steam-autoclaved and ethylene-oxide-treated implant surfaces adversely affected cellular and morphologic integration. However, the effects of these treatments on long-term biological responses including *in vivo* situations remain to be clarified.

Other more recently introduced techniques such as radiofrequency argon plasma cleaning treatments have succeeded in altering metal oxide chemistry and structure [Baier et al., 1984; Swart et al., 1992]. Numerous studies have demonstrated that PC treatments produce a relatively contaminant-free surface with improved surface energy (wettability), but conflicting biologic results have been reported with these surfaces. Recent *in vitro* studies have demonstrated that these highly energetic surfaces do not necessarily improve cellular responses such as attachment and cell expression. This has been confirmed by *in vivo*

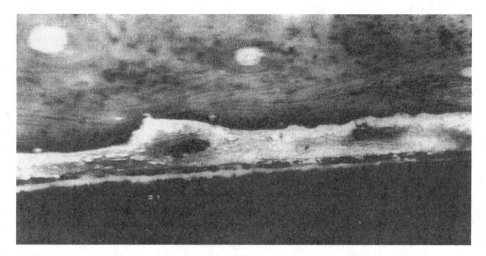

FIGURE 45.16   Light microscopic photomicrograph of a bone–smooth cpTi interface with intervening layer of soft connective tissue. This implant was mobile in the surgical site due to lack of tissue ingrowth. (Original magnification = 50×.)

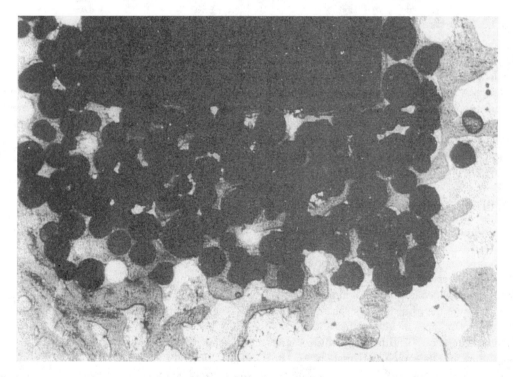

FIGURE 45.17   Light microscopic photomicrograph of a bone–porous Ti alloy implant interface. Note significant bone ingrowth in open porosity at the apical end of the implant. (Original magnification = 10×.)

studies which indicate that the overall histologic and ultrastructural morphology of the bone-implant interface is similar for plasma-cleaned and dry-heat-sterilized implant surfaces [Albrektsson et al., 1983]. Another promising technique for the sterilization of implant materials is the exposure of the implant surface to ultraviolet light [Singh and Schaff, 1989] or gamma irradiation [Keller et al., 1994]. Both these methods of sterilization produce a relatively contaminant-free thin oxide layer which fosters high levels of cell attachment [Keller et al., 1994] and inflammatory-free long-term *in vivo* responses [Hartman et al., 1989]. Currently, gamma irradiation procedures are widely used for the sterilization of metallic dental implant devices.

45.2.3.1 Metallic Corrosion

Throughout the history of the use of metals for biomedical implant applications, electrochemical corrosion with subsequent metal release has been problematic [Galante et al., 1991]. Of the biomedical metal systems available today, Ti and its major medical alloy, Ti–6A1–4V, are thought to be the most corrosion resistant; however, Ti metals are not totally inert *in vivo* [Woodman et al., 1984]. Release of Ti ions from Ti oxides can occur under relatively passive conditions [Ducheyne, 1988]. Whereas other factors such as positioning of the implant and subsequent biomechanical forces may play important roles in the overall tissue response to implants, it is not unreasonable to predict that electrochemical interactions between the implant surface and host tissue may affect the overall response of host bone [Blumenthal and Cosma, 1989]. For example, it has been shown by several groups [De Porter et al., 1986; Keller et al., 1987] that the percentages of intimate bony contact with the implant is inconsistent, at best, and generally averages approximately 50% over a 5-year period. Continued studies involving the effects of dissolution products on both local and systemic host responses are required in order to more fully understand the consequences of biologic interaction with metal implants.

45.2.3.2 Future Considerations for Implant Surfaces

It is clear that future efforts to improve the host tissue responses to implant materials will focus, in large part, on controlling cell and tissue responses at implant interfaces. This goal will require continued acquisition of fundamental knowledge of cell behavior and cell response to specific materials' characteristics. It is likely that a better understanding of the cellular-derived extracellular matrix-implant interface will offer a mechanism by which biologic response modifiers such as growth and attachment factors or hormones may be incorporated. Advancements of this type will likely shift the focus of future research from implant surfaces which as osseoconductive (permissive) to those which are osseoinductive (bioactive).

Defining Terms

Amorphous zone: A region of the tissue-implant interface immediately adjacent to the implant substrate. This zone is of variable thickness (usually <1000 Å), is free of collagen, and is comprised of proteoglycans of unknown composition.

Calcium phosphate: A family of calcium- and phosphate-containing materials of synthetic or natural origin which are utilized for implants and bone augmentation purposes. The most prominent materials are the tricalcium-phosphate- and hydroxyapatite-based materials, although most synthetic implants are a mixture of the various compositions.

Contact guidance: The theory by which cells attach to and migrate on substrates of specific microstructure and topographic orientation. The ability of the cell to attach and migrate on a substrate is related to the cytoskeletal and attachment molecules present on the cell membrane.

Junctional epithelium: The epithelial attachment mechanism which occurs with teeth, and has been observed infrequently with implants by some researchers. Less than 10 cell layers thick, the hemidesmosomal attachments of the basal cells to the implant surface provide a mechanical attachment for epithelium and prevent bacterial penetration into the sulcular area.

Osseointegration: A term developed by P.I. Branemark and his colleagues indicating the ability of host bone tissues to form a functional, mechanically immobile interface with the implant. Originally described for titanium only, several other materials are capable of forming this interface, which presumes a lack of connective tissue (foreign body) layer.

Plasma spray: A high-temperature process by which calcium-phosphate-containing materials are coated onto a suitable implant substrate. Although the target material may be of high purity, the high-temperature softening process can dramatically affect and alter the resultant composition of the coating.

References

Albrektsson, T., Branemark, P.I., Hansson, H.A. et al. 1983. The interface zone of inorganic implants *in vivo*: Titanium implants in bone. *Ann. Biomed. Eng.* 11: 1.

Albrektsson, T., Hansson, H.A., and Ivarsson, B. 1985. Interface analysis of titanium and zirconium bone implants. *Biomaterials* 6: 97.

Baier, R.E., Meyer, A.E., Natiella, J.R. et al. 1984. Surface properties determine bioadhesive outcomes. *J. Biomed. Mater. Res.* 18: 337.

Blumenthal, N.C. and Cosma, V. 1989. Inhibition of appetite formation by titanium and vanadium ions. *J. Biomed. Mater. Res.* 23: 13.

Bowers, K.T., Keller, J.C., Michaels, C.M. et al. 1992. Optimization of surface micromorphology for enhanced osteoblast responses *in vitro*. *Int. J. Oral Maxillofac. Implants* 7: 302.

Branemark, P.I. 1983. Osseointegration and its experimental background. *J. Pros. Dent.* 59: 399.

Brunski, J.B. 1992. Biomechanical factors affecting the bone-dental implant interface. *Clin. Mater.* 10: 153.

Chehroudi, B., Ratkay, J., and Brunette, D.M. 1992. The role of implant surface geometry on mineralization *in vivo* and *in vitro*: a transmission and scanning electron microscopic study. *Cells Mater.* 2: 89–104.

Cook, S.D., Kay, J.F., Thomas, K.A. et al. 1987. Interface mechanics and histology of titanium and hydroxylapatite coated titanium for dental implant applications. *Int. J. Oral Maxillofac. Implants* 2: 15.

Cook, S.D., Thomas, K.A., and Kay, J.F. 1991. Experimental coating defects in hydroxylapatite coated implants. *Clin. Orthop. Rel. Res.* 265: 280.

Davies, J.E., Lowenberg, B., and Shiga, A. 1990. The bone–titanium interface *in vitro*. *J. Biomed. Mater. Res.* 24: 1289–1306.

De Bruijn, J.D., Flach, J.S., deGroot, K. et al. 1993. Analysis of the bony interface with various types of hydroxyapatite *in vitro*. *Cells Mater.* 3: 115.

De Porter, D.A., Watson, P.A., Pilliar, R.M. et al. 1986. A histological assessment of the initial healing response adjacent to porous-surfaced, titanium alloy dental implants in dogs. *J. Dent. Res.* 65: 1064.

Driskell, T.D., Spungenberg, H.D., Tennery, V.J. et al. 1973. Current status of high density alumina ceramic tooth roof structures. *J. Dent. Res.* 52: 123.

Ducheyne, P. 1988. Titanium and calcium phosphate ceramic dental implants, surfaces, coatings and interfaces. *J. Oral Implantol.* 19: 325.

Filiaggi, M.J., Pilliar, R.M., and Coombs, N.A. 1993. Post-plasma spraying heat treatment of the HA coating/Ti–6A1–4V implant system. *J. Biomed. Mater. Res.* 27: 191.

Galante, J.O., Lemons, J., Spector, M. et al. 1991. The biologic effects of implant materials. *J. Orthop. Res.* 9: 760.

Groessner-Schreiber, B. and Tuan, R.S. 1992. Enhanced extracellular matrix production and mineralization by osteoblasts cultured on titanium surfaces *in vitro*. *J. Cell Sci.* 101: 209.

Hartman, L.C., Meenaghan, M.A., Schaaf, N.G. et al. 1989. Effects of pretreatment sterilization and cleaning methods on materials properties and osseoinductivity of a threaded implant. *Int. J. Oral Maxillofac. Implants* 4: 11.

Herman, H. 1988. Plasma spray deposition processes. *Mater. Res. Soc. Bull.* 13: 60.

Jansen, J.A., van der Waerden, J.P.C.M., and Wolke, J.G.C. 1993. Histological and histomorphometrical evaluation of the bone reaction to three different titanium alloy and hydroxyapatite coated implants. *J. Appl. Biomater.* 4: 213.

Jarcho, M., Kay, J.F., Gumaer, K.I. et al. 1977. Tissue, cellular and subcellular events at a bone-ceramic hydroxylapatite interface. *J. Bioeng.* 1: 79.

Jasty, M., Rubash, H.E., Paiemont, G.D. et al. 1992. Porous coated uncemented components in experimental total hip arthroplasty in dogs. *Clin. Orthop. Rel. Res.* 280: 300.

Johansson, C.B., Lausman, J., Ask, M. et al. 1989. Ultrastructural differences of the interface zone between bone and Ti-6A1-4V or commercially pure titanium. *J. Biomed. Eng.* 11: 3.

Katsikeris, N., Listrom, R.D., and Symington, J.M. 1987. Interface between titanium 6A1–4V alloy implants and bone. *Int. J. Oral Maxillofac. Surg.* 16: 473.

Kay, J.F. 1992. Calcium phosphate coatings for dental implants. *Dent. Clinic N. Am.* 36: 1.

Keller, J.C., Draughn, R.A., Wightman, J.P. et al. 1990. Characterization of sterilized cp titanium implant surfaces. *Int. J. Oral Maxillofac. Implants* 5: 360.

Keller, J.C. and Lautenschlager, E.P. 1986. Metals and alloys. In *Handbook of Biomaterials Evaluation*, A. Von Recon (Ed.), pp. 3–23, New York, Macmillan.

Keller, J.C., Niederauer, G.G., Lacefield, W.R. et al. 1992. Interaction of osteoblast-like cells with calcium phosphate ceramic materials. *Trans. Acad. Dent. Mater.* 5: 107.

Keller, J.C., Stanford, C.M., Wightman, J.P. et al. 1994. Characterization of titanium implant surfaces. *J. Biomed. Mater. Res.*

Keller, J.C., Young, F.A., Natiella, J.R. 1987. Quantitative bone remodeling resulting from the use of porous dental implants. *J. Biomed. Mater. Res.* 21: 305.

Koeneman, J., Lemons, J.E., Ducheyne, P. et al. 1990. Workshop of characterization of calcium phosphate materials. *J. Appl. Biomater.* 1: 79.

Lucas, L.C., Lemons, J.E., Lee, J., et al. 1987. *In vivo* corrosion characteristics of Co–Cr–Mu/ Ti–6A1–4V–Ti alloys. In *Quantitative Characterization and Performance of Porous Alloys for Hard Tissue Applications*, J.E. Lemons (Ed.), pp. 124–136, Philadelphia, ASTM.

Maxian, S.H., Zawadsky, J.P., and Durin, M.G. 1993. Mechanical and histological evaluation of amorphous calcium phosphate and poorly crystallized hydroxylapatite coatings on titanium implants. *J. Biomed. Mater. Res.* 27: 717.

Meenaghan, M.A., Natiella, J.R., Moresi, J.C. et al. 1979. Tissue response to surface treated tantalum implants: Preliminary observations in primates. *J. Biomed. Mater. Res.* 13: 631.

Orr, R.D., de Bruijn, J.D., and Davies, J.E. 1992. Scanning electron microscopy of the bone interface with titanium, titanium alloy and hydroxyapatite. *Cells Mater.* 2: 241.

Pilliar, R.M., DePorter, D.A., Watson, P.A. et al. 1991. Dental implant design — effect on bone remodeling. *J. Biomed. Mater. Res.* 25: 647.

Puleo, D.A., Holleran, L.A., Doremus, R.H. et al. 1991. Osteoblast responses to orthopedic implant materials *in vitro*. *J. Biomed. Mater. Res.* 25: 711.

Singh, S. and Schaaf, N.G. 1989. Dynamic sterilization of titanium implants with ultraviolet light. *Int. J. Oral Maxillofac. Implants* 4: 139.

Skalak, R. 1985. Aspects of biomechanical considerations. In *Tissue Integrated Prostheses*, P.I. Branemark, G. Zarb, and T. Albrektsson (Eds.), pp. 117–128, Chicago, Quintessence.

Smith, D.C. 1993. Dental implants: Materials and design considerations. *Int. J. Prosth.* 6: 106.

Stanford, C.M. and Keller, J.C. 1991. Osseointegration and matrix production at the implant surface. *CRC Crit. Rev. Oral Bio. Med.* 2: 83.

Stanford, C.M., Keller, J.C., and Solursh, M. 1994. Bone cell expression on titanium surfaces is altered by sterilization treatments. *J. Dent. Res.*

Steflik, D.E., McKinney, R.V., Koth, D.L. et al. 1984. Biomaterial-tissue interface: A morphological study utilizing conventional and alternative ultrastructural modalities. *Scanning Electron Microsc.* 2: 547.

Steflik, D.E., Sisk, A.L., Parr, G.R. et al. 1993. Osteogenesis at the dental implant interface: High voltage electron microscopic and conventional transmission electric microscopic observations. *J. Biomed. Mater. Res.* 27: 791.

Swart, K.M., Keller, J.C., Wightman, J.P. et al. 1992. Short term plasma cleaning treatments enhance *in vitro* osteoblast attachment to titanium. *J. Oral Implant* 18: 130.

Van Orden, A. 1985. Corrosive response of the interface tissue to 316L stainless steel, Ti-based alloy and cobalt-based alloys. In *The Dental Implant*, R. McKinney and J.E. Lemons (Eds.), pp. 1–25, Littleton, PSG.

Vezeau, P.J., Keller, J.C., and Koorbusch, G.F. 1991. Effects of multiple sterilization regimens on fibroblast attachment to titanium. *J. Dent. Res.* 70: 530.

Vrouwenvelder, W.C.A, Groot, C.G., and Groot, K. 1993. Histological and biochemical evaluation of osteoblasts cultured on bioactive glass, hydroxylapatite, titanium alloy and stainless steel. *J. Biomed. Mater. Res.* 27: 465–475.

Woodman, J.L., Jacobs, J.J., Galante, J.O. et al. Metal ion release from titanium-based prosthetic segmental replacements of long bones in baboons: A long term study. *J. Orthop. Res.* 1: 421–430.

Young, F.A. 1988. Future directions in dental implant materials research. *J. Dent. Ed.* 52: 770.

46

Controlling and Assessing Cell–Biomaterial Interactions at the Micro- and Nanoscale: Applications in Tissue Engineering

Jessica Kaufman
Joyce Y. Wong
Catherine Klapperich
Boston University

46.1 A Need for Understanding Cell–Biomaterial Interactions at the Micro- and Nanoscale

A long-standing goal of tissue engineering has been to create functional tissues, ideally by promoting the regenerative capacity of a patient's autologous cells by controlling cellular response. Regardless of whether this is achieved by using artificial scaffolds or naturally derived extracellular matrices, the engineered tissue must be able to support the necessary physiological loads during the remodeling processes that ultimately lead to generation of the functional tissue. While there has been tremendous progress in engineering a number of tissue systems, namely skin replacements [1–3], an incomplete understanding of the underlying mechanisms that control cell behavior has led to limited clinical success. Specifically, there are many open questions as to how cell–biomaterial interactions impact cellular and ultimately tissue phenotype [4,5].

In order to gain a mechanistic understanding of factors that control cell behavior, molecular and cell biologists have numerous methodologies to systematically unravel specific cell-signaling pathways involved in regulating cell behavior. It has been more difficult to control properties of biomaterials with analogous precision, but this is rapidly changing with recent enabling micro- and nanotechnologies that create scaffolds characterized by features that can now be controlled at length-scales that range from cellular dimensions all the way down to the molecular scale.

A solid base of research in both engineering and the biomedical sciences has demonstrated that tissue regeneration in synthetic environments is possible and often successful, but is difficult to predict and control. Design of these scaffolds has been conducted largely by trial and error, and little is known about how the chemical and mechanical properties of the scaffold affect the biological response of the seeded cells. Due to this lack of understanding, it has proven significantly more difficult to engineer complex tissues like cartilage, bone, nerves, and muscle [6,7] By considering the biological response of cells to scaffolds a material property that can be controlled by altering processing variables, we can begin to build the framework necessary for intelligent de novo design of new scaffold materials. However, in order for biological response to be a useful design variable, it must be quantifiable. Several of the approaches reviewed in this chapter are aimed at quantifying biological responses.

In most tissue engineering applications, a positive result is more likely if the scaffold material can provide the environmental stimuli necessary for healthy tissue regeneration. In most tissues, the molecular nature of these factors is unknown, but is likely some combination of mechanical, chemical, and biological stimuli take place on the micro- and nanoscale. It is largely unknown how mechanical forces and surface chemistry affect the physiology of cells, but this is a very active area of research [8–10]. Recently, many researchers have begun to focus on precisely how cells are responding to chemical and topological features at the micro- and nanoscale. Covered in this chapter are current issues involved in probing cell–biomaterials interactions on the molecular level and their implications for tissue engineering research. Discussed are methods to quantify cell response, engineer cell-surface molecules for targeted cell–biomaterials interactions, gain geometric and surface chemical control of cell fate, and directed movement of cells on substrates with mechanical gradients. We also discuss recent enabling technologies in materials processing that have yielded nanoscale biomaterials as tissue engineering scaffolds for various organ systems. Finally, we discuss the need for determining potential undesirable immunogenic responses to nano- and microsystems.

This review is by no means complete, and we apologize in advance to our colleagues for not including all of the excellent work in this area.

46.2 Genomic and Proteomic Data as a Measure of Cell–Biomaterials Interactions

By combining our ever increasing control over fabricating nanoscale features and the increased standardization of biochemical assays afforded by access to information about the human genome, we can now embark on intelligent tissue engineering scaffold design. Cell adhesion, migration, growth, and

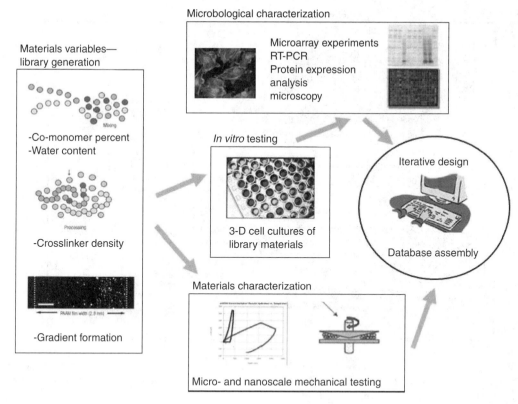

FIGURE 46.1   (See color insert following page **32**-14.) Schematic of the combinatorial approach using cell responses as variables in synthetic biomaterials design for tissue engineering applications. Libraries of chemically well-defined materials are generated combinatorially. The materials are characterized both chemically and mechanically at the nano- and microscale. *In vitro* cell-based assays are used to assess gene and protein expression. Cell–biomaterial interactions are visualized in 3-D culture using confocal microscopy. Finally, data is stored in an organized database for use in de novo materials design.

extracellular matrix synthesis are four major areas of cell responses that are relevant to tissue engineering applications. These responses can be probed on many levels including mRNA levels (gene expression) and protein levels (proteomics). A schematic of the general approach taken in one of our laboratories is included in Figure 46.1.

We have used the collagen–glycosaminoglycan (collagen–GAG) mesh scaffold to probe molecular level cell–biomaterials interactions [11]. We seeded IMR-90 human fibroblasts onto three-dimensional (3-D) collagen–GAG meshes and control surfaces of tissue culture polystyrene (TCPS). Nucleic acids (mRNA) from cells from each culture were isolated, amplified, and hybridized to human genome microarrays (U133A Gene Chip, Affymetrix, Santa Clara, CA).

Connective tissue growth factor (CTGF) and tissue inhibitor metalloproteinase 3 (TIMP3) were down regulated in 3-D collagen exposed fibroblasts compared to the tissue culture polystyrene grown cells. CTGF, which plays a role in the induction of collagen, has known involvement in matrix accumulation in fibrosis, as well as the development of excess fibrous connective tissue. TIMP3 inactivates metalloproteinases, which degrade components of the extracellular matrix thereby remodeling the tissue. By underexpressing TIMP3, it is suspected that collagen–GAG interaction encourages the reorganization of the fibroblasts extracellular matrix. The 3-D arrangement stimulated the expression of proangiogenic genes including vascular endothelial growth factor (VEGF) and angiopoietin (ANGPTL2). The 3-D mesh environment also yielded high expression levels of the mRNA for proteins involved in matrix remodeling such as type III collagen (COL3A1).

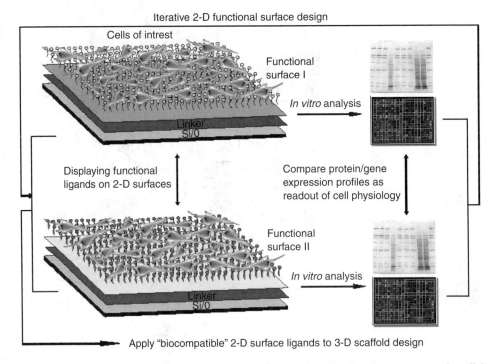

FIGURE 46.2 (See color insert following page **32**-14.) A functional surface-based strategy to probe cell–ligand interactions — an iterative tissue engineering scaffold design approach. (Reproduced from Song, J. et al., *J. Mater. Chem.*, 2004, **14**: 2643–8. With permission.)

These studies and complementary proteomic work are beginning to more precisely define material biocompatibility for tissue regeneration. We extended this approach to look at how surfaces conjugated with anionic peptides affected gene and protein expression in osteosarcoma cells (Figure 46.2) [12]. Other researchers have taken similar approaches to study the migration and spreading behavior of endothelial cells on small-gauge vascular prostheses [13]. Ku et al. [14] looked at global gene expression of osteoblasts grown on different Ti–6Al–4V surface treatments. They were able to detect differences in inflammatory response of cells on three different surface treatments. Once a more complete understanding of the molecular nature of biocompatibility is achieved, the cell-surface molecule modifications and advanced materials design techniques described later will become much more powerful tools.

46.3   Engineering the Cell Surface to Control Cell-Adhesion Events

Another approach to controlling cell–biomaterials interactions is to modify the cell surface. The surfaces of cells are decorated with polysaccharides, glycolipids, and glycoproteins. These cell-surface molecules are the handles through which cells communicate with their surroundings. Cell-adhesion events can trigger signaling events inside of the cell and lead to changes in gene expression and eventually cell fate. These properties make cell-surface molecules ideal engineering targets. By modifying the molecules presented on a cell surface, it may be possible to control a cell's phenotype and eventual fate.

One way to modify the cell-surface molecules is by introducing nonnatural monosugars into the biosynthetic pathways that build up polysaccharides (Figure 46.3) [15,16]. By introducing monosaccharides with synthetic ketone groups, Bertozzi et al. were able to engineer previously nonadherent Jurkat cells to adhere to lipid bilayers decorated with azides [17]. These researchers have also demonstrated that a

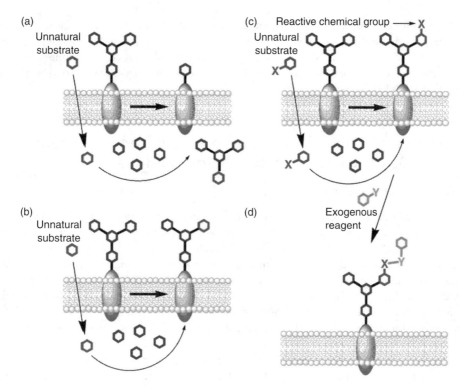

FIGURE 46.3 (See color insert following page **32**-14.) (Right) Modulating cell-surface glycosylation by metabolic interference. (a) Unnatural substrates fed to cells can divert oligosaccharide biosynthesis away from endogenous scaffolds, reducing the expression of specific carbohydrate structures. (b) Unnatural substrates can be used in biosynthetic pathways and incorporated into cell-surface glycoconjugates. (c) If the unnatural substrates possess unique functional groups, their metabolic products on the cell-surface can be chemically elaborated with exogenous reagents (d). (Reproduced from Bertozzi, C.R. and L.L. Kiessling, *Science*, 2001, **291**: 2357–64. With permission.)

modification of a cell-surface molecule, polysialic acid (PSA), in substrata cells supporting the growth of chick dorsal root ganglion sensory neurons were able to differentially affect the outgrowth and plasticity of those cells [18]. In this case a cell-surface molecule that inhibits adhesion and outgrowth of neurons was modified, but it is easy to imagine that engineering cell-surface molecules that encourage such outgrowth would benefit work in nerve tissue regeneration. Since these artificial sugars can be installed through metabolic pathways, the cell culture needs only to be fed the engineered sugar through the media. It has also been demonstrated that feeding these sugars to small animals orally leads to the desired cell-surface modifications in cells of the animal, indicating that these substances may be able to be administered as drugs to patients or injected directly into the site of artificial tissue repair.

Other methods of cell-surface engineering also look promising. Genetic methods have been used to transfect cells with genes that express unique or unnatural cell-surface protein [19,20]. Kato and Mrksich [21] describe a method to modify both the cell and the biomaterial surface in a complimentary manner to encourage specific cell adhesion. They transfected Chinese hamster ovary (CHO) cells to express a chimeric receptor with a carbonic anhydrase IV (CAIV) domain at its terminus. This domain binds selectively to benzenesulfonamide groups that were installed on self-assembled monolayers designed for the study. The study demonstrates the ability to control both sides of the receptor–ligand interaction, which suggests a potentially powerful tool for tissue engineering.

Since cell-adhesion events are almost always the first step in the regeneration of injured or destroyed tissues, the ability to control these events should lead to the generation of better artificial tissues. Complementary modifications of the cell and biomaterial surfaces could allow cells to be directed to a specific location for tissue regeneration. Current problems with cell seeding of artificial scaffolds could be ameliorated in this way. Of course it is essential to remain mindful that at this time only a patient's own cells can provide a preseeded tissue engineering scaffold that will not elicit an immune response. The advent of stem cell use in regenerative medicine and tissue engineering may solve some of these problems, but much research is left to be done [22,23].

46.4 Design of Model Micro- and Nanoenvironments to Probe and Direct Cell–Biomaterials Interactions

46.4.1 Geometric and Surface Chemical Control of Cell Fate

In order to sort out what cues cells are receiving from their three-dimensional extracellular environments, many groups have begun to make model environments with well-defined chemical and topological features. By maintaining control over the feature size and chemical character of the model system, changes in these variables can be made and the resulting cell responses can be measured using microbiological techniques. Most often, these features are made using photolithographic methods developed for the microelectronic industry [24]. Features approaching 1 μm in size are easily fabricated using these methods. In recent work, Dike et al. [25] demonstrated specific control over cell fate in vascular endothelial cells, showing that micropatterned surfaces can determine whether the cells would follow an angiogenic, apoptotic, or differentiation pathway.

Early work by Chen et al. [26] demonstrated that cells grown on subsequently smaller areas of microcontact printed extracellular matrix experienced different fates. In these experiments, changing the substrate extracellular matrix components and cell source, bovine or human, did not override the geometric effects. This work was expanded to three dimensions by examining how capillary endothelial cells grow in solution with fibronectin-coated beads [27]. Cells attached to single 10 μm beads did not improve viability whereas attaching cells to 25 μm beads did. The capillary epithelial cells undergo apoptosis unless the substrate is designed to allow them to adopt a relatively flat conformation by making multiple connections on a relatively planar surface.

Recently, Chen has used microneedle-like posts made of polydimethylsiloxane (PDMS) to measure the mechanical forces that smooth muscle cells exert on each other at cell adhesions (Figure 46.4) [28]. The researchers were also able to control the type of cell-adhesion molecules present on the tip of each elastomeric post. Using this approach of geometric control combined with precisely defined surface chemistries, they were able to demonstrate correlations between mechanical and chemical signals in these cells.

Just as Chen showed that cell fate can be determined by geometry of individual cells, Bhatia et al. [29] showed that the geometry of individual populations within a micropatterned coculture can also affect cell behavior. Cocultures were constructed by culturing hepatocytes on collagen-patterned wafers and then culturing fibroblasts directly on the substrate surrounding the wafers. In the experiment, the contact area between hepatocytes and fibroblasts and the contact area between individual hepatocytes were held constant. As the contact area between fibroblasts was increased, liver-specific functions in hepatocytes also increased. Work by Tang et al. [30] was a first step at using micropatterning techniques to create three-dimensional cocultures in collagen gels (Figure 46.5). Building up three-dimensional cultures with controlled geometries is a critical step toward multicellular tissue engineering constructs. Control of the local or microscale arrangement of cells in a tissue engineering scaffold will be a key to creating functional organs.

Cells do react to changes in their microscale environment, but cell–cell and cell–matrix adhesions are often nanoscale phenomena. Recently, techniques that yield nanoscale topography have emerged. As we are able to probe cells with smaller and smaller changes in surface topography and local surface chemistry, the closer we will come to mimicking the *in vivo* microenvironment. Andersson et al. [31] demonstrated that uroepithelial cells seeded onto substrates with nanoscale pillars expressed smaller amounts of the cytokines

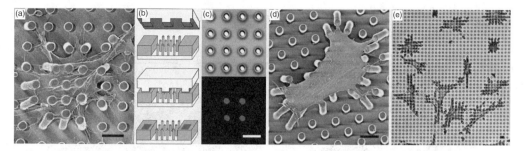

FIGURE 46.4 (See color insert following page **32**-14.) Cell culture on arrays of posts. (a) Scanning electron micrograph of a representative smooth muscle cell attached to an array of posts that was uniformly coated with fibronectin. Cells attached at multiple points along the posts as well as the base of the substrates. (b) Schematic of microcontact printing of protein (red), precoated on a PDMS stamp, onto the tips of the posts (gray). (c) Differential interference contrast (Upper) and immunofluorescence (Lower) micrographs of the same region of posts where a 2 × 2 array of posts has been printed with fibronectin. (d and e) Scanning electron micrograph (d) and phase-contrast micrograph (e) of representative smooth muscle cells attached to posts where only the tips of the posts have been printed with fibronectin by using a flat PDMS stamp. Cells deflected posts maximally during the 1 to 2-h period after plating, were fully spread after 2 h, and were fixed and critical point dried 4 h after plating. (Scale bars indicate 10 μm.) (Reproduced from Tan, J.L. et al., *Proc. Natl Acad. Sci. USA*, 2003, **100**: 1484–9. With permission.)

IL-6 and IL-8 than cells cultured on flat substrates of the same material. They saw no difference in cytokine production between cells grown on the flat substrate and one with parallel microscale grooves. Corneal epithelial cells were shown to exhibit significantly different phenotypes when seeded onto substrates with nanoscale features [32]. Focal adhesions and cytoskeleton proteins were found to align in the direction of the nanoscale features, a common result when cells are seeded on microscale surface topographies. This result was expected, since the surface of the corneal basal lamina is known to have features in the range of 20 to 200 nm.

46.4.2 Directed Movement of Cells on Mechanical Gradients

In addition to surface chemical micropatterning to control cell positioning, recently one of our laboratories has used micropatterning techniques to create mechanical gradient gels [33,34] (Figure 46.6). This phenomenon was first reported by Wang's and Dembo's groups [35] for 3T3 fibroblasts cultured on a substrate characterized with a step-gradient in mechanical properties. However, the method used to produce these substrates lacked precise control at the microscale, so we developed two methods based on photopolymerization to control substrate mechanical properties at the microscale. In one approach, mask patterns are used to control the degree of polymerization in polyacrylamide gels by controlling the UV light exposure time. Using this system, cell motility of bovine vascular smooth muscle cells were compared on mechanically patterned collagen-coated gels vs. uniformly compliant gels. The cells exhibited a clear migration from soft regions to stiff regions, durotaxis, when compared with cells grown on uniform hydrogels. Furthermore, the vascular smooth muscle cells accumulated in stiff regions of the gel, suggesting that mechanical patterning could be a powerful tool for creating complex cultures with multiple cell types that are stable over long periods of time.

The second approach involves the integration of a microfluidic gradient generator and photopolymerization to create substrate with well-defined compliance gradients [34]. An advantage of this approach is that more complex gradients can be achieved. In addition, variations in steepness of the gradient can be easily tuned in this system in order to quantify the range in which cells respond.

At this point, it is worth noting that there is limited data regarding the actual *local* mechanical properties of native and diseased tissues. Rather, our knowledge of tissue mechanical properties is largely based on *macroscopic* mechanical measurements. The lack of mechanical property characterization at the microscale

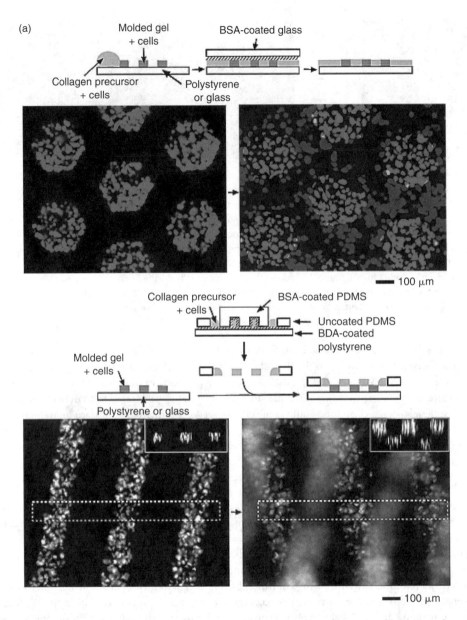

FIGURE 46.5   (See color insert following page **32**-14.) Schematic diagrams of the microfabrication of composite gels, and fluorescence images of cells in these gels. The shaded regions represent collagen gels in which fibroblasts are embedded. (a) (Left) An array of hexagonal gels (100 m on a side, 100 m thick) and cells on a glass coverslip. (Right) A composite structure that consists of an array of isolated hexagonal gels and a separate gel filling the spaces between the isolated gels on a glass coverslip. Fibroblasts in and between the hexagonal gels were prelabeled with green and red fluorescent dyes, respectively. (b) (Left) Lines (100 m wide, 100 m thick) of gel and cells formed by MIMIC on a glass coverslip. Nuclei of fibroblasts were labeled with the fluorescent dye Hoechst 33342 (1 g/ml; Molecular Probes). (Right) A bilayered structure that is composed of two layers of lines at a relative angle of ∼30 on a glass coverslip. The top layer is in focus, and the layer below is out-of-focus. (Insets) Cross-sectional views (corresponding to the regions outlined by dashed boxes) of deconvolved images. (Reproduced from Tang, M.D., A.P. Golden, and J. Tien, *J. Am. Chem. Soc.*, 2003, **125**: 12988-9. With permission.)

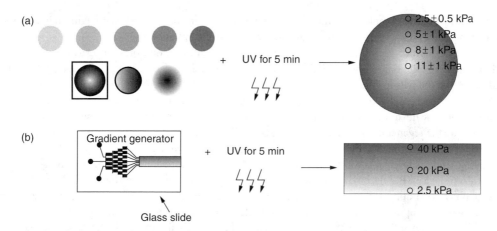

FIGURE 46.6 Methods for generating elastic substrata with gradients in mechanical properties. (a) Acrylamide is photopolymerized under transparency masks with varying degrees of opacity [33]. The radial gradient pattern boxed on the left can be used to create a substrate shown on the right with the 'map' of its mechanical properties (Young's modulus). (b) Acrylamide is photopolymerized using a combination of microfluidics and photopolymerization [34]. The gradient generator is used to create a gradient in the cross-linker (bis-acrylamide). The width of the gel is ~ 3 mm, and the gradient in the Young's modulus (as determined from atomic force microscopy) is approximately 12 Pa/μm. (Reproduced from Wong, J.Y., J.B. Leach, and Z.Q. Brown, *Surf. Sci.*, 2004, **570**: 119–33. With permission.)

is in part due to the limited number of techniques (e.g., modified atomic force microscopy [36]) that are able to measure the mechanical properties of hydrated tissues at this length-scale. Recently, we have developed a simple, inexpensive microindentation technique that is able to measure the local mechanical properties of hydrated biomaterials and tissue samples at the microscale [37]. While it is interesting that a number of different cell types have recently been shown to respond to changes in the mechanical properties of the substrate (see Reference 9), the measurement of the *local* mechanical properties of native and diseased tissues will be critical to establish clinical relevance when developing model *in vitro* biomaterial systems with physiologically matched mechanical properties.

46.4.3 Studies of Tissue Engineering Scaffolds with Nanoscale Features

Recently studies have been published that demonstrate enhanced cell growth, adhesion, and differentiation in the presence of nanoparticles or nanostructured coatings. In orthopedics, the fabrication of nanostructured ceramic coatings for total joint replacements has resulted in enhanced cell growth and bone remodeling *in vitro* [38]. Modified plasma spray processes have produced nanoscale hydroxyapatite coatings [39] for the same application. Hydrogel materials that either incorporate [40] or stimulate the nucleation of nanometer sized hydroxyapatite particles [41] have been demonstrated to form reasonable bone mimics. Tan and Saltzman [42] created a hierarchical bone-culture system employing microscale features coated with a nanoscale mineral phase. They were able to control both cell orientation and shape by modulating their surfaces. Further study will show if these materials will be successful as tissue engineering implants.

Several researchers focused on engineering soft tissues have also begun to employ nanostructured materials in the laboratory. Hydrogel materials with specific ligands for cell adhesion have been designed to affect desired cell-signaling events in native or implanted cells. A good review is provided by Boontheekul and Mooney [43]. Nerve tissue regeneration has been driven by the idea that if you can form a sheath of material of the appropriate size, then severed nerve endings will grow toward each other through it. Tubes have been made of silicone, collagen, and other synthetic and natural polymer materials. One common conclusion of much of this research is that not only do the regenerating axons need the mechanical cues provided by the artificial tube, but also most likely require the appropriate chemical signals at the nanoscale to drive complete and functional regeneration. Some researchers have begun to incorporate peptide sequences known to be neurotrophic in their tube-filling materials [44].

Hepatocytes, which are difficult to culture *in vitro* were cultured on gold nanoparticles to create a gold/hepatocyte colloidal solution [45]. The researchers were able to demonstrate increased proliferation and activity of the cells in culture.

Nanostructured poly(lactic-co-glycolic acid) (PGLA) created through chemical etching techniques was shown to increase the number and function of bladder smooth muscle cells in tissue engineering scaffolds intended for the regeneration of the bladder [46,47]. The authors attribute this result to the nanoscale surface topography, which they say more closely mimics the *in vitro* environment of soft tissue cells. Operating under similar assumptions, Zhang and Ma [48] developed a tissue engineering scaffold in poly(L-lactic acid) (PLLA) having micrometer scale pores with walls exhibiting nanofibrous features using a phase separation technique. These scaffolds were compared with scaffolds made from the same material with micropores that had smooth walls. Differences in adsorption of extracellular proteins into the scaffolds were studied using Western blot analysis [49]. The nanofibrous materials adsorbed more proteins than the smooth-walled scaffolds. Specifically, more fibronectin and vitronectin was adsorbed onto the nanostructured materials. The nanofibrous materials also enhanced adhesion of MC3T3-E1 osteoblasts when compared to the smooth-walled scaffolds.

Modified electrospray techniques have been used to produce polymer meshes for tissue scaffolds that have nanometer-scale fibers. This process involves injecting a polymer solution through a charged needle onto a substrate some distance away from the injection point. A mat of material can be made in varying thicknesses, and this mat can be cut or molded into the desired shape. Scaffolds of nanoscale fibers have been formed from poly(D,L-lactide-co-glycolide [50], collagen and elastin [51], and poly(D,L-lactide)-poly(ethylene glycol) (PLA-PEG) [52].

Nanoscale surface roughness can also affect cell differentiation. A recently developed technique for growing bone-like minerals on a hydrolyzed poly(lactide-co-glycolide) substrate by incubating in a salt-rich simulated body fluid was used to create bone mimics by Mooney et al. [53]. The resulting mineral layer displays a plate-like nanostructure similar to natural bone. Mesenchymal stem cells cultured under osteoblast inducing conditions were grown on both smooth substrate and mineralized substrate. Surprisingly, the mineralized substrate inhibited differentiation of the stem cells. In a similar work by Jansen et al. [54], surfaces roughness at the micron scale showed no effect on the differentiation of rat bone marrow cells under osteogenic conditions. Understanding both the chemical and nanoscale topographical signals necessary for differentiation will thus be essential for the development of stem-cell-based tissue-engineered constructs.

46.5   Impact of Nanoscale Processing on Biomaterial Properties

Recently there have been a number of reports of biomaterials that exploit molecular self-assembly processes. For example, repeating peptide sequences and synthetic polymers that form gels at neutral pH and body temperature are attractive materials for injectable scaffold materials [55]. A good review of these materials is found in Zhang et al. [56]. These materials will probably not be able to replace structural tissues in the near term, but are promising as materials for filling defects in these and other soft tissues. While these materials in general do not have nanoscale features, they are products of nanotechnology in that they are designed from the bottom up using solid-phase peptide synthesis. Stupp and coworkers [57] describe the formation of peptide amphiphiles that self-assemble to form nanostructures similar to extracellular matrix. They also demonstrated the ability of these nanostructures to nucleate hydroxyapatite nanocrystals from solution. Deming and coworkers [58] describe hydrogel formation from repeating polypeptide amphiphiles. By using these engineered materials in lieu of naturally occurring proteins, they describe enhanced control over the mechanical properties and processing of these biocompatible gels.

Some of the processing techniques described here require the application of either harsh chemicals or high temperatures. Before these materials can be exposed to cells or implanted into the body, they need to undergo extensive washing and in some cases sterilization. If nanostructured or micro/nanostructured materials prove to be advantageous for tissue engineering applications, more biocompatible manufacturing techniques will need to be developed.

46.6 Issues with Immune Response to Nanoparticles and Tissue Engineering Biomaterials

It has long been known in the orthopedic community that particles formed during the wear of total joint replacements will elicit an immune response in the body that can become chronic and systemic over the lifetime of an implant [59]. These particles are particularly troublesome when they are submicron in size and often lead to osteolysis, or pathological bone resorption [60–62] The cells responsible for digestion of these foreign particles, macrophages, initiate a more aggressive immune response to particles that are submicron in size [63,64] Total joint replacements are made of both polymer and metal components, and wear particles of both classes of materials have been found in tissues and organs throughout the bodies of patients wearing these devices [65].

Studies in the total joint replacement field should be a warning to those researchers attempting to use nanoparticles in imaging, detection, and tissue engineering applications. In fact, a recent study on polymer-based colloidal drug delivery systems found that nanoparticles from these injections are recognized and engulfed by the macrophages of the reticuloendothelial system [66] In addition, Akerman et al. [67] demonstrated that quantum dots (3–5 nm in size) used as fluorescent probes *in vivo* accumulated in the liver and the spleen of mice. This effect was eliminated by coating the quantum dots with polyethylene glycol. Given what we know about how submicron particle stimulate the immune system, it will be very important to consider what side effects nanoparticles of all types might have on all of the systems in the body.

One method of circumventing immune response is to encapsulate tissue-engineered constructs within immunoisolation membranes. By creating pores on the nanoscale, Desai et al. [68] have been able to prevent immune cells, antibodies, and complement from reaching the cells and biomaterials within the capsule, while allowing nutrients and products, such as insulin, to diffuse in and out of the capsule. Although, the cells and scaffold are not subject to an immune response, encapsulation devices, as with all implanted devices, will still have strong immune reactions at the biomaterial surface. To mitigate negative immune reactions, Desai et al. [69] have modified the outer surface of their biocapsule with PEG. *In vivo* studies suggest that the modified biocapsule elicits minimal fibrotic tissue development and no significant host response.

46.7 Summary

Recent advances in biomaterials science have allowed for greater control over materials chemistry and mechanical properties at smaller and smaller size scales. In addition to these advances, it is becoming more straightforward to test the molecular level response of cells to biomaterials. Only through the implementation of highly controlled biomaterials processing and characterization combined with a deeper understanding of cell response to synthetic microenvironments will the regeneration of more complicated tissues be possible.

Acknowledgments

Catherine M. Klapperich and Jessica D. Kaufman gratefully acknowledge the Whitaker Foundation for funding. Joyce Y. Wong gratefully acknowledges funding from the Whitaker Foundation, NSF (CAREER), NIH (NHLBI), and NASA.

References

[1] Jones, I., L. Currie, and R. Martin, A guide to biological skin substitutes. *Br. J. Plast. Surg.*, 2002, **55**: 185–93.

[2] Bello, Y.M., A.F. Falabella, and W.H. Eaglstein, Tissue-engineered skin. Current status in wound healing. *Am. J. Clin. Dermatol.*, 2001, **2**: 305–13.

[3] Boyce, S.T., Design principles for composition and performance of cultured skin substitutes. *Burns*, 2001, **27**: 523–33.

[4] Naughton, G.K., From lab bench to market: critical issues in tissue engineering. *Ann. NY Acad. Sci.*, 2002, **961**: 372–85.

[5] Mason, C., Automated tissue engineering: a major paradigm shift in health care. *Med. Device Technol.*, 2003, **14**: 16–8.

[6] Orban, J.M., K.G. Marra, and J.O. Hollinger, Composition options for tissue-engineered bone. *Tissue Eng.*, 2002, **8**: 529–39.

[7] Cancedda, R. et al., Tissue engineering and cell therapy of cartilage and bone. *Matrix Biol.*, 2003, **22**: 81–91.

[8] Guldberg, R.E., Consideration of mechanical factors. *Ann. NY Acad. Sci.*, 2002, **961**: 312–4.

[9] Wong, J.Y., J.B. Leach, and X.Q. Brown, Balance of chemistry, topography, and mechanics at the cell–biomaterial interface: issues and challenges for assessing the role of substrate mechanics on cell response. *Surf. Sci.*, 2004, **570**: 119–33.

[10] Brown, X.Q., K. Ookawa, and J.Y. Wong, Evaluation of polydimethylsiloxane scaffolds with physiologically-relevant elastic moduli: interplay of substrate mechanics and surface chemistry effects on vascular smooth muscle cell response. *Biomaterials*, 2005, **26**: 3123–9.

[11] Klapperich, C.M. and C.R. Bertozzi, Global gene expression of cells attached to a tissue engineering scaffold. *Biomaterials*, 2004, **25**: 5631–41.

[12] Song, J. et al., Functional glass slides for in vitro evaluation of interactions between osteosarcoma TE85 cells and mineral-binding ligands. *J. Mater. Chem.*, 2004, **14**: 2643–8.

[13] Gerritsen, M.E. et al., Branching out: a molecular fingerprint of endothelial differentiation into tube-like structures generated by affymetrix oligonucleotide arrays. *Microcirculation*, 2003, **10**: 63–81.

[14] Ku, C.H. et al., Large-scale gene expression analysis of osteoblasts cultured on three different Ti–6Al–4V surface treatments. *Biomaterials*, 2002, **23**: 4193–202.

[15] Mahal, L.K. and C.R. Bertozzi, Engineered cell surfaces: fertile ground for molecular landscaping. *Chem. Biol.*, 1997, **4**: 415–22.

[16] Mahal, L.K., K.J. Yarema, and C.R. Bertozzi, Engineering chemical reactivity on cell surfaces through oligosaccharide biosynthesis. *Science*, 1997, **276**: 1125–8.

[17] Yarema, K.J. et al., Metabolic delivery of ketone groups to sialic acid residues. Application to cell surface glycoform engineering. *J. Biol. Chem.*, 1998, **273**: 31168–79.

[18] Charter, N.W. et al., Differential effects of unnatural sialic acids on the polysialylation of the neural cell adhesion molecule and neuronal behavior. *J. Biol. Chem.*, 2002, **277**: 9255–61.

[19] Link, A.J., M.L. Mock, and D.A. Tirrell, Non-canonical amino acids in protein engineering. *Curr. Opin. Biotechnol.*, 2003, **14**: 603–9.

[20] Sampson, N.S., M. Mrksich, and C.R. Bertozzi, Surface molecular recognition. *Proc. Natl Acad. Sci. USA*, 2001, **98**: 12870–1.

[21] Kato, M. and M. Mrksich, Rewiring cell adhesion. *J. Am. Chem. Soc.*, 2004, **126**: 6504–5.

[22] Parenteau, N.L. and J. Hardin-Young, The use of cells in reparative medicine. *Ann. NY Acad. Sci.*, 2002, **961**: 27–39.

[23] Barry, F.P. and J.M. Murphy, Mesenchymal stem cells: clinical applications and biological characterization. *Int. J. Biochem. Cell Biol.*, 2004, **36**: 568–84.

[24] Desai, T.A., Micro- and nanoscale structures for tissue engineering constructs. *Med. Eng. Phys.*, 2000, **22**: 595–606.

[25] Dike, L.E. et al., Geometric control of switching between growth, apoptosis, and differentiation during angiogenesis using micropatterned substrates. *In Vitro Cell Dev. Biol. Anim.*, 1999, **35**: 441–8.

[26] Chen, C.S. et al., Geometric control of cell life and death. *Science*, 1997, **276**: 1425–8.

[27] Chen, C.S., M. Mrksich, S. Huang, G. M. Whitesides, and D. E. Ingber, Micropatterned surfaces for control of cell shape, position, and function. *Biotechnol. Prog.*, 1998. **14**: 356–63.

[28] Tan, J.L. et al., Cells lying on a bed of microneedles: an approach to isolate mechanical force. *Proc. Natl Acad. Sci. USA*, 2003, **100**: 1484–9.

[29] Bhatia, S.N., U.J. Balis, M.L. Yarmush, and M. Toner, Microfabrication of hepatocyte/fibroblast co-cultures: role of homotypic cell interactions. *Biotechnol. Prog.*, 1998, **14**: 378–87.

[30] Tang, M.D., A.P. Golden, and J. Tien, Molding of three-dimensional microstructures of gels. *J. Am. Chem. Soc.*, 2003, **125**: 12988–9.

[31] Andersson, A.S. et al., Nanoscale features influence epithelial cell morphology and cytokine production. *Biomaterials*, 2003, **24**: 3427–36.

[32] Teixeira, A.I. et al., Epithelial contact guidance on well-defined micro- and nanostructured substrates. *J. Cell Sci.*, 2003, **116**(Pt 10): 1881–92.

[33] Wong, J.Y., A. Velasco, P. Rajagopalan, and Q. Pham, Directed movement of vascular smooth muscle cells on gradient-compliant hydrogels. *Langmuir*, 2003, **19**: 1908–13.

[34] Zaari, N. et al., Hydrogels photopolymerized in a microfluidics gradient generator: tuning substrate compliance at the microscale to control cell response. *Adv. Mater.*, 2004, **15**: 2133–7.

[35] Lo, C.M. et al., Cell movement is guided by the rigidity of the substrate. *Biophys. J.*, 2000, **79**: 144–52.

[36] Dimitriadis, E.K. et al., Determination of elastic moduli of thin layers of soft material using the atomic force microscope. *Biophys. J.*, 2002, **82**: 2798–810.

[37] Jacot, J.G., S.W. Dianis, and J.Y. Wong, Probing microscale compliance of soft hydrated materials and tissues using simple microindentation. *Bio Phys. J.*, 2005: in review.

[38] Catledge, S.A. et al., Nanostructured ceramics for biomedical implants. *J. Nanosci. Nanotechnol.*, 2002, **2**: 293–312.

[39] Han, Y. et al., Evaluation of nanostructured carbonated hydroxyapatite coatings formed by a hybrid process of plasma spraying and hydrothermal synthesis. *J. Biomed. Mater. Res.*, 2002, **60**: 511–16.

[40] Liao, S.S. et al., Hierarchically biomimetic bone scaffold materials: nano-HA/collagen/PLA composite. *J. Biomed. Mater. Res.*, 2004, **69B**: 158–65.

[41] Song, J., E. Saiz, and C.R. Bertozzi, A new approach to mineralization of biocompatible hydrogel scaffolds: an efficient process toward 3-dimensional bonelike composites. *J. Am. Chem. Soc.*, 2003, **125**: 1236–43.

[42] Tan, J. and W.M. Saltzman, Biomaterials with hierarchically defined micro- and nanoscale structure. *Biomaterials*, 2004, **25**: 3593–601.

[43] Boontheekul, T. and D.J. Mooney, Protein-based signaling systems in tissue engineering. *Curr. Opin. Biotechnol.*, 2003, **14**: 559–65.

[44] Rekow, D., Informatics challenges in tissue engineering and biomaterials. *Adv. Dent. Res.*, 2003, **17**: 49–54.

[45] Gu, H.Y. et al., The immobilization of hepatocytes on 24 nm-sized gold colloid for enhanced hepatocytes proliferation. *Biomaterials*, 2004, **25**: 3445–51.

[46] Thapa, A. et al., Nano-structured polymers enhance bladder smooth muscle cell function. *Biomaterials*, 2003, **24**: 2915–26.

[47] Thapa, A., T.J. Webster, and K.M. Haberstroh, Polymers with nano-dimensional surface features enhance bladder smooth muscle cell adhesion. *J. Biomed. Mater. Res.*, 2003, **67A**: 1374–83.

[48] Zhang, R. and P.X. Ma, Synthetic nano-fibrillar extracellular matrices with predesigned macroporous architectures. *J. Biomed. Mater. Res.*, 2000, **52**: 430–8.

[49] Woo, K.M., V.J. Chen, and P.X. Ma, Nano-fibrous scaffolding architecture selectively enhances protein adsorption contributing to cell attachment. *J. Biomed. Mater. Res.*, 2003, **67A**: 531–7.

[50] Berkland, C., D.W. Pack, and K.K. Kim, Controlling surface nano-structure using flow-limited field-injection electrostatic spraying (FFESS) of poly(d,l-lactide-co-glycolide). *Biomaterials*, 2004, **25**: 5649–58.

[51] Boland, E.D. et al., Electrospinning collagen and elastin: preliminary vascular tissue engineering. *Front Biosci.*, 2004, **9**: 1422–32.

[52] Luu, Y.K. et al., Development of a nanostructured DNA delivery scaffold via electrospinning of PLGA and PLA–PEG block copolymers. *J. Control Release*, 2003, **89**: 341–53.

[53] Mooney, D.J., W.L. Murphy, S. Hsiong, T.P. Richardson, and C.A. Simmons, Effects of a bone-like mineral film on phenotype of adult human mesenchymal stem cells *in vitro*. *Biomaterials*, 2005, **26**: 303–10.

[54] Jansen, J.A., A.J.E. de Ruijter, P.H.M. Spauwen, and J. van den Dolder, Observations on the effect of BMP-2 on rat bone marrow cells cultured on titanium substrates of different roughness. *Biomaterials*, 2003, **24**: 1853–60.

[55] Zhang, S. et al., Design of nanostructured biological materials through self-assembly of peptides and proteins. *Curr. Opin. Chem. Biol.*, 2002, **6**: 865–71.

[56] Zhang, S., Emerging biological materials through molecular self-assembly. *Biotechnol. Adv.*, 2002, 20: 321–29.

[57] Hartgerink, J.D., E. Beniash, and S.I. Stupp, Self-assembly and mineralization of peptide-amphiphile nanofibers. *Science*, 2001, **294**: 1684–8.

[58] Nowak, A.P. et al., Rapidly recovering hydrogel scaffolds from self-assembling diblock copolypeptide amphiphiles. *Nature*, 2002, **417**: 424–8.

[59] Campbell, P., F.W. Shen, and H. McKellop, Biologic and tribologic considerations of alternative bearing surfaces. *Clin. Orthop.*, 2004 (418): 98–111.

[60] Ingham, E. and J. Fisher, Biological reactions to wear debris in total joint replacement. *Proc. Inst. Mech. Eng. [H]*, 2000, **214**: 21–37.

[61] Santerre, J.P., R.S. Labow, and E.L. Boynton, The role of the macrophage in periprosthetic bone loss. *Can. J. Surg.*, 2000, **43**: 173–9.

[62] Archibeck, M.J. et al., The basic science of periprosthetic osteolysis. *Instr. Course Lect.*, 2001, **50**: 185–95.

[63] Tomazic-Jezic, V.J., K. Merritt, and T.H. Umbreit, Significance of the type and the size of biomaterial particles on phagocytosis and tissue distribution. *J. Biomed. Mater. Res.*, 2001, **55**: 523–9.

[64] Bainbridge, J.A., P.A. Revell, and N. Al-Saffar, Costimulatory molecule expression following exposure to orthopaedic implants wear debris. *J. Biomed. Mater. Res.*, 2001, **54**: 328–34.

[65] Urban, R.M. et al., Dissemination of wear particles to the liver, spleen, and abdominal lymph nodes of patients with hip or knee replacement. *J. Bone Joint Surg. Am.*, 2000, **82**: 457–76.

[66] Moghimi, S.M. and A.C. Hunter, Capture of stealth nanoparticles by the body's defences. *Crit. Rev. Ther. Drug Carrier Syst.*, 2001, **18**: 527–50.

[67] Akerman, M.E. et al., Nanocrystal targeting *in vivo*. *Proc. Natl Acad. Sci. USA*, 2002, **99**: 12617–21.

[68] Tao, S.L. and T.A. Desai, Microfabricated drug delivery systems: from particles to pores. *Adv. Drug Delivery Rev.*, 2003, **55**: 315–28.

[69] Leoni, L. and T.A. Desai, Micromachined biocapsules for cell-based sensing and delivery. *Adv. Drug Delivery Rev.*, 2004, **56**: 211–29.

VI

Biomechanics

Donald R. Peterson
University of Connecticut Health Center

BIOMECHANICS IS DEEPLY ROOTED THROUGHOUT scientific history and has been influenced by the research work of early mathematicians, engineers, physicists, biologists, and physicians. Not one of these disciplines can claim sole responsibility for maturing biomechanics to its current state; rather, it has been a conglomeration and integration of these disciplines, involving the application of mathematics, physical principles, and engineering methodologies, that have been responsible for its advancement. Several examinations exist that offer a historical perspective on biomechanics in dedicated chapters within a variety of biomechanics textbooks. For this reason, a historical perspective is not presented within this brief introduction and it is left to the reader to discover the material within one of these textbooks. As an example, Fung (1993) provides a reasonably detailed synopsis of those who were influential to the progress of biomechanical understanding. A review of this material and similar material from other authors commonly shows that biomechanics has occupied the thoughts of some of the most conscientious minds involved in a variety of sciences.

The study of biomechanics, or biological mechanics, employs the principles of mechanics, which is a branch of the physical sciences that investigates the effects of energy and forces on matter or material systems. Biomechanics often embraces a broad range of subject matter that may include aspects of classical mechanics, material science, fluid mechanics, heat transfer, and thermodynamics, in an attempt to model and predict the mechanical behaviors of living systems. As such, it may be called the "liberal arts" of the biomedical engineering sciences.

The contemporary approach to solving problems in biomechanics typically follows a sequence of fundamental steps that are commonly defined as observation, experimentation, theorization, validation, and application. These steps are the basis of the engineering methodologies and their significance is emphasized within a formal education of the engineering sciences, especially biomedical engineering. Each step is considered to be equally important and an iterative relationship between steps, with mathematics serving as the common link, is often necessary in order to converge on a practical understanding of the system in question. An engineering education that ignores these interrelated fundamentals may produce engineers who are ignorant of the ways in which real-world phenomena differs from mathematical models. Since most biomechanical systems are inherently complex and cannot be adequately defined using only theory and mathematics, biomechanics should be considered as a discipline whose progress relies heavily on research and the careful implementation of this approach. When a precise solution is not obtainable, utilizing this approach will assist in identifying critical physical phenomena and obtaining approximate solutions that may provide a deeper understanding as well as improvements to the investigative strategy. Not surprisingly, the need to identify critical phenomena and obtain approximate solutions seems to be more significant in biomedical engineering than any other engineering discipline, which is primarily due to the complex biological processes involved.

Applications of biomechanics have traditionally focused on modeling the system-level aspects of the human body, such as the musculoskeletal system, the respiratory system, and the cardiovascular and cardiopulmonary systems. Technologically, most progress has been made on system-level device development and implementation, with obvious implications on athletic performance, work environment interaction, clinical rehabilitation, orthotics, prosthetics, and orthopaedic surgery. However, more recent biomechanics initiatives are now focusing on the mechanical behaviors of the biological subsystems, such as tissues, cells, and molecules, in order to relate subsystem functions across all levels by showing how mechanical function is closely associated with certain cellular and molecular processes. These initiatives have a direct impact on the development of biological nano- and microtechnologies involving polymer dynamics, biomembranes, and molecular motors. The integration of system and subsystem models will enhance our overall understanding of human function and performance and advance the principles of biomechanics. Even still, our modern understanding about certain biomechanic processes is limited, but through ongoing biomechanics research, new information that influences the way we think about biomechanics is generated and important applications that are essential to the betterment of human existence are discovered. As a result, our limitations are reduced and our understanding becomes more refined. Recent advances in biomechanics can also be attributed to advances in experimental methods and instrumentation, such as computational and imaging capabilities, which are also subject to constant progress. Therefore, the need to revise and add to the current selections presented within this section becomes obvious, ensuring the presentation of modern viewpoints and developments.

The third edition of this section presents a total of 20 chapters, 12 of which have been substantially updated and revised to meet this criterion. It also includes a new chapter introducing the importance of mechanics on a cellular level. These 20 selections present material from respected scientists with diverse backgrounds in biomechanics research and application. The presentation of the chapters within this section has been organized in an attempt to present the material in a systematic manner. The first group of chapters is related to musculoskeletal mechanics and includes hard and soft tissue mechanics, joint mechanics, and applications related to human function. The next group of chapters covers several aspects of biofluid mechanics and includes a wide range of circulatory dynamics, such as blood vessel and blood cell mechanics, and transport. It is followed by the new addition to this section, which introduces current methods and strategies for modeling cellular mechanics. The next group consists of two chapters introducing the mechanical functions and significance of the human ear. Finally, the remaining two chapters introduce performance characteristics of the human body system during exercise and exertion. It is the overall intention of this section to serve as a reference to the skilled professional as well as an introduction to the novice or student of biomechanics. Throughout all the editions of the biomechanics section, an attempt was made to incorporate material that covers a bulk of the biomechanics field; however, as biomechanics continues to grow, some topics may be inadvertently omitted causing a disproportionate presentation of the material. Suggestions and comments from readers are welcome on subject matter that may be considered for future editions.

Reference

Fung, Y.C. (1993). *Biomechanics: Mechanical Properties of Living Tissues*, 2nd ed. New York, Springer-Verlag.

47

Mechanics of
Hard Tissue

J. Lawrence Katz
University of Missouri-Kansas City

Hard tissue, *mineralized tissue*, and *calcified tissue* are often used as synonyms for bone when describing the structure and properties of bone or tooth. The *hard* is self-evident in comparison with all other mammalian tissues, which often are referred to as *soft tissues*. Use of the terms mineralized and calcified arises from the fact that, in addition to the principle protein, collagen, and other proteins, glycoproteins, and protein-polysaccherides, comprising about 50% of the volume, the major constituent of bone is a calcium phosphate (thus the term *calcified*) in the form of a crystalline carbonate **apatite** (similar to naturally occurring minerals, thus the term *mineralized*). Irrespective of its biological function, bone is one of the most interesting materials known in terms of structure–property relationships. Bone is an anisotropic, heterogeneous, inhomogeneous, nonlinear, thermorheologically complex viscoelastic material. It exhibits electromechanical effects, presumed to be due to streaming potentials, both *in vivo* and *in vitro* when wet. In the dry state, bone exhibits piezoelectric properties. Because of the complexity of the structure–property relationships in bone, and the space limitation for this chapter, it is necessary to concentrate on one aspect of the mechanics. Currey [1984] states unequivocally that he thinks, "the most important feature of bone material is its stiffness." This is, of course, the premiere consideration for the weight-bearing long bones. Thus, this chapter will concentrate on the elastic and viscoelastic properties of compact **cortical bone** and the elastic properties of trabecular bone as exemplar of mineralized tissue mechanics.

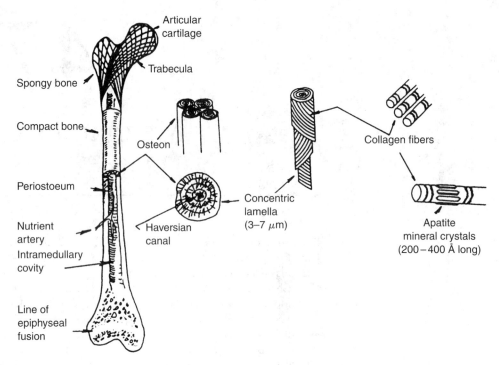

FIGURE 47.1   Hierarchical levels of structure in a human femur [Park, 1979]. (Courtesy of Plenum Press and Dr. J.B. Park.)

47.1 Structure of Bone

The complexity of bone's properties arises from the complexity in its structure. Thus it is important to have an understanding of the structure of mammalian bone in order to appreciate the related properties. Figure 47.1 is a diagram showing the structure of a human femur at different levels [Park, 1979]. For convenience, the structures shown in Figure 47.1 will be grouped into four levels. A further subdivision of structural organization of mammalian bone is shown in Figure 47.2 [Wainwright et al., 1982]. The individual figures within this diagram can be sorted into one of the appropriate levels of structure shown on Figure 47.1 as described in the following. At the smallest unit of structure we have the *tropocollagen* molecule and the associated apatite crystallites (abbreviated Ap). The former is approximately 1.5 by 280 nm, made up of three individual left-handed helical polypeptide (alpha) chains coiled into a right-handed triple helix. Ap crystallites have been found to be carbonate-substituted hydroxyapatite, generally thought to be nonstoichiometric. The crystallites appear to be about $4 \times 20 \times 60$ nm in size. This level is denoted the *molecular*. The next level we denote the *ultrastructural*. Here, the collagen and Ap are intimately associated and assembled into a microfibrilar composite, several of which are then assembled into fibers from approximately 3 to 5 μm thick. At the next level, the *microstructural*, these fibers are either randomly arranged (woven bone) or organized into concentric lamellar groups (**osteons**) or linear lamellar groups (**plexiform bone**). This is the level of structure we usually mean when we talk about bone *tissue* properties. In addition to the differences in lamellar organization at this level, there are also two different types of architectural structure. The dense type of bone found, for example, in the shafts of long bone is known as compact or *cortical bone*. A more porous or spongy type of bone is found, for example, at the articulating ends of long bones. This is called **cancellous bone**. It is important to note that the material and structural organization of collagen–Ap making up osteonic or *haversian* bone and plexiform bone are the same as the material comprising cancellous bone.

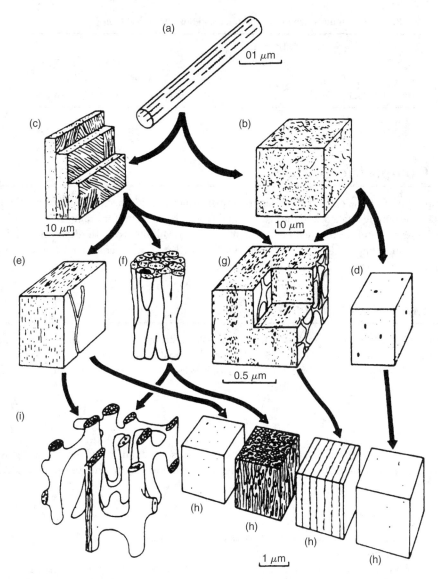

FIGURE 47.2 Diagram showing the structure of mammalian bone at different levels. Bone at the same level is drawn at the same magnification. The arrows show what types may contribute to structures at higher levels [Wainwright et al., 1982]. (Courtesy Princeton University Press.) (a) Collagen fibril with associated mineral crystals. (b) Woven bone. The collagen fibrils are arranged more or less randomly. Osteocytes are not shown. (c) Lamellar bone. There are separate lamellae, and the collagen fibrils are arranged in "domains" of preferred fibrillar orientation in each lamella. Osteocytes are not shown. (d) Woven bone. Blood channels are shown as large black spots. At this level woven bone is indicated by light dotting. (e) Primary lamellar bone. At this level lamellar bone is indicated by fine dashes. (f) **Haversian bone**. A collection of Haversian systems, each with concentric lamellae round a central blood channel. The large black area represents the cavity formed as a cylinder of bone is eroded away. It will be filled in with concentric lamellae and form a new Haversian system. (g) Laminar bone. Two blood channel networks are exposed. Note how layers of woven and lamellar bone alternate. (h) Compact bone of the types shown at the lower levels. (i) Cancellous bone.

Finally, we have the whole bone itself constructed of osteons and portions of older, partially destroyed osteons (called **interstitial lamellae**) in the case of humans or of osteons and/or plexiform bone in the case of mammals. This we denote the *macrostructural level*. The elastic properties of the whole bone results from the hierarchical contribution of each of these levels.

TABLE 47.1   Composition of Adult Human and Bovine Cortical Bone

Species	% H_2O	Ap	% Dry weight collagen	GAG^a	Reference
Bovine	9.1	76.4	21.5	$N.D^b$	Herring, 1977
Human	7.3	67.2	21.2	0.34	Pellagrino and Blitz, 1965; Vejlens, 1971

[a] Glycosaminoglycan.
[b] Not determined.

47.2   Composition of Bone

The composition of bone depends on a large number of factors: the species, which bone, the location from which the sample is taken, and the age, sex, and type of bone tissue, for example, woven, cancellous, cortical. However, a rough estimate for overall composition by volume is one-third Ap, one-third collagen and other organic components, and one-third H_2O. Some data in the literature for the composition of adult human and bovine cortical bone are given in Table 47.1.

47.3   Elastic Properties

Although bone is a viscoelastic material, at the quasi-static strain rates in mechanical testing and even at the ultrasonic frequencies used experimentally, it is a reasonable first approximation to model cortical bone as an anisotropic, linear elastic solid with Hooke's law as the appropriate constitutive equation. Tensor notation for the equation is written as:

$$\sigma_{ij} = C_{ijkl}\varepsilon_{kl} \tag{47.1}$$

where σ_{ij} and ε_{kl} are the second-rank stress and infinitesimal second rank strain tensors, respectively, and C_{ijkl} is the fourth-rank elasticity tenor. Using the reduced notation, we can rewrite Equation 47.1 as

$$\sigma_i = C_{ij}\epsilon_j \quad i,j = 1 \text{ to } 6 \tag{47.2}$$

where C_{ij} are the stiffness coefficients (elastic constants). The inverse of the C_{ij}, the S_{ij}, are known as the *compliance coefficients*.

The anisotropy of cortical bone tissue has been described in two symmetry arrangements. Lang [1969], Katz and Ukraincik [1971], and Yoon and Katz [1976a,b] assumed bone to be transversely isotropic with the bone axis of symmetry (the 3 direction) as the unique axis of symmetry. Any small difference in elastic properties between the radial (1 direction) and transverse (2 direction) axes, due to the apparent gradient in porosity from the periosteal to the endosteal sides of bone, was deemed to be due essentially to the defect and did not alter the basic symmetry. For a transverse isotropic material, the stiffness matrix $[C_{ij}]$ is given by

$$[C_{ij}] = \begin{bmatrix} C_{11} & C_{12} & C_{13} & 0 & 0 & 0 \\ C_{12} & C_{11} & C_{13} & 0 & 0 & 0 \\ C_{13} & C_{13} & C_{33} & 0 & 0 & 0 \\ 0 & 0 & 0 & C_{44} & 0 & 0 \\ 0 & 0 & 0 & 0 & C_{44} & 0 \\ 0 & 0 & 0 & 0 & 0 & C_{66} \end{bmatrix} \tag{47.3}$$

where $C_{66} = \frac{1}{2}(C_{11} - C_{12})$. Of the 12 nonzero coefficients, only 5 are independent.

However, Van Buskirk and Ashman [1981] used the small differences in elastic properties between the radial and tangential directions to postulate that bone is an **orthotropic** material; this requires that 9 of the 12 nonzero elastic constants be independent, that is,

$$[C_{ij}] = \begin{bmatrix} C_{11} & C_{12} & C_{13} & 0 & 0 & 0 \\ C_{12} & C_{22} & C_{23} & 0 & 0 & 0 \\ C_{13} & C_{23} & C_{33} & 0 & 0 & 0 \\ 0 & 0 & 0 & C_{44} & 0 & 0 \\ 0 & 0 & 0 & 0 & C_{55} & 0 \\ 0 & 0 & 0 & 0 & 0 & C_{66} \end{bmatrix} \tag{47.4}$$

Corresponding matrices can be written for the compliance coefficients, the S_{ij}, based on the inverse equation to Equation 47.2:

$$\varepsilon_i = S_{ij}\sigma_j \quad i, j = 1 \text{ to } 6 \tag{47.5}$$

where the S_{ij}th compliance is obtained by dividing the $[C_{ij}]$ stiffness matrix, minus the ith row and jth column, by the full $[C_{ij}]$ matrix and vice versa to obtain the C_{ij} in terms of the S_{ij}. Thus, although $S_{33} = 1/E_3$, where E_3 is Young's modulus in the bone axis direction, $E_3 \neq C_{33}$, since C_{33} and S_{33}, are not reciprocals of one another even for an isotropic material, let alone for **transverse isotropy** or orthotropic symmetry.

The relationship between the compliance matrix and the technical constants such as Young's modulus (E_i) shear modulus (G_i) and Poisson's ratio (ν_{ij}) measured in mechanical tests such as uniaxial or pure shear is expressed in Equation 47.6.

$$[S_{ij}] = \begin{bmatrix} \dfrac{1}{E_1} & \dfrac{-\nu_{21}}{E_2} & \dfrac{-\nu_{31}}{E_3} & 0 & 0 & 0 \\[2ex] \dfrac{-\nu_{12}}{E_1} & \dfrac{1}{E_2} & \dfrac{-\nu_{32}}{E_3} & 0 & 0 & 0 \\[2ex] \dfrac{-\nu_{13}}{E_1} & \dfrac{-\nu_{23}}{E_2} & \dfrac{1}{E_3} & 0 & 0 & 0 \\[2ex] 0 & 0 & 0 & \dfrac{1}{G_{23}} & 0 & 0 \\[2ex] 0 & 0 & 0 & 0 & \dfrac{1}{G_{31}} & 0 \\[2ex] 0 & 0 & 0 & 0 & 0 & \dfrac{1}{G_{12}} \end{bmatrix} \tag{47.6}$$

Again, for an orthotropic material, only 9 of the above 12 nonzero terms are independent, due to the symmetry of the S_{ij} tensor:

$$\frac{\nu_{12}}{E_1} = \frac{\nu_{21}}{E_2} \quad \frac{\nu_{13}}{E_1} = \frac{\nu_{31}}{E_3} \quad \frac{\nu_{23}}{E_2} = \frac{\nu_{32}}{E_3} \tag{47.7}$$

For the transverse isotropic case, Equation 47.5 reduces to only 5 independent coefficients, since

$$E_1 = E_2 \quad \nu_{12} = \nu_{21} \quad \nu_{31} = \nu_{32} = \nu_{13} = \nu_{23}$$

$$G_{23} = G_{31} \quad G_{12} = \frac{E_1}{2(1 + \nu_{12})} \tag{47.8}$$

In addition to the mechanical tests cited above, ultrasonic wave propagation techniques have been used to measure the anisotropic elastic properties of bone [Lang, 1969; Yoon and Katz, 1976a, b; Van Buskirk and Ashman, 1981]. This is possible, since combining Hooke's law with Newton's second law results in a wave equation which yields the following relationship involving the stiffness matrix:

$$\rho V^2 U_m = C_{mrns} N_r N_s U_n \tag{47.9}$$

where ρ is the density of the medium, V is the wave speed, and $\mathbf{U}$ and $\mathbf{N}$ are unit vectors along the particle displacement and wave propagation directions, respectively, so that U_m, N_r, etc. are direction cosines.

Thus to find the five transverse isotropic elastic constants, at least five independent measurements are required, for example, a dilatational longitudinal wave in the 2 and 1(2) directions, a transverse wave in the 13(23) and 12 planes, etc. The technical moduli must then be calculated from the full set of C_{ij}. For improved statistics, redundant measurements should be made. Correspondingly, for orthotropic symmetry, enough independent measurements must be made to obtain all 9 C_{ij}; again, redundancy in measurements is a suggested approach.

One major advantage of the ultrasonic measurements over mechanical testing is that the former can be done with specimens too small for the latter technique. Second, the reproducibility of measurements using the former technique is greater than for the latter. Still a third advantage is that the full set of either five or nine coefficients can be measured on one specimen, a procedure not possible with the latter techniques. Thus, at present, most of the studies of elastic anisotropy in both human and other mammalian bone are done using ultrasonic techniques. In addition to the bulk wave type measurements described above, it is possible to obtain Young's modulus directly. This is accomplished by using samples of small cross sections with transducers of low frequency so that the wavelength of the sound is much larger than the specimen size. In this case, an extensional longitudinal (bar) wave is propagated (which experimentally is analogous to a uniaxial mechanical test experiment), yielding

$$V^2 = \frac{E}{\rho} \tag{47.10}$$

This technique was used successfully to show that bovine plexiform bone was definitely orthotropic while bovine haversian bone could be treated as transversely isotropic [Lipson and Katz, 1984]. The results were subsequently confirmed using bulk wave propagation techniques with considerable redundancy [Maharidge, 1984].

Table 47.2 lists the C_{ij} (in GPa) for human (haversian) bone and bovine (both haversian and plexiform) bone. With the exception of Knet's [1978] measurements, which were made using quasi-static mechanical testing, all the other measurements were made using bulk ultrasonic wave propagation.

In Maharidge's study [1984], both types of tissue specimens, haversian and plexiform, were obtained from different aspects of the same level of an adult bovine femur. Thus the differences in C_{ij} reported between the two types of bone tissue are hypothesized to be due essentially to the differences in

TABLE 47.2   Elastic Stiffness Coefficients for Various Human and Bovine Bones

Experiments (bone type)	C_{11} (GPa)	C_{22} (GPa)	C_{33} (GPa)	C_{44} (GPa)	C_{55} (GPa)	C_{66} (GPa)	C_{12} (GPa)	C_{13} (GPa)	C_{23} (GPa)
Van Buskirk and Ashman [1981] (bovine femur)	14.1	18.4	25.0	7.00	6.30	5.28	6.34	4.84	6.94
Knets [1978] (human tibia)	11.6	14.4	22.5	4.91	3.56	2.41	7.95	6.10	6.92
Van Buskirk and Ashman [1981] (human femur)	20.0	21.7	30.0	6.56	5.85	4.74	10.9	11.5	11.5
Maharidge [1984] (bovine femur haversian)	21.2	21.0	29.0	6.30	6.30	5.40	11.7	12.7	11.1
Maharidge [1984] (bovine femur plexiform)	22.4	25.0	35.0	8.20	7.10	6.10	14.0	15.8	13.6

All measurements made with ultrasound except for Knets [1978] mechanical tests.

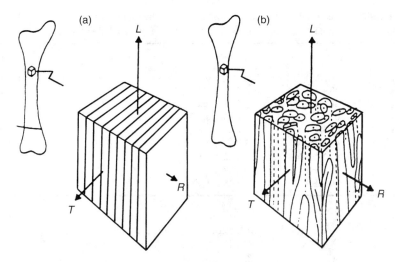

FIGURE 47.3 Diagram showing how laminar (plexiform) bone (a) differs more between radial and tangential directions (R and T) than does haversian bone (b). The arrows are vectors representing the various directions [Wainwright et al., 1982] (Courtesy Princeton University Press).

microstructural organization (Figure 47.3) [Wainwright et al., 1982]. The textural symmetry at this level of structure has dimensions comparable to those of the ultrasound wavelengths used in the experiment, and the molecular and ultrastructural levels of organization in both types of tissues are essentially identical. Note that while C_{11}, almost equals C_{22} and that C_{44} and C_{55} are equal for bovine haversian bone, C_{11} and C_{22} and C_{44} and C_{55} differ by 11.6 and 13.4%, respectively, for bovine plexiform bone. Similarly, although C_{66} and $\frac{1}{2}(C_{11} - C_{12})$ differ by 12.0% for the haversian bone, they differ by 31.1% for plexiform bone. Only the differences between C_{13} and C_{23} are somewhat comparable: 12.6% for haversian bone and 13.9% for plexiform. These results reinforce the importance of modeling bone as a hierarchical ensemble in order to understand the basis for bone's elastic properties as a composite material-structure system in which the collagen–Ap components define the material composite property. When this material property is entered into calculations based on the microtextural arrangement, the overall anisotropic elastic anisotropy can be modeled.

The human femur data [Van Buskirk and Ashman, 1981] support this description of bone tissue. Although they measured all nine individual C_{ij}, treating the femur as an orthotropic material, their results are consistent with a near transverse isotropic symmetry. However, their nine C_{ij} for bovine femoral bone clearly shows the influence of the orthotropic microtextural symmetry of the tissue's plexiform structure.

The data of Knets [1978] on human tibia are difficult to analyze. This could be due to the possibility of significant systematic errors due to mechanical testing on a large number of small specimens from a multitude of different positions in the tibia.

The variations in bone's elastic properties cited earlier above due to location is appropriately illustrated in Table 47.3, where the mean values and standard deviations (all in GPa) for all g orthotropic C_{ij} are given for bovine cortical bone at each aspect over the entire length of bone.

Since the C_{ij} are simply related to the "technical" elastic moduli, such as Young's modulus (E), shear modulus (G), bulk modulus (K), and others, it is possible to describe the moduli along any given direction. The full equations for the most general anisotropy are too long to present here. However, they can be found in Yoon and Katz [1976a]. Presented below are the simplified equations for the case of transverse isotropy. Young's modulus is

$$\frac{1}{E(\gamma_3)} = S'_{33} = (1 - \gamma_3^2)2S_{11} + \gamma_3^4 S_{33} + \gamma_3^2(1 - \gamma_3^2)(2S_{13} + S_{44}) \tag{47.11}$$

where $\gamma_3 = \cos\phi$, and ϕ is the angle made with respect to the bone (3) axis.

TABLE 47.3 Mean Values and Standard Deviations for the C_{ij} Measured by Van Buskirk and Ashman [1981] at Each Aspect Over the Entire Length of Bone (all Values in GPa)

	Anterior	Medial	Posterior	Lateral
C_{11}	18.7 ± 1.7	20.9 ± 0.8	20.1 ± 1.0	20.6 ± 1.6
C_{22}	20.4 ± 1.2	22.3 ± 1.0	22.2 ± 1.3	22.0 ± 1.0
C_{33}	28.6 ± 1.9	30.1 ± 2.3	30.8 ± 1.0	30.5 ± 1.1
C_{44}	6.73 ± 0.68	6.45 ± 0.35	6.78 ± 1.0	6.27 ± 0.28
C_{55}	5.55 ± 0.41	6.04 ± 0.51	5.93 ± 0.28	5.68 ± 0.29
C_{66}	4.34 ± 0.33	4.87 ± 0.35	5.10 ± 0.45	4.63 ± 0.36
C_{12}	11.2 ± 2.0	11.2 ± 1.1	10.4 ± 1.0	10.8 ± 1.7
C_{13}	11.2 ± 1.1	11.2 ± 2.4	11.6 ± 1.7	11.7 ± 1.8
C_{23}	10.4 ± 1.4	11.5 ± 1.0	12.5 ± 1.7	11.8 ± 1.1

The shear modulus (rigidity modulus or torsional modulus for a circular cylinder) is

$$\frac{1}{G(\gamma_3)} = \frac{1}{2}(S'_{44} + S'_{55}) = S_{44} + (S_{11} - S_{12}) - \frac{1}{2}S_{44}(1 - \gamma_3^2)$$
$$+ 2(S_{11} + S_{33} - 2S_{13} - S_{44})\gamma_3^2(1 - \gamma_3^2) \tag{47.12}$$

where, again $\gamma_3 = \cos\phi$.

The bulk modulus (reciprocal of the volume compressibility) is

$$\frac{1}{K} = S_{33} + 2(S_{11} + S_{12} + 2S_{13}) = \frac{C_{11} + C_{12} + 2C_{33} - 4C_{13}}{C_{33}(C_{11} + C_{12}) - 2C_{13}^2} \tag{47.13}$$

Conversion of Equation 47.11 and Equation 47.12 from S_{ij} to C_{ij} can be done by using the following transformation equations:

$$S_{11} = \frac{C_{22}C_{33} - C_{23}^2}{\Delta} \quad S_{22} = \frac{C_{33}C_{11} - C_{13}^2}{\Delta}$$

$$S_{33} = \frac{C_{11}C_{22} - C_{12}^2}{\Delta} \quad S_{12} = \frac{C_{13}C_{23} - C_{12}C_{33}}{\Delta} \tag{47.14}$$

$$S_{13} = \frac{C_{12}C_{23} - C_{13}C_{22}}{\Delta} \quad S_{23} = \frac{C_{12}C_{13} - C_{23}C_{11}}{\Delta}$$

$$S_{44} = \frac{1}{C_{44}} \quad S_{55} = \frac{1}{C_{55}} \quad S_{66} = \frac{1}{C_{66}}$$

where

$$\Delta = \begin{vmatrix} C_{11} & C_{12} & C_{13} \\ C_{12} & C_{22} & C_{23} \\ C_{13} & C_{23} & C_{33} \end{vmatrix} = C_{11}C_{22}C_{33} + 2C_{12}C_{23}C_{13} - (C_{11}C_{23}^2 + C_{22}C_{13}^2 + C_{33}C_{12}^2) \tag{47.15}$$

In addition to data on the elastic properties of cortical bone presented above, there is also available a considerable set of data on the mechanical properties of cancellous (trabecullar) bone including measurements of the elastic properties of single trabeculae. Indeed as early as 1993, Keaveny and Hayes [1993] presented an analysis of 20 years of studies on the mechanical properties of trabecular bone. Most of the earlier studies used mechanical testing of bulk specimens of a size reflecting a cellular solid, that is, of the order of cubic mm or larger. These studies showed that both the modulus and strength of trabecular bone are strongly correlated to the apparent density, where apparent density, ρ_a, is defined as the product of individual trabeculae density, ρ_t, and the volume fraction of bone in the bulk specimen, V_f, and is given by $\rho_a = \rho_t V_f$.

TABLE 47.4 Elastic Moduli of Trabecular Bone Material Measured by Different Experimental Methods

Study	Method	Average modulus	(GPa)
Townsend et al. [1975]	Buckling	11.4	(Wet)
	Buckling	14.1	(Dry)
Ryan and Williams [1989]	Uniaxial tension	0.760	
Choi et al. [1992]	4-point bending	5.72	
Ashman and Rho [1988]	Ultrasound	13.0	(Human)
	Ultrasound	10.9	(Bovine)
Rho et al. [1993]	Ultrasound	14.8	
	Tensile test	10.4	
Rho et al. [1999]	Nanoindentation	19.4	(Longitudinal)
	Nanoindentation	15.0	(Transverse)
Turner et al. [1999]	Acoustic microscopy	17.5	
	Nanoindentation	18.1	
Bumrerraj and Katz [2001]	Acoustic microscopy	17.4	

Elastic moduli, E, from these measurements generally ranged from approximately 10 MPa to the order of 1 GPa depending on the apparent density and could be correlated to the apparent density in g/cc by a power law relationship, $E = 6.13 P_a^{144}$, calculated for 165 specimens with an $r^2 = 0.62$ [Keaveny and Hayes, 1993].

With the introduction of micromechanical modeling of bone, it became apparent that in addition to knowing the bulk properties of trabecular bone it was necessary to determine the elastic properties of the individual trabeculae. Several different experimental techniques have been used for these studies. Individual trabeculae have been machined and measured in buckling, yielding a modulus of 11.4 GPa (wet) and 14.1 GPa (dry) [Townsend et al., 1975], as well as by other mechanical testing methods providing average values of the elastic modulus ranging from less than 1 GPa to about 8 GPa (Table 47.4). Ultrasound measurements [Ashman and Rho, 1988; Rho et al., 1993] have yielded values commensurate with the measurements of Townsend et al. [1975] (Table 47.4). More recently, acoustic microscopy and nanoindentation have been used, yielding values significantly higher than those cited above. Rho et al. [1999] using nanoindentation obtained average values of modulus ranging from 15.0 to 19.4 GPa depending on orientation, as compared to 22.4 GPa for osteons and 25.7 GPa for the interstitial lamellae in cortical bone (Table 47.4). Turner et al. [1999] compared nanoindentation and acoustic microscopy at 50 MHz on the same specimens of trabecular and cortical bone from a common human donor. While the nanoindentation resulted in Young's moduli greater than those measured by acoustic microscopy by 4 to 14%, the anisotropy ratio of longitudinal modulus to transverse modulus for cortical bone was similar for both modes of measurement; the trabecular values are given in Table 47.4. Acoustic microscopy at 400 MHz has also been used to measure the moduli of both human trabecular and cortical bone [Bumrerraj and Katz, 2001], yielding results comparable to those of Turner et al. [1999] for both types of bone (Table 47.4).

These recent studies provide a framework for micromechanical analyses using material properties measured on the microstructural level. They also point to using nano-scale measurements, such as those provided by atomic force microscopy (AFM), to analyze the mechanics of bone on the smallest unit of structure shown in Figure 47.1.

47.4 Characterizing Elastic Anisotropy

Having a full set of five or nine C_{ij} does permit describing the anisotropy of that particular specimen of bone, but there is no simple way of comparing the relative anisotropy between different specimens of the same bone or between different species or between experimenters' measurements by trying to relate individual C_{ij} between sets of measurements. Adapting a method from crystal physics

[Chung and Buessem, 1968] Katz and Meunier [1987] presented a description for obtaining two scalar quantities defining the compressive and shear anisotropy for bone with transverse isotropic symmetry. Later, they developed a similar pair of scalar quantities for bone exhibiting orthotropic symmetry [Katz and Meunier, 1990]. For both cases, the percentage compressive (Ac^*) and shear (As^*) elastic anisotropy are given, respectively, by

$$Ac^*(\%) = 100\frac{K^V - K_R}{K^V + K_R}$$
$$As^*(\%) = 100\frac{G_V - G_R}{G_V + G_R} \tag{47.16}$$

where K^V and K_R are the Voigt (uniform strain across an interface) and Reuss (uniform stress across an interface) bulk moduli, respectively, and G^V and G_R are the Voigt and Reuss shear moduli, respectively. The equations for K^V, K_R, G^V, and G_R are provided for both transverse isotropy and orthotropic symmetry in Appendix.

Table 47.5 lists the values of $As^*(\%)$ and $Ac^*(\%)$ for various types of hard tissues and apatites. The graph of $As^*(\%)$ vs. $Ac^*(\%)$ is given in Figure 47.4.

$As^*(\%)$ and $Ac^*(\%)$ have been calculated for a human femur, having both transverse isotropic and orthotropic symmetry, from the full set of Van Buskirk and Ashman [1981] C_{ij} data at each of the four aspects around the periphery, anterior, medial, posterior, and lateral, as denoted in Table 47.3, at fractional proximal levels along the femur's length, $Z/L = 0.3$ to 0.7. The graph of $As^*(\%)$ vs. Z/L, assuming transverse isotropy, is given in Figure 47.5. Note that the Anterior aspect, that is in tension during loading, has values of $As^*(\%)$ in some positions considerably higher than those of the other aspects. Similarly, the graph of $Ac^*(\%)$ vs. Z/L is given in Figure 47.6. Note here it is the posterior aspect that is in compression during loading, which has values of $Ac^*(\%)$ in some positions considerably higher than those of the other aspects. Both graphs are based on the transverse isotropic symmetry calculations; however, the identical trends were obtained based on the orthotropic symmetry calculations. It is clear that in addition to the moduli varying along the length and over all four aspects of the femur, the anisotropy varies as well, reflecting the response of the femur to the manner of loading.

Recently, Kinney et al. [2004] used the technique of resonant ultrasound spectroscopy (RUS) to measure the elastic constants (C_{ij}) of human dentin from both wet and dry samples. $As^*(\%)$ and $Ac^*(\%)$ calculated from these data are included in both Table 47.5 and Figure 47.4. Their data showed that the samples exhibited transverse isotropic symmetry. However, the C_{ij} for dry dentin implied even higher symmetry. Indeed, the result of using the average value for C_{11} and $C_{12} = 36.6$ GPa and the value for $C_{44} = 14.7$ GPa for dry dentin in the calculations suggests that dry human dentin is very nearly elastically isotropic. This isotropic-like behavior of the dry dentin may have clinical significance. There is independent experimental evidence to support this calculation of isotropy based on the ultrasonic data. Small angle x-ray diffraction

TABLE 47.5 $Ac*(\%)$ vs. $As*\%$ for Various Types of Hard Tissues and Apatites

Experiments (specimen type)	$Ac^*(\%)$	$As^*(\%)$
Van Buskirk et al. [1981] (bovine femur)	1.522	2.075
Katz and Ukraincik [1971] (OHAp)	0.995	0.686
Yoon (redone) in Katz [1984] (FAp)	0.867	0.630
Lang [1969,1970] (bovine femur dried)	1.391	0.981
Reilly and Burstein [1975] (bovine femur)	2.627	5.554
Yoon and Katz [1976] (human femur dried)	1.036	1.055
Katz et al. [1983] (haversian)	1.080	0.775
Van Buskirk and Ashman [1981] (human femur)	1.504	1.884
Kinney et al. [2004] (human dentin dry)	0.006	0.011
Kinney et al. [2004] (human dentin wet)	1.305	0.377

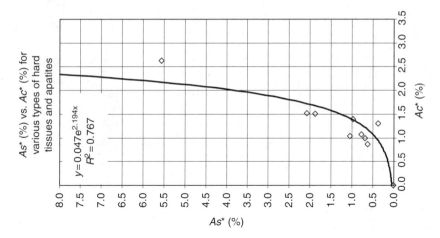

FIGURE 47.4 Values of $As^*(\%)$ vs. $Ac^*(\%)$ from Table 47.5 are plotted for various types of hard tissues and apatites.

of human dentin yielded results implying isotropy near the pulp and mild anisotropy in mid-dentin [Kinney et al., 2001].

It is interesting to note that haversian bones, whether human or bovine, have both their compressive and shear anisotropy factors considerably lower than the respective values for plexiform bone. Thus, not only is plexiform bone both stiffer and more rigid than haversian bone, it is also more anisotropic. These two scalar anisotropy quantities also provide a means of assessing whether there is the possibility either of systematic errors in the measurements or artifacts in the modeling of the elastic properties of hard tissues. This is determined when the values of $Ac^*(\%)$ and/or $As^*(\%)$ are much greater than the close range of lower values obtained by calculations on a variety of different ultrasonic measurements (Table 47.5). A possible example of this is the value of $As^*(\%) = 7.88$ calculated from the mechanical testing data of Knets [1978], Table 47.2.

47.5 Modeling Elastic Behavior

Currey [1964] first presented some preliminary ideas of modeling bone as a composite material composed of a simple linear superposition of collagen and Ap. He followed this later [1969] with an attempt to take into account the orientation of the Ap crystallites using a model proposed by Cox [1952] for fiber-reinforced composites. Katz [1971a] and Piekarski [1973] independently showed that the use of Voigt and Reuss or even Hashin–Shtrikman [1963] composite modeling showed the limitations of using linear combinations of either elastic moduli or elastic compliances. The failure of all these early models could be traced to the fact that they were based only on considerations of material properties. This is comparable to trying to determine the properties of an Eiffel Tower built using a composite material by simply modeling the composite material properties without considering void spaces and the interconnectivity of the structure [Lakes, 1993]. In neither case is the complexity of the structural organization involved. This consideration of hierarchical organization clearly must be introduced into the modeling.

Katz in a number of papers [1971b, 1976] and meeting presentations put forth the hypothesis that haversian bone should be modeled as a hierarchical composite, eventually adapting a hollow fiber composite model by Hashin and Rosen [1964]. Bonfield and Grynpas [1977] used extensional (longitudinal) ultrasonic wave propagation in both wet and dry bovine femoral cortical bone specimens oriented at angles of 5, 10, 20, 40, 50, 70, 80, and 85° with respect to the long bone axis. They compared their experimental results for Young's moduli with the theoretical curve predicted by Currey's model [1969]; this is shown in Figure 47.7. The lack of agreement led them to "conclude, therefore that an alternative model is required to account for the dependence of Young's modulus on orientation" [Bonfield and Grynpas, 1977].

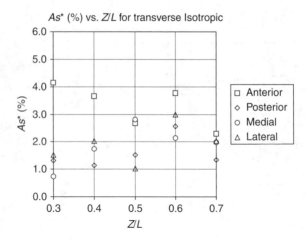

FIGURE 47.5 Values $As^*(\%)$ calculated from the data in Table 18.3 for human femoral bone, treated as having transverse isotropic symmetry, is plotted vs. Z/L for all four aspects, anterior, medial, posterior, lateral around the bone's periphery; Z/L is the fractional proximal distance along the femur's length.

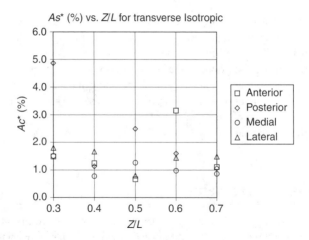

FIGURE 47.6 Values $Ac^*(\%)$ calculated from the data in Table 18.3 for human femoral bone, treated as having transverse isotropic symmetry, is plotted vs. Z/L for all four aspects, anterior, medial, posterior, lateral around the bone's periphery; Z/L is the fractional proximal distance along the femur's length.

Katz [1980, 1981], applying his hierarchical material-structure composite model, showed that the data in Figure 47.7 could be explained by considering different amounts of Ap crystallites aligned parallel to the long bone axis; this is shown in Figure 47.8. This early attempt at hierarchical micromechanical modeling is now being extended with more sophisticated modeling using either finite-element micromechanical computations [Hogan, 1992] or homogenization theory [Crolet et al., 1993]. Further improvements will come by including more definitive information on the structural organization of collagen and Ap at the molecular-ultrastructural level [Wagner and Weiner, 1992; Weiner and Traub, 1989].

47.6 Viscoelastic Properties

As stated earlier, bone (along with all other biologic tissues) is a viscoelastic material. Clearly, for such materials, Hooke's law for linear elastic materials must be replaced by a constitutive equation which

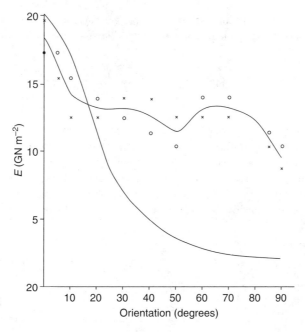

FIGURE 47.7 Variation in Young's modulus of bovine femur specimens (E) with the orientation of specimen axis to the long axis of the bone, for wet (o) and dry (x) conditions compared with the theoretical curve (———) predicted from a fiber-reinforced composite model [Bonfield and Grynpas, 1977] (Courtesy *Nature* 1977, 270: 453. ©Macmillan Magazines Ltd.).

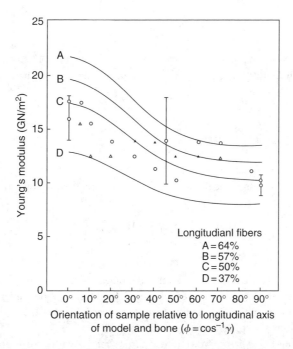

FIGURE 47.8 Comparison of predictions of Katz two-level composite model with the experimental data of Bonfield and Grynpas. Each curve represents a different lamellar configuration within a single osteon, with longitudinal fibers; A, 64%; B, 57%; C, 50%; D, 37%; and the rest of the fibers assumed horizontal. (From Katz J.L., *Mechanical Properties of Bone, AMD*, vol. 45, New York, American Society of Mechanical Engineers, 1981. With permission.)

includes the time dependency of the material properties. The behavior of an anisotropic linear viscoelastic material may be described by using the *Boltzmann superposition integral* as a constitutive equation:

$$\sigma_{ij}(t) = \int_{-\infty}^{t} C_{ijkl}(t - \tau) \frac{d\epsilon_{kl}(\tau)}{d\tau} d\tau \tag{47.17}$$

where $\sigma_{ij}(t)$ and $\epsilon_{kl}(\tau)$ are the time-dependent second rank stress and strain tensors, respectively, and $C_{ijkl}(t - \tau)$ is the fourth-rank relaxation modulus tensor. This tensor has 36 independent elements for the lowest symmetry case and 12 nonzero independent elements for an orthotropic solid. Again, as for linear elasticity, a reduced notation is used, that is, $11 \to 1, 22 \to 2, 33 \to 3, 23 \to 4, 31 \to 5,$ and $12 \to 6$. If we apply Equation 47.17 to the case of an orthotropic material, for example, plexiform bone, in uniaxial tension (compression) in the one direction [Lakes and Katz, 1974], in this case using the reduced notation, we obtain

$$\sigma_1(t) = \int_{-\infty}^{t} \left[C_{11}(t - \tau) \frac{d\epsilon_1(\tau)}{d\tau} + C_{12}(t - \tau) \frac{d\epsilon_2(\tau)}{d\tau} + C_{13}(t - \tau) \frac{d\epsilon_3(\tau)}{d\tau} \right] d\tau \tag{47.18}$$

$$\sigma_2(t) = \int_{-\infty}^{t} \left[C_{21}(t - \tau) \frac{d\epsilon_1(\tau)}{d\tau} + C_{22}(t - \tau) \frac{d\epsilon_2(\tau)}{d\tau} + C_{23}(t - \tau) \frac{d\epsilon_3(\tau)}{d\tau} \right] = 0 \tag{47.19}$$

for all t, and

$$\sigma_3(t) = \int_{-\infty}^{t} \left[C_{31}(t - \tau) \frac{d\epsilon_1(\tau)}{d\tau} + C_{32}(t - \tau) \frac{d\epsilon_2(\tau)}{d\tau} + C_{33}(t - \tau) \frac{d\epsilon_3(\tau)}{d\tau} \right] d\tau = 0 \tag{47.20}$$

for all t.

Having the integrands vanish provides an obvious solution to Equation 47.19 and Equation 47.20. Solving them simultaneously for $[d\epsilon_2^{(\tau)}]/d\tau$ and $[d\epsilon_3^{(\tau)}]/d\tau$ and and substituting these values in Equation 47.17 yields

$$\sigma_1(t) = \int_{-\infty}^{t} E_1(t - \tau) \frac{d\epsilon_1(\tau)}{d\tau} d\tau \tag{47.21}$$

where, if for convenience we adopt the notation $C_{ij} \equiv C_{ij}(t - \tau)$, then Young's modulus is given by

$$E_1(t - \tau) = C_{11} + C_{12} \frac{[C_{31} - (C_{21}C_{33}/C_{23})]}{[(C_{21}C_{33}/C_{23}) - C_{32}]} + C_{13} \frac{[C_{21} - (C_{31}C_{22}/C_{32})]}{[(C_{22}C_{33}/C_{32})/ - C_{23}]} \tag{47.22}$$

In this case of uniaxial tension (compression), only nine independent orthotropic tensor components are involved, the three shear components being equal to zero. Still, this time-dependent Young's modulus is a rather complex function. As in the linear elastic case, the inverse form of the Boltzmann integral can be used; this would constitute the compliance formulation.

If we consider the bone being driven by a strain at a frequency ω, with a corresponding sinusoidal stress lagging by an angle δ, then the complex Young's modulus $E^*(\omega)$ may be expressed as

$$E^*(\omega) = E'(\omega) + iE''(\omega) \tag{47.23}$$

where $E'(\omega)$, which represents the stress–strain ratio in phase with the strain, is known as the storage modulus, and $E''(\omega)$, which represents the stress–strain ratio 90 degrees out of phase with the strain, is known as the loss modulus. The ratio of the loss modulus to the storage modulus is then equal to tan δ. Usually, data are presented by a graph of the storage modulus along with a graph of tan δ, both against frequency. For a more complete development of the values of $E'(\omega)$ and $E''(\omega)$, as well as for the derivation of other viscoelastic technical moduli, see Lakes and Katz [1974]; for a similar development of the shear storage and loss moduli, see Cowin [1989].

Thus, for a more complete understanding of bone's response to applied loads, it is important to know its rheologic properties. There have been a number of early studies of the viscoelastic properties of various long bones [Sedlin, 1965; Smith and Keiper, 1965; Lugassy, 1968; Black and Korostoff, 1973; Laird and Kingsbury, 1973]. However, none of these was performed over a wide enough range of frequency (or time) to completely define the viscoelastic properties measured, for example, creep or stress relaxation. Thus it is not possible to mathematically transform one property into any other to compare results of three different experiments on different bones [Lakes and Katz, 1974].

In the first experiments over an extended frequency range, the biaxial viscoelastic as well as uniaxial viscoelastic properties of wet cortical human and bovine femoral bone were measured using both dynamic and stress relaxation techniques over eight decades of frequency (time) [Lakes et al., 1979]. The results of these experiments showed that bone was both nonlinear and thermorheologically complex, that is, time–temperature superposition could not be used to extend the range of viscoelastic measurements. A nonlinear constitutive equation was developed based on these measurements [Lakes and Katz, 1979a].

In addition, relaxation spectrums for both human and bovine cortical bone were obtained; Figure 47.9 shows the former [Lakes and Katz, 1979b]. The contributions of several mechanisms to the loss tangent of cortical bone is shown in Figure 47.10 [Lakes and Katz, 1979b]. It is interesting to note that almost all the major loss mechanisms occur at frequencies (times) at or close to those in which there are "bumps," indicating possible strain energy dissipation, on the relaxation spectra shown on Figure 47.9. An extensive review of the viscoelastic properties of bone can be found in the CRC publication *Natural and Living Biomaterials* [Lakes and Katz, 1984].

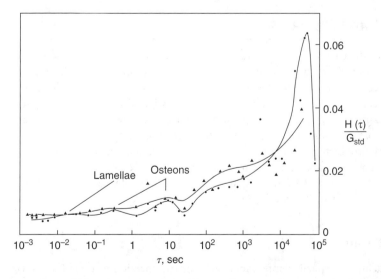

FIGURE 47.9 Comparison of relaxation spectra for wet human bone, specimens 5 and 6 [Lakes et al., 1979] in simple torsion; $T = 37°C$. First approximation from relaxation and dynamic data. • Human tibial bone, specimen 6. ▲ Human tibial bone, specimen 5, $G_{std} = G$ (10 sec). $G_{std}(5) = G$ (10 sec). $G_{std}(5) = 0.590 \times 10^6$ lb/in^2. $G_{std}(6) \times 0.602 \times 10^6$ lb/in^2. (Courtesy *Journal of Biomechanics*, Pergamon Press.)

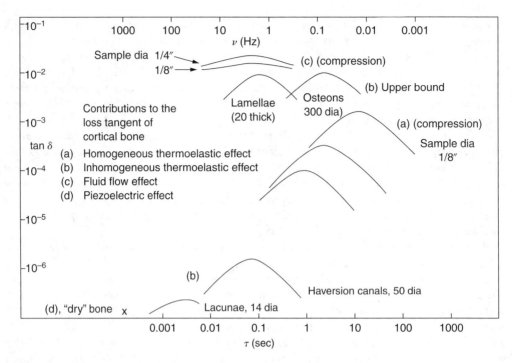

FIGURE 47.10   Contributions of several relaxation mechanisms to the loss tangent of cortical bone. (a) Homogeneous thermoelastic effect. (b) Inhomogeneous thermoelastic effect. (c) Fluid flow effect. (d) Piezoelectric effect [Lakes and Katz, 1984]. (Courtesy CRC Press)

Following on Katz's [1976, 1980] adaptation of the Hashin–Rosen hollow fiber composite model [1964], Gottesman and Hashin [1979] presented a viscoelastic calculation using the same major assumptions.

47.7   Related Research

As stated earlier, this chapter has concentrated on the elastic and viscoelastic properties of compact cortical bone and the elastic properties of trabecular bone. At present there is considerable research activity on the fracture properties of the bone. Professor William Bonfield and his associates at Queen Mary and Westfield College, University of London and Professor Dwight Davy and his colleagues at Case Western Reserve University are among those who publish regularly in this area. Review of the literature is necessary in order to become acquainted with the state of bone fracture mechanics.

An excellent introductory monograph which provides a fascinating insight into the structure–property relationships in bones including aspects of the two areas discussed immediately above is Professor John D. Currey's Bones Structure and Mechanics [2002], the 2nd edition of the book, *The Mechanical Adaptations of Bones*. Princeton University Press [1984].

Defining Terms

Apatite: Calcium phosphate compound, stoichiometric chemical formula $Ca_5(PO_4)_3 \cdot X$, where X is OH^- (hydroxyapatite), F^- (fluorapatite), Cl^- (chlorapatite), etc. There are two molecules in the basic crystal unit cell.

Cancellous bone: Also known as porous, spongy, trabecular bone. Found in the regions of the articulating ends of tubular bones, in vertebrae, ribs, etc.

Cortical bone: The dense compact bone found throughout the shafts of long bones such as the femur, tibia, etc. also found in the outer portions of other bones in the body.

Haversian bone: Also called osteonic. The form of bone found in adult humans and mature mammals, consisting mainly of concentric lamellar structures, surrounding a central canal called the haversian canal, plus lamellar remnants of older haversian systems (osteons) called interstitial lamellae.

Interstitial lamellae: See *Haversian bone* above.

Orthotropic: The symmetrical arrangement of structure in which there are three distinct orthogonal axes of symmetry. In crystals this symmetry is called orthothombic.

Osteons: See *Haversian bone* above.

Plexiform: Also called laminar. The form of parallel lamellar bone found in younger, immature nonhuman mammals.

Transverse isotropy: The symmetry arrangement of structure in which there is a unique axis perpendicular to a plane in which the other two axes are equivalent. The long bone direction is chosen as the unique axis. In crystals this symmetry is called hexagonal.

References

Ashman R.B. and Rho J.Y. 1988. Elastic modulus of trabecular bone material. *J. Biomech.* 21: 177.

Black J. and Korostoff E. 1973. Dynamic mechanical properties of viable human cortical bone. *J. Biomech.* 6: 435.

Bonfield W. and Grynpas M.D. 1977. Anisotropy of Young's modulus of bone. *Nature, London,* 270: 453.

Bumrerraj S. and Katz J.L. 2001. Scanning acoustic microscopy study of human cortical and trabecular bone. *Ann. Biomed. Eng.* 29: 1.

Choi K. and Goldstein S.A. 1992. A comparison of the fatigue behavior of human trabecular and cortical bone tissue. *J. Biomech.* 25: 1371.

Chung D.H. and Buessem W.R. 1968. In F.W. Vahldiek and S.A. Mersol (Eds.), *Anisotropy in Single-Crystal Refractory Compounds*, Vol. 2, p. 217. New York, Plenum Press.

Cowin S.C. 1989. *Bone Mechanics.* Boca Raton, FL, CRC Press.

Cowin S.C. 2001. *Bone Mechanics Handbook.* Boca Raton, FL, CRC Press.

Cox H.L. 1952. The elasticity and strength of paper and other fibrous materials. *Br. Appl. Phys.* 3: 72.

Crolet, J.M., Aoubiza B., and Meunier A. 1993. Compact bone: numerical simulation of mechanical characteristics. *J. Biomech.* 26: 677.

Currey J.D. 1964. Three analogies to explain the mechanical properties of bone. *Biorheology.* 1.

Currey J.D. 1969. The relationship between the stiffness and the mineral content of bone. *J. Biomech.*: 477.

Currey J.D. 1984. *The Mechanical Adaptations of Bones.* New Jersey, Princeton University Press.

Currey J.D. 2002. *Bone Structure and Mechanics.* New Jersey, Princeton University Press.

Gottesman T. and Hashin Z. 1979. Analysis of viscoelastic behavior of bones on the basis of microstructure. *J. Biomech.* 13: 89.

Hashin Z. and Rosen B.W. 1964. The elastic moduli of fiber reinforced materials. *J. Appl. Mech.*: 223.

Hashin Z. and Shtrikman S. 1963. A variational approach to the theory of elastic behavior of multiphase materials. *J. Mech. Phys. Solids*: 127.

Hastings G.W. and Ducheyne P. (Eds.). 1984. *Natural and Living Biomaterials.* Boca Raton, FL, CRC Press.

Herring G.M. 1977. Methods for the study of the glycoproteins and proteoglycans of bone using bacterial collagenase. Determination of bone sialoprotein and chondroitin sulphate. *Calcif. Tiss. Res.*: 29.

Hogan H.A. 1992. Micromechanics modeling of haversian cortical bone properties. *J. Biomech.* 25: 549.

Katz J.L. 1971a. Hard tissue as a composite material: I. Bounds on the elastic behavior. *J. Biomech.* 4:455.

Katz J.L. 1971b. Elastic properties of calcified tissues. *Isr. J. Med. Sci.* 7: 439.

Katz J.L. 1976. Hierarchical modeling of compact haversian bone as a fiber reinforced material. In R.E. Mates, and C.R. Smith (Eds), *Advances in Bioengineering*, pp. 17–18. New York, American Society of Mechanical Engineers.

Katz J.L. 1980. Anisotropy of Young's modulus of bone. *Nature* 283: 106.

Katz J.L. 1981. Composite material models for cortical bone. In S.C. Cowin (Ed.), *Mechanical Properties of Bone*, Vol. 45, pp. 171–184. New York, American Society of Mechanical Engineers.

Katz J.L. and Meunier A. 1987. The elastic anisotropy of bone. *J. Biomech.* 20: 1063.

Katz J.L. and Meunier A. 1990. A generalized method for characterizing elastic anisotropy in solid living tissues. *J. Mat. Sci. Mater. Med.* 1: 1.

Katz J.L. and Ukraincik K. 1971. On the anisotropic elastic properties of hydroxyapatite. *J. Biomech.* 4: 221.

Katz J.L. and Ukraincik K. 1972. A fiber-reinforced model for compact haversian bone. *Program and Abstracts of the 16th Annual Meeting of the Biophysical Society*, 28a FPM-C15, Toronto.

Keaveny T.M. and Hayes W.C. 1993. A 20-year perspective on the mechanical properties of trabecular bone. *J. Biomech. Eng.* 115: 535.

Kinney J.H., Pople J.A., Marshall G.W., and Marshall S.J. 2001. Collagen orientation and crystallite size in human dentin: A small angle x-ray scattering study. *Calcif. Tissue Inter.* 69: 31.

Kinney J.H., Gladden J.R., Marshall G.W., Marshall S.J., So J.H., and Maynard J.D. 2004. Resonant ultrasound spectroscopy measurements of the elastic constants of human dentin. *J. Biomech.* 37: 437.

Knets I.V. 1978. *Mekhanika Polimerov* 13: 434.

Laird G.W. and Kingsbury H.B. 1973. Complex viscoelastic moduli of bovine bone. *J. Biomech.* 6: 59.

Lakes R.S. 1993. Materials with structural hierarchy. *Nature* 361: 511.

Lakes R.S. and Katz J.L. 1974. Interrelationships among the viscoelastic function for anisotropic solids: Application to calcified tissues and related systems. *J. Biomech.* 7: 259.

Lakes R.S. and Katz J.L. 1979a. Viscoelastic properties and behavior of cortical bone. Part II. Relaxation mechanisms. *J. Biomech.* 12: 679.

Lakes R.S. and Katz J.L. 1979b. Viscoelastic properties of wet cortical bone: III. A nonlinear constitutive equation. *J. Biomech.* 12: 689.

Lakes R.S. and Katz J.L. 1984. Viscoelastic properties of bone. In G.W. Hastings and P. Ducheyne (Eds.), *Natural and Living Tissues*, pp. 1–87. Boca Raton, FL, CRC Press.

Lakes R.S., Katz J.L., and Sternstein S.S. 1979. Viscoelastic properties of wet cortical bone: I. Torsional and biaxial studies. *J. Biomech.* 12: 657.

Lang S.B. 1969. Elastic coefficients of animal bone. *Science* 165: 287.

Lipson S.F. and Katz, J.L. 1984. The relationship between elastic properties and microstructure of bovine cortical bone. *J. Biomech.* 4: 231.

Lugassy, A.A. 1968. Mechanical and Viscoelastic Properties of Bone and Dentin in Compression, thesis, Metallurgy and Materials Science, University of Pennsylvania.

Maharidge R. 1984. Ultrasonic properties and microstructure of bovine bone and Haversian bovine bone modeling, thesis, Rensselaer Polytechnic Institute, Troy, NY.

Park, J.B. 1979. *Biomaterials: An Introduction.* New York, Plenum.

Pellegrino, E.D. and Biltz, R.M. 1965. The composition of human bone in uremia. *Medicine* 44: 397.

Piekarski K. 1973. Analysis of bone as a composite material. *Int. J. Eng. Sci.* 10: 557.

Reuss A. 1929. Berechnung der fliessgrenze von mischkristallen auf grund der plastizitatsbedingung fur einkristalle, A. *Zeitschrift fur Angewandte Mathematik und Mechanik* 9: 49–58.

Rho J.Y., Ashman R.B., and Turner C.H. 1993. Young's modulus of trabecular and cortical bone material; ultrasonic and microtensile measurements. *J. Biomech.* 26: 111.

Rho J.Y., Roy M.E., Tsui T.Y., and Pharr G.M. 1999. Elastic properties of microstructural components of human bone tissue as measured by indentation. *J. Biomed. Mat. Res.* 45: 48.

Ryan S.D. and Williams J.L. 1989. Tensile testing of rodlike trabeculae excised from bovine femoral bone. *J. Biomech.* 22: 351.

Sedlin E. 1965. A rheological model for cortical bone. *Acta Orthop. Scand.* 36.

Smith R. and Keiper D. 1965. Dynamic measurement of viscoelastic properties of bone. *Am. J. Med. Elec.* 4: 156.

Townsend P.R., Rose R.M., and Radin E.L. 1975. Buckling studies of single human trabeculae. *J. Biomech.* 8: 199.

Turner C.H., Rho, J.Y., Takano Y, Tsui T.Y., and Pharr, G.M. 1999. The elastic properties of trabecular and cortical bone tissues are simular: results from two microscopic measurement techniques. *J. Biomech.* 32: 437.

Van Buskirk W.C. and Ashman R.B. 1981. The elastic moduli of bone. In S.C. Cowin (Ed.), *Mechanical Properties of Bone AMD*, Vol. 45, pp. 131–143. New York, American Society of Mechanical Engineers.

Vejlens L. 1971. Glycosaminoglycans of human bone tissue: I. Pattern of compact bone in relation to age. *Calcif. Tiss. Res.* 7: 175.

Voigt W. 1966. *Lehrbuch der Kristallphysik Teubner, Leipzig* 1910; reprinted (1928) with an additional appendix. Leipzig, Teubner, New York, Johnson Reprint.

Wagner, H.D. and Weiner S. 1992. On the relationship between the microstructure of bone and its mechanical stiffness. *J. Biomech.* 25: 1311.

Wainwright, S.A., Briggs, W.D., Currey, J.D., and Gosline, J.M. 1982. *Mechanical Design in Organisms.* Princeton NJ, Princeton University Press.

Weiner S. and Traub W. 1989. Crystal size and organization in bone. *Conn. Tissue Res.* 21: 259.

Yoon, H.S. and Katz, J.L. 1976a. Ultrasonic wave propagation in human cortical bone: I. Theoretical considerations of hexagonal symmetry. *J. Biomech.* 9: 407.

Yoon, H.S. and Katz, J.L. 1976b. Ultrasonic wave propagation in human cortical bone: II. Measurements of elastic properties and microhardness. *J. Biomech.* 9: 459.

Further Information

Several societies both in the United States and abroad hold annual meetings during which many presentations, both oral and poster, deal with hard tissue biomechanics. In the United States these societies include the Orthopaedic Research Society, the American Society of Mechanical Engineers, the Biomaterials Society, the American Society of Biomechanics, the Biomedical Engineering Society, and the Society for Bone and Mineral Research. In Europe there are alternate year meetings of the European Society of Biomechanics and the European Society of Biomaterials. Every four years there is a *World Congress of Biomechanics*; every three years there is a *World Congress of Biomaterials*. All of these meetings result in documented proceedings; some with extended papers in book form.

The two principal journals in which bone mechanics papers appear frequently are the *Journal of Biomechanics* published by Elsevier and the *Journal of Biomechanical Engineering* published by the American Society of Mechanical Engineers. Other society journals which periodically publish papers in the field are the *Journal of Orthopaedic Research* published for the Orthopaedic Research Society, the *Annals of Biomedical Engineering* published for the Biomedical Engineering Society, and the *Journal of Bone and Joint Surgery* (both American and English issues) for the American Academy of Orthopaedic Surgeons and the British Organization, respectively. Additional papers in the field may be found in the journal *Bone and Calcified Tissue International*.

The 1984 CRC volume, *Natural and Living Biomaterials* (Hastings G.W. and Ducheyne P., Eds.) provides a good historical introduction to the field. A recent more advanced book is *Bone Mechanics Handbook* (Cowin S.C., Ed. 2001), the 2nd ed. of *Bone Mechanics* (Cowin S.C., Ed. 1989).

Many of the biomaterials journals and society meetings will have occasional papers dealing with hard tissue mechanics, especially those dealing with implant–bone interactions.

Appendix

The Voigt and Reuss moduli for both transverse isotropic and orthotropic symmetry are given below:

Voigt transverse isotropic

$$K^V = \frac{2(C_{11} + C_{12}) + 4(C_{13} + C_{33})}{9}$$

$$G^V = \frac{(C_{11} + C_{12}) - 4C_{13} + 2C_{33} + 12(C_{44} + C_{66})}{30}$$

(47.A1)

Reuss transverse isotropic

$$K_R = \frac{C_{33}(C_{11} + C_{12}) - 2C_{13}^2}{(C_{11} + C_{12} - 4C_{13} + 2C_{33})}$$

$$G_R = \frac{5[C_{33}(C_{11} + C_{12}) - 2C_{13}^2]C_{44}C_{66}}{2\{[C_{33}(C_{11} + C_{12}) - 2C_{13}^2](C_{44} + C_{66}) + [C_{44}C_{66}(2C_{11} + C_{12}) + 4C_{13} + C_{33}]/3\}}$$

(47.A2)

Voigt orthotropic

$$K^V = \frac{C_{11} + C_{22} + C_{33} + 2(C_{12} + C_{13} + C_{23})}{9}$$

$$G^V = \frac{[C_{11} + C_{22} + C_{33} + 3(C_{44} + C_{55} + C_{66}) - (C_{12} + C_{13} + C_{23})]}{15}$$

(47.A3)

Reuss orthotropic

$$K_R = \frac{\Delta}{C_{11}C_{22} + C_{22}C_{33} + C_{33}C_{11}} - 2(C_{11}C_{23} + C_{22}C_{13} + C_{33}C_{12})$$

$$+ 2(C_{12}C_{23} + C_{23}C_{13} + C_{13}C_{12}) - (C_{12}^2 + C_{13}^2 + C_{23}^2)$$

$$G_R = 15/(4\{(C_{11}C_{22} + C_{22}C_{33} + C_{33}C_{11} + C_{11}C_{23} + C_{22}C_{13} + C_{33}C_{22})$$

$$- [C_{12}(C_{12} + C_{23}) + C_{23}(C_{23} + C_{13}) + C_{13}(C_{13} + C_{12})]\}/\Delta$$

$$+ 3(1/C_{44} + 1/C_{55} + 1/C_{66}))$$

(47.A4)

where Δ is given in Equation 47.15.

48

Musculoskeletal Soft Tissue Mechanics

Richard L. Lieber
University of California

Thomas J. Burkholder
Georgia Institute of Technology

Biological soft tissues are nonlinear, anisotropic, fibrous composites, and detailed description of their behavior is the subject of active research. One can separate these tissues based on their mode of loading: cartilage is generally loaded in compression; tendons and ligaments are loaded in tension; and muscles generate active tension. The structure and material properties differ to accommodate the tissue function, and this chapter outlines those features. Practical models of each tissue are described, with particular focus on active force generation by skeletal muscle and application to segmental modeling.

48.1 Structure of Soft Tissues

48.1.1 Cartilage

Articular cartilage is found at the ends of bones, where it serves as a shock absorber and lubricant between bones. It is best described as a hydrated proteoglycan gel supported by a sparse population of chondrocytes, and its composition and properties vary dramatically over its 1- to 2-mm thickness. The bulk composition of articular cartilage consists of approximately 20% collagen, 5% proteoglycan, primarily aggrecan bound to hyaluronic acid, with most of the remaining 75% water [Ker, 1999]. At the articular surface, collagen fibrils are most dense and arranged primarily in parallel with the surface. Proteoglycan content is very low and chondrocytes are rare in this region. At the bony interface, collagen fibrils are oriented perpendicular to the articular surface, chondrocytes are more abundant, but proteoglycan content is low. Proteoglycans are most abundant in the middle zone, where collagen fibrils lack obvious orientation in association with the transition from parallel to perpendicular alignment.

Collagen itself is a fibrous protein composed of tropocollagen molecules. Tropocollagen is a triple-helical protein, which self-assembles into the long collagen fibrils observable at the ultrastructural level. These fibrils, in turn, aggregate and intertwine to form the ground substance of articular cartilage. When cross-linked into a dense network, as in the superficial zone of articular cartilage, collagen has a low permeability to water and helps to maintain the water cushion of the middle and deep zones. Collagen fibrils arranged in a random network, as in the middle zone, structurally immobilize the large proteoglycan (PG) aggregates, creating the solid phase of the composite material.

Proteoglycans consist of a number of negatively charged glycosaminoglycan chains bound to an aggrecan protein core. Aggrecan molecules, in turn, bind to a hyaluronic acid backbone, forming a PG of 50 to 100 MDa, which carries a dense negative charge. This negative charge attracts positively charged ions (Na^+) from the extracellular fluid, and the resulting Donnan equilibrium results in rich hydration of the tissue creating an osmotic pressure that enables the tissue to act as a shock absorber.

The overall structure of articular cartilage is analogous to a jelly-filled balloon. The PG-rich middle zone is osmotically pressurized, with fluid restrained from exiting the tissue by the dense collagen network of the superficial zone and the calcified structure of the deep bone. The interaction between the mechanical loading forces and osmotic forces yields the complex material properties of articular cartilage.

48.1.2 Tendon and Ligament

The passive tensile tissues, tendon and ligament, are also composed largely of water and collagen, but contain very little of the PGs that give cartilage its unique mechanical properties. In keeping with the functional role of these tissues, the collagen fibrils are organized primarily in long strands parallel to the axis of loading (Figure 48.1) [Kastelic, et al., 1978]. The collagen fibrils, which may be hollow tubes [Gutsmann et al., 2003], combine in a hierarchical structure, with the 20–40-nm fibrils being bundled into 0.2–12-μm fibers. These fibers are birefringent under polarized light, reflecting an underlying wave or crimp structure with a periodicity between 20 and 100 μm. The fibers are bundled into fascicles, supported by fibroblasts or tenocytes, and surrounded by a fascicular membrane. Finally, multiple fascicles are bundled into a complete tendon or ligament encased in a reticular membrane.

As the tendon is loaded, the bending angle of the crimp structure of the collagen fibers can be seen to reversibly decrease, indicating that deformation of this structure is one source of elasticity. Individual

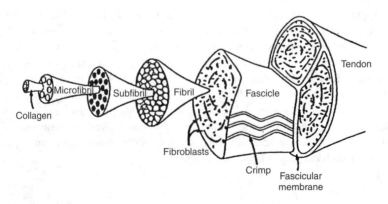

FIGURE 48.1 Tendons are organized in progressively larger filaments, beginning with molecular tropocollagen, and building to a complete tendon encased in a reticular sheath.

collagen fibrils also display some inherent elasticity, and these two features are believed to determine the bulk properties of passive tensile tissues.

48.1.3 Muscle

48.1.3.1 Gross Morphology

Muscles are described as running from a proximal origin to a distal insertion. While these attachments are frequently discrete, distributed attachments, and distinctly bifurcated attachments, are also common. Description of the subdomains of a muscle is largely by analogy to the whole body. The mass of muscle fibers can be referred to as the belly. In a muscle with distinctly divided origins, the separate origins are often referred to as heads, and in a muscle with distinctly divided insertions, each mass of fibers terminating on distinct tendons is often referred to as a separate belly.

A muscle generally receives its blood supply from one main artery, which enters the muscle in a single, or sometimes two branches. Likewise, the major innervation is generally by a single nerve, which carries both motor efferents and sensory afferents.

Some muscles are functionally and structurally subdivided into compartments. A separate branch of the principle nerve generally innervates each compartment, and motor units of the compartments do not overlap. Generally, a dense connective tissue, or fascial, plane separates the compartments.

48.1.3.2 Fiber Architecture

Architecture, the arrangement of fibers within a muscle, determines the relationship between whole muscle length changes and force generation. The stereotypical muscle architecture is fusiform, with the muscle originating from a small tendonous attachment, inserting into a discrete tendon, and having fibers running generally parallel to the muscle axis (Figure 48.2). Fibers of unipennate muscles run parallel to each other but at an angle (pennation angle) to the muscle axis. Bipennate muscle fibers run in two distinct directions. Multipennate or fan-like muscles have one distinct attachment and one broad attachment, and pennation angle is different for every fiber. Strap-like muscles have parallel fibers that run from a broad bony origin to a broad insertion. As the length of each of these muscles is changed, the change in length of its fibers depends on fiber architecture. For example, fibers of a strap-like muscle undergo essentially the same length change as the muscle, where the length change of highly pennate fibers is reduced by their angle.

48.1.3.3 Sarcomere

Force generation in skeletal muscle results from the interaction between myosin and actin proteins. These molecules are arranged in antiparallel filaments, a 2- to 3-nm diameter thin filament composed mainly of actin, and a 20-nm diameter thick filament composed mainly of myosin. Myosin filaments are arranged in a hexagonal array, rigidly fixed at the M-line, and are the principal constituents of the A-band (anisotropic, light bending). Actin filaments are arranged in a complimentary hexagonal array and rigidly fixed at the Z-line, comprising the l-band (isotropic, light transmitting). The sarcomere is a nearly crystalline structure, composed of an A-band and two adjacent l-bands, and is the fundamental unit of muscle force generation. Sarcomeres are arranged into arrays of myofibrils, and one muscle cell or myofiber contains many myofibrils. Myofibers themselves are multinucleated syncitia, hundreds of microns in diameter, and may be tens of millimeters in length that are derived during development by the fusion of myoblasts.

The myosin protein occurs in several different isoforms, each with different force-generating characteristics, and each associated with expression of characteristic metabolic and calcium-handling proteins. Broadly, fibers can be characterized as either fast or slow, with slow fibers having a lower rate of actomyosin ATPase activity, slower velocity of shortening, slower calcium dynamics, and greater activity of oxidative metabolic enzymes. The lower ATPase activity makes these fibers more efficient for generating force, while the high oxidative capacity provides a rich energy source, making slow fibers ideal for extended periods of activity. Their relatively slow speed of shortening results in poor performance during fast or ballistic motions.

48.2 Material Properties

48.2.1 Cartilage

The behavior of cartilage is highly viscoelastic. A compressive load applied to articular cartilage drives the positively charged fluid phase through the densely intermeshed and negatively charged solid phase while deforming the elastic PG-collagen structure. The mobility of the fluid phase is relatively low, and, for rapid changes in load, cartilage responds nearly as a uniform linear elastic solid with a Young's modulus of approximately 6 MPa [Carter and Wong, 2003].

At lower loading rates, cartilage displays more nonlinear properties. Ker [1999] reports that human limb articular cartilage stiffness can be described as $E = E_0(1 + \sigma^{0.366})$, with $E_0 = 3.0$ MPa and σ expressed in MPa.

48.2.2 Tendon and Ligament

At rest, the collagen fibrils are significantly crimped or wavy so that initial loading acts primarily to straighten these fibrils. At higher strains, the straightened collagen fibrils must be lengthened. Thus, tendons are more compliant at low loads and less compliant at high loads. The highly nonlinear low load region has been referred to as the "toe" region and occurs up to approximately 3% strain and 5 MPa [Butler et al., 1979; Zajac, 1989]. Typically, tendons have nearly linear properties from about 3% strain until ultimate strain, which ranges from 9 to 10% (Table 48.1). The tangent modulus in this linear

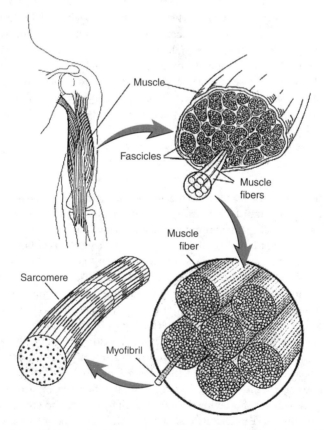

FIGURE 48.2 Skeletal muscle is organized in progressively larger filaments, beginning with molecular actin and myosin, arranged as myofibrils. Myofibrils assemble into sarcomeres and myofilaments. Myofilaments are assembled into myofibers, which are organized into the fascicles that form a whole muscle.

TABLE 48.1   Tendon Biomechanical Properties

Tendon	Ultimate stress (MPa)	Ultimate strain (%)	Stress under normal loads (MPa)	Strain under normal loads (%)	Tangent modulus (GPa)	References
Wallaby	40	9	15–40		1.56	Bennett et al. [1986]
Porpoise					1.53	Bennett et al. [1986]
Dolphin					1.43	Bennett et al. [1986]
Deer			28–74		1.59	Bennett et al. [1986]
Sheep					1.65	Bennett et al. [1986]
Donkey			22–44		1.25	Bennett et al. [1986]
Human leg			53		1.0–1.2	Bennett et al. [1986]
Cat leg					1.21	Bennett et al. [1986]
Pig tail					0.9	Bennett et al. [1986]
Rat tail					0.8–1.5	Bennett et al. [1986]
Horse				4–10		Ker et al. [1988]
Dog leg			84			Ker et al. [1988]
Camel ankle			18			Ker et al. [1988]
Human limb (various)	60–120					McElhaney et al. [1976]
Human calcaneal	55	9.5				McElhaney et al. [1976]
Human wrist	52–74	11–17	3.2–3.3	1.5–3.5		Loren and Lieber [1994]

region is approximately 1.5 GPa. Ultimate tensile stress reported for tendons is approximately 100 MPa [McElhaney et al., 1976]. However, under physiological conditions, tendons operate at stresses of only 5 to 10 MPa (Table 48.1) yielding a typical safety factor of 10.

48.2.3 Muscle

Tension generated by skeletal muscle depends on length, velocity, level of activation, and history. Performance characteristics of a muscle depend on both its intrinsic properties and the extrinsic organization of that tissue. Whole muscle maximum shortening velocity depends both upon the sliding velocity of its component sarcomeres and on the number of those sarcomeres arranged in series. Likewise, maximum isometric tension depends on both the intrinsic tension-generating capacity of the actomyosin crossbridges and on the number of sarcomeres arranged in parallel. The relationship between intrinsic properties and extrinsic function is further complicated by pennation of the fibers. Given the orthotropic nature of the muscle fiber, material properties should be considered relative to the fiber axis. That is, the relevant area for stress determination is not the geometric cross section, but the physiological cross section, perpendicular to the fiber axis. The common form for estimation of the physiological cross sectional area (PCSA) is:

$$\text{PCSA} = \frac{M \cdot \cos(\Theta)}{\rho \cdot \text{FL}}$$

where M is muscle mass, Θ is pennation angle, ρ is muscle density (1.06 g/cm^3), and FL is fiber length. Likewise, the relevant gage length for strain determination is not muscle length, but fiber length, or fascicle length in muscles composed of serial fibers.

Maximum muscle stress: Maximum active stress, or specific tension, varies somewhat among fiber types and species (Table 48.2) around a generally accepted average of 250 kPa. This specific tension can be determined in any system in which it is possible to measure force and estimate the area of contractile material. Given muscle PCSA, maximum force produced by a muscle can be predicted by multiplying this PCSA by specific tension (Table 48.2). Specific tension can also be calculated for isolated muscle fibers or motor units in which estimates of cross-sectional area have been made.

Maximum muscle contraction velocity: Muscle maximum contraction velocity is primarily dependent on the type and number of sarcomeres in series along the muscle fiber length [Gans, 1982]. The intrinsic

TABLE 48.2 Skeletal Muscle Specific Tension

Species	Muscle type	Preparation	Specific tension (kPa)	References
Various		Synthesis	300	Josephson [1989]
Rat	SO	Single fiber	134	Fitts et al. [1991]
Human	Slow	Single fiber	133	Fitts et al. [1991]
Rat	FOG	Single fiber	108	Fitts et al. [1991]
Rat	FG	Single fiber	108	Fitts et al. [1991]
Human	Fast	Single fiber	166	Fitts et al. [1991]
Cat	1	Motor unit	59	Dum et al. [1982]
Cat	S	Motor unit	172	Bodine et al. [1987]
Cat	2A	Motor unit	284	Dum et al. [1982]
Cat	FR	Motor unit	211	Bodine et al. [1987]
Cat	2B+2AB	Motor unit	343	Dum et al. [1982]
Cat	FF/FI	Motor unit	249	Bodine et al. [1987]
Human	Elbow	Whole muscle	230–420	Edgerton et al. [1990]
Human	Ankle	Whole muscle	45–250	Fukunaga et al. [1996]
Rat	TA	Whole muscle	272	Wells [1965]
Rat	Soleus	Whole muscle	319	Wells [1965]
Guinea pig	Hindlimb	Whole muscle	225	Powell et al. [1984]
Guinea pig	Soleus	Whole muscle	154	Powell et al. [1984]

TABLE 48.3 Muscle Dynamic Properties

Species	Muscle type	Preparation	V_{max}^{a}	a/Po	b/V_{max}	References
Rat	SO	single fiber	1.49 μ/sec			Fitts et al. [1991]
Human	slow	single fiber	0.86 μ/sec			Fitts et al. [1991]
Rat	FOG	single fiber	4.91 μ/sec			Fitts et al. [1991]
Rat	FG	single fiber	8.05 μ/sec			Fitts et al. [1991]
Human	Fast	single fiber	4.85 μ/sec			Fitts et al. [1991]
Mouse	Soleus	Whole muscle	31.7 μ/sec			Close [1972]
Rat	Soleus	Whole muscle	18.2 μ/sec			Close [1972]
Rat	Soleus	Whole muscle	5.4 cm/sec	0.214	0.23	Wells [1965]
Cat	Soleus	Whole muscle	13 μ/sec			Close [1972]
Mouse	EDL	Whole muscle	60.5 μ/sec			Close [1972]
Rat	EDL	Whole muscle	42.7 μ/sec			Close [1972]
Cat	EDL	Whole muscle	31 μ/sec			Close [1972]
Rat	TA	Whole muscle	14.4 cm/sec	0.356	0.38	Wells [1965]

[a] L/sec fiber or sarcomere lengths per second, μm/sec sarcomere velocity; cm/sec whole muscle velocity.

velocity of shortening has been experimentally determined for a number of muscle types (Table 48.3). Maximum contraction velocity of a given muscle can thus be calculated based on a knowledge of the number of serial sarcomeres within the muscle multiplied by the maximum contraction velocity of an individual sarcomere (Table 48.4 to Table 48.6). Sarcomere shortening velocity varies widely among species and fiber types (Table 48.3).

48.3 Modeling

48.3.1 Cartilage

Although cartilage can be modeled as a simple elastic element, more accurate results are obtained using a biphasic model [Mow et al., 1980], which describes the motion of the hydrating fluid relative to the charged organic matrix. The total stress acting on the cartilage is separated into independent solid and

TABLE 48.4   Architectural Properties of the Human Arm and Forearm[a,b]

Muscle	Muscle mass (g)	Muscle length (mm)	Fiber length (mm)	Pennation angle (o)	Cross-sectional area (cm^2)	FL/ML ratio
BR ($n = 8$)	16.6 ± 2.8	175 ± 8.3	121 ± 8.3	2.4 ± 6	1.33 ± 22	0.69 ± 0.062
PT ($n = 8$)	15.9 ± 1.7	130 ± 4.7	36.4 ± 1.3	9.6 ± 8	4.13 ± 52	0.28 ± 0.012
PQ ($n = 8$)	5.21 ± 1.0	39.3 ± 2.3	23.3 ± 2.0	9.9 ± 3	2.07 ± 33	0.58 ± 0.021
EDC I ($n = 8$)	3.05 ± 0.45	114 ± 3.4	56.9 ± 3.6	3.1 ± 5	0.52 ± 0.08	0.49 ± 0.024
EDC M ($n = 5$)	6.13 ± 1.2	112 ± 4.7	58.8 ± 3.5	3.2 ± 1.0	1.02 ± 0.20	0.50 ± 0.014
EDC R ($n = 7$)	4.70 ± 0.75	125 ± 10.7	51.2 ± 1.8	3.2 ± 54	0.86 ± 0.13	0.42 ± 0.023
EDC S ($n = 6$)	2.23 ± 0.32	121 ± 8.0	52.9 ± 5.2	2.4 ± 7	0.40 ± 0.06	0.43 ± 0.029
EDQ ($n = 7$)	3.81 ± 70	152 ± 9.2	55.3 ± 3.7	2.6 ± 6	0.64 ± 0.10	0.36 ± 0.012
EIP ($n = 6$)	2.86 ± 61	105 ± 6.6	48.4 ± 2.3	6.3 ± 8	0.56 ± 0.11	0.46 ± 0.023
EPL ($n = 7$)	4.54 ± 68	138 ± 7.2	43.6 ± 2.6	5.6 ± 1.3	0.98 ± 0.13	0.31 ± 0.020
PL ($n = 6$)	3.78 ± 82	134 ± 11.5	52.3 ± 3.1	3.5 ± 1.2	0.69 ± 0.17	0.40 ± 0.032
FDS I(P) ($n = 6$)	6.01 ± 1.1	92.5 ± 8.4	31.6 ± 3.0	5.1 ± 0.2	1.81 ± 0.83	0.34 ± 0.022
FDS I(D) ($n = 9$)	6.6 ± 0.8	119 ± 6.1	37.9 ± 3.0	6.7 ± 0.3	1.63 ± 0.22	0.32 ± 0.013
FDS I(C) ($n = 6$)	12.4 ± 2.1	207 ± 10.7	67.6 ± 2.8	5.7 ± 0.2	1.71 ± 0.28	0.33 ± 0.025
FDS M ($n = 9$)	16.3 ± 2.2	183 ± 11.5	60.8 ± 3.9	6.9 ± 0.7	2.53 ± 0.34	0.34 ± 0.014
FDS R ($n = 9$)	10.2 ± 1.1	155 ± 7.7	60.1 ± 2.7	4.3 ± 0.6	1.61 ± 0.18	0.39 ± 0.023
FDS S ($n = 9$)	1.8 ± 0.3	103 ± 6.3	42.4 ± 2.2	4.9 ± 0.7	0.40 ± 0.05	0.42 ± 0.014
FDP I ($n = 9$)	11.7 ± 1.2	149 ± 3.8	61.4 ± 2.4	7.2 ± 0.7	1.77 ± 0.16	0.41 ± 0.018
FDP M ($n = 9$)	16.3 ± 1.7	200 ± 8.2	68.4 ± 2.7	5.7 ± 0.3	2.23 ± 0.22	0.34 ± 0.011
FDP R ($n = 9$)	11.9 ± 1.4	194 ± 7.0	64.6 ± 2.6	6.8 ± 0.5	1.72 ± 0.18	0.33 ± 0.009
FDP S ($n = 9$)	13.7 ± 1.5	150 ± 4.7	60.7 ± 3.9	7.8 ± 0.9	2.20 ± 0.30	0.40 ± 0.015
FPL ($n = 9$)	10.0 ± 1.1	168 ± 10.0	45.1 ± 2.1	6.9 ± 0.2	2.08 ± 0.22	0.24 ± 0.10

[a] Data from Lieber et al., 1990, 1992.
[b] BR: brachioradialis; EDC 1, EDC M, EDC R, and EDC S: extensor digitorum communis to the index, middle, ring, and small fingers, respectively; EDQ: extensor digiti quinti; EIP: extensor indicis proprious; EPL: extensor pollicis longus; FDP I, FDP M, FDP R, and FDP S: flexor digitorum profundus muscles; FDS I, FDS M, FDS R, and FDS S: flexor digitorum superficialis muscles; FDS I (P) and FDS I (D): proximal and distal bellies of the FDS I; FDS I (C): the combined properties of the two bellies as if they were a single muscle; FPL: flexor pollicis longus; PQ: pronator quadratus; PS: palmaris longus; PT: pronator teres.

fluid phases:

$$\sigma^T = \sigma^s + \sigma^f$$

where s denotes the solid phase and f the fluid phase. The relative motion of the phases defines the equilibrium equations

$$\nabla \cdot \sigma^s = \frac{(v^s - v^f)}{k(1+\alpha)^2} = -\nabla \cdot \sigma^f$$

where α is tissue solid content and k the tissue permeability coefficient. In addition to the equilibrium equations, each phase is subject to separate constitutive relations:

$$\sigma^f = -p_a I \quad \text{and} \quad \sigma^s = -\alpha p_a I + De$$

where p_a is the apparent tissue stress, D is the material property tensor and e is the strain tensor. For a hyperelastic solid phase

$$De = \lambda \text{Tr}(e)I + 2\mu e$$

where λ and μ are the Lamé constants.

TABLE 48.5 Architectural Properties of Human Lower Limb[a,b]

Muscle	Muscle mass (g)	Muscle length (mm)	Fiber length (mm)	Pennation angle (o)	Cross-sectional area (cm^2)	FL/ML ratio
RF ($n = 3$)	84.3 ± 14	316 ± 5.7	66.0 ± 1.5	5.0 ± 0.0	12.7 ± 1.9	0.209 ± 0.002
VL ($n = 3$)	220 ± 56	324 ± 14	65.7 ± 0.88	5.0 ± 0.0	30.6 ± 6.5	0.203 ± 0.007
VM ($n = 3$)	175 ± 41	335 ± 15	70.3 ± 3.3	5.0 ± 0.0	21.1 ± 4.3	0.210 ± 0.005
VI ($n = 3$)	160 ± 59	329 ± 15	68.3 ± 4.8	3.3 ± 1.7	22.3 ± 8.7	0.208 ± 0.007
SM ($n = 3$)	108 ± 13	262 ± 1.5	62.7 ± 4.7	15 ± 2.9	16.9 ± 1.5	0.239 ± 0.017
BFl ($n = 3$)	128 ± 28	342 ± 14	85.3 ± 5.0	0.0 ± 0.0	12.8 ± 2.8	0.251 ± 0.022
BFs ($n = 3$)	—	271 ± 11	139 ± 3.5	23 ± 0.9	—	0.517 ± 0.032
ST ($n = 2$)	76.9 ± 7.7	317 ± 4	158 ± 2.0	5.0 ± 0.0	5.4 ± 1.0	0.498 ± 0.0
SOL ($n = 2$)	215 ($n = 1$)	310 ± 1.5	19.5 ± 0.5	25 ± 5.0	58.0 ($n = 1$)	0.063 ± 0.002
MG ($n = 3$)	150 ± 14	248 ± 9.9	35.3 ± 2.0	16.7 ± 4.4	32.4 ± 3.1	0.143 ± 0.010
LG ($n = 3$)	—	217 ± 11	50.7 ± 5.6	8.3 ± 1.7	—	0.233 ± 0.016
PLT ($n = 3$)	5.30 ± 14	85.0 ± 15	39.3 ± 6.7	3.3 ± 1.7	1.2 ± 0.4	0.467 ± 0.031
FHL ($n = 3$)	21.5 ± 3.3	222 ± 5.0	34.0 ± 1.5	10.0 ± 2.9	5.3 ± 0.6	0.154 ± 0.010
FDL ($n = 3$)	16.3 ± 2.8	260 ± 15	27.0 ± 0.58	6.7 ± 1.7	5.1 ± 0.7	0.104 ± 0.004
PL ($n = 3$)	41.5 ± 8.5	286 ± 17	38.7 ± 3.2	10.0 ± 0.0	12.3 ± 2.9	0.136 ± 0.010
PB ($n = 3$)	17.3 ± 2.5	230 ± 13	39.3 ± 3.5	5.0 ± 0.0	5.7 ± 1.0	0170 ± 0.006
TP ($n = 3$)	53.5 ± 7.3	254 ± 26	24.0 ± 4.0	11.7 ± 1.7	20.8 ± 3	0.095 ± 0.015
TA ($n = 3$)	65.7 ± 10	298 ± 12	77.3 ± 7.8	5.0 ± 0.0	9.9 ± 1.5	0.258 ± 0.015
EDL ($n = 3$)	35.2 ± 3.6	355 ± 13	80.3 ± 8.4	8.3 ± 1.7	5.6 ± 0.6	0.226 ± 0.024
EHL ($n = 3$)	12.9 ± 1.6	273 ± 2.4	87.0 ± 8.0	6.0 ± 1.0	1.8 ± 0.2	0.319 ± 0.030
SAR ($n = 3$)	61.7 ± 14	503 ± 27	455 ± 19	0.0 ± 0.0	1.7 ± 0.3	0.906 ± 0.017
GR ($n = 3$)	35.3 ± 7.4	335 ± 20	277 ± 12	3.3 ± 1.7	1.8 ± 0.3	0.828 ± 0.017
AM ($n = 3$)	229 ± 32	305 ± 12	115 ± 7.9	0.0 ± 0.0	18.2 ± 2.3	0.378 ± 0.013
AL ($n = 3$)	63.5 ± 16	229 ± 12	108 ± 2.0	6.0 ± 1.0	6.8 ± 1.9	0.475 ± 0.023
AB ($n = 3$)	43.8 ± 8.4	156 ± 12	103 ± 6.4	0.0 ± 0.0	4.7 ± 1.0	0.663 ± 0.036
PEC ($n = 3$)	26.4 ± 6.0	123 ± 4.5	104 ± 1.2	0.0 ± 0.0	2.9 ± 0.6	0.851 ± 0.040
POP ($n = 2$)	20.1 ± 2.4	108 ± 7.0	29.0 ± 7.0	0.0 ± 0.0	7.9 ± 1.4	0.265 ± 0.048

[a] Data from Wickiewicz et al. (1982).

[b] AB, adductor brevis; AL, adductor longus; AM, adductor magnus; BF$_1$, biceps femoris, long head; BF$_S$, biceps femoris, short head; EDL, extensor digitorum longus; EHL, extensor hallucis longus; FDL, flexor digitorum longus; GR, gracilis; FHL, flexor hallucis longus; LG, lateral gastrocnemius; MG, medical gastrocnemius; PEC, pectineus; PB, peroneus brevis; PL, peronius longus; PLT, plantaris; POP, popliteus; RF, rectus femoris; SAR, sartorius; SM, semimembranosus; SOL, soleus; ST, semitendinosus; TA, tibialis anterior; TP, tibialis posterior; VI, vastus intermedius; VL, vastus lateralis; VM, vastus medialis.

These equations can be solved analytically for the special case of confined compression against a porous platen [Mow et al., 1980]. The surface displacement during creep under an applied load f_0 is

$$\frac{u}{h} = \frac{f_0}{H_A}\left(1 - \frac{2}{\pi^2}\sum_{n=0}^{2}\left(n + \frac{1}{2}\right)^{-2}\exp\left\{-\pi^2\left(n + \frac{1}{2}\right)^2\frac{H_A k f}{(1 + 2a_0)h^2}\right\}\right)$$

where h is the tissue thickness, and H_A is the aggregate modulus ($\lambda + 2\mu$). Those authors estimate k as $7.6 \pm 3.0 \times 10^{-13}$ m^4/Nsec and H_A as 0.70 ± 0.09 MPa for bovine articular cartilage. Chen et al. [2001] report strongly depth-dependent values for H_A ranging between 1.16 ± 0.20 MPa in the superficial zone to 7.75 ± 1.45 MPa in the deep zone in human articular cartilage. The biphasic approach has been extended to finite element modeling, resulting in the u–p class of models [Wayne et al., 1991].

48.3.2 Tendon and Ligament

The composition and structure of the tensile soft tissues is quite similar to that of cartilage, and the biphasic theory can be applied to them as well. Fluid pressure serves a smaller role in tissues loaded

TABLE 48.6   Architectural Properties of Human Foot[a,b]

Muscle	Muscle volume (cm^3)	Muscle length (mm)	Fiber length (mm)	Cross-sectional area (cm^2)
ABDH	15.2 ± 5.3	115.8 ± 4.9	23.0 ± 5.5	6.68 ± 2.07
ABDM	8.8 ± 4.7	112.8 ± 19.0	23.9 ± 7.4	3.79 ± 1.83
ADHT	1.1 ± 0.6	24.8 ± 4.2	18.7 ± 5.2	0.62 ± 0.26
ADHO	9.1 ± 3.1	67.4 ± 4.6	18.6 ± 5.3	4.94 ± 1.36
EDB2	2.1 ± 1.2	69.8 ± 16.8	28.0 ± 6.5	0.79 ± 0.43
EDB3	1.3 ± 0.7	82.2 ± 20.7	26.4 ± 5.1	0.51 ± 0.30
EDB4	1.0 ± 0.7	70.4 ± 21.1	23.1 ± 3.8	0.44 ± 0.29
EHB	3.6 ± 1.5	65.7 ± 8.5	27.9 ± 5.7	1.34 ± 0.66
FDB2	4.5 ± 2.3	92.9 ± 15.0	25.4 ± 4.5	1.78 ± 0.79
FDB2	3.2 ± 1.5	98.8 ± 18.1	22.8 ± 4.0	1.49 ± 0.71
FDB4	2.6 ± 1.0	103.0 ± 9.2	20.8 ± 4.5	1.26 ± 0.47
FDB5	0.7 ± 0.3	83.2 ± 3.0	18.2 ± 2.2	0.35 ± 0.16
FDMB	3.4 ± 1.7	$.51.0 \pm 5.3$	17.7 ± 3.8	2.00 ± 1.02
FHBM	3.1 ± 1.3	76.0 ± 19.8	17.5 ± 4.8	1.80 ± 0.75
FHBL	3.4 ± 1.4	65.3 ± 7.1	16.5 ± 3.4	2.12 ± 0.84
DI1	2.7 ± 1.4	51.0 ± 4.9	16.1 ± 4.4	1.70 ± 0.64
DI2	2.5 ± 1.4	49.9 ± 5.1	15.3 ± 4.0	1.68 ± 0.80
DI3	2.5 ± 1.2	44.3 ± 5.6	15.6 ± 5.4	1.64 ± 0.58
DI4	4.2 ± 2.0	61.4 ± 4.5	16.0 ± 4.8	2.72 ± 1.33
LB2	0.6 ± 0.4	53.9 ± 11.8	22.4 ± 6.5	0.28 ± 0.17
LB3	0.5 ± 0.4	45.2 ± 8.7	22.3 ± 6.7	0.28 ± 0.09
LB4	0.6 ± 0.4	37.3 ± 19.9	21.1 ± 9.3	0.30 ± 0.32
LB5	0.4 ± 0.4	$41.0 + 12.1$	16.2 ± 7.0	0.18 ± 0.13
PI1	1.5 ± 0.5	46.2 ± 4.0	13.6 ± 3.7	1.23 ± 0.65
PI2	1.9 ± 0.7	56.6 ± 6.6	13.9 ± 3.5	1.41 ± 0.48
PI3	1.8 ± 0.6	48.8 ± 9.9	14.2 ± 5.9	$1.38 + 0.55$
QPM	5.6 ± 3.4	81.3 ± 20.1	27.5 ± 7.0	1.96 ± 0.94
QPL	2.4 ± 1.2	55.3 ± 3.9	$23.4 + 7.1$	1.00 ± 0.41

[a] Data from Kura et al. (1997).

[b] ABDH, abductor hallucis; FHBM flexor hallucis brevis medialis; FHBL, flexor hallucis brevis lateralis; ADHT, adductor hallucis transverse; ADHO, adductor hallucis oblique; ABDM, abductor digiti minimi; FDMB, flexor digiti minimi brevis; DI, dorsal interosseous; PI, plantar interosseous; FDB, flexor digitorum brevis; LB, lumbrical; QPM, quadratus plantaris medialis; QPL, quadratus plantaris lateralis; EHB, extensor hallucis brevis; EDB, extensor digitorum brevis.

in tension, and the complication of the biphasic model is generally unnecessary. For modeling of segmental mechanics, it is frequently sufficient to treat these structures according to a one-dimensional approximation.

While considering tendons and ligaments as simple nonlinear elastic elements (Table 48.6) are often sufficient, additional accuracy can be obtained by incorporating viscous damping. The quasi-linear viscoelastic approach [Fung, 1981] introduces a stress relaxation function, $G(t)$, that depends only on time, is convoluted with the elastic response, $T^e(\lambda)$, that depends only on the stretch ratio, to yield the complete stress response, $K(\lambda, t)$. To obtain the stress at any point in time requires that the contribution of all preceding deformations be assessed:

$$T(t) = \int_{-\infty}^{f} G(t - \tau) \frac{\partial T^e(\lambda)}{\partial \lambda} \frac{\partial \lambda}{\partial \tau} \, d\tau$$

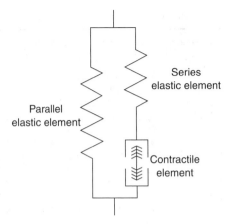

FIGURE 48.3 The Hill model of muscle separates the active properties of muscle into a contractile element, in series with a purely elastic element. The properties of the passive muscle are represented by the parallel elastic element.

Both the elastic response and the relaxation function are empirically determined. The common form for the relaxation function is a sum of exponentials

$$G(t) = A + \sum_i B_i e^{-t/\tau_i}$$

The form of the elastic response varies, but usually includes a power or exponential term to accommodate the toe region.

48.3.3 Muscle

48.3.3.1 Types of Muscle Models

There are three general classes of models for predicting muscle force: biochemical, or crossbridge, models; constitutive models; and phenomenological, or Hill, models. Crossbridge models [Huxley, 1957; Huxley and Simmons, 1971] attempt to determine force from the chemical reactions of the crossbridge cycle. Though accurate at the cross-bridge cycle, it is generally computationally prohibitive to model a whole muscle in this manner. Constitutive models, such as that described by Zahalak and Ma [1990], generally attempt to determine muscle behavior by describing populations of cross-bridges. A potentially powerful approach, this technique has not yet been widely adopted. The vanguard of muscle modeling remains the phenomenological model first described by Hill [1939], that describes the viscoelastic behavior of skeletal muscle using a framework analogous to the standard linear solid (Figure 48.3). Although the series elastic element represents primarily tendon, some series elasticity is found even in muscles lacking any external tendon or in segments of single fibers. The parallel elastic element represents the passive properties of the muscle, currently thought to reside primarily in titin. The contractile component is described by independent isometric force–length (Figure 48.4) and isotonic force–velocity relations (Figure 48.5) and an activation function [Zajac, 1989].

48.3.3.2 Muscle Force–Length Relationship

Under conditions of constant length, muscle force generated is proportional to the magnitude of the interaction between the actin and myosin contractile filaments. Myosin filament length in all species is approximately 1.6 μm, but actin filament length varies (Table 48.7). Optimal sarcomere length and maximum sarcomere length can be calculated using these filament lengths. For optimal force generation, each half myosin filament must completely overlap an actin filament, without opposing actin filaments overlapping. No active force is produced at sarcomere spacings shorter than the myosin filament length or longer than

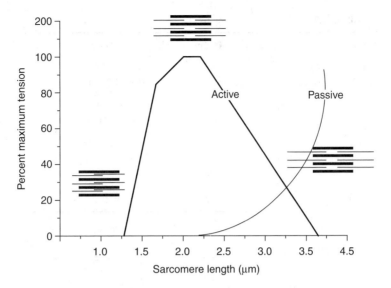

FIGURE 48.4 The force-generating capacity of a sarcomere depends strongly on the degree of overlap of myosin and actin filaments.

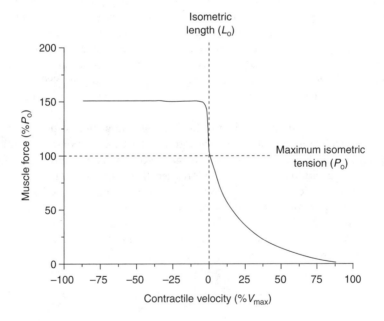

FIGURE 48.5 Active force generation depends strongly on shortening velocity.

the sum of the myosin and the pair of actin filament lengths. The range of operating sarcomere lengths varies among muscles, but generally covers a range of ±15% of optimal length [Burkholder and Lieber, 2003].

48.3.3.3 Muscle Force–Velocity Relationship

Under conditions of constant load the relationship between force and velocity is nearly hyperbolic [Hill, 1938]. The shortening force–velocity relation was can be described by:

$$(P + a)v = b(P_0 - P)$$

TABLE 48.7   Actin Filament Lengths

Species	Actin filament length (μm)	Optimal length (μm)	References
Cat	1.12	2.24	Herzog et al. [1992]
Rat	1.09	2.18	Herzog et al. [1992]
Rabbit	1.09	2.18	Herzog et al. [1992]
Frog	0.98	1.96	Page and Huxley [1963]
Monkey	1.16	2.32	Walker and Schrodt [1973]
Human	1.27	2.54	Walker and Schrodt [1973]
Hummingbird	1.75	3.50	Mathieu-Costello et al. [1992]
Chicken	0.95	1.90	Page [1969]
Wild rabbit	1.12	2.24	Dimery [1985]
Carp	0.98	1.92	Sosnicki et al. [1991]

while the lengthening relation can be described by:

$$F = 1.8 - 0.8 \frac{v_{\max} + v}{V_{\max} - 7.6\ V}$$

The dynamic parameters (a, b, and $V_{\max}$) vary across species and fiber types (Table 48.3).

It should be noted that this formulation omits several potentially important force-generating phenomena. Notable among these are the persistent extra tension obtained following stretch [Edman et al., 1982], the exaggerated short range stiffness [Rack and Westbury, 1974], and changes in the force–length relation associated with activation level [Rack and Westbury, 1969]. Some of these features can be accommodated by considering series elasticity and sarcomere length inhomogeneity [Morgan, 1990], and each represents a nonlinearity that substantially complicates modeling and may not be necessary for first approximations of muscle function.

Common applications of muscle modeling include forward simulation to predict output forces or motions and inverse analysis to estimate the muscle forces that produced an observed motion. In neither of these cases is it necessarily practical to determine muscle contractile properties empirically, and it is frequently necessary to resort to estimation of the force–length and force–velocity relations from muscle structure. If a muscle is considered to be a composition of uniform sarcomeres in series and in parallel, then the deformation of single sarcomeres can be estimated from whole muscle length changes. A simplified view of a muscle is an array of identical fibers of uniform length arranged at a common pennation angle to the line of force. Peak isometric tension can be estimated from PCSA. Pennation angle determines the relationship between muscle and fiber length changes:

$$\frac{\Delta L_{\mathrm{m}}}{L_{\mathrm{m}}} = \frac{\Delta L_{\mathrm{f}}}{L_{\mathrm{f}}} \cos(\theta)$$

If sarcomere length is known at any muscle length, it is then possible to scale the sarcomere length–tension and velocity–tension relations to the whole muscle. When reporting architectural data (Tables), muscle and fiber lengths should be normalized to optimal sarcomere length.

References

Butler, D.L., Grood, E.S., Noyes, F.R., and Zernicke, R.F. (1978). Biomechanics of ligaments and tendons. In *Exercise and Sport Sciences Reviews.* Vol. 6: pp. 125–181, Hutton, R.S. (Ed.). The Franklin Institute Press.

Fung, Y.C. (1981). *Biomechanics: Mechanical Properties of Living Tissues.* Springer-Verlag, New York.

Gans, C. (1982). Fiber architecture and muscle function. *Exerc. Sport Sci. Rev.* 10: 160–207.

Hill, A.V. (1938). The heat of shortening and the dynamic constants of muscle. *Proc. R. Soc. Lond. [Biol].* 126: 136–195.

Huxley, A.F. (1957). Muscle structure and theories of contraction. *Prog. Biophys. Mol. Biol.* 7: 255–318.

Huxley, A.F. and Simmons, R.M. (1971). Proposed mechanism of force generation in striated muscle. *Nature* 233: 533–538.

Kastelic, J., Galeski, A., and Baer, E. (1978). The multicomposite structure of tendon. *Connect. Tissue Res.* 6: 11–23.

Kura, H., Luo, Z., Kitaoka, H.B., and An, K. (1997). Quantitative analysis of the intrinsic muscles of the foot. *Anat. Rec.* 249: 143–151.

Lieber, R.L., Fazeli, B.M., and Botte, M.J. (1990). Architecture of selected wrist flexor and extensor muscles. *J. Hand Surg.* 15: 244–250.

Lieber, R.L., Jacobson, M.D., Fazeli, B.M., Abrams, R.A., and Botte, M.J. (1992). Architecture of selected muscles of the arm and forearm: anatomy and implications for tendon transfer. *J. Hand Surg.* 17: 787–798.

McElhaney, J.H., Roberts, V.L., and Hilyard, J.F. (1976) *Handbook of Human Tolerance.* Japan Automobile Research Institute, Inc. (JARI), Tokyo, Japan.

Mow, V.C., Kuei, S.C. Lai, W.M., and Armstrong, C.G. (1980). Biphasic creep and stress relaxation of articular cartilage in compression: theory and experiments. *Biomech. Eng.* 102: 73–84.

Powell, P.L., Roy, R.R., Kanim, P. Bello, M.A., and Edgerton, V.R. (1984). Predictability of skeletal muscle tension from architectural determinations in guinea pig hindlimbs. *J. Appl. Physiol.* 57: 1715–1721.

Wayne, J.S., Woo, S.L., and Kwan, M.K. (1991). Application of the u–p finite element method to the study of articular cartilage. *J. Biomech. Eng.* 113: 397–403.

Weiss, J.A. and Gardiner, J.C. (2001). Computational modeling of ligament mechanics. *Crit. Rev. Biomed. Eng.* 29: 303–371.

Wickiewicz, T.L., Roy, R.R., Powell, P.L. and Edgerton, V.R. (1983). Muscle architecture of the human lower limb. *Clin. Orthop. Rel. Res.* 179: 275–283.

Zahalak, G.I. and Ma, S.P. (1990). Muscle activation and contraction: constitutive relations based directly on cross-bridge kinetics. *J. Biomech. Eng.* 112: 52–62.

Zajac, F.E. (1989). Muscle and tendon: Properties, models, scaling and application to biomechanics and motor control. *Crit. Rev. Biomed. Eng.* 17: 359–411.

Joint-Articulating
Surface Motion

Kenton R. Kaufman
Kai-Nan An
Mayo Clinic

Knowledge of joint-articulating surface motion is essential for design of prosthetic devices to restore function; assessment of joint wear, stability, and degeneration; and determination of proper diagnosis and surgical treatment of joint disease. In general, kinematic analysis of human movement can be arranged into two separate categories (1) gross movement of the limb segments interconnected by joints, or (2) detailed analysis of joint articulating surface motion which is described in this chapter. Gross movement is the relative three-dimensional joint rotation as described by adopting the Eulerian angle system. Movement of this type is described in Chapter 51: Analysis of Gait. In general, the three-dimensional unconstrained rotation and translation of an articulating joint can be described utilizing the concept of the screw displacement axis. The most commonly used analytic method for the description of 6-degree-of-freedom

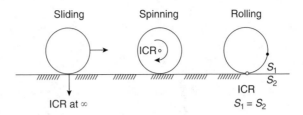

FIGURE 49.1   Three types of articulating surface motion in human joints.

displacement of a rigid body is the screw displacement axis [Kinzel et al., 1972; Spoor and Veldpaus, 1980; Woltring et al., 1985].

Various degrees of simplification have been used for kinematic modeling of joints. A hinged joint is the simplest and most common model used to simulate an anatomic joint in planar motion about a single axis embedded in the fixed segment. Experimental methods have been developed for determination of the instantaneous center of rotation for planar motion. The *instantaneous center of rotation* is defined as the point of zero velocity. For a true hinged motion, the instantaneous center of rotation will be a fixed point throughout the movement. Otherwise, loci of the instantaneous center of rotation or centrodes will exist. The center of curvature has also been used to define joint anatomy. The *center of curvature* is defined as the geometric center of coordinates of the articulating surface.

For more general planar motion of an articulating surface, the term *sliding, rolling,* and *spinning* are commonly used (Figure 49.1). Sliding (gliding) motion is defined as the pure translation of a moving segment against the surface of a fixed segment. The contact point of the moving segment does not change, while the contact point of the fixed segment has a constantly changing contact point. If the surface of the fixed segment is flat, the instantaneous center of rotation is located at infinity. Otherwise, it is located at the center of curvature of the fixed surface. Spinning motion (rotation) is the exact opposite of sliding motion. In this case, the moving segment rotates, and the contact points on the fixed surface does not change. The instantaneous center of rotation is located at the center of curvature of the spinning body that is undergoing pure rotation. Rolling motion occurs between moving and fixed segments where the contact points in each surface are constantly changing and the arc lengths of contact are equal on each segment. The instantaneous center of rolling motion is located at the contact point. Most planar motion of anatomic joints can be described by using any two of these three basic descriptions.

In this chapter, various aspects of joint-articulating motion are covered. Topics include the anatomical characteristics, joint contact, and axes of rotation. Joints of both the upper and lower extremity are discussed.

49.1   Ankle

The ankle joint is composed of two joints: the talocrural (ankle) joint and the talocalcaneal (subtalar joint). The talocrural joint is formed by the articulation of the distal tibia and fibula with the trochlea of the talus. The talocalcaneal joint is formed by the articulation of the talus with the calcaneus.

49.1.1   Geometry of the Articulating Surfaces

The upper articular surface of the talus is wedge-shaped, its width diminishing from front to back. The talus can be represented by a conical surface. The wedge shape of the talus is about 25% wider in front than behind with an average difference of 2.4 ± 1.3 mm and a maximal difference of 6 mm [Inman, 1976].

49.1.2   Joint Contact

The talocrural joint contact area varies with flexion of the ankle (Table 49.1). During plantarflexion, such as would occur during the early stance phase of gait, the contact area is limited and the joint is incongruous.

TABLE 49.1   Talocalcaneal (Ankle) Joint Contact Area

Investigators	Plantarflexion	Neutral	Dorsiflexion
Ramsey and Hamilton [1976]		4.40 ± 1.21	
Kimizuki et al. [1980]		4.83	
Libotte et al. [1982]	5.01 (30°)	5.41	3.60 (30°)
Paar et al. [1983]	4.15 (10°)	4.15	3.63 (10°)
Macko et al. [1991]	3.81 ± 0.93 (15°)	5.2 ± 0.94	5.40 ± 0.74 (10°)
Driscoll et al. [1994]	2.70 ± 0.41 (20°)	3.27 ± 0.32	2.84 ± 0.43 (20°)
Hartford et al. [1995]		3.37 ± 0.52	
Pereira et al. [1996]	1.49 (20°)	1.67	1.47 (10°)
Rosenbaum et al. [2003]		2.11 ± 0.72	

Note: The contact area is expressed in square centimeters.

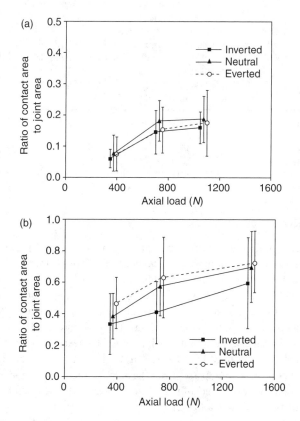

FIGURE 49.2   Ratio of total contact area to joint area in the (a) anterior/middle facet and (b) posterior facet of the subtalar joint as a function of applied axial load for three different positions of the foot. (From Wagner U.A., Sangeorzan B.J., Harrington R.M., and Tencer A.F. 1992. *J. Orthop. Res.* 10: 535. With permission.)

As the position of the joint progresses from neutral to dorsiflexion, as would occur during the midstance of gait, the contact area increases and the joint becomes more stable. The area of the subtalar articulation is smaller than that of the talocrural joint. The contact area of the subtalar joint is 0.89 ± 0.21 cm^2 for the posterior facet and 0.28 ± 15 cm^2 for the anterior and middle facets [Wang et al., 1994]. The total contact area (1.18 ± 0.35 cm^2) is only 12.7% of the whole subtalar articulation area (9.31 ± 0.66 cm^2)

TABLE 49.2   Axis of Rotation for the Ankle

Investigators	Axis[a]	Position
Elftman [1945]	Fix.	$67.6 \pm 7.4°$ with respect to sagittal plane
Isman and Inman [1969]	Fix.	8 mm anterior, 3 mm inferior to the distal tip of the lateral malleolus; 1 mm posterior, 5 mm inferior to the distal tip of the medial malleolus
Inman and Mann [1979]	Fix.	79° (68–88°) with respect to the sagittal plane
Allard et al. [1987]	Fix.	$95.4 \pm 6.6°$ with respect to the frontal plane, $77.7 \pm 12.3°$ with respect to the sagittal plane, and $17.9 \pm 4.5°$ with respect to the transverse plane
Singh et al. [1992]	Fix.	3.0 mm anterior, 2.5 mm inferior to distal tip of lateral malleolus; 2.2 mm posterior, 10 mm inferior to distal tip of medial malleolus
Sammarco et al. [1973]	Ins.	Inside and outside the body of the talus
D'Ambrosia et al. [1976]	Ins.	No consistent pattern
Parlasca et al. [1979]	Ins.	96% within 12 mm of a point 20 mm below the articular surface of the tibia along the long axis
Van Langelaan [1983]	Ins.	At an approximate right angle to the longitudinal direction of the foot, passing through the corpus tali, with a direction from anterolaterosuperior to posteromedioinferior
Barnett and Napier	Q-I	Dorsiflexion: down and lateral Plantarflexion: down and medial
Hicks [1953]	Q-I	Dorsiflexion: 5 mm inferior to tip of lateral malleolus to 15 mm anterior to tip of medial malleolus Plantarflexion: 5 mm superior to tip of lateral malleolus to 15 mm anterior, 10 mm inferior to tip of medial malleolus

[a] Fix. = fixed axis of rotation; Ins. = instantaneous axis of rotation; Q-I = quasi-instantaneous axis of rotation.

[Wang et al., 1994]. The contact area/joint area ratio increases with increases in applied load (Figure 49.2).

49.1.3 Axes of Rotation

Joint motion of the talocrural joint has been studied to define the axes of rotation and their location with respect to specific anatomic landmarks (Table 49.2). The axis of motion of the talocrural joint essentially passes through the inferior tibia at the fibular and tibial malleoli (Figure 49.3). Three types of motion have been used to describe the axes of rotation: fixed, quasi-instantaneous, and instantaneous axes. The motion that occurs in the ankle joints consists of dorsiflexion and plantarflexion. Minimal or no transverse rotation takes place within the talocrural joint. The motion in the talocrural joint is intimately related to the motion in the talocalcaneal joint which is described next.

The motion axes of the talocalcaneal joint have been described by several authors (Table 49.3). The axis of motion in the talocalcaneal joint passes from the anterior medial superior aspect of the navicular bone to the posterior lateral inferior aspect of the calcaneus (Figure 49.4). The motion that occurs in the talocalcaneal joint consists of inversion and eversion.

49.2 Knee

The knee is the intermediate joint of the lower limb. It is composed of the distal femur and proximal tibia. It is the largest and most complex joint in the body. The knee joint is composed of the tibiofemoral articulation and the patellofemoral articulation.

49.2.1 Geometry of the Articulating Surfaces

The shape of the articular surfaces of the proximal tibia and distal femur must fulfill the requirement that they move in contact with one another. The profile of the femoral condyles varies with the condyle

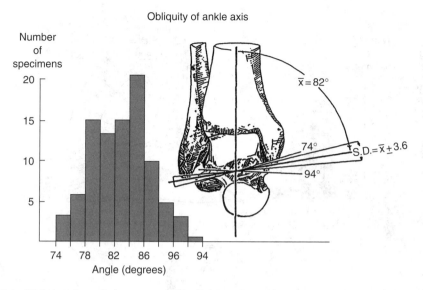

FIGURE 49.3 Variations in angle between middle of tibia and empirical axis of ankle. The histogram reveals a considerable spread of individual values. (From Inman V.T. 1976. *The Joints of the Ankle*, Baltimore, Williams and Wilkins. With permission.)

TABLE 49.3 Axis of Rotation for the Talocalcaneal (Subtalar) Joint

Investigators	Axis[a]	Position
Manter [1941]	Fix.	16° (8–24°) with respect to sagittal plane, and 42° (29–47°) with respect to transverse plane
Shephard [1951]	Fix.	Tuberosity of the calcaneus to the neck of the talus
Hicks [1953]	Fix.	Posterolateral corner of the heel to superomedial aspect of the neck of the talus
Root et al. [1966]	Fix.	17° (8–29°) with respect to sagittal plane, and 41° (22–55°) with respect to transverse plane
Isman and Inman [1969]	Fix.	23° ± 11° with respect to sagittal plane, and 41° ± 9° with respect to transverse plane
Kirby [1947]	Fix.	Extends from the posterolateral heel, posteriorly, to the first intermetatarsal space, anteriorly
Rastegar et al. [1980]	Ins.	Instant centers of rotation pathways in posterolateral quadrant of the distal articulating tibial surface, varying with applied load
Van Langelaan [1983]	Ins.	A bundle of axes that make an acute angle with the longitudinal direction of the foot passing through the tarsal canal having a direction from anteromediosuperior to posterolateroinferior
Engsberg [1987]	Ins.	A bundle of axes with a direction from anteromediosuperior to posterolateroinferior

[a] Fix. = fixed axis of rotation; Ins. = instantaneous axis of rotation.

examined (Figure 49.5 and Table 49.4). The tibial plateau widths are greater than the corresponding widths of the femoral condyles (Figure 49.6 and Table 49.6). However, the tibial plateau depths are less than those of the femoral condyle distances. The medial condyle of the tibia is concave superiorly (the center of curvature lies above the tibial surface) with a radius of curvature of 80 mm [Kapandji, 1987]. The lateral condyle is convex superiorly (the center of curvature lies below the tibial surface) with a radius of curvature of 70 mm [Kapandji, 1987]. The shape of the femoral surfaces is complementary to the shape of the tibial plateaus. The shape of the posterior femoral condyles may be approximated by spherical surfaces (Table 49.4).

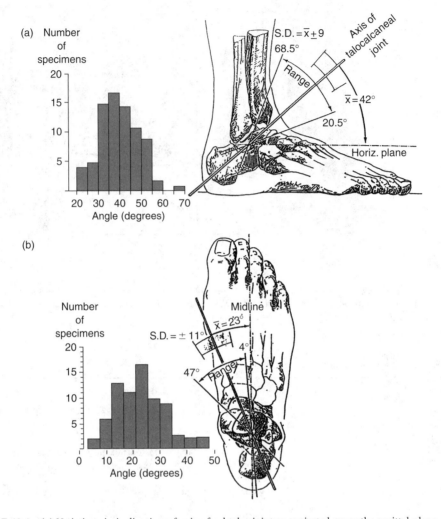

FIGURE 49.4 (a) Variations in inclination of axis of subtalar joint as projected upon the sagittal plane. The distribution of the measurements on the individual specimens is shown in the histogram. The single observation of an angle of almost 70° was present in a markedly cavus foot. (b) Variations in position of subtalar axis as projected onto the transverse plane. The angle was measured between the axis and the midline of the foot. The extent of individual variation is shown on the sketch and revealed in the histogram. (From Inman V.T. 1976. *The Joints of the Ankle*, Baltimore, Williams and Wilkins. With permission.)

The geometry of the patellofemoral articular surfaces remains relatively constant as the knee flexes. The knee sulcus angle changes only ±3.4° from 15 to 75° of knee flexion (Figure 49.7). The mean depth index varies by only ±4% over the same flexion range (Figure 49.7). Similarly, the medial and lateral patellar facet angles (Figure 49.8) change by less than a degree throughout the entire knee flexion range (Table 49.7). However, there is a significant difference between the magnitude of the medial and lateral patellar facet angles.

49.2.2 Joint Contact

The mechanism for movement between the femur and tibia is a combination of rolling and gliding. Backward movement of the femur on the tibia during flexion has long been observed in the human knee.

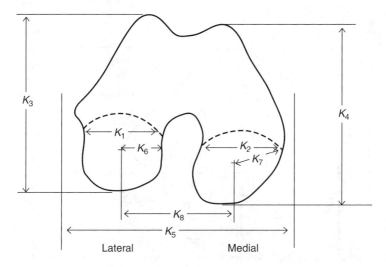

FIGURE 49.5 Geometry of distal femur. The distances are defined in Table 49.4.

TABLE 49.4 Geometry of the Distal Femur

Parameter	Symbol	Lateral Distance (mm)	Symbol	Medial Distance (mm)	Symbol	Overall Distance (mm)
Medial/lateral distance	K_1	31 ± 2.3 (male) 28 ± 1.8 (female)	K_2	32 ± 31 (male) 27 ± 3.1 (female)		
Anterior/posterior distance	K_3	72 ± 4.0 (male) 65 ± 3.7 (female)	K_4	70 ± 4.3 (male) 63 ± 4.5 (female)		
Posterior femoral condyle spherical radii	K_6	19.2 ± 1.7	K_7	20.8 ± 2.4		
Epicondylar width					K_5	90 ± 6 (male) 80 ± 6 (female)
Medial/lateral spacing of center of spherical surfaces					K_8	45.9 ± 3.4

Note: See Figure 49.5 for location of measurements.

Source: Yoshioka Y., Siu D., and Cooke T.D.V. 1987. *J. Bone Joint Surg.* 69A: 873–880. Kurosawa H., Walker P.S., Abe S., Garg A., and Hunter T. 1985. *J. Biomech.* 18: 487.

TABLE 49.5 Posterior Femoral Condyle Spherical Radius

	Normal knee	Varus knees	Valgus knees
Medial condyle	20.3 ± 3.4(16.1–28.0)	21.2 ± 2.1(18.0–24.5)	21.1 ± 2.0(17.84–24.1)
Lateral condyle	19.0 ± 3.0(14.7–25.0)	20.8 ± 2.1(17.5–30.0)	21.1* ± 2.1(18.4–25.5)

* Significantly different from normal knees ($p < 0.05$).

Source: Matsuda S., Miura H. Nagamine R., Mawatari T., Tokunaga M., Nabeyama R., and Iwamoto Y. Anatomical analysis of the femoral condyle in normal and osteoarthritic knees. *J. Ortho. Res.* 22: 104–109, 2004.

The magnitude of the rolling and gliding changes through the range of flexion. The tibial-femoral contact point has been shown to move posteriorly as the knee is flexed, reflecting the coupling of posterior motion with flexion (Figure 49.9). In the intact knee at full extension, the center of pressure is approximately 25 mm from the anterior edge of the tibial plateau [Andriacchi et al, 1986]. The medial femoral condyle rests

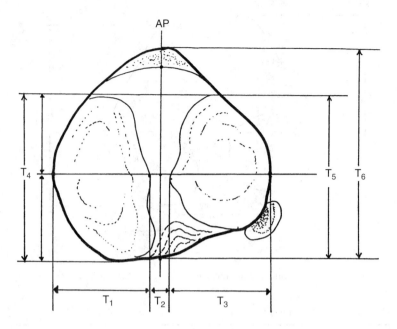

FIGURE 49.6   Contour of the tibial plateau (transverse plane). The distances are defined in Table 49.6.

TABLE 49.6   Geometry of the Proximal Tibia

Parameter	Symbols	All limbs	Male	Female
Tibial plateau with widths (mm)				
Medial plateau	T_1	32 ± 3.8	34 ± 3.9	30 ± 22
Lateral plateau	T_3	33 ± 2.6	35 ± 1.9	31 ± 1.7
Overall width	$T_1 + T_2 + T_3$	76 ± 6.2	81 ± 4.5	73 ± 4.5
Tibial plateau depths (mm)				
AP depth, medial	T_4	48 ± 5.0	52 ± 3.4	45 ± 4.1
AP depth, lateral	T_5	42 ± 3.7	45 ± 3.1	40 ± 2.3
Interspinous width (mm)	T_2	12 ± 1.7	12 ± 0.9	12 ± 2.2
Intercondylar depth (mm)	T_6	48 ± 5.9	52 ± 5.7	45 ± 3.9

Source: Yoshioka Y., Siu D., Scudamore R.A., and Cooke T.D.V. 1989. *J. Orthop. Res.* 7:
132.

further anteriorly on the tibial plateau than the lateral plateau. The medial femoral condyle is positioned 35 ± 4 mm from the posterior edge while the lateral femoral condyle is positioned 25 ± 4 mm from the posterior edge (Figure 49.9). During knee flexion to 90°, the medial femoral condyle moves back 15 ± 2 mm and the lateral femoral condyle moves back 12 ± 2 mm. Thus, during flexion the femur moves posteriorly on the tibia (Table 49.9).

The patellofemoral contact area is smaller than the tibiofemoral contact area (Table 49.10). As the knee joint moves from extension to flexion, a band of contact moves upward over the patellar surface (Figure 49.10). As knee flexion increases, not only does the contact area move superiorly, but it also becomes larger. At 90° of knee flexion, the contact area has reached the upper level of the patella. As the knee continues to flex, the contact area is divided into separate medial and lateral zones.

49.2.3   Axes of Rotation

The tibiofemoral joint is mainly a joint with two degrees of freedom. The first degree of freedom allows movements of flexion and extension in the sagittal plane. The axis of rotation lies perpendicular to the

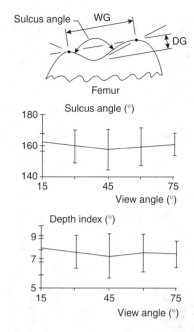

FIGURE 49.7 The trochlear geometry indices. The sulcus angle is the angle formed by the lines drawn from the top of the medial and lateral condyles to the deepest point of the sulcus. The depth index is the ratio of the width of the groove (WG) to the depth (DG). Mean and SD; $n = 12$. (From Farahmand et al. *J. Orthop. Res.* 16: 1, 140.)

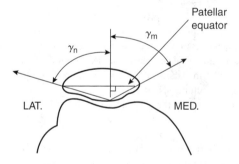

FIGURE 49.8 Medial (γ_m) and lateral (γ_n) patellar facet angles. (From Ahmed A.M., Burke D.L., and Hyder A. 1987. *J. Orthop. Res.* 5: 69–85.)

sagittal plane and intersects the femoral condyles. Both fixed axes and screw axes have been calculated (Figure 49.11). In Figure 49.11, the optimal axes are fixed axes, whereas the screw axis is an instantaneous axis. The symmetric optimal axis is constrained such that the axis is the same for both the right and left knee. The screw axis may sometimes coincide with the optimal axis but not always, depending upon the motions of the knee joint. The second degree of freedom is the axial rotation around the long axis of the tibia. Rotation of the leg around its long axis can only be performed with the knee flexed. There is also an automatic axial rotation which is involuntarily linked to flexion and extension. When the knee is flexed, the tibia internally rotates. Conversely, when the knee is extended, the tibia externally rotates.

During knee flexion, the patella makes a rolling/gliding motion along the femoral articulating surface. Throughout the entire flexion range, the gliding motion is clockwise (Figure 49.12). In contrast, the direction of the rolling motion is counter-clockwise between 0 and 90° and clockwise between 90 and 120° (Figure 49.12). The mean amount of patellar gliding for all knees is approximately 6.5 mm per 10° of

TABLE 49.7   Patellar Facet Angles

Facet angle	Knee Flexion Angle				
	0°	30°	60°	90°	120°
γ_m (deg)	60.88	60.96	61.43	61.30	60.34
	3.89[a]	4.70	4.12	4.18	4.51
γ_n (deg)	67.76	68.05	68.36	68.39	68.20
	4.15	3.97	3.63	4.01	3.67

[a] SD.

Source: Ahmed A.M., Burke D.L., and Hyder A. 1987. *J. Orthop. Res.* 5: 69–85.

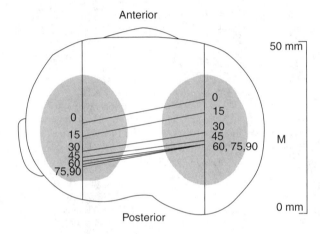

FIGURE 49.9   Diagram of the tibial plateau, showing the tibiofemoral contact pattern from 0° to 90° of knee flexion, in the loaded knee. In both medial and lateral compartments, the femoral condyle rolls back along the tibial plateau from 0° to 30°. Between 30° and 90° the lateral condyle continues to move posteriorly, while the medial condyle moves back little. (From Scarvell, J.M., Smith, P.N., Refshauge, K.M., Galloway, H.R., and Woods, K.R. Evaluation of a method to map tibiofemoral contact points in the normal knee using MRI. *J. Orthop. Res.* 22:788–793, 2004.)

flexion between 0 and 80° and 4.5 mm per 10° of flexion between 80 and 120°. The relationship between the angle of flexion and the mean rolling/gliding ratio for all knees is shown in Figure 49.13. Between 80 and 90° of knee flexion, the rolling motion of the articulating surface comes to a standstill and then changes direction. The reversal in movement occurs at the flexion angle where the quadriceps tendon first contacts the femoral groove.

49.3   Hip

The hip joint is composed of the head of the femur and the acetabulum of the pelvis. The hip joint is one of the most stable joints in the body. The stability is provided by the rigid ball-and-socket configuration.

49.3.1   Geometry of the Articulating Surfaces

The femoral head is spherical in its articular portion which forms twothirds of a sphere. The diameter of the femoral head is smaller for females than for males (Table 49.11). In the normal hip, the center of the femoral head coincides exactly with the center of the acetabulum. The rounded part of the femoral head is spheroidal rather than spherical because the uppermost part is flattened slightly. This causes

TABLE 49.8   Tibiofemoral Contact Area

Knee flexion (deg)	Contact area (cm^2)
−5	20.2
5	19.8
15	19.2
25	18.2
35	14.0
45	13.4
55	11.8
65	13.6
75	11.4
85	12.1

Source: Maquet P.G., Vandberg A.J., and Simonet J.C. 1975. *J. Bone Joint Surg.* 57A: 766.

TABLE 49.9   Posterior Displacement of the Femur Relative to the Tibia

Authors	Condition	A/P displacement (mm)
Kurosawa [1985]	*In vitro*	14.8
Andriacchi [1986]	*In vitro*	13.5
Draganich [1987]	*In vitro*	13.5
Nahass [1991]	*In vivo* (walking)	12.5
	In vivo (stairs)	13.9

TABLE 49.10   Patellofemoral Contact Area

Knee flexion (deg)	Contact area (cm^2)
20	2.6 ± 0.4
30	3.1 ± 0.3
60	3.9 ± 0.6
90	4.1 ± 1.2
120	4.6 ± 0.7

Source: Hubert H.H. and Hayes W.C. 1984. *J. Bone Joint Surg.* 66A: 715–725.

the load to be distributed in a ringlike pattern around the superior pole. The geometrical center of the femoral head is traversed by the three axes of the joint, the horizontal axis, the vertical axis, and the anterior/posterior axis. The head is supported by the neck of the femur, which joins the shaft. The axis of the femoral neck is obliquely set and runs superiorly, medially, and anteriorly. The angle of inclination of the femoral neck to the shaft in the frontal plane is the neck-shaft angle (Figure 49.14). In most adults, this angle is about 130° (Table 49.11). An angle exceeding 130° is known as *coxa valga*; an angle less than 130° is known as *coxa vara*. The femoral neck forms an acute angle with the transverse axis of the femoral condyles. This angle faces medially and anteriorly and is called the *angle of anteversion* (Figure 49.15). In the adult, this angle averages about 7.5° (Table 49.11).

The acetabulum receives the femoral head and lies on the lateral aspect of the hip. The acetabulum of the adult is a hemispherical socket. Its cartilage area is approximately 16 cm^2 [Von Lanz and Wauchsmuth, 1938]. Together with the labrum, the acetabulum covers slightly more than 50% of the femoral head

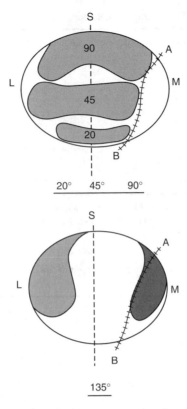

FIGURE 49.10 Diagrammatic representation of patella contact areas for varying degrees of knee flexion. (From Goodfellow J., Hungerford D.S., and Zindel M. *J. Bone Joint Surg.* 58-B: 3, 288. With permission.)

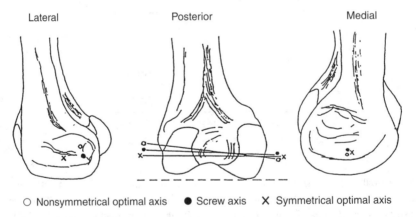

FIGURE 49.11 Approximate location of the optimal axis (case 1 — nonsymmetric, case 3 — symmetric), and the screw axis (case 2) on the medial and lateral condyles of the femur of a human subject for the range of motion of 0 to 90° flexion (standing to sitting, respectively). (From Lewis J.L. and Lew W.D. 1978. *J. Biomech. Eng.* 100: 187. With permission.)

[Tönnis, 1987]. Only the sides of the acetabulum are lined by articular cartilage, which is interrupted inferiorly by the deep acetabular notch. The central part of the cavity is deeper than the articular cartilage and is nonarticular. This part is called the *acetabular fossae* and is separated from the interface of the pelvic bone by a thin plate of bone.

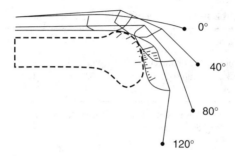

FIGURE 49.12   Position of patellar ligament, patella, and quadriceps tendon and location of the contact points as a function of the knee flexion angle. (From van Eijden T.M.G.J., Kouwenhoven E., Verburg J. et al. *J. Biomech.* 19: 227.)

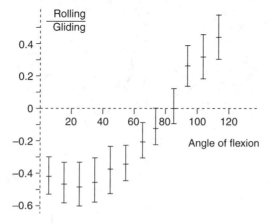

FIGURE 49.13   Calculated rolling/gliding ratio for the patellofemoral joint as a function of the knee flexion angle. (From van Eijden T.M.G.J., Kouwenhoven E., Verburg J. et al. *J. Biomech.* 19: 226.)

49.3.2 Joint Contact

Miyanaga et al. [1984] studied the deformation of the hip joint under loading, the contact area between the articular surfaces, and the contact pressures. They found that at loads up to 1000 N, pressure was distributed largely to the anterior and posterior parts of the lunate surface with very little pressure applied to the central portion of the roof itself. As the load increased, the contact area enlarged to include the outer and inner edges of the lunate surface (Figure 49.16). However, the highest pressures were still measured anteriorly and posteriorly. Of five hip joints studied, only one had a pressure maximum at the zenith or central part of the acetabulum.

Davy et al. [1989] utilized a telemetered total hip prosthesis to measure forces across the hip after total hip arthroplasty. The orientation of the resultant joint contact force varies over a relatively limited range during the weight-load-bearing portions of gait. Generally, the joint contact force on the ball of the hip prosthesis is located in the anterior/superior region. A three-dimensional plot of the resultant joint force during the gait cycle, with crutches, is shown in Figure 49.17.

49.3.3 Axes of Rotation

The human hip is a modified spherical (ball-and-socket) joint. Thus, the hip possesses three degrees of freedom of motion with three correspondingly arranged, mutually perpendicular axes that intersect at the geometric center of rotation of the spherical head. The transverse axis lies in the frontal plane and

TABLE 49.11   Geometry of the Proximal Femur

Parameter	Females	Males
Femoral head diameter (mm)	45.0 ± 3.0	52.0 ± 3.3
Neck shaft angle (deg)	133 ± 6.6	129 ± 7.3
Anteversion (deg)	8 ± 10	7.0 ± 6.8

Source: Yoshioka Y., Siu D., and Cooke T.D.V. 1987. *J. Bone Joint Surg.* 69A: 873.

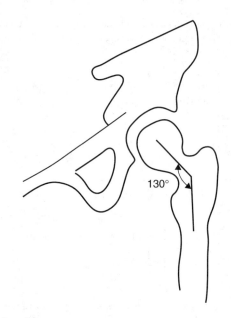

FIGURE 49.14   The neck-shaft angle.

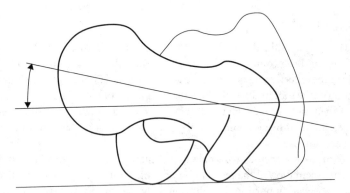

FIGURE 49.15   The normal anteversion angle formed by a line tangent to the femoral condyles and the femoral neck axis, as displayed in the superior view.

controls movements of flexion and extension. An anterior/posterior axis lies in the sagittal plane and controls movements of adduction and abduction. A vertical axis which coincides with the long axis of the limb when the hip joint is in the neutral position controls movements of internal and external rotation. Surface motion in the hip joint can be considered as spinning of the femoral head on the acetabulum. The

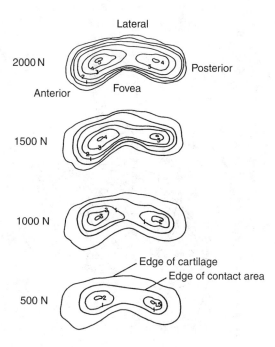

FIGURE 49.16 Pressure distribution and contact area of hip joint. The pressure is distributed largely to the anterior and posterior parts of the lunate surface. As the load increased, the contact area increased. (From Miyanaga Y., Fukubayashi T., and Kurosawa H. 1984. *Arch. Orth. Trauma Surg.* 103:13. With permission.)

pivoting of the bone socket in three planes around the center of rotation in the femoral head produces the spinning of the joint surfaces.

49.4 Shoulder

The shoulder represents the group of structures connecting the arm to the thorax. The combined movements of four distinct articulations — glenohumeral, acromioclavicular, sternoclavicular, and scapulothoracic — allow the arm to be positioned in space.

49.4.1 Geometry of the Articulating Surfaces

The articular surface of the humerus is approximately one-third of a sphere (Figure 49.18). The articular surface is oriented with an upward tilt of approximately 45° and is retroverted approximately 30° with respect to the condylar line of the distal humerus [Morrey and An, 1990]. The average radius of curvature of the humeral head in the coronal plane is 24.0 ± 2.1 mm [Iannotti et al., 1992]. The radius of curvature in the anteroposterior and axillary-lateral view is similar, measuring 13.1 ± 1.3 and 22.9 ± 2.9 mm, respectively [McPherson et al., 1997]. The humeral articulating surface is spherical in the center. However, the peripheral radius is 2 mm less in the axial plane than in the coronal plane. Thus the peripheral contour of the articular surface is elliptical with a ratio of 0.92 [Iannotti et al., 1992]. The major axis is superior to inferior and the minor axis is anterior to posterior [McPherson et al., 1997]. More recently, the three-dimensional geometry of the proximal humerus has been studied extensively. The articular surface, which is part of a sphere, varies individually in its orientation with respect to inclination and retroversion, and it has variable medial and posterior offsets [Boileau and Walch, 1997]. These findings have great impact in implant design and placement in order to restore soft-tissue function.

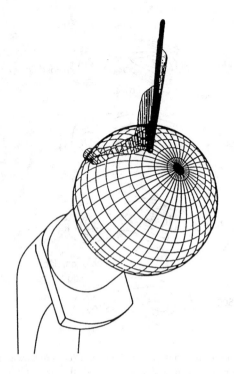

FIGURE 49.17   Scaled three-dimensional plot of resultant force during the gait cycle with crutches. The lengths of the lines indicate the magnitude of force. Radial line segments are drawn at equal increments of time, so the distance between the segments indicates the rate at which the orientation of the force was changing. For higher amplitudes of force during stance phase, line segments in close proximity indicate that the orientation of the force was changing relatively little with the cone angle between 30 and 40° and the polar angle between −25 and −15°. (From Davy D.T., Kotzar D.M., Brown R.H. et al. 1989. *J. Bone Joint Surg.* 70A: 45. With permission.)

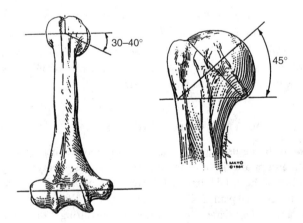

FIGURE 49.18   The two-dimensional orientation of the articular surface of the humerus with respect to the bicondylar axis. By permission of Mayo Foundation.

The glenoid fossa consists of a small, pear-shaped, cartilage-covered bony depression that measures 39.0 ± 3.5 mm in the superior/inferior direction and 29.0 ± 3.2 mm in the anterior/posterior direction [Iannotti et al., 1992]. The anterior/posterior dimension of the glenoid is pear-shaped with the lower half being larger than the top half. The ratio of the lower half to the top half is 1 : 0.80 ± 0.01 [Iannotti et al.,

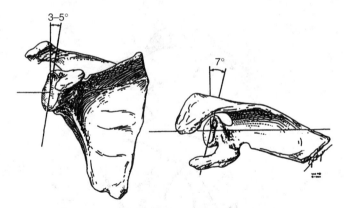

FIGURE 49.19   The glenoid faces slightly superior and posterior (retroverted) with respect to the body of the scapula. By permission of Mayo Foundation.

TABLE 49.12   Glenohumeral Contact Areas

Elevation angle (°)	Contact areas at SR (cm^2)	Contact areas at 20° internal to SR (cm^2)
0	0.87 ± 1.01	1.70 ± 1.68
30	2.09 ± 1.54	2.44 ± 2.15
60	3.48 ± 1.69	4.56 ± 1.84
90	4.95 ± 2.15	3.92 ± 2.10
120	5.07 ± 2.35	4.84 ± 1.84
150	3.52 ± 2.29	2.33 ± 1.47
180	2.59 ± 2.90	2.51 ± NA

SR = starting external rotation which allowed the shoulder to reach maximal elevation in the scapular plane ($\approx40° \pm 8°$); NA = not applicable.

Source: Soslowsky L.J., Flatow E.L., Bigliani L.U., Pablak R.J., Mow V.C., and Athesian G.A. 1992. *J. Orthop. Res.* 10: 524.

1992]. The glenoid radius of curvature is 32.2 ± 7.6 mm in the anteroposterior view and 40.6 ± 14.0 mm in the axillary–lateral view [McPherson et al., 1997]. The glenoid is therefore more curved superior to inferior (coronal plane) and relatively flatter in an anterior to posterior direction (sagittal plane). Glenoid depth is 5.0 ± 1.1 mm in the anteroposterior view and 2.9 ± 1.0 mm in the axillary–lateral [McPherson et al., 1997], again confirming that the glenoid is more curved superior to inferior. In the coronal plane the articular surface of the glenoid comprises an arc of approximately 75° and in the transverse plane the arc of curvature of the glenoid is about 50° [Morrey and An, 1990]. The glenoid has a slight upward tilt of about 5° [Basmajian and Bazant, 1959] with respect to the medial border of the scapula (Figure 49.19) and is retroverted a mean of approximately 7° [Saha, 1971]. The relationship of the dimension of the humeral head to the glenoid head is approximately 0.8 in the coronal plane and 0.6 in the horizontal or transverse plane [Saha, 1971]. The surface area of the glenoid fossa is only one-third to one-fourth that of the humeral head [Kent, 1971]. The arcs of articular cartilage on the humeral head and glenoid in the frontal and axial planes were measured [Jobe and Iannotti, 1995]. In the coronal plane, the humeral heads had an arc of 159° covered by 96° of glenoid, leaving 63° of cartilage uncovered. In the transverse plane, the humeral arc of 160° is opposed by 74° of glenoid, leaving 86° uncovered.

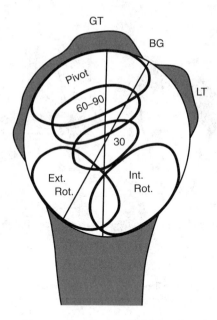

FIGURE 49.20 Humeral contact positions as a function of glenohumeral motion and positions. (From Morrey B.F. and An K.N. 1990. C.A. Rockwood and F.A. Matsen (Eds.), *The Shoulder*, pp. 208–245, Philadelphia, Saunders. With permission.)

49.4.2 Joint Contact

The degree of conformity and constraint between the humeral head and glenoid has been represented by conformity index (radius of head/radius of glenoid) and constraint index (arc of enclosure/360) [McPherson, 1997]. Based on the study of 93 cadaveric specimens, the mean conformity index was 0.72 in the coronal and 0.63 in the sagittal plane. There was more constraint to the glenoid in the coronal vs. sagittal plane (0.18 vs. 0.13). These anatomic features help prevent superior–inferior translation of the humeral head but allow translation in the sagittal plane. Joint contact areas of the glenohumeral joint tend to be greater at mid-elevation positions than at either of the extremes of joint position (Table 49.12). These results suggest that the glenohumeral surface is maximum at these more functional positions, thus distributing joint load over a larger region in a more stable configuration. The contact point moves forward and inferior during internal rotation (Figure 49.20). With external rotation, the contact is posterior/inferior. With elevation, the contact area moves superiorly. Lippitt and associates [1998] calculated the stability ratio, which is defined as a force necessary to translate the humeral head from the glenoid fossa divided by the compressive load times 100. The stability ratios were in the range of 50–60% in the superior–inferior direction and 30–40% in the anterior–posterior direction. After the labrum was removed, the ratio decreased by approximately 20%. Joint conformity was found to have significant influence on translations of humeral head during active positioning by muscles [Karduna et al., 1996].

49.4.3 Axes of Rotation

The shoulder complex consists of four distinct articulations: the glenohumeral joint, the acromioclavicular joint, the sternoclavicular joint, and the scapulothoracic articulation. The wide range of motion of the shoulder (exceeding a hemisphere) is the result of synchronous, simultaneous contributions from each joint. The most important function of the shoulder is arm elevation. Several investigators have attempted to relate glenohumeral and scapulothoracic motion during arm elevation in various planes

TABLE 49.13 Arm Elevation: Glenohumeral–Scapulothoracic Rotation

Investigator	Glenohumeral/scapulothoracic motion ratio
Inman et al. [1994]	2 : 1
Freedman and Munro [1966]	1.35 : 1
Doody et al. [1970]	1.74 : 1
Poppen and Walker [1976]	4.3 : 1 (<24° elevation)
	1.25 : 1 (>24° elevation)
Saha [1971]	2.3 : 1 (30–135° elevation)

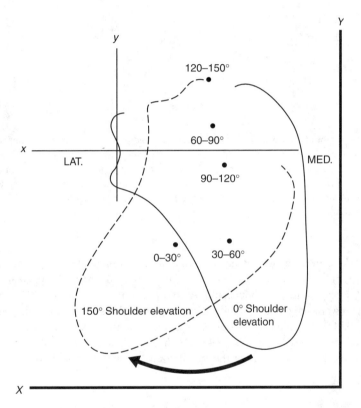

FIGURE 49.21 Rotation of the scapula on the thorax in the scapular plane. Instant centers of rotation (solid dots) are shown for each 30° interval of motion during shoulder elevation in the scapular plane from zero to 150°. The *x* and *y* axes are fixed in the scapula, whereas the *X* and *Y* axes are fixed in the thorax. From zero to 30° in the scapula rotated about its lower midportion; from 60° onward, rotation took place about the glenoid area, resulting in a medial and upward displacement of the glenoid face and a large lateral displacement of the inferior tip of the scapula. (From Poppen N.K. and Walker P.S. 1976. *J. Bone Joint Surg.* 58A:195. With permission.)

(Table 49.13). About two-thirds of the motion takes place in the glenohumeral joint and about one-third in the scapulothoracic articulation, resulting in a 2 : 1 ratio.

Surface motion at the glenohumeral joint is primarily rotational. The center of rotation of the glenohumeral joint has been defined as a locus of points situated within 6.0 ± 1.8 mm of the geometric center of the humeral head [Poppen and Walker, 1976]. However, the motion is not purely rotational. The humeral head displaces, with respect to the glenoid. From 0 to 30°, and often from 30 to 60°, the humeral head moves upward in the glenoid fossa by about 3 mm, indicating that rolling and/or gliding

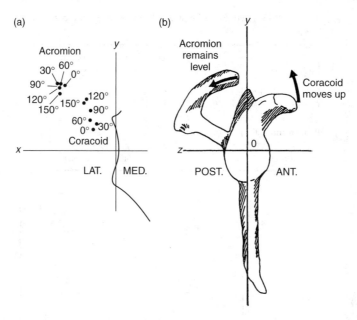

FIGURE 49.22   (a) A plot of the tips of the acromion and coracoid process on roentgenograms taken at successive intervals of arm elevation in the scapular plane shows upward movement of the coracoid and only a slight shift in the acromion relative to the glenoid face. This finding demonstrates twisting, or external rotation, of the scapula about the x-axis. (b) A lateral view of the scapula during this motion would show the coracoid process moving upward while the acromion remains on the same horizontal plane as the glenoid. (From Poppen N.K. and Walker P.S. 1976. *J. Bone Joint Surg.* 58A: 195. With permission.)

has taken place. Thereafter, the humeral head has only about 1 mm of additional excursion. During arm elevation in the scapular plane, the scapula moves in relation to the thorax [Poppen and Walker, 1976]. From 0 to 30° the scapula rotates about its lower mid portion, and then from 60° onward the center of rotation shifts toward the glenoid, resulting in a large lateral displacement of the inferior tip of the scapula (Figure 49.21). The center of rotation of the scapula for arm elevation is situated at the tip of the acromion as viewed from the edge on (Figure 49.22). The mean amount of scapular twisting at maximum arm elevation is 40°. The superior tip of the scapula moves away from the thorax, and the inferior tip moves toward it.

49.5   Elbow

The bony structures of the elbow are the distal end of the humerus and the proximal ends of the radius and ulna. The elbow joint complex allows two degrees of freedom in motion: flexion/extension and pronation/supination. The elbow joint complex is three separate synovial articulations. The humeral–ulnar joint is the articulation between the trochlea of the distal radius and the trochlear fossa of the proximal ulna. The humero–radial joint is formed by the articulation between the capitulum of the distal humerus and the head of the radius. The proximal radioulnar joint is formed by the head of the radius and the radial notch of the proximal ulna.

49.5.1   Geometry of the Articulating Surfaces

The curved, articulating portions of the trochlea and capitulum are approximately circular in a cross-section. The radius of the capitulum is larger than the central trochlear groove (Table 49.14). The centers of curvature of the trochlea and capitulum lie in a straight line located on a plane that slopes at 45 to 50°

TABLE 49.14   Elbow Joint Geometry

Parameter	Size (mm)
Capitulum radius	10.6 ± 1.1
Lateral trochlear flange radius	10.8 ± 1.0
Central trochlear groove radius	8.8 ± 0.4
Medial trochlear groove radius	13.2 ± 1.4
Distal location of flexion/extension axis from transepicondylar line:	
Lateral	6.8 ± 0.2
Medial	8.7 ± 0.6

Source: Shiba R., Sorbie C., Siu D.W., Bryant J.T., Cooke T.D.V., and Weavers H.W. 1988. *J. Orthop. Res.* 6: 897.

TABLE 49.15   Elbow Joint Contact Area

Position	Total articulating surface area of ulna and radial head (mm²)	Contact area (%)
Full extension	1598 ± 103	8.1 ± 2.7
90° flexion	1750 ± 123	10.8 ± 2.0
Full flexion	1594 ± 120	9.5 ± 2.1

Source: Goel V.K., Singh D., and Bijlani V. 1982. *J. Biomech. Eng.* 104: 169.

anterior and distal to the transepicondylar line and is inclined at 2.5° from the horizontal transverse plane [Shiba et al., 1988]. The curves of the ulnar articulations form two surfaces (coronoid and olecranon) with centers on a line parallel to the transepicondylar line but are distinct from it [Shiba et al., 1988]. The carrying angle is an angle made by the intersection of the longitudinal axis of the humerus and the forearm in the frontal plane with the elbow in an extended position. The carrying angle is contributed to, in part, by the oblique axis of the distal humerus and, in part, by the shape of the proximal ulna (Figure 49.23).

49.5.2 Joint Contact

The contact area on the articular surfaces of the elbow joint depends on the joint position and the loading conditions. Increasing the magnitude of the load not only increases the size of the contact area but shifts the locations as well (Figure 49.24). As the axial loading is increased, there is an increased lateralization of the articular contact [Stormont et al., 1985]. The area of contact, expressed as a percentage of the total articulating surface area, is given in Table 49.15. Based on a finite element model of the humero–ulnar joint, Merz et al. [1997] demonstrated that the humero–ulnar joint incongruity brings about a bicentric distribution of contact pressure, a tensile stress exists in the notch that is the same order of magnitude as the compressive stress [Merz, 1997].

49.5.3 Axes of Rotation

The axes of flexion and extension can be approximated by a line passing through the center of the trochlea, bisecting the angle formed by the longitudinal axes of the humerus and the ulna [Morrey and Chao, 1976]. The instant centers of flexion and extension vary within 2–3 mm of this axis (Figure 49.25). With the elbow fully extended and the forearm fully supinated, the longitudinal axes of humerus and ulna normally intersect at a valgus angle referred to as the *carrying angle*. In adults, this angle is usually 10–15° and

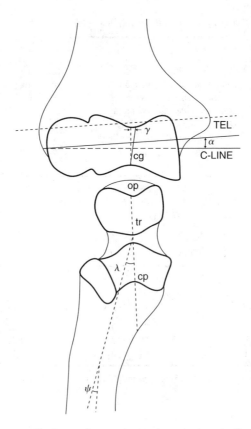

FIGURE 49.23 Components contributing to the carrying angles: $\alpha + \lambda + \psi$. Key: α, angle between C-line and TEL; γ, inclination of central groove (cg); λ, angle between trochlear notch (tn); ψ, reverse angulation of shaft of ulna; TLE, transepicondylar line; C-line, line joining centers of curvature of the trochlea and capitellum; cg, central groove; op, olecranon process; tr, trochlear ridge; cp, coronoid process. $\alpha = 2.5 \pm 0.0$; $\lambda = 17.5 \pm 5.0$ (females) and 12.0 ± 7.0 (males); $\psi = -6.5 \pm 0.7$ (females) and -9.5 ± 3.5 (males). (From Shiba R., Sorbie C., Siu D.W., Bryant J.T., Cooke T.D.V., and Weavers H.W. 1988. *J. Orthop. Res.* 6: 897. With permission.)

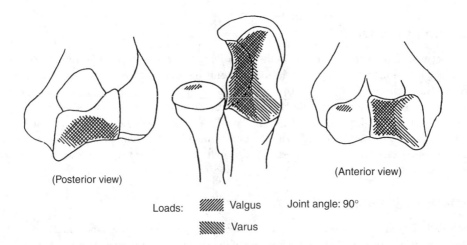

FIGURE 49.24 Contact of the ulnohumeral joint with varus and valgus loads and the elbow at 90°. Notice only minimal radiohumeral contact in this loading condition. (From Stormont T.J., An K.N., Morrey B.F., and Chae E.Y. 1985. *J. Biomech.* 18: 329. Reprinted with permission of Elsevier Science Inc.)

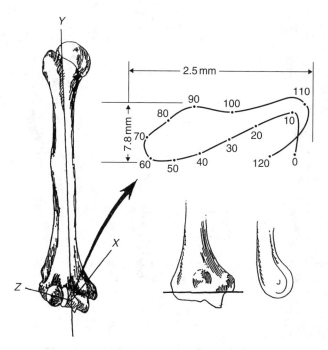

FIGURE 49.25 Very small locus of instant center of rotation for the elbow joint demonstrates that the axis may be replicated by a single line drawn from the inferior aspect of the medial epicondyle through the center of the lateral epicondyle, which is in the center of the lateral projected curvature of the trochlea and capitellum. (From Morrey B.F. and Chao E.Y.S. 1976. *J. Bone Joint Surg.* 58A: 501. With permission.)

normally is greater on average in women [Zuckerman and Matsen, 1989]. As the elbow flexes, the carrying angle varies as a function of flexion (Figure 49.26). In extension there is a valgus angulation of 10°; at full flexion there is a varus angulation of 8° [Morrey and Chao, 1976]. More recently, the three-dimensional kinematics of the ulno–humeral joint under simulated active elbow joint flexion–extension was obtained by using an electromagnetic tracking device [Tanaka et al., 1998]. The optimal axis to best represent flexion–extension motion was found to be close to the line joining the centers of the capitellum and the trochlear groove. Furthermore, the joint laxity under valgus–varus stress was also examined. With the weight of the forearm as the stress, a maximum of 7.6° valgus–varus and 5.3° of axial rotation laxity were observed.

49.6   Wrist

The wrist functions by allowing changes of orientation of the hand relative to the forearm. The wrist joint complex consists of multiple articulations of eight carpal bones with the distal radius, the structures of the ulnocarpal space, the metacarpals, and each other. This collection of bones and soft tissues is capable of a substantial arc of motion that augments hand and finger function.

49.6.1   Geometry of the Articulating Surfaces

The global geometry of the carpal bones has been quantified for grasp and active isometric contraction of the elbow flexors [Schuind et al., 1992]. During grasping there is a significant proximal migration of the radius of 0.9 mm, apparent shortening of the capitate, a decrease in the carpal height ratio, and an increase in the lunate uncovering index (Table 49.16). There is also a trend toward increase of the distal radioulnar joint with grasping. The addition of elbow flexion with concomitant grasping did not significantly change

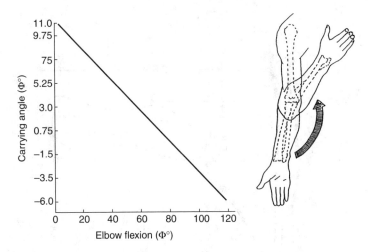

FIGURE 49.26 During elbow flexion and extension, a linear change in the carrying angle is demonstrated, typically going from valgus in extension to varus in flexion. (From Morrey B.F. and Chao E.Y.S. 1976. *J. Bone Joint Surg.* 58A: 501. With permission.)

TABLE 49.16 Changes of Wrist Geometry with Grasp

	Resting	Grasp	Analysis of variance ($p = $ level)
Distal radioulnar joint space (mm)	1.6 ± 0.3	1.8 ± 0.6	0.06
Ulnar variance (mm)	-0.2 ± 1.6	0.7 ± 1.8	0.003
Lunate, uncovered length (mm)	6.0 ± 1.9	7.6 ± 2.6	0.0008
Capitate length (mm)	21.5 ± 2.2	20.8 ± 2.3	0.0002
Carpal height (mm)	33.4 ± 3.4	31.7 ± 3.4	0.0001
Carpal ulnar distance (mm)	15.8 ± 4.0	15.8 ± 3.0	NS
Carpal radial distance (mm)	19.4 ± 1.8	19.7 ± 1.8	NS
Third metacarpal length (mm)	63.8 ± 5.8	62.6 ± 5.5	NS
Carpal height ratio	52.4 ± 3.3	50.6 ± 4.1	0.02
Carpal ulnar ratio	24.9 ± 5.9	25.4 ± 5.3	NS
Lunate uncovering index	36.7 ± 12.1	45.3 ± 14.2	0.002
Carpal radial ratio	30.6 ± 2.4	31.6 ± 2.3	NS
Radius — third metacarpal angle (deg)	-0.3 ± 9.2	-3.1 ± 12.8	NS
Radius — capitate angle (deg)	0.4 ± 15.4	-3.8 ± 22.2	NS

Note: 15 normal subjects with forearm in neutral position and elbow at 90° flexion.
Source: Schuind F.A., Linscheid R.L., An K.N., and Chao E.Y.S. 1992. *J. Hand Surg.* 17A: 698.

the global geometry, except for a significant decrease in the forearm interosseous space [Schuind et al., 1992].

49.6.2 Joint Contact

Studies of the normal biomechanics of the proximal wrist joint have determined that the scaphoid and lunate bones have separate, distinct areas of contact on the distal radius/triangular fibrocartilage complex surface [Viegas et al., 1987] so that the contact areas were localized and accounted for a relatively small fraction of the joint surface, regardless of wrist position (average of 20.6%). The contact areas shift from a more volar location to a more dorsal location as the wrist moves from flexion to extension. Overall, the scaphoid contact area is 1.47 times greater than that of the lunate. The

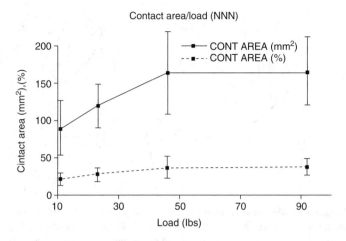

FIGURE 49.27   The nonlinear relation between the contact area and the load at the proximal wrist joint. The contact area was normalized as a percentage of the available joint surface. The load of 11, 23, 46, and 92 lbs was applied at the position of neutral pronation/supination, neutral radioulnar deviation, and neutral flexion/extension. (From Viegas S.F., Patterson R.M., Peterson P.D., Roefs J., Tencer A., and Choi S. 1989. *J. Hand Surg.* 14A: 458. With permission.)

TABLE 49.17   Force Transmission at the Intercarpal Joints

Joint	Force (N)
Radio-ulno-carpal	
Ulno-triquetral	12 ± 3
Ulno-lunate	23 ± 8
Radio-lunate	52 ± 8
Radio-scaphoid	74 ± 13
Midcarpal	
Triquetral-hamate	36 ± 6
Luno-capitate	51 ± 6
Scapho-capitate	32 ± 4
Scapho-trapezial	51 ± 8

Note: A total of 143 N axial force applied across the wrist.

Source: Horii E., Garcia-Elias M., An K.N., Bishop A.T., Cooney W.P., Linscheid R.L., and Chao E.Y. 1990. *J. Bone Joint Surg.* 15A: 393.

scapho-lunate contact area ratio generally increases as the wrist position is changed from radial to ulnar deviation and/or from flexion to extension. Palmer and Werner [1984] also studied pressures in the proximal wrist joint and found that there are three distinct areas of contact: the ulno-lunate, radio-lunate, and radio-scaphoid. They determined that the peak articular pressure in the ulno-lunate fossa is 1.4 N/mm^2, in the radio-ulnate fossa is 3.0 N/mm^2, and in the radio-scaphoid fossa is 3.3 N/mm^2. Viegas et al. [1989] found a nonlinear relationship between increasing load and the joint contact area (Figure 49.27). In general, the distribution of load between the scaphoid and lunate was consistent with all loads tested, with 60% of the total contact area involving the scaphoid and 40% involving the lunate. Loads greater than 46 lbs were found to not significantly increase the overall contact area. The overall contact area, even at the highest loads tested, was not more than 40% of the available joint surface.

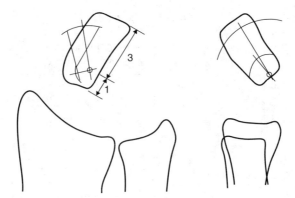

FIGURE 49.28 The location of the center of rotation during ulnar deviation (left) and extension (right), determined graphically using two metal markers embedded in the capitate. Note that during radial–ulnar deviation the center lies at a point in the capitate situated distal to the proximal end of this bone by a distance equivalent to approximately one-quarter of its total longitudinal length. During flexion–extension, the center of rotation is close to the proximal cortex of the capitate. (From Youm Y., McMurty R.Y., Flatt A.E., and Gillespie T.E. 1978. *J. Bone Joint Surg.* 60A: 423. With permission.)

Horii et al. [1990] calculated the total amount of force born by each joint with the intact wrist in the neutral position in the coronal plane and subjected to a total load of 143 N (Table 49.17). They found that 22% of the total force in the radio-ulno–carpal joint is dissipated through the ulna (14% through the ulno-lunate joint, and 18% through the ulno–triquetral joint) and 78% through the radius (46% through the scaphoid fossa and 32% through the lunate fossa). At the midcarpal joint, the scapho–trapezial joint transmits 31% of the total applied force, the scapho–capitate joint transmits 19%, the luno-capitate joint transmits 29%, and the triquetral-hamate joints transmits 21% of the load.

A limited amount of studies have been done to determine the contact areas in the midcarpal joint. Viegas et al. [1990] have found four general areas of contact: the scapho-trapezial-trapezoid (STT), the scapho-capitate (SC), the capito-lunate (CL), and the triquetral-hamate (TH). The high pressure contact area accounted for only 8% of the available joint surface with a load of 32 lbs and increased to a maximum of only 15% with a load of 118 lbs. The total contact area, expressed as a percentage of the total available joint area for each fossa was: STT = 1.3%, SC = 1.8%, CL = 3.1%, and TH = 1.8%.

The correlation between the pressure loading in the wrist and the progress of degenerative osteoarthritis associated with pathological conditions of the forearm was studied in a cadaveric model [Sato, 1995]. Malunion after distal radius fracture, tear of triangular fibrocartilage, and scapholunate dissociation were all responsible for the alteration of the articulating pressure across the wrist joint. Residual articular incongruity of the distal radius following intra-articular fracture has been correlated with early osteoarthritis. In an *in vitro* model, step-offs of the distal radius articular incongruity were created. Mean contact stress was significantly greater than the anatomically reduced case at only 3 mm of step-off [Anderson et al., 1996].

49.6.3 Axes of Rotation

The complexity of joint motion at the wrist makes it difficult to calculate the instant center of motion. However, the trajectories of the hand during radioulnar deviation and flexion/extension, when they occur in a fixed plane, are circular, and the rotation in each plane takes place about a fixed axis. These axes are located within the head of the capitate and are not altered by the position of the hand in the plane of rotation [Youm et al., 1978]. During radioulnar deviation, the instant center of rotation lies at a point in the capitate situated distal to the proximal end of this bone by a distance equivalent to approximately one-quarter of its total length (Figure 49.28). During flexion/extension, the instant center is close to the

TABLE 49.18 Individual Carpal Rotation Relative to the Radius (Deg) (Sagittal Plane Motion of the Wrist)

Wrist motion[a] carpal bone	X (+) Pronation; (−) Supination				Y (+) Flexion; (−) Extension				Z (+) Ulnar deviation; (−) Radial deviation			
	N-E60	N-E30	N-F30	N-F60	N-E60	N-E30	N-F60	N-E60	N-E60	N-E30	N-F30	N-F60
Trapezium ($N = 13$)	−0.9	−1.3	0.9	−1.4	−59.4	−29.3	28.7	54.2	1.2	0.3	−0.4	2.5
SD	2.8	2.2	2.6	2.7	2.3	1	1.8	3	4	2.7	1.3	2.8
Capitate ($N = 22$)	0.9	−1	1.3	−1.6	60.3	−30.2	21.5	63.5	0	0	0.6	3.2
SD	2.7	1.8	2.5	3.5	2.5	1.1	1.2	2.8	2	1.4	1.6	3.6
Hamate ($N = 9$)	0.4	−1	1.3	−0.3	−59.5	−29	28.8	62.6	2.1	0.7	0.1	1.8
SD	3.4	1.7	2.5	2.4	1.4	0.8	10.2	3.6	4.4	1.8	1.2	4.1
Scaphoid ($N = 22$)	−2.5	−0.7	1.6	2	−52.3	−26	20.6	39.7	4.5	0.8	2.1	7.8
SD	3.4	2.6	2.2	3.1	3	3.2	2.8	4.3	3.7	2.1	2.2	4.5
Lunate ($N = 22$)	1.2	0.5	0.3	−2.2	−29.7	−15.4	11.5	23	4.3	0.9	3.3	11.1
SD	2.8	1.8	1.7	2.8	6.6	3.9	3.9	5.9	2.6	1.5	1.9	3.4
Triquetrum ($N = 22$)	−3.5	−2.5	2.5	−0.7	−39.3	−20.1	15.5	30.6	0	−0.3	2.4	9.8
SD	3.5	2	2.2	3.7	4.8	2.7	3.8	5.1	2.8	1.4	2.6	4.3

[a] N-E60: neutral to 60° of extension; N-E30: neutral to 30° of extension; N-F30: neutral to 30° of flexion; N-F60: neutral to 60° of flexion.
SD = standard deviation.
Source: Kobayashi M., Berger R.A., Nagy L. et al. 1997. J. Biomech. 30: 8, 787.

proximal cortex of the capitate, which is somewhat more proximal than the location for the instant center of radioulnar deviation.

Normal carpal kinematics were studied in 22 cadaver specimens using a biplanar radiography method. The kinematics of the trapezium, capitate, hamate, scaphoid, lunate, and triquetrum were determined during wrist rotation in the sagittal and coronal plane [Kobagashi et al., 1997]. The results were expressed using the concept of the screw displacement axis and covered to describe the magnitude of rotation about and translation along three orthogonal axes. The orientation of these axes is expressed relative to the radius during sagittal plane motion of the wrist (Table 49.18). The scaphoid exhibited the greatest magnitude of rotation and the lunate displayed the least rotation. The proximal carpal bones exhibited some ulnar deviation in 60° of wrist flexion. During coronal plane motion (Table 49.19), the magnitude of radial–ulnar deviation of the distal carpal bones was mutually similar and generally of a greater magnitude than that of the proximal carpal bones. The proximal carpal bones experienced some flexion during radial deviation of the wrist and extension during ulnar deviation of the wrist.

49.7 Hand

The hand is an extremely mobile organ that is capable of conforming to a large variety of object shapes and coordinating an infinite variety of movements in relation to each of its components. The mobility of this structure is possible through the unique arrangement of the bones in relation to one another, the articular contours, and the actions of an intricate system of muscles. Theoretical and empirical evidence suggest that limb joint surface morphology is mechanically related to joint mobility, stability, and strength [Hamrick, 1996].

49.7.1 Geometry of the Articulating Surfaces

Three-dimensional geometric models of the articular surfaces of the hand have been constructed. The sagittal contours of the metacarpal head and proximal phalanx grossly resemble the arc of a circle

TABLE 49.19 Individual Carpal Rotation to the Radius (Deg) (Coronal Plane Motion of the Wrist)

| | Axis of rotation | | | | | | | | |
| Wrist motion[a] carpal bone | X (+) Pronation; (−) Supination | | | Y (+) Flexion; (−) Extension | | | Z (+) Ulnar deviation; (−) Radial deviation | | |
	N-RD15	N-UD15	N-UD30	N-RD15	N-UD15	N-UD30	N-RD15	N-UD15	N-UD30
Trapezium (N = 13)	−4.8	9.1	16.3	0	4.9	9.9	−14.3	16.4	32.5
S.D.	2.4	3.6	3.6	1.5	1.3	2.1	2.3	2.8	2.6
Capitate (N = 22)	−3.9	6.8	11.8	1.3	2.7	6.5	−14.6	15.9	30.7
S.D.	2.6	2.6	2.5	1.5	1.1	1.7	2.1	1.4	1.7
Hamate (N = 9)	−4.8	6.3	10.6	1.1	3.5	6.6	−15.5	15.4	30.2
S.D.	1.8	2.4	3.1	3	3.2	4.1	2.4	2.6	3.6
Scaphoid (N = 22)	0.8	2.2	6.6	8.5	−12.5	−17.1	−4.2	4.3	13.6
S.D.	1.8	2.4	3.1	3	3.2	4.1	2.4	2.6	3.6
Lunate (N = 22)	−1.2	1.4	3.9	7	−13.9	−22.5	−1.7	5.7	15
S.D.	1.6	0	3.3	3.1	4.3	6.9	1.7	2.8	4.3
Triquetrum (N = 22)	−1.1	−1	0.8	4.1	−10.5	−17.3	−5.1	7.7	18.4
S.D.	1.4	2.6	4	3	3.8	6	2.4	2.2	4

[a] N-RD15: neutral to 15° of radial deviation; N-UD30: neutral to 30° of ulnar deviation; N-UD15: neutral to 15° of ulnar deviation.

S.D. = standard deviation.

Source: Kobayashi M., Berger R.A., Nagy L., et al. 1997. *J. Biomech.* 30: 8, 787.

TABLE 49.20 Radius of Curvature of the Middle Sections of the Metacarpal Head and Proximal Phalanx Base

| | Radius (mm) | |
	Bony contour	Cartilage contour
MCH index	6.42 ± 1.23	6.91 ± 1.03
Long	6.44 ± 1.08	6.66 ± 1.18
PPB index	13.01 ± 4.09	12.07 ± 3.29
Long	11.46 ± 2.30	11.02 ± 2.48

Source: Tamai K., Ryu J., An K.N., Linscheid R.L., Cooney W.P., and Chao E.Y.S. 1988. *J. Hand Surg.* 13A: 521.

[Tamai et al., 1988]. The radius of curvature of a circle fitted to the entire proximal phalanx surface ranges from 11 to 13 mm, almost twice as much as that of the metacarpal head, which ranges from 6 to 7 mm (Table 49.20). The local centers of curvature along the sagittal contour of the metacarpal heads are not fixed. The locus of the center of curvature for the subchondral bony contour approximates the locus of the center for the acute curve of an ellipse (Figure 49.29). However, the locus of center of curvature for the articular cartilage contour approximates the locus of the obtuse curve of an ellipse.

The surface geometry of the thumb carpometacarpal (CMC) joint has also been quantified [Athesian et al., 1992]. The surface area of the CMC joint is significantly greater for males than for females (Table 49.21). The minimum, maximum, and mean square curvature of these joints is reported in Table 49.21. The curvature of the surface is denoted by κ and the radius of curvature is $\rho = 1/\kappa$. The curvature is negative when the surface is concave and positive when the surface is convex.

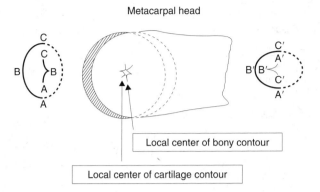

FIGURE 49.29 The loci of the local centers of curvature for subchondral bony contour of the metacarpal head approximates the loci of the center for the acute curve of an ellipse. The loci of the local center of curvature for articular cartilage contour of the metacarpal head approximates the loci of the bony center of the obtuse curve of an ellipse. (From Tamai K., Ryu J., An K.N., Linscheid R.L., Cooney W.P., and Chao E.Y.S. 1988. *J. Hand Surg.* 13A: 521. Reprinted with permission of Churchill Livingstone.)

TABLE 49.21 Curvature of Carpometacarpal Joint Articular Surfaces

	n	Area (cm^2)	$\bar{\kappa}_{min}$ (m^{-1})	$\bar{\kappa}_{max}$ (m^{-1})	$\bar{\kappa}_{rms}$ (m^{-1})
Trapezium					
Female	8	1.05 ± 0.21	-61 ± 22	190 ± 36	165 ± 32
Male	5	1.63 ± 0.18	-87 ± 17	114 ± 19	118 ± 6
Total	13	1.27 ± 0.35	-71 ± 24	161 ± 48	147 ± 34
Female vs. male		$p \leq 0.01$	$p \leq 0.05$	$p \leq 0.01$	$p \leq 0.01$
Metacarpal					
Female	8	1.22 ± 0.36	-49 ± 10	175 ± 25	154 ± 20
Male	5	1.74 ± 0.21	-37 ± 11	131 ± 17	116 ± 8
Total	13	1.42 ± 0.40	-44 ± 12	158 ± 31	140 ± 25
Female vs. male		$p \leq 0.01$	$p \leq 0.05$	$p \leq 0.01$	$p \leq 0.01$

Note: Radius of curvature: $\rho = 1/\kappa$.

Source: Athesian J.A., Rosenwasser M.P., and Mow V.C. 1992. *J. Biomech.* 25: 591.

49.7.2 Joint Contact

The size and location of joint contact areas of the metacarpophalangeal (MCP) joint changes as a function of the joint flexion angle (Figure 49.30) The radioulnar width of the contact area becomes narrow in the neutral position and expands in both the hyperextended and fully flexed positions [An and Cooney, 1991]. In the neutral position, the contact area occurs in the center of the phalangeal base, this area being slightly larger on the ulnar than on the radial side.

The contact areas of the thumb carpometacarpal joint under the functional position of lateral key pinch and in the extremes of range of motion were studied using a stereophotogrammetric technique [Ateshian et al., 1995]. The lateral pinch position produced contact predominately on the central, volar, and volar–ulnar regions of the trapezium and the metacarpals (Figure 49.31). Pelligrini et al. [1993] noted that the palmar compartment of the trapeziometacarpal joint was the primary contact area during flexion adduction of the thumb in lateral pinch. Detachment of the palmar beak ligament resulted in dorsal translation of the contact area producing a pattern similar to that of cartilage degeneration seen in the osteoarthritic joint.

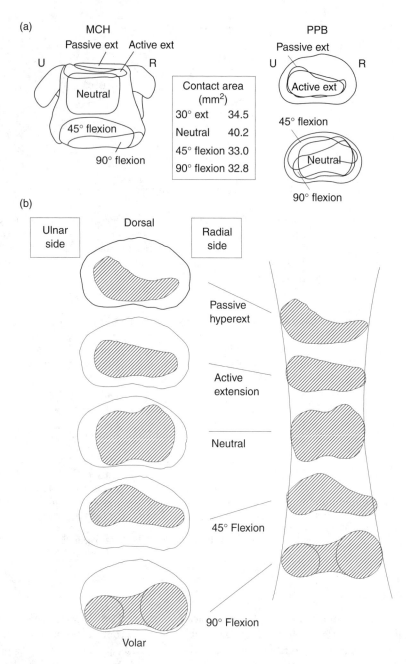

FIGURE 49.30   (a) Contact area of the MCP joint in five joint positions. (b) End on view of the contact area on each of the proximal phalanx bases. The radioulnar width of the contact area becomes narrow in the neutral position and expands in both the hyperextended and fully flexed positions. (From An K.N. and Cooney W.P. 1991. In B.F. Morrey (Ed.), *Joint Replacement Arthroplasty*, pp. 137–146, New York, Churchill Livingstone. By permission of Mayo Foundation.)

49.7.3   Axes of Rotation

Rolling and sliding actions of articulating surfaces exist during finger joint motion. The geometric shapes of the articular surfaces of the metacarpal head and proximal phalanx, as well as the insertion location

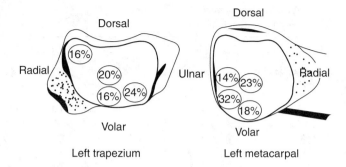

FIGURE 49.31 Summary of the contact areas for all specimens, in lateral pinch with a 25 N load. All results from the right hand are transposed onto the schema of a carpometacarpal joint from the left thumb. (From Ateshian G.A., Ark J.W., Rosenwasser M.P., et al. 1995. *J. Orthop. Res.* 13: 450.)

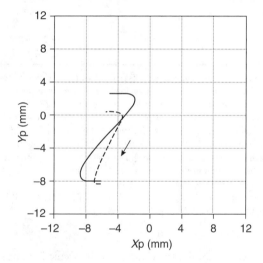

FIGURE 49.32 Intersections of the instantaneous helical angles with the metacarpal sagittal plane. They are relative to one subject tested twice in different days. The origin of the graph is coincident with the calibrated center of the metacarpal head. The arrow indicates the direction of flexion. (From Fioretti S. 1994. In F. Schuind et al. (Eds.). *Advances in the Biomechanics of the Hand and Wrist*, pp. 363–375, New York, Plenum Press. With permission.)

of the collateral ligaments, significantly govern the articulating kinematics, and the center of rotation is not fixed but rather moves as a function of the angle of flexion [Pagowski and Piekarski, 1977]. The instant centers of rotation are within 3 mm of the center of the metacarpal head [Walker and Erhman, 1975]. Recently the axis of rotation of the MCP joint has been evaluated *in vivo* by Fioretti [1994]. The instantaneous helical axis of the MCP joint tends to be more palmar and tends to be displaced distally as flexion increases (Figure 49.32).

The axes of rotation of the CMC joint have been described as being fixed [Hollister et al., 1992], but others believe that a polycentric center of rotation exists [Imaeda et al., 1994]. Hollister et al. [1992] found that axes of the CMC joint are fixed and are not perpendicular to each other, or to the bones, and do not intersect. The flexion/extension axis is located in the trapezium, and the abduction/adduction axis is on the first metacarpal. In contrast, Imaeda et al. [1994] found that there was no single center of rotation, but rather the instantaneous motion occurred reciprocally between centers of rotations within the trapezium and the metacarpal base of the normal thumb. In flexion/extension,

TABLE 49.22 Location of Center of Rotation of
Trapeziometacarpal Joint

	Mean $\pm$ SD (mm)
Circumduction	
X	0.1 ± 1.3
Y	-0.6 ± 1.3
Z	-0.5 ± 1.4
Flexion/extension (in x–y plane)	
X	
Centroid	-4.2 ± 1.0
Radius	2.0 ± 0.5
Y	
Centroid	-0.4 ± 0.9
Radius	1.6 ± 0.5
Abduction/adduction (in x–z plane)	
X	
Centroid	6.7 ± 1.7
Radius	4.6 ± 3.1
Z	
Centroid	-0.2 ± 0.7
Radius	1.7 ± 0.5

Note: The coordinate system is defined with the x-axis corresponding to internal/external rotation, the y-axis corresponding to abduction/adduction, and the z-axis corresponding to flexion/extension. The x-axis is positive in the distal direction, the y-axis is positive in the dorsal direction for the left hand and in the palmar direction for the right hand, and the z-axis is positive in the radial direction. The origin of the coordinate system was at the intersection of a line connecting the radial and ulnar prominences and a line connecting the volar and dorsal tubercles.

Source: Imaeda T., Niebur G., Cooney W.P., Linscheid R.L., and An K.N. 1994. *J. Orthop. Res.* 12: 197.

the axis of rotation was located within the trapezium, but for abduction/adduction the center of rotation was located distally to the trapezium and within the base of the first metacarpal. The average instantaneous center of circumduction was at approximately the center of the trapezial joint surface (Table 49.22).

The axes of rotation of the thumb interphalangeal and metacarpophalangeal joint were located using a mechanical device [Hollister et al., 1995]. The physiologic motion of the thumb joints occur about these axes (Figure 49.33 and Table 49.23). The interphalangeal joint axis is parallel to the flexion crease of the joint and is not perpendicular to the phalanx. The metacarpophalangeal joint has two fixed axes: a fixed flexion–extension axis just distal and volar to the epicondyles, and an abduction–adduction axis related to the proximal phalanx passing between the sesamoids. Neither axis is perpendicular to the phalanges.

49.8 Summary

It is important to understand the biomechanics of joint-articulating surface motion. The specific characteristics of the joint will determine the musculoskeletal function of that joint. The unique geometry of the joint surfaces and the surrounding capsule ligamentous constraints will guide the unique characteristics of the articulating surface motion. The range of joint motion, the stability of the joint, and the ultimate functional strength of the joint will depend on these specific characteristics. A congruent joint usually has a relatively limited range of motion but a high degree of stability, whereas a less

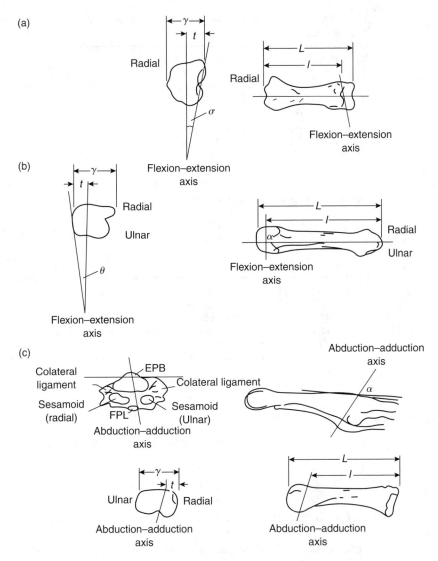

FIGURE 49.33   (a) The angles and length and breadth measurements defining the axis of rotation of the interphalangeal joint of the right thumb. (t/T = ratio of anatomic plane diameter; l/L = ratio of length). (b) The angles and length and breadth measurements of the metacarpophalangeal flexion–extension axis' position in the metacarpal. (c) The angles and length and breadth measurements that locate the metacarpophalangeal abduction–adduction axis. The measurements are made in the metacarpal when the metacapophalangeal joint is at neutral flexion extension. The measurements are made relative to the metacarpal because the axis passes through this bone, not the proximal phalanx with which it moves. This method of recording the abduction–adduction measurements allows the measurements of the axes to each other at a neutral position to be made. The metacarpophalangeal abduction–adduction axis passes through the volar plate of the proximal phalanx. (From Hollister A., Giurintano D.J., Buford W.L., et al. *Clin. Orthop. Relat. Res.* 320: 188, 1995.)

congruent joint will have a relatively larger range of motion but less degree of stability. The characteristics of the joint-articulating surface will determine the pattern of joint contact and the axes of rotation. These characteristics will regulate the stresses on the joint surface which will influence the degree of degeneration of articular cartilage in an anatomic joint and the amount of wear of an artificial joint.

TABLE 49.23   Measurement of Axis Location and Values for Axis Position in the Bone[a]

Interphalangeal joint flexion-extension axis (Figure 49.33a)	
t/T	$44 \pm 17\%$
l/L	$90 \pm 5\%$
Θ	$5 \pm 2°$
β	$83 \pm 4°$
Metacarpophalangeal joint flexion-extension axis (Figure 49.33b)	
t/T	$57 \pm 17\%$
l/L	$87 \pm 5\%$
α	$101 \pm 6°$
β	$5 \pm 2°$
Metacarpophalangeal joint abduction-adduction axis (Figure 49.33c)	
t/T	$45 \pm 8\%$
l/L	$83 \pm 13\%$
α	$80 \pm 9°$
β	$74 \pm 8°$
M	

[a] The angle of the abduction-adduction axis with respect to the flexion-extension axis is $84.8 \pm 12.2°$. The location and angulation of the K-wires of the axes with respect to the bones were measured (Θ, α, β) directly with a goniometer. The positions of the pins in the bones were measured (T, L) with a Vernier caliper.

Source: Hollister A., Giurintano D.J., Buford W.L. et al. 1995. *Clin. Orthop. Relat. Res.* 320: 188.

Acknowledgment

The authors thank Barbara Iverson-Literski for her careful preparation of the manuscript.

References

Ahmed A.M., Burke D.L., and Hyder A. 1987. Force analysis of the patellar mechanism. *J. Orthop. Res.* 5: 1, 69.

Allard P., Duhaime M., Labelle H., et al. 1987. Spatial reconstruction technique and kinematic modeling of the ankle. *IEEE Eng. Med. Biol.* 6: 31.

An K.N. and Cooney W.P. 1991. Biomechanics, Section II. The hand and wrist. In B.F. Morrey (Ed.), *Joint Replacement Arthroplasty*, pp. 137–146, New York, Churchill Livingstone.

Anderson D.D., Bell A.L., Gaffney M.B. et al. 1996. Contact stress distributions in malreduced intra-articular distal radius fractures. *J. Orthop. Trauma* 10: 331.

Andriacchi T.P., Stanwyck T.S., and Galante J.O. 1986. Knee biomechanics in total knee replacement. *J. Arthroplasty* 1: 211.

Ateshian G.A., Ark J.W., Rosenwasser M.D., et al. 1995. Contact areas in the thumb carpometacarpal joint. *J. Orthop. Res.* 13: 450.

Athesian J.A., Rosenwasser M.P., and Mow V.C. 1992. Curvature characteristics and congruence of the thumb carpometacarpal joint: differences between female and male joints. *J. Biomech.* 25: 591.

Barnett C.H. and Napier J.R. 1952. The axis of rotation at the ankle joint in man. Its influence upon the form of the talus and the mobility of the fibula. *J. Anat.* 86: 1.

Basmajian J.V. and Bazant F.J. 1959. Factors preventing downward dislocation of the adducted shoulder joint. An electromyographic and morphological study. *J. Bone Joint Surg.* 41A: 1182.

Boileau P. and Walch G. 1997. The three-dimensional geometry of the proximal humerus. *J. Bone Joint Surg.* 79B: 857.

D'Ambrosia R.D., Shoji H., and Van Meter J. 1976. Rotational axis of the ankle joint: comparison of normal and pathological states. *Surg. Forum* 27: 507.

Davy D.T., Kotzar D.M., Brown R.H. et al. 1989. Telemetric force measurements across the hip after total arthroplasty. *J. Bone Joint Surg.* 70A: 45.

Doody S.G., Freedman L., and Waterland J.C. 1970. Shoulder movements during abduction in the scapular plane. *Arch. Phys. Med. Rehabil.* 51: 595.

Draganich L.F., Andriacchi T.P., and Andersson G.B.J. 1987. Interaction between intrinsic knee mechanics and the knee extensor mechanism. *J. Orthop. Res.* 5: 539.

Driscoll H.L., Christensen J.C., and Tencer A.F. 1994. Contact characteristics of the ankle joint. *J. Am. Pediatr. Med. Assoc.* 84: 491.

Elftman H. 1945. The orientation of the joints of the lower extremity. *Bull. Hosp. Joint Dis.* 6: 139.

Engsberg J.R. 1987. A biomechanical analysis of the talocalcaneal joint *in vitro*. *J. Biomech.* 20: 429.

Farahmand F., Senavongse W., and Amis A.A. 1998. Quantitative study of the quadriceps muscles and trochlear groove geometry related to instability of the patellofemoral joint. *J. Orthop. Res.* 16: 136.

Fioretti S. 1994. Three-dimensional *in-vivo* kinematic analysis of finger movement. In F. Schuind et al. (Eds.), *Advances in the Biomechanics of the Hand and Wrist*, pp. 363–375, New York, Plenum.

Freedman L. and Munro R.R. 1966. Abduction of the arm in the scapular plane: scapular and glenohumeral movements. A roentgenographic study. *J. Bone Joint Surg.* 48A: 1503.

Goel V.K., Singh D., and Bijlani V. 1982. Contact areas in human elbow joints. *J. Biomech. Eng.* 104: 169–175.

Goodfellow J., Hungerford D.S., and Zindel M. 1976. Patellofemoral joint mechanics and pathology. *J. Bone Joint Surg.* 58B: 287.

Hamrick M.W. 1996. Articular size and curvature as detriments of carpal joint mobility and stability in strepsirhine primates. *J. Morphol.* 230: 113.

Hartford J.M., Gorczyca J.T., McNamara J.L. et al. 1985. Tibiotalar contact area. *Clin. Orthop.* 320: 82.

Hicks J.H. 1953. The mechanics of the foot. The joints. *J. Anat.* 87: 345–357.

Hollister A., Buford W.L., Myers L.M. et al. 1992. The axes of rotation of the thumb carpometacarpal joint. *J. Orthop. Res.* 10: 454.

Hollister A., Guirintano D.J., Bulford W.L., et al. 1995. The axes of rotation of the thumb interphalangeal and metacarpophalangeal joints. *Clin. Orthop.* 320: 188.

Horii E., Garcia-Elias M., An K.N., et al. 1990. Effect of force transmission across the carpus in procedures used to treat Kienböck's disease. *J. Bone Joint Surg.* 15A: 393.

Huberti H.H. and Hayes W.C. 1984. Patellofemoral contact pressures: the influence of Q-angle and tendofemoral contact. *J. Bone Joint Surg.* 66A: 715.

Iannotti J.P., Gabriel J.P., Schneck S.L., et al. 1992. The normal glenohumeral relationships: an anatomical study of 140 shoulders. *J. Bone Joint Surg.* 74A: 491.

Imaeda T., Niebur G., Cooney W.P., et al. 1994. Kinematics of the normal trapeziometacarpal joint. *J. Orthop. Res.* 12: 197.

Inman V.T., Saunders J.B. deCM, and Abbott L.C. 1944. Observations on the function of the shoulder joint. *J. Bone Joint Surg.* 26A: 1.

Inman V.T. 1976. *The Joints of the Ankle*, Baltimore, Williams and Wilkins.

Inman V.T. and Mann R.A. 1979. Biomechanics of the foot and ankle. In V.T. Inman (Ed.), *DuVrie's Surgery of the Foot*, St Louis, Mosby.

Iseki F. and Tomatsu T. 1976. The biomechanics of the knee joint with special reference to the contact area. *Keio. J. Med.* 25: 37.

Isman R.E. and Inman V.T. 1969. Anthropometric studies of the human foot and ankle. *Pros. Res.* 10–11: 97.

Jobe C.M. and Iannotti J.P. 1995. Limits imposed on glenohumeral motion by joint geometry. *J. Shoulder Elbow Surg.* 4: 281.

Kapandji I.A. 1987. *The Physiology of the Joints*, Vol. 2, Lower Limb, Edinburgh, Churchill-Livingstone, Edinburgh.

Karduna A.R., Williams G.R., Williams J.I. et al. 1996. Kinematics of the glenohumeral joint: influences of muscle forces, ligamentous constraints, and articular geometry. *J. Orthop. Res.* 14: 986.

Kent B.E. 1971. Functional anatomy of the shoulder complex. A review. *Phys. Ther.* 51: 867.

Kimizuka M., Kurosawa H., and Fukubayashi T. 1980. Load-bearing pattern of the ankle joint. Contact area and pressure distribution. *Arch. Orthop. Trauma Surg.* 96: 45–49.

Kinzel G.L., Hall A.L., and Hillberry B.M. 1972. Measurement of the total motion between two body segments: Part I. Analytic development. *J. Biomech.* 5: 93.

Kirby K.A. 1947. Methods for determination of positional variations in the subtalar and transverse tarsal joints. *Anat. Rec.* 80: 397.

Kobayashi M., Berger R.A., Nagy L., et al. 1997. Normal kinematics of carpal bones: a three-dimensional analysis of carpal bone motion relative to the radius. *J. Biomech.* 30: 787.

Kurosawa H., Walker P.S., Abe S. et al. 1985. Geometry and motion of the knee for implant and orthotic design. *J. Biomech.* 18: 487.

Lewis J.L. and Lew W.D. 1978. A method for locating an optimal "fixed" axis of rotation for the human knee joint. *J. Biomech. Eng.* 100: 187.

Libotte M., Klein P., Colpaert H. et al. 1982. Contribution à l'étude biomécanique de la pince malléolaire. *Rev. Chir. Orthop.* 68: 299.

Lippitts B., Vanderhooft J.E., Harris S.L. et al. 1993. Glenohumeral stability from concavity-compression: a quantitative analysis. *J. Shoulder Elbow Surg.* 2: 27.

Matsuda S., Miura H., Nagamine R., Mawatari T., Tokunaga M., Nabeyama R., and Iwamoto Y. 2004. Anatomical analysis of the femoral condyle in normal and osteoarthritic knees. *J. Orthop. Res.* 22: 104–109.

Macko V.W., Matthews L.S., Zwirkoski P. et al. 1991. The joint contract area of the ankle: the contribution of the posterior malleoli. *J. Bone Joint Surg.* 73A: 347.

Manter J.T. 1941. Movements of the subtalar and transverse tarsal joints. *Anat. Rec.* 80: 397–402.

Maquet P.G., Vandberg A.J., and Simonet J.C. 1975. Femorotibial weight bearing areas: experimental determination. *J. Bone Joint Surg.* 57A: 766–771.

McPherson E.J., Friedman R.J., An Y.H. et al. 1997. Anthropometric study of normal glenohumeral relationships. *J. Shoulder Elbow Surg.* 6: 105.

Merz B., Eckstein F., Hillebrand S. et al. 1997. Mechanical implication of humero-ulnar incongruity-finite element analysis and experiment. *J. Biomech.* 30: 713.

Miyanaga Y., Fukubayashi T., and Kurosawa H. 1984. Contact study of the hip joint: load deformation pattern, contact area, and contact pressure. *Arch. Orth. Trauma Surg.* 103: 13–17.

Morrey B.F. and An K.N. 1990. Biomechanics of the shoulder. In C.A. Rockwood and F.A. Matsen (Eds.), *The Shoulder*, pp. 208–245, Philadelphia, Saunders.

Morrey B.F. and Chao E.Y.S. 1976. Passive motion of the elbow joint: a biomechanical analysis. *J. Bone Joint Surg.* 58A: 501.

Nahass B.E., Madson M.M., and Walker P.S. 1991. Motion of the knee after condylar resurfacing — an *in vivo* study. *J. Biomech.* 24: 1107.

Paar O., Rieck B., and Bernett P. 1983. Experimentelle untersuchungen über belastungsabhängige Drukund Kontaktflächenverläufe an den Fussgelenken. *Unfallheilkunde* 85: 531.

Pagowski S. and Piekarski K. 1977. Biomechanics of metacarpophalangeal joint. *J. Biomech.* 10: 205.

Palmer A.K. and Werner F.W. 1984. Biomechanics of the distal radio–ulnar joint. *Clin. Orthop.* 187: 26.

Parlasca R., Shoji H., and D'Ambrosia R.D. 1979. Effects of ligamentous injury on ankle and subtalar joints. A kinematic study. *Clin. Orthop.* 140: 266.

Pellegrini V.S., Olcott V.W., and Hollenberg C. 1993. Contact patterns in the trapeziometacarpal joint: the role of the palmar beak ligament. *J. Hand Surg.* 18A: 238.

Pereira D.S., Koval K.J., Resnick R.B., et al. 1996. Tibiotalar contact area and pressure distribution: the effect of mortise widening and syndesmosis fixation. *Foot Ankle* 17: 269.

Poppen N.K. and Walker P.S. 1976. Normal and abnormal motion of the shoulder. *J. Bone Joint Surg.* 58A: 195.

Ramsey P.L. and Hamilton W. 1976. Changes in tibiotalar area of contact caused by lateral talar shift. *J. Bone Joint Surg.* 58A: 356.

Rastegar J., Miller N., and Barmada R. 1980. An apparatus for measuring the load-displacement and load-dependent kinematic characteristics of articulating joints — application to the human ankle. *J. Biomech. Eng.* 102: 208.

Rosenbaum D., Eils E., and Hillmann A. 2003. Changes in talocrural joint contact stress characteristics after simulated rotationplasty. *J. Biomech.* 36: 81–86.

Root M.L., Weed J.H., Sgarlato T.E., and Bluth D.R. 1966. Axis of motion of the subtalar joint. *J. Am. Pediatry Assoc.* 56: 149.

Saha A.K. 1971. Dynamic stability of the glenohumeral joint. *Acta Orthop. Scand.* 42: 491.

Sammarco G.J., Burstein A.J., and Frankel V.H. 1973. Biomechanics of the ankle: a kinematic study. *Orthop. Clin. North Am.* 4: 75–96.

Sato S. 1995. Load transmission through the wrist joint: a biomechanical study comparing the normal and pathological wrist. Nippon Seikeigeka Gakkai Zasshi-Journal of the Japanese *Orthopaedic Association* 69: 470–483.

Scarvell J.M., Smith P.N., Refshauge K.M., Galloway H.R., and Woods K.R. 2004. Evaluation of a method to map tibiofemoral contact points in the normal knee using MRI. *J. Orthop. Res.* 22: 788–793.

Schuind F.A., Linscheid R.L., An K.N. et al. 1992. Changes in wrist and forearm configuration with grasp and isometric contraction of elbow flexors. *J. Hand Surg.* 17A: 698.

Shephard E. 1951. Tarsal movements. *J. Bone Joint Surg.* 33B: 258.

Shiba R., Sorbie C., Siu D.W. et al. 1988. Geometry of the humeral–ulnar joint. *J. Orthop. Res.* 6: 897.

Singh A.K., Starkweather K.D., Hollister A.M. et al. 1992. Kinematics of the ankle: a hinge axis model. *Foot Ankle* 13: 439.

Soslowsky L.J., Flatow E.L., Bigliani L.U. et al. 1992. Quantitation of in situ contact areas at the glenohumeral joint: a biomechanical study. *J. Orthop. Res.* 10: 524.

Spoor C.W. and Veldpaus F.E. 1980. Rigid body motion calculated from spatial coordinates of markers. *J. Biomech.* 13: 391.

Stormont T.J., An K.A., Morrey B.F. et al. 1985. Elbow joint contact study: comparison of techniques. *J. Biomech.* 18: 329.

Tamai K., Ryu J., An K.N., et al. 1988. Three-dimensional geometric analysis of the metacarpophalangeal joint. *J. Hand Surg.* 13A: 521.

Tanaka S., An K.N., and Morrey B.F. 1998. Kinematics and laxity of ulnohumeral joint under valgus–varus stress. *J. Musculoskeletal Res.* 2: 45.

Tönnis D. 1987. *Congenital Dysplasia and Dislocation of the Hip and Shoulder in Adults*, pp. 1–12, Berlin, Springer-Verlag.

Van Eijden T.M.G.J., Kouwenhoven E., Verburg J., et al. 1986. A mathematical model of the patellofemoral joint. *J. Biomech.* 19: 219.

Van Langelaan E.J. 1983. A kinematical analysis of the tarsal joints. An x-ray photogrammetric study. *Acta Orthop. Scand.* 204: 211.

Viegas S.F., Tencer A.F., Cantrell J. et al. 1987. Load transfer characteristics of the wrist: Part I. The normal joint. *J. Hand Surg.* 12A: 971.

Viegas S.F., Patterson R.M., Peterson P.D. et al. 1989. The effects of various load paths and different loads on the load transfer characteristics of the wrist. *J. Hand Surg.* 14A: 458.

Viegas S.F., Patterson R.M., Todd P. et al. October 7, 1990. Load transfer characteristics of the midcarpal joint. Presented at *Wrist Biomechanics Symposium*, Wrist Biomechanics Workshop, Mayo Clinic, Rochester, MN.

Von Lanz D. and Wauchsmuth W. 1938. *Das Hüftgelenk, Praktische Anatomie* I Bd, pp. 138–175, Teil 4: Bein und Statik, Berlin, Springer-Verlag.

Wagner U.A., Sangeorzan B.J., Harrington R.M. et al. 1992. Contact characteristics of the subtalar joint: load distribution between the anterior and posterior facets. *J. Orthop. Res.* 10: 535.

Walker P.S. and Erhman M.J. 1975. Laboratory evaluation of a metaplastic type of metacarpophalangeal joint prosthesis. *Clin. Orthop.* 112: 349.

Wang C.-L., Cheng C.-K., Chen C.-W. et al. 1994. Contact areas and pressure distributions in the subtalar joint. *J. Biomech.* 28: 269.

Woltring H.J., Huiskes R., deLange A., and Veldpaus F.E. 1985. Finite centroid and helical axis estimation from noisy landmark measurements in the study of human joint kinematics. *J. Biomech.* 18: 379.

Yoshioka Y., Siu D., and Cooke T.D.V. 1987. The anatomy and functional axes of the femur. *J. Bone Joint Surg.* 69A: 873.

Yoshioka Y., Siu D., Scudamore R.A. et al. 1989. Tibial anatomy in functional axes. *J. Orthop. Res.* 7: 132.

Youm Y., McMurty R.Y., Flatt A.E. et al. 1978. Kinematics of the wrist: an experimental study of radioulnar deviation and flexion/extension. *J. Bone Joint Surg.* 60A: 423.

Zuckerman J.D. and Matsen F.A. 1989. Biomechanics of the elbow. In M. Nordine and V.H. Frankel (Eds.), *Basic Biomechanics of the Musculoskeletal System*, pp. 249–260, Philadelphia, Lea & Febiger.

50

Joint Lubrication

Michael J. Furey
Virginia Polytechnic Institute and State University

The Fabric of the Joints in the Human Body is a subject so much the more entertaining, as it must strike every one that considers it attentively with an Idea of fine Mechanical Composition. Wherever the Motion of one Bone upon another is requisite, there we find an excellent Apparatus for rendering that Motion safe and free: We see, for Instance, the Extremity of one Bone molded into an orbicular Cavity, to receive the Head of another, in order to afford it an extensive Play. Both are covered with a smooth elastic Crust, to prevent mutual Abrasion; connected with strong Ligaments, to prevent Dislocation; and inclosed in a Bag that contains a proper Fluid Deposited there, for lubricating the Two contiguous Surfaces. So much in general.

The above is the opening paragraph of the classic paragraph of the classic paper by the surgeon, Sir William Hunter, "Of the Structure and Diseases of Articulating Cartilages" which he read to a meeting of the Royal Society, June 2, 1743 [1]. Since then, a great deal of research has been carried out on the subject of synovial joint lubrication. However, the mechanisms involved are still unknown.

50.1 Introduction

The purpose of this article is twofold: (1) to introduce the reader to the subject of tribology — the study of friction, wear, and lubrication; and (2) to extend this to the topic of *biotribology*, which includes the lubrication of natural synovial joints. It is not meant to be an exhaustive review of joint lubrication theories; space does not permit this. Instead, major concepts or principles will be discussed not only in the light of what is known about synovial joint lubrication but perhaps more importantly what is not known. Several references are given for those who wish to learn more about the topic. It is clear that synovial joints are by far the most complex and sophisticated tribological systems that exist. We shall see that although numerous theories have been put forth to attempt to explain joint lubrication, the mechanisms involved are still far from being understood. And when one begins to examine possible connections between tribology and degenerative joint disease or osteoarthritis, the picture is even more complex and controversial. Finally, this article does not treat the (1) tribological behavior of artificial joints or partial joint replacements, (2) the possible use of elastic or poroplastic materials as artificial cartilage, and (3) new developments in cartilage repair using transplanted chondrocytes. These are separate topics, which would require detailed discussion and additional space.

50.2 Tribology

The word tribology, derived from the Greek "to rub," covers all frictional processes between solid bodies moving relative to one another that are in contact [2]. Thus tribology may be defined as the study of friction, wear, and lubrication.

Tribological processes are involved whenever one solid slides or rolls against another, as in bearings, cams, gears, piston rings and cylinders, machining and metalworking, grinding, rock drilling, sliding electrical contacts, frictional welding, brakes, the striking of a match, music from a cello, articulation of human synovial joints (e.g., hip joints), machinery, and in numerous less obvious processes (e.g., walking, holding, stopping, writing, and the use of fasteners such as nails, screws, and bolts).

Tribology is a multidisciplinary subject involving at least the areas of materials science, solid and surface mechanics, surface science and chemistry, rheology, engineering, mathematics, and even biology and biochemistry. Although tribology is still an emerging science, interest in the phenomena of friction, wear, and lubrication is an ancient one. Unlike thermodynamics, there are no generally accepted laws in tribology. But there are some important basic principles needed to understand any study of lubrication and wear and even more so in a study of biotribology or biological lubrication phenomena. These basic principles follow.

50.2.1 Friction

Much of the early work in tribology was in the area of friction — possibly because frictional effects are more readily demonstrated and measured. Generally, early theories of friction dealt with dry or unlubricated systems. The problem was often treated strictly from a mechanical viewpoint, with little or no regard for the environment, surface films, or chemistry.

In the first place, *friction may be defined as the tangential resistance that is offered to the sliding of one solid body over another*. Friction is the result of many factors and cannot be treated as something as singular as density or even viscosity. Postulated sources of friction have included (1) the lifting of one asperity over another (increase in potential energy), (2) the interlocking of asperities followed by shear, (3) interlocking followed by plastic deformation or plowing, (4) adhesion followed by shear, (5) elastic hysteresis and waves of deformation, (6) adhesion or interlocking followed by tensile failure, (7) intermolecular attraction, (8) electrostatic effects, and (9) viscous drag. The coefficient of friction, indicated in the literature by μ or f, is defined as the ratio F/W where F = friction force and W = the normal load. It is emphasized that friction is a force and not a property of a solid material or lubricant.

50.2.2 Wear and Surface Damage

One definition of wear in a tribological sense is that it is the *progressive loss of substance from the operating surface of a body as a result of relative motion at the surface.* In comparison with friction, very little theoretical work has been done on the extremely important area of wear and surface damage. This is not too surprising in view of the complexity of wear and how little is known of the mechanisms by which it can occur. Variations in wear can be, and often are, enormous compared with variations in friction. For example, practically all the coefficients of sliding friction for diverse dry or lubricated systems fall within a relatively narrow range of 0.1 to 1. In some cases (e.g., certain regimes of hydrodynamic or "boundary" lubrication), the coefficient of friction may be <0.1 and as low as 0.001. In other cases (e.g., very clean unlubricated metals in vacuum), friction coefficients may exceed one. Reduction of friction by a factor of two through changes in design, materials, or lubricant would be a reasonable, although not always attainable, goal. On the other hand, it is not uncommon for wear rates to vary by a factor of 100, 1000, or even more.

For systems consisting of common materials (e.g., metals, polymers, ceramics), there are at least four main mechanisms by which wear and surface damage can occur between solids in relative motion: (1) abrasive wear, (2) adhesive wear, (3) fatigue wear, and (4) chemical or corrosive wear. A fifth, fretting wear and fretting corrosion, combines elements of more than one mechanism. For complex biological materials such as articular cartilage, most likely other mechanisms are involved.

Again, wear is the removal of material. The idea that friction causes wear and therefore, low friction means low wear, is a common mistake. Brief descriptions of five types of wear; abrasive, adhesive, fatigue, chemical or corrosive, and fretting — may be found in Reference 2 as well as in other references in this article. Next, it may be useful to consider some of the major concepts of lubrication.

50.3 Lubrication

Lubrication is a process of reducing friction *and/or* wear (or other forms of surface damage) between relatively moving surfaces by the application of a solid, liquid, or gaseous substance (i.e., a lubricant). Since friction and wear do not necessarily correlate with each other, the use of the word *and* in place of *and/or* in the above definition is a common mistake to be avoided. The primary function of a lubricant is to reduce friction or wear or both between moving surfaces in contact with each other.

Examples of lubricants are wide and varied. They include automotive engine oils, wheel bearing greases, transmission fluids, electrical contact lubricants, rolling oils, cutting fluids, preservative oils, gear oils, jet fuels, instrument oils, turbine oils, textile lubricants, machine oils, jet engine lubricants, air, water, molten glass, liquid metals, oxide films, talcum powder, graphite, molybdenum disulfide, waxes, soaps, polymers, and the synovial fluid in human joints.

A few general principles of lubrication may be mentioned here:

1. The lubricant must be present at the place where it can function.
2. Almost any substance under carefully selected or special conditions can be shown to reduce friction or wear in a particular test, but that does not mean these substances are lubricants.
3. Friction and wear do not necessarily go together. This is an extremely important principle which applies to nonlubricated (dry) as well as lubricated systems. It is particularly true under conditions of "boundary lubrication," to be discussed later. An additive may reduce friction and increase wear, reduce wear and increase friction, reduce both or increase both. Although the reasons are not fully understood, this is an experimental observation. Thus, friction and wear should be thought of as separate phenomena — an important point when we discuss theories of synovial joint lubrication.
4. The effective or active lubricating film in a particular system may or may not consist of the original or bulk lubricant phase.

In a broad sense, it may be considered that the main function of a lubricant is to keep the surfaces apart so that interaction (e.g., adhesion, plowing, and shear) between the solids cannot occur; thus friction and wear can be reduced or controlled.

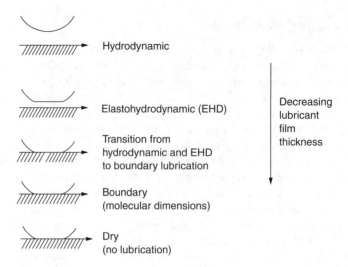

FIGURE 50.1   Regimes of lubrication.

The following regimes or types of lubrication may be considered in the order of increasing severity or decreasing lubricant film thickness (Figure 50.1):

1. Hydrodynamic lubrication
2. Elastohydrodynamic lubrication
3. Transition from hydrodynamic and elastohydrodynamic lubrication to boundary lubrication
4. Boundary lubrication

A fifth regime, sometimes referred to as *dry* or *unlubricated*, may also be considered as an extreme or limit. In addition, there is another form of lubrication that does not require relative movement of the bodies either parallel or perpendicular to the surface, that is, as in externally pressurized hydrostatic or aerostatic bearings.

50.3.1 Hydrodynamic Lubrication Theories

In hydrodynamic lubrication, the load is supported by the pressure developed due to relative motion and the geometry of the system. In the regime of hydrodynamic or fluid film lubrication, there is no contact between the solids. The film thickness is governed by the bulk physical properties of the lubricants, the most important being viscosity; friction arises purely from shearing of viscous lubricant.

Contributions to our knowledge of hydrodynamic lubrication, with special focus on journal bearings, have been made by numerous investigators including Reynolds. The classic Reynolds treatment considered the equilibrium of a fluid element and the pressure and shear forces on this element. In this treatment, eight assumptions were made (e.g., surface curvature is large compared to lubricant film thickness, fluid is Newtonian, flow is laminar, viscosity is constant through film thickness). Velocity distributions due to relative motion and pressure buildup were developed and added together. The solution of the basic Reynolds equation for a particular bearing configuration results in a pressure distribution throughout the film as a function of viscosity, film shape, and velocity.

The total load W and frictional (viscous) drag F can be calculated from this information. For rotating disks with parallel axes, the "simple" Reynolds equation yields:

$$\frac{h_o}{R} = 4.9\left(\frac{\eta U}{W}\right) \tag{50.1}$$

where h_o is the minimum lubricant film thickness, η is the absolute viscosity, U is the average velocity $(U_1 + U_2)/2$, W is the applied normal load per unit width of disk, and R is the reduced radius of curvature $(1/R = 1/R_1 + 1/R_2)$.

The dimensionless term $(\eta U/W)$ is sometimes referred to as the hydrodynamic factor. It can be seen that doubling either the viscosity or velocity doubles the film thickness, and that doubling the applied load halves the film thickness. This regime of lubrication is sometimes referred to as the *rigid isoviscous or classical Martin condition,* since the solid bodies are assumed to be perfectly rigid (non-deformable), and the fluid is assumed to have a constant viscosity.

At high loads with systems such as gears, ball bearings, and other high-contact-stress geometries, two additional factors have been considered in further developments of the hydrodynamic theory of lubrication. One of these is that the surfaces deform elastically; this leads to a localized change in geometry more favorable to lubrication. The second is that the lubricant becomes more viscous under the high pressure existing in the contact zone, according to relationships such as:

$$\eta/\eta_o = \exp \alpha(p - p_o) \tag{50.2}$$

where η is the viscosity at pressure p, η_o is the viscosity at atmospheric pressure p_o, and α is the pressure-viscosity coefficient (e.g., in Pa^{-1}). In this concept, the lubricant pressures existing in the contact zone approximate those of dry contact Hertzian stress. This is the regime of elastohydrodynamic lubrication, sometimes abbreviated as EHL or EHD. It may also be described as the elastic-viscous type or mode of lubrication, since elastic deformation exists and the fluid viscosity is considerably greater due to the pressure effect.

The comparable Dowson-Higginson expression for minimum film thickness between cylinders or disks in contact with parallel axes is:

$$\frac{h_o}{R} = 2.6 \left(\frac{\eta U}{W}\right)^{0.7} \left(\frac{\alpha W}{R}\right)^{0.54} \left(\frac{W}{RE'}\right)^{0.03} \tag{50.3}$$

The term E' represents the reduced modulus of elasticity:

$$\frac{1}{E'} = \frac{(1 - v_1^2)}{E_1} + \frac{(1 - v_2^2)}{E_2} \tag{50.4}$$

where E is the modulus, v is Poisson's ratio, and the subscripts 1 and 2 refer to the two solids in contact. All the other terms are the same as previously stated. In addition to the hydrodynamic factor $(\eta U/W)$, a pressure-viscosity factor $(\alpha W/R)$, and an elastic deformation factor (W/RE') can be considered. Thus, properties of both the lubricant and the solids as materials are included. In examining the elastohydrodynamic film thickness equations, it can be seen that the velocity U is an important factor ($h_o \propto U^{0.7}$) but the load W is rather unimportant ($h_o \propto W^{-0.13}$).

Experimental confirmation of the elastohydrodynamic lubrication theory has been obtained in certain selected systems using electrical capacitance, x-ray transmission, and optical interference techniques to determine film thickness and shape under dynamic conditions. Research is continuing in this area, including studies on micro-EHL or asperity lubrication mechanisms, since surfaces are never perfectly smooth. These studies may lead to a better understanding of not only lubricant film formation in high-contact-stress systems but lubricant film failure as well.

Two other possible types of hydrodynamic lubrication, rigid-viscous and elastic-isoviscous, complete the matrix of four, considering the two factors of elastic deformation and pressure-viscosity effects. In addition, *squeeze film lubrication* can occur when surfaces approach one another. For more information on hydrodynamic and elastohydrodynamic lubrication, see Cameron [3] and Dowson and Higginson [4].

50.3.2   Transition from Hydrodynamic to Boundary Lubrication

Although prevention of contact is probably the most important function of a lubricant, there is still much to be learned about the transition from hydrodynamic and elastohydrodynamic lubrication to boundary lubrication. This is the region in which lubrication goes from the desirable hydrodynamic condition of no contact to the less acceptable "boundary" condition, where increased contact usually leads to higher friction and wear. This regime is sometimes referred to as a condition of *mixed lubrication.*

Several examples of experimental approaches to thin-film lubrication have been reported [3]. It is important in examining these techniques to make the distinction between methods that are used to determine lubricant film thickness under hydrodynamic or elastohydrodynamic conditions (e.g., optical interference, electrical capacitance, or x-ray transmission), and methods that are used to determine the occurrence or frequency of contact. As we will see later, most experimental studies of synovial joint lubrication have focused on friction measurements, using the information to determine the lubrication regime involved; this approach can be misleading.

50.3.2.1   Boundary Lubrication

Although there is no generally accepted definition of boundary lubrication, it is often described as a condition of lubrication in which the friction and wear between two surfaces in relative motion are determined by the surface properties of the solids and the chemical nature of the lubricant rather than its viscosity. An example of the difficulty in defining boundary lubrication can be seen if the term *bulk viscosity* is used in place of viscosity in the preceding sentence — another frequent form. This opens the door to the inclusion of elastohydrodynamic effects which depend in part on the influence of pressure on viscosity. Increased friction under these circumstances could be attributed to increased viscous drag rather than solid-solid contact. According to another common definition, boundary lubrication occurs or exists when the surfaces of the bearing solids are separated by films of molecular thickness. That may be true, but it ignores the possibility that "boundary" layer surface films may indeed be very thick (i.e., 10, 20, or 100 molecular layers). The difficulty is that boundary lubrication is complex.

Although a considerable amount of research has been done on this topic, an understanding of the basic mechanisms and processes involved is by no means complete. Therefore, definitions of boundary lubrication tend to be nonoperational. This is an extremely important regime of lubrication because it involves more extensive solid-solid contact and interaction as well as generally greater friction, wear, and surface damage. In many practical systems, the occurrence of the boundary lubrication regime is unavoidable or at least quite common. The condition can be brought about by high loads, low relative sliding speeds (including zero for stop-and-go, motion reversal, or reciprocating elements) and low lubricant viscosity — factors that are important in the transition from hydrodynamic to boundary lubrication.

The most important factor in boundary lubrication is the chemistry of the tribological system — the contacting solids and total environment including lubricants. More particularly, the surface chemistry and interactions occurring with and on the solid surfaces are important. This includes factors such as physisorption, chemisorption, intermolecular forces, surface chemical reactions, and the nature, structure, and properties of thin films on solid surfaces. It also includes many other effects brought on by the process of moving one solid over another, such as (1) changes in topography and the area of contact, (2) high surface temperatures, (3) the generation of fresh reactive metal surfaces by the removal of oxide and other layers, (4) catalysis, (5) the generation of electrical charges, and (6) the emission of charged particles such as electrons.

In examining the action of boundary lubricant compounds in reducing friction or wear or both between solids in sliding contact, it may be helpful to consider at least the following five modes of film formation on or protection of surfaces: (1) physisorption, (2) chemisorption, (3) chemical reactions with the solid surface, (4) chemical reactions on the solid surface, and (5) mere interposition of a solid or other material. These modes of surface protection are discussed in more detail in Reference 2.

The beneficial and harmful effects of minor changes in chemistry of the environment (e.g., the lubric-ant) are often enormous in comparison with hydrodynamic and elastohydrodynamic effects. Thus, the

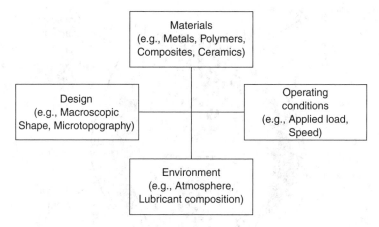

FIGURE 50.2   In any tribological system, friction, wear, and surface damage depend on four interrelated factors.

surface and chemical properties of the solid materials used in tribological applications become especially important. One might expect that this would also be the case in biological (e.g., human joint) lubrication where biochemistry is very likely an important factor.

50.3.2.2   General Comments on Tribological Processes

It is important to recognize that friction and wear depend upon four major factors, that is, materials, design, operating conditions, and total environment (Figure 50.2). This four-block figure may be useful as a guide in thinking about synovial joint lubrication either from a theoretical or experimental viewpoint — the topic discussed in the next section.

Readers are cautioned against the use of various terms in tribology which are either vaguely defined or not defined at all. These would include such terms as "lubricating ability," "lubricity," and even "boundary lubrication." For example, do "boundary lubricating properties" refer to effects on friction or effects on wear and damage? It makes a difference. It is emphasized once again that friction and wear are different phenomena. Low friction does not necessarily mean low wear. We will see several examples of this common error in the discussion of joint lubrication research.

50.4   Synovial Joints

Examples of natural synovial or movable joints include the human hip, knee, elbow, ankle, finger, and shoulder. A simplified representation of a synovial joint is shown in Figure 50.3. The bones are covered by a thin layer of articular cartilage bathed in synovial fluid confined by synovial membrane. Synovial joints are truly remarkable systems — providing the basis of movement by allowing bones to articulate on one another with minimal friction and wear. Unfortunately, various joint diseases occur even among the young — causing pain, loss of freedom of movement, or instability.

Synovial joints are complex, sophisticated systems not yet fully understood. The loads are surprisingly high and the relative motion is complex. Articular cartilage has the deceptive appearance of simplicity and uniformity. But it is an extremely complex material with unusual properties. Basically, it consists of water (approximately 75%) enmeshed in a network of collagen fibers and proteoglycans with high molecular weight. In a way, cartilage could be considered as one of Nature's composite materials. Articular cartilage also has no blood supply, no nerves, and very few cells (chondrocytes).

The other major component of an articular joint is *synovial fluid*, named by Paracelsus after "synovia" (egg-white). It is essentially a dialysate of blood plasma with added hyaluronic acid. Synovial fluid contains complex proteins, polysaccharides, and other compounds. Its chief constituent is water (approximately 85%). Synovial fluid functions as a joint lubricant, nutrient for cartilage, and carrier for waste products.

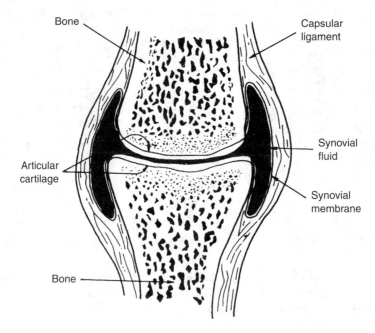

FIGURE 50.3   Representation of a synovial joint.

For more information on the biochemistry, structure, and properties of articular cartilage, Freeman [5], Sokoloff [6], Stockwell [7], and articles referenced in these works are suggested.

50.5   Theories on the Lubrication of Natural and Normal Synovial Joints

As stated, the word *tribology* means the study of friction, wear, and lubrication. Therefore, *biotribology* may be thought of as the study of biological lubrication processes, for example, as in synovial joints. A surprisingly large number of concepts and theories of synovial joint lubrication have been proposed [8–10] (as shown in Table 50.1). And even if similar ideas are grouped together, there are still well over a dozen fundamentally different theories. These have included a wide range of lubrication concepts, for example, hydrodynamic, hydrostatic, elasto-hydrodynamic, squeeze-film, "boundary," mixed-regime, "weeping," osmotic, synovial mucin gel, "boosted," lipid, electrostatic, porous layers, and special forms of boundary lubrication (e.g., "lubricating glycoproteins," structuring of boundary water "surface-active" phospholipids). This chapter will not review these numerous theories, but excellent reviews on the lubrication of synovial joints have been written by McCutchen [11], Swanson [12], and Higginsworth and Unsworth [13]. The book edited by Dumbleton is also recommended [14]. In addition, theses by Droogendijk [15] and Burkhardt [16] contain extensive and detailed reviews of theories of joint lubrication.

   McCutchen was the first to propose an entirely new concept of lubrication, "weeping lubrication," applied to synovial joint action [17,18]. He considered unique and special properties of cartilage and how this could affect flow and lubrication. The work of Mow et al. continued along a more complex and sophisticated approach in which a biomechanical model is proposed for the study of the dynamic interaction between synovial fluid and articular cartilage [19,20]. These ideas are combined in the more recent work of Ateshian [21] which uses a framework of the biphasic theory of articular cartilage to model interstitial fluid pressurization. Several additional studies have also been made of effects of porosity and compliance, including the behavior of elastic layers, in producing hydrodynamic and squeeze-film

TABLE 50.1 Examples of Proposed Mechanisms and Studies of Synovial Joint Lubrication

Mechanism	Authors	Date
1. Hydrodynamic	MacConnail	1932
2. Boundary	Jones	1934
3. Hydrodynamic	Jones	1936
4. Boundary	Charnley	1959
5. Weeping	McCutchen	1959
6. Floating	Barnett and Cobbold	1962
7. Elastohydrodynamic	Tanner	1966
	Dowson	1967
8. Thixotropic/elastic fluid	Dintenfass	1963
9. Osmotic (boundary)	McCutchen	1966
10. Squeeze-film	Fein	1966
	Higginson et al.	1974
11. Synovial gel	Maroudas	1967
12. Thin-film	Faber et al.	1967
13. Combinations of hydrostatic, boundary, & EHL	Linn	1968
14. Boosted	Walker et al.	1968
15. Lipid	Little et al.	1969
16. Weeping + boundary	McCutchen and Wilkins	1969
	McCutchen	1969
17. Boundary	Caygill and West	1969
18. Fat (or mucin)	Freeman et al.	1970
19. Electrostatic	Roberts	1971
20. Boundary + fluid squeeze-film	Radin and Paul	1972
21. Mixed	Unsworth et al.	1974
22. Imbibe/exudate composite model	Ling	1974
23. Complex biomechanical model	Mow et al.	1974
	Mansour and Mow	1977
24. Two porous layer model	Dinnar	1974
25. Boundary	Reimann et al.	1975
26. Squeeze-film + fluid film + boundary	Unsworth, Dowson et al.	1975
27. Compliant bearing model	Rybicki	1977
28. Lubricating glycoproteins	Swann et al.	1977
29. Structuring of boundary water	Sokoloff et al.	1979
30. Surface flow	Kenyon	1980
31. Lubricin	Swann et al.	1985
32. Micro-EHL	Dowson and Jin	1986
33. Lubricating factor	Jay	1992
34. Lipidic component	LaBerge et al.	1993
35. Constitutive modeling of cartilage	Lai et al.	1993
36. Asperity model	Yao et al.	1993
37. Bingham fluid	Tandon et al.	1994
38. Filtration/gel/squeeze film	Hlavacek et al.	1995
39. Surface-active phospholipid	Schwarz and Hills	1998
40. Interstitial fluid pressurization	Ateshian et al.	1998

lubrication. A good review in this area was given by Unsworth who discussed both human and artificial joints [22].

The following general observations are offered on the theories of synovial joint lubrication that have been proposed:

1. Most of the theories are strictly mechanical or rheological — involving such factors as deformation, pressure, and fluid flow.
2. There is a preoccupation with *friction*, which of course is very low for articular cartilage systems.

3. None of the theories consider *wear* — which is neither the same as friction nor related to it.
4. The detailed structure, biochemistry, complexity, and living nature of the total articular cartilage-synovial fluid system are generally ignored.

These are only general impressions. And although mechanical/rheological concepts seem dominant (with a focus on friction), wear and biochemistry are not completely ignored. For example, Simon [23] abraded articular cartilage from human patellae and canine femoral heads with a stainless steel rotary file, measuring the depth of penetration with time and the amount of wear debris generated. Cartilage wear was also studied experimentally by Bloebaum and Wilson [24], Radin and Paul [25], and Lipshitz, Etheredge, and Glimcher [26–28]. The latter researchers carried out several *in vitro* studies of wear of articular cartilage using bovine cartilage plugs or specimens in sliding contact against stainless steel plates. They developed a means of measuring cartilage wear by determining the hydroxyproline content of both the lubricant and solid wear debris. Using this system and technique, effects of variables such as time, applied load, and chemical modification of articular cartilage on wear and profile changes were determined. This work is of particular importance in that they addressed the question of *cartilage wear and damage* rather than friction, recognizing that wear and friction are different phenomena.

Special note is also made of two researchers, Swann and Sokoloff, who considered biochemistry as an important factor in synovial joint lubrication. Swann et al. very carefully isolated fractions of bovine synovial fluid using sequential sedimentation techniques and gel permeation chromatography. They found a high molecular weight glycoprotein to be the major constituent in the articular lubrication fraction from bovine synovial fluid and called this LGP-I (from lubricating glycoprotein). This was based on friction measurements using cartilage in sliding contact against a glass disc. An excellent summary of this work with additional references is presented in a chapter by Swann in *The Joints and Synovial Fluid: I* [6].

Sokoloff et al. [29] examined the "boundary lubricating ability" of several synovial fluids using a latex-glass test system and cartilage specimens obtained at necropsy from knees. Measurements were made of friction. The research was extended to other *in vitro* friction tests using cartilage obtained from the nasal septum of cows and widely differing artificial surfaces [30]. As a result of this work, a new model of boundary lubrication by synovial fluid was proposed — the structuring of boundary water. The postulate involves adsorption of one part of a glycoprotein on a surface followed by the formation of hydration shells around the polar portions of the adsorbed glycoprotein; the net result is a thin layer of viscous "structured" water at the surface. This work is of particular interest in that it involves not only a specific and more detailed mechanism of boundary lubrication in synovial joints but also takes into account the possible importance of water in this system.

In more recent research by Jay, an interaction between hyaluronic acid and a "purified synovial lubricating factor" (PSLF) was observed, suggesting a possible synergistic action in the boundary lubrication of synovial joints [31]. The definition of "lubricating ability" was based on friction measurements made with a latex-covered stainless steel stud in oscillating contact against polished glass.

The above summary of major synovial joint lubrication theories is taken from References 10 and 31 as well as the thesis by Burkhardt [33].

Two more recent studies are of interest since cartilage wear was considered although not as a part of a theory of joint lubrication. Stachowiak et al. [34] investigated the friction and wear characteristics of adult rat femur cartilage against a stainless steel plate using an environmental scanning microscope (ESM) to examine damaged cartilage. One finding was evidence of a load limit to lubrication of cartilage, beyond which high friction and damage occurred. Another study, by Hayes et al. [35] on the influence of crystals on cartilage wear, is particularly interesting not only in the findings reported (e.g., certain crystals can increase cartilage wear), but also in the full description of the biochemical techniques used.

A special note should be made concerning the doctoral thesis by Lawrence Malcom in 1976 [36]. This is an excellent study of cartilage friction and deformation, in which a device resembling a rotary plate rheometer was used to investigate the effects of static and dynamic loading on the frictional behavior of bovine cartilage. The contact geometry consisted of a circular cylindrical annulus in contact with a concave hemispherical section. It was found that dynamically loaded specimens in bovine synovial fluid yielded the more efficient lubrication based on friction measurements. The Malcom study is thorough and excellent in its attention to detail (e.g., specimen preparation) in examining the influence of type of loading and time effects on cartilage friction. It does not, however, consider cartilage wear and damage except in a very preliminary way. And it does not consider the influence of fluid biochemistry on cartilage friction, wear, and damage. In short, the Malcom work represents a superb piece of systematic research along the lines of mechanical, dynamic, rheological, and viscoelastic behavior — one important dimension of synovial joint lubrication.

50.6   *In Vitro* Cartilage Wear Studies

Over the past fifteen years, studies aimed at exploring possible connections between tribology and mechanisms of synovial joint lubrication and degeneration (e.g., osteoarthritis) have been conducted by the author and his graduate and undergraduate students in the Department of Mechanical Engineering at Virginia Polytechnic Institute and State University. The basic approach used involved *in vitro* tribological experiments using bovine articular cartilage, with an emphasis on the effects of fluid composition and biochemistry on cartilage wear and damage. This research is an outgrowth of earlier work carried out during a sabbatical study in the Laboratory for the Study of Skeletal Disorders, The Children's Hospital Medical Center, Harvard Medical School in Boston. In that study, bovine cartilage test specimens were loaded against a polished steel plate and subjected to reciprocating sliding for several hours in the presence of a fluid (e.g., bovine synovial fluid or a buffered saline reference fluid containing biochemical constituents kindly provided by Dr. David Swann). Cartilage wear was determined by sampling the test fluid and determining the concentration of 4-hydroxyproline — a constituent of collagen. The results of that earlier study have been reported and summarized elsewhere [37–40]. Figure 50.4 shows the average hydroxyproline contents of wear debris obtained from these *in vitro* experiments. These numbers are related to the cartilage wear which occurred. However, since the total quantities of collected fluids varied somewhat, the values shown in the bar graph should not be taken as exact or precise measures of fluid effects on cartilage wear.

The main conclusions of that study were as follows:

1. Normal bovine synovial fluid is very effective in reducing cartilage wear under these *in vitro* conditions as compared to the buffered saline reference fluid.
2. There is no significant difference in wear between the saline reference and distilled water.
3. The addition of hyaluronic acid to the reference fluid significantly reduces wear; but its effect depends on the source.
4. Under these tests conditions, Swann's LGP-I (Lubricating Glycoprotein-I), known to be extremely effective in reducing friction in cartilage-on-glass tests, does not reduce cartilage wear.

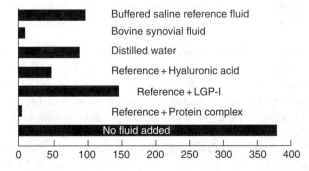

FIGURE 50.4   Relative cartilage wear based on hydroxyproline content of debris (*in vitro* tests with cartilage on stainless steel).

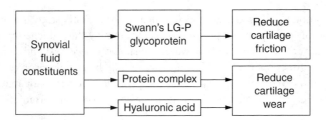

FIGURE 50.5   Friction and wear are different phenomena.

5. However, a protein complex isolated by Swann is extremely effective in reducing wear — producing results similar to those obtained with synovial fluid. The detailed structure of this constituent is complex and has not yet been fully determined.

6. Last, the lack of an added fluid in these experiments leads to extremely high wear and damage of the articular cartilage.

In discussing the possible significance of these findings from a tribological point of view, it may be helpful first of all to emphasize once again that friction and wear are different phenomena. Furthermore, as suggested by Figure 50.5, certain constituents of synovial fluid (e.g., Swann's Lubricating Glycoprotein) may act to reduce friction in synovial joints while other constituents (e.g., Swann's protein complex or hyaluronic acid) may act to reduce cartilage *wear*. Therefore, it is necessary to distinguish between biochemical anti-friction and anti-wear compounds present in synovial fluid.

In more recent years, this study has been greatly enhanced by the participation of interested faculty and students from the Virginia-Maryland College of Veterinary Medicine and Department of Biochemistry and Animal Science at Virginia Tech. One major hypothesis tested is a continuation of previous work showing that the detailed biochemistry of the fluid-cartilage system has a pronounced and possibly controlling influence on cartilage wear. A consequence of the above hypothesis is that a lack or deficiency of certain biochemical constituents in the synovial joint may be one factor contributing to the initiation and progression of cartilage damage, wear, and possibly osteoarthritis. A related but somewhat different hypothesis concerns synovial fluid constituents which may act to increase the wear and further damage of articular cartilage under tribological contact.

To carry out continued research on biotribology, a new device for studies of cartilage deformation, wear, damage, and friction under conditions of tribological contact was designed by Burkhardt [33] and later modified, constructed, and instrumented. A simplified sketch is shown in Figure 50.6. The key features of this test device are shown in Table 50.2. The apparatus is designed to accommodate cartilage-on-cartilage specimens. Motion of the lower specimen is controlled by a computer-driven x–y table, allowing simple oscillating motion or complex motion patterns. An octagonal strain ring with two full semi-conductor bridges is used to measure the normal load as well as the tangential load (friction). An LVDT, not shown in the figure, is used to measure cartilage deformation and linear wear during a test. However, hydroxyproline analysis of the wear debris and washings is used for the actual determination of total cartilage wear on a mass basis.

In one study by Schroeder [41], two types of experiments were carried out, that is, cartilage-on-stainless steel and cartilage-on-cartilage at applied loads up to 70 N — yielding an average pressure of 2.2 MPa in the contact area. Reciprocating motion (40 cps) was used. The fluids tested included (1) a buffered saline solution, (2) saline plus hyaluronic acid, and (3) bovine synovial fluid. In cartilage-on-stainless steel tests, scanning electron microscopy, and histological staining showed distinct effects of the lubricants on surface and subsurface damage. Tests with the buffered saline fluid resulted in the most damage, with large wear tracks visible on the surface of the cartilage plug, as well as subsurface voids and cracks. When hyaluronic acid, a constituent of the natural synovial joint lubricant, was added to the saline reference fluid, less severe damage was observed. Little or no cartilage damage was evident in tests in which the natural synovial joint fluid was used as the lubricant.

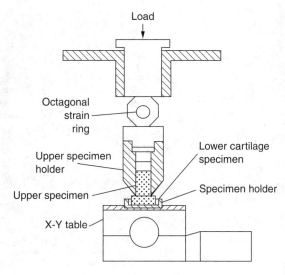

FIGURE 50.6   Device for *in vitro* cartilage-on-cartilage wear studies.

TABLE 50.2   Key Features of Test Device Designed for Cartilage Wear Studies [33]

Contact system	Cartilage-on-cartilage
Contact geometry	Flat-on-flat, convex-on-flat, irregular-on-irregular
Cartilage type	Articular, any source (e.g., bovine)
Specimen size	Upper specimen, 4 to 6 mm diam., lower specimen, ca. 15 to 25 mm diam.
Applied load	50–660 N
Average pressure	0.44–4.4 MPa
Type of motion	Linear, oscillating; circular, constant velocity; more complex patterns
Sliding velocity	0 to 20 mm/sec
Fluid temperature	Ambient (20∞C); or controlled humidity
Environment	Ambient or controlled humidity
Measurements	Normal load, cartilage deformation, friction; cartilage wear and damage, biochemical analysis of cartilage specimens, synovial fluid, and wear debris; sub-surface changes

These results were confirmed in a later study by Owellen [42] in which hydroxyproline analysis was used to determine cartilage wear. It was found that increasing the applied load from 20 to 65 N increased cartilage wear by eight-fold for the saline solution and approximately three-fold for synovial fluid. Furthermore, the coefficient of friction increased from an initial low value of 0.01 to 0.02 to a much higher value, for example, 0.20 to 0.30 and higher, during a normal test which lasted 3 h; the greatest change occurred during the first 20 min. Another interesting result was that a thin film of transferred or altered material was observed on the stainless steel disks — being most pronounced with the buffered saline lubricant and not observed with synovial fluid. Examination of the film with Fourier Transfer Infrared Microspectrometry shows distinctive bio-organic spectra which differs from that of the original bovine cartilage. We believe this to be an important finding since it suggests a possible bio-tribochemical effect [43].

In another phase of this research, the emphasis is on the cartilage-on-cartilage system and the influence of potentially beneficial as well as harmful constituents of synovial fluid on wear and damage. In cartilage-on-cartilage tests, the most severe wear and damage occurred during tests with buffered saline as the lubricant. The damage was less severe than in the stainless steel tests, but some visible wear tracks were detectable with scanning electron microscopy. Histological sectioning and staining of both the upper

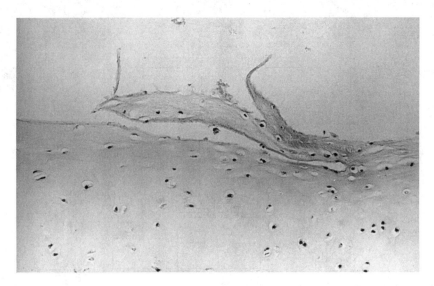

FIGURE 50.7   Cartilage damage produced by sliding contact.

and lower cartilage samples show evidence of elongated lacunae and coalesced voids that could lead to wear by delamination. An example is shown in Figure 50.7 (original magnification of 500× on 35 mm slide). The proteoglycan content of the subsurface cartilage under the region of contact was also reduced. When synovial fluid was used as the lubricant, no visible wear or damage was detected [44]. These results demonstrate that even in *in vitro* tests with bovine articular cartilage, the nature of the fluid environment can have a dramatic affect on the severity of wear and subsurface damage.

In a more recent study carried out by Berrien in the biotribology program at Virginia Tech, a different approach was taken to examine the role of joint lubrication in joint disease, particularly osteoarthritis. A degradative biological enzyme, collagenase-3, suspected of playing a role in a cartilage degeneration was used to create a physiologically adverse biochemical fluid environment. Tribological tests were performed with the same device and procedures described previously. The stainless steel disk was replaced with a 1 in. diameter plug of bovine cartilage to create a cartilage sliding on cartilage configuration more closely related to the in vivo condition. Normal load was increased to 78.6 N and synovial fluid and buffered saline were used as lubricants. Prior to testing, cartilage plugs were exposed to a fluid medium containing three concentrations of collagenase-3 for 24 h. The major discovery of this work was that exposure to the collagenase-3 enzyme had a substantial adverse effect on cartilage wear *in vitro*, increasing average wear values by three and one-half times those of the unexposed cases. Figure 50.8 shows an example of the effect of enzyme treatment when bovine synovial fluid was used as the lubricant. Scanning electron microscopy showed disruption of the superficial layer and collagen matrix with exposure to collagenase-3, where unexposed cartilage showed none. Histological sections showed a substantial loss of the superficial layer of cartilage and a distinct and abnormal loss of proteoglycans in the middle layer of collagenase-treated cartilage. Unexposed cartilage showed only minor disruption of the superficial layer [45].

This study indicates that some of the biochemical constituents that gain access to the joint space, during normal and pathological functions, can have a significant adverse effect on the wear and damage of the articular cartilage. Future studies will include determination of additional constituents that have harmful effects on cartilage wear and damage. This research, using bovine articular cartilage in *in vitro* sliding contact tests, raises a number of interesting questions:

1. Has "Nature" designed a special biochemical compound which has as its function the protection of articular cartilage?
2. What is the mechanism (or mechanisms) by which biochemical constituents of synovial fluid can act to reduce wear of articular cartilage?

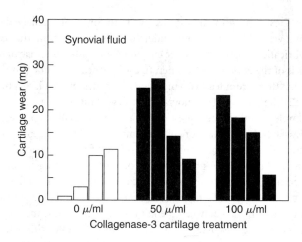

FIGURE 50.8   Effect of collagenase-3 on cartilage wear.

3. Could a lack of this biochemical constituent lead to increased cartilage wear and damage?
4. Does articular cartilage from osteoarthritic patients have reduced wear resistance?
5. Do any of the findings on the importance of synovial fluid biochemistry on cartilage wear in our *in vitro* studies apply to living or *in vitro* systems as well?
6. How does collagenase-3 treatment of cartilage lead to increased wear and does this finding have any significance in the *in vivo* situation? This question is addressed in the next section.

50.7   Biotribology and Arthritis: Are There Connections?

Arthritis is an umbrella term for more than 100 rheumatic diseases affecting joints and connective tissue. The two most common forms are osteoarthritis (OA) and rheumatoid arthritis (RA). Osteoarthritis — also referred to as *osteoarthrosis or degenerative joint disease* — is the most common form of arthritis. It is sometimes simplistically described as the "wear and tear" form of arthritis. The causes and progression of degenerative joint disease are still not understood. Rheumatoid arthritis is a chronic and often progressive disease of the synovial membrane leading to release of enzymes which attack, erode, and destroy articular cartilage. It is an inflammatory response involving the immune system and is more prevalent in females. Rheumatoid arthritis is extremely complex. Its causes are still unknown.

Sokoloff defines degenerative joint disease as "an extremely common, noninflammatory, progressive disorder of movable joints, particularly weight-bearing joints, characterized pathologically by deterioration of articular cartilage and by formation of new bone in the sub-chondral areas and at the margins of the "joint" [46]. As mentioned, osteoarthritis or osteoarthrosis is sometimes referred to as the "wear and tear" form of arthritis; but, wear itself is rarely a simple process even in well-defined systems.

It has been noted by the author that tribological terms occasionally appear in hypotheses which describe the etiology of osteoarthritis (e.g., "reduced wear resistance of cartilage" or "poor lubricity of synovial fluid"). It has also been noted that there is a general absence of hypotheses connecting normal synovial joint *lubrication* (or lack thereof) and synovial joint *degeneration*. Perhaps it is natural (and unhelpful) for a tribologist to imagine such a connection and that, for example, cartilage wear under certain circumstances might be due to or influenced by a lack of proper "boundary lubrication" by the synovial fluid. In this regard, it may be of interest to quote Swanson [12] who said in 1979 that "there exists at present no experimental evidence which certainly shows that a failure of lubrication is or is not a causative factor in the first stages of cartilage degeneration." A statement made by Professor Glimcher [52] may also be appropriate here. Glimcher fully recognized the fundamental difference between friction and wear as well as the difference between joint lubrication (one area of study) and joint degeneration (another area of study). Glimcher said that wearing or abrading cartilage with a steel file is not osteoarthritis; and neither is digesting cartilage in a test tube with an enzyme. But both forms of cartilage deterioration can occur in a living joint and in a way which is still not understood. It is interesting that essentially none of the many synovial joint lubrication theories consider enzymatic degradation of cartilage as a factor whereas practically all the models of the etiology of degenerative joint disease include this as an important factor.

It was stated earlier that there are at least two main areas to consider, that is, (1) mechanisms of synovial joint lubrication and (2) the etiology of synovial joint degeneration (e.g., as in osteoarthrosis). Both areas are extremely complex. And the key questions as to what actually happens in each have yet to be answered (and perhaps asked). It may therefore be presumptuous of the present author to suggest possible connections between two areas which in themselves are still not fully understood.

Tribological processes in a movable joint involve not only the contacting surfaces (articular cartilage), but the surrounding medium (synovial fluid) as well. Each of these depends on the synthesis and transport of necessary biochemical constituents to the contact region or interface. As a result of relative motion (sliding, rubbing, rolling, and impact) between the joint elements, friction and wear can occur.

It has already been shown and discussed — at least in *in vitro* tests with articular cartilage — that compounds which reduce friction do not necessarily reduce wear; the latter was suggested as being more important [10]. It may be helpful first of all to emphasize once again that friction and wear are different phenomena. Furthermore, certain constituents of synovial fluid (e.g., Swann's Lubricating Glycoprotein) may act to reduce *friction* in synovial joints while other constituents (e.g., Swann's protein complex or hyaluronic acid) may act to reduce cartilage *wear*.

A significant increase in joint friction could lead to a slight increase in local temperatures or possibly to reduce mobility. But the effects of cartilage wear would be expected to be more serious. When cartilage wear occurs, a very special material is lost and the body is not capable of regenerating cartilage of the same quality nor at the desired rate. Thus, there are at least two major tribological dimensions involved — one concerning the nature of the synovial fluid and the other having to do with the properties of articular cartilage itself. Changes in *either* the synovial fluid or cartilage could conceivably lead to increased wear or damage (or friction) as shown in Figure 50.9.

A simplified model or illustration of possible connections between osteoarthritis and tribology is offered in Figure 50.10 taken from Furey [53]. Its purpose is to stimulate discussion. There are other pathways to the disease, pathways which may include genetic factors.

In some cases, the body makes an unsuccessful attempt at repair, and bone growth may occur at the periphery of contact. As suggested by Figure 50.10, this process and the generation of wear particles could lead to joint inflammation and the release of enzymes which further soften and degrade the articular cartilage. This softer, degraded cartilage does not possess the wear-resistance of the original. It has been shown previously that treatment of cartilage with collagenase-3 increases wear significantly, thus supporting the idea of enzyme release as a factor in osteoarthritis. Thus, there exists a feedback process in which the occurrence of cartilage wear can lead to even more damage. Degradative enzymes can also be released by trauma, shock, or injury to the joint. Ultimately, as the cartilage is progressively thinned and bony growth occurs, a condition of osteoarthritis or degenerative joint disease may exist. There are other pathways to the disease, pathways which may include genetic factors. It is not argued that arthritis

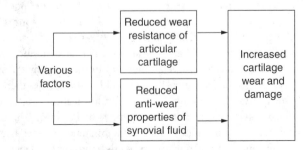

FIGURE 50.9   Two tribological aspects of synovial joint lubrication.

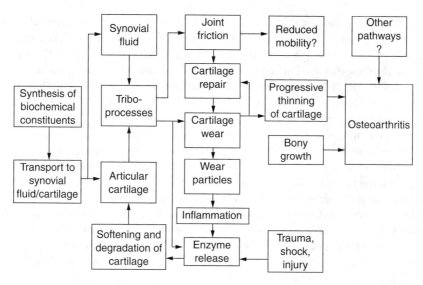

FIGURE 50.10   Osteoarthritis-tribology connections?

is a tribological problem. However, the inclusion of tribological processes in one set of pathways to osteoarthrosis would not seem strange or unusual.

A specific example of a different tribological dimension to the problem of synovial joint lubrication (i.e., third-body abrasion), was shown by the work of Hayes et al. [54]. In an excellent study of the effect of crystals on the wear of articular cartilage, they carried out *in vitro* tests using cylindrical cartilage sub-chondral bone plugs obtained from equine fetlock joints in sliding contact against a stainless steel plate. They examined the effects of three types of crystals (orthorhombic calcium pyrophosphate tetrahydrate, monoclinic calcium pyrophosphate dehydrate, and calcium hydroxyapatite) on wear using a Ringer's solution as the carrier fluid. Concentration of cartilage wear debris in the fluid was determined by analyzing for inorganic sulphate derived from the proteoglycans present. Several interesting findings were made, one of them being that the presence of the crystals roughly doubled cartilage wear. This is an important contribution which should be read by anyone seriously contemplating research on the tribology of articular cartilage. The careful attention to detail and potential problems, as well as the precise description of the biochemical procedures and diverse experimental techniques used, set a high standard.

50.8   Recapitulation and Final Comments

It is obvious from the unusually large number of theories of synovial joint lubrication proposed, that very little is known about the subject. Synovial joints are undoubtedly the most sophisticated and complex tribological systems that exist or will ever exist. It will require a great deal more research — possibly very different approaches — before we even begin to understand the processes involved.

Some general comments and specific suggestions are offered — not for the purpose of criticizing any particular study but hopefully to provide ideas which may be helpful in further research as well as in the re-interpretation of some past research.

50.8.1   Terms and Definitions

First of all, as mentioned earlier in this chapter, part of the problem has to do with the use and misuse of various terms in tribology — the study of friction, wear, and lubrication. A glance at any number of the published papers on synovial joint lubrication will reveal such terms and phrases as "lubricating ability," "lubricity," "lubricating properties," "lubricating component," and many others, all undefined. We also see terms like "boundary lubricant," "lubricating glycoprotein," or "lubricin." There is nothing inherently wrong with this but one should remember that lubrication is a process of reducing friction and/or wear between rubbing surfaces. Saying that a fluid is a "good" lubricant does not distinguish between friction and wear. And assuming that friction and wear are correlated and go together is the first pitfall in any tribological study. It cannot be overemphasized that friction and wear are different, though sometimes related, phenomena. Low friction does not mean low wear. The terms and phrases used are therefore extremely important. For example, in a brief and early review article by Wright and Dowson [55], it was stated that "Digestion of hyaluronate does not alter the boundary lubrication," referring to the work of Radin, Swann, and Weisser [56]. In another article, McCutchen re-states this conclusion in another way, saying "…the lubricating ability did not reside in the hyaluronic acid" and later asks the question "Why do the glycoprotein molecules (of Swann) lubricate?" [57] These statements are based on effects of various constituents on friction, not wear. The work of the present author showed that in tests with bovine articular cartilage, Swann's Lubricating Glycoprotein LGP-I which was effective in reducing friction did not reduce cartilage wear. However, hyaluronic acid — shown earlier not to be responsible for friction-reduction — did reduce cartilage wear. Thus, it is important to make the distinction between friction-reduction and wear-reduction. It is suggested that operational definitions be used in place of vague "lubricating ability," etc. terms in future papers on the subject.

50.8.2 Experimental Contact Systems

Secondly, some comments are made on the experimental approaches that have been reported in the literature on synovial joint lubrication mechanisms. Sliding contact combinations in *in vitro* studies have consisted of (1) cartilage-on-cartilage, (2) cartilage-on-some other surface (e.g., stainless steel, glass), and (3) solids other than cartilage sliding against each other in X-on-X or X-on-Y combinations.

The cartilage-on-cartilage combination is of course the most realistic and yet most complex contact system. But variations in shape or macroscopic geometry, microtopography, and the nature of contact present problems in carrying out well-controlled experiments. There is also the added problem of acquiring suitable specimens which are large enough and reasonably uniform.

The next combination — cartilage-on-another material — allows for better control of contact, with the more elastic, deformable cartilage loaded against a well-defined hard surface (e.g., a polished, flat solid made of glass or stainless steel). This contact configuration can provide useful tribological information on effects of changes in biochemical environment (e.g., fluids), on friction, wear, and sub-surface damage. It also could parallel the situation in a partial joint replacement in which healthy cartilage is in contact with a metal alloy.

The third combination, which appears in some of the literature on synovial joint lubrication, does not involve any articular cartilage at all. For example, Jay made friction measurements using a latex-covered stainless steel stud in oscillating contact against polished glass [31]. Williams et al., in a study of a lipid component of synovial fluid, used reciprocating contact of borosilicate glass-on-glass [58]. And in a recent paper on the action of a surface-active phospholipid as the "lubricating component of lubricin," Schwarz and Hills carried out friction measurements using two optically flat quartz plates in sliding contact [59]. In another study, a standard four-ball machine using alloy steel balls was used to examine the "lubricating ability" of synovial fluid constituents. Such tests, in the absence of cartilage, are easiest to control and carry out. However, they are not relevant to the study of synovial joint lubrication. With a glass sphere sliding against a glass flat, almost anything will reduce friction — including a wide variety of chemicals, biochemicals, semi-solids, and fluids. This has little if anything to do with the lubrication of synovial joints.

50.8.3 Fluids and Materials Used as Lubricants in *In Vitro* Biotribology Studies

Fluids used as lubricants in synovial joint lubrication studies have consisted of (1) "normal" synovial fluid (e.g., bovine), (2) buffered saline solution containing synovial fluid constituents (e.g., hyaluronic acid), and (3) various aqueous solutions of surface active compounds neither derived from nor present in synovial fluid. In addition, a few studies used synovial fluids from patients suffering from either osteoarthritis or rheumatoid arthritis.

The general comment made here is that the use of synovial fluids — whether derived from human or animal sources and whether "healthy" or "abnormal" — is important in *in vitro* studies of synovial joint lubrication. The documented behavior of synovial fluid in producing low friction and wear with articular cartilage sets a reference standard and demonstrates that useful information can indeed come from *in vitro* tests.

Studies that are based on adding synovial fluid constituents to a reference fluid (e.g., a buffered saline solution) can also be useful in attempting to identify which biochemical compound or compounds are responsible for reductions in frictions or wear. But if significant interactions between compounds exist, then such an approach may require an extensive program of tests. It should also be mentioned that in the view of the present author, the use of a pure undissolved constituent of synovial fluid, either derived or synthetic, in a sliding contact test is not only irrelevant but may be misleading. An example would be the use of a pure lipid (e.g., phospholipid) at the interface rather than in the concentration and solution form in which this compound would normally exist in synovial fluid. This is basic in any study of lubrication and particularly in the case of boundary lubrication where major effects on wear or friction can be brought on by minor, seemingly trivial, changes in chemistry.

50.8.4   The Preoccupation with Rheology and Friction

The synovial joint as a system — the articular cartilage and underlying bone structure as well as the synovial fluid as important elements — is extremely complex and far from being understood. It is noted that there is a proliferation of mathematical modeling papers stressing rheology and the mechanics of deformation, flow, and fluid pressures developed in the cartilage model. One recent example is the paper "The Role of Interstitial Fluid Pressurization and Surface Properties on the Boundary Friction of Articular Cartilage" by Ateshian et al. [21]. This study, a genuine contribution, grew out of the early work by Mow and connects also with the "weeping lubrication" model of McCutchen. Both McCutchen and Mow have made significant contributions to our understanding of synovial joint lubrication, although each approach is predominantly rheological and friction-oriented with little regard for biochemistry and wear. This is not to say that rheology is unimportant. It could well be that, as suggested by Ateshian, the mechanism of interstitial fluid pressurization that leads to low friction in cartilage could also lead to low wear rates [60].

50.8.5   The Probable Existence of Various Lubrication Regimes

In an article by Wright and Dowson, it is suggested that a variety of types of lubrication operate in human synovial joints at different parts of a walking cycle stating that, "At heel-strike a squeeze-film situation may develop, leading to elastohydrodynamic lubrication and possibly both squeeze-film and boundary lubrication, while hydrodynamic lubrication may operate during the free-swing phase of walking" [55].

In a simplified approach to examining the various regimes of lubrication that could exist in a human joint, it may be useful to look at Figure 50.11a which shows the variation in force (load) and velocity for a human hip joint at different parts of the walking cycle (taken from Graham and Walker [61]). As discussed earlier in this chapter, theories of hydrodynamic and elastohydrodynamic lubrication all include the hydrodynamic factor $(\eta U / W)$ as the key variable, where η = fluid viscosity, U = the relative sliding velocity, and W = the normal load. High values of $(\eta U / W)$ lead to thicker hydrodynamic films — a more desirable condition if one wants to keep surfaces apart. It can be seen from Figure 50.11a that there is considerable variation in load and velocity, with peaks and valleys occurring at different parts of the cycle. Note also that in this example, the loads can be quite high (e.g., up to three times body weight). The maximum load occurs at 20% of the walking cycle illustrated in Figure 50.11a, with a secondary maximum occurring at a little over the 50% point. The maximum angular velocity occurs at approximately 67% of the cycle. If one now creates a new curve of relative velocity/load or (U / W) from Figure 50.11a, the result

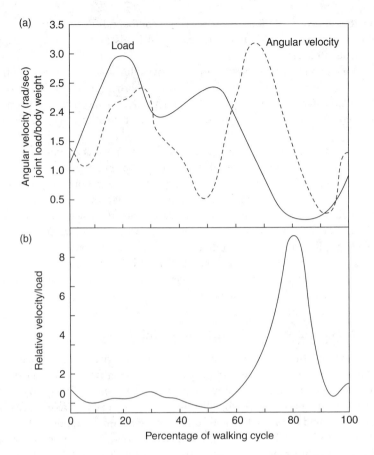

FIGURE 50.11 (a) Hip joint forces and angular velocities at different parts of the walking cycle (after Graham and Walker [61]). (b) Calculated ratio of velocity to force for the hip joint (from Figure 22.11a).

obtained is shown in Figure 50.11b. We see now a very different and somewhat simplified picture. There is a clear and distinct maximum in the ratio of velocity to load (U/W) at 80% of walking cycle, favoring the formation of a hydrodynamic film of maximum thickness. However, for most of the cycle (e.g., from 0 to 60%), the velocity/load ratio is significantly lower, thus favoring a condition of minimum film thickness and "boundary lubrication." However, we also know that synovial fluid is non-Newtonian; at higher rates of shear, its viscosity decreases sharply, approaching that of water. The shear rate is equal to the relative velocity divided by fluid film thickness (U/h) and is expressed in $\sec^{-1}$. This means that at the regions of low (U/W) ratios or thinner hydrodynamic films, the viscosity term in ($\eta U/W$) is even lower, thus pushing the minima to lower values favoring a condition of boundary lubrication. This is only a simplified view and does not consider those periods in which the relative sliding velocity is zero at motion reversal and where squeeze-film lubrication may come into play. A good example of the complexity of load and velocity variation in a human knee joint — including several zero-velocity periods — may be found in the chapter by Higginson and Unsworth [62] citing the work of Seedhom et al., which deals with biomechanics in the design of a total knee replacement [63].

The major point made here is that (1) there are parts of a walking cycle that would be expected to approach a condition of minimum fluid film thickness and boundary lubrication and (2) it is during these parts of the cycle that cartilage wear and damage resulting from contact is more likely to occur. Thus, approaches to reducing cartilage wear in a synovial joint could be broken down into two categories (i.e., promoting thicker hydrodynamic films and providing special forms of "boundary lubrication.")

50.8.6 Recent Developments

Recent developments in addressing some of the problems that involve cartilage damage and existing joint replacements include (1) progress in promoting cartilage repair [64], (2) possible use of artificial cartilage materials (e.g., synthetic hydrogels) [65,66], and (3) the development and application of more compliant joint replacement materials to promote a more favorable formation of an elastohydrodynamic film [67]. Although these are not strictly "lubricant-oriented" developments, they do and will involve important tribological aspects discussed in this chapter. For example, if new cartilage growth can be promoted by transplanting healthy chondrocytes to a platform in a damaged region of a synovial joint, how long will this cartilage last? If a hydrogel is used as an artificial cartilage, how long will it last? And if softer, elastomeric materials are used as partial joint replacements or coatings, how long will they last? These are questions of wear, not friction. And although the early fundamental studies of hydrogels as artificial cartilage measured only friction, and often only after a few moments of sliding, we know from recent work that even for hydrogels, low friction does not mean low wear [68].

50.9 Conclusions

The following main conclusions relating to the tribological behavior of natural, "normal" synovial joints are presented:

1. An unusually large number of theories and studies of joint lubrication have been proposed over the years. All of the theories focus on friction, none address wear, many do not involve experimental studies with cartilage, and very few consider the complexity and detailed biochemistry of the synovial-fluid articular-cartilage system.

2. It was shown by *in vitro* tests with bovine articular cartilage that the detailed biochemistry of synovial fluid has a significant effect on cartilage wear and damage. "Normal" bovine synovial fluid was found to provide excellent protection against wear. Various biochemical constituents isolated from bovine synovial fluid by Dr. David Swann, of the Shriners Burns Institute in Boston, showed varying effects on cartilage wear when added back to a buffered saline reference fluid. This research demonstrates once again the importance of distinguishing between friction and wear.

3. In a collaborative study of biotribology involving researchers and students in Mechanical Engineering, the Virginia-Maryland College of Veterinary Medicine, and Biochemistry, *in vitro* tribological tests using bovine articular cartilage demonstrated among other things that (1) normal synovial fluid provides better protection than a buffered saline solution in a cartilage-on-cartilage system, (2) tribological contact in cartilage systems can cause subsurface damage, delamination, changes in proteoglycan content, and in chemistry via a "biotribochemical" process not understood, and (3) pre-treatment of articular cartilage with the enzyme collagenase-3 — suspected as a factor in osteoarthritis — significantly increases cartilage wear.

4. It is suggested that these results could change significantly the way mechanisms of synovial joint lubrication are examined. Effects of biochemistry of the system on wear of articular cartilage are likely to be important; such effects may not be related to physical/rheological models of joint lubrication.

5. It is also suggested that connections between tribology/normal synovial joint lubrication and degenerative joint disease are not only possible but likely; however, such connections are undoubtedly complex. It is *not* argued that osteoarthritis is a tribological problem or that it is necessarily the result of a tribological deficiency. Ultimately, a better understanding of how normal synovial joints function from a tribological point of view could conceivably lead to advances in the prevention and treatment of osteoarthritis.

6. Several problems exist that make it difficult to understand and interpret many of the published works on synovial joint lubrication. One example is the widespread use of non-operational and vague terms such as "lubricating activity," "lubricating factor," "boundary lubricating ability," and

similar undefined terms which not only fail to distinguish between friction (which is usually measured) and cartilage wear (which is rarely measured), but tend to lump these phenomena together — a common error. Another problem is that a significant number of the published experimental studies of biotribology do not involve cartilage at all — relying on the use of glass-on-glass, rubber-on-glass, and even steel-on-steel. Such approaches may be a reflection of the incorrect view that "lubricating activity" is a property of a fluid and can be measured independently. Some suggestions are offered.

7. Last, the topic of synovial joint lubrication is far from being understood. It is a complex subject involving at least biophysics, biomechanics, biochemistry, and tribology. For a physical scientist or engineer, carrying out research in this area is a humbling experience.

Acknowledgments

The author wishes to acknowledge the support of the Edward H. Lane, G. Harold, and Leila Y. Mathers Foundations for their support during the sabbatical study at The Children's Hospital Medical Center. He also wishes to thank Dr. David Swann for his invaluable help in providing the test fluids and carrying out the biochemical analyses as well as Ms. Karen Hodgens for conducting the early scanning electron microscopy studies of worn cartilage specimens.

The author is also indebted to the following researchers for their encouraging and stimulating discussions of this topic over the years and for teaching a tribologist something of the complexity of synovial joints, articular cartilage, and arthritis: Drs. Leon Sokoloff, Charles McCutchen, Melvin Glimcher, David Swann, Henry Mankin, Clement Sledge, Helen Muir, Paul Dieppe, Heikki Helminen, as well as his colleagues at Virginia Tech — Hugo Veit, E. T. Kornegay, and E. M. Gregory.

Last, the author expresses his appreciation for and recognition of the valuable contributions made by students interested in biotribology over the years. These include graduate students Bettina Burkhardt, Michael Owellen, Matt Schroeder, Mark Freeman, and especially La Shaun Berrien, who contributed to this chapter, as well as the following summer undergraduate research students: Jean Yates, Elaine Ashby, Anne Newell, T. J. Hayes, Bethany Revak, Carolina Reyes, Amy Diegelman, and Heather Hughes.

References

[1] Hunter, W. Of the structure and diseases of articulating cartilages, *Phil. Trans.*, 42, 514–521, 1742–1743.

[2] Furey, M.J. "Tribology," *Encyclopedia of Materials Science and Engineering*, Pergamon Press, Oxford, 1986, pp. 5145–5158.

[3] Cameron, A. *The Principles of Lubrication*, Longmans Green & Co. Ltd, London, 1966.

[4] Dowson, D. and Higginson, G.R. *Elastohydrodynamic Lubrication*, SI Edition, Pergamon Press, Oxford, 1977.

[5] Freeman, M.A.R. *Adult Articular Cartilage*, Pitman Medical Publishing Co., Ltd., Tunbridge Wells, Kent, England, 2nd ed., 1979.

[6] Sokoloff, L., Ed. *The Joints and Synovial Fluid*, Vol. I, Academic Press, New York, 1978.

[7] Stockwell, R.A. *Biology of Cartilage Cells*, Cambridge University Press, Cambridge, 1979.

[8] Furey, M.J. Biochemical aspects of synovial joint lubrication and cartilage wear, European Society of Osteoarthrology. *Symposium on Joint Destruction in Arthritis and Osteoarthritis*, Noordwijkerhout, The Netherlands, May 24–27, 1992.

[9] Furey, M.J. Biotribology: cartilage lubrication and wear, *6th International Congress on Tribology*, EUROTRIB '93, Budapest, Hungary, August 30–September 2, 1993.

[10] Furey, M.J. and Burkhardt, B.M. Biotribology: friction, wear, and lubrication of natural synovial joints, *Lubrication Sci.* 255–271, 3–9, 1997.

[11] McCutchen, C.W. Lubrication of joints. *The Joints and Synovial Fluid*, Vol. I, Academic Press, New York, 1978, pp. 437–483.

[12] Swanson, S.A.V. *Friction, Wear and Lubrication*. In *Adult Articular Cartilage*, M.A.R. Freeman, Ed., Pitman Medical Publishing Co., Ltd., Tunbridge Wells, Kent, England, 2nd ed., 1979, pp. 415–460.

[13] Higginson, G.R. and Unsworth, T. The lubrication of natural joints. In *Tribology of Natural and Artificial Joints*, J. H. Dumbleton, Ed. Elsevier Scientific Publishing Co., Amsterdam and New York, 1981, pp. 47–73.

[14] Dumbleton, J.H. *Tribology of Natural and Artificial Joints*, Elsevier Scientific Publishing Co., Amsterdam, The Netherlands, 1981.

[15] Droogendijk, L. *On the Lubrication of Synovial Joints*, Ph.D. thesis, Twente University of Technology, The Netherlands, 1984.

[16] Burkhardt, B.M. *Development and Design of a Test Device for Cartilage Wear Studies*, M.S. thesis, Mechanical Engineering, Virginia Polytechnic Institute & State University, Blacksburg, VA, December 1988.

[17] McCutchen, C.W. Mechanisms of animal joints: sponge-hydrostatic and weeping bearings, *Nature*, (*Lond.*), 184, 1284–1285, 1959.

[18] McCutchen, C.W. The frictional properties of animal joints, *Wear* 5, 1–17, 1962.

[19] Torzilli, P.A. and Mow, V.C. On the fundamental fluid transport mechanisms through normal and pathological articular cartilage during friction-1. *The formulation. J. Biomech.* 9, 541–552, 1976.

[20] Mansour, J.M. and Mow, V.C. On the natural lubrication of synovial joints: normal and degenerated. *J. Lubrication Technol.*, 163–173, 1977.

[21] Ateshian, G. A., Wang, H., and Lai, W. M. The role of interstitial fluid pressurization and surface porosities on the boundary friction of articular cartilage, ASMS *J. Biomed. Eng.*, 120, 241–251, 1998.

[22] Unsworth, A. Tribology of human and artificial joints. Proc. I. Mech. E., Part II: *J. Eng. Med.* Vol. 205, 1991.

[23] Simon, W.H. Wear properties of articular cartilage. *In vitro*, Section on Rheumatic Diseases, Laboratory of Experimental Pathology, National Institute of Arthritis and Metabolic Diseases, National Institutes of Health, February 1971.

[24] Bloebaum, R.D. and Wilson, A.S. The morphology of the surface of articular cartilage in adult rats, *J. Anatomy*, 131, 333–346, 1980.

[25] Radin, E.L. and Paul, I.L. Response of joints to impact loading I. *In vitro* wear tests, *Arthritis Rheumatism* 14, 1971.

[26] Lipshitz, H. and Glimcher, M.J. A technique for the preparation of plugs of articular cartilage and subchondral bone, *J. Biomech.*, 7, 293–298.

[27] Lipshitz, H. and Etheredge, III, R. *In vitro* wear of articular cartilage. *J. Bone Joint Surg.*, 57-A, 527–534, 1975.

[28] Lipshitz, H. and Glimcher, M.J. *In vitro* studies of wear of articular cartilage, II. Characteristics of the wear of articular cartilage when worn against stainless steel plates having characterized surfaces. *Wear* 52, 297–337, 1979.

[29] Sokoloff, L. Davis, W.H., and Lee, S.L. Boundary lubricating ability of synovial fluid in degenerative joint disease, *Arthritis Rheumatism* 21, 754–760, 1978.

[30] Sokoloff, L., Davis, W.H., and Lee, S.L. A proposed model of boundary lubrication by synovial fluid: structuring of boundary water, *J. Biomech. Eng.*, 101, 185–192, 1979.

[31] Jay, D.J. Characterization of bovine synovial fluid lubricating factor, I. Chemical surface activity and lubrication properties, *Connective Tissue Res.*, 28, 71–88, 1992.

[32] Furey, M.J. Joint lubrication, in *The Biomedical Engineering Handbook*, Joseph D. Bronzino, Ed., CRC Press 1995, pp. 333–351.

[33] Burkhardt, B.M. *Development and Design of a Test Device for Cartilage Wear Studies*, M.S. thesis, Mechanical Engineering, Virginia Polytechnic Institute and State University, Blacksburg, VA, December 1988.

[34] Stachowiak, G.W., Batchelor, A.W., and Griffiths, L.J. Friction and wear changes in synovial joints, *Wear* 171, 135–142, 1994.

[35] Hayes, A., Harris, B., Dieppe, P.A., and Clift, S.E. Wear of articular cartilage: the effect of crystals, *IMechE* 41–58, 1993.

[36] Malcolm, L.L. An Experimental Investigation of the Frictional and Deformational Responses of Articular Cartilage Interfaces to Static and Dynamic Loading, Ph.D. thesis, University of California, San Diego, 1976.

[37] Furey, M.J. Biotribology: An *in vitro* study of the effects of synovial fluid constituents on cartilage wear. *Proc., XVth Symposium of the European Society of Osteoarthrology*, Kuopio, Finland, June 25–27, 1986, abstract in *Scandanavian Journal of Rheumatology*, Supplement.

[38] Furey, M.J. The influence of synovial fluid constituents on cartilage wear: a scanning electron microscope study. *Conference on Joint Destruction, XVth Symposium on the European Society of Osteoarthrology*, Sochi, USSR, September 28–October 3, 1987.

[39] Furey, M.J. Biochemical aspects of synovial joint lubrication and cartilage wear. European Society of Osteoarthrology. *Symposium on Joint Destruction in Arthritis and Osteoarthritis*, Noordwigkerhout, The Netherlands, May 24–27, 1992.

[40] Furey, M.J. Biotribology: cartilage lubrication and wear. *Proceedings of the 6th International Congress on Tribology EUROTRIB; '93*, Vol. 2, pp. 464–470, Budapest, Hungary, August 30–September 2, 1993.

[41] Schroeder, M.O. *Biotribology: Articular Cartilage Friction, Wear, and Lubrication*, M.S. thesis, Mechanical Engineering, Virginia Polytechnic Institute and State University, Blacksburg, VA, July 1995.

[42] Owellen, M.C. *Biotribology: The Effect of Lubricant and Load on Articular Cartilage Wear and Friction*, M.S. thesis, Mechanical Engineering, Virginia Polytechnic Institute and State University, Blacksburg, VA, July 1997.

[43] Furey, M.J., Schroeder, M.O., Hughes, H.L., Owellen, M.C., Berrien, L.S., Veit, H., Gregory, E.M., and Kornegay, E. T. Observations of subsurface damage and cartilage degradation in *in vitro* tribological tests using bovine articular cartilage, *21st Symposium of the European Society for Osteoarthrology*, Vol. 15, Gent, Belgium, September 1996, 5, 3.2.

[44] Furey, M.J., Schroeder, M.O., Hughes, H.L., Owellen, M.C., Berrien, L.S., Veit, H., Gregory, E.M., and Kornegay, E.T. *Biotribology, Synovial Joint Lubrication and Osteoarthritis*, Paper in Session W5 on Biotribology, *World Tribology Congress*, London, September 8–12, 1997.

[45] Berrien, L.S., Furey, M.J., Veit, H.P., and Gregory, E.M. The Effect of Collagenase-3 on the *In Vitro* Wear of Bovine Articular Cartilage, Paper, Biotribology Session, *Fifth International Tribology Conference*, Brisbane, Australia, December 6–9, 1998.

[46] Sokoloff, L. *The Biology of Degenerative Joint Disease*, University of Chicago Press, Chicago, IL, 1969.

[47] Kelley, W.N., Harris, Jr., E.D., Ruddy, S., and Sledge, C.B. *Textbook of Rheumatology*, W.B. Saunders Co., Philadelphia, 1981.

[48] Moskowitz, R.W., Howell, D.S., Goldberg, V.M., and Mankin, H.J. *Osteoarthritis: Diagnois and Management*, W.B. Saunders Co., Philadelphia, 1984.

[49] Verbruggen, G. and Veyes, E.M. Degenerative joints: test tubes, tissues, models, and man. *Proc. First Conference on Degenerative Joint Diseases*, Excerpta Medica, Amsterdam-Oxford-Princeton, 1982.

[50] Gastpar, H. Biology of the articular cartilage in health and disease. *Proc. Second Munich Symposium on Biology of Connective Tissue*, Munich, July 23–24, 1979; F.K. Schattauer Verlag, Stuttgart, 1980.

[51] Dieppe, P. and Calvert, P. *Crytals and Joint Disease*, Chapman and Hall, London, 1983.

[52] Discussions with M.J. Glimcher, The Children's Hospital Medical Center, Boston, MA, Fall 1983.

[53] Furey, M.J. Exploring possible connections between tribology and osteoarthritis, *Lubricat. Sci.* 273, May 1997.

[54] Hayes, A., Harris, B., Dieppe, P.A., and Clift, S.E. Wear of cartilage: the effect of crystals, *Proc. I.Mech.E.* 1993, 41–58.

[55] Wright, V. and Dowson, D. Lubrication and cartilage, *J. Anat.* 121, 107–118, 1976.

[56] Radin, E.L., Swann, D.A., and Weisser, P.A. Separation of a hyaluronate-free lubricating fraction from synovial fluid, *Nature* 228, 377–378, 1970.

[57] McCutchen, C.W. Joint Lubrication, *Bull. Hosp. Joint Dis. Orthop. Inst.* XLIII, 118–129, 1983.

[58] Williams, III, P.F., Powell, G.L., and LaBerge, M. Sliding friction analysis of phosphatidylcholine as a boundary lubricant for articular cartilage, *Proc. I.Mech.E.* 207, 41–166, 1993.

[59] Schwarz, I. M. and Hills, B. A. Surface-active phospholipid as the lubricating component of lubrician, *Br. J. Rheumatol.* 37, 21–26, 1998.

[60] Private communication, letter to Michael J. Furey from Gerard A. Ateshian, July 1998.

[61] Graham, J.D. and Walker, T.W. Motion in the hip: the relationship of split line patterns to surface velocities, a paper in *Perspectives in Biomedical Engineering*, R.M. Kenedi, Ed., University Park Press, Baltimore, MD, pp. 161–164, 1973.

[62] Higginson, G.R. and Unsworth, T. The lubrication of natural joints. In *Tribology by Natural and Artificial Joints*, J.H. Dumbleton, Ed., Elsevier Scientific Publishing Co., Amsterdam, pp. 47–73, 1981.

[63] Seedhom, B.B., Longton, E.B., Dowson, D., and Wright, V. Biomechanics background in the design of total replacement knee prosthesis. *Acta Orthop. Belgica* Tome 39, Fasc 1, 164–180, 1973.

[64] Brittberg, M. *Cartilage Repair*, a collection of five articles on cartilaginous tissue engineering with an emphasis on chondrocyte transplantation. Institute of Surgical Sciences and Department of Clinical Chemistry and Institute of Laboratory Medicine, Goteborg University, Sweden, 2nd ed., 1996.

[65] Corkhill, P.H., Trevett, A.S., and Tighe, B.J. The potential of hydrogels as synthetic articular cartilage. *Proc. Inst. Mech. Eng.* 204, 147–155, 1990.

[66] Caravia, L., Dowson, D., Fisher, J., Corkhill, P.H., and Tighe, B.J.A comparison of friction in hydrogel and polyurethane materials for cushion form joints. *J. Mater. Sci.: Mater. Med.* 4, 515–520, 1993.

[67] Caravia, L., Dowson, D., Fisher, J., Corkhill, P.H., and Tighe, B.J. Friction of hydrogel and polyurethane elastic layers when sliding against each other under a mixed lubrication regime. *Wear* 181–183, 236–240, 1995.

[68] Freeman, M.E., Furey, M.J., Love, B.J., and Hampton, J.M. Friction, wear, and lubrication of hydrogels as synthetic articular cartilage, paper, Biotribology Session, *Fifth International Tribology Conference, AUSTRIB '98*, Brisbane, Australia, December 6–9, 1998.

Further Information

For more information on synovial joints and arthritis, the following books are suggested: *The Biology of Degenerative Joint Disease* [46], *Adult Articular Cartilage* [5], *The Joints and Synovial Fluid: I* [6], *Textbook of Rheumatology* [47], *Osteoarthritis: Diagnosis and Management* [48], *Degenerative Joints: Test Tubes, Tissues, Models, and Man* [49], *Biology of the Articular Cartilage in Health and Disease* [50], and *Crystals and Joint Disease* [51].

51

Analysis of Gait

Roy B. Davis, III
Shriners Hospital for Children

Sylvia Õunpuu
Peter A. DeLuca
*University of Connecticut
Children's Medical Center*

Gait analysis is the quantitative measurement and assessment of human locomotion including both walking and running. A number of different disciplines use gait analysis techniques. Basic scientists seek a better understanding of the mechanisms that normal ambulators use to translate muscular contractions about articulating joints into functional accomplishment, for example, level walking [1] and stair climbing [2]. In sports biomechanics, athletes and their coaches use movement analysis techniques to investigate performance improvement while avoiding injury, for example, Ferber et al. [3], Hunter et al. [4], Kautz and Hull [5], and Tashman et al. [6]. Sports equipment manufacturers seek to quantify the perceived advantages of their products relative to a competitor's offering.

With respect to the analysis of gait in the clinical setting, or clinical gait analysis, medical professionals apply an evolving knowledge base in the interpretation of the walking patterns of impaired ambulators for the planning of treatment protocols, for example, orthotic prescription and surgical intervention. Clinical gait analysis is an evaluation tool that allows the clinician to determine the extent to which an individual's gait has been affected by an already diagnosed disorder [7]. Examples of clinical pathologies currently served by gait analysis include:

- Amputation [8]
- Cerebral palsy [9,10]
- Degenerative joint disease [11,12]
- Joint pain [13]
- Joint replacement [14]
- Poliomyelitis [15]

- Multiple sclerosis [16]
- Muscular dystrophy [17]
- Myelodysplasia [18,19]
- Rheumatoid arthritis [20]
- Spinal cord injury [21]
- Stroke [22]
- Traumatic brain injury [23]

Generally, gait analysis data collection protocols, measurement precision, and data reduction models have been developed to meet the requirements specific to the research, sport, or clinical setting. For example, gait measurement protocols in a research setting might include an extensive physical examination to characterize the anthropometrics of each subject. This time expenditure may not be possible in a clinical setting. The focus of this chapter is on the methods for the assessment of walking patterns of persons with locomotive impairment, that is, clinical gait analysis. The discussion includes a description of the available measurement technology, the components of data collection and reduction, the type of gait information produced for clinical interpretation, and the strengths and limitations of clinical gait analysis.

51.1 Fundamental Concepts

51.1.1 Clinical Gait Analysis Information

Gait is a cyclic activity for which certain discrete events have been defined as significant. Typically, the *gait cycle* is defined as the period of time from the point of *initial contact* (also referred to as *foot contact*) of the subject's foot with the ground to the next point of initial contact for that same limb. Dividing the gait cycle in stance and swing phases is the point in the cycle where the stance limb leaves the ground, called *toe off* or *foot off*. Gait variables that change over time such as the patient's joint angular displacements are normally presented as a function of the individual's gait cycle for clinical analysis. This is done to facilitate the comparison of different walking trials and the use of a normative database [24]. Data that are currently provided for the clinical interpretation of gait may include:

- A video recording of the individual's gait (before instrumentation) for qualitative review and quality control purposes
- Static physical examination measures, such as passive joint range of motion, muscle strength and tone, and the presence and degree of bony deformity
- Segment and joint angular positions associated with standing posture
- Stride and temporal parameters, such as step length and walking velocity
- Segment and joint angular displacements, commonly referred to as *kinematics*
- The forces and torque applied to the subject's foot by the ground, or ground reaction loads
- The reactive intersegmental moments produced about the lower extremity joints by active and passive soft tissue forces as well as the associated mechanical power of the intersegmental moment, collectively referred to as *kinetics*
- Indications of muscle activity, that is, voltage potentials produced by contracting muscles, known as dynamic *electromyography* (EMG)
- The dynamic pressure distributions on the plantar surface of the foot, referred to as *pedobarography*
- A measure of metabolic energy expenditure, for example, oxygen consumption, energy cost

51.1.2 Data Collection Protocol

The steps involved in the gathering of data for clinical gait analysis usually include a complete physical examination, biplanar videotaping, a static calibration of the "instrumented" subject, and multiple walks

TABLE 51.1   A Typical Gait Data Collection Protocol

Test component	Approximate time (min)
Pretest tasks: test explanation to the adult patient or the pediatric patient and parent, system calibration	10
Videotaping: brace, barefoot, close-up, standing	5–10
Clinical examination: range of motion, muscle strength, etc.	15–30
Motion marker placement	15–20
Motion data collection: subject calibration and multiple walks, per test condition (barefoot and orthosis)	10–60
Electromyography (surface electrodes and fine wire electrodes)	20–60
Data reduction of all trials	15–90
Data interpretation	20–30
Report dictation, generation, and distribution	120–180

along a walkway that is commonly both level and smooth. The time to complete these steps can range from one to three hours (Table 51.1). While the baseline for analysis is barefoot gait, subjects are tested in other conditions as well, for example, lower extremity orthoses and crutches. Requirements and constraints associated with clinical gait data gathering include the following:

- The patient should not be intimidated or distracted by the testing environment
- The measurement equipment and protocols should not alter the subject's gait
- Patient preparation and testing time must be minimized, and rest (or play) intervals must be included in the process as needed
- Data collection techniques must be reasonably repeatable
- Methodology must be sufficiently robust and flexible to allow the evaluation of a variety of gait abnormalities where the dynamic range of motion and anatomy may be significantly different from normal
- The collected data must be validated before the end of the test period, for example, raw data fully processed before the patient leaves the facility

51.2   Measurement Approaches and Systems

The purpose of this section is to provide an overview of the several technologies that are available to measure the dynamic gait variables listed earlier, including stride and temporal parameters, kinematics, kinetics, and dynamic EMG. Methods of data reduction will be described in a following section.

51.2.1   Stride and Temporal Parameters

The timing of the gait cycle events of initial contact and toe off must be measured for the computation of the stride and temporal quantities. These measures may be obtained through a wide variety of approaches ranging from the use of simple tools such as a stopwatch and tape measure to sophisticated arrays of photoelectric monitors. Foot switches may be applied to the plantar surface of the subject's foot over the bony prominences of the heel and metatarsal heads in different configurations depending on the information desired. A typical configuration is the placement of a switch on the heel, first and fifth metatarsal heads, and great toe. In a clinical population, foot switch placement is challenging because of the variability of foot deformities and the associated foot–ground contact patterns. This switch placement difficulty is avoided through the use of either shoe insoles instrumented with one or two large foot switches or entire contact sensitive walkways. These gait events may also be quantified using either the camera-based motion measurement or the force platform technology described below.

51.2.2 Motion Measurement

A number of alternative technologies are available for the measurement of body segment spatial position and orientation. These include the use of electrogoniometry, accelerometry, and video-based digitizers. These approaches are described below.

51.2.2.1 Electrogoniometry

A simple electrogoniometer consists of a rotary potentiometer with arms fixed to the shaft and base for attachment to the body segments juxtaposed to the joint of interest. Multiaxial goniometers extend this capability by providing additional, simultaneous, orthogonal measures of rotational displacement, more appropriate for human joint motion measurement. Electrogoniometers offer the advantages of real-time display and the rapid collection of single joint information on many subjects. These devices are limited to the measurement of relative angles and may be cumbersome in typical clinical applications such as the simultaneous, bilateral assessment of hip, knee, and ankle motion.

51.2.2.2 Accelerometry

Multiaxis accelerometers can be employed to measure both linear and angular accelerations (if multiple transducers are properly configured). Velocity and position data may then be derived through numerical integration although care must be taken with respect to the selection of initial conditions and the handling of gravitational effects.

51.2.2.3 Videocamera-Based Systems

This approach to human motion measurement involves the use of external markers that are placed on the subject's body segments and aligned with specific bony landmarks. Marker trajectories are then monitored by a system of motion capture cameras (generally from 6 to 12) placed around a measurement volume (Figure 51.1). In a frame-by-frame analysis, stereophotogrammetric techniques are then used to produce

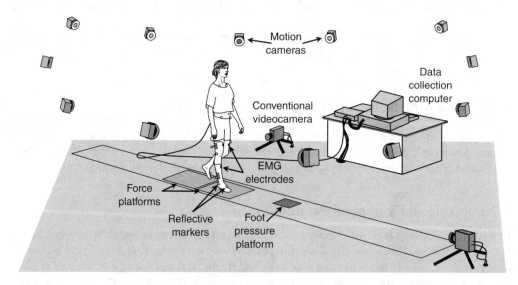

FIGURE 51.1   An "instrumented" patient with reflective spheres or markers and EMG electrodes. She walks along a level pathway while being monitored by 6–12 motion cameras (that monitor the displacement the reflective markers) and 2–4 force platforms (that measure ground reaction loads). She might also walk over a foot pressure platform that measures the plantar pressure distribution. Her walk is also videotaped with one or two conventional videocameras. All of these signals (from the motion cameras, force platforms, EMG electrodes, and foot pressure platform) are sent to the central data collection computer in the lab. These signals are then processed by the operator to produce the information used, along with the video recordings and other clinical examination data, to identify gait abnormalities and guide treatment planning.

the instantaneous three-dimensional (3-D) coordinates of each marker (relative to a fixed laboratory coordinate system) from the set of two-dimensional camera images. The processing of the 3-D marker coordinate data is described in a later section.

The videocamera-based systems employ either passive (retroreflective) or active (light-emitting diodes) markers. Passive marker camera systems incorporate strobe light sources (light-emitting diode [LED] rings around the camera lens). The cameras then capture the light returned from the highly reflective markers (usually small spheres). Active marker camera systems record the light that is produced by small LED markers that are placed directly on the subject. Advantages and disadvantages are associated with each approach. For example, the anatomical location (or identity) of each marker used in an active marker system is immediately known because the markers are sequentially pulsed by a controlling computer. User interaction is required currently for marker identification in passive marker systems although algorithms have been developed to expedite this process, that is, automatic tracking. The system of cables required to power and control the LED's of the active marker system may increase the possibility for subject distraction and gait alteration.

51.2.3 Ground Reaction Measurement

51.2.3.1 Force Platforms

The 3-D ground reaction force vector, the vertical ground reaction torque and the point of application of the ground reaction force vector (i.e., center of pressure) are measured with force platforms embedded in the walkway. Force plates with typical measurement surface dimensions of 0.5 × 0.5 m are comprised of several strain gauges or piezoelectric sensor arrays rigidly mounted together.

51.2.3.2 Pedobarography

The dynamic distributed load that corresponds to the vertical ground reaction force can be evaluated with the use of a flat, two-dimensional array of small piezoresistive sensors. Overall resolution of the transducer is dictated by the size of the individual sensor "cell." Sensor arrays configured as shoe insole inserts or flat plates offer the clinical user two measurement alternatives. Although the currently available technology does afford the clinical practitioner better insight into the qualitative force distribution patterns across the plantar surface of the foot, its quantitative capability is limited because of the challenge of calibration and signal drift (e.g., sensor creep).

51.2.4 Dynamic Electromyography (EMG)

Electrodes placed on the skin's surface and fine wires inserted into muscle are used to measure the voltage potentials produced by contracting muscles. The activity of the lower limb musculature is evaluated in this way with respect to the timing and the intensity of the contraction. Data collection variables that affect the quality of the EMG signal include the placement and distance between recording electrodes, skin surface conditions, distance between electrode and target muscle, signal amplification and filtering, and the rate of data acquisition. The phasic characteristics of the muscle activity may be estimated from the raw EMG signal. The EMG data may also be presented as a rectified and integrated waveform. To evaluate the intensity of the contraction, the dynamic EMG amplitudes are typically normalized by a reference value, for example, the EMG amplitude during a maximum voluntary contraction. This latter requirement is difficult to achieve consistently for patients who have limited isolated control of individual muscles, such as children with cerebral palsy (CP).

51.3 Gait Data Reduction

The predominant approach for the collection of clinical gait data involves the placement of external markers on the surface of body segments that are aligned with particular bony landmarks. These markers are commonly attached to the subject as either discrete units or in rigidly connected clusters. As described

(a)   (b)

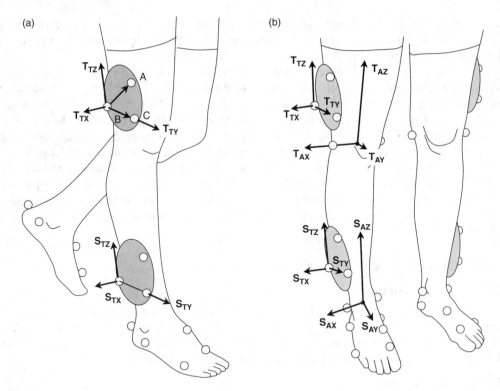

FIGURE 51.2 (a) Technical or marker-based coordinate systems "fixed" to the thigh and shank. A body fixed coordinate system may be computed for each cluster of three or more markers. On the thigh, for example, the vector cross product of the vectors from markers B to A and B to C produces a vector that is perpendicular to the cluster plane. From these vectors, the unit vectors T_{TX} and T_{TY} may be determined and used to compute the third orthogonal coordinate direction T_{TZ}. (b) A subject calibration relates technical coordinate systems with anatomical coordinate systems, for example, $\{T_T\}$ with $\{T_A\}$, through the identification of anatomical landmarks, for example, the medial and lateral femoral condyles and medial and lateral malleoli.

briefly above, the products of the data acquisition process are the 3-D coordinates (relative to an inertially fixed laboratory coordinate system) of each marker trajectory over a gait cycle. If at least three markers or reference points are identified for each body segment, then the six degrees-of-freedom associated with the translation and position of the segment may be determined. The following example illustrates this straightforward process.

Assume that a cluster of three markers has been attached to the thigh and shank of the test subject as shown in Figure 51.2a. A body-fixed coordinate system may be computed for each marker cluster. For example, for the thigh, the vector cross product of the vectors from markers B to A and B to C produces a vector that is perpendicular to the cluster plane. From these vectors, the unit vectors T_{TX} and T_{TY} may be determined and used to compute the third orthogonal coordinate direction T_{TZ}. In a similar manner, the marker-based, or technical, coordinate system may be calculated for the shank, that is, S_{TX}, S_{TY}, and S_{TZ}. At this point, one might use these two technical coordinate systems to provide an estimate of the absolute orientation of the thigh or shank or the relative angles between the thigh and shank. This assumes that the technical coordinate systems reasonably approximate the anatomical axes of the body segments, for example, that T_{TZ} approximates the long axis of the thigh. A more rigorous approach incorporates the use of a subject calibration procedure to relate technical coordinate systems with pertinent anatomical directions [25].

In a subject calibration, usually performed with the subject standing, additional data are collected by the measurement system that relates the technical coordinate systems to the underlying anatomical structure. For example, as shown in Figure 51.2b, the medial and lateral femoral condyles and the medial and lateral malleoli may be used as anatomical references with the application of additional markers. With the hip center location estimated from markers placed on the pelvis [26,27] and knee and ankle center locations based on the additional markers, anatomical coordinate systems may be computed, for example, $\{T_A\}$ and $\{S_A\}$. The relationship between the respective anatomical and technical coordinate system pairs as well as the location of the joint centers in terms of the appropriate technical coordinate system may be stored, to be recalled in the reduction of each frame of the walking data. In this way, the technical coordinate systems (shown in Figure 51.2b) are transformed into alignment with the anatomical coordinate systems.

Once anatomically aligned body-fixed coordinate systems have been computed for each body segment under investigation, one may compute the angular position of the joints and segments in a number of ways. The classical approach of Euler, or more specifically, Cardan angles is commonly used in clinical gait analysis to describe the motion of the thigh relative to the pelvis (or hip angles), the motion of the shank relative to the thigh (or knee angles), the motion of the foot relative to the shank (or ankle angles), as well as the absolute orientation of the pelvis and foot in space. The joint rotation sequence commonly used for the Cardan angle computation is flexion–extension, adduction–abduction, and transverse plane rotation [28]. Alternatively, joint motion has been described through the use of helical axes [29].

The intersegmental moments that soft tissue (e.g., muscle, ligaments, and joint capsule) forces produce about approximate joint centers may be computed through the use of inverse dynamics, that is, Newtonian mechanics. For example, the free body diagram of the foot shown in Figure 51.3 depicts the various external loads to the foot as well as the intersegmental reactions produced at the ankle. The mass, mass moments of inertia, and location of the center of mass may be estimated from regression-based anthropometric relationships [30–32], and linear and angular velocity and acceleration may be determined by numerical differentiation. If the ground reaction loads, F_G and T, are measured by a force platform, then the unknown ankle intersegmental force, F_A, may be solved for with Newton's translational equation of motion. It is noted that inverse dynamics underestimates the magnitude of the actual joint contact forces. Newton's rotational equation of motion may then be applied to compute the net ankle intersegmental moment, M_A. This process may then be repeated for the shank and thigh by using distal joint loads to solve for the proximal intersegmental reactions. The mechanical power associated with an intersegmental moment and the corresponding joint angular velocity may be computed from the vector dot product of the two vectors, for example, ankle power is computed through $M_A \cdot \omega_A$ where ω_A is the angular velocity of the foot relative to the shank. Readers are referred to descriptions by Õunpuu et al. [33] and Palladino and Davis [34] for more details associated with this process.

Although sometimes referred to as "muscle moments," these net intersegmental moments reflect the moments produced by several mechanisms, for example, ligamentous forces, passive muscle and tendon

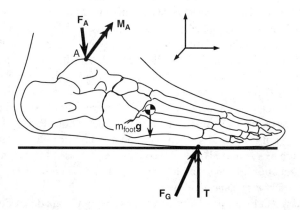

FIGURE 51.3   A free body diagram of the foot that illustrates the external loads to the foot, for example, the ground reaction loads, F_G and T, and the weight of the foot, $m_{foot}g$, as well as the unknown intersegmental reactions produced at the ankle, F_A and M_A, which may be solved for through the application of Newtonian mechanics.

force, and active muscle contractile force, in response to external loads. Currently, the evaluation of individual muscle forces in a patient population is not feasible because optimization strategies that may be successful for normal ambulation, for example, Chao and Rim [35], Anderson and Pandy [36], may not be appropriate for pathological muscle behavior, for example, spasticity, overactivity, hyper- or hypotonicity.

With respect to assumptions associated with these gait models, the body segments are assumed to be rigid, for example, soft tissue movement relative to underlying bony structures is small. The external markers are assumed to move with the underlying anatomical references. In this way, estimated joint center locations are assumed to remain fixed relative to the respective segmental coordinate systems, for example, the knee center is fixed relative to the thigh coordinate system. Moreover, the mass distribution changes during motion are assumed to be negligible. Consequently, marker or instrumentation attachment sites must be carefully selected, for example, over tendonous structures of the distal shank as opposed to the more proximal muscle masses of the gastrocnemius and soleus.

51.4   Illustrative Clinical Example

As indicated earlier, the information available for clinical gait interpretation may include static physical examination measures, stride and temporal data, segment and joint kinematics, joint kinetics, electromyograms, and a video record. With this information, the clinical team can assess the patient's gait deviations, attempt to identify the etiology of the abnormalities and recommend treatment alternatives. In this way, clinicians are able to isolate the biomechanical insufficiency that may produce a locomotive impairment and require a compensatory response from the patient. For example, a patient may excessively elevate a pelvis (compensatory) in order to gain additional foot clearance in swing, which is perhaps inadequate due to a weak ankle dorsiflexor (primary problem).

The following example illustrates how gait analysis data are used in the treatment decision-making process for a six-year-old child with cerebral palsy, left spastic hemiplegia. Initially, all gait and clinical examination data are reviewed and a list of primary problems and possible causes is generated. The reviewed data would include three-dimensional kinematic data (Figure 51.4), and kinetic data (Figure 51.5) and dynamic EMG data (Figure 51.6).

In the sagittal plane, increased left plantar flexion in stance and swing (Figure 51.4, Point A) is secondary to spasticity of the ankle plantar flexor muscles as the patient has normal passive range of motion of the ankle and can stand plantigrade. Premature plantar flexion of the right ankle in mid stance (Figure 51.4, Point B) is a vault compensation as the patient could isolate motion about the right ankle on clinical examination and produce an internal dorsiflexor moment during loading response (Figure 51.5, Point A). Increased left knee flexion at initial contact (Figure 51.4, Point C) is secondary to hamstring muscle spasticity/tightness (appreciated during the clinical examination) as well as overactivity of the hamstrings during gait (seen in the EMG data, Figure 51.6, Point A). Reduced left knee flexion in swing (Figure 51.4, Point D) is secondary to rectus femoris overactivity in mid swing (Figure 51.6, Point B), an absence of power generation at the ankle in terminal stance (Figure 51.5, Point B), reduced power generation at the hip in preswing (Figure 51.5, Point C), and out-of-plane positioning of the lower extremity due to internal hip rotation (Figure 51.4, Point E). Increasing anterior pelvic tilt during left side stance (Figure 51.4, Point F) is related to the patient's limited ability to isolate movement between the pelvis and femur on the left side. In the transverse plane, increased left internal hip rotation (Figure 51.4, Point E), increased left internal foot progression (Figure 51.4, Point G), and asymmetric pelvic rotation with the left side externally rotated (Figure 51.4, Point H) are all secondary to increased internal femoral torsion (noted during the clinical examination). In the coronal plane, asymmetrical hip rotations (Figure 51.4, Point I) are secondary to pelvic transverse plane asymmetry.

After all of the primary gait issues are identified and possible causes are determined, treatment options for each primary issue are proposed. For the child presented earlier here, treatment options include a left femoral derotation osteotomy to correct for internal femoral torsion and associated internal hip rotation. Expected secondary outcomes of this intervention include improved foot progression and symmetrical

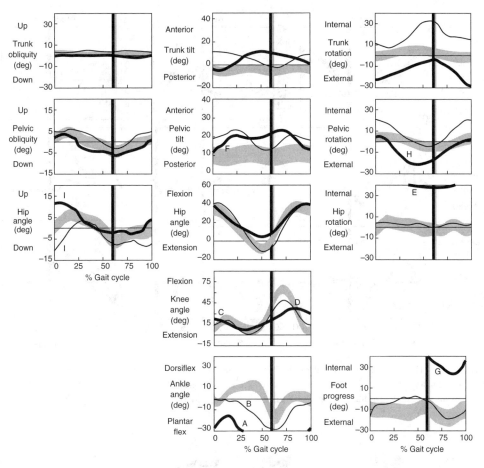

FIGURE 51.4 The left (thick lines) and right (thin lines) trunk, pelvic, and lower extremity kinematics for a six-year-old child with cerebral palsy, left spastic hemiplegia. Also shown are shaded bands that indicate one standard deviation about normal mean values. (Reproduced from Õunpuu, S., Gage, J.R., and Davis, R.B., *J. Pediatr. Orthop.*, 11, 341, 1991. With permission.)

pelvic position in the transverse plane. A left intramuscular plantar flexor muscle lengthening is recommended to provide more length to the ankle plantar flexors and reduce the impact of muscle stretch on the spastic plantar flexors, thereby reducing the excessive equinus in stance and swing and providing more stability in stance. A left hamstring muscle lengthening is also recommended to reduce the impact of muscle stretch on hamstring spasticity, thereby improving knee extension at initial contact and overall knee motion in stance. A rectus femoris muscle transfer is recommended to reduce the impact of inappropriate activity of the rectus femoris in mid swing and therefore improve peak knee flexion in swing. The premature plantar flexion of the right ankle in stance is secondary to a vault compensation and therefore, is predicted to resolve secondary to the surgery on the left side, that is, does not require any treatment. A standard protocol in most clinical gait laboratories is to repeat the gait analysis at about one year postsurgery. At this time, surgical hypotheses and progress with respect to resolution of gait abnormalities can be evaluated objectively.

51.5 Gait Analysis: Current Status

As indicated in the modeling discussion earlier, the utility of gait analysis information may be limited by sources of error such as soft tissue displacement relative to bone, estimates of joint center locations,

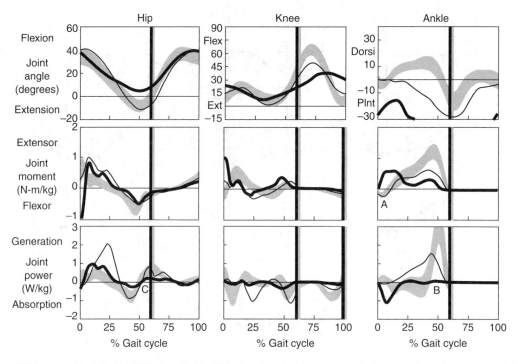

FIGURE 51.5 The left (thick lines) and right (thin lines) sagittal lower extremity kinetics for a six-year-old child with cerebral palsy, left spastic hemiplegia. Also shown are shaded bands that indicate one standard deviation about normal mean values. (Reproduced from Ōunpuu, S., Gage, J.R., and Davis, R.B., *J. Pediatr. Orthop.*, 11, 341, 1991. With permission.)

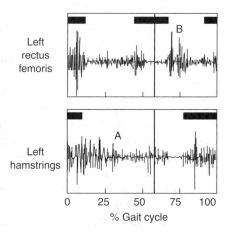

FIGURE 51.6 Electromyography tracing for the left rectus femoris and hamstring muscles for a six-year-old child with cerebral palsy, left spastic hemiplegia. The horizontal bars on the graphs indicate the approximate normal activity of these muscles during walking. (Reproduced from Bleck, E.E., *Orthopaedic Management in Cerebral Palsy*, Mac Keith Press, Philadelphia, PA, 1987, p. 87. With permission.)

approximations of the inertial properties of the body segments, and the numerical differentiation of noisy data. Other errors associated with data collection alter the results as well, for example, a marker improperly placed or a force platform inadvertently contacted by the swing limb. The evaluation of small subjects weakens the data because intermarker distances are reduced, thereby reducing the precision of angular computations, although recent improvements in technology have lessened this challenge to a degree. It is essential that the potential adverse effects of these errors on the gait information be understood and appreciated by the clinical team in the interpretation process.

Controversies related to gait analysis techniques include the use of individually placed markers versus clusters of markers and the application of helical or screw axes versus the use of Euler angles. Recent improvements in technology and computational techniques, for example, Leardini et al. [38], Piazza et al. [39], and Schwartz and Rozumalskia [40], have made the dynamic determination of the instantaneous joint center locations, suggested two decades ago by Cappozzo [25], more viable.

Despite these limitations, gait analysis facilitates the systematic quantitative documentation of walking patterns. With the various gait data, the clinician has the opportunity to separate the primary causes of a gait abnormality from compensatory gait mechanisms. Apparent contradictions between the different types of gait information can result in a more carefully developed understanding of the gait deviations. Gait analysis provides the clinical user the ability to more precisely (than observational gait analysis alone) plan complex multilevel surgeries and evaluate the efficacy of different interventions, for example, surgical approaches and orthotic designs. Through gait analysis, movement in planes of motion not easily observed, such as about the long axes of the lower limb segments, may be quantified. Finally, quantities that cannot be observed may be assessed, for example, muscular activity and joint kinetics. In the future, it is anticipated that our understanding of gait will be enhanced through the application of pattern recognition strategies, coupled dynamics, and the linkage of empirical kinematic and kinetic results with the simulations provided by forward dynamics modeling. The systematic and objective evaluation of gait both before and after intervention will ultimately lead to improved treatment outcome.

References

[1] Neptune, R.R., Zajac, F.E., and Kautz, S.A., Muscle force redistributes segmental power for body progression during walking, *Gait Posture*, 19, 194, 2004.

[2] Heller, M.O. et al., Musculo-skeletal loading conditions at the hip during walking and stair climbing, *J. Biomech.*, 34, 883, 2001.

[3] Ferber, R., Davis, I.M., and Williams, D.S. III, Gender differences in lower extremity mechanics during running, *Clin. Biomech.*, 18, 350, 2003.

[4] Hunter, J.P., Marshall, R.N., and McNair, P.J., Interaction of step length and step rate during sprint running, *Med. Sci. Sports Exerc.*, 36, 261, 2004.

[5] Kautz, S.A. and Hull, M.L., Dynamic optimization analysis for equipment setup problems in endurance cycling, *J. Biomech.*, 28, 1391, 1995.

[6] Tashman, S. et al., Abnormal rotational knee motion during running after anterior cruciate ligament reconstruction, *Am. J. Sports Med.*, 32, 975, 2004.

[7] Brand, R.A. and Crowninshield, R.D., Comment on criteria for patient evaluation tools, *J. Biomech.*, 14, 655, 1981.

[8] Sjodahl, C. et al., Pelvic motion in trans-femoral amputees in the frontal and transverse plane before and after special gait re-education, *Prosthet. Orthop. Int.*, 27, 227, 2003.

[9] Rodda, J.M. et al., Sagittal gait patterns in spastic diplegia, *J. Bone Joint Surg. Br.*, 86, 251, 2004.

[10] Schwartz, M.H. et al., Comprehensive treatment of ambulatory children with cerebral palsy: an outcome assessment, *J. Pediatr. Orthop.*, 24, 45, 2004.

[11] Kaufman, K.R. et al., Gait characteristics of patients with knee osteoarthritis, *J. Biomech.*, 34, 907, 2001.

[12] Kerrigan, D.C. et al., Effectiveness of a lateral-wedge insole on knee varus torque in patients with knee osteoarthritis, *Arch. Phys. Med. Rehabil.*, 83, 889, 2002.

[13] Powers, C.M. et al., The effect of bracing on patellofemoral joint stress during free and fast walking, *Am. J. Sports Med.*, 32, 224, 2004.

[14] Smith, A.J., Lloyd, D.G., and Wood, D.J., Pre-surgery knee joint loading patterns during walking predict the presence and severity of anterior knee pain after total knee arthroplasty, *J. Orthop. Res.*, 22, 260, 2004.

[15] Perry, J., Mulroy, S.J., and Renwick, S.E., The relationship of lower extremity strength and gait parameters in patients with post-polio syndrome, *Arch. Phys. Med. Rehabil.*, 74, 165, 1993.

[16] Benedetti, M.G. et al., Gait abnormalities in minimally impaired multiple sclerosis patients, *Mult. Scler.*, 5, 363, 1999.

[17] Sussman, M., Duchenne muscular dystrophy, *J. Am. Acad. Orthop. Surg.*, 10, 138, 2002.

[18] Õunpuu, S. et al., An examination of the knee function during gait in children with myelomeningocele, *J. Pediatr. Orthop.*, 20, 629, 2000.

[19] Dunteman, R.C., Vankoski, S.J., and Dias, L.S., Internal derotation osteotomy of the tibia: pre- and postoperative gait analysis in persons with high sacral myelomeningocele, *J. Pediatr. Orthop.*, 20, 623, 2000.

[20] Keenan, M.A. et al., Valgus deformities of the feet and characteristics of gait in patients who have rheumatoid arthritis, *J. Bone Joint Surg. Am.*, 73, 237, 1991.

[21] Patrick, J.H., Case for gait analysis as part of the management of incomplete spinal cord injury, *Spinal Cord*, 41, 479, 2003.

[22] Teixeira-Salmela, L.F. et al., Effects of muscle strengthening and physical conditioning training on temporal, kinematic and kinetic variables during gait in chronic stroke survivors, *J. Rehabil. Med.*, 33, 53, 2001.

[23] Perry, J., The use of gait analysis for surgical recommendations in traumatic brain injury, *J. Head Trauma Rehabil.*, 14, 116, 1999.

[24] Õunpuu, S., Gage, J.R., and Davis, R.B., Three-dimensional lower extremity joint kinetics in normal pediatric gait, *J. Pediatr. Orthop.*, 11, 341, 1991.

[25] Cappozzo, A., Gait analysis methodology, *Hum. Move. Sci.*, 3, 27, 1984.

[26] Bell, A.L., Pederson, D.R., and Brand, R.A., Prediction of hip joint center location from external landmarks, *Hum. Move. Sci.*, 8, 3, 1989.

[27] Davis, R.B. et al., A gait analysis data collection and reduction technique, *Hum. Move. Sci.*, 10, 575, 1991.

[28] Grood, E.S. and Suntay, W.J., A joint coordinate system for the clinical description of three-dimensional motions: application to the knee, *J. Biomech. Eng.*, 105, 136, 1983.

[29] Woltring, H.J., Huskies, R., and DeLange, A., Finite centroid and helical axis estimation from noisy landmark measurement in the study of human joint kinematics, *J. Biomech.*, 18, 379, 1985.

[30] Dempster, W.T., Space requirements of the seated operator: geometrical, kinematic, and mechanical aspects of the body with special reference to the limbs, WADC-55-159, AD-087-892, Wright Air Development Center, Wright-Patterson Air Force Base, Ohio, 1955.

[31] McConville, J.T. et al., Anthropometric relationships of body and body segment moments of inertia, Technical report AFAMRL-TR-80-119, Air Force Aerospace Medical Research Laboratory, Aerospace Medical Division, Air Force Systems Command, Wright-Patterson Air Force Base, Ohio, 1980.

[32] Jenson, R.K., Body segment mass, radius and radius of gyration proportions of children, *J. Biomech.*, 19, 359, 1986.

[33] Õunpuu, S., Davis, R.B., and DeLuca, P.A., Joint kinetics: methods, interpretation and treatment decision-making in children with cerebral palsy and myelomeningocele, *Gait Posture*, 4, 62, 1996.

[34] Palladino, J. and Davis, R.B., Biomechanics, in *Introduction to Biomedical Engineering*, Enderle, J., Blanchard, S., and Bronzino, J., Eds., Academic Press, San Diego, CA, 2000, p. 411.

[35] Chao, E.Y. and Rim, K., Application of optimization principles in determining the applied moments in human leg joints during gait, *J. Biomech.*, 6, 497, 1973.

[36] Anderson, F.C. and Pandy, M.G., Static and dynamic optimization solutions for gait are practically equivalent, *J. Biomech.*, 34, 153, 2001.

[37] Bleck, E.E., *Orthopaedic Management in Cerebral Palsy*, Mac Keith Press, Philadelphia, PA, 1987, p. 87.

[38] Leardini, A. et al., Validation of a functional method for the estimation of hip joint centre location, *J. Biomech.*, 32, 99, 1999.

[39] Piazza, S.J. et al., Assessment of the functional method of hip joint center location subject to reduced range of hip motion, *J. Biomech.*, 37, 349, 2004.

[40] Schwartz, M.H. and Rozumalskia, A., A new method for estimating joint parameters from motion data, *J. Biomech.*, 38, 107, 2005.

For Further Information on Gait Analysis Techniques

Berme, N. and Cappozzo, A., Eds., *Biomechanics of Human Movement: Applications in Rehabilitation, Sports and Ergonomics*, Bertec Corporation, Worthington, OH, 1990.

Whittle, M., *Gait Analysis: An Introduction*, Butterworth-Heinemann, Oxford, 1991.

Winter, D.A., *Biomechanics and Motor Control of Human Movement*, John Wiley & Sons, New York, 2005.

Allard, P., Stokes, I.A.F., and Blanchi, J.P., Eds., *Three-Dimensional Analysis of Human Movement*, Human Kinetics, Champaign, IL, 1995.

Harris, G.F. and Smith, P.A., Eds., *Human Motion Analysis*, IEEE Press, Piscataway, NJ, 1996.

For Further Information on Normal and Pathological Gait

Gage, J.R., *Gait Analysis in Cerebral Palsy*, Mac Keith Press, London, 1991.

Gage, J.R., Ed., *The Treatment of Gait Problems in Cerebral Palsy*, Mac Keith Press, London, 2004.

Perry, J., *Gait Analysis: Normal and Pathological Function*, Slack, Thorofare, NJ, 1992.

Sutherland, D.H. et al., *The Development of Mature Walking*, Mac Keith Press, London, 1988.

52

Mechanics of Head/Neck

Albert I. King
David C. Viano
Wayne State University

Injury is a major societal problem in the United States. Approximately 140,000 fatalities occur each year due to both intentional and unintentional injuries. Two thirds of these are unintentional, and of these, about one half are attributable to automotive-related injuries. In 1993, the estimated number of automotive-related fatalities dipped under 40,000 for the first time in the last three decades due to a continuing effort by both the industry and the government to render vehicles safer in crash situations. However, for people under 40 years of age, automotive crashes, falls, and other unintentional injuries are the highest risks of fatality in the United States in comparison with all other causes.

The principal aim of impact biomechanics is the prevention of injury through environmental modification, such as the provision of an airbag for automotive occupants to protect them during a frontal crash. To achieve this aim effectively, it is necessary that workers in the field have a clear understanding of the *mechanisms of injury,* be able to describe the *mechanical response* of the tissues involved, have some basic information on *human tolerance* to impact, and be in possession of tools that can be used as *human surrogates* to assess a particular injury [Viano et al., 1989]. This chapter deals with the biomechanics of blunt impact injury to the head and neck.

52.1 Mechanisms of Injury

52.1.1 Head Injury Mechanisms

Among the more popular theories of brain injury due to blunt impact are changes in intracranial pressure and the development of shear strains in the brain. Positive-pressure increases are found in the brain behind the site of impact on the skull. Rapid acceleration of the head, in-bending of the skull, and the propagation of a compressive pressure wave are proposed as mechanisms for the generation of intracranial compression that causes local contusion of brain tissue. At the contrecoup site, there is an opposite response in the form of a negative-pressure pulse that also causes bruising. It is not clear as to whether the injury is due to the negative pressure itself (tensile loading) or to a cavitation phenomenon similar to that seen on the surfaces of propellers of ships (compression loading). The pressure differential across the brain necessarily results in a pressure gradient that can give rise to shear strains developing within the deep structures of the brain. Furthermore, when the head is impacted, it not only translates but also rotates about the neck, causing relative motion of the brain with respect to the skull. Gennarelli [1983] has found that rotational acceleration of the head can cause a diffuse injury to the white matter of the brain in animal models, as evidenced by retraction balls developing along the axons of injured nerves. This injury was described by Strich [1961] as diffuse axonal injury (DAI) that she found in the white matter of autopsied human brains. Other researchers, including Lighthall et al. [1990], have been able to cause the development of DAI in the brain of an animal model (ferrets) by the application of direct impact to the brain without the associated head angular acceleration. Adams et al. [1986] indicated that DAI is the most important factor in severe head injury because it is irreversible and leads to incapacitation and dementia. It is postulated that DAI occurs as a result of the mechanical insult but cannot be detected by staining techniques at autopsy unless the patient survives the injury for at least several hours.

52.1.2 Neck Injury Mechanisms

The neck or the cervical spine is subjected to several forms of unique injuries that are not seen in the thoracolumbar spine. Injuries to the upper cervical spine, particularly at the atlanto-occipital joint, are considered to be more serious and life threatening than those at the lower level. The atlanto-occipital joint can be dislocated either by an axial torsional load or a shear force applied in the anteroposterior direction, or vice versa. A large compression force can cause the arches of Cl to fracture, breaking it up into two or four sections. The odontoid process of C2 is also a vulnerable area. Extreme flexion of the neck is a common cause of odontoid fractures, and a large percentage of these injuries are related to automotive accidents [Pierce and Barr, 1983]. Fractures through the pars interarticularis of C2, commonly known as "hangman's fractures" in automotive collisions, are the result of a combined axial compression and extension (rearward bending) of the cervical spine. Impact of the forehead and face of unrestrained occupants with the windshield can result in this injury. Garfin and Rothman [1983] discussed this injury in relation to hanging and traced the history of this mode of execution. It was estimated by a British judiciary committee that the energy required to cause a hangman's fracture was 1708 Nm (1260 ft lb).

In automotive-type accidents, the loading on the neck due to head contact forces is usually a combination of an axial or shear load with bending. Bending loads are almost always present, and the degree of axial or shear force depends on the location and direction of the contact force. For impacts near the crown of the head, compressive forces predominate. If the impact is principally in the transverse plane, there is less compression and more shear. Bending modes are infinite in number because the impact can come from any angle around the head. To limit the scope of the discussion, the following injury modes are considered: tension–flexion, tension–extension, compression–flexion, and compression–extension in the midsagittal plane and lateral bending.

52.1.2.1 Tension–Flexion Injuries

Forces resulting from inertial loading of the head–neck system can result in flexion of the cervical spine while it is being subjected to a tensile force. In experimental impacts of restrained subjects undergoing forward deceleration, Thomas and Jessop [1983] reported atlanto-occipital separation and C1–C2 separation occurring in subhuman primates at 120 g. Similar injuries in human cadavers were found at 34–38 g by Cheng et al. [1982], who used a preinflated driver airbag system that restrained the thorax but allowed the head and neck to rotate over the bag.

52.1.2.2 Tension–Extension Injuries

The most common type of injury due to combined tension and extension of the cervical spine is the "whiplash" syndrome. However, a large majority of such injuries involve the soft tissues of the neck, and the pain is believed to reside in the joint capsules of the articular facets of the cervical vertebrae [Wallis et al., 1997]. In severe cases, teardrop fractures of the anterosuperior aspect of the vertebral body can occur. Alternately, separation of the anterior aspect of the disk from the vertebral endplate is known to occur. More severe injuries occur when the chin impacts the instrument panel or when the forehead impacts the windshield. In both cases, the head rotates rearward and applies a tensile and bending load on the neck. In the case of windshield impact by the forehead, hangman's fracture of C2 can occur. Garfin and Rothman [1983] suggested that it is caused by spinal extension combined with compression on the lamina of C2, causing the pars to fracture.

52.1.2.3 Compression–Flexion Injuries

When a force is applied to the posterosuperior quadrant of the head or when a crown impact is administered while the head is in flexion, the neck is subjected to a combined load of axial compression and forward bending. Anterior wedge fractures of vertebral bodies are commonly seen, but with increased load, burst fractures and fracture-dislocations of the facets can result. The latter two conditions are unstable and tend to disrupt or injure the spinal cord, and the extent of the injury depends on the penetration of the vertebral body or its fragments into the spinal canal. Recent experiments by Pintar et al. [1989, 1990] indicate that burst fractures of lower cervical vertebrae can be reproduced in cadaveric specimens by a crown impact to a flexed cervical spine. A study by Nightingale et al. [1993] showed that fracture-dislocations of the cervical spine occur very early in the impact event (within the first 10 ms) and that the subsequent motion of the head or bending of the cervical spine cannot be used as a reliable indicator of the mechanism of injury.

52.1.2.4 Compression–Extension Injuries

Frontal impacts to the head with the neck in extension will cause compression–extension injuries. These involve the fracture of one or more spinous processes and, possibly, symmetrical lesions of the pedicles, facets, and laminae. If there is a fracture-dislocation, the inferior facet of the upper vertebra is displaced posteriorly and upward and appears to be more horizontal than normal on x-ray.

52.1.2.5 Injuries Involving Lateral Bending

If the applied force or inertial load on the head has a significant component out of the midsagittal plane, the neck will be subjected to lateral or oblique along with axial and shear loading. The injuries characteristic of lateral bending are lateral wedge fractures of the vertebral body and fractures to the posterior elements on one side of the vertebral column.

Whenever there is lateral or oblique bending, there is the possibility of twisting the neck. The associated torsional loads may be responsible for unilateral facet dislocations or unilateral locked facets [Moffat et al., 1978]. However, the authors postulated that pure torsional loads on the neck are rarely encountered in automotive accidents.

52.2 Mechanical Response

52.2.1 Mechanical Response of the Brain

Skull impact response was presented in the previous edition in which remarks were made regarding the unavailability of data on the response of the brain during an injury-producing impact. Such data are

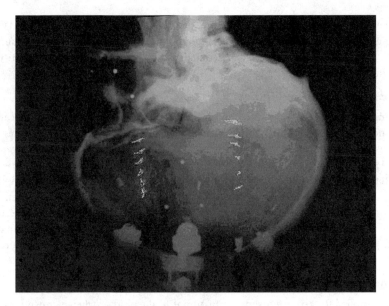

FIGURE 52.1 Brain response to blunt impact.

now available. For intact heads, the motion of the brain inside the skull has been recently studied by Hardy et al. [2001]. Isolated cadaveric heads were subjected to a combined linear and angular acceleration and exposed to a biplanar high-speed x-ray system. Neutral density targets made of tin or tungsten were preinserted into the brain. Video data collected from such impacts showed that most of the motion was in the center of the brain and that target motion was in the form of a figure 8, as shown in Figure 52.1. This motion was limited to ±5 mm regardless of the severity of the impact. Angular acceleration levels in excess of 10,000 rad/sec^2 were reached.

In another experiment, a Hybrid III dummy head and neck system was accelerated into a variety of plastic foams to assess head response with and without the use of a helmet used in American football. It was found that the helmet reduced the linear acceleration of the head substantially but did not change its angular acceleration significantly. However, it is believed by many that angular acceleration is the cause of brain injury. So if angular acceleration is the culprit, then how does the helmet protect the brain? In an attempt to answer this question, video data from NFL helmet impacts were analyzed and the helmet velocities were computed using stereophotogrammetric methods. The helmet impacts were reproduced in the laboratory by Newman et al. [1999] to yield head angular and linear accelerations, using helmeted Hybrid III dummies. These head accelerations were fed into a brain injury computer model developed by Zhang et al. [2001] to compute brain responses, such as strain (ε), strain rate ($d\varepsilon/dt$), and pressure. A total of 58 cases were studied, involving 25 cases of concussion or mild traumatic brain injury (MTBI), as reported by Pellman et al. [2003]. The results of the model were analyzed statistically to determine the best predictors of MTBI, using the logist analysis. It was found brain response parameters such as the product of strain and strain rate, were good predictors whereas angular acceleration was a poor predictor, as shown in Table 52.1. The chi square value is a measure of the ability of the parameter to predict injury and in this analysis, its ability to predict injury is high if the chi square value is high. These results are consistent with the findings of Viano and Lövsund [1999] who used animal data to determine the parameter most likely to cause DAI in a living brain. It was the product of the velocity (V) of the impactor and depth of penetration of the impactor as percentage of the brain depth (C). For the brain, the product, $V \cdot C$, is analogous to $\varepsilon \cdot d\varepsilon/dt$. Note that HIC is the current Head Injury Criterion used in Federal Motor Vehicle Safety Standard (FMVSS) 208 to assess head injury and GSI is the previous head injury criterion, now referred to as the Gadd Severity Index. The Cumulative Strain at 15% is measure of the volume of brain that experienced a strain of 15% or higher throughout the

TABLE 52.1 List of Best Predictors of MTBI

Rank order	Predictor variable	Chi square	p-value
1	$\varepsilon \cdot d\varepsilon/dt$	41.0	0.0000
2	$d\varepsilon/dt$	33.1	0.0000
3	HIC	31.5	0.0000
4	SI	31.2	0.0000
5	Linear acceleration	28.3	0.0000
6	ε_{max}	28.0	0.0000
7	Max. principal stress	27.3	0.0000
8	Cumulative strain at 15%	26.0	0.0000
9	Angular acceleration	24.9	0.0000

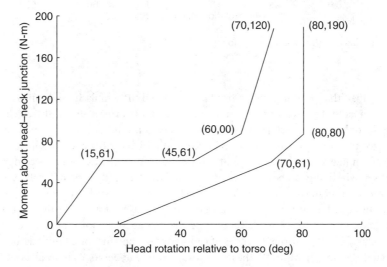

FIGURE 52.2 Loading corridor for neck flexion.

impact. It is concluded that response variable of the brain are better predictors of injury than input variables.

52.2.2 Mechanical Response of the Neck

The mechanical response of the cervical spine was studied by Mertz and Patrick [1967, 1971], Patrick and Chou [1976], Schneider et al. [1975], and Ewing et al. [1978]. Mertz et al. [1973] quantified the response in terms of rotation of the head relative to the torso as a function of bending moment at the occipital condyles. Loading corridors were obtained for flexion and extension, as shown in Figure 52.2 and Figure 52.3. An exacting definition of the impact environments to be used in evaluating dummy necks relative to the loading corridors illustrated in these figures is included in SAE J1460 [1985]. It should be noted that the primary basis for these curves is volunteer data and that the extension of these corridors to dummy tests in the injury-producing range is somewhat surprising.

The issue of whiplash is a controversial one principally because researchers in the field cannot agree on an injury mechanism. Currently, five such mechanisms have been proposed. It began with the hyperextension theory, which was discarded when the automotive headrest did not reduce the incidence of injury. The flexion theory is also considered untenable because head and neck flexion after the rear end collision is

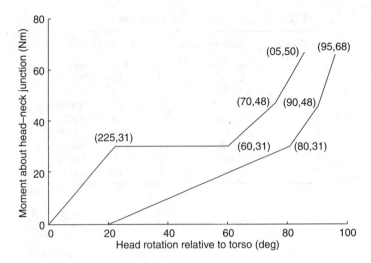

FIGURE 52.3   Loading corridor for neck extension.

much less severe than that resulting from a frontal impact and the whiplash syndrome is not frequently seen in frontal impacts. The theory that a momentary increase in pressure in the cerebrospinal fluid during whiplash could induce neck pain was also considered invalid because injury to the nerve roots require prolonged pressure and root compression leads to radiculopathy and not direct neck pain. The fourth theory of impingement of the facet joint surfaces was proposed but has not been demonstrated. It claims that the synovial lining can be trapped between the facets resulting in pain. Finally, the shear theory appears to be the most promising. A shear force is developed at every level of the cervical spine before the head and can be brought forward along with the torso, which is pushed forward by the seat back. This shear force causes relative motion between adjacent cervical vertebrae in the form of relative translation and rotation. Deng et al. [2000] performed a series of cadaveric tests and measured this relative displacement and also estimated the amount of stretch the facet capsules would undergo. Wallis et al. [1997] have shown that removal of nerve endings in the cervical facet capsules can relieve neck pain for an average of about nine months. Figure 52.4 shows the amount of forward motion of C5 relative to C4 and Figure 52.5 shows the estimated stretch of the C4–5 and C5–6 facet capsule. Of interest is the time of occurrence of these events. They occur before the head hits the headrest. It not only explains why the present headrest is in ineffective but also indicates to the safety engineer that the headrest needs to be much closer to the head if it is to be effective.

52.3   Regional Tolerance of the Head and Neck to Blunt Impact

52.3.1   Regional Tolerance of the Head

The most commonly measured parameter for head injury is acceleration. It is therefore natural to express human tolerance to injury in terms of head acceleration. The first known tolerance criterion is the Wayne State Tolerance Curve, proposed by Lissner et al. [1960] and subsequently modified by Patrick et al. [1965] by the addition of animal and volunteer data to the original cadaveric data. The modified curve is shown in Figure 52.6. The head can withstand higher accelerations for shorter durations and any exposure above the curve is injurious. When this curve is plotted on logarithmic paper, it becomes a straight line with a slope of −2.5. This slope was used as an exponent by Gadd [1961] in his proposed severity index, now

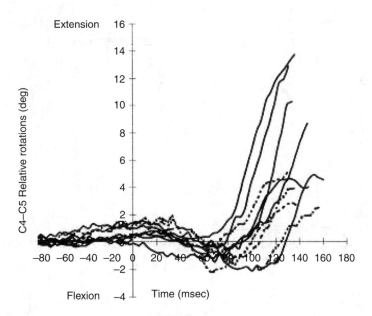

FIGURE 52.4 Relative displacement of C4 on C5 for 20° seat back angle tests (solid lines) and 0° seat back angle tests (dotted lines) simulating low-speed rear-end collisions, using a cadaver. (Reproduced from *Stapp Car Crash J.* 44: 171–188. With permission.)

known as the *Gadd Severity Index* (GSI):

$$\text{GSI} = \int_0^T a^{2.5}\,\mathrm{d}t \qquad\qquad (52.1)$$

where a is the instantaneous acceleration of the head, and T is the duration of the pulse.

If the integrated value exceeds 1000, a severe injury will result. A modified form of the GSI, now known as the *Head Injury Criterion* (HIC), was proposed by Versace [1970] to identify the most damaging part of the acceleration pulse by finding the maximum value of the following integral:

$$\text{HIC} = (t_2 - t_1)\left[(t_2 - t_1)^{-1}\int_{t_1}^{t_2} a(t)\,\mathrm{d}t\right]^{2.5}\Bigg|_{\max} \qquad\qquad (52.2)$$

where $a(t)$ is the resultant instantaneous acceleration of the head, and $t_2 - t_1$ is the time interval over which HIC is a maximum.

A severe but not life-threatening injury would have occurred if the HIC reached or exceeded 1000. Subsequently, Prasad and Mertz [1985] proposed a probabilistic method of assessing head injury and developed the curve shown in Figure 52.7. At an HIC of 1000, approximately 16% of the population would sustain a severe to fatal injury. It is apparent that this criterion is useful in automotive safety design and in the design of protective equipment for the head, such as football and bicycle helmets. However, there is another school of thought that believes in the injurious potential of angular acceleration in its ability to cause diffuse axonal injury and rupture of the parasagittal bridging veins between the brain and dura mater. The MTBI data referred to above show that this may not be case and that a strain related parameter should be designated as a brain injury criterion, regardless of the input. However, for the moment, HIC remains as the head injury criterion in FMVSS 208 and attempts to replace it have so far been unsuccessful.

As a matter of interest, tolerance data for MTBI, data obtained from the National Football League (NFL) data are presented in Table 52.2, taken from King et al. [2003].

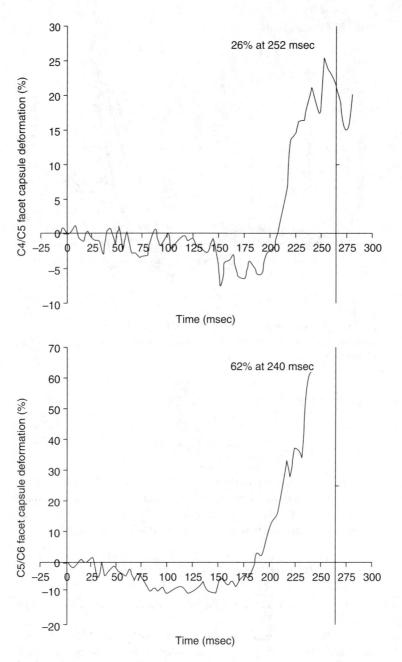

FIGURE 52.5   Estimated cervical facet capsule stretch during the simulated test described in Figure 52.4. (Reproduced from *Stapp Car Crash J.* 44:171–188. With Permission.)

52.3.2   Regional Tolerance of the Neck

Currently, there are no universally accepted tolerance values for the neck for the various injury modes. This is not due to a lack of data but rather to the many injury mechanisms and several levels of injury severity, ranging from life-threatening injuries to the spinal cord to minor soft-tissue injuries that cannot be identified on radiographic or magnetic scans. It is likely that a combined criterion of axial load and bending moment about one or more axes will be adopted as a future FMVSS.

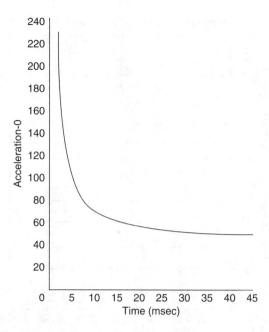

FIGURE 52.6   The Wayne State Tolerance Curve for head injury.

TABLE 52.2   Tolerance Estimates for MTBI

Variable	Tolerance estimate (Probability of injury)		
	25%	50%	75%
HIC	136	235	333
Linear acceleration (m/sec^2)	559	778	965
Angular acceleration (rad/sec^2)	4384	5757	7130
Max. principal strain, ε (%)	25	37	49
Max. principal strain rate, $d\varepsilon/dt$ (sec^{-1})	46	60	79
$\varepsilon \cdot d\varepsilon/dt$ (sec^{-1})	14	20	25

Source: King, A.I., Yang, K.H., Zhang, L. et al. 2003. Is head injury caused by linear or angular acceleration? In *Bertil Aldman Lecture, Proceedings of the 2003 International IRCOBI Conference on the Biomechanics of Impact*, pp. 1–12.

52.4   Human Surrogates of the Head and Neck

52.4.1   The Experimental Surrogate

The most effective experimental surrogate for impact biomechanics research is the unembalmed cadaver. This is also true for the head and neck, despite the fact that the cadaver is devoid of muscle tone because the duration of impact is usually too short for the muscles to respond adequately. It is true, however, that muscle pretensioning in the neck may have to be added under certain circumstances. Similarly, for the brain, the cadaveric brain cannot develop DAI, and the mechanical properties of brain change rapidly after death. If the pathophysiology of the central nervous system is to be studied, the ideal surrogate is an animal brain. Currently, the rat is frequently used as the animal of choice and there is some work in progress using the mini-pig.

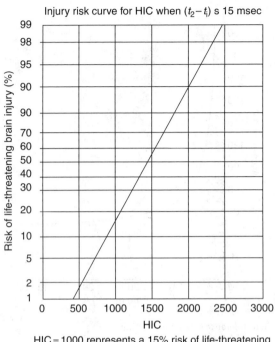

FIGURE 52.7   Head injury risk curve based on HIC.

52.4.2   The Injury-Assessment Tool

The response and tolerance data acquired from cadaveric studies are used to design human-like surrogates, known as *anthropomorphic test devices* (ATD). These surrogates are required not only to have biofidelity and the ability to simulate human response but also need to provide physical measurements that are representative of human injury. In addition, they are designed to be repeatable and reproducible. The current frontal impact dummy is the Hybrid III family of dummies ranging from the 95th percentile male to the 3-year-old infant. The 50th percentile male dummy is human like in many of its responses, including that of the head and neck. The head consists of an aluminum headform covered by an appropriately designed vinyl "skin" to yield human-like acceleration responses for frontal and lateral impacts against a flat, rigid surface. Two-dimensional physical models of the brain were proposed by Margulies et al. [1990] using a silicone gel in which preinscribed grid lines would deform under angular acceleration. No injury criterion is associated with this gel model.

The dummy neck was designed to yield responses in flexion and extension that would fit within the corridors shown in Figure 52.2 and Figure 52.3. The principal function of the dummy neck is to place the head in the approximate position of a human head in the same impact involving a human occupant.

52.4.3   Computer Models

Models of head impact first appeared over 50 years ago [Holbourn, 1943]. Extensive reviews of such models were made by King and Chou [1977] and Hardy et al. [1994]. The use of the finite-element method (FEM) to simulate the various components of the head appears to be the most effective and popular means of modeling brain response. A recent model by Zhang et al. [2001] is extremely detailed, with over 300,000 elements. It simulates the brain, the meninges, the cerebrospinal fluid and ventricles, the skull, scalp, and most of the facial bones and soft tissues. Validation was attempted against all available experimental data.

It has been used in many applications, including the prediction of MTBI for helmeted football players described earlier. Other less detailed models include those by Kleiven and Hardy [2002], Willinger et al. [1999], and Takhounts et al. [2003].

A large number of neck and spinal models also have been developed over the past four decades. A paper by Kleinberger [1993] provides a brief and incomplete review of these models. However, the method of choice for modeling the response of the neck is the finite-element method, principally because of the complex geometry of the vertebral components and the interaction of several different materials. A partially validated model for impact response was developed by Yang et al. [1998] to simulate both crown impact as well as the whiplash phenomenon due to a rear-end impact.

References

Adams, J.H., Doyle, D., Graham, D.I. et al. 1986. Gliding contusions in nonmissile head injury in humans. *Arch. Pathol. Lab. Med.* 110:485.

Cheng, R., Yang, K.H., Levine, R.S. et al. 1982. Injuries to the cervical spine caused by a distributed frontal load to the chest. In *Proceedings of the 26th Stapp Car Crash Conference*, pp. 1–40.

Deng, B., Begeman, P.C., Yang, K.H. et al. 2000. Kinematics of human cadaver cervical spine during low speed rear-end impacts. *Stapp Car Crash J.* 44: 171–188.

Ewing, C.L., Thomas, D.J., Lustick, L. et al. 1978. Effect of initial position on the human head and neck response to + Y impact acceleration. In *Proceedings of the 22nd Stapp Car Crash Conference*, pp. 101–138.

Gadd, C.W. 1961. Criteria for injury potential. In *Impact Acceleration Stress Symposium, National Research Council Publication No. 977*, pp. 141–144. Washington, National Academy of Sciences.

Garfin, S.R. and Rothman, R.H. 1983. Traumatic spondylolisthesis of the axis (Hangman's fracture). In R.W. Baily (Ed.), *The Cervical Spine*, pp. 223–232. Philadelphia, PA Lippincott.

Gennarelli, T.A. 1983. Head injuries in man and experimental animals: clinical aspects. *Acta Neurochir. Suppl.* 32: 1.

Hardy, W.N., Khalil, T.B., and King, A.I. 1994. Literature review of head injury biomechanics. *Int. J. Impact Eng.* 15: 561–586.

Hardy, W.N., Foster, C.D., Mason, M.J. et al. 2001. Investigation of head injury mechanisms using neutral density technology and high-speed biplanar x-ray. *Stapp Car Crash J.* 45: 337–368.

Holbourn, A.H.S. 1943. Mechanics of head injury. *Lancet* 2: 438.

King, A.I. and Chou, C. 1977. Mathematical modelling, simulation and experimental testing of biomechanical system crash response. *J. Biomech.* 9: 3–10.

King, A.I., Yang, K.H., Zhang, L. et al. 2003. Is head injury caused by linear or angular acceleration? In *Bertil Aldman Lecture, Proceedings of the 2003 International IRCOBI Conference on the Biomechanics of Impact*, pp. 1–12.

Kleinberger, M. 1993. Application of finite element techniques to the study of cervical spine mechanics. In *Proceedings of the 37th Stapp Car Crash Conference*, pp. 261–272.

Kleiven, S. and Hardy, W.N. 2002. Correlation of an FE model of the human head with experiments on localized motion of the brain — consequences for injury prediction. *Stapp Car Crash J.* 46: 123–144.

Lighthall, J.W., Goshgarian, H.G., and Pinderski, C.R. 1990. Characterization of axonal injury produced by controlled cortical impact. *J. Neurotrauma* 7(2): 65.

Lissner, H.R., Lebow, M., and Evans F.G. 1960. Experimental studies on the relation between acceleration and intracranial pressure changes in man. *Surg. Gynecol. Obstet.* 111: 329.

Margulies, S.S., Thibault, L.E., and Gennarelli, T.A. 1990. Physical model simulation of brain injury in the primate. *J. Biomech.* 23: 823.

Mertz, H.J. and Patrick, L.M. 1967. Investigation of the kinematics and kinetics of whiplash. In *Proceedings of the 11th Stapp Car Crash Conference*, pp. 267–317.

Mertz, H.J. and Patrick, L.M. 1971. Strength and response of the human neck. In *Proceedings of the 15th Stapp Car Crash Conference*, pp. 207–255.

Mertz, H.J., Neathery, R.F., and Culver, C.C. 1973. Performance requirements and characteristics of mechanical necks. In W.F. King and H.I. Mertz (Eds.), *Human Impact Response: Measurement and Simulations*, pp. 263–288. New York, Plenum Press.

Moffat, E.A., Siegel, A.W., and Huelke, D.F. 1978. The biomechanics of automotive cervical fractures. In *Proceedings of the 22nd Conference of American Association for Automotive Medicine*, pp. 151–168.

Newman, J., Beusenberg, M., Fournier, E. et al. 1999. A new biomechanical assessment of mild traumatic brain injury — part I:methodology. In *Proceedings of the 1999 International IRCOBI Conference on the Biomechanics of Impact*, pp. 17–36.

Nightingale, R.W., McElhaney, J.H., Best, T.M. et al. 1993. The relationship between observed head motion and cervical spine injury mechanism. In *Proceedings of the 39th Meeting of the Orthopedic Research Society*, p. 233.

Patrick, L.M. and Chou, C. 1976. Response of the human neck in flexion, extension, and lateral flexion, Vehicle Research Institute Report No. VRI-7-3. Warrendale, PA, Society of Automotive Engineers.

Patrick, L.M., Lissner, H.R., and Gurdjian, ES. 1965. Survival by design: head protection. In *Proceedings of the 7th Stapp Car Crash Conference*, pp. 483–499.

Pellman, E.J., Viano D.C., Tucker, A.M. et al. 2003. Concussion in professional football: reconstruction of game impacts and injuries. *Neurosurgery*, 53: 799–814.

Pierce, D.A. and Barr, J.S. 1983. Fractures and dislocations at the base of the skull and upper spine. In R.W. Baily (Ed.), *The Cervical Spine*, pp. 196–206. Philadelphia, PA, Lippincott.

Pintar, F.A., Yoganandan, N., Sances, A. Jr et al. 1989. Kinematic and anatomical analysis of the human cervical spinal column under axial loading. In *Proceedings of the 33rd Stapp Car Crash Conference*, pp. 191–214.

Pintar, F.A., Sances, A. Jr, Yoganandan, N. et al. 1990. Biodynamics of the total human cadaveric spine. In *Proceedings of the 34th Stapp Car Crash Conference*, pp. 55–72.

Prasad, P. and Mertz, H.J. 1985. The Position of the United States Delegation to the ISO Working Group 6 on the Use of HIC in the Automotive Environment, SAE Paper No. 851246. Warrendale, PA, Society of Automotive Engineers.

Schneider, L.W., Foust, D.R., Bowman, B.M. et al. 1975. Biomechanical properties of the human neck in lateral flexion. In *Proceedings of the 19th Stapp Car Crash Conference*, pp. 455–486.

Society of Automotive Engineers, Human Mechanical Response Task Force. 1985. Human Mechanical Response Characteristics, SAE J1460. Warrendale, PA, Society of Automotive Engineers.

Strich, S.J. 1961. Shearing of nerve fibres as a cause of brain damage due to head injury. *Lancet* 2: 443.

Takhounts, E.G., Eppinger, R.H., Campbell, J.Q. et al. 2003. On the development of the SIMon finite element head model. *Stapp Car Crash J.* 47: 107–134.

Thomas, D.J. and Jessop, M.E. 1983. Experimental head and neck injury. In C.L. Ewing et al. (Eds.), *Impact Injury of the Head and Spine*, pp. 177–217. Springfield, IL, Charles C Thomas.

Versace, J. 1970. A review of the severity index. In *Proceedings of the 15th Stapp Car Crash Conference*, pp. 771–796.

Viano, D.C., King, A.I., Melvin, J.W., and Weber, K. 1989. Injury biomechanics research: an essential element in the prevention of trauma. *J. Biomech.* 21: 403.

Viano, D.C. and Lövsund, P. 1999. Biomechanics of brain and spinal cord injury: analysis of neurophysiological experiments. *Crash Prevention and Injury Control*, 1: 35–43.

Wallis, B.J., Lord, S.M., and Bogduk, N. 1997. Resolution of psychological distress of whiplash patients following treatment by radiofrequency neurotomy: a randomized, double-blind, placebo controlled trial. *Pain* 73: 15–22.

Willinger, R., Kang, H.S., and Diaw, B. 1999. Three-dimensional human head finite-element model validation against two experimental impacts. *Ann. Biomed. Eng.* 27(3): 403–410.

Yang, K.H., Zhu, F., Luan, F. et al. 1998. Development of a finite element model of the human neck. In *Proceedings of the 42nd Stapp Car Crash Conference*, pp. 195–205.

Zhang, L., Yang, K.H., Dwarampudi, R. et al. 2001. Recent advances in brain injury research: a new human head model, development and validation. *Stapp Car Crash J.* 45: 369–394.

53
Biomechanics of Chest and Abdomen Impact

David C. Viano
Albert I. King
Wayne State University

53.1 Introduction

Injury is caused by energy transfer to the body by an impacting object. It occurs when sufficient force is concentrated on the chest or abdomen by striking a blunt object, such as a vehicle instrument panel or side interior, or being struck by a baseball or blunt ballistic mass. The risk of injury is influenced by the object's shape, stiffness, point of contact, and orientation. It can be reduced by energy absorbing padding or crushable materials, which allow the surfaces in contact to deform, extend the duration of impact, and reduce loads. The torso is viscoelastic, so reaction force increases with the speed of body deformation.

The biomechanical response of the body has three components, (1) inertial resistance by acceleration of body masses, (2) elastic resistance by compression of stiff structures and tissues, and (3) viscous resistance by rate-dependent properties of tissue. For low-impact speeds, the elastic stiffness protects from crush injuries; whereas, for high rates of body deformation, the inertial and viscous properties determine the force developed and limit deformation. The risk of skeletal and internal organ injury relates to energy stored or absorbed by the elastic and viscous properties. The reaction load is related to these responses and inertial resistance of body masses, which combine to resist deformation and prevent injury. When tissues are deformed beyond their recoverable limit, injuries occur.

53.2 Chest and Abdomen Injury Mechanisms

The primary mechanism of chest and abdomen injury is compression of the body at high rates of loading. This causes deformation and stretching of internal organs and vessels. When torso compression exceeds the rib-cage tolerance, fractures occur and internal organs and vessels can be contused or ruptured. In some chest impacts, internal injury occurs without skeletal damage. This can happen during high-speed loading, such as with a baseball impact causing ventricular fibrillation in a child without rib fractures. Injury is due to the viscous or rate-sensitive nature of human tissue as biomechanical responses differ for low- and high-speed impact.

When organs or vessels are loaded slowly, the input energy is absorbed gradually through deformation, which is resisted by elastic properties and pressure buildup in tissue. This is the situation when the shoulder belt loads the upper body in a frontal crash. When loaded rapidly, reaction force is proportional to the speed of tissue deformation as the viscous properties of the body resist deformation and provide a natural protection from impact. However, there is also a considerable inertial component to the reaction force. In this case, the body develops high internal pressure and injuries can occur before the ribs deflect much. The ability of an organ or other biological system to absorb impact energy without failure is called tolerance.

If an artery is stretched beyond its tensile strength, the tissue will tear. Organs and vessels can be stretched in different ways, which result in different types of injury. Motion of the heart during chest compression stretches the aorta along its axis from points of tethering in the body. This elongation generally leads to a transverse laceration when the strain limit is exceeded. In contrast, an increase in vascular pressure dilates the vessel and produces biaxial strain, which is larger in the transverse than axial direction. If pressure rises beyond the vessel's limit, it will burst. For severe impacts, intra-aortic pressure exceeds 500 to 1000 mm Hg, which is a significant, nonphysiological level, but is tolerable for short durations. When laceration occurs, the predominant mode of aortic failure is axial so the combined effects of stretch and internal pressure contribute to injury. Chest impact also compresses the rib cage causing tensile strain on the outer surface of the ribs. As compression increases, the risk of rib fracture increases. In both cases, the mechanism of injury is tissue deformation. Shah et al. [2001] found right-side impacts caused a higher risk of aortic injury than other impact directions.

The abdomen is more vulnerable to injury than the chest, because there is little bony structure below the ribcage to protect internal organs in front and lateral impact. Blunt impact of the upper abdomen can compress and injure the liver and spleen, before significant whole-body motion occurs. In the liver, compression increases intrahepatic pressure and generates tensile or shear strains. If the tissue is sufficiently deformed, laceration of the major hepatic vessels can result in hemoperitoneum. The injury tolerance of the solid organs in the abdomen is rate sensitive. Abdominal deformation also causes lobes of the liver to move relative to each other, stretching and shearing the vascular attachment at the hilar region.

Effective occupant restraints, safety systems, and protective equipment not only spread impact energy over the strongest body structures but also reduce contact velocity between the body and the impacted surface or striking object. The design of protective systems is aided by an understanding of injury mechanisms, quantification of human tolerance levels and development of numerical relationships between measurable engineering parameter, such as force, acceleration or deformation, and human injury. These relationships are called injury criteria.

53.3 Injury Criteria and Tolerances

53.3.1 Acceleration Injury

Stapp [1970] conducted rocket-sled experiments in the 1940s on belt-restraint systems and achieved a substantial human tolerance to long-duration, whole-body acceleration. Safety belts protected military personnel exposed to rapid but sustained acceleration. The experiments enabled Eiband [1959] to show in Figure 53.1 that the tolerance to whole-body acceleration increased as the exposure duration decreased. This linked human tolerance and acceleration for exposures of 2 to 1000 msec duration. The tolerance data is based on average sled acceleration rather than the acceleration of the volunteer subject, which would be higher due to compliance of the restraint system. Even with this limitation, the data provide useful early guidelines for the development of military and civilian restraint systems.

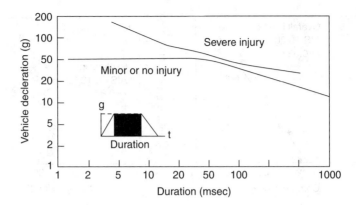

FIGURE 53.1 Whole-body human tolerance to vehicle acceleration based on impact duration. (Redrawn from Eiband A.M. Human Tolerance to Rapidly Applied Acceleration. A Survey of the Literature. National Aeronautics and Space Administration, Washington DC, NASA Memo No. 5-19-59E, 1959 and Viano D.C., *Bull. NY Acad. Med.*, 2nd Series, 64: 376–421, 1988. With permission.)

More recent side impact tests have led to other tolerance formulas for chest injury. Morgan et al. [1986] evaluated rigid, side-wall cadaver tests and developed TTI, a thoracic trauma index, which is the average rib and spine acceleration. TTI limits human tolerance to 85 to 90 g in vehicle crash tests. Better injury assessment was achieved by Cavanaugh et al. [1993] using average spinal acceleration (ASA), which is the average slope of the integral of spinal acceleration. ASA is the rate of momentum transfer during side impact, and a value of 30 g is proposed. In most cases, the torso can withstand 60 to 80 g peak, whole-body acceleration by a well-distributed load.

53.3.2 Force Injury

Whole-body tolerance is related to Newton's second law of motion, where acceleration of a rigid mass is proportional to the force acting on it, or $F = ma$. While the human body is not a rigid mass, a well-distributed restraint system allows the torso to respond as though it were fairly rigid when load is applied through the shoulder and pelvis. The greater the acceleration, the greater the force and risk of injury. For a high-speed frontal crash, a restrained occupant can experience 60 g acceleration. For a body mass of 76 kg, the inertial load is 44.7 kN (10,000 lb) and is tolerable if distributed over strong skeletal elements for a short period of time.

The ability to withstand high acceleration for short durations implies that tolerance is related to momentum transfer, because an equivalent change in velocity can be achieved by increasing the acceleration and decreasing its duration, as $\Delta V = a\Delta t$. The implication for occupant-protection systems is that the risk of injury can be decreased if the crash deceleration is extended over a greater period of time. For occupant restraint in 25 msec, a velocity change of 14.7 m/sec (32.7 mph) occurs with 60 g whole-body acceleration. This duration can be achieved by crushable vehicle structures and occupant restraints [Mertz and Gadd, 1971].

Prior to the widespread use of safety belts, safety engineers needed information on the tolerance of the chest to design energy-absorbing instrument panels and steering systems. The concept was to limit impact force below human tolerance by crushable materials and structures. Using the highest practical crush force, safety was extended to the greatest severity of vehicle crashes. GM Research and Wayne State University collaborated on the development of the first crash sled, which was used to simulate progressively more severe frontal impacts. Embalmed human cadavers were exposed to head, chest, and knee impact on 15 cm (6") diameter load cells until bone fracture was observed on x-ray. Patrick et al. [1965, 1967] demonstrated that blunt chest loading of 3.3 kN (740 lb) could be tolerated with minimal risk of serious injury. This is a pressure of 187 kPa. Gadd and Patrick [1968] later found a tolerance of 8.0 kN (1800 lb) if

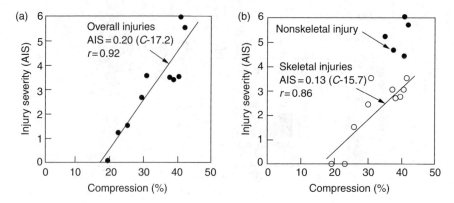

FIGURE 53.2 (a) Injury severity from blunt impact of human cadavers as a function of the maximum chest compression (from Viano [1988] with permission). (b) Severity of skeletal injury and incidence of internal organ injury as a function of maximum chest compression for blunt impacts of human cadavers. (From Viano D.C., *Bull. NY Acad. Med.*, 2nd Series, 64: 376–421, 1988. With permission).

the load was distributed over the shoulders and chest by a properly designed steering wheel and column. Cavanaugh et al. [1993] found side-impact tolerance is similar to frontal tolerance, and that shoulder contact is also an important load-path. However, for the abdomen, side padding needs to crush at lower force than the abdominal tolerance to protect the liver and spleen [Viano and Andrzejak, 1993].

53.3.3 Compression Injury

High-speed films of cadaver impacts show that whole-body acceleration does not describe torso impact biomechanics. Tolerance of the chest and abdomen must consider body deformation. Force acting on the body causes two simultaneous responses, (1) compression of the compliant structures of the torso, and (2) acceleration of body masses. The neglected mechanism of injury was compression, which causes the sternum to displace toward the spine as ribs bend and possibly fracture. Acceleration and force, per se, are not sufficient indicators of impact tolerance because they cannot discriminate between the two responses. Numerous studies have shown that acceleration is less related to injury than compression.

The importance of chest deformation was confirmed by Kroell et al. [1971,1974] in blunt thoracic impacts of unembalmed cadavers. Peak spinal acceleration and impact force were poorer injury predictors than the maximum compression of the chest, as measured by the percent change in the anteroposterior thickness of the body. A relationship was found between injury risk and compression and that it involves energy stored by elastic deformation of the body for moderate rates of chest compression. The stored energy (E_s) by a spring representing the ribcage and soft tissues is related to the displacement integral of force: $E_s = \int F dx$. Force in a spring is proportional to deformation: $F = kx$, where k is a spring constant representing the stiffness of the chest and is in the range of 26 kN/m. Stored energy is $E_s = k\int x dx = 0.5kx^2$. Over a compression range of 20 to 40%, stored energy is proportional to deformation or compression, so $E_s \approx C$.

Tests with human volunteers showed that compression up to 20% during moderate-duration loading was fully reversible. Cadaver impacts with compression greater than 20% showed (Figure 53.2a) an increase in rib fractures and internal organ injury as the compression increased to 40%. The deflection tolerance was originally set at 8.8 cm (3.5″) for moderate but recoverable injury. This represents 39% compression. However, at this level of compression, multiple rib fractures and serious injury can occur, so a more conservative tolerance of 32% has been used to avert the possibility of flail chest (Figure 53.2b). This reduces the risk of direct loading on the heart, lungs, and internal organs by a loss of the protective function of the ribcage.

53.3.4 Viscous Injury

The velocity of body deformation is an important factor in impact injury. For example, when a fluid-filled organ is compressed slowly, energy can be absorbed by tissue deformation without damage. When loaded rapidly, the organ cannot deform fast enough and rupture may occur without significant change in shape, even though the load is substantially higher than for the slow-loading condition. This situation depends on the viscous and inertial characteristics of the tissues.

The viscoelastic behavior of soft tissues becomes progressively more important as the velocity of body deformation exceeds 3 m/sec. For lower speeds, such as in slow-crushing loads or for a belt-restrained occupant in a frontal crash, tissue compression is limited by elastic properties resisting skeletal and internal organ injury. For higher speeds of deformation, such as occupant loading by the door in a side impact, an unrestrained occupant or pedestrian impact, or chest impact by a nonpenetrating bullet, maximum compression does not adequately address the viscous and inertial properties of the torso, nor the time of greatest injury risk. In these conditions, the tolerance to compression is progressively lower as the speed of deformation increases, and the velocity of deformation becomes a dominant factor in injury.

Insight on a rate-dependent injury mechanism came from over 20 years of research by Jonsson, Clemedson et al. [1979] on high-speed impact and blast-wave exposures. The studies confirmed that tolerable compression inversely varied with the velocity of impact. The concept was further studied in relation to the abdomen by Lau and Viano [1981] for frontal impacts in the range of 5 to 20 m/sec (10–45 mph). The liver was the target organ. Using a maximum compression of 16%, the severity of injury increased with the speed of loading, including serious mutilation of the lobes and major vessels in the highest-speed impacts. While the compression was within limits of volunteer loading at low speeds, the exposure produced critical injury at higher speeds. Subsequent tests on other animals and target organs verified an interrelationship between body compression, deformation velocity, and injury.

The previous observations led Viano and Lau [1988] to propose a viscous injury mechanism for soft biological tissues. The viscous response (VC) is defined as the product of velocity of deformation (V) and compression (C), which is a time-varying function in an impact. The parameter has physical meaning to absorbed energy (E_a) by a viscous dashpot under impact loading. Absorbed energy is related to the displacement integral of force: $E_a = \int F dx$, and force in a dashpot representing the viscous characteristics of the body is proportional to the velocity of deformation: $F = cV$, where c is a dashpot parameter in the range of 0.5 kN/m/sec for the chest. Absorbed energy is: $E_a = c \int V dx$, or a time integral by substitution: $E_a = c \int V^2 dt$. The integrand is composed of two responses, so: $E_a = c(\int d(Vx) - \int ax dt)$, where a is acceleration across the dashpot. The first term is the viscous response and the second an inertial term related to the deceleration of fluid set in motion. Absorbed energy is given by: $E_a = c(Vx - \int ax dt)$. The viscous response is proportional to absorbed energy, or $E_a \approx VC$, during the rapid phase of impact loading prior to peak compression.

Subsequent tests by Lau and Viano [1986,1988] verified that serious injury occurred at the time of peak VC, much earlier than peak compression. For blunt chest impact, peak VC occurs in about half the time for maximum compression. Rib fractures also occur progressively with chest compression, as early as 9 to 14 msec — at peak VC — in a cadaver impact requiring 30 msec to reach peak compression. Upper-abdominal injury by steering wheel contact also relates to viscous loading. Lau, Horsch et al. [1987] showed that limiting the viscous response by a self-aligning steering wheel reduced the risk of liver injury, as does force limiting an armrest in side impacts. Animal tests have also shown that VC is a good predictor of functional injury to heart and respiratory systems. In these experiments, Stein et al. [1982] found that the severity of cardiac arrhythmia and traumatic apnea was related to VC. This situation is important to baseball impact protection of children, Viano et al. [1992], and in the definition of human biomechanical responses used in the assessment of bullet-proof protective vests and blunt ballistics [Bir et al., 2004].

With the increasing use of bullet-proof vests and nonpenetrating munitions by the police and military, blunt, high-velocity impacts are occurring to the chest. Although rarely lethal, there has been a concern for improving the understanding of injury mechanisms and means to establish standards for the technology.

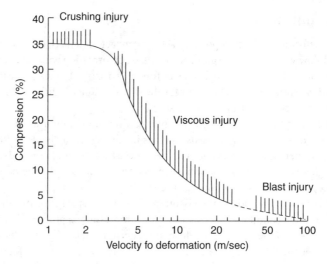

FIGURE 53.3   Biomechanics of chest injury by a crushing injury mechanism limited by tolerable compression at $C_{max} = 35\%$, a viscous injury mechanism limited by the product of velocity and extent of deformation at $VC_{max} = 1.0$ m/sec, and a blast injury mechanism for shock wave loading.

Behind-body-armor standards use the depth of the cavity created in clay after a bullet is stopped by the vest. The roots of this approach involve military research. However, the clay may not adequately simulate the human viscoelastic properties and biomechanical responses. Recent research has defined the blunt ballistic characteristics of the chest and the mechanisms for ventricular fibrillation [Bir and Viano, 1999; Bir et al., 2004].

Sturdivan et al. [2004] developed the Blunt Criterion (BC) in the 1970s. It is energy based and assesses vulnerability to blunt weapons, projectile impacts and behind-body-armor exposures. $BC = \ln[E/(W^{0.33} TD)]$, where $E = \frac{1}{2} MV^2$ is the kinetic energy of the projectile at impact in Joules, M is the projectile mass in kg, V is projectile velocity in m/sec, D is the projectile diameter in cm, W is the mass of the individual in kg and T is body-wall thickness in cm. BC is an energy ratio. The numerator is the striking kinetic energy of the blunt projectile, the energy available to cause injury. The denominator is a semiempirical expression of the capacity of the body to absorb the impact energy without lethal damage to the vulnerable organs, scaled by the mass of the individual. The viscous and blunt criteria are both energy-based and have been correlated for chest and abdominal impacts.

Figure 53.3 summarizes injury mechanisms associated with torso impact deformation. For low speeds of deformation, the limiting factor is crush injury from compression of the body (C). This occurs at $C = 35$–40% depending on the contact area and orientation of loading. For deformation speeds above 3 m/sec, injury is related to a peak viscous response of $VC = 1.0$ m/sec. In a particular situation, injury can occur by a compression or viscous responses, or both, as these responses occur at different times in an impact. At extreme rates of loading, such as in a blast-wave exposure, injury occurs with less than 10–15% compression by high-energy transfer to viscous elements of the body.

53.4   Biomechanical Responses During Impact

The reaction force developed by the chest varies with the velocity of deformation, and biomechanics is best characterized by a family of force-deflection responses. Figure 53.4 summarizes frontal and lateral chest biomechanics for various impact speeds. The dynamic compliance is related to viscous, inertial, and elastic properties of the body. The initial rise in force is due to inertia as the sternal mass, which is rapidly accelerated to the impact speed as the chest begins to deform. The plateau force is related to the viscous component, which is rate-dependent, and a superimposed elastic stiffness, which increases force

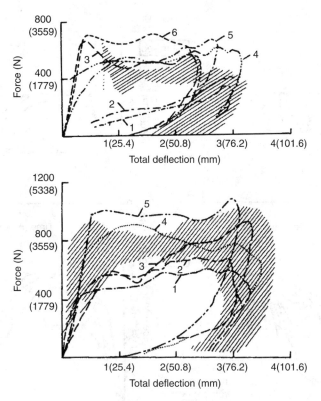

FIGURE 53.4 Frontal and lateral force-deflection response of the human cadaver chest at various speeds of blunt pendulum impact. The initial stiffness is followed by a plateau force until unloading. (From Kroell et al., *Proceedings of the 18th Stapp Car Crash Conference*, pp. 383–457, SAE Paper No. 741187, Society of Automotive Engineers, Warrendale PA, 1974, and Viano, *Proceedings of the 33rd Stapp Car Crash Conference*, pp. 113–142, SAE Paper No. 892432, Society of Automotive Engineers, Warrendale, PA, 1989, summarized by Cavanaugh J.M., The Biomechanics of Thoracic Trauma, In *Accidental Injury: Biomechanics and Prevention*, Nahum A.M. and Melvin J.W., (Eds.), pp. 362–391, Springer-Verlag, New York, 1993. With permission.)

with chest compression. Unloading provides a hysterisis loop representing the energy absorbed by body deformation.

Melvin et al. [1988] analyzed frontal biomechanics of the chest. The dynamic compliance is related to viscous, inertial, and elastic properties of the body. There is an initial rise in force, which is related to the inertia of the sternal mass, which is rapidly accelerated to the impact speed. This is followed by a plateau in force, which is related to the viscous properties and is rate dependent. There is also an elastic stiffness component from chest compression that adds to the force. The force-deflection response can be modeled as an initial stiffness $k = 0.26 + 0.60(V - 1.3)$ and a plateau force $F = 1.0 + 0.75(V - 3.7)$, where k is in kN/cm, F is in kN, and the velocity of impact V is in m/sec. The force F reasonably approximates the plateau level for lateral chest and abdominal impact, but the initial stiffness is lower at $F = 0.12(V - 1.2)$ for side loading [Melvin and Weber, 1988].

The reaction force developed by the chest varies with the velocity of impact, so biomechanics is best characterized by the force-deflection response of the torso (25.6). The dynamic compliance is related to viscous, inertial, and elastic properties of the body. There is an initial rise in force, which is related to inertial responses as the sternal mass is rapidly accelerated to the impact speed. This is followed by a plateau in force, which is related to the viscous response and is rate dependent, and a superimposed stiffness component related to chest compression. By analyzing frontal biomechanics, the chest response can be modeled as an initial stiffness $k = 0.26 + 0.60(V - 1.3)$ and a plateau force $F = 1.0 + 0.75(V - 3.7)$, where k is in kN/cm, F is in kN, and the velocity of impact V is in m/sec. The force F reasonably approximates the

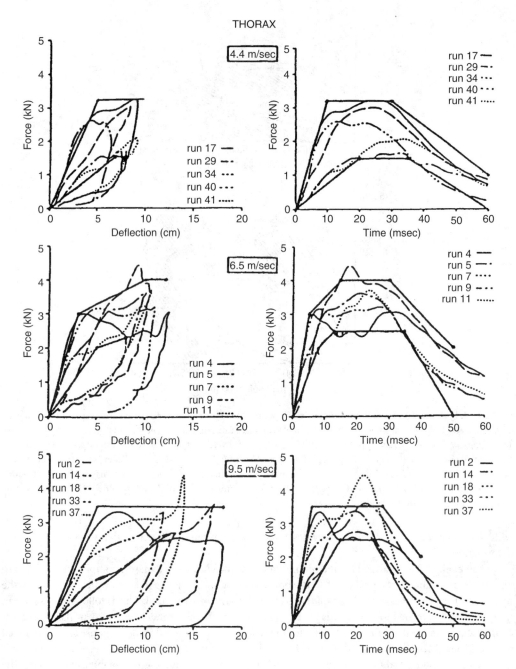

FIGURE 53.4 Continued.

plateau level for lateral chest and abdominal impact, but the initial stiffness is lower at $F = 0.12(V - 1.2)$ for side loading.

A simple, but relevant, lumped-mass model of the chest was developed by Lobdell et al. [1973] and is shown in Figure 53.5. The impacting mass is m_1 and skin compliance is represented by k_{12}. An energy-absorbing interface was added by Viano [1987] to evaluate protective padding. Chest structure is represented by a parallel Voigt and Maxwell spring-dashpot system, which couples the sternal m_2 and spinal m_3 masses. When subjected to a blunt sternal impact, the model follows established force-deflection corridors. The biomechanical model is effective in studying compression and viscous responses.

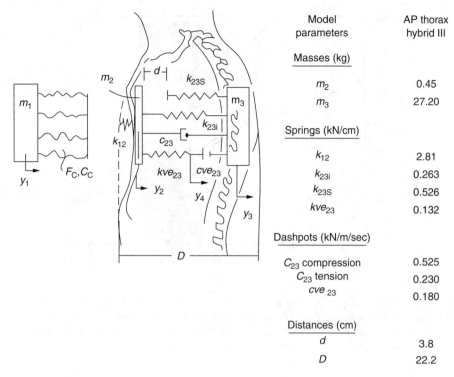

Model parameters	AP thorax hybrid III
Masses (kg)	
m_2	0.45
m_3	27.20
Springs (kN/cm)	
k_{12}	2.81
k_{23i}	0.263
k_{23S}	0.526
kve_{23}	0.132
Dashpots (kN/m/sec)	
C_{23} compression	0.525
C_{23} tension	0.230
cve_{23}	0.180
Distances (cm)	
d	3.8
D	22.2

FIGURE 53.5 Lumped-mass model of the human thorax with impacting mass and energy-absorbing material interface. The biomechanical parameters are given for mass, spring, and damping characteristics of the chest in blunt frontal impact. (Modified from Lobdell et al. Impact Response of the Human Thorax, In *Human Impact Response Measurement and Simulation*, King W.F. and Mertz H.J., (Eds.), Plenum Press, New York, pp. 201–245, 1973 by Viano, D.C., *Proceedings of the 31st Stapp Car Crash Conference*, pp. 185–224, SAE Paper No. 872213, Society of Automotive Engineers, Warrendale, PA, 1987. With permission.)

It also simulates military exposures to high-speed, nonpenetrating projectiles (Figure 53.6), even though the loading conditions are quite different from the cadaver database used to develop the model. This mechanical system characterizes the elastic, viscous, and inertial components of the torso.

The Hybrid III dummy was the first to demonstrate humanlike chest responses typical of the biomechanical data for frontal impacts [Foster et al., 1977]. Rouhana [1989] developed a frangible abdomen, useful in predicting injury for lap-belt submarining. More recent work by Schneider et al. [1992] led to a new prototype frontal dummy. Lateral impact tests of cadavers against a rigid wall and blunt pendulum led to side-impact dummies, such as the Eurosid and Biosid [Mertz, 1993]. Even more recently, a small female-sized side-impact dummy has been developed [Scherer et al., 1998].

53.5 Injury Risk Assessment

Over years of study, tolerances have been established for most responses of the chest and abdomen. Table 53.1 provides tolerance levels from reviews by Cavanaugh [1993], and Rouhana [1993], Viano et al. [1989]. While these are single thresholds, they are commonly used to evaluate safety systems. The implication is that for biomechanical responses below tolerance, there is no injury, and for responses above tolerance, there is injury. An additional factor is biomechanical response scaling for individuals of different size and weight. The commonly accepted procedure involves equal stress and velocity, which enabled Mertz et al. [1989] to predict injury tolerances and biomechanical responses for different size adult dummies.

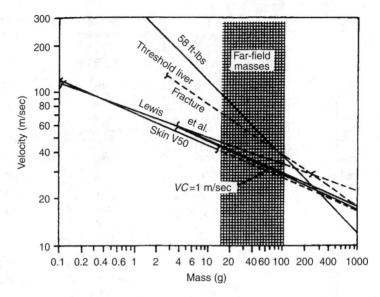

FIGURE 53.6 Tolerance levels for blunt loading as a function of impact mass and velocity. The plot includes information from automotive impact situations and from high-speed military projectile impacts. The Lobdell model is effective over the entire range of impact conditions. (Modified from Quatros J.H., *Proceedings of the 14th International Symposium on Ballistics*, Quebec, Canada, September 26–29, 1993. With permission.)

TABLE 53.1 Human Tolerance for Chest and Abdomen Impact

Criteria	Chest		Abdomen		Criteria
	Frontal	Lateral	Frontal	Lateral	
Acceleration					*Acceleration*
3 msec limit	60 g				
TTI		85–90 g			
ASA		30 g			
AIS 4+		45 g		39 g	AIS 4+
Force					*Force*
Sternum	3.3 kN				
Chest + shoulder	8.8 kN	10.2 kN			
AIS 3+			2.9 kN	3.1 kN	AIS 3+
AIS 4+		5.5 kN	3.8 kN	6.7 kN	AIS 4+
Pressure					*Pressure*
	187 kPa		166 kPa		AIS 3+
			216 kPa		AIS 4+
Compression					*Compression*
Rib fracture	20%				
Stable ribcage	32%		38%		AIS 3+
Flail chest	40%	38%	48%	44%	AIS 4+
Viscous					*Viscous*
AIS 3+	1.0 m/sec				AIS 3+
AIS 4+	1.3 m/sec	1.47 m/sec	1.4 m/sec	1.98 m/sec	AIS 4+

Source: (Adapted from Cavanaugh J.M., The Biomechanics of Thoracic Trauma, In *Accidental Injury: Biomechanics and Prevention*, Nahum A.M. and Melvin J.W., (Eds.), pp. 362–391, Springer-Verlag, New York, 1993 and Rouhana S.W., Biomechanics of Abdominal Trauma, In *Accidental Injury: Biomechanics and Prevention*, Nahum A.M. and Melvin J.W., (Eds.), pp. 391–428, Springer-Verlag, New York, 1993.)

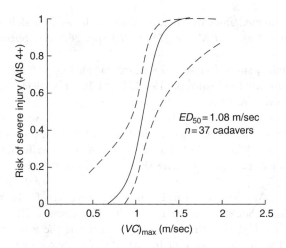

FIGURE 53.7 Typical Logist injury probability function relating the risk of serious injury to the viscous response of the chest. (From Viano D.C., *Bull. NY Acad. Med.*, 2nd Series, 64: 376–421, 1988. With permission.)

TABLE 53.2 Injury Probability Functions for Blunt Impact

Body region	$ED_{25\%}$	α	β	x^2	p	R
	Frontal impact					
Chest (AIS 4+)						
VC	1.0 m/sec	11.42	11.56	25.6	0.000	0.68
C	34%	10.49	0.277	15.9	0.000	0.52
	Lateral impact					
Chest (AIS 4+)						
VC	1.5 m/sec	10.02	6.08	13.7	0.000	0.77
C	38%	31.22	0.79	13.5	0.000	0.76
Abdomen (AIS 4+)						
VC	2.0 m/sec	8.64	3.81	6.1	0.013	0.60
C	47%	16.29	0.35	4.6	0.032	0.48
Pelvis (pubic ramus facture)						
C	27%	84.02	3.07	11.5	0.001	0.91

Source: Modified from Viano et al. *J. Biomech.* 22: 403–417, 1989.

Injury risk assessment is frequently used. It evaluates the probability of injury as a continuous function of a biomechanical response. A Logist function relates injury probability p to a biomechanical response x by $p(x) = [1 + \exp(\alpha - \beta x)]^{-1}$ where α and β are parameters derived from statistical analysis of biomechanical data. This function provides a sigmoidal relationship with three distinct regions in Figure 53.7. For low biomechanical response levels, there is a low probability of injury. Similarly, for very high levels, the risk asymptotes to 100%. The transition region between the two extremes involves risk, which is proportional to the biomechanical response. A sigmoidal function is typical of human tolerance because it represents the distribution in weak through strong subjects in a population exposed to impact. Table 53.2 summarizes available parameters for chest and abdominal injury risk assessment.

References

Bir, C. and Viano, D.C., Biomechanics of Commotio Cordis. *J. Trauma*, 47(3): 468–473, 1999.

Bir, C., Viano, D.C., and King, A.I., Human Response of the Thorax to Blunt Ballistic Impacts. *J. Biomech.*, 37(1): 73–79, 2004.

Cavanaugh, J.M., The Biomechanics of Thoracic Trauma, In *Accidental Injury: Biomechanics and Prevention*, Nahum A.M. and Melvin J.W. (Eds.), pp. 362–391, Springer-Verlag, New York, 1993.

Cavanaugh, J.M. et al., Injury and Response of the Thorax in Side Impact Cadaveric Tests, *Proceedings of the 37th Stapp Car Crash Conference*, pp. 199–222, SAE Paper No. 933127, Society of Automotive Engineers, Warrendale, PA, 1993.

Eiband, A.M., Human Tolerance to Rapidly Applied Acceleration. A Survey of the Literature. National Aeronautics and Space Administration, Washington DC, NASA Memo No. 5-19-59E, 1959.

Foster, J.K., Kortge, J.O., and Wolanin, M.J., Hybrid III-A Biomechanically-Based Crash Test Dummy, *Stapp Car Crash Conference*, pp. 975–1014, SAE Paper No. 770938, Society of Automotive Engineers, Warrendale, PA, 1977.

Gadd, C.W. and Patrick, L.M., Systems Versus Laboratory Impact Tests for Estimating Injury Hazards, SAE Paper No. 680053, Society of Automotive Engineers, Warrendale, PA, 1968.

Jonsson, A., Clemedson, C.J. et al., Dynamic Factors Influencing the Production of Lung Injury in Rabbits Subjected to Blunt Chest Wall Impact, *Aviation, Space Environ. Med.*, 50: 325–337, 1979.

King, A.I., Regional Tolerance to Impact Acceleration, In SP-622, SAE 850852, Society of Automotive Engineers, Warrendale, PA, 1985.

Kroell, C.K., Schneider, D.C., and Nahum, A.M., Impact Tolerance and Response to the Human Thorax, *Proceedigns of the 15th Stapp Car Crash Conference*, pp. 84–134, SAE Paper No. 710851, Society of Automotive Engineers, Warrendale, PA, 1971.

Kroell, C.K., Schneider, D.C., and Nahum, A.M., Impact Tolerance and Response to the Human Thorax II, *Proceedings of the 18th Stapp Car Crash Conference*, pp. 383–457, SAE Paper No. 741187, Society of Automotive Engineers, Warrendale PA, 1974.

Lau, I.V. and Viano, D.C., Influence of Impact Velocity on the Severity of Nonpenetrating Hepatic Injury, *J. Trauma*, 21(2): 115–123, 1981.

Lau, I.V. and Viano, D.C., The Viscous Criterion-Bases and Application of an Injury Severity Index for Soft Tissue, *Proceedings of the 30th Stapp Car Crash Conference*, pp. 123–142, SAE Paper No. 861882, Society of Automotive Engineers, Warrendale, PA, 1986.

Lau, I.V., Horsch, J.D. et al., Biomechanics of Liver Injury by Steering Wheel Loading, *J. Trauma*, 27: 225–237, 1987.

Lau, I.V. and Viano, D.C., How and When Blunt Injury Occurs: Implications to Frontal and Side Impact Protection. *Proceedings of the 32nd Stapp Car Crash Conference*, pp. 81–100, SAE Paper No. 881714, Society of Automotive Engineers, Warrendale, PA, 1988.

Lobdell, T.E., Kroell, C.K., Schneider, D.C., Hering, W.E., and Nahum, A.M., Impact Response of the Human Thorax, In *Human Impact Response Measurement and Simulation*, King W.F. and Mertz H.J. (Eds.), Plenum Press, New York, pp. 201–245, 1973.

Melvin, J.W., King, A.I., and Alem, N.M., AATD System Technical Characteristics, Design Concepts, and Trauma Assessment Criteria, AATD task E-F Final Report, DOT-HS-807-224, US Department of Transportation, National Highway Traffic Safety Administration, Washington DC, 1988.

Melvin, J.W. and Weber, K. (Eds.), Review of Biomechanical Response and Injury in the Automotive Environment, AATD Task B Final Report, DOT-HS-807-224, US Department of Transportation, National Highway Traffic Safety Administration, Washington, DC, 1988.

Mertz, H.J. and Gadd, C.W., Thoracic Tolerance to Whole-Body Deceleration, *Proceedings of the 15th Stapp Car Crash Conference*, pp. 135–157, SAE Paper No. 710852, Society of Automotive Engineers, Warrendale, PA, 1971.

Mertz, H.J., Irwin, A. et al., Size, Weight and Biomechanical Impact Response Requirements for Adult Size Small Female and Large Male Dummies, SAE Paper No. 890756, Society of Automotive Engineers, Warrendale PA, 1989.

Mertz, H.J., Anthropomorphic Test Devices, In *Accidental Injury: Biomechanics and Prevention*, Nahum A.M. and Melvin J.W. (Eds.), pp. 66–84, Springer-Verlag, New York, 1993.

Morgan, R.M., Marcus, J.H., and Eppinger, R.H., Side Impact — The Biofidelity of NHTSA's Proposed ATD and Efficacy of TTI, *Proceedings of the 30th Stapp Car Crash Conference*, pp. 27–40, SAE Paper No. 861877, Society of Automotive Engineers, Warrendale PA, 1986.

Patrick, L.M., Kroell, C.K., and Mertz, H.J., Forces on the Human Body in Simulated Crashes, *Proceedings of the 9th Stapp Car Crash Conference*, SAE, pp. 237–260, Society of Automotive Engineers, Warrendale, PA, 1965.

Patrick, L.M., Mertz, H.J., and Kroell, C.K., Cadaver Knee, Chest, and Head Impact Loads, *Proceedings of the 11th Stapp Car Crash Conference*, pp. 168–182, SAE Paper No. 670913, Society of Automotive Engineers, Warrendale, PA, 1967.

Quatros, J.H., Terminal Ballistics of Non-lethal Projectiles, *Proceedings of the 14th International Symposium on Ballistics*, Quebec, Canada, September 26–29, 1993.

Rouhana, S.W. et al., Assessing Submarining and Abdominal Injury Risk in the Hybrid III Family of Dummies, *Proceedings of the 33rd Stapp Car Crash Conference*, pp. 257–279, SAE Paper No. 892440, Society of Automotive Engineers, Warrendale, PA, 1989.

Rouhana, S.W., Biomechanics of Abdominal Trauma, In *Accidental Injury: Biomechanics and Prevention*, Nahum A.M. and Melvin J.W. (Eds.), pp. 391–428, Springer-Verlag, New York, 1993.

Scherer, R.D., Kirkish, S.L., McCleary, J.P., Rouhana, S.W. et al., SIDS-IIs Beta\u+− prototype dummy biomechanical responses. SAE 983151, *Proceedings of the 42nd Stapp Car Crash Conference*, Society of Automotive Engineers, Warrendale, PA, 1998.

Schneider, L.W., Haffner, M.P. et al., Development of an Advanced ATD Thorax for Improved Injury Assessment in Frontal Crash Environments, *Porceedings of the 36th Stapp Car Crash Conference*, pp. 129–156, SAE Paper No. 922520, Society of Automotive Engineers, Warrendale, PA, 1992.

Shah, C.S., Yang, K.H., Hardy, W.N., Wang, H.K., and King, A.I., Development of a Computer Model to Predict Aortic Rupture due to Impact Loading. SAE 2001-22-0007, Society of Automotive Engineers, Warrendale, PA, *Stapp Car Crash J.*, 45: 161–182, 2001.

Society of Automotive Engineers, *Human Tolerance to Impact Conditions as Related to Motor Vehicle Design*, SAE J885, Society of Automotive Engineers, Warrendale, PA 1986.

Stapp, J.P., Voluntary Human Tolerance Levels, In *Impact Injury and Crash Protection*, Gurdjian, E.S., Lange, W.A., Patrick, L.M., and Thomas, L.M. (Eds.), pp. 308–349, Charles C Thomas, Springfield IL, 1970.

Stein, P.D., Sabbah, H.N. et al., Response of the Heart to Nonpenetrating Cardiac Trauma. *J. Trauma*, 22(5): 364–373, 1982.

Sturdivan, L.M., Viano, D.C., and Champion, H., Analysis of Injury Criteria to Assess Chest and Abdominal Injury Risks in Blunt and Ballistic Impacts. *J. Trauma*, 56: 651–663, 2004.

Viano, D.C., King, A.I. et al., Injury Biomechanics Research: An Essential Element in the Prevention of Trauma, *J. Biomech.*, 22: 403–417, 1989.

Viano, D.C. and Lau, I.V., A Viscous Tolerance Criterion for Soft Tissue Injury Assessment, *J. Biomech.*, 21: 387–399, 1988.

Viano, D.C., Cause and Control of Automotive Trauma, *Bull. NY Acad. Med.*, 2nd Series, 64: 376–421, 1988.

Viano, D.C., Biomechanical Responses and Injuries in Blunt Lateral Impact, *Proceedings of the 33rd Stapp Car Crash Conference*, pp. 113–142, SAE Paper No. 892432, Society of Automotive Engineers, Warrendale, PA, 1989.

Viano, D.C., Evaluation of the Benefit of Energy-Absorbing Materials for Side Impact Protection, *Proceedings of the 31st Stapp Car Crash Conference*, pp. 185–224, SAE Paper No. 872213, Society of Automotive Engineers, Warrendale, PA, 1987.

Viano, D.C., Andrzejak, D.V., Polley, T.Z., and King, A.I., Mechanism of Fatal Chest Injury by Baseball Impact: Development of an Experimental Model, *Clin. J. Sport Med.*, 2: 166–171, 1992.

Viano, D.C. and Andrzejak, D.V., Biomechanics of Abdominal Injury by Armrest Loading. *J. Trauma*, 34(1): 105–115, 1993.

54

Cardiac Biomechanics

Andrew D. McCulloch
University of California-San Diego

54.1 Introduction

The primary function of the heart, to pump blood through the circulatory system, is fundamentally mechanical. In this chapter, cardiac function is discussed in the context of the mechanics of the ventricular walls from the perspective of the determinants of myocardial stresses and strains (Table 54.1). Many physiological, pathophysiological, and clinical factors are directly or indirectly affected by myocardial stress and strain (Table 54.2). Of course, the factors in Table 54.1 and Table 54.2 are closely interrelated — most of the factors affected by myocardial stress and strain in turn affect the stress and strain in the ventricular wall. For example, changes in wall stress due to altered hemodynamic load may cause ventricular remodeling, which in turn alters geometry, structure, and material properties. This chapter is organized around the governing determinants in Table 54.1, but mention is made where appropriate to some of the factors in Table 54.2.

54.2 Cardiac Geometry and Structure

The mammalian heart consists of four pumping chambers, the left and right atria and ventricles communicating through the atrioventricular (mitral and tricuspid) valves, which are structurally connected by chordae tendineae to papillary muscles that extend from the anterior and posterior aspects of the right and left ventricular lumens. The muscular cardiac wall is perfused via the coronary vessels that originate at the left and right coronary ostia located in the sinuses of Valsalva immediately distal to the aortic valve leaflets. Surrounding the whole heart is the collagenous parietal pericardium that fuses with

TABLE 54.1 Basic Determinants of Myocardial Stress and Strain

Geometry and structure	
Three-dimensional shape	Wall thickness
	Curvature
	Stress-free and unloaded reference configurations
Tissue structure	Muscle fiber architecture
	Connective tissue organization
	Pericardium, epicardium, and endocardium
	Coronary vascular anatomy
Boundary/initial conditions	
Pressure	Filling pressure (preload)
	Arterial pressure (afterload)
	Direct and indirect ventricular interactions
	Thoracic and pericardial pressure
Constraints	Effects of inspiration and expiration
	Constraints due to the pericardium and its attachments
	Valves and fibrous valve annuli, chordae tendineae
	Great vessels, lungs
Material properties	
Resting or passive	Nonlinear finite elasticity
	quasilinear viscoelasticity
	Anisotropy
	Biphasic poroelasticity
Active dynamic	Activation sequence
	Myofiber isometric and isotonic contractile dynamics
	Sarcomere length and length history
	Cellular calcium kinetics and metabolic energy supply

TABLE 54.2 Factors Affected by Myocardial Stress and Strain

Direct factors	Regional muscle work
	Myocardial oxygen demand and energetics
	Coronary blood flow
Electrophysiological responses	Action potential duration (QT interval)
	Repolarization (T wave morphology)
	Excitability
	Risk of arrhythmia
Development and morphogenesis	Growth rate
	Cardiac looping and septation
	Valve formation
Vulnerability to injury	Ischemia
	Arrhythmia
	Cell dropout
	Aneurysm rupture
Remodeling, repair, and adaptation	Eccentric and concentric hypertrophy
	Fibrosis
	Scar formation
Progression of disease	Transition from hypertrophy to failure
	Ventricular dilation
	Infarct expansion
	Response to reperfusion
	Aneurysm formation

TABLE 54.3   Representative Left Ventricular Minor-Axis Dimensions[a]

Species	Comments	Inner radius (mm)	Outer radius (mm)	Wall thickness: inner radius
Dog (21 kg)	Unloaded diastole (0 mmHg)	16	26	0.62
	Normal diastole (2–12 mmHg)	19	28	0.47
	Dilated diastole (24–40 mmHg)	22	30	0.36
	Normal systole (1–9 mmHg EDP)	14	26	0.86
	Long axis, apex-equator (normal diastole)	42	47	0.12
Young rats	Unloaded diastole (0 mmHg)	1.4	3.5	1.50
Mature rats	Unloaded diastole (0 mmHg)	3.2	5.8	0.81
Human	Normal	24	32	0.34
	Compensated pressure overload	27	42	0.56
	Compensated volume overload	32	42	0.33

[a] Dog data from Ross et al., *Circ. Res.*, 21, 409–421, 1967 [129], and Streeter and Hanna, *Circ. Res.*, 33, 639–655, 1973 [2]. Human data from Grossman, *Am. J. Med.*, 69, 576–583, 1980 [130] Grossman, et al., *J. Clin. Invest.*, 56, 56–64, 1975 [131]. Rat data are from unpublished observations in the author's laboratory.

the diaphragm and great vessels. These are the anatomical structures that are most commonly studied in the field of cardiac mechanics. Particular emphasis in this chapter is given to the ventricular walls, which are the most important for the pumping function of the heart. Most studies of cardiac mechanics have focused on the left ventricle, but many of the important conclusions apply equally to the right ventricle.

54.2.1 Ventricular Geometry

From the perspective of engineering mechanics, the ventricles are three-dimensional thick-walled pressure vessels with substantial variations in wall thickness and principal curvatures both regionally and temporally through the cardiac cycle. The ventricular walls in the normal heart are thickest at the equator and base of the left ventricle and thinnest at the left ventricular apex and right ventricular free wall. There are also variations in the principal dimensions of the left ventricle with species, age, phase of the cardiac cycle, and disease (Table 54.3). But, in general, the ratio of wall thickness to radius is too high to be treated accurately by all but the most sophisticated thick-wall shell theories [1].

Ventricular geometry has been studied in most quantitative detail in the dog heart [2,3]. Geometric models have been very useful in the analysis, especially the use of confocal and nonconfocal ellipses of revolution to describe the epicardial and endocardial surfaces of the left and right ventricular walls (Figure 54.1). The canine left ventricle is reasonably modeled by a thick ellipsoid of revolution truncated at the base. The crescentic right ventricle wraps about 180° degrees around the heart wall circumferentially and extends longitudinally about two-thirds of the distance from the base to the apex. Using a truncated ellipsoidal model, left ventricular geometry in the dog can be defined by the major and minor radii of two surfaces, the left ventricular endocardium, and a surface defining the free wall epicardium and the septal endocardium of the right ventricle. Streeter and Hanna [2] described the position of the basal plane using a truncation factor f_b defined as the ratio between the longitudinal distances from equator-to-base and equator-to-apex. Hence, the overall longitudinal distance from base to apex is $(1 + f_b)$ times the major radius of the ellipse. Since variations in f_b between diastole and systole are relatively small (0.45 to 0.51), they suggested a constant value of 0.5.

The focal length d of an ellipsoid is defined from the major and minor radii (a and b) by $d^2 = a^2 - b^2$, and varies only slightly in the dog from endocardium to epicardium between end-diastole (37.3 to 37.9 mm) and end-systole (37.7 to 37.1 mm) [2]. Hence, within the accuracy that the boundaries of the left ventricular wall can be treated as ellipsoids of revolution, the assumption that the ellipsoids are confocal appears to be a good one. This has motivated the choice of prolate spheroidal (elliptic-hyperbolic-polar) coordinates

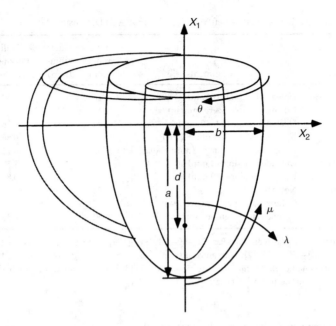

FIGURE 54.1 Truncated ellipsoid representation of ventricular geometry, showing major left ventricular radius (a), minor radius (b), focal length (d) and prolate spheroidal coordinates (λ, μ, θ).

(λ, μ, θ) as a system for economically representing ventricular geometries obtained postmortem or by noninvasive tomography [3,4]. The Cartesian coordinates of a point are given in terms of its prolate spheroidal coordinates by

$$x_1 = d \cosh \lambda \cos \mu$$
$$x_2 = d \sinh \lambda \sin \mu \cos \theta \tag{54.1}$$
$$x_3 = d \sinh \lambda \sin \mu \sin \theta$$

Here, the focal length d defines a family of coordinate systems that vary from spherical polar when $d = 0$ to cylindrical polar in the limit when $d \to \infty$. A surface of constant transmural coordinate λ (Figure 54.1) is an ellipse of revolution with major radius $a = d \cosh \lambda$ and minor radius $b = d \sinh \lambda$. In an ellipsoidal model with a truncation factor of 0.5, the longitudinal coordinate μ varies from zero at the apex to 120° at the base. Integrating the Jacobian in prolate spheroidal coordinates gives the volume of the wall or cavity:

$$d^3 \int_0^{2\pi} \int_0^{\mu_2} \int_{\lambda_1}^{\lambda_2} ((\sinh^2 \lambda + \sin^2 \mu) \sinh \lambda \sin \mu) d\lambda \, d\mu \, d\theta$$
$$= \frac{2\pi d^3}{3} \left|(1 - \cos \mu_2) \cosh^3 \lambda - (1 - \cos^3 \mu_2) \cosh \lambda \right|_{\lambda_1}^{\lambda_2} \tag{54.2}$$

The scaling between heart mass M_H and body mass M within or between species is commonly described by the allometric formula,

$$M_H = kM^\alpha \tag{54.3}$$

Using combined measurements from a variety of mammalian species with M expressed in kilograms, the coefficient k is 5.8 g and the power α is close to unity (0.98) [5]. Within individual species, the ratio of heart weight to body weight is somewhat lower in mature rabbits and rats (about 2 g/kg) than in humans (5 g/kg) and higher in horses and dogs (8 g/kg) [6]. The rate α of heart growth with body weight decreases with age in most species but not in humans. At birth, left and right ventricular weights are similar, but the left ventricle is substantially more massive than the right by adulthood.

54.2.2 Myofiber Architecture

The cardiac ventricles have a complex three-dimensional muscle fiber architecture (for a comprehensive review see Streeter) [7]. Although the myocytes are relatively short, they are connected such that at any point in the normal heart wall there is a clear predominant fiber axis that is approximately tangent with the wall (within 3 to 5° in most regions, except near the apex and papillary muscle insertions). Each ventricular myocyte is connected via gap junctions at intercalated disks to an average of 11.3 neighbors, 5.3 on the sides and 6.0 at the ends [8]. The classical anatomists dissected discrete bundles of fibrous swirls, though later investigations showed that the ventricular myocardium could be unwrapped by blunt dissection into a single continuous muscle "ban" [9]. However, more modern histological techniques have shown that in the plane of the wall, the mean muscle fiber angle makes a smooth transmural transition from epicardium to endocardium (Figure 54.2). About the mean, myofiber angle dispersion is typically 10 to 15° [10] except in certain pathologies. Similar patterns have been described for humans, dogs, baboons, macaques, pigs, guinea pigs, and rats. In the left ventricle of humans or dogs, the muscle fiber angle typically varies continuously from about −60° (i.e., 60° clockwise from the circumferential axis) at the epicardium to about +70° at the endocardium. The rate of change of fiber angle is usually greatest at the epicardium, so that circumferential (0°) fibers are found in the outer half of the wall, and begins to slow approaching the inner third near the trabeculata–compacta interface. There are also small increases in fiber orientation from end-diastole to systole (7 to 19°), with greatest changes at the epicardium and apex [11].

Regional variations in ventricular myofiber orientations are generally smooth except at the junction between the right ventricular free wall and septum. A detailed study in the dog that mapped fiber angles throughout the entire right and left ventricles described the same general transmural pattern in all regions including the septum and right ventricular free wall, but with definite regional variations [3]. Transmural differences in fiber angle were about 120 to 140° in the left ventricular free wall, larger in the septum (160 to 180°) and smaller in the right ventricular free wall (100 to 120°). A similar study of fiber angle distributions in the rabbit left and right ventricles has recently been reported [12]. For the most part, fiber angles in the rabbit heart were very similar to those in the dog, except for on the anterior wall, where average fiber orientations were 20 to 30° counterclockwise of those in the dog. While the most reliable reconstructions of ventricular myofiber architecture have been made using quantitative histological techniques, diffusion tensor magnetic resonance imaging (MRI) has proven to be a reliable technique for estimating fiber orientation nondestructively in fixed [13,14] and even intact beating human hearts [15].

The locus of fiber orientations at a given depth in the ventricular wall has a spiral geometry that may be modeled as a general helix by simple differential geometry. The position vector **x** of a point on a helix inscribed on an ellipsoidal surface that is symmetric about the x_1 axis and has major and minor radii, a and b, is given by the parametric equation,

$$\mathbf{x} = a \sin t \mathbf{e}_1 + b \cos t \sin wt \mathbf{e}_2 + b \cos t \cos wt \mathbf{e}_3 \tag{54.4}$$

where the parameter is t, and the helix makes $w/4$ full turns between apex and equator. A positive w defines a left-handed helix with a positive pitch. The fiber angle or helix pitch angle η, varies along the arc length:

$$\sin \eta = \sqrt{\frac{a^2 \cos^2 t + b^2 \sin^2 t}{(a^2 + b^2 w^2) \cos^2 t + b^2 \sin^2 t}} \tag{54.5}$$

Epicardium

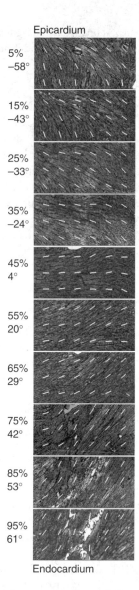

Endocardium

FIGURE 54.2 Cardiac muscle fiber orientations vary continuously through the left ventricular wall from a negative angle at the epicardium (0%) to near zero (circumferential) at the midwall (50%) and to increasing positive values toward the endocardium (100%). (Courtesy Jyoti Rao, Micrographs of murine myocardium from the author's laboratory.)

If another, deformed configuration $\hat{\mathbf{x}}$ is defined in the same way as Equation 54.4, the fiber-segment-extension ratio $d\hat{s}/ds$ associated with a change in the ellipsoid geometry [16] can be derived from

$$\frac{d\hat{s}/dt}{ds/dt} = \frac{|d\hat{x}/dt|}{|dx/dt|} \tag{54.6}$$

Although the traditional notion of discrete myofiber bundles has been revised in view of the continuous transmural variation of muscle fiber angle in the plane of the wall, there is a transverse laminar structure in the myocardium that groups fibers together in sheets an average of 4 ± 2 myocytes thick ($48 \pm 20\ \mu$m), separated by histologically distinct cleavage planes [17–19]. LeGrice and colleagues [19] investigated these structures in a detailed morphometric study of four dog hearts. They describe an ordered laminar arrangement of myocytes with extensive cleavage planes running approximately radially from endocardium toward epicardium in transmural section. Like the fibers, the sheets also have a branching pattern with the number of branches varying considerably through the wall thickness. Recent reports suggest that, in addition to fiber orientations, diffusion tensor MRI may be able to detect laminar sheet orientations [20]. The tensor of diffusion coefficients in the myocardium detected by MRI has shown to be orthotropic, and the principal axis of slowest diffusion was seen to coincide with the direction normal to the sheet planes.

The fibrous architecture of the myocardium has motivated models of myocardial material symmetry as transversely isotropic. The transverse laminae are the first structural evidence for material orthotropy and have motivated the development of models describing the variation of fiber, sheet, and sheet-normal axes throughout the ventricular wall [21]. This has led to the idea that the laminar architecture of the ventricular myocardium affects the significant transverse shears [22] and myofiber rearrangement [18] described in the intact heart during systole. By measuring three-dimensional distributions of strain across the wall thickness using biplane radiography of radiopaque markers, LeGrice and colleagues [23] found that the cleavage planes coincide closely with the planes of maximum shearing during ejection, and that the consequent reorientation of the myocytes may contribute 50% or more of normal systolic wall thickening. Arts et al. [24] showed that the distributions of sheet orientations measured within the left ventricular wall of the dog heart coincided closely with those predicted from observed three-dimensional wall strains using the assumption that laminae are oriented in planes that contain the muscle fibers and maximize interlaminar shearing. This assumption also leads to the conclusion that two families of sheet orientations may be expected. Indeed, a retrospective analysis of the histology supported this prediction and more recent observations confirm the presence of two distinct populations of sheet plane in the inner half of the ventricular wall.

A detailed description of the morphogenesis of the muscle fiber system in the developing heart is not available but there is evidence of an organized myofiber pattern by day 12 in the fetal mouse heart that is similar to that seen at birth (day 20) [25]. Abnormalities of cardiac muscle fiber patterns have been described in some disease conditions. In hypertrophic cardiomyopathy, which is often familial, there is substantial myofiber disarray, typically in the interventricular septum [10,26].

54.2.3 Extracellular Matrix Organization

The cardiac extracellular matrix consists primarily of the fibrillar collagens, type I (85%) and III (11%), synthesized by the cardiac fibroblasts, the most abundant cell type in the heart. Collagen is the major structural protein in connective tissues, but only comprises 2 to 5% of the myocardium by weight, compared with the myocytes, which make up 90% [27]. The collagen matrix has a hierarchical organization (Figure 54.3), and has been classified according to conventions established for skeletal muscle into endomysium, perimysium, and epimysium [28,29]. The endomysium is associated with individual cells and includes a fine weave surrounding the cell and transverse structural connections 120 to 150 nm long connecting adjacent myocytes, with attachments localized near the z-line of the sarcomere. The primary purpose of the endomysium is probably to maintain registration between adjacent cells. The perimysium groups cells together and includes the collagen fibers that wrap bundles of cells into the laminar sheets described above as well as large coiled fibers typically 1 to 3μm in diameter composed of smaller collagen fibrils (40 to 50 nm) [30]. The helix period of the coiled perimysial fibers is about 20μm and the convolution index (ratio of fiber arclength to midline length) is approximately 1.3 in the unloaded state of the ventricle [31,32]. These perimysial fibers are most likely to be the major structural elements of the collagen extracellular matrix though they probably contribute to myocardial strain energy by uncoiling rather than stretching [31]. Finally, a thick epimysial collagen sheath surrounds the entire myocardium forming the protective epicardium (visceral pericardium) and endocardium.

Collagen content, organization, cross-linking and ratio of types I to III change with age and in various disease conditions including myocardial ischemia and infarction, hypertension and hypertrophy

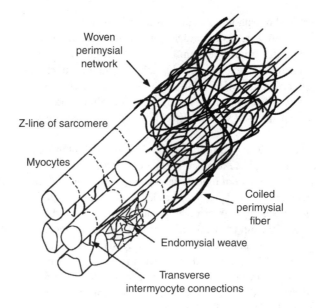

FIGURE 54.3 Schematic representation of cardiac tissue structure showing the association of endomysial and perimysial collagen fibers with cardiac myocytes. (Courtesy Dr. Deidre MacKenna.)

TABLE 54.4 Changes in Ventricular Collagen Structure and Mechanics with Age and Disease

Condition	Collagen morphology	Types and crosslinking	Passive stiffness	Other
Pressure overload hypertrophy	[Hydroxyproline]: ⇑-⇑⇑⇑ [132,133] Area fraction: ⇑⇑⇑ [133,134]	Type III: ⇑ [135] Cross-links: no change [136]	Chamber: ⇑-⇑⇑ [133,134] Tissue: ⇑⇑ [137]	Perivascular fibrosis ⇑⇑ [133] Focal scarring: [138,139]
Volume overload hypertrophy	[Hydroxyproline]: no change-⇓: [140,141] Area Fraction: no change [132,142]	Cross-links: ⇑ [136,141] Type III/I: ⇑ [141]	Chamber: ⇓ [143] Tissue: no change/⇑ [143]	Parallel changes
Acute ischemia/stunning	[Hydroxyproline]: ⇓ [Charney 1992 #1118] Light microscopy: no change/⇓ [144] ⇓⇓ endomysial fibers [145]		⇓ early [146] ⇑ late [147]	Collagenase activity: ⇑ [148,149]
Chronic myocardial infarction	[Hydroxyproline]: ⇑⇑⇑ [150,151] Loss of birefringence [152]	Type III: ⇑ [153]	Chamber: ⇑ early [154] Chamber: ⇓ late [154]	Organization: ⇑-⇑⇑⇑ [155,156]
Age	[Hydroxyproline]: ⇑-⇑⇑⇑ [148,157] Collagen fiber diameter ⇑ [157]	Type III/I: ⇓ [158] Cross-links: ⇑ [158]	Chamber: ⇑ [159] Papillary muscle: ⇑ [160]	Light microscopy: fibril diameter ⇑ [157]

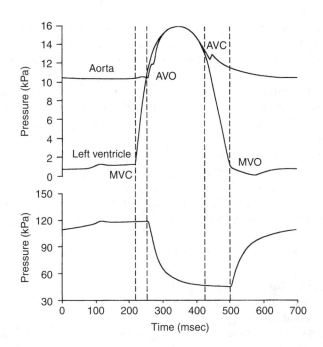

FIGURE 54.4 Left ventricular pressure, aortic pressure, and left ventricular volume during a single cardiac cycle showing the times of mitral valve closure (MVC), aortic valve opening (AVO), aortic valve closure (AVC) and mitral valve opening (MVO).

(Table 54.4). Changes in myocardial collagen content and organization coincide with alterations in diastolic myocardial stiffness [33]. Collagen intermolecular cross-linking is mediated by two separate mechanisms. The formation of enzymatic hydroxylysyl pyridinoline cross-links is catalyzed by lysyl oxidase, which requires copper as a cofactor. Nonenzymatic collagen cross-links known as advanced glycation endproducts can be formed in the presence of reducing sugars. This mechanism has been seen to significantly increase ventricular wall stiffness independent of changes in tissue collagen content, not only in diabetics, but also in an animal model of volume overload hypertrophy [34]. Hence the collagen matrix plays an important role in determining the elastic material properties of the ventricular myocardium.

54.3 Cardiac Pump Function

54.3.1 Ventricular Hemodynamics

The most basic mechanical parameters of the cardiac pump are blood pressure and volume flowrate, especially in the major pumping chambers, the ventricles. From the point of view of wall mechanics, the ventricular pressure is the most important boundary condition. Schematic representations of the time-courses of pressure and volume in the left ventricle are shown in Figure 54.4. Ventricular filling immediately following mitral valve opening (MVO) is initially rapid because the ventricle produces a diastolic suction as the relaxing myocardium recoils elastically from its compressed systolic configuration below the resting chamber volume. The later slow phase of ventricular filling (diastasis) is followed finally by atrial contraction. The deceleration of the inflowing blood reverses the pressure gradient across the valve leaflets and causes them to close mital valve closure (MVC). Valve closure may not, however, be completely passive, because the atrial side of the mitral valve leaflets, which unlike the pulmonic and aortic valves are cardiac in embryological origin, have muscle and nerve cells, and are electrically coupled to atrial conduction [35].

Ventricular contraction is initiated by excitation, which is almost synchronous (the duration of the QRS complex of the ECG is only about 60 msec in the normal adult) and begins about 0.1 to 0.2 sec after atrial depolarization. Pressure rises rapidly during the isovolumic contraction phase (about 50 msec in adult humans), and the aortic valve opens (AVO) when the developed pressure exceeds the aortic pressure (afterload). Most of the cardiac output is ejected within the first quarter of the ejection phase before the pressure has peaked. The aortic valve closes (AVC) 20 to 30 msec after AVO when the ventricular pressure falls below the aortic pressure owing to the deceleration of the ejecting blood. The dichrotic notch, a characteristic feature of the aortic pressure waveform and a useful marker of aortic valve closure, is caused by pulse wave reflections in the aorta. Since the pulmonary artery pressure against which the right ventricle pumps is much lower than the aortic pressure, the pulmonic valve opens before and closes after the aortic valve. The ventricular pressure falls during isovolumic relaxation, and the cycle continues. The rate of pressure decay from the value P_0 at the time of the peak rate of pressure fall until MVO is commonly characterized by a single exponential time constant, that is,

$$P(t) = P_0 e^{-t/\tau} + P_\infty \tag{54.7}$$

where P_∞ is the (negative) baseline pressure to which the ventricle would eventually relax if MVO were prevented [36]. In dogs and humans, τ is normally about 40 msec, but it is increased by various factors including elevated afterload, asynchronous contraction associated with abnormal activation sequence or regional dysfunction, and slowed cytosolic calcium reuptake to the sarcoplasmic reticulum associated with cardiac hypertrophy and failure. The pressure and volume curves for the right ventricle look essentially the same; however, the right ventricular and pulmonary artery pressures are only about a fifth of the corresponding pressures on the left side of the heart. The intraventricular septum separates the right and left ventricles and can transmit forces from one to the other. An increase in right ventricular volume may increase the left ventricular pressure by deformation of the septum. This direct interaction is most significant during filling [37].

The phases of the cardiac cycle are customarily divided into systole and diastole. The end of diastole — the start of systole — is generally defined as the time of MVC. Mechanical end-systole is usually defined as the end of ejection, but Brutsaert and colleagues proposed extending systole until the onset of diastasis (see the review by Brutsaert and Sys [38]), since there remains considerable myofilament interaction and active tension during relaxation. The distinction is important from the point of view of cardiac muscle mechanics: the myocardium is still active for much of diastole and may never be fully relaxed at sufficiently high heart rates (over 150 beats per minute). Here, we will retain the traditional definition of diastole, but consider the ventricular myocardium to be "passive" or "resting" only in the final slow-filling stage of diastole.

54.3.2 Ventricular Pressure–Volume Relations and Energetics

A useful alternative to Figure 54.4 for displaying ventricular pressure and volume changes is the pressure–volume loop shown in Figure 54.5a. During the last 20 years, the ventricular pressure–volume relationship has been explored extensively, particularly by Sagawa, and colleagues [39], who wrote a comprehensive book on the approach. The isovolumic phases of the cardiac cycle can be recognized as the vertical segments of the loop, the lower limb represents ventricular filling, and the upper segment is the ejection phase. The difference on the horizontal axis between the vertical isovolumic segments is the stroke volume, which expressed as a fraction of the end-diastolic volume is the ejection fraction. The effects of altered loading on the ventricular pressure–volume relation have been studied in many preparations, but the best controlled experiments have used the isolated cross-circulated canine heart in which the ventricle fills and ejects against a computer-controlled volume servo-pump.

Changes in the filling pressure of the ventricle (preload) move the end-diastolic point along the unique end-diastolic pressure–volume relation (EDPVR), which represents the passive filling mechanics of the chamber that are determined primarily by the thick-walled geometry and nonlinear elasticity of the resting

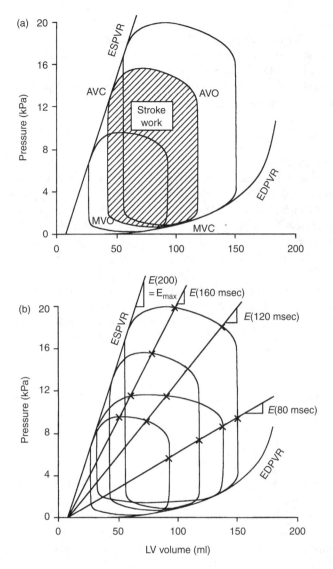

FIGURE 54.5 Schematic diagram of left ventricular pressure–volume loops: (a) End-systolic pressure–volume relation (ESPVR), end-diastolic pressure–volume relation (EDPVR) and stroke work. The three P–V loops show the effects of changes in preload and afterload. (b) Time-varying elastance approximation of ventricular pump function (see text).

ventricular wall. Alternatively, if the afterload seen by the left ventricle is increased, stroke volume decreases in a predictable manner. The locus of end-ejection points (AVC) forms the end-systolic pressure–volume relation (ESPVR), which is approximately linear in a variety of conditions and also largely independent of the ventricular load history. Hence, the ESPVR is almost the same for isovolumic beats as for ejecting beats, although consistent effects of ejection history have been well characterized [40]. Connecting pressure–volume points at corresponding times in the cardiac cycle also results in a relatively linear relationship throughout systole with the intercept on the volume axis V_0 remaining nearly constant (Figure 54.5b). This leads to the valuable approximation that the ventricular volume $V(t)$ at any instance during systole is simply proportional to the instantaneous pressure $P(t)$ through a time-varying elastance $E(t)$:

$$P(t) = E(t)\{V(t) - V_0\} \tag{54.8}$$

The maximum elastance E_{max}, the slope of the ESPVR, has acquired considerable significance as an index of cardiac contractility that is independent of ventricular loading conditions. As the inotropic state of the myocardium increases, for example with catecholamine infusion, E_{max} increases, and with a negative inotropic effect such as a reduction in coronary artery pressure, it decreases.

The area of the ventricular pressure–volume loop is the external work (EW) performed by the myocardium on the ejecting blood:

$$EW = \int_{EDV}^{ESV} P(t)dV \qquad (54.9)$$

Plotting this stroke work against a suitable measure of preload gives a ventricular function curve, which illustrates the single most important intrinsic mechanical property of the heart pump. In 1914, Patterson and Starling [41] performed detailed experiments on the canine heart–lung preparation, and Starling summarized their results with his famous "Law of the Heart," which states that the work output of the heart increases with ventricular filling. The so-called Frank–Starling mechanism is now well recognized to be an intrinsic mechanical property of cardiac muscle (see Section 54.4).

External stroke work is closely related to cardiac energy utilization. Since myocardial contraction is fueled by ATP, 90 to 95% of which is normally produced by oxidative phosphorylation, cardiac energy consumption is often studied in terms of myocardial oxygen consumption, VO_2 (ml $O_2.g^{-1}.beat^{-1}$). Since energy is also expended during nonworking contractions, Suga and colleagues [42] defined the pressure–volume area (PVA) ($J.g^{-1}.beat^{-1}$) as the loop area (external stroke work) plus the end-systolic potential energy (internal work), which is the area under the ESPVR left of the isovolumic relaxation line (Figure 54.5a),

$$PVA = EW + PE \qquad (54.10)$$

The PVA has strong linear correlation with VO_2 independent of ejection history. Equation 54.11 has typical values for the dog heart:

$$VO_2 = 0.12(PVA) + 2.0 \times 10^{-4} \qquad (54.11)$$

The intercept represents the sum of the oxygen consumption for basal metabolism and the energy associated with activation of the contractile apparatus, which is primarily used to cycle intracellular Ca^{2+} for excitation–contraction coupling [42]. The reciprocal of the slope is the contractile efficiency [43,44]. The VO_2–PVA relation shifts its elevation but not its slope with increments in E_{max} with most positive and negative inotropic interventions [43,45–48]. However, ischemic-reperfused viable but "stunned" myocardium has a smaller O_2 cost of PVA [49].

Although the PVA approach has also been useful in many settings, it is fundamentally phenomenological. Because the time-varying elastance assumptions ignores the well-documented load-history dependence of cardiac muscle tension, [50–52] theoretical analyses that attempt to reconcile PVA with crossbridge mechanoenergetics [53] are usually based on isometric or isotonic contractions. So that regional oxygen consumption in the intact heart can be related to myofiber biophysics, regional variations on the pressure–volume area have been proposed, such as the tension-area area [54], normalization of E_{max} [55], and the fiber stress-strain area [56].

In mammals, there are characteristic variations in cardiac function with heart size. In the power law relation for heart rate as a function of body mass (analogous to Equation 54.3), the coefficient k is 241 beats.min^{-1} and the power α is -0.25 [5]. In the smallest mammals, like soricine shrews that weigh only a few grams, maximum heart rates exceeding 1000 beats.min^{-1} have been measured [57]. Ventricular cavity volume scales linearly with heart weight, and ejection fraction and blood pressure are reasonably invariant from rats to horses. Hence, stroke work also scales directly with heart size [58], and thus work rate and energy consumption would be expected to increase with decreased body size in the same manner as heart rate. However, careful studies have demonstrated only a twofold increase in myocardial heat production as body mass decreases in mammals ranging from humans to rats, despite a 4.6-fold increase in heart rate [59]. This suggests that cardiac energy expenditure does not scale in proportion to heart rate and that cardiac metabolism is a lower proportion of total body metabolism in the smaller species.

The primary determinants of the EDPVR are the material properties of resting myocardium, the chamber dimensions and wall thickness, and the boundary conditions at the epicardium, endocardium, and valve annulus [60]. The EDPVR has been approximated by an exponential function of volume (see e.g., chapter 9 in Gaasch and Lewinter [61]), though a cubic polynomial also works well. Therefore, the passive chamber stiffness dP/dV is approximately proportional to the filling pressure. Important influences on the EDPVR include the extent of relaxation, ventricular interaction and pericardial constraints, and coronary vascular engorgement. The material properties and boundary conditions in the septum are important since they determine how the septum deforms [62,63]. Through septal interaction, the EDPVR of the left ventricle may be directly affected by changes in the hemodynamic loading conditions of the right ventricle. The ventricles also interact indirectly since the output of the right ventricle is returned as the input to the left ventricle via the pulmonary circulation. Slinker and Glantz [64], using pulmonary artery and venae caval occlusions to produce direct (immediate) and indirect (delayed) interaction transients, concluded that the direct interaction is about half as significant as the indirect coupling. The pericardium provides a low friction mechanical enclosure for the beating heart that constrains ventricular overextension [65] Since the pericardium has stiffer elastic properties than the ventricles [66], it contributes to direct ventricular interactions. The pericardium also augments the mechanical coupling between the atria and ventricles [67]. Increasing coronary perfusion pressure has been seen to increase the slope of the diastolic pressure–volume relation (an "erectile" effect) [68,69].

54.4 Myocardial Material Properties

54.4.1 Muscle Contractile Properties

Cardiac muscle mechanics testing is far more difficult than skeletal muscle testing mainly owing to the lack of ideal test specimens like the long single fiber preparations that have been so valuable for studying the mechanisms of skeletal muscle mechanics. Moreover, under physiological conditions, cardiac muscle cannot be stimulated to produce sustained tetanic contractions due to the absolute refractory period of the myocyte cell membrane. Cardiac muscle also exhibits a mechanical property analogous to the relative refractory period of excitation. After a single isometric contraction, some recovery time is required before another contraction of equal amplitude can be activated. The time constant for this mechanical restitution property of cardiac muscle is about 1 sec [70].

Unlike skeletal muscle, in which maximal active force generation occurs at a sarcomere length that optimizes myofilament overlap ($\sim$2.1 μm), the isometric twitch tension developed by isolated cardiac muscle continues to rise with increased sarcomere length in the physiological range (1.6 to 2.4 μm) (Figure 54.6a). Early evidence for a descending limb of the cardiac muscle isometric length–tension curve was found to be caused by shortening in the central region of the isolated muscle at the expense of stretching at the damaged ends where specimen was tethered to the test apparatus. If muscle length is controlled so that sarcomere length in the undamaged part of the muscle is indeed constant, or if the developed tension is plotted against the instantaneous sarcomere length rather than the muscle length, the descending limb is eliminated [71]. Thus, the increase with chamber volume of end-systolic pressure and stroke work is reflected in isolated muscle as a monotonic increase in peak isometric tension with sarcomere length (Figure 54.6b). Note that the active tension shown in Figure 54.6 is the total tension minus the resting tension, which, unlike in skeletal muscle, becomes very significant at sarcomere lengths over 2.3 μm. The increase in slope of the ESPVR associated with increased contractility is mirrored by the effects of increased calcium concentration in the length–tension relation. The duration as well as the tension developed in the active cardiac twitch also increases substantially with sarcomere length (Figure 54.6a).

The relationship between cytosolic calcium concentration and isometric muscle tension has mostly been investigated in muscle preparations in which the sarcolemma has been chemically permeabilized. Because

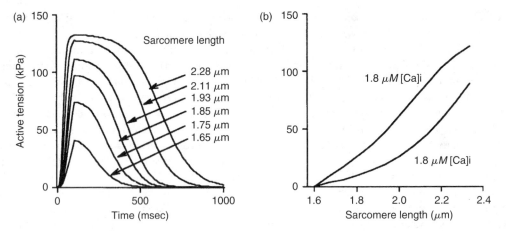

FIGURE 54.6 Cardiac muscle isometric twitch tension generated by a model of rat cardiac contraction (courtesy Dr. Julius Guccione): (a) Developed twitch tension as a function of time and sarcomere length; (b) Peak isometric twitch tension vs. sarcomere length for low and high calcium concentration.

there is evidence that this chemical "skinning" alters the calcium sensitivity of myofilament interaction, recent studies have also investigated myofilament calcium sensitivity in intact muscles tetanized by high-frequency stimulation in the presence of a compound such as ryanodine that open calcium release sites in the sarcoplasmic reticulum. Intracellular calcium concentration was estimated using calcium-sensitive optical indicators such as Fura. The myofilaments are activated in a graded manner by micromolar concentrations of calcium, which binds to troponin-C according to a sigmoidal relation [72]. Half-maximal tension in cardiac muscle is developed at intracellular calcium concentrations of 10^{-6} to 10^{-5} M (the C_{50}) depending on factors such as species and temperature [70]. Hence, relative isometric tension T_0/T_{max} may be modeled using [73,74].

$$\frac{T_0}{T_{max}} = \frac{[Ca]^n}{[Ca]^n + C_{50}^n} \tag{54.12}$$

The Hill coefficient (n) governs the steepness of the sigmoidal curve. A wide variety of values have been reported but most have been in the range 3 to 6 [75–78]. The steepness of the isometric length–tension relation (Figure 54.6b), compared with that of skeletal muscle is due to length-dependent calcium sensitivity. That is, the C_{50} (M) and n both change with sarcomere length, L (μm). Hunter et al. [74] used the following approximations to fit the data of Kentish et al. [76] from rat right ventricular trabeculae:

$$n = 4.25\{1 + 1.95(L/L_{ref} - 1)\}, \quad pC_{50} = -\log_{10}C_{50} = 5.33\{1 + 0.31(L/L_{ref} - 1)\} \tag{54.13}$$

where the reference sarcomere length L_{ref} was taken to be 2.0 μm.

The isotonic force–velocity relation of cardiac muscle is similar to that of skeletal muscle, and A.V. Hill's well-known hyperbolic relation is a good approximation except at larger forces greater than about 85% of the isometric value. The maximal (unloaded) velocity of shortening is essentially independent of preload, but does change with time during the cardiac twitch and is affected by factors that affect contractile ATPase activity and hence crossbridge cycling rates. deTombe and colleagues [79] using sarcomere length-controlled isovelocity release experiments found that viscous forces imposes a significant internal load-opposing sarcomere shortening. If the isotonic shortening response is adjusted for the confounding effects of passive viscoelasticity, the underlying crossbridge force–velocity relation is found to be linear.

Cardiac muscle contraction also exhibits other significant length-history-dependent properties. An important example is "deactivation" associated with length transients. The isometric twitch tension redeveloped following a brief length transient that dissociates crossbridges, reaches the original isometric value when the transient is imposed early in the twitch before the peak tension is reached. But following transients applied at times after the peak twitch tension has occurred, the fraction of tension redeveloped declines progressively since the activator calcium has fallen to levels below that necessary for all crossbridges to reattach [80].

There have been many model formulations of cardiac muscle contractile mechanics, too numerous to summarize here. In essence they may be grouped into three categories. Time-varying elastance models include the essential dependence of cardiac active force development on muscle length and time. These models would seem to be well suited to the continuum analysis of whole heart mechanics [1,81,82] by virtue of the success of the time-varying elastance concept of ventricular function (see Section 54.3.2). In "Hill" models the active fiber stress development is modified by shortening or lengthening according to the force–velocity relation, so that fiber tension is reduced by increased shortening velocity [83,84]. Fully history-dependent models are more complex and are generally based on A.F. Huxley's crossbridge theory [52,85–87]. A statistical approach known as the distribution moment model has also been shown to provide an excellent approximation to crossbridge theory [88]. An alternative more phenomenological approach is Hunter's fading memory theory, which captures the complete length-history dependence of cardiac muscle contraction without requiring all the biophysical complexity of crossbridge models [74]. The appropriate choice of model will depend on the purpose of the analysis. For many models of global ventricular function, a time-varying elastance model will suffice, but for an analysis of sarcomere dynamics in isolated muscle or the ejecting heart, a history-dependent analysis is more appropriate.

Although Hill's basic assumption that resting and active muscle fiber tension are additive is axiomatic in one-dimensional tests of isolated cardiac mechanics, there remains little experimental information on how the passive and active material properties of myocardium superpose in two or three dimensions. The simplest and commonest assumption is that active stress is strictly one-dimensional and adds to the fiber component of the three-dimensional passive stress. However, even this addition will indirectly affect all the other components of the stress response, since myocardial elastic deformations are finite, nonlinear and approximately isochoric (volume conserving). In an interesting and important new development, biaxial testing of tetanized and barium-contracted ventricular myocardium has shown that developed systolic stress also has a large component in directions transverse to the mean myofiber axis that can exceed 50% of the axial fiber component [89]. The magnitude of this transverse active stress depended significantly on the biaxial loading conditions. Moreover, evidence from osmotic swelling and other studies suggests that transverse strain can affect contractile tension development along the fiber axis by altering myofibril lattice spacing [90,91]. The mechanisms of transverse active stress development remain unclear but two possible contributors are the geometry of the crossbridge head itself, which is oriented oblique to the myofilament axis [92], and the dispersion of myofiber orientation [10].

54.4.2 Resting Myocardial Properties

Since, by the Frank–Starling mechanism, end-diastolic volume directly affects systolic ventricular work, the mechanics of resting myocardium also have fundamental physiological significance. Most biomechanics studies of passive myocardial properties have been conducted in isolated, arrested whole heart or tissue preparations. Passive cardiac muscle exhibits most of the mechanical properties characteristic of soft tissues in general [93]. In cyclic uniaxial loading and unloading, the stress–strain relationship is nonlinear with small but significant hysteresis. Depending on the preparation used, resting cardiac muscle typically requires from 2 to 10 repeated loading cycles to achieve a reproducible (preconditioned) response. Intact cardiac muscle experiences finite deformations during the normal cardiac cycle, with maximum Lagrangian strains (which are generally radial and endocardial) that may easily exceed 0.5 in magnitude. Hence, the classical linear theory of elasticity is quite inappropriate for resting myocardial mechanics. The hysteresis of the tissue is consistent with a viscoelastic response, which is undoubtedly

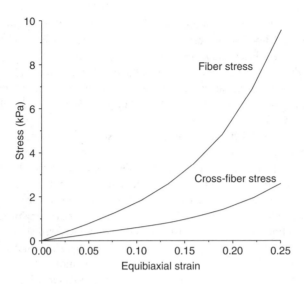

FIGURE 54.7 Representative stress–strain curves for passive rat myocardium computed using Equation 17 and Equation 19. Fiber and crossfiber stress are shown for equibiaxial strain. (Courtesy Dr. Jeffrey Omens.)

related to the substantial water content of the myocardium (about 80% by mass). Changes in water content, such as edema, can cause substantial alterations in the passive stiffness and viscoelastic properties of myocardium. The viscoelasticity of passive cardiac muscle has been characterized in creep and relaxation studies of papillary muscle from cat and rabbit. In both species, the tensile stress in response to a step in strain relaxes 30 to 40% in the first 10 seconds [94,95]. The relaxation curves exhibit a short exponential time constant (<0.02 sec) and a long one (about 1000 sec), and are largely independent of the strain magnitude, which supports the approximation that myocardial viscoelasticity is quasilinear. Myocardial creep under isotonic loading is 2 to 3% of the original length after 100 sec of isotonic loading and is also quasilinear with an exponential timecourse. There is also evidence that passive ventricular muscle exhibits other anelastic properties such as maximum-strain-dependent "strain softening" [96,97], a well-known property in elastomers first described by Mullins [98].

Since the hysteresis of passive cardiac muscle is small and only weakly affected by changes in strain rate, the assumption of pseudoelasticity [93] is often appropriate. That is, the resting myocardium is considered to be a finite elastic material with different elastic properties in loading vs. unloading. Although various preparations have been used to study resting myocardial elasticity, the most detailed and complete information has come from biaxial and multiaxial tests of isolated sheets of cardiac tissue, mainly from the dog [99–101]. These experiments have shown that the arrested myocardium exhibits significant anisotropy with substantially greater stiffness in the muscle fiber direction than transversely. In equibiaxial tests of muscle sheets cut from planes parallel to the ventricular wall, fiber stress was greater than the transverse stress (Figure 54.7) by an average factor of close to 2.0 [102]. Moreover, as suggested by the structural organization of the myocardium described in Section 54.2, there may also be significant anisotropy in the plane of the tissue transverse to the fiber axis.

The biaxial stress–strain properties of passive myocardium display some heterogeneity. Recently, Novak et al. [103] measured regional variations of biaxial mechanics in the canine left ventricle. Specimens from the inner and outer thirds of the left ventricular free wall were stiffer than those from the midwall and interventricular septum, but the degree of anisotropy was similar in each region. Significant species variations in myocardial stiffness have also been described. Using measurements of two-dimensional regional strain during left ventricular inflation in the isolated whole heart, a parameter optimization approach showed that canine cardiac tissue was several times stiffer than that of the rat, though the nonlinearity and anisotropy were similar [104]. Biaxial testing of the collagenous parietal pericardium and epicardium have shown that these tissues have distinctly different properties than the myocardium being very compliant and isotropic at low-biaxial strains (<0.1 to 0.15) but rapidly becoming very stiff and anisotropic as the strain is increased [66,100].

Various constitutive models have been proposed for the elasticity of passive cardiac tissues. Because of the large deformations and nonlinearity of these materials, the most useful framework has been provided by the pseudostrain-energy formulation for hyperelasticity. For a detailed review of the material properties of passive myocardium and approaches to constitutive modeling, the reader is referred to chapters 1 to 6 of Glass et al [105]. In hyperelasticity, the components of the stress* are obtained from the strain energy W as a function of the Lagrangian (Green's) strain E_{RS}.

The myocardium is generally assumed to be an incompressible material, which is a good approximation in the isolated tissue, although in the intact heart there can be a significant redistribution of tissue volume associated with phasic changes in regional coronary blood volume. Incompressibility is included as a kinematic constraint in the finite elasticity analysis, which introduces a new pressure variable that is added as a Lagrange multiplier in the strain energy. The examples that follow are various strain–energy functions, with representative parameter values (for W in kPa, i.e., mJ.ml^{-1}) that have been suggested for cardiac tissues. For the two-dimensional properties of canine myocardium, Yin and colleagues [102] obtained reasonable fits to experimental data with an exponential function,

$$W = 0.47 e^{(35E_{11}^{1.2} + 20E_{22}^{1.2})} \tag{54.14}$$

where E_{11} is the fiber strain and E_{22} is the crossfiber in-plane strain. Humphrey and Yin [106] proposed a three-dimensional form for W as the sum of an isotropic exponential function of the first principal invariant I_1 of the right Cauchy–Green deformation tensor and another exponential function of the fiber stretch ratio λ_F:

$$W = 0.21 \left(e^{9.4(I_1 - 3)} - 1 \right) + 0.35 \left(e^{66(\lambda_F - 1)^2} - 1 \right) \tag{54.15}$$

The isotropic part of this expression has also been used to model the myocardium of the embryonic chick heart during the ventricular looping stages, with coefficients of 0.02 kPa during diastole and 0.78 kPa at end-systole, and exponent parameters of 1.1 and 0.85, respectively [107]. Another related transversely isotropic strain-energy function was used by Guccione et al. [108] and Omens et al. [109] to model material properties in the isolated mature rat and dog hearts:

$$W = 0.6(e^Q - 1) \tag{54.16}$$

where, in the dog

$$Q = 26.7E_{11}^2 + 2.0(E_{22}^2 + E_{33}^2 + E_{23}^2 + E_{32}^2) + 14.7(E_{12}^2 + E_{21}^2 + E_{13}^2 + E_{31}^2) \tag{54.17}$$

and, in the rat

$$Q = 9.2E_{11}^2 + 2.0(E_{22}^2 + E_{33}^2 + E_{23}^2 + E_{32}^2) + 3.7(E_{12}^2 + E_{21}^2 + E_{13}^2 + E_{31}^2) \tag{54.18}$$

In Equation 54.17 and Equation 54.18, normal and shear strain components involving the radial (x_3) axis are included. Humphrey and colleagues [110] determined a new polynomial form directly from biaxial tests. Novak et al. [103] gave representative coefficients for canine myocardium from three layers of the left ventricular free wall. For the outer third, they obtained

$$W = 4.8(\lambda_F - 1)^2 + 3.4(\lambda_F - 1)^3 + 0.77(I_1 - 3) - 6.1(I_1 - 3)(\lambda_F - 1) + 6.2(I_1 - 3)^2 \tag{54.19}$$

---

* In a hyperelastic material, the *second Piola Kirchhoff* stress tensor is given by, $P_{RS} 1/2((\partial W / \partial E_{RS}) + (\partial W / \partial E_{SR}))$.

for the midwall region

$$W = 5.3(\lambda_F - 1)^2 + 7.5(\lambda_F - 1)^3 + 0.43(I_1 - 3) - 7.7(I_1 - 3)(\lambda_F - 1) + 5.6(I_1 - 3)^2 \qquad (54.20)$$

and for the inner layer of the wall

$$W = 0.51(\lambda_F - 1)^2 + 27.6(\lambda_F - 1)^3 + 0.74(I_1 - 3) - 7.3(I_1 - 3)(\lambda_F - 1) + 7.0(I_1 - 3)^2 \qquad (54.21)$$

A power law strain–energy function expressed in terms of circumferential, longitudinal and transmural extension ratios (λ_1, λ_2, and λ_3) was used [111] to describe the biaxial properties of sheep myocardium 2 weeks after experimental myocardial infarction, in the scarred infarct region:

$$W = 0.36 \left(\frac{\lambda_1^{32}}{32} + \frac{\lambda_2^{30}}{30} + \frac{\lambda_3^{31}}{31} - 3 \right) \qquad (54.22)$$

and in the remote, noninfarcted tissue:

$$W = 0.11 \left(\frac{\lambda_1^{22}}{22} + \frac{\lambda_2^{26}}{26} + \frac{\lambda_3^{24}}{24} - 3 \right) \qquad (54.23)$$

Finally, based on the observation that resting stiffness rises steeply at strains that extend coiled collagen fibers to the limit of uncoiling, Hunter and colleagues have proposed a pole-zero constitutive relation in which the stresses rise asymptotically as the strain approaches a limiting elastic strain [74].

The strain in the constitutive equation must generally be referred to the stress-free state of the tissue. However, the unloaded state of the passive left ventricle is not stress-free; residual stress exists in the intact, unloaded myocardium, as shown by Omens and Fung [112]. Cross-sectional equatorial rings from potassium-arrested rat hearts spring open elastically when the left ventricular wall is resected radially. The average opening angle of the resulting curved arc is $45 \pm 10°$ in the rat. Subsequent radial cuts produce no further change. Hence, a slice with one radial cut is considered to be stress-free, and there is a nonuniform distribution of residual strain across the intact wall, being compressive at the endocardium and tensile at the epicardium, with some regional differences. Stress analyses of the diastolic left ventricle have shown that residual stress acts to minimize the endocardial stress concentrations that would otherwise be associated with diastolic loading [108]. An important physiological consequence of residual stress is that sarcomere length is nonuniform in the unloaded resting heart. Rodriguez et al. [113] showed that sarcomere length is about 0.13 μm greater at epicardium than endocardium in the unloaded rat heart, and this gradient vanishes when residual stress is relieved. Three-dimensional studies have also revealed the presence of substantial transverse residual shear strains [114]. Residual stress and strain may have an important relationship to cardiac growth and remodeling. Theoretical studies have shown that residual stress in tissues can arise from growth fields that are kinematically incompatible [115,116].

54.5   Regional Ventricular Mechanics: Stress and Strain

Although ventricular pressures and volumes are valuable for assessing the global pumping performance of the heart, myocardial stress and strain distributions are needed to characterize regional ventricular function, especially in pathological conditions, such as myocardial ischemia and infarction, where profound localized changes may occur. The measurement of stress in the intact myocardium involves resolving the local forces acting on defined planes in the heart wall. Attempts to measure local forces [117,118] have had limited success because of the large deformations of the myocardium and the uncertain nature of the mechanical coupling between the transducer elements and the tissue. Efforts to measure intramyocardial pressures using miniature implanted transducers have been more successful but have also raised controversy over the extent to which they accurately represent changes in interstitial fluid pressure. In all cases, these methods provide an incomplete description of three-dimensional wall stress distributions. Therefore, the most common approach for estimating myocardial stress distributions is the use of mathematical models based on the laws of continuum mechanics. Although there is no room to review these analyses here, the important elements of such models are the geometry and structure, boundary conditions, and material properties, described in the foregoing sections. An excellent review of ventricular wall stress analysis is given by Yin [119]. The most versatile and powerful method for ventricular stress analysis is the finite element method, which has been used in cardiac mechanics for over 20 years [120]. However, models must also be validated with experimental measurements. Since the measurement of myocardial stresses is not yet reliable, the best experimental data for model validation are measurements of strains in the ventricular wall.

The earliest myocardial strain gauges were mercury-in-rubber transducers sutured to the epicardium. These days, local segment length changes are routinely measured with various forms of the piezoelectric crystal sonomicrometer. However, since the ventricular myocardium is a three-dimensional continuum, the local strain is only fully defined by all the normal and shear components of the myocardial strain tensor. Villarreal et al. [121] measured two-dimensional midwall strain components by arranging three piezoelectric crystals in a small triangle so that three segment lengths could be measured simultaneously. They showed that the principal axis of greatest shortening is not aligned with circumferential midwall fibers, and that this axis changes with altered ventricular loading and contractility. Therefore, uniaxial segment measurements do not reveal the full extent of alterations in regional function caused by an experimental intervention. Another approach to measuring regional myocardial strains is the use of clinical imaging techniques, such as contrast ventriculography, high-speed x-ray tomography, MRI or two-dimensional echocardiography. But the conventional application of these techniques is not suitable for measuring regional strains because they cannot be used to identify the motion of distinct myocardial points. They only produce a profile or silhouette of a surface, except in the unusual circumstance when radiopaque markers are implanted in the myocardium during cardiac surgery or transplantation [122]. Hunter and Zerhouni [123] describe the prospects for noninvasive imaging of discrete points in the ventricular wall. The most promising method is the use of MRI tagging methods, which are now being used to map three-dimensional ventricular strain fields in conscious subjects [4].

In experimental research, implantable radiopaque markers are used for tracking myocardial motions with high spatial and temporal resolution. Meier et al. [124,125] placed triplets of metal markers 10 to 15 mm apart near the epicardium of the canine right ventricle and reconstructed their positions from biplane cinéradiographic recordings. By polar decomposition, they obtained the two principal epicardial strains, the principal angle, and the local rotation in the region. The use of radiopaque markers was extended to three dimensions by Waldman and colleagues [22], who implanted three closely separated columns of 5 to 6 metal beads in the ventricular wall. With this technique, it is possible to find all six components of strain and all three rigid-body rotation angles at sites through the wall. For details of this method, see the review by Waldman in chapter 7 of Glass et al [105]. An enhancement to this method uses high-order finite element interpolation of the marker positions to compute continuous transmural distributions of myocardial deformation [126].

Studies and models such as these are producing an increasingly detailed picture of regional myocardial stress and strain distributions. Of the many interesting observations, there are some useful generalizations, particularly regarding the strain. Myocardial deformations are large and three dimensional, and hence the nonlinear finite strain tensors are more appropriate measures than the linear infinitesimal Cauchy strain. During filling in the normal heart, the wall stretches biaxially but nonuniformly in the plane of the wall, and thins in the transmural direction. During systole, shortening is also two dimensional and the wall thickens. There are substantial regional differences in the timecourse, magnitude, and pattern of myocardial deformations. In humans and dogs, in-plane systolic myocardial shortening and diastolic lengthening vary with longitudinal position on the left and right ventricular free walls generally increasing in magnitude from base to apex.

Both during systole and diastole, there are significant shear strains in the wall. In-plane (torsional) shears are negative during diastole, consistent with a small left-handed torsion of the left ventricle during filling, and positive as the ventricular twist reverses during ejection. Consequently, the principal axes of greatest diastolic segment lengthening and systolic shortening are not circumferential or longitudinal but at oblique axes, which are typically rotated 10 to 60° clockwise from circumferential. There are circumferential variations in regional left ventricular strain. The principal axes of greatest diastolic lengthening and systolic shortening tend to be more longitudinal on the posterior wall and more circumferentially oriented on the anterior wall. Perhaps the most significant regional variations are transmural. In-plane and transmural, normal or principal strains, are usually significantly greater in magnitude at the endocardium than the epicardium both in filling and ejection. However, when the strain is resolved in the local muscle fiber direction, the transmural variation of fiber strain becomes insignificant. The combination of torsional deformation and the transmural variation in fiber direction means that systolic shortening and diastolic lengthening tend to be maximized in the fiber direction at the epicardium and minimized at the endocardium. Hence, whereas maximum shortening and lengthening are closely aligned with muscle fibers at the subepicardium, they are almost perpendicular to the fibers at the subendocardium. In the left ventricular wall there are also substantial transverse shear strains (i.e., in the circumferential-radial and longitudinal-radial planes) during systole, though during filling they are smaller. Their functional significance remains unclear, though they change substantially during acute myocardial ischemia or ventricular pacing and are apparently associated with the transverse laminae described earlier [23].

Sophisticated continuum mechanics models are needed to determine the stress distributions associated with these complex myocardial deformations. With modern finite element methods it is now possible to include in the analysis the three-dimensional geometry and fiber architecture, finite deformations, nonlinear material properties, and muscle contraction of the ventricular myocardium. Some models have included other factors such as viscoelasticity, poroelasticity, coronary perfusion, growth and remodeling, regional ischemia, residual stress and electrical activation. To date, continuum models have provided some valuable insight into regional cardiac mechanics. These include the importance of muscle fiber orientation, torsional deformations and residual stress, and the substantial inhomogeneities associated with regional variations in geometry and fiber angle or myocardial ischemia and infarction. A new arena in which models promise to make important contributions is the rapidly growing field of cardiac resynchronization therapy [127]. The use of biventricular pacing in cases of congestive heart failure that are accompanied by electrical conduction asynchrony has been seen to significantly improve ventricular pump function. However the improvement in mechanical function is not well predicted by the improvement in electrical synchrony. New electromechanical models promise to provide insights into the mechanisms of cardiac resynchronization therapy and potentially to optimize the pacing protocols used [128].

Acknowledgments

I am indebted to many colleagues and students, past and present, for their input and perspective of cardiac biomechanics. Owing to space constraints, I have relied on much of their work without adequate citation, especially in the final section. Special thanks to Drs. Jeffrey Omens, Deidre MacKenna, Julius Guccione, and Jyoti Rao.

References

[1] Taber, L.A., On a nonlinear theory for muscle shells. Part II — application to the beating left ventricle, *ASME J. Biomech. Eng.*, 113, 63–71, 1991.

[2] Streeter, D.D., Jr. and Hanna, W.T., Engineering mechanics for successive states in canine left ventricular myocardium: I. Cavity and wall geometry, *Circ. Res.*, 33, 639–655, 1973.

[3] Nielsen, P.M.F., Le Grice, I.J., Smaill, B.H. et al., Mathematical model of geometry and fibrous structure of the heart, *Am. J. Physiol.*, 260, H1365–H1378, 1991.

[4] Young, A.A. and Axel, L., Three-dimensional motion and deformation in the heart wall: estimation from spatial modulation of magnetization — a model-based approach, *Radiology*, 185, 241–247, 1992.

[5] Stahl, W.R., Scaling of respiratory variable in mammals, *J. Appl. Physiol.*, 22, 453–460, 1967.

[6] Rakusan, K., Cardiac growth, maturation and aging, in *Growth of the Heart in Health and Disease*, R. Zak, Ed. Raven Press, New York: 1984, pp. 131–164.

[7] Streeter, D.D., Jr., Gross morphology and fiber geometry of the heart, in *Handbook of Physiology, Section 2: The Cardiovascular System, Chapter 4*, I, B.R.M, Ed. American Physiological Society, Bethesda, MD: 1979, pp. 61–112.

[8] Saffitz, J.E., Kanter, H.L., Green, K.G. et al., Tissue-specific determinants of anisotropic conduction velocity in canine atrial and ventricular myocardium, *Circ. Res.*, 74, 1065–1070, 1994.

[9] Torrent-Guasp, F., *The Cardiac Muscle*, Juan March Foundation, 1973.

[10] Karlon, W.J., Covell, J.W., McCulloch, A.D. et al., Automated measurement of myofiber disarray in transgenic mice with ventricular expression of ras, *Anat. Rec.*, 252, 612–625, 1998.

[11] Streeter, D.D., Jr., Spotnitz, H.M., Patel, D.P. et al., Fiber orientation in the canine left ventricle during diastole and systole, *Circ. Res.*, 24, 339–347, 1969.

[12] Vetter, F.J. and McCulloch, A.D., Three-dimensional analysis of regional cardiac function: a model of rabbit ventricular anatomy, *Prog. Biophys. Mol. Biol.*, 69, 157–183, 1998.

[13] Hsu, E.W., Muzikant, A.L., Matulevicius, S.A. et al., Magnetic resonance myocardial fiber-orientation mapping with direct histological correlation, *Am. J. Physiol.*, 274, H1627–H1634, 1998.

[14] Scollan, D.F., Holmes, A., Winslow, R. et al., Histological validation of myocardial microstructure obtained from diffusion tensor magnetic resonance imaging, *Am. J. Physiol.*, 275, H2308–H2318, 1998.

[15] Dou, J., Tseng, W.Y., Reese, T.G. et al., Combined diffusion and strain MRI reveals structure and function of human myocardial laminar sheets *in vivo*, *Magn. Reson. Med.*, 50, 107–113, 2003.

[16] McCulloch, A.D., Smaill, B.H., and Hunter, P.J., Regional left ventricular epicardial deformation in the passive dog heart, *Circ. Res.*, 64, 721–733, 1989.

[17] Smaill, B.H. and Hunter, P.J., Structure and function of the diastolic heart, in *Theory of Heart*, L. Glass, P. J. Hunter, and A. D. McCulloch, Eds. Springer-Verlag, New York: 1991, pp. 1–29.

[18] Spotnitz, H.M., Spotnitz, W.D., Cottrell, T.S., et al., Cellular basis for volume related wall thickness changes in the rat left ventricle, *J. Mol. Cell Cardiol.*, 6, 317–331, 1974.

[19] LeGrice, I.J., Smaill, B.H., Chai, L.Z., et al., Laminar structure of the heart: ventricular myocyte arrangement and connective tissue architecture in the dog, *Am. J. Physiol.*, 269, H571–H582, 1995.

[20] Tseng, W.Y., Wedeen, V.J., Reese, T.G., et al., Diffusion tensor MRI of myocardial fibers and sheets: correspondence with visible cut-face texture, *J. Magn. Reson. Imaging*, 17, 31–42, 2003.

[21] Legrice, I.J., Hunter, P.J., and Smaill, B.H., Laminar structure of the heart: a mathematical model, *Am. J. Physiol.*, 272, H2466–H2476, 1997.

[22] Waldman, L.K., Fung, Y.C., and Covell, J.W., Transmural myocardial deformation in the canine left ventricle: normal *in vivo* three-dimensional finite strains, *Circ. Res.*, 57, 152–163, 1985.

[23] LeGrice, I.J., Takayama, Y., and Covell, J.W., Transverse shear along myocardial cleavage planes provides a mechanism for normal systolic wall thickening, *Circ. Res.*, 77, 182–193, 1995.

[24] Arts, T., Costa, K.D., Covell, J.W. et al., Relating myocardial laminar architecture to shear strain and muscle fiber orientation, *Am. J. Physiol. Heart Circ. Physiol.*, 280, H2222–H2229, 2001.

[25] McLean, M., Ross, M.A., and Prothero, J., Three-dimensional reconstruction of the myofiber pattern in the fetal and neonatal mouse heart, *Anat. Rec.*, 224, 392–406, 1989.

[26] Maron, B.J., Bonow, R.O., Cannon, R.O.D. et al., Hypertrophic cardiomyopathy. Interrelations of clinical manifestations, pathophysiology, and therapy (1), *N. Engl. J. Med.*, 316, 780–789, 1987.

[27] Weber, K.T., Cardiac interstitium in health and disease: the fibrillar collagen network, *J. Am. Coll. Cardiol.*, 13, 1637–165, 1989.

[28] Robinson, T.F., Cohen-Gould, L., and Factor, S.M., Skeletal framework of mammalian heart muscle: arrangement of inter- and pericellular connective tissue structures, *Lab. Invest.*, 49, 482–498, 1983.

[29] Caulfield, J.B. and Borg, T.K., The collagen network of the heart, *Lab. Invest.*, 40, 364–371, 1979.

[30] Robinson, T.F., Geraci, M.A., Sonnenblick, E.H. et al., Coiled perimysial fibers of papillary muscle in rat heart: morphology, distribution, and changes in configuration, *Circ. Res.*, 63, 577–592, 1988.

[31] MacKenna, D.A., Omens, J.H., and Covell, J.W., Left ventricular perimysial collagen fibers uncoil rather than stretch during diastolic filling, *Basic Res. Cardiol.*, 91, 111–22, 1996.

[32] MacKenna, D.A., Vaplon, S.M., and McCulloch, A.D., Microstructural model of perimysial collagen fibers for resting myocardial mechanics during ventricular filling, *Am. J. Physiol.*, 273, H1576–H1586, 1997.

[33] MacKenna, D.A. and McCulloch, A.D., Contribution of the collagen extracellular matrix to ventricular mechanics, in *Systolic and Diastolic Function of the Heart*, N.B. Ingels, G.T. Daughters, J. Baan, J.W. Covell, R.S. Reneman, and F.C.-P. Yin, Eds. IOS Press, Amsterdam: 1996, pp. 35–46.

[34] Herrmann, K.L., McCulloch, A.D., and Omens, J.H., Glycated collagen cross-linking alters cardiac mechanics in volume-overload hypertrophy, *Am. J. Physiol. Heart Circ. Physiol.*, 284, H1277–H1284, 2003.

[35] Sonnenblick, E.H., Napolitano, L.M., Daggett, W.M. et al., An intrinsic neuromuscular basis for mitral valve motion in the dog, *Circ. Res.*, 21, 9–15, 1967.

[36] Yellin, E.L., Hori, M., Yoran, C. et al., Left ventricular relaxation in the filling and nonfilling intact canine heart, *Am. J. Physiol.*, 250, H620–H629, 1986.

[37] Janicki, J.S. and Weber, K.T., The pericardium and ventricular interaction, distensibility and function, *Am. J. Physiol.*, 238, H494–H503, 1980.

[38] Brutsaert, D.L. and Sys, S.U., Relaxation and diastole of the heart, *Physiol. Rev.*, 69, 1228, 1989.

[39] Sagawa, K., Maughan, L., Suga, H. et al., *Cardiac Contraction and the Pressure–Volume Relationship*. Oxford University Press, 1988.

[40] Hunter, W.C., End-systolic pressure as a balance between opposing effects of ejection, *Circ. Res.*, 64, 265–275, 1989.

[41] Patterson, S.W. and Starling, E.H., On the mechanical factors which determine the output of the ventricles, *J. Physiol.*, 48, 357–379, 1914.

[42] Suga, H., Hayashi, T., and Shirahata, M., Ventricular systolic pressure–volume area as predictor of cardiac oxygen consumption, *Am. J. Physiol.*, 240, H39–H44, 1981.

[43] Suga, H. and Goto, Y., Cardiac oxygen costs of contractility (Emax) and mechanical energy (PVA): new key concepts in cardiac energetics, in *Recent Progress in Failing Heart Syndrome*, S. Sasayama and H. Suga, Eds. Springer-Verlag, Tokyo: 1991, pp. 61–115.

[44] Suga, H., Goto, Y., Kawaguchi, O. et al., Ventricular perspective on efficiency, *Basic Res. Cardiol.*, 88 (Suppl 2), 43–65, 1993.

[45] Suga, H., Ventricular energetics, *Physiol. Rev.*, 70, 247–277, 1990.

[46] Suga, H., Goto, Y., Yasumura, Y. et al., O2 consumption of dog heart under decreased coronary perfusion and propranolol, *Am. J. Physiol.*, 254, H292–H303, 1988.

[47] Zhao, D.D., Namba, T., Araki, J. et al., Nipradilol depresses cardiac contractility and O2 consumption without decreasing coronary resistance in dogs, *Acta. Med. Okayama.*, 47, 29–33, 1993.

[48] Namba, T., Takaki, M., Araki, J. et al., Energetics of the negative and positive inotropism of pentobarbitone sodium in the canine left ventricle, *Cardiovascular. Res.*, 28, 557–564, 1994.

[49] Ohgoshi, Y., Goto, Y., Futaki, S. et al., Increased oxygen cost of contractility in stunned myocardium of dog, *Circulat. Res.*, 69, 975–988, 1991.

[50] Burkhoff, D., Schnellbacher, M., Stennett, R.A. et al., Explaining load-dependent ventricular performance and energetics based on a model of E-C coupling, in *Cardiac Energetics: from Emax*

to Pressure–Volume Area, M.M. LeWinter, H. Suga, and M.W. Watkins, Eds. Kluwer Academic Publishers, Boston: 1995.

[51] ter Keurs, H.E. and de Tombe, P.P., Determinants of velocity of sarcomere shortening in mammalian myocardium, *Adv. Exp. Med. Biol.*, 332, 649–664; discussion 664–665, 1993.

[52] Guccione, J.M. and McCulloch, A.D., Mechanics of active contraction in cardiac muscle: part I — constitutive relations for fiber stress that describe deactivation, *J. Biomech. Eng.*, 115, 72–81, 1993.

[53] Taylor, T.W., Goto, Y., and Suga, H., Variable cross-bridge cycling-ATP coupling accounts for cardiac mechanoenergetics, *Am. J. Physiol.*, 264, H994–H1004, 1993.

[54] Goto, Y., Futaki, S., Kawaguchi, O. et al., Coupling between regional myocardial oxygen consumption and contraction under altered preload and afterload, *J. Am. Coll. Cardiol.*, 21, 1522–1531, 1993.

[55] Sugawara, M., Kondoh, Y., and Nakano, K., Normalization of Emax and PVA, in *Cardiac Energetics: From Emax to Pressure–Volume Area*, M.M. LeWinter, H. Suga, and M.W. Watkins, Eds. Kluwer Academic Publishers, Boston: 1995, pp. 65–78.

[56] Delhaas, T., Arts, T., Prinzen, F.W. et al., Regional fibre stress–fibre strain area as an estimate of regional blood flow and oxygen demand in the canine heart, *J. Physiol. (Lond.)*, 477, 481–496, 1994.

[57] Vornanen, M., Maximum heart rate of sorcine shrews: correlation with contractile properties and myosin composition, *Am. J. Physiol.*, 31, R842–R851, 1992.

[58] Holt, J.P., Rhode, E.A., Peoples, S.A. et al., Left ventricular function in mammals of greatly different size, *Circ. Res.*, 10, 798–806, 1962.

[59] Loiselle, D.S. and Gibbs, C.L., Species differences in cardiac energetics, *Am. J. Physiol.*, 237, 1979.

[60] Gilbert, J.C. and Glantz, S.A., Determinants of left ventricular filling and of the diastolic pressure–volume relation, *Circ. Res.*, 64, 827–852, 1989.

[61] Gaasch, W.H. and LeWinter, M.M., *Left Ventricular Diastolic Dysfunction and Heart Failure.* Lea & Febiger, Philadelphia, PA: 1994.

[62] Glantz, S.A., Misbach, G.A., Moores, W.Y. et al., The pericardium substantially affects the left ventricular diastolic pressure–volume relationship in the dog, *Circ. Res.*, 42, 433–441, 1978.

[63] Glantz, S.A. and Parmley, W.W., Factors which affect the diastolic pressure–volume curve, *Circ. Res.*, 42, 171–180, 1978.

[64] Slinker, B.K. and Glantz, S.A., End-systolic and end-diastolic ventricular interaction, *Am. J. Physiol.*, 251, H1062–H1075, 1986.

[65] Mirsky, I. and Rankin, J.S., The effects of geometry, elasticity, and external pressures on the diastolic pressure–volume and stiffness–stress relations: How important is the pericardium? *Circ. Res.*, 44, 601–611, 1979.

[66] Lee, M.C., Fung, Y.C., Shabetai, R. et al., Biaxial mechanical properties of human pericardium and canine comparisons, *Am. J. Physiol.*, 253, H75–H82, 1987.

[67] Maruyama, Y., Ashikawa, K., Isoyama, S. et al., Mechanical interactions between the four heart chambers with and without the pericardium in canine hearts, *Circ. Res.*, 50, 86–100, 1982.

[68] May-Newman, K., Omens, J.H., Pavelec, R.S. et al., Three-dimensional transmural mechanical interaction between the coronary vasculature and passive myocardium in the dog, *Circ. Res.*, 74, 1166–1178, 1994.

[69] Salisbury, P.F., Cross, C.E., and Rieben, P.A., Influence of coronary artery pressure upon myocardial elasticity, *Circ. Res.*, 8, 794–800, 1960.

[70] Bers, D.M., *Excitation-Contraction Coupling and Cardiac Contractile Force.* Kluwer, 1991.

[71] ter Keurs, H.E.D.J., Rijnsburger, W.H., van Heuningen, R. et al., Tension development and sarcomere length in rat cardiac trabeculae: evidence of length-dependent activation, *Circ. Res.*, 46, 703–713, 1980.

[72] Rüegg, J.C., *Calcium in Muscle Activation: A Comparative Approach*, 2nd ed. Springer-Verlag, 1988.

[73] Tözeren, A., Continuum rheology of muscle contraction and its application to cardiac contractility, *Biophys. J.*, 47, 303–309, 1985.

[74] Hunter, P.J., McCulloch, A.D., and ter Keurs, H.E., Modelling the mechanical properties of cardiac muscle, *Prog. Biophys. Mol. Biol.*, 69, 289–331, 1998.

[75] Backx, P.H., Gao, W.D., Azan-Backx, M.D. et al., The relationship between contractile force and intracellular $[Ca^{2+}]$ in intact rat cardiac trabeculae, *J. Gen. Physiol.*, 105, 1–19, 1995.

[76] Kentish, J.C., Ter Keurs, H.E.D.J., Ricciari, L. et al., Comparisons between the sarcomere length–force relations of intact and skinned trabeculae from rat right ventricle, *Circ. Res.*, 58, 755–768, 1986.

[77] Yue, D.T., Marban, E., and Wier, W.G., Relationship between force and intracellular $[Ca^{2+}]$ in tetanized mammalian heart muscle, *J. Gen. Physiol.*, 87, 223–242, 1986.

[78] Gao, W.D., Backx, P.H., Azan-Backx, M. et al., Myofilament Ca^{2+} sensitivity in intact versus skinned rat ventricular muscle, *Circ. Res.*, 74, 408–415, 1994.

[79] de Tombe, P.P. and ter Keurs, H.E., An internal viscous element limits unloaded velocity of sarcomere shortening in rat myocardium, *J. Physiol. (Lond.)*, 454, 619–642, 1992.

[80] ter Keurs, H.E.D.J., Rijnsburger, W.H., and van Heuningen, R., Restoring forces and relaxation of rat cardiac muscle, *Eur. Heart J.*, 1, 67–80, 1980.

[81] Arts, T., Reneman, R.S., and Veenstra, P.C., A model of the mechanics of the left ventricle, *Ann. Biomed. Eng.*, 7, 299–318, 1979.

[82] Chadwick, R.S., Mechanics of the left ventricle, *Biophys. J.*, 39, 279–288, 1982.

[83] Nevo, E. and Lanir, Y., Structural finite deformation model of the left ventricle during diastole and systole, *J. Biomech. Eng.*, 111, 342–349, 1989.

[84] Arts, T., Veenstra, P.C., and Reneman, R.S., Epicardial deformation and left ventricular wall mechanics during ejection in the dog, *Am. J. Physiol.*, 243, H379–H390, 1982.

[85] Panerai, R.B., A model of cardiac muscle mechanics and energetics, *J. Biomech.*, 13, 929–940, 1980.

[86] Landesberg, A., Markhasin, V.S., Beyar, R. et al., Effect of cellular inhomogeneity on cardiac tissue mechanics based on intracellular control mechanisms, *Am. J. Physiol.*, 270, H1101–H1114, 1996.

[87] Landesberg, A. and Sideman, S., Coupling calcium binding to troponin C and cross-bridge cycling in skinned cardiac cells, *Am. J. Physiol.*, 266, H1260–H1271, 1994.

[88] Ma, S.P. and Zahalak, G.I., A distribution-moment model of energetics in skeletal muscle [see comments], *J. Biomech.*, 24, 21–35, 1991.

[89] Lin, D.H.S. and Yin, F.C.P., A multiaxial constitutive law for mammalian left ventricular myocardium in steady-state barium contracture or tetanus, *J. Biomech. Eng.*, 120, 504–517, 1998.

[90] Schoenberg, M., Geometrical factors influencing muscle force development. I. The effect of filament spacing upon axial forces, *Biophys. J.*, 30, 51–67, 1980.

[91] Zahalak, G.I., Non-axial muscle stress and stiffness, *J. Theor. Biol.*, 182, 59–84, 1996.

[92] Schoenberg, M., Geometrical factors influencing muscle force development. II. Radial forces, *Biophys. J.*, 30, 69–77, 1980.

[93] Fung, Y.C., *Biomechanics: Mechanical Properties of Living Tissues*, 2nd ed. Springer-Verlag, Inc., 1993.

[94] Pinto, J.G. and Patitucci, P.J., Creep in cardiac muscle, *Am. J. Physiol.*, 232, H553–H563, 1977.

[95] Pinto, J.G. and Patitucci, P.J., Visco-elasticity of passive cardiac muscle, *J. Biomech. Eng.*, 102, 57–61, 1980.

[96] Emery, J.L., Omens, J.H., and McCulloch, A.D., Strain softening in rat left ventricular myocardium, *J. Biomech. Eng.*, 119, 6–12, 1997.

[97] Emery, J.L., Omens, J.H., and McCulloch, A.D., Biaxial mechanics of the passively overstretched left ventricle, *Am. J. Physiol.*, 272, H2299–H2305, 1997.

[98] Mullins, L., Effect of stretching on the properties of rubber, *J. Rubber Res.*, 16, 275–289, 1947.

[99] Halperin, H.R., Chew, P.H., Weisfeldt, M.L. et al., Transverse stiffness: a method for estimation of myocardial wall stress, *Circ. Res.*, 61, 695–703, 1987.

[100] Humphrey, J.D., Strumpf, R.K., and Yin, F.C.P., Biaxial mechanical behavior of excised ventricular epicardium, *Am. J. Physiol.*, 259, H101–H108, 1990.

[101] Demer, L.L. and Yin, F.C.P., Passive biaxial mechanical properties of isolated canine myocardium, *J. Physiol.*, 339, 615–630, 1983.

[102] Yin, F.C.P., Strumpf, R.K., Chew, P.H. et al., Quantification of the mechanical properties of noncontracting canine myocardium under simultaneous biaxial loading, *J. Biomech.*, 20, 577–589, 1987.

[103] Novak, V.P., Yin, F.C.P., and Humphrey, J.D., Regional mechanical properties of passive myocardium, *J. Biomech.*, 27, 403–412, 1994.

[104] Omens, J.H., MacKenna, D.A., and McCulloch, A.D., Measurement of strain and analysis of stress in resting rat left ventricular myocardium, *J. Biomech.*, 26, 665–676, 1993.

[105] Glass, L., Hunter, P., and McCulloch, A.D., Theory of heart: biomechanics, biophysics and nonlinear dynamics of cardiac function, in *Institute for Nonlinear Science*, H. Abarbanel, Ed. Springer-Verlag, New York: 1991.

[106] Humphrey, J.D. and Yin, F.C.P., A new constitutive formulation for characterizing the mechanical behavior of soft tissues, *Biophys. J.*, 52, 563–570, 1987.

[107] Lin, I.-E. and Taber, L.A., Mechanical effects of looping in the embryonic chick heart, *J. Biomech.*, 27, 311–321, 1994.

[108] Guccione, J.M., McCulloch, A.D., and Waldman, L.K., Passive material properties of intact ventricular myocardium determined from a cylindrical model, *J. Biomech. Eng.*, 113, 42–55, 1991.

[109] Omens, J.H., MacKenna, D.A., and McCulloch, A.D., Measurement of two-dimensional strain and analysis of stress in the arrested rat left ventricle, *Adv. Bioeng.*, BED-20, 635–638, 1991.

[110] Humphrey, J.D., Strumpf, R.K., and Yin, F.C.P., Determination of a constitutive relation for passive myocardium: I. A new functional form, *J. Biomech. Eng.*, 112, 333–339, 1990.

[111] Gupta, K.B., Ratcliff, M.B., Fallert, M.A. et al., Changes in passive mechanical stiffness of myocardial tissue with aneurysm formation, *Circulation*, 89, 2315–2326, 1994.

[112] Omens, J.H. and Fung, Y.C., Residual strain in rat left ventricle, *Circ. Res.*, 66, 37–45, 1990.

[113] Rodriguez, E.K., Omens, J.H., Waldman, L.K. et al., Effect of residual stress on transmural sarcomere length distribution in rat left ventricle, *Am. J. Physiol.*, 264, H1048–H1056, 1993.

[114] Costa, K., May-Newman, K., Farr, D. et al., Three-dimensional residual strain in canine mid-anterior left ventricle, *Am. J. Physiol.*, 273, H1968–H1976, 1997.

[115] Skalak, R., Dasgupta, G., Moss, M. et al., Analytical description of growth, *J. Theor. Biol.*, 94, 555–577, 1982.

[116] Rodriguez, E.K., Hoger, A., and McCulloch, A.D., Stress-dependent finite growth in soft elastic tissues, *J. Biomech.*, 27, 455–467, 1994.

[117] Feigl, E.O., Simon, G.A., and Fry, D.L., Auxotonic and isometric cardiac force transducers, *J. Appl. Physiol.*, 23, 597–600, 1967.

[118] Huisman, R.M., Elzinga, G., Westerhof, N. et al., Measurement of left ventricular wall stress, *Cardiovasc. Res.*, 14, 142–153, 1980.

[119] Yin, F.C.P., Ventricular wall stress, *Circ. Res.*, 49, 829–842, 1981.

[120] Yin, F.C.P., Applications of the finite-element method to ventricular mechanics, *CRC Crit. Rev. Biomed. Eng.*, 12, 311–342, 1985.

[121] Villarreal, F.J., Waldman, L.K., and Lew, W.Y.W., Technique for measuring regional two-dimensional finite strains in canine left ventricle, *Circ. Res.*, 62, 711–721, 1988.

[122] Ingels, N.B., Jr., Daughters, G.T., II, Stinson, E.B. et al., Measurement of midwall myocardial dynamics in intact man by radiography of surgically implanted markers, *Circulation*, 52, 859–867, 1975.

[123] Hunter, W.C. and Zerhouni, E.A., Imaging distinct points in left ventricular myocardium to study regional wall deformation, in *Innovations in Diagnostic Radiology*, J.H. Anderson, Ed. Springer-Verlag, New York: 1989, pp. 169–190.

[124] Meier, G.D., Bove, A.A., Santamore, W.P. et al., Contractile function in canine right ventricle, *Am. J. Physiol.*, 239, H794–H804, 1980.

[125] Meier, G.D., Ziskin, M.C., Santamore, W.P. et al., Kinematics of the beating heart, *IEEE Trans. Biomed. Eng.*, 27, 319–329, 1980.

[126] McCulloch, A.D. and Omens, J.H., Non-homogeneous analysis of three-dimensional transmural finite deformations in canine ventricular myocardium, *J. Biomech.*, 24, 539–548, 1991.

[127] Leclercq, C., Faris, O., Tunin, R. et al., Systolic improvement and mechanical resynchronization does not require electrical synchrony in the dilated failing heart with left bundle-branch block, *Circulation*, 106, 1760–1763, 2002.

[128] Usyk, T.P. and McCulloch, A.D., Electromechanical model of cardiac resynchronization in the dilated failing heart with left bundle branch block, *J. Electrocardiol.*, 36, 57–61, 2003.

[129] Ross, J., Jr., Sonnenblick, E.H., Covell, J.W. et al., The architecture of the heart in systole and diastole: technique of rapid fixation and analysis of left ventricular geometry, *Circ. Res.*, 21, 409–421, 1967.

[130] Grossman, W., Cardiac hypertrophy: useful adaptation or pathologic process? *Am. J. Med.*, 69, 576–583, 1980.

[131] Grossman, W., Jones, D., and McLaurin, L.P., Wall stress and patterns of hypertrophy in the human left ventricle, *J. Clin. Invest.*, 56, 56–64, 1975.

[132] Medugorac, I., Myocardial collagen in different forms of hypertrophy in the rat, *Res. Exp. Med. (Berl.)*, 177, 201–211, 1980.

[133] Weber, K.T., Janicki, J.S., Shroff, S.G. et al., Collagen remodeling of the pressure-overloaded, hypertrophied nonhuman primate myocardium, *Circ. Res.*, 62, 757–65, 1988.

[134] Jalil, J.E., Doering, C.W., Janicki, J.S. et al., Structural vs. contractile protein remodeling and myocardial stiffness in hypertrophied rat left ventricle, *J. Mol. Cell. Cardiol.*, 20, 1179–87, 1988.

[135] Mukherjee, D. and Sen, S., Collagen phenotypes during development and regression of myocardial hypertrophy in spontaneously hypertensive rats, *Circ. Res.*, 67, 1474–1480, 1990.

[136] Harper, J., Harper, E., and Covell, J.W., Collagen characterization in volume-overload- and pressure-overload-induced cardiac hypertrophy in minipigs, *Am. J. Physiol.*, 265, H434–H438, 1993.

[137] Omens, J.H., Milkes, D.E., and Covell, J.W., Effects of pressure overload on the passive mechanics of the rat left ventricle, *Ann. Biomed. Eng.*, 23, 152–163, 1995.

[138] Contard, F., Koteliansky, V., Marotte, F. et al., Specific alterations in the distribution of extracellular matrix components within rat myocardium during the development of pressure overload, *Lab. Invest.*, 64, 65–75, 1991.

[139] Silver, M.A., Pick, R., Brilla, C.G. et al., Reactive and reparative fibrillar collagen remodelling in the hypertrophied rat left ventricle: two experimental models of myocardial fibrosis, *Cardiovasc. Res.*, 24, 741–747, 1990.

[140] Michel, J.B., Salzmann, J.L., Ossondo Nlom, M. et al., Morphometric analysis of collagen network and plasma perfused capillary bed in the myocardium of rats during evolution of cardiac hypertrophy, *Basic Res. Cardiol.*, 81, 142–154, 1986.

[141] Iimoto, D.S., Covell, J.W., and Harper, E., Increase in crosslinking of type I and type III collagens associated with volume overload hypertropy, *Circ. Res.*, 63, 399–408, 1988.

[142] Weber, K.T., Pick, R., Silver, M.A. et al., Fibrillar collagen and remodeling of dilated canine left ventricle, *Circulation*, 82, 1387–1401, 1990.

[143] Corin, W.J., Murakami, T., Monrad, E.S. et al., Left ventricular passive diastolic properties in chronic mitral regurgitation, *Circulation*, 83, 797–807, 1991.

[144] Whittaker, P., Boughner, D.R., Kloner, R.A. et al., Stunned myocardium and myocardial collagen damage: differential effects of single and repeated occlusions, *Am. Heart J.*, 121, 434–441, 1991.

[145] Zhao, M., Zhang, H., Robinson, T.F. et al., Profound structural alterations of the extracellular collagen matrix in postischemic dysfunctional ("tunned") but viable myocardium, *J. Am. Coll. Cardiol.*, 10, 1322–1334, 1987.

[146] Forrester, J.S., Diamond, G., Parmley, W.W. et al., Early increase in left ventricular compliance after myocardial infarction, *J. Clin. Invest.*, 51, 598–603, 1972.

[147] Pirzada, F.A., Ekong, E.A., Vokonas, P.S. et al., Experimental myocardial infarction XIII. Sequential changes in left ventricular pressure–length relationships in the acute phase, *Circulation*, 53, 970–975, 1976.

[148] Takahashi, S., Barry, A.C., and Factor, S.M., Collagen degradation in ischaemic rat hearts, *Biochem. J.*, 265, 233–241, 1990.

[149] Charney, R.H., Takahashi, S., Zhao, M. et al., Collagen loss in the stunned myocardium, *Circulation*, 85, 1483–1490, 1992.

[150] Connelly, C.M., Vogel, W.M., Wiegner, A.W. et al., Effects of reperfusion after coronary artery occlusion on post-infarction scar tissue, *Circ. Res.*, 57, 562–577, 1985.

[151] Jugdutt, B.I. and Amy, R.W., Healing after myocardial infarction in the dog: changes in infarct hydroxyproline and topography, *J. Am. Coll. Cardiol.*, 7, 91–102, 1986.

[152] Whittaker, P., Boughner, D.R., and Kloner, R.A., Analysis of healing after myocardial infarction using polarized light microscopy, *Am. J. Pathol.*, 134, 879–893, 1989.

[153] Jensen, L.T., Hørslev-Petersen, K., Toft, P. et al., Serum aminoterminal type III procollagen peptide reflects repair after acute myocardial infarction, *Circulation*, 81, 52–57, 1990.

[154] Pfeffer, J.M., Pfeffer, M.A., Fletcher, P.J. et al., Progressive ventricular remodeling in rat with myocardial infarction, *Am. J. Physiol.*, 260, H1406–H1414, 1991.

[155] Whittaker, P., Boughner, D.R., and Kloner, R.A., Role of collagen in acute myocardial infarct expansion, *Circulation*, 84, 2123–2134, 1991.

[156] Holmes, J.W., Yamashita, H., Waldman, L.K. et al., Scar remodeling and transmural deformation after infarction in the pig, *Circulation*, 90, 411–420, 1994.

[157] Eghbali, M., Robinson, T.F., Seifter, S. et al., Collagen accumulation in heart ventricles as a function of growth and aging, *Cardiovasc. Res.*, 23, 723–729, 1989.

[158] Medugorac, I. and Jacob, R., Characterisation of left ventricular collagen in the rat, *Cardiovasc. Res.*, 17, 15–21, 1983.

[159] Borg, T.K., Ranson, W.F., Moslehy, F.A. et al., Structural basis of ventricular stiffness, *Lab. Invest.*, 44, 49–54, 1981.

[160] Anversa, P., Puntillo, E., Nikitin, P. et al., Effects of age on mechanical and structural properties of myocardium of Fischer 344 rats, *Am. J. Physiol.*, 256, H1440–H1449, 1989.

55

Heart Valve Dynamics

Ajit P. Yoganathan

Jack D. Lemmon

Jeffrey T. Ellis

Georgia Institute of Technology

The heart has four valves that control the direction of blood flow through the heart, permitting forward flow and preventing back flow. On the right side of the heart, the tricuspid and pulmonic valves regulate the flow of blood that is returned from the body to the lungs for oxygenation. The mitral and aortic valves control the flow of oxygenated blood from the left side of the heart to the body. The aortic and pulmonic valves allow blood to be pumped from the ventricles into arteries on the left and right side of the heart, respectively. Similarly, the mitral and tricuspid valves lie between the atria and ventricles of the left and right sides of the heart, respectively. The aortic and pulmonic valves open during systole when the ventricles are contracting, and close during diastole when the ventricles are filling through the open mitral and tricuspid valves. During isovolumic contraction and relaxation, all four valves are closed (Figure 55.1).

When closed, the pulmonic and tricuspid valves must withstand a pressure of approximately 30 mmHg. However, the closing pressures on the left side of the heart are much higher. The aortic valve withstands pressures of approximately 100 mmHg, while the mitral valve closes against pressures up to 150 mmHg. Since diseases of the valves on the left side of the heart are more prevalent, most of this chapter will focus on the aortic and mitral valves. Where pertinent, reference will be made to the pulmonic and tricuspid valves.

55.1 Aortic and Pulmonic Valves

The aortic valve is composed of three semilunar cusps, or leaflets, contained within a connective tissue sleeve. The valve cusps are attached to a fibrous ring embedded in the fibers of the ventricular septum and the anterior leaflet of the mitral valve. Each of the leaflets is lined with endothelial cells and has a dense collagenous core adjacent to the high pressure aortic side. The side adjacent to the aorta is termed the fibrosa and is the major fibrous layer within the belly of the leaflet. The layer covering the ventricular side of the valve is called the ventricularis and is composed of both collagen and elastin. The ventricularis is thinner than the fibrosa and presents a very smooth surface to the flow of blood [Christie, 1990]. The central portion of the valve, called the spongiosa, contains variable loose connective tissue and proteins and is normally not vascularized. The collagen fibers within the fibrosa and ventricularis are unorganized in the unstressed state. When a stress is applied, they become oriented primarily in

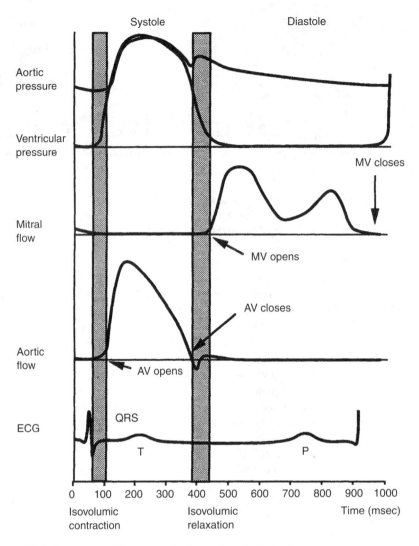

FIGURE 55.1   Typical pressure and flow curves for the aortic and mitral valves.

the circumferential direction with a lower concentration of elastin and collagen in the radial direction [Christie, 1990; Thubrikar, 1990].

The fibrous annular ring of the aortic valve separates the aorta from the left ventricle and superior to this ring is a structure called the sinus of Valsalva, or aortic sinus. The sinus is comprised of three bulges at the root of the aorta, with each bulge aligned with the belly or central part of the specific valve leaflet. Each valve cusp and corresponding sinus is named according to its anatomical location within the aorta. Two of these sinuses give rise to coronary arteries that branch off the aorta, providing blood flow to the heart itself. The right coronary artery is based at the right or right anterior sinus, the left coronary artery exits the left or left posterior sinus, and the third sinus is called the non-coronary or right posterior sinus. Figure 55.2 shows the configuration of the normal aortic sinuses and valve in the closed position. Because the length of the aortic valve cusps is greater than the annular radius, a small overlap of tissue from each leaflet protrudes and forms a coaptation surface within the aorta when the valve is closed [Emery and Arom, 1991]. This overlapped tissue, called the lunula, may help to ensure that the valve is sealed. When the valve is open, the leaflets extend to the upper edge of the sinuses of Valsalva. The anatomy of the pulmonic valve is similar to that of the aortic valve, but the surrounding structure is slightly different.

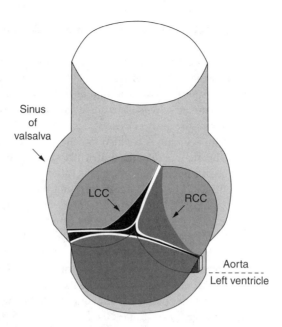

FIGURE 55.2 The aortic sinuses and valve in the closed position. The noncoronary cusp (NCC) is in front. The left and right coronary cusps (LCC and RCC) are positioned as marked. The aorta is above the closed valve in this orientation and the left ventricle is below the dashed line.

The main differences are that the sinuses are smaller in the pulmonary artery and the pulmonic valve annulus is slightly larger than that of the aortic valve.

The dimensions of the aortic and pulmonic valves and their leaflets have been measured in a number of ways. Before noninvasive measurement techniques such as echocardiography became available, valve measurements were recorded from autopsy specimens. An examination of 160 pathologic specimens revealed the aortic valve diameter to be 23.2 ± 3.3 mm, whereas the diameter of the pulmonic valve was measured at 24.3 ± 3.0 mm [Westaby et al., 1984]. However, according to M-mode echocardiographic measurements, the aortic root diameter at end systole was 35 ± 4.2 mm and 33.7 ± 4.4 mm at the end of diastole [Gramiak and Shah, 1970]. The differences in these measurements reflect the fact that the autopsy measurements were not performed under physiologic pressure conditions and that intrinsic differences in the measurement techniques exist. On average, pulmonic leaflets are thinner than aortic leaflets: 0.49 vs. 0.67 mm [David et al., 1994], although the leaflets of the aortic valve show variable dimensions depending on the respective leaflet. For example, the posterior leaflet tends to be thicker, have a larger surface area, and weigh more than the right or left leaflet [Silver and Roberts, 1985; Sahasakul et al., 1988], and the average width of the right aortic leaflet is greater than that of the other two [Vollebergh and Becker, 1977].

55.1.1 Mechanical Properties

Due to the location and critical function of the aortic valve, it is difficult to obtain measurements of its mechanical properties *in vivo*; however, reports are available from a small number of animal studies. This section will reference the *in vivo* data whenever possible and defer to the *in vitro* data when necessary. Since little mathematical modeling of the aortic valve's material properties has been reported, it will be sufficient to describe the known mechanical properties of the valve. Like most biological tissues, the aortic valve is anisotropic, inhomogeneous, and viscoelastic. The collagen fibers within each valve cusp are aligned along the circumferential direction. Vesely and Noseworthy [1992] found that both the ventricularis and fibrosa were stiffer in the circumferential direction than in the radial direction. However, the ventricularis was more extensible radially than circumferentially, while the fibrosa had uniform extensibility in both directions.

There are also elastin fibers, at a lesser concentration, that are oriented orthogonal to the collagen. It is this fiber structure that accounts for the anisotropic properties of the valve. The variation in thickness and composition across the leaflets is responsible for their inhomogeneous material properties. Although the aortic valve leaflet as a whole is asymmetric in its distensibility, the basal region tends to be relatively isotropic while the central region shows the greatest degree of anisotropy [Lo and Vesely, 1995]. The role and morphology of elastin and how elastin is coupled to collagen remain points of investigation. Scott and Vesely [1996] have shown that the elastin in the ventricularis consists of continuous amorphous sheets or compact meshes, while elastin in the fibrosa consists of complex arrays of large tubes that extend circumferentially across the leaflet. These tubes may surround the large circumferential collagen bundles in the fibrosa. Mechanical testing of elastin structures from the fibrosa and ventricularis separately have shown that the purpose of elastin in the aortic valve leaflet is to maintain a specific collagen fiber configuration and return the fibers to that state during cyclic loading [Vesely, 1998]. The valve's viscoelastic properties are actually dominated by the elastic component (over the range of *in vitro* testing) so that the viscous effects, which are largely responsible for energy losses, are small [Thubrikar, 1990]. In addition to the collagen and elastin, clusters of lipids have been observed in the central spongiosa of porcine aortic valves. Vesely et al. [1994] have shown that the lipids tend to be concentrated at the base of the valve leaflets, while the coaptation regions and free edges of the leaflets tend to be devoid of these lipids. In addition, the spatial distribution of the lipids within the spongiosal layer of the aortic leaflets corresponded to areas in which calcification is commonly observed on bioprosthetic valves suggesting that these lipid clusters may be potential nucleation sites for calcification. In contrast, pulmonic leaflets showed a substantially lower incidence of lipids [Dunmore-Buyze et al., 1995]. The aortic valve leaflets have also been shown to be slightly stiffer than pulmonary valve leaflets, although the extensibilities and relaxation rates of the two tissues are similar [Leeson-Dietrich et al., 1995].

Using marker fluoroscopy, in which the aortic valve leaflets were surgically tagged with radio-opaque markers and imaged with high speed x-rays, the leaflets have been shown to change length during the cardiac cycle [Thubrikar, 1990]. The cusps are longer during diastole than systole in both the radial and circumferential direction. The variation in length is greatest in the radial direction, approximately 20%, while the strain in the circumferential direction is about 10% of the normal systolic length [Lo and Vesely, 1995]. The difference in strain is due to the presence of the compliant elastin fibers aligned in this radial direction. The length change in both directions results in an increased valve surface area during diastole. During systole, the shortening of the valve leaflets helps to reduce obstruction of the aorta during the systolic ejection of blood. It should be noted that this change in area is by no means an active mechanism within the aortic valve; the valve simply reacts to the stresses it encounters in a passive manner.

In addition to this change in surface area, the aortic valve leaflets also undergo bending in the circumferential direction during the cardiac cycle. In diastole when the valve is closed, each leaflet is convex toward the ventricular side. During systole when the valve is open, the curvature.changes and each leaflet is concave toward the ventricle. This bending is localized on the valve cusp near the wall of the aorta. This location is often thicker than the rest of the leaflet. The total diastolic stress in a valve leaflet has been estimated at 2.5×10^6 dyn/cm^2 for a strain of 15% [Thubrikar, 1990]. The stress in the circumferential direction was found to be the primary load bearing element in the aortic valve. Due to the collagen fibers oriented circumferentially, the valve is relatively stiff in this direction. The strain that does occur circumferentially is primarily due to scissoring of the fibrous matrix and straightening of collagen fibers that are kinked or crimped in the presence of no external stress. However, in the radial direction, because elastin is the primary element, the valve can undergo a great deal of strain, ranging from 20 to 60% in tissue specimens [Christie, 1990; Lo and Vesely, 1995]. In the closed position, the radial stress levels are actually small compared to those in the circumferential direction. This demonstrates the importance of the lunula in ensuring that the valve seals tightly to prevent leakage. Because of their anatomical location, the lunula cause these high circumferential stress levels by enabling the aortic pressure to pull each leaflet in the circumferential direction towards the other leaflets.

The composition, properties, and dimensions of the aortic valve change with age and in the presence of certain diseases. The valve leaflets become thicker, the lunula become fenestrated, or mesh-like, and in later stages of disease the central portion of the valve may become calcified [Davies, 1980]. This thickening of the valve typically occurs on the ventricular side of the valve, in the region where the tips of the leaflets come together. Another site of calcification and fibrosis is the point of maximum cusp flexion and is thought to be a response to fatigue in the normal valve tissue.

55.1.2 · Valve Dynamics

The aortic valve opens during systole when the ventricle is contracting and then closes during diastole as the ventricle relaxes and fills from the atrium. Systole lasts about one third of the cardiac cycle and begins when the aortic valve opens, which typically takes only 20 to 30 msec [Bellhouse, 1969]. Blood rapidly accelerates through the valve and reaches a peak velocity after the leaflets have opened to their full extent and start to close again. Peak velocity is reached during the first third of systole and the flow begins to decelerate rapidly after the peak is reached, albeit not as fast as its initial acceleration. The adverse pressure gradient that is developed affects the low momentum fluid near the wall of the aorta more than that at the center; this causes reverse flow in the sinus region [Reul and Talukdar, 1979]. Figure 55.2 illustrates the pressure and flow relations across the aortic valve during the cardiac cycle. During systole, the pressure difference required to drive the blood through the aortic valve is on the order of a few millimeters of mercury; however, the diastolic pressure difference reaches 80 mmHg in normal individuals. The valve closes near the end of the deceleration phase of systole with very little reverse flow through the valve.

During the cardiac cycle the heart undergoes translation and rotation due to its own contraction pattern. As a result, the base of the aortic valve varies in size and also translates, mainly along the axis of the aorta. Using marker fluoroscopy to study the base of the aortic valve in dogs, Thubrikar et al. [1993] found that the base perimeter is at its largest at end diastole and decreases in size during systole; it then reaches a minimum at the end of systole and increases again during diastole. The range of this perimeter variation during the cardiac cycle was 22% for an aortic pressure variation of 120/80 mmHg. The valve annulus also undergoes translation, primarily parallel to the aortic axis. The aortic annulus moves downward toward the ventricle during systole and then recoils back toward the aorta as the ventricle fills during diastole. The annulus also experiences a slight side-to-side translation with its magnitude approximately one half the displacement along the aortic axis.

During systole, vortices develop in all three sinuses behind the leaflets of the aortic valve. The function of these vortices was first described by Leonardo da Vinci in 1513, and they have been researched extensively in this century primarily through the use of *in vitro* models [Bellhouse, 1969; Reul and Talukdar, 1979]. It has been hypothesized that the vortices help to close the aortic valve so that blood is prevented from returning to the ventricle during the closing process. These vortices create a transverse pressure difference that pushes the leaflets toward the center of the aorta and each other at the end of systole, thus minimizing any possible closing volume. However, as shown *in vitro* by Reul and Talukdar [1979], the axial pressure difference alone is enough to close the valve. Without the vortices in the sinuses, the valve still closes but its closure is not as quick as when the vortices are present. The adverse axial pressure difference within the aorta causes the low inertia flow within the developing boundary layer along the aortic wall to decelerate first and to reverse direction. This action forces the belly of the leaflets away from the aortic wall and toward the closed position. When this force is coupled with the vortices that push the leaflet tips toward the closed position, a very efficient and fast closure is obtained. Closing volumes have been estimated to be less than 5% of the forward flow [Bellhouse and Bellhouse, 1969].

The parameters that describe the normal blood flow through the aortic valve are the velocity profile, time course of the blood velocity or flow, and magnitude of the peak velocity. These are determined in part by the pressure difference between the ventricle and aorta and by the geometry of the aortic valve complex. As seen in Figure 55.3, the velocity profile at the level of the aortic valve annulus is relatively flat. However there is usually a slight skew toward the septal wall (less than 10% of the center-line velocity) which is caused by the orientation of the aortic valve relative to the long axis of the left ventricle. This skew

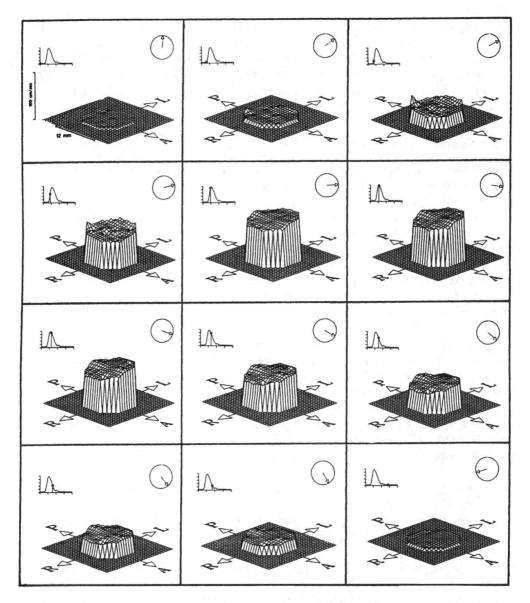

FIGURE 55.3 Velocity profiles measured 2 cm downstream of the aortic valve with hot film anemometry in dogs [Paulsen and Hasenkam, 1983]. The timing of the measurements during the cardiac cycle is shown by the marker on the aortic flow curve.

in the velocity profile has been shown by many experimental techniques, including hot film anemometry, Doppler ultrasound, and MRI [Paulsen and Hasenkam, 1983; Rossvol et al., 1991; Kilner et al., 1993]. In healthy individuals, blood flows through the aortic valve at the beginning of systole and then rapidly accelerates to its peak value of 1.35 ± 0.35 m/sec; for children this value is slightly higher at 1.5 ± 0.3 m/sec [Hatle and Angelson, 1985]. At the end of systole there is a very short period of reverse flow that can be measured with Doppler ultrasound. This reverse flow is probably either a small closing volume or the velocity of the valve leaflets as they move toward their closed position. The flow patterns just downstream of the aortic valve are of particular interest because of their complexity and relation to arterial disease. Highly skewed velocity profiles and corresponding helical flow patterns have been observed in the human aortic arch using magnetic resonance phase velocity mapping [Kilner et al., 1993].

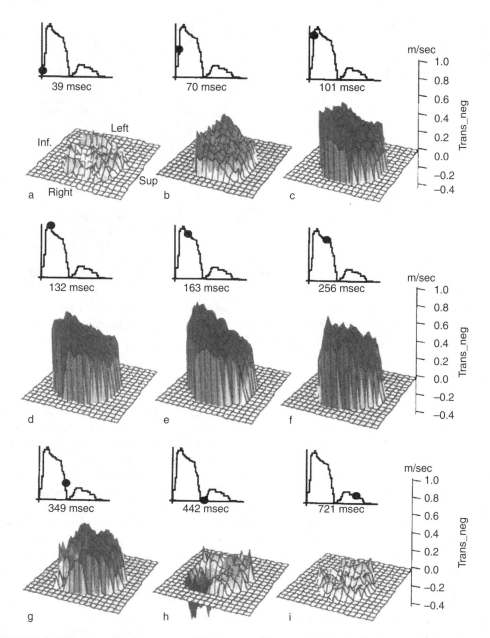

FIGURE 55.4 Velocity profiles downstream of the human pulmonary valve obtained with magnetic resonance phase velocity mapping [Sloth, 1994]. Again the timing of the measurements is shown by the market on the flow curve.

The pulmonic valve flow behaves similarly to that of the aortic valve, but the magnitude of the velocity is not as great. Typical peak velocities for healthy adults are 0.75 ± 0.15 m/sec; again these values are slightly higher for children at 0.9 ± 0.2 m/sec [Weyman, 1994]. As seen in Figure 55.4 a rotation of the peak velocity can be observed in the pulmonary artery velocity profile. During acceleration, the peak velocity is observed inferiorly with the peak rotating counterclockwise throughout the remainder of the ejection phase [Sloth et al., 1994]. The mean spatial profile is relatively flat, however, although there is a region of reverse flow that occurs in late systole which may be representative of flow separation. Typically, there is only a slight skew to the profile. The peak velocity is generally within 20% of the spatial mean throughout the cardiac cycle. Secondary flow patterns can also be observed in the pulmonary artery and

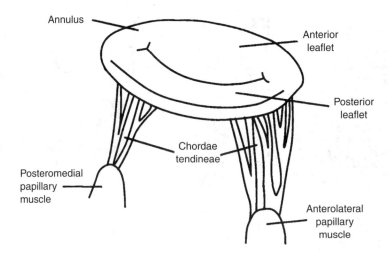

FIGURE 55.5 Schematic of the mitral valve showing the valve leaflets, papillary muscles, and chordae tendineae.

its bifurcation. *In vitro* laser Doppler anemometry experiments have shown that these flow patterns are dependent on the valve geometry and thus can be used to evaluate function and fitness of the heart valve and [Sung and Yoganathan, 1990].

55.2 Mitral and Tricuspid Valves

The mitral (Figure 55.5) and tricuspid valves are similar in structure with both valves composed of four primary elements (1) the valve annulus, (2) the valve leaflets, (3) the papillary muscles, and (4) the chordae tendineae. The base of the mitral leaflets form the mitral annulus, which attaches to the atrial and ventricular walls, and aortic root. At the free edge of the leaflets, the chordae tendinae insert at multiple locations and extend to the tips of the papillary muscles. This arrangement provides continuity between the valve and ventricular wall to enhance valvular function. The valvular apparatus, or complex, requires an intricate interplay between all components throughout the cardiac cycle.

The mitral annulus is an elliptical ring composed of dense collagenous tissue surrounded by muscle. It goes through dynamic changes during the cardiac cycle by not only changing in size, but also by moving three-dimensionally. The circumference of the mitral annulus ranges from 8 to 12 cm during diastole. Recent studies involving the measurement of annular shape have also shown that the mitral annulus is not planar, but instead has a three-dimensional form. The annulus actually forms a saddle, or ski-slope shape [Levine et al., 1987; Komoda et al., 1994; Pai et al., 1995; Glasson et al., 1996]. This three-dimensional shape must be taken into account when non-invasively evaluating valvular function.

The mitral valve is a bileaflet valve comprised of an anterior and posterior leaflet. The leaflet tissue is primarily collagen-reinforced endothelium, but also contains striated muscle cells, non-myelinated nerve fibers, and blood vessels. The anterior and posterior leaflets of the valve are actually one continuous piece of tissue, as shown in Figure 55.6. The free edge of this tissue shows several indentations of which two are regularly placed, called the commisures. The commisures separate the tissue into the anterior and posterior leaflets. The location of the commisures can be identified by the fan-like distribution of chordae tendinae and the relative positioning of the papillary muscles. The combined surface area of both leaflets is approximately twice the area of the mitral orifice; this extra surface area permits a large line of coaptation and ample coverage of the mitral orifice during normal function and provides compensation in cases of disease [He, 1997, 1999]. The posterior leaflet encircles roughly two-thirds of the mitral annulus and is essentially an extension of the mural endocardium from the free walls of the left atrium. The anterior leaflet portion of the annulus is a line of connection, for the leaflet, the wall of the ascending aorta, the aortic valve, and the atrial septum. The anterior leaflet is slightly larger than the posterior leaflet,

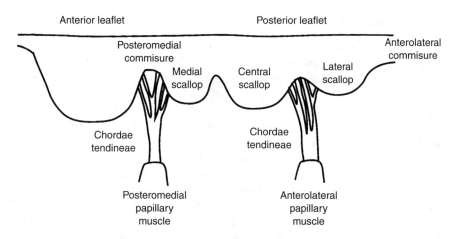

FIGURE 55.6 Diagram of the mitral valve as a continuous piece of tissue. The posterior and anterior leaflets are indicated, as are the scallops, chordae tendineae, and papillary muscles.

and is roughly semi-lunar in shape as opposed to the quadrangular shaped posterior leaflet. The normal width and height of the anterior leaflet is approximately 3.3 and 2.3 cm, respectively. The height of the posterior leaflet is 1.3 cm, while the commisure height is less than 1.0 cm. The posterior leaflet typically has indentations, called scallop, that divide the leaflet into three regions (1) the medial, (2) central, and (3) lateral scallop [Silverman and Hurst, 1968; Raganathan et al., 1970; Roberts, 1983; Barlow, 1987; Kunzelmar et al., 1994].

The mitral leaflet tissue can be divided into both a rough and clear zone. The rough zone is the thicker part of the leaflet and is defined from the free edge of the valve to the valve's line of closure. The term "rough" is used to denote the texture of the leaflet due to the insertion of the chordae tendineae in this area. The clear zone is thinner and translucent and extends from the line of closure to the annulus in the anterior leaflet and to the basal zone in the posterior leaflet. Unlike the mitral valve, the tricuspid valve has three leaflets (1) an anterior leaflet, (2) a posterior leaflet with a variable number of scallops, and (3) a septal leaflet. The tricuspid valve is larger and structurally more complicated than the mitral valve and the separation of the valve tissue into distinct leaflets is less pronounced than with the mitral valve. The surface of the leaflets is similar to that of the mitral valve; however, the basal zone is present in all of the leaflets [Silver et al., 1971].

Chordae tendineae from both leaflets attach to each of the papillary muscles. The chordae tendineae consist of an inner core of collagen surrounded by loosely meshed elastin and collagen fibers with an outer layer of endothelial cells. In the mitral complex structure, there are marginal and basal chordae that insert into the mitral leaflets. From each papillary muscle, several chordae originate and branch into the marginal and basal chordae. The thinner marginal chordae insert into the leaflet free edge at multiple insertion points, while the thicker basal chordae insert into the leaflets at a higher level towards the annulus. The marginal chordae function to keep the leaflets stationary while the basal chordae seem to act more as supports [Kunzelman, 1994].

The left side of the heart has two papillary muscles, called anterolateral and posteromedial, that attach to the ventricular free wall and tether the mitral valve in place via the chordae tendinae. This tethering prevents the mitral valve from prolapsing into the atrium during ventricular ejection. On the right side of the heart, the tricuspid valve has three papillary muscles. The largest one, the anterior papillary muscle, attaches to the valve at the commissure between the anterior and posterior leaflets. The posterior papillary muscle is located between the posterior and septal leaflets. The smallest papillary muscle, called the septal muscle, is sometimes not even present. Improper tethering of the leaflets will result in valve prolapse during ventricular contraction, permitting the valve leaflets to extend into the atrium. This incomplete apposition of the valve leaflets can cause regurgitation, which is leaking of the blood being ejected back into the atrium.

55.2.1 Mechanical Properties

Studies on the mechanical behavior of the mitral leaflet tissue have been conducted to determine the key connective tissue components which influence the valve function. Histological studies have shown that the tissue is composed of three layers which can be identified by differences in cellularity and collagen density. Analysis of the leaflets under tension indicated that the anterior leaflet would be more capable of supporting larger tensile loads than the posterior leaflet. The differences between the mechanical properties between the two leaflets may require different material selection for repair or replacement of the individual leaflets [Kunzelman et al., 1993a,b].

Studies have also been done on the strength of the chordae tendinae. The tension of chordae tendineae in dogs was monitored throughout the cardiac cycle by Salisbury and co-workers [1963]. They found that the tension only paralleled the left ventricular pressure tracings during isovolumic contraction, indicating slackness at other times in the cycle. Investigation of the tensile properties of the chordae tendineae at different strain rates by Lim and Bouchner [1975] found that the chordae had a non-linear stress–strain relationship. They found that the size of the chordae had a more significant effect on the development of the tension than did the strain rate. The smaller chordae with a cross-sectional area of 0.001 to 0.006 cm^2 had a modulus of 2×10^9 dyn/cm^2, while larger chordae with a cross-sectional area of 0.006 to 0.03 cm^2 had a modulus of 1×10^9 dyn/cm^2.

A theoretical study of the stresses sustained by the mitral valve was performed by Ghista and Rao [1972]. This study determined that the stress level can reach as high as 2.2×10^6 dynes/cm^2 just prior to the opening of the aortic valve, with the left ventricular pressure rising to 150 mmHg. A mathematical model has also been created for the mechanics of the mitral valve. It incorporates the relationship between chordae tendineae tension, left ventricular pressure, and mitral valve geometry [Arts et al., 1983]. This study examined the force balance on a closed valve, and determined that the chordae tendinae force was always more than half the force exerted on the mitral valve orifice by the transmitral pressure gradient. During the past 10 years, computational models of mitral valve mechanics have been developed, with the most advanced modeling being three-dimensional finite element models (FEM) of the complete mitral apparatus. Kunzelman and co-workers [1993, 1998] have developed a model of the mitral complex that includes the mitral leaflets, chordae tendinae, contracting annulus, and contracting papillary muscles. From these studies, the maximum principal stresses found at peak loading (120 mmHg) were 5.7×10^6 dyn/cm^2 in the annular region, while the stresses in the anterior leaflet ranged from 2×10^6 to 4×10^6 dyn/cm^2. This model has also been used to evaluate mitral valve disease, repair in chordal rupture, and valvular annuloplasty.

55.2.2 Valve Dynamics

The valve leaflets, chordae tendineae, and papillary muscles all participate to ensure normal functioning of the mitral valve. During isovolumic relaxation, the pressure in the left atrium exceeds that of the left ventricle, and the mitral valve cusps open. Blood flows through the open valve from the left atrium to the left ventricle during diastole. The velocity profiles at both the annulus and the mitral valve tips have been shown to be skewed [Kim et al., 1994] and therefore are not flat as is commonly assumed. This skewing of the inflow profile is shown in Figure 55.7. The initial filling is enhanced by the active relaxation of the ventricle, maintaining a positive transmitral pressure. The mitral velocity flow curve shows a peak in the flow curve, called the E-wave, which occurs during the early filling phase. Normal peak E-wave velocities in healthy individuals range from 50 to 80 cm/sec [Samstad et al., 1989; Oh et al., 1997]. Following active ventricular relaxation, the fluid begins to decelerate and the mitral valve undergoes partial closure. Then the atrium contracts and the blood accelerates through the valve again to a secondary peak, termed the A-wave. The atrium contraction plays an, important role in additional filling of the ventricle during late diastole. In healthy individuals, velocities during the A-wave are typically lower than those of the E-wave, with a normal E/A velocity ratio ranging from 1.5 to 1.7 [Oh et al., 1997]. Thus, normal diastolic filling of

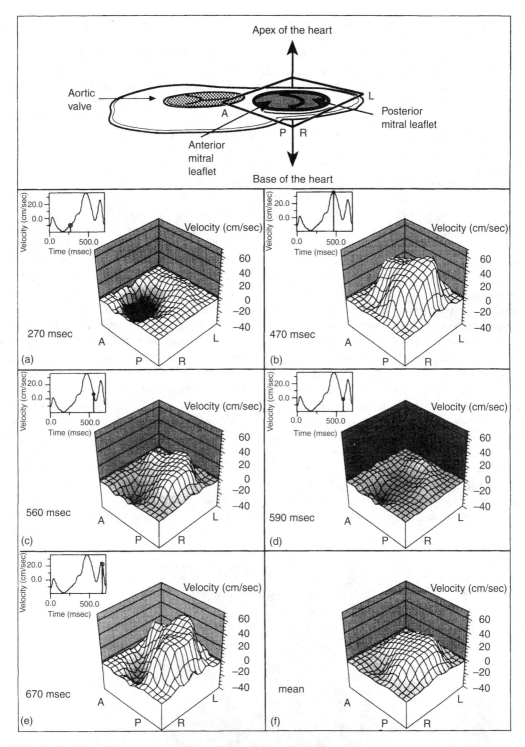

FIGURE 55.7 Two-dimensional transmitral velocity profiles recorded at the level of the mitral annulus in a pig [Kim et al., 1994]. (a) systole; (b) peak E-wave; (c) deceleration phase of early diastole; (d) mid-diastolic period (diastasis); (e) peak A-wave; (f) time averaged diastolic cross-sectional mitral velocity profile. (Reprinted with permission from the American College of Cardiology, *J. Am. Coll. Cardiol.* 24: 532–545.)

the left ventricle shows two distinct peaks in the flow curve with no flow leaking back through the valve during systole.

The tricuspid flow profile is similar to that of the mitral valve, although the velocities in the tricuspid valve are lower because it has a larger valve orifice. In addition, the timing of the valve opening is slightly different. Since the peak pressure in the right ventricle is less than that of the left ventricle, the time for right ventricular pressure to fall below the right atrial pressure is less than the corresponding time period for the left side of the heart. This leads to a shorter right ventricular isovolumic relaxation and thus an earlier tricuspid opening. Tricuspid closure occurs after the mitral valve closes since the activation of the left ventricle precedes that of the right ventricle [Weyman, 1994].

A primary focus in explaining the fluid mechanics of mitral valve function has been understanding the closing mechanism of the valve. Bellhouse [1972] first suggested that the vortices generated by ventricular filling were important for the partial closure of the mitral valve following early diastole. Their *in vitro* experiments suggested that without the strong outflow tract vortices, the valve would remain open at the onset of ventricular contraction, thus resulting in a significant amount of mitral regurgitation before complete closure. Later *in vitro* experiments by Reul and Talukdar [1981] in a left ventricle model made from silicone suggested that an adverse pressure differential in mid-diastole could explain both the flow deceleration and the partial valve closure, even in the absence of a ventricular vortex. Thus, the studies by Reul and Talukdar suggest that the vortices may provide additional closing effects at the initial stage; however, the pressure forces are the dominant effect in valve closure. A more unified theory of valve closure put forth by Yellin and co-workers [1981] includes the importance of chordal tension, flow deceleration, and ventricular vortices, with chordal tension being a necessary condition for the other two. Their animal studies indicated that competent valve closure can occur even in the absence of vortices and flow deceleration. Recent studies using magnetic resonance imaging to visualize the three-dimensional flow field in the left ventricle showed that in normal individuals a large anterior vortex is present at initial partial closure of the valve, as well as following atrial contraction [Kim et al., 1995]. Studies conducted in our laboratory using magnetic resonance imaging of healthy individuals clearly show the vortices in the left ventricle [Walker et al., 1996], which may be an indication of normal diastolic function. An example of these vortices is presented in Figure 55.8.

Another area of interest has been the motion of the mitral valve complex. The heart moves throughout the cardiac cycle; similarly, the mitral apparatus moves and changes shape. Recent studies have been conducted which examined the three-dimensional dynamics of the mitral annulus during the cardiac cycle [Ormiston et al., 1981; Komoda et al., 1994; Pai et al., 1995; Glasson et al., 1996]. These studies

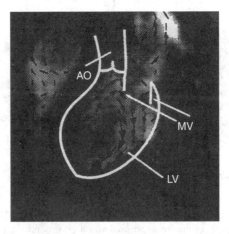

FIGURE 55.8   Magnetic resonance image of a healthy individual during diastole. An outline of the interior left ventricle (LV) is indicated in white as are the mitral valve leaflets (MV) and the aorta (AO). Velocity vectors were obtained from MRI phase velocity mapping and superimposed on the anatomical image.

have shown that during systole the annular circumference decreases from the diastolic value due to the contraction of the ventricle, and this reduction in area ranges from 10 to 25%. This result agrees with an animal study of Tsakiris and co-workers [1971] that looked at the difference in the size, shape, and position of the mitral annulus at different stages in the cardiac cycle. They noted an eccentric narrowing of the annulus during both atrial and ventricular contractions that reduced the mitral valve area by 10 to 36% from its peak diastolic area. This reduction in the annular area during systole is significant, resulting in a smaller orifice area for the larger leaflet area to cover. Not only does the annulus change size, but it also translates during the cardiac cycle. The movement of the annulus towards the atrium has been suggested to play a role in ventricular filling, possibly increasing the efficiency of blood flow into the ventricle. During ventricular contraction, there is a shortening of the left ventricular chamber along its longitudinal axis, and the mitral and tricuspid annuli move towards the apex [Simonson and Schiller, 1989; Hammarström et al., 1991; Alam and Rosenhamer, 1992; Pai et al., 1995].

The movement of the papillary muscles is also important in maintaining proper mitral valve function. The papillary muscles play an important role in keeping the mitral valve in position during ventricular contraction. Abnormal strain on the papillary muscles could cause the chordae to rupture, resulting in mitral regurgitation. It is necessary for the papillary muscles to contract and shorten during systole to prevent mitral prolapse; therefore, the distance between the apex of the heart to the mitral apparatus is important. The distance from the papillary muscle tips to the annulus was measured in normal individuals during systole and was found to remain constant [Sanfilippo et al., 1992]. In patients with mitral valve prolapse, however, this distance decreased, corresponding to a superior displacement of the papillary muscle towards the annulus.

The normal function of the mitral valve requires a balanced interplay between all of the components of the mitral apparatus, as well as the interaction of the atrium and ventricle. Engineering studies into mitral valve function have provided some insight into its mechanical properties and function. Further fundamental and detailed studies are needed to aid surgeons in repairing the diseased mitral valve and in understanding the changes in function due to mitral valve pathologies. In addition, these studies are crucial for improving the design of prosthetic valves that more closely replicate native valve function.

References

Alam, M. and Rosenhamer, G. 1992. Atrioventricular plane displacement and left ventricular function. *J. Am. Soc. Echocardiogr.* 5: 427–433.

Arts, T., Meerbaum, S., Reneman, R., and Corday, E. 1983. Stresses in the closed mitral valve: a model study. *J. Biomech.* 16: 539–547.

Barlow, J.B. 1987. *Perspectives on the Mitral Valve.* F.A. Davis Company, Philadelphia, PA.

Bellhouse, B.J. and Bellhouse, F. 1969. Fluid mechanics of model normal and stenosed aortic valves. *Circ. Res.* 25: 693–704.

Bellhouse, B.J. 1969. Velocity and pressure distributions in the aortic valve. *J. Fluid. Mech.* 37: 587–600.

Bellhouse, B.J. 1972. The fluid mechanics of a model mitral valve and left ventricle. *Cardiovasc. Res.* 6: 199–210.

Christie, G.W. 1990. Anatomy of aortic heart valve leaflets: the influence of glutaraldehyde fixation on function. *Eur. J. Cardio-Thorac. Surg.* 6[Supp 1]: S25–S33.

David, H., Boughner, D.R., Vesely, I., and Gerosa, G. 1994. The pulmonary valve: is it mechanically suitable for use as an aortic valve replacement? *ASAIO J.* 40: 206–212.

Davies, M.J. 1980. *Pathology of Cardiac Valves.* Butterworths, London.

Dunmore-Buyze, J., Boughner, D.R., Macris, N., and Vesely, I. 1995. A comparison of macroscopic lipid content within porcine pulmonary and aortic valves: implications for bioprosthetic valves. *J. Thorac. Cardiovasc. Surg.* 110: 1756–1761.

Emery, R.W. and Arom, K.V. 1991. *The Aortic Valve.* Hanley & Belfus, Philadelphia, PA.

Glasson, J.R., Komeda, M., Daughters, G.T., Niczyporuk, M.A., Bolger, A.F., Ingels, N.B., and Miller, D.C. 1996. Three-dimensional regional dynamics of the normal mitral annulus during left ventricular ejection. *J. Thorac. Cardiovasc. Surg.* 111: 574–585.

Gramiak, R. and Shah, P.M. 1970. Echocardiography of the normal and diseased aortic valve. *Radiology* 96: 1.

Ghista, D.N. and Rao, A.P. 1972. Structural mechanics of the mitral valve: stresses sustained by the valve; non-traumatic determination of the stiffness of the *in vivo* valve. *J. Biomech.* 5: 295–307.

Hammarström, E., Wranne, B., Pinto, F.J., Puryear, J., and Popp, R.L. 1991. Tricuspict annular motion. *J. Am. Soc. Echocardiogr.* 4: 131–139.

Hatle, L. and Angelsen, B. 1985. *Doppler Ultrasound in Cardiology: Physical Principals and Clinical Applications.* Lea and Febiger, Philadelphia, PA.

He, S., Fontaine, A.A., Schwammenthal, E., Yoganathan, A.P., and Levine, R.A. 1997. Integrated mechanism for functional mitral regurgitation: leaflet elongation versus coapting force: *in vitro* study. *Circulation* 96: 1826–1834.

He, S., Lemmon, J.D., Weston, M.W., Jensen, M.O., Levine, R.A., and Yoganathan, A.P. 1999. Mitral valve compensation for annular dilatation: *in vitro* study into the mechanisms of functional mitral regurgitation with an adjustable annulus model. *J. Heart Valve Dis.* 8: 294–302.

Kilner, P.J., Yang, G.Z., Mohiaddin, R.H., Firmin, D.N., and Longmore, D.B. 1993. Helical and retrograde secondary flow patterns in the aortic arch studied by three-directional magnetic resonance velocity mapping. *Circulation* 88[part I]: 2235–2247.

Kim, W.Y., Bisgaard, T., Nielsen, S.L., Poulsen, J.K., Pederson, E.M., Hasenkam, J.M., and Yoganathan, A.P. 1994. Two-dimensional mitral flow velocity profiles in pig models using epicardial echo-Doppler-cardiography. *J. Am. Coll. Cardiol.* 3: 673–683.

Kim, W.Y., Walker, P.G., Pederson, E.M., Poulsen, J.K., Houlind, K.C., and Oyre, S. 1995. Left ventricular blood flow patterns in normal subjects: a quantitative analysis of three-dimensional magnetic resonance velocity mapping. 4: 422–438.

Komoda, T., Hetzer, R., Uyama, C., Siniawski, H., Maeta, H., Rosendahl, P., and Ozaki, K. 1994. Mitral annular function assessed by 3D imaging for mitral valve surgery. *J. Heart Valve Dis.* 3: 483–490.

Kunzelman, K.S., Cochran, R.P., Murphee, S.S., Ring, W.S., Verrier, E.D., and Eberhart, R.C. 1993a. Differential collagen distribution in the mitral valve and its influence on biomechanical behaviour. *J. Heart Valve Dis.* 2: 236–244.

Kunzelman, K.S., Cochran, R.P., Chuong, C., Ring, W.S., Verner, E.D., and Eberhart, R.D. 1993b. Finite element analysis of the mitral valve. *J. Heart Valve Dis.* 2: 326–340.

Kunzelman, K.S., Reimink, M.S., and Cochran, R.P. 1998. Flexible versus rigid ring annuloplasty for mitral valve annular dilatation: a finite element model. *J. Heart Valve Dis.* 7: 108–116.

Kunzelman, K.S., Cochran, R.P., Verner, E.D., and Eberhart, R.D. 1994. Anatomic basis for mitral valve modeling. *J. Heart Valve Dis.* 3: 491–496.

Leeson-Dietrich, J., Boughner, D., and Vesely, I. 1995. Porcine pulmonary and aortic valves: a comparison of their tensile viscoelastic properties at physiological strain rates. *J. Heart Valve Dis.* 4: 88–94.

Levine, R.A., Trivizi, M.O., Harrigan, P., and Weyman, A.E. 1987. The relationship of mitral annular shape to the diagnosis of mitral valve prolapse. *Circulation* 75: 756–767.

Lim, K.O. and Bouchner, D.P. 1975. Mechanical properties of human mitral valve chordae tendineae: variation with size and strain rate. *Can. J. Physiol. Pharmacol.* 53: 330–339.

Lo, D. and Vesely, I. 1995. Biaxial strain analysis of the porcine aortic valve. *Ann. Thorac. Surg.* 60(Suppl II): S374–S378.

Oh, J.K., Appleton, C.P., Hatle, L.K., Nishimura, R.A., Seward, J.B., and Tajik, A.J. 1997. The noninvasive assessment of left ventricular diastolic function with two-dimensional and doppler echocardiography. *J. Am. Soc. Echocardiogr.* 10: 246–270.

Ormiston, J.A., Shah, P.M., Tei, C., and Wong, M. 1981. Size and motion of the mitral valve annulus in man: a two-dimensional echocardiographic method and findings in normal subjects. *Circulation* 64: 113–120.

Pai, R.G., Tanimoto, M., Jintapakorn, W., Azevedo, J., Pandian, N.G., and Shah, P.M. 1995. Volume-rendered three-dimensional dynamic anatomy of the mitral annulus using a transesophageal echocardiographic technique. *J. Heart Valve Dis.* 4: 623–627.

Paulsen, P.K. and Hasenkam, J.M. 1983. Three-dimensional visualization of velocity profiles in the ascending aorta in dogs, measured with a hot film anemometer. *J. Biomech.* 16: 201–210.

Raganathan, N., Lam, J.H.C., Wigle, E.D., and Silver, M.D. 1970. Morphology of the human mitral valve: the valve leaflets. *Circulation* 41: 459–467.

Reul, H. and Talukdar, N. 1979. Heart valve mechanics. In *Quantitative Cardiovascular Studies Clinical and Research Applications of Engineering Principles.* Hwang, N.H.C., Gross, D.R., and Patel, D.J., Eds. University Park Press, Baltimore, MD, pp. 527–564.

Roberts, W.C. 1983. Morphologic features of the normal and abnormal mitral valve. *Am. J. Cardiol.* 51: 1005–1028.

Rossvoll, O., Samstad, S., Torp, H.G., Linker, D.T., Skjærpe, T., Angelsen, B.A.J., and Hatle, L. 1991. The velocity distribution in the aortic annulus in normal subjects: a quantitative analysis of two-dimensional Doppler flow maps. *J. Am. Soc. Echocardiogr.* 4: 367–378.

Sahasakul, Y., Edwards, W.D., Naessens, J.M., and Tajik, A.J. 1988. Age-related changes in aortic and mitral valve thickness: implications for two-dimensional echocardiography based on an autopsy study of 200 normal human hearts. *Am. J. Cardiol.* 62: 424–430.

Salisbury, P.F., Cross, C.E., and Rieben, P.A. 1963. Chordae tendinea tension. *Am. J. Physiol.* 25: 385–392.

Samstad, O., Gorp, H.G., Linker, D.T., Rossvoll, O., Skjaerpe, T., Johansen, E., Kristoffersen, K., Angelson, B.A.J., and Hatle, L. 1989. Cross-sectional early mitral flow velocity profiles from colour Doppler. *Br. Heart J.* 62: 177–84.

Sanfilippo, A.J., Harrigan, P., Popovic, A.D., Weyman, A.E., and Levine, R.A. 1992. Papillary muscle traction in mitral valve prolapse: quantitation by two-dimensional echocardiography. *J. Am. Coll. Cardiol.* 19: 564–571.

Scott, M.J. and Vesely, I. 1996. Morphology of porcine aortic valve cusp elastin. *J. Heart Valve Dis.* 5: 464–471.

Silver, M.D., Lam, J.H.C., Raganathan, N., and Wigle, E.D. 1971. Morphology of the human tricuspid valve. *Circulation* 43: 333–348.

Silver, M.A. and Roberts, W.C. 1985. Detailed anatomy of the normally functioning aortic valve in hearts of normal and increased weight. *Am. J. Cardiol.* 55: 454–461.

Silverman, M.E. and Hurst, J.W. 1968. The mitral complex: interaction of the anatomy, physiology, and pathology of the mitral annulus, mitral valve leaflets, chordae tendineae and papillary muscles. *Am. Heart J.* 76: 399–418.

Simonson, J.S. and Schiller, N.B. 1989. Descent of the base of the left ventricle: an echocardiogiaphic index of left ventricular function. *J. Am. Soc. Echocardiogr.* 2: 25–35.

Sloth, E., Houlind, K.C., Oyre, S., Kim, Y.K., Pedersen, E.M., Jørgensen, H.S., and Hasenkam, J.M. 1994. Three-dimensional visualization of velocity profiles in the human main pulmonary artery using magnetic resonance phase velocity mapping. *Am. Heart J.* 128: 1130–1138.

Sung, H.W. and Yoganathan, A.P. 1990. Axial flow velocity patterns in a normal human pulmonary artery model: pulsatile *in vitro* studies. *J. Biomech.* 23: 210–214.

Thubrikar, M. 1990. *The Aortic Valve.* CRC Press, Boca Raton, FL.

Thubrikar, M., Heckman, J.L., and Nolan, S.P. 1993. High speed cine-radiographic study of aortic valve leaflet motion. *J. Heart Valve Dis.* 2: 653–661.

Tsakiris, A.G., von Bernuth, G., Rastelli, G.C., Bourgeois, M.J., Titus, J.L., and Wood, E.H. 1971. Size and motion of the mitral valve annulus in anesthetized intact dogs. *J. Appl. Physiol.* 30: 611–618.

Vesely, I. and Noseworthy, R. 1992. Micromechanics of the fibrosa and the ventricularis in aortic valve leaflets. *J. Biomech.* 25: 101–113.

Vesely, I., Macris, N., Dunmore, P.J., and Boughner, D. 1994. The distribution and morphology of aortic valve cusp lipids. *J. Heart Valve Dis.* 3: 451–456.

Vesely, I. 1998. The role of elastin in aortic valve mechanics. *J. Biomech.* 31: 115–123.

Vollebergh, F.E.M.G. and Becker, A.E. 1977. Minor congenital variations of cusp size in tricuspid aortic valves: possible link with isolated aortic stenosis. *Br. Heart J.* 39: 106–111.

Walker, P.G., Cranney, G.B., Grimes, R.Y., Delatore, J., Rectenwald, J., Pohost, G.M., and Yoganathan, A.P. 1996. Three-dimensional reconstruction of the flow in a human left heart by magnetic resonance phase velocity encoding. *Ann. Biomed. Eng.* 24: 139–147.

Westaby, S., Karp, R.B., Blackstone, E.H., and Bishop, S.P. 1984. Adult human valve dimensions and their surgical significance. *Am. J. Cardiol.* 53: 552–556.

Weyman, A.E. 1994. *Principles and Practices of Echocardiography.* Lea & Febiger, Philadelphia, PA.

Yellin, E.L., Peskin, C., Yoran, C., Koenigsberg, M., Matsumoto, M., Laniado, S., McQueen, D., Shore, D., and Frater, R.W.M. 1981. Mechanisms of mitral valve motion during diastole. *Am. J. Physiol.* 241: H389–H400.

56

Arterial Macrocirculatory Hemodynamics

Baruch B. Lieber
State University
of New York-Buffalo

The arterial circulation is a multiply branched network of compliant tubes. The geometry of the network is complex, and the vessels exhibit nonlinear **viscoelastic** behavior. Flow is pulsatile, and the blood flowing through the network is a suspension of red blood cells and other particles in plasma which exhibits complex *non-Newtonian* properties. Whereas the development of an exact biomechanical description of arterial hemodynamics is a formidable task, surprisingly useful results can be obtained with greatly simplified models.

The geometrical parameters of the canine **systemic** and **pulmonary** circulations are summarized in Table 56.1. Vessel diameters vary from a maximum of 19 mm in the proximal aorta to 0.008 mm (8 μm) in the capillaries. Because of the multiple branching, the total cross-sectional area increases from 2.8 cm^2 in the proximal aorta to 1357 cm^2 in the capillaries. Of the total blood volume, approximately 83% is in the systemic circulation, 12% is in the pulmonary circulation, and the remaining 5% is in the heart. Most of the systemic blood is in the venous circulation, where changes in compliance are used to control mean circulatory blood pressure. This chapter will be concerned with flow in the larger arteries, classes 1 to 5 in the systemic circulation and 1 to 3 in the pulmonary circulation in Table 56.1. Flow in the microcirculation is discussed in Chapter 59, and venous hemodynamics is covered in Chapter 60.

56.1 Blood Vessel Walls

The detailed properties of blood vessels were described earlier in this section, but a few general observations are made here to facilitate the following discussion. Blood vessels are composed of three layers, the intima, media, and adventitia. The inner layer, or intima, is composed primarily of **endothelial** cells, which line

TABLE 56.1   Model of Vascular Dimensions in 20-kg Dog

Class	Vessels	Mean diameter (mm)	Number of vessels	Mean length (mm)	Total cross-section (cm²)	Total blood volume (ml)	Percentage of total volume
				Systemic			
1	Aorta	(19–4.5)	1		(2.8–0.2)	60	
2	Arteries	4.000	40	150.0	5.0	75	
3	Arteries	1.300	500	45.0	6.6	30	
4	Arteries	0.450	6000	13.5	9.5	13	11
5	Arteries	0.150	110,000	4.0	19.4	8	
6	Arterioles	0.050	2.8×10^6	1.2	55.0	7	
7	Capillaries	0.008	2.7×10^9	0.65	1357.0	88	5
8	Venules	0.100	1.0×10^7	1.6	785.4	126	
9	Veins	0.280	660,000	4.8	406.4	196	
10	Veins	0.700	40,000	13.5	154.0	208	
11	Veins	1.800	2,100	45.0	53.4	240	
12	Veins	4.500	110	150.0	17.5	263	67
13	Venae cavae	(5–14)	2		(0.2–1.5)	92	
Total						1406	
				Pulmonary			
1	Main artery	1.600	1	28.0	2.0	6	
2	Arteries	4.000	20	10.0	2.5	25	3
3	Arteries	1.000	1550	14.0	12.2	17	
4	Arterioles	0.100	1.5×10^6	0.7	120.0	8	
5	Capillaries	0.008	2.7×10^9	0.5	1357.0	68	4
6	Venules	0.110	2.0×10^6	0.7	190.0	13	
7	Veins	1.100	1650	14.0	15.7	22	
8	Veins	4.200	25	100.0		35	5
9	Main veins	8.000	4	30.0		6	
Total						200	
				Heart			
	Atria		2			30	
	Ventricles		2			54	5
Total						84	
Total circulation						1690	100

Source: Milnor, W.R. 1989. *Hemodynamics*, 2nd ed., p. 45. Baltimore, Williams and Wilkins. With permission.

the vessel and are involved in control of vessel diameter. The media, composed of **elastin, collagen,** and smooth muscle, largely determines the elastic properties of the vessel. The outer layer, or adventitia, is composed mainly of connective tissue. Unlike in structures composed of passive elastic materials, vessel diameter and elastic modulus vary with smooth-muscle tone. Dilation in response to increases in flow and **myogenic** constriction in response to increases in pressure have been observed in some arteries. Smooth-muscle tone is also affected by circulating **vasoconstrictors** such as norepinephrine and **vasodilators** such as nitroprusside. Blood vessels, like other soft biological tissues, generally do not obey Hooke's law, becoming stiffer as pressure is increased. They also exhibit viscoelastic characteristics such as hysteresis and creep. Fortunately, for many purposes a linear elastic model of blood vessel behavior provides adequate results.

56.2   Flow Characteristics

Blood is a complex substance containing water, inorganic ions, proteins, and cells. Approximately 50% is plasma, a nearly **Newtonian** fluid consisting of water, ions, and proteins. The balance contains erythrocytes (red blood cells), leukocytes (white blood cells), and platelets. Whereas the behavior of blood in vessels smaller than approximately 100 μm exhibits significant non-Newtonian effects, flow in larger vessels can be described reasonably accurately using the Newtonian assumption. There is some evidence suggesting that in blood analog fluids wall shear stress distributions may differ somewhat from Newtonian values [Liepsch et al., 1991].

Flow in the arterial circulation is predominantly laminar with the possible exception of the proximal aorta and main pulmonary artery. In steady flow, transition to turbulence occurs at Reynolds numbers (N_R) above approximately 2300

$$N_R = \frac{2rV}{v} \qquad (56.1)$$

where r = vessel radius, V = velocity, v = kinematic viscosity = viscosity/density.

Flow in the major systemic and pulmonary arteries is highly pulsatile. Peak-to-mean flow amplitudes as high as 6 to 1 have been reported in both human and dog [Milnor, 1989, p. 149]. Womersley's [1957] analysis of incompressible flow in rigid and elastic tubes showed that the importance of pulsatility in the velocity distributions depended on the parameter

$$N_w = r\sqrt{\frac{\omega}{v}} \qquad (56.2)$$

where ω = frequency.

This is usually referred to as the *Womersley number* (N_w) or *α-parameter*. Womersley's original report is not readily available; however, Milnor provides a reasonably complete account [Milnor, 1989, pp. 106–121].

Mean and peak Reynolds numbers in human and dog are given in Table 56.2, which also includes mean, peak, and minimum velocities as well as the Womersley number. Mean Reynolds numbers in the entire systemic and pulmonary circulations are below 2300. Peak systolic Reynolds numbers exceed 2300 in the aorta and pulmonary artery, and some evidence of transition to turbulence has been reported. In dogs, distributed flow occurs at Reynolds numbers as low as 1000, with higher Womersley numbers increasing the transition Reynolds number [Nerem and Seed, 1972]. The values in Table 56.2 are typical for individuals at rest. During exercise, cardiac output and hence Reynolds numbers can increase severalfold. The Womersley number also affects the shape of the instantaneous velocity profiles as discussed below.

TABLE 56.2 Normal Average Hemodynamics Values in Man and Dog

	Dog (20 kg)			Man (70 kg, 1.8 m²)		
	N_w	Velocity (cm/sec)	N_R	N_w	Velocity (cm/sec)	N_R
Systemic Vessels						
Ascending aorta	16	15.8 (89/0)[a]	870 (4900)[b]	21	18 (112/0)[a]	1500 (9400)[a]
Abdominal aorta	9	12 (60.0)	370 (1870)	12	14 (75/0)	640 (3600)
Renal artery	3	41 (74/26)	440 (800)	4	40 (73/26)	700 (1300)
Femoral artery	4	10 (42/1)	130 (580)	4	12 (52/2)	200 (860)
Femoral vein	5	5	92	7	4	104
Superior vena cava	10	8 (20/0)	320 (790)	15	9 (23/0)	550 (1400)
Inferior vena cava	11	19 (40/0)	800 (1800)	17	21 (46/0)	1400 (3000)
Pulmonary vessels						
Main artery	14	18 (72/0)	900 (3700)	20	19 (96/0)	1600 (7800)
Main vein[c]	7	18 (30/9)	270 (800)	10	19 (38/10)	800 (2200)

[a] Mean (systolic/diastolic).
[b] Mean (peak).
[c] One of the usually four terminal pulmonary veins.
Source: Milnor, W.R. 1989. *Hemodynamics*, 2nd ed., p. 148, Baltimore, Williams and Wilkins. With permission.

TABLE 56.3 Pressure Wave Velocities in Arteries[a,b]

Artery	Species	Wave velocity (cm/sec)
Ascending Aorta	Man	440–520
	Dog	350–472
Thoracic aorta	Man	400–650
	Dog	400–700
Abdominal aorta	Man	500–620
	Dog	550–960
Iliac	Man	700–880
	Dog	700–800
Femoral	Man	800–1800
	Dog	800–1300
Popliteal	Dog	1220–1310
Tibial	Dog	1040–1430
Carotid	Man	680–830
	Dog	610–1240
Pulmonary	Man	168–182
	Dog	255–275
	Rabbit	100
	Pig	190

[a]All data are apparent pressure wave velocities (although the average of higher frequency harmonics approximates the true velocity in many cases), from relatively young subjects with normal cardiovascular systems, at approximately normal distending pressures.
[b]Ranges for each vessel and species taken from Table 9.1 of source.
Source: Milnor, W.R. 1989. *Hemodynamics*, 2nd ed., p. 235, Baltimore, Williams and Wilkins. With permission.

56.3 Wave Propagation

The viscoelasticity of blood vessels affects the hemodynamics of arterial flow. The primary function of arterial elasticity is to store blood during systole so that forward flow continues when the aortic valve is closed. Elasticity also causes a finite wave propagation velocity, which is given approximately by the Moens–Korteweg relationship

$$c = \sqrt{\frac{Eh}{2\rho r}} \tag{56.3}$$

where E = wall elastic modulus, h = wall thickness, ρ = blood density, r = vessel radius.

Although Moens [1878] and Korteweg [1878] are credited with this formulation, Fung [1984, p. 107] has pointed out that the formula was first derived much earlier [Young, 1808]. Wave speeds in arterial blood vessels from several species are given in Table 56.3. In general, wave speeds increase toward the periphery as vessel radius decreases and are considerably lower in the main pulmonary artery than in the aorta owing primarily to the lower pressure and consequently lower elastic modulus.

Wave reflections occur at branches where there is not perfect **impedance** matching of parent and daughter vessels. The input impedance of a network of vessels is the ratio of pressure to flow. For rigid vessels with laminar flow and negligible inertial effects, the input impedance is simply the resistance and is independent of pressure and flow rate. For elastic vessels, the impedance is dependent on the frequency of the fluctuations in pressure and flow. The impedance can be described by a complex function expressing the amplitude ratio of pressure to flow oscillations and the phase difference between the peaks.

$$\bar{Z}_i(\omega) = \frac{\bar{P}(\omega)}{\bar{Q}(\omega)}$$

$$|\bar{Z}_i(\omega)| = \left|\frac{\bar{P}(\omega)}{\bar{Q}(\omega)}\right| \tag{56.4}$$

$$\theta_i(\omega) = \theta[(\bar{P}(\omega))] - \theta[(\bar{Q}(\omega))]$$

where $\bar{Z}_i$ is the complex impedance, $|\bar{Z}_i|$ is the amplitude, and θ_i is the phase.

For an infinitely long straight tube with constant properties, input impedance will be independent of position in the tube and dependent only on vessel and fluid properties. The corresponding value of input impedance is called the *characteristic impedance Z_0* given by

$$Z_0 = \frac{\rho c}{A} \tag{56.5}$$

where A = vessel cross-sectional area.

In general, the input impedance will vary from point to point in the network because of variations in vessel sizes and properties. If the network has the same impedance at each point (perfect impedance matching), there will be no wave reflections. Such a network will transmit energy most efficiently. The reflection coefficient R, defined as the ratio of reflected to incident wave amplitude, is related to the relative characteristic impedance of the vessels at a junction. For a parent tube with characteristic impedance Z_0 branching into two daughter tubes with characteristic impedances Z_1 and Z_2, the reflection coefficient is given by

$$R = \frac{Z_0^{-1} - (Z_1^{-1} + Z_2^{-1})}{Z_0^{-1} + (Z_1^{-1} + Z_2^{-1})} \tag{56.6}$$

and perfect impedance matching requires

$$\frac{1}{Z_0} = \frac{1}{Z_1} + \frac{1}{Z_2} \tag{56.7}$$

The arterial circulation exhibits partial impedance matching; however, wave reflections do occur. At each branch point, local reflection coefficients typically are less than 0.2. Nonetheless, global reflection coefficients, which account for all reflections distal to a given site, can be considerably higher [Milnor, 1989, p. 217].

In the absence of wave reflections, the input impedance is equal to the characteristic impedance. Womersley's analysis predicts that impedance modulus will decrease monotonically with increasing frequency, whereas the phase angle is negative at low frequency and becomes progressively more positive with increasing frequency. Typical values calculated from Womersley's analysis are shown in Figure 56.1. In the actual circulation, wave reflections cause oscillations in the modulus and phase. Figure 56.2 shows input impedance measured in the ascending aorta of a human. Measurements of input resistance, characteristic impedance, and the frequency of the first minimum in the input impedance are summarized in Table 56.4.

56.4 Velocity Profiles

Typical pressure and velocity fluctuations throughout the cardiac cycle in man are shown in Figure 56.3 Although mean pressure decreases slightly toward the periphery due to viscous effects, peak pressure shows small increases in the distal aorta due to wave reflection and vessel taper. A rough estimate of mean

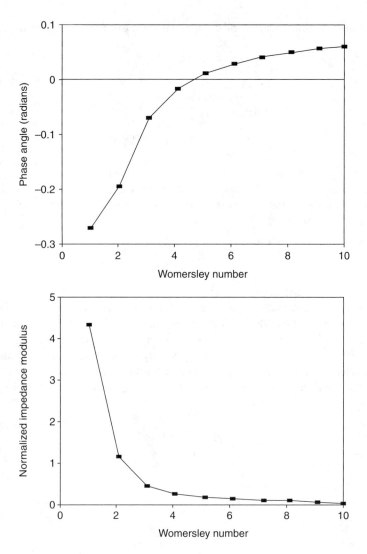

FIGURE 56.1 Characteristic impedance calculated from Womersley's analysis. The top panel contains the phase of the impedance and the bottom panel the modulus, both plotted as a function of the Womersley number N_W, which is proportional to frequency. The curves shown are for an unconstrained tube and include the effects of wall viscosity. The original figure has an error in the scale of the ordinate which has been corrected. (From Milnor, W.R. 1989. *Hemodynamics*, 2nd ed., p. 172, Baltimore, Williams and Wilkins. With permission.)

pressure can be obtained as 1/3 of the sum of systolic pressure and twice the diastolic pressure. Velocity peaks during systole, with some backflow observed in the aorta early in diastole. Flow in the aorta is nearly zero through most of the diastole; however, more peripheral arteries such as the iliac and renal show forward flow throughout the cardiac cycle. This is a result of capacitive discharge of the central arteries as arterial pressure decreases.

Velocity varies across the vessel due to viscous and inertial effects as mentioned earlier. The velocities in Figure 56.3 were measured at one point in the artery. Velocity profiles are complex because the flow is pulsatile and vessels are elastic, curved, and tapered. Profiles measured in the thoracic aorta of a dog at normal arterial pressure and cardiac output are shown in Figure 56.4. Backflow occurs during diastole, and profiles are flattened even during peak systolic flow. The shape of the profiles varies considerably with mean aortic pressure and cardiac output [Ling et al., 1973].

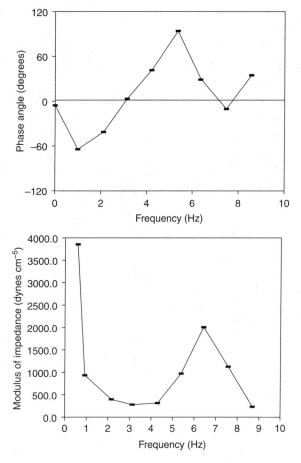

FIGURE 56.2 Input impedance derived from the pressure and velocity data in the ascending aorta of Figure 56.3. The top panel contains the modulus and the bottom panel the phase, both plotted as functions of frequency. The peripheral resistance (DC impedance) for this plot was 16,470 dyne sec/cm^5. (From Mills C.J., Gabe I.T., Gault J.N. et al. 1970. Pressure–flow relationships and vascular impedance in man. *Cardiovasc. Res.* 4: 405. With permission.)

TABLE 56.4 Characteristic Arterial Impedances in Some Mammals: Average ($\pm$SE)[a,b]

Species	Artery	R_{in}	Z_0	f_{min}
Dog	Aorta	2809–6830	125–288	6–8
Dog	Pulmonary	536–807	132–295	2–3.5
Dog	Femoral	110–162[c]	4.5–15.8[c]	8–13
Dog	Carotid	69[c]	7.0–9.4[c]	8–11
Rabbit	Aorta	20–50[c]	1.8–2.1[c]	4.5–9.8
Rabbit	Pulmonary		1.1[c]	3.0
Rat	Aorta	153[c]	11.2[c]	12

Abbreviations: R_{in}, input resistance (mean arterial pressure/flow) in dyn sec/cm^5; Z_0, characteristic impedance, in dyn sec/cm^5, estimated by averaging high-frequency input impedances in aorta and pulmonary artery; value at 5Hz for other arteries, f_{min}, frequency of first minimum of Z_i.
[a]Values estimated from published figures if averages were not reported.
[b]Ranges for each species and vessel taken from values in Table 7.2 of source.
[c]10^3 dyn sec/cm^5.

Source: Milnor, W.R. 1989. Hemodynamics, 2nd ed., p. 183, Baltimore, Williams and Wilkins. With permission.

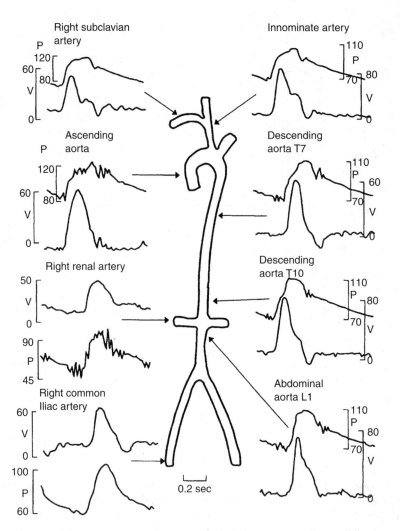

FIGURE 56.3 Simultaneous pressure and blood velocity patterns recorded at points in the systemic circulation of a human. Velocities were recorded with a catheter-tip electromagnetic flowmeter probe. The catheter included a lumen for simultaneous pressure measurement V is the velocity (cm/sec), P is the pressure (mmHg). (From Mills, C.J., Gabe, I.T., Gault, J.N. et al., 1970. *Cardiovasc. Res.* 40: 405. With permission.)

In more peripheral arteries the profiles are resembling parabolic ones as in fully developed laminar flow. The general features of these fully developed flow profiles can be modeled using Womersley's approach, although nonlinear effects may be important in some cases. The qualitative features of the profile depend on the Womersley number N_w. Unsteady effects become more important as N_w increases. Below a value of about 2 the instantaneous profiles are close to the steady parabolic shape. Profiles in the aortic arch are skewed due to curvature of the arch.

56.5 Pathology

Atherosclerosis is a disease of the arterial wall which appears to be strongly influenced by hemodynamics. The disease begins with a thickening of the intimal layer in locations which correlate with the shear stress distribution on the endothelial surface [Friedman et al., 1993]. Over time the lesion continues to grow until a significant portion of the vessel lumen is occluded. The peripheral circulation will dilate

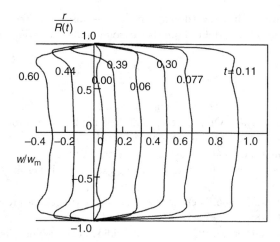

FIGURE 56.4 Velocity profiles obtained with a hot-film anemometer probe in the descending thoracic aorta of a dog at normal arterial pressure and cardiac output. The velocity at t = time/(cardiac period) is plotted as a function of radial position. Velocity w is normalized by the maximum velocity w_m and radial position at each time by the instantaneous vessel radius $R(t)$. The aortic valve opens at $t = 0$. Peak velocity occurs 11% of the cardiac period after aortic valve opening. (From Ling, S.C., Atabek, W.G., Letzing, W.G. et al. 1973. *Circ. Res.* 33: 198. With permission.)

to compensate for the increase in resistance of the large vessels, compromising the ability of the system to respond to increases in demand during exercise. Eventually the circulation is completely dilated, and resting flow begins to decrease. A blood clot may form at the site or lodge in a narrowed segment, causing an acute loss of blood flow. The disease is particularly dangerous in the coronary and carotid arteries due to the critical oxygen requirements of the heart and brain.

In addition to intimal thickening, the arterial wall properties also change with age. Most measurements suggest that arterial elastic modulus increases with age (hardening of the arteries); however, in some cases arteries to become more compliant (inverse of elasticity) [Learoyd and Taylor, 1966]. Local weakening of the wall may also occur, particularly in the descending aorta, giving rise to an **aneurysm**, which, if ruptures, can cause sudden death.

Defining Terms

Aneurysm: A ballooning of a blood vessel wall caused by weakening of the elastic material in the wall.

Atherosclerosis: A disease of the blood vessels characterized by thickening of the vessel wall and eventual occlusion of the vessel.

Collagen: A protein found in blood vessels which is much stiffer than elastin.

Elastin: A very elastic protein found in blood vessels.

Endothelial: The inner lining of blood vessels.

Impedance: A (generally) complex number expressing the ratio of pressure to flow.

Myogenic: A change in smooth-muscle tone due to stretch or relaxation, causing a blood vessel to resist changes in diameter.

Newtonian: A fluid whose stress-rate-of-strain relationship is linear, following Newton's law. The fluid will have a viscosity whose value is independent of rate of strain.

Pulmonary: The circulation which delivers blood to the lungs for reoxygenation and carbon dioxide removal.

Systemic: The circulation which supplies oxygenated blood to the tissues of the body.

Vasoconstrictor: A substance which causes an increase in smooth-muscle tone, thereby constricting blood vessels.

Vasodilator: A substance which causes a decrease in smooth-muscle tone, thereby dilating blood vessels.
Viscoelastic: A substance which exhibits both elastic (solid) and viscous (liquid) characteristics.

References

Chandran, K.B. 1992. *Cardiovascular Biomechanics.* New York, New York University Press.

Friedman, M.H., Brinkman, A.M., Qin, J.J. et al. 1993. Relation between coronary artery geometry and the distribution of early sudanophilic lesions. *Atherosclerosis* 98:193.

Fung, Y.C. 1984. *Biodynamics: Circulation.* New York, Springer-Verlag.

Korteweg, D.J. 1878. Uber die Fortpflanzungsgeschwindigkeit des Schalles in elastischen. *Rohren. Ann. Phys. Chem.* (NS) 5: 525.

Learoyd, B.M., and Taylor, M.G. 1966. Alterations with age in the viscoelastic properties of human arterial walls. *Circ. Res.* 18: 278.

Liepsch, D., Thurston, G., and Lee, M. 1991. Studies of fluids simulating blood-like rheological properties and applications in models of arterial branches. *Biorheology* 28: 39.

Ling, S.C., Atabek, W.G., Letzing, W.G. et al. 1973. Nonlinear analysis of aortic flow in living dogs. *Circ. Res.* 33: 198.

Mills, C.J., Gabe, I.T., Gault, J.N. et al. 1970. Pressure–flow relationships and vascular impedance in man. *Cardiovasc. Res.* 4: 405.

Milnor, W.R. 1989. *Hemodynamics*, 2nd ed., Baltimore, Williams and Wilkins.

Moens, A.I. 1878. *Die Pulskurve*, Leiden.

Nerem, R.M., and Seed, W.A. 1972. An *in-vivo* study of aortic flow disturbances. *Cardiovasc. Res.* 6: 1.

Womersley, J.R. 1957. The mathematical analysis of the arterial circulation in a state of oscillatory motion. Wright Air Development Center Technical Report WADC-TR-56-614.

Young, T. 1808. Hydraulic investigations, subservient to an intended Croonian lecture on the motion of the blood. *Phil. Trans. R. Soc. Lond.* 98: 164.

Further Information

A good introduction to cardiovascular biomechanics, including arterial hemodynamics, is provided by K.B. Chandran in *Cardiovascular Biomechanics.* Y. C. Fung's *Biodynamics — Circulation* is also an excellent starting point, somewhat more mathematical than Chandran. Perhaps the most complete treatment of the subject is in *Hemodynamics* by W.R. Milnor, from which much of this chapter was taken. Milnor's book is quite mathematical and may be difficult for a novice to follow.

Current work in arterial hemodynamics is reported in a number of engineering and physiological journals, including the *Annals of Biomedical Engineering, Journal of Biomechanical Engineering, Circulation Research,* and *The American Journal of Physiology, Heart and Circulatory Physiology.* Symposia sponsored by the American Society of Mechanical Engineers, Biomedical Engineering Society, American Heart Association, and the American Physiological Society contain reports of current research.

57

Mechanics of Blood Vessels

Thomas R. Canfield
Argonne National Laboratory

Philip B. Dobrin
*Hines VA Hospital and Loyola
University Medical Center*

57.1 Assumptions

This chapter is concerned with the mechanical behavior of blood vessels under static loading conditions and the methods required to analyze this behavior. The assumptions underlying this discussion are for *ideal* blood vessels that are at least regionally homogeneous, incompressible, elastic, and cylindrically orthotropic. Although physiologic systems are *nonideal*, much understanding of vascular mechanics has been gained through the use of methods based upon these ideal assumptions.

57.1.1 Homogeneity of the Vessel Wall

On visual inspection, blood vessels appear to be fairly homogeneous and distinct from surrounding connective tissue. The inhomogeneity of the vascular wall is realized when one examines the tissue under a low-power microscope, where one can easily identify two distinct structures: the media and adventitia. For this reason the assumption of vessel wall homogeneity is applied cautiously. Such an assumption may be valid only within distinct macroscopic structures. However, few investigators have incorporated macroscopic inhomogeneity into studies of vascular mechanics [1].

57.1.2 Incompressibility of the Vessel Wall

Experimental measurement of wall compressibility of 0.06% at 270 cm of H_2O indicates that the vessel can be considered incompressible when subjected to physiologic pressure and load [2]. In terms of the mechanical behavior of blood vessels, this is small relative to the large magnitude of the distortional strains that occur when blood vessels are deformed under the same conditions. Therefore, vascular compressibility may be important to understanding other physiologic processes related to blood vessels, such as the transport of interstitial fluid.

57.1.3 Inelasticity of the Vessel Wall

That blood vessel walls exhibit inelastic behavior such as length-tension and pressure-diameter hysteresis, stress relaxation, and creep has been reported extensively [3,4]. However, blood vessels are able to maintain stability and contain the pressure and flow of blood under a variety of physiologic conditions. These conditions are dynamic but slowly varying with a large static component.

57.1.4 Residual Stress and Strain

Blood vessels are known to retract both longitudinally and circumferentially are excision. This retraction is caused by the relief of distending forces resulting from internal pressure and longitudinal tractions. The magnitude of retraction is influenced by several factors. Among these factors are growth, aging, and hypertension. Circumferential retraction of medium-caliber blood vessels, such as the carotid, iliac, and bracheal arteries, can exceed 70% following reduction of internal blood pressure to zero. In the case of the carotid artery, the amount of longitudinal retraction tends to increase during growth and to decrease in subsequent aging [5]. It would seem reasonable to assume that blood vessels are in a nearly stress-free state when they are fully retracted and free of external loads. This configuration also seems to be a reasonable choice for the reference configuration. However, this ignores residual stress and strain effects that have been the subject of current research [6–11].

Blood vessels are formed in a dynamic environment which gives rise to imbalances between the forces that tend to extend the diameter and length and the internal forces that tend to resist the extension. This imbalance is thought to stimulate the growth of elastin and collagen and to effectively reduce the stresses in the underlying tissue. Under these conditions it is not surprising that a residual stress state exists when the vessel is fully retracted and free of external tractions. This process has been called *remodeling* [7]. Striking evidence of this remodeling is found when a cylindrical slice of the fully retracted blood vessel is cut longitudinally through the wall. The cylinder springs open, releasing bending stresses kept in balance by the cylindrical geometry [11].

57.2 Vascular Anatomy

A blood vessel can be divided anatomically into three distinct cylindrical sections when viewed under the optical microscope. Starting at the inside of the vessel, they are the intima, the media, and the adventitia. These structures have distinct functions in terms of the blood vessel physiology and mechanical properties.

The intima consists of a thin monolayer of endothelial cells that line the inner surface of the blood vessel. The endothelial cells have little influence on blood vessel mechanics but do play an important role in hemodynamics and transport phenomena. Because of their anatomical location, these cells are subjected to large variations in stress and strain as a result of pulsatile changes in blood pressure and flow.

The media represents the major portion of the vessel wall and provides most of the mechanical strength necessary to sustain structural integrity. The media is organized into alternating layers of interconnected smooth muscle cells and elastic lamellae. There is evidence of collagen throughout the media. These small collagen fibers are found within the bands of smooth muscle and may participate in the transfer of forces between the smooth muscle cells and the elastic lamellae. The elastic lamellae are composed principally of the fiberous protein elastin. The number of elastic lamellae depends upon the wall thickness and the anatomical location [12]. In the case of the canine carotid, the elastic lamellae account for a major component of the static structural response of the blood vessel [13]. This response is modulated

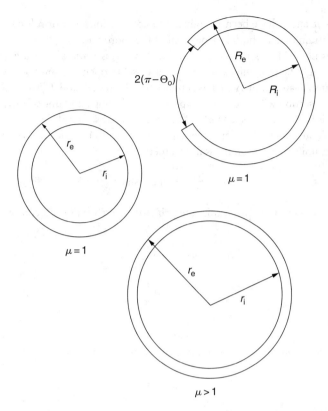

FIGURE 57.1 Cylindrical geometry of a blood vessel: *top:* stress-free reference configuration; *middle:* fully retracted vessel free of external traction; *bottom:* vessel *in situ* under longitudinal tether and internal pressurization.

by the smooth-muscle cells, which have the ability to actively change the mechanical characteristics of the wall [14].

The adventitia consists of loose, more disorganized fiberous connective tissue, which may have less influence on mechanics.

57.3   Axisymmetric Deformation

In the following discussion we will concern ourselves with deformation of cylindrical tubes, see Figure 57.1. Blood vessels tend to be nearly cylindrical *in situ* and tend to remain cylindrical when a cylindrical section is excised and studied *in vitro*. Only when the vessel is dissected further does the geometry begin to deviate from cylindrical. For this deformation there is a unique coordinate mapping

$$(R, \Theta, Z) \rightarrow (r, \theta, z) \tag{57.1}$$

where the undeformed coordinates are given by (R, Θ, Z) and the deformed coordinates are given by (r, θ, z). The deformation is given by a set of restricted functions

$$r = r(R) \tag{57.2}$$

$$\theta = \beta\Theta \tag{57.3}$$

$$z = \mu Z + C_1 \tag{57.4}$$

where the constants μ and β have been introduced to account for a uniform longitudinal strain and a symmetric residual strain that are both independent of the coordinate Θ.

If $\beta = 1$, there is no residual strain. If $\beta \neq 1$, residual stresses and strains are present. If $\beta > 1$, a longitudinal cut through the wall will cause the blood vessel to open up, and the new cross-section will form a c-shaped section of an annulus with larger internal and external radii. If $\beta < 1$, the cylindrical shape is unstable, but a thin section will tend to overlap itself. In Choung and Fung's formulation, $\beta = \pi/\Theta_o$, where the angle Θ_o is half the angle spanned by the open annular section [6].

For cylindrical blood vessels there are two assumed constraints. The first assumption is that the longitudinal strain is uniform through the wall and therefore

$$\lambda_z = \mu = \text{a constant} \tag{57.5}$$

for any cylindrical configuration. Given this, the principal stretch ratios are computed from the above function as

$$\lambda_r = \frac{dr}{dR} \tag{57.6}$$

$$\lambda_\theta = \beta \frac{r}{R} \tag{57.7}$$

$$\lambda_z = \mu \tag{57.8}$$

The second assumption is wall incompressibility, which can be expressed by

$$\lambda_r \lambda_\theta \lambda_z \equiv 1 \tag{57.9}$$

or

$$\beta \mu \frac{r}{R} \frac{dr}{dR} = 1 \tag{57.10}$$

and therefore

$$r\,dr = \frac{1}{\beta \mu} R\,dR \tag{57.11}$$

Integration of this expression yields the solution

$$r^2 = \frac{1}{\beta \mu} R^2 + c_2 \tag{57.12}$$

where

$$c_2 = r_e^2 - \frac{1}{\beta \mu} R_e^2 \tag{57.13}$$

As a result, the principal stretch ratios can be expressed in terms of R as follows:

$$\lambda_r = \frac{R}{\sqrt{\beta \mu (R^2 + \beta \mu c_2)}} \tag{57.14}$$

$$\lambda_\theta = \sqrt{\frac{1}{\beta \mu} + \frac{c_2}{R^2}} \tag{57.15}$$

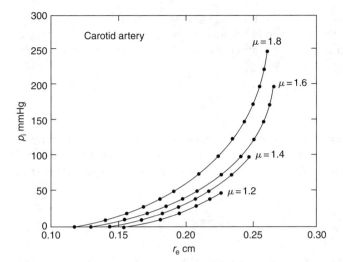

FIGURE 57.2 Pressure–radius curves for the canine carotid artery at various degrees of longitudinal extension.

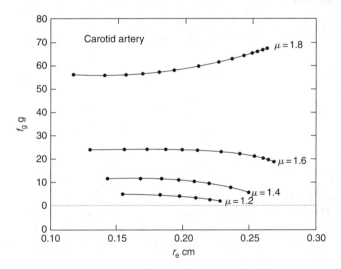

FIGURE 57.3 Longitudinal distending force as a function of radius at various degrees of longitudinal extension.

57.4 Experimental Measurements

The basic experimental setup required to measure the mechanical properties of blood vessels *in vitro* is described in Reference 14. It consists of a temperature-regulated bath of physiologic saline solution to maintain immersed cylindrical blood vessel segments, devices to measure diameter, an apparatus to hold the vessel at a constant longitudinal extension and to measure longitudinal distending force, and a system to deliver and control the internal pressure of the vessel with 100% oxygen. Typical data obtained from this type of experiment are shown in Figure 57.2 and Figure 57.3.

57.5 Equilibrium

When blood vessels are excised, they retract both longitudinally and circumferentially. Restoration to natural dimensions requires the application of internal pressure, p_i, and a longitudinal tether force,

F_T. The internal pressure and longitudinal tether are balanced by the development of forces within the vessel wall. The internal pressure is balanced in the circumferential direction by a wall tension, T. The longitudinal tether force and pressure are balanced by the retractive force of the wall, F_R

$$T = p_i r_i \tag{57.16}$$

$$F_R = F_T + p_i \pi r_i^2 \tag{57.17}$$

The first equation is the familiar law of Laplace for a cylindrical tube with internal radius r_i. It indicates that the force due to internal pressure, p_i, must be balanced by a tensile force (per unit length), T, within the wall. This tension is the integral of the circumferentially directed force intensity (or stress, σ_θ) across the wall:

$$T = \int_{r_i}^{r_e} \sigma_\theta \, dr = \bar{\sigma}_\theta h \tag{57.18}$$

where $\bar{\sigma}_\theta$ is the mean value of the circumferential stress and h is the wall thickness. Similarly, the longitudinal tether force, F_T, and extending force due to internal pressure are balanced by a retractive internal force, F_R, due to axial stress, σ_z, in the blood vessel wall:

$$F_R = 2\pi \int_{r_i}^{r_e} \sigma_z r \, dr = \bar{\sigma}_z \pi h (r_e + r_i) \tag{57.19}$$

where $\bar{\sigma}_z$ is the mean value of this longitudinal stress. The mean stresses are calculated from the above equation as

$$\bar{\sigma}_\theta = p_i \frac{r_i}{h} \tag{57.20}$$

$$\bar{\sigma}_z = \frac{F_T}{\pi h (r_e + r_i)} + \frac{p_i}{2} \frac{r_i}{h} \tag{57.21}$$

The mean stresses are a fairly good approximation for thin-walled tubes where the variations through the wall are small. However, the range of applicability of the thin-wall assumption depends upon the material properties and geometry. In a linear elastic material, the variation in σ_θ is less than 5% for $r/h > 20$. When the material is nonlinear or the deformation is large, the variations in stress can be more severe (see Figure 57.10).

The stress distribution is determined by solving the equilibrium equation,

$$\frac{1}{r} \frac{d}{dr} (r \sigma_r) - \frac{\sigma_\theta}{r} = 0 \tag{57.22}$$

This equation governs how the two stresses are related and must change in the cylindrical geometry. For uniform extension and internal pressurization, the stresses must be functions of a single radial coordinate, r, subject to the two boundary conditions for the radial stress:

$$\sigma_r(r_i, \mu) = -p_i \tag{57.23}$$

$$\sigma_r(r_e, \mu) = 0 \tag{57.24}$$

57.6 Strain Energy Density Functions

Blood vessels are able to maintain their structural stability and contain steady oscillating internal pressures. This property suggests a strong elastic component, which has been called the *pseudoelasticity* [4]. This elastic response can be characterized by a single potential function called the *strain energy density*. It is a scalar function of the strains that determines the amount of stored elastic energy per unit volume. In the case of a cylindrically orthotropic tube of incompressible material, the strain energy density can be written in the following functional form:

$$W = W^\star(\lambda_r, \lambda_\theta, \lambda_z) + \lambda_r \lambda_\theta \lambda_z p \tag{57.25}$$

where p is a scalar function of position, R. The stresses are computed from the strain energy by the following:

$$\sigma_i = \lambda_i \frac{\partial W^\star}{\partial \lambda_i} + p \tag{57.26}$$

We make the following transformation [15]

$$\lambda = \frac{\beta r}{\sqrt{\beta \mu (r^2 - c_2)}} \tag{57.27}$$

which upon differentiation gives

$$r \frac{d\lambda}{dr} = \beta^{-1}(\beta\lambda - \mu\lambda^3) \tag{57.28}$$

After these expressions and the stresses in terms of the strain energy density function are introduced into the equilibrium equation, we obtain an ordinary differential equation for p

$$\frac{dp}{d\lambda} = \frac{\beta W^\star_{,\lambda_\theta} - W^\star_{,\lambda_r}}{\beta\lambda = \mu\lambda^3} - \frac{dW^\star_{,\lambda_r}}{d\lambda} \tag{57.29}$$

subject to the boundary conditions

$$p(R_i) = p_i \tag{57.30}$$

$$p(R_e) = 0 \tag{57.31}$$

57.6.1 Isotropic Blood Vessels

A blood vessel generally exhibits anisotropic behavior when subjected to large variations in internal pressure and distending force. When the degree of anisotropy is small, the blood vessel may be treated as isotropic. For isotropic materials it is convenient to introduce the strain invariants:

$$I_1 = \lambda_r^2 + \lambda_\theta^2 + \lambda_z^2 \tag{57.32}$$

$$I_2 = \lambda_r^2\lambda_\theta^2 + \lambda_\theta^2\lambda_z^2 + \lambda_z^2\lambda_r^2 \tag{57.33}$$

$$I_3 = \lambda_r^2\lambda_\theta^2\lambda_z^2 \tag{57.34}$$

These are measures of strain that are independent of the choice of coordinates. If the material is incompressible

$$I_3 = j^2 \equiv 1 \tag{57.35}$$

and the strain energy density is a function of the first two invariants, then

$$W = W(I_1, I_2) \tag{57.36}$$

The least complex form for an incompressible material is the first-order polynomial, which was first proposed by Mooney to characterize rubber:

$$W^* = \frac{G}{2}[(I_1 - 3) + k(I_2 - 3)] \tag{57.37}$$

It involves only two elastic constants. A special case, where $k = 0$, is the neo-Hookean material, which can be derived from thermodynamics principles for a simple solid. Exact solutions can be obtained for the cylindrical deformation of a thick-walled tube. In the case where there is no residual strain, we have the following:

$$P = -G(1 + k\mu^2)\left[\frac{\log \lambda}{\mu} + \frac{1}{2\mu^2\lambda^2}\right] + c_0 \tag{57.38}$$

$$\sigma_r = G\left[\frac{1}{\lambda^2\mu^2} + k\left(\frac{1}{\mu^2} + \frac{1}{\lambda^2}\right)\right] + p \tag{57.39}$$

$$\sigma_\theta = G\left[\lambda^2 + k\left(\frac{1}{\mu^2} + \lambda^2\mu^2\right)\right] + p \tag{57.40}$$

$$\sigma_z = G\left[\mu^2 + k\left(\lambda^2\mu^2 + \frac{1}{\lambda^2}\right)\right] + p \tag{57.41}$$

However, these equations predict stress softening for a vessel subjected to internal pressurization at fixed lengths, rather than the stress stiffening observed in experimental studies on arteries and veins (see Figure 57.4 and Figure 57.5).

An alternative isotropic strain energy density function which can predict the appropriate type of stress stiffening for blood vessels is an exponential where the arguments is a polynomial of the strain invariants.

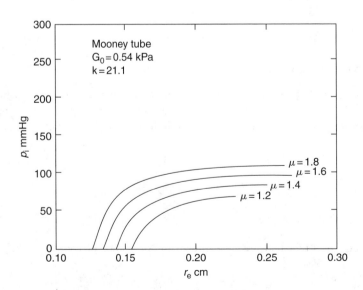

FIGURE 57.4 Pressure–radius curves for a Mooney–Rivlin tube with the approximate dimensions of the carotid.

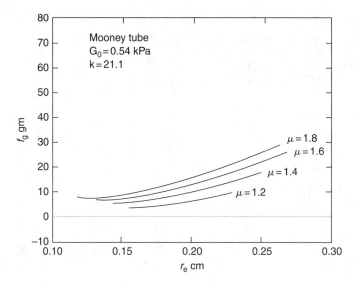

FIGURE 57.5   Longitudinal distending force as a function of radius for the Mooney–Rivlin tube.

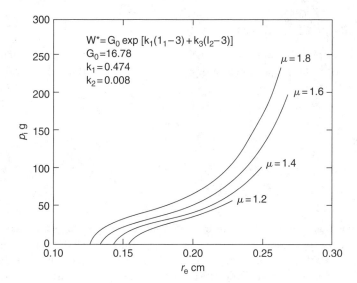

FIGURE 57.6   Pressure–radius curves for tube with the approximate dimensions of the carotid calculated using an isotropic exponential strain energy density function.

The first-order form is given by

$$W^\star = \frac{G_0}{2k_1} \exp[k_1(I_1 - 3) + k_2(I_2 - 3)] \tag{57.42}$$

This requires the determination of only two independent elastic constants. The third, G_0, is introduced to facilitate scaling of the argument of the exponent (see Figure 57.6 and Figure 57.7). This exponential form is attractive for several reasons. It is a natural extension of the observation that biologic tissue stiffness is proportional to the load in simple elongation. This stress stiffening has been attributed to a statistical recruitment and alignment of tangled and disorganized long chains of proteins. The exponential forms resemble statistical distributions derived from these same arguments.

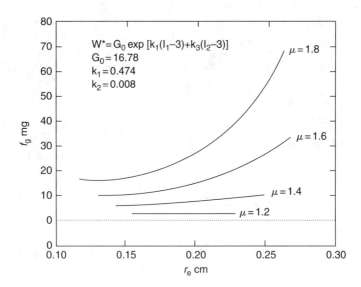

FIGURE 57.7   Longitudinal distending force as a function of radius for the isotropic tube.

57.6.2 Anisotropic Blood Vessels

Studies of the orthotropic behavior of blood vessels may employ polynomial or exponential strain energy density functions that include all strain terms or extension ratios. In particular, the strain energy density function can be of the form

$$W^\star = q_n(\lambda_r, \lambda_\theta, \lambda_z) \tag{57.43}$$

or

$$W^\star = e^{q_n(\lambda_r, \lambda_\theta, \lambda_z)} \tag{57.44}$$

where q_n is a polynomial of order n. Since the material is incompressible, the explicit dependence upon λ_r can be eliminated either by substituting $\lambda_r = \lambda_\theta^{-1}\lambda_z^{-1}$ or by assuming that the wall is thin and hence that the contribution of these terms is small. Figure 57.8 and Figure 57.9 illustrate how well the experimental data can be fitted to an exponential strain density function whose argument is a polynomial of order $n = 3$.

Care must be taken to formulate expressions that will lead to stresses that behave properly. For this reason it is convenient to formulate the strain energy density in terms of the Lagrangian strains

$$e_i = 1/2(\lambda_i^2 - 1) \tag{57.45}$$

and in this case we can consider polynomials of the lagrangian strains, $q_n(e_r, e_\theta, e_z)$.

Vaishnav et al. [16] proposed using a polynomial of the form

$$W^\star = \sum_{i=2}^{n}\sum_{j=0}^{i} a_{ij-i} e_\theta^{i-j} e_z^j \tag{57.46}$$

to approximate the behavior of the canine aorta. They found better correlation with order-three polynomials over order-two, but order-four polynomials did not warrant the addition work.

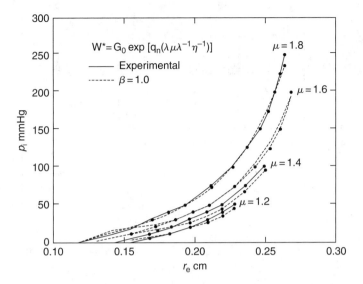

FIGURE 57.8 Pressure–radius curves for a fully orthotropic vessel calculated with an exponential strain energy density function.

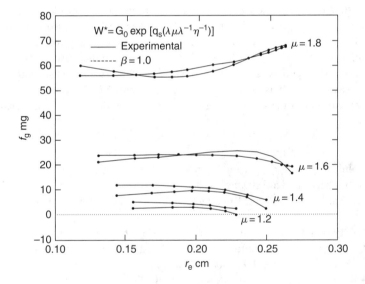

FIGURE 57.9 Longitudinal distending force as a function of radius for the orthotropic vessel.

Later, Fung et al. [4] found very good correlation with an expression of the form

$$W - \frac{C}{2} \exp[a_1(e_\theta^2 - e_z^{\star 2}) + a_2(e_z^2 - e_z^{\star 2}) + 2a_4(e_\theta e_z - e_\theta^\star e_z^\star)] \tag{57.47}$$

for the canine carotid artery, where $e_\theta^\star$ and $e_z^\star$ are the strains in a reference configuration at *in situ* length and pressure. Why should this work? One answer appears to be related to residual stresses and strains.

When residual stresses are ignored, large-deformation analysis of thick-walled blood vessels predicts steep distributions in σ_θ and σ_z through the vessel wall, with the highest stresses at the interior. This prediction is considered significant because high tensions in the inner wall could inhibit vascularization and oxygen transport to vascular tissue.

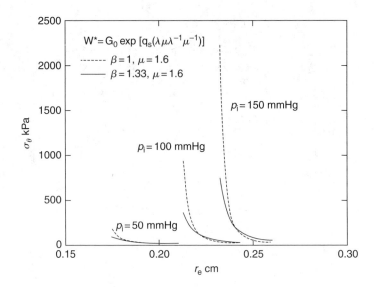

FIGURE 57.10 Stress distributions through the wall at various pressures for the orthotropic vessel.

When residual stresses are considered, the stress distributions flatten considerably and become almost uniform at *in situ* length and pressure. Figure 57.10 shows the radial stress distributions computed for a vessel with $\beta = 1$ and $\beta = 1.11$. Takamizawa and Hayashi have even considered the case where the strain distribution is uniform *in situ* [9]. The physiologic implications are that vascular tissue is in a constant state of flux. New tissue is synthesized in a state of stress that allows it to redistribute the internal loads more uniformly. There probably is no stress-free reference state [7,8,17]. Continuous dissection of the tissue into smaller and smaller pieces would continue to relieve residual stresses and strains [10].

References

[1] Von Maltzahn, W.-W., Desdo, D., and Wiemier, W. 1981. Elastic properties of arteries: a nonlinear two-layer cylindrical model. *J Biomech*. 4: 389.

[2] Carew, T.E., Vaishnav, R.N., and Patel, D.J. 1968. Compressibility of the arterial walls. *Circ. Res.* 23:61.

[3] Bergel, D.H. 1961. The static elastic properties of the arterial wall. *J. Physiol.* 156:445.

[4] Fung, Y.C., Fronek, K., and Patitucci, P. 1979. Pseudoelasticity of arteries and the choice of its mathematical expression. *Am. J. Physiol.* 237:H620.

[5] Dobrin, P.B. 1978. Mechanical properties of arteries. *Physiol. Rev.* 58:397.

[6] Choung, C.J. and Fung, Y.C. 1986. On residual stresses in arteries. *J. Biomed. Eng.* 108:189.

[7] Fung, Y.C., Liu, S.Q., and Zhou, J.B. 1993. Remodeling of the constitutive equation while a blood vessel remodels itself under strain. *J. Biomech. Eng.* 115:453.

[8] Rachev, A., Greenwald, S., Kane, T., Moore, J., and Meister J.-J. 1994. Effects of age-related changes in the residual strains on the stress distribution in the arterial wall. In J. Vossoughi (Ed.), *Proceedings of the Thirteenth Society of Biomedical Engineering Recent Developments*, pp. 409–412, Washington, DC, University of District of Columbia.

[9] Takamizawa, K. and Hayashi, K. 1987. Strain energy density function and the uniform strain hypothesis for arterial mechanics. *J. Biomech.* 20:7.

[10] Vassoughi, J. 1992. Longitudinal residual strain in arteries. *Proceedings of the 11th South Biomed Engrg Conf*, Memphis, TN.

[11] Vaishnav, R.N. and Vassoughi, J. 1983. Estimation of residual stresses in aortic segments. In C.W. Hall (Ed.), *Biomedical Engineering II, Recent Developments*, pp. 330–333, New York, Pergamon Press.

[12] Wolinsky, H. and Glagov, S. 1969. Comparison of abdominal and thoracic aortic media structure in mammals. *Circ. Res.* 25:677.

[13] Dobrin, P.B. and Canfield, T.R. 1984. Elastase, collagenase, and the biaxial elastic properties of dog carotid artery. *Am. J. Physiol.* 2547:H124.

[14] Dobrin, P.B. and Rovick, A.A. 1969. Influence of vascular smooth muscle on contractile mechanics and elasticity of arteries. *Am. J. Physiol.* 217:1644.

[15] Chu, B.M. and Oka, S. 1973. Influence of longitudinal tethering on the tension in thick-walled blood vessels in equilibrium. *Biorheology* 10:517.

[16] Vaishnav, R.N., Young, J.T., Janicki, J.S., and Patel, D.J. 1972. Nonlinear anisotropic elastic properties of the canine aorta. *Biophys. J.* 12:1008.

[17] Dobrin, P.D., Canfield, T., and Sinha, S. 1975. Development of longitudinal retraction of carotid arteries in neonatal dogs. *Experientia* 31:1295.

[18] Doyle, J.M. and Dobrin, P.B. 1971. Finite deformation of the relaxed and contracted dog carotid artery. *Microvasc. Res.* 3:400.

58

The Venous System

Artin A. Shoukas
Johns Hopkins University School of Medicine

Carl F. Rothe
Indiana University

The venous system not only serves as a conduit for the return of blood from the capillaries to the heart but also provides a dynamic, variable blood storage compartment that influences cardiac output. The systemic (noncardiopulmonary) venous system contains more than 75% of the blood volume of the entire systemic circulation. Although the heart is the source of energy for propelling blood throughout the circulation, filling of the right heart before the subsequent beat is primarily passive. The subsequent amount of blood ejected is exquisitely sensitive to the transmural filling pressure (e.g., a change of right heart filling pressure of 1 cm water can cause the cardiac output to change by about 50%).

Because the blood vessels are elastic and have smooth muscle in their walls, contraction or relaxation of the smooth muscle can quickly redistribute blood between the periphery and the heart to influence cardiac filling and thus cardiac output. Even though the right ventricle is not essential for life, its functioning acts to reduce the central venous pressure to facilitate venous return [1]. It largely determines the magnitude of the cardiac output by influencing the degree of filling of the left heart. Dynamic changes in venous tone, by redistributing blood volume, can thus, at rest, change cardiac output over a range of more than ±20%. The dimensions of the vasculature influence both blood flow — by way of their resistive properties — and contained blood volume — by way of their capacitive properties. The arteries have about 10 times the resistance of the veins, and the veins are more than 10 times as compliant as the arteries.

The conduit characteristics of the venous system primarily depend on the anatomy of the system. Valves in the veins of the limbs are crucial for reducing the pressure in dependent parts of the body. Even small movements from skeletal muscle activity tend to compress the veins and move blood toward the heart. A competent valve then blocks back flow, thus relieving the pressure when the movement stops. Even a few steps can reduce the transmural venous pressure in the ankle from as much as 100 mmHg to about 20 mmHg. Without this mechanism, transcapillary movement of fluid into the extravascular spaces results in edema. Varicose (swollen) veins and peripheral pooling of blood can result from damage to the venous valves. During exercise, the rhythmic contraction of the skeletal muscles, in conjunction with venous valves, provides an important mechanism — the skeletal muscle pump — aiding the large increases in blood flow through the muscles without excessive increases in capillary pressure and blood pooling in the veins of the muscles. Without this mechanism, the increase in venous return leading to the dramatic increases in cardiac output would be greatly limited.

58.1   Definitions

58.1.1   Capacitance

Capacitance is a general term that relates the magnitude of contained volume to the transmural pressure across the vessel walls and is defined by the pressure–volume relationship. In living blood vessels, the pressure–volume relationship is complex and nonlinear. At transmural pressure near zero, there is a finite volume within the vessels (see definition of *unstressed volume*). If this volume is then removed from the vessels, there is only a small decrease in transmural pressure as the vessel collapses from a circular cross-section to an elliptical one. This is especially true for superficial or isolated venous vessels. However, for vessels which are tethered or embedded in tissue a negative pressure may result without appreciably changing the shape of the vessels. With increases in contained volume, the vessel becomes distended, and there is a concomitant increase in transmural pressure. The incremental change in volume to incremental change in transmural pressure is often relatively constant. At very high transmural pressures vessels become stiffer, and the incremental volume change to transmural pressure change is small. Because all blood vessels exhibit these nonlinearities, no single parameter can describe capacitance; instead the entire pressure-volume relationship must be considered.

58.1.2   Compliance

Vascular compliance (C) is defined as the slope of the pressure-volume relationship. It is the ratio of the change in incremental volume (ΔV) to a change in incremental transmural pressure (ΔP). Thus $C = \Delta V / \Delta P$. Because the pressure-volume relationship is nonlinear, the slope of the relationship is not constant over its full range of pressures, and so the compliance should be specified at a given pressure. Units of compliance are those of volume divided by pressure, usually reported in ml/mmHg. Values are typically normalized to wet tissue weight or to total body weight. When the compliance is normalized by the total contained blood volume, it is termed the *vascular distensibility* and represents the fractional change in volume ($\Delta V / V$) per change in transmural pressure; $D = (\Delta V / V)\, \Delta P$, where V is the volume at control or at zero transmural pressure.

58.1.3   Unstressed Volume

Unstressed volume (V_0) is the volume in the vascular system when the transmural pressure is zero. It is a calculated volume obtained by extrapolating the relatively linear segment of the pressure-volume relationship over the normal operating range to zero transmural pressure. Many studies have shown that reflexes and drugs have quantitatively more influence on V_0 than on the compliance.

58.1.4   Stressed Volume

The *stressed volume* (V_s) is the volume of blood in the vascular system that must be removed to change the computed transmural pressure from its prevailing value to zero transmural pressure. It is computed as the product of the vascular compliance and transmural distending pressure: $V_s = C \times P$. The total contained blood volume at a specific pressure (P) is the sum of stressed and unstressed volume. The unstressed volume is then computed as the total blood volume minus the stressed volume. Because of the marked nonlinearity around zero transmural pressure and the required extrapolation, both V_0 and V_s are virtual volumes.

58.1.5 Capacity

Capacity refers to the amount of blood volume contained in the blood vessels at a specific distending pressure. It is the sum of the unstressed volume and the stressed volume, $V = V_0 + V_s$.

58.1.6 Mean Filling Pressure

If the inflow and outflow of an organ are suddenly stopped, and blood volume is redistributed so that all pressures within the vasculature are the same, this pressure is the *mean filling pressure* [2]. This pressure can be measured for the systemic or pulmonary circuits or the body as a whole. The arterial pressure often does not equal the venous pressure as flow is reduced to zero, because blood must move from the distended arterial vessels to the venous beds during the measurement maneuver, and flow may stop before equilibrium occurs. This is because smooth-muscle activity in the arterial vessels, rheological properties of blood, or high interstitial pressures act to impede the flow. Thus corrections must often be made [2,3]. The experimentally measured mean filling pressure provides a good estimate of P_v (the pressure in the minute venules), for estimating venous stressed volume.

58.1.7 Venous Resistance

Venous resistance (R) refers to the hindrance to blood flow through the venous vasculature caused by friction of the moving blood along the venous vascular wall. By definition it is the ratio of the pressure gradient between the entrance of the venous circulation, namely the capillaries, and the venous outflow divided by the venous flow rate. Thus

$$R = \frac{(P_c = P_{ra})}{F} \tag{58.1}$$

where R is the venous resistance, P_c is the capillary pressure, P_{ra} is the right atrial pressure, and F is the venous flow. As flow is decreased to zero, arterial closure may occur, leading to a positive perfusion pressure at zero flow. With partial collapse of veins, a Starling resistor like condition is present in which an increase in outlet pressure has no influence on flow until the outlet pressure is greater than the "waterfall" pressure.

58.1.8 Venous Inertance

Venous inertance (I_v) is the opposition to a change in flow rate related to the mass of the bolus of blood that is accelerated or decelerated. The inertance I_v for a cylindrical tube with constant cross-sectional area is $I_v = L\rho/A$, where L is the length of the vessel, ρ is the density of the blood, and A is the cross-sectional area [4].

58.2 Methods to Measure Venous Characteristics

Our knowledge of the nature and role of the capacitance characteristics of the venous system has been limited by the difficulty of measuring the various variables needed to compute parameter values. State-of-the-art equipment is often needed because of the low pressures and many disturbing factors present. Many of the techniques that have been used to measure venous capacitance require numerous assumptions that may not be correct or are currently impossible to evaluate [3].

58.2.1 Resistance

For the estimate of vascular resistance, the upstream to outflow pressure gradient across the tissues must be estimated along with a measure of flow. Pressures in large vessels are measured with a catheter connected to a pressure transducer, which typically involves measurement of minute changes in resistance elements attached to a stiff diaphragm which flexes proportionally to the pressure. For the veins in tissue, the upstream pressure, just downstream from the capillaries, is much more difficult to measure because of the minute size ($\sim$15 μm) of the vessels. For this a servo-null micropipette technique may be used. A glass micropipette with a tip diameter of about 2 μm is filled with a 1 to 2 mol saline solution. When the pipette is inserted into a vein, the pressure tends to drive the lower conductance blood plasma into the pipette. The conductance is measured using an AC-driven bridge. A servosystem, driven by the imbalance signal, is used to develop a counter pressure to maintain the interface between the low-conductance filling solution and the plasma near the tip of the pipette. This counter pressure, which equals the intravascular pressure, is measured with a pressure transducer. Careful calibration is essential.

Another approach for estimating the upstream pressure in the veins is to measure the mean filling pressure of the organ (see above) and assume that this pressure is the upstream venous pressure. Because this venous pressure must be less than the capillary pressure and because most of the blood in an organ is in the small veins and venules, this assumption, though tenuous, is not unreasonable. To measure flow many approaches are available including electromagnetic, transit-time ultrasonic, or Doppler ultrasonic flowmeters. Usually the arterial inflow is measured with the assumption that the outflow is the same. Indicator dilution techniques are also used to estimate average flow. They are based on the principle that the reduction in concentration of infused indicator is inversely proportional to the rate of flow. Either a bolus injection or a continuous infusion may be used. Adequacy of mixing of indicator across the flow stream, lack of collateral flows, and adequately representative sampling must be considered [5].

58.2.2 Capacitance

For estimating the capacitance parameters of the veins, contained volume, rather than flow, and transmural pressure, rather than the longitudinal pressure gradient, must be measured. Pressures are measured as described above. For the desired pressure-volume relationship the total contained volume must be known.

Techniques used to measure total blood volume include *indicator dilution.* The ratio of the integral of indicator concentration time to that of concentration is used to compute the mean transit time (MIT) following the sudden injection of a bolus of indicator [3,5]. The active volume is the product of MTT and flow, with flow measured as outlined above. Scintigraphy provides an image of the distribution of radioactivity in tissues. A radioisotope, such as technicium 99 that is bound to red blood cells which in turn are contained within the vasculature, is injected and allowed to equilibrate. A camera, with many collimating channels sensitive to the emitted radiation, is placed over the tissue. The activity recorded is proportional to the volume of blood. Currently it is not possible to accurately calibrate the systems to provide measures of blood volume because of uncertain attenuation of radiation by the tissue and distance. Furthermore, delimiting a particular organ within the body and separating arterial and venous segments of the circulation are difficult.

58.2.3 Compliance

To estimate compliance, changes in volume are needed. This is generally easier than measuring the total blood volume. Using *plethysmography,* a rigid container is placed around the organ, and a servo system functions to change the fluid volume in the chamber to maintain the chamber pressure-constant. The consequent volume change is measured and assumed to be primarily venous, because most of the vascular volume is venous. With a tight system and careful technique, at the end of the experiment both inflow and outflow blood vessels can be occluded and then the contained blood washed out and measured to provide a measure of the total blood volume [6].

58.2.4 Gravimetric Techniques

Gravimetric techniques can be used to measure changes in blood volume. If the organ can be isolated and weighed continuously with the blood vessels intact, changes in volume can be measured in response to drugs or reflexes. With an important modification, this approach can be applied to an organ or the systemic circulation; the tissues are perfused at a constant rate, and the outflow is emptied at a constant pressure into a reservoir. Because the reservoir is emptied at a constant rate for the perfusion, changes in reservoir volume reflect an opposite change in the perfused tissue blood volume [7]. To measure compliance, the outflow pressure is changed (2 to 5 mmHg) and the corresponding change in reservoir volume noted. With the inflow and outflow pressure held constant, the pressure gradients are assumed to be constant so that 100% of an outflow pressure change can be assumed to be transmitted to the primary capacitance vessels. Any reflex or drug-induced change in reservoir volume may be assumed to be inversely related to an active change in vascular volume [7–9]. If resistances are also changed by the reflex or drug, then corrections are needed and the interpretations are more complex.

58.2.5 Outflow Occlusion

If the outflow downstream from the venous catheter is suddenly occluded, the venous pressure increases, and its rate of increase is measured. The rate of inflow is also measured so that the compliance can be estimated as the ratio flow to rate of pressure rise: Compliance in ml/mmHg = (flow in ml/min)/(rate of venous pressure rise in mmHg/min). The method is predicated on the assumption that the inflow continues at a constant rate and that there is no pressure gradient between the pressure measuring point and the site of compliance for the first few seconds of occlusion when the rate of pressure rise is measured.

58.2.6 Integral of Inflow Minus Outflow

With this technique both inflow and outflow are measured and the difference integrated to provide the volume change during an experimental forcing. If there is a decrease in contained volume, the outflow will be transiently greater than the inflow. The volume change gives a measure of the response to drugs or reflexes. Following a change in venous pressure, the technique can be used to measure compliance. Accurate measures of flow are needed. Serious errors can result if the inflow is not measured but is only assumed to be constant during the experimental protocol. With all methods dependent on measured or controlled flow, small changes in zero offset, which is directly or indirectly integrated, leads to serious error after about 10 min, and so the methods are not useful for long-term or slow responses.

58.3 Typical Values

Cardiac output, the sine qua non of the cardiovascular system, averages about 100 ml/(min-kg). It is about 90 in humans, is over 110 ml/(min-kg) in dogs and cats, and is even higher on a body weight basis in small animals such as rats and mice. The mean arterial blood pressure in relaxed, resting, conscious mammals averages about 90 mmHg. The mean circulatory filling pressure averages about 7 mmHg, and the central venous pressure just outside the right heart about 2 mmHg. The blood volume of the body is about 75 ml/kg, but in humans it is about 10% less, and it is larger in small animals. It is difficult to measure accurately because the volume of distribution of the plasma is about 10% higher than that of the red blood cells.

Vascular compliance averages about 2 ml (mmHg-kg body weight). The majority is in the venules and veins. Arterial compliance is only about 0.05 ml/mmHg-kg. Skeletal muscle compliance is less than that of the body as a whole, whereas the vascular compliance of the liver is about 10 times that of other organs. The stressed volume is the product of compliance and mean filling pressure and so is about 15 ml/kg. By difference, the unstressed volume is about 60 ml/kg.

As flow is increased through a tissue, the contained volume increases even if the outflow pressure is held constant, because there is a finite pressure drop across the veins which is increased as flow increases. This increase in upstream distending pressure acts to increase the contained blood volume. The volume sensitivity to flow averages about 0.1 ml per 1 ml/min change in flow [10]. For the body as a whole, the sensitivity is about 0.25 ml per 1 ml/min with reflexes blocked, and with reflexes intact it averages about 0.4 ml/min^3. Using similar techniques, it appears that the passive compensatory volume redistribution from the peripheral toward the heart during serious left heart failure is similar in magnitude to a reflex-engendered redistribution from activation of venous smooth muscle [6].

The high-pressure carotid sinus baroreceptor reflex system is capable of changing the venous capacitance [9]. Over the full operating range of the reflex it is capable of mobilizing up to 7.5 ml/kg of blood by primarily changing the unstressed vascular volume with little or no changes in venous compliance [7,8]. Although this represents only a 10% change in blood volume, it can cause nearly a 100% change in cardiac output. It is difficult to say with confidence what particular organ and/or tissue is contributing to this blood volume mobilization. Current evidence suggests that the splanchnic vascular bed contributes significantly to the capacitance change, but this also may vary between species [11].

Acknowledgments

This work was supported by National Heart Lung and Blood Institute grants HL 19039 and HL 07723.

References

[1] Furey, S.A.I., Zieske, H., and Levy, M.N. 1984. The essential function of the right heart. *Am. Heart J.* 107: 404.

[2] Rothe, C.F. 1993. Mean circulatory filling pressure: its meaning and measurement. *J. Appl. Physiol.* 74: 499.

[3] Rothe, C.F. 1983. Venous system: physiology of the capacitance vessels. In J.T. Shepherd, and F.M. Abboud (Eds.), *Handbook of Physiology: The Cardiovascular System*, sec. 2, Vol 3, pt 1, pp. 397–452, Bethesda, MD, American Physiology Society.

[4] Rose, W. and Shoukas, A.A. 1993. Two-port analysis of systemic venous and arterial impedances. *Am. J. Physiol.* 265 (*Heart Circ. Physiol.* 34): H1577.

[5] Lassen, N.A. and Perl, W. 1979. *Tracer Kinetic Methods in Medical Physiology*. New York, Raven Press.

[6] Zink, J., Delaive, J., Mazerall, E., and Greenway, C.V. 1976. An improved plethsmograph with servo control of hydrostatic pressure. *J. Appl. Physiol.* 41: 107.

[7] Shoukas, A.A. and Sagawa, K. 1973. Control of total systemic vascular capacity by the carotid sinus baroreceptor reflex. *Circ. Res.* 33: 22.

[8] Shoukas, A.A., MacAnespie, C.L., Brunner, M.J. et al. 1981. The importance of the spleen in blood volume shifts of the systemic vascular bed caused by the carotid sinus baroreceptor reflex in the dog. *Circ. Res.* 49: 759.

[9] Shoukas, A.A. 1993. Overall systems analysis of the carotid sinus baroreceptor reflex control of the circulation. *Anesthesiology* 79: 1402.

[10] Rothe, C.F. and Gaddis, M.L. 1990. Autoregulation of cardiac output by passive elastic characteristics of the vascular capacitance system. *Circulation* 81: 360.

[11] Haase, E. and Shoukas, A.A. 1991. The role of the carotid sinus baroreceptor reflex on pressure and diameter relations of the microvasculature of the rat intestine. *Am. J. Physiol.* 260: H752.

[12] Numao, Y. and Iriuchijima J. 1977. Effect of cardiac output on circulatory blood volume. *Jpn. J. Physiol.* 27: 145.

59

Mechanics, Molecular Transport, and Regulation in the Microcirculation

Aleksander S. Popel
Johns Hopkins University

Roland N. Pittman
Medical College of Virginia

59.1 Introduction

The microcirculation is comprised of blood vessels (arterioles, capillaries, and venules) with diameters of less than approximately 150 μm. The importance of the microcirculation is underscored by the fact that most of the hydrodynamic resistance of the circulatory system lies in the microvessels (especially in arterioles) and most of the exchange of nutrients and waste products occurs at the level of the smallest microvessels. The subjects of microcirculatory research are blood flow and molecular transport in microvessels, mechanical interactions and molecular exchange between these vessels and the surrounding tissue, and regulation of blood flow and pressure and molecular transport. Quantitative knowledge of microcirculatory mechanics and mass transport has been accumulated primarily in the past 30 years owing to significant innovations in methods and techniques to measure microcirculatory parameters and methods to analyze microcirculatory data. The development of these methods has required joint efforts of physiologists and biomedical engineers. Key innovations include significant improvements in intra-vital microscopy, the dual-slit method (Wayland–Johnson) for measuring velocity in microvessels, the servo-null method (Wiederhielm–Intaglietta) for measuring pressure in microvessels, the recessed oxygen microelectrode (Whalen) for polarographic measurements of partial pressure of oxygen, and the micro-spectrophotometric method (Pittman–Duling) for measuring oxyhemoglobin saturation in microvessels. The single-capillary cannulation method (Landis–Michel) has provided a powerful tool for studies of transport of water and solutes through the capillary endothelium. In the last decade, new experimental techniques have appeared, many adapted from cell biology and modified for *in vivo* studies, that are having a tremendous impact on the field. Examples include confocal and multiphoton microscopy for better three-dimensional resolution of microvascular structures, methods of optical imaging using fluorescent labels (e.g., labeling blood cells for velocity measurements) and fluorescent dyes (e.g., calcium ion and nitric oxide sensitive dyes for measuring their dynamics in vascular smooth muscle, endothelium, and surrounding tissue cells *in vivo*), development of sensors (glass filaments, optical and magnetic tweezers) for measuring forces in the nanonewton range that are characteristic of cell–cell interactions, phosphorescence decay measurements as an indicator of oxygen tension, and methods of manipulating receptors on the surfaces of blood cells and endothelial cells. In addition to the dramatic developments in experimental techniques, quantitative knowledge and understanding of the microcirculation have been significantly enhanced by theoretical studies, perhaps having a larger impact than in other areas of physiology. Extensive theoretical work has been conducted on the mechanics of the red blood cell (RBC) and leukocyte; mechanics of blood flow in single microvessels and microvascular networks, oxygen (O_2), carbon dioxide (CO_2), and nitric oxide (NO) exchange between microvessels and surrounding tissue; and water and solute transport through capillary endothelium and the surrounding tissue [1,2]. These theoretical studies not only aid in the interpretation of experimental data, but in many cases also serve as a framework for quantitative testing of working hypotheses and as a guide in designing and conducting further experiments. The accumulated knowledge has led to significant progress in our understanding of mechanisms of regulation of blood flow and molecular exchange in the microcirculation in many organs and tissues under a variety of physiolo-gical and pathological conditions (e.g., hypoxia, hypertension, sickle cell anemia, diabetes, inflammation, hemorrhage, ischemia/reperfusion, sepsis, cancer). Discussions are under way to organize the enormous amount of information on the microcirculation in the form of a database or a network of databases encompassing anatomical and functional data, and conceptual (pathway) and computational models. This effort is referred to as the Microcirculation Physiome Project, a subset of the Physiome Project [3].

The goal of this chapter is to give an overview of the current status of research on the systemic microcirculation. Issues of pulmonary microcirculation are not discussed. Because of space limitations, it is not possible to recognize numerous important contributions to the field of microcirculatory mechanics and mass transport. In most cases we refer to recent reviews, when available, and journal articles where earlier references can be found. We discuss experimental and theoretical findings and point out gaps in our understanding of microcirculatory flow phenomena.

59.2 Mechanics of Microvascular Blood Flow

Vessel dimensions in the microcirculation are small enough so that the effects of the particulate nature of blood are significant [2]. Blood is a suspension of formed elements (red blood cells, white blood cells [leukocytes], and platelets) in plasma. Plasma is an aqueous solution of mostly proteins (albumin, globulins, and fibrinogen) and electrolytes. Under static conditions, human RBCs are biconcave discs with a diameter of approximately 7–9 μm. The main function of the RBC is delivery of O_2 to tissue. Most of the O_2 carried by the blood is chemically bound to hemoglobin inside the RBCs. The mammalian RBC is comprised of a viscoelastic membrane filled with a viscous fluid, concentrated hemoglobin solution. The membrane consists of the plasma membrane and underlying cytoskeleton. The membrane can undergo deformations without changing its surface area, which is nearly conserved locally. RBCs are so easily deformable that they can flow through small pores with a diameter of <3 μm. Leukocytes (grouped into several categories: granulocytes, monocytes, lymphocytes, macrophages, and phagocytes) are spherical cells with a diameter of approximately 10–20 μm. They are stiffer than RBCs. The main function of these cells is immunologic, that is, protection of the body against microorganisms causing disease. In contrast to mammalian RBCs, leukocytes are nucleated and are endowed with an internal structural cytoskeleton. Leukocytes are capable of active ameboid motion, the property which allows their migration from the blood stream into the tissue. Platelets are disc-shaped blood elements with diameter of approximately 2–3 μm. Platelets play a key role in thrombogenic processes and blood coagulation. The normal volume fraction of RBCs (hematocrit) in humans is 40–45%. The total volume of RBCs in blood is much greater than the volume of leukocytes and platelets. Rheological properties of blood in arterioles and venules and larger vessels are determined primarily by RBCs; however, leukocytes play an important mechanical role in capillaries and small venules.

Blood plasma is a Newtonian fluid with viscosity of approximately 1.2 cP. The viscosity of whole blood in a rotational viscometer or a large-bore capillary viscometer exhibits shear-thinning behavior, that is, viscosity decreases when shear rate increases. At shear rates >100 s^{-1} and a hematocrit of 40%, typical viscosity values are 3–4 cP. The dominant mechanism of the non-Newtonian behavior is RBC aggregation and the secondary mechanism is RBC deformation under shear forces. The cross-sectional distribution of RBCs in vessels is nonuniform, with a core of concentrated RBC suspension and a cell-free or cell-depleted marginal layer, typically 2–5 μm thick, adjacent to the vessel wall. The nonuniform RBC distribution results in the **Fahraeus effect** (the microvessel hematocrit is smaller than the feed or discharge hematocrit) due to the fact that, on the average, RBCs move with a higher velocity than blood plasma, and the concomitant **Fahraeus–Lindqvist effect** (the **apparent viscosity** of blood is lower than the bulk viscosity measured with a rotational viscometer or a large-bore capillary viscometer at a high shear rate). The **apparent viscosity** of a fluid flowing in a cylindrical vessel of radius R and length L under the influence of a pressure difference ΔP is defined as

$$\eta_a = \frac{\pi \Delta P R^4}{8QL}$$

where Q is the volumetric flow rate. For a Newtonian fluid the apparent viscosity becomes the dynamic viscosity of the fluid and the above equation represents **Poiseuille's Law**. The apparent viscosity is a function of hematocrit, vessel radius, blood flow rate, and other parameters. In the microcirculation, blood flows through a complex branching network of arterioles, capillaries, and venules. Arterioles are typically 10–150 μm in diameter, capillaries are 4–8 μm, and venules are 10–200 μm. Now we will discuss vascular wall mechanics and blood flow in vessels of different sizes in more detail.

59.2.1 Mechanics of the Microvascular Wall

The wall of arterioles is comprised of the intima that contains a single layer of contiguous endothelial cells, the media that contains a single layer of smooth muscle cells in terminal and medium-size arterioles or several layers in the larger arterioles, and the adventitia that contains collagen fibers with occasional fibroblasts and mast cells. Fibers situated between the endothelium and the smooth muscle cells comprise the basement membrane. The single layer of smooth muscle cells terminates at the capillaries and reappears at the level of small venules; the capillary wall is devoid of smooth muscle cells. Venules typically have a larger diameter and smaller wall thickness-to-diameter ratio than arterioles of the corresponding branching order.

Most of our knowledge of the mechanics of the microvascular wall comes from *in vivo* or *in vitro* measurements of vessel diameter as a function of transmural pressure [4]. Development of isolated microvessel preparations has made it possible to precisely control the transmural pressure during experiments. In addition, these preparations allow one to separate the effects of metabolic factors and blood flow rate from the effect of pressure by controlling both the chemical environment and the flow rate through the vessel. Arterioles and venules exhibit vascular tone, that is, their diameter is maximal when smooth muscle is completely relaxed (inactivated). When the vascular smooth muscle is constricted, small arterioles may even completely close their lumen to blood flow, presumably by buckling endothelial cells. Arterioles exhibit a **myogenic response** not observed in other blood vessels, with the exception of cerebral arteries: within a certain physiological pressure range the vessels constrict in response to elevation of transmural pressure and dilate in response to reduction of transmural pressure; in other words, in a certain range of pressures the slope of the pressure–diameter relationship is negative. Arterioles of different size exhibit different degrees of myogenic responsiveness. This effect has been documented in many tissues both *in vivo* and *in vitro* (in isolated arterioles) and has been shown to play an important role in regulation of blood flow and capillary pressure (see the section on Regulation of Blood Flow below).

The stress–strain relationship for a thin-walled microvessel can be derived from the experimentally obtained pressure–diameter relationship using the Law of Laplace. Stress in the vessel wall can be decomposed into passive and active components. The passive component corresponds to the state of complete vasodilation. The active component determines the vascular tone and the myogenic response. Steady-state stress–strain relationships are, generally, nonlinear. For arterioles, diameter variations of 50% or even 100% under physiological conditions are not unusual, so that finite deformations have to be considered in formulating the constitutive relationship for the wall (relationship between stress, strain, and their temporal derivatives). Pertinent to the question of microvascular mechanics is the mechanical interaction of a vessel with its environment, which consists of connective tissue, parenchymal cells, and extracellular fluid. There is ultrastructural evidence that blood vessels are tethered to the surrounding tissue, so that mechanical forces can be generated when the vessels constrict or dilate, or when the tissue is moving, for example, in contracting striated muscle, myocardium, or intestine. Little quantitative information is currently available about the magnitude of these forces, chiefly because of the difficulty of such measurements. Magnetic tweezers make it possible to probe the mechanics of the microvascular wall *in vivo* and its interaction with the surrounding tissue [5].

Under time-dependent conditions microvessels exhibit viscoelastic behavior. In response to a stepwise change in the transmural pressure, arterioles typically respond with a fast "passive" change in diameter followed by a slow "active" response with a characteristic time of the order of tens of seconds. For example, when the pressure is suddenly increased, the vessel diameter will quickly increase, with subsequent vasoconstriction that may result in a lower value of steady-state diameter than that prior to the increase in pressure. Therefore, to accurately describe the time-dependent vessel behavior, the constitutive relationship between stress and strain or pressure and diameter must also contain temporal derivatives of these variables. Theoretical analysis of the resulting nonlinear equations shows that such constitutive equations lead to predictions of spontaneous oscillations of vessel diameter (**vasomotion**) under certain conditions [6,7]. Theoretical analysis of Ca^{2+} oscillations in vascular smooth muscle cells also predicts spontaneous oscillations [8]. Vasomotion has been observed *in vivo* in various tissues and under various physiological conditions. Whether experimentally observed vasomotion and its effect on blood flow (flow motion) can be quantitatively described by the theoretical studies remains to be established. It should be noted that other mechanisms leading to spontaneous flow oscillations have been reported that are associated with blood rheology and not with vascular wall mechanics [9,10].

For most purposes, capillary compliance is not taken into account. However, in some situations, such as analysis of certain capillary water transport experiments or leukocyte motion in a capillary, this view is not adequate and capillary compliance has to be accounted for. Since the capillary wall is devoid of smooth muscle cells, much of this compliance is passive, and its magnitude is small. However, the presence of contractile proteins in the cytoskeleton of capillary endothelial cells and associated pericytes opens a possibility of active capillary constriction or dilation.

59.2.2 Capillary Blood Flow

Progress in this area is closely related to studies of mechanics of blood cells described elsewhere in this book. In narrow capillaries, RBCs flow in single file, separated by gaps of plasma. They deform and assume a parachute-like shape, generally non-axisymmetric, leaving a submicron plasma sleeve between the RBC and endothelium. In the smallest capillaries, their shape is sausage-like. The hemoglobin solution inside an RBC is a Newtonian fluid. The constitutive relationship for the membrane is accurately expressed by the Evans–Skalak finite-deformations model; molecular-based models considering spectrin, actin, and other RBC cytoskeleton constituents have also been formulated [11]. The coupled mechanical problem of membrane and fluid motion has been extensively investigated using both analytical and numerical approaches [12]. An important result of the theoretical studies is the prediction of the apparent viscosity of blood. While these predictions are in good agreement with *in vitro* studies in glass tubes, they underestimate a few available *in vivo* capillary measurements of apparent viscosity. In addition, *in vivo* capillary hematocrit in some tissues is lower than predicted from *in vitro* studies with tubes of the same size. To explain the low values of hematocrit, RBC interactions with the endothelial glycocalyx have been implicated [13]. Recent direct measurements of microvascular resistance and theoretical analyses provide further evidence of the role of the glycocalyx [14,15].

The motion of leukocytes through blood capillaries has also been studied thoroughly in recent years. Because leukocytes are larger and stiffer than RBCs, under normal flow conditions an increase in capillary resistance caused by a single leukocyte may be orders of magnitude greater than that caused by a single RBC [16]. Under certain conditions, flow stoppage may occur caused by leukocyte plugging. After a period of ischemia, red blood cell and leukocyte plugging may prevent tissue reperfusion (ischemia-reperfusion injury) [17]. Chemical bonds between membrane-bound receptors and endothelial adhesion molecules play a crucial role in leukocyte–endothelium interactions. Methods of cell and molecular biology permit manipulation of the receptors and thus make it possible to study leukocyte microcirculatory mechanics at the molecular level. More generally, methods of cell and molecular biology open new and powerful ways to study cell micromechanics and cell–cell interactions.

59.2.3 Arteriolar and Venular Blood Flow

The cross-sectional distribution of RBCs in arterioles and venules is nonuniform. A concentrated suspension of RBCs forms a core surrounded by a cell-free or cell-depleted layer of plasma. This "lubrication" layer of lower viscosity fluid near the vessel wall results in lower values of the apparent viscosity of blood compared to its bulk viscosity, resulting in the Fahraeus–Lindqvist effect [2,18]. There is experimental evidence that velocity profiles of RBCs are generally symmetric in arterioles, except very close to vascular bifurcations, but may be asymmetric in venules; the profiles are close to parabolic in arterioles at normal flow rates, but are blunted in venules [19,20]. Moreover, flow in the venules may be stratified as the result of converging blood streams that do not mix rapidly. The key to understanding the pattern of arteriolar and venular blood flow is the mechanics of flow at vascular bifurcations, diverging for arteriolar flow and converging for venular flow [21]. An important question is under what physiological or pathological conditions does RBC aggregation affect arteriolar and venular velocity distribution and vascular resistance. Much is known about aggregation *in vitro*, but *in vivo* knowledge is incomplete [2,18,22,23].

Problems of leukocyte distribution in the microcirculation and their interaction with the microvascular endothelium have attracted considerable attention in recent years [17]. Leukocyte rolling along the walls of venules, but not arterioles, has been demonstrated. This effect results from differences in the microvascular endothelium, mainly attributed to the differential expression of adhesion molecules on the endothelial surface [24]. Platelet distribution in the lumen is important because of platelets' role in blood coagulation. Detailed studies of platelet distribution in arterioles and venules show that the cross-sectional distribution of these disk-shaped blood elements is dependent on the blood flow rate and vessel hematocrit [25]; molecular details of platelet–endothelium interactions are available [26]. Considerable progress has been made in computational modeling of leukocytes in microvessels and their interaction with red blood cells [27–29].

To conclude, many important features of blood flow through arterioles and venules are qualitatively known and understood; however, a rigorous theoretical description of flow as a suspension of discrete particles is not yet available. Such description is necessary for a quantitative understanding of the mechanisms of the nonuniform distribution of blood cells in microvessels.

59.2.4 Microvascular Networks: Structure and Hemodynamics

Microvascular networks in different organs and tissues differ in their appearance and structural organization. Methods have been developed to quantitatively describe network architectonics and hemodynamics [30]. The microvasculature is an adaptable structure capable of changing its structural and functional characteristics in response to various stimuli [31]. **Angiogenesis**, rarefaction, and microvascular remodeling are important examples of this adaptive behavior that play important physiological and pathophysiological roles. Methods of fractal analysis have been applied to interpret experimental data on angioarchitecture and blood flow distribution in the microcirculation; these methods explore the property of geometrical and flow similarity that exist at different scales in the network [32]. Microvascular hydraulic pressure varies systematically between consecutive branching orders, decreasing from the systemic values down to 20–25 mmHg in the capillaries and decreasing further by 10–15 mmHg in the venules. Mean microvascular blood flow rate in arterioles decreases toward the capillaries, in inverse proportion to the number of "parallel" vessels, and increases from capillaries through the venules. In addition to this longitudinal variation of blood flow and pressure among different branching orders, there are significant variations among vessels of the same branching order, referred to as flow heterogeneity. The heterogeneity of blood flow and RBC distribution in microvascular networks has been well-documented in a variety of organs and tissues. This phenomenon may have important implications for tissue exchange processes, so significant efforts have been devoted to the quantitative analysis of blood flow in microvascular networks. A mathematical model of blood flow in a network can be formulated as follows: First, network topology or vessel interconnections have to be specified. Second, the diameter and length of every vascular segment have to be known. Alternatively, vessel diameter can be specified as a function of transmural pressure and perhaps some other parameters; these relationships are discussed in the preceding section on wall mechanics. Third, the apparent viscosity of blood has to be specified as a function of vessel diameter, local hematocrit, and shear rate. Fourth, a relationship between RBC flow rates and bulk blood flow rates at diverging bifurcations has to be specified; this relationship is often referred to as the "bifurcation law." Finally, at the inlet vessel branches boundary conditions have to be specified: bulk flow rate as well as RBC flow rate or hematocrit; alternatively, pressure can be specified at both inlet and outlet branches. This set of generally nonlinear equations can be solved to yield pressure at each bifurcation, blood flow rate through each segment, and discharge or microvessel hematocrit in each segment. These equations also predict vessel diameters if vessel compliance is taken into account. The calculated variables can then be compared with experimental data. Such a detailed comparison was reported for rat mesentery [30]. The authors found a good agreement between theoretical and experimental data when histograms of parameter distributions were compared, but poor agreement, particularly for vessel hematocrit, when comparison was done on a vessel-by-vessel basis. In these calculations, the expression for apparent viscosity was taken from *in vitro* experiments. The agreement was improved when the apparent viscosity was increased substantially from its *in vitro* values, particularly in the smallest vessels. Thus, a working hypothesis was put forward that *in vivo* apparent viscosity in small vessels is higher than the corresponding *in vitro* viscosity in glass tubes. Recent experimental and theoretical studies support this hypothesis and attribute the difference to the effect of the endothelial glycocalyx and its associated macromolecules, which are often referred to, collectively, as the endothelial surface layer (ESL) [14]. The ESL appears to be exquisitely controlled, and it is affected by a variety of biochemical and mechanical factors [33,34].

59.3 Molecular Transport in the Microcirculation

59.3.1 Transport of Oxygen, Carbon Dioxide, and Nitric Oxide

One of the most important functions of the microcirculation is the delivery of O_2 to tissue and the removal of waste products, particularly of CO_2, from tissue. O_2 is required for aerobic intracellular respiration for the production of adenosine triphosphate (ATP). CO_2 is produced as a by-product of these biochemical reactions. Tissue metabolic rate can change drastically, for example, in aerobic muscle in the transition from rest to exercise, which necessitates commensurate changes in blood flow and O_2 delivery. One of the major issues studied is how O_2 delivery is matched to O_2 demand under different physiological and pathological conditions. This question arises for short-term or long-term regulation of O_2 delivery in an individual organism, organ, or tissue, as well as in the evolutionary sense, in phylogeny. The hypothesis of symmorphosis, a fundamental balance between structure and function, has been formulated for the respiratory and cardiovascular systems and tested in a number of animal species [35].

In the smallest exchange vessels (capillaries and small arterioles and venules), O_2 molecules are released from hemoglobin inside RBCs, diffuse through the plasma, cross the endothelium, the extravascular space, and parenchymal cells until they reach mitochondria where they are utilized in the process of oxidative phosphorylation. The nonlinear relationship between hemoglobin saturation with O_2 and the local O_2 tension (PO_2) is described by the **oxyhemoglobin dissociation curve** (ODC). The theory of O_2 transport from capillaries to tissue was conceptually formulated by August Krogh in 1918 and it has dominated the thinking of physiologists for eight decades. The model he formulated considered a cylindrical tissue volume supplied by a single central capillary; this element was considered the building block for the entire tissue. A constant metabolic rate was assumed and PO_2 at the capillary–tissue interface was specified. The solution to the corresponding transport equation is the Krogh–Erlang equation describing the radial variation of O_2 tension in tissue. Over the years, the **Krogh Tissue Cylinder model** has been modified by many investigators to include transport processes in the capillary and PO_2-dependent consumption. However, in the past few years new conceptual models of O_2 transport have emerged. First, it was discovered experimentally and subsequently corroborated by theoretical analysis that capillaries are not the only source of oxygen, but arterioles (**precapillary O_2 transport**) and to a smaller extent venules (postcapillary O_2 transport), also participate in tissue oxygenation; in fact, a complex pattern of O_2 exchange may exist among arterioles, venules and adjacent capillary networks [36,37]. Second, theoretical analysis of intracapillary transport suggested that a significant part of the resistance to O_2 transport, on the order of 50%, is located within the capillary, primarily due to poor diffusive conductance of the plasma gaps between the erythrocytes. Third, the effect of **myoglobin-facilitated O_2 diffusion** in red muscle fibers and cardiac myocytes has been re-evaluated, however, its significance must await additional experimental studies. Fourth, geometric and hemodynamic heterogeneities in O_2 delivery have been quantified experimentally and modeled theoretically. Theoretical analyses of oxygen transport have been applied to a variety of tissues and organs [38–40]. One important emerging area of application of this knowledge is artificial oxygen carriers, hemoglobin-based and nonhemoglobin-based [41].

Transport of CO_2 is coupled to O_2 through the Bohr effect (effect of CO_2 tension on the blood O_2 content) and the Haldane effect (effect of PO_2 on the blood CO_2 content). Diffusion of CO_2 is faster than that of O_2 because CO_2 solubility in tissue is higher; theoretical studies predict that countercurrent exchange of CO_2 between arterioles and venules is of major importance so that equilibration of CO_2 tension with surrounding tissue should occur before capillaries are reached. Experiments are needed to test these theoretical predictions.

Nitric oxide (NO) is a diatomic gas that is enzymatically synthesized from l-arginine by several isoforms of NO synthase (NOS). The isoforms of NO synthase are divided into inducible NOS (iNOS or NOS2) and constitutive NOS (cNOS), based on their nondependent and dependent, respectively, control of activity from intracellular calcium/calmodulin. Constitutive NOS are further classified as neuronal NOS (nNOS or NOS1) and endothelial NOS (eNOS or NOS3). Nitric oxide plays an important role in both autocrine and paracrine manners in a myriad of physiological processes including regulation of blood pressure and blood flow, platelet aggregation and leukocyte adhesion. In smooth muscle cells, NO activates the enzyme soluble guanylate cyclase (sGC) that catalyzes the conversion of guanosine triphosphate (GTP) to cyclic guanosine monophosphate (cGMP), thus causing vasodilation [42]. Traditionally, eNOS has been considered the principal source of bioavailable microvascular NO under most physiological conditions. Evidence is mounting that nNOS expressed in nerve fibers, which innervate arterioles, together with nNOS positive mast cells are also major sources of NO [43]. NO produced by endothelial cells diffuses to vascular smooth muscle and to the flowing blood, where it rapidly reacts with hemoglobin in RBCs and free hemoglobin present in pathological conditions, such as sickle cell disease, or during administration of free hemoglobin as a blood substitute. Other non-neuronal cell types, including cardiac and skeletal myocytes, also express nNOS. Direct measurements of NO concentration in the microcirculation with high spatial resolution have been performed with porphyrinic-based microsensors and optical dyes. Mathematical models of NO transport have been developed that describe the transport of NO synthesized by eNOS and nNOS in and around microvessels [44–50]. In addition to the mechanism of free diffusion of NO, another mechanism has been proposed and is under intense scrutiny whereby NO reacts with thiols in blood to form long-lived *S*-nitrosothiols (SNOs) with vasodilatory activity [51]. No theoretical work has been attempted to simulate this mechanism.

59.3.2 Transport of Solutes and Water

The movement of solute molecules across the capillary wall occurs primarily by two mechanisms: diffusion and solvent drag. Diffusion is the passive mechanism of transport that rapidly and efficiently transports small solutes over the small distances (tens of microns) between the blood supply (capillaries) and tissue cells. Solvent drag refers to the movement of solute that is entrained in the bulk flow of fluid across the capillary wall and is generally negligible, except in cases of large molecules with small diffusivities and high transcapillary fluid flow.

The capillary wall is composed of a single layer of endothelial cells about 1 μm thick. Lipid soluble substances (e.g., O_2) can diffuse across the entire wall surface, whereas water soluble substances are restricted to small aqueous pathways equivalent to cylindrical pores 8 to 9 nm in diameter (e.g., glucose in most capillaries; in capillaries with tight junctions and few fenestrations (brain, testes), glucose is predominantly transported). Total pore area is about 0.1% of the surface area of a capillary. The permeability of the capillary wall to a particular substance depends upon the relative size of the substance and the pore ("restricted" diffusion). The efficiency of diffusive exchange can be increased by increasing the number of perfused capillaries (e.g., heart and muscle tissue from rest to exercise), since this increases the surface area available for exchange and decreases the distances across which molecules must diffuse.

The actual pathways through which small solutes traverse the capillary wall appear to be in the form of clefts between adjacent endothelial cells. Rather than being open slits, these porous channels contain a matrix of small cylindrical fibers (primarily glycosaminoglycans) that occupy about 5% of the volume of these pathways. The permeability properties of the capillary endothelium are modulated by a number of factors, among which are plasma protein concentration and composition, rearrangement of the endothelial cell glycocalyx, calcium influx into the endothelial cell, and endothelial cell membrane potential. Many of the studies that have established our current understanding of the endothelial exchange barrier have been carried out on single perfused capillaries in the frog and in mammalian tissues [52,53]. There could be, in addition to the porous pathways, nonporous pathways that involve selective uptake of solutes and subsequent transcellular transport (of particular importance in endothelium barriers). In order to study such pathways, one must try to minimize the contributions to transcapillary transport from solvent drag.

The processes whereby water passes back and forth across the capillary wall are called filtration and absorption. The flow of water depends upon the relative magnitude of hydraulic and osmotic pressures across the capillary wall and is described quantitatively by the Kedem–Katchalsky equations (the particular form of the equations applied to capillary water transport is referred to as **Starling's Law**). Recently, the physical mechanism of Starling's Law has been re-assessed [54]. Overall, in the steady state there is an approximate balance between hydraulic and osmotic pressures which leads to a small net flow of water. Generally, more fluid is filtered than is reabsorbed; the overflow is carried back to the vascular system by the lymphatic circulation. The lymphatic network is composed of a large number of small vessels, the terminal branches of which are closed. Flap valves (similar to those in veins) ensure unidirectional flow of lymph back to the central circulation. The smallest (terminal) vessels are very permeable, even to proteins that occasionally leak from systemic capillaries. Lymph flow is determined by interstitial fluid pressure and the lymphatic "pump" (oneway flap valves and skeletal muscle contraction). Control of interstitial fluid protein concentration is one of the most important functions of the lymphatic system. If more net fluid is filtered than can be removed by the lymphatics, the volume of interstitial fluid increases.

This fluid accumulation is called edema. This circumstance is important clinically since solute exchange (e.g., O_2) decreases due to the increased diffusion distances produced when the accumulated fluid pushes the capillaries, tethered to the interstitial matrix, away from each other.

59.4   Regulation of Blood Flow

The cardiovascular system controls blood flow to individual organs (1) by maintaining arterial pressure within narrow limits and (2) by allowing each organ to adjust its vascular resistance to blood flow so that each receives an appropriate fraction of the cardiac output. There are three major mechanisms that control the function of the cardiovascular system: neural, humoral, and local [55]. The sympathetic nervous system and circulating hormones both provide overall vasoregulation, and thus coarse flow control, to all vascular beds. The local mechanisms provide finer regional control within a tissue, usually in response to local changes in tissue activity or local trauma. The three mechanisms can work independently of each other, but there are also interactions among them.

The classical view of blood flow control involved the action of vasomotor influences on a set of vessels called the "resistance vessels," generally arterioles and small arteries smaller than about 100 to 150 μm in diameter, which controlled flow to and within an organ [56]. The notion of "precapillary sphincters" that control flow in individual capillaries has been abandoned in favor of the current notion that the terminal arterioles control the flow in small capillary networks that branch off of these arterioles. In recent years, it has become clear that the resistance to blood flow is distributed over a wider range of vessel branching orders with diameters up to 500 μm. There are mechanisms to be discussed in Section 59.4.2 that are available for coordinating the actions of local control processes over wider regions.

59.4.1   Neurohumoral Regulation of Blood Flow

The role of neural influences on the vasculature varies greatly from organ to organ. Although all organs receive sympathetic innervation, regulation of blood flow in the cerebral and coronary vascular beds occurs mostly through intrinsic local (metabolic) mechanisms. The circulations in skeletal muscle, skin, and some other organs, however, are significantly affected by the sympathetic nerves. In general, the level of intrinsic myogenic activity and sympathetic discharge sets the state of vascular smooth muscle contraction (basal vascular tone) and hence vascular resistance in organs. This basal tone is modulated by circulating and local vasoactive influences, for example, endothelium-derived relaxing factor (EDRF), identified as nitric oxide, endothelium-derived hyperpolarizing factor (EDHF) [57], prostacyclin (PGI_2), endothelin, and vasoactive substances released from parenchymal cells.

59.4.2   Local Regulation of Blood Flow

In addition to neural and humoral mechanisms for regulating the function of the cardiovascular system, there are mechanisms intrinsic to the various tissues that can operate independently of neurohumoral influences. The site of local regulation is the microcirculation. Examples of local control processes are autoregulation of blood flow, reactive hyperemia, and active (or functional) hyperemia. The mechanisms of local regulation have been identified as (1) the myogenic mechanism based on the ability of vascular smooth muscle to actively contract in response to stretch; (2) the metabolic mechanism, based on a link between blood flow and tissue metabolism; (3) the flow-dependent mechanism, primarily based on the release of NO by endothelial cells in response to shear forces. The effects are coordinated and integrated in the microvascular network via chemical and electrical signals propagating through gap junctions. Experimental evidence and theoretical models are discussed in [55,56,58–60].

Cells have a continuous need for O_2 and also continuously produce metabolic wastes, some of which are vasoactive (usually vasodilators). Under normal conditions there is a balance between O_2 supply and demand, but imbalances give rise to adjustments in blood flow that bring supply back into register with demand. Consider exercising skeletal muscle as an example. With the onset of exercise, metabolite production and O_2 requirements increase. The metabolites diffuse away from their sites of production and reach the vasculature. Vasodilation ensues, lowering resistance to blood flow. The resulting increase in blood flow increases the O_2 supply and finally a new steady state is achieved in which O_2 supply and demand are matched. This scenario operates for other tissues in which metabolic activity changes.

The following O_2-linked metabolites have been implicated as potential chemical mediators in the metabolic hypothesis: adenosine (from ATP hydrolysis: ATP $\rightarrow$ ADP $\rightarrow$ AMP $\rightarrow$ adenosine), H^+, and lactate (from lactic acid generated by glycolysis). Their levels are increased when there is a reduction in O_2 supply relative to demand (i.e., tissue hypoxia). The production of more CO_2 as a result of increased tissue activity (leading to increased oxidative metabolism) leads to vasodilation through increased H^+ concentration. Increased potassium ion and interstitial fluid osmolarity (i.e., more osmotically active particles) transiently cause vasodilation under physiological conditions associated with increased tissue activity.

It has also been established that the RBC itself could act as a mobile sensor for hypoxia [61]. The mechanism works as follows: Under conditions of low oxygen and pH, the RBC releases ATP, which binds to purinergic receptors on the endothelial cells. This leads to the production in the endothelial cells of the vasodilator NO. Since the most likely location for hypoxia would be in or near the venular network, the local vasodilatory response to NO is propagated to upstream vessels causing arteriolar vasodilation (see the following section on Coordination of Vasomotor Responses).

59.4.3 Coordination of Vasomotor Responses

Communication via gap junctions between the two active cell types in the blood vessel wall, smooth muscle, and endothelial cells plays an important role in coordinating the responses among resistance elements in the vascular network [55,56,62]. There is chemical and electrical coupling between the cells of the vessel wall, and this signal, in response to locally released vasoactive substances (e.g., from vessel wall, RBCs or parenchymal cells), can travel along a vessel in either direction with a length constant of about 2 mm. There are two immediate consequences of this communication. A localized vasodilatory stimulus of metabolic origin will be propagated to contiguous vessels, thereby lowering the resistance to blood flow in a larger region. In addition, this more generalized vasodilation should increase the homogeneity of blood flow in response to the localized metabolic event. The increase in blood flow produced as a result of this vasodilation will cause flow as well to increase at upstream sites. The increased shear stress on the endothelium as a result of the flow increase will lead to vasodilation of these larger upstream vessels. Thus, the neurohumoral and local responses are linked together in a complex control system that matches regional perfusion to the local metabolic needs.

59.4.4 Angiogenesis and Vascular Remodeling

In addition to short-term regulation of blood flow operating on the timescale of tens of seconds to minutes, there are mechanisms that operate on the scales of hours, days, and weeks that result in angiogenesis (capillary growth from the preexisting microvessels) and microvascular remodeling or adaptation (structural and geometric changes in the vascular wall) [31]. Stimuli for angiogenesis and microvascular remodeling could be hypoxia, injury, inflammation, or neoplasia. The processes of angiogenesis and vascular remodeling are complex and knowledge at the molecular, cellular, and tissue level is being accumulated at a fast rate. Briefly, it is understood that low cellular oxygen is sensed through a transcription factor HIF1 (Hypoxia-Inducible Factor) pathway, leading to activation of dozens of genes [63]. Among them is vascular endothelial growth factor (VEGF) — one of the most potent inducers of angiogenesis. VEGF is secreted by parenchymal and stromal cells and diffuses through the extracellular space. Once it reaches endothelial cells, it activates them causing hyperpermeability and expression of metalloproteinases (MMPs) that then participate in the proteolysis of the extracellular matrix. The activated endothelial cells migrate, proliferate, and differentiate, resulting in the formation of a capillary sprout. Subsequently, the endothelial cells secrete platelet-derived growth factor (PDGF) that participates in recruiting stromal fibroblasts and progenitor cells to the new capillaries. When these cells reach the vessels, they differentiate into pericytes and smooth muscle cells, thus stabilizing the vessels. Many of these processes are poorly understood. At this point, quantitative computational approaches are particularly useful in gaining a better understanding of these processes; research in this area is rapidly evolving [60,64–66].

Defining Terms

Angiogenesis: The growth of new capillaries from the preexisting microvessels.

Apparent viscosity: The viscosity of a Newtonian fluid that would require the same pressure difference to produce the same blood flow rate through a circular vessel as the blood.

Fahraeus effect: Microvessel hematocrit is smaller than hematocrit in the feed or discharge reservoir.

Fahraeus–Lindqvist effect: Apparent viscosity of blood in a microvessel is smaller than the bulk viscosity measured with a rotational viscometer or a large-bore capillary viscometer.

Krogh tissue cylinder model: A cylindrical volume of tissue supplied by a central cylindrical capillary.

Myogenic response: Vasoconstriction in response to elevated transmural pressure and vasodilation in response to reduced transmural pressure.

Myoglobin-facilitated O_2 diffusion: An increase of O_2 diffusive flux as a result of myoglobin molecules acting as a carrier for O_2 molecules.

Oxyhemoglobin dissociation curve: The equilibrium relationship between hemoglobin saturation and O_2 tension.

Poiseuille's Law: The relationship between volumetric flow rate and pressure difference for steady flow of a Newtonian fluid in a long circular tube.

Precapillary O_2 transport: O_2 diffusion from arterioles to the surrounding tissue.

Starling's Law: The relationship between water flux through the endothelium and the difference between the hydraulic and osmotic transmural pressures.

Vasomotion: Spontaneous rhythmic variation of microvessel diameter.

Acknowledgments

This work was supported by National Heart, Lung, and Blood Institute grants HL 18292, HL 52684, HL 79087, and HL 79653.

References

[1] Popel A.S. Mathematical and computational models of the microcirculation. In *Microvascular Research: Biology and Pathology*, Shepro D. Ed., Elsevier, 2005, pp. 1123–1129.

[2] Popel A.S. and Johnson P.C. Microcirculation and hemorheology. *Ann. Rev. Fluid Mech.* 37: 43–69, 2005.

[3] Hunter P.J. and Borg T.K. Integration from proteins to organs: the Physiome Project. *Nat. Rev. Mol. Cell. Biol.* 4: 237–243, 2003.

[4] Davis M.J. and Hill M.A. Signaling mechanisms underlying the vascular myogenic response. *Physiol. Rev.* 79: 387–423, 1999.

[5] Guilford W.H. and Gore R.W. The mechanics of arteriole–tissue interaction. *Microvasc. Res.* 50: 260–287, 1995.

[6] Regirer S.A. and Shadrina N. A simple model of a vessel with a wall sensitive to mechanical stimuli. *Biophysics* 47: 845–850, 2002.

[7] Ursino M., Colantuoni A., and Bertuglia S. Vasomotion and blood flow regulation in hamster skeletal muscle microcirculation: a theoretical and experimental study. *Microvasc. Res.* 56: 233–252, 1998.

[8] Parthimos D., Edwards D.H., and Griffith T.M. Minimal model of arterial chaos generated by coupled intracellular and membrane Ca^{2+} oscillators. *Am. J. Physiol.* 277: H1119–H1144, 1999.

[9] Carr R.T. and Lacoin M. Nonlinear dynamics of microvascular blood flow. *Ann. Biomed. Eng.* 28: 641–652, 2000.

[10] Kiani M.F., Pries A.R., Hsu L.L., Sarelius I.H., and Cokelet G.R. Fluctuations in microvascular blood flow parameters caused by hemodynamic mechanisms. *Am. J. Physiol.* 266: H1822–H1828, 1994.

[11] Discher D.E. New insights into erythrocyte membrane organization and microelasticity. *Curr. Opin. Hematol.* 7: 117–122, 2000.

[12] Secomb T.W. Mechanics of red blood cells and blood flow in narrow tubes. In *Modeling and Simulation of Capsules and Biological Cells*, Pozrikidis C. (Ed.), Boca Raton, FL, Chapman & Hall/CRC, 2003, pp. 163–196.

[13] Desjardins C. and Duling B.R. Heparinase treatment suggests a role for the endothelial cell glycocalyx in regulation of capillary hematocrit. *Am. J. Physiol.* 258: H647–H654, 1990.

[14] Pries A.R., Secomb T.W., and Gaehtgens P. The endothelial surface layer. *Pflugers Arch.* 440: 653–666, 2000.

[15] Secomb T.W., Hsu R., and Pries A.R. Blood flow and red blood cell deformation in nonuniform capillaries: effects of the endothelial surface layer. *Microcirculation* 9: 189–196, 2002.

[16] Schmid-Schonbein G.W. Biomechanics of microcirculatory blood perfusion. *Ann. Rev. Biomed. Eng.* 1: 73–102, 1999.

[17] Schmid-Schonbein G.W. and Granger D.N. *Molecular Basis for Microcirculatory Disorders.* Springer-Verlag, Berlin, 2003.

[18] Lipowsky H.H. Microvascular rheology and hemodynamics. *Microcirculation* 12: 5–15, 2005.

[19] Bishop J.J., Nance P.R., Popel A.S., Intaglietta M., and Johnson P.C. Effect of erythrocyte aggregation on velocity profiles in venules. *Am. J. Physiol. Heart Circ. Physiol.* 280: H222–H236, 2001.

[20] Ellsworth M.L. and Pittman R.N. Evaluation of photometric methods for quantifying convective mass transport in microvessels. *Am. J. Physiol.* 251: H869–H879, 1986.

[21] Das B., Enden G., and Popel A.S. Stratified multiphase model for blood flow in a venular bifurcation. *Ann. Biomed. Eng.* 25: 135–153, 1997.

[22] Baskurt O.K. and Meiselman H.J. Blood rheology and hemodynamics. *Semin. Thromb. Hemost.* 29: 435–450, 2003.

[23] Cabel M., Meiselman H.J., Popel A.S., and Johnson P.C. Contribution of red blood cell aggregation to venous vascular resistance in skeletal muscle. *Am. J. Physiol.* 272: H1020–H1032, 1997.

[24] Ley K. The role of selectins in inflammation and disease. *Trends Mol. Med.* 9: 263–268, 2003.

[25] Woldhuis B., Tangelder G.J., Slaaf D.W., and Reneman R.S. Concentration profile of blood platelets differs in arterioles and venules. *Am. J. Physiol.* 262: H1217–H1223, 1992.

[26] Tailor A., Cooper D., and Granger D. Platelet–vessel wall interactions in the microcirculation. *Microcirculation* 12: 275–285, 2005.

[27] Jadhav S., Eggleton C.D., and Konstantopoulos K. A 3-D computational model predicts that cell deformation affects selectin-mediated leukocyte rolling. *Biophys. J.* 88: 96–104, 2005.

[28] N'Dri N.A., Shyy W., and Tran-Son-Tay R. Computational modeling of cell adhesion and movement using a continuum-kinetics approach. *Biophys. J.* 85: 2273–2286, 2003.

[29] Sun C. and Munn L.L. Particulate nature of blood determines macroscopic rheology: a 2-D lattice Boltzmann analysis. *Biophys. J.* 88: 1635–1645, 2005.

[30] Pries A.R., Secomb T.W., and Gaehtgens P. Biophysical aspects of blood flow in the microvasculature. *Cardiovasc. Res.* 32: 654–667, 1996.

[31] Skalak T.C. Angiogenesis and microvascular remodeling: a brief history and future roadmap. *Microcirculation* 12: 47–58, 2005.

[32] Baish J.W. and Jain R.K. Fractals and cancer. *Cancer Res.* 60: 3683–3688, 2000.

[33] Mulivor A.W. and Lipowsky H.H. Inflammation- and ischemia-induced shedding of venular glycocalyx. *Am. J. Physiol. Heart Circ. Physiol.* 286: H1672–H1680, 2004.

[34] Platts S.H. and Duling B.R. Adenosine A3 receptor activation modulates the capillary endothelial glycocalyx. *Circ. Res.* 94: 77–82, 2004.

[35] Weibel E.R. and Hoppeler H. Exercise-induced maximal metabolic rate scales with muscle aerobic capacity. *J. Exp. Biol.* 208: 1635–1644, 2005.

[36] Pittman R.N. Oxygen transport and exchange in the microcirculation. *Microcirculation* 12: 59–70, 2005.

[37] Tsai A.G., Johnson P.C., and Intaglietta M. Oxygen gradients in the microcirculation. *Physiol. Rev.* 83: 933–963, 2003.

[38] Beard D.A., Schenkman K.A., and Feigl E.O. Myocardial oxygenation in isolated hearts predicted by an anatomically realistic microvascular transport model. *Am. J. Physiol. Heart Circ. Physiol.* 285: H1826–H1836, 2003.

[39] Goldman D. and Popel A.S. A computational study of the effect of capillary network anastomoses and tortuosity on oxygen transport. *J. Theor. Biol.* 206: 181–194, 2000.

[40] Secomb T.W., Hsu R, Park E.Y., and Dewhirst M.W. Green's function methods for analysis of oxygen delivery to tissue by microvascular networks. *Ann. Biomed. Eng.* 32: 1519–1529, 2004.

[41] Alayash A.I. Oxygen therapeutics: can we tame haemoglobin? *Nat. Rev. Drug Discov.* 3: 152–159, 2004.

[42] Ignarro L.J. Signal transduction mechanisms involving nitric oxide. *Biochem. Pharmacol.* 41: 485–490, 1991.

[43] Kashiwagi S., Kajimura M., Yoshimura Y., and Suematsu M. Nonendothelial source of nitric oxide in arterioles but not in venules: alternative source revealed in vivo by diaminofluorescein microfluorography. *Circ. Res.* 91: e55–e64, 2002.

[44] Buerk D.G. Can we model nitric oxide biotransport? A survey of mathematical models for a simple diatomic molecule with surprisingly complex biological activities. *Ann. Rev. Biomed. Eng.* 3: 109–143, 2001.

[45] Buerk D.G., Lamkin-Kennard K., and Jaron D. Modeling the influence of superoxide dismutase on superoxide and nitric oxide interactions, including reversible inhibition of oxygen consumption. *Free Radic. Biol. Med.* 34: 1488–1503, 2003.

[46] Kavdia M. and Popel A.S. Contribution of nNOS- and eNOS-derived NO to microvascular smooth muscle NO exposure. *J. Appl. Physiol.* 97: 293–301, 2004.

[47] Kavdia M. and Popel A.S. Wall shear stress differentially affects NO level in arterioles for volume expanders and Hb-based O_2 carriers. *Microvasc. Res.* 66: 49–58, 2003.

[48] Tsoukias N.M., Kavdia M., and Popel A.S. A theoretical model of nitric oxide transport in arterioles: frequency- vs. amplitude-dependent control of cGMP formation. *Am. J. Physiol. Heart Circ. Physiol.* 286: H1043–H1056, 2004.

[49] Tsoukias N.M. and Popel A.S. A model of nitric oxide capillary exchange. *Microcirculation* 10: 479–495, 2003.

[50] Vaughn M.W., Kuo L., and Liao J.C. Estimation of nitric oxide production and reaction rates in tissue by use of a mathematical model. *Am. J. Physiol.* 274: H2163–H2176, 1998.

[51] Singel D.J. and Stamler J.S. Chemical physiology of blood flow regulation by red blood cells: the role of nitric oxide and S-nitrosohemoglobin. *Ann. Rev. Physiol.* 67: 99–145, 2005.

[52] Curry F.R. Microvascular solute and water transport. *Microcirculation* 12: 17–31, 2005.

[53] Michel C.C. and Curry F.E. Microvascular permeability. *Physiol. Rev.* 79: 703–761, 1999.

[54] Hu X. and Weinbaum S. A new view of Starling's hypothesis at the microstructural level. *Microvasc. Res.* 58: 281–304, 1999.

[55] Segal S.S. Regulation of blood flow in the microcirculation. *Microcirculation* 12: 33–45, 2005.

[56] Segal S.S. Integration of blood flow control to skeletal muscle: key role of feed arteries. *Acta Physiol. Scand.* 168: 511–518, 2000.

[57] Busse R., Edwards G., Feletou M., Fleming I., Vanhoutte P.M., and Weston A.H. EDHF: bringing the concepts together. *Trends Pharmacol. Sci.* 23: 374–380, 2002.

[58] Cornelissen A.J., Dankelman J., VanBavel E., and Spaan J.A. Balance between myogenic, flow-dependent, and metabolic flow control in coronary arterial tree: a model study. *Am. J. Physiol. Heart Circ. Physiol.* 282: H2224–H2237, 2002.

[59] Pohl U. and de Wit C. A unique role of NO in the control of blood flow. *News Physiol. Sci.* 14: 74–80, 1999.

[60] Pries A.R. and Secomb T.W. Control of blood vessel structure: insights from theoretical models. *Am. J. Physiol. Heart Circ. Physiol.* 288: H1010–H1015, 2005.

[61] Ellsworth M.L. Red blood cell-derived ATP as a regulator of skeletal muscle perfusion. *Med. Sci. Sports Exerc.* 36: 35–41, 2004.

[62] Figueroa X.F., Isakson B.E., and Duling B.R. Connexins: gaps in our knowledge of vascular function. *Physiology (Bethesda)* 19: 277–284, 2004.

[63] Semenza G.L. Hydroxylation of HIF-1: oxygen sensing at the molecular level. *Physiology (Bethesda)* 19: 176–182, 2004.

[64] Karagiannis E.D. and Popel A.S. Distinct modes of collagen type I proteolysis by matrix metallo-proteinase (MMP) 2 and membrane type I MMP during the migration of a tip endothelial cell: Insights from a computational model. *J. Theor. Biol.* 238: 124–145, 2006.

[65] Mac Gabhann F. and Popel A.S. Differential binding of VEGF isoforms to VEGF Receptor 2 in the presence of Neuropilin-1: a computational model. *Am. J. Physiol. Heart Circ. Physiol.* 288: H2851–H2860, 2005.

[66] Peirce S.M., Van Gieson E.J., and Skalak T.C. Multicellular simulation predicts microvascular patterning and in silico tissue assembly. *FASEB J.* 18: 731–733, 2004.

Further Information

Two-Volume set and CD: Microvascular Research: Biology and Pathology. D. Shepro, Editor-in-Chief. Elsevier, New York, 2005.

Two-Volume set: Handbook of Physiology. Section 2: The Cardiovascular System. Volume IV, Parts 1 & 2: Microcirculation. Edited by E.M. Renkin and C.C. Michel. 1984 American Physiological Society. The book remains a useful overview of the field.

Original research articles on microcirculation can be found in academic journals: Microcirculation, Microvascular Research, *American Journal of Physiology* (Heart and Circulatory Physiology), *Journal of Vascular Research*, Biorheology.

60

Mechanics and Deformability of Hematocytes

Richard E. Waugh
University of Rochester Medical Center

Robert M. Hochmuth
Duke University

60.1 Introduction

The term hematocytes refers to the circulating cells of the blood. These are divided into two main classes: erythrocytes, or red cells, and leukocytes, or white cells. In addition to these there are specialized cell-like structures called platelets. The mechanical properties of these cells are of special interest because of their physiological role as circulating corpuscles in the flowing blood. The importance of the mechanical properties of these cells and their influence on blood flow is evident in a number of hematological pathologies. The properties of the two main types of hematocytes are distinctly different. The essential character of a red cell is that of an elastic bag enclosing a Newtonian fluid of comparatively low viscosity. The essential behavior of white cells is that of a highly viscous fluid drop with a more or less constant cortical (surface) tension. Under the action of a given force, red cells deform much more readily than white cells. In this chapter we focus on descriptions of the behavior of the two cell types separately, concentrating on the viscoelastic characteristics of the red cell membrane, and the fluid characteristics of the white cell cytosol.

60.2 Fundamentals

60.2.1 Stresses and Strains in Two Dimensions

The description of the mechanical deformation of the membrane is cast in terms of principal **force resultants** and **principal extension ratios** of the surface. The force resultants, like conventional three-dimensional strains, are generally expressed in terms of a tensorial quantity, the components of which depend on coordinate rotation. For the purposes of describing the constitutive behavior of the surface, it is convenient to express the surface resultants in terms of rotationally invariant quantities. These can be either the principal force resultants N_1 and N_2, or the isotropic resultant $\bar{N}$ and the maximum shear resultant N_s. The surface strain is also a tensorial quantity, but may be expressed in terms of the principal extension ratios of the surface λ_1 and λ_2. The rate of surface shear deformation is given by [Evans and Skalak, 1979]:

$$V_s = \left(\frac{\lambda_1}{\lambda_2}\right)^{1/2} \frac{d}{dt}\left(\frac{\lambda_1}{\lambda_2}\right)^{1/2} \tag{60.1}$$

The membrane deformation is calculated from observed macroscopic changes in cell geometry, usually with the use of simple geometric shapes to approximate the cell shape. The membrane force resultants are calculated from force balance relationships. For example, in the determination of the **area expansivity modulus** of the red cell membrane or the **cortical tension** in neutrophils, the force resultants in the plane of the membrane of the red cell or the cortex of the white cell are isotropic. In this case, as long as the membrane surface of the cell does not stick to the pipette, the membrane force resultant can be calculated from the law of Laplace:

$$\Delta P = 2\bar{N}\left(\frac{1}{R_p} - \frac{1}{R_c}\right) \tag{60.2}$$

where R_p is the radius of the pipette, R_c is the radius of the spherical portion of the cell outside the pipette, $\bar{N}$ is the isotropic force resultant (tension) in the membrane, and ΔP is the aspiration pressure in the pipette.

60.2.2 Basic Equations for Newtonian Fluid Flow

The constitutive relations for fluid flow in a sphere undergoing axisymmetric deformation can be written:

$$\sigma_{rr} = -p + 2\eta\frac{\partial V_r}{\partial r} \tag{60.3}$$

$$\sigma_{r\theta} = \eta\left[\frac{1}{r}\frac{\partial V_r}{\partial \theta} + r\frac{\partial}{\partial r}\left(\frac{V_\theta}{r}\right)\right] \tag{60.4}$$

where σ_{rr} and $\sigma_{r\theta}$ are components of the stress tensor, p is the hydrostatic pressure, r is the radial coordinate, θ is the angular coordinate in the direction of the axis of symmetry in spherical coordinates, and V_r and V_θ are components of the fluid velocity vector. These equations effectively define the material viscosity, η. In general, η may be a function of the strain rate. The second term in Equation 60.3 contains the radial strain rate $\dot{\varepsilon}_{rr}$ and the bracketed term in Equation 60.4 corresponds to $\dot{\varepsilon}_{r\theta}$. For the purposes of evaluating this dependence, it is convenient to define the mean shear rate $\dot{\gamma}_m$ averaged over the cell volume and duration of the deformation process t_e:

$$\dot{\gamma}_m = \left(\frac{3}{4}\frac{1}{t_e}\int_0^{t_e}\int_0^{R(t)}\int_0^\pi \frac{r^2}{R^3}\left(\dot{\varepsilon}_{ij}\dot{\varepsilon}_{ij}\right)\sin\theta\, d\theta\, dr\, dt\right)^{1/2} \tag{60.5}$$

where repeated indices indicate summation.

60.3 Red Cells

60.3.1 Size and Shape

The normal red cell is a biconcave disk at rest. The average human cell is approximately 7.7 μm in diameter and varies in thickness from ~2.8 μm at the rim to ~1.4 μm at the center [Fung et al., 1981]. However, red cells vary considerably in size even within a single individual. The mean surface area is ~130 μm^2 and the mean volume is 98 μm^3 (Table 60.1), but the range of sizes within a population is Gausian distributed with standard deviations of ~15.8 μm^2 for the area and ~16.1 μm^3 for the volume [Fung et al., 1981]. Cells from different species vary enormously in size, and tables for different species have been tabulated elsewhere [Hawkey et al., 1991].

Red cell deformation takes place under two important constraints: fixed surface area and fixed volume. The constraint of fixed volume arises from the impermeability of the membrane to cations. Even though the membrane is highly permeable to water, the inability of salts to cross the membrane prevents significant water loss because of the requirement for colloidal osmotic equilibrium [Lew and Bookchin, 1986]. The constraint of fixed surface area arises from the large resistance of bilayer membranes to changes in area per molecule [Needham and Nunn, 1990]. These two constraints place strict limits on the kinds of deformations that the cell can undergo and the size of the aperture that the cell can negotiate. Thus, a major determinant of red cell deformability is its ratio of surface area to volume. One measure of this parameter is the *sphericity*, defined as the dimensionless ratio of the two-thirds power of the cell volume to the cell area times a constant that makes its maximum value 1.0:

$$S = \frac{4\pi}{(4\pi/3)^{2/3}} \cdot \frac{V^{2/3}}{A} \tag{60.6}$$

The mean value of sphericity of a normal population of cells was measured by interference microscopy to be 0.79 with a standard deviation (S.D.) of 0.05 at room temperature [Fung et al., 1981]. Similar values were obtained using micropipettes: mean = 0.81, S.D. = 0.02 [Waugh and Agre, 1988]. The membrane area increases with temperature, and the membrane volume decreases with temperature, so the sphericity at physiological temperature is expected to be somewhat smaller. Based on measurements of the thermal area expansivity of 0.12%/°C [Waugh and Evans, 1979], and a change in volume of −0.14%/°C [Waugh and Evans, 1979], the mean sphericity at 37°C is estimated to be 0.76 to 0.78 (see Table 60.1).

60.3.2 Red Cell Cytosol

The interior of a red cell is a concentrated solution of hemoglobin, the oxygen-carrying protein, and it behaves as a Newtonian fluid [Cokelet and Meiselman, 1968]. In a normal population of cells there is a distribution of hemoglobin concentrations in the range 29 to 39 g/dl. The viscosity of the cytosol depends

TABLE 60.1 Parameter Values for a Typical Red Blood Cell (37°C)

Area	132 μm^2
Volume	96 μm^3
Sphericity	0.77
Membrane area modulus	400 mN/m
Membrane shear modulus	0.006 mN/m
Membrane viscosity	0.00036 mN sec/m
Membrane bending stiffness	0.2×10^{-18} J
Thermal area expansivity	0.12%/°C
$\frac{1}{V}\frac{dV}{dT}$	−0.14%/°C

TABLE 60.2 Viscosity of Red Cell Cytosol (37°C)

Hemoglobin concentration (g/l)	Measured viscosity[1] (mPa sec)	Best fit viscosity[2] (mPa sec)
290	4.1–5.0	4.2
310	5.2–6.6	5.3
330	6.6–9.2	6.7
350	8.5–13.0	8.9
370	10.8–17.1	12.1
390	15.0–23.9	17.2

[1]Data taken from Cokelet, G.R. and Meiselman, H.J. 1968. *Science* 162: 275–277; Chien, S., Usami, S. and Bertles, J.F. 1970. *J. Clin. Invest.* 49: 623–634.
[2]Fitted curve from Ross, P.D. and Minton, A.P. 1977. *Biochem. Biophys. Res. Commun.* 76: 971–976.

on the hemoglobin concentration as well as temperature (see Table 60.2). Based on theoretical models [Ross and Minton, 1977], the temperature dependence of the cytosolic viscosity is expected to be the same as that of water, that is, the ratio of cytosolic viscosity at 37°C to the viscosity at 20°C is the same as the ratio of water viscosity at those same temperatures. In most cases, even in the most dense cells, the resistance to flow of the cytosol is small compared with the viscoelastic resistance of the membrane when membrane deformations are appreciable.

60.3.3 Membrane Area Dilation

The large resistance of the membrane to area dilation has been characterized in micromechanical experiments. The changes in surface area that can be produced in the membrane are small, and so they can be characterized in terms of a simple Hookean elastic relationship between the isotropic force resultant $\bar{N}$ and the fractional change in surface area $\alpha = A/A_0 - 1$:

$$\bar{N} = K\alpha \tag{60.7}$$

The proportionality constant K is called the *area compressibility modulus* or the *area expansivity modulus*. Early estimates placed its value at room temperature at ~450 mN/m [Evans and Waugh, 1977] and showed a dependence of the modulus on temperature, its value changing from ~300 mN/m at 45°C to a value of ~600 mN/m at 5°C [Waugh and Evans, 1979]. Subsequently it was shown that the measurement of this parameter using micropipettes is affected by extraneous electric fields, and the value at room temperature was corrected upward to ~500 mN/m [Katnik and Waugh, 1990]. The values in Table 60.3 are based on this measurement, and the fractional change in the modulus with temperature is based on the original micropipette measurements [Waugh and Evans, 1979].

60.3.4 Membrane Shear Deformation

The shear deformations of the red cell surface can be large, and so a simple linear relationship between force and extension is not adequate for describing the membrane behavior. The large resistance of the membrane composite to area dilation led early investigators to postulate that the membrane maintained constant surface density during shear deformation, that is, that the surface was two-dimensionally incompressible. Most of what exists in the literature about the shear deformation of the red cell membrane is based on this assumption. In the mid-1990s, experimental evidence emerged that this assumption is an oversimplification of the true cellular behavior, and that deformation produces changes in the local surface

TABLE 60.3   Temperature Dependence of Viscoelastic
Coefficients of the Red Cell Membrane

Temperature (°C)	K (mN/m)[1]	μ_m (mN/m)[2]	η (mN sec/m)[3]
5	660	0.0078	0.0021
15	580	0.0072	0.0014
25	500	0.0065	0.00074
37	400	0.0058	0.00036
45	340	0.0053	—

[1] Based on a value of the modulus at 25°C of 500 mN/m and the
fractional change in modulus with temperature measured by Waugh,
R. and Evans, E.A. 1979. *Biophys. J.* 26: 115–132.
[2] Based on linear regression to the data of Waugh, R. and Evans, E.A.
1979. *Biophys. J.* 26: 115–132.
[3] Data from Hochmuth, R.M., Buxbaum, K.L. and Evans, E.A. 1980.
Biophys. J. 29: 177–182.

density of the membrane elastic network [Discher et al., 1994]. Nevertheless, the older simpler relationships provide a relatively simple description of the cell behavior that can be useful for many applications,
and so the properties of the cell defined under that assumption are summarized here.

For a simple, two-dimensional, incompressible, hyperelastic material, the relationship between the
membrane shear force resultant N_s and the material deformation is [Evans and Skalak, 1979]

$$N_s = \frac{\mu_m}{2}\left(\frac{\lambda_1}{\lambda_2} - \frac{\lambda_2}{\lambda_1}\right) + 2\eta_m V_s \tag{60.8}$$

where λ_1 and λ_2 are the principal extension ratios for the deformation and V_s is the rate of surface shear
deformation (Equation 60.1). The *membrane shear modulus* μ_m and the *membrane viscosity* η_m are defined
by this relationship. Values for these coefficients at different temperatures are given in Table 60.3.

60.3.5 Stress Relaxation and Strain Hardening

Subsequent to these original formulations, a number of refinements to these relationships have been
proposed. Observations of persistent deformations after micropipette aspiration for extended periods of
time formed the basis for the development of a model for long-term stress relaxation [Markle et al., 1983].
The characteristic times for these relaxations were on the order of 1 to 2 h, and they were thought to
correlate with permanent rearrangements of the membrane elastic network.

Another type of stress relaxation is thought to occur over very short times ($\sim$0.1 sec) after rapid
deformation of the membrane either by micropipette [Chien et al., 1978] or in cell extension experiments
(Waugh and Bisgrove, unpublished observations). This phenomenon is thought to be due to transient
entanglements within the deforming network. Whether or not the phenomenon actually occurs remains
controversial. The stresses relax rapidly, and it is difficult to account for inertial effects of the measuring
system and to reliably assess the intrinsic cellular response.

Finally, there has been some evidence that the coefficient for shear elasticity may be a function of the
surface extension, increasing with increasing deformation. This was first proposed by Fischer in an effort
to resolve discrepancies between theoretical predictions and observed behavior of red cells undergoing
dynamic deformations in fluid shear [Fischer et al., 1981]. Increasing elastic resistance with extension has
also been proposed as an explanation for discrepancies between theoretical predictions based on a constant
modulus and measurements of the length of a cell projection into a micropipette [Waugh and Marchesi,
1990]. However, due to the approximate nature of the mechanical analysis of cell deformation in shear
flow, and the limits of optical resolution in micropipette experiments, the evidence for a dependence of
the modulus on extension is not clear-cut, and this issue remains unresolved.

60.3.6 New Constitutive Relations for the Red Cell Membrane

The most modern picture of membrane deformation recognizes that the membrane is a composite of two layers with distinct mechanical behavior. The membrane bilayer, composed of phospholipids and integral membrane proteins, exhibits a large elastic resistance to area dilation but is fluid in surface shear. The membrane skeleton, composed of a network of structural proteins at the cytoplasmic surface of the bilayer, is locally compressible and exhibits an elastic resistance to surface shear. The assumption that the membrane skeleton is locally incompressible is no longer applied. This assumption had been challenged over the years on the basis of theoretical considerations, but only very recently has experimental evidence emerged that shows definitively that the membrane skeleton is compressible. This has led to a new constitutive model for membrane behavior [Mohandas and Evans, 1994]. The principal stress resultants in the membrane skeleton are related to the membrane deformation by:

$$N_1 = \mu_{\mathrm{N}} \left(\frac{\lambda_1}{\lambda_2} - 1 \right) + K_{\mathrm{N}} \left(\lambda_1 \lambda_2 - \frac{1}{(\lambda_1 \lambda_2)^n} \right) \qquad (60.9)$$

and,

$$N_2 = \mu_{\mathrm{N}} \left(\frac{\lambda_2}{\lambda_1} - 1 \right) + K_{\mathrm{N}} \left(\lambda_1 \lambda_2 - \frac{1}{(\lambda_1 \lambda_2)^n} \right) \qquad (60.10)$$

where μ_{N} and K_{N} are the shear and isotropic moduli of the membrane skeleton respectively, and n is a parameter to account for molecular crowding of the skeleton in compression. The original modulus based on the two-dimensionally incompressible case is related to these moduli by:

$$\mu_{\mathrm{m}} \approx \frac{\mu_{\mathrm{N}} K_{\mathrm{N}}}{\mu_{\mathrm{N}} + K_{\mathrm{N}}} \qquad (60.11)$$

Values for the coefficients determined from fluorescence measurements of skeletal density distributions during micropipette aspiration studies are $\mu_{\mathrm{N}} \approx 0.01$ mN/m and $K_{\mathrm{N}} \approx 0.02$ mN/m. The value for n is estimated to be $\sim$2 [Discher et al., 1994].

These new concepts for membrane constitutive behavior have yet to be thoroughly explored. The temperature dependence of these moduli is unknown, and the implications that such a model will have on interpretation of dynamic deformations of the membrane remain to be resolved.

60.3.7 Bending Elasticity

Even though the membrane is very thin, it has a high resistance to surface dilation. This property, coupled with the finite thickness of the membrane gives the membrane a small but finite resistance to bending. This resistance is characterized in terms of the **membrane bending modulus**. The bending resistance of biological membranes is inherently complex because of their lamellar structure. There is a local resistance to bending due to the inherent stiffness of the individual leaflets of the membrane bilayer. (Because the membrane skeleton is compressible, it is thought to contribute little if anything to the membrane bending stiffness.) In addition to this local stiffness, there is a **nonlocal bending resistance** due to the net compression and expansion of the adjacent leaflets resulting from the curvature change. The nonlocal contribution is complicated by the fact that the leaflets may be redistributed laterally within the membrane capsule to equalize the area per molecule within each leaflet. The situation is further complicated by the likely possibility that molecules may exchange between leaflets to alleviate curvature-induced dilation/compression. Thus, the bending stiffness measured by different approaches probably reflects contributions from both local and nonlocal mechanisms, and the measured values may differ because of different contributions from the two mechanisms. Estimates based on buckling instabilities during micropipette aspiration give a value of $\sim 0.18 \times 10^{-18}$ J [Evans, 1983]. Measurements based on the mechanical formation of lipid tubes from the cell surface give a value of 0.2 to 0.25×10^{-18} J [Hwang and Waugh, 1997].

60.4 White Cells

Whereas red cells account for approximately 40% of the blood volume, white cells occupy less than 1% of the blood volume. Yet because white cells are less deformable, they can have a significant influence on blood flow, especially in the microvasculature. Unlike red cells, which are very similar to each other, as are platelets, there are several different kinds of white cells or *leukocytes*. Originally, leukocytes were classified into groups according to their appearance when viewed with the light microscope. Thus, there are *granulocytes, monocytes,* and *lymphocytes* [Alberts et al., 1989]. The granulocytes with their many internal granules are separated into *neutrophils, basophils,* and *eosinophils* according to the way each cell stains. The neutrophil, also called a *polymorphonuclear leukocyte* because of its segmented or "multilobed" nucleus, is the most common white cell in the blood (see Table 60.4). The lymphocytes, which constitute 20 to 40% of the white cells and which are further subdivided into *B lymphocytes* and *killer* and *helper T lymphocytes,* are the smallest of the white cells. The other types of leukocytes are found with much less frequency. Most of the geometric and mechanical studies of white cells reported below have focused on the neutrophil because it is the most common cell in the circulation, although the lymphocyte has also received attention.

60.4.1 Size and Shape

White cells at rest are spherical. The surfaces of white cells contain many folds, projections, and "microvilli" to provide the cells with sufficient membrane area to deform as they enter capillaries with diameters much smaller than the resting diameter of the cell. (Without the reservoir of membrane area in these folds, the constraints of constant volume and membrane area would make a spherical cell essentially undeformable.) The excess surface area of the neutrophil, when measured in a wet preparation, is slightly more than twice the apparent surface area of a smooth sphere with the same diameter [Evans and Yeung, 1989; Ting-Beall et al., 1993]. It is interesting to note that each type of white cell has its own unique surface topography, which allows one to readily determine if a cell is, for example, either a neutrophil or monocyte or lymphocyte [Hochmuth et al., 1995].

TABLE 60.4 Size and Appearance of White Cells in the Circulation

Granulocytes	Occurrence[1] (% of WBC's)	Cell volume[2] (μm^3)	Cell diameter[2] (μm)	Nucleus[3] % cell volume	Cortical tension (mN/m)
Neutrophils	50–70	300–310	8.2–8.4	21	0.024–0.035 [4]
Basophils	0–1	—			—
Eosinophils	1–3	—		18	—
Monocytes	1–5	400	9.1	26	0.06[5]
Lymphocytes	20–40	220	7.5	44	0.035[5]

[1] Diggs, L.W., Sturm, D. and Bell, A. 1985. 5th ed. Abbott Laboratories, Abbott Park, Illinois.
[2] Ting-Beall, H.P., Needham, D. and Hochmuth, R.M. 1993. *Blood* 81: 2774–2780. (Diameter calculated from the volume of a sphere).
[3] Schmid-Schönbein, G.W., Shih, Y.Y. and Chien, S. 1980. *Blood* 56: 866–875.
[4] Evans, E., and Yeung, A. 1989. *Biophys. J.* 56: 151–160, Needham, D., and Hochmuth, R.M. 1992. *Biophys. J.* 61: 1664–1670 Tsai, M.A., Frank, R.S. and Waugh, R.E. 1993. *Biophys. J.* 65: 2078–2088, Tsai, M.A., Frank, R.S. and Waugh, R.E. 1994. *Biophys. J.* 66: 2166–2172.
[5] Preliminary data, Hochmuth, Zhelev and Ting-Beall.

The cell volumes listed in Table 60.4 were obtained with the light microscope, either by measuring the diameter of the spherical cell or by aspirating the cell into a small glass pipette with a known diameter and then measuring the resulting length of the cylindrically shaped cell. Other values for cell volume obtained using transmission electron microscopy are somewhat smaller, probably because of cell shrinkage due to fixation and drying prior to measurement [Schmid-Schönbein et al., 1980; Ting-Beall et al., 1995]. Although the absolute magnitude of the cell volume measured with the electron microscope may be erroneous, if it is assumed that all parts of the cell dehydrate equally when they are dried in preparation for viewing, then this approach can be used to determine the volume occupied by the nucleus (Table 60.4) and other organelles of various white cells. The volume occupied by the granules in the neutrophil and eosinophil (recall that both are granulocytes) is 15 and 23%, respectively, whereas the granular volume in monocytes and lymphocytes is less than a few percent.

60.4.2 Mechanical Behavior

The early observations of Bagge et al. [1977] led them to suggest that the neutrophil behaves as a simple viscoelastic solid with a Maxwell element (an elastic and viscous element in series) in parallel with an elastic element. This elastic element in the model was thought to pull the unstressed cell into its spherical shape. Subsequently, Evans and Kukan [1984] and Evans and Yeung [1989] showed that the cells flow continuously into a pipette, with no apparent approach to a static limit, when a constant suction pressure was applied. Thus, the cytoplasm of the neutrophil should be treated as a liquid rather than a solid, and its surface has a persistent *cortical tension* that causes the cell to assume a spherical shape.

60.4.3 Mechanical Behavior

Using a micropipette and a small suction pressure to aspirate a hemispherical projection from a cell body into the pipette, Evans and Yeung measured a value for the cortical tension of 0.035 mN/m. Needham and Hochmuth [1992] measured the cortical tension of individual cells that were driven down a tapered pipette in a series of equilibrium positions. In many cases the cortical tension increased as the cell moved further into the pipette, which means that the cell has an apparent area expansion modulus (Equation 60.7). They obtained an average value of 0.04 mN/m for the expansion modulus and an extrapolated value for the cortical tension (at zero area dilation) in the resting state of 0.024 mN/m. The importance of the actin cytoskeleton in maintaining cortical tension was demonstrated by Tsai et al. [1994]. Treatment of the cells with a drug that disrupts actin filament structure (CTB = cytochalasin B) resulted in a decrease in cortical tension from 0.027 to 0.022 mN/m at a CTB concentration of 3 μM and to 0.014 mN/m at 30 μM.

Preliminary measurements in one of our laboratories (RMH) indicate that the value for the cortical tension of a monocyte is about double that for a granulocyte, that is, 0.06 mN/m, and the value for a lymphocyte is about 0.035 mN/m.

60.4.4 Bending Rigidity

The existence of a cortical tension suggests that there is a cortex — a relatively thick layer of F-actin filaments and myosin — that is capable of exerting a finite tension at the surface. If such a layer exists, it would have a finite thickness and bending rigidity. Zhelev et al. [1994] aspirated the surface of neutrophils into pipettes with increasingly smaller diameters and determined that the surface had a bending modulus of about 1 to 2×10^{-18} J, which is 5 to 50 times the bending moduli for erythrocyte or lipid bilayer membranes. The thickness of the cortex should be smaller than the radius of smallest pipette used in this study, which was 0.24 μm.

60.4.5 Apparent Viscosity

Using their model of the neutrophil as a Newtonian liquid drop with a constant cortical tension and (as they showed) a negligible surface viscosity, Yeung and Evans [1989] analyzed the flow of neutrophils into a micropipette and obtained a value for the **cytoplasmic viscosity** of about 200 Pa sec. In their experiments, the aspiration pressures were on the order of 10 to 1000 Pa. Similar experiments by Needham and Hochmuth [1990] using the same Newtonian model (with a negligible surface viscosity) but using higher aspiration pressures (ranging from 500 to 2000 Pa) gave an average value for the cytoplasmic viscosity of 135 Pa sec for 151 cells from five individuals. The apparent discrepancy between these two sets of experiments was resolved to a large extent by Tsai et al. [1993], who demonstrated that the neutrophil viscosity decreases with increasing rate of deformation. They proposed a model of the cytosol as a **power law fluid**:

$$\eta = \eta_c \left(\frac{\dot{\gamma}_m}{\dot{\gamma}_c} \right)^{-b} \tag{60.12}$$

where $b = 0.52$, $\dot{\gamma}_m$ is defined by Equation 60.5, and η_c is a characteristic viscosity of 130 Pa sec when the characteristic mean shear rate, $\dot{\gamma}_c$, is 1 sec^{-1}. These values are based on an approximate method for calculating the viscosity from measurements of the total time it takes for a cell to enter a micropipette. Because of different approximations used in the calculations, the values of viscosity reported by Tsai et al. [1993] tend to be somewhat smaller than those reported by Evans et al. or Hochmuth et al. Nevertheless, the shear rate dependence of the viscosity is the same, regardless of the method of calculation. Values for the viscosity are given in Table 60.5.

In addition to the dependence of the viscosity on shear rate, there is also evidence that it depends on the extent of deformation. In micropipette experiments the initial rate at which the cell enters the pipette is significantly faster than predicted, even when the shear rate dependence of the viscosity is taken into account. In a separate approach, the cytosolic viscosity was estimated from observation of the time course of the cell's return to a spherical geometry after expulsion from a micropipette. When the cellular deformations were large, a viscosity of 150 Pa sec was estimated [Tran-Son-Tay et al., 1991], but when the deformation was small, the estimated viscosity was only 60 Pa sec [Hochmuth et al., 1993]. Thus, it appears that the viscosity is smaller when the magnitude of the deformation is small, and increases as deformations become large.

An alternative attempt to account for the initial rapid entry of the cell into micropipettes involved the application of a **Maxwell fluid** model with a constant cortical tension. Dong et al. [1988] used this model to analyze both the shape recovery of neutrophils following small, complete deformations in pipettes and the small-deformation aspiration of neutrophils into pipettes. Another study by Dong et al. [1991], they used a finite-element, numerical approach and a Maxwell model with constant cortical tension to describe

TABLE 60.5 Viscous Parameters of White Blood Cells

Cell type	Range of viscosities (Pa sec)[1]		Characteristic viscosity (Pa sec)	Shear rate dependence (b)
	Minimum	Maximum		
Neutrophil	50	500	130[2]	0.52[2]
(30 M CTB)	41	52	54[2]	0.26[2]
Monocyte	70	1000	—	—
HL60 (G1)	—	—	220[3]	0.53[3]
HL60 (S)	—	—	330[3]	0.56[3]

[1] Evans, E., and Yeung, A. 1989. *Biophys. J.* 56: 151–160, Needham, D., and Hochmuth, R.M. 1992. *Biophys. J.* 61: 1664–1670 Tsai, M.A., Frank, R.S. and Waugh, R.E. 1993. *Biophys. J.* 65: 2078–2088, Tsai, M.A., Frank, R.S. and Waugh, R.E. 1994. *Biophys. J.* 66: 2166–2172.

[2] Tsai, M.A., Frank, R.S. and Waugh, R.E. 1993. *Biophys. J.* 65: 2078–2088, Tsai, M.A., Frank, R.S. and Waugh, R.E. 1994. *Biophys. J.* 66: 2166–2172.

[3] Tsai, M.A., Waugh, R.E. and Keng, P.C. 1996b *Biophys. J.* 70: 2023–2029.

the continuous, finite-deformation flow of a neutrophil into a pipette. However, in order to fit the theory to the data for the increase in length of the cell in the pipette with time, Dong et al. [1991] had to steadily increase both the elastic and viscous coefficients in their finite-deformation Maxwell model. This shows that even a Maxwell model is not adequate for describing the rheological properties of the neutrophil.

Although it is clear that the essential behavior of the cell is fluid, the simple fluid drop model with a constant and uniform viscosity does not match the observed time course of cell deformation in detail. Many of these discrepancies have been resolved by Drury and Dembo, who developed a finite element analysis of a cell using a model having substantial cortical dissipation with shear thinning and a shear thinning cytoplasm [Drury and Dembo 2001]. Their model matches cellular behavior during micropipette aspiration over a wide range of pipette diameters and entry rates. Only the initial rapid entry phase of the deformation is not predicted. Thus, the fluid drop model including shear thinning and elevated viscosity at the cell cortex captures the essential behavior of the cell, and when it is applied consistently (that is, for similar rate and extent of deformation) it provides a sound basis for predicting cell behavior and comparing the behaviors of different types of cells.

Although the mechanical properties of the neutrophil have been studied extensively as discussed above, the other white cells have not been studied in depth. Preliminary unpublished results from one of our laboratories (RMH) indicate that monocytes are somewhat more viscous (from roughly 30% to a factor of two) than neutrophils under similar conditions in both recovery experiments and experiments in which the monocyte flows into a pipette. A lymphocyte, when aspirated into a small pipette so that its relatively large nucleus is deformed, behaves as an elastic body in that the projection length into the pipette increases linearly with the suction pressure. This elastic behavior appears to be due to the deformation of the nucleus, which has an apparent area elastic modulus of 2 mN/m. A lymphocyte recovers its shape somewhat more quickly than the neutrophil does, although this recovery process is driven both by the cortical tension and by the elastic nucleus. These preliminary results are discussed by Tran-Son-Tay et al. [1994]. Finally, the properties of a human myeloid leukemic cell line (HL60) thought to resemble immature neutrophils of the bone marrow have also been characterized, as shown in Table 60.5. The apparent cytoplasmic viscosity varies both as a function of the cell cycle and during maturation toward a more neutrophil-like cell. The characteristic viscosity ($\dot{\gamma}_c = 1 \text{ sec}^{-1}$) is 200 Pa sec for HL60 cells in the G1 stage of the cell cycle. This value increases to 275 Pa sec for cells in the S phase, but decreases with maturation, so that 7 days after induction the properties approach those of neutrophils (150 Pa sec) [Tsai et al., 1996a, b].

It is important to note in closing that the characteristics described above apply to passive leukocytes. It is the nature of these cells to respond to environmental stimulation and engage in active movements and shape transformations. **White cell activation** produces significant heterogeneous changes in cell properties. The cell projections that form as a result of stimulation (called pseudopodia) are extremely rigid, whereas other regions of the cell may retain the characteristics of a passive cell. In addition, the cell may produce large protrusive or contractile forces. The changes in cellular mechanical properties that result from cellular activation are complex and only beginning to be formulated in terms of mechanical models. One notable recent contribution to this field was made by Herant et al., who developed a two-phase model of the cell interior accounting for different properties of the cytoskeleton and the cytosol, and estimating possible effects of swelling and polymerization forces [Herant et al., 2003].

60.5 Summary

Constitutive equations that capture the essential features of the responses of red blood cells and passive leukocytes have been formulated, and material parameters characterizing the cellular behavior have been measured. The red cell response is dominated by the cell membrane which can be described as a hyper-viscoelastic, two-dimensional continuum. The passive white cell behaves like a highly viscous fluid drop, and its response to external forces is dominated by the large viscosity of the cytosol. Refinements of these constitutive models and extension of mechanical analysis to activated white cells is anticipated as the ultrastructural events that occur during cellular deformation are delineated in increasing detail.

Defining Terms

Area expansivity modulus: A measure of the resistance of a membrane to area dilation. It is the proportionality between the isotropic force resultant in the membrane and the corresponding fractional change in membrane area. (Units: 1 mN/m = 1 dyn/cm)

Cortical tension: Analogous to surface tension of a liquid drop, it is a persistent contractile force per unit length at the surface of a white blood cell. (Units: 1 mN/m = 1 dyn/cm)

Cytoplasmic viscosity: A measure of the resistance of the cytosol to flow. (Units: 1 Pa sec = 10 poise)

Force resultant: The stress in a membrane integrated over the membrane thickness. It is the two-dimensional analog of stress with units of force/length. (Units: 1 mN/m = 1 dyn/cm)

Maxwell fluid: A constitutive model in which the response of the material to applied stress includes both an elastic and viscous response in series. In response to a constant applied force, the material will respond elastically at first, then flow. At fixed deformation, the stresses in the material will relax to zero.

Membrane bending modulus: The intrinsic resistance of the membrane to changes in curvature. It is usually construed to exclude nonlocal contributions. It relates the moment resultants (force times length per unit length) in the membrane to the corresponding change in curvature (inverse length). (Units: 1 Nm = 1 J = 10^7 erg)

Membrane shear modulus: A measure of the elastic resistance of the membrane to surface shear deformation; that is, changes in the shape of the surface at constant surface area (Equation 60.8). (Units: 1 mN/m = 1 dyn/cm)

Membrane viscosity: A measure of the resistance of the membrane to surface shear flow, that is to the rate of surface shear deformation (Equation 60.8). (Units: 1 mN sec/m = 1 m Pa sec m = 1 dyn sec/cm = 1 surface poise)

Nonlocal bending resistance: A resistance to bending resulting from the differential expansion and compression of the two adjacent leaflets of a lipid bilayer. It is termed nonlocal because the leaflets can move laterally relative to one another to relieve local strains, such that the net resistance to bending depends on the integral of the change in curvature of the entire membrane capsule.

Power law fluid: A model to describe the dependence of the cytoplasmic viscosity on rate of deformation (Equation 60.12).

Principal extension ratios: The ratios of the deformed length and width of a rectangular material element (in principal coordinates) to the undeformed length and width.

Sphericity: A dimensionless ratio of the cell volume (to the 2/3 power) to the cell area. Its value ranges from near zero to one, the maximum value corresponding to a perfect sphere (Equation 60.6).

White cell activation: The response of a leukocyte to external stimuli that involves reorganization and polymerization of the cellular structures and is typically accompanied by changes in cell shape and cell movement.

References

Alberts, B., Bray, D., Lewis, J., Raff, M., Roberts, K., and Watson, J.D. 1989. *Molecular Biology of The Cell*, 2nd ed. Garland Publishing, Inc., New York and London.

Bagge, U., Skalak, R., and Attefors, R. 1977. Granulocyte rheology. *Adv. Microcirc.* 7: 29–48.

Chien, S., Sung, K.L.P., Skalak, R., and Usami, S. 1978. Theoretical and experimental studies on viscoelastic properties of erythrocyte membrane. *Biophys. J.* 24: 463–487.

Chien, S., Usami, S., and Bertles, J.F. 1970. Abnormal rheology of oxygenated blood in sickle cell anemia. *J. Clin. Invest.* 49: 623–634.

Cokelet, G.R. and Meiselman, H.J. 1968. Rheological comparison of hemoglobin solutions and erythrocyte suspensions. *Science* 162: 275–277.

Diggs, L.W., Sturm, D., and Bell, A. 1985. *The Morphology of Human Blood Cells*, 5th ed. Abbott Laboratories, Abbott Park, Illinois.

Discher, D.E., Mohandas, N., and Evans, E.A., 1994. Molecular maps of red cell deformation: hidden elasticity and in situ connectivity. *Science* 266: 1032–1035.

Dong, C., Skalak, R., and Sung, K.-L.P. 1991. Cytoplasmic rheology of passive neutrophils. *Biorheology* 28: 557–567.

Dong, C., Skalak, R., Sung, K.-L.P., Schmid-Schönbein, G.W. and Chien, S. 1988. Passive deformation analysis of human leukocytes. *J. Biomech. Eng.* 110: 27–36.

Drury, J.L. and Dembo, M. 2001. Aspiration of human neutrophils: effects of shear thinning and cortical dissipation. *Biophys. J.* 81: 3166–3177.

Evans, E.A. 1983. Bending elastic modulus of red blood cell membrane derived from buckling instability in micropipet aspiration tests. *Biophys. J.* 43: 27–30.

Evans E. and Kukan, B. 1984. Passive material behavior of granulocytes based on large deformation and recovery after deformation tests. *Blood* 64: 1028–1035.

Evans, E.A. and Skalak, R. 1979. Mechanics and thermodynamics of biomembrane. *CRC Crit. Rev. Bioeng.* 3: 181–418.

Evans, E.A. and Waugh, R. 1977. Osmotic correction to elastic area compressibility measurements on red cell membrane. *Biophys. J.* 20: 307–313.

Evans, E. and Yeung, A. 1989. Apparent viscosity and cortical tension of blood granulocytes determined by micropipet aspiration. *Biophys. J.* 56: 151–160.

Fischer, T.M., Haest, C.W.M., Stohr-Liesen, M., Schmid-Schonbein, H., and Skalak, R. 1981. The stress-free shape of the red blood cell membrane. *Biophys. J.* 34: 409–422.

Fung, Y.C., Tsang, W.C.O., and Patitucci, P. 1981. High-resolution data on the geometry of red blood cells. *Biorheology* 18: 369–385.

Hawkey, C.M., Bennett, P.M., Gascoyne, S.C., Hart, M.G., and Kirkwood, J.K. 1991. Erythrocyte size, number and haemoglobin content in vertebrates. *Br. J. Haematol.* 77: 392–397.

Hochmuth, R.M., Buxbaum, K.L., and Evans, E.A. 1980. Temperature dependence of the viscoelastic recovery of red cell membrane. *Biophys. J.* 29: 177–182.

Hochmuth, R.M., Ting-Beall, H.P., Beaty, B.B., Needham, D., and Tran-Son-Tay, R. 1993. Viscosity of passive human neutrophils undergoing small deformations. *Biophys. J.* 64: 1596–1601.

Hochmuth, R.M., Ting-Beall, H.P., and Zhelev, D.V. 1995. The mechanical properties of individual passive neutrophils *in vitro*. In *Physiology and Pathophysiology of Leukocyte Adhesion*, D.N. Granger and G.W. Schmid-Schönbein, eds. Oxford University Press, London.

Hwang, W.C. and Waugh, R.E. 1997. Energy of dissociation of lipid bilayer from the membrane skeleton of red blood cells. *Biophys. J.* 72: 2669–2678.

Katnik, C. and Waugh, R. 1990. Alterations of the apparent area expansivity modulus of red blood cell membrane by electric fields. *Biophys. J.* 57: 877–882.

Lew, V.L. and Bookchin, R.M. 1986. Volume, pH and ion content regulation human red cells: analysis of transient behavior with an integrated model. *J. Membr. Biol.* 10: 311–330.

Markle, D.R., Evans, E.A., and Hochmuth, R.M. 1983. Force relaxation and permanent deformation of erythrocyte membrane. *Biophys. J.* 42: 91–98.

Mohandas, N. and Evans, E. 1994. Mechanical properties of the red cell membrane in relation to molecular structure and genetic defects. *Ann. Rev. Biophys. Biomol. Struct.* 23: 787–818.

Needham, D. and Hochmuth, R.M. 1990. Rapid flow of passive neutrophils into a 4 μm pipet and measurement of cytoplasmic viscosity. *J. Biomech. Eng.* 112: 269–276.

Needham, D. and Hochmuth, R.M. 1992. A sensitive measure of surface stress in the resting neutrophil. *Biophys. J.* 61: 1664–1670.

Needham, D. and Nunn, R.S. 1990. Elastic deformation and failure of lipid bilayer membranes containing cholesterol. *Biophys. J.* 58: 997–1009.

Ross, P.D. and Minton, A.P. 1977. Hard quasispherical model for the viscosity of hemoglobin solutions. *Biochem. Biophys. Res. Commun.* 76: 971–976.

Schmid-Schönbein, G.W., Shih, Y.Y., and Chien, S. 1980. Morphometry of human leukocytes. *Blood* 56: 866–875.

Ting-Beall, H.P., Needham, D., and Hochmuth, R.M. 1993. Volume, and osmotic properties of human neutrophils. *Blood* 81: 2774–2780.

Ting-Beall, H.P., Zhelev, D.V., and Hochmuth, R.M. 1995. Comparison of different drying procedures for scanning electron microscopy using human leukocytes. *Microscopy Research of Technique* 32: 357–361.

Ting-Beall, H.P, Zhelev, D.V., Needham, D. Ghazi, Y., and Hochmuth, R.M. 1994b. The volume of white cells. *Blood* to be submitted.

Tran-Son-Tay, R., Needham, D., Yeung, A., and Hochmuth, R.M. 1991. Time-dependent recovery of passive neutrophils after large deformation. *Biophys. J.* 60: 856–866.

Tran-Son-Tay, R., Kirk, T.F. III, Zhelev, D.V., and Hochmuth, R.M. 1994. Numerical simulation of the flow of highly viscous drops down a tapered tube. *J. Biomech. Eng.* 116: 172–177.

Tsai, M.A., Frank, R.S., and Waugh, R.E. 1993. Passive mechanical behavior of human neutrophils: power-law fluid. *Biophys. J.* 65: 2078–2088.

Tsai, M.A., Frank, R.S., and Waugh, R.E. 1994. Passive mechanical behavior of human neutrophils: effect of Cytochalasin B. *Biophys. J.* 66: 2166–2172.

Tsai, M.A., Waugh, R.E., and Keng, P.C. 1996a. Changes in HL-60 cell deformability during differentiation induced by DMSO. *Biorheology* 33: 1–15.

Tsai, M.A., Waugh, R.E., and Keng, P.C. 1996b. Cell cycle dependence of HL-60 deformability. *Biophys. J.* 70: 2023–2029.

Waugh, R.E. and Agre, P. 1988. Reductions of erythrocyte membrane viscoelastic coefficients reflect spectrin deficiencies in hereditary spherocytosis. *J. Clin. Invest.* 81: 133–141.

Waugh, R. and Evans, E.A. 1979. Thermoelasticity of red blood cell membrane. *Biophys. J.* 26: 115–132.

Waugh, R.E. and Marchesi, S.L. 1990. Consequences of structural abnormalities on the mechanical properties of red blood cell membrane. In *Cellular and Molecular Biology of Normal and Abnormal Erythrocyte Membranes*, C.M. Cohen and J. Palek, eds. pp. 185–199, Alan R. Liss, New York, NY.

Yeung, A. and Evans, E. 1989. Cortical shell-liquid core model for passive flow of liquid-like spherical cells into micropipets. *Biophys. J.* 56: 139–149.

Zhelev, D.V., Needham, D., and Hochmuth, R.M., 1994. Role of the membrane cortex in neutrophil deformation in small pipets. *Biophys. J.* 67: 696–705.

Further Information

Basic information on the mechanical analysis of biomembrane deformation can be found in Evans and Skalak [1979], which also appeared as a book under the same title (CRC Press, Boca Raton, FL, 1980). A more recent work that focuses more closely on the structural basis of the membrane properties is Berk et al., chapter 15, pp. 423–454, in the book *Red Blood Cell Membranes: Structure, Function, Clinical Implications* edited by Peter Agre and John Parker, Marcel Dekker, New York, 1989. More detail about the membrane structure can be found in other chapters of that book.

Basic information about white blood cell biology can be found in the book by Alberts et al. [1989]. A more thorough review of white blood cell structure and response to stimulus can be found in two reviews by T.P. Stossel, one entitled, "The mechanical response of white blood cells," in the book, *Inflammation: Basic Principles and Clinical Correlates*, edited by J.I. Galin et al., Raven Press, New York, 1988, pp. 325–342, and the second entitled, "The molecular basis of white blood cell motility," in the book, *The Molecular Basis of Blood Diseases*, edited by G. Stamatoyannopoulos et al., W. B. Saunders, Philadelphia, 1994, pp. 541–562. The most recent advances in white cell rheology can be found in the book, *Cell Mechanics and Cellular Engineering*, edited by Van C. Mow et al., Springer Verlag, New York, 1994.

61

Mechanics of Tissue/Lymphatic Transport

Geert W. Schmid-Schönbein
Alan R. Hargens
University of California-San Diego

61.1 Introduction

Transport of fluid and metabolites from blood to tissue is critically important for maintaining the viability and function of cells within the body. Similarly, transport of fluid and waste products from tissue to the **lymphatic system** of vessels and nodes is also crucial to maintain tissue and organ health. Therefore, it is important to understand the mechanisms for transporting fluid containing micro- and macromolecules from blood to tissue and the drainage of this fluid into the lymphatic system. Because of the succinct nature of this chapter, readers are encouraged to consult more complete reviews of blood/tissue/lymphatic transport by Aukland and Reed [1993], Bert and Pearce [1984], Casley-Smith [1982], Curry [1984], Hargens [1986], Jain [1987], Lai-Fook [1986], Levick [1984], Reddy [1986], Schmid-Schönbein [1990], Schmid-Schönbein and Zweifach [1994], Staub [1988], Staub et al. [1987], Taylor and Granger [1984], Wei et al. [2003], Zweifach and Lipowsky [1984], and Zweifach and Silverberg [1985].

Most previous studies of blood/tissue/lymphatic transport have used isolated organs or whole animals under general anesthesia. Under these conditions, transport of fluid and metabolites is artificially low in comparison to animals that are actively moving. In some cases, investigators employed passive motion by connecting an animal's limb to a motor in order to facilitate studies of blood to lymph transport and lymphatic flow. However, new methods and technology allow studies of physiologically active animals so that a better understanding of the importance of transport phenomena in moving tissues is now apparent, especially in skeletal muscle, skin, and subcutaneous tissue. Therefore, the major focus of this chapter emphasizes recent developments in the understanding of the mechanics of tissue/lymphatic transport.

The majority of the fluid that is filtered from the microcirculation into the interstitial space is carried out of the tissue via the lymphatic network. This unidirectional transport system originates with a set of blind channels in distal regions of the microcirculation. It carries a variety of interstitial molecules, proteins, metabolites, colloids, and even cells along channels deeply embedded in the tissue parenchyma toward a set of sequential lymph nodes and eventually back into the venous system via the right and left thoracic ducts. The lymphatics are the pathways for immune surveillance by the lymphocytes and thus, they are one of the important pathways of the immune system [Wei et al., 2003].

In the following sections, we describe basic transport and tissue morphology as related to lymph flow. We also present recent evidence for a two-valve system in lymphatics that offers an updated view of lymph transport.

61.2 Basic Concepts of Tissue/Lymphatic Transport

61.2.1 Transcapillary Filtration

Because lymph is formed from fluid filtered from the blood, an understanding of transcapillary exchange must be gained first. Usually pressure parameters favor filtration of fluid across the **capillary** wall to the **interstitium** (J_c) according to the Starling–Landis equation:

$$J_c = L_p A [(P_c - P_t) - \sigma_p (\pi_c - \pi_t)] \tag{61.1}$$

where J_c is the net transcapillary fluid transport, L_p is hydraulic conductivity of capillary wall, A is capillary surface area, P_c is capillary blood pressure, P_t is interstitial fluid pressure, σ_p is reflection coefficient for protein, π_c is capillary blood **colloid osmotic pressure**, and π_t is the interstitial fluid colloid osmotic pressure.

In many tissues, fluid transported out of the capillaries is passively drained by the initial lymphatic vessels so that:

$$J_c = J_l \tag{61.2}$$

where J_l is the lymph flow and pressure within the initial lymphatic vessels P_l depends on higher interstitial fluid pressure P_t for establishing lymph flow:

$$P_t \geq P_l \tag{61.3}$$

61.2.2 Starling Pressures and Edema Prevention

Hydrostatic and *colloid osmotic pressures* within the blood and interstitial fluid primarily govern transcapillary fluid shifts (Figure 61.1). Although input arterial pressure averages about 100 mmHg at heart level, capillary blood pressure P_c is significantly reduced due to resistance R, according to the Poiseuille's equation:

$$R = \frac{8\eta l}{\pi r^4} \tag{61.4}$$

where η is the blood viscosity, l is the vessel length between feed artery and capillary, and r is the radius.

Therefore, normally at the heart level, P_c is approximately 30 mmHg. However, during upright posture, P_c at foot level is about 90 mmHg and only about 25 mmHg at head level [Parazynski et al., 1991].

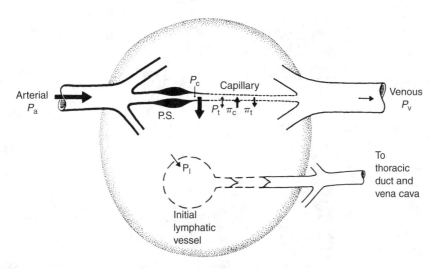

FIGURE 61.1 Starling pressures that regulate transcapillary fluid balance. Pressure parameters which determine direction and magnitude of transcapillary exchange include capillary blood pressure P_c, interstitial fluid pressure P_t (directed into capillary when positive or directed into tissue when negative), plasma colloidal osmotic pressure π_c, and interstitial fluid colloidal osmotic pressure π_t. Precapillary sphincters (P.S.) regulate P_c, capillary flow, and capillary surface area A. It is generally agreed that a hydrostatic pressure gradient ($P_t >$ lymph pressure P_l) drains off excess interstitial fluid under conditions of net filtration. Relative magnitudes of pressures are depicted by the size of arrows. (From Hargens A.R. 1986. In R. Skalak and S. Chien (Eds.), *Handbook of Bioengineering*, vol. 19, pp. 1–35, New York, McGraw-Hill. With permission.)

Differences in P_c between capillaries of the head and feet are due to gravitational variation of the blood pressure such that the pressure $p = \rho g h$. For this reason, volumes of transcapillary filtration and lymph flows are generally higher in tissues of the lower body as compared to those of the upper body. Moreover, one might expect much more sparse distribution of lymphatic vessels in upper body tissues. The brain has no lymphatics, but most other vascular tissues have lymphatics. In fact, tissues of the lower body of humans and other tall animals have efficient skeletal muscle pumps, prominent lymphatic systems, and noncompliant skin and fascial boundaries to prevent dependent **edema** [Hargens et al., 1987].

Other pressure parameters in the Starling–Landis equation such as P_t, π_c, and π_t are not as sensitive to changes in body posture as is P_c. Typical values for P_t range from -2 to 10 mmHg depending on the tissue or organ under investigation [Wiig, 1990]. However, during movement, P_t in skeletal muscle increases to 150 mmHg or higher [Murthy et al., 1994], providing a mechanism to promote lymphatic flow and venous return via the skeletal pump (Figure 61.2). Blood colloid osmotic pressure π_c usually ranges between 25 and 35 mmHg and is the other major force for retaining plasma within the vascular system and preventing edema. Interstitial π_t depends on the reflection coefficient of the capillary wall (σ_p ranges from 0.5 to 0.9 for different tissues) as well as washout of interstitial proteins during high filtration rates [Aukland and Reed, 1993]. Typically π_t ranges between 8 and 15 mmHg with higher values in upper body tissues compared to those in the lower body [Parazynski et al., 1991; Aukland and Reed, 1993]. Precapillary sphincter activity (see Figure 61.1) also decreases blood flow, decreases capillary filtration area A, and reduces P_c in dependent tissues of the body to help prevent edema during upright posture [Aratow et al., 1991].

61.2.3 Interstitial Fluid Transport

Interstitial flow of proteins and other macromolecules occurs by two mechanisms, diffusion and convection. During simple diffusion according to Fick's equation:

$$J_p = -D\frac{\partial c_p}{\partial x} \tag{61.5}$$

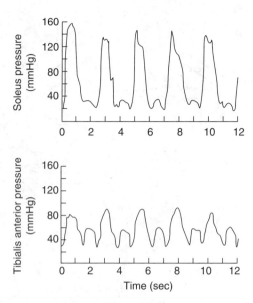

FIGURE 61.2 Simultaneous intramuscular pressure oscillations in the soleus (top panel) and the tibialis anterior (bottom panel) muscles during plantar- and dorsiflexion exercise. Soleus muscle is an integral part of the calf muscle pump. (From Murthy, G., Watenpaugh, D.E., Ballard, R.E. et al., 1994. *J. Appl. Physiol.* 76: 2742. With permission.)

where J_p is the one-dimensional protein flux, D is diffusion coefficient, and $\partial c_p / \partial x$ is the concentration gradient of protein through interstitial space.

For most macromolecules such as proteins, the diffusional transport is limited. It serves to disperse molecules, but it does not effectively serve to transport large molecules especially if their diffusion is restricted by interstitial matrix proteins, membrane barriers, or other structures that limit their free thermal motion. Instead, both experimental and theoretical evidence highlights the dependence of volume and solute flows on hydrostatic and osmotic pressure gradients [Hargens and Akeson, 1986; Hammel, 1994] and suggests that convective flow plays the dominating role in interstitial flow and transport of nutrients to tissue cells. For example, in the presence of osmotic or hydrostatic pressure gradients, protein transport J_p is coupled to fluid transport according to:

$$J_p = \bar{c}_p J_v \qquad (61.6)$$

where $\bar{c}_p$ is the average protein concentration and J_v is the volume flow of fluid.

Transport of interstitial fluid toward the lymphatics requires convective flow, since it needs to be focused on relatively few channels in the interstitium. Diffusion cannot serve such a purpose because diffusion merely disperses fluid and proteins. Lymph formation and flow greatly depend upon tissue movement or activity related to muscle contraction and tissue deformations. It is also generally agreed that formation of initial lymph depends solely on the composition of nearby interstitial fluid and pressure gradients across the interstitial/lymphatic boundary [Zweifach and Lipowsky, 1984; Hargens, 1986]. For this reason, lymph formation and flow can be quantified by measuring disappearance of isotope-labeled albumin from subcutaneous tissue or skeletal muscle [Reed et al., 1985].

61.2.4 Lymphatic Architecture

To understand lymph transport in engineering terms it is paramount that we develop a detailed picture of the lymphatic network topology and vessel morphology. This task is facilitated by a number of morphological and ultrastructural studies from past decades that give a general picture of the morphology

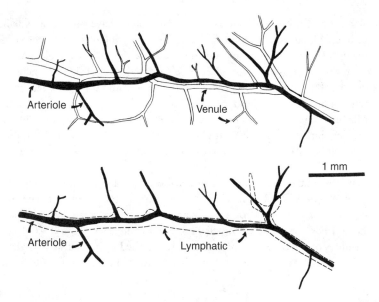

FIGURE 61.3 Tracing of a typical lymphatic channel (bottom panel) in rat spinotrapezius muscle after injection with a micropipette of a carbon contrast suspension. All lymphatics are of the initial type and are closely associated with the arcade arterioles. Few lymphatics follow the path of the arcade venules, or their side branches, the collecting venules or the transverse arterioles. (From Skalak et al., 1986. In A.R. Hargens (Ed.) *Tissue Nutrition and Viability*, pp. 243–262, Springer-Verlag, New York. With permission.)

and location of lymphatic vessels in different tissues. Lymphatics are studied by injections of macroscopic and microscopic contrast media and by light and electron microscopic sections. The display of the lymphatics is organ specific and there are many variations in lymphatic architecture [Schmid-Schönbein, 1990]. In this chapter, we will focus our discussion predominantly on skeletal muscle, intestine, and skin. However, the mechanisms outlined below may in part be also relevant to other tissues and organs.

In skeletal muscle, lymphatics are positioned in *immediate* proximity of the arterioles [Skalak et al., 1984]. The majority of feeder arteries in skeletal muscle and most, but not all, of the arcade arterioles are closely accompanied by a lymphatic vessel (Figure 61.3). Lymphatics can be traced along the entire length of the arcade arterioles, but they can be traced only over relatively short distances (less than about 50 μm) into the side branches of the arcades, the transverse (terminal) arterioles, which supply the blood into the capillary network. Systematic reconstructions of the lymphatics in skeletal muscle have yielded little evidence for lymphatic channels that enter into the capillary network per se [Skalak et al., 1984]. Thus, the network density of lymphatics is quite low compared to the high density of the capillary network in muscle, a characteristic feature of lymphatics in most organs [Skalak et al., 1986]. The close association between lymphatics and the vasculature is also present in skin [Ikomi and Schmid-Schönbein, 1995] and in other organs and may extend into the central vasculature. Recently, Saharinen et al. [2004] reviewed lymphatic vasculature development and molecular regulation in tumor metastasis and inflammation. It is apparent that current understandings of lymphatic growth factors and strategies to limit lymphatic vessel growth may allow manipulation of lymphatic growth in disease.

61.2.5 Lymphatic Morphology

Histological sections of the lymphatics permit the classification into two distinct subsets, *initial* lymphatics and *collecting* lymphatics. The initial lymphatics (sometimes also denoted as terminal or capillary lymphatics) form a set of blind endings in the tissue that feed into the collecting lymphatics, and that in turn, are the conduits into the lymph nodes. While both initial and collecting lymphatics are lined by a highly attenuated endothelium, only the collecting lymphatics have smooth muscle in their media. In accordance, contractile lymphatics exhibit spontaneous narrowing of their lumen, while there is no evidence for contractility (in the sense of a smooth muscle contraction) in the initial lymphatics. Contractile lymphatics are capable of peristaltic smooth muscle contractions that, in conjunction with periodic opening and closing of intraluminal valves, permit unidirectional fluid transport. The lymphatic smooth muscle has adrenergic innervation [Ohhashi et al., 1982], it exhibits myogenic contraction [Hargens and Zweifach, 1977; Mizuno et al., 1997], and reacts to a variety of vasoactive stimuli [Ohhashi et al., 1978; Benoit, 1997], including signals that involve nitric oxide [Ohhashi and Takahashi, 1991; Bohlen and Lash, 1992; Yokoyama and Ohhashi, 1993]. None of these contractile features has been documented in initial lymphatics.

The lymphatic endothelium has a number of similarities with vascular endothelium. It forms a continuous lining and has typical cytoskeletal fibers such as microtubules, intermediate fibers, and actin in both fiber bundle form and matric form. There are numerous caveolae, Weibel-Palade bodies, but lymphatic endothelium has fewer interendothelial adhesion complexes and a discontinuous basement membrane. The residues of the basement membrane are attached to interstitial collagen via anchoring filaments [Leak and Burke, 1968] that provide relatively firm attachment of the endothelium to interstitial structures.

61.2.6 Lymphatic Network Display

One of the interesting aspects regarding lymphatic transport in skeletal muscle is the fact that all lymphatics *inside* the muscle parenchyma are of the noncontractile, *initial* type [Skalak et al., 1984]. *Collecting* lymphatics can only be observed outside the muscle fibers as conduits to adjacent lymph nodes. The fact that all lymphatics inside the tissue parenchyma are of the initial type is not unique to skeletal muscle, but has been demonstrated in other organs [Unthank and Bohlen, 1988; Yamanaka et al., 1995]. The initial lymphatics are positioned in the adventitia of the arcade arterioles surrounded by collagen fibers (Figure 61.4). Thus, the initial lymphatics are in immediate proximity to the arteriolar smooth muscle, and adjacent to myelinated nerves fibers and a set of mast cells that accompany the arterioles. The initial lymphatics are frequently sandwiched between arteriolar smooth muscle and their paired venules, and they in turn are embedded between the skeletal muscle fibers [Skalak et al., 1984]. The initial lymphatics are firmly attached to the adjacent basement membrane and collagen fibers via anchoring filaments [Leak and Burke, 1968]. The basement membrane of the lymphatic endothelium is discontinuous, especially at the interendothelial junctions, so that macromolecules and even cells and particles enter the initial lymphatics [Casley-Smith, 1962; Bach and Lewis, 1973; Strand and Persson, 1979; Bollinger et al., 1981; Ikomi et al., 1996].

The lumen cross section of initial lymphatics is highly irregular in contrast to the overall circular cross section of collecting lymphatics (Figure 61.4). Luminal cross sections of initial lymphatics are partially or completely collapsed and may frequently span around the arcade arteriole. In fact, we have documented cases in which the arcade arteriole is completely surrounded by an initial lymphatic channel, highlighting the fact that the activity of the lymphatics is closely linked to that of the arterioles [Ikomi and Schmid-Schönbein, 1995].

61.2.7 The Intraluminal (Secondary) Lymphatic Valves

Initial lymphatics in skeletal muscle have intraluminal valves that consist of bileaflets and a funnel structure [Mazzoni et al., 1987]. The leaflets are flexible structures and are opened and closed by a viscous pressure drop along the valve funnel. In closed position, these leaflets can support considerable pressures [Eisenhoffer et al., 1995; Ikomi et al., 1997]. This arrangement preserves normal valve function even in initial lymphatics with irregularly shaped lumen cross sections.

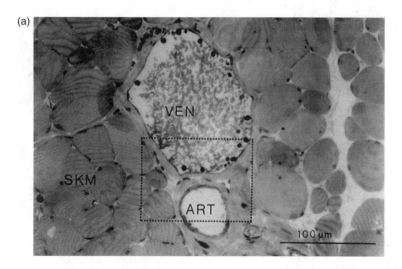

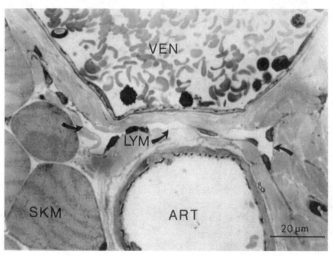

FIGURE 61.4 Histological cross sections of lymphatics (LYM) in rat skeletal muscle before (a) and after (b) contraction of the paired arcade arterioles (ART). The lymphatic channel is of the initial type with a single attenuated endothelial layer (curved arrows). Note, that in the dilated arteriole, the lymphatic is essentially compressed (a) while the lymphatic is expanded after arteriolar contraction (b) which is noticeable by the folded endothelial cells in the arteriolar lumen. In both cases, the lumen cross-sectional shape of the initial lymphatic channels is highly irregular. All lymphatics in skeletal muscle have these characteristic features. (From Skalak T.C., Schmid-Schönbein G.W., and Zweifach B.W. 1984. *Microvasc. Res.* 28: 95.)

61.2.8 The Primary Lymphatic Valves

The lymphatic endothelial cells are attenuated and have many of the morphological characteristics of vascular endothelium, including expression of P-selectin, von Willebrand factor [Di Nucci et al., 1996], and factor VIII [Schmid-Schönbein, 1990]. An important difference between vascular and lymphatic endothelium lies in the arrangement of the endothelial junctions. In the initial lymphatics, the endothelial cells lack tight junctions [Schneeberger and Lynch, 1984] and are frequently encountered in an overlapping but open position, so that proteins, large macromolecules, and even chylomicron particles can readily pass through the junctions [Casley-Smith, 1962, 1964; Leak, 1970]. Examination of the junctions with scanning electron microscopy shows that there exists a periodic *interdigitating* arrangement of endothelial extensions. Individual extensions are attached via anchoring filaments to the underlying basement membrane

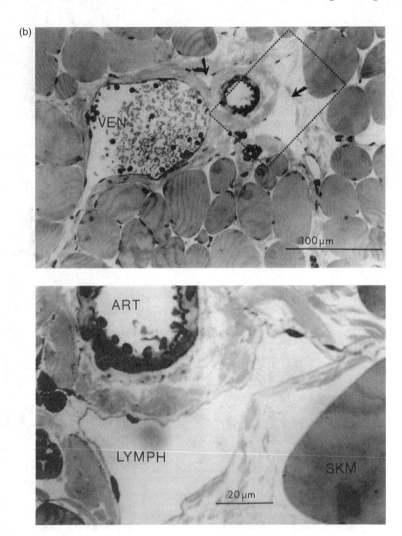

FIGURE 61.4 Continued.

and connective tissue, but the two extensions of adjacent endothelial cells resting on top of each other are not attached by interendothelial adhesion complexes. Mild mechanical stretching of the initial lymphatics shows that the endothelial extensions can be separated in part from each other, indicating that the membranes of two neighboring lymphatic endothelial cells are not attached to each other, but are firmly attached to the underlying basement membrane [Castenholz, 1984]. Lymphatic endothelium does not exhibit continuous junctional complexes, and instead has a "streak and dot" like immunostaining pattern of VE-cadherin and associated intracellular proteins desmoplakin and plakoglobulin [Schmelz et al., 1994]. However the staining pattern is not uniform for all lymphatics, and in larger lymphatics a more continuous pattern is present. This highly specialized arrangement has been referred to as the *lymphatic endothelial microvalves* [Schmid-Schönbein, 1990] or primary lymphatic valves. They are "*primary*" because fluid from the interstitium must first pass across these valves before entering the lymphatic lumen and then pass across the intraluminal, that is, secondary, valves. Particles deposited into the interstitial space adjacent to initial lymphatics pass across the endothelium of the initial lymphatics. However once the particles are inside the initial lymphatic lumen, they cannot return back into the interstitial space unless the endothelium is injured. Indeed, the endothelial junctions of the initial lymphatics serve as a functional valve system [Trzewik et al., 2001].

61.2.9 Mechanics of Lymphatic Valves

In contrast to the central large valves in the heart that are closed by inertial fluid forces, the lymphatic valves are small and the fluid Reynolds number is almost zero. Thus, because no inertial forces are available to open and close these valves, unique valve morphology has evolved in these small valves. The valves form long funnel-shaped channels, which are inserted into the lymph conduits and attached at their base. The funnel is prevented from inversion by attachment via a buttress to the lymphatic wall. The valve wall structure consists of a collagen layer sandwiched between two endothelial layers, and the entire structure is quite deformable under mild physiological fluid pressures. The funnel structure allows a *viscous pressure gradient* that is sufficient to generate a pressure drop during forward fluid motion to open, and upon flow reversal to close the valves [Mazzoni et al., 1987]. The primary lymphatic valves also open as passive structures at the peripheral endothelial cell extensions. They require sites where they are free to bend into the lumen of the initial lymphatics and where they are *not* attached by anchoring filaments to the adjacent extracellular matrix [Mendoza et al., 2003].

61.2.10 Lymph Formation and Pump Mechanisms

One of the important questions fundamental to lymphology is: How do fluid and large particles in the interstitium find their way into initial lymphatics? In light of the relative sparse existence of initial lymphatics, a directed convective transport is required that can be provided by either a hydrostatic or a colloid osmotic pressure drop [Zweifach and Silberberg, 1979]. However, the exact mechanism of this unidirectional flow has remained an elusive target. Several proposals have been advanced and these are discussed in detail in Schmid-Schönbein [1990]. Briefly, a number of authors have postulated that there exists a constant pressure drop from the interstitium into the initial lymph, which may support a steady fluid flow into the lymphatics. Nevertheless, repeated measurements with different techniques have uniformly failed to provide supporting evidence for a *steady* pressure drop to transport fluid into the initial lymphatics [Zweifach and Prather, 1975; Clough and Smaje, 1978]. Under steady-state conditions, no steady pressure drop exists in the vicinity of the initial lymphatics in skeletal muscle within the resolution of the measurement technique (about 0.2 cm H_2O) [Skalak et al., 1984]. An order of magnitude estimate of the pressure drop expected at the relatively slow flow rates of the lymphatics shows, however, that the pressure drop from the interstitium may be significantly lower [Schmid-Schönbein, 1990]. Furthermore, the assumption of a *steady* pressure drop is not in agreement with the substantial evidence that lymph flow rate is enhanced under unsteady conditions (see below). Some investigators have postulated an osmotic pressure in the lymphatics to aspirate fluid into the initial lymphatics [Casley-Smith, 1972] due to ultrafiltration across the lymphatic endothelium, a mechanism referred to as "bootstrap effect" [Perl, 1975]. Critical tests of this hypothesis, such as the microinjection of hyperosmotic protein solutions, have not led to a uniformly accepted hypothesis for lymph formation involving an osmotic mechanism. Others have suggested a retrograde aspiration mechanism, such that the recoil in the collecting lymphatics serves to lower the pressure in the initial lymphatics upstream of the collecting lymphatics [Reddy, 1986; Reddy and Patel, 1995], or an electric charge difference across lymphatic endothelium [O'Morchoe et al., 1984].

61.2.11 Tissue Mechanical Motion and Lymphatic Pumping

An intriguing feature of lymphatic pressure is that lymphatic flow rates depend on tissue motion. In a resting tissue, the lymph flow rate is relatively small. However, different forms of tissue motion serve to enhance lymph flow. This was originally demonstrated for pulsatile pressures in the rabbit ear. Perfusion of the ear with steady pressure (even at the same mean pressure) stops lymph transport, while pulsatile pressures promote lymph transport [Parsons and McMaster, 1938]. In light of the paired arrangement of the arterioles and lymphatics, periodic expansion of the arterioles compresses adjacent lymphatics, and vice versa, a reduction of arteriolar diameter during the pressure reduction phase expands adjacent lymphatics [Skalak et al., 1984] (Figure 61.4). Vasomotion, associated with a slower contraction of the arterioles, but with a larger amplitude than pulsatile pressure, increases lymph formation

[Intaglietta and Gross, 1982; Colantuoni et al., 1984]. In addition, muscle contractions, simple walking [Olszewski and Engeset, 1980], respiration, intestinal peristalsis, skin compression [Ohhashi et al., 1991], and other tissue motions are associated with increased lymph flow rates. Periodic tissue motions are significantly more effective to enhance the lymph flow than elevation of the venous pressure [Ikomi et al., 1996), which is also associated with enhanced fluid filtration (Renkin et al., 1977].

A requirement for lymph fluid flow is the periodic expansion and compression of the initial lymphatics. Because initial lymphatics do not have their own smooth muscle, the expansion and compression of initial lymphatics depend on the motion of tissue in which they are embedded. In skeletal muscle, the strategic location of the initial lymphatics in the adventitia of the arterioles provides the milieu for expansion and compression via several mechanisms: arteriolar pressure pulsations or vasomotion, active or passive skeletal muscle contractions, or external muscle compression. Direct measurements of the cross-sectional area of the initial lymphatics during arteriolar contractions or during skeletal muscle shortening support this hypothesis [Skalak et al., 1984; Mazzoni et al., 1990] (Figure 61.5). The different lymph pump mechanisms are additive. Resting skeletal muscle has much lower lymph flow rates (provided largely by the arteriolar pressure pulsation and vasomotion) than skeletal muscle during exercise (produced by a combination of intramuscular pressure pulsations and skeletal muscle shortening) [Ballard et al., 1998].

Measurements of lymph flow rates in an afferent lymph vessel (diameter about 300 to 500 μm, proximal to the popliteal node) in the hind leg [Ikomi and Schmid-Schönbein, 1996] demonstrate that lymph fluid formation is influenced by passive or active motion of the surrounding tissue. Lymphatics in this tissue region drain muscle and skin of the hind leg, and the majority is of the *initial* type, whereas collecting lymphatics are detected outside the tissue parenchyma in the fascia proximal to the node. Without whole leg rotation, lymph flow remains at low but nonzero values. If the pulse pressure is stopped, lymph flow falls to values below detectable limits (less than about 10% of the values during pulse pressure). Introduction of whole leg passive movement causes strong, frequency-dependent lymph flow rates that increase linearly with the logarithm of frequency between 0.03 and 1.0 Hz (Figure 61.6). Elevation of venous pressure, which enhances fluid filtration from the vasculature and elevates the flow rates, does not significantly alter the dependency of lymph flow on periodic tissue motion [Ikomi et al., 1996].

Similarly, application of passive tissue compression on the skin elevates lymph flow rate in a frequency-dependent manner. Lymph flow rates are determined to a significant degree by the *local* action of the lymph pump, because arrest of the heartbeat and reduction of the central blood pressure to zero does not

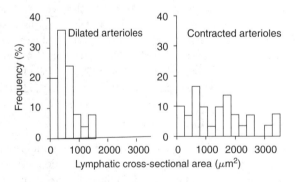 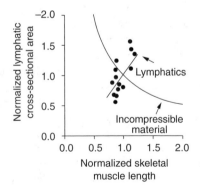

FIGURE 61.5   Histograms of initial lymphatic cross-sectional area in rat spinotrapezius muscle before (left) and after (middle) contraction of the paired arteriole with norepinephrine. Lymphatic cross-sectional area as a function of muscle length during active contraction or passive stretch (right). Cross-sectional area and muscle length are normalized with respect to the values *in vivo* in resting muscle. Note the expansion of the initial lymphatics with contraction of the arterioles or muscle stretch. (From Skalak T.C., Schmid-Schönbein G.W., and Zweifach B.W. 1984. *Microvasc. Res.* 28: 95; Mazzoni M.C., Skalak T.C., and Schmid-Schönbein G.W. 1990. *Am. J. Physiol.* 259: H1860.)

stop lymph flow. Instead, cardiac arrest reduces lymph flow rate only about 50% during continued leg motion or application of periodic shear stress to the skin for several hours [Ikomi and Schmid-Schönbein, 1996]. Periodic compression of the initial lymphatics also enhances proteins and lymphocyte counts in the lymphatics [Ikomi et al., 1996] (Figure 61.7). Thus either arteriolar smooth muscle or parenchymal skeletal muscle activity expands and compresses the initial lymphatics in skeletal muscle. These mechanisms serve to adjust lymph flow rates according to organ activity such that a resting skeletal muscle has a very low lymph flow rate. During normal daily activity or mild or strenuous exercise, lymph flow rates as well as protein and cell transport into the lymphatics increases [Olszewski et al., 1977].

61.2.12 A Lymph Pump Mechanism with Primary and Secondary Valves

Regular expansion and compression of initial lymphatic channels require a set of valves to achieve uni-directional flow. Such valves open and close with each expansion and compression of the lymphatics to permit entry at the upstream end of the lymphatics and discharge downstream toward the lymph nodes. There is a cycle of valve opening and closing with every expansion and compression of the lymphatic channels. During expansion, the upstream primary lymphatics are open and permit entry of interstitial fluid. The secondary valves are closed to prevent retrograde flow along the lymphatic channels. During compression, the primary valves are closed, while the secondary valves are open to permit discharge along the lymphatic channels into the contractile lymphatics and toward the lymph nodes.

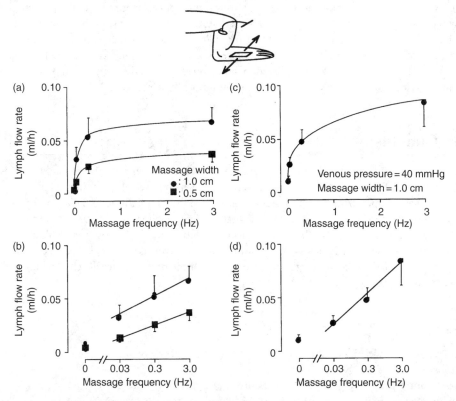

FIGURE 61.6 Lymph flow rates in a prenodal afferent lymphatic draining the hind leg as a function of the frequency of a periodic surface shear motion (massage) without (panels a, b) and with (panels c, d) elevation of the venous pressure by placement of a cuff. Zero frequency refers to a resting leg with a lymph flow rate, which depends on pulse pressure. The amplitudes of the tangential skin shear motion were 1 and 0.5 cm (panels a, b) and 1 cm in the presence of the elevated venous pressure (panels c, d). Note that the ordinates in panels c and d are larger than those in panels a and b. (From Ikomi F., Hunt J., Hanna G. et al. 1996. *J. Appl. Physiol.* 81: 2060.)

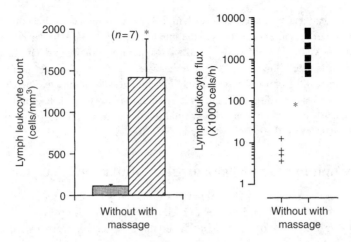

FIGURE 61.7   Lymph leukocyte count (left) and leukocyte flux (right) before and after application of periodic hind leg skin shear motion (massage) at a frequency of about 1 Hz and amplitude of 1 cm. The flux rates were computed from the product of lymph flow rates and the lymphocyte counts. *Statistically significant different from case without massage. (Adapted from Ikomi F., Hunt J., Hanna G. et al. 1996. *J. Appl. Physiol.* 81: 2060.)

Thus, we view lymphatic transport as having a robust mechanism that requires the presence of two-valve systems. In fact, all compartments that rely on a repeated cycle of expansion and compression require two-valve systems, the lymphangions along the contractile lymphatics, and even larger structures such as the ventricles of the heart, the blower in the fireplace, or even the shipping locks in the Panama Canal. None of these structures can provide unidirectional transport if one of the valves is removed, irrespective of whether it is located upstream or downstream [Schmid-Schönbein, 2003].

61.3   Conclusion

The lymphatic vessel is a unique transport system that is present even in primitive physiological systems. These vessels carry out a multitude of functions, many of which have yet to be discovered. Lymphatics have a two-valve system, a primary valve system at the level of the lymphatic endothelium and a secondary valve system in the lumen of the lymphatics, facilitating unidirectional transport toward the lymphatic nodes and thoracic duct. Details of lymphatic growth kinetics are subject to initial molecular analysis designed to identify key growth factors and their molecular control [Lohela et al., 2003; Saharinen et al., 2004]. A more detailed bioengineering analysis, especially at the molecular level [Jeltsch et al., 1997] is a fruitful area for future exploration.

Defining Terms

Capillary: The smallest blood vessel of the body that provides oxygen and other nutrients to nearby cells and tissues.

Colloid osmotic pressure: A negative pressure that depends on protein concentration (mainly of albumin and globulins) and prevents excess filtration across the capillary wall.

Edema: Excess fluid or swelling within a given tissue.

Interstitium: The space between cells of various tissues of the body. Normally fluid and proteins within this space are transported from the capillary to the initial lymphatic vessel.

Lymphatic System: The clear network of vessels which return excess fluid and proteins to the blood via the thoracic duct.

Acknowledgments

This work was supported by NASA grants NAG9-1425 and NNJ04HF71G as well as NIH grants HL 10881 and 43026.

References

Aratow M., Hargens A.R., Meyer J.-U. et al. 1991. Postural responses of head and foot cutaneous microvascular flow and their sensitivity to bed rest. *Aviat. Space Environ. Med.* 62: 246.

Aukland K. and Reed R.K. 1993. Interstitial-lymphatic mechanisms in the control of extracellular fluid volume. *Physiol. Rev.* 73: 1.

Bach C. and Lewis G.P. 1973. Lymph flow and lymph protein concentration in the skin and muscle of the rabbit hind limb. *J. Physiol. (Lond.)* 235: 477.

Ballard R.E., Watenpaugh D.E., Breit G.A. et al. 1998. Leg intramuscular pressures during locomotion in humans. *J. Appl. Physiol.* 84: 1976.

Benoit J.N. 1997. Effects of alpha-adrenergic stimuli on mesenteric collecting lymphatics in the rat. *Am. J. Physiol.* 273: R331.

Bert J.L. and Pearce R.H. 1984. The interstitium and microvascular exchange. In E. Renkin and C. Michel (Eds.), *Handbook of Physiology: The Cardiovascular System: Microcirculation*, sec. 2, Vol. 4, pt 1, pp. 521–547, Bethesda, MD, American Physiological Society.

Bohlen H.G. and Lash J.M. 1992. Intestinal lymphatic vessels release endothelial-dependent vasodilators. *Am. J. Physiol.* 262: H813.

Bollinger A., Jäger K., Sgier F. et al. 1981. Fluorescence microlymphography. *Circulation* 64: 1195.

Casley-Smith J.R. 1962. The identification of chylomicra and lipoproteins in tissue sections and their passage into jejunal lacteals. *J. Cell Biol.* 15: 259.

Casley-Smith J.R. 1964. Endothelial permeability — the passage of particles into and out of diaphragmatic lymphatics. *Q. J. Exp. Physiol.* 49: 365.

Casley-Smith J.R. 1972. The role of the endothelial intercellular junctions in the functioning of the initial lymphatics. *Angiologica* 9: 106.

Casley-Smith J.R. 1982. Mechanisms in the formation of lymph. In A.C. Guyton and J.E. Hall (Eds.), *Cardiovascular Physiology IV, International Review of Physiology*, pp. 147–187, Baltimore, University Park Press.

Castenholz A. 1984. Morphological characteristics of initial lymphatics in the tongue as shown by scanning electron microscopy. *Scanning Electr. Microsc.* 1984: 1343.

Clough G. and Smaje L.H. 1978. Simultaneous measurement of pressure in the interstitium and the terminal lymphatics of the cat mesentery. *J. Physiol. (Lond.)* 283: 457.

Colantuoni A., Bertuglia S., and Intaglietta M. 1984. A quantitation of rhythmic diameter changes in arterial microcirculation. *Am. J. Physiol.* 246: H508.

Curry F.-R.E. 1984. Mechanics and thermodynamics of transcapillary exchange. In E. Renkin and C. Michel (Eds.), *Handbook of Physiology: The Cardiovascular System: Microcirculation*, sec. 2, Vol. 4, pt 1, pp. 309–374, Bethesda, MD, American Physiological Society.

Di Nucci A., Marchetti C., Serafini S. et al. 1996. P-selectin and von Willebrand factor in bovine mesenteric lymphatics: an immunofluorescent study. *Lymphology* 29: 25.

Eisenhoffer J., Kagal A., Klein T. et al. 1995. Importance of valves and lymphangion contractions in determining pressure gradients in isolated lymphatics exposed to elevations in outflow pressure. *Microvasc. Res.* 49: 97.

Hammel H.T. 1994. How solutes alter water in aqueous solutions. *J. Phys. Chem.* 98: 4196.

Hargens A.R. and Akeson W.H. 1986. Stress effects on tissue nutrition and viability, In A.R. Hargens (Ed.), *Tissue Nutrition and Viability*, pp. 1–24, New York, Springer-Verlag.

Hargens A.R. and Zweifach B.W. 1977. Contractile stimuli in collecting lymph vessels. *Am. J. Physiol.* 233: H57.

Hargens A.R., Millard R.W., Pettersson K. et al. 1987. Gravitational haemodynamics and oedema prevention in the giraffe. *Nature* 329: 59.

Hargens A.R. 1986. Interstitial fluid pressure and lymph flow. In R. Skalak and S. Chien (Eds.), *Handbook of Bioengineering*, Vol. 19, pp. 1–35, New York, McGraw-Hill.

Ikomi F. and Schmid-Schönbein G.W. 1995. Lymph transport in the skin. *Clin. Dermatol.*, 13: 419, Elsevier Science Inc.

Ikomi F. and Schmid-Schönbein G.W. 1996. Lymph pump mechanics in the rabbit hind leg. *Am. J. Physiol.* 271: H173.

Ikomi F., Hunt J., Hanna G. et al. 1996. Interstitial fluid, protein, colloid and leukocyte uptake into interstitial lymphatics. *J. Appl. Physiol.* 81: 2060.

Ikomi F., Zweifach B.W., and Schmid-Schönbein G.W. 1997. Fluid pressures in the rabbit popliteal afferent lymphatics during passive tissue motion. *Lymphology* 30: 13.

Intaglietta M. and Gross J.F. 1982. Vasomotion, tissue fluid flow and the formation of lymph. *Int. J. Microcirc. Clin. Exp.* 1: 55.

Jain R.K. 1987. Transport of molecules in the tumor interstitium: a review. *Cancer Res.* 47: 3039.

Jeltsch M., Kaipainen A., Joukov V. et al. 1997. Hyperplasia of lymphatic vessels in VEGF-C transgenic mice. *Science* 276: 1423.

Lai-Fook S.J. 1986. Mechanics of lung fluid balance. *Crit. Rev. Biomed. Eng.* 13: 171.

Leak L.V. 1970. Electron microscopic observations on lymphatic capillaries and the structural components of the connective tissue-lymph interface. *Microvasc. Res.* 2: 361.

Leak L.V. and Burke J.F. 1968. Ultrastructural studies on the lymphatic anchoring filaments. *J. Cell Biol.* 36: 129.

Levick J.R. 1984. E. Renkin and C. Michel (Eds.), *Handbook of Physiology: The Cardiovascular System: Microcirculation*, sec. 2, Vol. 4, pt 1, pp. 917–947, Bethesda, MD, American Physiological Society.

Lohela M., Saaristo A., Veikkola T., and Alitalo K. 2003 Lymphangiogenic growth factors, receptors and therapies. *Thromb. Haemost.* 90: 167–184.

Mazzoni M.C., Skalak T.C., and Schmid-Schönbein G.W. 1987. The structure of lymphatic valves in the spinotrapezius muscle of the rat. *Blood Vessels* 24: 304.

Mazzoni M.C., Skalak T.C., and Schmid-Schönbein G.W. 1990. The effect of skeletal muscle fiber deformation on lymphatic volume. *Am. J. Physiol.* 259: H1860.

Mendoza, E. and Schmid-Schönbein G.W. 2003. A model for mechanics of primary lymphatic valves. *J. Biomech. Eng.* 125: 407–413.

Mizuno R., Dornyei G., Koller A. et al. 1997. Myogenic responses of isolated lymphatics: modulation by endothelium. *Microcirculation* 4: 413.

Murthy G., Watenpaugh D.E., Ballard R.E. et al. 1994. Supine exercise during lower body negative pressure effectively simulates upright exercise in normal gravity. *J. Appl. Physiol.* 76: 2742.

O'Morchoe C.C.C., Jones W.R.I., Jarosz H.M. et al. 1984. Temperature dependence of protein transport across lymphatic endothelium *in vitro*. *J. Cell Biol.* 98: 629.

Ohhashi T. and Takahashi N. 1991. Acetylcholine-induced release of endothelium-derived relaxing factor from lymphatic endothelial cells. *Am. J. Physiol.* 260: H1172.

Ohhashi T., Kawai Y., and Azuma T. 1978. The response of lymphatic smooth muscles to vasoactive substances. *Plügers Arch.* 375: 183.

Ohhashi T., Kobayashi S., and Tsukahara S. et al. 1982. Innervation of bovine mesenteric lymphatics: from the histochemical point of view. *Microvasc. Res.* 24: 377.

Ohhashi T., Yokoyama S., and Ikomi F. 1991. Effects of vibratory stimulation and mechanical massage on micro- and lymph-circulation in the acupuncture points between the paw pads of anesthetized dogs. In H. Niimi and F.Y. Zhuang (Eds.), *Recent Advances in Cardiovascular Diseases*, pp. 125–133, Osaka, National Cardiovascular Center.

Olszewski W.L. and Engeset A. 1980. Intrinsic contractility of prenodal lymph vessels and lymph flow in human leg. *Am. J. Physiol.* 239: H775.

Olszewski W.L., Engeset A., Jaeger P.M. et al. 1977. Flow and composition of leg lymph in normal men during venous stasis, muscular activity and local hyperthermia. *Acta Physiol. Scand.* 99: 149.

Parazynski S.E., Hargens A.R., Tucker B. et al. 1991. Transcapillary fluid shifts in tissues of the head and neck during and after simulated microgravity. *J. Appl. Physiol.* 71: 2469.

Parsons R.J. and McMaster P.D. 1938. The effect of the pulse upon the formation and flow of lymph. *J. Exp. Med.* 68: 353.

Perl W. 1975. Convection and permeation of albumin between plasma and interstitium. *Microvasc. Res.* 10: 83

Reddy N.P. and Patel K. 1995. A mathematical model of flow through the terminal lymphatics. *Med. Eng. Phys.* 17: 134.

Reddy N.P. 1986. Lymph circulation: physiology, pharmacology, and biomechanics. *Crit. Rev. Biomed. Sci.* 14: 45.

Reed R.K., Johansen S., and Noddeland H. 1985. Turnover rate of interstitial albumin in rat skin and skeletal muscle. Effects of limb movements and motor activity. *Acta Physiol. Scand.* 125: 711.

Renkin E.M., Joyner W.L., Sloop C.H. et al. 1977. Influence of venous pressure on plasma-lymph transport in the dog's paw: convective and dissipative mechanisms. *Microvasc. Res.* 14: 191.

Schmelz M., Moll R., Kuhn C. et al. 1994. Complex adherentes, a new group of desmoplakin-containing junctions in endothelial cells: II. Different types of lymphatic vessels. *Differentiation* 57: 97.

Saharinen P., Tammela T., Karkkainen M.J., and Alitalo K. 2004. Lymphatic vasculature: development, molecular regulation and role in tumor metastasis and inflammation. *Trends Immunol.* 25: 387.

Schmid-Schönbein G.W. 1990. Microlymphatics and lymph flow. *Physiol. Rev.* 70: 987.

Schmid-Schönbein G.W. and Zweifach B.W. 1994. Fluid pump mechanisms in initial lymphatics. *News Physiol. Sci.* 9: 67.

Schmid-Schönbein G.W. 2003. The second valve system in lymphatics. *Lymph. Res. Biol.* 1: 25–31.

Schneeberger E.E. and Lynch R.D. 1984. Tight junctions: their structure, composition and function. *Circ. Res.* 5: 723.

Skalak T.C., Schmid-Schönbein G.W., and Zweifach B.W. 1984. New morphological evidence for a mechanism of lymph formation in skeletal muscle. *Microvasc. Res.* 28: 95.

Skalak T.C., Schmid-Schönbein G.W., and Zweifach B.W. 1986. Lymph transport in skeletal muscle. In A.R. Hargens (Ed.), *Tissue Nutrition and Viability*, pp. 243–262, New York, Springer-Verlag.

Staub N.C. 1988. New concepts about the pathophysiology of pulmonary edema. *J. Thorac. Imaging* 3: 8.

Staub N.C., Hogg J.C., and Hargens A.R. 1987. *Interstitial–Lymphatic Liquid and Solute Movement*, pp. 1–290, Basel, Karger.

Strand S.-E. and Persson B.R.R. 1979. Quantitative lymphoscintigraphy I: basic concepts for optimal uptake of radiocolloids in the parasternal lymph nodes of rabbits. *J. Nucl. Med.* 20: 1038.

Taylor A.E. and Granger D.N. 1984. Exchange of macromolecules across the microcirculation. In E. Renkin and C. Michel (Eds.), *Handbook of Physiology: The Cardiovascular System: Microcirculation*, sec. 2, Vol. 4, pt 1, pp. 467–520, Bethesda, MD, American Physiological Society.

Trzewik J., Mallipattu S.R., Artmann G.M. et al. 2001. Evidence for a second valve system in lymphatics: Endothelial microvalves. *FASEB J.* 15: 1711.

Unthank J.L. and Bohlen H.G. 1988. Lymphatic pathways and role of valves in lymph propulsion from small intestine. *Am. J. Physiol.* 254: G389.

Wei S.H., Parker I., Miller M.J., and Cahalan M.D. 2003. A stochastic view of lymphocyte motility and trafficking within the lymph node. *Immunol. Rev.* 195: 136.

Wiig H. 1990. Evaluation of methodologies for measurement of interstitial fluid pressure (Pi): physiological implications of recent Pi data. *Crit. Rev. Biomed. Eng.* 18: 27.

Yamanaka Y., Araki K., and Ogata T. 1995. Three-dimensional organization of lymphatics in the dog small intestine: a scanning electron microscopic study on corrosion casts. *Arch. Hist. Cytol.* 58: 465.

Yokoyama S. and Ohhashi T. 1993. Effects of acetylcholine on spontaneous contractions in isolated bovine mesenteric lymphatics. *Am. J. Physiol.* 264: H1460.

Zweifach B.W. and Silberberg A. 1979. The interstitial-lymphatic flow system. In A.C. Guyton, D.B. Young (Eds.), *International Review of Physiology — Cardiovascular Physiology III*, pp. 215–260, Baltimore, University Park Press.

Zweifach B.W. and Silverberg A. 1985. The interstitial-lymphatic flow system. In M.G. Johnston and C.C. Michel (Eds.), *Experimental Biology of the Lymphatic Circulation*, pp. 45–79, Amsterdam, Elsevier.

Zweifach B.W. and Lipowsky H.H. 1984. Pressure–flow relations in blood and lymph microcirculation. In E. Renkin and C. Michel (Eds.), *Handbook of Physiology: The Cardiovascular System: Microcirculation*, sec. 2, Vol. 4, pt 1, pp. 251–307, Bethesda, MD, American Physiological Society.

Zweifach B.W. and Prather J.W. 1975. Micromanipulation of pressure in terminal lymphatics of the mesentary. *J. Appl. Physiol.* 228: 1326.

Further Information

Drinker C.K. and Yoffey J.M. 1941. *Lymphatics, Lymph and Lymphoid Tissue: Their Physiological and Clinical Significance.* Harvard University Press, Cambridge, MA. This is a classic treatment of the lymphatic circulation by two pioneers in the field of lymphatic physiology.

Yoffey J.M. and Courtice F.C. 1970. *Lymphatics, Lymph and the Lymphomyeloid Complex.* Academic Press. London, New York. This is a classic book in the field of lymphatic physiology. The book contains a comprehensive review of pertinent literature and experimental physiology on the lymphatic system.

62

Modeling in Cellular Biomechanics

Alexander A. Spector
Johns Hopkins University

Roger Tran-Son-Tay
University of Florida

62.1 Introduction

Mechanical forces, stresses, strains, and velocities play a critical role in many important aspects of cell physiology, such as cell adhesion, motility, and signal transduction. The modeling of cell mechanics is a challenging task because of the interconnection of mechanical, electrical, and biochemical processes; involvement of different structural cellular components; and multiple timescales. It can involve nonlinear mechanics and thermodynamics, and because of its complexity, it is most likely that it will require the use of computational techniques. Typical steps in the development of a cell modeling include *constitutive relations* describing the state or evolution of the cell or its components, *mathematical solution or transformation* of the corresponding equations and boundary conditions, and *computational implementation* of the model.

Modeling is a powerful tool in the simulation of processes in cells dealing with different time and spatial scales, and in the mechanical characterization of cellular parameters. It is also effective in the interpretation and design of experiments, as well as in the prediction of new effects and phenomena. It is clear that modeling would play an increasing role in improving our understanding of the biological and physiological processes in cells, under both normal and pathological conditions.

In this chapter, we focus on several important features of the cell physiology where mechanical models have been developed. All the presented analyses are based on the cell constitutive relations, in which parameters are extracted from the experiments. We also discuss different forms of cell motility, including rolling, crawling, swimming, and gliding. The topic of cell adhesion is presented in the context of cell rolling. Finally, we review various forms of mechanotransduction in cells. Some areas where mechanics also plays an important role, such as cell growth and division, are left for further reading in the recommended literature.

62.2   Mechanical Properties of the Cell

62.2.1   Constitutive Relations

The basis of cell modeling is the relationships that exist between the applied forces (stresses) and the corresponding cellular response in terms of strains or velocities. Under appropriate timescales, the cellular material can be considered elastic. In this case, the constitutive relations express the stresses in terms of strains (displacement gradients). If a cell undergoes a large deformation (e.g., in the micropipette aspiration experiment), the corresponding equation is nonlinear. If a cell composition and the applied external forces are such that cellular properties are direction-independent then the cell is considered isotropic. If the properties of a cell or its cytoskeleton are different depending on the direction (e.g., the cylindrical cochlear outer hair cell's composite membrane is softer in the longitudinal direction) then the cell is considered anisotropic. Cells that are naturally isotropic can acquire anisotropy as a result of a directional application of an external load (e.g., a reorganization of the cytoskeleton in endothelial cells in response to blood-flow shear stresses). If stresses or (and) strains relax during the process under consideration, or there is a significant frequency effect on the cellular response, models of viscoelastic materials are used. Maxwell and Voigt models describe, respectively, fluid-type and solid-type behavior. The standard linear solid model combines the properties of both, Maxwell and Voigt models, includes two relaxation times, and can describe both stress and strain relaxation. Recently, a more general viscoelastic model for cells has been proposed [Fabry et al., 2001]. The feature of this model is a power dependence of the viscoelastic moduli on the frequency with Voigt-type and Maxwell-type behavior for low and high frequencies, respectively. Purely elastic or viscoelastic models treat the cellular material as a single phase. While the cell has several components, its content can be treated as a two-phase medium where one phase is associated with the cytoskeleton and the other is related to the cytoplasm.

Long molecules that compose the cellular cytoskeleton can be treated from the standpoint of polymer mechanics where the response of the material to the application of a force is associated with changes in entropy (transition from disorder to more order). The cytoskeletal fibers are treated either as chains of segments that are completely free to move in three directions (freely joined chain model) or as flexible slender rods (worm-like chain model). The same approaches are applied to cellular components, such as the cytoskeleton, membrane, and nucleus. There is an important distinction in the models of relatively thin cellular membranes. They are considered either as shells with a certain stress distribution across the thickness or as intrinsically two-dimensional continua. In both cases, the mechanical parameters are split into two groups: moduli characterizing the in-plane properties and those characterizing the out-of-plane bending and twist of the membrane.

62.2.2   Interpretation of Experiments

There are several major techniques that are used to extract the mechanical properties of cells. The models and experiments are interconnected: the experiments provide parameters for the models and, in turn, the models are the basis for the interpretation of the experiments. One common technique is micropipette aspiration, where a pipette is sealed on the surface of a cell, negative pressure is applied inside the pipette, and a portion of the cell is aspirated into the pipette. The height of the aspirated portion is considered as an inverse measure of the cell stiffness. The same technique is used to observe the time response of the cell to the application of pressure, and in this case, the corresponding relaxation time is a measure of the cell's viscoelastic properties. The experiment with the micropipette aspiration of a red blood cell was interpreted by considering the cell membrane (including the cytoskeleton) as a nonlinear elastic half-space

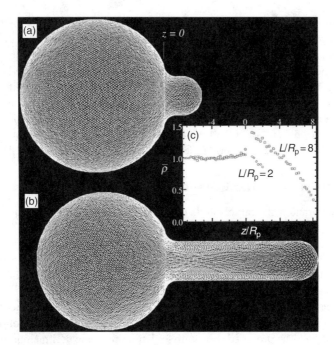

FIGURE 62.1   Simulation of the micropipette aspiration of the red blood cell cytoskeletal network for different ratios, (a) and (b), of the aspiration length L to the radius of the pipette R_p; (c) shows the profiles of the network element density $\bar{\rho}$ along the z-axis of the pipette. (From Discher, D.E., Boal, D.H., and Boey, S.K. *Biophys. J.*, 75, 1584, 1998. With permission.)

characterized by two parameters, an area expansion modulus and a shear modulus. This approach was extended to include the viscoelasticity of the cell membrane. Earlier continuum thermodynamic models of the red blood cell membrane were summarized in the monograph by Evans and Skalak [1980]. Later, Discher et al. [1998] developed an analysis of the micropipette aspiration experiment by considering the red blood cell cytoskeleton as a polymer network. Each spectrin molecule was treated as a worm-like chain, and the state of the whole network inside the micropipette was determined by a Monte Carlo simulation (Figure 62.1).

White blood cells have also been extensively studied with the micropipette, and many models have been developed to describe the cell rheological properties [Tran-Son-Tay et al., 2004; Kan et al., 1999a].

Theret et al. [1988] analyzed the micropipette experiment with endothelial cell. The cell was interpreted as a linear elastic isotropic half-space, and the pipette was considered as an axisymmetric rigid punch. This approach was later extended to a viscoelastic material of the cell and to the model of the cell as a deformable layer. The solutions were obtained both analytically by using the Laplace transform and numerically by using the finite element method. Spector et al. [1998] analyzed the application of the micropipette to a cylindrical cochlear outer hair cell. The cell composite membrane (wall) was treated as an orthotropic elastic shell, and the corresponding problem was solved in terms of Fourier series. Recently, Hochmuth [2000] reviewed the micropipette technique applied to the analysis of the cellular properties.

Another technique widely used in the estimation of the properties of cells and their components is atomic force microscopy, where the sample is probed by a sharp tip located at the end of a cantilever of a prescribed stiffness, and the corresponding indentation is tracked with a laser. The force/indentation relationship is a characterization of the cell (cellular component) properties. A traditional interpretation of this experiment is based on Hertz theory of a frictionless contact of a rigid tip with an elastic isotropic half-space [Radmacher et al., 1996]. The finite thickness of the cell can be taken into account by considering an elastic layer adhered to a substrate. More details of cell geometry and rheology can be considered by using the finite element method.

Magnetocytometry is also a popular method of the characterization of the cell mechanical properties. In this method, a magnetic bead specifically coated to adhere to a targeted area is perturbed by a magnetic field. The properties of the cell are extracted by using the resulting (force or moment)/(displacement or rotation) of the bead. Wang and Ingber [1994] used this technique to analyze how the viscoelastic properties of the cytoskeleton of endothelial cells are controlled by cell shape and the cell's interaction with the extracellular matrix. In a recent study, Karcher et al. [2003] considered a bead under the action of a magnetic force on the surface of a cellular monolayer. On the basis of a linear viscoelastic model and finite element solutions, the authors found the force/displacement relationship for the bead. Van Vilet et al. [2003] have presented a broad review of the techniques used to probe living cells.

62.2.3 Properties of Cellular Components

The cell plasma membrane is critical for mechanotransduction and cellular metabolism, and its mechanical properties have been estimated by a number of experimental techniques. The major features of biomembranes are their fluidity, bending elasticity, and the local surface area preservation. Helfrich [1973] proposed and Evans [1974] established a thermodynamic basis for a strain energy function for such membranes. Recently, Steigmann [1999] derived the most general form of the model for a two-dimensional fluid with bending resistance. For a finer analysis, another mechanical characteristic of biomembranes, nonlocal bending, was introduced [Evans, 1980; Waugh and Hochmuth, 1987; Bo and Waugh, 1989]. This parameter comes from differential area expansions and compressions of two layers of the membrane that slip relative to each other. The proposed constitutive relations for biological membranes were applied to the interpretation of important experiments, such as pulling tethers and aspiration into the micropipette.

The mechanical properties of the nucleus, the stiffest component of the cell, are important for the overall cellular response. It is, probably, even more significant that forces transmitted from the cell surface and acting on the nucleus can alter gene expression and protein synthesis. Kan et al. (1999a) have modeled the nucleus as a viscous fluid and analyzed the effect of the nucleus on the leukocyte recovery. Guilak et al. [2000] have estimated the linear viscoelastic properties of nuclei of chondrocytes. Caille et al. [2002] used a model of nonlinear elastic material to estimate Young's modulus of endothelial cell nuclei. Recently, Dahl et al. [2004], by using the micropipette technique, have estimated the mechanical properties of the cell's nuclear envelope.

62.3 Cell Motility

62.3.1 Cell Rolling and Adhesion

Cell rolling can be described as a decrease in velocity of cells (occurring only with leukocytes) in preparation to adhere to an endothelial wall. It is an essential part of a larger process of the immune system which allows leukocytes to travel and bind to trauma-induced tissues. A factor that influences the effectiveness of rolling is cell velocity. As leukocyte velocity decreases (slow rolling), the chance for adhesion rises. Another contributing factor to this phenomenon is time. Leukocytes are viscoelastic bodies, which mean that they are susceptible to deformation when a given force is applied over a specific time. As this interval grows, the shape of the leukocyte changes even more, causing an increase in the contact area of the cell. As the contact area increases, so does its chance of adhesion.

As noted earlier, there is much evidence to support the statement that rolling is an absolute prerequisite to leukocyte adhesion. This is certainly true for muscle and skin tissue. However, this is not conclusive for all tissues. The liver, lung, and heart are examples where rolling may not be necessary for leukocyte recruitment. In the lung's alveolar capillaries and the liver's sinusoids, rolling is not observed because the vessel lumen or interstitial gap is extremely small, which allows for adhesion to occur straight from tethering.

The recent cell adhesion paradigm has been developed to emphasize the role of kinetics. Conceptualized by Bell [1978] and refined by several authors [Hammer and Lauffenburger, 1987; Dembo et al., 1988], the reaction kinetics approach integrates the adhesive interaction of the cells with the surface into the adhesion mechanism. Several physicochemical properties can affect the adhesion of a cell, such as rates of reaction, affinity, mechanical elasticity, kinetic response to stress, and length of adhesion molecules.

Several models have been proposed for describing the interaction of the leukocyte with the endothelium cells. Mathematical models of cell rolling/adhesion can be classified into two classes based on equilibrium [Evans, 1985; Alon et al., 1995] and kinetics concepts [Dembo et al., 1988; Alon et al., 1998; Kan et al., 1999b]. The kinetics approach is more capable of handling the dynamics of cell adhesion and rolling. In this approach, formation and dissociation of bonds occur according to the reverse and forward rate constants.

Using this concept, Hammer and Lauffenburger [1987] studied the effect of external flow on cell adhesion. The cell is modeled as a solid sphere, and the receptors at the surface of the sphere are assumed to diffuse and to convect into the contact area. The main finding is that the adhesion parameters, such as the reverse and forward reaction rates and the receptor number, have a strong influence on the peeling of the cell from the substrate.

Dembo et al. [1988] developed a model based on the ideas of Evans [1985] and Bell [1978]. In this model, a piece of membrane is attached to the wall, and a pulling force is exerted on one end while the other end is held fixed. The cell membrane is modeled as a thin inextensible membrane. The model of Dembo et al. [1988] was subsequently extended via a probabilistic approach for the formation of bonds by Coezens-Roberts et al. [1990]. Other authors used the probabilistic approach and Monte Carlo simulation to study the adhesion process as reviewed by Zhu [2000]. Dembo's model has also been extended to account for the distribution of microvilli on the surface of the cell and to simulate the rolling and the adhesion of a cell on a surface under shear flow. Hammer and Apte [1992] modeled the cell as a microvilli-coated hard sphere covered with adhesive springs. The binding and breakage of bonds and the distribution of the receptors on the tips of the microvilli are computed using a probabilistic approach.

In order to take into account the cell deformability, which has shown to be necessary for calculating the magnitude of the adhesion force, Dong and Lei [2000] have modeled the cell as a liquid drop encapsulated into an elastic ring. They show how the deformability and the adhesion parameters affect the leukocyte and adhesion process in shear flow. However, only a small portion of the adhesion length is allowed to peel away from the vessel wall. This constraint is not physically sound, and a more sophisticated model was developed by N'Dri et al. [2003].

Chang et al. [2000] used computer simulation of cell adhesion to study the initial tethering and rolling process based on Bell's model, and constructed a state diagram for cell adhesion under viscous flows under an imposed shear rate of 100 $\sec^{-1}$. This shear rate corresponds to the experimental value where rolling of the cell occurs. To create the state diagrams, the ratio V/V_H of rolling velocity V to the hydrodynamic velocity V_H (velocity of nonadherent cells translating near the wall) is computed as a function of the reverse reaction rate, k_{ro}, for a given value of r_0 as using the Bell equation

$$k_r = k_{ro} \exp\left(\frac{r_0 f}{k_b T}\right) \tag{62.1}$$

where k_{ro} is the unstressed dissociation rate constant, $k_b T$ the thermal energy, r_0 the reactive compliance, and f the bond force. From the graph of V/V_H vs. k_{ro}, the values of k_{ro} for a given value of r_0 are estimated. The estimated values are used to plot k_{ro} as a function of r_0 for a given ratio of V/V_H. From these curves, different dynamic states of adhesion can be identified. The first state, where cells move at a velocity greater than 95% of the hydrodynamic velocity V_H, is defined as no adhesion state. The second state, where $0 < V/V_H < 0.5$, is considered as the rolling domain and consists of fast and transient adhesion regimes. The firm adhesion state, where $V/V_H = 0.0$ for a given period of time, defines the final state. Figure 62.2 shows the computed values of k_{ro} as a function of r_0.

Adhesion occurs for high values of k_{ro} and low values of r_0, as indicated by the wide area between the no- and firm-adhesion zones in Figure 62.3. As r_0 increases, k_{ro} has to decrease in order for adhesion to take place. In the simulation (Figure 62.3), both association rate k_f and wall shear rate are kept constant. Varying k_f does not change the shape of the state diagram but shifts the location of the rolling envelope

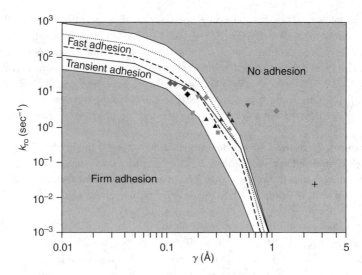

FIGURE 62.2 State diagram for adhesion. Four different states are shown. The dotted curve represents velocity of 0.3 V_H and the dashed curve represents velocity of 0.1 V_H. (From Chang, K.C., Tees, D.F.J., and Hammer, D.A. *Proc. Natl Acad. Sci. USA*, 97, 11262, 2000. With permission.)

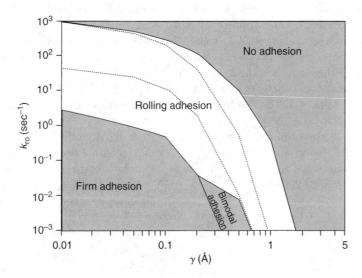

FIGURE 62.3 State of diagram for shear rate ranging from 30 to 400 sec^{-1}. The dotted curves indicate the boundaries of the rolling state at shear rate $G = 100$ sec^{-1}. The rolling adhesion area represents the region where rolling motion occurs over shear rate ranging from 30 to 400 sec^{-1}. In the bimodal-adhesion regime, cells display either firm adhesion or no adhesion, without rolling motion, as the applied shear rate is altered from 100 to 400 sec^{-1}. (From Chang, K.C., Tees, D.F.J., and Hammer, D.A. *Proc. Natl Acad. Sci. USA*, 97, 11262, 2000. With permission.)

in the k_{ro}–r_0 plane. The shear rate used in Chang et al. [2000] is in the range of the physiological flow for postcapillary venules and lies between 30 and 400 sec^{-1}. They found that as the shear rate increases, there is an abrupt change from firm adhesion to no adhesion without rolling motion. As r_0 increases, k_{ro} has to decrease in order for adhesion to take place. In the simulation, both association rate k_f and wall shear rate are kept constant. For values of r_0 less than 0.1 Å and high reverse rate constant values k_{ro}, the rolling velocity is independent of the spring constant.

Tees et al. [2002] used the approach described in Chang et al. [2000] to study the effect of particle size on the adhesion. They observed that an increase of the particle size raises the rolling velocity. This is consistent with the experimental finding of Shinde Patil et al. [2001]. In both studies, the Bell model is used to construct the state diagram but same results can be achieved using the spring model.

Using leukocytes, Alon et al. [1995] showed that the Bell equation and the spring model both fit the experimental data better than the linear relationship, suggesting an exponential dependence of k_r on F_b. Chen and Springer [1990] studied the principles that govern the formation of bonds between a cell moving freely over a substrate in shear flow and those governing the bond dissociation due to hydrodynamic forces, and found that bond formation is governed by shear rate whereas bond breakage is governed by shear stress. Their experimental data are well described by the Bell equation.

In the study of Smith et al. [1999], a high temporal and spatial resolution microscopy is used to reveal features that previous studies could not capture [Alon et al., 1995]. They found that the measured dissociation constants for neutrophil tethering events at 250 pN/bond are lower than the values predicted by the Bell and Hookean spring models. The plateau observed in the graph of the shear stress vs. the reaction rate k_r suggests that there is a force value above which the Bell and spring models are not valid. Since the model proposed so far considers the cell as a rigid body, whether the plateau is due to molecular, mechanical or cell deformation is not clear at this time.

Cell rolling and adhesion have been extensively studied over the years. However, it is clear that much further studies are needed. Table 62.1 summarizes some of the efforts reported in the literature.

62.3.2 Cell Crawling

The process of cell crawling consists of three major stages (1) extension of the leading edge, (2) establishing new adhesions in the front area and weakening of the exiting adhesions in the trailing area, and (3) pulling the back of the cell. Polymerization of the actin fibers in the protruded area of the crawling cell is considered the main mechanism of pushing the cell ahead. Thus, the modeling of the production of the pushing force is based on the polymerization/depolymerization analysis of actin fibers. There are two main approaches to the modeling of the polymerization-based active forces. In the first approach, the kinetics of a single fiber or array of fibers is considered. In the second, which is the continuum-type model, the fibers are treated as one phase of a two-phase reacting cytosol.

Peskin et al. [1993] have proposed the Brownian ratchet theory to describe the active force production. The main component of that theory was the interaction between a rigid protein and a diffusing object in front of it. If the object undergoes a Brownian motion, and the fiber undergoes polymerization, there are rates at which the polymer can push the object and overcome the external resistance. The problem was formulated in terms of a system of reaction-diffusion equations for the probabilities of the polymer to have certain number of monomers. Two limiting cases, fast diffusion and fast polymerization, were treated analytically that resulted in explicit force/velocity relationships. This theory was subsequently extended to elastic objects and to the transient attachment of the filament to the object. The correspondence of these models to recent experimental data is discussed in the article by Mogilner and Oster [2003].

Mogilner and Edelstein-Keshet [2002] modeled the protrusion of the leading edge of a cell by considering an array of actin fibers inclined with respect to the cell membrane. The authors have considered the main sequence of events associated with the actin dynamics, including polymerization of the barbed edge of the actin polymer and depolymerization at the protein pointed edge. The barbed edges assemble actin monomers with molecules of adenosine triphosphate (ATP) attached. The new barbed edges are activated by Arp2/3 complexes and they branch to start new actin filaments. The rate of polymerization is controlled by capping of the barbed edges. The problem reduced to a system of reaction-diffusion equations and was solved in the steady-state case. As a result of this solution, the force/velocity relationships corresponding to different regimes were obtained. Recently, Bindschadler et al. [2004] have constructed a comprehensive model of the actin cycle that can be used in various problems of cell motility. The authors took into account the major actin-binding protein regulating actin assembly and disassembly and solved the problem in a steady-state case.

TABLE 62.1   Overview of Some Fundamental Adhesion Kinetic Models

Kinetic model	Main assumptions/features	Major findings
Point attachment [Hammer and Lauffenberger, 1987]	Bonds are equally stressed in the contact area (flat) Binding and dissociation occur according to characteristic rate constants Receptors diffuse and convect into the binding area of contact	Adhesion occurrence depends on values of dimensionless quantities that characterize the interaction between the cell and the surface
Peeling [Dembo et al., 1988]	Clamped elastic membrane Bond stress and chemical rate constants are related to bond strain Bonds are linear springs fixed in the plane of the membrane Chemical reaction of bond formation and breakage is reversible Diffusion of adhesion molecules is negligible	Critical tension to overcome the tendency of the membrane to spread over the surface can be calculated Predictions of model depend whether the bonds are catch-bonds or slip-bonds If adhesion is mediated by catch-bonds, then no matter how much tension is applied, it is impossible to separate membrane and surface
Microvilli-coated hard sphere covered with adhesive springs [Hammer and Apte, 1992]	Combined point attachment model with peeling model Binding determined by a random statistical sampling of a probability distribution that describes the binding (or unbinding)	Model can describe rolling, transit attachment, and firm adhesion A critical adhesion modulator is the spring slippage (it relates the strain of a bond to its rate of breakage; the higher the slippage, the faster the breakage for the same strain)
Two-dimensional elastic ring [Dong et al., 1999]	Bond density related to the kinetics of bond formation Bonds are elastic springs Interaction between moving fluid and adherent cell	Shear forces acting on the entire cortical shell of the cell are transmitted on a relatively small "peeling zone" at the cell's trailing edge
Two-dimensional cell modeled as a liquid and a compound drop [N'Dri et al., 2003]	Cell deforms with nucleus inside Bonds are elastic springs Macro/micro model for cell deformation Kinetics model based on Dembo [1988]. Nano scale model for ligand-receptor Uniform flow at the inlet as in parallel-flow chamber assay	Results compare well with numerical and experimental results found in the literature for simple liquid drop Cell viscosity and surface tension affect Leukocyte rolling velocity Nucleus increases the bond lifetime and decreases leukocyte rolling velocity Cell with larger diameter rolls faster Uniform flow at the inlet as in parallel flow chamber assay

An alternative to the explicit analysis of actin fibers is a continuum approach where the cytoskeletal fibers are treated as one of two phases of the cytosol. Dembo and Harlow [1986] have proposed a general model of contractile biological polymer networks based on the analysis of reactive interpenetrating flow. In that model, the cytoplasm was viewed as a mixture of a contractile network of randomly oriented cytoskeletal filaments and an aqueous solution. Both phases were treated as homogeneous Newtonian fluids. Later, Alt and Dembo [1999] have applied a similar approach to the modeling of the motion of ameboid cells. The authors paid a special attention to the boundary conditions. They introduced three boundary surfaces: the area of contact between the cell and the substrate, the surface separating the cell

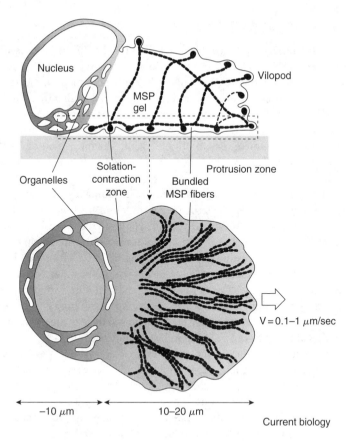

FIGURE 62.4 The model of locomotion of the nematode sperm cell. At the leading edge of the cell, the growing MSP filaments bundle into thick fibers that push the cell front out, and at the same time, store elastic energy. In the acidic environment at the rear part of the cell, the interfilament interactions weaken, the filaments unbundled and contract providing the contractile force to pull up the cell body. (From Mogilner, A. and Oster, G. *Curr. Biol.*, 13, R721, 2003. With permission.)

body and the lamellapodium, and the surface of the lamellapodium, and they specified particular boundary conditions along each of these surfaces. Numerical solution of the problem resulted in cellular responses in the form of waves along the direction of the cellular movement. Recently, a two-phase continuum model has been applied to two problems of motility of the active neutrophil. In the first problem, the neutrophil was stimulated with the chemoattractant fMLP and the generation of the pseudopod was modeled, and in the second, the cell moved inside the micropipette toward the same chemoattractant. Two models, a cytoskeletal swelling force and a polymerization force, were used for the active force production. A finite difference method in terms of the time variable and a Galerkin finite element treatment in terms of the special variables were used to obtain numerical solutions.

Bottino et al. [2002] used a version of the continuum two-phase method and studied the crawling of nematode sperm. This process is also driven by polymerization of another (not actin) protein, called the major sperm protein (MSP). The proposed model considers the major stages of crawling, including filament polymerization and generation of the force for the lamellapodial extension, storage of elastic energy, and finally the production of the contraction that pulls the rear of the cell. The total stresses consisted of two parts, the passive elastic stresses and active tensile stresses. In the acidic environment near the leading edge of the cell, the cytosol solates, and the elastic energy is released to push the cell forward. The solation was modeled by the removal of the active stresses. The solation rate was modeled by a pH gradient with lower pH at the rear part of the cell (Figure 62.4). The finite element method was used in the implementation of a two-dimensional version of the model.

62.3.3   Cell Swimming and Gliding

Most bacteria move by swimming for which they use helical flagella. In the bacteria with a left-handed helix (e.g., *Escherichia coli* and *Salmonella*), counterclockwise rotation generates a force pushing the cell forward. In contrast, clockwise rotation results in instability of the cell motion: the flagella fly apart, and the cell is not pushed in any particular direction. In the former case, the cell movement looks like smooth swimming, and in the latter case, the cell tumbles. In general, bacteria alternate between these two regimes of movement. The rotation of flagella is controlled by the molecular motor embedded in the bacterial membrane and driven by the transmembrane proton gradient. The movement of the bacterium can be changed by addition of chemoattractants, which results in suppression of tumbling and swimming toward a food source.

In contrast to bacterial swimming, many microorganisms, including myxobacteria, cyanobacteria, and flexobacteria, move via gliding. Nozzle-like structures were found in some of these bacteria. Slime is extruded through the nozzle pores, and this fact leads to a hypothesis that the bacterial sliding is driven by a slime-related propulsion mechanism. In earlier models of torque and switching in the bacterial flagellar motor, the motor consisted of two, rotating and stationary, parts. The rotating part had tilted positively and negatively charged strips along its surface. The stationary part of the motor included several channels conducting protons. Each channel had two binding sites, and therefore, could be in four states. The electrostatic energy of the interaction between the charges along the rotating part and protons bound to the channels was converted into the corresponding torque acting on the moving part. Further development and review of the models of this type can be found in Elston and Oster [1996].

CheY is one of the proteins controlling the motor in the flagella in chemotaxis. Phosphorylation of this protein results in tumbling of the bacterium. Mogilner et al. [2002] have modeled the process of switching of the bacterial molecular motor in response to binding CheY. The motor was assumed being in one of two states that correspond to the two directions of rotation of the flagella. The kinetic equations for the probabilities of the motor being in each state included a rate constant proportional to the concentration of CheY. In addition, the free energy profile with two minima that depend on the CheY concentration was introduced. As a result, the fraction of time that the motor rotates clockwise was found as a function of the CheY concentration. This function described by a sigmoidal curve was checked against experimental data and good agreement was found. Wolgemuth et al. [2002] have proposed a model of myxobacteria gliding. The authors assumed that the area inside the cell near the nozzle is filled with a polyelectrolyte gel that consists of cross-linked fibers. When the bacterium interacts with its liquid environment, the gel swells and releases from the nozzle. This results in the generation of a propulsive force pushing the bacterium forward. The authors showed that the extrusion of the gel through 50 nozzles produces a force sufficient to drive the bacterium through the viscous environment at the velocities observed in the experiment.

62.4   Mechano-, Mechanoelectrical, and Electromechanical Transduction

62.4.1   Mechanotransduction

Cells of all types are constantly exposed to external forces within their physiological environment. In mechanotransduction, cells convert the external mechanical signals into biochemical, morphological, biophysical, and the like responses. As an example, endothelial cells respond to shear stresses acting on the cell's membrane. Under physiological conditions, these stresses are associated with blood flow. In another example, the external stress (compression) causes mechanotransduction in chondrocytes, which is important, both for the functioning of natural cartilage and for design of artificial cartilage. Adhesion (traction) forces along the area of interaction of a cell with the extracellular matrix determine cell shape, which is critically important for cell's fate, including growth, division, and apoptosis (Chen et al., 1997, 2004, for review). Recently, Nelson et al. (2005) have found that cell growth is controlled by stress gradients in the cellular layer. General models that include biochemical aspect of signaling are complex; and their philosophy is discussed in the article by Asthagiri and Lauffenburger [2000]. Here we concentrate on several biomechanical aspects of the problem. One of them is the remodeling of the cytoskeleton in endothelial cells resulting from the action of external shear stress.

Suciu et al. [1997] have modeled the process of a reorientation of the actin filaments in response to shear stress acting on the membrane of endothelial cells. The authors assumed that the filament angular drift velocity is proportional to the applied shear stress and reduced the problem to a system of integrodifferential equations in terms of the partial concentrations of actin filaments being in different states (free, attached to the membrane, etc.). The same mathematical approach was later used to model a reorganization of the actin filaments in endothelial cells subjected to a cyclic stretch (simulation of the effect of the circumferential cyclic stretch of blood vessel). The reorganization of the cytoskeleton results in overall changes in cellular mechanical properties. Thoumine et al. [1999] have analyzed such changes that occur during fibroblast spreading and they found a significant stiffening of the cell. Sato et al. [2000] have shown significant changes in the viscoelastic properties of endothelial cells as a result of the action of shear stresses.

One of the hypothesis of mechanotransduction is based on force transmission from the cell surface (cell membrane or adhesion sites) through the cytoskeleton to the nucleus, the ultimate site of biochemical signals where this pathway ends with alteration of gene expression and protein synthesis [Thomas et al., 2002]. The forces deforming the nucleus can have a severalfold effect: first, they can change the binding rates of the molecules involved in DNA synthesis and gene transcription; second, these forces can cause changes in DNA molecules and chromatin fibers; and third, they can affect transport on mRNA molecules through the nuclear pores. Jean et al. [2004, 2005], by using analytical and computational approaches, have analyzed the adhesion–cytoskeleton–nucleus mechanical pathway during the rounding of endothelial cells.

62.4.2 Mechanoelectrical Transduction, Mechanosensitive Channels, and Electromechanical Transduction

During mechanoelectrical transduction, the mechanical stimuli applied to the cell membrane result in (in-) activation of ionic currents through mechanosensitive channels. In eukaryotic cells, such channels are typically connected to the cell cytoskeleton. In several examples, stretch-activated channels modulate cell volume in cardiac ventricular myocytes, have a functional role in electrical and mechanical activity of smooth muscles, are involved in bone response to mechanical loading, produce a Ca^{++} influx that leads to waves of calcium-induced calcium release, and so on. One of the features of mechanosensitive channels is the sensing not only of the stimulus itself but also of its time history [Sachs and Morris, 1998]. The main technique of studying the physiology of mechanosensitive channels is the patch pipette, and it was found that a full opening of the channel requires several cmHg of pressure, or several thousandths of Newton per meter of the equivalent membrane force (resultant). In the modeling of mechanosensitive channels, the channel has several states, and the probability of the channel of being open is determined by free energy barriers that depend on the mechanical stimulus. Usually, this stimulus is represented by isotropic tension in the cell membrane, which, in the expression of free energy, is multiplied by a typical change in the area of the channel. Bett and Sachs [2000] have analyzed the mechanosensitive channels in the chick heart, and, to reflect the observed inactivation of ionic current, used a three — closed, open, and inactivated — state model of the channel. The authors have also proposed that inactivation consists of two stages: reorganization of the cytoskeleton and blocking action of an agent released by the cell. A quantitative description of this two-step process was based on a viscoelastic-type model that reflected the mechanical properties of the cortical layer underlying the channel. Auditory hair cells and vestibular cells receive mechanical stimuli and sense them via transducer channels located in the stereocilia bundle. The channels in hair cells receiving acoustic signal are extremely fast, typical time up to 10 μsec [Corey and Hudspeth, 1979], and there is recent evidence that they can provide an active amplification of the mechanical stimulus applied to the stereocilia. A theoretical interpretation of the behavior of these channels is based on gating-spring models that state that there is an elastic element (gating spring) whose tension determines the transition of the channel from a closed to an open state.

Electromechanical transduction, a novel form of signal transduction, was found in outer hair cells of the mammalian cochlea. The hearing process in vertebrates is associated only with the mechanoelectrical form of transduction via transducer channels in the stereocilia of a single type of sensory cells. However, mammals have a special arrangement with two types of sensory cells, inner and outer hair cells. The outer hair cells provide a positive feedback in the processing of sound via a unique form of motility, named electromotility, when unconstrained cells change their length and constrained cells generate active forces in response to changes in the cell membrane potential. Deformation of the cell causes displacement current in the cell membrane. These features constitute the direct and converse piezoelectric-type effects, and a nonlinear thermodynamically consistent piezoelectric model has been proposed to describe mechanics and electromotility of the outer hair cell [Spector, 2001; Spector and Jean, 2004].

Acknowledgments

The authors are thankful to Drs. Robert Hochmuth and Alex Mogilner for their comments on the chapter.

References

Alon, R., Hammer D.A., and Springer T.A. Lifetime of the P-selectin-carbohydrate bond and its response to tensile force in hydrodynamic flow, *Nature (London)*, 374, 539, 1995.

Alon, R., Chen, S., Fuhlbrigge, R., Puri, K.D. et al. The kinetics and shear threshold of transient and rolling interactions of L-selectin with its ligand on leukocytes, *Proc. Natl Acad. Sci. USA*, 95, 11631, 1998.

Alt, W. and Dembo, M. Cytoplasm dynamics and cell motion: two-phase flow model. *Math. Biosci.*, 156, 207, 1999.

Asthagiri, A.R. and Lauffenburger, D.A. Bioengineering models of cell signaling, *Ann. Biomed. Eng.*, 2, 31, 2000.

Bell, G.I. Models for the specific adhesion of cells to cells, *Science*, 200, 618, 1978.

Bett, G.C.L. and Sachs, F. Activation and inactivation of mechanosensitive currents in the chick heart, *J. Membr. Biol.*, 173, 237, 2000.

Bindschadler, M., Osborn, E.A., Dewey, C.F. et al. A mechanistic model of the actin cycle, *Biophys. J.*, 86, 2720, 2004.

Bo, L. and Waugh, R.E. Determination of bilayer membrane bending stiffness by tether formation from giant, thin-walled vesicles, *Biophys. J.*, 55, 509, 1989.

Bottino, D., Mogilner, A., Roberts, T. et al. How nematode sperm crawl, *Cell Sci.*, 115, 367, 2002.

Caille, N., Thuomine, O., Tardy, Y. et al. Contribution of the nucleus to the mechanical properties of endothelial cells, *J. Biomech.*, 33, 177, 2002.

Chang, K.C., Tees, D.F.J., and Hammer, D.A. The state diagram for cell adhesion under flow: leukocyte rolling and firm adhesion, *Proc. Natl Acad. Sci. USA*, 97, 11262, 2000.

Cheng Zhu. Kinetics and mechanics of cell adhesion, *J. Biomech.*, 33, 23, 2000.

Chen, S. and Springer, T.A. An automatic breaking system that stabilizes leukocyte rolling by an increase in selectin bond number with shear, *J. Cell Biol.*, 144, 185, 1999.

Chen, C.S., Mrksich, M., Huang, S. et al. Geometric control of cell life and death, *Science*, 276, 1425, 1997.

Chen, C.S., Tan, J., and Tien, J. Mechanotransduction at cell-matrix and cell–cell contacts, *Annu. Rev. Biomed. Eng.*, 6, 275, 2004.

Corey, D.P. and Hudspeth, A.J. Response latency of vertebrate hair cells, *Biophys. J.*, 26, 499, 1979.

Cozens-Roberts, C., Lauffenburger, D.A., and Quinn, J.A. A receptor-mediated cell attachment and detachment kinetics: I. Probabilistic model and analysis, *Biophys. J.*, 58, 841, 1990.

Dahl, K.N., Kahn, S.M., Wilson, K.L. et al. The nuclear envelope lamina network has elasticity and a compressibility limit suggestive of a molecular shock absorber. *J. Cell Sci.* 117, 4779, 2004.

Dembo, M. and Harlow, F. Cell motion, contractile networks, and the physics of interpenetrating reactive flow, *Biophys. J.*, 50, 109, 1986.

Dembo, M., Torney, D.C., Saxaman, K. et al. The reaction-limited kinetics of membrane-to-surface adhesion and detachment, *Proc. R. Soc. Lond. B*, 234, 55, 1988.

Discher, D.E., Boal, D.H., and Boey, S.K. Simulation of the erythrocyte cytoskeleton at large deformation. II. Micropipette aspiration, *Biophys. J.*, 75, 1584, 1998.

Dong, C. and Lei, X.X. Biomechanics of cell rolling: shear flow, cell-surface adhesion, and cell deformability, *J. Biomech.*, 33, 35, 2000.

Elston, T.C. and Oster, G., Protein turbines! The bacterial flagellar motor, *Biophys. J.*, 73, 703, 1996.

Evans, E.A. Bending resistance and chemically induced moments in membrane bilayers, *Biophys. J.*, 14, 923, 1974.

Evans, E.A. Minimum energy analysis of membrane deformation applied to pipet aspiration and surface adhesion of red blood cells, *Biophys. J.*, 30, 265, 1980.

Evans, E.A. Detailed mechanics of membrane–membrane adhesion and separation. I. Continuum of molecular cross-bridges, *Biophys. J.*, 48, 175, 1985.

Evans, E.A. and Skalak, R. *Mechanics and Thermodynamics of Biomembranes*, CRC Press, Boca Raton, FL, 1980.

Fabry, B., Maksym, G.N., Butler J.P. et al. Scaling the microrheology of living cells, *Physiol. Rev. Lett.*, 87, 148102, 2001.

Guilak, F., Tedrow, J.R., and Burgkart, R. Viscoelastic properties of the cell nucleus, *Biochem. Biophys. Res. Commun.*, 269, 781, 2000.

Hammer, D.A. and Apte, S.M. Simulation of cell rolling and adhesion on surfaces in shear-flow — general results and analysis of selectin-mediated neutrophil adhesion, *Biophys. J.*, 63, 35, 1992.

Hammer, D.A. and Lauffenburger, D.A. A dynamical model for receptor-mediated cell adhesion to surfaces, *Biophys. J.*, 52, 475, 1987.

Helfrich, W., Elastic properties of lipid bilayers: theory and possible experiments, *Z. Naturforsch.*, C28, 693, 1973.

Hochmuth, R.M. Micropipette aspiration of living cells, *J. Biomech.*, 33, 15, 2000.

Jean, R.P., Chen, C.S., and Spector, A.A. Finite element analysis of the adhesion — cytoskeleton–nucleus mechano transduction pathway during endothelial cell rounding, axisymmetric model, *J. Biomech. Eng.*, 127, 594, 2005.

Jean, R.P., Gray, D.S., Spector, A.A. et al. Characterization of the nuclear deformation caused by changes in endothelial cell shape, *J. Biomech. Eng.*, 126, 552, 2004.

Kan, H.-C., Udaykumar, H.S., Shyy, W., and Vigneron, P., Tran-Son-Tay, R., Effects of nucleus on leukocyte recovery. *Ann. Biomed. Eng.*, 27, 648, 1999a.

Kan, H.-C., Udaykumar, H.S., Shyy, W. et al. Numerical analysis of the deformation of an adherent drop under shear flow, *J. Biomech. Eng.*, 121, 160, 1999b.

Karcher, H., Lammerding, J., Huang, H. et al. A three-dimensional viscoelastic model for cell deformation with experimental verification, *Biophys. J.*, 85, 3336, 2003.

Mogilner, A. and Edelstein-Keshet, L. Regulation of actin dynamics in rapidly moving cells: a quantitative analysis, *Biophys. J.*, 83, 1237, 2002.

Mogilner, A., Elston, T.C., Wang, H. et al. Switching in the bacterial flagellar motor, in *Computational Cell Biology*, Fall, C.P., Marland, E.S., Wagner, J.M. et al., Eds. Springer, New York, 2002, chap. 13.

Mogilner, A. and Oster, G. Polymer motors: pushing out the front and pulling up the back, *Curr. Biol.*, 13, R721, 2003.

N'Dri, N.A., Shyy, W., and Tran-Son-Tay, R. Computational modeling of cell adhesion and movement using a continuum-kinetics approach. *Biophys. J.*, 85, 2273, 2003.

Nelson, C.M., Jean, R.P., and Tan, J.L. Emerging patterns of growth controlled by multicellular form and mechanics, *Proc. Natl. Acad. Sci. USA*, 102, 11594, 2005.

Peskin, C.S., Odell, G.M., and Oster, G. Cellular motors and thermal fluctuation: the Brownian ratchet, *Biophys. J.*, 65, 316, 1993.

Radmacher, M., Fritz, M., Kacher, C.M. et al. Measuring the viscoelastic properties of human platelets with the atomic force microscope, *Biophys. J.*, 70, 556, 1996.

Sacks, F. and Morris, C.E. Mechanosensitive ion channels in non-specialized cell's, in *Reviews of Physiology, Biochemistry, and Pharmacology*, 132, 1, 1998.

Sato, M., Nagayama, K., Kataoka, N. et al., Local mechanical properties measured by atomic force microscopy for cultured bovine endothelial cells exposed to shear stress, *J. Biomech.*, 33, 127, 2000.

Shinde Patil, V.R., Campbell, C.J., Yun, Y.H. et al. Particle diameter influences adhesion under flow, *Biophys. J.*, 80, 1733, 2001.

Smith Mcrae, J., Berg, E.L., and Lawrence, M.B., A direct comparison of selectin-mediated transient, adhesive events using high temporal resolution, *Biophys. J.*, 77, 3371, 1999.

Spector, A.A. A nonlinear electroelastic model of the auditory outer hair cell, *Int. J. Solids Struct.*, 38, 2115, 2001.

Spector, A.A., Brownell, W.E., and Popel, A.S. Analysis of the micropipette experiment with the anisotropic outer hair cell wall, *J. Acoust. Soc. Am.*, 103, 1001, 1998.

Spector, A.A. and Jean, R.P. Modes and balance of energy in the piezoelectric cochlear outer hair cell wall, *J. Biomech. Eng.*, 126, 17, 2004.

Steigmann, D.J. Fluid films with curvature elasticity, *Arch. Ration. Mech. Anal.*, 150, 127, 1999.

Suciu, A., Civelekoglu, G., Tardy, Y. et al. Model of the alignment of actin filaments in endothelial cells subjected to fluid shear stress, *Bull. Math. Biol.*, 59, 1029, 1997.

Tees, D.F.J., Chang, K.C., Rodgers, S.D., et al. Simulation of cell adhesion to bioreactive surfaces in shear: the effect of cell size, *Ind. Eng. Chem. Res.*, 41, 486, 2002.

Theret, D.P., Levesque, M.J., Sato, M. et al. The application of a homogeneous half-space model in the analysis of endothelial cell micropipette measurements, *J. Biomech. Eng.*, 110, 190, 1988.

Thomas, C.H., Colllier, J.H., Sfeir, C. et al. Engineering gene expression and protein synthesis by modulation of nuclear shape, *Proc. Natl Acad. Sci. USA*, 99, 1972, 2002.

Thoumine, O., Cardoso, O., and Meister J.J. Changes in the mechanics of fibroblast during spreading: a micromanipulation study, *Eur. Biophys. J.*, 28, 222, 1999.

Tran-Son-Tay, R., Ting-Beall, H.P., Zheler, D.V. et al. Viscous behaviour of leukocytes in cell mechanics and cellular engineering, Mow, V.C., Guilak, F., Tran-Son-Tay, R.A. (Eds.), Spinger, New York, 1994, pp. 22–32.

Van Vilet, K.J., Bao, G., and Suresh, S. The biomechanics toolbox: experimental approaches for living cells and biomolecules. *Acta Material.* 51, 5881, 2003.

Wang, N. and Ingber, D.E. Control of cytoskeletal mechanics by extracellular matrix, cell shape, and mechanical tension, *Biophys. J.*, 66, 2181, 1994.

Waugh, R.E. and Hochmuth, R.M. Mechanical equilibrium of thick, hollow, liquid membrane cylinders, *Biophys. J.*, 52, 391, 1987.

Wolgemuth, C., Holczyk, E., Kaiser, D. et al. How myxobacteria glide, *Curr. Biol.*, 12, 369, 2002.

Further Information

Howard, *Journal of Mechanics of Motor Proteins and the Cytoskeleton*. Sinauer Ass. Inc., Sunderland, Massachusetts, 2001 (analysis of the molecular motors, cytoskeleton, and cells as a whole by using basic physical principles; can be used for the development of undergraduate or graduate courses).

Cell Mechanics and Cellular Engineering, Van C. Mow, Guilak, F., Tran-Son-Tay, R., and Hochmuth, R.M., Eds. Springer, New York, 1994 (collection of original papers on the topics close to the scope of the present chapter).

Computational Cell Biology, Fall, C.P., Marland, E.S., Wagner, J.M., and Tyson, J.J., Eds. Springer, New York, 2002 (book consists of several sections written by leading experts in the mathematical and computational analysis of cell physiology; the material includes exercises, necessary mathematics and software, and it can be used for teaching advanced graduate courses).

Physics of Bio-Molecules and Cells, Flyvbjerg, H., Julicher, F., Ormos, P., and David, F., Eds. EDP Sciences; Springer, Berlin, 2002 (collection of advanced lectures that provides active researches with a review of several important areas in cellular and molecular biophysics).

63

Cochlear Mechanics

Charles R. Steele
Gary J. Baker
Jason A. Tolomeo
Deborah E. Zetes-Tolomeo
Stanford University

63.1 Introduction

The inner ear is a transducer of mechanical force to appropriate neural excitation. The key element is the receptor cell, or hair cell, which has cilia on the apical surface and afferent (and sometimes efferent) neural synapses on the lateral walls and base. Generally for hair cells, mechanical displacement of the cilia in the forward direction toward the tallest cilia causes the generation of electrical impulses in the nerves, while backward displacement causes inhibition of spontaneous neural activity. Displacement in the lateral direction has no effect. For moderate frequencies of sinusoidal ciliary displacement (20 to 200 Hz), the neural impulses are in synchrony with the mechanical displacement, one impulse for each cycle of excitation. Such impulses are transmitted to the higher centers of the brain and can be perceived as sound. For lower frequencies, however, neural impulses in synchrony with the excitation are apparently confused with the spontaneous, random firing of the nerves. Consequently, there are three mechanical devices in the inner ear of vertebrates that provide perception in the different frequency ranges. At zero frequency, that is, linear acceleration, the otolith membrane provides a constant force acting on the cilia of hair cells. For low frequencies associated with rotation of the head, the semicircular canals provide the proper force on cilia. For frequencies in the hearing range, the cochlea provides the correct forcing of hair cell cilia. In nonmammalian vertebrates, the equivalent of the cochlea is a bent tube, and the upper frequency of hearing is around 7 kHz. For mammals, the upper frequency is considerably higher, 20 kHz for man but extending to almost 200 kHz for toothed whales and some bats. Other creatures, such as certain insects, can perceive high frequencies, but do not have a cochlea nor the frequency discrimination of vertebrates.

Auditory research is a broad field [Keidel and Neff, 1976]. The present article provides a brief guide of a restricted view, focusing on the transfer of the input sound pressure into correct stimulation of hair cell cilia in the cochlea. In a general sense, the mechanical functions of the semicircular canals and the otoliths are clear, as are the functions of the outer ear and middle ear; however, the cochlea continues to elude a reasonably complete explanation. Substantial progress in cochlear research has been made in the past decade, triggered by several key discoveries, and there is a high level of excitement among workers in the area. It is evident that the normal function of the cochlea requires a full integration of mechanical, electrical, and chemical effects on the milli-, micro-, and nanometer scales. Recent texts, which include details of the anatomy, are by Pickles [1988] and Gulick and coworkers [1989]. A summary of analysis and data related to the macromechanical aspect up to 1982 is given by Steele [1987], and more recent surveys specifically on the cochlea are by de Boer [1991], Dallos [1992], Hudspeth [1989], Ruggero [1993], and Nobili and colleagues [1998].

63.2 Anatomy

The cochlea is a coiled tube in the shape of a snail shell (Cochlea = Schnecke = Snail), with length about 35 mm and radius about 1 mm in man. There is not a large size difference across species: the length is 60 mm in elephant and 7 mm in mouse. There are two and one-half turns of the coil in man and dolphin, and five turns in guinea pig. Despite the correlation of coiling with hearing capability of land animals [West, 1985], no significant effect of the coiling on the mechanical response has yet been identified.

63.2.1 Components

The cochlea is filled with fluid and divided along its length by two partitions. The main partition is at the center of the cross-section and consists of three segments (1) on one side — the *bony shelf*, (or *primary spiral osseous lamina*), (2) in the middle, an elastic segment (*basilar membrane*) (shown in Figure 63.1) and (3) on the other side, a thick support (*spiral ligament*). The second partition is *Reissner's membrane*, attached at one side above the edge of the bony shelf and attached at the other side to the wall of the cochlea. *Scala media* is the region between Reissner's membrane and the basilar membrane, and is filled with *endolymphatic fluid*. This fluid has an ionic content similar to intracellular fluid, high in potassium and low in sodium, but with a resting positive electrical potential of around +80 mV. The electrical potential is supplied by the *stria vascularis* on the wall in scala media. The region above Reissner's membrane is *scala vestibuli*, and the region below the main partition is *scala tympani*. Scala vestibuli and scala tympani are connected at the apical end of the cochlea by an opening in the bony shelf, the *helicotrema*, and are filled with *perilymphatic fluid*. This fluid is similar to extracellular fluid, low in potassium and high in sodium with zero electrical potential. Distributed along the scala media side of the basilar membrane is the sensory epithelium, the *organ of Corti*. This contains one row of *inner hair cells* and three rows of *outer hair cells*. In humans, each row contains about 4000 cells. Each of the inner hair cells has about twenty afferent synapses; these are considered to be the primary receptors. In comparison, the outer hair cells are sparsely innervated but have both afferent (5%) and efferent (95%) synapses.

The basilar membrane is divided into two sections. Connected to the edge of the bony shelf, on the left in Figure 63.1, is the *arcuate zone*, consisting of a single layer of transverse fibers. Connected to the edge of the spiral ligament, on the right in Figure 63.1, is the *pectinate zone*, consisting of a double layer of transverse fibers in an amorphous ground substance. The *arches of Corti* form a truss over the arcuate zone, which consist of two rows of *pillar cells*. The foot of the inner pillar is attached at the point of connection of the bony shelf to the arcuate zone, while the foot of the outer pillar cell is attached at the common border of the arcuate zone and pectinate zone. The heads of the inner and outer pillars are connected and form the support point for the *recticular lamina*. The other edge of the recticular lamina is attached to the top of *Henson cells*, which have bases connected to the basilar membrane. The inner hair cells are attached on the bony shelf side of the inner pillars, while the three rows of outer hair cells are attached to

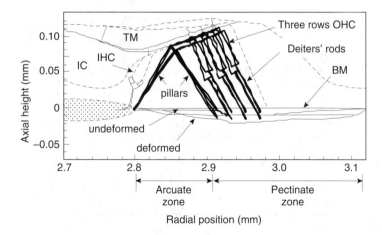

FIGURE 63.1   Finite element calculation for the deformation of the cochlear partition due to pressure on the basilar membrane (BM). Outer hair cell (OHC) stereocilia are sheared by the motion of the pillars of Corti and reticular lamina relative to the tectorial membrane (TM). The basilar membrane is supported on the left by the bony shelf and on the right by the spiral ligament. The inner hair cells (IHC) are the primary receptors, each with about 20 afferent synapses. The inner sulcus (IC) is a fluid region in contact with the cilia of the inner hair cells.

the recticular lamina. The region bounded by the inner pillar cells, the recticular lamina, the Henson cells, and the basilar membrane forms another fluid region. This fluid is considered to be perilymph, since it appears that ions can flow freely through the arcuate zone of the basilar membrane. The cilia of the hair cells protrude into the endolymph. Thus the outer hair cells are immersed in perilymph at 0 mV, have an intracellular potential of −70 mV, and have cilia at the upper surface immersed in endolymph at a potential of +80 mV. In some regions of the ears of some vertebrates [Freeman and Weiss, 1990], the cilia are free standing. However, mammals always have a *tectorial membrane*, originating near the edge of the bony shelf and overlying the rows of hair cells parallel to the recticular lamina. The tallest rows of cilia of the outer hair cells are attached to the tectorial membrane. Under the tectorial membrane and inside the inner hair cells is a fluid space, the *inner sulcus,* filled with endolymph. The cilia of the inner hair cells are not attached to the overlying tectorial membrane, so the motion of the fluid in the inner sulcus must provide the mechanical input to these primary receptor cells. Since the inner sulcus is found only in mammals, the fluid motion in this region generated by acoustic input may be crucial to high frequency discrimination capability.

   With a few exceptions of specialization, the dimensions of all the components in the cross section of the mammalian cochlea change smoothly and slowly along the length, in a manner consistent with high stiffness at the base, or input end, and low stiffness at the apical end. For example, in the cat the basilar membrane width increases from 0.1 to 0.4 mm while the thickness decreases from 13 to 5 μm. The density of transverse fibers decreases more than the thickness, from about 6000 fibers per μm at the base to 500 per μm at the apex [Cabezudo, 1978].

63.2.2   Material Properties

Both perilymph and endolymph have the viscosity and density of water. The bone of the wall and the bony shelf appear to be similar to compact bone, with density approximately twice that of water. The remaining components of the cochlea are soft tissue with density near that of water. The stiffnesses of the components vary over a wide range, as indicated by the values of Young's modulus listed in Table 63.1. These values are taken directly or estimated from many sources, including the stiffness measurements in the cochlea by Békésy [1960], Gummer and coworkers [1981], Strelioff and Flock [1984], Miller [1985], Zwislocki and Cefaratti [1989], and Olson and Mountain [1994].

TABLE 63.1   Typical Values and Estimates for Young's Modulus E

Compact bone	20	GPa
Keratin	3	GPa
Basilar membrane fibers	1.9	GPa
Microtubules	1.2	GPa
Collagen	1	GPa
Reissner's membrane	60	MPa
Actin	50	MPa
Red blood cell, extended (assuming thickness = 10 nm)	45	MPa
Rubber, elastin	4	MPa
Basilar membrane ground substance	200	kPa
Tectorial membrane	30	kPa
Jell-O	3	kPa
Henson's cells	1	kPa

63.3   Passive Models

The anatomy of the cochlea is complex. By modeling, one attempts to isolate and understand the essential features. Following is an indication of proposition and controversy associated with a few such models.

63.3.1   Resonators

The ancient Greeks suggested that the ear consisted of a set of tuned resonant cavities. As each component in the cochlea was discovered subsequently, it was proposed to be the tuned resonator. The most well known resonance theory is Helmholtz's. According to this theory, the transverse fibers of the basilar membrane are under tension and respond like the strings of a piano. The short strings at the base respond to high frequencies and the long strings toward the apex respond to low frequencies. The important feature of the Helmholz theory is the *place principle*, according to which the receptor cells at a certain *place* along the cochlea are stimulated by a certain frequency. Thus the cochlea provides a real-time frequency separation (Fourier analysis) of any complex sound input. This aspect of the Helmholtz theory has since been validated, since each of the some 30,000 fibers exiting the cochlea in the auditory nerve is sharply tuned to a particular frequency. A basic difficulty with such a resonance theory is that sharp tuning requires small damping, which is associated with a long ringing after the excitation ceases. Yet, the cochlea is remarkable for combining sharp tuning with short time delay for the onset of reception and the same short time delay for the cessation of reception.

A particular problem with the Helmholtz theory arises from the equation for the resonant frequency for a string under tension:

$$f = \frac{1}{2b}\sqrt{\frac{T}{\rho h}} \tag{63.1}$$

in which T is the tensile force per unit width, ρ is the density, b is the length, and h is the thickness of the string. In man, the frequency range over which the cochlea operates is $f = 200$ to $20,000$ Hz, a factor of 100, while the change in length b is only a factor of 5 and the thickness of the basilar membrane h varies the wrong way by a factor of 2 or so. Thus to produce the necessary range of frequency, the tension T would have to vary by a factor of about 800. In fact the spiral ligament, which would supply such tension, varies in area by a factor of only 10.

63.3.2   Traveling Waves

No theory anticipated the actual behavior found in the cochlea in 1928 by Békésy [1960]. He observed *traveling waves* moving along the cochlea from base toward apex which have a maximum amplitude at a certain place. The place depends on the frequency, as in the Helmholz theory, but the amplitude envelope in not very localized. In Békésy's experimental models, and in subsequent mathematical and experimental models, the anatomy of the cochlea is greatly simplified. The coiling, Reissner's membrane, and the organ of Corti are all ignored, so the cochlea is treated as a straight tube with a single partition. (An exception is in Fuhrmann and colleagues [1986]). A gradient in the partition stiffness similar to that in the cochlea, gives beautiful traveling waves in both experimental and mathematical models.

63.3.3 One-Dimensional Model

A majority of work has been based on the assumption that the fluid motion is one-dimensional. With this simplification the governing equations are similar to those for an electrical transmission line and for the long wavelength response of an elastic tube containing fluid. The equation for the pressure p in a tube with constant cross-sectional area A and with constant frequency of excitation is:

$$\frac{\mathrm{d}^2 p}{\mathrm{d}x^2} + \frac{2\rho\omega^2}{AK}p = 0 \tag{63.2}$$

in which x is the distance along the tube, ρ is the density of the fluid, ω is the frequency in radians per second, and K is the generalized partition stiffness, equal to the net pressure divided by the displaced area of the cross-section. The factor of 2 accounts for fluid on both sides of the elastic partition. Often K is represented in the form of a single degree-of-freedom oscillator:

$$K = k + \mathrm{i}\omega d - m\omega^2 \tag{63.3}$$

in which k is the static stiffness, d is the damping, and m is the mass density:

$$m = \rho_P \frac{h}{b} \tag{63.4}$$

in which ρ_P is the density of the plate, h is the thickness, and b is the width. Often the mass is increased substantially to provide better curve fits. A good approximation is to treat the pectinate zone of the basilar membrane as transverse beams with simply supported edges, for which

$$k = \frac{10Eh^3 c_{\mathrm{f}}}{b^5} \tag{63.5}$$

in which E is the Young's modulus, and c_f is the volume fraction of fibers. Thus for the moderate changes in the geometry along the cochlea as in the cat, h decreasing by a factor of 2, c_f decreasing by a factor of 12, b increasing by a factor of 5, the stiffness k from Equation 63.4 decreases by five orders of magnitude, which is ample for the required frequency range. Thus it is the bending stiffness of the basilar membrane pectinate zone and not the tension which governs the frequency response of the cochlea. The solution of Equation 63.2 can be obtained by numerical or asymptotic (called WKB or CLG) methods. The result is traveling waves for which the amplitude of the basilar membrane displacement builds to a maximum and then rapidly diminishes. The parameters of K are adjusted to obtain agreement with measurements of the dynamic response in the cochlea. Often all the material of the organ of Corti is assumed to be rigidly attached to the basilar membrane so that h is relatively large and the effect of mass m is large. Then the maximum response is near the *in vacua* resonance of the partition given by

$$\omega^2 = \frac{b}{h}\frac{k}{\rho} \tag{63.6}$$

The following are objections to the 1-D model [Siebert, 1974] (1) The solutions of Equation 63.2 show wavelengths of response in the region of maximum amplitude that are small in comparison with the size of the cross section, violating the basic assumption of 1-D fluid flow. (2) In the drained cochlea, Békésy [1960] observed no resonance of the partition, so there is no significant partition mass. The significant mass is entirely from the fluid and therefore Equation 63.6 is not correct. This is consistent with the observations of experimental models. (3) In model studies by Békésy [1960] and others, the localization of response is independent of the area A of the cross-section. Thus Equation 63.2 cannot govern the most interesting part of the response, the region near the maximum amplitude for a given frequency. (4) Mechanical and neural measurements in the cochlea show dispersion which is incompatible with the 1-D model [Lighthill, 1991]. (5) The 1-D model fails badly in comparison with experimental measurements in models for which the parameters of geometry, stiffness, viscosity, and density are known.

Nevertheless, the simplicity of Equation 63.2 and the analogy with the transmission line have made the 1-D model popular. We note that there is interest in utilizing the principles in an analog model built on a silicon chip, because of the high performance of the actual cochlea. Watts [1993] reports on the first model with an electrical analog of 2-D fluid in the scali. An interesting observation is that the transmission line hardware models are sensitive to failure of one component, while the 2-D model is not. In experimental models, Békésy found that a hole at one point in the membrane had little effect on the response at other points.

63.3.4 Two-Dimensional Model

The pioneering work with two-dimensional fluid motion was begun in 1931 by Ranke, as reported in Ranke [1950] and discussed by Siebert [1974]. Analysis of 2-D and 3-D fluid motion without the *a priori* assumption of long or short wavelengths and for physical values of all parameters is discussed by Steele [1987]. The first of two major benefits derived from the 2-D model is the allowance of short wavelength behavior, that is, the variation in fluid displacement and pressure in the duct height direction. Localized fluid motion near the elastic partition generally occurs near the point of maximum amplitude and the exact value of A becomes immaterial. The second major benefit of a 2-D model is the admission of a stiffness-dominated elastic partition (i.e., massless) which better approximates the physiological properties of the basilar membrane. The two benefits together address all the objections the 1-D model discussed previously.

Two-dimensional models start with the Navier-Stokes and continuity equations governing the fluid motion, and an anisotropic plate equation governing the elastic partition motion. The displacement potential φ for the incompressible and inviscid fluid must satisfy Laplace's equation:

$$\varphi_{,xx} + \varphi_{,zz} = 0 \tag{63.7}$$

where x is the distance along the partition and z the distance perpendicular to the partition, and the subscripts with commas denote partial derivatives. The averaged potential and the displacement of the partition are:

$$\bar{\varphi} = \frac{1}{H} \int_0^H \varphi \, dz \quad w = \varphi_z(x, 0) \tag{63.8}$$

so Equation 63.7 yields the "macro" continuity condition (for constant H):

$$\bar{\varphi}_{,xx} - w = 0 \tag{63.9}$$

An approximate solution is

$$\bar{\varphi}(x, z, t) = F(x) \cosh[n(x)(z - H)]e^{i\omega t} \tag{63.10}$$

where F is an unknown amplitude function, n is the local wave number, H is the height of the duct, t is time, and ω is the frequency. This is an exact solution for constant properties and is a good approximation when the properties vary slowly along the partition. The conditions at the plate fluid interface yield the dispersion relation:

$$n \tanh(nH) = \frac{2\rho\omega^2}{AK} H \tag{63.11}$$

The averaged value Equation 63.8 of the approximate potential Equation 63.10 is:

$$\bar{\bar{\varphi}} = \frac{F \sinh nH}{nH} \tag{63.12}$$

so the continuity condition Equation 63.9 yields the equation:

$$\bar{\bar{\varphi}}_{,xx} = n^2 \bar{\bar{\varphi}} = 0 \tag{63.13}$$

For small values of the wave number n, the system Equation 63.11 and Equation 63.13 reduce to the 1-D problem Equation 63.2.

For physiological values of the parameters, the wave number for a given frequency is small at the stapes and becomes large (i.e., short wave lengths) toward the end of the duct. With this formulation, the form of the wave is not assumed. It is clear that for large n the WKB solution will give excellent approximation to the solution of Equation 63.13 in exponential form. So it is possible to integrate Equation 63.13 numerically for small n for which the solution is not exponential and match the solution with the WKB approximation. This provides a uniformly valid solution for the entire region of interest without an *a prior* assumption of the wave form.

For a physically realistic model, the mass of the membrane can be neglected and K written as:

$$K = k(1 + i\varepsilon) \tag{63.14}$$

in which k is the static stiffness. For many polymers, the material damping ε is nearly constant. If the damping comes from the viscous boundary layer of the fluid, then ε is approximated by

$$\varepsilon \approx n \sqrt{\frac{\mu}{2\rho\omega}} \tag{63.15}$$

in which μ is the viscosity. For water, ε is small with a value near 0.05 at the point of maximum amplitude. The actual duct is tapered, so $H = H(x)$ and additional terms must be added to Equation 63.13.

The best verification of the mathematical model and calculation procedure comes from comparison with measurements in experimental models for which the parameters are known. Zhou and coworkers [1994] provide the first life-sized experimental model, designed to be similar to the human cochlea, but with fluid viscosity 28 times that of water to facilitate optical imaging. Results are shown in Figure 63.2 and Figure 63.3. Equation 63.13 gives rough agreement with the measurements.

63.3.5 Three-Dimensional Model

A further improvement in the agreement with experimental models can be obtained by adding the component of fluid motion in the direction across the membrane for a full 3-D model. The solution by direct numerical means is computationally intensive, and was first carried out by Raftenberg [1990], who reports a portion of his results for the fluid motion around the organ of Corti. Böhnke and colleagues [1996] use the finite element code ANSYS for the most accurate description to date of the structure of the organ of Corti. However, the fluid is not included and only a restricted segment of the cochlea considered. The fluid is also not included in the finite element calculations of Zhang and colleagues [1996]. A "large finite element method," which combines asymptotic and numerical methods for shell analysis, can be

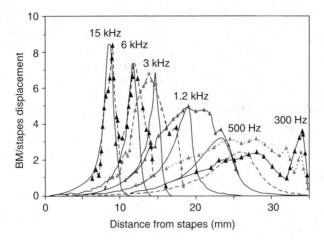

FIGURE 63.2 Comparison of 3-D model calculations (solid curves) with experimental results of Zhou and co-workers [1994] (dashed curves) for the amplitude envelopes for different frequencies. This is a life-sized model, but with an isotropic BM and fluid viscosity 28 times that of water. The agreement is reasonable, except for the lower frequencies.

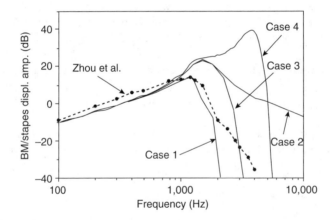

FIGURE 63.3 Comparison of 3-D model calculations with experimental results of Zhou and coworkers [1994] for amplitude at the place $x = 19$ mm as a function of frequency. The scales are logarithmic (20 dB is a factor of 10 in amplitude). Case 1 shows a direct comparison with the physical parameters of the experiment, with isotropic BM and viscosity 28 times that of water. Case 2 is computed for the viscosity reduced to that of water. Case 3 is computed for the BM made of transverse fibers. Case 4 shows the effect of active OHC feed-forward, with the pressure gain $\alpha = 0.21$ and feed-forward distance $\dot{y}x$ 25 μm. Thus lower viscosity, BM orthotropy, and active feed-forward all contribute to higher amplitude and increased localization of the response.

used for an efficient computation of all the structural detail as shown in Figure 63.1. Both the fluid and the details of the structure are considered with a simplified element description and simplified geometry by Kolston and Ashmore [1996], requiring some 10^5 degrees of freedom and hours of computing time (on a 66 MHz PC) for the linear solution for a single frequency. The asymptotic WKB solution, however, provides the basis for computing the 3-D fluid motion [Steele, 1987] and yields excellent agreement with older measurements of the basilar membrane motion in the real cochlea (with a computing time of 1 sec per frequency). The 2-D analysis Equation 63.13 can easily be extended to 3-D. The 3-D WKB calculations are compared with the measurements of the basilar membrane displacement in the experimental model of Zhou and coworkers [1994] in Figure 63.2 and Figure 63.3. As shown by Taber and Steele [1979], the 3-D fluid motion has a significant effect on the pressure distribution. This is confirmed by the measurements by Olson [1998] for the pressure at different depths in the cochlea, that show a substantial increase near the partition.

63.4   The Active Process

Before around 1980, it was thought that the processing may have two levels. First the basilar membrane and fluid provide the correct place for a given frequency (a purely mechanical "first filter"). Subsequently, the micromechanics and electrochemistry in the organ of Corti, with possible neural interactions, perform a further sharpening (a physiologically vulnerable "second filter").

A hint that the two-filter concept had difficulties was in the measurements of Rhode [1971], who found significant nonlinear behavior of the basilar membrane in the region of the maximum amplitude at moderate amplitudes of tone intensity. Passive models cannot explain this, since the usual mechanical nonlinearities are significant only at very high intensities, that is, at the threshold of pain. Russell and Sellick [1977] made the first *in vivo* mammalian intracellular hair cell recordings and found that the cells are as sharply tuned as the nerve fibers. Subsequently, improved measurement techniques in several laboratories found that the basilar membrane is actually as sharply tuned as the hair cells and the nerve fibers. Thus the sharp tuning occurs at the basilar membrane. No passive cochlear model, even with physically unreasonable parameters, has yielded amplitude and phase response similar to such measurements. Measurements in a damaged or dead cochlea show a response similar to that of a passive model. Further evidence for an active process comes from Kemp [1978], who discovered that sound pulses into the ear caused echoes coming from the cochlea at delay times corresponding to the travel time to the place for the frequency and back. Spontaneous emission of sound energy from the cochlea has now been measured in the external ear canal in all vertebrates [Probst, 1990]. Some of the emissions can be related to the hearing disability of tinnitus (ringing in the ear). The conclusion drawn from these discoveries is that normal hearing involves an active process in which the energy of the input sound is greatly enhanced. A widely accepted concept is that spontaneous emission of sound energy occurs when the local amplifiers are not functioning properly and enter some sort of limit cycle [Zweig and Shera, 1995]. However, there remains doubt about the nature of this process [Allen and Neely (1992), Hudspeth (1989), Nobili and coworkers (1998)].

63.4.1   Outer Hair Cell Electromotility

Since the outer hair cells have sparse afferent innervation, they have long been suspected of serving a basic motor function, perhaps beating and driving the subtectorial membrane fluid. Nevertheless, it was surprising when Brownell and colleagues [1985] found that the outer hair cells have *electromotility*: the cell expands and contracts in an oscillating electric field, either extra- or intracellular. The electromotility exists at frequencies far higher than possible for normal contractile mechanisms [Ashmore, 1987]. The sensitivity is about 20 nm/mV (about 10^5 better than PZT-2, a widely used piezoelectric ceramic). It has not been determined if the electromotility can operate to the 200 kHz used by high frequency mammals. However, a calculation of the cell as a pressure vessel with a fixed charge in the wall [Jen and Steele, 1987] indicates that, despite the small diameter (10 μm), the viscosity of the intra- and extracellular fluid is not a limitation to the frequency response. In a continuation of the work reported by Hemmert and coworkers [1996], the force generation is found to continue to 80 kHz in the constrained cell. In contradiction, however, the same laboratory [Preyer and coworkers (1996)] finds that the intracellular voltage change due to displacement of the cilia drops off at a low frequency.

The motility appears to be due to a passive piezoelectric behavior of the cell plasma membrane [Kalinec and colleagues, 1992]. Iwasa and Chadwick [1992] measured the deformation of a cell under pressure loading and voltage clamping and computed the elastic properties of the wall, assuming isotropy. It appears that for agreement with both the pressure and axial stiffness measurements, the cell wall must be

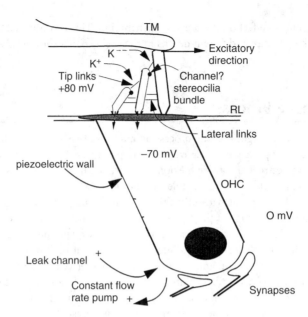

FIGURE 63.4 Model of outer hair cell. The normal pumping of ions produces negative intracellular electrical potential. Displacement of the cilia in the excitatory direction causes an opening of the ion channels in the cilia. There is evidence that the channels are located at the point of closest proximity of the two cilia. The tip and lateral links are important to maintain the correct stiffness and position. The opening of the channels decreases the intracellular potential, causing a piezoelectric contraction of the cell and excitation of the neural synapses. This can be modeled by a constant flow rate pump, leak channel, and spring controlled gate. The mechanical effect of the flow on the gate is important. The inner hair cell also has cilia, no piezoelectric property, but about twenty afferent synapses.

orthotropic, similar to a filament reinforced pressure vessel with close to the optimum filament angle of 38° [Tolomeo and Steele, 1995]. Holley [1990] finds circumferential filaments of the cytoskeleton with an average nonzero angle of about 26°. Mechanical measurements of the cell wall by Tolomeo and coworkers [1996] directly confirm the orthotropic stiffness.

63.4.2 Hair Cell Gating Channels

In 1984, Pickles and colleagues discovered tip links connecting the cilia of the hair cell, as shown in Figure 63.4, that are necessary for the normal function of the cochlea. These links are about 6 nm in diameter and 200 nm long [Pickles, 1988]. Subsequent work by Hudspeth [1989] and Assad and Corey [1992] shows convincingly that there is a resting tension in the links. A displacement of the ciliary bundle in the excitatory direction causes an opening of ion channels in the cilia, which in turn decreases the intracellular potential. This depolarization causes neural excitation, and in the piezoelectric outer hair cells, a decrease of the cell length.

A purely mechanical analog model of the gating is in Steele [1992], in which the ion flow is replaced by viscous fluid flow and the intracellular pressure is analogous to the voltage. A constant flow-rate pump and leak channel at the base of the cell establish the steady-state condition of negative intracellular pressure, tension in the tip links, and a partially opened gate at the cilia through which there is an average magnitude of flow. The pressure drop of the flow through the gate has a nonlinear negative spring effect on the system. If the cilia are given a static displacement, the stiffness for small perturbation displacement is dependent on the amplitude of the initial displacement, as observed by Hudspeth [1989]. For oscillatory forcing of the cilia, the fluid analog shows that a gain in power is possible, as in an electrical or fluidic amplifier, and that a modest change in the parameters can lead to instability.

Thus it appears that amplification in the cochlea resides in the gating of the outer hair cell cilia, while the motility is due to passive piezoelectric properties of the cell wall. The flow through the gate has significant nonlinearity at small amplitudes of displacement of the cilia (10 nm). Sufficiently high amplitudes of displacement of the cilia will cause the tip links to buckle. We estimate that this will occur at around 70 dB sound pressure level, thereby turning off the active process for higher sound intensity.

There is evidence reported by Hackney and colleagues [1996] that the channels do not occur at either end of the tip links, but at the region of closest proximity of the cilia, as shown in Figure 63.4. Mechanical models such as in Furness and colleagues [1997], indicate that the channels at such a location can also be opened by force on the cilia. More elaborate models show that the stiffness of the tip links remains important to the mechanism.

There may be a connection between the gating channels and the discovery by Canlon and coworkers [1988]. They found that acoustic stimulation of the wall of the isolated outer hair cell caused a tonic (DC) expansion of the cell over a narrow frequency band, which is related to the place for the cell along the cochlea. Khanna and coworkers [1989] observe a similar tonic displacement of the whole organ of Corti.

63.5 Active Models

De Boer, [1991], Geisler [1993], and Hubbard [1993] discuss models in which the electromotility of the outer hair cells feeds energy into the basilar membrane. The partition stiffness K is expanded from Equation 35.3 into a transfer function, containing a number of parameters and delay times. These are classed as phenomenological models, for which the physiological basis of the parameters is not of primary concern. The displacement gain may be defined as the ratio of ciliary shearing displacement to cell expansion. For these models, the gain used is larger by orders of magnitude than the maximum found in laboratory measurements of isolated hair cells.

Another approach [Steele and colleagues (1993)], which is physiologically based, appears promising. The outer hair cells are inclined in the propagation direction. Thus the shearing of the cilia at the distance x causes a force from the hair cells acting on the basilar membrane at the distance $x+\Delta x$. This "feed-forward" law can be expressed in terms of the pressure as

$$p_{ohc}(x + \Delta x) = \alpha p(x) = \alpha[2p_f(x) + p_{ohc}(x)] \qquad (63.16)$$

where p, the total pressure acting on the basilar membrane, consists of the effective pressure acting on the basilar membrane from the hair cells p_{ohc} and the pressure from the fluid p_f. The coefficient α is the force gain supplied by the outer hair cells. With this law, Equation 63.11 is replaced by:

$$(1 - e^{in\Delta x})n \tanh nH = 2\frac{\rho\omega^2}{AK}H \qquad (63.17)$$

from which the local wave number n must be computed numerically. Only two new parameters are needed, the gain α and the spacing Δx. With physiologically reasonable gain $\alpha = 0.18$ and spacing $\Delta x = 20~\mu m$, the result is an increase of the response of the basilar membrane for higher frequencies by a factor of 10^2 in a narrow sector, apical to the passive peak. The simple feed-forward addition in Equation 63.17 enhances a narrow band of wave lengths without a closed control loop. At this time, it appears that much of the elaborate structure of the organ of Corti is for the purpose of such a "feed-forward." This approach is also found to work well for the 1-D model by Geisler and Sang [1995]. The results from the 3-D model for the effect of adding some feed-forward are shown in Figure 63.3. One defect of the current feed-forward results is that the shift of the maximum response point is about one octave, as seen in Figure 63.3, rather than one-half octave consistently shown in normal cochlear measurements of mechanical and neural response.

The significant nonlinear effect is the saturation of the active process at high amplitudes. This can be computed by letting the gain α be a function of the amplitude.

In the normal, active cochlea, it was first observed by Khanna and colleagues [1989] and subsequently by Gummer and colleagues [1996], that the tectorial membrane (TM in Figure 63.1) has a substantially higher amplitude than the basilar membrane. Presumably, the electromotile expansion of the outer hair cells encounters less resistance from the tectorial membrane than the basilar membrane. This shows the importance of getting the correct stiffness and geometry into a model.

63.6 Fluid Streaming

Békésy [1960] and many others have observed significant fluid streaming in the actual cochlea and in experimental models. Particularly for the high frequencies, it is tempting to seek a component of steady streaming as the significant mechanical stimulation of the inner hair cells [Lighthill, 1992]. Passive models indicated that such streaming occurs only at high sound intensity. Among the many open questions is whether or not the enhancement of amplitude provided by the feed-forward of energy by the outer hair cells and the mechanical nonlinearity at low amplitudes of displacement provided by the ciliary gating can trigger significant streaming. It is clear from the anatomy Figure 63.1, that the motion and corresponding pressure in the fluid of the inner sulcus is the primary source of excitation for the inner hair cells. The DC pressure associated with DC streaming would be an important effect.

63.7 Clinical Possibilities

A better understanding of the cochlear mechanisms would be of clinical value. Auditory pathology related to the inner ear is discussed by Pickles [1988] and Gulick and colleagues [1989]. The spontaneous and stimulated emissions from the cochlea raise the possibility of diagnosing local inner ear problems, which is being pursued at many centers around the world. The capability for more accurate, physically realistic modeling of the cochlea should assist in this process. A significant step is provided by Zweig and Shera [1995], who find that a random distribution of irregularities in the properties along the cochlea explains much of the emissions.

A patient with a completely nonfunctioning cochlea is referred to as having "nerve deafness." In fact, there is evidence that in many cases the nerves may be intact, while the receptor cells and organ of Corti are defective. For such patients, a goal is to restore hearing with cochlear electrode implants to stimulate the nerve endings directly. Significant progress has been made. However, despite electrode stimulation of nerves at the correct place along the cochlea for a high frequency, the perception of high frequency has not been achieved. So, although substantial advance in cochlear physiology has been made in the recent past, several such waves of progress may be needed to adequately understand the functioning of the cochlea.

References

Allen J.B. and Neely S.T. 1992. Micromechanical models of the cochlea. *Phys. Today*, 45: 40–47.
Ashmore J.F. 1987. A fast motile response in guinea-pig outer hair cells: the cellular basis of the cochlear amplifier. *J. Physiol.* 388: 323–347.
Assad J.A. and Corey D.P. 1992. An active motor model for adaptation by vertebrate hair cells. *J. Neurosci.* 12(9): 3291–3309.
Békésy G. von. 1960. *Experiments in Hearing.* McGraw-Hill, New York.
Böhnke F., von Mikusch-Buchberg J., and Arnold W. 1996. 3D Finite Elemente Modell des cochleären Verstärkers. *Biomedizinische Technik.* 42: 311–312.
Brownell W.E., Bader C.R., Bertrand D., and de Ribaupierre Y. 1985. Evoked mechanical responses of isolated cochlear outer hair cells. *Science* 227: 194–196.
Canlon B., Brundlin L., and Flock Å. 1988. Acoustic stimulation causes tonotopic alterations in the length of isolated outer hair cells from the guinea pig hearing organ. *Proc. Natl Acad. Sci. USA* 85: 7033–7035.

Cabezudo L.M. 1978. The ultrastructure of the basilar membrane in the cat. *Acta Otolaryngol.* 86: 160–175.

Dallos P. 1992. The active cochlea. *J. Neurosci.* 12(12): 4575–4585.

De Boer E. 1991. Auditory physics. Physical principles in hearing theory. III. *Phys. Rep.* 203(3): 126–231.

Freeman D.M. and Weiss T.F. 1990. Hydrodynamic analysis of a two-dimensional model for micromechanical resonance of free-standing hair bundles. *Hearing Res.* 48: 37–68.

Fuhrmann E., Schneider W., and Schultz M. 1987. Wave propagation in the cochlea (inner ear): effects of Reissner's membrane and non-rectangular cross-section. *Acta Mech.*, 70: 15–30.

Furness D.N., Zetes D.E., Hackney C.M., and Steele C.R. 1997. Kinematic analysis of shear displacement as a means for operating mechanotransduction channels in the contact region between adjacent stereocilia of mammalian cochlear hair cells. *Proc. R. Soc. Lond. B* 264: 45–51.

Geisler C.D. 1993. A realizable cochlear model using feedback from motile outer hair cells. *Hearing Res.* 68: 253–262.

Geisler C.D. and Sang C. 1995. A cochlear model using feed-forword outer-hair-cell forces, *Hearing Res.* 85: 132–146.

Gulick W.L., Gescheider G.A., and Fresina R.D. 1989. *Hearing: Physiological Acoustics, Neural Coding, and Psychoacoustics.* Oxford University Press, London.

Gummer A.W., Johnston B.M., and Armstrong N.J. 1981. Direct measurements of basilar membrane stiffness in the guinea pig. *J. Acoust. Soc. Am.* 70: 1298–1309.

Gummer A.W., Hemmert W., and Zenner H.P. 1996. Resonant tectorial membrane motion in the inner ear: its crucial role in frequency tuning. *Proc. Natl Acad. Sci. USA* 93: 8727–8732.

Hackney C.M., Furness D.N., and Katori Y. 1996. Stereociliary ultrastructure in relation to mechanotransduction: tip links and the contact region. *Diversity in Auditory Mechanics.* University of California, Berkeley, pp. 173–180.

Hemmert W., Schauz C., Zenner H.P., and Gummer A.W. 1996. Force generation and mechanical impedance of outer hair cells. *Diversity in Auditory Mechanics.* University of California, Berkeley, pp. 189–196.

Holley M.D. 1990. Cell biology of hair cells. *Semin. Neurosci.* 2: 41–47.

Hubbard A.E. 1993. A traveling wave-amplifier model of the cochlea. *Science* 259: 68–71.

Hudspeth A.J. 1989. How the ears work. *Nature* 34: 397–404.

Iwasa K.H. and Chadwick R.S. 1992. Elasticity and active force generation of cochlear outer hair cells. *J. Acoust. Soc. Am.* 92: 3169–3173.

Jen D.H. and Steele C.R. 1987. Electrokinetic model of cochlear hair cell motility. *J. Acoust. Soc. Am.* 82: 1667–1678.

Kalinec F., Holley M.C., Iwasa K.H., Lim D., and Kachar B. 1992. A membrane-based force generation mechanism in auditory sensory cells. *Proc. Natl Acad. Sci. USA* 89: 8671–8675.

Keidel W.D. and Neff W.D., Eds. 1976. *Handbook of Sensory Physiology, Volume V: Auditory System.* Springer-Verlag, Berlin.

Kemp D.T. 1978. Stimulated acoustic emissions from within the human auditory system. *J. Acoust. Soc. Am.* 64: 1386–1391.

Khanna S.M., Flock Å, and Ulfendahl M. 1989. Comparison of the tuning of outer hair cells and the basilar membrane in the isolated cochlea. *Acta Otolaryngol. [Suppl] Stockholm* 467: 141–156.

Kolston P.J. and Ashmore J.F. 1996. Finite element micromechanical modeling of the cochlea in three dimensions. *J. Acoust. Soc. Am.* 99: 455–467.

Lighthill J. 1991. Biomechanics of hearing sensitivity. *J. Vibr. Acoust.* 113: 1–13.

Lighthill J. 1992. Acoustic streaming in the ear itself. *J. Fluid Mech.* 239: 551–606.

Miller C.E. 1985. Structural implications of basilar membrane compliance measurements. *J. Acoust. Soc. Am.* 77: 1465–1474.

Nobili R., Mommano F., and Ashmore J. 1998. How well do we understand the cochlea? *TINS* 21(4): 159–166.

Olson E.S. and Mountain D.C. 1994. Mapping the cochlear partition's stiffness to its cellular architecture. *J. Acoust. Soc. Am.* 95(1): 395–400.

Olson E.S. 1998. Observing middle and inner ear mechanics with novel intracochlear pressure sensors. *J. Acoust. Soc. Am.* 103(6): 3445–3463.

Pickles J.O. 1988. *An Introduction to the Physiology of Hearing*, 2nd ed. Academic Press, London.

Preyer S., Renz S., Hemmert W., Zenner H., and Gummer A. 1996. Receptor potential of outer hair cells isolated from base to apex of the adult guinea-pig cochlea: implications for cochlear tuning mechanisms. *Auditory Neurosci.* 2: 145–157.

Probst R. 1990. Otoacoustic emissions: an overview. *Adv. Oto-rhino-laryngol.* 44: 1–9.

Raftenberg M.N. 1990. Flow of endolymph in the inner spiral sulcus and the subtectorial space. *J. Acoust. Soc. Am.* 87(6): 2606–2620.

Ranke O.F. 1950. Theory of operation of the cochlea: a contribution to the hydrodynamics of the cochlea. *J. Acoust. Soc. Am.* 22: 772–777.

Rhode W.S. 1971. Observations of the vibration of the basilar membrane in squirrel monkeys using the Mössbauer technique. *J. Acoust. Soc. Am.* 49: 1218–1231.

Ruggero M.A. 1993. Distortion in those good vibrations. *Curr. Biol.* 3(11): 755–758.

Russell I.J. and Sellick P.M. 1977. Tuning properties of cochlear hair cells. *Nature* 267: 858–860.

Siebert W.M. 1974. Ranke revisited — a simple short-wave cochlear model. *J. Acoust. Soc. Am.* 56(2): 594–600.

Steele C.R. 1987. Cochlear mechanics. In *Handbook of Bioengineering*, R. Skalak and S. Chien, Eds., pp. 30.11–30.22, McGraw-Hill, New York.

Steele C.R. 1992. Electroelastic behavior of auditory receptor cells. *Biomimetics* 1(1): 3–22.

Steele C.R., Baker G, Tolomeo J.A., and Zetes D.E. 1993. Electro-mechanical models of the outer hair cell, *Biophysics of Hair Cell Sensory Systems*, In H. Duifhuis, J.W. Horst, P. van Dijk, and S.M. van Netten, Eds., World Scientific.

Strelioff D. and Flock Å. 1984. Stiffness of sensory-cell hair bundles in the isolated guinea pig cochlea. *Hearing Res.* 15: 19–28.

Taber L.A. and Steele C.R. 1979. Comparison of "WKB" and experimental results for three-dimensional cochlear models. *J. Acoust. Soc. Am.* 65: 1007–1018.

Tolomeo J.A. and Steele C.R. 1995. Orthotropic piezoelectric propeties of the cochlear outer hair cell wall. *J. Acoust. Soc. Am.* 95(5): 3006–3011.

Tolomeo J.A., Steele C.R., and Holley M.C. 1996. Mechanical properties of the lateral cortex of mammalian auditory outer hair cells. *Biophys. J.* 71: 421–429.

Watts L. 1993. *Cochlear Mechanics: Analysis and Analog VLSI.* Ph.D. Thesis, California Institute of Technology.

West C.D. 1985. The relationship of the spiral turns of the cochlea and the length of the basilar membrane to the range of audible frequencies in ground dwelling mammals. *J. Acoust. Soc. Am.* 77(3): 1091–1101.

Zhang L., Mountain D.C., and Hubbard A.E. 1996. Shape changes from base to apex cannot predict characteristic frequency changes. *Diversity in Auditory Mechanics.* University of California, Berkeley, pp. 611–618.

Zhou G., Bintz L., Anderson D.Z., and Bright K.E. 1994. A life-sized physical model of the human cochlea with optical holographic readout. *J. Acoust. Soc. Am.* 93(3): 1516–1523.

Zweig G. and Shera C.A. 1995. The origin of periodicity in the spectrum of evoked otoacoustic emissions. *J. Acoust. Soc. Am.* 98(4): 2018–2047.

Zwislocki J.J. and Cefaratti L.K. 1989. Tectorial membrane II: stiffness measurements *in vivo*. *Hearing Res.,* 42: 211–227.

Further Information

The following are workshop proceedings that document many of the developments.

De Boer E, and Viergever MA, Eds. 1983. *Mechanics of Hearing.* Nijhoff, The Hague.

Allen JB, Hall JL, Hubbard A, Neely ST, and Tubis A, Eds. 1985. *Peripheral Auditory Mechanisms.* Springer, Berlin.

Wilson JP and Kemp DT, Eds. 1988. *Cochlear Mechanisms: Structure, Function, and Models.* Plenum, New York.

Dallos P, Geisler CD, Matthews JW, Ruggero MA, and Steele CR, Eds. 1990. *The Mechanics and Biophysics of Hearing.* Springer, Berlin.

Duifhuis H, Horst JW, van Kijk P, and van Netten SM, Eds. 1993. *Biophysics of Hair Cell Sensory Systems.* World Scientific, Singapore.

Lewis ER, Long GR, Lyon RF, Narins PM, Steele CR, and Hecht-Poinar E, Eds. 1997. *Diversity in Auditory Mechanics.* World Scientific, Singapore.

64

Vestibular Mechanics

Wallace Grant
*Virginia Polytechnic Institute and
State University*

64.1   Introduction

The vestibular system is responsible for sensing motion and gravity and using this information for control of posture and body motion. This sense is also used to control eye position during head movement, allowing for a clear visual image. Vestibular function is rather inconspicuous, and for this reason it is frequently not recognized for its vital roll in maintaining balance and equilibrium, and in visual fixation with eye movements. It is truly a sixth sense, different from the five originally defined by Greek physicians.

The vestibular system is named for its position within the vestibule of the temporal bone of the skull. It is located in the inner ear along with the auditory sense. The vestibular system has both central and peripheral components. This chapter deals with the mechanical sensory function of the peripheral end organ and its ability to measure linear and angular inertial motion of the skull over the frequency ranges encountered in normal activities. The transduction process used to convert the mechanical signals into neural ones is also described.

64.2   Structure and Function

The vestibular system in each ear consists of the *otolith* and *saccule* (collectively by called the *otolithic organs*), which are the linear motion sensors, and the three *semicircular canals* (SCCs), which sense rotational motion. The SCCs are oriented in three nearly mutually perpendicular planes so that angular motion about any axis may be sensed. The otoliths and SCCs consist of membranous structures that are situated in hollowed-out sections and passageways in the vestibule of the temporal bone. This hollowed-out section of the temporal bone is called the bony labyrinth and the membranous labyrinth, composed of cell lined soft tissue membrane, lies within this bony structure. The membranous labyrinth is filled with a fluid called *endolymph*, which is high in potassium, and the volume between the membranous and bony labyrinths is filled with a fluid called perilymph, which is similar to blood plasma.

The utricular otolith sits in the utricle and the saccular otolith is located within membranous saccule. Each of these organs is rigidly attached to the temporal bone of the skull with connective tissue. The three semicircular canals terminate on the utricle forming a complete circular fluid path and the membranous canals are also rigidly attached to the bony skull. This rigid attachment is vital to the roll of measuring inertial motion of the skull.

Each SCC has a bulge called the *ampulla* near one end, and inside the ampulla is the *cupula*, which is composed of saccharide gel, and forms a complete hermetic seal with the ampulla. The cupula sits on top of the *crista* which contains the sensory receptor cells called *hair cells*. These hair cells have small *stereocilia* (hairs) which extend into the cupula and sense its deformation. When the head is rotated the endolymph fluid, which fills the canal, tends to remain at rest due to its inertia, the relative flow of fluid in the canal deforms the cupula like a diaphragm and the hair cells transduce the deformation into nerve signals.

The otolithic organs are flat-layered structures covered above with endolymph. The top layer consists of calcium carbonate crystals called *otoconia* which are bound together by a saccharide gel. The middle layer consists of pure saccharide gel and the bottom layer consists of receptor hair cells which have stereocilia that extend into the gel layer. When the head is accelerated the dense otoconial crystals tend to remain at rest due to their inertia as the sensory layer tends to move away from the otoconial layer. This relative motion between the otoconial layer and the sensory layer deforms the gel layer. The hair cell stereocilia sense this deformation and the receptor cells transduce this deformation into nerve signals. When the head is tilted the weight acting on the otoconial layer also will deform the gel layer in shear and deflect the hair cell stereocilia. The hair cell stereocilia also have directional sensitivity which allows them to determine the direction of the acceleration acting in the plane of the otolith and saccule. The planes of the two organs are arranged perpendicular to each other so that linear acceleration in any direction can be sensed. These organs also respond to gravity and are used to measure head tilt. The *vestibular nerve*, which forms half of the *VIII cranial nerve*, innervates all of the receptor cells of the vestibular apparatus.

64.3   Otolith Distributed Parameter Model

The otoliths are an overdamped second-order system whose structure is shown in Figure 64.1a. In this model the otoconial layer is assumed to be rigid and nondeformable, the gel layer is a deformable layer of isotropic viscoelastic material, and the fluid endolymph is assumed to be Newtonian fluid. A small element of the layered structure with surface area dA is cut from the surface and a vertical view of this surface element, of width dx, is shown in Figure 64.1b. To evaluate the forces that are present, free body diagrams are constructed of each elemental layer of the small differential strip. See the nomenclature table for a description of all variables used in the following formulas (for derivation details see Grant et al., 1984 and 1991).

Otolith Variables

x	=	coordinate direction in the plane of the otoconial layer
y_g	=	coordinate direction normal to the plane of the otolith with origin at the gel base
y_f	=	coordinate direction normal to the plane of the otolith with origin at the fluid base
t	=	time
$u(y_f, t)$	=	velocity of the endolymph fluid measured with respect to the skull
$v(t)$	=	velocity of the otoconial layer measured with respect to the skull
$w(y_g, t)$	=	velocity of the gel layer measured with respect to the skull

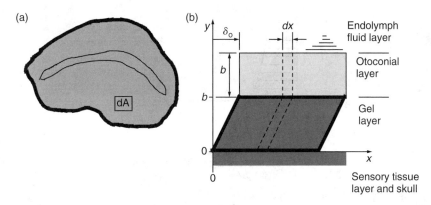

FIGURE 64.1 Schematic of the otolith organ: (a) Top view showing the peripheral region with differential area dA where the model is developed, and the striolar area that makes a arch through the center of the otolith. (b) Cross section showing the layered structure where dx is the width of the differential area dA shown in the top view.

δ = displacement of the otoconial layer measured with respect to the skull
V_s = skull velocity in the x-direction measured with respect to an inertial reference frame
V = a characteristic velocity of the skull in the problem (e.g., magnitude of a step change)
ρ_o = density of the otoconial layer
ρ_f = density of the endolymph fluid
τ_g = gel shear stress in the x-direction
μ_g = viscosity of the gel material
μ_f = viscosity of the endolymph fluid
G = shear modulus of the gel material
b = gel layer and otoconial layer thickness (assumed equal)
g_x = gravity component in the x-direction

In the equation of motion for the endolymph fluid, the force τ_fdA acts on the fluid at the fluid–otoconial layer interface (Figure 64.2). This shear stress τ_f is responsible for driving the fluid flow. The linear Navier-Stokes equation for an incompressible fluid are used to describe this endolymph flow. Expressions for the pressure gradient, the flow velocity of the fluid measured with respect to an inertial reference frame, and the force due to gravity (body force) are substituted into the Navier-Stokes equation for flow in the x-direction yielding

$$\rho_f \frac{\partial u}{\partial t} = \mu_f \frac{\partial^2 u}{\partial y_f^2} \tag{64.1}$$

with boundary and initial conditions: $u(0, t) = v(t)$; $u(\infty, t) = 0$; and $u(y_f, 0) = 0$.

The gel layer is treated as a *Kelvin–Voight viscoelastic material* where the gel shear is acting in parallel. This viscoelastic material stress has both an elastic and viscous component acting in parallel. This viscoelastic material model was substituted into the momentum equation and the resulting gel layer equation of motion is

$$\rho_f \frac{\partial w}{\partial t} = G \int_0^t \left(\frac{\partial^2 w}{\partial y_f^2} \right) dt + \mu_f \frac{\partial^2 w}{\partial y_f^2} \tag{64.2}$$

with boundary and initial conditions: $w(b, t) = v(t)$; $w(0, t) = 0$; $w(y_g, 0) = 0$; and $\delta_g(y_g, 0) = 0$. The elastic term in the equation is written in terms of the integral of velocity with respect to time, instead of displacement, so the equation is in terms of a single dependent variable, the velocity.

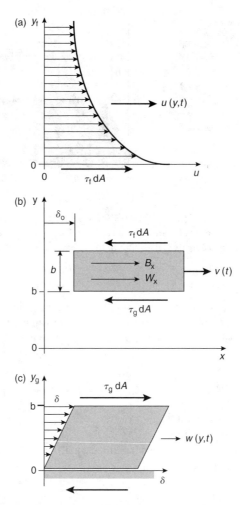

FIGURE 64.2 The free-body diagrams of each layer of the otolith with the forces that act on each layer. The interfaces are coupled by shear stresses of equal magnitudes that act in opposite directions at each surface. The τ_g shear stress acts between the gel–otoconial layer and the τ_f acts between the fluid–otoconial layer. The forces acting at these interfaces are the product of shear stress τ and area dA. The B_x and W_x forces are the components of the buoyant and weight forces acting in the plane of the otoconial layer, respectively. See the nomenclature table for definitions of other variables. (a) *Endolymph fluid layer:* The spatial coordinate in the vertical direction is y_f and the velocity of the endolymph fluid is $u(y_f, t)$, a function of the fluid depth y_f and time t. (b) *Otoconial layer:* The otoconial layer with thickness b and at a height b above the gel layer vertical coordinate origin. The velocity of the otoconial layer is $v(t)$, which is a function of time only. (c) *Gel layer:* Gel layer of thickness b, vertical coordinate y_g, and horizontal coordinate δ_g the gel deflection. The gel deflection is a function of both y_g and time t. The velocity of the gel is $w(y_g, t)$, a function of y_g and t.

The otoconial layer equation was developed using Newton's second law of motion, equating the forces that act on the otoconial layer: fluid shear, gel shear, buoyant, and weight to the product of mass and inertial acceleration. The resulting otoconial layer equation is

$$\rho_o b \frac{\partial v}{\partial t} + (\rho_o - \rho_f)\left[\frac{\partial V_s}{\partial t} - g_x\right] = \mu_f \left(\frac{\partial u}{\partial y_f}\bigg|_{y_f=0}\right) - G \int_0^t \left(\frac{\partial w}{\partial y_g}\bigg|_{y_g=b}\right) dt + \mu_g \left(\frac{\partial w}{\partial y_g}\bigg|_{y_g=b}\right)$$

$$(64.3)$$

with the following initial conditions $v(0) = 0$. The otoconial layer displacement can be calculated by integrating the velocity of this layer with respect to time

$$\delta = \int_0^t v \, dt \tag{64.4}$$

Displacement of the otoconial layer is the variable of importance, it is proportional to acceleration, and is the variable transduced into a neural signal.

64.4 Nondimensionalization of the Otolith Motion Equations

The equations of motion are then nondimensionalized to reduce the number of physical and dimensional parameters, and combine them into some useful nondimensional numbers. The following nondimensional variables, which are indicated by overbars, are introduced into the motion equations:

$$\bar{y}_f = \frac{y_f}{b} \quad \bar{y}_g = \frac{y_g}{b} \quad \bar{t} = \left(\frac{\mu_f}{\rho_o b^2}\right) t \quad \bar{u} = \frac{u}{V} \quad \bar{v} = \frac{v}{V} \quad \bar{w} = \frac{w}{V} \tag{64.5}$$

Several nondimensional parameters occur naturally as a part of the nondimensionalization process; these parameters are

$$R = \frac{\rho_f}{\rho_o} \quad \varepsilon = \frac{Gb^2 \rho_o}{\mu_f^2} \quad M = \frac{\mu_g}{\mu_f} \quad \bar{g}_x = \left(\frac{\rho_o b^2}{V \mu_f}\right) g_x \tag{64.6}$$

These parameters represent the following: R is the density ratio and represents the system nondimentional mass, ε is a nondimensional elastic parameter and represents the system elasticity, M is the viscosity ratio and represents the system damping, and $\bar{g}_x$ is the nondimensional gravity.

The governing equations of motion in nondimensional form are then as follows:

$$\textit{Endolymph Fluid Layer} \quad R\frac{\partial \bar{u}}{\partial \bar{t}} = \frac{\partial^2 \bar{u}}{\partial \bar{y}_f^2} \tag{64.7}$$

$$\textit{Boundary Conditions} \quad \bar{u}(0, \bar{t}) = \bar{v}(\bar{t}) \qquad \bar{u}(\infty, \bar{t}) = 0$$

$$\textit{Initial Conditions} \quad \bar{u}(\bar{y}_f, 0) = 0$$

$$\textit{Otoconial Layer} \quad \frac{\partial \bar{v}}{\partial \bar{t}} + (1 - R)\left[\frac{\partial \bar{V}_s}{\partial \bar{t}} - \bar{g}_x\right] = \left(\frac{\partial \bar{u}}{\partial \bar{y}_f}\bigg|_0\right) - \varepsilon \int_0^{\bar{t}} \left(\frac{\partial \bar{w}}{\partial \bar{y}_g}\bigg|_1\right) dt - M\left(\frac{\partial \bar{w}}{\partial \bar{y}_g}\bigg|_1\right) \tag{64.8}$$

$$\textit{Initial Condition} \quad \bar{v}(0) = 0$$

$$\textit{Gel Layer} \quad R\frac{\partial \bar{w}}{\partial \bar{t}} = \varepsilon \int_0^{\bar{t}} \left(\frac{\partial^2 \bar{w}}{\partial \bar{y}_g^2}\right) dt + M\left(\frac{\partial^2 \bar{w}}{\partial \bar{y}_g^2}\right) \tag{64.9}$$

$$\textit{Boundary Conditions} \quad \bar{w}(1, \bar{t}) = \bar{v}(\bar{t}) \qquad \bar{w}(0, \bar{t}) = 0$$

$$\textit{Initial Conditions} \quad \bar{w}(\bar{y}_g, 0) = 0 \qquad \bar{\delta}_g(\bar{y}_g, 0) = 0$$

The nondimensional otoconial layer displacement becomes

$$\bar{\delta} = \left(\frac{V\rho_0 b^2}{\mu_f}\right) \int_0^{\bar{t}} \bar{v}\, d\bar{t} \tag{64.10}$$

These equations can be solved numerically for the case of a step change in acceleration or velocity of the skull [Grant and Cotton, 1991]. Solutions for both step change in acceleration and velocity are shown in Figure 64.3.

64.5 Otolith Transfer Function

A transfer function of otoconial layer deflection re. (related to) skull acceleration can be obtained from the governing equations [Grant et al., 1994]. Starting with the nondimensional fluid and gel layer equations, taking the Laplace transform with respect to time and using the initial conditions, gives two ordinary differential equations. These equations can then be solved, using the boundary conditions. Taking the Laplace transform of the otoconial layer motion equation, combining with the two differential equation solutions, and integrating otoconial layer velocity to get deflection produces the transfer function for displacement re. acceleration

$$\frac{\bar{\delta}}{\bar{A}}(s) = \frac{(1-R)}{s[s + \sqrt{Rs} + (\varepsilon/s + M)\sqrt{Rs/(\varepsilon/s + M)}\coth(\sqrt{Rs/(\varepsilon/s + M)})]} \tag{64.11}$$

s is the Laplace transform variable, and a general acceleration term A is defined as

$$\bar{A} = -\left(\frac{\partial \bar{V}_s}{\partial \bar{t}} - \bar{g}_x\right) \tag{64.12}$$

64.6 Otolith Frequency Response

This transfer function can now be studied in the frequency domain. It should be noted that these are linear partial differential equations and that the process of frequency domain analysis is appropriate. The range of values of $\varepsilon = 0.01$ to 0.2, $M = 5$ to 20, and $R = 0.75$ have been established [Grant and Cotton, 1991] in a numerical finite difference solution of the governing equations. Having established these values the frequency response can be completed.

In order to construct a magnitude and phase vs. frequency plot of the transfer function, the nondimensional time will be converted back to real time for use on the frequency axis. For the conversion to real time the following physical variables will be used: $\rho_0 = 1350$ kg/m^3, $b = 15\ \mu$m, and $\mu_f = 0.85$ mPa/sec. The general frequency response is shown in Figure 64.4. The flat response from DC up to the first corner frequency establishes this system as an accelerometer. This is the range of motion frequencies encountered in normal motion environments where this transducer is expected to function.

The range of flat response can be easily controlled with the two parameters and ε and M. It is interesting to note that both the elastic term and the system damping are controlled by the gel layer, thus an animal can easily control the system response by changing the parameters of this saccharide gel layer. The cross-linking of saccharide gels is extremely variable yielding vastly different elastic and viscous properties of the resulting structure. The density ratio R has the effect of changing the magnitude of the response, and the parameters ε and M control the dynamics of the response.

The otoconial layer transfer function can be compared to recent data from single fiber neural recording. The only discrepancy between the experimental data and theoretical model is a low-frequency phase lead and accompanying amplitude reduction. This has been observed in most experimental single-fiber recordings and has been attributed to the hair cell.

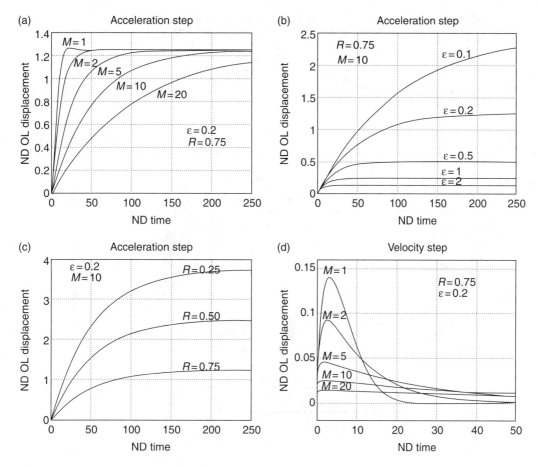

FIGURE 64.3 Solution of the otolith governing equations for the stimulus cases of a step change in acceleration and a step change in the velocity (impulse in acceleration). Scale label abbreviations used: ND = nondimensional, OL = otoconial layer. These solutions are shown for various values of the nondimensional elastic parameters ε, M, and R. In each case two of the nondimensional parameters were held constant and the remaining one was varied. These solutions reflect the general system behavior. The nondimensional time and displacement scales can be converted to real time and displacement for human physical variables as follows: nondimensional time of $1 = 0.36$ msec, and nondimensional displacement of $1 = 36\ \mu m$ (human physical variables used: $b = 15\ \mu m$, $\mu_f = 0.85$ mPa/sec, $\rho_f = 1000$ kg/m^3, $\rho_o = 1350$ kg/m^3, $G = 10$ Pa, $V = 0.1$ m/sec).

(a) Solution for a step change in acceleration for various values of the nondimensional system damping parameter M. The value of $M = 1$ shows a slight displacement overshoot. Note that as M is increased the displacement rise time is increased.

(b) Solution for a step change in acceleration of the head for various values of the nondimensional system elastic parameter ε. Note that as ε is increased the displacement magnitude decreases along with the rise time.

(c) Solution for a step change in acceleration of the head for various values of the nondimensional density ratio R. Since $R = \rho_f/\rho_o$, as it is increased the amplitude of displacement is decreases (the effect of increasing R is to lower the density of the otoconial layer). This parameter only changes the displacement amplitude with no effect on the dynamics.

(d) Solution for a step change in velocity of the head (impulse in acceleration) for various values of the nondimensional damping parameter M. Note that as M is increased the amplitude peak is decreased and the settling time is increased. In this case the otoconial layer does not settle to a permanent fixed displacement, but returns to its equilibrium position. Again with $M = 1$ a slight overshoot on the return to equilibrium.

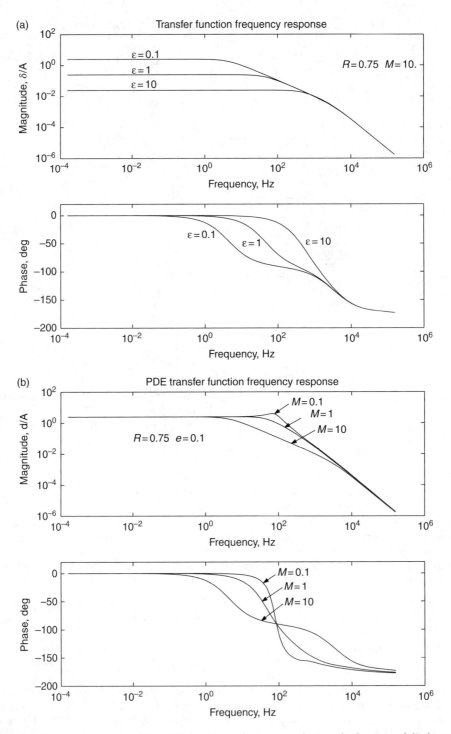

FIGURE 64.4 Frequency response of the utricular system shown using the transfer function of displacement re. acceleration. (a) Showing the effects of the nondimensional stiffness parameter term ε, while R and M are held constant. (b) Showing the effects of the nondimensional damping parameter term M, while R and ε are held constant. Note that the system is slightly underdamped when $M = 0.1$ as is denoted by the increase in magnitude at the corner frequency (slightly less than 10^2 Hz). This underdamped response is entirely possible since no restrictions were placed on the system during model formulation.

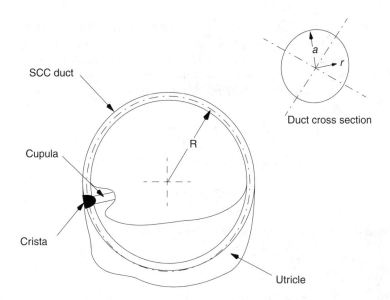

FIGURE 64.5 Schematic structure of the semicircular canal showing a cross section through the canal duct and utricle. Also shown in the upper right-hand corner is a cross section of the duct. R is the radius of curvature of the semicircular canal, a is the inside radius to the duct wall, and r is the spatial coordinate in the radial direction of the duct.

64.7 Semicircular Canal Distributed Parameter Model

The membranous SCC duct is modeled as a section of a rigid torus filled with an incompressible Newtonian fluid. The governing equations of motion for the fluid are developed from the Navier-Stokes equation. Refer to the nomenclature section for definition of all variables, and Figure 64.5 for a cross section of the SCC and membranous utricle sack.

Semicircular Canal Variables

$u(r, t)$ = velocity of endolymph fluid measured with respect to the canal wall
r = radial coordinate of canal duct
a = inside radius of the canal duct
R = radius of curvature of semicircular canal
ρ_f = density of the endolymph fluid
μ_f = viscosity of the endolymph fluid
α = angular acceleration of the canal wall measured with respect to an inertial frame
ω = angular velocity of the canal wall measured with respect to an inertial frame
ϕ = angular displacement of the canal wall measured with respect to an inertial frame
Ω = magnitude of a step change of angular velocity of the head or canal wall
K = pressure–volume modulus of the cupula = $\Delta p / \Delta V$
Δp = differential pressure across the cupula
ΔV = volumetric displacement of endolymph fluid
β = angle subtended by the canal in radians ($\beta = \pi$ for a true semicircular canal)
λ_n = roots of $J_0(x) = 0$, where J_0 is Bessel's function of order 0 ($\lambda_1 = 2.405, \lambda_2 = 5.520, \ldots$)

We are interested in the flow of endolymph fluid with respect to the duct wall and this requires that the inertial motion of the duct wall $R\Omega$ be added to the fluid velocity u measured with respect to the duct wall.

The curvature of the duct can be shown to be negligible since $a \ll R$, and no secondary flow is induced, thus the curve duct can be treated as straight. Pressure gradients arise from two sources in the duct (1) presence of the utricle and (2) from the cupula. The cupula, when deflected, exerts a restoring force on the endolymph. The cupula can be modeled as a membrane with a linear pressure–volume modulus $K = \Delta p / \Delta V$, where Δp is the pressure difference across the cupula, which is produced by a volumetric displacement ΔV, where

$$\Delta V = 2\pi \int_0^t \int_0^a u(r,t)r\,dr\,dt \tag{64.13}$$

If the angle subtended by the membranous duct is denoted by β, the pressure gradient in the duct produced by the cupula is

$$\frac{\partial p}{\partial z} = \frac{K \Delta V}{\beta R} \tag{64.14}$$

The utricle pressure gradient can be approximated by [VanBuskirk, 1977]

$$\frac{\partial p}{\partial z} = \frac{2\pi - \beta}{\beta} \rho R\alpha \tag{64.15}$$

When this information is substituted into the Navier-Stokes equation the following governing equation for endolymph flow relative to the duct wall is obtained

$$\frac{\partial u}{\partial t} + \left(\frac{2\pi}{\beta}\right) R\alpha = -\frac{2\pi K}{\rho \beta R} \int_0^t \int_0^a u(r\,dr)dt + \frac{\mu_f}{\rho_f}\left[\frac{1}{r}\frac{\partial}{\partial r}\left(r\frac{\partial u}{\partial r}\right)\right] \tag{64.16}$$

This equation can be nondimensionalized using the following nondimensional variables denoted by overbars

$$\bar{r} = \frac{r}{a} \qquad \bar{t} = \left(\frac{\mu_f}{\rho_f a^2}\right)t \qquad \bar{u} = \frac{u}{R\Omega} \tag{64.17}$$

In terms of the nondimensional variables the governing equation for endolymph flow velocity becomes

$$\frac{\partial \bar{u}}{\partial \bar{t}} + \left(\frac{2\pi}{\beta}\right)\alpha(\bar{t}) = -\varepsilon \int_0^{\bar{t}} \int_0^1 (\bar{u}\bar{r}d\bar{r})dt + \frac{1}{r}\frac{\partial}{\partial \bar{r}}\left(\bar{r}\frac{\partial \bar{u}}{\partial \bar{r}}\right) \tag{64.18}$$

where the nondimensional parameter

$$\varepsilon = \frac{2K\pi a^6 \rho_f}{\beta R\mu_f^2} \tag{64.19}$$

which contains physical parameters for the system mass, stiffness, and damping. This ε parameter governs the response of the canals to angular acceleration. The boundary and initial conditions for this equation are a follows

Boundary conditions $\bar{u}(1,\bar{t}) = 0$ $\dfrac{\partial \bar{u}}{\partial \bar{r}}(0,\bar{t}) = 0$

Initial condition $\bar{u}(\bar{r},0) = 0$

64.8 Semicircular Canal Frequency Response

To examine the frequency response of the SCC, a transfer function must be developed that relates the mean angular displacement of endolymph to head motion. The objective of this analysis is to see if the SCCs are angular acceleration, velocity, or displacement sensors. To achieve this, a relationship between α = angular acceleration, ω = angular velocity, and ϕ = angular displacement of the head, all measured with respect to an inertial reference frame, is developed. This relationship in terms of the Laplace transform variable s is

$$\alpha(s) = s\omega(s) = s^2\phi(s) \tag{64.20}$$

To relate these to the mean angular displacement of endolymph, the volumetric displacement $\Delta V = \int_0^t (\int_0^a (u(r,t)2\pi r\, dr))dt$ is calculated from the distributed parameter solution and this is related to the mean angular displacement of the endolymph θ as

$$\theta = \frac{\Delta V}{\pi a^2 R} \tag{64.21}$$

Using the solution to the distributed parameter formulation for the SCC, for $\varepsilon \ll 1$, and for a step change in angular velocity of the canal wall Ω, the volumetric displacement becomes

$$\Delta V = \left(\frac{\pi \rho_f a^4}{8\mu_f}\right)\left(\frac{2\pi}{\beta}\right)R\Omega\sum_{n=1}^{\infty}\frac{1}{\lambda_n^4}\left(1 - e^{-(\lambda_n^2\mu_f/a^2\rho_f)t}\right) \tag{64.22}$$

where λ_n represents the roots of the equation $J_0(x) = 0$, where J_0 is the Bessel function of zero order ($\lambda_1 = 2.405, \lambda_2 = 5.520, \ldots$) [VanBuskirk et al., 1976; VanBuskirk and Grant, 1987].

A transfer function in terms of s can now be developed for frequency response analysis. This starts by developing an ordinary differential equation in θ for the system, using a moment sum about the SCC center, and developing terms for the inertia, damping, restoring moment created by the cupula incorporating ΔV. Using this relationship and Equation 64.20, the transfer function of mean angular displacement of endolymph θ re. ω the angular velocity of the canal wall (or head) is

$$\frac{\theta}{\omega}(s) = \left(\frac{\rho_f a^2}{8\mu_f}\right)\left(\frac{2\pi}{\beta}\right)\left(\frac{s}{(s + 1/\tau_L)(s + 1/\tau_S)}\right) \tag{64.23}$$

where the two time constants, one long (τ_L) and one short (τ_s) are given by:

$$\tau_S \cong \frac{a^2\rho_f}{\lambda_1^2\mu_f} \qquad \tau_L = \frac{8\mu_f\beta R}{K\pi a^4} \tag{64.24}$$

where $\tau_L \gg \tau_S$. Here the angular velocity of the head is used instead of the angular acceleration or angular displacement because, in the range of frequencies encountered by humans in normal motion, the canals are angular velocity sensors. This is easily seen if the other two transfer functions are plotted.

The utility of the above transfer function is apparent when used to generate the frequency response of the system. The values for the various parameters for humans are as follows: $a = 0.15$ mm, $R = 3.2$ mm, the dynamic viscosity of endolymph $\mu = 0.85$ mPa sec, $\rho_f = 1000$ kg/m^3, $\beta = 1.4\pi$, and $K = 3.4$ GPa/m^3. This produces values of the two time constants of $\tau_L = 20.8$ sec and $\tau_s = 0.00385$ sec. The frequency response of the system is shown in Figure 64.6. The range of frequencies from 0.01 to 30 Hz establishes the SCCs as angular velocity transducers of head motion. This range includes those encountered in everyday movement. Environments such a aircraft flight, automobile travel, and shipboard travel can produce frequencies outside the linear range for these transducers.

Rabbitt and Damino [1992] have modeled the flow of endolymph in the ampulla and its interaction with the cupula. This model indicates that the cupula adds a high frequency gain enhancement as well as phase lead over previous mechanical models. This is consistent with measurements of vestibular nerve recordings of gain and phase. Prior to this work, this gain and phase enhancement were thought to be of hair cell origin.

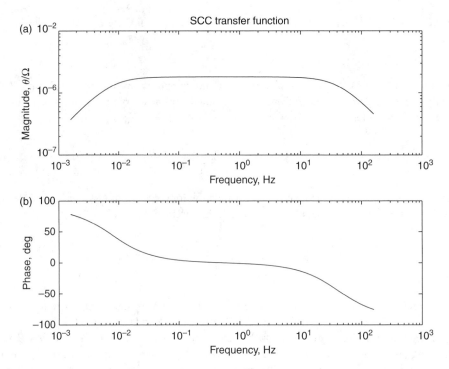

FIGURE 64.6 Frequency response of the human semicircular canals for the transfer function of mean angular displacement of endolymph fluid θ re. angular velocity of the head ω.

64.9   Hair Cell Structure and Transduction

As can be seen from the two frequency response diagrams for the otolith and SCC, the sensed variables, linear acceleration in the case of the otolith and angular velocity for the SCC, are transduced into a displacements. These displacements are cupula displacement for the SCC and otoconial layer displacement for the otolith. These displacements are then further transduced into neural signals by the hair cells in each sensory organ. The hair cells project small cilia or hairs, called *stereocilia*, from the apical surface of the cell body into the otolith gel layer and cupula (see Figure 64.7 and Figure 64.8). Figure 64.7 shows the geometry of a single stereocilium, which is cylindrical in shape and has a tapered base. Each stereocilium has an internal core of actin, which deforms when a force is applied to its top. Because of the tapered base, most of the deformation in a stereocilium is bending in this tapered section with a top force applied. Both bending and shear deformation take place throughout the entire stereocilia when they are deflected.

The stereocilia of a single hair cell form a bundle, with definite regular spacing in an hexagonal array when viewed form the top (see Figure 64.7). The height of each stereocilium in a bundle increases, in a stepwise fashion, to form an organ pipe arrangement. Stereocilia in a bundle are bound together by a set of links the run from stereocilia to stereocilia. These bundle links are what forms a bundle into a single functional unit. These links come in many types; however, there are two main structural types, *tip links* that run up at an angle from the tip of the stereocilia to its next taller neighbor, and *upper lateral links* that run horizontally in sets. The lateral links extend from one stereocilia to its six neighbors, forming six sets associated with each stereocilia.

A set is composed of a group of links that are spaced up and down the height of the stereocilia. The protein composition of these links is unknown, but each type of link is believed to have a different structure. The tip links are stiff and resist elongation more than the lateral links. The tallest cilia in the bundle is called a *kinocilium*, which is a true cilia with 9+2 tubule structure, different from the stereocilia, and it is linked to its neighboring stereocilia by a third type of link called a *stereocilia–kinocilium link*. Other link

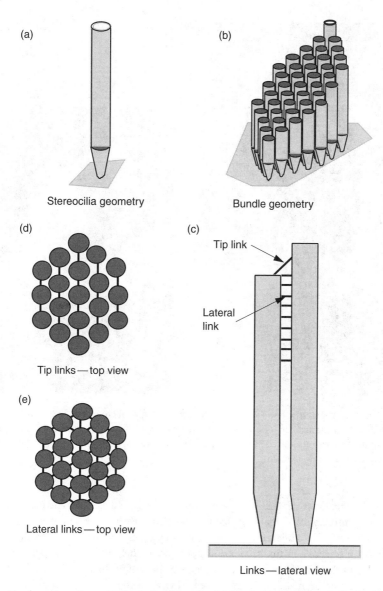

FIGURE 64.7   Configuration of a vestibular hair cell bundle. (a) Stereocilia geometry of circular shaft with tapered base. These stereocilia are composed of actin surrounded by the cell membrane. (b) Bundle geometry for a typical vestibular stereocilia bundle, showing the staircase arrangement of increasing height of the stereocilia in the bundle. The tallest cilia in the bundle is different in structure from the stereocilia and is called a kinocilium, which has the 9+2 microtubule structure of a true cilium. The microtubule structure lacks the biochemical ability to be mobile and it appears to be present for structural rigidity only. (c) Lateral view of two stereocilia connected by tip and lateral links. (d) Top view of the stereocilia showing the locations of orientation of the tip links. (e) Top view of the stereocilia showing the locations and orientation of the lateral links.

structures have been identified in the bundle but will not be discussed here, as these are thought to be insignificant structural links. These interconnected stereocilia and kinocilium form a complete vestibular bundle.

Kinocilia are attached to the cupula and otoconial gel layer so that when these are deflected the kinocilia are also deflected pulling the entire hair cell bundle with it. When a hair cell bundle is deflected by a force applied to the kinocilium in a direction away from the bundle, the resulting deflection stretches the tip

(a)   (b)

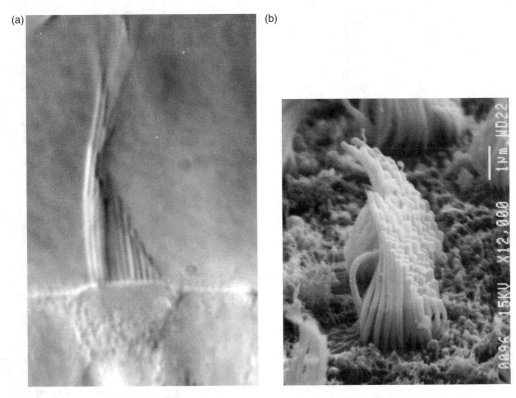

FIGURE 64.8 Photomicrographs of real hair cell bundles. (a) Light micrograph (DIC). (b) Scanning electron microscope of a bundle in the striolar region of the utricle (×12,000). Due to the fixation and drying for electron microscopy many artifacts are introduced in the bundle. (Photomicrographs taken by Dr. Ellengene Peterson, Ohio University, and used here with permission.)

links increasing their tension. In addition, lateral links are tensioned as well. The increased tension in a tip link increases the probability that an ion channel attached to the tip link will open. These ion channels are imbedded in the outer lipid bilayer of the hair cell and there is evidence that there are as many as two channels on each tip link. When tip link tension opens a channel, it allows free positive ions from the surrounding endolymph fluid to flow into the intercellular space of the hair cell. This influx of positive ions decreases the resting membrane potential of the cell. This starts the cascade of events that are associated with the depolarization of any sensory receptor cell, which ends with the release of neurotransmitter, and firing of the nerve that is in contact with the cell. In this fashion the mechanical deflection of the hair cell's bundle is converted into a neural signal. This process is termed *mechanotransduction*, and when linked with the extracellular structure of otoconial layer deflection and cupula deflection, the entire organ function becomes a complex inertial motion sensor of the head.

64.10 Hair Cell Mechanical Model

Mechanical deformation behavior of the hair cell bundles has been analyzed using finite element analysis (FEA). This analysis was done using a custom-written program that will accommodate any hair bundle configuration [Cotton and Grant, 2000]. The resulting model is a three-dimensional, distributed parameter formulation which ramps up any applied force in incremental steps. Each force step considers the new, deformed geometry and recalculates displacements, link tensions, and internal force directions, until each of these values converges. This incremental ramp loading is a nonlinear computational process.

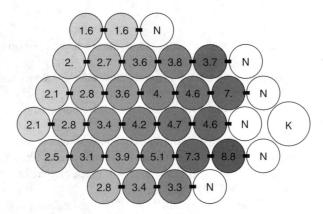

FIGURE 64.9   Circle plots of a bundle showing the tip link tensions in pN. These plots are topviews of the bundle where each stereocilia and kinocilium in the bundle is represented by a circle. The arrangement is to scale and represents the organization of cilia studied. The tip links are represented as solid lines connecting the circles. The number inside each circle represents the tension in the tip link attached to the top of that stereocilium which runs to the side of the next taller stereocilium. The shading is a relative designation of the tip link tension within that bundle, with dark indicating maximum tension. Stereocilia with an N designation indicates the absence of a tip link due to the absence of a taller stereocilium for attachment. The kinocilium is shown with a K in its circle. In the figure the bundle has a point loaded force applied at the top of the kinocilium. The magnitude of the applied force was adjusted to produce a bundle deflection of 50 nm. The force magnitude to produce the 50 nm deflection is 8 pN.

The model uses shear deformable beam elements for cilia. Tip links and lateral links are modeled as two-force members with linear spring-like behavior in tension. Lateral links can buckle and are not allowed to support compressive loads. Tip links are almost always in tension, they are treated similarly to lateral links and are not allowed to support a compressive load.

The program allows input specifications of material and geometric properties. Geometric properties include cilia and link diameters, tapering at the base of stereocilia, and cilia locations on the hair cell's apical surface. Material properties include elastic moduli for cilia and links, and the shear moduli for cilia.

In order to formulate a realistic bundle model, geometric data was gathered using light microscope and SEM photomicrographs. Material properties were determined from reference materials and using parametric studies. Figure 64.9 illustrates the pattern of tip link tensions generated in a bundle which is loaded with a force of sufficient magnitude to produce a 50-nm deflection, a typical large physiologic deflection (for details see Silber et al., 2004). In this figure, circles represent the configuration of stereocilia and kinocilium (K) on the apical surface of each hair cell (bundle viewed from top). The number inside each circle is the magnitude of tension in pN (peco Newtons) for the tip link attached to the top of that stereocilium; shading is scaled to this magnitude. The simulations shows that tensions are highest close to the kinocilium, and they drop steadily with distance from the kinocilium. Note also that higher tensions generally tend to occur in the middle columns of the bundle; peripheral columns have relatively low tensions, even those close to the kinocilium.

64.11   Concluding Remark

The mechanical signal of inertial head motion has been followed and quantified through the vestibular organs to neural signals that are generated in the receptor hair cells. As stated in the introduction, the central nervous system uses these signals for eye positioning during periods of motion and to coordinate muscular activity. The biggest problem for people who have lost their vestibular function is not being able to see during periods of body motion. Implantable artificial vestibules are being developed for future medical application.

References

Cotton, J.R. and Grant, J.W. 2000. A finite element method for mechanical response of hair cell ciliary bundles. *J. Biomech. Eng., Trans. ASME* 122: 44–50.

Grant, J.W., Huang, C.C., and Cotton, J.R. 1994. Theoretical mechanical frequency response of the otolith organs. *J. Vestib. Res.* 4: 137–151.

Grant, J.W. and Cotton, J.R. 1991. A model for otolith dynamic response with a viscoelastic gel layer. *J. Vestib. Res.* 1: 139–151.

Grant, J.W., Best, W.A., and Lonegro, R. 1984. Governing equations of motion for the otolith organs and their response to a step change in velocity of the skull. *J. Biomech. Eng.* 106: 302–308.

Rabbitt, R.D. and Damino, E.R. 1992. A hydroelastic model of macromechanics in the endolymphatic vestibular canal. *J. Fluid Mech.* 238: 337–369.

Silber, J., Cotton, J., Nam, J., Peterson, E., and Grant, W. 2004. Computational models of hair cell bundle mechanics: III. 3-D utricular bundles. *Hearing Res.* (in press).

Van Buskirk, W.C. and Grant, J.W. 1987. Vestibular mechanics. In *Handbook of Bioengineering*, Eds. R. Skalak and S. Chien, pp. 31.1–31.17. McGraw-Hill, New York.

Van Buskirk, W.C. 1977. The effects of the utricle on flow in the semicircular canals. *Ann. Biomed. Eng.* 5: 1–11.

Van Buskirk, W.C., Watts, R.G., and Liu, Y.K. 1976. Fluid mechanics of the semicircular canal. *J. Fluid Mech.* 78: 87–98.

65

Exercise Physiology

Arthur T. Johnson
Cathryn R. Dooly
University of Maryland

The study of exercise is important to medical and biological engineers. Cognizance of acute and chronic responses to exercise gives an understanding of the physiological stresses to which the body is subjected. To appreciate exercise responses requires a true systems approach to physiology, because during exercise all physiological responses become a highly integrated, total supportive mechanism for the performance of the physical stress of exercise. Unlike the study of pathology and disease, the study of exercise physiology leads to a wonderful understanding of the way the body is supposed to work while performing at its healthy best.

For exercise involving resistance, physiological and psychological adjustments begin even before the start of the exercise. The central nervous system (CNS) sizes up the task before it, assessing how much muscular force to apply and computing trial limb trajectories to accomplish the required movement. Heart rate may begin rising in anticipation of increased oxygen demands and respiration may also increase.

65.1 Muscle Energetics

Deep in muscle tissue, key components have been stored for this moment. Adenosine triphosphate (ATP), the fundamental energy source for muscle cells, is at maximal levels. Also stored are significant amounts of creatine phosphate and glycogen.

When the actinomyocin filaments of the muscles are caused to move in response to neural stimulation, ATP reserves are rapidly used, and ATP becomes adenosine diphosphate (ADP), a compound with much less energy density than ATP. Maximally contracting mammalian muscle uses approximately 1.7×10^{-5} mole of ATP per gram per second [White et al., 1959]. ATP stores in skeletal muscle tissue amount to 5×10^{-6} mole per gram of tissue, or enough to meet muscle energy demands for no more than 0.5 sec.

Initial replenishment of ATP occurs through the transfer of creatine phosphate (CP) into creatine. The resting muscle contains 4 to 6 times as much CP as it does ATP, but the total supply of high-energy phosphate cannot sustain muscle activity for more than a few seconds.

Glycogen is a polysaccharide present in muscle tissues in large amounts. When required, glycogen is decomposed into glucose and pyruvic acid, which, in turn, becomes lactic acid. These reactions form ATP and proceed without oxygen. They are thus called **anaerobic.**

When sufficient oxygen is available (aerobic conditions), either in muscle tissue or elsewhere, these processes are reversed. ATP is reformed from ADP and AMP (adenosine monophosphate), CP is reformed from creatine and phosphate (P), and glycogen is reformed from glucose or lactic acid. Energy for these processes is derived from the complete oxidation of carbohydrates, fatty acids, or amino acids to form carbon dioxide and water. These reactions can be summarized by the following equations:

Anaerobic:

$$ATP \leftrightarrow ADP + P + free\ energy \tag{65.1}$$

$$CP + ADP \leftrightarrow creatine + ATP \tag{65.2}$$

$$glycogen\ or\ glucose + P + ADP \rightarrow lactate + ATP \tag{65.3}$$

Aerobic:

$$Glycogen\ or\ fatty\ acids + P + ADP + O_2 \rightarrow CO_2 + H_2O + ATP \tag{65.4}$$

All conditions:

$$2ADP \leftrightarrow ATP + AMP \tag{65.5}$$

The most intense levels of exercise occur anaerobically [Molé, 1983] and can be maintained for only a minute or two (Figure 65.1).

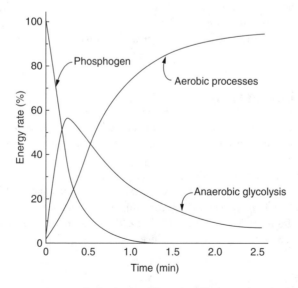

FIGURE 65.1   Muscle energy sources at the beginning of exercise. (Redrawn from Molé, 1983. In A.A. Bove and D.T. Lowenthal [Eds.], *Exercise Medicine*, pp. 43–88. New York, Academic Press. With permission.)

65.2 Cardiovascular Adjustments

Mechanoreceptors in the muscles, tendons, and joints send information to the CNS that the muscles have begun movement, and this information is used by the CNS to increase heart rate via the sympathetic autonomic nervous system. Cardiac output, the rate of blood pumped by the heart, is the product of heart rate and stroke volume (amount of blood pumped per heart beat). Heart rate increases nearly exponentially at the beginning of exercise with a time constant of about 30 s. Stroke volume does not change immediately but lags a bit until the cardiac output completes the loop back to the heart.

During rest a large volume of blood is stored in the veins, especially in the extremities. When exercise begins, this blood is transferred from the venous side of the heart to the arterial side. Attempting to push extra blood flow through the resistance of the arteries causes a rise in both systolic (during heart ventricular contraction) and diastolic (during the pause between contractions) blood pressures. The increased blood pressures are sensed by baroreceptors located in the aortic arch and carotid sinus (Figure 65.2).

As a consequence, small muscles encircling the entrance to the arterioles (small arteries) are caused to relax by the CNS. Since, by Poiseuille's Law:

$$R = \frac{8L\mu}{\pi r^4} \tag{65.6}$$

where

R = resistance of a tube, N·sec/m^5
L = length of the tube, m
μ = viscosity of the fluid, kg/(m·sec) or N·sec/m^2
r = radius of the tube lumen, m

increasing the arteriole radius by 19% will decrease its resistance to one-half. Thus, systolic pressure returns to its resting value, and diastolic pressure may actually fall. Increased blood pressures are called *afterload* on the heart.

To meet the oxygen demand of the muscles, blood is redistributed from tissues and organs not directly involved with exercise performance. Thus, blood flows to the gastrointestinal tract and kidneys are reduced, whereas blood flows to skeletal muscle, cardiac muscle, and skin are increased.

The heart is actually two pumping systems operated in series. The left heart pumps blood throughout the systemic blood vessels. The right heart pumps blood throughout the pulmonary system. Blood pressures in the systemic vessels are higher than blood pressures in the pulmonary system.

Two chambers comprise each heart. The atrium is like an assist device that produces some suction and collects blood from the veins. Its main purpose is to deliver blood to the ventricle, which is the more

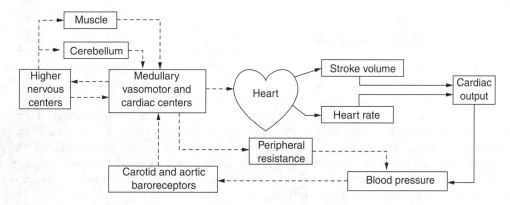

FIGURE 65.2   General scheme for blood pressure regulation. Dashed lines indicate neural communication, and solid lines indicate direct mechanical effect.

powerful chamber that develops blood pressure. The myocardium (heart muscle) of the left ventricle is larger and stronger than the myocardium of the right ventricle. With two hearts and four chambers in series, there could be a problem matching flow rates from each of them. If not properly matched, blood could easily accumulate downstream from the most powerful chamber and upstream from the weakest chamber.

Myocardial tissue exerts a more forceful contraction if it is stretched before contraction begins. This property (known as *Starling's law of the heart*) serves to equalize the flows between the two hearts by causing a more powerful ejection from the heart in which more blood accumulates during diastole. The amount of initial stretching of the cardiac muscle is known as *preload*.

65.3 Maximum Oxygen Uptake

The heart has been considered to be the limiting factor for delivery of oxygen to the tissues. As long as oxygen delivery is sufficient to meet demands of the working muscles, exercise is considered to be aerobic. If oxygen delivery is insufficient, anaerobic metabolism continues to supply muscular energy needs, but lactic acid accumulates in the blood. To remove lactic acid and reform glucose requires the presence of oxygen, which must usually be delayed until exercise ceases or exercise level is reduced.

Fitness of an individual is characterized is characterized by a mostly reproducible measurable quantity known as maximal oxygen uptake ($V_{O_{2max}}$) that indicates a person's capacity for aerobic energy transfer and the ability to sustain high-intensity exercise for longer than 4 or 5 min (Figure 65.3). The more fit, the higher is$V_{O_{2max}}$. Typical values are 2.5 l/min for young male nonathletes, 5.0 l/min for well-trained male athletes; women have $V_{O_{2max}}$ values about 70 to 80% as large as males. Maximal oxygen uptake declines with age steadily at 1% per year.

Exercise levels higher than those that result in $V_{O_{2max}}$ can be sustained for various lengths of time. The accumulated difference between the oxygen equivalent of work and $V_{O_{2max}}$ is called the **oxygen deficit** incurred by an individual (Figure 65.4). There is a maximum oxygen deficit that cannot be exceeded by an individual. Once this maximum deficit has been reached, the person must cease exercise.

The amount of oxygen used to repay the oxygen deficit is called the **excess postexercise oxygen consumption** (EPOC). EPOC is always larger than the oxygen deficit because (1) elevated body temperature immediately following exercise increases bodily metabolism in general, which requires more than resting levels of oxygen to service, (2) increased blood epinephrine levels increase general bodily metabolism, (3) increased respiratory and cardiac muscle activity requires oxygen, (4) refilling of body oxygen stores requires excess oxygen, and (5) there is some thermal inefficiency in replenishing muscle chemical stores. Considering only lactic acid oxygen debt, the total amount of oxygen required to return the body to its normal resting state is about twice the oxygen debt; the efficiency of anaerobic metabolism is about 50% of aerobic metabolism.

65.4 Respiratory Responses

Respiratory also increases when exercise begins, except that the time constant for respiratory response is about 45 sec instead of 30 sec for cardiac responses (Table 65.1). Control of respiration (Figure 65.5) appears to begin with chemoreceptors located in the aortic arch, in the carotid bodies (in the neck), and in the ventral medula (in the brain). These receptors are sensitive to oxygen, carbon dioxide, and acidity levels but are most sensitive to carbon dioxide and acidity. Thus, the function of the respiratory system appears to be remove excess carbon dioxide and, secondarily, to supply oxygen. Perhaps this is because excess CO_2 has narcotic effects, but insufficient oxygen does not produce severe reactions until oxygen levels in the inhaled air fall to one-half of normal. There is no well-established evidence that respiration limits oxygen delivery to the tissues in normal individuals.

Oxygen is conveyed by convection in the upper airways and by diffusion in the lower airways to the alveoli (lower reaches of the lung where gas exchange with the blood occurs). Oxygen must diffuse from

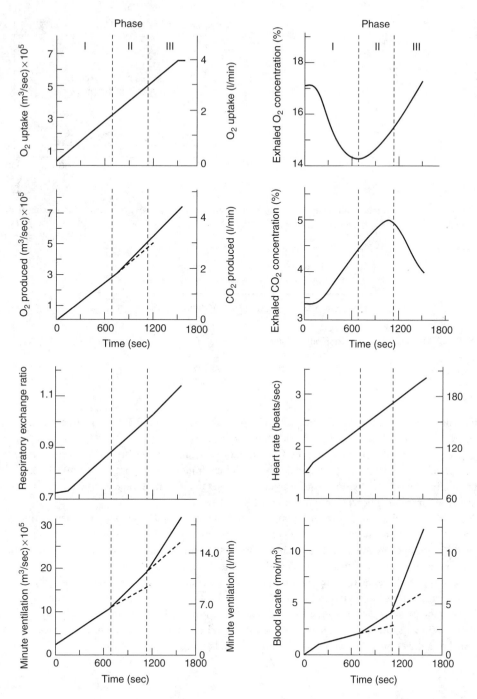

FIGURE 65.3 Concurrent typical changes in blood and respiratory parameters during exercise progressing from rest to maximum. (Adapted and redrawn from Skinner, J.S. and McLellan, T.H. 1980, by permission of the American Alliance for Health, Physical Education, Recreation and Dance.)

the alveoli, through the extremely thin alveolocapillary membrane into solution in the blood. Oxygen diffuses further into red blood cells where it is bound chemically to hemoglobin molecules. The order of each of these processes is reversed in the working muscles where the concentration gradient of oxygen is in the opposite direction. Complete equilibration of oxygen between alveolar air and pulmonary blood

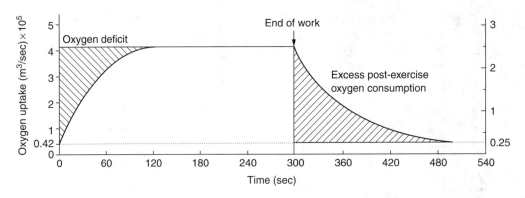

FIGURE 65.4 Oxygen uptake at the beginning of constant-load exercise increases gradually, accumulating an oxygen deficit that must be repaid at the end of exercise.

TABLE 65.1 Comparison of Response Time Constants for Three Major Systems of the Body

System	Dominant time constant, sec
Heart	30
Respiratory system	45
Oxygen uptake	49
Thermal system	3600

requires about 0.75 sec. Carbon dioxide requires somewhat less, about 0.50 sec. Thus, alveolar air more closely reflects levels of blood carbon dioxide than oxygen.

Both respiration rate and tidal volume (the amount of air moved per breath) increase with exercise, but above the anaerobic threshold the tidal volume no longer increases (remains at about 2 to 2.5 l). From that point, increases in ventilation require greater increases in respiration rate. A similar limitation occurs for stroke volume in the heart (limited to about 120 ml).

The work of respiration, representing only about 1 to 2% of the body's oxygen consumption at rest, increases to 8 to 10% or more of the body's oxygen consumption during exercise. Contributing greatly to this is the work to overcome resistance to movement of air, lung tissue, and chest wall tissue. Turbulent airflow in the upper airways (those nearest and including the mouth and nose) contributes a great deal of pressure drop. The lower airways are not as rigid as the upper airways and are influenced by the stretching and contraction of the lung surrounding them. High exhalation pressures external to the airways coupled with low static pressures inside (due to high flow rates inside) tend to close these airways somewhat and limit exhalation airflow rates. Resistance of these airways becomes very high, and the respiratory system appears like a flow source, but only during extreme exhalation.

65.5 Optimization

Energy demands during exercise are so great that optimal courses of action are followed for many physiological responses (Table 65.2). Walking occurs most naturally at a pace that represents the smallest energy expenditure; the transition from walking to running occurs when running expends less energy than walking; ejection of blood from the left ventricle appears to be optimized to minimize energy expenditure; respiratory rate, breathing waveforms, the ratio of inhalation time to exhalation time, airways resistance, tidal volume, and other respiratory parameters all appear to be regulated to minimize energy expenditure [Johnson, 1993].

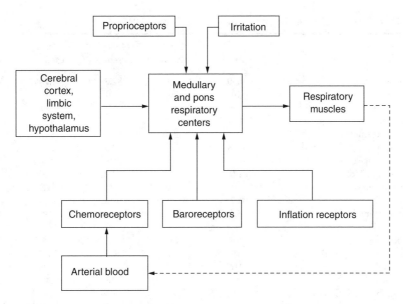

FIGURE 65.5   General scheme of respiratory control.

65.6   Thermal Response

When exercise extends for a long enough time, heat begins to build up in the body. In order for heat accumulation to become important, exercise must be performed at a relatively low rate. Otherwise, performance time would not be long enough for significant amounts of heat to be stored.

Muscular activities are at most 20–25% efficient, and, in general, the smaller the muscle, the less efficient it is. Heat results from the other 75–80% of the energy supplied to the muscle.

Thermal challenges are met in several ways. Blood sent to the limbs and blood returning from the limbs are normally conveyed by arteries and veins in close proximity deep inside the limb. This tends to conserve heat by countercurrent heat exchange between the arteries and veins. Thermal stress causes blood to return via surface veins rather than deep veins. Skin surface temperature increases and heat loss by convection and radiation also increases. In addition, vasodilation of cutaneous blood vessels augments surface heat loss but puts an additional burden on the heart to deliver added blood to the skin as well as the muscles. Heart rate increases as body temperature rises.

Sweating begins. Different areas of the body begin sweating earlier than others, but soon the whole body is involved. If sweat evaporation occurs on the skin surface, then the full cooling power of evaporating sweat (670 W·h/kg) is felt. If the sweat is absorbed by clothing, then the full benefit of sweat evaporation is not realized at the skin. If the sweat falls from the skin, no benefit accrues.

Sweating for a long time causes loss of plasma volume (plasma shift), resulting in some hemoconcentration (2% or more). This increased concentration increases blood viscosity, and cardiac work becomes greater.

65.7   Applications

Knowledge of exercise physiology imparts to the medical or biological engineer the ability to design devices to be used with or by humans or animals, or to borrow ideas from human physiology to apply to other situations. There is need for engineers to design the many pieces of equipment used by sports and health enthusiasts, to modify prostheses or devices for the handicapped to allow for performance of greater than light levels of work and exercise, to alleviate physiological stresses caused by personal protective equipment and other occupational ergonometric gear, to design human-powered machines

TABLE 65.2   Summary of Exercise Responses for a Normal Young Male

	Rest	Light exercise	Moderate exercise	Heavy exercise	Maximal exercise
Oxygen uptake (l/min)	0.30	0.60	2.2	3.0	3.2
Maximal oxygen uptake (%)	10	20	70	95	100
Physical work rate (W)	0	10	140	240	430
Aerobic fraction (%)	100	100	98	85	50
Performance time (min)	α	480	55	9.3	3.0
Carbon dioxide production (l/min)	0.18	1.5	2.3	2.8	3.7
Respiratory exchange ratio	0.72	0.84	0.94	1.0	1.1
Blood lactic acid (mMol/l)	1.0	1.8	4.0	7.2	9.6
Heart rate (beats/min)	70	130	160	175	200
Stroke volume (l)	0.075	0.100	0.105	0.110	0.110
Cardiac output (l/min)	5.2	13	17	19	22
Minute volume (l/min)	6	22	50	80	120
Tidal volume (l)	0.4	1.6	2.3	2.4	2.4
Respiration rate (breaths/min)	15	26	28	57	60
Peak flow (l/min)	216	340	450	480	480
Muscular efficiency (%)	0	5	18	20	20
Aortic hemoglobin saturation (%)	98	97	94	93	92
Inhalation time (sec)	1.5	1.25	1.0	0.7	0.5
Exhalation time (sec)	3.0	2.0	1.1	0.75	0.5
Respiratory work rate (W)	0.305	0.705	5.45	12.32	20.03
Cardiac work rate (W)	1.89	4.67	9.61	11.81	14.30
Systolic pressure (mmHg)	120	134	140	162	172
Diastolic pressure (mmHg)	80	85	90	95	100
End-inspiratory lung volume (l)	2.8	3.2	4.6	4.6	4.6
End-expiratory lung volume (l)	2.4	2.2	2.1	2.1	2.1
Gas partial pressures (mmHg)					
Arterial pCO_2	40	41	45	48	50
pO_2	100	98	94	93	92
Venous pCO_2	44	57	64	70	72
pO_2	36	23	17	10	9
Alveolar pCO_2	32	40	28	20	10
pO_2	98	94	110	115	120
Skin conductance [watts/($m^2 \cdot °C$)]	5.3	7.9	12	13	13
Sweat rate (kg/sec)	0.001	0.002	0.008	0.007	0.002
Walking/running speed (m/sec)	0	1.0	2.2	6.7	7.1
Ventilation/perfusion of the lung	0.52	0.50	0.54	0.82	1.1
Respiratory evaporative water loss (l/min)	1.02×10^{-5}	4.41×10^{-5}	9.01×10^{-4}	1.35×10^{-3}	2.14×10^{-3}
Total body convective heat loss (W)	24	131	142	149	151
Mean skin temperature (°C)	34	32	30.5	29	28
Heat production (W)	105	190	640	960	1720
Equilibrium rectal temperature (°C)	36.7	38.5	39.3	39.7	500
Final rectal temperature (°C)	37.1	38.26	39.3	37.4	37

that are compatible with the capabilities of the operators, and to invent systems to establish and maintain locally benign surroundings in otherwise harsh environments. Recipients of these efforts include athletes, the handicapped, laborers, firefighters, space explorers, military personnel, farmers, power-plant workers, and many others. The study of exercise physiology, especially in the language used by medical and biological engineers, can result in benefits to almost all of us.

Defining Terms

Anaerobic threshold: The transition between exercise levels that can be sustained through nearly complete aerobic metabolism and those that rely on at least partially anaerobic metabolism. Above the anaerobic threshold, blood lactate increases and the relationship between ventilation and oxygen uptake becomes nonlinear.

Excess postexercise oxygen consumption (EPOC): The difference between resting oxygen consumption and the accumulated rate of oxygen consumption following exercise termination.

Maximum oxygen consumption: The maximum rate of oxygen use during exercise. The amount of maximum oxygen consumption is determined by age, sex, and physical condition.

Oxygen deficit: The accumulated difference between actual oxygen consumption at the beginning of exercise and the rate of oxygen consumption that would exist if oxygen consumption rose immediately to its steady-state level corresponding to exercise level.

References

Johnson, A.T. 1993. How much work is expended for respiration? *Front. Med. Biol. Eng.* 5: 265.

Molé, P.A. 1983. Exercise metabolism. In A.A. Bove and D.T. Lowenthal (Eds.), *Exercise Medicine*, pp. 43–88. New York, Academic Press.

Skinner, J.S. and McLellan, T.H. 1980. The transition from aerobic to anaerobic metabolism. *Res. Q. Exerc. Sport* 51: 234.

White, A., Handler, P., Smith, E.L. et al. 1959. *Principles of Biochemistry.* New York, McGraw-Hill.

Further Information

A comprehensive treatment of quantitative predictions in exercise physiology is presented in *Biomechanics and Exercise Physiology* by Arthur T. Johnson (John Wiley & Sons, 1991). There are a number of errors in the book, but an errata sheet is available from the author.

P.O. Astrand and K. Rodahl's *Textbook of Work Physiology* (McGraw-Hill, 1970) contains a great deal of exercise physiology and is probably considered to be the standard textbook on the subject.

Biological Foundations of Biomedical Engineering, edited by J. Kline (Little Brown, Boston), is a very good textbook of physiology written for engineers.

66

Factors Affecting Mechanical Work in Humans

Ben F. Hurley
Arthur T. Johnson
University of Maryland

High technology has entered our diversions and leisure activities. Sports, exercise, and training are no longer just physical activities but include machines and techniques attuned to individual capabilities and needs. This chapter considers several factors related to exercise and training that help in understanding human performance.

Physiological work performance is determined by energy transformation that begins with the process of photosynthesis and ends with the production of biological work (Figure 66.1). Energy in the form of nuclear transformations is converted to radiant energy, which then transforms the energy from carbon dioxide and water into oxygen and glucose through photosynthesis. In plants, the glucose can also be converted to fats and proteins. Upon ingesting plants or other animals that eat plants, humans convert this energy through cellular respiration (the reverse of photosynthesis) to chemical energy in the form of adenosine triphosphate (ATP). The endergonic reactions (energy absorbed from the surroundings) that produce ATP are followed by exergonic reactions (energy released to surroundings) that release energy through the breakdown of ATP to produce chemical and mechanical work in the human body. The steps involved in the synthesis and breakdown of carbohydrates, fats, and proteins produce chemical work and provide energy for the mechanical work produced from muscular contractions. The purpose of this chapter is to provide a brief summary of some factors that can affect mechanical work in humans.

66.1 Exercise Biomechanics

66.1.1 Equilibrium

Anybody, including the human body, remains in stable equilibrium if the vectorial sum of all forces and torques acting on the body is zero. An unbalanced force results in linear acceleration, and an unbalanced

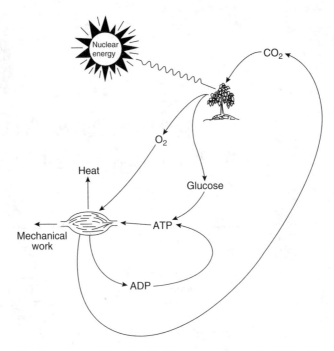

FIGURE 66.1   Schematic of energy transformations leading to muscular mechanical work.

TABLE 66.1   Fraction of Body Weights for Various Parts of the Body

Body part	Fraction
Head and neck	0.07
Trunk	0.43
Upper arms	0.07
Forearms and hands	0.06
Thighs	0.23
Lower legs and feet	0.14
	1.00

torque results in rotational acceleration. Static equilibrium requires that:

$$\sum F = 0 \qquad (66.1)$$

$$\sum T = 0 \qquad (66.2)$$

where F is vectorial forces, N, and T is vectorial torques, N m.

Some sport activities, such as wrestling, weight lifting, and fencing, require stability, whereas other activities, including running, jumping, and diving, cannot be performed unless there is managed instability. Shifting body position allows for proper control. The mass of the body is distributed as in Table 66.1, and the center of mass is located at approximately 56% of a person's height and midway from side-to-side and front-to-back. The center of mass can be made to shift by extending the limbs or by bending the torso.

66.1.2 Muscular Movement

Mechanical movement results from contraction of muscles that are attached at each end to bones that can move relative to each other. The arrangement of this combination is commonly known as a class 3

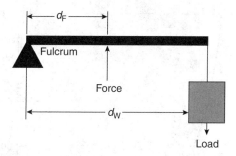

FIGURE 66.2   A class 3 lever is arranged with the applied force interposed between the fulcrum and the load. Most skeletal muscles are arranged in this fashion.

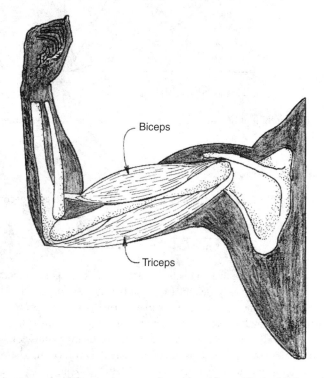

FIGURE 66.3   The biceps muscle of the arm is arranged as a class 3 lever. The load is located at the hand and the fulcrum at the elbow.

lever (Figure 66.2), where one joint acts as the fulcrum (Figure 66.3), the other bone acts as the load, and the muscle provides the force interposed between fulcrum and load. This arrangement requires that the muscle force be greater than the load, sometimes by a very large amount, but the distance through which the muscle moves is made very small. These characteristics match muscle capabilities well (muscles can produce 7×10^5 N/m^2, but cannot move far). Since the distance is made smaller, the speed of shortening of the contracting muscle is also slower than it would be if the arrangement between the force and the load were different:

$$\frac{S_L}{S_M} = \frac{d_L}{d_M}$$ (66.3)

where S is speed, m/sec; d is distance from fulcrum, m; and L, M denotes load and muscle.

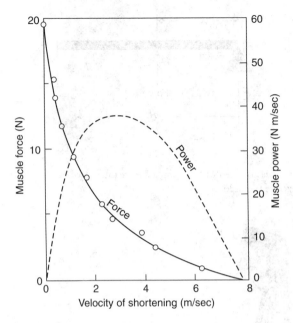

FIGURE 66.4   Force and power output of a muscle as a function of velocity. (Adapted and used with permission from Milsum, 1966.)

66.1.3 Muscular Efficiency

Efficiency relates external, or physical, work produced to the total chemical energy consumed:

$$\eta = \frac{\text{External work produced}}{\text{Chemical energy consumed}} \tag{66.4}$$

Muscular efficiencies range from close to zero to about 20 to 25%. The larger numbers would be obtained for leg exercises that involve lifting body weight. In carpentry and foundry work, where both arms and legs are used, average mechanical efficiency is approximately 10% [Johnson, 1991]. For finer movements that require exquisite control, small muscles are often arranged in antagonistic fashion, that is, the final movement is produced as a result of the difference between two or more muscles working against each other. In this case, efficiencies approach zero. Isometric muscular contraction, where a force is produced but no movement results, has an efficiency of zero [Johnson et al. 2002].

Muscles generally are able to exert the greatest force when the velocity of muscle contraction is zero. Power produced by this muscle would be zero. When the velocity of muscle contraction is about 8 m/sec the force produced by the muscle becomes zero, and the power produced by this muscle again becomes zero. Somewhere in between the above conditions stated, the power produced and the efficiency become the maximum (Figure 66.4).

The isometric length–tension relationship of a muscle shows that the maximum force developed by a muscle is exerted at its resting length (the length of a slightly stretched muscle attached by its tendons to the skeleton) and decreases to zero at twice its resting length. Maximum force also decreases to zero at the shortest possible muscular length. Since muscular contractile force depends on the length of the muscle and length changes during contraction, muscular efficiency is always changing (Figure 66.5).

Negative (eccentric) work is produced by a muscle when it maintains a force against an external force tending to stretch the muscle. An example of negative work is found as the action of the leg muscle during a descent of a flight of stairs. Since the body is being lowered, external work is less than zero. The muscles are using physiological energy to control the descent and prevent the body from accumulating kinetic energy as it descends.

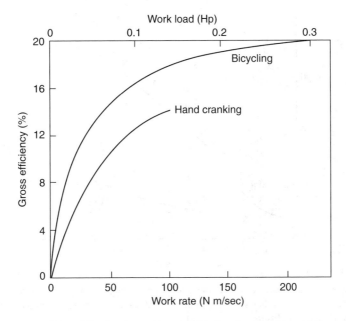

FIGURE 66.5 The gross efficiency for hand cranking or bicycling is a function of the rate of work. (From Goldman, R.F., 1978. Computer models in manual materials handling. In Drury, C.G. (Ed.), *Safety in Manual Materials Handling*, National Institute for Occupational Safety and Health (NIOSH), Cincinnati, Ohio, pp. 110–116.)

Muscular efficiencies for walking downhill approach 120% [McMahon, 1984]. Since heat produced by the muscle is the difference between 100% and the percent efficiency, heat produced by muscles walking downhill is about 220% of their energy expenditure. Energy expenditure of muscles undergoing negative work is about one-sixth that of a muscle doing positive work [Johnson, 1991], so a leg muscle going uphill produces about twice as much heat as a leg muscle going downhill.

66.1.4 Locomotion

The act of locomotion involves both positive and negative work. There are four successive stages of a walking stride. In the first stage, both feet are on the ground, with one foot ahead of the other. The trailing foot pushes forward, and the front foot is pushing backward. In the second stage, the trailing foot leaves the ground and the front foot applies a braking force. The center of mass of the body begins to lift over the front foot. In the third stage, the trailing foot is brought forward and the supporting foot applies a vertical force. The body center of mass is at its highest point above the supporting foot. In the last stage, the body's center of mass is lowered and the trailing foot provides an acceleration force.

This alteration of the raising and lowering of the body center of mass, along with the pushing and braking provided by the feet, makes walking a low-efficiency maneuver. Walking has been likened to alternatively applying the brakes and accelerator while driving a car. Just as the fuel efficiency of the car would suffer from this mode of propulsion, so the energy efficiency of walking suffers from the way walking is performed.

There is an optimum speed of walking. Faster than this speed, additional muscular energy is required to propel the body forward. Moving slower than the optimal speed requires additional muscular energy to retard leg movement. Thus, the optimal speed is related to the rate at which the leg can swing forward. Simple analysis of the leg as a physical pendulum shows that the optimal walking speed is related to leg length:

$$S \propto \sqrt{L} \qquad\qquad (66.5)$$

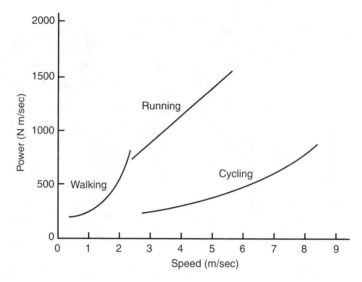

FIGURE 66.6 Power required for walking, running, and cycling by an adult male. Curves for walking and running interact at about 2.3 m/sec and show that walking is more efficient below the intersection and running is more efficient above. (Redrawn with permission from Alexander, 1984.)

Unlike walking, there is a stage of running during which both feet leave the ground. The center of mass of the body does not rise and fall as much during running as during walking, so the efficiency for running can be greater than for walking.

At a speed of about 2.5 m/sec, running appears to be more energy efficient than walking, and the transition is usually made between these forms of locomotion (Figure 66.6). Unlike walking, there does not appear to be a functional relationship between speed and leg length, so running power expenditure is linearly related to speed alone.

Why would anyone want to propel the extra weight of a bicycle in addition to body weight? On the surface it would appear that cycling would cost more energy than running or walking. However, the center of mass of the body does not move vertically as long as the cyclist sits on the seat. Without the positive and negative work associated with walking or running, cycling is a much more efficient form of locomotion than the other two (Figure 66.6), and the cost of moving the additional weight of the bicycle can easily be supplied.

Many sports or leisure activities have a biomechanical basis. Understanding of the underlying biomechanical processes can lead to improved performance. Yet, there are limits to performance that cause frustrations for competitive athletes. Hence, additional factors are sometimes employed to expand these limits. A brief discussion of some of these factors is given here.

66.1.5 Effects of Age

It is well established that the maximal capacity to exercise declines with age. However, many factors that change with age also affect maximal capacity to exercise. Examples of these factors include a gain in body fat, a decrease in lean body mass, onset of disease, and a decline in the level of physical activity. For this reason, it is difficult to determine exactly how much of the loss in capacity to exercise with age can really be attributed solely to the effects of aging. Nevertheless, the decline in cardiovascular or aerobic capacity with advanced aging is substantial. Aerobic capacity is assessed by measuring the maximal amount of oxygen that can be utilized during exercise and is known as V_{O_2max}. Pollock et al. [1997] reported more than a 30% decline in V_{O_2max} per decade of aging in a 20-year longitudinal study in those who did not maintain high levels of physical activity as they aged. This age-related decline was reduced substantially ($\sim$5 to 8% per decade) when exercise training was maintained throughout aging. Thus, there is no doubt that maximal work capacity declines with advancing age. Although regular exercise (training) appears to reduce this decline substantially, it cannot completely prevent the detrimental effects of age on aerobic capacity.

Muscular strength (maximal force production) is maintained for a much longer time period throughout aging. Knee extensor strength, for example, does not become significantly reduced in men until they reach their 60s [Lynch et al., 1999]. These losses then occur at a rate of ~12 to 14% per decade. Loss of muscle mass occurs at a rate of ~6% per decade [Lynch et al., 1999]. There is some uncertainty about the magnitude of muscle power (product of force and velocity) loss with age [Martin et al., 2000], but it is believed to occur at a faster rate than strength [Skeleton et al., 1994]. There is also a loss of ~8% per decade in force per unit of muscle mass (muscle quality) [Lynch et al., 1999], indicating that the loss of strength is more than can be accounted for by strength alone.

66.1.6 Effects of Exercise Training

For the purpose of this review, exercise training will be divided into two training modalities, aerobic exercise training and strength training. Aerobic exercise training consists of regular muscular activities that use large amounts of oxygen to produce energy and include exercises such as walking, jogging, swimming, and cycling. Strength training (ST) refers to the type of regular muscular activity that cause muscles to contract (e.g., isotonic or so-called concentric exercise) or attempt to contract (e.g., isometric or eccentric exercise) against resistance. Hence, this type of training is often called resistance or resistive training and it can be performed with weight plates, machines, or by just using one's body weight for resistance, such as is done with certain kinds of calisthenics.

66.1.6.1 Aerobic Exercise Training

Many compensatory reactions allow the body to adapt to minor stresses, such as mild aerobic exercise, so that homeostasis (equilibrium) can be maintained. For example, the increased energy demands of aerobic exercise stimulate an increase in heart rate, respiration, blood flow, and many other cardiovascular and metabolic reactions that allow the body to maintain homeostasis. As the intensity of exercise increases it becomes more difficult for compensatory mechanisms to maintain homeostasis. After exceeding about 80% of an untrained person's maximal exercise capacity homeostasis can no longer be maintained for more than a few minutes before exhaustion results.

Regular aerobic exercise (training) elevates the threshold level so that a single exercise session can be performed before disturbing and eventually losing homeostasis. It does this by elevating the maximal physiological capacity for homeostasis so that the same intensity of aerobic exercise may no longer disrupt homeostasis because it is a lower percentage of maximal capacity. In addition, training produces specific adaptations during submaximal exercise that permit greater and longer amounts of work before losing homeostasis [Hurley and Hagberg, 1998]. A good example of this is when blood lactate rises with increased intensity of exercise. Prior to training, blood lactate concentration rises substantially when the intensity of exercise exceeds about 75% of maximal oxygen consumption (V_{O_2max}).

Following training, the same intensity of exercise results in a lower concentration of blood lactate, so exercise can now be performed at a higher fraction of the untrained V_{O_2max} before blood lactate reaches the same level as before training. This adaptation is so profound that blood lactate levels are often only slightly above resting values after training when performing submaximal exercise (e.g., <65% of V_{O_2max}). Thus, exercise training allows an individual to perform a much greater amount of work during exercise before homeostasis is disturbed to the point at which muscular exhaustion results.

66.1.6.2 Strength Training

Muscular strength declines with age [Lindle et al., 1997; Lynch et al., 1999; Roth et al., 2001], disease [Singh, 2002], and as a consequence of the administration of some medications [Singh, 2002] and can be increased substantially in a relatively short time period with ST [Hurley and Roth, 2000; Hurley and Kostek, 2001]. Muscle power can also be increased with ST, but the magnitude of increase depends on the movement velocity of training during the muscle-shortening phase of exercise. Typical training modalities of ~2 sec during the shortening phase and ~4 sec during the muscle-lengthening phase of movement result in ~30% increase in strength [Lemmer et al., 2000] and ~25% increase in power [Jozsi et al., 1999]. However, increases of almost 100% have been reported when fast-velocity training has been incorporated [Fielding et al., 2002]. Our group has reported increases in muscle mass of ~12% with ST, within the first couple of months of training, based on measurements made by magnetic resonance imaging of the entire volume of the muscle being trained [Ivey et al., 2000]. The amount of force per unit of muscle volume also increases substantially with ST [Tracey et al., 1999]. We have shown that ~3 decades of age-related strength loss and two decades of age-related muscle mass loss can be recovered/reversed within the first couple of months of ST [Ivey et al., 2000; Lemmer et al., 2000].

66.1.7 Effects of Gender

Cardiovascular fitness and muscular strength are substantially higher in men compared to women. The aerobic capacity in men is about 40 to 50% higher than women. In addition, upper body strength is ~100% higher and lower body strength is ~50% higher in men [Lynch et al., 1999]. However, these differences are diminished substantially when body composition is taken into consideration. For example, when V_{O_2max} is expressed with reference to body mass (ml/kg of body weight/min) this difference narrows to ~20% and to ~10% when differences in muscle mass are taken into consideration. Differences in muscular strength between men and women are also narrowed when normalized for fat free mass [Lynch et al., 1999]. There does not appear to be any significant difference in responses to training between men and women when expressed on a relative basis (% change), but men appear to have greater muscle mass gains than women in response to ST when expressed in absolute terms [Ivey et al., 2000].

66.1.8 Effects of Genetics

We have observed great inter-individual variability in both the loss of muscle strength and mass with age, known as sarcopenia [Lindle et al., 1997; Lynch et al., 1999], as well as the gain in muscle strength and muscle mass with exercise training [Ivey et al., 2000; Lemmer et al., 2000]. For example, in a large number of ST studies performed in our laboratory, the increases in strength for individual subjects range from <5 to >100% and muscle mass changes range from no appreciable change to >25% increase. These ST-induced changes in strength and muscle mass are also highly variable in both young and older men and women. In this context, after only nine weeks of a highly standardized quadriceps ST program in a healthy and homogeneous group of young (20–30 yrs) and older (65–75 yrs) men and women, knee extension strength gains ranged from 9 to 45 kg in the young group and from 2 to 39 kg in the older group [Ivey et al., 2000]. These strength changes amounted to a 10–51% increase in the young group and a 5–59% increase in the older group. In this same study, the increases in MRI measured quadriceps muscle volume ranged from 19 to 344 cm^3 in the older subjects and 60 to 481 cm^3 in the young subjects. On a relative basis these increases ranged from <1 to 20% of the initial muscle volume of these subjects, further demonstrating the wide range of inter-individual changes in the trained muscle mass resulting from this highly standardized, short-term ST intervention. Others have observed similar large variations in strength and muscle mass changes with training [Buchner et al., 1993]. Collectively, these data strongly support the notion that genetic factors are involved in determining muscle strength and muscle mass responses to strength training.

The hypothesis that genetic factors may influence muscular strength is also supported by data from both animals [Biesiadecki et al., 1998] and humans [Reed et al., 1991]. Biesiadecki et al. [1998] observed a 1.5–5.2 fold divergence between the muscular strength of male rat strains with the lowest- and highest-strength levels, and Reed et al. [1991] observed significant genetic effects for absolute grip strength normalized for body weight in 127 identical and 130 fraternal twin pairs. Heredity accounted for 65% of the variance in grip strength, even after adjusting for the effects of weight, height, and age. Furthermore, Seeman et al. [1996] reported that genetic factors accounted for 60–80% of the inter-individual differences in lean body mass. More recently, Huygens et al. [2004] reported heritability of skeletal muscle mass of up to 90%. In addition, Thomis et al. [1998] found evidence for a significant role of heredity in strength responses to strength training. These responses were independent of the influence of genetic factors on baseline strength values. These data provide strong support that genetic factors may influence sarcopenia (i.e., alterations in strength and muscle mass with age) and strength and muscle mass response to strength training. However, none of these studies assessed the effects of specific candidate genes or candidate gene variations (polymorphisms) on strength or muscle mass response to training.

The heritability of muscle mass and strength indicate that specific genes contribute to differences in muscle phenotype. More importantly, specific polymorphisms could at least partly explain the inter-individual variability in sarcopenia and muscle response to ST. We recently explored the relationship of gene polymorphisms to muscle phenotypes in genes thought to have a plausible physiological connection to changes in strength and muscle mass. We identified several candidate gene polymorphisms that were associated with changes in strength or muscle mass with either age or ST. These included genes that code for ciliary neurotrophic factor, insulin-like growth factors I and II, growth and differentiation factor 8 (myostatin), Vitamin D, and androgen receptors. At the time of this writing, studies are ongoing to assess the role of these genes in determining the extent to which strength and muscle mass respond to aging and ST. Based on the substantial heritability of muscle phenotype, future research will likely find other gene variants that help explain the inter-individual variability in both sarcopenia and muscle adaptation in response to both aerobic and strength training. This information is likely to provide a basis for individualizing exercise prescriptions for the prevention and treatment of sarcopenia and help explain why some people make substantial adaptations to training, whereas others do not. Moreover, it will provide specific explanations from a mechanistic perspective as to how genetics can influence mechanical and biological work in humans.

References

Alexander, R.M. Walking and running. *Am. Sci.* 72: 348, 1984.

Biesiadecki, B.J., Brand, P.H., Metting, P.J., Koch, L.G., and Britton, S.L. Phenotypic variation in strength among eleven inbred strains of rats. *Proc. Soc. Exp. Biol. Med.* 219: 126–131, 1998.

Buchner, D.M., Cress, M.E., de Lateur, B.J., and Wagner, E.H. Variability in the effect of strength training on skeletal muscle strength in older adults. *J. Gerontol.* 7: 143–153, 1993.

Fiatarone-Singh, M.A. Exercise comes of age: rationale and recommendations for a geriatric exercise prescription. *J. Gerontol.: Med. Sci.* 57A: M262–M282, 2002.

Fielding, R.A., LeBrasseur, N.K., Cuoco, A., Bean, J., Mizer, K., and Fiatarone-Singh, M.A. High-velocity resistance training increases skeletal muscle peak power in older women. *J. Am. Geriatr. Soc.* 50: 655–662, 2002.

Goldman, R.F. Computer models in manual materials handling. In Drury, C.G. (Ed.), *Safety in Manual Materials Handling*, National Institute for Occupational Safety and Health (NIOSH), Cincinnati, OH, 110–116, 1978.

Hurley, B.F. and Hagberg, J.M. Optimizing health in older persons: aerobic or strength training? In *Exercise and Sport Sciences Reviews*, Vol. 26, Williams & Wilkins, Baltimore, MD, pp. 61–89, 1998.

Hurley, B.F. and Kostek, M.C. Exercise interventions for seniors. What training modality is best for health? *Orthop. Phys. Ther. Clin. N. Am.* 10: 213–225, 2001.

Hurley, B.F. and Roth, S.M. Strength training in the elderly: effects on risk factors for age-related diseases. *Sports Med.* 30: 249–268, 2000.

Huygens, W., Thomis, M.A., Peeters, M.W., Vlietinck, R.F., and Beunen, G.P. Determinants and upper-limit heritabilities of skeletal muscle mass and strength. *Can. J. Appl. Physiol.* 29: 186–200, 2004.

Ivey, F.M., Tracy, B.L., Lemmer, J.T., Hurlbut, D.E., Martel, G.F., Roth, S.M., Fozard, J.L., Metter, E.J., and Hurley, B.F. The effects of age, gender and myostatin genotype on the hypertrophic response to heavy resistance strength training. *J. Gerontol.: Med. Sci.* 55A: M641–M648, 2000.

Johnson, A.T. *Biomechanics and Exercise Physiology*, John Wiley, New York, 1991.

Johnson, A.T., Benjamin, M.B., and Silverman, N. Oxygen consumption, heat production, and muscular efficiency during uphill and downhill walking. *Appl. Ergon.*, 33: 485–491, 2002.

Jozsi, A.C., Campbell, W.W., Joseph, L., Davey, S.L., and Evans, W.J. Changes in power with resistance training in older and younger men and women. *J. Gerontol.* 54A: M591–M596, 1999.

Lemmer, J.T., Hurbut, D.E., Martel, G.F., Tracy, B.L., Ivey, F.M., Metter, E.J., Fozard, J.L., Fleg, J.L., and Hurley, B.F. Age and gender responses to strength training and detraining. *Med. Sci. Sports Exer.* 32: 1505–1512, 2000.

Lindle, R., Metter, E., Lynch, N., Fleg, J., Fozard, J., Tobin, J., Roy, T., and Hurley, B. Age and gender comparisons of muscle strength in 654 women and men aged 20–93. *J. Appl. Physiol.* 83: 1581–1587, 1997.

Lynch, N.A., Metter, E.J., Lindle, R.S., Fozard, J.L., Tobin, J.D., Roy, T.A., Fleg, J.L., and Hurley, B.F. Muscle quality I: age-associated differences in arm vs. leg muscle groups. *J. Appl. Physiol.* 86: 188–194, 1999.

Martin, J.C., Farrar, R.P., Wagner, B.M., and Spinduso, W.W. Maximal power across the lifespan. *J. Gerontol.: Med. Sci.* 55A: M311–M316, 2000.

McMahon, T.A. *Muscles, Reflexes, and Locomotion*, Princeton University Press, Princeton, NJ, 1984.

Milsum, J.H. *Biological Control Systems Analysis*, McGraw-Hill, New York, 1966.

Pollock, M.L., Mengelkoch, L.F., Graves, J.S., Lowenthal, D.T., Limacher, M.C., Foster, C., and Wilmore, J.H. Twenty year follow-up of aerobic power and body composition of older track athletes. *J. Appl. Physiol.* 82: 1508–1516, 1997.

Reed, T., Babsitz, R., Selby, J., and Carmelli, D. Genetic influences and grip strength norms in the NHLBI twin study males aged 50–69. *Ann. Hum. Biol.* 18: 425–432, 1991.

Roth, S.M., Schrager, M.A., Ferrell, R.E., Reichman, Metter, S.E., Lynch, N.A., Lindle, R.S., and Hurley, B.F. Ciliary neurotrophic factor genotype is associated with muscular strength and quality in humans across the adult age span. *J. Appl. Physiol.* 90: 1205–1210, 2001.

Seeman, E., Hopper, J., Young, N., Formica, C., Goss, P., and Tsalamandris, C. Do genetic factors explain associations between muscle strength, lean mass, and bone density? A twin study. *Am. J. Physiol.* 270: E320–E327, 1996.

Skeleton, D.A., Greig, C.A., Davies, J.M., and Young, A. Power and related functional ability of healthy people aged 65–89 years. *Age Aging* 23: 371–377, 1994.

Thomis, M.A., Beunen, G.P., Maes, H.H., Blimkie, C.J., Leemputte, M.V., Claessens, A.L., Marchal, G., Willems, E., and Vlietinck, R.F. Strength training: importance of genetic factors. *Med. Sci. Sports Exer.* 30: 724–731, 1998.

Tracy, B.L., Ivey, F.M., Hurlbut, D., Martel, G.F., Lemmer, J.T., Siegel, E.L., Metter, E.J., Fozard, J.L., Fleg, J.L., and Hurley, B.F. Muscle quality II: effects of strength training in 65–75 year old men and women. *J. Appl. Physiol.* 86: 195–201, 1999.

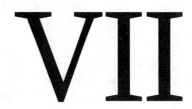

VII

Rehabilitation Engineering

Charles J. Robinson
Clarkson University and the Syracuse VA Medical Center

E NGINEERING ADVANCES HAVE RESULTED in enormous strides in the field of rehabilitation. Individuals with reduced or no vision can be given "sight"; those with severe or complete hearing loss can "hear" by being provided with a sense of their surroundings; those unable to talk can be aided to "speak" again; and those without full control of a limb (or with the limb missing) can, by artificial means, "walk" or regain other movement functions. But the present level of available functional restoration for seeing, hearing, speaking, and moving still pales in comparison to the capabilities of individuals without disability. As is readily apparent from the content of many of the chapters in this handbook, the human sensory and motor (movement) systems are marvelously engineered, both within a given system and integrated across systems. The rehabilitation engineer thus faces a daunting task in trying to design augmentative or replacement systems when one or more of these systems is impaired.

Rehabilitation engineering had its origins in the need to provide assistance to individuals who were injured in World War II. Rehabilitation engineering can be defined in a number of ways. Perhaps the most encompassing (and the one adopted here) is that proposed by Reswick [1982] — Rehabilitation engineering is the application of science and technology to ameliorate the handicaps of individuals with disabilities. With this definition, any device, technique, or concept used in rehabilitation that has a technological basis falls under the purview of rehabilitation engineering. This contrasts with the much narrower view that is held by some that rehabilitation engineering is only the design and production phase of a broader field called Assistive Technology. Lest one consider this distinction trivial, consider that the U.S. Congress has mandated that rehabilitation engineering and technology services be provided by all states; and an argument has ensued among various groups of practitioners about who can legally provide such services because of the various interpretations of what rehabilitation engineering is.

There is a core body of knowledge that defines each of the traditional engineering disciplines. Biomedical engineering is less precisely defined; but, in general, a biomedical engineer must be proficient in a traditional engineering discipline and have a working knowledge of things biological or medical. The rehabilitation engineer is a biomedical engineer who must not only be technically proficient as an engineer and know biology and medicine, but must also integrate artistic, social, financial, psychological, and physiological considerations to develop or analyze a device, technique, or concept that meets the needs of the population the engineer is serving. In general, rehabilitation engineers deal with musculo-skeletal or sensory disabilities. They often have a strong background in biomechanics. Most work in a multidisciplinary team setting.

Rehabilitation engineering deals with many aspects of rehabilitation including applied, scientific, clinical, technical, and theoretical. Various topics include, but are not limited to, assistive devices and other aids for those with disability, sensory augmentation and substitution systems, functional electrical stimulation (for motor control and sensory-neural prostheses), orthotics and prosthetics, myoelectric devices and techniques, transducers (including electrodes), signal processing, hardware, software, robotics, systems approaches, technology assessment, postural stability, wheelchair seating systems, gait analysis, biomechanics, biomaterials, control systems (both biological and external), ergonomics, human performance, and functional assessment [Robinson, 1993].

In this section of the handbook, we focus only on applications of rehabilitation engineering. The concepts of rehabilitation engineering, rehabilitation science, and rehabilitation technology are outlined in Chapter 67. Chapter 69 discusses the importance of personal mobility and various wheeled modes of transportation (wheelchairs, scooters, cars, vans, and public conveyances). Chapter 70 looks at other non-wheeled ways to enhance mobility and physical performance. Chapter 71 covers techniques available to augment sensory impairments or to provide a substitute to input sensory information. Conversely, Chapter 72 looks at the output side.

For the purposes of this handbook, many topics that partially fall under the rubric of rehabilitation engineering are covered elsewhere. These include chapters on Electrical Stimulation (Durand), Hard

Tissue Replacement — Long-Bone Repair and Joints (Goel), Biomechanics (Schneck), Musculoskeletal Soft Tissue Mechanics (Lieber), Analysis of Gait (Davis), Sports Biomechanics/Kinesiology (Johnson), Biodynamics (Diggs), Cochlear Mechanics (Steele), Measurement of Neuromuscular Performance Capabilities (Smith), Human Factors Applications in Rehabilitation Engineering (Strauss and Gunderson), Electrical Stimulators (Peckham), Prostheses and Artificial Organs (Galletti), Nerve Guidance Channels (Valentini), and Tracheal, Laryngeal, and Esophageal Replacement Devices (Shimizu).

Rehabilitation engineering can be described as an engineering systems discipline. Imagine being the design engineer on a project that has an unknown, highly nonlinear plant, with coefficients whose variations in time appear to follow no known or solvable model, where time (yours and your client's) and funding are severely limited, where no known solution has been developed (or if it has, will need modification for nearly every client so no economy of scale exists). Further, there will be severe impedance mismatches between available appliances and your client's needs. Or, the low residual channel capacity of one of your client's senses will require enormous signal compression to get a signal with any appreciable information content through it. Welcome to the world of the rehabilitation engineer!!

References

Reswick, J. 1982. What is a rehabilitation engineer?, in *Annual Review of Rehabilitation*, Vol. 2, E.L. Pan, T.E. Backer, and C.L. Vash, Eds., Springer-Verlag, New York.

Robinson, C.J., 1993. Rehabilitation engineering — an editorial, *IEEE Trans. Rehab. Eng.*, 1: 1–2.

67

Rehabilitation Engineering, Science, and Technology

Charles J. Robinson
Clarkson University and the
Syracuse VA Medical Center

67.1   Introduction

Rehabilitation engineering requires a multidisciplinary effort. To put rehabilitation engineering into its proper context, we need to review some of the other disciplines with which rehabilitation engineers must be familiar. Robinson [1993] has reviewed or put forth the following working definitions and discussions: *Rehabilitation is the (re)integration of an individual with a* **disability** *into society.* This can be done either by enhancing existing capabilities or by providing alternative means to perform various functions or to substitute for specific sensations.

Rehabilitation engineering is the "*application* of science and technology to ameliorate the handicaps of individuals with disabilities" [Reswick, 1982]. In actual practice, many individuals who say that they practice "rehabilitation engineering" are not engineers by training. While this leads to controversies from practitioners with traditional engineering degrees, it also has the *de facto* benefit of greatly widening the scope of what is encompassed by the term "rehabilitation engineering."

Rehabilitation medicine is a clinical *practice* that focuses on the physical aspects of functional recovery, but that also considers medical, neurological and psychological factors. *Physical therapy, occupational therapy,* and *rehabilitation counseling* are professions in their own right. On the sensory-motor side, other medical and therapeutical specialties practice rehabilitation in vision, audition, and speech.

Rehabilitation technology (or *assistive technology*) narrowly defined is the selection, design, or manufacture of augmentative or assistive devices that are appropriate for the individual with a disability. Such devices are selected based on the specific disability, the function to be augmented or restored, the user's wishes, the clinician's preferences, cost, and the environment in which the device will be used.

Rehabilitation science is the *development* of a body of knowledge, gleaned from rigorous basic and clinical research, that describes how a disability alters specific physiological functions or anatomical structures, and that details the underlying principles by which residual function or capacity can be measured and used to restore function of individuals with disabilities.

67.2   Rehabilitation Concepts

Effective rehabilitation engineers must be well versed in all of the areas described above since they generally work in a team setting, in collaboration with physical and occupational therapists, orthopedic surgeons, physical medicine specialists and/or neurologists. Some rehabilitation engineers are interested in certain activities that we do in the course of a normal day that could be summarized as **activities of daily living** (ADL). These include eating, toileting, combing hair, brushing teeth, reading, etc. Other engineers focus on *mobility* and the limitations to mobility. Mobility can be personal (e.g., within a home or office) or public (automobile, public transportation, accessibility questions in buildings). Mobility also includes the ability to move functionally through the environment. Thus, the question of mobility is not limited to that of getting from place to place, but also includes such questions as whether one can reach an object in a particular setting or whether a paralyzed urinary bladder can be made functional again. Barriers that limit mobility are also studied. For instance, an ill-fitted wheelchair cushion or support system will most assuredly limit mobility by reducing the time that an individual can spend in a wheelchair before he or she must vacate it to avoid serious and difficult-to-heal pressure sores. Other groups of rehabilitation engineers deal with *sensory disabilities*, such as sight or hearing, or with *communications disorders*, both in the production side (e.g., the nonvocal) or in the comprehension side. For any given client, a rehabilitation engineer might have all of these concerns to consider (i.e., ADLs, mobility, sensory and communication dysfunctions).

A key concept in physical or sensory rehabilitation is that of **residual function or residual capacity.** Such a concept implies that the function or sense can be quantified, that the performance range of that function or sense is known in a nonimpaired population, and that the use of residual capacity by a disabled individual should be encouraged. These measures of human performance can be made subjectively by clinicians or objectively by some rather clever computerized test devices.

A rehabilitation engineer asks three key questions: Can a diminished function or sense be successfully augmented? Is there a substitute way to return the function or to restore a sense? And is the solution appropriate and cost-effective? These questions give rise to two important rehabilitation concepts: orthotics and prosthetics. An **orthosis** is an appliance that aids an existing function. A **prosthesis** provides a substitute.

An artificial limb is a *prosthesis,* as is a wheelchair. An ankle brace is an *orthosis.* So are eyeglasses. In fact, eyeglasses might well be the consumate rehabilitation device. They are inexpensive, have little social stigma, and are almost completely unobtrusive to the user. They have let many millions of individuals with correctable vision problems lead productive lives. But in essence, a pair of eyeglasses is an optical device, governed by traditional equations of physical optics. Eyeglasses can be made out of simple glass (from a raw material as abundant as the sands of the earth!) or complex plastics such as those that are ultraviolet sensitive. They can be ground by hand or by sophisticated computer-controlled optical grinders. Thus, crude technology can restore functional vision. Increasing the technical content of the eyeglasses (either by material or manufacturing method) in most cases will not increase the amount of function restored, but it might make the glasses cheaper, lighter and more prone to be used.

67.3 Engineering Concepts in Sensory Rehabilitation

Of the five traditional senses, vision and hearing most define the interactions that permit us to be human. These two senses are the main input channel through which data with high information content can flow. We read; we listen to speech or music; we view art. A loss of one or the other of these senses (or both) can have a devastating impact on the individual affected. Rehabilitation engineers attempt to restore the functions of these senses either through augmentation or via sensory substitution systems. Eyeglasses and hearing aids are examples of augmentative devices that can be used if some residual capacity remains. A major area of rehabilitation engineering research deals with *sensory substitution systems* [Kaczmarek, Chapter 72].

The visual system has the capability to detect a single photon of light, yet also has a dynamic range that can respond to intensities many orders of magnitude greater. It can work with high contrast items and with those of almost no contrast, and across the visible spectrum of colors. Millions of parallel data channels form the optic nerve that comes from an eye; each channel transmits an asynchronous and quasi-random (in time) stream of binary pulses. While the temporal coding on any one of these channels is not fast (on the order of 200 bits/sec or less), the capacity of the human brain to parallel process the entire image is faster than any supercomputer yet built.

If sight is lost, how can it be replaced? A simple pair of eyeglasses will not work, since either the sensor (the retina), the communication channel (the optic nerve and all of its relays to the brain), or one or more essential central processors (the occipital part of the cerebral cortex for initial processing; the parietal and other cortical areas for information extraction) has been damaged. For replacement within the system, one must determine where the visual system has failed and whether a stage of the system can be artificially bypassed. If one uses another sensory modality (e.g., touch or hearing) as an alternate input channel, one must determine whether there is sufficient bandwidth in that channel and whether the higher-order processing hierarchy is plastic enough to process information coming via a different route.

While the above discussion might seem just philosophical, it is more than that. We normally read printed text with our eyes. We recognize words from their (visual) letter combinations. We comprehend what we read via a mysterious processing in the parietal and temporal parts of the cerebral cortex. Could we perhaps read and comprehend this text or other forms of writing through our fingertips with an appropriate interface? The answer surprisingly is yes! And, the adaptation actually goes back to one of the earliest applications of coding theory — that of the development of Braille. Braille condenses all text characters to a raised matrix of 2 by 3 dots (2^6 combinations), with certain combinations reserved as indicators for the next character (such as a number indicator) or for special contractions. Trained readers of Braille can read over 250 words per minute of grade 2 Braille (as fast as most sighted readers can read printed text!). Thus, the Braille code is in essence a rehabilitation engineering concept where an alternate sensory channel is used as a substitute and where a recoding scheme has been employed.

Rehabilitation engineers and their colleagues have designed other ways to read text. To replace the retina as a sensor element, a modern high resolution, high sensitivity, fast imaging sensor (CCD, etc.) is employed to capture a visual image of the text. One method, used by various page scanning devices, converts the scanned image to text by using optical character recognition schemes, and then outputs the text as speech via text-to-speech algorithms. This machine essentially recites the text, much as a sighted helper might do when reading aloud to the blind individual. The user of the device is thus freed of the absolute need for a helper. Such *independence* is often the goal of rehabilitation.

Perhaps the most interesting method presents an image of the scanned data directly to the visual cortex or retina via an array of implantable electrodes that are used to electrically activate nearby cortical or retinal structures. The visual cortex and retina are laid out in a topographic fashion such that there is an orderly mapping of the signal from different parts of the visual field to the retina, and from the retina to corresponding parts of the occipital cortex. The goal of stimulation is to mimic the neural activity that would have been evoked had the signal come through normal channels. And, such stimulation does produce the sensation of light. Since the "image" stays within the visual system, the rehabilitation solution is said to be **modality-specific.** However, substantial problems dealing with biocompatibility and image processing and reduction remain in the design of the electrode arrays and processors that serve to interface the electronics and neurological tissue.

Deafness is another manifestation of a loss of a communication channel, this time for the sense of hearing. Totally deaf individuals use vision as a substitute input channel when communicating via sign language (also a substitute code), and can sign at information rates that match or exceed that of verbal communication. Hearing aids are now commercially available that can adaptively filter out background noise (a predictable signal) while amplifying speech (unpredictable) using autoregressive, moving average (ARMA) signal processing. With the recent advent of powerful digital signal processing chips, true digital hearing aids are now available. Previous analog aids, or digitally programable analog aids, provided a set of tunable filters and amplifiers to cover the low, mid and high frequency ranges of the hearing spectrum. But the digital aids can be specifically and easily tailored (i.e., programmed) to compensate for the specific losses of each individual client across the frequency continuum of hearing, and still provide automatic gain control and one or more user-selectable settings that have been adjusted to perform optimally in differing noise environments.

An exciting development is occurring outside the field of rehabilitation that will have a profound impact on the ability of the deaf to comprehend speech. Electronics companies are now beginning to market universal translation aids for travellers, where a phrase spoken in one language is captured, parsed, translated, and restated (either spoken or displayed) in another language. The deaf would simply require that the visual display be in the language that they use for writing.

Deafness is often brought on (or occurs congenitally) by damage to the cochlea. The cochlea normally transduces variations in sound pressure intensity at a given frequency into patterns of neural discharge. This neural code is then carried by the auditory (eighth cranial) nerve to the brainstem where it is preprocessed and relayed to auditory cortex for initial processing and on to the parietal and other cortical areas for information extraction. Similar to the case for the visual system, the cochlea, auditory nerve, auditory cortex and all relays in between maintain a topological map, this time based on tone frequency (tonotopic). If deafness is solely due to cochlear damage (as is often the case) and if the auditory nerve is still intact, a cochlear implant can often be substituted for the regular transducer array (the cochlea) while still sending the signal through the normal auditory channel (to maintain modality-specificity).

At first glance, the design of a cochlear prosthesis to restore hearing appears daunting. The hearing range of a healthy young individual is 20 to 16,000 Hz. The transducing structure, the cochlea, has 3,500 inner and 12,000 outer hair cells, each best activated by a specific frequency that causes a localized mechanical resonance in the basilar membrane of the cochlea. Deflection of a hair cell causes the cell to fire an all-or-none (i.e., pulsatile) neuronal discharge, whose rate of repetition depends to a first approximation on the amplitude of the stimulus. The outputs of these hair cells have an orderly convergence on the 30,000 to 40,000 fibers that make up the auditory portion of the eighth cranial nerve. These afferent fibers in turn go to brainstem neurons that process and relay the signals on to higher brain centers [Klinke, 1983]. For many causes of deafness, the hair cells are destroyed, but the eighth nerve remains intact. Thus, if one could elicit activity in a specific output fiber by means other than the hair cell motion, perhaps some sense of hearing could be restored. The geometry of the cochlea helps in this regard as different portions of the nerve are closer to different parts of the cochlea.

Electrical stimulation is now used in the cochlear implant to bypass hair cell transduction mechanisms [Loeb, 1985; Clark et al., 1990]. These sophisticated devices have required that complex signal processing, electronic and packaging problems be solved. One current cochlear implant has 22 stimulus sites along the scala tympani of the cochlea. Those sites provide excitation to the peripheral processes of the cells of the eighth cranial nerve, which are splayed out along the length of the scala. The electrode assembly itself has 22 ring electrodes spaced along its length and some additional guard rings between the active electrodes and the receiver to aid in securing the very flexible electrode assembly after it is snaked into the cochlea's very small (a few mm) round window (a surgeon related to me that positioning the electrode was akin to pushing a piece of cooked spaghetti through a small hole at the end of a long tunnel). The electrode is attached to a receiver that is inlaid into a slot milled out of the temporal bone. The receiver contains circuitry that can select any electrode ring to be a source and any other electrode to be a sink for the stimulating current, and that can rapidly sequence between various pairs of electrodes. The receiver is powered and controlled by a radiofrequency link with an external transmitter, whose alignment is maintained by means of a permanent magnet imbedded in the receiver.

A digital signal processor stores information about a specific user and his or her optimal electrode locations for specific frequency bands. The object is to determine what pair of electrodes best produces the subjective perception of a certain pitch *in the implanted individual,* and then to associate a particular filter with that pair via the controller. An enormous amount of compression occurs in taking the frequency range necessary for speech comprehension and reducing it to a few discrete channels. At present, the optimum compression algorithm is unknown, and much fundamental research is being carried out in speech processing, compression and recognition. But, what is amazing is that a number of totally deaf individuals can relearn to comprehend speech exceptionally well without speech-reading through the use of these implants. Other individuals find that the implant aids in speech-reading. For some only an awareness of environmental sounds is apparent; and for another group, the implant appears to have had little effect. But, if you could (as I have been able to) finally converse in unaided speech with an individual who had been rendered totally blind and deaf by a traumatic brain injury, you begin to appreciate the power of rehabilitation engineering.

67.4   Engineering Concepts in Motor Rehabilitation

Limitations in mobility can severely restrict the quality of life of an individual so affected. A wheelchair is a prime example of a prosthesis that can restore personal mobility to those who cannot walk. Given the proper environment (fairly level floors, roads, etc.), modern wheelchairs can be highly efficient. In fact, the fastest times in one of man's greatest tests of endurance, the Boston Marathon, are achieved by the wheelchair racers. Although they do gain the advantage of being able to roll, they still must climb the same hills, and do so with only one-fifth of the muscle power available to an able-bodied marathoner.

While a wheelchair user could certainly go down a set of steps (not recommended), climbing steps in a normal manual or electric wheelchair is a virtual impossibility. Ramps or lifts are engineered to provide accessibility in these cases, or special climbing wheelchairs can be purchased. Wheelchairs also do not work well on surfaces with high rolling resistance or viscous coefficients (e.g., mud, rough terrain, etc.), so alternate mobility aids must be found if access to these areas is to be provided to the physically disabled. Hand-controlled cars, vans, tractors and even airplanes are now driven by wheelchair users. The design of appropriate control modifications falls to the rehabilitation engineer.

Loss of a limb can greatly impair functional activity. The engineering aspects of artificial limb design increase in complexity as the amount of residual limb decreases, especially if one or more joints are lost. As an example, a person with a mid-calf amputation could use a simple wooden stump to extend the leg, and could ambulate reasonably well. But such a leg is not cosmetically appealing and completely ignores any substitution for ankle function.

Immediately following World War II, the United States government began the first concerted effort to foster better engineering design for artificial limbs. Dynamically lockable knee joints were designed for artificial limbs for above-knee amputees. In the ensuing years, energy-storing artificial ankles have been designed, some with prosthetic feet so realistic that beach thongs could be worn with them! Artificial hands, wrists and elbows were designed for upper limb amputees. Careful design of the actuating cable system also provided for a sense of hand grip force, so that the user had some feedback and did not need to rely on vision alone for guidance.

Perhaps the most transparent (to the user) artificial arms are the ones that use electrical activity generated by the muscles remaining in the stump to control the actions of the elbow, wrist and hand [Stein et al., 1988]. This electrical activity is known as myoelectricity, and is produced as the muscle contraction spreads through the muscle. Note that these muscles, if intact, would have controlled at least one of these joints (e.g., the biceps and triceps for the elbow). Thus, a high level of modality-specificity is maintained since the functional element is substituted only at the last stage. All of the batteries, sensor electrodes, amplifiers, motor actuators and controllers (generally analog) reside entirely within these myoelectric arms. An individual trained in the use of a myoelectric arm can perform some impressive tasks with this arm. Current engineering research efforts involve the control of simultaneous multi-joint movements (rather than the single joint movement now available) and the provision for sensory feedback from the end effector of the artificial arm to the skin of the stump via electrical means.

67.5 Engineering Concepts in Communications Disorders

Speech is a uniquely human means of interpersonal communication. Problems that affect speech can occur at the initial transducer (the larynx) or at other areas of the vocal tract. They can be of neurological (due to cortical, brainstem or peripheral nerve damage), structural, and/or cognitive origin. A person might only be able to make a halting attempt at talking, or might not have sufficient control of other motor skills to type or write.

   If only the larynx is involved, an externally applied artificial larynx can be used to generate a resonant column of air that can be modulated by other elements in the vocal tract. If other motor skills are intact, typing can be used to generate text, which in turn can be spoken via text-to-speech devices described above. And the rate of typing (either whole words or via coding) might be fast enough so that reasonable speech rates could be achieved.

   The rehabilitation engineer often becomes involved in the design or specification of augmentative communication aids for individuals who do not have good muscle control, either for speech or for limb movement. A whole industry has developed around the design of symbol or letter boards, where the user can point out (often painstakingly) letters, words or concepts. Some of these boards now have speech output. Linguistics and information theory have been combined in the invention of acceleration techniques intended to speed up the communication process. These include alternative language representation systems based on semantic (iconic), alphanumeric, or other codes; and prediction systems, which provide choices based on previously selected letters or words. A general review of these aids can be found in Chapter 73, while Goodenough-Trepagnier [1994] edited a good publication dealing with human factors and cognative requirements.

   Some individuals can produce speech, but it is dysarthric and very hard to understand. Yet the utterance does contain information. Can this limited information be used to figure out what the individual wanted to say, and then voice it by artificial means? Research labs are now employing neural network theory to determine which pauses in an utterance are due to content (i.e., between a word or sentence) and those due to unwanted halts in speech production.

67.6 Appropriate Technology

Rehabilitation engineering lies at the interface of a wide variety of technical, biological and other concerns. A user might (and often does) put aside a technically sophisticated rehabilitation device in favor of a simpler device that is cheaper, and easier to use and maintain. The cosmetic appearance of the device (or cosmesis) sometimes becomes the overriding factor in acceptance or rejection of a device. A key design factor often lies in the use of the **appropriate technology** to accomplish the task adequately given the extent of the resources available to solve the problem and the residual capacity of the client. Adequacy can be verified by determining that increasing the technical content of the solution results in disproportionately diminishing gains or escalating costs. Thus, a rehabilitation engineer must be able to distinguish applications where high technology is required from those where such technology results in an incremental gain in cost, durability, acceptance and other factors. Further, appropriateness will greatly depend on location. What is appropriate to a client near a major medical center in a highly developed country might not be appropriate to one in a rural setting or in a developing country.

This is not to say that rehabilitation engineers should shun advances in technology. In fact, a fair proportion of rehabilitation engineers work in a research setting where state-of-the-art technology is being applied to the needs of the disabled. However, it is often difficult to transfer complex technology from a laboratory to disabled consumers not directly associated with that laboratory. Such devices are often designed for use only in a structured environment, are difficult to repair properly in the field, and often require a high level of user interaction or sophistication.

Technology transfer in the rehabilitation arena is difficult, due to the limited and fragmented market. Advances in rehabilitation engineering are often piggybacked onto advances in commercial electronics. For instance, the exciting developments in text-to-speech and speech-to-text devices mentioned above are being driven by the commercial marketplace, and not by the rehabilitation arena. But such developments will be welcomed by rehabilitation engineers no less.

67.7 The Future of Engineering in Rehabilitation

The traditional engineering disciplines permeate many aspects of rehabilitation. Signal processing, control and information theory, materials design, computers are all in widespread use from an electrical engineering perspective. Neural networks, microfabrication, fuzzy logic, virtual reality, image processing and other emerging electrical and computer engineering tools are increasingly being applied. Mechanical engineering principles are used in biomechanical studies, gait and motion analysis, prosthetic fitting, seat cushion and back support design, and the design of artificial joints. Materials and metalurgical engineers provide input on newer biocompatable materials. Chemical engineers are developing implantable sensors. Industrial engineers are increasingly studying rehabilitative ergonomics.

The challenge to rehabilitation engineers is to find advances in *any* field, engineering or otherwise, that will aid their clients who have a disability.

Defining Terms

Note: All terms with * have been proposed by the National Center for Medical Rehabilitation and Research (NCMRR) of the US National Institutes of Health (NIH).

Activities of daily living (ADL): Personal activities that are done by almost everyone in the course of a normal day including eating, toileting, combing hair, brushing teeth, reading, etc. ADLs are distinguished from hobbies and from work-related activities (e.g., typing).

Appropriate technology: the technology that will accomplish a task adequately given the resources available. Adequacy can be verified by determining that increasing the technological content of the solution results in diminishing gains or increasing costs.

Disability: Inability or limitation in performing tasks, activities, and roles to levels expected within physical and social contexts.

Functional limitation: Restriction or lack of ability to perform an action in the manner or within the range consistent with the purpose of an organ or organ system.

Impairment: Loss or abnormality of cognitive, emotional, physiological, or anatomical structure or function, including all losses or abnormalities, not just those attributed to the initial pathophysiology.

Modality-specific: A task that is specific to a single sense or movement pattern.

Orthosis: A modality-specific appliance that aids the performance of a function or movement by augmenting or assisting the residual capabilities of that function or movement. An orthopaedic brace is an orthosis.

Pathophysiology: Interruption or interference with normal physiological and developmental processes or structures.

Prosthesis: an appliance that substitutes for the loss of a particular function, generally by involving a different modality as an input and/or output channel. An artificial limb, a sensory substitution system, or an augmentative communication aid are prosthetic devices.

Residual function or residual capacity: Residual function is a measure of the ability to carry out one or more general tasks using the methods normally used. Residual capacity is a measure of the ability to carry out these tasks using any means of performance. These residual measures are generally more subjective than other more quantifiable measures such as residual strength.

*****Societal limitation:**   Restriction, attributable to social policy or barriers (structural or attitudinal), which limits fulfillment of roles, or denies access to services or opportunities that are associated with full participation in society.

References

Clark, G.M., Y.C. Tong, and J.F. Patrick, 1990. *Cochlear Prostheses*, Edinburgh, Churchill Livingstone.

Goodenough-Trepagnier, C., 1994. Guest Editor of a special issue of *Assistive Technology* 6(1) dealing with mental loads in augmentative communication.

Kaczmarek, K.A., J.G. Webster, P. Bach-y-Rita, and W.J. Tompkins, 1991. Electrotactile and Vibrotactile Displays for Sensory Substitution, *IEEE Trans. Biomed. Eng.*, 38: 1–16.

Klinke, R. 1983. Physiology of the Sense of Equilibrium, Hearing and Speech. In *Human Physiology* (Eds. R.F. Schmidt and G. Thews), Berlin, Springer-Verlag, Chap. 12.

Loeb, G.E. 1985. The Functional Replacement of the Ear, *Sci. Am.*, 252: 104–111.

Reswick, J. 1982. What is a Rehabiliation Engineer? In *Annual Review of Rehabiltation*, Vol. 2. (Eds. E.L. Pan, T.E. Backer, and C.L. Vash), New York, Springer-Verlag.

Robinson, C.J. 1993. Rehabilitation Engineering — An Editorial, *IEEE Trans. Rehabil. Eng.*, 1(1): 1–2.

Stein, R.B., D. Charles, and K.B. James, 1988. Providing Motor Control for the Handicapped: A Fusion of Modern Neuroscience, Bioengineering, and Rehabilitation, *Advances in Neurology, Vol. 47: Functional Recovery in Neurological Disease* (Ed. S.G. Waxman), Raven Press, New York.

Further Information

Readers interested in rehabilitation engineering can contact RESNA — an interdisciplinary association for the advancement of rehabilitation and assistive technologies, 1101 Connecticut Ave., N.W., Suite 700, Washington, D.C. 20036. RESNA publishes a quarterly journal called Assistive Technology.

The United States Department of Veterans Affairs puts out a quarterly Journal of Rehabilitation R&D. The January issue of each year contains an overview of most of the rehabilitation engineering efforts occurring in the U.S. and Canada, with over 500 listings.

The IEEE Engineering in Medicine and Biology Society publishes the IEEE Transactions on Neural Systems and Rehabilitation Engineering. The reader should contact the IEEE at PO Box 1331, 445 Hoes Lane, Piscataway, NJ 08855-1331 U.S.A. for further details.

68

Orthopedic Prosthetics and Orthotics in Rehabilitation

Marilyn Lord
Alan Turner-Smith
King's College Hospital-London

An *orthopedic prosthesis* is an internal or external device that *replaces* lost parts or functions of the **neuroskeletomotor system**. In contrast, a *orthopedic orthosis* is a device that *augments* a function of the skeletomotor system by controlling motion or altering the shape of body tissue. For example, an artificial leg or hand is a prosthesis, whereas a calliper (or brace) is an orthosis. This chapter addresses only orthoses and external orthopedic prostheses; internal orthopedic prostheses, such as artificial joints, are a subject on their own.

When a human limb is lost through disease or trauma, the integrity of the body is compromised in so many ways that an engineer may well feel daunted by the design requirements for a prosthetic replacement. Consider the losses from a lower limb amputation. Gone is the structural support for the upper body in standing, along with the complex joint articulations and muscular motor system involved in walking. Lost also is the multimode sensory feedback, from *inter alia* pressure sensors on the sole of the foot, length and force sensors in the muscles, and position sensors in the joints, which closed the control loop around the skeletomotor system. The body also has lost a significant percentage of its weight and is now asymmetrical and unbalanced.

We must first ask if it is desirable to attempt to replace all these losses with like-for-like components. If so, we need to strive to make a bionic limb of similar weight embodying anthropomorphic articulations with equally powerful motors and distributed sensors connected back into the wearer's residual neuromuscular system. Or, is it better to accept the losses and redefine the optimal functioning of the new unit of person-plus-technology? In many cases, it may be concluded that a wheelchair is the optimal solution for lower limb loss. Even if engineering could provide the bionic solution, which it certainly cannot at present despite huge inroads made into aspects of these demands, there remain additional problems inherent to prosthetic replacements to consider. Of these, the unnatural mechanical interface between the external environment and the human body is one of the most difficult. Notable, in place of weight bearing through the structures of the foot that are well adapted for this purpose, load must now be transferred to the skeletal structures via intimate contact between the surface of residual limb and prosthesis; the exact distribution of load becomes critical. To circumvent these problems, an alternative direct **transcutaneous** fixation to the bone has been attempted in limited experimental trials, but this brings its own problems of materials **biocompatability** and prevention of infection ingress around the opening through the skin. Orthotic devices are classified by acronyms that describe the joint which they cross. Thus an AFO is an ankle-foot orthosis, a CO is a cervical orthosis (neck brace or collar), and a TLSO is a thoracolumbosacral orthosis (spinal brace or jacket). The main categories are braces for the cervix (neck), upper limb, trunk, lower limb, and foot. Orthoses are generally simpler devices than prostheses, but because orthoses are constrained by the existing body shape and function, they can present an equally demanding design challenge. Certainly the interaction with body function is more critical, and successful application demands an in-depth appreciation of both residual function and the probable reaction to external interference. External orthotics are often classified as structural or functional, the former implying a static nature to hold an unstable joint and the latter a flexible or articulated system to promote the correct alignment of the joints during dynamic functioning. An alternative orthotic approach utilizes functional electrical stimulation (FES) of the patient's own muscles to generate appropriate forces for joint motion; this is dealt with in Chapter 70.

68.1 Fundamentals

Designers of orthotic and prosthetic devices are aware of the three cardinal considerations — function, structure, and **cosmesis**.

For requirements of function, we must be very clear about the objectives of treatment. This requires first an understanding of the clinical condition. **Functional prescription** is now a preferred route for the medical practitioner to specify the requirements, leaving the implementation of this instruction to the prosthetist, orthotist, or rehabilitation technologist. The benefits of this distinction between client specific-ation and final hardware will be obvious to design engineers. Indeed, the influence of design procedures on the supply process is a contribution from engineering that is being appreciated more and more.

The second requirement for function is the knowledge of the biomechanics that underlies both the dysfunction in the patient and the function of proposed device to be coupled to the patient. Kinematics, dynamics, energy considerations, and control all enter into this understanding of function. Structure is the means of carrying the function, and finally both need to be embodied into a design that is cosmetically acceptable. Some of the fundamental issues in these concepts are discussed here.

To function well, the device needs an effective coupling to the human body. To this end, there is often some part that is molded to the contours of the wearer. Achieving a satisfactory mechanical interface of a molded component depends primarily on the shape. The internal dimensions of such components are not made an exact match to the external dimensions of the limb segment, but by a process of **rectification**, the shape is adjusted to relieve areas of skin with low load tolerance. The Shapes are also evolved to achieve appropriate load distribution for stability of coupling between prosthetic socket and limb or, in orthotic design, a system of usually three forces that generates a moment to stabilize a collapsing joint (Figure 68.1). Alignment is a second factor influencing the interface loading. For lower limb prostheses particularly, the alignment of the molded socket to the remainder of the structural components also will be critical in determining the moments and forces transmitted to the interface when the foot is flat on the ground. The same is true for lower limb orthoses, where the net action of the ground reaction forces and consequent

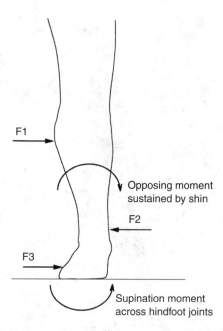

F1

Opposing moment
sustained by shin

F2

F3

Supination moment
across hindfoot joints

FIGURE 68.1 Three-force system required in an orthosis to control a valgus hindfoot due to weakness in the hindfoot supinators.

moments around the natural joints are highly dependent on the alignment taken up by the combination of orthosis and shoe. Adjustability may be important, particularly for children or progressive medical conditions. Functional components that enable desirable motions are largely straightforward engineering mechanisms such as hinges or dampers, although the specific design requirements for their dynamic performance may be quite complex because of the biomechanics of the body. An example of the design of knee joints is expanded below. These motions may be driven from external power sources but more often are passive or body-powered mechanisms. In orthoses where relatively small angular motions are needed, these may be provided by material flexibility rather than mechanisms.

The structural requirements for lower-limb prosthetics have been laid down at a consensus meeting [1978] bases on biomechanical measurement of forces in a gait laboratory, referred to as the *Philadelphia standards* and soon to be incorporated into an ISO standard (ISO 13404,5; ISO 10328). Not only are the load level and life critical, but so is the mode of failure. Sudden failure of an ankle bolt resulting in disengagement of an artificial foot is not only potentially life-threatening to an elderly amputee who falls and breaks a hip but also can be quite traumatic to unsuspecting witnesses of the apparent event of autoamputation. Design and choice of materials should ensure a controlled slow yielding, not brittle fracture. A further consideration is the ability of the complete structure to absorb shock loading, either the repeated small shocks of walking at the heel strike or rather more major shocks during sports activities or falls. This minimizes the shock transmitted through the skin to the skeleton, known to cause both skin lesions and joint degeneration. Finally, the consideration of hygiene must not be overlooked; the user must be able to clean the orthosis or prosthesis adequately without compromising its structure or function.

Added to the two elements of structure and function, the third element of *cosmesis* completes the trilogy. Appearance can be of great psychological importance to the user, and technology has its contribution here, too. As examples, special effects familiar in science fiction films also can be harnessed to provide realistic cosmetic covers for hand or foot prostheses. Borrowing from advanced manufacturing technology, optical shape scanning linked to three-dimensional (3D) computer-aided design, and **CNC machining** can be pressed into service to generate customized shapes to match a contralateral remaining limb. Up-to-date materials and component design each contribute to minimize the "orthopedic appliance" image of the devices (Figure 68.2). In providing cosmesis, the views of the user must remain paramount. The wearer

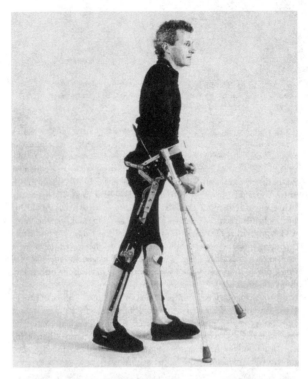

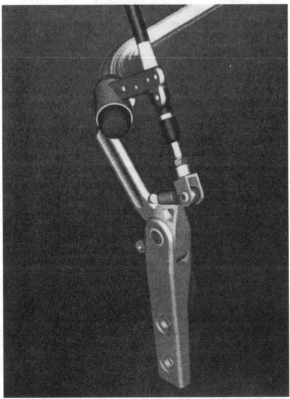

FIGURE 68.2   The ARGO reciprocating-gait orthosis, normally worn under the clothing, with structural components produced from 3D CAD. (Courtesy of Hugh Steeper, Ltd., U.K.)

will often choose an attractive functional design in preference to a life like design that is not felt to be part of his or her body.

Upper limb prostheses are often seen as a more interesting engineering challenge than lower limb, offering the possibilities for active motor/control systems and complex articulations. However, the market is an order of magnitude smaller and cost/benefit less easy to prove — after all, it is possible to function fairly well with one arm, but try walking with one leg. At the simplest end, an arm for a below-elbow amputee might comprise a socket with a terminal device offering a pincer grip (hand or hook) that can be operated through a Bowden cable by shrugging the shoulders. Such body-powered prostheses may appear crude, but they are often favored by the wearer because of a sense of position and force feedback from the cable, and they do not need a power supply. Another, more elegant method of harnessing body power is to take a muscle made redundant by an amputation and tether its tendon through an artificially fashioned loop of skin: the cable can then be hooked through the loop [Childress, 1989].

Externally powered devices have been attempted using various power sources with degrees of success. Pneumatic power in the form of a gas cylinder is cheap and light, but recharging is a problem that exercised the ingenuity of early suppliers: where supplies were not readily available, even schemes to involve the local fire services with recharging were costed. Also, contemplate the prospect of bringing a loaded table fork toward your face carried on the end of a position-controlled arm powered with spongy, low-pressure pneumatic actuators, and you will appreciate another aspect of difficulties with this source. Nevertheless, gas-powered grip on a hand can be a good solution. Early skirmishes with stiffer hydraulic servos were largely unsuccessful because of power supply and actuator weight and oil leakage. Electric actuation, heavy and slow at first, has gradually improved to establish its premier position. Input control to these powered devices can be from surface electromyography or by mechanical movement of, for example, the shoulder or an ectromelic limb. Feedback can be presented as skin pressure, movement of a sensor over the skin, or electric stimulation. Control strategies range from position control around a single joint or group of related joints through combined position and force control for hand grip to computer-assisted coordination of entire activities such as feeding.

The physical designs in prosthetic and orthotic devices has changed substantially over the past decade. One could propose that this is solely the introduction of new materials. The sockets of artificial limbs have always been fashioned to suit the individual patient, historically by carving wood, shaping leather, or beating sheet metal. Following the introduction of thermosetting fiber-reinforced plastics hand-shaped over a plaster cast of the limb residuum, substitution of thermoforming plastics that could be automatically vacuum-formed made a leap forward to give light, rapidly made, and cosmetically improved solutions. Polypropylene is the favored material in this application. The same materials permitted the new concept of custom-molded orthoses. Carbon fiber composites substituted for metal have certainly improved the performance of structural components such as limb shanks. But some of the progress owes much to innovative thinking. The flex foot is a fine example, where a traditional anthropomorphic design with imitation ankle joint and metatarsal break is completely abandoned and a functional design adopted to optimize energy storage and return. This is based on two leaf springs made from Kevlar, joined together at the ankle with one splaying down toward the toes to form the forefoot spring and the other rearward to form the heel spring (Figure 68.3). Apart from the gains for the disabled athletes for whom the foot was designed — and these are so remarkable that there is little point in competing now without this foot — clients across all age groups have benefited from the adaptability to rough ground and shock-absorption capability.

68.2 Applications

68.2.1 Computer-Aided Engineering in Customized Component Design

Computer-aided engineering has found a fertile ground for exploitation in the process of design of customized components to match to body shape. A good example is in sockets for artificial limbs. What prosthetists particularly seek is the ability to produce a well-fitting socket during the course of a single

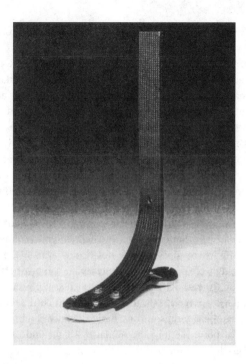

FIGURE 68.3   The flex foot.

patient consultation. Traditional craft methods of casting the residual limb in plaster of paris, pouring a positive mold, manual rectification, and then socket fabrication over the **rectified** cast takes too long.

By using advanced technology, residual limb shapes can be captured in a computer, rectified by computer algorithms, and CNC machined to produce the rectified cast in under an hour so that with the addition of vacuum-formed machinery to pull a socket rapidly over the cast, the socket can be ready for trial fitting in one session. There are added advantages too, in that the shape is now stored in digital form in the computer and can be reproduced or adjusted whenever and wherever desired. Although such systems are still in an early stage of introduction, many practicing prosthetists in the United States have now had hands-on experience of this technology, and a major evaluation by the Veterans Administration has been undertaken [Houston et al., 1992].

Initially, much of the engineering development work went into the hardware components, a difficult brief in view of the low cost target for a custom product. Requirements are considerably different from those of standard engineering, for example, relaxation in the accuracies required (millimeters, not microns); a need to measure limb or trunk parts that are encumbered by the attached body, which may resist being orientated conveniently in a machine and which will certainly distort with the lightest pressure; and a need to reproduce fairly bulky items with strength to be used as a sacrificial mold. Instrumentation for body shape scanning has been developed using methods of silhouettes, Moiré fringes, contact probes measuring contours of plaster casts, and light triangulation. Almost universally the molds are turned by "milling on a spit" [Duncan and Mair, 1983], using an adapted lathe with a milling head to spiral down a large cylindrical plug of material such as plaster of paris mix. Rehabilitation engineers watch with great interest, some with envy, the developments in rapid prototyping manufacture, which is so successful in reducing the cycle time for one-off developments elsewhere in industry, but alas the costs of techniques such as stereolithography are as yet beyond economic feasibility for our area.

Much emphasis also has been placed on the graphics and algorithms needed to achieve rectification. Opinions vary as to what extent the computer should simply provide a more elegant tool for the prosthetist to exercise his or her traditional skills using 3D modeling and on-screen sculpting as a direct replacement for manual plaster rectification or to what extent the computer system should take over the bulk of the

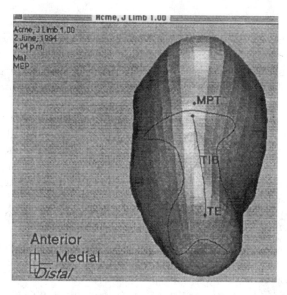

FIGURE 68.4 A rectification requirement defined over the tibia of lower limb stump using the Shapemaker application for computer-aided socket design.

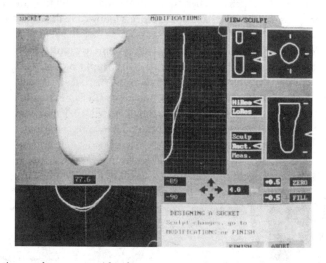

FIGURE 68.5 Adjusting a socket contour with reference to 3D graphics and cross-sectional profiles in the UCL CASD system. (Reproduced from Reynolds, D.P. and Lord, M. 1992. *Med. Biol. Eng. Comput.* 30: 419. With permission.)

process by an expert systems approach. Systems currently available tend to do a little of each. A series of rectification maps can be held as templates, each storing the appropriate relief or buildup to be applied over a particular anatomic area of the limb. Thus the map might provide for a ridge to be added down the front of the shin of a lower limb model so that the eventual socket will not press against the vulnerable bony prominence of the tibia (Figure 68.4). Positioning of the discrete regions to match individual anatomy might typically be anchored to one or more anatomic features indicated by the prosthetist. The prosthetist is also able to free-form sculpt a particular region by pulling the surface interactively with reference to graphic representation (Figure 68.5); this is particularly useful where the patient has some unusual feature not provided for in the templates.

As part of this general development, finite-element analysis has been employed to model the soft tissue distortion occurring during limb loading and to look at the influence of severity of rectification in the resultant distribution of interface stress [Reynolds and Lord, 1992] (Figure 68.6). In engineering terms, this modeling is somewhat unusual and decidedly nonlinear. For a start, the tissues are highly deformable but nearly incompressible, which raises problems of a suitable Poisson ratio to apply in the modeling. Values of $n = 0.3$ to $n = 0.49$ have been proposed, based on experimental matching of stress-strain curves from indentation of limb tissue in vivo. In reality, though, compression (defined as a loss of volume) may be noted in a limb segment under localized external pressure due to loss of mass as first the blood is rapidly evacuated and then interstitial fluids are more slowly squeezed out. Also, it is difficult to define the boundaries of the limb segment at the proximal end, still attached to the body, where **soft tissues** can easily bulge up and out. This makes accurate experimental determination of the stress-strain curves for the tissue matrix difficult. A nonlinear model with interface elements allowing slip to occur between skin and socket at the limit of static friction may need to be considered, since the frictional conditions at the interface will determine the balance between shear and direct stresses in supporting body weight against the sloping sidewalls. Although excessive shear at the skin surface is considered particularly damaging, higher pressures would be required in its complete absence.

In a similar vein, computer-aided design (CAD) techniques are also finding application in the design of bespoke orthopedic footwear, using CAD techniques from the volume fashion trade modified to suit the one-off nature of bespoke work. This again requires the generation of a customized mold, or shoe last, for each foot, in addition to the design of patterns for the shoe uppers [Lord et al., 1991]. The philosophy of design of shoe lasts is quite different from that of sockets, because last shapes have considerable and fundamental differences from foot shapes. In this instance, a library of reference last shapes is held, and a suitable one is selected both to match the client's foot shape and to fulfill the shoemaking needs for the particular style and type of shoe. The schematic of the process followed in development of the Shoemaster system is shown in Figure 68.7.

Design of shoe inserts is another related application, with systems to capture, manipulate, and reproduce underfoot contours now in commercial use. An example is the Ampfit system, where the foot is placed on

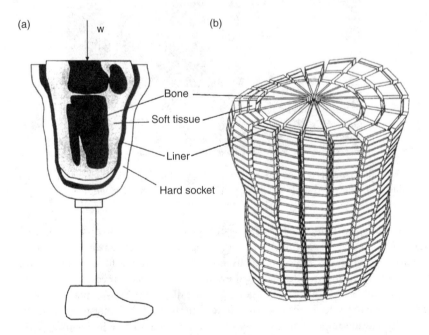

FIGURE 68.6 Finite-element analysis employed to determine the sensitivity of interface pressure to socket shape rectification: (a) limb and socket; (b) elements in layers representing idealized geometry of bone, soft tissue, and socket liner; (c) rectification map of radial differences between the external free shape of the limb and the internal dimensions of socket; and (d) FE predictions of direct pressure. (Courtesy of Zhang Ming, King's College London.)

(c)

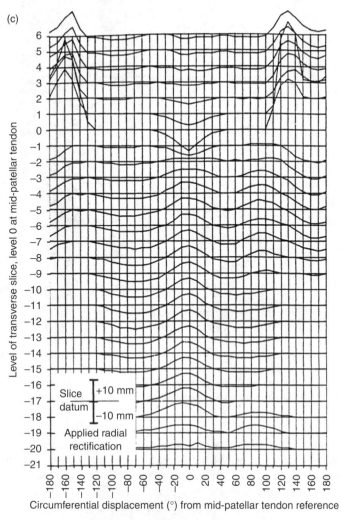

(d)

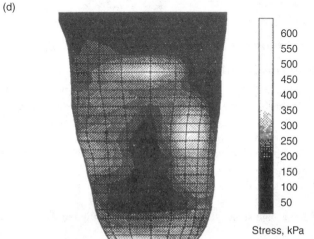

FIGURE 68.6 Continued

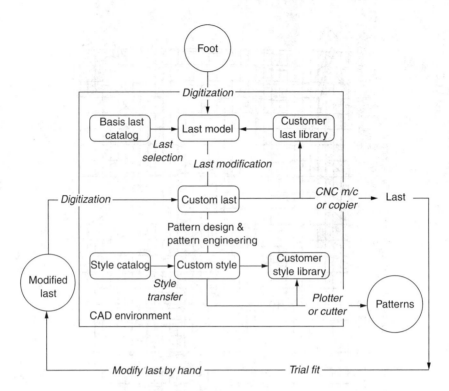

FIGURE 68.7 Schematic of operation of the Shoemaster shoe design system based on selection of a basis last from a database of model lasts. A database of styles is also employed to generate the upper patterns.

a platform to which preshaped arch supports or other wedges or domes may first be attached. A matrix of round-ended cylinders is then forced up by gas pressure through both platform and supports, supporting the foot over most of the area with an even load distribution. The shape is captured from the cylinder locations and fed into a computer, where rectification can be made similar to that described for prosthetic sockets. A benchtop CNC machine then routs the shoe inserts from specially provided blanks while the client waits.

68.2.2 Examples of Innovative Component Design

68.2.2.1 An Intelligent Prosthetic Knee

The control of an artificial lower limb turns out to be most problematic during the swing phase, during which the foot is lifted off the ground to be guided into contact ahead of the walker. A prosthetic lower limb needs to be significantly lighter than its normal counterpart because the muscular power is not present to control it. Two technological advances have helped. First, carbon fiber construction has reduced the mass of the lower limb, and second, pneumatic or hydraulically controlled damping mechanisms for the knee joint have enabled adjustment of the swing phase to suit an individual's pattern of walking.

Swing-phase control of the knee should operate in three areas:

1. Resistance to flexion at late stance during toe-off controls any tendency to excessive heel rise at early swing
2. Assistance to extension after midswing ensures that the limb is fully extended and ready for heel strike
3. Resistance before a terminal impact at the end of the extension swing dampens out the inertial forces to allow a smooth transition from flexed to extended knee position

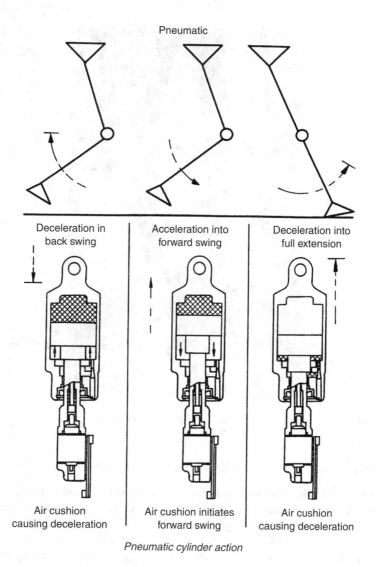

FIGURE 68.8 Pneumatic cylinder action in a swing phase controller. (Reprinted with permission from S. Zahedi, The Results of the Field Trial of the Endolite Intelligent Prosthesis, Internal publication, Chas. A. Blatchford & Sons, U.K.)

In conventional limbs, parameters of these controls are determined by fixed components (springs, bleed valves) that are set to optimum for an individual's normal gait at one particular speed, for example, the pneumatic controller in Figure 68.8. If the amputee subsequently walks more slowly, the limb will tend to lead, while if the amputee walks more quickly, the limb will tend to fall behind; the usual compensatory actions are, respectively, an unnatural tilting of the pelvis to delay heel contact or abnormal kicking through of the leg.

In a recent advance, intelligence is built into the swing-phase controller to adjust automatically for cadence variations (Figure 68.9). A 4-bit microprocessor is used to adjust a needle valve, via a linear stepper motor, according to duration of the preceding swing phase [Zahedi, 1995]. The unit is programmed by the prosthetist to provide optimal damping for the particular amputee's swing phase at slow, normal, and fast walking paces. Thereafter, the appropriate damping is automatically selected for any intermediate speed.

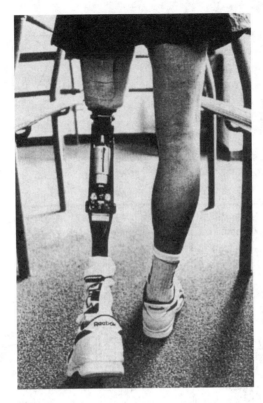

FIGURE 68.9   The Endolite intelligent prosthesis in use, minus its cosmetic covers.

68.2.3   A Hierarchically Controlled Prosthetic Hand

Control of the intact hand is hierarchical. It starts with the owner's intention, and an action plan is formulated based on knowledge of the environment and the object to be manipulated. For gross movements, the numerous articulations rely on "preprogrammed" coordination from the central nervous system. Fine control leans heavily on local feedback from force and position sensors in the joints and tactile information about loading and slip at the skin. In contrast, conventional prostheses depend on the conscious command of all levels of control and so can be slow and tiring to use.

Current technology is able to provide both the computing power and transducers required to recreate some of a normal hand's sophisticated proprioceptive control. A concept of extended physiologic proprioception (EPP) was introduced for control of gross arm movement [Simpson and Kenworthy, 1973] whereby the central nervous system is retrained through residual proprioception to coordinate gross actions applying to the geometry of the new extended limb. This idea can be applied to initiate gross hand movements while delegating fine control to an intelligent controller.

Developments by Chappell and Kyberd [1991] and others provide a fine example of the possibilities. A suitable mechanical configuration is shown in Figure 68.10. Four 12-V dc electric motors with gearboxes control, respectively, thumb adduction, thumb flexion, forefinger flexion, and flexion of digits 3, 4, and 5. Digits 3, 4, and 5 are linked together by a double-swingletree mechanism that allows all three to be driven together. When one digit touches an object the other two can continue to close until they also touch or reach their limit of travel. The movement of the digits allows one of several basic postures:

- *Three-point chuck:* Precision grip with digits 1, 2, and 3 (thumb set to oppose the midline between digits 2 and 3); digits 4 and 5 give additional support

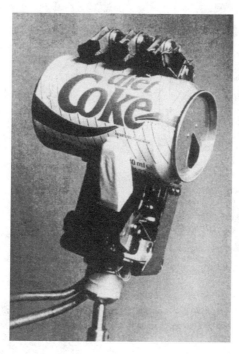

FIGURE 68.10 The Southampton hand prosthesis with four degrees of freedom in a power grip. An optical/acoustic sensor is mounted on the thumb. (Reprinted from Chappell, P.H. and Kyberd, P.J. 1991. *J. Biomed. Eng.* 13: 363, Figure 1.)

- *Two-point grip:* Precision grip with digits 1 and 2 (thumb set to oppose forefinger); digits 3, 4, and 5 fully flexed and not used or fully extended
- *Fist:* As two-point grip but with thumb fully extended to allow large objects to be grasped
- *Small Fist:* As fist but with thumb flexed and abducted to oppose side of digit 2
- *Side, or key:* Digits 2 to 5 half fully flexed with thumb opposing side of second digit
- *Flat hand:* Digits 2 to 5 fully extended with thumb abducted and flexed, parked beside digit 2

The controller coordinates the transition between these positions and ensures that trajectories do not tangle. Feedback to the controller is provided by several devices. Potentiometers detect the angles of flexion of the digits; touch sensors detect pressure on the palmer surfaces of the digits; and a combined contact force (Hall effect) and slip sensor (from acoustic frequency output of force sensor) is mounted at the fingertips. The latter detects movement of an object and so controls grip strength appropriate to the task — whether holding a hammer or an egg [Kyberd and Chappell, 1993].

The whole hand may be operated by electromyographic signals from two antagonistic muscles in the supporting forearm stump, picked up at the skin surface. In response to tension in one muscle, the hand opens progressively and then closes to grip with an automatic reflex. The second muscle controls the mode of operation as the hand moves between the states of touch, hold, squeeze, and release.

68.2.4 A Self-Aligning Orthotic Knee Joint

Knee orthosis are often supplied to resist knee flexion during standing and gait at an otherwise collapsing joint. The rigid locking mechanisms on these devices are manually released to allow knee flexion during sitting. Fitting is complicated by the difficulty of attaching the orthosis with its joint accurately aligned to that of the knee. The simple diagram in Figure 68.11 shows how misplacement of a simple hinged orthosis with a notional fixed knee axis would cause the cuffs on the thigh and calf to press into the soft tissues of the limb (known as pistoning).

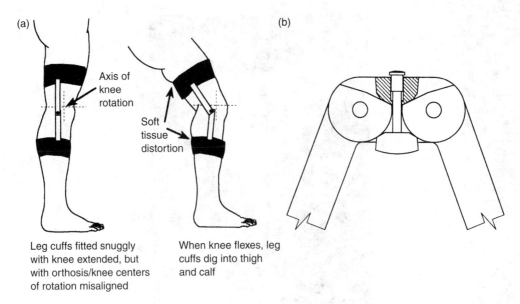

FIGURE 68.11   The problem caused by misplacement of a single-axis orthotic joint (a) is overcome by an orthosis (b) with a self-aligning axis. (The Laser system, courtesy of Hugh Steeper, Ltd., U.K.)

The human knee does not have a fixed axis, though, but is better represented as a polycentric joint. In a sagittal (side) view, it is easy to conceptualize the origin of these kinematics from the anatomy of the cruciate ligaments running crisscross across the joint, which together with the base of the femur and the head of the tibia form a classic four-bar linkage. The polycentric nature of the motion can therefore be mimicked by a similar geometry of linkage on the orthosis.

The problem of alignment still remains, however, and precision location of attachment points is not possible when gripping through soft tissues. In one attempt to overcome this specific problem, the knee mechanism has been designed with not one but two axes (Figure 68.11). The center of rotation is then free to self-align. This complexity of the joint while still maintaining the ability to fixate the knee and meeting low weight requirements is only achieved by meticulous design in composite materials.

68.3   Summary

The field of prosthetics and orthotics is one where at present traditional craft methods sit alongside the application of high technology. Gradually, advanced technology is creeping into most areas, bringing vast improvements in hardware performance specifications and aesthetics. This is, however, an area where the clinical skills of the prosthetist and orthotist will always be required in specification and fitting and where many of the products have customized components. The successful applications of technology are those which assist the professional to exercise his or her judgment, providing him or her with good tools and means to realize a functional specification.

Since the demand for these devices is thankfully low, their design and manufacture are small scale in terms of volume. This taxes the skills of most engineers, both to design the product at reasonable up-front costs and to manufacture it economically in low volume. For bespoke components, we are moving from a base of craft manufacture through an era when modularization was exploited to allow small-batch production toward the use of CAD. In the latter, the engineering design effort is then embodied in the CAD system, leaving the prosthetist or orthotist to incorporate clinical design for each individual component.

Specific examples of current applications have been described. These can only represent a small part of the design effort that is put into prosthetics and orthotics on a continuing basis, making advances in materials and electronics in particular available.

We are also aware that in the space available, it has not been possible to include a discussion of the very innovative work that is being done in intermediate technology for the third world, for which the International Society of Prosthetics and Orthotics (address below) currently has a special working group.

Defining Terms

Biocompatability: Compatibility with living tissue, for example, in consideration of toxicity, degradability, and mechanical interfacing.

CNC machining: Use of a computer numerically controlled machine.

Cosmesis: Aesthetics of appearance.

Ectromelia: Congenital gross shortening of the long bones of a limb.

Functional prescription: A doctor's prescription for supply of a device written in terms of its function as opposed to embodiment.

Neuroskeletomotor system: The skeletal frame of the body with the muscles, peripheral nerves, and central nervous system of the spine and brain, which together participate in movement and stabilization of the body.

Rectified, rectification: Adjustment of a model of body shape to achieve a desirable load distribution in a custom-molded prosthesis or orthosis.

Soft tissues: Skin, fat, connective tissues, and muscles which, along with the hard tissues of bone, teeth, etc. and the fluids, make up the human body.

Transcutaneous: Passing through the skin.

References

Chappell, P.H. and Kyberd, P.J. 1991. Prehensile control of a hand prosthesis by a microcontroller. *J. Biomed. Eng.* 13: 363.

Childress, D.S. 1989. Control philosophies for limb prostheses. In J. Paul et al. (Eds.), *Progress in Bioengineering*, pp. 210–215. New York, Adam Hilger.

Duncan, J.P. and Mair, S.G. 1983. *Sculptured Surfaces in Engineering and Medicine*. Cambridge, England, Cambridge University Press.

Houston, V.L., Burgess, E.M., Childress, D.S. et al. 1992. Automated fabrication of mobility aids (AFMA): below-knee CASD/CAM testing and evaluation. *J. Rehabil. Res. Dev.* 29: 78.

Kyberd, P.J. and Chappell, P.H. 1993. A force sensor for automatic manipulation based on the Hall effect. *Meas. Sci. Technol.* 4: 281.

Lord, M., Foulston, J., and Smith, P.J. 1991. Technical evaluation of a CAD system for orthopaedic shoe-upper design. *Eng. Med. Proc. Instrum. Mech. Eng.* 205: 109.

Reynolds, D.P. and Lord, M. 1992. Interface load analysis for computer-aided design of below-knee prosthetic sockets. *Med. Biol. Eng. Comput.* 30: 419.

Simpson, D.C. and Kenworthy, G. 1973. The design of a complete arm prosthesis. *Biomed. Eng.* 8: 56.

Zahedi, S. 1995. Evaluation and biomechanics of the intelligent prosthesis: a two-year study. *Orthop. Tech.* 46: 32–40.

Further Information

Bowker, P., Condie, D.N., Bader, D.L., and Pratt, D.J. (Eds.). 1993. *Biomechanical Basis of Orthotic Management*. Oxford, Butterworth-Heinemann.

Murdoch, G. and Donovan, R.G. (Eds.). 1988. *Amputation Surgery and Lower Limb Prosthetics*. Boston, Blackwell Scientific Publications.

Nordin, M. and Frankel, V. 1980. *Basic Mechanics of the Musculoskeletal System*, 2nd ed. Philadelphia, Lea & Febiger.

Smidt, G.L. (ed). 1990. *Gait in Rehabilitation*. New York, Churchill-Livingstone.

Organizations

International Society of Prosthetics and Orthotics (ISPO), Borgervaenget 5,2100 Copenhagen Ø, Denmark [tel (31) 20 72 60].

Department of Veterans Affairs, VA Rehabilitation Research and Development Service, 103 Gay Street, Baltimore, MD 21202-4051.

Rehabilitation Engineering Society of North America (RESNA), Suite 1540, 1700 North Moore Street, Arlington, VA 22209-1903.

69

Wheeled Mobility: Wheelchairs and Personal Transportation

Rory A. Cooper
University of Pittsburgh

69.1 Introduction

Centuries ago, people with disabilities who survived for an extended period of time were transported on hammocks slung between poles which were carried by others. This was the preferred means of transportation of the upper class and thus carried no stigma. Later the wheelbarrow was developed and soon became a common mode of transportation for people with disabilities. Because wheelbarrows were used to transport materials, during this period in history, people with disabilities were looked upon as outcasts from society. During the renaissance, the French court popularized the first wheelchairs. Wheelchairs were overstuffed arm chairs with wheels placed upon them. This enabled movement, with assistance, indoors. Later the wooden wheelchair with wicker matting was developed. This type of chair remained the standard until the 1930s. Franklin D. Roosevelt was not satisfied with the wooden wheelchair and had many common metal kitchen chairs modified with wheels. In the 1930s a young mining engineer, named Everest experienced an accident that left him mobility impaired. He worked with a fellow engineer Jennings to develop steel wheelchairs. Within a few years, they formed a company Everest & Jennings to manufacture wheelchairs. Following World War II, medical advances saved the lives of many veterans with spinal cord injuries or lower limb amputations, who would have otherwise died. Veterans medical centers issued these veterans steel framed wheelchairs with 18 inch seat widths. These wheelchairs were designed to provide the veteran some mobility within the hospital and home, and not to optimize ergonomic variables. Just as among the ambulatory population, mobility among people with disabilities varies. Mobility is more of a functional limitation than a disability related condition. Powered mobility can have tremendous positive psycho-social effects on an individual. Power wheelchairs provide greater independence to thousands of people with severe mobility impairments.

Power wheelchairs began in the 1940s as standard cross-brace folding manual wheelchairs adapted with automobile starter motors and an automobile battery. The cross-braced wheelchair remained the standard for a number of years. When the rigid power wheelchair frame was developed, space became available under the seat for electronic controls, respirators, communication systems, and reclining devices. By the mid-1970s, wheelchairs had evolved to the point where people had acquired a significant level of mobility.

A personal automobile has a profound effect on a persons' mobility and ability to participate in society. A wheelchair is suitable for short distances, and for many situations where an unimpaired person would walk. Modifications to vehicles may be as simple as a lever attached to the brake and accelerator pedals or as complex as a complete joystick controlled fly-by-wire system. Modifications to other components of the vehicle may be required to provide wheelchair access. An automobile may not be appropriate for some people who travel distances too long to be convenient with a wheelchair, but not long enough to warrant an adapted automobile. Micro-cars, enlarged wheelchairs which travel at bicycle speeds, are convenient for many people who wish only to travel to the local grocery store or post office. Micro-cars are also useful for people who like to travel along bicycle paths or drive short distances off-road.

69.2   Categories of Wheelchairs

There are two basic classes of wheelchairs: manually powered and externally powered. For practical purposes, externally powered wheelchairs are electrically powered wheelchairs. There are approximately 200,000 wheelchairs sold annually within the United States of which about 20,000 are powered wheelchairs. Most wheelchairs are purchased by third-party-payers (e.g., insurance companies, government agencies). This requires the market to be responsive to wheelchairs user's needs, prescriber expertise and experience, third-party-payer purchase criteria, and competition from other manufacturers. Despite the complicated interaction between these components, and the regulation of products by several government agencies, a variety of wheelchairs and options are available.

Depot wheelchairs are intended for institutional use where several people may use the same wheelchair. Generally, these wheelchairs are inappropriate for active people who use wheelchairs for personal mobility. Depot wheelchairs are designed to be inexpensive, accommodate large variations in body size, to be low maintenance, and often to be attendant propelled. They are heavy and their performance is limited. A typical depot wheelchair will have swing away footrests, removable armrests, a single cross-brace frame and solid tires.

People who have impairment of an arm and one or both lower extremities may benefit from a one-arm drive wheelchair that uses a linkage connecting the rear wheels. This allows the user to push upon the pushrim of one wheel and to propel both wheels. To effectively turn the wheelchair, the user must have the ability to disengage the drive mechanism.

Some people have weakness of the upper and lower extremities and can gain maximal benefit from wheelchair propulsion by combining the use of their arms and legs or by using only their legs. The design and selection of a foot-drive wheelchair depends greatly upon how the user can take greatest advantage of their motor abilities.

Indoor spaces are more limited and one is often required to get close to furnishings and fixtures to use them properly. Indoor wheelchairs often use rear casters because of the manueverability of these designs.

However, rear caster designs make the wheelchair less stable in lateral directions. Indoor wheelchairs typically have short wheelbases.

All wheelchairs are not propelled by the person sitting in the wheelchair. In many hospitals and long-term care facilities, wheelchairs are propelled by attendants. Attendant propelled wheelchair designs must consider the rider and the attendant as users. The rider must be transported safely and comfortably. The attendant must be able to operate and easily maneuver safely and with minimum physical strain.

Active users often prefer highly maneuverable and responsive wheelchairs which fit their physical and psychosocial character. The ultralight wheelchair evolved from the desire of wheelchair users to develop functional ergonomic designs for wheelchairs. Ultralight wheelchairs are made of such materials as aluminum, alloy steel, titanium, or composites. The design of ultralight wheelchairs allows a number of features to be customized by the user or be specified for manufacture. The most common features of all are the light weight, the high quality of materials used in their construction, and their functional design. Many people can benefit from ultralight wheelchair designs.

The desire to achieve better performance has led wheelchair users, inventors, and manufacturers to constantly develop specialized wheelchairs for sports. There is no real typical sports wheelchair as the design depends heavily on the sport. Basketball and tennis wheelchairs are often thought to typify sports wheelchair design. However, racing, field events or shooting wheelchairs have little in common with the former.

Some wheelchairs are made to change configuration from reclining to sitting, and from sitting to standing. Most stand-up wheelchairs cannot be driven in the stand-up setting in order to insure safe and stable operation. Standing gives the user the ability to reach cabinet and counter spaces otherwise inaccessible. Standing has the additional advantage of providing therapeutic benefits, that is, hemodynamic improvements, and amelioration of osteoporosis.

Stairs and other obstacles persist despite the progress made in universal design. Stair-climbing wheelchairs are electrically powered wheelchairs designed to ascend and descend stairs safely under the occupant's control. Stair-climbing wheelchairs are quite complicated, and often reconfigure themselves while climbing stairs. The additional power required to climb stairs often reduces the range of the wheelchair when compared to standard power wheelchairs.

69.3   Wheelchair Structure and Component Design

Several factors must be considered when designing a wheelchair frame: what are the intended uses, what are the abilities of the user, what are the resources available, and what are the existing products available. These factors determine if and how the frame will be designed and built. Successful designs of wheelchairs can only be accomplished with continuous input from and interaction with wheelchair users. The durability, aesthetics, function, ride comfort, and cost of the frame are dependent on the materials for construction, the frame geometry, and fabrication methods. One of the issues that makes wheelchair design more complicated is the fact that many users are dependent upon wheeled mobility everyday, nearly all day.

69.3.1   Materials

Most wheelchairs are made of either aluminum or steel. Some chairs are made of titanium or advanced composite materials, primarily carbon fiber, and in the future composite frames will probably begin to become more available. All of these materials have their strengths and weaknesses.

Common aluminum wheelchairs are Tungsten Inert Gas (TIG) welded (i.e., electrically welded together in a cloud of inert gas). They are sometimes bolted together using lugs. Most aluminum wheelchair frames are constructed of round drawn 6061 aluminum tubing. This is one of the least expensive and most versatile of the heat treatable aluminum alloys. It has most of the desirable qualities of aluminum, has good mechanical properties and high corrosion resistance. It can be fabricated using most standard techniques.

Most steel wheelchairs are made of mild steel (1040 or 1060) or chromium-molybdenum alloy (4130 or 4140) seamless tubing commonly called chro-moly. Mild steel is very inexpensive and easy to work with. It is wildly available, and performs well for many applications. However, it has a low strength to weight ratio compared to other materials. Chro-moly is widely used because of its weldability, ease of fabrication, mild hardenability, and high fatigueability. Commonly wheelchairs are made of tubing 0.028 to 0.035 in. in wall thickness but diameters vary depending on the expected loads between 0.25 and 1.25 in.

More and more of the high-end wheelchairs are made of titanium. Titanium is a lightweight, strong, nonferrous metal. Titanium wheelchair frames are TIG welded. Titanium is the most exotic of the metals used in production wheelchairs and the most expensive. Titanium requires special tooling and skill to be machined and welded. It has very good mechanical properties and high corrosion resistance. It is resilient to wear and abrasion. Titanium is used because of its availability, appearance, corrosion resistance, very good strength and light weight. A drawback of titanium, besides cost, is that titanium once worn or if flawed may break rapidly (i.e., it has a tendency towards brittle fractures).

Advanced composites have been in use in aerospace and industrial applications for a number of years. These materials include Kevlar, carbon fiber, and polyester limestone composite. These materials are now making the transition to wheelchair design. Kevlar is an organic fiber which is yellow in color and soft to the touch. It is extremely strong and tough. It is one of the lightest structural fabrics on today's market. Kevlar is highly resistant to impact, but its compression strength is poor. Carbon fibers are made by changing the molecular structure of rayon fibers by extreme stretching and heating. Carbon fiber is very stiff (high modulus of elasticity), very strong (high tensile strength) and has very low density (weight for a given volume). Composites come as cloth or yarn. Composite cloth is woven into bidirectional or unidirectional cloth. Unidirectional weaves can add strength along a particular direction. Composites must be bound together by resin or epoxy. Generally, polyester resins or various specialty epoxies (e.g., Safe-T-Poxy) are used. To achieve greatest strength a minimum amount of epoxy must be used while wetting all of the fibers. This is often achieved through a process called bagging. To increase the strength and stiffness of structural components a foam (e.g., styrofoam, urethane or PVC) core is used. The strengthening occurs because of the separation of the cloth layers (it now becomes more like a tube than a flat sheet). Polyester limestone composites have been used widely in industrial high voltage electrical component enclosures. A blend of polyester and limestone are used to form a mixture which can be molded under pressure and heated to form a stiff and durable finished product. Polyester limestone composites have high impact strength, and hold tolerances well, but have substantially lower strength to weight ratios than other composites. Their primary advantage is cost, polyester limestone composites are very inexpensive and readily available. Composites can be molded into elaborate shapes which opens a multitude of possibilities for wheelchair design.

69.3.2 Frame Design

Presently all common wheelchair frames center around tubular construction. The tubing can either be welded together, or bolted together using lugs. There are two basic common frame styles: box frame and the cantilever frame. The box frame is named such because of its rectangular shape, and that tubes outline the edges of the "box." Box frames can be very strong and very durable. A cantilever frame is named so because the front and rear wheels, when viewing the chair from the side, appear to be connected by only one tube; this is similar to having the front wheels attached to a cantilever beam fixed at the rear wheels. Both frame types require cross bracing to provide adequate strength and stiffness.

The box frame provides great strength and rigidity. If designed and constructed properly the frame only deflects minimally during normal loading, and most of the suspension is provided by the seat cushion, the wheels and the wheel mounting hardware. Many manufacturers do not triangulate their box frame designs to allow some flexibility. The cantilever frame is based upon a few basic principles (1) the frame can act as a suspension, (2) there are fewer tubes and they are closer to the body which may make the chair less conspicuous, and (3) there are fewer parts and fewer welds which makes the frame easier to construct.

69.3.3 Wheels and Casters

Casters can be as small as 2 in. in diameter or as large as 12 in. in diameter for wheelchairs designed for daily use. Casters are either pneumatic, semi-pneumatic, or solid (polyurethane). Pneumatic casters offer a smoother ride at the cost of increased maintenance, whereas polyurethane casters are very durable. Semi-pneumatic tires offer a compromise. Most active users prefer 5 in. polyurethane casters or 8 in. pneumatic casters for daily use. An 8-in. caster offers a better ride comfort at the expense of foot clearance. Caster foot clearance is maximized with a 2-in. "Roller Blade" caster often used for court sports (e.g., basketball, tennis, and racquetball). Rear wheels come in three common sizes 22, 24, and 26 in. They come in two styles: spoked and MAG. MAG wheels are typically made of plastic and are die cast. MAG wheels require minimal maintenance, and wear well. However, spoked wheels are substantially lighter, more responsive, and are generally preferred by active manual wheelchair users. Rear tires can be two types; pneumatic or puncture proof. Pneumatic tires can either use a separate tube and tire or a combined tube and tire (sew-up). Commonly, a belted rubber tire with a Butyl tube (65 psi) is used. However, those desiring higher performance prefer sew-up tires or Kevlar belted tires with high pressure tubes (180 psi). Puncture proof tires are heavier, provide less suspension, and are less lively than pneumatic tires.

The chair must be designed to optimize the interaction of the wheels with the ground. Four critical performance factors need to be considered (1) Caster Flutter, (2) Caster Float, (3) Tracking, and (4) Alignment. Caster flutter is the shimmy (rapid vibration of the front wheels) that may occur on some surfaces above certain speeds. When one of the casters does not touch the floor when on level ground, the wheelchair has caster float. Caster float decreases the stability and performance of the wheelchair. A manual wheelchair uses rear wheel steering via differential propulsion torque. Tracking is the tendency of the wheelchair/rider to maintain its course once control has been relinquished. Tracking is important, as the rider propels the handrims periodically (about every second) and if the chair does not track well it will drift from its course between pushes and force the rider to correct heading. This will waste valuable energy and reduce control over the chair. Alignment generally refers to the orientation of the rear wheels with respect to one another. Typically, it is desirable to have the rear wheels parallel to one another without any difference between the distance across the two rear wheels at the front and back. Misalignment on the order of 1/8 in. can cause a noticeable increase in the effort required to propel the wheelchair.

69.4 Ergonomics of Wheelchair Propulsion

The most important area of wheelchair design and prescription is determining the proper interaction between the wheelchair and the user. This can lead to reducing the risk of developing repetitive strain injury while maximizing mobility. Cardiovascular fitness can be improved through exercise which requires a properly fitted wheelchair.

69.4.1 Kinematics

Kinematic data by itself does not provide sufficient information for the clinician to implement appropriate rehabilitation intervention strategies or for the engineer to incorporate this information into wheelchair design changes. Kinematic data are commonly collected at 60 Hz, which is the maximum frequency of many videotape-based systems. Kinematic data analysis shows that experienced wheelchair users contact the pushrim behind top-dead-center and push to nearly 90° in front of top-dead-center. This is significantly longer than non-wheelchair users. Lengthening the stroke permits lowering the propulsion moment and may place less stress on the users' joints.

An important aspect of the evaluation, and possible retraining of wheelchair users is to determine the optimal stroke kinetics and kinematics [2]. However, there is typically some degree of variation from one stroke to another. Wheelchair propulsion kinematic data are typically cyclic (i.e., a person repeats or nearly repeats his/her arm motions over several strokes). Each marker of the kinematic model (e.g., shoulder, elbow, wrist, knuckle) of each subject generates an x and y set of data which is periodic. The frequencies of the x and y data are dependent upon the anthropometry of the individual, the construction of the wheelchair, and the speed of propulsion. The periodic nature of the kinematic data for wheelchair propulsion can be exploited to develop a characteristic stroke from a set of kinematic data (with the rear hub of the wheelchair chosen as the origin) including several strokes.

69.4.2 Kinetics

The SMART[wheel] was developed to measure the pushrim forces required for evaluating net joint forces and moments to allow the clinician and researcher to study the level of stress experienced by the joint structures during wheelchair propulsion. The SMART[wheel] uses a standard wheelchair wheel fitted with three beams 120° apart and each has two full strain gage bridges. The strain gage bridges are each interfaced through an instrumentation amplifier to a micro-controller which transmits the data through a mercury slip-ring to the serial port of a computer. Kinetics of wheelchair propulsion are affected by speed of propulsion, injury level, user experience, and wheelchair type and fit. Van Der Woude et al. have reported on an ergometer which detected torque by way of a force transducer located in the wheel center and attached to what is referred to as the "wheel/hand rim construction" [7]. The ergometer was adjusted for each subject's anthropometric measurements. Data were sampled at 100 Hz for 7.5 sec periods with a digital filter cut-off frequency of 10 Hz. Mean and peak torque increased with mean velocity, a maximum mean peak torque of 31 N-m occurred at 1.27 m/sec. Torque curves of inexperienced subjects showed an initial negative deflection and a dip in the rising portion of the curve. Torque curves were reported to be in agreement with results of previous investigations [8–10].

Brauer and Hertig [12] measured the static torque produced on push-rims which were rigidly restrained by springs and mounted independent of the tires and rims of the wheelchair. The spring system was adjustable for the subject's strength. The wheels were locked in a fixed position. Torque was measured using slide-wire resistors coupled to the differential movements between the push-rim and wheels and recorded using a strip chart recorder. Subjects were asked to grasp the push-rim at six different test positions (−10, 0, 10, 20, 30, and 40 degrees relative to vertical) and to use maximal effort to turn both wheels forward. Male subjects (combined ambulatory and wheelchair users) produced torques of 27.9 to 46.6 N-m and female subjects produced torques of 17.1 to 32.1 N-m [12]. Grip location, handedness, grip strength, and how well the test wheelchair fit the anthropometric measurements of the individual affected the torque generated. Problems encountered were slipperiness of the push-rims due to a polished finish and limited contact due to the small diameter of the push-rim tubing (12.7 mm or 1/2 in). The use of one wheelchair for all subjects presented the problem of variations due to inappropriate fit for some individuals.

Brubaker, Ross, and McLaurin [13] examined the effect of horizontal and vertical seat position (relative to the wheel position) on the generation of static push-rim force. Force was measured using a test platform with a movable seat and strain gauged beams to which the push-rims were mounted. Pushing and pulling forces were recorded using a strip chart recorder. Static force was measured for four grip positions (−30, 0, 30, and 60 degrees) with various seat positions. Push-rim force ranged from approximately 500 to 750 N and varied considerably with seat position and rim position [13].

69.4.3 Net Joint Forces and Moments

Net joint forces and moments acting at the wrist, elbow and shoulder during wheelchair propulsion provide scientists and clinicians with information related to the level of stress borne by the joint structure. Joint moments and forces are calculated using limb segment and joint models, anthropometric data, kinetic data, and kinematic data. Joint moments data shows that forces at each joint vary among subjects in terms of peak forces, where they occur during the propulsion phase, and how quickly they develop. Peak net joint moments occur at different joint angles for different subjects, and conditions (e.g., speed, resistance). Convention for joint angles is that 180 degrees at the elbow represents full extension; while at the wrist, this is the hand in the neutral position (flexion less than 180 degrees and extension greater than 180 degrees). Joint angles at the shoulder are determined between the arm and the trunk, with zero measured at the point where the trunk and arm are aligned. Wheelchair users show maximum net shoulder moment between 20° and 40° of extension. Some wheelchair users also show a rapid rise in the elbow extensor moment at the beginning of the stroke with the elbow at about 120°. This moment value begins to decrease between 150° and 170°. At the wrist, the peak moments occur between 190° and 220°. Net joint moments and force models need to account for hand center of pressure, inaccuracies in anthropometric data, and joint models related to clinical variables.

69.5   Power Wheelchair Electrical Systems

Some people are impaired to an extent that they would have no mobility without a power wheelchair. However, some people may have limited upper body mobility and may have the ability to propel a manual wheelchair for short distances. These people may liken using a power wheelchair to admitting defeat. However, a power wheelchair may provide greater mobility. In such cases it may be best to suggest a power wheelchair for longer excursions, and a manual wheelchair for in home and recreational use.

69.5.1   User Interface

Power wheelchairs are often used in conjunction with a number of other adaptive devices. For people with severe mobility impairments, power wheelchairs may be used with communication devices, computer access devices, respirators, and reclining seating systems. The integration of the users' multiple needs must also be considered when designing or prescribing a power wheelchair.

The joystick is the most common control interface between the user and the wheelchair. Joysticks produce voltage signals proportional to displacement, force, or switch closures. Displacement joysticks are most popular. Displacement joysticks may use either potentiometers, variable inductors (coils) or optical sensors to convert displacement to voltage. Inductive joysticks are most common as they wear well and they can be made quite sensitive. Joysticks can be modified to be used for chin, foot, elbow, tongue or shoulder control. Typically, short throw joysticks are used for these applications. Force sensing joysticks use three basic transducers: simple springs and dampeners on a displacement joystick, cantilever beams with strain gages, and fluid with pressure sensors. Force sensing joysticks which rely on passive dampeners or fluid pressure generally require the user to have a range of motion within normal values for displacement joysticks users. Beam-based force sensing joysticks require negligible motion, and hence may be used for people with limited motion abilities.

People who exhibit intention or spastic tremor or with multiple sclerosis may require special control considerations. Signal processing techniques are often required to grant the user greater control over the wheelchair. Typically, signal averaging or a low pass filter with a cut-off frequency of below 5 Hz is used. The signal processing is typically incorporated into the controller.

Some people lack the fine motor control to effectively use a joystick. An alternative for these people is to use a switch control or a head position control. A switch control simply uses either a set of switches or a single switch and a coded input, that is, Morse code or some other simple switch code. The input of the user is latched by the controller and the wheelchair performs the task commanded by the user. The user may latch the chair to repeatedly perform a task a specified number of times, for example, continue straight until commanded to do otherwise. Switch control is quite functional, but it is generally slower than joystick control. Switch inputs can be generated in many ways. Typically, low pressure switches are used. The input can come from a sip-and-puff mechanism which works off of a pressure transducer. A switch contact is detected when the pressure exceeds or drops below a threshold. The pressure sensor may be configured to react to pressure generated by the user blowing into or sipping from an input or by the user simply interrupting the flow in or out of a tube. Sip-and-puff may also be used as a combination of proportional and switch control. For example, the user can put the control in the "read speed" mode and then the proportional voltage output from the pressure transducer will be latched as the user-desired speed.

Simple switches of various sizes can be used to control the chair using many parts of the body. Switches may be mounted on the armrests or a lap tray for hand or arm activation, on the footrest(s) for foot activation, or on a head rest for head activation. The motion of the head can also be used for proportional control by using ultrasonic sensors. Ultrasonic sensors can be mounted in an array about the headrest. The signal produced by the ultrasonic sensors is related to the position of the head. Hence, motion of the head can be used to create a proportional control signal. Ultrasonic head control and switch control can be combined to give some users greater mastery over their power wheelchair. Switches can be used to select the controller mode, whereas the ultrasonic sensors give a proportional input signal.

A critical consideration when selecting or designing a user interface is that the ability of the user to accurately control the interface is heavily dependent upon the stability of the user within the wheelchair. Often custom seating and postural support systems are required for a user interface to be truly effective. The placement of the user interface is also critical to its efficacy as a functional control device.

69.5.2 Integrated Controls

People with severe physical impairments may only be able to effectively manipulate a single input device. Integrated controls are used to facilitate using a single input device (e.g., joystick, head switches, voice recognition system) to control multiple actuators (e.g., power wheelchair, environmental control unit, manipulator). This provides the user with greater control over the environment. The M3S-Multiple Master Multiple Slave bus is designed to provide simple, reliable access to a variety of assistive devices. Assistive devices include input devices, actuators, and end-effectors. M3S is based on the Computer Area Network (CAN) standard.

A wide range of organizations provide assistive devices which offer the opportunity of functioning in a more independent manner. However, many of these devices and systems are developed without coordination resulting in incompatible products. Clinicians and users often desire to combine products from various sources to achieve maximal independence. The result is to have several devices with their own input devices and overlapping functions. Integrated controls provide access to various end-effectors with a single input device. The M3S provides an electronic communication protocol so that the system operates properly.

M3S is an interface specification with a basic hardware architecture, a bus communication protocol, and a configuration method. The M3S standard incorporates CAN plus two additional lines for greater security (i.e., 7 wire bus, 2 power lines, 2 CAN lines, safety lines, 1 shield, and 1 harness line). The system can be configured to each individual's needs. An M3S system consists of a microcontroller in each device and a control and configuration module (CCM). The CCM insures proper signal processing, system configuration, and safety monitoring. The CCM is linked to a display (e.g., visual, auditory, tactile) which allows the user to select and operate each end-effector. Any M3S compatible device can communicate with another M3S compatible device. M3S is an International Organization of Standards (ISO) open system communication implementation.

69.5.3 Power System

To implement a motor controller, a servo-amplifier is required to convert signal level power (volts at milliamps) to motor power (volts at amps). Typically, a design requirement for series, shunt, and brushless motor drives is to control torque and speed, and hence, power. Voltage control can often be used to control speed for both shunt and series motors. Series motors require feedback to achieve accurate control.

Either a linear servo-amplifier or a chopper can be used. Linear servo amplifiers are not generally used with power wheelchairs primarily because of their lower efficiency than chopper circuits. A motor can be thought of as a filter to a chopper circuit, in this case, the switching unit can be used as part of a speed and current control loop. The torque ripple and noise associated with phase control drives can be avoided by the use of high switching frequencies. The response of the speed control loop is likewise improved with increasing switching frequency.

Motor torque is proportional to the armature current in shunt motors and to the square of the current in series motors. The conduction loss of the motor and servo-amplifier are both proportional to the current squared. Optimal efficiency is achieved by minimizing the form factor (I_{rms}/I_{mean}). This can be done by increasing the switching frequency to reduce the amplitude of the ripple. Benefits of increased efficiency are increased brush life, gear life, and lower probability of field permanent magnet demagnetization.

Switching or chopper drives are classified as either unidirectional or bi-directional. They are further divided by whether they use dynamic braking. Typically, power wheelchairs use bi-directional drives without dynamic braking. However, scooters may use unidirectional drives. The average voltage delivered to the motor from a switching drive is controlled by varying the duty cycle of the input waveform. There are two common methods of achieving this goal (1) fixed pulse width, variable repetition rate, and (2) pulse-width modulation (PWM). Power wheelchair servo-amplifiers typically employ PWM.

Pulse width modulation at a fixed frequency has no minimum on-time restriction. Therefore, current peaking and torque ripple can be minimized. For analysis, a d.c. motor can be modeled as a RL circuit, resistor and inductor, or in series with a voltage source. If the motor current is assumed continuous, then the minimum and maximum motor current can be represented by the following equation:

$$I_{min} = \frac{e^{-(R/L)t_{off}}\left(1 - e^{-(R/L)t_{on}}\right)}{1 - e^{-(R/L)(t_{on}-t_{off})}}\frac{V_s}{R} - \frac{V_{gen}}{R}$$

$$I_{max} = \frac{1 - e^{-(R/L)t_{on}}}{1 - e^{-(R/L)(t_{on}-t_{off})}}\frac{V_s}{R} - \frac{V_{gen}}{R}$$

Two basic design principles are used when designing switching servo-amplifiers (1) I_{max} should be limited to five times the rated current of the motor to ensure that demagnetization does not occur, (2) the ripple, ($I_{max}-I_{min}$)/I_{avg}, should be minimized to improve the form factor, and reduce the conduction loss in the switching devices. To achieve low ripple, either the inductance has to be large or the switching frequency has to be high. Permalloy powder cores can be used to reduce core loss at frequencies above a few kilohertz. However, this comes at the cost of the electrical time constant of the motor, degrading the motor response time. Hence, raising the switching frequency is most desirable. A power MOSFET has the ability to switch rapidly without the use of load-shaping components.

There are several motor types that may be suitable for use with power wheelchairs. Most current designs use permanent magnet direct current motors. These motors provide high torque, high starting torque and are simplest to control. Permanent magnet direct current motors can either be controlled in what are commonly called current mode or voltage mode. These modes developed out of designs based upon controlling torque and speed, respectively.

Alternating current motors can be designed to be highly efficient and can be controlled with modern power circuitry. Because of the development and wide spread dissemination of switching direct current converters, it is quite feasible to use alternating current motors with a battery supply. To date, alternating current motors have only been used in research on power wheelchairs. The output of the motor is controlled by varying the phase or the frequency.

The battery energy storage system is recognized as one of the most significant limiting factors in powered wheelchair performance. Battery life and capacity are important. If battery life can be improved, the powered wheelchair user will have longer, reliable performance from his/her battery. An increase in battery capacity will allow powered wheelchair users to travel greater distances with batteries that weigh and measure the same as existing wheelchair batteries. Most importantly, increases in battery capacity will enable the use of smaller and lighter batteries. Because batteries account for such a large proportion of both the weight and volume of current powered wheelchair systems, wheelchair manufacturers must base much of their design around the battery package.

TABLE 69.1 Standard Power Wheelchair Battery Group Sizes

Group number	Length	Width	Height
U1	7–3/4	5–3/16	7–5/16
22NF	9–7/16	5–1/2	8–15/16
24	10–1/4	6–13/16	8–7/8
27	12–1/16	6–13/16	8–7/8

Note: Units are in inches.

Power wheelchairs typically incorporate 24 V d.c. energy systems. The energy for the wheelchair is provided by two, deep cycle lead-acid batteries connected in series. Either wet cell or gel cell batteries are used. Wet cell batteries also cost about one-half as much as gel cell batteries. Gel cells may be required for transport by commercial air carriers.

Battery technology for wheelchair users remains unchanged despite the call for improvements by power wheelchair users. This may be in part due to the relatively low number of units purchased, about 500,000 per annum, when compared to automotive applications with about 6.6 million per annum by a single manufacturer. Wheelchair batteries are typically rated at 12 V and 30 to 90 ampere-h capacity at room temperature. A power wheelchair draws about 10 A during use. The range of the power wheelchair is directly proportional to the ampere-hour rating for the operating temperature.

Batteries are grouped by size. Group size is indicated by a standard number. The group size defines the dimensions of the battery as shown in Table 69.1. The ampere-hour rating defines the battery's capacity.

It is important that the appropriate charger be used with each battery set. Many battery chargers automatically reduce the amount of current delivered to the battery as the battery reaches full charge. This helps to prevent damage to the battery from boiling. The rate at which wet and gel cell batteries charge is significantly different. Some chargers are capable of operating with both types of batteries. Many require setting the charger for the appropriate battery type. Most wheelchair batteries connected in series are charged simultaneously with a 24 V battery charger.

69.5.4 Electromagnetic Compatibility

Powered wheelchairs have been reported to exhibit unintended movement. Wheelchair manufacturers and the US Food and Drug Administration Center for Devices and Radiological Health (FDA-CDRH) have examined the susceptibility of powered wheelchairs and scooters to interference from radio and microwave transmissions. These devices are tested at frequencies ranging from 26 MHz to 1 GHz, which is common for transmissions (e.g., radio, TV, microwave, telephones, mobile radios). Power wheelchairs incorporate complex electronics and microcontrollers which are sensitive to electromagnetic (EM) radiation, electrostatic discharge (ESD), and other energy sources.

Electric powered wheelchairs may be susceptible to electromagnetic interference (EMI) present in the ambient environment. Some level of EMI immunity is necessary to ensure the safety of power wheelchair users. Electromagnetic compatibility (EMC) is the term used to describe how devices and systems behave in an electromagnetic environment. Because of the complexity of power wheelchairs and scooters, and the interaction with an electromagnetic environment, susceptibility to interference cannot be calculated or estimated reliably. A significant number of people attach accessories (e.g., car stereos, computers, communication systems) to their power wheelchairs which also share the batteries. This may increase the susceptibility of other system components to EMI. A number of companies make electric powered devices designed to operate on power wheelchairs to provide postural support, pressure relief, environmental control, and motor vehicle operation. These devices may alter the EMI compatibility of power wheelchairs as provided by the original equipment manufacturer (OEM). Wheelchairs and accessories can be made to function properly within EM environments through testing.

Field strengths have been measured at 20 V/m from a 15 W hand held cellular telephone, and 8 V/m from a 1 W hand held cellular telephone [2]. The FDA-CDRH has tested power wheelchairs and scooters in a Gigahertz Transverse Electromagnetic (GTEM) cell, and in an anechoic chamber with exposure strengths from 3 to 40 V/m. The US FDA requires that a warning sticker be placed on each power wheelchair or scooter indicating the risk due to EMI.

Two tests are commonly performed on chairs: brake release and variation in wheel speed. The device(s) used for measuring wheel speed and brake release must not significantly alter the field. The brakes shall not release or the wheels are not to move with a wheel torque equivalent to a 1:6 slope with a 100 kg rider when the wheelchair is exposed to EM radiation. Non-electrical contact methods (e.g., audio sensing, optical sensing) of measuring brake release or wheelchair movement are preferable. Nominal wheel speed may drift over the length of the test. This drift is primarily due to drop in battery charge over the test interval. Wheel speed must be recorded without EM interference between test intervals. The percentage change in wheel speed during exposure to EM interference shall be referenced to the nominal wheel speed for that test interval. The variation in absolute forward speed, $(v_{emR} + v_{emL})/2$, is to be within 30% of the nominal forward speed, $(v_{nomR} + v_{nomL})/2$. The differential speed between the two wheels should be within 30% of each other, $2 \cdot (v_{emR} - v_{emL})/(v_{nomR} + v_{nomL})$. The test frequency must be held long enough to accommodate the slowest time constant (time required to reach 63% of maximum or minimum) of parameters related to wheelchair driving behavior. Currently two seconds is used by the FDA-CDRH test laboratory.

69.6 Personal Transportation

Special adaptive equipment requirements increase with the degree of impairment and desired degree of independence in areas such as personal care, mobility, leisure, personal transportation, and employment. People are concerned that they receive the proper equipment for them to safely operate their vehicle. Access and egress equipment have the greatest maintenance requirements. Other devices such as hand controls, steering equipment, securement mechanisms, and interior controls require less maintenance. Most users of adaptive driving equipment are satisfied with the performance of such equipment. Most frequent equipment problems are minor and are repaired by consumers themselves.

Physical functional abilities such as range of motion, manual muscle strength, sensation, grip strength, pinch strength, fine motor dexterity, and hand-eye coordination all may be related to driving potential. Driving characteristics must also be evaluated when determining an individual's potential to safely operate a motor vehicle. Throttle force, brake force, steering force, brake reaction time, and steering reaction time are all factors which influence an individual's driving potential.

69.6.1 Vehicle Selection

While it is often a difficult task to find an automobile which meets the specific needs of a particular wheelchair user, currently, no automobile meets the needs of all wheelchair users. Automotive consumers with disabilities are also concerned about ease of entry, stowage space for the wheelchair, and seat positioning. Reduced size, increasingly sloping windshields, lower roofs, and higher sills of new cars make selecting a new vehicle difficult for wheelchair users. The ability to load the wheelchair into a vehicle is essential. Some individuals with sufficient strength and a suitable vehicle are able to stow their wheelchairs inside the vehicle without the use of assistive devices. Many people must rely on an external loading device. The selection of the appropriate vehicle should be based upon the client's physical abilities and social needs.

An approach some people have used to overcome the problems associated with a smaller car is to use a car-top wheelchair carrying device. These devices lift the wheelchair to the top of the car, fold, and stow it. They have been designed to work with four door sedans, light trucks, and compact automobiles.

TABLE 69.2 Typical Ranges of
Accessibility Dimensions for
Sedans

Wheelbase	93–108
Door height	33–47
Door width	41–47
Headroom	36–39
Max. Space behind seat	9–19
Min. Space behind seat	4–9
Seat-to-ground distance	18–22
Width of door opening	38–51

Note: Units in inches.

There are several critical dimensions to an automobile when determining wheelchair accessibility. The wheelbase of the automobile is often used by auto manufacturers to determine vehicle size (e.g., full-size, mid-size, compact). Typical ranges for passenger vehicles are presented in Table 69.2.

69.6.2 Lift Mechanisms

Many wheelchair users who cannot transfer into a passenger vehicle seat or prefer a larger vehicle, drive vans equipped with wheelchair lifts. Platform lifts may use a lifting track, a parallelogram lifting linkage, or a rotary lift. Lift devices are either electromechanically or electrohydraulically powered. The platform often folds into the side doorway of the van. Crane lifts, also called swing-out lifts, have a platform which elevates and folds or rotates into the van. Lifts may either be semi-automatic or automatic. In many cases semi-automatic lifts require the user to initiate various stages (e.g., unlocking door, door opening, lowering lift) of the lifting process. Automatic lifts are designed to perform all lift functions. They usually have an outside key operated control box, or an interior radio controlled control box.

Some lifts use electrohydraulic actuators to lift and fold, with valves and gravity used to lower the lift. Crane lifts may swing out from a post at the front or rear of the side door. Interlocking mechanisms are available with some lifts to prevent the lift from being operated while the door is closed. The Society of Automotive Engineers (SAE) has developed guidelines for the testing of wheelchair lift devices for entry and exit from a personal vehicle. The standards are intended to set an acceptable level of reliability and performance for van lifts.

69.6.3 Wheelchair Restraint Mechanisms

Securement systems are used to temporarily attach wheelchairs to vehicles during transport. Many wheelchair users can operate a motor vehicle from their wheelchair, but are unable to transfer into a vehicle seat. Auto safety standards have reduced the number of U.S. automobile accident fatalities despite an increase in the number of vehicles. The crash pulse determines the severity of the collision of the test sled, and hence, simulates real-world conditions. Securement systems are tested with a surrogate wheelchair at 30 miles per h (48 +2/−0 km per h) with a 20g deceleration. Wheelchairs must be safely restrained when experiencing an impact of this magnitude and no part of the wheelchair shall protrude into the occupant space where it might cause injury.

Proper use of lap and shoulder belts is critical to protecting passengers in automobiles seats. A similar level of crash protection is required for individuals who remain in their wheelchairs during transportation. Wheelchairs are flexible, higher than a standard automobile seat, and not fixed to the vehicle. The passenger is restrained using a harness of at least one belt to provide pelvic restraint and two shoulder or torso belts that restrain both shoulders. A head support may also be used to prevent rearward motion of the head during impact or rebound. A three point restraint is the combination of a lap belt and a shoulder belt (e.g., pelvic torso restraint, lap-sash restraint, lap-shoulder restraint).

The relationship between injury criteria and the mechanics of restraint systems are important to insure the safety of wheelchair users in motor vehicles. Hip and head deflection are often used criteria for determining potential injury. The automotive industry has invested considerable effort for research and development to protect vehicle passengers. Research is not nearly extensive for the passenger who remains seated in a wheelchair while traveling. Many wheelchair and occupant restraint systems copy the designs used for standard automobile seats. However, this type of design may not be appropriate.

Crash tests have shown that for 10 or 20 g impacts of 100 msec duration, people may sustain injuries despite being restrained. When shoulder belts mounted 60 in. above the floor were used to restrain a 50th percentile male dummy, it was found that the torso was well controlled, and head and chest excursions were limited. When shoulder belts were anchored 36 in. above the floor they were ineffective in controlling torso movement. Kinematic results and head injury criteria (HIC) can be used to estimate the extent of injury sustained by a human passenger. A HIC of 1000 or greater indicates a serious or fatal head injury. Generally, a HIC value approaching or exceeding 1000 is indicative of head impact with some portion of the vehicle interior. The open space typically surrounding a wheelchair user in a public bus precludes impact with the buses' interior. High HIC values may occur when the torso is effectively restrained and there is a high degree of neck flexion. If the chin strikes the chest then there may be an impact great enough to cause head injury.

69.6.4 Hand Controls

Hand-controls are available for automatic and manual transmission vehicles. However, hand-controls for manual transmission automobiles must be custom made. There are also portable hand-controls, and long-term hand controls. Portable hand-controls are designed to easily attach to most common automobiles with a minimal number of tools. Hand-controls are available for either left or right hand control.

Many hand controls are attached to the steering column. Hand-controls either clamp to the steering column or are attached to a bracket which is bolted to the steering column or dash, typically where the steering column bolts to the dash. Installation of the hand-controls should not interfere with driver safety features (e.g., air bags, collapsible steering columns). The push rods of the hand-control either clamp directly to the pedals or the levers connected to them.

Most systems activate the brakes by having the driver push forward on a lever with a hand grip. This allows the driver to push against the back of the seat, creating substantial force, and braces the driver in the event of a collision. The throttle, or gas pedal, is operated in a number of ways. Some systems use a twist knob or motorcycle type throttle. Other systems actuate the throttle by pulling on the brake throttle lever. Another method is to rotate the throttle-brake lever downwards (i.e., pull the lever towards the thigh at a right angle to the brake application to operate the throttle). It is common to have the same vehicle driven by multiple people which may require the vehicle to be safely operated with hand-controls, and the OEM foot controls. Care must be taken to insure that the lever and brackets of the hand-controls do not restrict the driving motions of foot control drivers.

Many people have the motor control necessary to operate a motor vehicle, but they do not have the strength required to operate manual hand-controls. Automatic or Fly-By-Wire hand-controls use external actuators (e.g., air motors, servo mechanisms, hydraulic motors) to reduce the force required to operate various vehicle primary controls. Power steering, power brakes, six-way power seats, and power adjustable steering columns can be purchased as factory options on many vehicles.

Six-way power seats are used to provide greater postural support and positioning than standard automotive seats. They can be controlled by a few switches to move fore-aft, incline-recline, and superior-inferior. This allows the user to position the seat for easy entry and exit, and for optimal driving comfort. Power adjustable steering columns also make vehicles more accessible. By using a few buttons, the steering column can be tilted upwards or downwards allowing positioning for entry/exist into the vehicle, and for optimal driving control.

Custom devices are available for people who require more than the OEM options for power assistance. Microprocessor and electronic technology have dramatically changed how motor vehicles are designed.

Many functions of an automobile are controlled electronically or with electromechanical-electrohydraulic controls. This change in vehicle design has made a wide variety of options available for people who require advanced vehicle controls. Many automobiles use electronic fuel injection. Electronic fuel injection systems convert the position of the accelerator pedal to a serial digital signal which is used by a microcontroller to inject the optimal fuel-air mixture into the automobile at the proper time during the piston stroke. The electronic signal for the accelerator position can be provided by another control device (e.g., joystick, slide-bar).

References

[1] Adams, T.C. and Reger, S.I. 1993, Factors affecting wheelchair occupant injury in crash simulation. *Proceedings of the 16th Annual RESNA Conference*, Las Vegas, NV, pp. 80–82.

[2] Adams, T.C., Sauer, B., and Reger, S.I. 1992, Kinematics of the wheelchair seated body in crash simulation. *Proceedings of the RESNA International '92*, Toronto, Ontario, Canada, pp. 360–362.

[3] Asato, K.T., Cooper, R.A., Robertson, R.N., and Ster, J.F. 1993, SMART^{Wheels}: development and testing of a system for measuring manual wheelchair propulsion dynamics, *IEEE Trans. Biomed. Eng.*, 40: 1320–1324.

[4] Aylor, J.H., Thieme, A., and Johnson, B.W. 1992, A battery state-of-charge indicator, *IEEE Trans. Ind. Electr.*, 39: 398–409.

[5] Boninger, M.L., Cooper, R.A., Robertson, R.N., and Shimada, S.D. 1997, Three-dimensional pushrim forces during two speeds of wheelchair propulsion, *Am. J. Phys. Med. Rehabil.*, 76: 420–426.

[6] Brauer, R.L. and Hertig, B.A. 1981, Torque generation on wheelchair handrims, *Proceedings of the 1981 Biomechanics Symposium, ASME/ASCE Mechanics Conference*, pp. 113–116.

[7] Brienza, D.M., Cooper, R.A., and Brubaker, C.E. 1996, Wheelchairs and seating, *Curr. Opin. Orthop.*, 7:82–86.

[8] Brubaker, C.E., Ross, S., and McLaurin, C.A. 1982, Effect of seat position on handrim force, *Proceedings of the 5th Annual Conference on Rehabilitation Engineering*, p. 111.

[9] Cooper, R.A. 1998, *Wheelchair Selection and Configuration*, Demos Medical Publishers, New York, NY.

[10] Gray, D.B., Quatrano, L.A., and Lieberman, M.L. 1998, *Designing and Using Assistive Technology*, Brookes Publishing Company, Baltimore, MD.

[11] Cooper, R.A., Trefler E., and Hobson D.A. 1996, Wheelchairs and seating: issues and practice, *Technol. Disability*, 5:3–16.

[12] Cooper, R.A. 1995, Intelligent control of power wheelchairs, *IEEE Eng. Med. Biol. Mag.*, 15:423–431.

[13] Cooper, R.A. 1995, *Rehabilitation Engineering Applied to Mobility and Manipulation*, Institute of Physics Publishing, Bristol, United Kingdom.

[14] Cooper, R.A., Gonzalez, J.P., Lawrence, B.M., Rentschler, A., Boninger, M.L., and VanSickle, D.P. 1997, Performance of selected lightweight wheelchairs on ANSI/RESNA tests, *Arch. Phys. Med. Rehabil.*, 78:1138–1144.

[15] Cooper, R.A. 1996, A perspective on the ultralight wheelchair revolution, *Technol. Disabil.*, 5:383–392.

[16] Cooper, R.A., Robertson, R.N., Lawrence, B., Heil, T., Albright S.J., VanSickle, D.P., and Gonzalez J.P. 1996, Life-cycle analysis of depot versus rehabilitation manual wheelchairs, *J. Rehab. Res. Dev.*, 33:45–55.

[17] Cooper, R.A. 1993, Stability of a wheelchair controlled by a human pilot, *IEEE Trans. Rehabil. Eng.*, 1:193–206.

[18] Cooper, R.A., Baldini, F.D., Langbein, W.E., Robertson R.N., Bennett P., and Monical, S. 1993, Prediction of pulmonary function in wheelchair users, *Paraplegia*, 31:560–570.

[19] Cooper, R.A., Horvath, S.M., Bedi, J.F., Drechsler-Parks D.M., and Williams R.E. 1992, Maximal exercise responses of paraplegic wheelchair road racers, *Paraplegia*, 30:573–581.

[20] Cooper, R.A. 1991, System identification of human performance models, *IEEE Trans. Syst., Man, Cybern.*, 21:244–252.

[21] Cooper, R.A. 1991, High tech wheelchairs gain the competetive edge, *IEEE Eng. Med. Biol. Mag.*, 10:49–55.

[22] Kauzlarich, J.J., Ulrich, V., Bresler, M., and Bruning, T. 1983, Wheelchair batteries: driving cycles and testing, *J. Rehabil. Res. Dev.*, 20:31–43.

[23] MacLeish, M.S., Cooper, R.A., Harralson, J., and Ster, J.F. 1993, Design of a composite monocoque frame racing wheelchair, *J. Rehabil. Res. Dev.*, 30:233–249.

[24] Powell, F. and Inigo, R.M. 1992, Microprocessor based D.C. brushless motor controller for wheelchair propulsion. *Proceedings of the RESNA International '92*, Toronto, Canada, pp. 313–315.

[25] Riley, P.O. and Rosen M.J. 1987, Evaluating manual control devices for those with tremor disability, *J. Rehabil. Res. Dev.*, 24:99–110.

[26] Sprigle, S.H., Morris, B.O., and Karg, P.E. 1992, Assessment of transportation technology: survey of driver evaluators. *Proceedings of the RESNA International '92*, Toronto, Ontario, Canada, pp. 351–353.

[27] Sprigle, S.H., Morris, B.O., and Karg, P.E. 1992, Assessment of transportation technology: survey of equipment vendors. *Proceedings of the RESNA International '92*, Toronto, Ontario, Canada, pp. 354–356.

[28] Schauer, J., Kelso, D.P., and Vanderheiden, G.C. 1990, Development of a serial auxiliary control interface for powered wheelchairs. *Proceedings of the RESNA 13th Annual Conference* Washington, D.C., pp. 191–192.

70

Externally Powered and Controlled Orthoses and Prostheses

Dejan B. Popović

University of Belgrade and Aalborg University

Rehabilitation of humans with sensory–motor disability requires effective assistive systems that would allow their fast and maximal reintegration into the normal life. The cost-benefit functions that humans with disability likely appreciate and optimize comprise elements, such as (1) the quality of life measured by reintegration into the social and work environments; (2) reliability of the assistive system; (3) energy rate and cost with respect to the one used for accomplishing the same task with alternative methods; (4) disruption of normal activities when employing the assistive system; (5) cosmetics; (6) maintenance; and (7) cost. The same elements are considered, but, in a different order by the developers of the rehabilitation technology, practitioners of physical medicine, and rehabilitation and health-care providers.

Here we present technical aspects of the available externally powered orthoses and prostheses that interface directly or indirectly with the human neuro-musculo-skeletal system. We elaborate here two methods for the restoration of movements in humans with paralysis: functional activation of paralyzed muscles termed functional electrical stimulation (FES) or functional neuromuscular stimulation (FNS or NMS), and parallel application of FES and a mechanical orthosis called hybrid assistive system (HAS). We also describe externally controlled and powered leg and arm/hand prostheses.

70.1 Neural Prostheses Based on FES

Assistive systems that apply FES to restore sensory or motor function are called neural prostheses. A **neural prosthesis** (NP) could improve sensory or motor function in subjects after cerebro-vascular accident (CVA), spinal cord injury (SCI), and some other diseases of the central nervous (CNS) [1]. A motor NP applies electrical stimulation to artificially generate muscle contractions required for executing of a functional task in subjects who have lost voluntary control because of a disease or injury. The basic phenomena of the FES are the contraction of a muscle due to the direct stimulation of motorneurons, and reflexive responses due to the activation of sensory pathways and CNS. A NP sends a burst of short electric pulses (pulse duration: 0 to 250 μsec, pulse amplitude: 10 to 150 mA) to generate a function. The key element for achieving functional movement is the appropriate sequencing of bursts of electrical pulses. To achieve a smooth contraction of the extremity the burst of pulses has to have a frequency of about 20 pulses/sec. If less than 20 pulses/sec are induced into the motor nerve the muscle generates a series of twitches, instead of a fused smooth contraction of the muscle. In order to generate stronger force (tetanic contraction) higher frequencies (e.g., 30 to 50 pulses/sec) need to be applied. The higher the stimulation, the more the fatigue that will be developed in the stimulated muscle. Other types of stimulation (e.g., intermittent stimulation, use of doublets or n-plets) could improve the force vs. fatigue ratio. If the motor nerve is missing, then the muscle becomes denervated and it cannot generate functional force by means of NP. Recently, new methods were suggested that claim to be applicable for stimulation of denervated muscles [2,3]. The motor nerves can be stimulated using monophasic and biphasic current or voltage pulses. The monophasic pulses are used only with the surface electrodes because they lead to unbalanced charge delivery to the tissues, potentially causing the damage. Most NPs implement monophasic compensated current or voltage pulses.

The motor nerves can be stimulated using either surface (transcutaneous), percutaneous, or implanted electrodes. The transcutaneous stimulation is performed with self-adhesive or nonadhesive electrodes that are placed on the subject's skin in the vicinity of the motor point of the muscle that needs to be stimulated. Recently, new technology that uses electrode arrays positioned on the skin instead of single-filed electrodes was suggested [4]. This electrode array allows variation of the stimulation effects without moving of the electrode (e.g., simultaneous control of agonist and antagonistic muscles resulting with the variable stiffness of the joint, in parallel with the strong activation of the prime movers needed for the desired movement, and dynamic adaptation to the change of the position of the muscle vs. electrode during the movement) [5].

The alternative to surface electrodes is the implantable electrodes. One type of electrodes are wire electrodes that are applied percutaneously, that is, the electrode connects to the stimulator outside of the body, while the stimulation point is close to the motor point (inside the body). Another option is fully implantable electrodes that are sutured to the fascia placed close to the entry point of the motor nerve (epimysial electrodes). More recently, cuff electrodes have been introduced as the NP interface to the tissues. The cuff electrode allows selective stimulation of specific nerve fascicles. Implanted electrodes compared to surface electrodes guarantee higher stimulation selectivity with much less electrical charge applied, both being desired characteristics of NPs. The technology that was introduced few years ago use miniature implantable stimulator that communicates with the external unit via radio-frequency electromagnetic field. The current version of the small implants called Bion comprises the rechargeable battery that is charged when not used and is discharged during operation [6–8].

70.1.1 Restoration of Hand Functions

During the last 50 years several NPs for grasping have been designed and tested; yet, only few were brought to the market [9–11]. An important recent finding is that NPs have therapeutic effects if applied appropriately and timely [12]. The proof of the long-term therapeutic effect of NPs could be the milestone for the health-care providers to change their attitude and start paying for this important rehabilitation modality.

The neural prosthesis for grasping is most frequently used to help tetraplegic subjects to restore or hemiplegic patients to promote the recovery of the grasping function. Among tetraplegic subjects, the patients who benefit the most have a complete C5/C6 spinal lesion. Typically, these patients have preserved proximal upper limb muscles allowing them to perform limited reaching and manipulation, while their wrist and finger movements are greatly compromised. In hemiplegic subjects one arm is often fully functional, while the other arm is paretic or paralyzed because of the CVA. Hemiplegic subjects feel unpleasant stimulation because the sensory mechanisms are intact. One can decrease the unpleasant sensation by applying stimulation at higher frequency (e.g., 50 pulses/sec). The unpleasant sensation can also be decreased by using the pulses with the exponential rising edge.

The NP for grasping restores the two most frequently used grasp types: the palmar and the lateral grasp. The palmar grasp provides the opposition of the palm and the thumb; hence, allows holding bigger and heavier objects such as cans and bottles. The lateral grasp provides the opposition of the flexed index finger and the thumb and it is used to hold thinner objects such as keys, paper, etc. Finger flexion is performed by stimulating the *Flexor Digitorum Superficialis m.* and the *Flexor Digitorum Profundus m.* Finger extension is obtained by stimulating the *Extensor Communis Digitorum m.* Stimulation of the thumb's Thenar muscle or the median nerve produces thumb flexion. The FES can also be applied to generate elbow extension by stimulating the *Triceps Brachii m.* Such elbow extension in combination with the voluntary *Biceps Brachii m.* contraction can be used to augment the reaching. The FES could be used to stimulate elbow flexion (*Biceps Brachii m.*), or even the shoulder muscles to provide upper arm movements, yet these systems have not been developed into practical devices.

The NPs for grasping can be classified upon the source of control signals that trigger or regulate the stimulation pattern to the following groups: shoulder control [13], voice control [14,15], respiratory control [16], joystick control [13], position transducers [18,19], and trigger [11,20]. The classification can also be made upon the interface between the stimulator and the tissues to the following groups : one or two channel surface electrode systems [17–20], multichannel surface stimulation system [11,15,17], multichannel percutaneous systems with intramuscular electrodes [10,13,14,16], and fully implanted systems [10].

The first grasping system used to provide prehension and release [21] used a splint with a spring for closure and electrical stimulation of the thumb extensor for release. Rudel et al. [22] suggested the use of a simple two-channel stimulation system and a position transducer (sliding potentiometer). The shift of the potentiometer generated by the user controlled the opening and closing of the hand. This technique was used for the therapy of hemiplegic patients and as an orthosis for tetraplegic patients.

The approach taken at Ben Gurion University, Israel [15] used a voice controlled multichannel surface electrode system. Up to 12 bipolar stimulation channels, and a splint were used to control elbow, wrist, and hand functions. Daily mounting and fitting of the system were complex; but the experience lead to the commercial device called Handmaster NMS1 [23]. The Handmaster is a NP for grasping with three surface-stimulation channels. One stimulation channel is used to stimulate the finger extensors, the second for finger flexors, and the third generates the thumb opposition. The Handmaster is controlled with a push-button switch that triggers the hand opening and closing functions. One of the major advantages of the Handmaster in comparison with other surface stimulation systems is that it is easy to don and doff. The second feature is that Handmaster stabilizes the wrist being important for effective grasping, yet also limiting from some movements (e.g., supination and pronation).

Prochazka [18] introduced an assistive system that enhances tenodesis grasp that was controlled by a wrist flexion and extension. This, so called Bionic glove comprised three channels of stimulation to interface the paralyzed sensory–motor systems. The self-adhering surface electrodes, with the metal pin contacting the flexible garment, were positioned over the prime movers contributing to finger flexors, finger extensors, and thumb opposition/flexion. The wrist joint angle sensor triggered the "close the hand" pattern once the wrist extension was bigger than the selected threshold and vice versa, that is, the "open the hand" stimulation pattern was triggered once the sensor measured the wrist flexion bigger than the preset threshold. Clinical evaluation of the Bionic glove [24] indicated that the 6 months of use of the

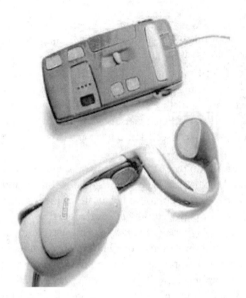 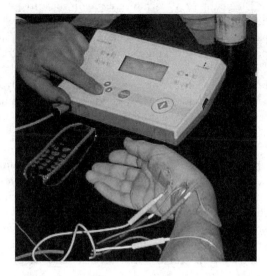

FIGURE 70.1 Handmaster NMS1 (NESS, Israel) grasping device for tetraplegic and hemiplegic patients (left). Actigrip CS (Neurodan A/S, Denmark) is the surface functional electrical therapy system (right). (See text for details.)

Bionic glove was beneficial for tetraplegic patients both therapeutically and as an orthosis, yet, the overall acceptance rate remained insufficient.

Recently, an assistive system called Actigrip CS® (Figure 70.1, right panel) was brought to the market by the company Neurodan A/S, Denmark [11]. This device follows the development of the system introduced as the Belgrade Grasping-Reaching System (BGS®) [17]. The BGS had four stimulation channels, three of which were used to control the hand, while the fourth channel was used to control the elbow extension (stimulation of the *triceps brachii m.*) allowing a tetraplegic subject to reach objects that he/she was not able to do without of the NP. The grasping function was controlled by a push button switch that triggered the hand opening and closing. The grasping was separated into three phases: prehension that forms the correct aperture; relaxation that allows the hand to get in good contact with the object; and closing the hand by opposing either the palm and the thumb, or the side of the index finger and the thumb. The releasing function included two stages, opening of the hand and resting. The reaching function was controlled by implementing the synergy typical for able-bodied humans between the shoulder flexion/extension and elbow flexion/extension.

The Actigrip CS uses four channels of stimulation to control the hand functions. The novelty is the use of the life-like control: the use of triphasic pattern of agonist and antagonistic muscles and use of parallel stimulation of agonist and antagonistic muscles to control the joint stiffness [5]. Clinical studies with the Actigrip CS in poststroke humans suggested excellent recovery compared with the recovery following the conventional therapy.

The ETHZ-ParaCare NP was designed to improve grasping and walking functions in SCI and stroke patients [25]. This surface NP is fully programmable. The system has four stimulation channels, and can be interfaced with many sensors or sensory systems. The ETHZ-ParaCare neural prosthesis for grasping provides both palmar and lateral grasps. The system can be controlled with proportional EMG (electromyography), discrete EMG, push button, and sliding resistor control strategies [25–27].

The group at the Institute for Biokybernetik, Karlsruhe, Germany, suggested the use of EMG recordings from the muscle that is stimulated [28]. The aim of this device was to enhance grasping using weak muscles. It was possible to use retained recordings from the volar side of the forearm to trigger on and off the stimulation of the same muscle groups. In this case, it was essential to eliminate the stimulation artifact and the evoked potential caused by the stimulus in order to eliminate positive feedback effects, which could generate a tetanic contraction that could not be turned off. Sennels et al. (1997) [29] have further developed this approach. In order to implement EMG control the NP has to include electrodes positioned over the muscle that can be voluntarily controlled [30]. The electrodes should be connected to low-noise, high-impedance, high common mode rejection ratio preamplifier. The output from the preamplifier should be fed to a blanking device in order to eliminate the stimulation artifact. The obtained integrated signal can be used as a trigger (switch), or as an input to a state machine. If the EMG recordings are to be used only as a trigger, a comparator that is connected to the reference voltage at the second input can achieve effective operation [30]. A state control relying on a multi-threshold detection could be used to allow the user to vary the strength of the grasp or select other modalities of grasping.

The alternatives to surface electrodes are implantable electrodes or fully implantable systems. In the early 1980s the FES group in Sendai developed a microcomputer-controlled NP for grasping by means of implanted electrodes [31]. The system comprised several intramuscular electrodes that were positioned by the hypodermal needles. These external parts comprised the NEC PC-98LT personal computer, and an external microcontroller-based stimulator. The stimulation patterns were "cloned" from the muscle activities recorded during voluntary grasping movements of able-bodied subjects. The stimulation sequences were triggered with a push button or a pneumatic pressure sensor. The subsequent version of the same system had 30 stimulation channels. This system demonstrated that post-SCI subjects with complete C4–C6 spinal cord lesion could achieve both reaching and grasping functions. Since 1994, in collaboration with NEC Inc. the Sendai FES team has developed a fully implantable 16-channel electric stimulator NEC FESMate. Two hundred of these stimulators were manufactured [32]. The operation of the NEC FESMate system is similar to the earlier Sendai stimulator.

The Freehand system (NeuroControl Co, Cleveland, OH, USA) (Figure 70.2) has eight implanted epimysial stimulation electrodes and an implanted stimulator [33]. The stimulation electrodes are used to generate flexion and extension of the fingers and the thumb in C5 and C6 SCI subjects in order to provide them with lateral (key pinch) or palmar grasp. The stimulation sequences that are used to generate both palmar and lateral grasps are individually tuned and are preprogrammed in the form of a "muscle contraction map." The hand closure and the hand opening are commanded using a position sensor that is placed on the shoulder of the subject's opposite arm. The position sensor monitors two axes of shoulder motion, protraction/retraction and elevation/depression. Typically, the protraction/retraction motion of the shoulder is used as a proportional signal for hand opening and closing. The shoulder elevation/depression motion is used to generate logic commands that are used to establish a zero level for the protraction/retraction command and to "freeze" the stimulation levels until the next logic command is issued. An additional switch is also provided to allow a user to choose between palmar and lateral grasp strategies. The shoulder position sensor and the controller are not implanted. Besides this sensor configuration, the Freehand system also allows one to use either external or implanted transducer mounted on ipsilateral wrist. This transducer measures the dorsal/volar flexion of the wrist and uses this motion to control hand opening and closing in a way similar to the shoulder position sensor [34,35]. The output of the shoulder or the wrist sensor is sent to an external control unit that generates an appropriate stimulation sequence for each stimulation electrode. This sequence is then sent via an inductive link to an implanted stimulator that generates the stimulation trains for each implanted stimulation electrode. More than 250 tetraplegic subjects have received the Freehand neural prosthesis at more than a dozen sites around the world. The subjects have demonstrated the ability to grasp and release objects and performing of typical daily activities more independently when using the neural prosthesis compared with no NP.

The idea of controlling the whole arm and assist manipulation in humans lacking shoulder and elbow control is getting more attention recently by the research team at the Case Western Reserve University (CWRU) in Cleveland, OH [36–39]. The system was designed to combine a fully implantable grasping system with some additional channels to control elbow extension, flexion, and shoulder movements. The control of reaching, unlike the control in the BGS NP, measures the position of the arm in space and for certain arm positions automatically triggers stimulation of the *triceps brachii m.*

Scott et al. [40] suggested the use of EMG recordings from sternocleidomastoid (SCM) muscles to control a FES system for hand control of tetraplegic individuals. Surface electrodes were applied over the

Implantable components of the freehand system

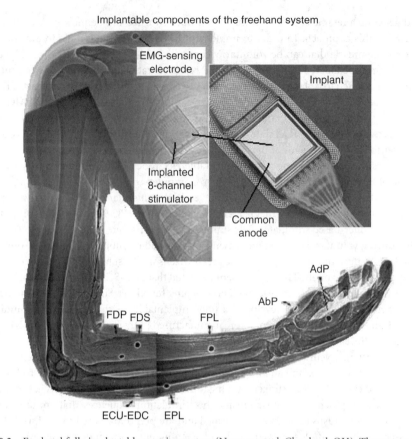

FIGURE 70.2　Freehand fully implantable grasping system (Neurocontrol, Cleveland, OH). The system comprises 8 epimysial electrodes for interfacing the muscles. The device is driven and controlled by an external unit that transmits energy and control signals to the implantable unit.

SCM muscles to record the EMG. The control could be described as a three-state machine (1) Strong flexion of the ipsilateral SCM opens the hand, (2) weaker flexion closes the hand, and (3) no flexion (below a selected threshold) locks the grasp. This is to say that three levels of EMG recordings trigger the controller to activate the following programs (1) increase the stimulation of the muscles that are contributing to the opening of the hand, (2) increase the stimulation of the muscles that are contributing to the closing of the hand, and (3) keep the activation of the muscles at the selected level. The control has been implemented using a fully implantable Freehand® grasping system. The use of SCM muscles could be of specific importance for bilateral application of commercial open-loop FES systems to improve hand grasp since the contralateral shoulder could be used for the control of the respective hand.

The development of implantable cuff electrodes to be used for sensing contact, slippage, and pressure [41–43] opened a new prospective in controlling grasping devices; and the Center for Sensory Motor Interactions in Aalborg, Denmark was pursuing a series of experiments combining their sensing technique with the fully implantable CWRU system.

70.1.2　Restoration of Standing and Walking

The application of NP to the restoration of gait was first investigated systematically in Ljubljana, Slovenia [44]. Currently, NP for gait rehabilitation is used in a clinical setting in several rehabilitation centers [45–51], and there is a growing trend for the design of devices for home use (see Figure 70.3).

Current surface NP systems use various numbers of stimulation channels. The simplest one, from a technical point, is a single channel stimulation system. This system is only suitable for hemiplegic

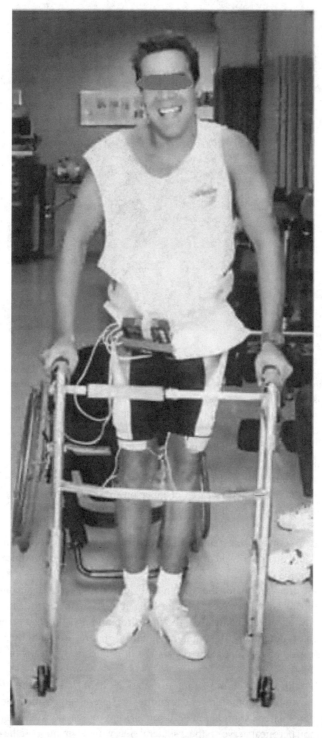

FIGURE 70.3 A complete paraplegic subject walking assisted with the Parastep I (Sigmedics, Chicago, IL). The walking assist comprises six channels that stimulate hip and knee extensors and withdrawal reflex bilaterally. Patient is wearing an ankle–foot orthosis and uses the rolling walker instrumented with the switches for control of stepping.

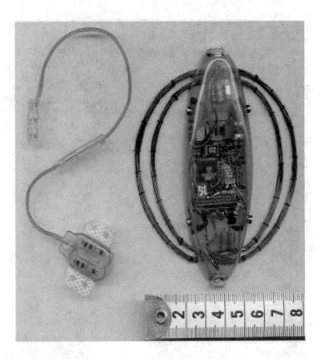

FIGURE 70.4 The components of the prototype of the Actigait system. The Actigait is an implantable foot-drop preventor for poststroke hemiplegic patients. The picture shows the cuff electrode that selectively stimulates the peroneal nerve connected to the implantable two-channel stimulator (left side of the image). The right side of the image shows the external unit with the cooper winding (transmitting antenna).

patients, and a limited group of incomplete paraplegic patients. These individuals can perform limited ambulation with assistance of the upper extremities without NP. The NP in these humans is used to activate a single muscle group. The first demonstrated application of this technique was in hemiplegic patients [52] following the patent and research of Liberson [53]. The stimulation was applied to ankle dorsiflexors so the "foot-drop" can be eliminated. Several versions of foot-drop stimulators with the shoe trigger-switch were developed and tested with various levels of success [54–56]. A commercial system was designed by Stein et al. [57] integrating a single-channel stimulator and a tilt sensor that replaced the foot trigger-switch. Single- and dual-channel correcting foot-drop is now a regular clinical treatment in some rehabilitation institution [58].

A version of the foot-drop stimulator that is being introduced is called Actigait, and it was brought to the market by the company Neurodan A/S, DK. The Actigait uses a cuff electrode to selectively stimulate peroneal nerve; thereby, effectively controlling the foot-drop and assisting the paretic limb during the swing. The heel switch or, potentially, the implantable sensor that records activity from a sensory nerve innervating the lateral side of the foot [59] triggers the dorsiflexion by means of a multichannel cuff electrode (see Figure 70.4).

A multichannel NP with a minimum of four stimulation channels is required for ambulation of a patient with a complete motor lesion of lower extremities and preserved balance and upper body motor control [44]. Appropriate bilateral stimulation of the quadriceps muscles locks the knees during standing. Stimulating the common peroneal nerve on the ipsilateral side, while switching off the quadriceps stimulation on that side, produces a withdrawal of that leg. This withdrawal (flexion) combined with an adequate movement of the upper body and use of the upper extremities for propulsion and support allow ground clearance. This withdrawal is considered as the swinging of the leg. Hand or foot switches can provide the flexion–extension alternation needed for a slow forward or backward progression. Sufficient arm strength must be available to provide balance in parallel bars, rolling walker, or crutches. These systems evolved into a commercial six-channel assistive system called Parastep-1R (Sigmedics, Chicago, IL) approved for home usage by the Food and Drugs Administration (FAD) in 1994.

Multichannel percutaneous systems for gait restoration, with many channels, were suggested [60–62]. The main advantage of these systems is the plausibility to selectively activate many muscle groups. The implantable system also activates deep muscles that are not accessible by surface stimulation. A preprogrammed stimulation pattern that is a replica of the EMG pattern typical for humans with no motor disorders is delivered to muscles controlling the ankle, knee, and hip joints as well as to some trunk muscles. The experience of the Cleveland research team suggested that 48 channels are required for a complete paraplegic patient to achieve an acceptable and effective walking pattern. More recently the Cleveland group changed their stimulation strategy and are suggesting limited external bracing to operate in parallel to the electrical stimulation. Fine-wire intramuscular electrodes are cathodes positioned close to the motor point within selected muscles. Knee extensors (rectus femoris, vastus medialis, vastus lateralis, vastus intermedius), hip flexors (sartorius, tensor fasciae latae, gracilis, iliopsoas), hip extensors (semimembranosus, gluteus maximus), hip abductors (gluteus medius), ankle dorsiflexors (tibialis anterior, peroneus longus), ankle plantar flexors (gastrocnemius lateralis and medialis, plantaris and soleus), and paraspinal muscles are selected for activation. A surface electrode is used as a common anode. Interleaved pulses are delivered with a multichannel, battery-operated, portable stimulator. The hand controller allows the selection of gait activity. These systems were limited to the clinical environment. The application was investigated in complete spinal cord lesions and in stroke patients. The same strategy and selection criteria for implantation were used for both stroke and SCI patients. Recent developments use the CWRU system with eight channels per leg to be activated and improved control.

A multichannel totally implanted FES system [51] was proposed and tested in few subjects. This system uses a 16-channel implantable stimulator and attached to the epineurium electrodes. Femoral and gluteal nerves were stimulated for hip and knee extension. The so-called round-about stimulation was applied in which four electrodes were located around the nerve and stimulated intermittently. This stimulation method reduces muscle fatigue.

The development of the stimulation technology is giving new hopes. Two new techniques are especially important (1) application of remotely controlled wireless micro-stimulators [63,64], and (2) so-called stimulator for all seasons [65]. There are several attempts to design effective wireless stimulator that are believed to be capable of selectively stimulating fascicles [66,67]. Using the technology of cochlear implants is finding its way for standing and walking restoration [68].

Some essentials limit effectiveness of FES based NPs: muscle fatigue caused by nonphysiological activation of sensory-motor systems, reduced muscle forces compared with the forces in naturally controlled muscles, modified reflex activities, spasticity, etc. From the engineering point of view the further development of NPs has to address the following issues: the interface between a FES system and neuromuscular structures in the organism, biocompatibility of the FES system, and overall practicality. The least resolved solution in FES based motor NPs is automatic control (see Chapter 15 of this book).

70.1.3 Hybrid Assistive Systems for Walking

The combination of FES and external skeleton for restoring motor functions in humans with sensory-motor disability is called hybrid assistive system (HAS) [69–71]. Several HAS designs have been proposed that combine relatively simple rigid mechanical structures for passive stabilization of lower limbs during stance phase and FES systems. These systems combine use of a **reciprocating gait orthosis** with multichannel stimulation, the use of an ankle–foot orthosis or an extended ankle–foot orthosis with a knee cage or the use of a **self-fitting modular orthosis** [72–78]. Each trend in the design of HAS implies different applications as well as specific hardware and control problems. On the basis of accumulated experience, the following features can serve as criteria for a closer description of various HAS designs (1) partial mechanical support, (2) parallel operation of the biological and mechanical system, (3) sequential operation of the biological and the mechanical system. The partial mechanical support refers to the use of braces to assist FES only at specific events within a walking cycle [75]. The advanced version of powered orthoses to be used with FES is being developed by Goldfarb and colleagues [76]. Control of joints in mechanical orthosis is becoming again a target of research and development mainly because of new technological tools [77,78].

70.2   Active Prostheses

The role of active prosthesis is to extend the function provided by a "nonexternally" powered and controlled artificial organ (see Chapter 137 of previous edition), hence to improve the over all performance of motor function, ultimately providing better quality of life.

70.2.1   Externally Controlled Transfemoral Prostheses

Effective restoration of walking and standing of handicapped humans is an important element to improve the quality of life. Artificial legs of different kinds have been in use for a long time, but in many cases they are inadequate for the needs of amputees, specifically for high transfemoral (above the knee) amputees (e.g., hip disarticulation), bilateral amputees, and highly active patients (e.g., subjects involved in sport).

Modern technology has led to greatly improved design of transtibial (below the knee) prostheses (TTP). Below-knee amputees perform many normal locomotor activities, and participate in many sports requiring running, jumping, and other jerky movements [79]. The biggest progress was made using readily available and easy-to-work-with plastic and graphite alloys for building the artificial skeletal portion of the shank and foot [80]. TTP are light, easy to assemble, and over-all very reliable. TTP provide good support and excellent energy absorption leading to reduced impacts and jerks; yet, allowing storing of the energy that helps in the push-off phase in the gait cycle. Existing TTP, although without ankle joints, duplicate closely the dynamics of the normal foot–ankle complex during swing and stance phases of the step cycle.

The same technology has been introduced into the design of transfemoral prostheses (TFP). The requirements for a TFP were stated by Wagner and Catranis [81]. The prosthesis must support the body weight of the amputee like the normal limb during the stance phase of level walking, on slopes and on soft or rough terrain. This implies that the prosthesis provides "stability" during weight bearing: that is, it prevents sudden or uncontrolled flexion of the knee during weight bearing. The second requirement is that the body is supported such that undesirable socket/stump interface pressures and gait abnormalities due to painful socket/stump contact are prevented. The analysis of biomechanical factors that influence the shaping, fitting, and alignment of the socket is a problem in itself. If the fitting has been accomplished, allowing the amputee to manipulate and control the prosthesis in an active and comfortable manner, the socket and stump can be treated as one single body. The third requirement, which is somewhat controversial, is that the prosthesis should duplicate as nearly as possible the kinematics and dynamics of normal gait. The amputee should walk with a normal-looking gait over a useful range of speeds associated with typical activities for normal persons of similar age. The latter requirement has received attention in recent years and fully integrated systems, so-called self-contained active TFPs are being incorporated into modern rehabilitation. The self-contained principle implies that the artificial leg contains the energy source, actuator, controller, and sensors.

The externally controlled knee is a recent development that provides some solutions that fulfill the said requirements. Two microprocessor controlled pneumatic knee prosthesis using the Kobe technology [82] are available: the Endolite Intelligent Prosthesis (Blatchford and Sons, London, UK) and the Seattle Limb Systems Power Knee (Seattle Limb Systems, Seattle, WA). Intelligent Prosthesis was first developed in 1993 and an improved version was further introduced in 1995 (Intelligent Prosthesis Plus) and 1998 (Adaptive Prosthesis) [83].

The Adaptive Prosthesis uses two microprocessor-controlled motor valves to control a hybrid hydraulic and pneumatic system. The hydraulic system controls stance, flexion, and terminal impact. The pneumatic portion of the system control both swing phase and knee extension. The Adaptive Prosthesis also offers a

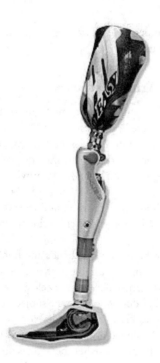

FIGURE 70.5 The C-leg. The C-leg is a transfemoral prosthesis that incorporates intelligent knee mechanism allowing controlled swing and stance phases of the gait cycle.

voluntary locking mechanism for extended standing and a stumble control that responds to prevent knee buckling. The Adaptive Prosthesis has batteries that power the system for several months and a software design that prevents memory loss during battery replacement [83–85].

The C-leg® produced by Otto Bock was introduced in 1997. The C-leg® comprises the microprocessor-controlled knee with both hydraulic stance and swing phase control [86]. It has force sensors in the shin that use heel, toe, and axial loading data to determine stance phase stability. A knee-angle sensor provides data for control of swing phase, angle, velocity, and direction of the moment created by the knee. Sensor technology adapts to movement by measuring angles and moments 50 times per second. The unit transfers information to the hydraulic valve allowing reaction to changing conditions. This mechanism results in an individual's gait that resembles natural walking on many different types of terrain. The C-leg® uses a rechargeable battery that lasts 25 to 30 h. When the battery drains of power, the knee goes into safety mode [86]. The company claims that C-leg® immediately adapts to different walking speeds and provides knee stability (see Figure 70.5).

The application of prostheses starts to be more complex when subjects are to walk stairs, slope, and uneven terrain. Walking downstairs and down the slope requires the controlled flexion of the knee joint, and the flexion is totally dependent on the environmental conditions. James et al. [87] introduced a microcomputer control of the hydraulic system effecting stiffness in both flexion and extension from free to lock states. C-leg from Otto Bock, Germany is the first microprocessor-controlled knee joint which incorporates some of these features. Electronic sensors supply basic data for stance-phase stability and stance-phase control. This is the closest approximation to natural gait where subjects no longer have to think about walking. Walking upstairs and up slopes requires a powered knee joint, which is still not commercially available and has not been developed even for experimental purposes to the satisfaction of researchers, clinical, and over all potential users. Powered transfemoral prostheses have been suggested [88,89] but the technology and control have not been adequate.

There are two groups of patients who will benefit greatly from the powered leg: patients with hip disarticulation and bilateral amputees. In both cases, amputees are not able to generate movement of the thigh that is required to drive the underpowered system; hence, the externally powered knee joint will compensate for lack of power by the user.

70.2.2 Powered Hand and Arm Prostheses

The power for active hand and arm prostheses can come form the body (Body-powered Prosthesis), or from external sources (Externally-powered prosthesis) [90–97]. Gross body movement controls a body-powered prosthesis. The movement of the shoulder, upper arm, or chest is captured by a harness system, which is attached to a cable that is connected to a terminal device (hook or hand). For some levels of amputation or deficiency, an elbow system can be added to provide the amputee additional function. An amputee must possess at least one or more of the following gross body movements: glenohumeral flexion, scapular abduction or adduction, shoulder depression and elevation, and chest expansion in order to control body-powered prosthesis. In addition, sufficient residual limb length and sufficient musculature must exist.

There are two types of controls for body-powered hands and hooks, voluntary opening and voluntary closing: voluntary opening gives the subject grasping control even when he/she is relaxed. The tradeoff for this is limited grip force, often less than 30 N. Voluntary closing allows the subject to have substantially greater grip force, often over 150 N, but does not allow the subject to relax without losing grasp.

Many amputees who wear a body-powered prosthesis develop increased control due to a phenomenon called extended proprioception [90]. Extended proprioception gives the wearer feedback as to the position of the terminal device. The subject will know whether the hook is open or closed by the extent of pressure the harness is exerting on his or her shoulder area without having to visually inspect the operation. Many amputees do not like the cosmetic appearance of the hook and control cables and they request a "natural-like" part of the body replacement.

Externally powered prostheses use electrical power to provide function. The electrical power is applied via motors located in the terminal device (hand or hook), wrist, and elbow. The grip force of the hand can be in excess of 100 N. Command signals are generated either by voluntary contraction of muscles, so-called **myoelectric control**, or by using switches of different kinds. For applications that are more complex, both the command signals are used for different operations (e.g., control of several degrees of freedom).

Myoelectric control is a very popular command method [95]. It relies on the ability of the amputee to generate voluntary contraction of a muscle that he or she would normally use for the same function before the disability, or some other synergistic muscle at his/her subconscious level. Muscle contraction can be registered by recording of the electrical activity of muscles (Electromyogram — EMG). Electrodes that contact the skin capture EMG signal. The EMG can be recorded accurately if the appropriate technology is used. EMG has to be carefully extracted from "electrical noise." Many individuals prefer this type of control because it only requires the wearer to contract his muscles. This eliminates the need for a tight, often uncomfortable control harness. Another advantage of a myoelectric prosthesis is that because it does not require a control cable or harness, a cosmetic skin can be applied in either latex or silicone, greatly enhancing the cosmetic restoration.

An example of the profound designs is the Utah Arm 2 for the transhumeral amputees (see Figure 70.6) [92]. The Utah arm and hand system for transhumeral amputees allows sensitive control of elbow, hand, and wrist (optional) using only EMG signals from two muscles. The exclusive myoelectric system eliminates cables, letting the amputee move the arm and hand slowly or quickly in any position, ultimately leading to a more natural response with less effort. The Utah Arm, combined with its high performance hand control, supplies the wearer with superior cosmetic appearance. Smooth exterior hand covers provide natural look. For rugged tasks, the hand can be changed to another hand or terminal device. The optional electrically driven wrist joint allows hand pronation and supination. Proportional or on–off myoelectric controls are both available based on the subject's request and abilities.

The ServoPro, an exclusive feature of the Utah Arm, is designed for amputees with shoulder disarticulation, interscapulothorasic, or brachial plexus injuries. The ServoPro eliminates the electrodes normally

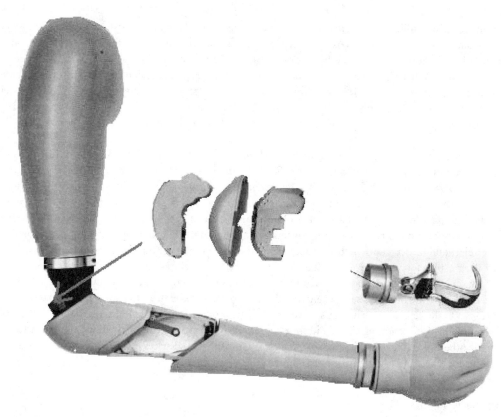

FIGURE 70.6 The Utah arm is a self-contained battery powered artificial arm–hand complex. The system comprises myoelectric control of the elbow, wrist, and grasping movements.

required to operate the Utah Arm. The system may be the only option, which can provide functional control of both elbow and hand. The ServoPro is based on a harness, but instead of cables, electronic components are pushed and pulled to generate command signals that will control the electrically powered prosthesis. The ServoPro requires much smaller excursion of movement and less effort compared with body-powered cables in equivalent mechanical systems. The servo control is accurate and it uses feedback from sensors in the elbow and hand.

Hybrid prosthesis utilizes a body-powered elbow and a myoelectrically controlled terminal device — hook or hand. Most important ability provided to the patient is to simultaneously control elbow flexion and extension while opening or closing the electric hand/hook or while rotating the wrist. The other prosthetic options generally require the wearer to control one function at a time (flex the elbow, lock the elbow, open or close the terminal device). The hybrid prosthesis weighs less and is less expensive than a similar prosthesis with an electrically powered elbow and hand. An example is the Ergo arm from Otto Bock that uses the new elbow system that can be unlocked or locked in any position, even under loads up to 250 N. A slight pull on the cable lowers the forearm gradually. Releasing the cable immediately locks the elbow in that position. For normal locking or unlocking, the cable has to be pulled stronger. The elbow is designed to support myoelectric hand. When the prosthetic arm is extended, the system stores the energy to facilitate flexion. The arm swings smoothly while walking. Subject-adjustable counterbalance makes the arm feel lighter, even with an electric wrist and terminal device.

Otto Bock Sensor Hand provides secure grasps of various objects. The system frees the user from constant watch on the objects in the hand since the automatic grasping feature senses when an object is about to slip and makes necessary adjustments. The Flexi-Grip function gives the amputee a natural look and flexible grip. The hand is controlled by volitional contraction of muscles that are touching the socket.

The electrodes are built into the socket. This hand is used with the passive wrist rotation with ratchet mechanism or optional friction wrist. The Sensor Hand senses the change in the center of gravity and readjusts its grip automatically. The hand closes at maximum speed and grips an object with the least amount of force. When the contact of fingers and the object are sensed, the control changes to grip-force control and increases the force to its maximum. Two programs can be executed, namely, (1) controlling the opening speed by the strength of the muscle signal (contraction) in addition to controlling the closing speed based on a decrease in muscle tension and (2) controlling both speed by the strength of the muscle contraction.

The current commercial hand prostheses have extremely limited performance compared with the able-bodied arm and hand. The Southampton Artificial Hand has been in existence for several decades and is based upon the original hypothesis for the development of a hierarchically controlled myoelectric prosthesis. The mechanics of the Southampton hand has undergone several stages; however, the main hypothesis remains the same. Vast quantities of information are utilized to form a stable and comfortable grip in able-bodied humans. The grip is constantly adjusted to prevent the slip, deforming or crushing of the object and incorrect orientation (e.g., spilling the content of a container). In all systems described above the grasping force is preselected based on experience, and rarely voluntarily adjusted based on visual feedback. The philosophy behind the development of the Southampton hand is to come with the adaptive, mechanical structure that uses sensors and intelligent control to generate optimum grip. The basis of the control is a finite state of modeling and use of synergistic model of movement of fingers and the thumb. The hand has five functioning digits and four degrees of freedom. The index finger acts independently from the other three fingers, which move in tandem. The other two degrees of freedom are in the thumb. Slip transducers are built in the pads of the fingers.

Defining Terms

Artificial reflex control: A sensory-driven control algorithm based on knowledge representation (production rule based system).

Externally controlled assistive system: Assistive system for restoration of motor functions with automatic control.

Externally powered assistive system: Assistive system for restoration of motor functions that uses external power to control muscles of drive actuators.

Hybrid assistive systems: Combination of a functional electrical stimulation and a mechanical orthosis.

Myoelectric (EMG) control: Use of voluntary generated myoelectric activity as control signals for an externally controlled and powered assistive system.

Neural Prosthesis — Assistive systems for replacing or augmenting sensory–motor funcion Functional electrical stimulation or Functional neuromuscular stimulation: Patterned electrical stimulation of neuromuscular structures dedicated to restore motor functions.

Reciprocating gait orthosis: A walking and standing assistive system with a reciprocating mechanism for hip joints, which extends the contralateral hip when the ipsilateral hip is flexed.

Self-fitting modular orthosis: A modular, self-fitting, mechanical orthosis with a soft interface between human body and the orthosis.

Transfemoral prosthesis: Artificial leg for amputees with the amputation between the knee and hip joint (transfemur).

Transtibial prosthesis: Artificial leg for amputees with the amputation between the ankle and the knee joints (transtibia)

References

[1] Popović, D.B. and Sinkjær, T., *Control of Movement for the Physically Disabled*. Springer, London, 2000.

[2] Salmons, S., Ashley, H. et al., FES of denervated muscles: basic issues, In Bijak, M., Mayr, W., and Pichler, M. (Eds.) *Proceedings of 8th International Workshop on FES*, Vienna, Austria, Sept. 10–13, pp. 52–57, 2004.

[3] Kern, H., Mödlin, M., and Fostner, C., The RISE patient study: FES in the treatment of flaccid paraplegia. In Bijak, M., Mayr, W., and Pichler, M. (Eds.) *Proceedings of 8th International Workshop on FES*, Vienna, Austria, Sept. 10–13, pp. 27–31, 2004.

[4] Popović-Bijelić, A., Bijelić, G. et al., Multi-field surface electrode for selective electrical stimulation. In Bijak, M., Mayr, W., and Pichler, M. (Eds.) *Proceedings of 8th International Workshop on FES*, Vienna, Austria, Sept. 10–13, pp. 195–198, 2004.

[5] Popović, M.B. and Popović, D.B., Hierarchical hybrid control for therapeutic electrical stimulation of upper extremities. In Bijak, M., Mayr, W., and Pichler, M. (Eds.) *Proceedings of 8th International Workshop on FES*, Vienna, Austria, Sept. 10–13, pp. 142–145, 2004.

[6] Loeb, G., Implantable device having an electrolytic storage electrode, United States Patent 5,312,439, www.uspto.gov/patfv/index.html, 1994.

[7] Schulman, J. et al., Implantable microstimulator, United States Patent 5,324,316, www.uspto.gov/patfv/index.html, 1995.

[8] Cameron, T., Loeb, G.E., Peck, R. et al., Micromodular implants to provide electrical stimulation of paralyzed muscles and limbs, *IEEE Trans. Biomed. Eng.* BME-44: 781–790, 1997.

[9] Nathan, R., Device for generating hand function, Patent application 5,330,516, www.uspto.gov/patfv/index.html, 1994.

[10] Peckham, P.H. et al., Functional neuromuscular stimulation system, United States Patent 5,167,229. www.uspto.gov/patfv/index.html, 1992.

[11] Sinkjær, T. and Popović, D.B., Functional Electrical Therapy Systems (FETS). United States Patent Application US2004147975, www.uspto.gov/patfv/index.html, 2004.

[12] Popović D.B., Popović M.B., Sinkjær T., Stefanović A., and Schwirtlich L., Therapy of paretic arm in hemiplegic subjects augmented with a neural prosthesis: a cross-over study, *Can. J. Physio. Pharmacol.* 82: 749–756, 2004.

[13] Buckett, J.R., Peckham, H.P. et al., A flexible, portable system for neuro-muscular stimulation in the paralyzed upper extremities, *IEEE Trans. Biomed. Eng.* BME-35: 897–904, 1988.

[14] Handa, Y., Handa, T. et al., Functional electrical stimulation (FES) systems for restoration of motor function of paralyzed muscles — versatile systems and a portable system, *Front. Med. Biol. Eng.* 4: 241–255, 1992.

[15] Nathan, R.H. Control strategies in FNS systems for the upper extremities, *Crit. Rev. Biomed. Eng.* 21: 485–568, 1993.

[16] Hoshimiya, N., Naito, N., Yajima, M., and Handa, Y., A multichannel FES system for the restoration of motor functions in high spinal cord injury patients: a respiration-controlled system for multijoint upper extremity, *IEEE Trans. Biomed. Eng.* BME-36: 754–760, 1989.

[17] Popović, D., Popović, M. et al., Clinical evaluation of the Belgrade grasping system. *Proceedings of 5th Vienna International Workshop on Functional Electrical Stimulation*, Vienna, 1998.

[18] Prochazka, A., Gauthier, M., Wieler, M., and Kenwell, Z., The bionic glove: an electrical stimulator garment that provides controlled grasp and hand opening in quadriplegia, *Arch Phys. Med. Rehabil.* 78: 608–614, 1997.

[19] Rebersek, S. and Vodovnik, L., Proportionally controlled functional electrical stimulation of hand, *Arch. Phys. Med. Rehabil.* 54: 378–382, 1973.

[20] Nathan, R., Handmaster NMS — present technology and the next generation. In Popović, D. (Ed.) *Proceedings of 2nd International Symposium on FES*, Burnaby, pp. 139–140, 1997.

[21] Long, C. II and Masciarelli, C.V., An electrophysiologic splint for the hand, *Arch. Phys. Med. Rehabil.* 44: 499–503, 1963.

[22] Rudel, D., Bajd, T., Rebersek, S., and Vodovnik, L., FES assisted manipulation in quadriplegic patients. In Popović, D. (Ed.) *Advances in External Control of Human Extremities VIII*, pp. 273–282, ETAN, Belgrade, 1984.

[23] Ijzerman, M., Stoffers, T. et al., The NESS Handmaster orthosis: restoration of hand function in C5 and stroke patients by means of electrical stimulation, *J. Rehab. Sci.* 9: 86–89, 1996.

[24] Popović, D., Stojanović, A. et al., Clinical evaluation of the bionic glove, *Arch. Phys. Med. Rehabil.* 80: 299–304, 1999.

[25] Keller, T., Curt, A. et al., Grasping in high lesioned tetraplegic subjects using the EMG controlled neural prosthesis, *J. NeuroRehab.* 10: 251–255, 1998.

[26] Popović, M.R., Keller, T. et al., Surface stimulation technology for grasping and walking neural prosthesis, *IEEE Engng. Med. Biol. Mag.* 20: 82–93, 2001.

[27] Keller, T. and Popović, M.R., Real-time stimulation artifact removal in EMG signals for neural prosthesis control applications. *Proceedings of 6th Annual IFESS Conference*, Cleveland, OH, June 10–13, pp. 208–210, 2001.

[28] Holländer, H.J., Huber, M., and Vossius, G., An EMG controlled multichannel stimulator. In Popović, D. (Ed.) *Advances in External Control of Human Extremities IX*, pp. 291–295, Published by ETAN, Belgrade, 1987.

[29] Sennels, S., Biering-Soerensen, F., Anderson, O.T., and Hansen, S.D., Functional neuromuscular stimulation control by surface electromyographic signals produced by volitional activation of the same muscle: adaptive removal of the muscle response from the recorded EMG-signal, *IEEE Trans. Rehab. Eng.* TRE-5:195: 206, 1997.

[30] Saxena, S., Nikolić, S., and Popović, D., An EMG controlled FES system for grasping in tetraplegics, *J. Rehabil. Res. Dev.* 32: 17–23, 1995.

[31] Hoshimiya, N. and Handa, Y., A master–slave type multichannel functional electrical stimulation (FES) system for the control of the paralyzed upper extremities, *Automedica* 11: 209–220, 1989.

[32] Takahashi, K., Hoshimiya, N., Matsuki, H., and Handa, Y., Externally powered implantable FES system, *Jap. J. Med. Electron. Biol. Engng.* 37: 43–51, 1999.

[33] *The Neurocontrol Freehand System*, Manual, NeuroControl, Cleveland, OH, USA, 1998.

[34] Hart, R.L., Kilgore, K.L., and Peckham, P.H., A comparison between control methods for implanted FES hand-grasp systems, *IEEE Trans. Rehab. Engng.* 6: 208–218, 1998.

[35] Kilgore, K.L., Peckham, P.H. et al., An implanted upper-extremity neural prosthesis: follow-up of five patients, *J. Bone Joint Surg. Am.* 79: 533–541, 1997.

[36] Grill, J.H. and Peckham, P.H., Functional neuromuscular stimulation for combined control of elbow extension and hand grasp in C5 and C6 quadriplegics, *IEEE Trans. Rehab. Eng.* TRE-6: 190–199, 1998.

[37] Crago, P.E., Memberg, W.D., Usey, M.K. et al., An elbow extension neuroprosthesis for individuals with tetraplegia, *IEEE Trans. Rehab. Eng.* TRE-6: 1–6, 1998.

[38] Johnson, M.W. and Peckham, P.H., Evaluation of shoulder movement as a command control source, *IEEE Trans. Biomed. Engng.* BME-37: 876–885, 1990.

[39] Smith, B.T., Mulcahey, M.J., and Betz, R.R., Development of an upper extremity FES system for individuals with C4 tetraplegia, *IEEE Trans. Rehab. Eng.* TRE-4: 264–270, 1996.

[40] Scott, T.R.D., Peckham, P.H., and Kilgore, K.L., Tri-state myoelectric control of bilateral upper extremity neuroprosthesis for tetraplegic individuals, *IEEE Trans. Rehab. Eng.* TRE-4: 251–263, 1996.

[41] Haugland, M., Lickel, A., Haase, J., and Sinkjær, T., Control of FES thumb force using slip information obtained from the cutaneous electroneurogram in quadriplegic man, *IEEE Trans. Rehab. Eng.* TRE-7: 215–227, 1999.

[42] Haugland, M.K. and Hoffer, J.A., Slip information provided by nerve cuff signals: application in closed-loop control of functional electrical stimulation, *IEEE Trans. Rehab. Eng.* TRE-2: 29–37, 1994.

[43] Haugland, M.K., Hoffer, J.A., and Sinkjaer, T., Skin contact force information in sensory nerve signals recorded by implanted cuff electrodes, *IEEE Trans. Rehab. Eng.* TRE-2: 18–27, 1994.

[44] Kralj, A. and Bajd, T., *Functional Electrical Stimulation, Standing and Walking After Spinal Cord Injury*, CRC Press, Boca Raton, FL, 1989.

[45] Andrews, B.J., Baxendale, R.H. et al., Hybrid FES orthosis incorporating closed loop control and sensory feedback, *J. Biomed. Engng.* 10: 189–195, 1988.

[46] Brindley, G.S., Polkey, C.E., and Rushton, D.N., Electrical splinting of the knee in paraplegia, *Paraplegia* 16: 428–435, 1978.

[47] Jaeger, R., Yarkony, G.Y., and Smith, R., Standing the spinal cord injured patient by electrical stimulation: refinement of a protocol for clinical use, *IEEE Trans. Biomed. Eng.* BME-36: 720–728, 1989.

[48] Mizrahi, J., Braun, Z., Najenson, T., and Graupe, D., Quantitative weight bearing and gait evaluation of paraplegics using functional electrical stimulation, *Med. Biol. Eng. Comput.* 23: 101–107, 1985.

[49] Petrofsky, J.S. and Phillips, C.A., Computer controlled walking in the paralyzed individual, *J. Neurol. Orthop. Surg.* 4: 153–164, 1983.

[50] Solomonow, M., Biomechanics and physiology of a practical powered walking orthosis for paraplegics. In Stein, R.B., Peckham, H.P., and Popović, D. (Eds.) *Neural Prostheses: Replacing Motor Function After Disease or Disability*, Oxford University Press, New York, pp. 202–230, 1992.

[51] Thoma, H., Frey, M. et al., Functional neurostimulation to substitute locomotion in paraplegia patients, In Andrade, D. et al. (Eds.), *Artificial Organs*, VCH Publishers, pp. 515–529, 1987.

[52] Graćanin, F., Prevec, T., and Trontelj, J., Evaluation of use of functional electronic peroneal brace in hemiparetic patients. In *Advances in External Control of Human Extremities III*, ETAN, Belgrade, pp. 198–210, 1967.

[53] Liberson, W.T., Holmquest, H.J., Scott, D., and Dow, A., Functional electrotherapy. stimulation of the peroneal nerve synchronized with the swing phase of the gait of hemiplegic patients, *Arch. Phys. Med. Rehab.* 42: 101–105, 1961.

[54] Burridge, J.H., Taylor, P.N. et al., The effect of common peroneal stimulation on the effort and speed of walking. A randomised controlled trial of chronic hemiplegic patients, *Clin. Rehab.* 11: 201–210, 1997.

[55] Taylor, P.N., Burridge, J.H. et al., Clinical use of the Odstock dropped foot stimulator: its effect on the speed and effort of walking, *Arch. Phys. Med. Rehab.* 80: 1577–1583, 1999.

[56] Waters, R.L., McNeal, D.R., Fallon, W., and Clifford, B., Functional electrical stimulation of the peroneal nerve for hemiplegia, *J. Bone Joint Surg.* 67: 792–793, 1985.

[57] Dai, R., Stein, R.B. et al., Application of tilt sensors in functional electrical stimulation, *IEEE Trans. Rehab. Eng.* TRE-4: 63–72, 1996.

[58] Taylor, P., Burridge, J.H. et al., Clinical audit of 5 years provision of the Odstock dropped foot stimulator, *Artif. Organs* 23: 440–442, 1999.

[59] Childs, C., *Application of Selective Stimulation in Human Peripheral Nerves*, Ph.D. Thesis, Aalborg University, Denmark, 2004.

[60] Marsolais, E.B. and Kobetic, R., Implantation techniques and experience with percutaneous intramuscular electrode in the lower extremities, *J. Rehab. Res.* 23: 1–8, 1987.

[61] Kobetic, R. and Marsolais, E.B., Synthesis of paraplegic gait with multichannel functional electrical stimulation, *IEEE Trans. Rehab. Eng.* TRE-2: 66–79, 1994.

[62] Abbas, J.J. and Triolo, R.J., Experimental evaluation of an adaptive feedforward controller for use in functional neuromuscular stimulation systems, *IEEE Trans. Rehab. Eng.* TRE-5: 12–22, 1997.

[63] Cameron, T., Liinama, T., Loeb, G.E., and Richmond, F.J.R., Long term biocompatibility of a miniature stimulator implanted in feline hind limb muscles, *IEEE Trans. Biomed. Eng.* BME-45: 1024–1035, 1998.

[64] Cameron, T., Richmond, F.J.R., and Loeb, G.E., Effects of regional stimulation using a miniature stimulator implanted in feline posterior bicpes femoris, *IEEE Trans. Biomed. Eng.* BME-45: 1036–1045, 1998.

[65] Strojnik, P., Whitmoyer, D., and Schulman, J., An implantable stimulator for all season, In Popović, D. (Ed.) *Advances in External Control of Human Extremities X*, Nauka, Belgrade, pp. 335–344, 1990.

[66] Ziaie, B., Nardin, M.D., Coghlan, A.R., and Najafi, K., A single channel implantable microstim-ulator for functional neuromuscular stimulation, *IEEE Trans. Biomed. Eng.* BME-44: 909–920, 1997.

[67] Haugland, M.K., A miniature implantable nerve stimulator. In Popović, D. (Ed.) *Proceedings of 2nd International Symposium on FES*, Burnaby, pp. 221–222, 1997.

[68] Houdayer, T., Davis, R. et al., Prolonged closed-loop standing in paraplegia with implanted cochlear FES-22 stimulator and Andrews ankle-foot orthosis. In Popović, D. (Ed.) *Proceedings of 2nd International Symposium on FES*, Burnaby, pp. 168–169, 1997.

[69] Andrews, B.J., Baxendale, R.M. et al., A hybrid orthosis for paraplegics incorporating feedback control. In *Advances in External Control of Human Extremities IX*, ETAN, Belgrade, pp. 297–310, 1987.

[70] Popović, D., Tomović, R., and Schwirtlich, L., Hybrid assistive system — Neuroprosthesis for motion, *IEEE Trans. Biomed. Eng.* BME-37: 729–738, 1989.

[71] Solomonow, M., Baratta, R. et al., Evaluation of 70 paraplegics fitted with the LSU RGO/FES. In Popović, D. (Ed.) *Proceedings of 2nd International Symposium on FES*, Burnaby, p. 159, 1997.

[72] Andrews, B.J., Barnett, R.W. et al., Rule-based control of a hybrid FES orthosis for assisting paraplegic locomotion, *Automedica* 11: 175–199, 1989.

[73] Schwirtlich, L. and Popović, D., Hybrid orthoses for deficient locomotion. In Popović, D. (Ed.) *Advances in External Control of Human Extremities VIII*, ETAN, Belgrade, pp. 23–32, 1984.

[74] Phillips, C.A., An interactive system of electronic stimulators and gait orthosis for walking in the spinal cord injured, *Automedica* 11: 247–261, 1989.

[75] Popović, D., Schwirtlich, L., and Radosavljević, S., Powered hybrid assistive system. In Popović, D. (Ed.) *Advances in External Control of Human Extremities X*, Nauka, Belgrade, pp. 191–200, 1990.

[76] Goldfarb, M. and Durfee, W.K., Design of a controlled-brake orthosis for FES-aided gait, *IEEE Trans. Rehab. Eng.* TRE-4: 13–24, 1996.

[77] Irby, S.E., Kaufman, K.R., and Sutherland, D.H., A digital logic controlled electromechanical long leg brace. In *Proceedings of 15th Southern Biomedical Engineering Conference*, Dayton, OH, p. 28, 1996.

[78] Kaufman, K.R., Irby, S.E., Mathewson, J.W. et al., Energy efficient knee-ankle-foot orthosis, *J. Prosthet. Orthot.* 8: 79–85, 1996.

[79] Inman, V.T., Ralston, J.J., and Todd, F., *Human Walking*. Williams & Wilkins, Baltimore, London, 1981.

[80] Doane, N.E. and Holt, L.E., A comparison of the SACH foot and single axis foot in the gait of the unilateral below-knee amputee, *Prosthet. Orthot. Int.* 7: 33–36, 1983.

[81] Wagner, E.M. and Catranis, J.G., New developments in lower-extremity prostheses. In Klopsteg, P.E., Wilson, P.D. et al. (Eds.) *Human Limbs and Their Substitutes*, McGraw-Hill Book Company, New York, (Reprinted 1968), 1954.

[82] Michael, J.W., Modern prosthetic knee mechanisms, *Clin. Orthop. Relat. Res.* 361: 39–47, 1999.

[83] The adaptive prosthesis: for transfemoral amputees. From http://www. blatchford.co.uk /products/products.

[84] Pike, A., The new high tech prostheses. From www.amputee-coalition.orq/inmotion/mav iun 99/hitech.html

[85] Schuch, C.M., A guide to lower limb prosthetics. Part I — prosthetic design: basic concepts. From www.amputeecoalition.orq/inmotion/mar apr 98/pros primer/paqe2.html

[86] 3C100 C-leg system. New generation leg system revolutionizes lower limb prosthesis. From www.ottobockus.com/products/op lower cleg.asp

[87] James, K., Stein, R.B., Rolf, R., and Tepavac, D., Active suspension above-knee prosthesis. In Goh, D. and Nathan, A. (Eds.) *Proceedings of 6th International Conference on Biomedical Engineering*, pp. 317–320, 1991.

[88] Tomović, R., Popović, D., Turajlić S., and McGhee, R.B., Bioengineering actuator with non-numerical control. In *Proceedings of IFAC Conference Orthotics and Prosthetics*, Columbus, OH, Pergamon Press, pp. 145–151, 1982.

[89] Popović, D. and Schwirtlich, L., Belgrade active A/K prosthesis. In deVries J. (Ed.) *Electrophysiological Kinesiology*, Excerpta Medica, Amsterdam, *Intern. Cong. Ser*, 804: 337–343, 1988.

[90] Simpson, D.C., The choice of control system for the multi-movement prosthesis: extended physiological proprioception (e.p.p.). In *The Control of Upper-Extremity Prostheses and Orthoses* Ch. 15, pp. 146–150, 1973.

[91] Sheridan, T.B. and Mann, R.W., Design of control devices for people with severe motor impairment, *Hum. Factors* 20: 312–338, 1978.

[92] Jacobsen, S.C., Knutti, F.F., Johnson, R.T., and Sears, H.H., Development of the Utah artificial arm, *IEEE Trans. Biomed. Eng.* BME-29: 249–269, 1982.

[93] Gibbons, D.T., O'Riain, M.D., and Philippe-Auguste, J.S., An above-elbow prosthesis employing programmed linkages, *IEEE Trans. Biomed. Eng.* BME-34: 251–258, 1987.

[94] Kyberd, P.J., Holland, O.E., Chappel, P.H. et al., MARCUS: a two degree of freedom hand prosthesis with hierarchical grip control, *IEEE Trans. Rehab. Eng.* TRE-3: 70–76, 1995.

[95] Park, E. and Meek, S.G., Adaptive filtering of the electromyographic signal for prosthetic and force estimation, *IEEE Trans. Biomed. Eng.* BME-42: 1044–1052, 1995.

[96] Kurtz, I., Programmable prosthetic controller. In *Proceedings of MEC '97*, Frederciton, NB, p. 33, 1997.

[97] Bertos, Y.A., Hechathorne, C.H., Weir, R.F., and Childress, D.S., Microprocessor based EPP position controller for electric powered upper limb prostheses. In *Proceedings of IEEE Internatinal Conference on EMBS*, Chicago, 1997.

Further Reading

Agnew, W.V. and McCreery, D.B., *Neural Prostheses: Fundamental Studies*, Prentice Hall, Englewood Cliffs, NJ, 1990.

Dhilon, G. and Horch, K. (Eds.) *Neuroprosthetics: Theory and Practice*, World Science Publications, 2004.

Popović, D. and Sinkjær, T., *Control of Movement for the Physically Disabled*, Springer, 2000.

Popović, D. (Ed.) *Advances in External Control of Human Extremities I-X*, Aalborg University, 2002, ISSN (Electronic version of the 10 Proceedings from Dubrovnik meetings 1963–1990).

Stein, R.B., Peckham, H.P., and Popović, D., *Neural Prostheses: Replacing Motor Function After Disease or Disability*, Oxford University Press, New York, 1992.

71
Sensory Augmentation and Substitution

Kurt A. Kaczmarek
University of Wisconsin-Madison

This chapter will consider methods and devices used to present visual, auditory, and tactual (touch) information to persons with sensory deficits. **Sensory augmentation systems** such as eyeglasses and hearing aids enhance the existing capabilities of a functional human sensory system. **Sensory substitution** is the use of one human sense to receive information normally received by another sense. Braille and speech synthesizers are examples of systems that substitute touch and hearing, respectively, for information that is normally visual (printed or displayed text).

The following three sections will provide theory and examples for aiding the visual, auditory, and tactual systems. Because capitalizing on an *existing* sensory capability is usually superior to substitution, each section will consider first augmentation and then substitution, as shown below:

Human Sensory Systems

Visual	Auditory	Tactual
Visual augmentation	Auditory augmentation	Tactual augmentation
Tactual vision substitution	Visual auditory substitution	Tactual substitution
Auditory vision substitution	Tactual auditory substitution	

71.1   Visual System

With a large number of receptive channels, the human visual system processes information in a parallel fashion. A single glimpse acquires a wealth of information; the field of view for two eyes is 180 degrees horizontally and 120 vertically [Mehr and Shindell, 1990]. The spatial resolution in the central (foveal) part of the visual field is approximately 0.5–1.0 min of arc [Shlaer, 1937], although Vernier acuity, the specialized task of detecting a misalignment of two lines placed end to end, is much finer, approximately 2 sec of arc [Stigmar, 1970]. Low-contrast presentations substantially reduce visual acuity.

The former resolution figure is the basis for the standard method of testing visual acuity, the Snellen chart. Letters are considered to be "readable" if they subtend approximately 5 min of arc and have details one-fifth this size. Snellen's 1862 method of reporting visual performance is still used today. The ratio 20/40, for instance, indicates that a test was conducted at 20 ft and that the letters that were recognizable at that distance would subtend 5 min of arc of 40 ft (the distance at which a normally sighted, or "20/20," subject could read them). Although the standard testing distance is 20, 10 and even 5 ft may be used, under certain conditions, for more severe visual impairments [Fonda, 1981].

Of the approximately 6 to 11.4 million people in the United States who have visual impairments, 90% have some useful vision [NIDRR, 1993]. In the United States, *severe visual impairment* is defined to be 20/70 vision in the better eye with best refractive correction (see below). Legal blindness means that the best corrected acuity is 20/200 or that the field of view is very narrow (<20 degrees). People over 65 years of age account for 46% of the legally blind and 68% of the severely visually impaired. For those with some useful vision, a number of useful techniques and devices for visual augmentation can allow performance of many everyday activities.

71.1.1   Visual Augmentation

People with certain eye disorders see better with higher- or lower-than-normal light levels; an **illuminance** from 100 to 4000 lux may promote comfortable reading [Fonda, 1981]. Ideal illumination is diffuse and directed from the side at a 45-degree angle to prevent glare. The surrounding room is preferably 20% to 50% darker than the object of interest.

Refractive errors cause difficulties in focusing on an object at a given distance from the eye [Mountcastle, 1980]. Myopia (near-sightedness), hyperopia (far-sightedness), astigmatism (focus depth that varies with radial orientation), and presbyopia (loss of ability to adjust focus, manifested as far-sightedness) are the most common vision defects. These normally can be corrected with appropriate eyeglasses or contact lenses and are rarely the cause of a disability.

Magnification is the most useful form of image processing for vision defects that do not respond to refractive correction. The simplest form of image magnification is getting closer; halving the distance to an object doubles its size. Magnifications up to 20 times are possible with minimal loss of field of view. At very close range, eyeglasses or a loupe may be required to maintain focus [Fonda, 1981]. Hand or stand magnifiers held 18–40 cm (not critical) from the eye create a virtual image that increases rapidly in size as the object-to-lens distance approaches the focal length of the lens. Lenses are rated in diopters ($D = 1/f$, where f is the focal length of the lens in centimeters). The useful range is approximately 4–20 D; more powerful lenses are generally held close to the eye as a loupe, as just mentioned, to enhance field of view. For distance viewing, magnification of 2–10 times can be achieved with hand-held telescopes at the expense of a reduced field of view.

Closed-circuit television (CCTV) systems magnify print and small objects up to 60 times, with higher effective magnifications possible by close viewing. Users with vision as poor as 1/400 (20/8000) may be able to read ordinary print with CCTV [Fonda, 1981]. Some recent units are portable and contain black/white image reversal and contrast enhancement features.

Electrical (or, more recently, magnetic) stimulation of the visual cortex produces perceived spots of light called *phosphenes*. Some attempts, summarized in Webster et al. [1985], have been made to map these sensations and display identifiable patterns, but the phosphenes often do not correspond spatially with the specific location on the visual cortex. Although the risk and cost of this technique do not yet justify the minimal "vision" obtained, future use cannot be ruled out.

71.1.2 Tactual Vision Substitution

With sufficient training, people without useful vision can acquire sufficient information via the tactile sense for many activities of daily living, such as walking independently and reading. The traditional long cane, for example, allows navigation by transmitting surface profile, roughness, and elasticity to the hand. Interestingly, these features are *perceived* to originate at the tip of the cane, not the hand where they are transduced; this is a simple example of **distal attribution** [Loomis, 1992]. Simple electronic aids such as the hand-held Mowat sonar sensor provide a tactile indication of range to the nearest object.

Braille reading material substitutes raised-dot patterns on 2.3-mm centers for visual letters, enabling reading rates up to 30 to 40 words per minute (wpm). Contracted Braille uses symbols for common words and affixes, enabling reading at up to 200 wpm (125 wpm is more typical).

More sophisticated instrumentation also capitalizes on the spatial capabilities of the tactile sense. The Optacon (*op*tical-to-*tac*tile *con*verter) by TeleSensory, Inc. (Mountain View, Calif.) converts the outline of printed letters recorded by a small, hand-held camera to enlarged **vibrotactile** letter outlines on the user's fingerpad. The camera's field of view is divided into 100 or 144 pixels (depending on the model), and the reflected light intensity at each pixel determines whether a corresponding vibrating pin on the fingertip is active or not. Ordinary printed text can be read at 28 (typical) or 90 (exceptional) wpm.

Spatial orientation and recognition of objects beyond the reach of a hand or long cane are the objective of experimental systems that convert an image from a television-type camera to a matrix of **electrotactile** or vibrotactile stimulators on the abdomen, forehead, or fingertip. With training, the user can interpret the patterns of tingling or buzzing pints to identify simple, high-contrast objects in front of the camera, as well as experience visual phenomena such as looming, perspective, parallax, and distal attribution [Bach-y-Rita, 1972; Collins, 1985].

Access to graphic or spatial information that cannot be converted into text is virtually impossible for blind computer users. Several prototype devices have been built to display computer graphics to the fingers via vibrating or stationary pins. A fingertip-scanned display tablet with embedded electrodes, under development in our laboratory [Kaczmarek et al., 1997], eliminates all moving parts; ongoing tests will determine if the spatial performance and reliability are adequate.

71.1.3 Auditory Vision Substitution

Electronic speech synthesizers allow access to electronic forms of text storage and manipulation. Until the arrival of graphic user interfaces such as those in the Apple Macintosh® and Microsoft Windows® computer operating systems, information displayed on computer screens was largely text-based. A number of products appeared that converted the screen information to speech at rates of up to 500 wpm, thereby giving blind computer users rapid access to the information revolution. Fortunately, much of the displayed information in graphic operating systems is not essentially pictorial; the dozen or so common graphic features (e.g., icons, scroll bars, buttons) can be converted to a limited set of words, which can then be spoken. Because of the way information is stored in these systems, however, the screen-to-text conversion process is much more complex, and the use of essentially spatial control features such as the mouse await true spatial display methods [Boyd et al., 1990].

Automated optical character recognition (OCR) combined with speech synthesis grants access to the most common printed materials (letters, office memorandums, bills), which are seldom available in Braille or narrated-tape format. First popularized in the Kurzweil reading machine, this marriage of technologies is combined with a complex set of lexical, phonetic, and syntactic rules to produce understandable speech from a wide variety of, but not all, print styles.

Mobility of blind individuals is complicated, especially in unfamiliar territory, by hazards that cannot be easily sensed with a long cane, such as overhanging tree limbs. A few devices have appeared that convert the output of sonar-like ultrasonic ranging sensors to discriminable audio displays. For example, the Wormald Sonicguide uses interaural intensity differences to indicate the azimuth of an object and frequency to indicate distance [Cook, 1982]; subtle information such as texture can sometimes also be discriminated.

71.2 Auditory System

The human auditory system processes information primarily serially; having at best two receptive channels, spatial information must be built up by integration over time. This later capability, however, is profound. Out of a full orchestra, a seasoned conductor can pinpoint an errant violinist by sound alone.

Human hearing is sensitive to sound frequencies from approximately 16 to 20,000 Hz and is most sensitive at 1000 Hz. At this frequency, a threshold root-mean-square pressure of 20 Pa (200 μbar) can be perceived by normally hearing young adults under laboratory conditions. **Sound pressure level** (SPL) is measured in decibels relative to this threshold. Some approximate benchmarks for sound intensity are a whisper at 1 m (30 dB), normal conversion at 1 m (60 dB), and a subway train at 6 m (90 dB). Sounds increasing from 100 to 140 dB become uncomfortable and painful, and short exposures to a 160-dB level can cause permanent hearing impairment, while continuous exposure to sound levels over 90 dB can cause slow, cumulative damage [Sataloff et al., 1980].

Because hearing sensitivity falls off drastically at lower frequencies, clinical audiometric testing uses somewhat different scales. With the DIN/ANSI reference threshold of 6.5 dB SPL at 1 kHz, the threshold rises to 24.5 dB at 250 Hz and 45.5 dB at 125 Hz [Sataloff et al., 1980]. Hearing loss is then specified in decibels relative to the reference threshold, rather than the SPL directly, so that a normal audiogram would have a flat threshold curve at approximately 0 dB.

71.2.1 Auditory Augmentation

Loss of speech comprehension, and hence interpersonal communication, bears the greatest effect on daily life and is the main reason people seek medical attention for hearing impairment. Functional impairment begins with 21- to 35-dB loss in average sensitivity, causing difficulty in understanding faint speech [Smeltzer, 1993]. Losses of 36–50 dB and 51–70 dB cause problems with normal and loud speech. Losses greater than 90 dB are termed *profound* or *extreme* and cannot be remedied with any kind of hearing aid; these individuals require auditory substitution rather than augmentation.

Hearing loss can be caused by conduction defects in the middle ear (tympanic membrane and ossicles) or by sensorineural defects in the inner ear (cochlear transduction mechanisms and auditory nerve). Conduction problems often can be corrected medically or surgically. If not, hearing aids are often of benefit because the hearing threshold is elevated uniformly over all frequencies, causing little distortion of the signal. Sensorineural impairments differentially affect different frequencies and also cause other forms of distortion that cannot be helped by amplification or filtering. The dynamic range is also reduced, because while loud sounds ($>$100 dB) are often still perceived as loud, slightly softer sounds are lost. Looked at from this perspective, it is easy to understand why the amplification and automatic gain control of conventional hearing aids do not succeed in presenting the 30-dB or so dynamic range of speech to persons with 70 + dB of sensorineural impairment.

Most hearing aids perform three basic functions (1) Amplification compensates for the reduced sensitivity of the damaged ear. (2) Frequency-domain filtering compensates for hearing loss that is not spectrally uniform. For example, most sensorineural loss disproportionately affects frequencies over 1 kHz or so, so high-frequency preemphasis may be indicated. (3) Automatic gain control (ACG) compresses the amplitude range of desired sounds to the dynamic range of the damaged ear. Typical AGC systems respond to loud transients in 2–5 msec (attack time) and reduce their effect in 100–300 msec (recovery time).

Sophisticated multiband AGC systems have attempted to normalize the ear's amplitude/frequency response, with the goal of preserving intact the usual intensity relationships among speech elements. However, recent research has shown that only certain speech features are important for intelligibility

[Moore, 1990]. The fundamental frequency (due to vocal cord vibration), the first and second formants (the spectral peaks of speech that characterize different vowels), and place of articulation are crucial to speech recognition. In contrast, the overall speech envelope (the contour connecting the individual peaks in the pressure wave) is not very important; articulation information is carried in second-formant and high-frequency spectral information and is not well-represented in the envelope [Van Tasell, 1993]. Therefore, the primary design goal for hearing aids should be to preserve and make audible the individual spectral components of speech (formants and high-frequency consonant information).

The cochlear implant could properly be termed an auditory augmentation device because it utilizes the higher neural centers normally used for audition. Simply stated, the implant replaces the function of the (damaged) inner ear by electrically stimulating the auditory nerve in response to sound collected by an external microphone. Although the auditory percepts produced are extremely distorted and noiselike due to the inadequate coding strategy, many users gain sufficient information to improve their lipreading and speech-production skills. The introductory chapter in this section provides a detailed discussion of this technology.

71.2.2 Visual Auditory Substitution

Lipreading is the most natural form of auditory substitution, requiring no instrumentation and no training on the part of the speaker. However, only about one-third to one-half of the 36 or so phonemes (primary sounds of human speech) can be reliably discriminated by this method. The result is that 30% to 50% of the words used in conversational English look just like, or very similar to, other words (homophenes) [Becker, 1972]. Therefore, word pairs such as buried/married must be discriminated by grammar, syntax, and context.

Lipreading does not provide information on voice fundamental frequency or formants. With an appropriate hearing aid, any residual hearing (less than 90-dB loss) often can supply some of this missing information, improving lipreading accuracy. For the profoundly deaf, technological devices are available to supply some or all of the information. For example, the Upton eyeglasses, an example of a cued-speech device, provide discrete visual signals for certain speech sounds such as fricatives (letters like *f* of *s*, containing primarily high-frequency information) that cannot be readily identified by sight.

Fingerspelling, a transliteration of English alphabet into hand symbols, can convey everyday words at up to 2 syllables per second, limited by the rate of manual symbol production [Reed et al., 1990]. American Sign Language uses a variety of upper body movements to convey words and concepts rather than just individual letters, at the same effective rate as ordinary speech, 4 to 5 syllables per second.

Closed captioning encodes the full text of spoken words on television shows and transmits the data in a nonvisible part of the video signal (the vertical blanking interval). Since July of 1993, all new television sets sold in the United States with screens larger than 33 cm diagonal have been required to have built-in decoders that can optionally display the encoded text on the screen. Over 1000 h per week of programming is closed captioned [National Captioning Institute, 1994].

Automatic speech-recognition technology may soon be capable of translating ordinary spoken discourse accurately into visually displayed text, at least in quiet environments; this may eventually be a major boon for the profoundly hearing impaired. Presently, such systems must be carefully trained on individual speakers and/or must have a limited vocabulary [Ramesh et al., 1992]. Because there is much commercial interest in speech command of computers and vehicle subsystems, this field is advancing rapidly.

71.2.3 Tactual Auditory Substitution

Tadoma is a method of communication used by a few people in the deaf-blind community and is of theoretical importance for the development of tactual auditory substitution devices. While sign language requires training by both sender and receiver, in Tadoma, the sender speaks normally. The trained receiver places his or her hands on the face and neck of the sender to monitor lip and jaw movements, airflow at the lips, and vibration of the neck [Reed et al., 1992]. Experienced users achieve 80% keyword recognition of everyday speech at a rate of 3 syllables per second. Using no instrumentation, this the highest speech communication rate recorded for any tactual-only communication system.

Alternatively, tactile vocoders perform a frequency analysis of incoming sounds, similarly to the ear's cochlea [Békésy, 1955], and adjust the stimulation intensity of typically 8 to 32 tactile stimulators (vibrotactile or electrotactile) to present a linear spectral display to the user's abdominal or forehead skin. Several investigators [Saunders et al., 1981; Blamey and Clark, 1985; Brooks and Frost, 1986; Boothroyd and Hnath-Chisolm, 1988] have developed laboratory and commercial vocoders. Although vocoder users cannot recognize speech as well as Tadoma users, research has shown that vocoders can provide enough "auditory" feedback to improve the speech clarity of deaf children and to improve auditory discrimination and comprehension in some older patients [Szeto and Riso, 1990] and aid in discrimination of phonemes by lipreading [Hughes, 1989; Rakowski et al., 1989]. An excellent review of earlier vocoders appears in Reed et al. [1982]. The most useful information provided by vocoders appears to be the second-formant frequency (important for distinguishing vowels) and position of the high-frequency plosive and fricative sounds that often delineate syllables [Bernstein et al., 1991].

71.3 Tactual System

Humans receive and combine two types of perceptual information when touching and manipulating objects. *Kinesthetic* information describes the relative positions and movements of body parts as well as muscular effort. Muscle and skin receptors are primarily responsible for kinesthesis; joint receptors serve primarily as protective limit switches [Rabischong, 1981]. Tactile information describes spatial pressure patterns on the skin given a fixed body position. Everyday touch perception combines tactile and kinesthetic information; this combination is called **tactual** or **haptic perception**. Loomis and Lederman [1986] provide an excellent review of these perceptual mechanisms.

Geldard [1960] and Sherrick [1973] lamented that as a communication channel, the tactile sense is often considered inferior to sight and hearing. However, the tactile system possess some of the same spatial and temporal attributes as both of the "primary" senses [Bach-y-Rita, 1972]. With over 10,000 parallel channels (receptors) [Collins and Saunders, 1970], the tactile system is capable of processing a great deal of information if it is properly presented.

The human kinesthetic and tactile senses are very robust and, in the case of tactile, very redundant. This is fortunate, considering their necessity for the simplest of tasks. Control of movement depends on kinesthetic information; tremors and involuntary movements can result from disruption of this feedback control system. Surgically repaired fingers may not have tactile sensation for a long period or at all, depending on the severity of nerve injuries; it is known that insensate digits are rarely used by patients [Tubiana, 1988]. Insensate fingers and toes (due to advanced Hansen's disease or diabetes) are often injured inadvertently, sometimes requiring amputation. Anyone who has had a finger numbed by cold realizes that it can be next to useless, even if the range of motion is normal.

The normal sensitivity to touch varies markedly over the body surface. The threshold forces in dynes for men (women) are lips, 9 (5); fingertips, 62 (25); belly 62 (7); and sole of foot, 343 (79) [Weinstein, 1968]. The fingertip threshold corresponds to 10-μm indentation. Sensitivity to vibration is much higher and is frequency-and area-dependent [Verillo, 1985]. A 5-cm^2 patch of skin on the palm vibrating at 250 Hz can be felt at 0.16-μm amplitude; smaller areas and lower frequencies require more displacement. The minimal separation for two nonvibrating points to be distinguished is 2–3 mm on the fingertips, 17 mm on the forehead, and 30–50 mm on many other locations. However, size and localization judgments are considerably better than these standard figures might suggest [Vierck and Jones, 1969].

71.3.1 Tactual Augmentation

Although we do not often think about it, kinesthetic information is reflected to the user in many types of human-controlled tools and machines, and lack of this feedback can make control difficult. For example, an automobile with power steering always includes some degree of "road feel" to allow the driver to respond reflexively to minor bumps and irregularities without relying on vision. Remote-control robots (telerobots) used underwater or in chemical- or radiation-contaminated environments are slow and cumbersome to operate, partly because most do not provide force feedback to the operator; such feedback enhances task performance [Hannaford and Wood, 1992].

Tactile display of spatial patterns on the skin uses three main types of transducers [Kaczmarek et al., 1991; Kaczmarek and Bach-y-Rita, 1995]. **Static tactile** displays use solenoids, shape-memory alloy actuators, and scanned air or water jets to indent the skin. Vibrotactile displays encode stimulation intensity as the amplitude of a vibrating skin displacement (10–500 Hz); both solenoids and piezoelectric transducers have been used. *Electrotactile* stimulation uses $1–100$ mm^2-area surface electrodes and careful waveform control to electrically stimulate the afferent nerves responsible for touch, producing a vibrating or tingling sensation.

Tactile rehabilitation has received minimal attention in the literature or medical community. One research device sensed pressure information normally received by the fingertips and displayed it on the forehead using electrotactile stimulation [Collins and Madey, 1974]. Subjects were able to estimate surface roughness and hardness and detect edges and corners with only one sensor per fingertip. Phillips [1988] reviews prototype tactile feedback systems that use the intact tactile sense to convey hand and foot pressure and elbow angle to users of powered prosthetic limbs, often with the result of more precise control of these devices.

Slightly more attention has been given to tactile augmentation in special environments. Astronauts, for example, wear pressurized gloves that greatly diminish tactile sensation, complicating extravehicular repair and maintenance tasks. Efforts to improve the situation range from mobile tactile pins in the fingertips to electrotactile stimulation on the abdomen of the information gathered from fingertip sensors [Bach-y-Rita et al., 1987].

71.3.2 Tactual Substitution

Because of a paucity of adequate tactual display technology, spatial pressure information from a robot or remote manipulator is usually displayed to the operator visually. A three-dimensional bar graph, for example, could show the two-dimensional pressure pattern on the gripper. While easy to implement, this method suffers from two disadvantages (1) the visual channel is required to process more information (it is often already heavily burdened), and (2) reaction time is lengthened, because the normal human tactual reflex systems are inhibited. An advantage of visual display is that accurate measurements of force and pressure may be displayed numerically or graphically.

Auditory display of tactual information is largely limited to warning systems, such as excessive force on a machine. Sometimes such feedback is even inadvertent. The engine of a bulldozer will audibly slow down when a heavy load is lifted; by the auditory and vibratory feedback, the operator can literally "feel" the strain.

The ubiquity of such tactual feedback systems suggests that the human-machine interface on many devices could benefit from intentionally placed tactual feedback systems. Of much current interest is the **virtual environment**, a means by which someone can interact with a mathematic model of a place that may or may not physically exist. The user normally controls the environment by hand, head, and body movements; these are sensed by the system, which correspondingly adjusts the information presented on a wide-angle visual display and sometimes also on a spatially localized sound display. The user often describes the experience as "being there," a phenomenon known as *telepresence* [Loomis, 1992]. One can only imagine how much the experience could be enhanced by adding kinesthetic and tactile feedback [Shimoga, 1993], quite literally putting the user in touch with the virtual world.

Defining Terms

Distal attribution: The phenomenon whereby events are normally perceived as occurring external to our sense organs — but also see Loomis' [1992] engaging article on this topic. The environment or transduction mechanism need not be artificial; for example, we visually perceive objects as distant from our eyes.

Electrotactile: Stimulation that evokes tactile (touch) sensations within the skin at the location of the electrode by passing a pulsatile, localized electric current through the skin. Information is delivered by varying the amplitude, frequency, etc. of the stimulation waveform. Also called *electrocutaneous stimulation.*

Illuminance: The density of light falling on a surface, measured in lux. One lux is equivalent to 0.0929 foot-candles, an earlier measure. Illuminance is inversely proportional to the square of the distance form a point light source. A 100-W incandescent lamp provides approximately 1280 lux at a distance of 1 ft (30.5 cm). Brightness is a different measure, depending also on the reflectance of the surrounding area.

Kinesthetic perception: Information about the relative positions of and forces on body parts, possibly including efference copy (internal knowledge of muscular effort).

Sensory augmentation: The use of devices that assist a functional human sense; eyeglasses are one example.

Sensory substitution: The use of one human sense to receive information normally received by another sense. For example, Braille substitutes touch for vision.

Sound pressure level (SPL): The root-mean-square pressure difference from atmospheric pressure (≈ 100 kPa) that characterizes the intensity of sound. The conversion SPL $= 20 \log(P/P_0)$ expresses SPL in decibels, where P_0 is the threshold pressure of approximately 20 Pa at 1 kHz.

Static tactile: Stimulation that is a slow local mechanical deformation of the skin. It varies the deformation amplitude directly rather than the amplitude of vibration. This is "normal touch" for grasping objects, etc.

Tactile perception: Information about spatial pressure patterns on the skin with a fixed kinesthetic position.

Tactual (haptic) perception: The seamless, usually unconscious combination of tactile and kinesthetic information; this is "normal touch."

Vibrotactile: Stimulation that evokes tactile sensations using mechanical vibration of the skin, typically at frequencies of 10 to 500 Hz. Information is delivered by varying the amplitude, frequency, etc. of the vibration.

Virtual environment: A real-time interactive computer model that attempts to display visual, auditory, and tactual information to a human user as if he or she were present at the simulated location. The user controls the environment with head, hand, and body motions. A airplane cockpit simulator is one example.

References

Bach-y-Rita, P. 1972. *Brain Mechanisms in Sensory Substitution.* New York, Academic Press.

Bach-y-Rita, P., Webster, J.G., Tompkins, W.J., and Crabb, T. 1987. Sensory substitution for space gloves and for space robots. In *Proceedings of the Workshop on Space Telerobotics, Jet Propulsion Laboratory, Publication* 87-13, pp. 51–57.

Bach-y-Rita, P., Kaczmarek, K.A., Tyler, M., and Garcia-Lara, M. 1998. Form perception with a 49-point electrotactile stimulus array on the tongue. *J. Rehab. Res. Dev.* 35:427–430.

Barfield, W., Hendrix, C., Bjorneseth, O., Kaczmarek, K.A., and Lotens, W. 1996. Comparison of human sensory capabilities with technical specifications of virtual environment equipment. *Presence* 4: 329–356.

Becker, K.W. 1972. *Speechreading: Principles and Methods.* Baltimore, MD, National Educational Press.

Békésy, G.V. 1955. Human skin perception of traveling waves similar to those of the cochlea. *J. Acoust. Soc. Am.* 27:830.

Bernstein, L.E., Demorest, M.E., Coulter, D.C., and O'Connell, M.P. 1991. Lipreading sentences with vibrotactile vocoders: performance of normal-hearing and hearing-impaired subjects. *J. Acoust. Soc. Am.* 90:2971.

Blamey, P.J. and Clark, G.M. 1985. A wearable multiple-electrode electrotactile speech processor for the profoundly deaf. *J. Acoust. Soc. Am.* 77:1619.

Boothroyd, A. and Hnath-Chisolm, T. 1988. Spatial, tactile presentation of voice fundamental frequency as a supplement to lipreading: results of extended training with a single subject. *J. Rehab. Res. Dev.* 25(3):51.

Boyd, L.H., Boyd, W.L., and Vanderheiden, G.C. 1990. *The Graphical User Interface Crisis: Danger and Opportunity.* September, Trace R&D Center, University of Wisconsin–Madison.

Brooks, P.L. and Frost, B.J. 1986. The development and evaluation of a tactile vocoder for the profoundly deaf. *Can. J. Public Health* 77:108.

Collins, C.C. 1985. On mobility aids for the blind. In D.H. Warren and E.R. Strelow (Eds.), *Electronic Spatial Sensing for the Blind.* pp 35–64. Dordrecht, The Netherlands, Matinus Nijhoff.

Collins, C.C. and Madey, J.M.J. 1974. Tactile sensory replacement. In *Proceedings of the San Diego Biomedical Symposium,* pp. 15–26.

Collins, C.C. and Saunders, F.A. 1970. Pictorial display by direct electrical stimulation of the skin. *J. Biomed. Syst.* 1:3–16.

Cook, A.M. 1982. Sensory and communication aids. In A.M. Cook and J.G. Webster (Eds.), *Therapeutic Medical Devices: Application and Design,* pp. 152–201. Englewood Cliffs, NJ, Prentice-Hall.

Fonda, G.E. 1981. *Management of Low Vision.* New York, Thieme-Stratton.

Geldard, F.A. 1960. Some neglected possibilities of communication. *Science* 131:1583.

Hannaford, B. and Wood L. 1992. Evaluation of performance of a telerobot. *NASA Tech. Briefs* 16(2): item 62.

Hughes, B.G. 1989. A new electrotactile system for the hearing impaired. National Science Foundation final project report, ISI-8860727, Sevrain-Tech, Inc.

Kaczmarek, K.A. and Bach-y-Rita, P. 1995. Tactile displays. In W. Barfield and T. Furness (Eds.), *Virtual Environments and Advanced Interface Design.* New York, Oxford University Press.

Kaczmarek, K.A., Webster, J.G., Bach-y-Rita, P., and Tompkins, W.J. 1991. Electrotactile and vibrotactile displays for sensory substitution systems. *IEEE Trans. Biomed. Eng.* 38:1.

Kaczmarek, K.A., Tyler, M.E., and Bach-y-Rita, P. 1997. Pattern identification on a fingertip-scanned electrotactile display. *Proceedings of the 19th Annual International Conference on IEEE Engineering Medical Biological Society,* pp. 1694–1697.

Loomis, J.M. 1992. Distal attribution and presence. *Presence: Teleoper. Virtual Environ.* 1(1):113.

Loomis, J.M. and Lederman, S.J. 1986. Tactual perception. In K.R. Boff et al. (Eds.), *Handbook of Perception and Human Performance, vol II: Cognitive Processes and Performance,* pp. 31.1–31.41. New York, Wiley.

Mehr, E. and Shindell, S. 1990. Advances in low vision and blind rehabilitation. In M.G. Eisenberg and R.C. Grzesiak (Eds.), *Advances in Clinical Rehabilitation,* Vol. 3, pp. 121–147. New York, Springer.

Moore, B.C.J. 1990. How much do we gain by gain control in hearing aids? *Acta Otolaryngol. (Stockh)* Suppl. 469:250.

Mountcastle, V.B. (Ed.). 1980. *Medical Physiology.* St. Louis, Mosby.

National Captioning Institute, Falls Church, VA, 1994. Personal communication.

NIDRR. 1993. Protocols for choosing low vision devices. U.S. Department of Education. Consensus Statement 1(1–28).

Phillips, C.A. 1988. Sensory feedback control of upper- and lower-extremity motor prostheses. *CRC Crit. Rev. Biomed. Eng.* 16:105.

Rabischong, P. 1981. Physiology of sensation. In R. Tubiana (Ed.), *The Hand,* pp. 441–467. Philadelphia, PA, Saunders.

Rakowski, K., Brenner, C., and Weisenberger, J.M. 1989. Evaluation of a 32-channel electrotactile vocoder (abstract). *J. Acoust. Soc. Am.* 86 (Suppl.1):S83.

Ramesh, P., Wilpon, J.G., McGee, M.A. et al. 1992. Speaker independent recognition of spontaneously spoken connected digits. *Speech Commun.* 11:229.

Reed, C.M., Durlach, N.I., and Bradia, L.D. 1982. Research on tactile communication of speech: a review. *AHSA Monogr.* 20:1.

Reed, C.M., Delhorne, L.A., Durlach, N.I., and Fischer, S.D. 1990. A study of the tactual and visual reception of fingerspelling. *J. Speech Hear. Res.* 33:786.

Reed, C.M., Rabinowitz, W.M., Durlach, N.I. et al. 1992. Analytic study of the Tadoma method: improving performance through the use of supplementary tactile displays. *J. Speech Hear. Res.* 35:450.

Sataloff, J., Sataloff, R.T., and Vassallo, L.A. 1980. *Hearing Loss*, 2nd ed. Philadelphia, PA, Lippincott.

Saunders, F.A., Hill, W.A., and Franklin, B. 1981. A wearable tactile sensory aid for profoundly deaf children. *J. Med. Syst.* 5:265.

Sherrick, C.E. 1973. Current prospects for cutaneous communication. In *Proceedings of the Conference on Cutaneous Communication System Development*, pp. 106–109.

Shimoga, K.B. 1993. A survey of perceptual feedback issues in dextrous telemanipulation: II. Finger touch feedback. In *IEEE Virtual Reality Annual International Symposium*, pp. 271–279.

Shlaer, S. 1937. The relation between visual acuity and illumination. *J. Gen. Physiol.* 21:165.

Smeltzer, C.D. 1993. Primary care screening and evaluation of hearing loss. *Nurse Pract.* 18:50.

Stigmar, G. 1970. Observation on vernier and stereo acuity with special reference to their relationship. *Acta Ophthalmol.* 48:979.

Szeto, A.Y.J. and Riso, R.R. 1990. Sensory feedback using electrical stimulation of the tactile sense. In R.V. Smith and J.H. Leslie, Jr (Eds.), *Rehabilitation Engineering*, pp. 29–78. Boca Raton, FL, CRC Press.

Tubiana, R. 1988. Fingertip injuries. In R. Tubiana (Ed.), *The Hand*, pp. 1034–1054. Philadelphia, PA Saunders.

Van Tasell, D.J. 1993. Hearing loss, speech, and hearing aids. *J. Speech Hear. Res.* 36:228.

Verrillo, R.T. 1985. Psychophysics of vibrotactile stimulation. *J. Acoust. Soc. Am.* 77:225.

Vierck, C.J. and Jones, M.B. 1969. Size discrimination on the skin. *Science* 163:488.

Webster, J.G., Cook, A.M., Tompkins, W.J., and Vanderheiden, G.C. (Eds.). 1985. *Electronic Devices for Rehabilitation.* New York, Wiley.

Weinstein, S. 1968. Intensive and extensive aspects of tactile sensitivity as a function of body part, sex and laterality. In D.R. Kenshalo (Ed.), *The Skin Senses*, pp. 195–218. Springfield, IL, Charles C Thomas.

Further Information

Presence: Teleoperators and Virtual Environments is a bimonthly journal focusing on advanced human-machine interface issues. In an effort to develop tactile displays without moving parts, our laboratory has demonstrated simple pattern recognition on the fingertip [Kaczmarek et al., 1997] and tongue [Bach-y-Rita et al., 1998] using electrotactile stimulation.

The Trace Research and Development Center, Madison, Wisc., publishes a comprehensive resource book on commercially available assistive devices, organizations, etc. for communication, control, and computer access for individuals with physical and sensory impairments.

Electronic Devices for Rehabilitation, edited by J.G. Webster [Wiley, 1985], summarizes the technologic principles of electronic assistive devices for people with physical and sensory impairments.

72

Augmentative and Alternative Communication

Barry Romich
Prentke Romich Company

Gregg Vanderheiden
University of Wisconsin

Katya Hill
Edinboro University of Pennsylvania

72.1 Introduction

The inability to express oneself through either speech or writing is perhaps the most limiting of physical disabilities. Meaningful participation in life requires the communication of basic information, desires, needs, feelings, and aspirations. The lack of full interpersonal communication substantially reduces an individual's potential for education, employment, and independence.

Today, through multidisciplinary contributions, individuals who cannot speak or write effectively have access to a wide variety of techniques, therapies and systems designed to ameliorate challenges to verbal communication. The field of augmentative and alternative communication (AAC) consists of many different professions, including speech-language pathology, regular and special education, occupational and physical therapy, engineering, linguistics, technology, and others. Experienced professionals now can become certified as Assistive Technology practitioners and/or suppliers [Minkel, 1996]. Individuals who rely on AAC, as well as their families and friends, also contribute to the field [Slesaransky-Poe, 1998].

Engineering plays a significant role in the development of the field of AAC and related assistive technology. Engineering contributions range from relatively independent work on product definition and design to the collaborative development and evaluation of tools to support the contributions of other professions, such as classical and computational linguistics and speech-language pathology.

Augmentative communication can be classified in a variety of ways ranging from unaided communication techniques, such as gestures, signs, and eye pointing, to highly sophisticated electronic devices employing the latest technology. This chapter focuses on the review of technology-aided techniques and related issues.

Technology-based AAC systems have taken two forms: hardware designed specifically for this application and software that runs on mass market computer hardware. Three basic components comprise AAC systems. These are the language representation method (including acceleration techniques), the user interface, and the outputs. Generally, a multidisciplinary team evaluates the current and projected skills and needs of the individual, determines the most effective language representation method(s) and physical access technique(s), and then selects a system with characteristics that are a good match.

72.2 Language Representation Methods and Acceleration Techniques

The ultimate goal of AAC intervention is functional, interactive communication. The four purposes that communication fulfills are (1) communication of needs/wants, (2) information transfer, (3) social closeness, and (4) social etiquette [Light, 1988]. From the perspective of the person who uses AAC, communicative competence involves the ability to transmit messages efficiently and effectively in all four of the interaction categories, based on individual interests, circumstances, and abilities [Buekelman and Miranda, 1998]. To achieve communication competence, the person using an AAC system must have access to language representation methods capable of handling the various vocabulary and message construction demands of the environment. Professionals rely on the theoretical models of language development and linguistics to evaluate the effectiveness of an AAC language representation method.

Language is defined as an abstract system with rules governing the sequencing of basic units (sounds, morphemes, words, and sentences), and rules governing meaning and use [McCormick and Schiefelbusch, 1990]. An individual knows a language when he or she understands and follows its basic units and rules. Knowledge of language requires both linguistic competence (understanding the rules), and linguistic performance (using these rules). Most language models identify the basic rules as phonology, semantics, morphology, syntax and pragmatics. The basic rules of language apply to AAC. For example, AAC research on vocabulary use has documented the phenomenon of core and fringe vocabulary [Yorkston et al., 1988] and the reliance on a relatively limited core vocabulary to express a majority of communication utterances [Vanderheiden and Kelso, 1987]. Research on conversations has documented topic and small talk patterns [Stuart et al., 1993; King et al., 1995]. An awareness of how a given AAC system handles these basic rules enables one to be critical of AAC language representation methods.

In addition to the language representation method, the acceleration technique(s) available in an AAC system contribute(s) to communication competence. Communication by users of AAC systems is far slower than that of the general population. Yet the speed of communication is a significant factor influencing the perceptions of the user's communication partner, and potential for personal achievement for the person relying on AAC. The development and application of techniques to accelerate communication rates is critical. Further, these techniques are most effective when developers pay attention to human factors design principles [Goodenough-Trepagnier, 1994].

Alphabet-based language representation methods involve the use of traditional orthography and acceleration techniques that require spelling and reading skills. AAC systems using orthography require the user to spell each word using a standard keyboard or alphabet overlay on a static or dynamic display. A standard or customized alphabet overlay provides use for all the rules and elements of a natural language; however, spelling letter-by-letter is a slow and inefficient AAC strategy without acceleration techniques.

Abbreviation systems represent language elements using a number of keystrokes typically smaller than that required by spelling. For example, words or sentences are abbreviated using principled approaches based on vowel elimination or the first letters of salient words. Abbreviation systems can be fast, but require not only spelling and reading skills, but memory of abbreviation codes. Typically, people with spelling and reading skills have large vocabulary needs and increased demands on production of text. Demasco [1994] offers additional background and proposes some interesting work in this area.

Word prediction is another acceleration technique available from many sources. Based on previously selected letters and words, the system presents the user with best guess choices for completing the spelling of a word. The user then chooses one of the predictions or continues spelling, resulting in yet another set of predictions. Prediction systems have demonstrated a reduction in the number of keystrokes, but recent research [Koester and Levine, 1994] reports that the actual communication rate does not represent a statistical improvement over spelling. The reason for word predication's failure to improve rate is that increased time is needed to read and select the word table choices. The cost of discontinuity and increased cognitive load in the task seems to match the benefits of reduced keystrokes.

Picture Symbol-based language representation methods involve the use of graphic or line drawn symbols to represent single word vocabulary or messages (phrases, sentences, and paragraphs). A variety of AAC symbol sets are available on devices or software depict the linguistics elements available through the system. Picture Communication Symbols (PCS), DynaSyms, and Blissymbols are popular symbol sets used in either dedicated or computer-aided systems. One taxonomy differentiates symbols according to several subordinate levels including static/dynamic, iconic/opaque, and set/system [Fuller et al., 1998].

Universal considerations regarding the selection of a symbol set include research on symbol characteristics such as size, transparency, complexity and iconicity [Romski and Sevcik, 1988; Fuller et al., 1997]. Understanding symbol characteristics is necessary to make clinical decisions about vocabulary organization and system selection. The choice of picture communication language representation methods is facilitated when teams use a goal-driven graphic symbol selection process [Schlosser et al., 1996]. For example, identification of vocabulary and language outcomes assists the selection of an AAC graphic symbol system.

Vocabulary size and representation of linguistic rules (grammar) are concerns for users relying on graphic symbol sets. Users of static display systems have a limited number of symbols available on any one overlay; however, they have ready access to that vocabulary. Dynamic display users have an almost unlimited number of symbols available as vocabulary for message generation; however, they must navigate through pages or displays to locate a word. Frequently, morphology and syntax are not graphically represented. Since research has strongly supported the need for users to construct spontaneous, novel utterances [Beukelman et al., 1984], neither method is efficient for interactive communication.

Semantic Compaction or Minspeak is perhaps the most commonly used AAC language representation method [Baker, 1994]. With this method, language is represented by a relatively small set of multi-meaning icons. The specific meaning of each icon is a function of the context in which it is used. Semantic compaction makes use of a meaningful relationship between the icon and the information it represents; it does not require spelling and reading skills, and yet is powerful even for people with these skills. The performance of Minspeak stems from its ability to handle both vocabulary and linguistic structures as found in the Minspeak Application Programs (MAPS) of Words Strategy and Unity. Both MAPS support the concept of a core and fringe vocabulary. They provide the architecture for handling rules of grammar and morphology. The number of required keystrokes is reduced relative to spelling.

Predictive selection is an acceleration technique used with Minspeak. When this feature is enabled, only those choices that complete a meaningful sequence can be selected. With scanning, for example, the selection process can be significantly faster because the number of possible choices is automatically reduced.

72.3   User Interface

Most AAC systems employ a user interface based on the selection of items that will produce the desired output [Vanderheiden and Lloyd, 1986]. Items being selected may be individual letters, as used in spelling, or whole words or phrases expressing thoughts, or symbols that represent vocabulary. The numerous techniques for making selections are based on either direct selection or scanning.

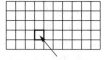

FIGURE 72.1   Direct selection.

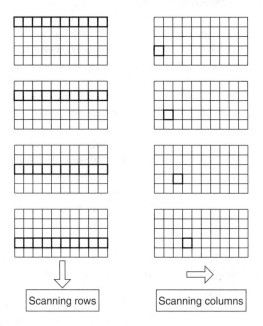

FIGURE 72.2   Row–column scanning.

Direct selection refers to techniques by which a single action from a set of choices indicates the desired item. A common example of this method is the use of a computer keyboard. Each key is directly selected by finger. Expanded keyboards accommodate more gross motor actions, such as using the fist or foot. In some cases, pointing can be enhanced through the use of technology. Sticks are held in the mouth or attached to the head using a headband or helmet. Light pointers are used to direct a light beam at a target. Indirect pointing systems might include the common computer mouse, trackball, or joystick. Alternatives to these for people with disabilities are based on the movement of the head or other body part. Figure 72.1 depicts direct selection in that the desired location is pointed to directly.

Scanning refers to techniques in which the individual is presented with a time sequence of choices and indicates when the desired choice appears. A simple linear scanning system might be a clock face type display with a rotating pointer to indicate a letter, word, or picture. Additional dimensions of scanning can be added to reduce the selection time when the number of possible choices is larger. A common technique involves the arrangement of choices in a matrix of rows and columns. The selection process has two steps. First, rows are scanned to select the row containing the desired element. The selected row is then scanned to select the desired element. This method is called row–column scanning. See Figure 72.2. Either by convention or by the grouping of the elements, the order might be reversed. For example, in the United Kingdom, column–row scanning is preferred over row–column scanning. Other scanning techniques also exist and additional dimensions can be employed.

Both direct selection and scanning are used to select elements that might not of themselves define an output. In these cases the output may be defined by a code of selected elements. A common example is Morse code by which dots and dashes are directly selected but must be combined to define letters and numbers. Another example, more common to AAC, has an output defined by a sequence of two or more pictures or icons.

Scanning, and to some degree direct selection, can be faster when the choices are arranged such that those most frequently used are easiest to access. For example, in a row–column scanning spelling system that scans top to bottom and left to right, the most frequently used letters are usually grouped toward the upper left corner.

Generally the selection technique of choice should be that which results in the fastest communication possible. Consideration of factors such as cognitive load [Cress and French, 1994], environmental changes, fatigue, aesthetics, and stability of physical skill often influence the choice of the best selection technique.

72.4 Outputs

AAC system outputs in common use are speech, displays, printers, beeps, data, infrared, and other control formats. Outputs are used to facilitate the interactive nature of "real time" communication. Users may rely on auditory and visual feedback to enhance vocabulary selection and the construction of messages. The speech and display outputs may be directed toward the communication partner to support the exchange of information. Auditory feedback such as beeps and key clicks, while useful to the individual using the system, also provide the communication partner with the pragmatic information that a user is in the process of generating a message. Finally, outputs may be used to control other items or devices such as printers.

AAC speech output normally consists of two types: synthetic and digitized.

Synthetic speech usually is generated from text input following a set of rules. Synthetic speech is usually associated with AAC systems that are able to generate text. These systems have unlimited vocabulary and are capable of speaking any word or expression that can be spelled. Commonly used synthetic speech systems like DECtalk™ offer a variety of male, female, and child voices. Intelligibility has improved over recent years to the point that it is no longer a significant issue. With some systems it is actually possible to sing songs, again a feature that enhances social interaction. Most synthetic speech systems are limited to a single language, although bilingual systems are available. Further limitations relate to the expression of accent and emotion. Research and development in artificial speech technology is attacking these limitations.

Digitized speech is essentially speech that has been recorded into digital memory. Relatively simple AAC systems typically use digitized speech. The vocabulary is entered by speaking into the system through a microphone. People who use these systems can say only what someone else said in programming them. They are independent of language and can replicate the song, accent, and emotion of the original speaker.

RS-232c serial data output is used to achieve a variety of functional outcomes. Serial output permits the AAC system to replace the keyboard and mouse for computer access, a procedure known as emulation. The advantage of emulation is that the language representation method and physical access method used for speaking is used for writing and other computer tasks [Buning and Hill, 1998]. Another application for the serial output is environmental control. Users are able to operate electrical and electronic items in their daily-living surroundings. Particular sequences of characters, symbols or icons are used to represent commands such as answering the telephone, turning off the stereo, and even setting a thermostat. In addition, the serial output also may be used to monitor the language activity for purposes of clinical intervention, progress reporting, and research.

Infrared communication now is available in many AAC devices. Infrared output supports the same functions as the RS-232c serial data output, but without requiring direct wiring or linking between operating devices. Infrared interfaces providing computer access improve the independence of AAC users because no physical connection needs to be manipulated to activate the system. Infrared interfaces can perform as environmental control units by learning the codes of entertainment and other electronic systems.

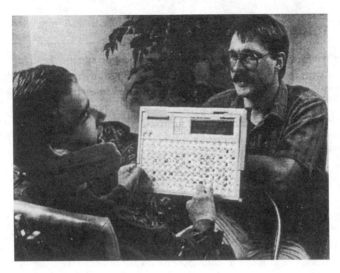

FIGURE 72.3   Individual using an electronic communication system. (Photo courtesy of Prentke Romich Company, Wooster, OH.)

72.5   Outcomes, Intervention, and Training

The choice of an AAC system should rely primarily on the best interests of the person who will be using the system. Since outcomes and personal achievement will be related directly to the ability to communicate, the choice of a system will have lifelong implications. The process of choosing the most appropriate system is not trivial and can be accomplished best with a multidisciplinary team focusing on outcomes. Team members should realize that the interests of the individual served professionally are not necessarily aligned with those of the providers and/or payers of AAC services. The temptation to select a system that is easy to apply or inexpensive to purchase frequently exists, especially with untrained teams. Teams that identify outcomes and have the goal of achieving interactive communication make informed decisions.

Following the selection (and funding) of a system, the next step is the actual intervention program. For successful outcomes to be achieved, intervention must go beyond the technical use of the AAC system and include objectives for language development and communication pragmatics. Early in the history of AAC, Rodgers postulates [1984] that AAC systems are more like tools than appliances. To be effective, there is a need for much more than simply "plugging them in and turning them on." The individual who relies on AAC must develop the skills to become a communication craftsperson. In general, as well as specific to AAC, the fastest, most efficient use of a system occurs when the individual operates from knowledge that is in the head, rather than knowledge that must be gathered from the world [Norman, 1980]. The implication for AAC is that an intervention program must include a significant training component to assure that the needed knowledge is put into the head [Romich, 1994]. Further, a drill component of training develops automaticity [Treviranus, 1994].

Perhaps the single factor limiting the widespread use of assistive technology in general and AAC in particular is the lack of awareness of its availability and the impact it can have on the lives of the people who could benefit [Romich, 1993]. This situation exists within not only the general public but also in many of the professions providing services to this population. Training opportunities continue to be limited for a majority of professionals working with persons who could benefit from AAC technology. University programs have lagged behind in their integration of this information into professional curricula.

Intervention and training should extend beyond the initial application of the system. People who rely on AAC frequently live unstable lives. Consequently they have a need for on-going services. For people with congenital (from birth) conditions, developmental delays may have occurred that result in educational and training needs past the normal age of public school services. For people with progressive neurological disorders, such as Lou Gehrig's disease, the physical skill level will change and additional accommodations will need to be evaluated and implemented.

72.6 Future

Technological development in and of itself will not solve the problems of people with disabilities. Technology advancements, however, will continue to provide more powerful tools allowing the exploration of new and innovative approaches to support users and professionals. As access to lower cost, more powerful computer systems increases, the availability of alternative sources of information, technical support and training is possible either through software or the internet. Users and professionals will have increased opportunities to learn and exchange ideas and outcomes.

A related development is the collection and analysis of data describing the actual long term use of AAC devices. Currently, clinicians and researchers have not utilized this information in the clinical intervention process, progress reporting, or research. Tools for monitoring, editing, and analyzing language activity are just now becoming available [Hill and Romich, 1998].

References

Baker, B.R. 1994. Semantic compaction: an approach to a formal definition. *Proceedings of the Sixth Annual European Minspeak Conference,* Swinstead, Lincs, UK, Prentke Romich Europe.

Beukelman, D.R., Yorkson, K., Poblete, M., and Naranjo, C. 1984. Frequency of word occurrence in communication samples produced by adult communication aid users, *J. Speech Hearing Dis.,* 49, 360–367.

Beukelman, D.R. and Mirenda, P. 1998. *Augmentative and Alternative Communication: Management of Severe Communication Disorders in Children and Adults,* Baltimore, MD, Paul H. Brookes Publishing Co.

Buning, M.E. and Hill, K. 1999. An A.A.C device as a computer keyboard: more bang for the buck. *AOTA Annual Conference,* Indianapolis.

Cress, C.J. and French, G.J. 1994. The relationship between cognitive load measurements and estimates of computer input control skills, *Ass. Tech.* 6.1, 54–66.

Demasco, P. 1994. Human factors considerations in the design of language interfaces in AAC, *Ass. Tech.* 6.1, 10–25.

Fuller, D., Lloyd, L., and Schlosser, R. 1992. Further development of an augmentative and alterntive communication symbol taxonomy, *Aug. Alt. Comm.* 8, 67–74.

Fuller, D., Lloyd, L., and Stratton, M. 1997. Aided A.A.C symbols. In L. Lloyd, D. Fuller, and H. Arvidson (Eds.), *Augmentative and Alternative Communication: Principles and Practice,* pp. 48–79, Needham Heights, MA, Allyn & Bacon.

Goodenough-Trepagnier, D. 1994. Design goals for augmentative communication, *Ass. Tech.* 6.1, 3–9.

Hill, K. and Romich, B. 1998. Language research needs and tools in AAC, *Ann. Biomed. Eng.* 26, 131.

Horstmann Koester, H. and Levine, S.P. 1994. Learning and performance of able-bodied individuals using scanning systems with and without word prediction, *Ass. Tech.* 6.1, 42–53.

King, J., Spoeneman, T., Stuart, S., and Beukelman, D. 1995. Small talk in adult conversations, *Aug. Alt. Comm.* 11, 244–248.

Light, J. 1988. Interaction involving individuals using augmentative and alternative communication systems: state of the art and future directions, *Aug. Alt. Comm.* 4, 66–82.

McCormick, L. and Schiefelbusch, R.L. 1990. *Early Language Intervention: An Introduction,* 2nd ed., Columbus, Merrill Publishing Company.

Minkel, J. 1996. Credentialing in assistive technology: myths and realities, *RESNA News* 8(5), 1.

Norman, D.A. 1980. *The Psychology of Everyday Things,* New York, Basic Books, Inc.

Rodgers, B. 1984. Presentation at Discovery '84 Conference, Chicago, IL.

Romich, B. 1993. Assistive technology and AAC: an industry perspective, *Ass. Tech.* 5.2, 74–77.

Romich, B. 1994. Knowledge in the world vs. knowledge in the head: the psychology of AAC systems, *Comm. Out.* 14(4).

Romski, M. and Sevcik, R. 1988. Augmentative and alternative communication systems: considerations for individuals with severe intellectual disabilities, *Aug. Alt. Comm.* 4, 83–93.

Schlosser, R.W., Lloyd, L.L., and McNaughton, S. 1996. Graphic symbol selection in research and practice: making the case for a goal-driven process, communication... naturally: theoretical and methodological issues. In: E. Bjorck-Akesson and P. Lindsay (Eds.), *Proceedings of the Forth, ISAAC Research Symposium,* pp. 126–139.

Slesaransky-Poe, G. 1998. ACOLUG: the communication on-line user's group, *ISAAC Proc.* 51–52.

Stuart, S., Vanderhoof, D., and Beukelman, D. 1993. Topic and vocabulary use patterns of elderly women, *Aug. Alt. Comm.* 9, 95–110.

Treviranus, J. 1994. Mastering alternative computer access: the role of understanding, trust, and automaticity, *Ass. Tech.* 6.1, 26–41.

Vanderheiden, G.C. and Lloyd, L.L. 1986. In S.W. Blackstone (Ed.), *Augmentative Communication: An Introduction,* Rockville, MD: American Speech–Language–Hearing Association.

Vanderheiden, G.C. and Kelso, D. 1987. Comparative analysis of fixed-vocabulary comunication acceleration techniques, *Aug. Alt. Comm.* 3, 196–206.

Yorkston, K.M., Dowden, P.A., Honsinger, M.J., Marriner, N., and Smith K. 1988. A comparison of standard and user vocabulary list, Aug. Alt. Comm. 4, 189–210.

Further Information

There are a number of organizations and publications that relate to AAC.

AAC (Augmentative and Alternative Communication) is the quarterly refereed journal of ISAAC. It is published by Decker Periodicals Inc., PO Box 620, L.C.D. 1, Hamilton, Ontario, L8N 3K7 CANADA, Tel. 905-522-7017, Fax. 905-522-7839. http://www.isaac-online.org

ACOLUG (Augmentative Communication On-Line User Group) is a listserve with primary participants being people who rely on AAC. Topics include a wide range of issues of importance to this population, their relatives, and friends, and those who provide AAC services. http://nimbus.ocis.temple.edu/~kcohen/listserv/homeacolug.html

American Speech-Language-Hearing Association (ASHA) is the professional organization of speech-language pathologists. ASHA has a Special Interest Division on augmentative communication. ASHA, 10801 Rockville Pike, Rockville, MD, 20852, Tel. 301-897-5700, Fax. 301-571-0457. http://www.asha.org.

Augmentative Communication News is published bi-monthly by Augmentative Communication, Inc., 1 Surf Way, Suite #215, Monterey, CA, 93940, Tel. 408-649-3050, Fax. 408-646-5428.

CAMA (Communication Aid Manufacturers Association) is an organization of manufacturers of AAC systems marketed in North America. CAMA, 518-526 Davis St., Suite 211-212, Evanston, IL, 60201, Tel. 800-441-2262, Fax. 708-869-5689. http://www.aacproducts.org.

Communicating Together is published quarterly by Sharing to Learn as a means of sharing the life experiences and communication systems of augmentative communicators with other augmentative communicators, their families, their communities, and those who work with them. Sharing to Learn, PO Box 986, Thornhill, Ontario, L3T 4A5, CANADA, Tel. 905-771-1491, Fax. 905-771-7153. http://www.isaac-online.org.

Communication Outlook is an international quarterly addressed to the community of individuals interested in the application of technology to the needs of persons who experience communication handicaps. It is published by the Artificial Language Laboratory, Michigan State University, 405 Computer Center, East Lansing, MI, 48824-1042, Tel. 517-353-0870, Fax. 517-353-4766. http://www.msu.edu/~artlang/CommOut.html.

ISAAC is the International Society for Augmentative and Alternative Communication). USSAAC is the United States chapter. Both can be contacted at PO Box 1762 Station, R., Toronto, Ontario, M4G 4A3, Canada, Tel. 905-737-9308, Fax 905-737-0624. http://www.isaac-online.org.

RESNA is an interdisciplinary association for the advancement of rehabilitation and assistive technologies. RESNA has many Special Interest Groups including those on Augmentative and Alternative Communication and Computer Applications. RESNA, 1700 North Moore Street, Suite 1540, Arlington, VA, 22209-1903, Tel. 703-524-6686.

Trace Research & Development Center, University of Wisconsin — Madison. http://www.trace.wisc.edu.

73

Measurement Tools and Processes in Rehabilitation Engineering

George V. Kondraske
University of Texas-Arlington

In every engineering discipline, measurement facilitates the use of structured **procedures** and decision-making processes. In rehabilitation engineering, the presence of "a human," the only or major component of *the system of interest*, has presented a number of unique challenges with regard to measurement. This is especially true with regard to the routine processes of rehabilitation that either do or could incorporate and rely on measurements. This, in part, is due to the complexity of the human system's architecture, the variety of ways in which it can be adversely affected by disease or injury, and the versatility in the way it can be used to accomplish various **tasks** of interest to an individual.

Measurement supports a wide variety of assistive device design and prescription activities undertaken within rehabilitation engineering (e.g., Webster et al. [1985], Smith and Leslie [1990], and other chapters within this section). In addition, rehabilitation engineers contribute to the specification and design of measurement instruments that are used primarily by other service providers (such as physical and occupational therapists). As measurements of human **structure**, **performance**, and **behavior** become more rigorous and instruments used have taken advantage of advanced technology, there is also a growing role for rehabilitation engineers to assist these other medical professionals with the proper application of measurement instruments (e.g., for determining areas that are most deficient in an individual's performance profile, objectively documenting progress during rehabilitation, etc.). This is in keeping with the team approach to rehabilitation that has become popular in clinical settings. In short, the role of measurement in rehabilitation engineering is dynamic and growing.

In this chapter, a top-down overview of measurement tools and processes in rehabilitation engineering is presented. Many of the measurement concepts, processes, and devices of relevance are common to applications outside the rehabilitation engineering context. However, the nature of the human population with which rehabilitation engineers must deal is arguably different in that each individual must be assumed to be unique with respect to at least a subset of his or her performance capacities and/or structural parameters; that is, population reference data cannot be assumed to be generally applicable. While there are some exceptions, population labels frequently used such as "head-injured" or "spinal cord-injured" represent only a gross classification that should not be taken to imply homogeneity with regard to parameters such as range of motion, strength, movement speed, information processing speed, and other performance capacities. This is merely a direct realization that many different ways exist in which the human system can be adversely affected by disease or injury and recognition of the continuum that exists with regard to the degree of any given effect. The result is that in rehabilitation engineering, compared with standard human factors design tasks aimed at the average healthy population, many measurement values must be acquired directly for the specific client.

Measurement in the present context encompasses actions that focus on (1) the human (e.g., structural aspects and performance capacities of subsystems at different hierarchical levels ranging from specific neuromuscular subsystems to the total person and his or her activities in daily living, including work), (2) assistive devices (e.g., structural aspects and demands placed on the human), (3) tasks (e.g., distances between critical points, masses of objects involved, etc.), and (4) overall systems (e.g., performance achieved by a human-assistive device-task combination, patterns of electrical signals representing the timing of muscle activity while performing a complex maneuver, behavior of an individual before and after being fitted with a new prosthetic devices, etc.). Clearly, an exhaustive treatment is beyond the scope of this chapter. Measurements are embedded in every specialized subarea of rehabilitation engineering. However, there are also special roles served by measurement in a broader and more generic sense, as well as principles that are common across the many special applications. Emphasis here is placed on these.

There is no lack of other literature regarding the types of measurement outlined to be of interest here and their use. However, it is diffusely distributed, and gaps exist with regard to how such tools can be integrated to accomplish **goals** beyond simply the acquisition of numeric data for a given parameter. With rapidly changing developments over the last decade, there is currently no comprehensive source that describes the majority of instruments available, their latest implementations, procedures for their use, evaluation of effectiveness, etc. While topics other than measurement are discussed, Leslie and Smith [1990] produced what is perhaps the single most directly applicable source with respect to rehabilitation engineering specifically, although it too is not comprehensive with regard to measurement, nor does it attempt to be.

73.1 Fundamental Principles

Naturally, the fundamental principles of human physiology manifest themselves in the respective sensory, neuromuscular, information-processing, and life-sustaining systems and impact approaches to measurement. In addition, psychological considerations are vital. Familiarization with this material is essential to measurement in rehabilitation; however, treatment here is far beyond the scope of this chapter. The numerous reference works available may be most readily found by consulting relevant chapters in this *Handbook* and the works that they reference. In this section, key principles that are more specific to measurement and of general applicability are presented.

73.1.1 Structure, Function, Performance, and Behavior

It is necessary to distinguish between structure, **function**, performance, and behavior and measurements thereof for both human and artificial systems. In addition, hierarchical systems concepts are necessary both to help organize the complexity of the systems involved and to help understand the various needs that exist.

Structural measures include dimensions, masses (of objects, limb segments), moments of inertia, circumferences, contours, compliances, and any other aspects of the physical system. These may be considered hierarchically as being pertinent to the total human (e.g., height, weight, etc.), specific body segments (e.g., forearm, thigh, etc.), or components of basic systems such as tendons, ligaments and muscles.

Function is the *purpose* of the system of interest (e.g., to move a limb segment, to communicate, to feed and care for oneself). Within the human, there are many single-purpose systems (e.g., those that function to move specific limb segments, process specific types of information, etc.). As one proceeds to higher levels, such as the total human, systems that are increasingly more multifunctional emerge. These can be recognized as higher-level configurations of more basic systems that operate to feed oneself, to conduct personal hygiene, to carry out task of a job, etc. This multilevel view of just functions begins to help place into perspective the scope over which measurement can be applied.

In rehabilitation in general, a good deal of what constitutes measurement involves the application of structured subjective observation techniques (see also the next subsection) in the form of a wide range of rating scales [e.g., Granger and Greshorn, 1984; Potvin et al., 1985; Fuhrer, 1987]. These are often termed **functional assessment scales** and are typically aimed at obtaining a global index of an individual's ability to function independently in the world. The global index is typically based on a number of items within a given scale, each of which addresses selected, relatively high-level functions (e.g., personal hygiene, mobility, etc.). The focus of measurement for a given item is often in estimate of the *level* of independence or dependence that the subject exhibits or needs to carry out the respective function. In addition, inventories of functions that an individual is able or not able to carry out (with and without assistance) are often included. The large number of such scales that have been proposed and debated is a consequence of the many possible functions and combinations thereof that exist on which to base a given scale. Functional assessment scales are relatively quick and inexpensive to administer and have a demonstrated role in rehabilitation. However, the nature and levels of measurements obtained are not sufficient for many rehabilitation engineering purposes. This latter class of applications generally begins with a function at the level and of the type used as a constituent component of functional assessment scales, considers the level of performance at which that function is executed more quantitatively, and incorporates one or more lower levels in the hierarchy (i.e., the human subsystems involved in achieving the specific functions of daily life that are of interest and their capacities for performance).

Where functions can be described and inventoried, *performance* measures directly characterize *how well* a physical system of interest executes its intended function. Performance is multidimensional (e.g., strength, range, speed, accuracy, steadiness, endurance, etc.). Of special interest are the concepts of **performance capacity** and **performance capacity measurement**. Performance capacity represents the *limits* of a given system's ability to operate in its corresponding multidimensional performance space. In this chapter, a resource-based model for both human and artificial system performance and measurement of their performance capacities is adopted [e.g., Kondraske, 1990, 1995]. Thus the *maximum* knee flexor strength available (i.e., the resource availability) under a stated set of conditions represents one unique performance capacity of the knee flexor system. In rehabilitation, the terms *impairment, disability,* and *handicap* (World Health Organization, 1980) have been prominently applied and are relevant to the concept of performance. While these terms place an emphasis on what is missing or what a person cannot do and imply not only a measurement but also the incorporation of an assessment or judgment based on one or more observations the resource-based performance perspective focuses on "what is present" or "what is right". (i.e., performance resource availability). From this perspective, an impairment can be determined to exist if a given performance capacity is found to be less than a specified level (e.g., less than 5th percentile value of a health reference population). A disability exists when performance resource insufficiency exists in a specified task.

While performance relates more to what a system can do (i.e., a challenge or maximal stress is implied), *behavior* measurements are used to characterize what a system does naturally. Thus a given variable such as movement speed can relate to both performance and behavior depending on whether the system (e.g., human subsystem) was maximally challenged to respond "as fast as possible" (performance) or simply observed in the course of operation (behavior). It is also possible to observe a system that it is behaving at one or more of its performance capacities (e.g., at the maximum speed possible, etc.) (see Table 73.1).

73.1.2   Subjective and Objective Measurement Methods

Subjective measurements are made by humans without the aid of instruments and objective measurements result from the use of instruments. However, it should be noted that the mere presence of an instrument does not guarantee complete objectivity. For example, the use of a ruler requires a human judgment in reading the scale and thus contains a subjective element. A length-measurement system with an integral data-acquisition system would be more objective. However, it is likely that that even this system would involve human intervention in its use, for example, the alignment of the device and making the decision as to exactly what is to be measured with it by selection of reference points. Measures with more objectivity (less subjectivity) are preferred to minimize questions of bias. However, measurements that are intrinsically more objective are frequently more costly and time-consuming to obtain. Well-reasoned tradeoffs must be made to take advantage of the ability of a human (typically a skilled professional) to quickly "measure" many different items subjectively (and often without recording the results but using them internally to arrive at some decision).

It is important to observe that identification of the variable of interest is not influenced by whether it is measured subjectively or objectively. This concept extends to the choice of instrument used for objective measurements. This is an especially important concept in dealing with human performance and behavior, since variables of interest can be much more abstract than simple lengths and widths (e.g., coordination, postural stability, etc.). In fact, many measurement variables in rehabilitation historically have tended to be treated as if they were inextricably coupled with the measurement method, confounding debate regarding *what should be measured with what should be used to measure it* in a given context.

73.1.3   Measurements and Assessments

The basic representation of a measurement itself in terms of the actual units of measure is often referred to as the *raw form*. For measures of performance, the term *raw score* is frequently applied. Generally, some form of *assessment* (i.e., judgment or interpretation) is typically required. Assessments may be applied to (or, viewed from a different perspective, may require) either a single measure of groups of them. Subjective assessments are frequently made that are based on the practitioner's familiarity with values for a given parameter in a particular context. However, due to the large number of parameters and the amount of experience that would be required to gain a sufficient level of familiarity, a more formal and objective realization of the process that takes place in subjective assessments is often employed. This process combines the measured value with objectively determined reference values to obtain new metrics, or scores, that facilitate one or more steps in the assessment process.

For aspects of performance, *percent normal scores* are computed by expressing subject Y's availability of performance resource $k[R_{A_k}(Y)]$ as a fraction of the mean availability of that resource in a specified reference population $[R_{A_k}(\text{pop})]$. Ideally, the reference population is selected to match the characteristics of the individual as closely as possible (e.g., age range, gender, handedness, etc.).

$$\text{Percent normal} = \frac{R_{A_k}(Y)}{R_{A_k}(\text{pop})} \times 100 \qquad (73.1)$$

TABLE 73.1 The Scope of Measurement in Rehabilitation Is Broad

Hierarchical level	Structure	Function	Performance	Behavior
Global/composite • Total human • Human with artificial systems	• Height • Weight • Postures • Subjective and instrumented methods	• Multifunction, reconfigurable system • High-level functions: tasks of daily life (working, grooming, recreation, etc.) • Functional assessment scales • Single-number global index • Level of indep. estimates	• No single-number direct measurement is possible • Possible models to integrate lower-level measures • Direct measurement (subjective and instrumented) of selected performance attribute for selected functions	• Subjective self- and family reports • Instrumented ambulatory activity monitors (selected attributes) • See notes under "function"
Complex body systems • Cognitive • Speech • Lifting, gait • Upper extremity • Cardiovascular/respiratory • Etc.	• Dimensions • Shape • Etc. • Instrumented methods	• Multifunction, reconfigurable systems • System-specific functions	• Function specific subjective rating scales Often based on impairment/disability concepts Relative metrics • Some instrumented performance capacity measures Known also as "functional capacity" (misnomer)	• Subjective and automated (objective) videotape evaluation • Instrumented measures of physical quantities vs. time (e.g., forces, angles, motions) • Electromyography (e.g., muscle timing patterns, coordination)
Basic systems • Visual information processors • Flexors, extensors • Visual sensors • Auditory sensors • Lungs • Etc.	• Dimensions • Shape • Masses • Moments of inertia • Instrumented methods	• Single function • System-specific functions	• Subjective estimates by clinician for diagnostic and routine monitoring purposes • Instrumented measures of performance capacities (e.g., strength, extremes/range of motion, speed, accuracy, endurance, etc.)	• Instrumented systems Measure and log electrophysiologic biomechanical, and other variables vs. time Post-hoc parameterization
Components of basic systems • Muscle • Tendon • Nerve • Etc.	• Mechanical properties • Instrumented methods/imaging	• Generally single-function • Component-specific functions	• Difficult to assess for individual subjects • Infer from measures at "basic system level" • Direct measurement methods with lab samples, research applications	• Difficult to assess for individual subject • Direct measurement methods with lab samples, research applications

Note: Structure, function, performance, and behavior are encompassed at multiple hierarchical levels. Both subjective and objective, instrumented methods of measurement are employed.

Aside from the benefit of placing all measurements on a common scale, a percent normal representation of a performance capacity score can be loosely interpreted as a probability. Consider grip strength as the performance resource. Assume that there is a uniform distribution of demands of demands placed on grip strength across a representative sample of tasks of daily living, with requirements ranging from zero to the value representing mean grip strength availability in the reference population. Further assuming that grip strength was the only performance resource that was in question for subject Y (i.e., all other were available in nonlimiting amounts), the percent normal score would represent the probability that a task involving grip strength, randomly selected from those which average individuals in the reference population could execute (i.e., those for which available grip strength would be adequate), could be successfully executed by subject Y. While the assumptions stated here are unlikely to be perfectly true, this type of interpretation helps place measurements that are most commonly made in the laboratory into daily-life contexts.

In contrast to percent normal metrics, *z-scores* take into account variability within the selected reference population. Subject Y's performance is expressed in terms of the difference between it and the reference population mean, normalized by a value corresponding to one standard deviation unit (σ) of the reference population distribution:

$$z = \frac{R_{A_k}(Y) - R_{A_k}(\text{pop})}{\sigma} \tag{73.2}$$

It is important to note that valid z-scores assume that the parameter in question exhibit a normal distribution in the reference population. Moreover, z-scores are useful in assessing measures of structure, performance, and behavior. With regard to performance (and assuming that measures are based on a resource construct, that is, a larger numeric value represents better performance), a z-score of zero is produced when the subject's performance equals that of the mean performance in the reference population. Positive z-scores reflect performance that is better than the population mean. In a normal distribution, 68.3% of the samples fall between z-scores of -1.0 and $+1.0$, while 95.4% of these samples fall between z-scores of -2.0 and $+2.0$. Due to variability of a given performance capacity within a healthy population (e.g., some individuals are stronger, faster, more mobile than others), a subject with a raw performance capacity score that produces a percent normal score of 70% could easily produce a z-score of -1.0. Whereas this percent normal score might raise concern regarding the variable of interest, the z-score of -1.0 indicates that a good fraction of healthy individuals exhibit lower level of performance capacity.

Both percent normal and z-scores require reference population data to compute. The best reference (i.e., most sensitive) is data for that specific individual (e.g., preinjury or predisease onset). In most cases, these data do not exist. However, practices such as preemployment screenings and regular checkups are beginning to provide individualized reference data in some rehabilitation contexts.

In yet another alternative, it is frequently desirable to use values representing demands imposed by tasks $[R_{D_k}(\text{task A})]$ as the reference for assessment of performance capacity measures. Demands on performance resources can be envisioned to vary over the time course of a task. In practice, an estimate of the worst-case value (i.e., highest demand) would be used in assessments that incorporate task demands as reference values. In one form, such assessments can produce binary results. For example, availability can be equal to or exceed demand (resource sufficiency), or it can be less than demand (resource insufficiency). These rule-based assessments are useful in identifying limiting factors, that is, those performance resources that inhibit a specified type of task from being performed successfully or that prevent achievement of a higher level of performance in a given type of task.

$$\text{If } R_{A_k}(\text{subject Y}) \geq R_{D_k}(\text{task A}), \quad \text{then } R_{A_k}(\text{subject Y}) \text{ is sufficient,}$$
$$\text{else } R_{A_k}(\text{subject Y}) \text{ is insufficient} \tag{73.3}$$

These rule-based assessments represent the basic process often applied (sometimes subliminally) by experienced clinicians in making routine decisions, as evidenced by statements such as "not enough strength," "not enough stability," etc. It is natural to extend and build on these strategies for use with objective measures. Extreme care must be employed. It is often possible, for example, for an individual to substitute another performance resource that is not insufficient for one that is. Clinicians take into account many such factors, and objective components should be combined with subjective assessments that provide the required breadth that enhances validity of objective components of a given assessment.

Using the same numeric values employed in rule-based binary assessments, a *preference capacity stress* metric can be computed:

$$\text{Performance capacity stress (\%)} = \frac{R_{D_k}(\text{task A})}{R_{A_k}(\text{subject Y})} \times 100 \tag{73.4}$$

Binary assessments also can be made using this metric and a threshold of 100%. However, the stress value provides additional information regarding how far (or close) a given performance capacity value is from the sufficiency threshold.

73.2 Measurement Objectives and Approaches

73.2.1 Characterizing the Human System and Its Subsystems

Figure 73.1 illustrates various points at which measurements are made over the course of a disease or injury, as well as some of the purposes for which they are made. The majority of measurements made in rehabilitation are aimed at characterizing the human system.

Measurements of human structure [Pheasant, 1986] play a critical role in the design and prescription of components such as seating, wheelchairs, workstations, artificial limbs, etc. Just like clothing, these items must "fit" the specific individual. Basic tools such as measuring tapes and rulers are becoming supplemented with three-dimensional digitizers and devices found in computer-aided manufacturing. Measurements of structure (e.g., limb segment lengths, moments of inertia, etc.) are also used with computer models [Vasta and Knodraske, 1995] in the process of analyzing tasks to determine demands in terms of performance capacity variables associated with basic systems such as flexors and extensors.

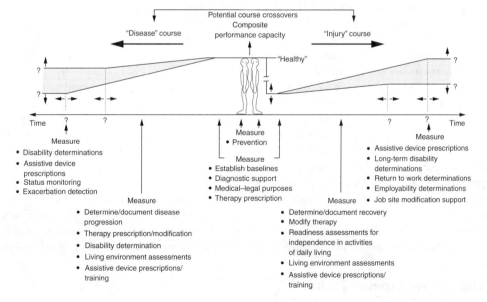

FIGURE 73.1 Measurements of structure, performance, and behavior serve many different purposes at different points over the course of a disease or injury that results in the need for rehabilitation services.

After nearly 50 years, during which a plethora of mostly disease- and injury-specific functional assessment scales were developed, the *functional independence measure* (FIM) [Hamilton et al., 1987; Keith et al., 1987] is of particular note. It is the partial result of a task-force effort to produce a systematic methodology (Uniform Data System for Medical Rehabilitation) with the specific intent of achieving standardization throughout the clinical service-delivery system. This broad methodology uses subjective judgements exclusively, based on rigorous written guidelines, to categorize demographic, diagnostic, functional, and cost information for patients within rehabilitation settings. Its simplicity to use once learned and its relatively low cost of implementation have helped in gaining a rather widespread utilization for tracking progress of individuals from admission to discharge in rehabilitation programs and evaluating effectiveness of specific therapies within and across institutions.

In contrast, many objective measurement tools of varying degrees of technological sophistication exist [Potvin et al., 1985; Smith and Leslie, 1990; Jones, 1995; Kondraske, 1995; Smith, 1995] (also see Further Information below). A good fraction of these have been designed to accomplish the same purposes as corresponding subjective methods, but with increased resolution, sensitivity, and repeatability. The intent is not always to replace subjective methods completely but to make available alternatives with the advantages noted for situations that demand superior performance in the aspects noted. There are certain measurement needs, however, that cannot be accomplished via subjective means (e.g., measurement of a human's visual information-processing speed, which involves the measurement of times of less than 1 sec with millisecond resolution). These needs draw on the latest technology in a wide variety of ways, as demonstrated in the cited material.

With regard to instrumented measurements that pertain to a specific individual, performance capacity measures at both complex body system and basic system levels (Figure 73.1) constitute a major area of activity. A prime example is methodology associated with the implementation of industrial lifting standards [NIOSH, 1981]. Performance-capacity measures reflect the limits of availability of one or more selected resources and require test strategies in which the subject is commanded to perform at or near a maximum level under controlled conditions. Performance tests typically last only a short time (seconds or minutes). To improve estimates of capacities, multiple trials are usually included in a given "test" from which a final measure is computed according to some established reduction criterion (e.g., average across five trials, best of three trials). This strategy also tends to improve test-retest repeatability. Performance capacities associated with basic and intermediate-level systems are important because they are "targets of therapy" [Tourtellotte, 1993], that is, the entities that patients and service providers want to increase to enhance the chance that enough will be available to accomplish the tasks of daily life. Thus measurements of baseline levels and changes during the course of a rehabilitation program provide important documentation (for medical, legal, insurance, and other purposes) as well as feedback to both the rehabilitation team and the patient.

Parameters of human behavior are also frequently acquired, often to help understand an individual's response to a therapy or new circumstance (e.g., obtaining a new wheelchair or prosthetic device). Behavioral parameters reflect what the subject does normally and are typically recorded over longer time periods (e.g., hours or days) compared with that required for a performance capacity measurement under conditions that are more representative of the subject's natural habitat (i.e., less laboratory-like). The general approach involves identifying the behavior (i.e., an event such as "head flexion," "keystrokes," "steps," "repositionings," etc.) and at least one parametric attribute of it. Frequency, with units of "events per unit time," and time spent in a given behavioral or activity state [Ganapathy and Kondraske, 1990] are the most commonly employed behavioral metrics. States may be detected with electromyographic means or electronic sensors that respond to force, motion, position, or orientation. Behavioral measures can be used as feedback to a subject as a means to encourage desired behaviors or discourage undesirable behaviors.

73.2.2 Characterizing Tasks

Task characterization or *task analysis*, like the organization of human system parameters, is facilitated with a hierarchical perspective. A highly objective, algorithmic approach could be delineated for task analysis in any given situation [Imrhan, 1995; Maxwell, 1995]. The basic objective is to obtain both descriptive and quantitative information for making decisions about the interface of a system (typically a human) to a given task. Specifically, function, procedures, and goals are of special interest. *Function* represents the purpose of a task (e.g., to flex the elbow, to lift an object, to communicate). In contrast, task goals relate to performance, or how well the function is to be excuted, and are quantifiable (e.g., the mass of an object to be lifted, the distance over which the lift must occur, the speed at which the lift must be performed, etc.). In situations with human and artificial systems, the term **overall task goals** is used to distinguish between goals of the combined human-artificial system and goals associated with the task of operating the artificial system. Procedures represent the process by which goals are achieved. Characterization of procedures can include descriptive and quantitative components (e.g., location of a person's hands at beginning and end points of a task, path in three-dimensional space between beginning and end points). Partial or completely unspecified procedures allow for variations in **style**. *Goals* and *procedures* are used to obtain numeric estimates of task demands in terms of the performance resources associated with the systems anticipated to be used to execute the task. Task demands are time dependent. Worst-case demands, which may occur only at specific instants in time, are of primary interest in task analysis.

Estimates of task demand can be obtained (1) direct measurement (i.e., of goals and procedures), (2) the use of physics-based models to map direct measurements into parameters that relate more readily to measurable performance capacities of human subsystems, or (3) inference. Examples of direct measurement include key dimensions and mass of objects, three-dimensional spatial locations between "beginning" and "end points" of objects in tasks involving the movement of objects, etc. Instrumentation supporting task analysis is available (e.g., load cells, video and other systems for measuring human position and orientation in real-time during dynamic activities), but it is not often integrated into systems for task analysis per se. Direct measurements of forces based on masses of objects and gravity often must be translated (to torques about a given body joint): this requires the use of static and dynamic models and analysis [Winter, 1990; Vasta and Kondraske, 1995].

An example of an inferential task-analysis approach that is relatively new is nonlinear causal resource analysis (NCRA) [Kondraske, 1998, 1999; Kondraske et al., 1997]. This method was motivated by human performance analysis situations where direct analysis is not possible (e.g., determination of the amount of visual information-processing speed required to drive safely on a highway). Quantitative task demands, in terms of performance variables that characterize the involved subsystems, are inferred from a population data set that includes measures of subsystem performance, resource availabilities (e.g., speed, accuracy, etc.), and overall performance on the task in question. This method is based on the simple observation that the individual with the *least amount* of the given resource (i.e., the lowest performance capacity) who is still able to accomplish a given goal (i.e., achieve a given level of performance in the specified high-level task) provides the key clue. That amount of availability is used to infer the amount of demand imposed by the task.

The ultimate goal to which task characterization contributes is to identify limiting factors or unsafe conditions when a specific subject undertakes the task in question; this goal must not be lost while carrying out the basic objectives of task analysis. While rigorous algorithmic approaches are useful to make evident the true detail of the process, they are generally not performed in this manner in practice at present. Rather, the skill and experience of individuals performing the analysis are used to simplify the process, resulting in a judicious mixture of subjectives estimates and objective measurements. For example, some limiting factors (e.g., grip strength) may be immediately identified without measurement of the human or the task requirements because the margin between availability and demand is so great that quick subjective "measurements" followed by an equally quick "assessment" can be used to arrive at the proper conclusion (e.g., "grip strength is a limiting factor in this task").

73.2.3 Characterizing Assistive Devices

Assistive devices can be viewed as artificial systems that either completely or partially bridge a gap between a given human (with his or her unique profile of performance capacities, i.e., available performance resources) and a particular task or class of tasks (e.g., communication, mobility, etc.). It is thus possible to consider the aspects of the device that constitute the user-device interface and those aspects which constitute, more generally, the device-task interface. In general, measurements supporting assessment of the user-device interface can be viewed to consist of (1) those which characterize the human and (2) those which characterize tasks (i.e., "operating" the assistive device). Each of these was described earlier. Measurements that characterize the device-task interface are often carried out in the context of the complete system, that is, the human-assistive device-task combination (see next subsection).

73.2.4 Characterizing Overall Systems in High-Level-Task Situations

This situation generally applies to a human-artificial system-task combination. Examples include an individual using a communication aid to communicate, an individual using a wheelchair to achieve mobility, etc. Here, concern is aimed at documenting how well the task (e.g., communication, mobility, etc.) is achieved by the composite or overall system. Specific aspects or *dimensions of performance* associated with the relevant function should first be identified. Examples include speech, accuracy, stability, efficiency, etc. The total system is then maximally challenged (tempered by safety considerations) to operate along one or more of these dimensions of performance (usually not more than two dimensions are maximally challenged at the same time). For example, a subject with a communication device may be challenged to generate a single selected symbol "as fast as possible" (stressing speed without concern for accuracy). Speed is measured (e.g., with units of symbols per second) over the course of short trial (so as not to be influenced by fatigue). Then the "total system" may be challenged to generate a subset of specific symbols (chosen at random from the set of those available with a given device) one at a time, "as accurately as possible" (stressing accuracy while minimizing stress on speed capacities). Accuracy is then measured after a representative number of such trials are administered (in terms of "percent correct," for example). To further delineate the speed-accuracy performance envelope, "the system" may be challenge to select symbols at a fixed rate while accuracy is measured. Additional dimensions can be evaluated similarly. For example, endurance (measure in units of time) can be determined by selecting an operating point (e.g., by reference to the speed-accuracy performance envelope) and challenging the total system "to communicate" for "as long as possible" under the selected speed-accuracy condition.

In general, it is more useful if these types of characterizations consider all relevant dimensions with some level of measurements (i.e., subjective or objective) than it would be to apply a high resolution, objective measurement in a process that considers only one aspect of performance.

73.3   Decision-Making Processes

Measurements that characterize the human, task, assistive device, or combination thereof are themselves only means to an end; the end is typically a decision. As noted previously, decisions are often the result of assessment processes involving one or more measurements. Although not exhaustive, many of the different types of assessments encountered are related to the following questions (1) Is a particular aspect of performance normal (or impaired)? (2) Is a particular aspect of performance improving, stable, or getting worse? How should therapy be modified? (3) Can a given subject utilize (and benefit from) a particular assistive device? (4) Does a subject possess the required capacity to accomplish a given higher level task (e.g., driving, a particular job after a work-related injury, etc.)?

In Figure 73.2, several of the basic concepts associated with measurement are used to illustrate how they enter into and facilitate systematic decision-making processes. The upper section shows raw score values as well as statistics for a healthy normal reference population in tabular form (left). It is difficult to reach any decision by simple inspection of just the raw performance capacity values. Tabular data are used to obtain percent normal (middle) and z-score (right) assessments. Both provide a more directly interpretable result regarding subject A's impairments. By examining the "right shoulder flexion extreme of motion" item in the figure, it can be seen that a raw score value corresponding to 51.2% normal yields a very large-magnitude, negative z-score (-10.4). This z-score indicates that virtually no one in the reference population would have a score this low. In contrast, consider similar scores for the "grip strength" item (56.2% normal, z-score $= -1.99$). On the basis of percent normal scores, it would appear that both of these resources are similarly affected, whereas the z-score basis provides a considerably different perspective due to the fact that grip strength is *much more variable* in healthy populations than the extreme angle obtained by a given limb segment about a joint, relatively speaking. As noted, z-scores account for this variability.

The lower section of Figure 73.2 considers a situation in which the issue is a specific individual (subject A) considered in a specific task. Tabular data now include raw score values (which are the same as in upper section of the figure) and quantitative demands (typically worst case) imposed on the respective performance resources by task X. The lower-middle plot illustrates the process of individually assessing sufficiency of each performance resource in this task context using a rule-based assessment that incorporates the idea of a threshold (i.e., availability must exceed demand for sufficiency). The lower-right plot illustrates an analogous assessment process that is executed after computation of a stress metric for each of the performance capacities. Here, any demand that corresponds to more than a 100% stress level is obviously problematic. In addition to binary conclusions regarding whether a given capacity is or is not a limiting factor, it is possible to observe that of the two **limiting resources** (e.g., grip strength and right shoulder flexion extreme of motion), the former is more substantial. This might suggest, for example, that the task be modified so as to decrease the grip-strength demand (i.e., gains in performance capacity required would be substantial to achieve sufficiency) and the use of focused exercise therapy to increase shoulder flexion mobility (i.e., gains in mobility required are relatively small).

73.4 Current Limitations

73.4.1 Quality of Measurements

Key issues are measurement validity, reliability (or repeatability), accuracy, and discriminating power. At issue in terms of current limitations is not necessarily the quality of measurements but limitations with regard to methods employed to determine the quality of measurements and their interpretability.

A complete treatment of these complex topics is beyond the present scope. However, it can be said that standards are such [Potvin et al., 1985] that most published works regarding measurement instruments do address quality of measurements to some extent. Validity (i.e., how well does the measurement reflect the intended quantity) and reliability are most often addressed. However, one could easily be left with the impression that these are binary conditions (i.e., measurement is or is not reliable or valid), when in fact a continuum is required to represent these constructs. Of all attributes that relate to measurement quality, reliability is most commonly expressed in quantitative terms. This is perhaps because statistical methods have been defined and promulgated for the computation of so-called reliability coefficients [Winer, 1971]. Reliability coefficients range from 0.0 to 1.0, and the implication is that 1.0 indicates a perfectly reliable or repeatable measurement process. Current methods are adequate, at best, for making inferences regarding the relative quality of two or more methods of quantifying "the same thing." Even these comparisons require great care. For example, measurement instruments that have greater intrinsic resolving power have a great opportunity to yield smaller-reliability coefficients simply because they are capable of measuring the true variability (on repeated measurement) of the parameter in question within the system under test. While there has been widespread determination or reliability coefficients, there has been little or no effort directed toward determination of what value of a reliability coefficient is "good enough" for a particular application. In fact, reliability coefficients are relatively abstract to most practitioners.

Methods for determining the quality of a measurement process (including the instrument, procedures, examiner, and actual noise present in the variable of interest) that allow a practitioner to easily reach decisions regarding the use of a particular measurement instrument in a specific application and limitations thereof are currently lacking. At the use of different measurements increases and the number of options available for obtaining a given measurement grows, this topic will undoubtedly receive additional

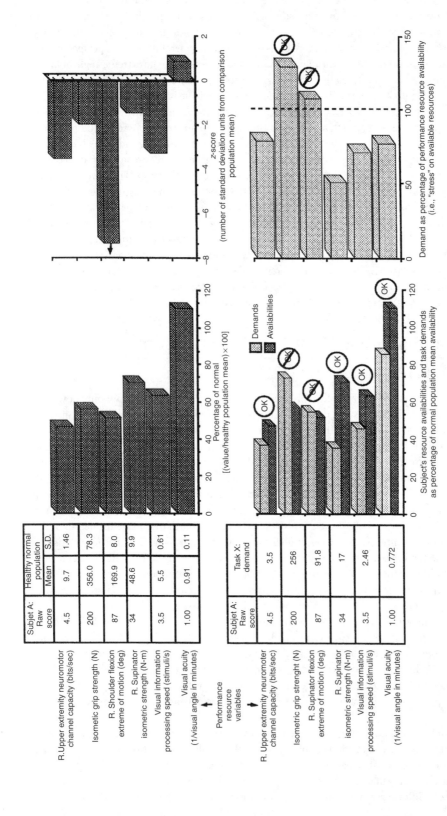

FIGURE 73.2 Examples of different types of assessments that can be performed by combining performance capacity measures and reference values of different types. The upper section shows raw score values as well as statistics for a healthy normal reference population in tabular form (*left*). It is difficult to reach any decision by simple inspection of just the raw performance capacity values. Tabular data are used to obtain a percent normal assessment (*middle*) and a z-score assessment (*right*). Both of these provide a more directly interpretable result regarding subject A's impairments. The lower section shows raw score values (same as in upper section) and quantitative demands (typically worst case) imposed on the respective performance resources by task X. The lower-middle plot illustrates the process of individually assessing sufficiency of each performance resource in this task context using a threshold rule (i.e., availability must exceed demand for sufficiency). The lower-right plot illustrates a similar assessment process after computation of a stress metric for each of the performance capacities. Here, any demand that corresponds to more than a 100% stress level is obviously problematic.

attention. Caution in interpreting literature, common sense, and the use of simple concepts such as "I need to measure range of motion to within 2 degrees in my application" are recommended in the meantime [Mayer et al., 1997].

73.4.1.1 Standards

Measurements, and concepts with which they are associated, can contribute to a shift from experience-based knowledge acquisition to rule-based, engineering-like methods. This requires (1) a widely accepted conceptual framework (i.e., known to assistive device manufacturers, rehabilitation engineers, and other professionals within the rehabilitation community), (2) a more complete set of measurement tools that are at least standardized with regard to the definition of the quantity measured, (3) special analysis and assessment software (that removes the resistance to the application of more rigorous methods by enhancing the quality of decisions as well as the speed with which they can be reached), and (4) properly trained practitioners. Each is a necessary *but not sufficient* component. Thus balanced progress is required in each of these areas.

73.4.2 Rehabilitation Service Delivery and Rehabilitation Engineering

In a broad sense, it has been argued that all engineers can be considered rehabilitation engineers who merely work at different levels along a comprehensive spectrum of human performance, which itself can represent a common denominator among all humans. Thus an automobile is a mobility aid, a telephone is a communication aid, and so on. Just as in other engineering disciplines, measurement must be recognized not only as an important end in itself (in appropriate instances) but also as an integral component or means within the overall scope of rehabilitation and rehabilitation engineering processes. The service-delivery infrastructure must provide for such means. At present, one should anticipate and be prepared to overcome potential limitations associated with factors such as third-party reimbursement for measurement procedures, recognition of equipment and maintenance costs associated with obtaining engineering-quality measurements, and education of administrative staff and practitioners with regard to the value and proper use of measurements.

Defining Terms

Behavior: A general term that relates to what a human or artificial system does while carrying out its function(s) under given conditions. Often, behavior is characterized by measurement of selected parameters or identification of unique system states over time.

Function: The purpose of a system. Some systems map to a single primary function (e.g., process visual information). Others (e.g., the human arm) map to multiple functions, although at any given time multifunction systems are likely to be executing a single function (e.g., polishing a car). Functions can be described and inventoried, whereas level of performance of a given function can be measured.

Functional assessment: The process of determining, from a relatively global perspective, an individual's ability to carry out tasks in daily life. Also, the result of such a process. Functional assessments typically cover a range of selected activity areas and include (at a minimum) a relatively gross indication (e.g., can or cannot do; with or without assistance) of status in each area.

Goal: A desired endpoint (i.e., result) typically characterized by multiple parameters, at least one of which is specified. Examples include specified task goals (e.g., move an object of specified mass from point A to point B in 3 sec) or estimated task performance (maximum mass, range, speed of movement obtainable given a specified elemental performance resource availability profile), depending on whether a reverse or forward analysis problem is undertaken. Whereas function describes the general process of task, the goal directly relates to performance and is quantitative.

Limiting resource: A performance resource at any hierarchical level (e.g., vertical lift strength, knee flexor speed) that is available in an amount that is less than the worst-case demand imposed by a task. Thus a given resource can be "limiting" only when considered in the context of a specific task.

Overall task goals: Goals associated with a task to be executed by a human-artificial system combination (to be distinguished from goals associated with the task of operating the artificial system).

Performance: Unique qualities of a human or artificial system (e.g., strength, speed, accuracy, endurance) that pertain to how well that system executes its function.

Performance capacity: A quantity in finite availability that is possessed by a system or subsystem, drawn on during tasks, and limits some aspect (e.g., speed, force, production, etc.) of a system's ability to execute tasks, or, the limit of that aspect itself.

Performance capacity measurement: A general class of measurements, performed at different hierarchical levels, intended to quantify one or more performance capacities.

Procedure: A set of constraints placed on a system in which flexibility exists regarding how a goal (or set of goals) associated with a given function can be achieved. Procedure specification requires specification of initial intermediate, and/or final states or conditions dictating how the goal is to be accomplished. Such specification can be thought of in terms of removing some degrees of freedom.

Structure: Physical manifestation and attributes of a human or artificial system and the object of one type of measurements at multiple hierarchical levels.

Style: Allowance for variation within a procedure, resulting in the intentional incomplete specification of a procedure or resulting from either international or unintentional incomplete specification of procedure.

Task: That which results from (1) the combination of specified functions, goals, and procedures or (2) the specification of function and goals and the observation of procedures utilized to achieve the goals.

References

Fuhrer, M.J. 1987. *Rehabilitation Outcomes: Analysis and Measurement.* Baltimore, MD, Brookes.

Ganapathy, G. and Kondraske, G.V. 1990. Microprocessor-based instrumentation for ambulatory behavior monitoring. *J. Clin. Eng.* 15(16): 459.

Granger, C.V. and Greshorn, G.E. 1984. *Functional Assessment in Rehabilitation Medicine.* Baltimore, MD, Williams & Wilkins.

Hamilton, B.B., Granger, C.V., Sherwin, F.S. et al. 1987. A uniform national data system for medical rehabilitation. In M.J. Fuhrer (Ed.), *Rehabilitation Outcomes: Analysis and Measurement*, pp. 137–147. Baltimore, MD, Brookes.

Imrhan, S. 2000. Task analysis and decomposition: physical components. In J.D. Bronzino (Ed.), *Handbook of Biomedical Engineering*, 2nd ed. Boca Raton, FL, CRC Press.

Jones, R.D. 1995. Measurement of neuromotor control performance capacities. In J.D. Bronzino (Ed.), *Handbook of Biomedical Engineering.* Boca Raton, FL, CRC Press.

Keith, R.A., Granger, C.V., Hamilton, B.B., and Sherwin, F.S. 1987. The functional independence measure: a new tool for rehabilitation. In M.G. Eisenberg and R.C. Grzesiak (Eds.), *Advances in Clinical Rehabilitation*, Vol. 1, pp. 6–18. New York, Springer-Verlag.

Kondraske, G.V. 1988. Experimental evaluation of an elemental resource model for human performance. In *Proceedings of the Tenth Annual IEEE Engineering in Medicine and Biology Society Conference*, pp. 1612–1613, New Orleans.

Kondraske, G.V. 1990. Quantitative measurement and assessment of performance. In R.V. Smith and J.H. Leslie (Eds.), *Rehabilitation Engineering*, pp. 101–125. Boca Raton, FL, CRC Press.

Kondraske, G.V. 2000. A working model for human system–task interfaces. In J.D. Bronzino (Ed.), *Handbook of Biomedical Engineering*, 2nd ed. Boca Raton, FL, CRC Press.

Kondraske, G.V. and Vasta, P.J. 2000. Measurement of information processing performance capacities. In J.D. Bronzino (Ed.), *Handbook of Biomedical Engineering*, 2nd ed. Boca Raton, FL, CRC Press.

Kondraske, G.V., Johnston, C., Pearson, A., and Tarbox, L. 1997. Performance prediction and limiting resource identification with nonlinear causal resource analysis. In *Proceedings of the 19th Annual Engineering in Medicine and Biology Society Conference*, pp. 1813–1816.

Maxwell, K.J. 2000. High-level task analysis: mental components. In J.D. Bronzino (Ed.), *Handbook of Biomedical Engineering*, 2nd ed. Boca Raton, FL, CRC Press.

Mayer, T., Kondraske, G.V., Brady Beals, S., and Gatchel, R.J. 1997. Spinal range of motion: accuracy and sources of error with inclinometric measurement. *Spine* 22(17): 1976–1984.

National Institute of Occupational Safety and Health (NIOSH). 1981. *Work Practices Guide for Manual Lifting* (DHHS Publication No. 81122). Washington, US Government Printing Office.

Pheasant, S.T. 1986. *Bodyspace: Anthropometry, Ergonomics and Design*. Philadelphia, PA, Taylor & Francis.

Potvin, A.R., Tourtellotte, W.W., Potvin, J.H. et al. 1985. *The Quantitative Examination of Neurologic Function*. Boca Raton, FL, CRC Press.

Smith, R.V. and Leslie, J.H. 1990. *Rehabilitation Engineering*. Boca Raton, FL, CRC Press.

Smith, S.S. 2000. Measurement of neuromuscular performance capacities. In J.D. Bronzino (Ed.), *Handbook of Biomedical Engineering*, 2nd ed. Boca Raton, FL, CRC Press.

Tourtellotte, W.W. 1993. Personal communication.

Vasta, P.J. and Kondraske, G.V. 1994. Performance prediction of an upper extremity reciprocal task using non-linear causal resource analysis. In *Proceedings of the Sixteenth Annual IEEE Engineering in Medicine and Biology Society Conference*, Baltimore, MD.

Vasta, P.J. and Kondraske, G.V. 2000. Human performance engineering: computer based design and analysis tools. In J.D. Bronzino (Ed.), *Handbook of Biomedical Engineering*, 2nd ed. Boca Raton, FL, CRC Press.

Webster, J.G., Cook, A.M., Tompkin, W.J., and Vanderheiden, G.C. 1985. *Electronic Devices for Rehabilitation*. New York, Wiley.

Winer, B.J. 1971. *Statistical Principles in Experimental Design*, 2nd ed. New York, McGraw-Hill.

Winter, D.A. 1990. *Biomechanics and Motor Control of Human Movement*, 2nd ed. New York, Wiley.

World Health Organization. 1980. *International Classification of Impairments, Disabilities, and Handicaps*. Geneva, World Health Organization.

Further Information

The section of this *Handbook* entitled "*Human Performance Engineering*" contains chapters that address human performance modeling and measurement in considerably more detail.

Manufacturers of instruments used to characterize different aspects of human performance often provide technical literature and bibliographies with conceptual backgrounds, technical specifications and application examples. A partial list of such sources is included below. (No endorsement of products is implied.)

Baltimore Therapeutic Equipment Co.
7455-L New Ridge Road
Hanover, MD 21076-3105
http://www.bteco.com/

Chattanooga Group
4717 Adams Road
Hixson, TN 37343
http://www.chattanoogagroup.com/

Henley Healthcare
120 Industrial Blvd.
Sugarland, TX 77478
http://www.henleyhealth.com/

Human Performance Measurement, Inc.
P.O. Box 1996
Arlington, TX 76004-1996
http://www.flash.net/~hpm/

Lafayette Instrument
3700 Sagamore Parkway North
Lafayette, IN 47904-5729
http://www.lafayetteinstrument.com

The National Institute on Disability and Rehabilitation Research (NIDRR), part of the Department of Education, funds a set of Rehabilitation Engineering Research Centers (RERCs) and Research and Training Centers (RTCs). Each has a particular technical focus; most include measurements and measurements issues. Contact NIDRR for a current listing of these centers.

Measurement devices, issues, and application examples specific to rehabilitation are included in the following journals:

IEEE Transactions on Rehabilitation Engineering
IEEE Service Center
445 Hoes Lane
P.O. Box 1331
Piscataway, N.J. 08855-1331
http://www.ieee.org/index.html

Journal of Rehabilitation Research and Development
Scientific and Technical Publications Section
Rehabilitation Research and Development Service
103 South Gay St., 5th floor
Baltimore, MD 21202-4051
http://www.vard.org/jour/jourindx.htm

Archives of Physical Medicine and Rehabilitation
Suite 1310
78 East Adams Street
Chicago, IL 60603-6103
American Journal of Occupational Therapy
The American Occupational Therapy Association, Inc.
4720 Montgomery Ln.,
Bethesda, MD 20814-3425
http://www.aota.org/

Physical Therapy
American Physical Therapy Association
1111 North Fairfax St.
Alexandria, VA 22314
http://www.apta.org/

Journal of Occupational Rehabilitation
Subscription Department
Plenum Publishing Corporation
233 Spring St.
New York, NY 10013
http://www.plenum.com/

74

Rehabilitation Engineering Technologies: Principles of Application

Douglas Hobson
Elaine Trefler
University of Pittsburgh

Rehabilitation engineering is the branch of *biomedical engineering* that is concerned with the application of science and technology to improve the quality of life of individuals with disabilities. Areas addressed within rehabilitation engineering include wheelchairs and seating systems, access to computers, sensory aids, prosthetics and orthotics, alternative and augmentative communication, home and work-site modifications, and universal design. Because many products of rehabilitation engineering require careful selection to match individual needs and often require custom fitting, rehabilitation engineers have necessarily become involved in service delivery and application as well as research, design, and development. Therefore, as we expand on later, it is not only engineers that practice within the field of rehabilitation engineering.

As suggested above, and as in many other disciplines, there are really two career tracks in the field of rehabilitation engineering. There are those who acquire qualifications and experience to advance the state of knowledge through conducting research, education, and product development, and there are others who are engaged in the application of technology as members of service delivery teams. At one time it was possible for a person to work in both arenas. However, with the explosion of technology and the growth of the field over the past decade, one must now specialize not only within research or service delivery but often within a specific area of technology.

One can further differentiate between rehabilitation and assistive technology. *Rehabilitation technology* is a term most often used to refer to technologies associated with the acute-care rehabilitation process. Therapy evaluation and treatment tools, clinical dysfunction measurement and recording instrumentation, and prosthetic and orthotic appliances are such examples. *Assistive technologies* are those devices and services that are used in the daily lives of people in the community to enhance their ability to function independently, examples being specialized seating, wheelchairs, environmental control devices, workstation access technologies and services are now communication aids. Recognition and support of assistive technology devices and services are now embedded in all the major disability legislation that has been enacted over the last decade.

The primary focus of this chapter is on the role of the rehabilitation engineering practitioner as he or she carries out the responsibilities demanded by the application of assistive technology.

Before launching into the primary focus of this chapter, let us first set a conceptual framework for the *raison d'etre* for assistive technology and the role of the assistive technology professional.

74.1 The Conceptual Frameworks

The application of assistive technology can be conceptualized as minimizing the functional gap between the person and his or her environment. This reality is what technology does for all of us to varying degrees. For example, if you live in a suburban area that has been designed for access only by car and your car breaks down, you are handicapped. If your house has been designed to be cooled by air conditioning in the "dog days" of summer and you lose a compressor, your comfort is immediately compromised by your incompatibility with your environment. Similarly, if you live in a home that has only access by steps and you have an impairment requiring the use of a wheelchair, you are handicapped because you no longer have abilities that are compatible with your built environment. Because our environments, homes, workplaces, schools, and communities have been designed to be compatible with the abilities of the norm, young children, persons with disabilities, and many elderly people experience the consequences of their mismatch as a matter of course. The long-term utopian solution would be to design environments and their contents so that they can be used by all people of all ages, which is the essence of the universal design concept. However, given that today we do not have very many products and environments that have been universally designed, rehabilitation engineers attempt to minimize the effects of the mismatch by designing, developing, and providing technologies that will allow persons with disabilities to pursue their life goals in a manner similar to any other person. Of course, the rehabilitation engineer cannot accomplish this working in isolation but rather must function as a part of a consumer-responsive team that can best deal with the multiplicity of factors that usually impact on the successful application of assistive technology.

Let us now move to another conceptual framework, one that conceptualizes how people actually interact with technology.

The following conceptualization has been adapted from the model proposed by Roger Smith [1992]. In Figure 74.1, Smith suggests that there are three cyclic elements that come into play when humans interact with technology: the human and his or her innate sensory, cognitive, and functional abilities; the human factor's characteristics of the interface between the human and the technology; and the technical characteristics of the technology itself in terms of its output as a result of a specific input by the user. People with disabilities may have varying degrees of dysfunction in their sensory, cognitive, and functional abilities. The interface will have to be selected or adapted to these varying abilities in order to allow the person to effectively interact with the technology. The technology itself will need to possess

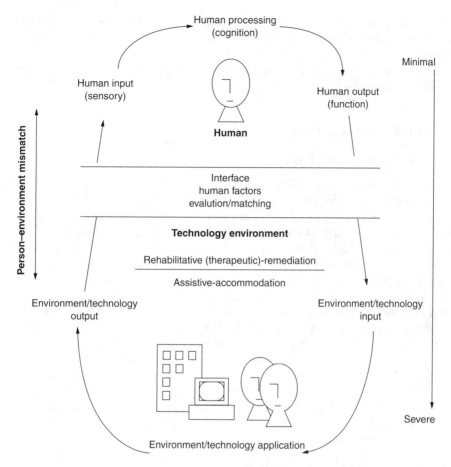

FIGURE 74.1   Conceptual framework of technology and disability. (Modified from Smith, R.O. 1992. *AJOT* 1:22.)

specific electronic or mechanical capabilities in order to yield the desired outcome. The essence of assistive technology applications is to integrate all three of these element into a functional outcome that meets the specific needs of a user. This is usually done by selecting commercially available devices and technologies at a cost that can be met by either the individual or his or her third-party payment source. When technologies are not available, then they must be modified from existing devices or designed and fabricated as unique custom solutions. It is particularly in these latter activities that a rehabilitation engineer can make his or her unique contribution to team process.

Cook and Hussey [1995], published an excellent text, *Assistive Technologies — Principles and Practice*. As well as comprehensively addressing many of the assistive technologies briefly covered in this chapter, they also present a conceptual framework which builds on the one developed by Smith above. They introduce the additional concepts of activity and context. That is, understanding of a person's activity desires and the context (social, setting, physical) in which they are to be carried out are essential components to successful assistive technology intervention.

It should be realized that there are several levels of assistive technology. The first level might be termed *fundamental technology* in contrast to advanced technology. Fundamental technologies, such as walkers, crutches, many wheelchairs, activities of daily living (ADL) equipment, etc., usually do not require the involvement of the rehabilitation engineer in their application. Others on the team can better assess the need, confirm the interface compatibility, and verify that the outcome is appropriate. The rehabilitation engineer is most often involved in the application of advanced technologies, such as powered wheelchairs, computerized workstation designs, etc., that require an understanding of the underlying technological principles in order to achieve the best match with the abilities and needs of the user, especially if custom modifications or integration of devices are required to the original equipment. The rehabilitation engineer is usually the key person if a unique solution is necessary.

Let's now discuss a few fundamental concepts related to the process by which assistive technology is typically provided in various service delivery programs.

74.2   The Provision Process

74.2.1   The Shifting Paradigm

In the traditional rehabilitation model of service delivery, a multidisciplinary team of professionals is already in place. Physicians, therapists, counselors, and social worker meet with the client and, based on the findings of a comprehensive evaluation, plan a course of action. In the field of assistive technology, the rules of the team are being charted anew. First, the decision making often takes place in a nonmedical environment and often without a physician as part of the team. Second, the final decision is rapidly moving into the hands of the consumer, not the professionals. The third major change is the addition of a rehabilitation engineer to the team. Traditional team members have experience working in groups and delegating coordination and decision making to colleagues depending on the particular situation. They are trained to be team players and are comfortable working in groups. Most engineers who enter the field of rehabilitation engineering come with a traditional engineering background. Although well versed in design and engineering principles, they often do not receive formal training in group dynamics and need to learn these skills if they are to function effectively. As well, engineers are trained to solve problems with technical solutions. The psychosocial aspects of assisting people with disabilities to make informed choices must be learned most often outside the traditional education stream. Therefore, for the engineer to be a contributing member of the team, not only must he or she bring engineering expertise, but it must be integrated in such a manner that it supports the overall objectives of the technology delivery process, which is to respond to the needs and desires of the consumer.

People with disabilities want to have control over the process and be informed enough to make good decisions. This is quite different from the traditional medical or rehabilitation model, in which well-meaning professionals often tell the individual what is best for him or her. Within this new paradigm, the role is to inform, advise, and educate, not to decide. The professional provides information as to the technical options, prices, etc. and then assists the person who will use the technology to acquire it and learn how to use it.

74.2.2   The Evaluation

An evaluation is meant to guide decision-making for the person with a disability toward appropriate and cost-effective technology. Often, more than one functional need exists for which assistive technology could be prescribed. Costly, frustrating, and time-consuming mistakes often can be avoided if a thorough evaluation based on a person's total functional needs is performed before any technology is recommended. Following the evaluation, a long-range plan for acquisition and training in the chosen technology can be started.

For example, suppose a person needs a seating system, both a powered and manual wheelchair, an augmentative communication device, a computer workstation, and an environmental control unit (ECU). Where does one begin? Once a person's goals and priorities have been established, the process can begin. First, a decision would likely be made about the seating system that will provide appropriate support in the selected manual chair. However, the specifications of seating system should be such that the components also can be interfaced into the powered chair. The controls for the computer and augmentative communication device must be located so that they do not interfere with the display of the communication device and must in some way be compatible wit the controls for the ECU. Only if all functional needs are addressed can the technology be acquired in a logical sequence and in such a manner that all components will be compatible. The more severely disabled the individual, the more technology he or she will need, and the more essential is the process of setting priorities and ensuring compatibility of technical components.

In summary, as suggested by the conceptual model, the process begins by gaining an understanding of the person's sensory, cognitive, and functional abilities, combined with clarification of his or her desires and needs. These are then filtered through the technology options, both in terms of how the interface will integrate with the abilities of the user and how the technology itself will be integrated to meet the defined needs. This information and the associated pros and cons are conveyed to the user, or in some cases their caregiver, who then has the means to participate in the ultimate selection decisions.

74.2.3 Service Delivery Models

People with disabilities can access technology through a variety of different service delivery models. A team of professionals might be available in a university setting where faculty not only teach but also deliver technical services to the community. More traditionally, the team of rehabilitation professionals, including a rehabilitation engineer, might be available at a hospital or rehabilitation facility. More recently, technology professionals might be in private practice either individually, as a team, or part of the university, hospital, or rehabilitation facility structure. Another option is the growing number of rehabilitation technology suppliers (RTSs) who offer commercial technology services within the community. They work in conjunction with an evaluation specialist and advise consumers as to the technical options available to meet their needs. They then sell and service the technology and train the consumer in its use. Local chapters of national disability organizations such as United Cerebral Palsy and Easter Seals also may have assistive technology services. In recent years, a growing number of centers for independent living (CILs) have been developed in each state with federal support. Some of these centers have opted to provide assistive technology services, in addition to their information and referral services, which are common to all CILs. And finally, there are volunteers, either in engineering schools or community colleges (student supervised projects) or in industry (high-technology industries often have staff interested in doing community service), such as the Telephone Pioneers. Each model has its pros and cons for the consumer, and only after thoroughly researching the options will the person needing the service make the best choice as to where to go with his or her need in the community. A word of caution. Only if there is timely provision and follow-up available is a service delivery system considered appropriate, even if the cost of the service is less.

A more extensive description of service delivery options may be reviewed in a report that resulted from a RESNA-organized conference on service delivery [ANSI/RESNA, 1987].

74.3 Education and Quality Assurance

Professionals on the assistive technology team have a primary degree and credential in their individual professions. For example, the occupational or physical therapist will have a degree and most often state licensure in occupational or physical therapy. The engineer will have recognized degrees in mechanical, electrical, biomedical, or some other school of engineering. However, in order to practice effectively in the field of assistive technology, almost all will need advanced training. A number of occupational therapy curriculums provide training in assistive technology, but not all. The same is true of several of the others. Consumers and payers of assistive technology need to know that professionals practicing in the field of assistive technology have a certain level of competency. For this reason, all professionals, including rehabilitation engineers, are pursuing the ATP (assistive technology practitioner) credential through RESNA.

74.3.1 RESNA

RESNA, an interdisciplinary association of persons dedicated to the advancement of assistive technology for people with disabilities, has a credentialing program that credentials individuals on the assistive technology team. As part of the process, the minimum skills and knowledge base for practitioners is tested. Ties with professional organizations are being sought so that preservice programs will include at least some of the knowledge and skills base necessary. Continuing education efforts by RESNA and others also will assist in building the level of expertise of practitioners and consumers. At this time RESNA has a voluntary credentialling process to determine if a person meets a predetermined minimal standard of practice in the field of Assistive Technology. Persons who meet the prerequisite requirements, pass a written exam, and agree to abide by the RESNA Standards of Practice can declare themselves as RESNA certified. They can add the ATP if they are practitioners or ATS if they are suppliers of assistive technology.

Payment for technology and the services required for its application is complex and changing rapidly as health care reform evolves. It is beyond the scope of this discussion to detail the very convoluted and individual process required to ensure that people with disabilities receive what they need. However, there are some basic concepts to be kept in mind. Professionals need to be competent. The documentation of need and the justification of selection must be comprehensive. Time for a person to do this must be allocated if there is to be success. Persistence, creativity, education of the payers, and documentation of need and outcomes are the key issues.

74.4   Specific Impairments and Related Technologies

Current information related to specific technologies is best found in brochures, trade magazines (*Report Rehab*), exhibit halls of technology-related conferences, and databases such as ABLEDATA. Many suppliers and manufacturers are now maintaining Websites, which provides a quick means to locate information on current products. What follows is only a brief introduction to specific disabilities areas to which assistive technology applications are commonly used.

74.4.1   Mobility

Mobility technologies include wheelchairs, walkers, canes, orthotic devices, FES (functional electrical stimulation), laser canes, and any other assistive device that would assist a person with a mobility impairment, be it motor or sensory, to move about in his or her environment. There are very few people who have a working knowledge of all the possible commercial options. Therefore, people usually acquire expertise in certain areas, such as wheelchairs. There are hundreds of varieties of wheelchairs, each offering a different array of characteristics that need to be understood as part of the selection process. Fortunately, there are now several published ways that the practitioner and the consumer can obtain useful information. A classification system has been developed that sets a conceptual framework for understanding the different types of wheelchairs that are produced commercially [Hobson, 1990]. *Paraplegic News and Sports and Spokes* annually publish the specifications on most of the manual and powered wheelchairs commonly found in the North American marketplace. These reviews are based on standardized testing that is carried out by manufacturers following the ANSI/RESNA wheelchair standards [ANSI/RESNA, 1990]. Since the testing and measurements of wheelchairs are now done and reported in a standard way, it is possible to make accurate comparisons between products, a tremendous recent advancement for the wheelchair specialist and the users they serve [Axelson et al., 1994].

Possibly the most significant advancement in wheelchairs is the development and application of industry, on an international scale, for testing the safety and durability of their products. These standards also mandate what and how the test information should be made available in the manufacturer's presale literature. The Rehabilitation Engineering Research Center and University of Pittsburgh [RERC, 1999] maintains a large Website, where among its many resources is a listing of wheelchair research publications and a general reference site, termed Wheelchairnet [Wheelchairnet, 1999]. The RERC site also tracks the current activities occurring in many of the wheelchair standards working groups. Finally, Cooper [1995, 1998] has published two excellent reference texts on rehabilitation engineering with emphasis on wheeled mobility.

74.4.2 Sitting

Many people cannot use the wheelchairs as they come from the manufacturer. Specialized seating is required to help persons to remain in a comfortable and functional seated posture for activities that enable them to access work and attend educational and recreational activities. Orthotic supports, seating systems in wheelchairs, chairs that promote dynamic posture in the workplace, and chairs for the elderly that fit properly, are safe, and encourage movement all fit into the broad category of sitting technology.

74.4.3 Sensation

People with no sensation are prone to skin injury. Special seating technology can assist in the preventions of tissue breakdown. Specially designed cushions and backs for wheelchairs and mattresses that have pressure-distributing characteristics fall into this category. Technology also has been developed to measure the interface pressure. These tools are now used routinely to measure and record an individual's pressure profile, making cushion selection and problem solving more of a science than an art.

Again, a classification system of specialized seating has been developed that provides a conceptual framework for understanding the features of the various technologies and their potential applications. The same reference also discusses the selection process, evaluation tools, biomechanics of supported sitting, and materials properties of weight-relieving materials [Hobson, 1990].

74.4.4 Access (Person–Machine Interface)

In order to use assistive technology, people with disabilities need to be able to operate the technology. With limitations in motor and/or sensory systems, often a specially designed or configured interface system must be assembled. It could be as simple as several switches or a miniaturized keyboard or as complex as an integrated control system that allows a person to drive a wheelchair and operate a computer and a communication device using only one switch.

74.4.5 Communication

Because of motor or sensory limitations, some individuals cannot communicate with spoken or written word. There are communication systems that enable people to communicate using synthesized voice or printed output. Systems for people who are deaf allow them to communicate over the phone or through computer interfaces. Laptop computers with appropriate software can enable persons to communicate faster and with less effort than previously possible. Some basic guidelines for selecting an augmentative communication system, including strategies for securing funding, have been proposed in an overview chapter by James Jones and Winifred Jones [Jones and Jones, 1990].

74.4.6 Transportation

Modified vans and cars enable persons with disabilities to independently drive a vehicle. Wheelchair tie-downs and occupant restraints in personal vehicles and in public transportation vehicles are allowing people to be safely transported to their chosen destination. Fortunately, voluntary performance standards for restraint and tie-down technologies have been developed by a task group within the Society for Automotive Engineers (SAE). Standards for car hand controls, van body modifications, and wheelchair lifts are also available from SAE. These standards provide the rehabilitation engineer with a set of tools that can be used to confirm safety compliance of modified transportation equipment. Currently in process and still requiring several more years of work are transport wheelchair and vehicle power control standards.

74.4.7 Activities of Daily Living (ADL)

ADL technology enables a person to live independently as much as possible. Such devices as environmental control units, bathroom aids, dressing assists, automatic door openers, and alarms are all considered aids to daily living. Many are inexpensive and can be purchased through careful selection in stores or through catalogues. Others are quite expensive and must be ordered through vendors who specialize in technology for independent living.

Ron Mace, now deceased and creator of the Center for Universal Design at the North Carolina State University, is widely acknowledged as the father of the Universal Design concept. The concept of universal design simply means that if our everyday built environments and their contained products could be designed to meet the needs of a wider range of people, both young and old, then the needs of more persons with disabilities would be met without the need for special adaptions [Center for Universal Design, 1999]. Others like Paul Grayson have also published extensively regarding the need to re-think how we design our living environments [Grayson, 1991]. Vanderheiden and Denno have prepared human factors guidelines that provide design information to allow improved access by the elderly and persons with disabilities [Vanderheiden and Vanderheiden, 1991; Denno et al., 1992; Trace Center, 1999].

74.4.8 School and Work

Technology that supports people in the workplace or in an educational environment can include such applications as computer workstations, modified restrooms, and transportation to and from work or school. Students need the ability to take notes and do assignments, and people working have a myriad of special tasks that may need to be analyzed and modified to enable the employee with the disability to be independent and productive. Weisman has presented an extensive overview of rehabilitation engineering in the workplace, which includes a review of different types of workplaces, the process of accommodation, and many case examples [Weisman, 1990].

74.4.9 Recreation

A component of living that is often overlooked by the professional community is the desire and, in fact, need of people with disabilities to participate in recreational activities. Many of the adaptive recreational technologies have been developed by persons with disabilities themselves in their effort to participate and be competitive in sports. Competitive wheelchair racing, archery, skiing, bicycles, and technology that enables people to bowl, play pool, and fly their own airplanes are just a few areas in which equipment has been adapted for specific recreational purposes.

74.4.10 Community and Workplace Access

There is probably no other single legislation that is having a more profound impact on the lives of people with disabilities then the Americans with Disabilities Act (ADA), signed into law by President Bush in August of 1990. This civil rights legislation mandates that all people with disabilities have access to public facilities and that reasonable accommodations must be made by employers to allow persons with disabilities to access employment opportunities. The impact of this legislation is now sweeping America and leading to monumental changes in the way people view the rights of persons with disabilities.

74.5 Future Developments

The field of rehabilitation engineering, both in research and in service delivery, is at an important crossroad in its young history. Shifting paradigms of services, reduction in research funding, consumerism, credentialing, health care reform and limited formal educational options all make speculating on what the future may bring rather hazy. Given all this, it is reasonable to say that one group of rehabilitation engineers will continue to advance the state of the art through research and development, while another group will be on the front lines as members of clinical teams working to ensure that individuals with disabilities receive devices and services that are most appropriate for their particular needs.

The demarcation between researchers and service providers will become clearer, since the latter will become credentialed. RESNA and its professional specialty group (PSG) on rehabilitation engineering are working out the final credentialing steps for the Rehabilitation Engineer RE and the Rehabilitation Engineering Technologist RET. Both must also be an ATP. They will be recognized as valued members of the clinical team by all members of the rehabilitation community, including third-party payers, who will reimburse them for the rehabilitation engineering services that they provide. They will spend as much or more time working in the community as they will in clinical settings. They will work closely with consumer-managed organizations who will be the gatekeepers of increasing amounts of government-mandated service dollars.

If these predictions come to pass, the need for rehabilitation engineering will continue to grow. As medicine and medical technology continue to improve, more people will survive traumatic injury, disease, and premature birth, and many will acquire functional impairments that impede their involvement in personal, community, educational, vocational, and recreational activities. People continue to live longer lives, thereby increasing the likelihood of acquiring one or more disabling conditions during their lifetime. This presents an immense challenge for the field of rehabilitation engineering. As opportunities grow, more engineers will be attracted to the field. More and more rehabilitation engineering education programs will develop that will support the training of qualified engineers, engineers who are looking for exciting challenges and opportunities to help people live more satisfying and productive lives.

References

ANSI/RESNA. 1990. *Wheelchair Standards.* RESNA Press, RESNA, 1700 Moore St., Arlington, VA 22209-1903.

Axelson, P., Minkel, J., and Chesney, D. 1994. A Guide to Wheelchair Selection: How to Use the ANSI/RESNA Wheelchair Standards to Buy a Wheelchair. Paralyzed Veterans of America (PVA).

Bain, B.K. and Leger, D. 1997. *Assistive Technology. An Interdisciplinary Approach.* Churchill Livingstone, New York.

Center for Universal Design, 1999. http://www.design.ncsu.edu/cud/

Cook, A.M. and Hussey, S.M. 1995. *Assistive Technologies: Principles and Practice.* Mosby, St. Louis, MO.

Cooper, R.A. 1995. *Rehabilitation Engineering Applied to Mobility and Manipulation.* Institute of Physics Publishing, Bristol, U.K.

Cooper, R.A. 1998. *Wheelchair Selection and Configuration.* Demos Medical Publishing, New York.

Deno, J.H. et al. 1992. *Human Factors Design Guidelines for the Elderly and People with Disabilities.* Honeywell, Inc., Minneapolis, MN 55418 (Brian Isle, MN65-2300).

Galvin, J.C. and Scherer, M.J. 1996. *Evaluating, Selecting, and Using Appropriate Assistive Technology,* Aspen Publishers, Gaithersburg, MD.

Hobson, D.A. 1990. Seating and mobility for the severely disabled. In R. Smith and J. Leslie (Eds.), *Rehabilitation Engineering*, pp. 193–252. CRC Press, Boca Raton, FL.

Jones, D. and Jones, W. 1990. Criteria for selection of an augmentative communication system. In R. Smith and J. Leslie (Eds.), *Rehabilitation Engineering*, pp. 181–189. CRC Press, Boca Raton, FL.

Medhat, M. and Hobson, D. 1992. *Standardization of Terminology and Descriptive Methods for Specialized Seating.* RESNA Press, RESNA, 1700 Moore St., Arlington, VA 22209-1903.

Rehabilitation Technology Service Delivery — A Practical Guide. 1987. RESNA Press, RESNA, 1700 Moore St., Arlington, VA 22209-1903.

Smith, R.O. 1992. Technology and disability. *AJOT* 1: 22.

Society for Automotive Engineers. 1994. Wheelchair Tie-Down and Occupant Restraint Standard (committee draft). SAE. Warrendale, PA.

Trace Center, 1999. http://trace.wisc.edu/

Vanderheiden, G. and Vanderheiden, K. 1991. Accessibility Design Guidelines for the Design of Consumer Products to Increase their Accessibility to People with Disabilities or Who Are Aging. Trace R&D Center, University of Wisconsin, Madison, WI.

Weisman, G. 1990. Rehabilitation engineering in the workplace. In R. Smith and J. Leslie (Eds.), *Rehabilitation Engineering*, pp. 253–297. CRC Press, Boca Raton, FL.

WheelchairNet, 1999. http://www.wheelchairnet.org

Further Information

ABLEDATA, 8455 Colesville Rd., Suite 935, Silver Spring, Md. 20910–3319.

VIII

Human Performance Engineering

George V. Kondraske
University of Texas-Arlington

T HE ULTIMATE GOAL OF HUMAN PERFORMANCE engineering is the enhancement of performance and safety of humans in the execution of tasks. The more formalized conception of this field was fueled initially by military needs. It has steadily evolved to become an important component in industrial and other settings as well. In a biomedical engineering context, the scope of definition applied to the term "human" not only encompasses individuals with capabilities that differ from those of a typical healthy individual in many possible different ways (e.g., individuals who are disabled, injured, unusually endowed, etc.), but also includes those who are simply "healthy" (e.g., healthcare professionals). Consequently, one finds a wide range of problems in which human performance engineering and associated methods are employed. Just a few examples include:

- Evaluation of an individual's performance capacities to determine the efficacy of new therapeutic interventions, or so-called "level of disability" for worker's compensation and other medical–legal purposes.
- Design of assistive devices and work sites in such a way that a person with some deficiency in their performance resource profile will be able to accomplish a given task to a specified level of performance.
- Design of operator interfaces for medical instruments that promote efficient, safe, and error-free use.

But human performance engineering is not only concerned with situations that are directly linked to a medical context or motivated by a medical problem. Evaluation and optimization of performance in specific sport tasks, work tasks, playing musical instruments, and even education represent relevant application targets. Human performance engineering encompasses the exciting prospect of helping individuals achieve their personal best in selected endeavors. In general, the field encompasses applications in medical and nonmedical contexts.

In basic and most general terms, each of the representative application situations noted involves one or more of the following: (1) a human, (2) a task(s), and (3) the interface of a human to a task(s). Human performance engineering emphasizes concepts, methods, and tools that strive toward treatment of each of these areas with the same engineering rigor that is routinely applied to artificial systems (e.g., mechanical, electronic, etc.). Importance is thus placed on models (a combination of cause-and-effect and statistical), measurements (of varying degrees of sophistication that are selected to fit needs of a particular circumstance), and diverse types of analyses. Many specialty areas within biomedical engineering begin with an emphasis on a specific subsystem and then proceed to deal with it at *lower* levels of detail (sometimes even at the molecular level) to determine how it functions and often why it malfunctions. One way of characterizing human performance engineering is to note that it emphasizes subsystems and their performance capacities (i.e., *how well* a system functions), the integration of these into a whole and their interactions, and their operation in the execution of tasks that are of ultimate concern to humans. These include tasks of daily living, work, and recreation. In recent years, there has been an increased concern within medical communities on issues such as quality of life, treatment outcome measures, and treatment cost-effectiveness. By linking human subsystems into the "whole" and discovering objective quantitative relationships between the human and tasks, human performance engineering can play the lead role in addressing these and other related concerns.

Human performance engineering combines knowledge, expertize, concepts, and methods from across many disciplines (e.g., biomechanics, neuroscience, psychology, physiology — and many others), which, in their overlapping aspect, essentially deal with similar types of problems. To capture the essence of the problems addressed by human performance engineering and the knowledge base that is unique to it, a conceptual framework is necessary. Few candidate frameworks exist even within the relevant disciplines. The Elemental Resource Model is presented in Chapter 75, including concepts of General Systems Performance Theory, to serve this role. Introduced initially almost two decades ago, its utility and appropriateness have been demonstrated in a variety of situations and has garnered wider acceptance than any other such framework known. In a further attempt to enhance continuity across this section, authors of other chapters have been requested to consider the Elemental Resource Model and to incorporate basic concepts and terms where applicable.

Chapter 76 through Chapter 78 look "toward the human" and focus on measurement of performance capacities of specific groups of human subsystem and related issues. Due to a combination of the complexity of the human system (even when viewed as a collection of rather high-level subsystems) and limited space available, treatment is not comprehensive. For example, measurement of sensory performance capacities (e.g., tactile, visual, auditory) is not included. Both systems and tasks can be viewed at various hierarchical levels. Chapter 76 and Chapter 77 focus on a rather "low" systems level and discuss basic functional units such as actuator, processor, and memory systems. Chapter 78 moves to a more intermediate level where speech, postural control, gait, and hand-eye coordination systems could be considered. Measurement of structural parameters, which play important roles in both performance measurement and many analyses, is also not allocated the separate chapter it deserves (as a minimum) due to space limitations. Chapter 79 and Chapter 80 then shift focus to consider the analysis of different types of tasks in a similar, representative fashion.

Chapter 81 through Chapter 83 are included to provide insight into a representative selection of application types. Space constraints, the complexity of human performance, and the great variety of tasks that can be considered limit the level of detail with which such material can be reasonably presented. Work in all application areas is now benefiting from computer-based tools; this is the theme of Chapter 84. The section concludes with a look to the future (Chapter 85), including a summary of selected limitations, identification of some corresponding research and development needs, and speculation regarding the nature of the anticipated evolution of the field.

Many have contributed their talents to this exciting field in terms of both research and applications, yet much remains to be done. I am indebted to the authors not only for their contributions and cooperation during the preparation of this section, but also for their willingness to accept the burdens of communicating complex subject matter reasonably, selectively, and as accurately as possible within the imposed constraints.

75

The Elemental Resource Model for Human Performance

George V. Kondraske
University of Texas-Arlington

75.1 Introduction

Humans are complex **systems**. Our natural interest in things and ourselves that we do has given rise to the study of this complex system at every conceivable level ranging from genetic, through cellular and organ systems, to interactions of the total human with the environment in the conduct of purposeful activities. At each level, there are corresponding practitioners who attempt to discover and rectify or prevent problems at the respective level. Some practitioners are concerned with specific individuals, while others (e.g., biomedical scientists and product designers) address populations as a whole. Problems dealt with span medical and nonmedical contexts, often with interaction between the two. Models play a key role not only in understanding the key issues at each level, but also in describing relationships between various levels and in providing frameworks that allow practitioners to obtain reasonably predictable results in a systematic and efficient fashion. In this chapter, a working model for human system–**task** interfaces is presented. Any such model must, of course, consider not only the interface per se, but also representations of the human system and tasks. The model presented here, the Elemental Resource Model

(ERM), represents the most recent effort in a relatively small family of models that attempt to address similar needs.

75.1.1 Background

The interface of a human to a task of daily living (e.g., work, recreation, or other) represents a level that is quite high in the hierarchy noted above. One way in which to summarize previous efforts directed at this level, across various application contexts, is to recognize two different lines along which study has evolved (1) bottom-up and (2) top-down. Taken together, these relative terms imply a focus of interest at a particular level of convergence, which, here, is the human–task interface level. It is emphasized that these terms are used here to characterize the general course of development and not specific approaches applied at a particular instant of time. A broad view is necessary to grapple with the many previous efforts that either are, or could be, construed to be pertinent.

The biomedical community has approached the human–task interface largely along the "bottom-up" path. This is not surprising given the historical evolution of interest first in anatomy (human structure) and then physiology (**function**). The introduction of chemistry, giving rise to biochemistry, and the refinement of the microscope provided motivations to include even lower hierarchical levels of inquiry and of a substantially different character. Models in this broad "bottom-up" category begin with *anatomical components* and include muscles, nerves, tendons (or subcomponents thereof), or subsets of organs (e.g., heart, lungs, vasculature, etc.). They often focus on relationships between components and exhibit a scope that stays within the confines of the human system. Many cause-and-effect models have been developed at these lower levels for specific purposes (e.g., to understand lines of action of muscle forces and their changes during motion about a given joint).

As a natural consequence of linkages that occur between hierarchical levels and our tendency to utilize that which exists, consideration of an issue at any selected level (in this case, the human–task interface level) brings into consideration *all lower levels* and all models that have been put forth with the stated purpose of understanding problems or behaviors at the original level of focus. The amount of detail that is appropriate or required at these original, lower levels results in great complexity when applied to the total human at the human–task interface level. In addition, many lower-level modeling efforts (even those which are quantitative) are aimed primarily at obtaining a basic scientific understanding of human physiology or specific pathologies (i.e., pertaining to *populations* of humans). In such circumstances, highly specialized, invasive, and cumbersome laboratory procedures for obtaining the necessary data to populate models are justified. However, it is difficult and sometimes impossible to obtain data describing *a specific individual* to be utilized in analyses when such models are extended to the human–task interface level. Another result of drawing lower-level models (and their approaches) into the human–task interface context is that the results have a specific and singular character (e.g., biomechanical vs. neuromuscular control vs. psychologic, etc.) [e.g., Card et al., 1986; Hemami, 1988; Schoner and Kelso, 1988; Gottlieb et al., 1989; Delp, 1990]. Models that incorporate most or all of the multiple aspects of the human system or frameworks for integrating multiple lower-level modeling approaches have been lacking. Lower-level models that serve meaningful purposes at the original level of focus have provided and will continue to provide insights into specific issues related to human **performance** at multiple levels of consideration. However, their direct extension to serve general needs at the human–task interface level has inherent problems; a different approach is suggested.

A "top-down" progression can be observed over the major history in human factors/ergonomic [Taylor, 1911; Gilbreth and Gilbreth, 1917] and vocational assessment [e.g., Botterbusch, 1987] fields (although the former has more recently emphasized a "human-centered" concept with regard to design applications). In contrast to the bottom-up path in which anatomical components form the initial basis of modeling efforts, the focus along the top-down developmental path begins with consideration of the *task or job* which is to be performed by the total human. The great variety in the full breadth of activities in which humans can be engaged gives rise to one aspect of complexity at this level that pertains to taxonomies for job and task classification [e.g., Fleishman and Quaintance, 1984; Meister, 1989; U.S. Department of Labor, 1992].

Another enigmatic aspect that quickly adds complexity with respect to modeling concerns the appropriate level to be used to dissect the items (e.g., jobs) at the highest level into lower level components (e.g., tasks and subtasks). In fact, the choice of level is complicated by the fact that no clear definition has evolved for a set of levels from which to choose.

After progressing through various levels at which all model elements represent tasks and are completely outside the confines of the human body, a level is eventually reached where one encounters the human. Attempts to go further have been motivated, for example, by desires to predict performance of a human in a given task (e.g., lifting an object, assembling a product, etc.) from a set of measures that characterizes the human. From the human–task interface, difficulty is encountered with regard to the strategy for approaching a system as complex, multifaceted, and multipurpose as a human [Fleishman and Quaintance, 1984; Wickens, 1984]. In essence, the full scope of options that have emerged from the bottom-up development path are now encountered from the opposite direction. Options range from relatively gross analyses (e.g., estimates of the "fraction" of a task that is physical or mental) to those which are much more detailed and quantitative. The daunting prospect of considering a "comprehensive quantitative model" has led to approaches and models, argued to be "more practical," in which sets of parameters are often selected in a somewhat mysterious fashion based on experience (including previous research) and intuition. The selected parameters are then used to develop predictive models, most of which have been based primarily on statistical methods (i.e., regression models) [Fleishman, 1967; Fleishman and Quaintance, 1984]. Although the basic modeling tools depend only on correlation, it is usually possible to envision a causal link between the independent variables selected (e.g., visual acuity) and the dependent variable to be predicted (e.g., piloting an aircraft). Models (one per task) are then tested in a given population and graded with regard to their prediction ability, the best of which have performed marginally [Kondraske and Beehler, 1994]. Another characteristic associated with many of the statistically-based modeling efforts from the noted communities is the almost exclusive use of healthy, "normal" subjects for model development (i.e., humans with impairments were excluded). Homogeneity is a requirement of such statistical models, leading to the need for one model per task per population (at best). Moreover, working with a mindset that considers only normal subjects can be observed to skew estimates regarding which of the many parameters that one might choose for incorporation in a model are "most important." The relatively few exceptions that employ cause-and-effect models (e.g., based on physical laws) at some level of fidelity [e.g., Chaffin and Andersson, 1991] often adopt methods that have emerged from the bottom-up path and are, as noted above, limited in character at the "total human" level (e.g., "biomechanical" in the example cited).

It is critical to note that the issue is *not* that no useful models have emerged from previous efforts but rather that no clear comprehensive strategy has emerged for modeling at the human–task interface level. A National Research Council panel on human performance modeling [Baron et al., 1990] considered the fundamental issues discussed here and also underscored needs for models at the human–task interface level. While it was concluded that an all-inclusive model might be desirable (i.e., high fidelity, in the sense that biomechanical, information processing, sensory and perceptual aspects, etc. are represented), such a model was characterized as being highly unlikely to achieve and perhaps ultimately not useful because it would be overly complex for many applications. The basic recommendation made by this panel was to pursue development of more limited scope submodels. The implication is that two or more submodels could be integrated to achieve a broader range of fidelity, with the combination selected to meet the needs of particular situations. The desire to divide efforts due to inherent complexity of the problem also surfaces within the histories of the bottom-up and top-down development paths discussed above. While a reasonable concept in theory, one component in the division of effort that has consistently been underrepresented is the part that ties together the so-called submodels. Without a conceptual framework for integration of relatively independent modeling efforts and a set of common modeling constructs, prospects for long-term progress are difficult to envision. This, along with the recognition that enough work had been undertaken in the submodel areas so that key issues and common denominators could be identified, motivated development of the ERM.

The broad objectives of the ERM are most like those of Fleishman and colleagues [Fleishman, 1966, 1972, 1982; Fleishman and Quaintance, 1984], whose efforts in human performance are generally well known in many disciplines. These are the only two efforts known that (1) focus on the total human in a task situation (i.e., directly address the human–task interface level); (2) consider tasks in general, and not only a specific task such as gait, lifting, reading, and so on; (3) incorporate all aspects of the total human system (e.g., sensory, biomechanical, information processing, etc.); and (4) aim at quantitative models. There are also some similarities with regard to the incorporation of the ideas of "abilities" (of humans) and "requirements" (of tasks). The work of Fleishman and colleagues has thus been influential in shaping the ERM either directly or indirectly through its influence of others. However, there are several substantive conceptual differences that have resulted in considerably different end-points. Fleishman's work emerged from "the task" perspective and is rooted in psychology, whereas the ERM emerges from the perspective of "human system architecture" and is rooted in engineering methodology with regard to quantitative aspects of system performance and also incorporates psychology *and* physiology. Both approaches address humans *and* tasks and both efforts contain aspects identifiable with psychology and engineering, as they ultimately must. These different perspectives, however, may explain in part some of the major differences. Aspects unique to the ERM include (1) it is based on modeling and measurement of *all* aspects of a system's performance using **resource constructs**; (2) the use of cause-and-effect **resource economic principles** (i.e., the idea of threshold "costs" for achieving a given level of performance in any given high-level task); (3) the concept of monadology (i.e., the use of a finite set of "elements" to explain a complex phenomenon); and (4) a consistent strategy for identifying performance elements at different hierarchical levels.

The ERM attempts to provide a quantitative and relatively straightforward framework for characterizing the human system, tasks, and the interface of the human to tasks. It depends in large part on, and evolves directly from, a separate body of material collectively referred to as general systems performance theory (GSPT). GSPT was developed first and independently; that is, removed from the human system context. It incorporates resource constructs exclusively for modeling of the abstract idea of *system performance*, including specific rules for measuring performance resource availability, and resource economic principles to provide a cause-and-effect analysis of the interface of any system (e.g., humans) to tasks. The concept of a "performance model" is emphasized and distinguished from other model types.

75.2 Basic Principles

The history of the ERM and the context in which it was developed are described elsewhere [Kondraske, 1987a, 1990b; 1995]. It is important to note that the ERM is derived from the combination of GSPT with the philosophy of monadology and their application to the human system. As such, these two constituents are briefly reviewed before presenting and discussing the actual ERM.

75.2.1 General Systems Performance Theory

The concept of "performance" now pervades all aspects of life, especially decision-making processes that involve both human and artificial systems. Yet, it has not been well-understood theoretically, and systematic techniques for modeling and its measurement have been lacking. While a considerable body of material applicable to general systems theory exists, the concept of performance has not been incorporated in it nor has performance been addressed in a general fashion elsewhere. Most of the knowledge that exists regarding performance and its quantitative treatment has evolved within individual application contexts, where generalizations can easily be elusive.

Performance is multifaceted, pertaining to how well a given system executes an intended function and the various factors that contribute to this. It differs from **behavior** of a system in that "the best of something" is implied. The broad objectives of GSPT are:

1. To provide a common conceptual basis for defining and measuring all aspects of the performance of any *system*
2. To provide a common conceptual basis for the analysis of any *task* in a manner that facilitates system–task interface assessments and decision-making

3. To identify cause-and-effect principles, or laws, that explain what occurs when any given system is used to accomplish any given task

While GSPT was motivated by needs in situations where the human is "the system" of interest and it was first presented in this context [Kondraske, 1987a], application of it has been extended to the context of artificial systems. These experiences range from computer vision and sensor fusion [Yen and Kondraske, 1992] to robotics [Kondraske and Standridge, 1988; Kondraske and Khoury, 1992].

A succinct statement of GSPT designed to emphasize key constructs is presented below in a step-like format. The order of steps is intended to suggest how one might approach any system or system–task interface situation to apply GSPT. While somewhat terse and "to-the-point," it is nonetheless an essential prerequisite for a reasonably complete understanding of the ERM:

1. Within a domain of interest, select any level of abstraction and identify the system(s) of interest (i.e., the physical **structure**) and its *function* (i.e., purpose).

2. Consider "the system" and "the task" separately.

3. Use a *resource construct* to model the system's *performance*. First, consider the unique intangible qualities that characterize *how well a system executes its function*. Each of these is considered to represent a unique **performance resource** associated with a specific **dimension of performance**(e.g., speed, accuracy, stability, smoothness, "friendliness," etc.) of that system. Each performance resource is recognized as a *desirable* item (e.g., endurance vs. fatigue, accuracy vs. error, etc.) "possessed" by the system in a certain quantitative amount. Thus, one can consider *quantifying* the amount of given *quality* available. As illustrated, an important consequence of using the resource construct at this stage is that confusion associated with duality of terms is eliminated.

4. Looking toward the system, identify all "I" dimensions of performance associated with it. In situations where the system does not yet exist (i.e., design contexts), it is helpful to note that dimensions of performance of the system are the same as those of the task.

5a. Keeping the resource construct in mind, define a parameterized metric for each dimension of performance (e.g., speed, accuracy, etc.). If the resource construct is followed, values will be produced with these metrics that are always nonnegative. Furthermore, a larger numerical value will consistently represent *more* of a given resource and therefore *more* **performance capacity**.

5b. Measure system performance with the system *removed from* the specific intended task. This is a reinforcement of step (2). The general strategy is to *maximally stress* the system (within limits of comfort and/or safety, when appropriate) to define its **performance envelope**; or more specifically, the envelope that defines *performance resource availability*, $R_{A_S}(t)$. Note that $R_{A_S}(t)$ is a continuous surface in the system's nonnegative, multidimensional performance space. Also note that unless all dimensions of performance and parameterized metrics associated with each are defined using the resource construct, a performance envelope cannot be guaranteed. Addressing the issue of measurement more specifically, consider resource availability values, $R_{A_i}|_{Q_{i,k}}(t)$ for $i = 1$ to I, associated with each of the "I" dimensions of performance. Here, each $Q_{i,k}$ represents a unique condition, in terms of a set of values R_i along *other* identified dimensions of performance, under which a specific resource availability (R_{A_i}) is measured; that is, $Q_{i,k} = \{R_{1,k}, R_{2,k}, \ldots, R_{p,k}\}$ for all $p \neq i$ ($1 \geq p \geq I$). The subscript "k" is used to distinguish several possible conditions under which a given resource availability (R_{A_1}) can be measured. These values are measured using a set of "test-tasks," each of which is designed to *maximally stress* the system (within limits of comfort and safety, when appropriate) (a) along each dimension of performance individually (where $Q_{i,k} = Q_{i,0} = \{0, 0, \ldots, 0\}$), or (b) along selected subsets of dimensions of performance simultaneously (i.e., $Q_{i,k} = Q_{i,n}$, where each possible $Q_{i,n}$ has one or more nonzero elements). The points obtained ($R_{A_i}|_{Q_{i,k}}(t)$) provide the basis to estimate the performance envelope, $R_{A_S}(t)$. Note that if only on-axis points are obtained (e.g., maximally stress one specific performance resource availability with minimal or no stress on other performance resources, or the $Q_{i,0}$ condition), a rectangular or idealized performance envelope is obtained. A more accurate representation, which would be contained within the idealized envelope, can be obtained at the expense of making additional measurements or the use of known mathematical functions that define the shape of envelope in two or more dimensions.

5c. Define estimates of single-number *system figures-of-merit*, or *composite performance capacities*, as the mathematical product of all or any selected subset of $R_{A_i}|_{Q_{i,0}}(t)$. If more accuracy is desired and a sufficient number of data points is available from the measurement process described in (5b), composite performance capacities can be determined by integration over $R_{A_S}(t)$ to determine the volume enclosed by the envelope. The *composite performance capacity* is a measure of performance at a higher level of abstraction than any individual dimension of performance at the "system" level, representing the capacity of the system to perform tasks which place demands on *those performance resources availabilities included in the calculation*. Different composite performance capacities can be computed for a given system by selecting different combinations of dimensions of performance. Note that the definition of a composite performance capacity used here preserves dimensionality; for example, if speed and accuracy dimensions are included in the calculation, the result has units of speed × accuracy. (This step is used only when needed; e.g., when two general-purpose systems of the same type are to be compared. However, if decision making that involves the interface of a specific system to a specific task is the issue at hand, a composite performance capacity is generally not of any use.)

6. Assess the "need for detail." This amounts to a determination of the number of hierarchical levels included in the analysis. If the need is to determine whether the currently identified "system" can work in the given task or how well it can execute its function, go to step (7) now. If the need is to determine the *contribution of one or more constituent subsystems* or why a desired level of performance is not achieved at the system level, repeat 1 => 5 for all "J" functional units (subsystems), or a selected subset thereof based on need, that form the system that was originally identified in step (1); that is, go to the next lowest hierarchical level.

7. At the "system" level, look toward the task(s) of interest. Measure, estimate, or calculate *demands* on system performance resources (e.g., the speed, accuracy, etc. required), $R_{D_i}|_{Q'_{i,k}}(t)$, where the notation here is analogous to that employed in step (5b). This represents the quantitative definition and communication of **goals**, or the set of values (P_{HLT}) representing level of performance (P) desired in a specific high-level task (HLT). Use a worst-case or other less-conservative strategy (with due consideration of the impact of this choice) to summarize variations over time. This will result in a set of "M" points (R_{D_m}, for $m = 1$ to M) that lie in the multidimensional space defined by the set of "I" dimensions of performance. Typically, $M \geq I$.

8. Use *resource economic principles* (i.e., require $R_A \geq R_D$ for "success") at the system level *and* at all system–task interfaces at the subsystem level (if included) to evaluate success/failure at each interface. More specifically, for a given system–task interface, all task-demand points (i.e., the set of R_{D_m}-associated with a given task or subtask) must lie within the performance resource envelope, $R_{A_S}(t)$, of the corresponding system. This is the key law that governs system–task interfaces. If a two-level model is used (i.e., "system" and "subsystem" levels are incorporated), map system level demands to demands on constituent subsystems. That is, functional relationships between P_{HLT} and demands imposed on constituent subsystems (i.e., $R_{D_{ij}}(t, P_{HLT})$) must be determined. The nature of these mappings depends on the type of systems in question (e.g., mechanical, information processing, etc.). The basic process includes application of step (7) to the subtasks associated with each subsystem. If **resource utilization flexibility** (i.e., redundancy in subsystems of similar types) exists, select the "best" or optimal subsystem configuration (handled in GSPT with the concept of **performance resource substitution**) and **procedure** (i.e., use of performance resources over time) as that which allows *accomplishment of goals* with *minimization of stress* on available performance resources across all subsystems and over the time of task execution. Thus, redundancy is addressed in terms of a constrained performance resource optimization problem. Stress on individual performance resources is defined as $0 \leq R_{D_{ij}}(t, P_{HLT})/R_{A_{ij}}(t) \leq 1$. It is also useful to define and take note of reserve capacity; that is, the margin between available and utilized performance resources.

The above statement is intended to reflect the true complexity that exists in systems, tasks, and their interfaces when viewed primarily from the perspective of performance. This provides a basis for the judicious decision making required to realize "the best" *practical implementation* in a given situation where many engineering trade-offs must be considered. While a two-level approach is described above, it should be apparent that it could be applied with any number of hierarchical levels by repeating the steps outlined in an iterative fashion starting at a different level each time. A striking feature of GSPT is the *threshold effect* associated with the resource economic principle. This nonlinearity has important implications in quantitative human performance modeling, as well as interesting ramifications in practical applications such as rehabilitation, sports, and education. Note also no distinction is made as to whether a given performance resource is derived from a human or artificial system; both types of systems, or subcomponents thereof, can be incorporated into models and analyses.

75.2.2 Monadology

Monadology dates back to 384 BC [Neel, 1977] but was formalized and its importance emphasized by Gottfried Wilhelm Leibniz, inventor of calculus, in his text *Monadologia* in 1714. This text presents what is commonly called *Leibniz's Monadology* and has been translated and incorporated into contemporary philosophy texts [Leibniz and Montgomery, 1992]. It is essentially the idea of "basic elements" *vis a vis* chemistry, alphabets, genetic building blocks, etc. The concept is thus already well accepted as being vital to the systematic description of human systems from certain perspectives (i.e., chemical, genetic). Success associated with previous application of monadology, whether intentional or unwitting (i.e., discovered to be at play *after* a given taxonomy has emerged), compels its serious *a priori* consideration for other problems.

Insight into how monadology is applied to human performance modeling is perhaps more readily obtained with reference to a widely known example in which monadology is evident, such as chemistry. Prior to modern chemistry (i.e., prior to the introduction of the periodic table), alchemy existed. The world was viewed as being composed of an infinite variety of unique *substances*. The periodic table captured the notion that this infinite variety of substances could all be defined in terms of a finite set of basic elements. Substances have since been analyzed using the "language" of chemistry and organized into categories of various complexity, that is, elements, simple compounds, complex compounds, etc. Despite the fact that this transition occurred approximately 200 years ago, compounds remain, which have yet to be analyzed. Furthermore, the initial periodic table was incorrect and has undergone revision up to relatively recent times. Analogously, in the alchemy of human performance the world is viewed as being composed of an infinite variety of unique tasks. A "chemistry" can be envisioned that first starts with the identification of the "basic elements," or more specifically, *basic elements of performance*. Simple and complex tasks are thus analogous to simple and complex compounds, respectively. The analogy carries over to quantitative aspects of GSPT as well. Consider typical equations of chemical reactions with resources on the left and products (i.e., tasks) on the right. Simple compounds (tasks) are realized by drawing upon basic elements in the proper combination and amounts. The amount of "product" (level of performance in a high-level task) obtained depends on availability of the **limiting resource**.

Another informative aspect of this analogy is the issue of how to deal with the treatment of hierarchical level. Clearly, the chemical elements are made up of smaller particles (e.g., protons, neutrons, and electrons). Physicists have identified even smaller, more elusive entities such as bosons, quarks, and so on. Do we need to consider items at this lowest level of abstraction each time a simple compound such as hydrochloric acid is made? Likewise, the term "basic" in basic elements of performance is clearly relative and requires the choice of a particular hierarchical level of abstraction for the identification of systems or basic functional units; a level which is considered to be both natural and useful for the purpose at hand. Just as it is possible but not always necessary or practical to map chemical elements down to the atomic particle level, it is possible to consider mapping a basic element of performance (see latter) such as elbow flexor torque production capacity down to the level of muscle fibers, biochemical reactions at neuromuscular junctions, and so forth.

75.2.3 The Elemental Resource Model

The resource and resource economic constructs used in GSPT specifically to address performance have employed and have become well-established in some segments of the human performance field, specifically with regard to attention and information processing [Navon and Gopher, 1979; Wickens, 1984]. However, in these cases the term "resource" is used mostly conceptually (in contrast to quantitatively), somewhat softly defined, and applied to refer in various instances to systems (e.g., different processing centers), broad functions (e.g., memory vs. processing), and sometimes to infer a particular aspect of performance (e.g., attentional resources). In the ERM, through the application of GSPT, these constructs are incorporated universally (i.e., applied to all human subsystems) and specifically to model "performance" at both conceptual and quantitative levels. In addition to the concept of monadology, the insights of others [Turvey et al., 1978; Shoner and Kelso, 1988] were valuable in reinforcing the basic "systems architecture" employed in the ERM and in refining description of more subtle, but important aspects.

As illustrated in Figure 75.1, the ERM contains multiple hierarchical levels. Specifically, three levels are defined (1) the basic element level; (2) the **generic intermediate level**, and (3) the high level. GSPT is to define performance measures at any hierarchical level. This implies that to measure performance, one must isolate the desired system and then stress it maximally along one dimension of performance (or more, if interaction effects are desired) to determine performance resource availability. For example, consider the human "posture stabilizing" system (at the generic intermediate level), which is stressed maximally along a stability dimension. As further illustrated below, the basic element level contains represents measurable stepping-stones in the human system hierarchy between lower-level systems (i.e., ligaments, tendons, nerves, etc.) and higher-level tasks.

A summary representation emphasizing the basic element level of the ERM is depicted in Figure 75.2. While this figure is intended to be more or less self-explanatory, a brief walk-through is warranted.

75.2.3.1 Looking Toward the Human

The entire human (lower portion of Figure 75.2) is modeled as a pool of elemental *performance resources*, which are grouped into one of the four different domains (1) life sustaining, (2) environmental interface (containing purely sensory and sensorimotor components), (3) the central processing, and (4) information. Within each of the first three domains, physical subsystems referred to as *functional units* are identified (see labels along horizontal aspect of grids) through application of fairly rigorous criteria [Kondraske, 1990b]. GSPT is applied to each functional unit, yielding first a set of dimensions of performance (defined using a resource construct) for each unit. A single **Basic Element of Performance** (BEP) is defined by specifying two items (1) the basic functional unit and (2) one of its dimensions of performance. Within a domain, not every dimension of performance indicated in Figure 75.2 is applicable to every functional unit in that domain. However, there is an increasing degree of "likeness" among functional units (i.e., fewer fundamentally different types) in this regard as one moves from life sustaining, to environmental interface, to central processing domains. The fourth domain, the information domain, is substantially different from the other three. Whereas the first three represent physical systems and their intangible performance resources, the information domain simply represents information. Thus, while memory functional units are located within the central processing domain, the contents of memory (e.g., motor programs and associated reference information) are partitioned into the information domain. As illustrated, information is grouped but within each group there are many specific skills. The set of available performance resources $(R_{A_{ij}}(t)|\mathbf{Q})$ consist of both BEPs (i = dimension of performance, j = functional unit) and information sets (e.g., type "i" within group "j"). Although intrinsically different, both fit the resource construct. This approach permits even the most abstract items such as motivation and friendliness to be considered with the same basic framework as strength and speed.

Note that resource availability in GSPT and thus in the ERM is potentially a function of time, allowing quantitative modeling of dynamic processes such as child development, aging, disuse atrophy, and rehabilitation. The notation further implies that availability of a given resource must be evaluated at a specific operating point, denoted as $\mathbf{Q}$. At least conceptually, many parameters can be used to characterize

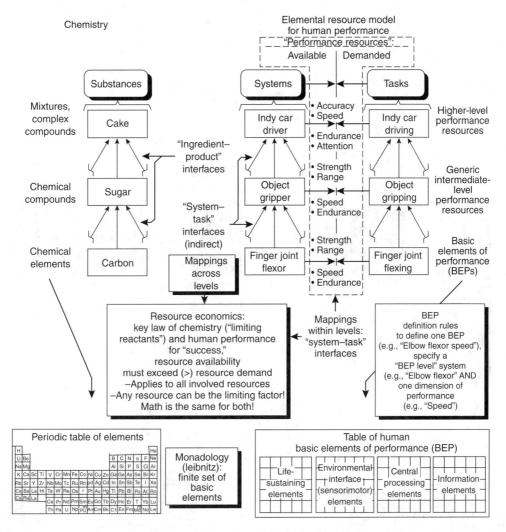

FIGURE 75.1   The Elemental Resource Model contains multiple hierarchical levels. Performance resources (i.e., the basic elements) at the "basic element level" are finite in number, as dictated by the finite set of human subsystems and the finite set of their respective dimensions of performance. At higher levels, new "systems" can be readily created by configuration of systems at the basic element level. Consequently, there are in infinite number of performance resources (i.e., higher-level elements) at these levels. However, rules of General Systems Performance Theory (refer to text) are applied at any level in the same way resulting in the identification of the system, its function, dimensions of performance, performance resource availabilities (system attributes), and performance resource demands (task attributes).

this **Q** point. In general, the goal of measurement when looking "toward the human" is to isolate functional units and maximally stress (safely) individual performance resources to determine availability. Such measures reflect performance capacities. The simplest **Q** point is one in which there is stress along only one dimension of performance (i.e., that corresponding to the resource being stressed). Higher fidelity representation is possible at the expense of additional measurements. The degree to which isolation can be achieved is of practical concern in humans. Nonetheless, it is felt that reasonable isolation can be achieved in most situations [Kondraske, 1990a, b]. Moreover, this and similar issues of practical concern should be addressed as separate problems; that is, they should not be permitted to obfuscate or thwart efforts to explain phenomenon at the human–task interface.

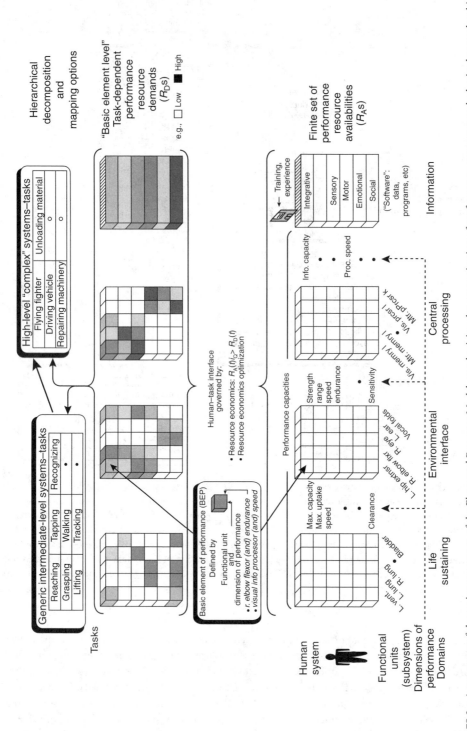

FIGURE 75.2 A summary of the major constructs of the Elemental Resource Model, emphasizing the categorization of performance resources at the basic element level into four: life-sustaining, environmental interface, central processing, and information domains.

75.2.3.2 Looking Toward the Task

The mid-portion of Figure 75.2 suggests the representation of any given task in terms of the unique set of demands ($R_{D_{ij}}(t)$) imposed on the pool of BEPs and information resources; that is, this is the elemental level of task representation. Shading implies that demands can be represented quantitatively in terms of amount. The upper portion of the figure defines hierarchical mapping options, where mapping is the process of translating what happens in tasks typically executed by humans to the elemental level. Two such additional levels (for a total of three, including the elemental level) are included as part of the ERM (1) generic intermediate-level tasks, and (2) higher-level complex tasks. At all three levels (Figure 75.1 and Figure 75.2) tasks are processes which occur over time and can be characterized by specific goals (e.g., in terms of speed, force, etc.) and related to systems at the same level that possess performance resources. Using established analytic techniques, even the most complex task can be divided into discrete task segments. Then mapping analyses, which take into account task procedures (e.g., a squatting subject with two hands on the side of a box . . .), are applied to each task segment to determine $R_{D_{ij}}(t)$. Once this is found, the worst case or a selected percentile point in the resource demand distribution (over a time period corresponding to a selected task segment) can be used to obtain a single numerical value representation of demand for a given resource *and* the conditions under which the given demand occurs; that is, the **Q′** point (e.g., at what speed and position angle does the worst-case demand on elbow flexor torque occur?). This reduction process requires parameterization algorithms that are similar to those used to process time series data collected during tests designed to measure performance resource availability.

75.2.3.3 The Human–Task Interface

Using GSPT, success in achieving the goals of a given task segment is governed by resource economic principles requiring that $R_{A_{ij}}(t)|_Q \geq R_{D_{ij}}(t)$ for all is and js (i.e., $R_{A_{11}} \geq R_{D_{11}}$ AND $R_{A_{12}} \geq R_{D_{12}}$ AND $R_{A_{13}} \geq R_{D_{13}} \cdots$). In other words, all task demands, when translated to the individual subsystems involved, must fit within the envelopes that define performance resource availability. Adequacy associated with any one resource is a *necessary, but not sufficient condition* for success. Concepts and observations in human performance referred to as "compensation" or "redundancy" are explained in terms of *resource utilization flexibility,* which includes the possibility of substituting one performance resource (of the same dimensionality) for another (i.e., *resource substitution*). It has been hypothesized [Kondraske, 1990b] that an optimal performance resource utilization is achieved through learning. Furthermore, the optimization rule suggested by GSPT is that the human system is driven to accomplish task goals and use procedures that minimize performance resource stress (i.e., the fraction of available performance resources utilized) over the duration of a given task segment and across all BEPs involved. Minimizing stress is equivalent to maximizing the margin between available and utilized performance resources. Thus, optimization is highly dependent on the resource availability profile and it would be predicted, for instance, that two individuals with different resource availability profiles would not optimally accomplish the same task goals by using identical procedures.

75.3 Application Issues

Implications of the ERM and what it demonstrates regarding intrinsic demands imposed by nature and methods for creatively navigating these demands over both the short and long terms are considered. The ERM offers a number of flexibilities with regard to how it can be applied (e.g., "in whole" or "in part," "conceptually" or "rigorously," with "low-tech" or sophisticated "high-tech" tools, and to define perform-ance measures or to develop predictive models). While immediate application is possible at a conceptual level of application, it also provides the motivation and potential to consider coordinated, collaborative developments that allow rigorous and efficient solutions to complex problems by practitioners without extraordinary training.

The ERM provides a basis for obtaining insight into the nature of routine tasks that clinicians and other practitioners are expected to perform; there are both "troublesome" and "promising" insights in this regard. Perhaps the most obvious troublesome aspect is that the ERM makes it painfully evident that *many* BEPs are typically called into play in tasks of daily living, work, or recreation and that resource insufficiency associated with *any one* of this subset of BEPs can be the factor which limits performance in the higher-level task. The further implication is that for rigorous application, one must know (via measurement and analyses) the availability and demand associated with each and every one of these unique resources. An additional complexity with which practitioners must cope is the high degree of specificity and complexity of resources in the information domain (i.e., the "software"). There is no simple, rapid way to probe into this domain of the ERM to determine if the information required for a given task is correct; it requires methods analogous to those used to debug software source code.

The aspects that hold promise are associated with (1) the nature of hierarchical systems; (2) the threshold mathematics of resource economics; and (3) the fact that when "n" resources combine to address a single task, the mathematics of logical combination is employed to arrive at an overall assessment. That is, the individual "$R_A \geq R_D$?" questions result in a set of "OK" or "Not OK" results that are combined with logical "AND" operations to obtain the final "OK" or "Not OK" assessment (*Note*: the "OR" operator is used when resource substitution is possible.).

75.3.1 Conceptual, Low-Tech, Practical Application

The ERM description alone can be used simply to provide a common conceptual basis for discussing the wide range of concepts, measurements, methods, and processes of relevance in human performance or a particular application area [Mayer and Gatchel, 1988; Syndulko et al., 1988; Frisch, 1993] It can also be used at this level as a basis for structured assessment [Kondraske, 1988b, 1994b, 1995] of individuals in situations including therapy prescription, assistive device prescription, independent living decision making (e.g., self-feeding, driving, etc.), age or gender discrimination issues in work or recreational tasks, etc. At points in such processes, it is often more important to consider the full scope of different performance resources involved in a task using even a crude level of quantification than it is to consider just a select few in great depth. A "checklist" approach is recommended. The professional uses only his or her judgment and experience to consider both the specific individual and the specific task of interest to make quantitative but relatively gross assessments of resource adequacy using a triage-like categorization process (e.g., with "definitely limiting," "definitely not limiting," or "not sure" categories). This is feasible because of the threshold nature of the system–task interface; in cases where R_A and R_D are widely and separately instrumented, high resolution measurements are not required to determine if a given performance resource is limiting. Any resource(s) so identified as "definitely limiting" becomes an immediate focus of interest. If none is categorized as such, concern moves to those in the "not sure" category in which case more sensitive measurements may be required. Purely subjective methods of measuring resource availability and demands can be augmented with selected, more objective, and higher-resolution measurements in "hybrid applications."

75.3.2 Conceptual, Theoretical Application

The ERM can be used in its broadest conceptual sense as a basis for formulating context-dependent models for specific situations involving human performance. Dillon et al. [2000] utilized ERM constructs to propose approaches to deal with outcome assessment in engineering education, Chesky et al. [2002] applied the ERM as a basis for a conceptual understanding of medical problems of musicians, and Olson and Kondraske [2005] incorporated it into pain management.

It can also be employed in a theoretical fashion to reconsider previous work in human performance. For example, it can be employed to reason why Fleishman [Fleishman and Quaintance, 1984] (as well as others) achieve promising, but limited, success with statistically based predictions of performance in higher-level tasks using regression models with independent variables, which can now be viewed as representing lower-level performance resources (in most cases). Specifically, regression models rely funda-mentally on an assumption that there exists some correlation between dependent and each independent variable, the latter of which typically represent scores from maximal performance tasks and therefore reflect resource availability (using GSPT and ERM logic). Brief reflection results in the realization that correlation is not to be anticipated between the level of performance attainable in a "higher-level task" and *availability* of one of the many performance resources essential to the task (e.g., if four cups of flour are needed for a given cake, having 40 cups available will not *alone* result in a larger cake of equal quality — availability of another ingredient may in fact be limiting). Rather, correlation *is* expected between high-level task performance and the amount of resource *utilization.* Unfortunately, as noted above, the independent variables used typically reflect resource availability. The incomplete labeling of performance variables in such studies reflects the general failure to distinguish between utilization and availability. Why not, then, just use measures of resource utilization in such statistical models? Resource availability measures are simple to obtain in the laboratory without requiring that the individual execute *the* high-level task of interest. Resource utilization measures can only be obtained experimentally by requiring the subject to execute the task in question, which is counterproductive with respect to the goal of using a set of laboratory measurements to extrapolate to performance in one or more higher-level task situations. Regression models based on linear combination of resource *availability* measures do not reflect the nonlinear threshold effect accounted for with resource economic, GSPT-based performance models. One potential alternative based on GSPT and termed nonlinear causal resource analysis (NCRA) has been proposed [Kondraske, 1988a; Vasta and Kondraske, 1994]. NCRA application examples are cited in Section 75.3.4.

75.3.3 Application "In Part"

In this approach, whole domains (i.e., many BEPs) are assessed simultaneously resulting in an estimate or well-founded assumption, which states that "all performance resources in Domain X are nonlimiting in Task(s) Y." Such assumptions are often well justified. For example, it would be reasonable to assume that a young male with a sport-related knee injury would have only a reduction in performance resource availability in the environmental interface domain. More specifically, it is reasonable to assume that the scope of interest can be confined to a smaller subset of functional units, as in gait or speech. These can then be addressed with rigorous application. Examples of this level and manner of applying the ERM have been or are being developed for head/neck control in the context of assistive communication device prescription [Carr, 1989]; workplace design [Kondraske, 1988c]; evaluating worksites and individuals with disabilities for employment [Parnianpour and Marras, 1993]; gait [Carollo and Kondraske, 1987]; measurement of upper extremity motor control [Behbehani et al., 1988]; speech production performance [Jafari, 1989; Jafari et al., 1989]; and to illustrate changes in performance capacity associated with aging [Kondraske, 1989]. Additionally, in some applications only the Generic Intermediate Level need be considered. For example, one may only need to know how well an individual can walk, lift, etc. While it is sometimes painfully clear just how complex is the execution of even a relatively simple task; it can also be recognized that relatively simple, justifiable, and efficient strategies can be developed to maintain a reasonable degree of utility in a given context.

75.3.4 Rigorous, High-Tech Application

While this path may offer the greatest potential for impact, it also presents the greatest challenge. The ultimate *goal* would be to capture the analytic and modeling capability (as implied by the above discussions) for a "total human" (single subject or populations) and "any task" in a desktop computer system (used along with synergistic "peripherals" that adopt the same framework, such as measurement tools [Kondraske, 1990a]). This suggests a long-term, collaborative effort. However, intermediate tools that provide significant utility are feasible [e.g., Vasta and Kondraske, 1994] and needed [Allard et al., 1994; Vasta and Kondraske, 1995]. A promising example of such tools based directly on GSPT and the ERM is NCRA [Vasta and Kondraske, 1994; Kondraske et al., 1997]. This inferential method has recently been used [Kondraske et al., 1997] to develop models that relate performance resource demands on various human subsystems to the level of performance attained in higher level mobility tasks (e.g., gait and stair climbing). In turn, these models have used to predict level of performance in these higher level tasks with success that exceeds that which has been obtained with regression models. Furthermore, the NCRA method inherently provides not only a prediction of high-level task performance, but also identifies which performance resources are most likely to be preventing better performance (i.e., which ones are the "limiting performance resources"). Similar applications of NCRA have been used to develop models of laparoscopic surgical performance [Gettman et al., 2003; Johnson et al., 2004], driving performance [Fischer et al., 2002], and to understand falls in elderly subjects [Murphy, 2000]. A special NCRA software package has been developed to facilitate model development and use. While such tools that are useful to practitioners are desirable, they are almost essential for the efficient conduct of in-depth experimental work with the ERM.

The issue of biologic variability and its influence on numerical analyses can be raised in the context of rigorous numerical application. In this regard, the methods underlying GSPT and the ERM (or any similar cause-and-effect model) are noted to be analogous with those used to design artificial systems. In recent years, conceptual approaches and mathematical tools widely known as Taguchi methods [Bendell et al., 1988] have shown to be effective for understanding and managing a very similar type of variability that surfaces in the manufacture of artificial systems (e.g., variability associated with performance of components of larger systems and the effect on aspects of performance of the final "product"). Such tools may prove useful in working through engineering problems such as those associated with variability.

75.4 Conclusion

The ERM is a step toward the goal of achieving an application-independent approach to modeling any human–task interface. It provides a systematic and generalizable (across all subsystem types) means of identifying performance measures that characterize human subsystems, as well as a consistent basis for performance measurement definition (and task analysis). It has also served to stimulate focus on a standardized, distinct set of variables, which facilitates clear communication of an individual's status among professionals.

After the initial presentation, refinements in both GSPT and the ERM were made. However, the basic approaches, terminology, and constructs used in each have remained quite stable. More recent work has focused on development of various components required for application of the ERM in nontrivial situations. This entails using GSPT and basic ERM concepts to guide a full "fleshing out" of the details of measurement parameterizations and models for different types of human subsystems, definition of standard conventions and notations, and development of computer-based tools. In addition, experimental studies designed to evaluate key constructs of the ERM and to demonstrate the various ways in which it can be applied are being conducted. A good portion of the developmental work is aimed at building a capability to conduct more complex, nontrivial experimental studies. Collaborations with other research groups have also emerged and are being supported to the extent possible. Experiences with it in various contexts and at various levels of application have been productive and encouraging.

The ERM is one, relatively young attempt at organizing and dealing with the complexity of some major aspects of human performance. There is no known alternative that, in a specific sense, attempts to accomplish the same goals as the working model presented here. Is it good enough? For what purposes? Is a completely different approach or merely refinement required? The process of revision is central to the natural course of the history of ideas. Needs for generalizations in human performance persist.

Defining Terms

Basic element of performance (BEP): A modeling item at the basic element level in the ERM defined by identification of a specific system at this level and one of its dimensions of performance (e.g., functional unit = visual information processor, dimension of performance = speed, BEP = visual information processor speed).

Behavior: A general term that relates to what a human or artificial system does while carrying out its function(s) under given conditions. Often, behavior is characterized by measurement of selected parameters or identification of unique system states over time.

Composite performance capacity: A performance capacity at a higher level of abstraction, formed by combining two or more lower-level performance capacities (e.g., via integration to determine the area or volume within a performance envelope).

Dimension of performance: A unique quality that characterizes how well a system executes its function (e.g., speed, accuracy, and torque production); one of axes or the label associated with one of the axes in a multidimensional performance space.

Function: The purpose of a system. Some systems map to a single primary function (e.g., process visual information). Others (e.g., the human arm) map to multiple functions , although at any given time multifunction systems are likely to be executing a single function (e.g., polishing a car). Functions can be described and inventoried, whereas level of performance of a given function can be measured.

Generic intermediate level: One of three major hierarchical levels for systems and tasks identified in the elemental resource model. The generic intermediate level represents new systems (e.g., postural maintenance system, object gripper, object lifter, etc.) formed by the combination of functional units at the basic element level (e.g., flexors, extensors, processors, etc.). The term "generic" is used to imply the high frequency of use of systems at this level in tasks of daily life (i.e., items at the "high level" in the ERM).

Goal: A desired end-point (i.e., result) typically characterized by multiple parameters, at least one of which is specified. Examples include specified task goals (e.g., move an object of specified mass from point A to point B in 3 sec) or estimated task performance (maximum mass, range, speed of movement obtainable given a specified elemental performance resource availability profile), depending on whether a reverse or forward analysis problem is undertaken. Whereas function describes the general process of a task, the goal directly relates to performance and is quantitative.

Limiting resource: A performance resource at any hierarchical level (e.g., vertical lift strength, and knee flexor speed) that is available in an amount that is less than the worst case demand imposed by a task. Thus, a given resource can only be "limiting" when considered in the context of a specific task.

Performance: Unique qualities of a human or artificial system (e.g., strength, speed, accuracy, and endurance) that pertain to how well that system executes its function.

Performance capacity: A quantity in finite availability that is possessed by a system or subsystem, drawn on during the execution of tasks, and limits some aspects (e.g., speed, force production, etc.) of a system's ability to execute tasks; or, the limit of that aspect itself.

Performance envelope: The surface in a multidimensional performance space, formed with a selected subset of a system's dimensions of performance, that defines the limits of a systems performance. Tasks represented by points which fall within this envelope can be performed by the system in question.

Performance resource: A unique quality of a system's performance modeled and quantified using a resource construct.

Performance resource substitution: The term used in GSPT to describe the manner in which intelligent system's, such as humans, utilize redundancy or adapt to unusual circumstances (e.g., injuries) to obtain optimal procedures for executing a task.

Procedure: A set of constraints placed on a system in which flexibility exists regarding how a goal (or set of goals) associated with a given function can be achieved. Procedure specification requires specification of initial, intermediate and final states, or conditions dictating how the goal is to be accomplished. Such specification can be thought of in terms of removing some degrees of freedom.

Resource construct: The collective set of attributes that define and uniquely characterize a resource. Usually, the term is applied to only tangible items. A resource is desirable, measurable in terms of amount (from zero to some finite positive value) in such a manner that a larger numerical value indicates a greater amount of the resource.

Resource economic principle: The principle, observable in many contexts, which states that the amount of a given resource that is available (e.g., money) must exceed the demand placed on it (e.g., cost of an item) if a specified goal (e.g., purchase of the item) is to be achieved.

Resource utilization flexibility: A term used in GSPT to describe situations in which there is more than one possible source of a given performance resource type, that is, redundant supplies exist.

Structure: Physical manifestation and attributes of a human or artificial system and the object of one type of measurements at multiple hierarchical levels.

Style: Allowance for variation within a procedure, resulting in the intentional incomplete specification of a procedure or resulting from either intentional or unintentional incomplete specification of procedure.

System: A physical structure, at any hierarchical level of abstraction, that executes one or more functions.

Task: That which results from (1) the combination of specified functions, goals and procedures, or (2) the specification of function and goals and the observation of procedures utilized to achieve the goals.

References

Allard, P., Stokes, I.A.F., and Blanchi, J.P. 1994. *Three-Dimensional Analysis of Human Movement*, Human Kinetics, Champaign, IL.

Baron, S., Kruser, D.S., and Huey, B.M., Eds. 1990. *Quantitative Modeling of Human Performance in Complex, Dynamic Systems*, National Academy Press, Washington, DC.

Behbehani, K., Kondraske, G.V., and Richmond, J.R. 1988. Investigation of upper extremity visuomotor control performance measures. *IEEE Trans. Biomed. Eng.*, 35: 518–525.

Bendell, A., Disney, J., and Pridmore, W.A. 1988. *Taguchi Methods: Applications in World Industry*, IFS Publishing, London.

Botterbusch, K.F. *Vocational Assessment and Evaluation Systems: A Comparison*. Stout Vocational Rehabiltation Institute, Unversity of Wisconsin, Menomonie, WI.

Card, S.K., Moran, T.P., and Newell, A. 1986. The model human processor. In Boff, K.R., Kaufman, L., and Thomas, J.P. (Eds.), *Handbook of Perception and Human Performance*, Vol. II, Wiley, New York, pp. 45.1–45.35.

Carollo, J.J. and Kondraske, G.V. 1987. The prerequisite resources for walking: characterization using a task analysis strategy. In Leinberger, J. (Ed.), *Proceedings of the 9th Annual IEEE Engineering in Medical and Biological Society Conference*, p. 357.

Carr, B. 1989. *Head/neck control performance measurement and task interface model*. M.S. Thesis, University of Texas at Arlington, Arlington, TX.

Chaffin, D.B. and Andersson, G.B.J. 1991. *Occupational Biomechanics*, John Wiley and Sons, New York.

Chesky, K., Kondraske, G.V., Henoch, M., and Rubin, B. 2002. Musicians' health. In Colwell, R. and Richardson, C. (Eds.), *The New Handbook of Research on Music Teaching and Learning*, Oxford University Press, New York, pp. 1023–1039.

Delp, S.L., Loan, J.P., Hoy, M.G., Zajac, F.E., Topp, E.L., and Rosen, J.M. 1990. An interactive graphics-based model of the lower extremity to study orthopaedic surgical procedures. *IEEE Trans. Biomed. Eng.* 37: 757–767.

Dillon, W.E., Kondraske, G.V., Everett, L.J., and Volz, R.A. 2000. Performance theory based outcome measurement in engineering education and training. *IEEE Trans. Eng. Edu.* 43: 92–99.

Fischer, C.A., Kondraske, G.V., and Stewart, R.M. 2002. Prediction of driving performance using nonlinear causal resource analysis. *CD-ROM Proceedings of the 24th International Conference on IEEE Engineering in Medicine and Biological Society*, Houston, October 23–26, pp. 2473–2474.

Fleishman, E.A. 1956. Psychomotor selection tests: research and application in the United States Air Force. *Personnel Psychol.* 9: 449–467.

Fleishman, E.A. 1966. Human abilities and the acquisition of skill. In Bilodeau, E.A. (Ed.), *Acquisition of Skill*, Academic Press, New York, pp. 147–167.

Fleishman, E.A. 1967. Performance assessment based on an empirically derived task taxonomy. *Hum. Factors* 9: 349–366.

Fleishman, E.A. 1972. Structure and measurement of psychomotor abilities. In Singer, R.N. (Ed.), *The Psychomotor Domain: Movement Behavior*, Lea and Febiger, Philadelphia, pp. 78–106.

Fleishman, E.A. 1982. Systems for describing human tasks. *Am. Psychol.* 37: 821–824.

Fleishman, E.A. and Quaintance, M.K. 1984. *Taxonomies of Human Performance*, Academic Press, Orlando, FL.

Frisch, H.P. 1993. Man/machine interaction dynamics and performance analysis. In *Proceedings of the NATO-Army-NASA Advanced Study Institute on Concurrent Engineering Tools and Technologies for Mechanical System Design*, Springer-Verlag, New York.

Gettman, M.T., Kondraske, G.V., Traxer, O., Ogan, K., Napper, C., Jones, D.B., Pearle, M.S., and Cadeddu, J. 2003. Assessment of basic human performance resources predicts operative performance of laparoscopic surgery. *J. Am. Coll. Surg.* 197: 489–496.

Gilbreth, F.B. and Gilbreth, F.M. 1917. *Applied Motion Study.* Sturgis and Walton Co., New York.

Gottlieb, G.L., Corcos, D.M., and Agarwal, G.C. 1989. Strategies for the control of voluntary movements with one mechanical degree of freedom, *Behav. Brain Sci.* 12: 189–250.

Hemami, H. 1988. Modeling, control, and simulation of human movement, *CRC Crit. Rev. Bioeng.* 13: 1–34.

Jafari, M. 1989a. *Modeling and Measurement of Human Speech Performance Toward Pathology Pattern Recognition, Dissertation*, The University of Texas at Arlington, Arlington, TX.

Jafari, M., Wong, K.H., Behbehani, K., and Kondraske, G.V. 1989b. Performance characterization of human pitch control system: an acoustic approach. *J. Acoust. Soc. Am.* 85: 1322–1328.

Johnson, D.B., Kondraske, G.V., Wilhelm, D.M., Jacomides, L., Ogan, K., Pearle, M.S., and Cadeddu, J.A. 2004. Assessment of basic human performance resources predicts performance of virtual ureterorenoscopy. *J. Urol.* 171: 80–84.

Kondraske, G.V. 1987a. Human performance: science or art? In Foster, K. (Ed.), *Proceedings of 13th Northeast Bioengineering Conference*, pp. 44–47.

Kondraske, G.V. 1987b. Looking at the study of human performance. *SOMA: Eng. Hum. Body (ASME)* 2: 50.

Kondraske, G.V. 1988a. Experimental evaluation of an elemental resource model for human performance. In Harris, G. and Walker, C. (Eds.), *Proceedings of the 10th Annual IEEE Engineering in Medicine and Biological Society Conference*, IEEE, New York, pp. 1612–1613.

Kondraske, G.V. 1988b. Human performance measurement and task analysis, In Enders, A. (Ed.), *Technology for Independent Living Sourcebook*, 2nd ed., RESNA, Washington, DC.

Kondraske, G.V. 1988c. Workplace design: an elemental resource approach to task analysis and human performance measurements. *Proceedings of the International Conference on Association in Advances Rehabilitation Technology*, pp. 608–611.

Kondraske, G.V., Beehler, P.J.H., Behbehani, K., Chwialkowski, M., Imrhan, S., Mooney, V., Pape, E., Richmond, J., Smith, S., and von Maltzahn, W. 1988. Measuring human performance: concepts, methods, and application examples. *SOMA: Eng. Hum. Body (ASME)* Jan: 6–13.

Kondraske, G.V. and Standridge, R. 1988. Robot performance: conceptual strategies. In *Conference of Digest IEEE Midcon/88 Technological Conference*, IEEE, New York, pp. 359–362.

Kondraske, G.V. 1989. Neuromuscular performance: resource economics and product-based composite indices. *Proceedings of the 11th Annual IEEE Engineering in Medicine and Biological Society Conference*, IEEE, New York, pp. 1045–1046.

Kondraske, G.V. 1990a. A PC-based performance measurement laboratory system. *J. Clin. Eng.* 15: 467–477.

Kondraske, G.V. 1990b. Quantitative measurement and assessment of performance. In Smith, R.V. and Leslie, J.H. (Eds.), *Rehabilitation Engineering*, CRC Press, Boca Raton, FL, pp. 101–125.

Kondraske, G.V. and Khoury, G.J. 1992. Telerobotic system performance measurement: motivation and methods. In *Cooperative Intelligent Robotics in Space III*, SPIE, Vol. 1829, pp. 161–172.

Kondraske, G.V. 1993. *The HPI Shorthand Notation System for Human System Parameters*, Technical Report 92–001R V1.5, Human Performance Institute, The University of Texas at Arlington, Arlington, TX.

Kondraske, G.V. 1995. An elemental resource model for the human–task interface. *Int. J. Technol. Asses. Health Care* 11: 153–173.

Kondraske, G.V. and Beehler, P.J.H. 1994. Applying general systems performance theory and the elemental resource model to gender-related issues in physical education and sport. *Women Sport Physical Activity J.* 3: 1–19.

Kondraske, G.V. 1995. Measurement tools and processes in rehabilitation engineering. In Bronzino, J.D. (Ed.), *Handbook of Biomedical Engineering*, CRC Press, Boca Raton, FL.

Kondraske, G.V., Johnston, C., Pearson, A., and Tarbox, L. (1997). Performance prediction and limiting resource identification with nonlinear causal resource analysis. *Proceedings, 19th Annual Engineering in Medicine and Biology Society Conference*, pp. 1813–1816.

Leibniz, G.W. and Montgomery, G.R. *Discourse on Metaphysics and the Monadology*. Prometheus Books, 1992.

Mayer, T.G. and Gatchel, R.J. 1991. *Functional Restoration for Spinal Disorders: The Sports Medicine Approach*, Lea & Febeger, Philadelphia, pp. 66–77.

Meister, D. 1989. *Conceptual Aspects of Human Performance*, The Johns Hopkins University Press, Baltimore.

Murphy, M. 2002. The fall factor. *Rehab. Manag.* 15: 34–38.

Navon, D. and Gopher, D. 1979. On the economy of the human processing system. *Psych. Rev.* 86: 214–253.

Neel, A. 1977. *Theories of Psychology: A Handbook*, Schenkman Publishing Co., Cambridge, MA.

Olson, S. and Kondraske, G.V. 2005, in press. Clinical applications of the elemental resource model and performance theory. In Simmonds, M.J. (Ed.), *Measuring and Managing Pain, Patients, and Practitioners. Assessment, Outcomes and Evidence.* Elsevier Press, New York.

Parnianpour, M. and Marras, W.S. 1993. Development of clinical protocols based on ergonomics evaluation in response to American Disability Act (1992), In *Rehabilitation Engineering Center Proposal to National Institute on Disability and Rehabilitation Research*, Ohio State University, Columbus, OH.

Schoner, G. and Kelso, J.A.S. 1988. Dynamic pattern generation in behavioral and neural systems. *Science* 239: 1513–1520.

Syndulko, K., Tourtellotte, W.W., and Richter, E. 1988. Toward the objective measurement of central processing resources, *Med. Biol. Soc. Mag.* 7: 17–20.

Taylor, F.W. 1911. *The Principles of Scientific Management.* Harper and Brothers, New York.

Turvey, M.T., Shaw, R.E., and Mace, W. 1978. Issues in the theory of action: degrees of freedom, coordinative structures, and coalitions. In Requin, J. (Ed.), *Attention and Performance VII*, Lawrence Earlbaum Assoc., Hillsdale, NJ.

U.S. Department of Labor. 1992. *Dictionary of Occupation Titles*, 4th ed., Claitor's Publishing Div., Baton Rouge, LA, pp. 1–1404.

Vasta, P.J. and Kondraske, G.V. 1994. Performance prediction of an upper extremity reciprocal task using non-linear causal resource analysis, In *Proceedings of 16th Annual IEEE Engineering in Medicine and Biology Society Conference*, IEEE, New York, pp. ?–?.

Wickens, C.D. 1984. *Engineering Psychology and Human Performance*, Charles E. Merrill Publishing Co, Columbus, OH.

World Health Organization (WHO). 1980. International classification of impairments, disabilities, and handicaps, *WHO Chronicle*, 34: 376.

Yen, S.S. and Kondraske, G.V. 1992. Machine shape perception: object recognition based on need-driven resolution flexibility and convex-hull carving. In *Proc. Conf. Intelligent Robots Computer Vision X: Algorithms Techniques*, SPIE, 1607: 176–187.

Further Information

General discussions of major issues associated with human performance modeling can be found in the following texts:

Fleishman, E.A. and Quaintance, M.K. 1984. *Taxonomies of Human Performance*, Academic Press, Orlando, FL.

Meister, D. 1989. *Conceptual Aspects of Human Performance*, The Johns Hopkins University Press, Baltimore.

Neel, A. 1977. *Theories of Psychology: A Handbook*, Schenkman Publishing Co., Cambridge, MA.

Requin, J. 1978. *Attention and Performance VII*, Lawrence Earlbaum Assoc., Hillsdale, NJ.

Wickens, C.D. 1984. *Engineering Psychology and Human Performance*, Charles E. Merrill Publishing Co, Columbus, OH.

More detailed information regarding general systems performance theory, the elemental resource model, and their application is available from the Human Performance Institute, P.O. Box 19180, University of Texas at Arlington, Arlington, TX 76019–0180 and at the HPI web site: http://www-ee.uta.edu/hpi

76

Measurement of Neuromuscular Performance Capacities

Susan S. Smith
Texas Women's University

Movements allow us to interact with our environment, express ourselves, and communicate with each other. Life is movement. Movement is constantly occurring at many hierarchical levels including cellular and subcellular levels. By using the adjective "human" to clarify the term "movement," we are not only defining the species of interest, but also limiting the study to observable performance and its more overt causes. Study of human performance is of interest to a broad range of professionals including rehabilitation engineers, orthopedic surgeons, therapists, biomechanists, kinesiologists, psychologists, and so on. Because of the complexity of human performance and the variety of investigators, the study of human performance is conducted from several theoretical perspectives including (1) anatomical, (2) purpose or character of the movement (such as locomotion), (3) physiological, (4) biomechanical, (5) psychological, (6) socio-cultural, and (7) integrative. The elemental resource model (ERM), presented at the beginning of this section, is an integrative model that incorporates aspects of the other models into a singular system accounting for the human, the task, and the human–task interface [Kondraske, 2005].

The purposes of this chapter are to (1) provide reasons for measuring four selected variables of human performance: extremes/**range of motion**, strength, **speed of movement**, and **endurance**; (2) briefly define and discuss these variables; (3) overview selected instruments and methods used to measure these variables; and (4) discuss interpretation of performance for a given neuromuscular subsystem.

76.1   Neuromuscular Functional Units

While the theoretical perspectives listed previously may be useful within specific contexts or within specific disciplines, the broader appreciation of human performance and its control can be gained from the perspective of an integrative model such as the ERM [Kondraske, 2005]. This model organizes performance resources into four different domains. Basic movements, such as elbow flexion, are executed by **neuromuscular functional units** in the environmental interface domain. Intermediate and complex tasks, such as walking and playing the piano, utilize multiple basic functional units. The human performing a movement operates the involved functional units along different dimensions of performance according to the demands of the task. Dimensions of performance are factors such as joint motion, strength, speed of movement, and endurance. Lifting a heavy box off the floor requires, among other things, a specific amount of strength associated with neuromuscular functional units of the back, legs, and arms according to the weight and size of the box. Reaching for a light-weight box from the top shelf of a closet requires that the shoulder achieve certain **extremes of motion** according to the height of the shelf.

Whereas four dimensions of performance are considered individually in this chapter, they are *highly interdependent*. For example, strength availability during a movement is partly dependent on joint angle. Despite interdependence, considering the variables as different dimensions is essential to studying human performance. The components limiting the human's ability to complete a task can only be identified and subsequently enhanced by determining, for example, that the reason the human cannot reach the box off the top shelf is not because of insufficient range of motion of the shoulder, but because of insufficient strength of the shoulder musculature required to lift the arm through the range of motion. Isolating the subsystems involved in a task and maximally stressing them along one or more "isolated" dimensions of performance is a key concept in the ERM. "Maximally stressing" the subsystems means that the maximum amount of the resource available is being determined. This differs from determining the amount of the resource that happened to be used while performing a particular task. Often the distinction between obtaining maximal performance from a human and submaximal performance is in the instructions given the subject. For example, when measuring speed, we say, "move as fast as you can."

76.1.1 Purposes of Measuring Selected Neuromuscular Performance Capacities

Range of motion, strength, speed of movement, and endurance can be measured for one or more of the following purposes:

1. To determine the amount of the resource available and to compare it to the normal value for that individual. "Normal" is frequently determined by comparisons with the opposite extremity or with normative data when available. This information can be used to develop goals and a program to change the performance.
2. To assist in determining the possible affects of insufficient or imbalanced amounts of the variable on a person's performance of activities of daily living, work, sport, and leisure pursuits. In this case the amount of the variable is compared to the demands of the task, rather than to norms or to the opposite extremity.
3. To assist in diagnosis of medical conditions and the nature of movement dysfunctions.
4. To reassess status in order to determine the effectiveness of a program designed to change the amount of the variable.
5. To motivate persons to comply with treatment or training regimes.
6. To document status and the results of treatment or training and to communicate with other involved persons.
7. To assist in ergonomically designed furniture, equipment, techniques, and environments.
8. To provide information that when combined with other measures of human performance can be used to predict functional capabilities.

76.2 Range of Motion and Extremes of Motion

Range of motion (ROM) is the amount of movement that occurs at a joint. ROM is typically measured by noting the *extremes of motion (EOM)*. The designated reference or zero position must be specified for measurements of the two extremes of motion. For example, to measure elbow (radiohumeral joint) flexion and extension, the preferred starting position is with the subject supine with the arm parallel to the lateral midline of the body with the palm facing upward [Norkin and White, 2003; Reese and Bandy, 2003]. Measurements are taken with the elbow in the fully flexed position and with the elbow in the fully extended position.

76.2.1 Movement Terminology

Joint movements are described using a coordinate system with the human body in anatomical position. Anatomical position of the body is an erect position, face forward, arms at sides, palms facing forward, and fingers and thumbs in extension. The central coordinate system consists of three cardinal planes and axes with its origin located between the cornua of the sacrum [Panjabi, et al., 1974]. Figure 76.1 demonstrates the planes and axes of the central coordinate system. The same coordinate system can parallel the master system at any joint in the body by relocating the origin to any defined point.

The sagittal plane is the y, z plane; and the frontal (or coronal) plane is the y, x plane; and the horizontal (or transverse) plane is the x, z plane. Movements are described in relation to the origin of the coordinate system. The arrows indicate the positive direction of each axis. An anterior translation is $+z$; a posterior translation is $-z$. Clockwise rotations are $+\theta$, and counterclockwise rotations are $-\theta$.

Joints are described as having degrees of freedom (DOF) of movement; DOF, that is, the number of axes associated with a joint each of which allows motion in a plane in three-dimensional space. If a motion occurs in one plane and around one axis, the joint is defined as having one DOF. Joints with movements in two planes occurring around two different axes, have two DOF, and so on.

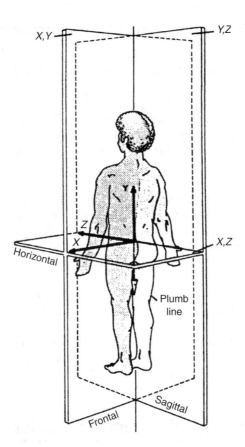

FIGURE 76.1   Planes and axes are illustrated in anatomical position. The central coordinate system with its origin between the cornua of the sacrum is shown. (From White III A.A. and Panjabi M.M. 1990. *Clinical Biomechanics of the Spine*, 2nd ed., p. 87. Philadelphia, JB Lippincott Company. With permission.)

Angular movements refer to motions that cause an increase or decrease in the angle between the articulating bones. Angular movements are flexion, extension, abduction, adduction, and lateral flexion (see Table 76.1). Rotational movements generally occur around a longitudinal (or vertical) axis except for movements of the clavicle and scapula. The rotational movements occurring around the longitudinal axis (internal rotation, external rotation, opposition, horizontal abduction, and horizontal adduction) are described in Table 76.1. Rotation of the scapula is described in terms of the direction of the inferior angle. Movement of the inferior angle of the scapula toward the midline is a medial (or downward) rotation, and movement of the inferior angle away from the midline is lateral (or upward) rotation. In the extremities, the anterior surface of the extremity is used as the reference area. Because the head, neck, trunk, and pelvis rotate about a midsagittal, longitudinal axis, rotation of these parts is designated as right or left.

A communications problem often exists in describing motion using the terms defined in Table 76.1. A body segment can be in a position such as flexion, but can be moving toward extension. This confusion is partially remedied by using the form of the word with the suffix, *-ion*, to indicate a static position and using the suffix, *-ing*, to denote a movement. Thus, an elbow can be in a position of 90° flex*ion* and also extend*ing*.

76.2.2   Factors Influencing ROM/EOM and ROM/EOM Measurements

The ROM and EOM available at a joint are determined by morphology and the soft tissues surrounding and crossing a joint, including the joint capsule, ligaments, tendons, and muscles. Other factors such as

TABLE 76.1 Movement Terms, Planes, Axes, and Descriptions of Movements

Movement term	Plane	Axis	Description of movement
Flexion	Sagittal	Frontal	Bending of a part such that the anterior surfaces approximate each other. However, flexion of the knee, ankle, foot, and toes refers to movement in the posterior direction.
Extension	Sagittal	Frontal	Opposite of flexion; involves straightening a body part.
Abduction	Frontal	Sagittal	Movement away from the midline of the body or body part; abduction of the wrist is sometimes called *radial deviation*.
Adduction	Frontal	Sagittal	Movement toward the midline of the body or body part; adduction of the wrist is sometimes called *ulnar deviation*.
Lateral flexion	Frontal	Sagittal	Term used to denote lateral movements of the head, neck, and trunk.
Internal (medial) rotation	Horizontal	Longitudinal	Turning movement of the anterior surface of a part towards the midline of the body; internal rotation of the forearm is referred to as *pronation*.
External (lateral) rotation	Horizontal	Longitudinal	Turning movement of the anterior surface of a part away from the midline of the body; external rotation of the forearm is referred to as *supination*.
Opposition	Multiple	Multiple	Movement of the tips of the thumb and little finger toward each other.
Horizontal abduction	Horizontal	Longitudinal	Movement of the arm in a posterior direction away from the midline of the body with the shoulder joint in 90° of either flexion or abduction.
Horizontal adduction	Horizontal	Longitudinal	Movement of the arm in an anterior direction toward the midline of the body with the shoulder joint in 90° of either flexion or abduction.
Tilt	Depends on joint	Depends on joint	Term used to describe certain movements of the scapula and pelvis. In the scapula, an anterior tilt occurs when the coracoid process moves in an anterior and downward direction while the inferior angle moves in a posterior and upward direction. A posterior tilt of the scapula is the opposite of an anterior tilt. In the pelvis, an anterior tilt is rotation of the anterior superior spines (ASISs) of the pelvis in an anterior and downward direction; a posterior tilt is movement of the ASISs in a posterior and upward direction. A lateral tilt of the pelvis occurs when the pelvis is not in level from side to side, but one ASIS is higher than the other one.
Gliding	Depends on joint	Depends on joint	Movements that occur when one articulating surface slides on the opposite surface.
Elevation	Frontal		A gliding movement of the scapula in an upward direction as in shrugging the shoulders.
Depression	Frontal		Movement of the scapula downward in a direction reverse of elevation.

age, gender, swelling, muscle mass development, body fat, passive insufficiency (change in the ROM/EOM available at one joint in a two-joint muscle complex caused by the position of the other joint), and time of day (diurnal effect) also affect the amount of motion available. Some persons, because of posture, genetics, body type, or movement habits, normally demonstrate hypermobile or hypomobile joints. Dominance has not been found to significantly affect available ROM. See discussion in Miller [1985]. The shapes of joint surfaces, which are designed to allow movement in particular directions, can become altered by disease, trauma, and posture, thereby increasing or decreasing the ROM/EOM. Additionally, the soft tissues crossing a joint can become short (contracted) or overstretched altering the ROM/EOM.

The type of movement, active or passive, also affects ROM/EOM. When measuring active ROM (AROM), the person voluntarily contracts muscles and moves the body part through the available motion. When measuring passive ROM (PROM), the examiner moves the body part through the ROM. PROM is usually slightly greater than AROM due to the extensibility of the tissues crossing and comprising the joint. AROM can be decreased because of restricted joint mobility, muscle weakness, pain, unwillingness to move, or inability to follow instructions. PROM is assessed to clinically determine the integrity of the joint and the extent of structural limitation.

76.2.3 Instrumented Systems Used to Measure ROM/EOM

The most common instrument used to measure joint ROM/EOM is a goniometer. The universal goniometer, shown in Figure 76.2a, is most widely used clinically. A variety of universal goniometers have been developed for specific applications. Two other types of goniometers are also shown in Figure 76.2.

Table 76.2 lists and compares several goniometric instruments used to measure ROM/EOM. Choice of the instrument used to measure ROM/EOM depends upon the degree of accuracy required, time available to the examiner, the measurement environment, the body segment being measured, and the equipment available.

Non-goniometric methods of joint measurement are available. Tape measures, radiographs, photography, cinematography, videotape, and various optoelectric movement-monitoring systems can also be used to measure or calculate the motion available at various joints. These methods are beyond the scope of this chapter.

76.2.4 Key Concepts in Goniometric Measurement

Numerous textbooks [Palmer and Epler, 1998; Clarkson, 2000; Reese and Bandy, 2002; Norkin and White, 2003] are available that describe precise procedures for goniometric measurements of each joint. Unfortunately, there is a lack of standardization among these references.

In general, the anatomical position of zero degrees (*preferred starting position*) is the desired starting position for all ROM/EOM measurements except rotation at the hip, shoulder, and forearm. The arms of the goniometer are usually aligned parallel and lateral to the long axis of the moving and the fixed-body segments in line with the appropriate landmarks. In the past, some authors contended that placement of the axis of the goniometer should be congruent with the joint axis for accurate measurement [Wiechec and Krusen, 1939; West, 1945]. However, the axis of rotation for joints changes as the body segment moves through its ROM; therefore, a goniometer cannot be placed in a position in line with the joint axis during movement. Robson [1966] described how variations in the placement of the goniometer's axis could affect the accuracy of ROM measurements. Miller [1985] suggested that the axis problem could be handled by ignoring the goniometer's axis and concentrating on the accurate alignment of the arms of the goniometer with the specified landmarks. Potentially some accuracy may be sacrificed, but the technique is simplified and theoretically more reproducible. When using devices such as the APM I, pictured in Figure 76.2c, the manufacturer's user's manual [Human Performance Measurement, Inc., 1998–2003] recommends placing the alignment guide of the device *along* the side of body segments vs. placing the device directly on body segments (as is frequently done when using the fluid goniometer pictured in Figure 76.2b). Placing

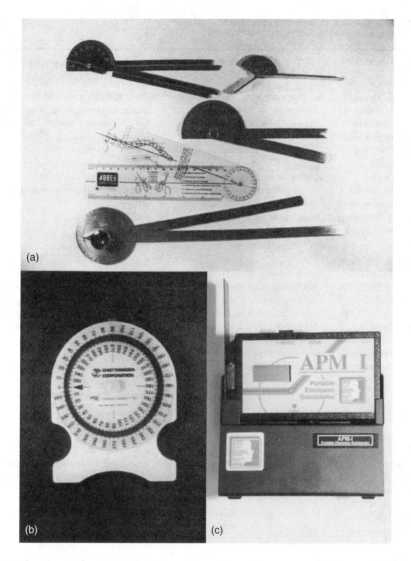

FIGURE 76.2 Three types of goniometric instruments used to measure range and extremes of motion are shown: (a) typical 180- and 360-degree universal goniometers of various sizes; (b) a fluid goniometer, which is activated by the effects of gravity; (c) an APM I digital electronic device that works similarly to a pendulum goniometer, but is not limited by gravity dependency.

the device along the body segment avoids minimizes procedural measurement noise caused by varying pressure on the soft tissue and interindividual differences in soft tissue structure (which can be relevant when establishing norms or comparing a given subject to norms). In any case, the subject's movement is observed during testing for unwanted motions that could result in inaccurate measurement. For example, a subject might attempt to increase forearm supination by laterally flexing the trunk.

76.2.5 Numerical Notation Systems

Three primary systems exist for expressing joint motion in terms of degrees. These are the *0–180 System*, the *180–0 System*, and the *360 System*. The 0–180 System is the most widely accepted system in medical applications and may be the easiest system to interpret. In the 0–180 System, the starting position for all movements is considered to be 0°, and movements proceed toward 180°. As the joint motion increases, the

TABLE 76.2   Comparison of Various Goniometers Commonly Used to Measure Joint Range and Extremes of Motion

Type of goniometer	Advantages/uses	Disadvantages/limitations
Universal goniometer A protractor-like device with one arm considered movable and the other arm stationary; protractor can have a 180 or 360° scale and is usually numbered in both directions; available in a range of sizes and styles to accommodate different joints (see Figure 76.2a)	Inexpensive; portable; familiar devices; size of the joint being measured determines size of the goniometer used; clear plastic goniometers have a line through the center of the arms to make alignment easier and more accurate; finger goniometers can be placed over the dorsal aspect of the joint being measured	Several goniometers of different sizes may be required, especially if digits are measured; full-circle models may be difficult to align when the subject is recumbent and axis alignment is inhibited by the protractor bumping the surface; the increments on the protractors may vary from 1, 2, or 5°; placement of the arms is a potential source of error
Fluid (or bubble) goniometer A device with a fluid-filled channel with a 360° scale that relies on the effects of gravity (see Figure 76.2b); dial turns allowing the goniometer to be "zeroed"; some models are strapped on and others must be held against the body part	Quick and easy to use because it is not usually aligned with bony landmarks; does not have to conform to body segments; useful for measuring neck and spinal movements; using a pair of fluid goniometers permits distinguishing regional spinal motion	More expensive than universal goniometers; using a pair of goniometers is awkward; useless for motions in the horizontal plane; error can be induced by slipping, skin movement, variations in amount of soft tissue owing to muscle contraction, swelling, or fat, and the examiner's hand pressure changing body segment contour; reliability may be sacrificed from lack of orientation to landmarks and difficulty with consistent realignment [Miller, 1985]
Pendulum goniometer A scaled, inclinometer-like device with a needle or pointer (usually weighted); some models are strapped on and others must be held against the body part (not shown)	Inexpensive; same advantages as for the fluid goniometer described above	Some models cannot be "zeroed"; useless for motions in the horizontal plane; same soft tissue error concerns as described above for the fluid goniometer
"Myrin" OB goniometer A fluid-filled, rotatable container consisting of compass needle that responds to the earth's magnetic field (to measure horizontal motion), a gravity-activated inclination needle (to measure frontal and sagittal motion), and a scale (not shown)	Can be strapped on the body part allowing the hands free to stabilize and move the body part; not necessary to align the goniometer with the joint axis; permits measurements in all three planes	Expensive and bulky compared with universal goniometer; not useful for measuring small joints of hand and foot; susceptible to magnetic fields [Clarkson, 2000]; subject to same soft tissue error concerns described above under fluid goniometer
Arthrodial protractor A large, flat, clear plastic protractor without arms that has a level on the straight edge (not shown)	Does not need to conform to body segments; most useful for measuring joint rotation and axioskeletal motion	Not useful for measuring smaller joints, especially those with lesser ROMs; usually scaled in large increments only

TABLE 76.2   Continued

Type of goniometer	Advantages/uses	Disadvantages/limitations
APM I		
Computerized goniometer with digital sensing and electronics; can either perform continuous monitoring or calculate individual ROM/EOM from a compound motion function (see Figure 76.2c)	Easy to use; provides rapid digital read-out; measures angles in *any* plane of motion (by using an "inertial" type of sensor gravity dependency is eliminated allowing for easier measurement of rotary movements, such as trunk rotation); one hand is free to stabilize and move body segments; particularly easy for measuring regional spinal movements	Expensive compared to most other instruments described; device must be rotated perpendicular to the direction of segment motion only; unit must stabilize prior to measurement; excessive delays in recording must be avoided; subject to the same soft tissue error concerns as described above under fluid goniometer, unless the device is aligned along (versus on) the body segment
Electrogoniometer		
Arms of a goniometer are attached to a potentiometer and are strapped to the proximal and distal body parts; movement from the device causes resistance in the potentiometer, which measures the ROM (not shown)	More useful for dynamic ROM, especially for determining kinematic variables during activities such as gait; provides immediate data; some electrogoniometers permit measurement in one, two, or three dimensions	Aligning and attaching the device is time-consuming and not amenable to all body segments; device and equipment needed to use it are moderately expensive; essentially laboratory equipment; less accurate for measurement of absolute limb position; device itself is cumbersome and may alter the movement being studied

numbers on the goniometric scale increase. In the 180–0 System, movements toward flexion approach 0° and movements toward extension approach 180°. Different rules are used for the other planes of motion. The 360 System is similar to the 180–0 System, which movements are frequently performed from a starting position of 180°. Movements of extension or adduction, which go beyond the neutral position, approach 360°. Joint motion can be reported in tables, charts, graphs, or pictures. In the 0–180 System, the starting and ending ranges are recorded separately, as 0–130°. If a joint cannot be started in the 0° position, the actual starting position is recorded, as 10–130°.

76.3   Strength

Muscle strength implies the force or torque production capacity of muscles. However, to measure strength, the term must be operationally defined. One definition modified from Clarkson [2000] states that muscular strength is the maximal amount of torque or force that a muscle or muscle groups can voluntarily exert in one maximal effort, when type of muscle contraction, limb velocity, and joint angle(s) are specified.

76.3.1   Strength Testing and Muscle Terminology

Physiologically, skeletal muscle strength is the ability of muscle fibers to generate maximal tension for a brief time interval. A muscle's ability to generate maximal tension and to sustain tension for differing time intervals is dependent on the muscle's cross-sectional area (the larger the cross-sectional area, the greater the strength), geometry (including the muscle fiber arrangement, length, moment arm, and angle of pennation), and physiology. Characteristics of muscle fibers have been classified based on twitch tension and fatigability. Different fiber types have different metabolic traits. Different types of muscle fibers are differentially stressed depending on the intensity and duration of the contraction. Ideally, strength tests should measure the ability of the muscle to develop tension rapidly and to sustain the tension for brief time intervals. In order to truly measure muscle tension, a measurement device must be directly attached to the muscle or tendon. Whereas this direct procedure has been performed [Komi, 1990], it is hardly useful as a routine clinical measure. Indirect measures are used to estimate the strength of muscle groups performing a given function, such as elbow flexion.

Muscles work together in groups and may be classified according to the major role of the group in producing movement. The *prime mover*, or *agonist*, is a muscle or muscle group that makes the major contribution to movement at a joint. The *antagonist* is a muscle or muscle group that has an opposite action to the prime mover(s). The antagonist relaxes as the agonist moves the body part through the ROM. *Synergists* are accessory muscles that contract and work with the agonist to produce the desired movement. Synergists may work by stabilizing proximal joints, preventing unwanted movement, and joining with the prime mover to produce a movement that one muscle group acting alone could not produce.

A number of terms and concepts are important toward understanding the nature and scope of strength capacity testing. Several of these terms are defined below; however, there are no universally accepted definitions for these terms.

Dynamic contraction — the output of muscles moving body segments [Kroemer, 1991].
Isometric — tension develops in a muscle, but the muscle length does not change and no movement occurs.
Static — same as isometric.
Isotonic — a muscle develops constant tension against a load or resistance. Kroemer [1991] suggests the term, *isoforce*, more aptly describes this condition.
Concentric — a contraction in which a muscle develops internal force that exceeds the external force of resistance, the muscle shortens, and movement is produced [Gowitzke et al., 1980].
Eccentric — a contraction in which a muscle lengthens while continuing to maintain tension [Gowitzke et al., 1980].
Isokinetic — a condition where the angular velocity is held constant. Kroemer [1991] prefers the term, *isovelocity*, to describe this type of muscle exertion.
Isoinertial — a static or dynamic muscle contraction where the external load is held constant [Kroemer, 1983].

76.3.2 Factors Influencing Muscle Strength and Strength Measurement

In addition to the anatomical and physiological factors affecting strength, other factors must be considered when strength testing. The ability of a muscle to develop tension depends on the type of muscle contraction. Per unit of muscle, the greatest tension can be generated eccentrically, less can be developed isometrically, and the least can be generated concentrically. These differences in tension-generating capacity are so great that the type of contraction being strength-tested requires specification.

Additionally, strength is partially determined by the ability of the nervous system to cause more motor units to fire synchronously. As one trains, practices an activity, or learns test expectations, strength can increase. Therefore, strength is affected by previous training and testing. This is an important consideration in standardizing testing and in retesting.

A muscle's attachments define the angle of pull of the tendon on the bone and thereby the mechanical leverage at the joint center. Each muscle has a moment arm length, which is the length of a line normal to the muscle passing through the joint center. This moment arm length changes with the joint angle, which changes the muscle's tension output. Optimal tension is developed when a muscle is pulling at a 90° angle to the bony segment.

Changes in muscle length alter the force-generating capacity of muscle. This is called the *length–tension relationship*. *Active* tension decreases when a muscle is either lengthened or shortened relative to its resting length. However, applying a precontraction stretch, or slightly lengthening a muscle and the series elastic component (connective tissue), prior to a contraction causes a greater amount of *total* tension to be developed [Soderberg, 1992]. Of course, excessive lengthening would reduce the tension-generating capacity.

A number of muscles cross over more than one joint. The length of these muscles may be inadequate to permit complete ROM of all joints involved. When a multijoint muscle simultaneously shortens at all joints it crosses, further effective tension development is prevented. This phenomena is called *active insufficiency*. For example, when the hamstrings are tested as knee flexors with the hip extended, less tension can be developed than when the hamstrings are tested with the hip flexed. Therefore, when testing the strength of multijoint muscles, the position of all involved joints must be considered.

The *load–velocity relationship* is also important in testing muscle strength. A load–velocity curve can be generated by plotting the velocity of motion of the muscle lever arm against the external load. With concentric muscle contractions, the least tension is developed at the highest velocity of movement and vice versa. When the external load equals the maximal force that the muscle can exert, the velocity of shortening reaches zero and the muscle contracts isometrically. When the load is increased further, the muscle lengthens eccentrically. During eccentric contractions, the highest tension can be achieved at the highest velocity of movement [Komi, 1973].

The force generated by a muscle is proportional to the contraction time. The longer the contraction time, the greater the force development up to the point of maximum tension. Slower contraction leads to greater force production because more time is allowed for the tension produced in contractile elements to be transferred through the noncontractile components to the tendon. This is the *force–time relationship*. Tension in the tendon will reach the maximum tension developed by the contractile tissues only if the active contraction process is of adequate (even up to 300 msec) duration [Sukop and Nelson, 1974].

Subject effort or motivation, gender, age, fatigue, time of day, temperature, occupation, and dominance can also affect force or torque production capacity. Important additional considerations may be changes in muscle function as a result of pain, overstretching, immobilization, trauma, paralytic disorders, neurologic conditions, and muscle transfers.

76.3.3 Grading Systems and Parameters Measured

Clinically, the two most frequently used methods of strength testing are actually noninstrumented tests: the manual muscle test (MMT) and the functional muscle test (see Amundsen [1990] for more information on functional muscle tests). In each of these cases interval scaled grading criteria are operationally defined. However, a distinct advantage of using instruments to measure strength is that quantifiable units can be obtained.

Deciding whether to measure force (a translational quantity) or torque (a rotational quantity) is an important issue in testing strength. Even when the functional units of interest produce rotational motion, force measurement at some point along the moment arm is common. This is due to the evolution from manual muscle tests to the use of objective measurements where a force sensor replaces the human examiner sense of force resisted or generated. If d is the distance from the point of rotation to the point of force measurement and the force vector is tangent to the arc of motion, then

$$T = Fd \tag{76.1}$$

Therefore, when force are measured, unless the measurement devices are applied at the same anatomical position for each test, force measurements can differ substantially even though the torque production capacity about the selected DOF is the same. Torque can be measured directly if the strength-testing device has an axis of rotation that can be aligned with the anatomical axis of rotation and a torque sensor is used, as in many isokinetic test devices. When this is not the case, the moment arm can be measured and torque calculated. Thus, for neuromuscular systems producing rotational motion, torque measures make the most sense and are preferred. The use of force measurements is the result of clinical traditional and these measures can be easily converted to torque units using knowledge of the applicable moment arm. Force measures are appropriate in whole-body exertions, such as lifting, where the motion is fundamentally translational. Another issue is whether to measure and record peak or averaged values. However, if strength is defined as maximum torque production capacity, peak values are implied.

In addition to single numerical values, some strength measurement systems display and print force or torque (vs. time) curves, angle-torque curves, and graphs. Computerized systems frequently compare the "involved" with the "uninvolved" extremity calculating "percent deficits." As strength is considered proportional to body weight (perhaps erroneously, see Delitto [1990]), force and torque measurements are frequently reported as a peak torque-to-body-weight ratio. This is seemingly to facilitate use of normative data where present, as the normalization results in a reduction in the variance of the data distribution.

76.3.4 Methods and Instruments Used to Measure Muscle Strength

There are two broad categories of testing force or torque production capacity: one category consists of measuring the capacity of defined, local muscle groups (e.g., elbow flexors); the second category of tests consists of measuring several muscle groups on a whole–body basis performing a higher-level task (e.g., lifting). The purpose of the test, required level of sensitivity, and expense are primary factors in selecting the method of strength testing. No single method has emerged as being clearly superior or more widely applicable. Like screwdrivers, different types and different sizes are needed depending upon job demands.

Many of the instrumented strength-testing techniques, which are becoming more standardized clinically and which are almost exclusively used in engineering applications, are based on the concepts and methods of MMT. Although not used for performance capacity tests, because of the ease, practicality, and speed of manual testing, it is still considered a useful tool, especially diagnostically to localize lesions and confirm weakness. Several MMT grading systems prevail. These differ in the actual test positions and premises upon which muscle grading is based. For example, the approach promoted by Kendall et al. [2005] tests a specific muscle (e.g., brachioradialis) rather than a motion. The Daniels and Worthingham method [Hislop and Montgomery, 2002] tests motions (e.g., elbow flexion) that involve all the agonists and synergists used to perform the movement. The latter is considered more functional and less time-consuming, but less specific. The reader is advised to consult these references directly for more information about MMT methods. Further discussion of noninstrumented tests is beyond the scope of this chapter.

An argument can be made for using isometric strength testing because the force or torque reflects actual muscle tension as the position of the body part is held constant and the muscle mechanics do not change. Additionally, good stabilization is easier to achieve, and muscle actions can be better isolated. However, some clinicians prefer dynamic tests, perceiving them as more reflective of function. An unfortunate fact is that neither static nor dynamic strength measurements alone can reveal whether strength is adequate for functional activities. However, strength measurements can be used with models and engineering analyses for such assessments.

Selected instrumented methods of measuring force or torque production capacity are listed and compared in Table 76.3. Table 76.3 is by no means comprehensive. More in-depth review and comparisons of various methods can be found in Amundsen [1990] and Mayhew and Rothstein [1985]. Figure 76.3 illustrates three common instruments used to measure strength.

76.3.5 Key Concepts in Measuring Strength

Because of the number of factors influencing strength and strength testing (discussed in Section 76.3.2), one can become discouraged rather than challenged when faced with the need to measure strength. Optimally, strength testing would be based on the "worst-case" functional performance demands required by an individual in his or her daily life. "Worst-case" testing requires knowing the performance demands of tasks including the positions required, types of muscle contractions, and so on.

In the absence of such data, current strategy is to choose the instruments and techniques that maximally stress the system under a set of representative conditions that either (a) seem logical based on knowledge of the task, or (b) have been reported as appropriate and reliable for the population of interest. An attempt

TABLE 76.3 Comparison of Various Instrumented Methods Used to Measure Muscle Strength

Instrument/method	Advantages/uses	Disadvantages/limitations
Repetition maximum Amount of weight a subject can lift a given number of times and no more; one determines either a one-repetition maximum (1-RM) or a ten-repetition maximum (10-RM). A 1-RM is the maximum amount of weight a subject can lift once; a 10-RM is the amount of weight a subject can lift 10 times; a particular protocol to determine RMs is defined [DeLorme and Watkins, 1948]; measures dynamic strength in terms of weight (pounds or kilograms) lifted	Requires minimal equipment (weights); inexpensive and easy to administer; frequently used informally to assess progress in strength training	Uses serial testing of adding weights that may invalidate subsequent testing; no control for speed of contraction or positioning; minimal information available on the reliability and validity of this method
Hand-held dynamometer Device held in the examiner's hand used to test strength; devices use either hydraulics, strain gauges (load–cells), or spring systems (see Figure 76.3a); used with a "break test" (the examiner exerts a force against the body segment to be tested until the part gives way) or a "make test" (the examiner applies a constant force while the subject exerts a maximum force against it); "make tests" are frequently preferred for use with hand-held dynamometers [Smidt, 1984; Bohannon, 1990] measures force; unclear whether test measures isometric or eccentric force (this may depend on whether a "make test" or a "break test" is used)	Similar to manual muscle testing (MMT) in test positions and sites for load application; increased objectivity over MMT; portable; easy to administer; relatively inexpensive; commercially available from several suppliers; adaptable for a variety of test sites; provide immediate output; spring and hydraulic systems are nonelectrical; load–cell based systems provide more precise digital measurements	Stabilization of the device and body segment can be difficult; results can be affected by the examiner's strength; limited usefulness with large muscle groups; spring-based systems fatigue over time becoming inaccurate; range and sensitivity of the systems vary; shape of the unit grasped by the examiner and shape of the end-piece vary in comfort, and therefore the force a subject or examiner is willing to exert; more valuable for testing subjects with weakness than for less involved or healthy subjects due to range limits within the device (see discussion in Bohannon [1990])
Cable tensiometer One end of a cable is attached to an immovable object and the other end is attached to a limb segment; the tensiometer is placed between the sites of fixation; as the cable is pulled, it presses on the tensiometer's riser which is connected to a gauge (see discussion in Mayhew and Rothstein [1985]); measures isometric force	Mostly used in research settings; evidence presented on reliability when used with normal subjects [Clarke, 1952; Clarke et al., 1954]; relatively inexpensive	Requires special equipment for testing; testing is time-consuming and some tests require two examiners; unfamiliar to most clinicians; not readily available; less sensitive at low force levels
Strain gauge Electroconductive material applied to metal rings or rods; a load applied to the ring or bar deforms the metal and a gauge; deformation of the gauge changes the electrical resistance of the gauge causing a voltage variation; this change can be converted and displayed using a strip chart recorder or digital display; measures isometric force	Mostly used in research settings; increased sensitivity for testing strong and weak muscles	Strain gauges require frequent calibration and are sensitive to temperature variations; to be accurate the body part must pull or push against the gauge in the same line that the calibration weights were applied; unfamiliar to most clinicians; not commercially available; difficult to interface the device comfortably with the subject

Continued

TABLE 76.3 Continued

Instrument/method	Advantages/uses	Disadvantages/limitations
Isokinetic dynamometer Constant velocity loading device; several models marketed by a number of different companies; most consist of a movable lever arm controlled by an electronic servomotor that can be preset for selected angular velocities usually between 0 and 500° per second; when the subject attempts to accelerate beyond the pre-set machine speed, the machine resists the movement; a load cell measures the torque needed to prevent body part acceleration beyond the selected speed; computers provide digital displays and printouts (see typical device in Figure 76.3b); measures isokinetic-concentric (and in some cases, isokinetic-eccentric) and isometric strength; provides torque (or occasionally force) data; debate exists about whether data are ratio-scaled or not; accounting for the weight of the segment permits ratio-scaling [Winter et al., 1981]	Permits dynamic testing of most major body segments; especially useful for stronger movements; most devices provide good stabilization; measures reciprocal muscle contractions; widespread clinical acceptance; also records angular data, work, power, and endurance-related measures; provides a number of different reporting options; also used as exercises devices	Devices are large and expensive; need calibration with external weights or are "self-calibrating"; signal damping and "windowing" may affect data obtained; angle-specific measurements may not be accurate if a damp is used because torque readings do not relate to the goniometric measurements; joints must be aligned with the mechanical axis of the machine; inferences about muscle function in daily activities from isokinetic test results have not been validated; data obtained between different brands are not interchangeable; adequate stabilization may be difficult to achieve for some movements; may not usable with especially tall or short persons
Hand dynamometer Instruments to measure gripping or pinching strength specifically for the hand; usually use a spring scale or strain-gauge system (see typical grip strength testing device in Figure 76.3c); measures isometric force	Readily available from several suppliers; easy to use; relatively inexpensive; widespread use; some normative data available	Only useful for the hand; different brands not interchangeable; normative data only useful when reported for the same instrument and when measurements are taken with the same body position and instrument setting; must be recalibrated frequently

is made to standardize the testing in terms of contraction type, test administration instructions, feedback, warm-up, number of trials, time of day, examiner, duration of contraction (usually 4 to 6 sec), method and location of application of force, testing order, environmental distractions, subject posture and position of testing, degree of stabilization, and rest intervals between exertions (usually 30 sec to 2 min) [Chaffin, 1975; Smidt and Rogers, 1982]. In addition, the subject must be observed for muscle group substitutions and "trick" movements.

76.4 Speed of Movement

Speed of movement refers to the rate of movement of the body or body segments. The maximum movement speed that can be achieved represents another unique performance capacity of an identified system that is responsible for producing motion. Everyday living, work, and sport tasks are commonly described in terms of the speed requirements (e.g., repetitions per minute or per hour). For physical tasks, such descriptions translate to translational motion speeds (e.g., as in lifting) as well as rotational motion speeds (i.e., movement about a DOF of the joint systems involved). Thus, there is important motivation to characterize this capacity.

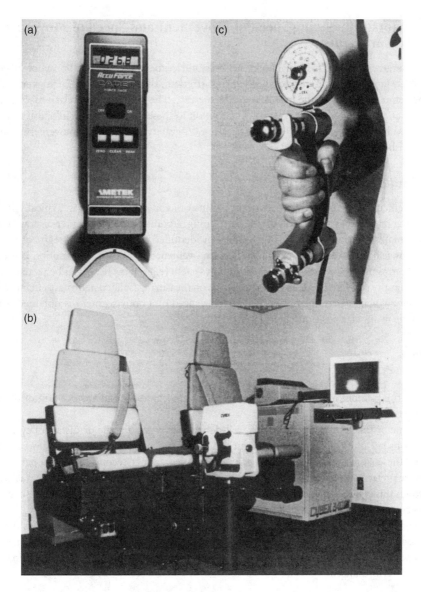

FIGURE 76.3 Three types of instrumented strength testing devices are shown (a) a representative example of a typical hand-held dynamometer; (b) an example of an isokinetic strength testing device; and (c) a hand dynamometer used to measure grip strength.

76.4.1 Speed of Movement Terminology

Speed of movement must be differentiated from *speed of contraction*. Speed of contraction refers to how fast a muscle generates tension. Two body parts may be moving through an arc with the same speed of movement; however, if one part has a greater mass, its muscles must develop more tension per unit of time to move the heavier body part at the same speed as the lighter body part.

Speed, velocity, and acceleration also can be distinguished. The terms velocity and speed are often used interchangeably; however, the two quantities are frequently not identical. Velocity means the rate of motion *in a particular direction. Acceleration* results from a change in velocity over time. General velocity and acceleration measurements are beyond the intent of this chapter. Reaction speed and response speed are other related variables also not considered.

76.4.2   Factors Influencing Speed of Movement and Speed of Movement Measurements

Muscles with larger moment arms, longer muscle fibers, and less pennation tend to be capable of generating greater speed. Many of the same factors influencing strength, discussed earlier, such as muscle length, fatigue, and temperature affect the muscle's contractile rate. The load–velocity relationship is especially important when testing speed of movement. In addition to these and other physiological factors, speed can be reduced by factors such as friction, air resistance, gravity, unnecessary movements, and inertia [Jensen and Fisher, 1979].

76.4.3   Parameters Measured

Speed of movement can be measured as a linear quantity or as an angular quantity. Typically, if the whole body is moving linearly in space as in walking or running, a point such as the center of gravity is picked, and translational motion is measured. Also, when an identified point on a body segment (e.g., the tip of the index finger) is moved in space, translational movement is observed, and motion is measured in translational terms. If the speed of a rotational motion system (e.g., elbow flexors) is being measured, then the angular quantity is determined. As the focus here is on measuring isolated neuromuscular performance capacities, the angular metric is emphasized. Angular speed of a body segment is obtained by: angular speed = change in angular position/change in time,

$$\partial = \frac{\Delta\phi}{\Delta t} \qquad (76.2)$$

Thus, speed of movement may be expressed in revolutions, degrees, or radians per unit of time, such as degrees per second (deg/sec).

Another type of speed measure applies to well-defined (over fixed angle or distance) cyclic motions. Here repetitions per unit time or cycles per unit time measures are sometimes used. However, in almost every one of these situations, speed can be expressed in degrees per second or meters per second. The latter units are preferred because they allow easier comparison of speeds across a variety of tasks. The only occasion when this is difficult is when translation motion is not in a simple straight line, such as when a person is performing a complex assembly task with multiple subtasks.

The issue of whether to express speed as maximum, averaged, or instantaneous values must also be decided, based on which measure is a more useful indicator of the performance being measured. In addition to numerical reporting of speed data, time-history graphs of speed may be helpful in comparing some types of performance.

76.4.4   Instruments Used to Measure Speed of Movement

When movement time is greater than a few seconds and the distance is known, speed can be measured with a stopwatch or with switch plates, such as the time elapsed in moving between two points or over a specified angle. With rapid angular joint movements, switch plates or electrogoniometers with electronic timing devices are required. Speeds can also be computed from the distance or angle and time data available from cinematography, optoelectric movement monitoring systems, and videotape systems. Some dynamic strength testing devices involve presetting a load and measuring the speed of movement.

In addition, accelerometers can be used to measure acceleration directly, and speed can be derived through integration. However, piezoelectric models have no steady-state response and may not be useful for slower movements. Single accelerometers are used to measure linear motion. Simple rotary motions require two accelerometers. Triaxial accelerometers are commercially available that contain three pre-mounted accelerometers perpendicular to each other. Multiple accelerometer outputs require appropriate processing to resolve the vector component corresponding to the desired speed. Accelerometers are most appropriately used to measure acceleration when they are mounted on rigid materials. Accelerometers have the advantage of continuously and directly measuring acceleration in an immediately usable form. They can also be very accurate if well-mounted. Because they require soft tissue fixation and cabling or telemetry, they may alter performance and further error may be induced by relative motion of the device and tissues. The systems are moderately expensive (see discussion of accelerometers in Robertson and Sprigings [1987]).

76.4.5 Key Concepts in Speed of Movement Measurement

As discussed, maximum speed is determined when there is little stress on torque production resources. As resistance increases, speed will decrease. Therefore, the load must be considered and specified when testing speed. Because speed of movement data are calculated from displacement and temporal data, a key issue is minimizing error that might result from collecting this information. Error can result from inaccurate identification of anatomical landmarks, improper calibration, perspective error, instrument synchronization error, resolution, digitization error, or vibration. The sampling rate of some of the measurement systems may become an issue when faster movements are being analyzed. In addition, the dynamic characteristics of signal conditioning systems should be reported.

76.5 Endurance

Endurance is the ability of a system to sustain an activity for a prolonged time (static endurance) or to perform repeatedly (dynamic endurance). Endurance can apply to the body as a whole, a particular body system, or to specific neuromuscular functional units. High levels of endurance imply that a given level of performance can be continued for a long time period.

76.5.1 Endurance Terminology

General endurance of the body as a whole is traditionally considered cardiovascular endurance, or aerobic capacity. Cardiovascular endurance is most frequently viewed in terms of $V_{O2\,max}$. This chapter considers only endurance of neuromuscular systems. Although many central and peripheral anatomic sites and physiologic processes contribute to a loss of endurance, endurance of neuromuscular functional units is also referred to as *muscular endurance*.

Absolute muscle endurance is defined as the amount of time that a neuromuscular system can continue to accomplish a specified task against a constant resistance (load and rate) without relating the resistance to the muscle's strength. Absolute muscle endurance and strength are highly correlated. Conversely, strength and *relative muscle endurance* are inversely related. That is, when resistance is adjusted to the person's strength, a weaker person tends to demonstrate more endurance than a stronger person. Furthermore, the same relationships between absolute and relative endurance and strength are correlated by type of contraction; in other words, there is a strong positive correlation between isotonic strength and *absolute* isotonic endurance and vice versa for strength and *relative* isotonic endurance. The same types of relationships exist for isometric strength and isometric endurance [Jensen and Fisher, 1979].

76.5.2 Factors Influencing Neuromuscular Endurance and Measurement of Endurance

Specific muscle fiber types, namely fast-twitch fatigue-resistant fibers (FR), generate intermediate levels of tension and are resistant to short-term fatigue (a duration of about 2 min or intermittent stimulation). Slow-twitch fibers (S) generate low levels of tension slowly, and are highly resistant to fatigue. Muscle contractions longer than 10 sec, but less than 2 min, will reflect local muscle endurance [Åstrand et al., 2003]. For durations longer than 2 min, the S fibers will be most stressed. A submaximal isometric contraction to the point of voluntary fatigue will primarily stress the FR and S fibers [Thorstensson and Karlsson, 1976]. Repetitive, submaximal, dynamic contractions continued for about 2 to 6 min will measure the capacity of FR and S fibers. Strength testing requires short duration and maximal contractions; therefore, to differentiate strength and endurance testing, the duration and intensity of the contractions must be considered.

Because strength affects endurance, all of the factors discussed previously as influencing strength, also influence endurance. In addition to muscle physiology and muscle strength, endurance is dependent upon the extensiveness of the muscle's capillary beds, the involved neuromuscular mechanisms, contraction force, load, and the rate at which the activity is performed.

Endurance time, or the time for muscles to reach fatigue, is a function of the contraction force or load [von Rohmert, 1960]. As the load (or torque required) increases, endurance time decreases. Also, as speed increases, particularly with activities involving concentric muscle contractions, endurance decreases.

76.5.3 Parameters Measured

Endurance is *how long* an activity can be performed at the required load and rate level. Thus, the basic unit of measure is time. Time is the only measure of how long it takes to complete a task. If the focus is on a given variable (e.g., strength, speed, or endurance), it is necessary to either control or measure the others. When the focus is endurance, the other factors of force or torque, speed, and joint angle, can be described as conditions under which endurance is measured. Because of the interactions of endurance and load or endurance and time (as e.g.), a number of *endurance-related* measures have evolved. These endurance-related measures have clouded endurance testing.

One endurance-related measure uses either the number of repetitions that can be performed at 20, 25, or 50% of maximum peak torque or force. The units used to reflect endurance in this case are number of repetitions at a specified torque or force level. One difficulty with this definition has been described previously, that is, the issue of relative vs. absolute muscle endurance. Rothstein and Rose [1982] demonstrated that elderly subjects with selected muscle fiber type atrophy were able to maintain 50% of their peak torque longer than young subjects. However, if a high force level is required to perform the task, then the younger subject would have more endurance in that particular activity [Rothstein, 1982]. Another difficulty is that the "repetition method" can be used only for dynamic activities. If isometric activities are involved, then the time an activity can be sustained at a specified force or torque level is measured. Why have different units of endurance? Time could be used in both cases. Furthermore, the issue of absolute vs. relative muscle endurance becomes irrelevant if the demands of the task are measured.

Yet another method used to reflect endurance is to calculate an endurance-related work ratio. Many isokinetic testing devices, such as the one shown in Figure 76.3b, will calculate work (integrate force or torque over displacement). In this case, the total amount of work performed in the first five repetitions is compared with the total amount of work performed in the last five repetitions of a series of repetitions (usually 25 or more). Work degradation *reflects* endurance and is reported as percentage. An additional limitation of using these endurance ratios is that work cannot be determined in isometric test protocols. Mechanically there is no movement, and no work is being performed.

Overall, the greatest limitation with most *endurance-related* approaches is that the measures obtained cannot be used to perform task-related assessments. In a workplace assessment, for example, one can determine how long a specific task (defined by the conditions of load, range, and speed) needs to be performed. Endurance-related metrics can be used to reflect changes over time in a subject's available endurance capacity; however, endurance-related metrics cannot be compared to the demands of the task. Task demands are measured in time or repetitions (e.g., 10 h) with a given rate (e.g., 1/0.5 h) from which total time (e.g., 5 h) can be calculated. A true endurance measure (vs. an endurance-related measure) can serve both purposes. Time reflects changes in endurance as the result of disease, disuse, training, or rehabilitation and also can be linked to task demands.

76.5.4 Methods and Instruments Used to Measure Neuromuscular Endurance

Selection of the method or instrument used to measure endurance depends on the purpose of the measurement and whether endurance or endurance-related measures will be obtained. As in strength testing, endurance tests can involve simple, low-level tasks or whole-body, higher-level activities. The simplest method of measuring endurance is to define a task in terms of performance criteria and then time the performance with a stopwatch. A subject is given a load and a posture and asked to hold it "as long as possible" or to move from one point to another point at a specific rate of movement for "as long as possible."

An example of a static endurance test is the Sorensen test used to measure endurance of the trunk extensors [Biering-Sorensen, 1984]. This test measures how long a person can sustain his or her torso in a suspended prone posture. The individual is not asked to perform a maximal voluntary contraction, but an indirect calculation of load is possible [Smidt and Blanpied, 1987].

An example of a dynamic endurance test is either a standardized or nonstandardized, dynamic isoinertial (see description in Section 76.3.1 on strength testing) repetition test. In other words, the subject is asked to lift a known load with a specified body part or parts until defined conditions can no longer be met. Conditions such as acceleration, distance, method of performance, or speed may or may not be controlled. The more standardized of these tests, particularly those that involve lifting capacity, are reported and projections about performance capacity over time are estimated [Snook, 1978]. Ergometers and some of the isokinetic dynamometers discussed earlier measure work, and several can calculate endurance-related ratios. These devices could be adapted to measure endurance in time units.

76.5.5 Key Concepts in Measuring Muscle Endurance

Of the four variables of human performance discussed in this chapter, endurance testing is the least developed and standardized. Except for test duration and rest intervals, attention to the same guidelines as described for strength testing is currently recommended.

76.6 Reliability, Validity, and Limitations in Testing

Space does not permit a complete review of these important topics. However, a few key comments are in order. First, it is important to note that reliability and validity are not inherent qualities of instruments, but exist in the measurements obtained only within the context in which they are tested. Second, reliability and validity are not either present or absent but are present or absent along a continuum. Third, traditional quantitative measures of reliability might indicate how much reliability a given measurement method demonstrates, but not how much reliability is actually needed. Fourth, technology has advanced to the extent that it is generally possible to measure physical variables such as time, force, torque, angles, and speed accurately, repeatably, and with high resolution. Finally, clinical generalizability of human performance capacity ultimately measures results from looking at the body of literature on reliability as a whole and not from single studies.

For these types of variables, results of reliability studies basically report that (1) if the instrumentation is good, and (2) if established, optimal procedures are carefully followed, then results of repeat testing will usually be in the range of about 5 to 20% of each other. This range of repeatability depends on (1) the particular variable being measured (i.e., repeated endurance measures will differ more than repeated measures of hinge joint EOM), and (2) the magnitude of the given performance capacity (i.e., errors are often in fixed amounts such as 3° for ROM; thus, 3° out of 180° is smaller percentage-wise than 3° out of 20°). One can usually determine an applicable working value (e.g., 5 or 20%) by careful review of the relevant reliability studies. Much of the difference obtained in test–retest is because of limitations in how well one can reasonably control procedures and the actual variability of the parameter being measured, even in the most ideal test subjects. Measurements should be used with these thoughts in mind. If a specific application requires extreme repeatability, then a reliability study should be conducted under conditions that most closely match those in which the need arises. Reliability discussions specific to the some of the focal measures of this chapter are presented in Amundsen [1990], Hellebrandt et al. [1949], Mayhew and Rothstein [1985], and Miller [1985].

Measurements can be reliable, but useless, without validity. Most validity studies have compared the results of one instrument to another instrument or to known quantities. This is the classical type of validity testing, which is an effort to determine whether the measurement reflects the variable being measured. In the absence of a "gold standard" this type of testing is of limited value. In addition to traditional studies of the validity of measurements, the issue of the *validity of the inferences* based on the measurements is becoming increasingly important [Rothstein and Echternach, 1993]. That is, can the measurements be used to make inferences about human performance in real-life situations? Unfortunately, measurements that have not demonstrated more than content validity are frequently used as though they are predictive. The validity of the inferences made from human performance data needs to be rigorously addressed.

Specific measurement limitations were briefly addressed in Table 76.2 and Table 76.3 and in the written descriptions of various measurement techniques and instruments. Other limitations have more to do with interpreting the data. A general limitation is that performance variables are not fixed human attributes. Another limitation is that population data are limited, and available normative data are, unfortunately, frequently extrapolated to women, older persons, and so on [Chaffin et al., 1999]. Some normative data suggest the amount of resources, such as strength, ROM, speed of movement, and endurance, *required* for given activities; other data suggest the amount *available*. As previously mentioned, these are two different issues. Performance measurements may yield information about the current status of performance, but testing rarely indicates the *cause* or the nature of dysfunction. More definitive, diagnostic studies are used to answer these questions. While, considerable information exists with regard to measuring performance capacities of human systems, much less energy has been directed to understanding requirements of tasks. The link between functional performance in tasks and laboratory-acquired measurements is a critical question and a major limitation in interpreting test data. The ERM addresses several of these limitations by using a multidimensional, individualized, cause-and-effect model.

76.7 Performance Capacity Space Representations

In both the study and practice, performance of neuromuscular systems has been characterized along one or two dimensions of performance at a time. However, human subsystems function within a *multi-dimensional* performance space. ROM/EOM, strength, movement speed, and endurance capacities are not only interdependent, but may also vary uniquely within individuals. Multiple measurements are necessary to characterize a person's performance capacity space, and performance capacity is dependent on the task to be performed. Therefore, both the individual and the task must be considered when selecting measurement tools and procedures [Chaffin et al., 1999].

In many of the disciplines in which human performance is of interest, traditional thinking has often focused on single number measures of ROM, strength, speed, and so forth. More recent systems engineering approaches [Kondraske, 2005] emphasize consideration of the performance envelope of a given system and suggest ways to integrate single measurement points that define the limits of performance of a given system [Vasta and Kondraske, 1997]. Figure 76.4 illustrates a three-dimensional performance envelope derived from torque, angle, and velocity data for the knee extensor system. The additional dimension of endurance can be represented by displaying this envelope after performing an activity for different lengths of time. A higher-level, composite performance capacity, as is sometimes needed, could be derived by computing the volume enclosed by this envelope. Such representations also facilitate assessment of the given system in a specific task; that is, a task is defined as a point in this space that will either fall inside or outside the envelope.

Åstrand P.-O., Rodahl K., Dahl H.A., and Stromme S.B. 2003. *Textbook of Work Physiology: Physiological Bases of Exercise*, 4th ed. Champaign, IL, Human Kinetics Publishers.

Biering-Sorensen F. 1984. Physical measurements as risk indicators for low back trouble over a one year period. *Spine* 9: 106–119.

Bohannon R.W. 1990. Muscle strength testing with hand-held dynamometers. In L.R. Amundsen (Ed.), *Muscle Strength Testing: Instrumented and Non-Instrumented Systems*, pp. 69–88. New York, Churchill Livingstone.

Chaffin D.B. 1975. Ergonomics guide for the assessment of human strength. *Am. Ind. Hyg. J.* 36: 505–510.

Chaffin D.B., Andersson G.B.J., and Martin B.J. 1999. *Occupational Biomechanics*, 3rd ed. New York, Wiley-Interscience.

Clarke H.H. 1954. Comparison of instruments for recording muscle strength. *Res. Q.* 25: 398–411.

Clarke H.H., Bailey T.L., and Shay C.T. 1952. New objective strength tests of muscle groups by cable-tension methods. *Res. Q.* 23: 136–148.

Clarkson H.M. 2000. *Musculoskeletal Assessment: Joint Range of Motion and Manual Muscle Strength*, 2nd ed. Philadelphia, Lippincott, Williams & Wilkins.

Delitto, A. 1990. Trunk strength testing. In L.R. Amundsen (Ed.), *Muscle Strength Testing: Instrumented and Non-Instrumented Systems*, pp. 151–162. New York, Churchill Livingstone.

DeLorme T.L. and Watkins A.L. 1948. Technics of progressive resistive exercise. *Arch. Phys. Med. Rehabil.* 29: 263–273.

Gowitzke B.A., Milner M., and O'Connel A.L., 1980. *Understanding the Scientific Bases of Human Movement*, 2nd ed. Baltimore, Williams & Wilkins.

Hellebrandt F.A., Duvall E.N., and Moore M.L. 1949. The measurement of joint motion: part III — reliability of goniometry. *Phys. Ther. Rev.* 29: 302–307.

Hislop H.J. and Montgomery J. 2002. *Daniels and Worthingham's Muscle Testing: Techniques of Manual Examination*, 7th ed. Philadelphia, WB Saunders Company.

Human Performance Measurement, Inc. 1998–2003. *APM I Portable Electronic Goniometer: User's Manual.* PO Box 1996, Arlington, TX 76004-1996.

Jensen C.R. and Fisher A.G. 1979. *Scientific Basis of Athletic Conditioning*, 2nd ed. Philadelphia, Lea & Febiger.

Kendall F.P., McCreary E.K., Provance P.G., Rodgers M., and Romani W. 2005. *Muscles: Testing and Function with Posture and Pain.* Philadelphia, Lippincott, Williams & Wilkins.

Komi P.V. 1973. Measurement of the force–velocity relationship in human muscle under concentric and eccentric contractions. In S. Cerquiglini, A. Venerando, and J. Wartenweiler (Eds.), *Biomechanics III*, pp. 224–229. Baltimore, University Park Press.

Komi P.V. 1990. Relevance of *in vivo* force measurements to human biomechanics. *J. Biomech.* 23: 23–34.

Kondraske G.V. 2005. A working model for human system–task interfaces. In J.D. Bronzino (Ed.), *Biomedical Engineering Handbook*, 3rd ed. Boca Raton, FL, CRC Press, Inc.

Kroemer K.H.E. 1983. An isoinertial technique to assess individual lifting capability. *Hum. Factors* 25: 493–506.

Kroemer K.H.E. 1991. A taxonomy of dynamic muscle exertions. *J. Hum. Muscle Perform.* 1: 1–4.

Mayhew T.P. and Rothstein J.M. 1985. Measurement of muscle performance with instruments. In J.M. Rothstein (Ed.), *Measurement in Physical Therapy*, pp 57–102. New York, Churchill Livingstone.

Miller P.J. 1985. Assessment of joint motion. In J.M. Rothstein (Ed.), *Measurement in Physical Therapy*, pp. 103–136. New York, Churchill Livingstone.

Norkin C.C. and White D.J. 2003. *Measurement of Joint Motion: A Guide to Goniometry*, 3rd ed. Philadelphia, FA Davis Company.

Palmer M.L. and Epler M.E. 1998. *Fundamentals of Musculoskeletal Assessment Techniques*, 2nd ed. Philadelphia, JB Lippincott Company.

Panjabi M.M., White III A.A., and Brand R.A. 1974. A note on defining body parts configurations. *J. Biomech.* 7: 385–387.

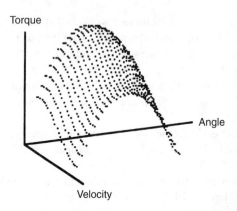

FIGURE 76.4   An example of a torque–angle–velocity performance envelope for the knee extensor system. (I Vasta P.J. and Kondraske G.V. 1994. Technical Report 94-001R p. 11. University of Texas at Arlington, Hu Performance Institute, Arlington, Texas. With permission.)

76.8   Conclusion

In conclusion, human movement is so essential that it demands interest and awe from the most ca observer to the most sophisticated scientists. The complexity of performance is truly inspiring. We challenged to understand it. We want to reduce it to comprehensible units and then enhance it, repro it, restore it, and predict it. To do so, we must be able to define and quantify the variables. Hence, an a of instruments and methods has emerged to measure various aspects of human performance. To (measurement of neuromuscular performance capacities along the dimensions of ROM/EOM, stren speed of movement, and endurance represents a giant stride but only the "tip of the iceberg." Prog in developing reliable, accurate, and valid instruments and in understanding the factors influencing measurements cannot be permitted to discourage us from the larger issues of applying the measurem toward a purpose. Yet, single measurements will not suffice; multiple measurements of different asp of performance will be necessary to fully characterize human movement.

Defining Terms

Endurance: The amount of time a body or body segments can sustain a specified static or repeti activity.

Extremes of motion (EOM):   The end ranges of motion at a joint measured in degrees.

Muscle strength: The maximal amount of torque or force production capacity that a muscle or mu groups can voluntarily exert in one maximal effort, when type of muscle contraction, movem velocity, and joint angle(s) are specified.

Neuromuscular functional units: Systems (that is, the combination of nerves, muscles, tend(ligaments, and so on) responsible for producing basic movements.

Range of motion (ROM):   The amount of movement that occurs at a joint, typically measured degrees. ROM is usually measured by noting the extremes of motion, or as the difference betw(the extreme motion and the reference position.

Speed of movement: The rate of movement of the body or body segments.

References

Amundsen L.R. 1990. *Muscle Strength Testing: Instrumented and Non-Instrumented Systems.* New Yo Churchill Livingstone.

Reese N.B. and Bandy W.D. 2002. *Joint Range of Motion and Muscle Length Testing*. Philadelphia, WB Saunders Company.

Robertson G. and Sprigings E. 1987. Kinematics. In D.A. Dainty and R.W. Norman (Eds.), *Standardizing Biomechanical Testing in Sport*, pp. 9–20. Champaign, Ill, Human Kinetics Publishers, Inc.

Robson P. 1966. A method to reduce the variable error in joint range measurement. *Ann. Phys. Med.* 8: 262–265.

Rothstein J.M. 1982. Muscle biology: clinical considerations. *Phys. Ther.* 62: 1823–1830.

Rothstein J.M. and Echternach J.L. 1993. *Primer on Measurement: An Introductory Guide to Measurement Issues*. Alexandria, VA, American Physical Therapy Association.

Rothstein J.M. and Rose S.J. 1982. Muscle mutability — part II: adaptation to drugs, metabolic factors, and aging. *Phys. Ther.* 62: 1788–1798.

Soderberg G.L. 1992. Skeletal muscle function. In D.P. Currier and R.M. Nelson (Eds.), *Dynamics of Human Biologic Tissues*, pp. 74–96. Philadelphia, FA Davis Company.

Smidt G.L. 1984. *Muscle Strength Testing: A System Based on Mechanics*. Iowa City Ia, SPARK Instruments and Academics, Inc.

Smidt G.L. and Blanpied P.R. 1987. Analysis of strength tests and resistive exercises commonly used for low-back disorders. *Spine* 12: 1025–1034.

Smidt G.L and Rogers M.R. 1982. Factors contributing to the regulation and clinical assessment of muscular strength. *Phys. Ther.* 62: 1284–1290.

Snook S.H. 1978. The design of manual handling tasks. *Ergonomics* 21: 963–985.

Sukop J. and Nelson R.C. 1974. Effects of isometric training in the force-time characteristics of muscle contractions. In R.C. Nelson, and C.A. Morehouse (Eds.), *Biomechanics IV*, pp. 440–447. Baltimore, University Park Press.

Thorstensson A. and Karlsson J. 1976. Fatiguability and fibre composition of human skeletal muscle. *Acta Physiol. Scand.* 98: 318–322.

Vasta P.J. and Kondraske G.V. 1994. A multi-dimensional performance space model for the human knee extensor, Technical Report 94-001R. University of Texas at Arlington, Human Performance Institute, Arlington, Texas.

Vasta P.J. and Kondraske G.V. 1997. An approach to estimating performance capacity envelopes: knee extensor system example. *Proceedings of the 19th Annual Engineering in Medicine and Biology Society Conference*, pp. 1713–1716.

von Rohmert W. 1960. Ermittlung von erholungspausen fur statische arbeit des menschen. *Int. Z. Angew. Physiol.* 18: 123–124.

West C.C. 1945. Measurement of joint motion. *Arch. Phys. Med.* 26: 414–425.

White III A.A. and Panjabi M.M. 1990. *Clinical Biomechanics of the Spine*, 2nd ed. Philadelphia, JB Lippincott Company.

Wiechec F.J. and Krusen F.H. 1939. A new method of joint measurement and a review of the literature. *Am. J. Surg.* 43: 659–668.

Winter D.A., Wells R.P., and Orr G.W. 1981. Errors in the use of isokinetic dynamometers. *Eur. J. Appl. Physiol.* 46: 397–408.

Further Information

Journals: *Clinical Biomechanics, Journal of Biomechanics, Medicine and Science in Sports and Exercise, Physical Therapy.*

Smith S.S. and Kondraske G.V. 1987. Computerized system for quantitative measurement of sensorimotor aspects of human performance. *Phys. Ther.* 67: 1860–1866.

Task Force on Standards for Measurement in Physical Therapy. 1991. Standards for tests and measurements in physical therapy practice. *Phys. Ther.* 71: 589–622.

77

Measurement of Sensory-Motor Control Performance Capacities: Tracking Tasks

Richard D. Jones
Christchurch Hospital

77.1 Introduction

The human nervous system is capable of simultaneous and integrated control of 100 to 150 mechanical degrees of freedom of movement in the body via tensions generated by about 700 muscles. In its widest context, movement is carried out by a sensory-motor system comprising multiple sensors (visual, auditory, proprioceptive), multiple actuators (muscles and skeletal system), and an intermediary processor which can be summarized as a multiple-input multiple-output nonlinear dynamic time-varying control system. This grand control system comprises a large number of interconnected processors and sub-controllers at various sites in the central nervous system of which the more important are the cerebral cortex, thalamus, basal ganglia, cerebellum, and spinal cord. It is capable of responding with remarkable accuracy, speed (when necessary), appropriateness, versatility, and adaptability to a wide spectrum of continuous and discrete stimuli and conditions. Certainly, by contrast, it is orders of magnitude more complex and sophisticated than the most advanced robotic systems currently available — although the latter also have what are often highly desirable attributes such as precision and repeatability and a much greater immunity from factors such as fatigue, distraction, and lack of motivation!

This chapter addresses the control function. First, it introduces several important concepts relating to **sensory-motor control**, accuracy of movement, and **performance resources**/capacities. Second, it provides an overview of apparatuses and methods for the *measurement* and *analysis* of complex sensory-motor performance. The overview focuses on measurement of sensory-motor control performance capacities of the *upper-limbs* and by means of *tracking tasks*.

77.2 Basic Principles

77.2.1 Sensory-Motor Control and Accuracy of Movement

From the perspective of Kondraske's [Kondraske, 1995a,b] *elemental resource model* of human perform-ance, sensory-motor control is the function of the overall sensory-motor control system. This system can be considered as a hierarchy of multiple interconnected sensory-motor controllers cited in the *central processing and skills ("software") domains* (cf. environmental interface domain, comprising sensors and actuators, and life sustaining domains) of the elemental resource model. These controllers range from low-level elemental level controllers for control of movement around single joints, through intermediate-level controllers needed to generate integrated movements of an entire limb and involving multiple joints and degrees of freedom, and high-level controllers and processors to enable coordinated synergistic multi-limb movements and the carrying out of *central executive* functions concerned with allocation and switching of resources for execution of multiple tasks simultaneously.

Each of these controllers is considered to possess limited *performance resources (PRs)* — or *perform-ance capacities* — necessary to carry out their control functions. PRs are characterized by dimensions of performance, which for controllers are *accuracy of movement* (including steadiness and stability) and *speed of movement*. Accuracy is the most important of these and can be divided into four major classes:

1. Spatial accuracy — Required by tasks which are *self-paced* and for which time taken is of secondary or minimal importance and includes tracing (e.g., map-tracking), walking, reaching, and, in fact, most activities of daily living. Limitation in speed PRs should have no influence on this class of accuracy.
2. Spatial accuracy with time constraints — Identical to "spatial accuracy" except that, in addition to accuracy, speed of execution of task is also of importance. Because maximal performance capacities for accuracy and speed of movement cannot, in general, be realized simultaneously, the carrying out of such tasks must necessarily involve speed-accuracy tradeoffs [Fitts, 1954; Fitts and Posner, 1967]. The extent to which accuracy is sacrificed for increased speed of execution, or vice versa, is dependent on the perceived relative importance of accuracy and speed.
3. Temporal accuracy — Required by tasks which place minimal demands on positional accuracy and includes single and multi-finger tapping and foot tapping.
4. **Spatiotemporal accuracy** — Required by tasks which place considerable demand on attainment of simultaneous spatial and temporal accuracy. This includes *paced* positional tasks such as tracking, driving a vehicle, ball games and sports, and video games. It should be stressed, however, that most of the above self-paced tasks also involve a considerable interrelationship between space and time.

Tracking tasks have become well established as being able to provide one of the most accurate and flexible means for laboratory-based measurement of spatiotemporal accuracy and, thus, of the **performance capacity** of sensory-motor control or sensory-motor coordination. In addition, they provide an unsurpassed framework for studies of the underlying control mechanisms of motor function [e.g., Lynn et al., 1979; Cooper et al., 1989; Neilson et al., 1993, 1995, 1998] — the potential for which was recognized as early as 1943 as seen in writings by Craik [1966]. They have achieved this status through their (a) ability to maximally stress the accuracy **dimension of performance** and, hence, the corresponding control PR, (b) the continuous nature and wide range of type and characteristics of input target signals they permit, (c) facility for a wide range of 1-D and 2-D *sensors* for measuring a subject's motor output, and (d) measure of continuous performance (cf. reaction time tests).

From this perspective, it will be of little surprise to find that tracking tasks are the primary thrust of this chapter.

77.2.2 The Influence of Lower-Level Performance Resources on Higher-Level Control Performance Resources

By their very nature, tasks which enable one to measure spatiotemporal accuracy are complex or higher-level sensory-motor tasks. These place demands on a large number of lower-level PRs such as visual acuity, dynamic visual perception, range of movement, strength, simple reaction times, acceleration/deacceleration, static steadiness, dynamic steadiness, prediction, memory, open-loop movements, concentration span, attention switching, that is, central executive function or supervisory attentional system (multitask abilities), utilization of preview, and learning.

It is, therefore, important to ask: If there are so many PRs involved in tracking, can tracking performance provide an accurate estimate of sensory-motor control performance capacities? Or, if differences are seen in tracking performance between subjects, do these necessarily indicate comparable differences in control performance capacities? Yes, they can, but only if the control resource is the *only* resource being maximally stressed during the **tracking task**. Confirmation that the other PRs are not also being maximally stressed for a particular subject can be ascertained by two means. First, by independently measuring the capacity of the other PRs and confirming that these are considerably greater than that determined as necessary for the tracking task in question. For example, if the speed range for a certain reference group on a nontarget speed test is 650 to 1250 mm/sec and the highest speed of a tracking target signal is 240 mm/sec, then one can be reasonably confident that intra-group differences in performance on the tracking task are unrelated to intra-group differences in speed. Second, where this process is less straightforward or not possible, it may be possible to alter the demands imposed by the task on the PR in question. For example, one could see whether visual acuity was being maximally stressed in a tracking task (and hence, be a significant limiting factor to the performance obtained) by increasing or decreasing the eye-screen distance. Similarly, one could look at strength in this context by altering the friction, damping, or inertia of the **sensor**, or at range of movement by altering the gain of the sensor.

The conclusion that a task and a PR are unrelated for a particular group does not, of course, mean that this can necessarily be extrapolated to some other group. For example, strength may be completely uncorrelated with tracking performance in normal males yet be the primary factor responsible for poor tracking performance by the paretic arm of subjects who have suffered a stroke.

The foregoing discussion is based on the concept of a assumption that if a task requires less than the absolute maximum available of a particular PR then performance on that task will be independent of that PR. Not surprisingly, the situation is unlikely to be this simplistic or clear-cut! If, for example, a tracking task places moderate sub-maximal demands on several PRs, these PRs will be stressed to varying levels such that the subject may tend to optimize the utilization of those resources [Kondraske, 1995a,b] so as to achieve an acceptable balance between accuracy, speed, stress/effort, and fatigue (physical and cognitive). Thus, although strength available is much greater than strength needed (i.e., Resource available ≫ Resource demand) for both males and females, could the differential in strength be responsible for males performing better on tracking tasks than females? [Jones et al., 1986].

77.3 Measurement of Sensory-Motor Control Performance

77.3.1 Techniques: An Overview

Tracking tasks are the primary methodological approach outlined in this chapter for measurement of sensory-motor control performance. There are, however, a large number of other approaches, each with their own set of apparatuses and methods, which can provide similar or different data on control performance. It is possible to give only a cursory mention of these other techniques in this chapter (see also Further Information).

Hand and foot test boards comprising multiple touch-plate sensors provide measures of accuracy and speed of lateral reaching-tapping abilities [Kondraske et al., 1984, 1988].

Measurement of steadiness and tremor in an upper-limb, lower-limb, or segment of either, particularly when sustended, can be made using variable size holes, accelerometers, or force transducers [Potvin et al., 1975]. A dual-axis capacitive transducer developed by Kondraske et al. [1984] provides an improved means of quantifying steadiness and tremor due to it requiring no mechanical connection to the subject (i.e., no added inertia) and by providing an output of limb position as opposed to less informative measures of acceleration or force. Interestingly, tests of steadiness can be appropriately considered as a category of tracking tasks in which the target is static. The same is also true for measurement of postural stability using force balance platforms, whether for standing [Kondraske et al., 1984; Milkowski et al., 1993] or sitting [Riedel et al., 1992] (see also Further Information).

77.3.2 Tracking Tasks: An Overview

A tracking task is a laboratory-based test apparatus characterized by a continuous input signal — the target — which a subject must attempt to match as closely as possible by his/her output response by controlling the position of (or force applied to) some sensor. It provides unequalled opportunities for wide-ranging experimental control over sensors, displays, target signals, dimensionality (degrees of freedom), control modes, controlled system dynamics, and sensor-display compatibility, as well as the application of a vast armamentarium of linear and non-linear techniques for response signal analysis and systems identification. Because of this, the tracking task has proven to be *the* most powerful and versatile tool for assessing, studying, and modelling higher-level functioning of the human "black-box" sensory-motor system.

There are three basic categories of tracking tasks differing primarily in their visual display and in the corresponding control system (Figure 77.1). The pursuit task displays both the present input and output signals, whereas the compensatory task displays only the difference or error signal between these. The preview task [Poulton, 1964; Welford, 1968; Jones and Donaldson, 1986] (Figure 77.2) is similar to the pursuit task except that the subject can see in advance where the input signal is going to be and plan accordingly to minimize the resultant error signal. Tracing tasks [Driscoll, 1975; Stern et al., 1983; Hocherman and Aharon-Peretz, 1994] are effectively self-paced 2-D preview tracking tasks.

The input-output nature of tracking tasks has made them most suitable for analysis using engineering control theories. This has led to the common view of pursuit tracking as a task involving continuous negative feedback [Notterman et al., 1982] but there is evidence that tracking viewed as a series of discrete events would be more appropriate [Bösser, 1984; Neilson et al., 1988]. The inclusion of preview of the input signal greatly complicates characterization of the human controller and Sheridan [1966] has suggested three models of preview control which employ the notions of constrained preview and nonuniform importance of input. Lynn et al. [1979] and Neilson et al. [1992] have also demonstrated how, by treating the neurologically impaired subject as a black-box, control analysis can lead to further information on underlying neurological control mechanisms.

Despite the wide-spread utilization and acceptance of tracking tasks as a powerful and versatile means for quantifying and studying sensory-motor control capacities, there is little available on the market in this area. The most obvious exception to this is the photoelectric pursuit rotor which is ubiquitous in the motor behavior laboratories of university psychology departments and has been available since the 1950s

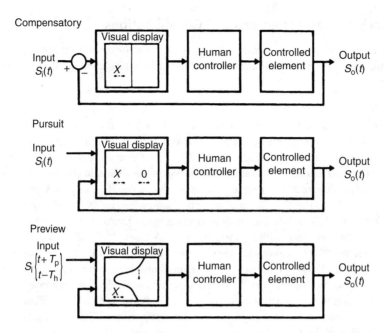

FIGURE 77.1 Modes of tracking (i) Compensatory: subject aims to keep resultant error signal X (= input signal–output signal = $s_i(t) - s_o(t)$) on stationary vertical line. (ii) Pursuit: subject aims to keep his output signal X, $s_o(t)$, on the target input signal O, $s_i(t)$. (iii) Preview: subject aims to keep his output signal X, $s_o(t)$, on the descending target input signal, $[s_i(t + T_p) - s_i(t - T_h)]$ (where t = present time, T_p = preview time, T_h = history or postview time).

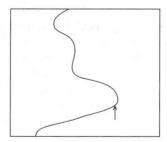

FIGURE 77.2   Visual display for random tracking with a preview of 8.0 sec and postview of 1.1 sec.

[Welford, 1968; Schmidt, 1982; Siegel, 1985]. It is a paced 2-D task with a target with the periodic on each revolution. Although inexpensive, the pursuit rotor is a crude tracking task allowing limited control over target signals and possessing a very gross performance analysis in terms of time on target. Thus nearly all of the many and varied tracking tasks which have been used in countless experimental studies around the world have been developed by the users themselves for their specific objectives.

An improvement in this situation has occurred recently with the arrival on the market of a number of tracking devices from Human Performance Measurement, Inc. (Arlington, TX). These devices are a natural extension of those developed by Kondraske et al. [1984]. Off-the-shelf availability of computer-based tracking tests, including sensors for both upper- and lower-limbs, opens up the possibility of a much broader and widespread use of tracking tasks. In particular, one can look forward to a much greater utilization of tracking tasks outside of traditional research areas and in more routine assessment applications in clinical, rehabilitative, vocational, sports, and other environments.

77.3.3 Tracking Tasks: Options and Considerations

Whatever the reasons for needing quantification of sensory-motor control capacity via a tracking task, there are a number of options available and factors to be considered in choosing or designing a tracking task.

77.3.3.1 Sensors

Sensors for measuring a subject's motor output in 1-D tracking tasks can be categorized under (a) movements involving a single degree of freedom such as flexion-extension rotation around a single joint including elbow [Lynn et al., 1977; Deuschl et al., 1996; O'Dwyer et al., 1996; Soliveri et al., 1997], wrist [Johnson et al., 1996], or a finger, or pronation-supination of the wrist, and (b) movements involving two or more degrees of freedom of a body part (e.g., hand) — that is, coordinated movement at multiple joints — which are either 1-D, such as some form of linear transducer [Patrick and Mutlusoy, 1982; Baroni et al., 1984; van den Berg et al., 1987] or 2-D, such as steering wheel [Buck, 1982; Ferslew et al., 1982; Jones and Donaldson, 1986; Jones et al., 1993], stirring wheel [De Souza et al., 1980], position stick (i.e., 1-D joystick) [Potvin et al., 1977; Neilson and Neilson, 1980; O'Dwyer and Neilson, 1998], joystick [Kondraske et al., 1984; Miall et al., 1985; Jones et al., 1993], finger-controlled rotating knob [Neilson et al., 1993], and light-pen [Neilson and Neilson, 1980]. Force sticks, utilizing strain-gauge transducers mounted on a cantilever, are also commonly used as sensors [Garvey, 1960; Potvin et al., 1977; Miller and Freund, 1980; Barr et al., 1988; Stelmach and Worrington, 1988]. Isometric integrated EMG (i.e., full-wave rectification and low-pass filtering of the raw EMG) can also be used to control the tracking response cursor, as was done by Neilson et al. [1990] to help show that impairment of sensory-motor learning is the primary cause of functional disability in cerebral palsy.

Sensors for 2-D tasks must, of course, be capable of moving with and recording two degrees of freedom. Joysticks are commonly used for this and range in size from small, for finger movement [Anderson, 1986] and wrist/forearm movement [Bloxham et al., 1984; Frith et al., 1986; Neilson et al., 1998], up to large floor-mounted joysticks for arm movements primarily involving shoulder and elbow function [Kondraske et al., 1984; Anderson, 1986; Behbehani et al., 1988; Jones et al., 1993; Dalrymple-Alford et al., 1994; Watson et al., 1997; Watson and Jones, 1998]. Other 2-D task sensors include a hand-held stylus for the photoelectric pursuit rotor [Schmidt, 1982; Siegel, 1985], plexiglass tracing [Driscoll, 1975], and tasks utilizing sonic digitizers [Stern et al., 1984; Viviani and Mounoud, 1990; Hocherman and Aharon-Peretz, 1994]. Abend et al. [1982] and Flash and Hogan [1985] used a two-joint mechanical arm to restrict hand movements to the horizontal plane in the investigation of CNS control of two-joint (shoulder and elbow) movements in trajectory formation. Stern et al. [1983] simply used the subject's finger as the sensor for a tracing task on a vertical plexiglass "screen"; a video camera behind the screen recorded finger movements. Novel "whole-body" 2-D tracking is also possible by having subjects alter their posture while standing on a dual-axis force platform [Kondraske et al., 1984].

1-D sensors can also be used in 2-D tasks by way of bimanual tracking. For example, O'Dwyer and Neilson [1995] used two 1-D joysticks to investigate dynamic synergies between the right and left arms.

77.3.3.2 Displays

Early tracking devices used mechanical-based displays such as a rotating smoked drum [Vince, 1948], the ubiquitous pursuit rotor, and a paper-strip preview task [Poulton, 1964; Welford, 1968]. An oscilloscope was, and still is to a much less degree, used in a large number of tracking tasks, initially driven by analog circuitry [Flowers, 1976; Anderson, 1986] but later by D/A outputs on digital computers [Kondraske et al., 1984; Miall et al., 1985; Sheridan, M.R. et al., 1987; Cooper et al., 1989]. Standard raster-based television screens have been used by some workers [Potvin et al., 1977; Beppu et al., 1984]. Non-raster vector graphics displays, such as Digital Equipment's VT11 dynamic graphics unit, proved valuable during the PDP-era as a means for generating more complex dynamic stimuli such as squares [Neilson and Neilson, 1980; Frith et al., 1986] and preview [Jones and Donaldson, 1986] (Figure 77.2). More recently, raster-based color graphics boards have allowed impressive static displays and simple dynamic tracking displays to be generated on PCs. However, such boards are not, in general, immediately amenable for the generation of flawless dynamic displays involving more complex stimuli, such as required for preview tracking. Jones et al. [1993] have overcome this drawback by the use of specially-written high-speed assembly-language routines for driving their display. These generate a display of the target and the subject's response marker by considering the video memory (configured in EGA mode) as four overlapping planes, each switchable (via a mask), and each capable of displaying the background color and a single color from a palette. Two planes are used to display the target, with the remaining two being used to display the subject's pointer. The current target is displayed on one target plane, while the next view of the target, in its new position, is being drawn on the other undisplayed target plane. The role of the two planes is reversed when the computer receives a vertical synchronization interrupt from the graphics controller indicating the completion of a raster. Through a combination of a high update-rate of 60.34 Hz (i.e., the vertical interrupt frequency), assembly language, and dual display buffers, it has been possible to obtain an extremely smooth dynamic color display. Their system for tracking and other quantitative sensory-motor assessments is further enhanced through its facility to generate dynamic color graphics on two high-resolution monitors simultaneously: one for the tracking display, and one for use by the assessor for task control and analysis. The monitors are driven by a ZX1000 graphic controller (Artist Graphics Inc), at 800×600, and a standard VGA controller, respectively.

In contrast to the above CRT-based displays, Warabi et al. [1986] used a laser-beam spot to indicate a subject's hand position together with a row of LEDs for displaying a step target. Similarly, Gibson et al. [1987] used a galvonometer-controlled laser spot to display smooth and step stimuli on a curved screen together with a white-light spot controlled by subject. Leist et al. [1987], Viviani and Mounoud [1990], and Klockgether [1994] also used galvonometer-controlled spots but via back-projection onto a curved screen, transparent digitizing table, and plexiglass surface respectively. Van den Berg et al. [1987] used two rows of 240 LEDs each to display target and response. 2-D arrays of LEDs have also been used to indicate step targets in 2-D tracking tasks [Abend et al., 1982; Flash and Hogan, 1985].

77.3.3.3 Target Signals

Tracking targets cover a spectrum from smoothly-changing (low-bandwidth) targets, such as sinusoidal and random, through constant velocity ramp targets, to abrupt changing step targets.

77.3.3.4 Sinusoidal Targets

The periodicity, constancy of task complexity (over cycles), and spectral purity of sine targets make them valuable for measurement of within-run changes in performance (e.g., learning, lapses in concentration) [Jones and Donaldson, 1981], the study of ability to make use of the periodicity to improve tracking performance [Jones and Donaldson, 1989], and the study of the human frequency response [Leist et al., 1987]. Several other workers have also used sine targets in their tracking tasks [Potvin et al., 1977; Miller and Freund, 1980; Ferslew et al., 1982; Notterman et al., 1982; Johnson et al., 1996; Soliveri et al., 1997].

Bloxham et al. [1984] and Frith et al. [1986] extended the use of sinewaves into a 2-D domain by having subjects track a moving circle on the screen.

77.3.3.5 Random Targets

These are commonly generated via a sum of sines approach in which a number of harmonically or non-harmonically related sinusoids of random phase are superimposed [Cassell, 1973; Neilson and Neilson, 1980; Miall et al., 1985; Baddeley et al., 1986; Frith et al., 1986; van den Berg et al., 1987; Barr et al., 1988; Cooper et al., 1989; Jones et al., 1993; Hufschmidt and Lücking, 1995; Watson et al., 1997; Watson and Jones, 1998]. If harmonically related, this can effectively give a flat spectrum target out to whatever bandwidth is required. Thus, in Jones et al.'s [Jones et al., 1993; Watson et al., 1997; Watson and Jones, 1998] system the random signal generation program asks the user for the required signal bandwidth and then calculates the number of equal amplitude harmonics that must be summed together to give this bandwidth, each harmonic being assigned a randomly selected phase from a uniform phase distribution. Each target comprises 4096 (2^{12}) or more samples, a duration of at least 68 sec (4096 samples/60.34 Hz), and a fundamental frequency of 0.0147 Hz (i.e., period of 68 sec). By this means it is possible to have several different pseudo-random target signals that are non-periodic up to 68 sec duration, have flat spectra within a user specified bandwidth, no components above this bandwidth, and whose spectra can be accurately computed by FFT from any 68 sec block of target (or response). Another common approach to the generation of random targets is to digitally filter a sequence of pseudo-random numbers [Lynn et al., 1977; Potvin et al., 1977; Kondraske et al., 1984; van den Berg et al., 1987; Neilson et al., 1993] although this method gives less control over the spectral characteristics of the target. B'sser [1984] summed a number of these filtered sequences in such a way as to generate a target having an approximate 1/f spectrum. Another smooth pursuit target was generated by linking together short segments of sinewaves with randomly selected frequencies up to some maximum [Gibson et al., 1987] and was thus effectively a hybrid sinusoidal-random target.

77.3.3.6 Ramp Targets

These have been used in conjunction with sensory gaps of target or response to study predictive tracking and ability to execute smooth constant velocity movements in the absence of immediate visual cues in normal subjects [Flowers, 1978b] and subjects with cerebellar disorders [Beppu et al., 1987], stroke [Jones et al., 1989], and Parkinson's disease [Cooke et al., 1978; Flowers, 1978a].

77.3.3.7 Step Targets

These have been used in many applications and studies to measure and investigate subjects' abilities to predict, program, and execute ballistic (open-loop) movements. To enable this, spatial and temporal unpredictability have been incorporated into step tasks in various ways:

- Temporal predictability — The time of onset of steps has ranged from (a) explicitly predictable, with preview of the stimulus [Day et al., 1984; Jones et al., 1993], (b) implicitly predictable, with fixed interval between steps [Potvin et al., 1977; Cooke et al., 1978; Flowers, 1978; Abend et al., 1982; Deuschl et al., 1996; Johnson et al., 1996], to (c) unpredictable, with intervals between steps varied randomly over spans lying somewhere between 1.5 and 7.0 sec [Angel et al., 1970; Flowers, 1976; Baroni et al., 1984; Kondraske et al., 1984; Anderson, 1986; Jones and Donaldson, 1986; Warabi et al., 1986; Gibson et al., 1987; Sheridan et al., 1987; Jones et al., 1993; Neilson et al., 1995; Watson et al., 1997; O'Dwyer and Neilson, 1998].
- Amplitude predictability — The amplitude of steps has ranged from (a) explicitly predictable, where the endpoint of the step is shown explicitly before it occurs [Abend et al., 1982; Baroni et al., 1984; Sheridan et al., 1987; Jones et al., 1993; Deuschl et al., 1996; Watson et al., 1997], (b) implicitly predictable, where all steps have the same amplitude [Angel et al., 1970; Potvin et al., 1977; Cooke et al., 1978; Day et al., 1984; Kondraske et al., 1984; Anderson, 1986; Johnson et al., 1996; O'Dwyer and Neilson, 1998] or return-to-centre steps in variable-amplitude step tasks [Flowers, 1976; Jones and Donaldson, 1986; Jones et al., 1993], to (c) unpredictable, with between 2 and 8 randomly distributed amplitudes [Flowers, 1976; Jones and Donaldson, 1986; Warabi et al., 1986; Gibson et al., 1987; Sheridan et al., 1987; Jones et al., 1993].
- Direction predictability — Previous step tasks have had steps whose direction of steps has ranged from (a) all steps explicitly predictable, alternating between right and left [Flowers, 1976; Potvin et al., 1977; Cooke et al., 1978; Baroni et al., 1984; Kondraske et al., 1984; Deuschl et al., 1996; Johnson et al., 1996; O'Dwyer and Neilson, 1998], or all in one direction (i.e., a series of discontinuous steps) [Sheridan et al., 1987], or between corners of an invisible square [Anderson, 1986], or having preview [Abend et al., 1982; Jones et al., 1993], (b) most steps predictable but with occasional "surprises" for studying anticipation [Flowers, 1978a], (c) a combination of unpredictable (outward) and predictable (back-to-center) steps [Angel et al., 1970; Jones and Donaldson, 1986; Jones et al., 1993; Watson et al., 1997], and (d) all steps unpredictable, with multiple endpoints [Warabi et al., 1986; Gibson et al., 1987] or resetting between single steps [Day et al., 1984].

TABLE 77.1 Unpredictability in Step Tracking Tasks

		Temporal			Spatial–Amplitude			Spatial–Direction			Overall Full
		Full	Partial	None	Full	Partial	None	Full	Partial	None	
Angel et al. [1970][a]	1-D	•				•		•		•	
Flowers [1976][a]	1-D	•			•	•				•	
Potvin et al. [1977]	1-D		•			•				•	
Cooke et al. [1978]	1-D		•			•				•	
Flowers [1978a]	1-D		•			•			•		
Baroni et al. [1984]	1-D	•					•			•	
Day et al. [1984]	1-D			•		•		•			
Kondraske et al. [1984]	1-D	•				•				•	
Warabi et al. [1986]	1-D	•			•			•		•	•
Jones and Donaldson [1986][a]	1-D	•			•	•		•		•	•
Gibson et al. [1987][a]	1-D	•			•			•			•
Sheridan et al. [1987][a]	1-D	•			•		•			•	
Jones et al. [1993][a]	1-D	•		•	•	•		•		•	•
Deuschl et al. [1996]	1-D		•				•			•	
Johnson et al. [1996][a]	1-D		•			•				•	
O'Dwyer and Neilson [1998]	1-D	•				•				•	
Abend et al. [1982]	2-D		•				•			•	
Anderson [1986]	2-D	•				•				•	
Watson et al. [1997]	2-D	•					•	•			

[a] Several authors have several variations of unpredictability within one task or between multiple tasks.

The three elements of unpredictability can be combined in various ways to generate tasks ranging from completely predictable to completely unpredictable (Table 77.1). Several groups have implemented several variations of unpredictability both within and between step tracking tasks to investigate the possible loss of ability to use predictability to improve performance in, for example, Parkinson's disease [Flowers, 1978; Sheridan et al., 1987; Watson et al., 1997]. In addition to unpredictability, other characteristics can be built into step tasks including explicit target zones [Sheridan et al., 1987] and visual gaps in target [Flowers, 1976; Warabi et al., 1986].

An example of a 1-D step tracking task possessing full spatial and temporal unpredictability is that of Jones and colleagues [Jones and Donaldson, 1986; Jones et al., 1993] (Figure 77.3a). The task comprises 32 abrupt steps alternating between displacement from and return to center screen. In the non-preview form, spatial unpredictability is present in the outward steps through four randomly distributed amplitude/direction movements (large and small steps requiring 90 and 22.5 deg. on a steering wheel respectively, and both to right and left of center) with temporal unpredictability achieved via four randomly distributed durations between steps (2.8, 3.4, 4.0, 4.6 sec). This task has been used, together with preview random tracking, to demonstrate deficits in sensory-motor control in the asymptomatic arm of subjects who have had a unilateral stroke [Jones et al., 1989].

Watson and Jones [1997] also provide an example of a 2-D step tracking task with spatial and temporal unpredictability. In this task the subject must move a cross from within a central starting square to within one of eight 10 mm × 10 mm target squares that appear on the screen with temporal and spatial unpredictability (Figure 77.3b). The centers of the eight surrounding targets are positioned at the vertices and midway along the perimeter of an imaginary 100 mm × 100 mm square centered on the central square. To initiate the task, the subject places the cross within the perimeter of the central target. After a 2–5 sec delay, one of the surrounding blue targets turns green and the subject moves the cross to within the green target square as quickly and as accurately as possible. After a further delay, the central target turns green indicating onset of the spatially predictive "back-to-center" target. The task, which comprises ten outward and ten return targets, was used to show that Parkinsonian subjects perform worse than

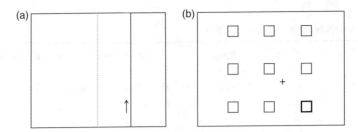

FIGURE 77.3 Visual displays for (a) 1-D step tracking task and (b) 2-D step tracking task (bottom-right square is current target).

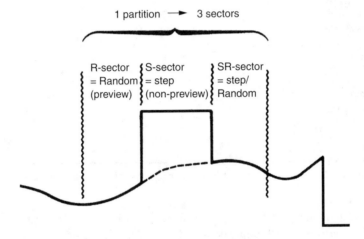

FIGURE 77.4 Section of input waveform in combination tracking in which the target alternates between preview-random and nonpreview-step.

matched controls on all measures of step tracking but are not impaired in their ability to benefit from spatial predictability to improve performance.

Step tasks with explicit target zones, in 1-D [Sheridan et al., 1987] or 2-D [Watson et al., 1997], provide the possibility of altering task difficulty by varying the size of the target. On the basis that subjects need only aim to get their marker somewhere within target zone (cf. close to center) then, according to Fitt's [1954] ratio rule, the difficulty of the primary movement is proportional to $\log_2(2A/W)$, where A is the amplitude of the movement and W is the width of the target.

77.3.3.8 Combination Targets

Jones et al. [1986, 1989, 1993] have combined two quite different modes of tracking within a single task. Combination tracking involves alternating between preview random and non-preview step tracking over 11 sec cycles (Figure 77.4). Thus, while tracking the random target, the preview signal is abruptly and unpredictably replaced by a stationary vertical line at some distance from the random signal, and vice versa. Although the steps occur with a fixed foreperiod (as with the step tasks listed above with implicit temporal predictability) of 7.3 sec, subjects are not informed of this and, irrespective, Weber's law [Fitts and Posner, 1967] indicates the accuracy of prediction of steps with such a long pre-stimulus warning is very low. Combination tracking allows the study of ability to change *motor set* [Robertson and Flowers, 1990] between quite different modes of tracking and is analogous to having to quickly and appropriately respond to an unexpected obstacle, such as a child running onto the road, while driving a vehicle.

77.3.3.9 Dimensionality

The number of dimensions of a tracking task usually refers to the number of cartesian coordinates over which the *target* moves, rather than those of the response marker or sensor handle, or the number of degrees of freedom of the target or of the upper-limb. Some examples (1) Most tasks with a 2-D joystick sensor or light-pen are 2-D but, if the target moves in the vertical direction only [Neilson and Neilson, 1980; Kondraske et al., 1984; Miall et al., 1985; Jones et al., 1993], the task is only considered 1-D, irrespective of whether the response marker is confined to vertical movements on the screen or not; (2) If the target trajectory is a circle [Bloxham et al., 1984], the task is 2-D despite the target having only one degree of freedom (i.e., radius r is constant); (3) A pursuit rotor is a 2-D task as it has a target which moves in two dimensions (whether cartesian or polar) as well as doing so with two degrees of freedom.

Watson and Jones [1998] compared random 2-D with 1-D performance but in doing so scaled their 2-D target down so as to have an average displacement and velocity equal to that of its 1-D horizontal and vertical components. By this means they were able to unequivocally demonstrate that there is poorer performance on 2-D tasks and that is due to both the increased dimensionality and increased position/speed demands of an unscaled 2-D task.

Dual-axis tracking is a variant of 2-D tracking in which the 2-D task comprises two simultaneous orthogonal 1-D tasks in which one or more of the target, input device, control dynamics, and on-line feedback are different between the two axes. It has been used to investigate mechanisms and characteristics of 2-D tracking, such as whether it is a single task or two separate orthogonal tasks [Navon et al., 1984; Fracker and Wickens, 1989].

77.3.3.10 Tracking Mode

The two primary modes of tracking — compensatory and pursuit — have been introduced above. The majority of tasks are of the pursuit type which is appropriate in that has a more direct parallel with real-world sensory-motor tasks than the more artificial compensatory task [Vince, 1948; Garvey, 1960; Potvin et al., 1977; Miller and Freund, 1980; B'sser, 1984; Barr et al., 1988] in which the subject is only shown the instantaneous value of the error signal. The compensatory mode may be preferentially chosen for control-theory modelling due to its simpler set of defining equations [Potvin et al., 1977]. The preview task [Welford, 1968; Jones and Donaldson, 1986] is an important variation of pursuit tracking in which a still greater correspondence with everyday tasks is achieved.

77.3.3.11 Controlled System Dynamics

It has been well established that subjects can deal satisfactorily with a variety of tracking systems incorporating different control characteristics [Poulton, 1974; Neilson et al., 1995]. That notwithstanding, the majority of tracking tasks have a zero-order controlled system in which the position of the response marker is proportional to the position of the sensor and the mechanical characteristics of friction, inertial mass, and velocity damping are simply those of the input device. Van den Berg et al. [1987] eliminated even these by feeding back a force signal from a strain gauge on the tracking handle to the power amplifier of a torque motor connected to their sensor. Conversely, Neilson et al. [1993] artificially introduced mechanical characteristics into the movement of their response marker by having a linear 2nd-order filter as the controlled system; by an appropriate transfer function ($H(z) = 0.4060/(1 - 1.0616z^{-1} + 0.4610z^{-2})$), they were able to introduce inertial lag and underdamping (resonant peak at 2.0 Hz). Miall et al. [1985] introduced an analog delay of 500 msec between their joystick and display so that they could study the effect of delayed visual feedback on performance. Soliveri et al. [1997] used both 1st-order (velocity) and zero-order (position) linear control dynamics to investigate differences in learning between parkinsonian and control subjects and between on- and off-medication. Navon et al. [1984] used a combination of velocity and acceleration control dynamics in their study on dual-axis tracking. Nonlinear transfer functions, such as 2nd-order Volterra (fading memory) nonlinearities, have also been used in tracking controlled systems, primarily as a means for investigating adaptive inverse modelling mechanisms in the brain relating to voluntary movement [Sriharan, 1997; Davidson et al., 1999].

Controlled system dynamics can also be changed during a task. In "critical tracking," a novel variation of pursuit tracking conceived by Jex [1966], the delay of the controlled system increases during the task. There is no external target but instead the subject's own instability acts as an input to an increasingly unstable controlled system, $Y(s) = K8/(s-8)$, in which the level of instability, represented by the root $8(=1/T)$, is steadily increased during the task until a preset error is exceeded. The task has been described as analogous to driving a truck with no brakes down a hill on a winding road [Potvin et al., 1977]. The task has been applied clinically by Potvin et al. [1977] and Kondraske et al. [1984] and shown to be a reliable measure of small changes in neurological function [Potvin et al., 1977]. Alternatively, "gain-change step tracking" [Neilson et al., 1995], in which the gain of the control-display relation is increased or decreased without warning, has been used to investigate adaptive mechanisms in the brain [O'Dwyer and Neilson, 1998].

Having a torque motor as part of the sensor opens up several new possibilities. It can be operated as a "torque servo," in which applied torque is independent of position [Kondraske et al., 1984], or a "position servo," in which applied torque is proportional to position error (together with velocity damping if desired) [Thomas et al., 1976]. By adding external force perturbations, it is possible to measure and study neuromuscular reflexes and limb transfer function (i.e., stiffness, viscosity, and inertia), such as by applying constant velocity movements [Kondraske et al., 1984] or pulsatile [van den Berg et al., 1987], sinusoidal [Gottlieb et al., 1984], or random [Kearney and Hunter, 1983; van den Berg et al., 1987] force perturbations. Alternatively, the torque motor can be used to alter controlled system characteristics in tracking tasks for studies and/or improvement of voluntary movement. For example, van den Berg et al. [1987] cancelled unwanted controller characteristics. Chelette et al. [1995] used "force reflection" to improve tracking performance in both normal subjects and those with spasticity, and Johnson et al. [1996] used anti-viscous loading to investigate the cause of poor tracking in patients with Parkinson's disease.

77.3.3.12 Sensor-Display Compatibility

It is generally accepted that the level of compatibility between sensor and display in continuous tracking tasks influences the accuracy of performance [Neilson and Neilson, 1980]. The perfectly compatible sensor is the display marker itself [Poulton, 1974] where the subject holds and moves the response marker directly such as with a light-pen in tracking [Neilson and Neilson, 1980], rotary pursuit [Schmidt, 1982; Welford, 1968], handle on a two-joint mechanical arm [Abend et al., 1982], or in self-paced 2-D tracing tasks [Driscoll, 1975; Stern et al., 1984; Hocherman and Aharon-Peretz, 1994]. Similarly, van den Berg et al. [1987] achieve a high sensor-display compatibility by having the LED arrays for target and response displayed directly above a horizontally-moving handle. However, the majority of tracking tasks have sensors which are quite separate from the response marker displayed on an oscilloscope or computer screen. Sensor-display compatibility can be maximized in this case by having the sensor physically close to the display, moving in the same direction as the marker, and with a minimum of controlled system dynamics (e.g., zero-order). In the case of a joystick in a 2-D task, for example, direct compatibility (*Left–Right → Left–Right*) is easier than inverse compatibility (*Left–Right → Right–Left*), which is easier than non-compatibility (*Left–Right → Up–Down*). In contrast, fore-aft movements on a joystick appear to possess bidirectional compatibility in that *Fore–aft → Up–Down* seems as inherently natural as *Fore–aft → Down–Up* (i.e., no obvious inverse).

Sensor-display compatibility may not, however, be overly critical to performance. For example, Neilson and Neilson [1980] found no decrement in performance on random tracking of overall error scores, such as mean absolute error, between a light pen and a 1-D joystick; nevertheless, the latter did result in a decrease in gain, an increase in phase lag, and an increase in the non-coherent response component. Conversely, normal subjects find incompatible 2-D tracking very difficult to perform, taking up to 4 h of practice to reach a level of performance equal to that seen on prepractice 2-D compatible tracking [Neilson et al., 1998].

77.3.3.13   Response Sampling Rates

Although some workers have manually analyzed tracking data from multichannel analog chart recordings [Flowers, 1976; Beppu et al., 1984] or analog processed results [Potvin et al., 1977], the majority have used computers, sometimes via a magnetic tape intermediary [Day et al., 1984; Miall et al., 1985], to digitize data for automated analyses. Sampling rates used have varied from 10 Hz [Neilson and Neilson, 1980], through 20 Hz [Cooper et al., 1989; Neilson et al., 1993; Neilson et al., 1998], 28.6 Hz [Jones and Donaldson, 1986], 30.2 Hz [Watson et al., 1997; Watson and Jones, 1998], 40 Hz [Frith et al., 1986], 60 Hz [Viviani and Mounoud, 1990], 60.3 Hz (= screen's vertical interrupt rate) [Jones et al., 1993], 66.7 Hz [O'Dwyer and Neilson, 1998], 100 Hz (all 2-D tasks) [Abend et al., 1982; Stern et al., 1984; Hocherman and Aharon-Peretz, 1994], to as high as 250 Hz [Day et al., 1984].

For the most part, a relatively low sampling rate is quite satisfactory for analysis of tracking performance as long as the Nyquist criterion is met and there is appropriate analog or digital low-pass filtering to prevent aliasing. Spectral analysis indicates that the fastest of voluntary arm movements have no power above about 8.7 Hz [Jones and Donaldson, 1986]. This is very similar to the maximal voluntary oscillations of the elbow of 4-6 Hz [Neilson, 1972; Leist et al., 1987] and to maximum finger tapping rates of 6-7 Hz [Muir et al., 1995]. The sampling rate can be reduced still further if the primary interest is only in *coherent* performance, whose bandwidth is only of the order of 2 Hz for both kinesthetic stimuli [Neilson, 1972] and visual stimuli [Leist et al., 1987; Neilson et al., 1993]; that is, performance above 2 Hz must be open-loop and, hence, learned and preprogrammed [Neilson, 1972]. Thus, from an information theory point of view, there is no need to sample tracking performance beyond, say, 20 Hz. However, a higher rate may well be justified on the grounds of needing better temporal resolution than 50 ms for transient or cross-correlation analysis, unless one is prepared to regenerate the signal between samples by some form of non-linear interpolation (e.g., sinc, spline, polynomial).

77.3.3.14   Other Measures

Several researchers have further extended the information which can be derived from upper-limb tracking performance by comparison with other simultaneously recorded biosignals. The most common of these is the EMG, particularly integrated EMG due to its close parallel to force of contraction [Neilson, 1972] and where the tracking movement is constrained to be around a single joint. The EMG has been used together with step tracking for fractionating reaction times into premotor and motor components [Anson, 1987; Sheridan et al., 1987] and confirmation of open-loop primary movements [Sittig et al., 1985; Sheridan et al., 1987]. In smooth tracking, correlation/cross-spectral analysis between the EMG and limb position has been used to study limb dynamics [Neilson, 1972; Barr et al., 1988].

In contrast, Cooper et al. [1989] measured the EEG at four sites during 2-D random tracking to show that slow changes in the EEG (equivalent to the Bereitschaftspotential preceding self-paced voluntary movement), particularly at the vertex, are correlated with the absolute velocity of the target.

Simultaneous measurement of hand and eye movements has been carried out by Warabi et al. [1986] and Leist et al. [1987] using EOG to measure horizontal eye movements and by Gibson et al. [1987] who used an infra-red limbus reflection technique. Interestingly, Leist et al. [1987] found that ocular pursuit and self-paced oscillations were limited to about 1 and 2.2 Hz, respectively, whereas the equivalent values for arm movements are 2 and 4-6 Hz, respectively.

77.3.3.15   Standard Assessment Procedures

Having designed and constructed a tracking task or set of tracking tasks with the characteristics necessary to allow measurement of the sensory-motor control performance capacities under investigation, it is essential that this process be complemented by a well formulated set of standard assessment procedures. These must include (a) standard physical setup, in which positioning of subject, sensor, and screen are tightly specified and controlled, as well as factors such as screen brightness, room lighting, etc., and (b) standardized instructions. The latter are particularly important in tasks where speed-accuracy tradeoff [Fitts, 1954; Welford, 1968; Agarwal and Logsdon, 1990] is possible. This applies particularly to step tracking in which leaving the tracking strategy completely up to subjects introduces the possibility of misinterpretation of differences in performance on certain measures, such as reaction time, risetime, and mean absolute error. For example, subjects need to know if it is more important to have the initial movement end up close to the target (i.e., emphasis on accuracy of primary movement) or to get within the vicinity of the target as soon as possible (i.e., emphasis on speed of primary movement); the latter results in greater under/overshooting but also tends to result in lower mean errors). The most common approach taken is to stress the importance of both speed and accuracy with an instruction to subjects of the form: "Follow the target as fast and as accurately as possible."

77.3.3.16   Test and Experimental Protocols

The design of appropriate test and experimental protocols is also a crucial component of the tracking task design process [Roscoe, 1975; Pitrella and Kruger, 1983]. When comparisons are made between different subjects, tasks, and/or conditions, careful consideration needs to be given to the paramount factors of *matching* and *balancing* to minimize the possibility of significant differences being due to some bias or confounding variable other than that under investigation. Matching can be achieved between experimental and control subjects in an inter-subject design by having average or one-to-one equivalence on age, gender, education, etc., or through an intra-subject design in which the subject acts as his/her own control in, say, a study of dominant versus non-dominant arm performance. Balancing is primarily needed to offset *order effects* due to learning which pervade much of sensory-motor performance [Welford, 1968; Poulton, 1974; Schmidt, 1982; Frith et al., 1986; Jones et al., 1990]. A study by Jones and Donaldson [1989] provides a good example of the application of these principles. Their study, aimed at investigating the effect of Parkinson's disease on predictive motor planning, involved 16 Parkinsonian subjects and 16 age and sex matched control subjects. These were then divided into 8 subgroups in a 3-way randomized cross-over design so as to eliminate between- and within-session order effects in determining the effect of target type, target preview, and medication on tracking performance.

77.4   Analysis of Sensory-Motor Control Performance

77.4.1   Accuracy

Analyses of raw tracking data can provide performance information which is objective and quantitative and which can be divided into two broad classes:

Measures of Global Accuracy of Performance: Measures of global (or overall or integrated) sensory-motor control capacities have proven invaluable for:

- *Vocational screening* of minimum levels of sensory-motor skills: Tracking tasks, in fact, have their origins in this area during World War II when they were used to help screen and train aircraft pilots [Welford, 1968; Poulton, 1974].
- *Clinical screening* for sensory-motor deficits (arising from one or more lesions in one or more sites in the sensory-motor system): An excellent example of the application of this in clinical practice is the provision of objective measures in off-road driving assessment programs [Jones et al., 1983; Croft and Jones, 1987].
- *Clinical and rehabilitation research* by measurement of longitudinal changes in sensory-motor function: There are many examples of subjects being assessed repeatedly on tracking tasks for periods up to 12 or more months. This has been done to quantify recovery following head injury [Jones and Donaldson, 1981] and stroke [Lynn et al., 1977; De Souza et al., 1980; Jones and Donaldson, 1981; Jones et al., 1990] as well as for studies of learning in tracking performance [Poulton, 1974; Jones and Donaldson, 1981; Schmidt, 1982; Frith et al., 1986; Jones et al., 1990]. They can also be used to quantify changes due to medication, such as in Parkinson's disease [Baroni et al., 1984; Johnson et al., 1996; Jones et al., 1996; Soliveri et al., 1997].

Measures of Characteristics of Performance: Measures of global accuracy of tracking performance can detect and quantify the presence of abnormal sensory-motor control performance capacities with considerable sensitivity [Potvin et al., 1977; Jones et al., 1989]. Conversely, they are unable to give any indication of which of the many subsystems or performance resources in the overall sensory-motor system are, or may be, responsible for the abnormal performance. Nor can they provide any particular insight into the underlying neuromuscular control mechanisms of normal or abnormal performance.

Four approaches can be taken to provide information necessary to help identify the sensory-motor subsystems and their properties responsible for the *characteristics* of observed normal and abnormal performance:

- Batteries of neurologic sensory-motor tests — These tests can be used to, at least ideally, isolate and quantify the various sensory, motor, cognitive, and integrative functions and subsystems involved in sensory-motor control performance as measured globally by, for example, tracking tasks.
- Functional decomposition — Fractionation of the various performance resources contributing to tracking performance.
- Traditional signal processing approaches — Time domain (ballistic and nonballistic) and frequency domain techniques.
- Graphical analysis — This has primarily been developed for measurement and investigation of changes in performance and underlying PRs over time.

77.4.2 Measures of Global Accuracy of Performance

The most commonly used measure of global or overall accuracy is the *mean absolute error* (MAE) [Jones and Donaldson, 1986] which indicates the average distance the subject was away from the target irrespective of side; it is also variously called average absolute error [Poulton, 1974], modulus mean error [Poulton, 1974], mean rectified error [Neilson and Neilson, 1980], or simply tracking error [Kondraske et al., 1984; Behbehani et al., 1988]. In contrast, the mean error, or constant position error, is of little value as it simply indicates only the extent to which the response is more on one side of the target than the other [Poulton, 1974]. Measures of overall performance which give greater weighting to larger errors include mean square error [Neilson et al., 1993], root mean square error [McRuer and Krendel, 1959; Poulton, 1974; Navon et al., 1984; O'Dwyer and Neilson, 1995], variance of error [Neilson and Neilson, 1980], and standard deviation of error [Poulton, 1974]. Relative or normalized error score equivalents of these can be calculated by expressing the raw error scores as a percentage of the respective scores obtained had subject simply held the response marker stationary at the mean target position [Poulton, 1974; Neilson and Neilson, 1980; Day et al., 1984]; that is, noresponse = 100%. Alternatively, the relative root mean square error, defined as the square root of the ratio of the mean square value of the error signal to the mean square value of the target signal expressed as a percentage, allows tracking errors to be compared across tests using different target signals [Neilson et al., 1998].

Overall coherence is an important alternative to the above measures when it is wished to assess the similarity between target and response waveforms but there is a substantial delay between them. It provides an estimate of the proportion of the response that is correlated with the target over all frequencies [O'Dwyer and Neilson, 1995; O'Dwyer et al., 1996].

An issue met in viewing error scores from the perspective of Kondraske's [Kondraske, 1995a,b] elemental resource model is the unifying requirement of its associated *general systems performance theory (GSPT)* that all dimensions of performance must be in a form for which a higher numerical value indicates a superior performance. Thus scores which state that a *smaller* score indicates a superior performance, including reaction times, movement times, and all error scores, need to be transformed into *performance scores* [Kondraske, 1988]. For example:

- *Central response speed = 1/(reaction time)*
- *Information processing speed = 1/(8-choice reaction time)*
- *Movement speed = 1/(movement time)*
- *Tracking accuracy = 1/(tracking error)*

As transformation via inversion is non-linear, the distributions of raw error scores and derived performance will be quite different. This has no effect on ordinal analyses, such as non-parametric statistics, but will have some effect on linear analyses, such as parametric statistics, linear regression/correlation, etc., and may include improvements due to a possible greater normality of the distributions of derived performances. An alternative transformation which would retain a linear relationship with the error scores is:

Tracking accuracy = 100 − *Relative tracking error*. However, while this gives a dimension of performance with the desired 'bigger is better' characteristic, it also raises the possibility of negative values, implying an accuracy worse than zero! — the author can attest to the fact that some subjects do indeed end up with error scores worse than the "hands off" score. Irrespective of GSPT, there is no doubt that it is beneficial to deal conceptually and analytically with multiple performance measures when *all* measures are consistently defined in terms of "bigger is better."

Time on target is a much cruder measure of tracking performance than all of the above but it has been used reasonably widely due to it being the result obtained from the pursuit rotor. The crudeness generally reflects (a) a lack of spatiotemporal sampling during a task (i.e., simple integration of time on target only) preventing the possibility of further analysis of any form, and (b) a task's performance *ceiling* due to the target having a finite zone within which greater accuracy, relative to center of zone, is unrewarded. This latter factor can, however, be used to advantage for the case where the investigator wishes to have control over the *difficulty* of a task, to gain, for example, similar levels of task difficulty across subjects irrespective of individual ability. This attribute has been used very effectively with 2-D random tracking tasks to minimize the confounding effects of major differences in task load between experimental and control subjects in dual task studies of impairment of central executive function in subjects with Alzheimer's disease [Baddeley et al., 1986] and Parkinson's disease [Dalrymple-Alford et al., 1994].

77.4.3 Measures of Characteristics of Performance

77.4.3.1 Batteries of Neurologic Sensory-Motor Tests

Potvin and associates [Potvin and Tourtellotte, 1975; Potvin et al., 1985], now led by Kondraske et al. [1984, 1988], have developed what is by far the most comprehensive battery of tests available for quantitative evaluation of neurologic function covering a number of sensory, motor, cognitive, and sensory-motor functions or performance resources. Similarly, Jones et al. [1989, 1993] have developed a battery of *component* function tests, most of which have been specifically designed to isolate and quantify the various performance resources involved in their tracking tasks. There is, therefore, a close resemblance between the component and tracking tests so as to maximize the validity of comparisons made between them.

77.4.3.2 Functional Decomposition of Tracking Performance

There are three main approaches whereby tracking performance can be fractionated or decomposed into its functional components: sensory, perceptual, cognitive, motor planning, and motor execution.

The first involves breaking the ballistic response in step tracking into reaction time, movement time, overshoot, and settling time [Flowers, 1976; Evarts et al., 1981; Jones and Donaldson, 1986; Behbehani et al., 1988; Kondraske et al., 1988] (see "Time domain (ballistic) analysis" below). This allows indirect deductions about cognitive, motor planning, and motor execution functions, although the distinction between cognitive and motor elements often remains imprecise.

The second involves calculation of differentials in tracking performance from inter-trial alterations in target and/or controlled system dynamics. This has been successfully used to study predictive motor planning [Flowers, 1976; Flowers, 1978; Bloxham et al., 1984; Day et al., 1984; Jones and Donaldson, 1989], acquisition/modification of motor sets [Frith et al., 1986], and reliance on visual feedback [Flowers, 1976; Cooke et al., 1978; Frith et al., 1986] in Parkinson's disease.

The third approach allows a more direct identification of the contribution of certain elemental resources to tracking performance during a specific tracking run. For example, by introducing the concept of a visuoperceptual buffer-zone, it is possible to estimate the contribution of visuoperceptual function to tracking performance [Jones et al., 1996]. This technique has been used to demonstrate that impaired visuoperceptual function in Parkinsonian subjects plays only a minor role in their poor tracking perform-ance [Jones et al., 1996] but, conversely, that impaired tracking performance in stutterers is predominantly due to reduced dynamic visuospatial perception [A.J. White, R.D. Jones, K.H.C. Lawson, and T.J. Ander-son, unpublished observations]. Furthermore, the visuoperceptual function can itself be fractionated into visual acuity, static perception, and dynamic perception [Jones and Donaldson, 1995].

In contrast to fractionation of performance on a high level task (e.g., tracking, driving), Kondraske et al. [1995a,b] have developed techniques for the reverse process. They have shown how their hierarchical elemental resource model can be used to *predict* performance on high level tasks from performance on a number of lower level tasks [Kondraske, 1987; Vasta and Kondraske, 1994; Kondraske, 1995b; Kondraske et al., 1997]. This approach has considerable potential in application areas such as rehabilitation. For example, it could be used in driving assessment programs to predict on-road driving ability by off-road measurement of performance on several key lower level tasks pertinent to driving, such as reaction time, visuospatial, cognitive, and tracking.

77.4.3.3   Time Domain (Non-Ballistic) Analysis of Tracking Performance

There are several run-averaged biases which can indicate the general form of errors being made, particu-larly when the tracking performance is subnormal. Positive *side of target* (%) and *direction of target* (%) biases reflect a greater proportion of errors occurring to the right of the target or while the target is moving to the right respectively [Jones and Donaldson, 1986] which, if substantial, may indicate the presence of some visuoperceptual deficit. Similarly, the *side of screen* bias (assuming mean target pos-ition is mid-screen) [Jones and Donaldson, 1986] is identical to the mean error or constant position error.

Perhaps the single most important measure of performance, other than mean absolute error, for non-transient targets is that of the average time delay, or *lag*, of a subject's response with respect to the target signal. The lag is most commonly defined as being the shift, τ, corresponding to the peak of the cross-correlation function, calculated directly in the time domain or indirectly via the inverse of the cross-spectrum in the frequency domain. Although simulation studies indicate that these techniques are at least as accurate and as robust to noise/remnants as the alternatives listed below [Watson, 1994], one needs to be aware of a bias leading to underestimation of the magnitude of the lag (or lead) due to distortion of the standard cross-correlation function, but specifically of the peak towards zero shift. The distortion arises due to the varying overlap of two truncated signals (i.e., the target and the response) resulting in the multiplication of the cross-correlation function by a triangle (maximum at $\tau = 0$ and zero at $\tau = NT_S$, assuming signals of equal length NT_S). This effect is minimal as long as both signals have a mean value of zero (i.e., zero d.c.). Temporal resolution is another factor deserving consideration. If desired, greater resolution than that of the sampling period can be obtained by interpolation of the points around the peak of the cross-correlation function by some form of curve fitting (e.g., parabola [Jones et al., 1993]).

An alternative estimate of the lag, which has proven accurate on simulated responses, can be gained from the *least squares time delay estimation* by finding the time shift between the response and target at which the mean square error is minimized [Fertner and Sjölund, 1986; Jones et al., 1993]. Another approach, *phase shift time delay* estimation, calculates lag from the gradient of the straight line providing a best least-squares to the phase points in the cross-spectrum [Watson et al., 1997]. This technique has, however, proven more sensitive to non-correlated remnants in the response than the other procedures [Watson, 1994].

Several measures used to help characterize within-run variability in performance include variance of error [Neilson and Neilson, 1980], standard deviation of error [Poulton, 1974], and inconsistency [Jones and Donaldson, 1986].

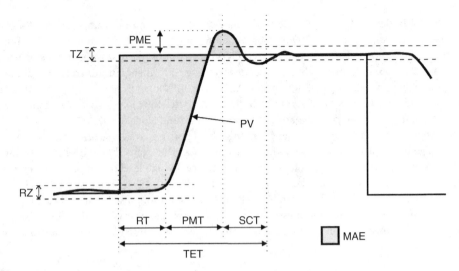

FIGURE 77.5 Transient response analysis. Tolerance zones: RZ is the reaction zone, and TZ is the target zone. Performance parameters: RT is the reaction time, PMT is the primary movement time, SCT is the secondary correction time, TET is the target entry time, PV is the peak velocity, PME is the primary movement error, and MAE is the mean absolute error over a fixed interval following stimulus.

77.4.3.4 Time Domain (Ballistic) Analysis of Tracking Performance

Whether or not any of the above nonballistic analyses, evaluation of step tracking performance usually involves separate ballistic or transient analysis of each of the step responses. This generally takes the form of breaking up each response into three phases (Figure 77.5) (1) reaction time phase, or the time between onset of step stimulus and initiation of movement defined by exit from a visible or invisible reaction zone, (2) primary movement phase, or the open-loop ballistic movement made by most normal subjects aiming to get within the vicinity of the target as quickly as possible, the end of which is defined as the first stationary point, and (3) secondary correction phase, comprising one or more adjustments and the remaining time needed to enter and stay within target zone. The step measures from individual steps can then be grouped into various step categories to allow evaluation of the effect of step size, spatial predictability, arm dominance, etc., on transient performance.

Accuracy of the primary aimed movement can also be characterized in terms of a constant error and a variable error (standard deviation of error), which are considered to be indices of accuracy of central motor programming and motor execution respectively [Guiard et al., 1983].

Phase-plane (velocity vs. position) plots provide an alternative means for displaying and examining the qualitative characteristics of step tracking responses. In particular, they have proven valuable for rapid detection of gross abnormalities [Potvin et al., 1985]. Behbehani et al. [1988] have introduced a novel quantitative element to phase-plane analysis by deriving an index of coordination: $I_C = V_m^2/A$, where V_m is the maximum velocity during an outward and return step and A is the area within the resultant loop on the phase-plane plot.

77.4.3.5 Frequency Domain Analysis of Tracking Performance

Cross-correlation and spectral analysis have proven invaluable tools for quantifying the frequency dependent characteristics of the human subject. The cross-spectral density function, or cross-spectrum $S_{xy}(f)$, can be obtained from the random target $x(t)$ and random response $y(t)$ by taking the Fourier transform of the cross-correlation function $r_{xy}(\tau)$, that is, $S_{xy}(f) = F\{r_{xy}(\tau)\}$, or in the frequency domain via $S_{xy}(f) = X(f)Y(f)^*$, or by a nonparametric system identification approach (e.g., "spa.m" in MATLAB®). The cross-spectrum provides estimates of the relative amplitude (i.e., gain) and phase-lag at each frequency. Gain, phase, and remnant frequency response curves provide objective measures of pursuit tracking behavior, irrespective of linearity, and are considered a most appropriate "quasi-linear" tool for obtaining a quantitative assessment of pursuit tracking behaviour [Neilson and Neilson, 1980]. From the cross-spectrum one can also derive the *coherence function* which gives the proportion of the response signal linearly related to the target at each frequency: $(xy^2 =^* S_{xy}(f)^*2/S_x(f)S_y(f)$. Lynn et al. [1977] emphasize, however, that one must be cognizant of the difficulty representing tracking performance by a quasi-linear time-invariant transfer function, especially if the run is of short duration or if the target waveform is of limited bandwidth, as the results can be so statistically unreliable as to make description by a 2nd- or 3rd-order transfer function quite unrealistic. Van den Berg et al. [1987] chose four parameters to characterize tracking performance: low-frequency performance via the mean gain of transfer function at the 3 lowest of 8 frequencies in target signal, high-frequency performance via the frequency at which the gain has dropped to less than 0.4, mean delay via shift of peak of cross-correlation function, and remnant via power in frequencies introduced by subject relative to total power. Spectral and coherence analysis have been used to demonstrate that the human bandwidth is about 2 Hz for both kinaesthetic tracking [Neilson, 1972] and visual tracking [Neilson et al., 1993], a much greater relative amplitude of second harmonic in the response of cerebellar subjects in sine tracking [Miller and Freund, 1980], a near constant lag except at low frequencies in normal subjects [Cassell, 1973], adaptation to time-varying signals [Bösser, 1984], 2-D asymmetry in postural steadiness [Milkowski et al., 1993], and that normal subjects can form non-dynamic and dynamic inter-limb synergies in a bimanual tracking task [O'Dwyer and Neilson, 1995].

77.4.3.6 Graphical Analysis of Tracking Performance

Most of the of the above analyses give quantitative estimates of some aspect of performance which is effectively assumed to be constant over time, other than for random fluctuations. This is frequently not the case, especially for more complex sensory-motor tasks such as tracking. Changes in performance over time can be divided into two major classes: class I: those for which the underlying PRs remain unchanged (these are due to factors such as practice, fatigue, lapses in concentration, lack of practice, and changes in task complexity) and class II: those for which one or more underlying PRs have changed (these are due to abrupt or gradual alterations at one or more sites in the sensory-motor system and include normal changes, such as due to age, and abnormal changes, due to trauma or pathology).

Studies of class I factors using tracking tasks are complicated most by the intra-run *difficulty* of a task not being constant. Changes in tracking accuracy *during* a run can be viewed via graphs of target, response, and errors [Jones et al., 1993]. The latter is particularly informative for sinusoidal targets for which the mean absolute errors can be calculated over consecutive epochs, corresponding to sine-wave cycles, and plotted both in a histogram form and as a smoothed version of this [Jones and Donaldson, 1986]. As complexity of task is constant over epochs (cf. random pursuit task), the error graph gives an accurate measure of a subject's time-dependent spatiotemporal accuracy that is not confounded by changes in task difficulty and, therefore, gives a true indication of changes in performance due to factors such as learning, fatigue, and lapses in concentration. Attempts by the author to derive an instantaneous or short epoch (up to several seconds) function or *index of task difficulty* which would allow equivalent graphs to be generated for random targets were unsuccessful.

Neilson et al. [1998] devised an alternative procedure for intra-run analysis, termed micromovement analysis. This involves segmentation of the X and Y deflections of the response cursor on the basis of discontinuities, flat regions, and changes in direction of the response. They used this to identify changes in visual-motor coupling during the first 4 min of tracking on a 2-D compatible task following 4 h of practice on a 2-D incompatible task. They propose that these changes are evidence of rapid switching between different sensory-motor models in the brain.

By comparison, as long as the task remains unchanged over successive runs, studies of class II factors using tracking tasks are complicated most by inter-run *learning*. Although most learning occurs over the first one or two runs or sessions, tracking performance can continue to improve over extended periods as evidenced by, for example, significant improvements still being made by normal subjects after nine weekly sessions [Jones and Donaldson, 1981]. Consequently, a major difficulty met in the interpretation of serial measures of performance following acute brain damage is differentiation of neurologic recovery from normal learning. Furthermore, it is not simply a matter of subtracting off the degree of improved performance due to learning seen in normal control subjects. Jones et al. [1990] have developed graphical analysis techniques which provide for the removal of the learning factor, as much as is possible, and which can be applied to generating recovery curves for individual subjects following acute brain damage such as stroke. They demonstrated that, for tracking, percentage improvement in performance (PIP) graphs give more reliable evidence of neurologic recovery than absolute improvement in performance (PIA) graphs due to the former's greater independence from what are often considerably different absolute levels of performance.

77.4.4 Statistical Analysis

Parametric statistics (t-test, ANOVA) are by far the most commonly used in studies of sensory-motor/psychomotor performance due, in large part, to their availability and ability to draw out interactions between dependent variables. However, there is also a strong case for the use of non-parametric statistics. For example, the Wilcoxon matched-pairs statistic may be preferable for both between-group and within-subject comparisons due to its greater robustness over its parametric paired t-test equivalent, with only minimal loss of power. This is important due to many sensory-motor measures having very non-Gaussian skewed distributions as well as considerably different variances between normal and patient groups.

Defining Terms

Basic element of performance (BEP): Defined by a *functional unit* and a *dimension of performance*, for example, right elbow flexor + speed.

Dimension of performance: A basic measure of performance such as speed, range of movement, strength, spatial perception, spatiotemporal accuracy.

Functional unit: A subsystem such as right elbow flexor, left eye, motor memory.

Performance capacity: The maximal level of performance possible on a particular dimension of performance.

Performance resource (PR): One of a pool of elemental resources, from which the entire human is modelled (Kondraske, 1995b), and which is available for performing tasks. These resources can be subdivided into life sustaining, environmental interface, central processing, and skills domains, and have a parallel with *basic elements of performances*.

Sensor: [in context of tracking tasks] A device for measuring/transducing a subject's motor output.

Sensory-motor control: The primary (but not only) performance resource responsible for accuracy of movement.

Spatiotemporal accuracy: The class of accuracy most required by tasks which place considerable demand on attainment of simultaneous spatial and temporal accuracy; this refers particularly to *paced* tasks such as tracking, driving, ball games, and video games.

Tracking task: A laboratory apparatus and associated procedures which have proven one of the most versatile means for assessing and studying the human "black-box" sensory-motor system by providing a continuous record of a subject's response, via some *sensor*, to any one of a large number of continuous and well-controlled stimulus or *target* signals.

References

Abend, W., Bizzi, E., and Morasso, P. 1982. Human arm trajectory formation. *Brain* 105: 331–348.

Agarwal, G.C. and Logsdon, J.B. 1990. Optimal principles for skilled limb movements and speed accuracy tradeoff. *Proc. Ann. Int. Conf. IEEE Eng. Med. Biol. Soc.* 12: 2318–2319.

Anderson, O.T. 1986. A system for quantitative assessment of dyscoordination and tremor. *Acta Neurol. Scand.* 73: 291–294.

Angel, R.W., Alston, W., and Higgins, J.R. 1970. Control of movement in Parkinson's disease. *Brain* 93: 1–14.

Anson, J.C. 1987. Fractionated simple reaction time as a function of movement direction and level of pre-stimulus muscle tension. *Int. J. Neurosci.* 35: 140.

Baddeley, A., Logie, R., Bressi, S., Della Salla, S., and Spinnler, H. 1986. Dementia and working memory. *Quart. J. Exp. Psychol.* 38A: 603–618.

Baroni, A., Benvenuti, F., Fantini, L., Pantaleo, T., and Urbani, F. 1984. Human ballistic arm abduction movements: effects of L-dopa treatment in Parkinson's disease. *Neurology* 34: 868–876.

Barr, R.E., Hamlin, R.D., Abraham, L.D., and Greene, D.E. 1988. Electromyographic evaluation of operator performance in manual control tracking. *Proc. Ann. Int. Conf. IEEE Eng. Med. Biol. Soc.* 10: 1608–1609.

Behbehani, K., Kondraske, G.V., and Richmond, J.R. 1988. Investigation of upper extremity visuomotor control performance measures. *IEEE Trans. Biomed. Eng.* 35: 518–525.

Beppu, H., Suda, M., and Tanaka, R. 1984. Analysis of cerebellar motor disorders by visually-guided elbow tracking movement. *Brain* 107: 787–809.

Beppu, H., Nagaoka, M., and Tanaka, R. 1987. Analysis of cerebellar motor disorders by visually-guided elbow tracking movement: 2. Contributions of the visual cues on slow ramp pursuit. *Brain* 110: 1–18.

Bloxham, C.A., Mindel, T.A., and Frith, C.D. 1984. Initiation and execution of predictable and unpredictable movements in Parkinson's disease. *Brain* 107: 371–384.

Bösser, T. 1984. Adaptation to time-varying signals and control-theory models of tracking behaviour. *Psychol. Res.* 46: 155–167.

Buck, L. 1982. Location versus distance in determining movement accuracy. *J. Mot. Behav.* 14: 287–300.

Cassell, K.J. 1973. The usefulness of a temporal correlation technique in the assessment of human motor performance on a tracking task. *Med. Biol. Eng.* 11: 755–761.

Chelette, T.L., Repperger, D.W., and Phillips, C.A. 1995. Enhanced metrics for identification of forearm rehabilitation. *IEEE Trans. Rehabil. Eng.* 3: 122–131.

Cooke, J.D., Brown, J.D., and Brooks, V.B. 1978. Increased dependence on visual information for movement control in patients with Parkinson's disease. *Can. J. Neurol. Sci.* 5: 413–415.

Cooper, R., McCallum, W.C., and Cornthwaite, S.P. 1989. Slow potential changes related to the velocity of target movement in a tracking task. *Electroenceph. Clin. Neurophysiol.* 72: 232–239.

Craik, K.J.W. 1966. The mechanism of human action. In Sherwood, S.L. (Ed.), *The Nature of Psychology — A Selection of Papers, Essays, and Other Writings by the Late Kenneth J.W. Craik*, Cambridge, Cambridge University Press.

Croft, D. and Jones, R.D. 1987. The value of off-road tests in the assessment of driving potential of unlicensed disabled people. *Br. J. Occup. Ther.* 50: 357–361.

Dalrymple-Alford, J.C., Kalders, A.S., Jones, R.D., and Watson, R.W. 1994. A central executive deficit in patients with Parkinson's disease. *J. Neurol. Neurosurg. Psychiatr.* 57: 360–367.

Davidson, P.R., Jones, R.D., Sirisena, H.R. et al., 1999. Evaluation of nonlinear generalizations of the Adaptive Model Theory. *Proc. Int. Conf. IEEE Eng. Med. Biol. Soc.* 21.

Day, B.L., Dick, J.P.R., and Marsden, C.D. 1984. Patient's with Parkinson's disease can employ a predictive motor strategy. *J. Neurol. Neurosurg. Psychiatr.* 47: 1299–1306.

De Souza, L.H., Langton Hewer, R., Lynn, P.A., Mller, S., and Reed, G.A.L. 1980. Assessment of recovery of arm control in hemiplegic stroke patients: 2. Comparison of arm function tests and pursuit tracking in relation to clinical recovery. *Int. Rehabil. Med.* 2: 10–16.

Deuschl, G., Toro, C., Zeffiro, T. et al., 1996. Adaptation motor learning of arm movements in patients with cerebellar disease. *J. Neurol. Neurosurg. Psychiatr.* 60: 515–519.

Driscoll, M.C. 1975. Creative technological aids for the learning-disabled child. *Am. J. Occup. Ther.* 29: 102–105.

Ferslew, K.E., Manno, J.E., Manno, B.R., Vekovius, W.A., Hubbard, J.M., and Bairnsfather, L.E. 1982. Pursuit meter II, a computer-based device for testing pursuit-tracking performance. *Percep. Mot. Skills* 54: 779–784.

Fertner, A. and Sj'lund, S.J. 1986. Comparison of various time delay estimation methods by computer simulation. *IEEE Trans. Acoust. Speech Signal Proc.* 34: 1329–1330.

Fitts, P.M. 1954. The information capacity of the human motor system in controlling the amplitude of movement. *J. Exp. Psychol.* 47: 381–391.

Fitts, P.M. and Posner, M.I. 1967. *Human Performance*, California, Brooks/Cole.

Flash, T. and Hogan, N. 1985. The coordination of arm movements: an experimentally confirmed mathematical model. *J. Neurosci.* 5: 1688–1703.

Flowers, K.A. 1976. Visual "closed-loop" and "open-loop" characteristics of voluntary movement in patients with Parkinsonism and intention tremor. *Brain* 99: 269–310.

Flowers, K.A. 1978a. Lack of prediction in the motor behaviour of Parkinsonism. *Brain* 101: 35–52.

Flowers, K.A. 1978b. The predictive control of behaviour: appropriate and inappropriate actions beyond the input in a tracking task. *Ergonomics* 21: 109–122.

Frith, C.D., Bloxham, C.A., and Carpenter, K.N. 1986. Impairments in the learning and performance of a new manual skill in patients with Parkinson's disease. *J. Neurol. Neurosurg. Psychiatr.* 49: 661–668.

Garvey, W.D. 1960. A comparison of the effects of training and secondary tasks on tracking behavior. *J. Appl. Psychol.* 44:370–375.

Gibson, J.M., Pimlott, R., and Kennard, C. 1987. Ocular motor and manual tracking in Parkinson's disease and the effect of treatment. *Neurology* 50:853–860.

Gottlieb, G.L., Agarwal, G.C., and Penn, R. 1984. Sinusoidal oscillation of the ankle as a means of evaluating the spastic patient. *J. Neurol. Neurosurg. Psychiatr.* 41:32–39.

Guiard, Y., Diaz, G., and Beaubaton, D. 1983. Left-hand advantage in right-handers for spatial constant error: preliminary evidence in a unimanual ballistic aimed movement. *Neuropsychologica* 21: 111–115.

Hocherman, S. and Aharon-Peretz, J. 1994. Two-dimensional tracing and tracking in patients with Parkinson's disease. *Neurology* 44: 111–116.

Hufschmidt, A and Lücking, C. 1995. Abnormalities of tracking behavior in Parkinson's disease. *Mov. Disord.* 10: 267–276.

Jex, H.R. 1966. A "critical" tracking task for manual control research. *IEEE Trans. Hum. Factors Electron.* 7: 138–145.

Johnson, M.T.V., Kipnis, A.N., Coltz, J.D. et al. 1996. Effects of levodopa and viscosity on the velocity and accuracy of visually guided tracking in Parkinson's disease. *Brain* 119: 801–813.

Jones, R.D. and Donaldson, I.M. 1981. Measurement of integrated sensory-motor function following brain damage by a preview tracking task. *Int. Rehabil. Med.* 3: 71–83.

Jones, R.D. and Donaldson, I.M. 1986. Measurement of sensory-motor integrated function in neurological disorders: three computerized tracking tasks. *Med. Biol. Eng. Comput.* 24: 536–540.

Jones, R.D. and Donaldson, I.M. 1989. Tracking tasks and the study of predictive motor planning in Parkinson's disease. *Proc. Ann. Int. Conf. IEEE Eng. Med. Biol. Soc.* 11: 1055–1056.

Jones, R.D. and Donaldson, I.M. 1995. Fractionation of visuoperceptual dysfunction in Parkinson's disease. *J. Neurol. Sci.* 131: 43–50.

Jones, R.D., Donaldson, I.M., and Sharman, N.B. 1996. A technique for the removal of the visuospatial component from tracking performance and its application to Parkinson's disease. *IEEE Trans. Biomed. Eng.* 43: 1001–1010.

Jones, R., Giddens, H., and Croft, D. 1983. Assessment and training of brain-damaged drivers. *Am. J. Occup. Ther.* 37: 754–760.

Jones, R.D., Williams, L.R.T., and Wells, J.E. 1986. Effects of laterality, sex, and age on computerized sensory-motor tests. *J. Hum. Mot. Stud.* 12: 163–182.

Jones, R.D., Donaldson, I.M., and Parkin, P.J. 1989. Impairment and recovery of ipsilateral sensory-motor function following unilateral cerebral infarction. *Brain* 112: 113–132.

Jones, R.D., Donaldson, I.M., Parkin, P.J., and Coppage, S.A. 1990. Impairment and recovery profiles of sensory-motor function following stroke: single-case graphical analysis techniques. *Int. Disabil. Stud.* 12: 141–148.

Jones, R.D., Sharman, N.B., Watson, R.W., and Muir, S.R. 1993. A PC-based battery of tests for quantitative assessment of upper-limb sensory-motor function in brain disorders. *Proc. Ann. Int. Conf. IEEE Eng. Med. Biol. Soc.* 15: 1414–1415.

Kearney, R.E. and Hunter, I.W. 1983. System identification of human triceps surae stretch reflex dynamics. *Exp. Brain Res.* 51: 117–127.

Kondraske, G.V. 1988. Experimental evaluation of an elemental resource model for human performance. *Proc. Ann. Int. Conf. IEEE Eng. Med. Biol. Soc.* 10: 1612–1613.

Kondraske, G.V. 1995a. An elemental resource model for the human-task interface. *Int. J. Technol. Assess. Health Care* 11: 153–173.

Kondraske, G.V. 1995b. A working model for human system–task interfaces. In Bronzino, J.D. (Ed.), *The Biomedical Engineering Handbook*, pp. 2157–2174. Boca Raton, FL, CRC Press.

Kondraske, G.V., Johnson, C., Pearson, A., and Tarbox, L. 1997. Performance prediction and limited resource identification with nonlinear causal resource analysis. *Proc. Ann. Int. Conf. IEEE Eng. Med. Biol. Soc.* 19: 1813–1816.

Kondraske, G.V., Potvin, A.R., Tourtellotte, W.W., and Syndulko, K. 1984. A computer-based system for automated quantitation of neurologic function. *IEEE Trans. Biomed. Eng.* 31: 401–414.

Kondraske, G.V., Behbehani, K., Chwialkowski, M., Richmond, R., and van Maltzahn, W. 1988. A system for human performance measurement. *IEEE Eng. Med. Biol. Mag.* March:23–27.

Leist, A., Freund, H.J., and Cohen, B. 1987. Comparative characteristics of predictive eye–hand tracking. *Hum. Neurobiol.* 6: 19–26.

Lynn, P.A., Reed, G.A.L., Parker, W.R., and Langton Hewer, R. 1977. Some applications of human-operator research to the assessment of disability in stroke. *Med. Biol. Eng.* 15: 184–188.

Lynn, P.A., Parker, W.R., Reed, G.A.L., Baldwin, J.F., and Pilsworth, B.W. 1979. New approaches to modelling the disabled human operator. *Med. Biol. Eng. Comput.* 17: 344–348.

McRuer, D.T. and Krendel, E.S. 1959. The human operator as a servo element. *J. Franklin Inst.* 267: 381–403.

Miall, R.C., Weir, D.J., and Stein, J.F. 1985. Visuomotor tracking with delayed visual feedback. *Neuroscience* 16: 511–520.

Milkowski, L.M., Prieto, T.E., Myklebust, J.B., lovett, and Klebust, B.M. 1993. Two-dimensional coherence: a measure of asymmetry in postural steadiness. *Proc. Ann. Int. Conf. IEEE Eng. Med. Biol. Soc.* 15: 1181.

Miller, R.G. and Freund, H.J. 1980. Cerebellar dyssynergia in humans — a quantitative analysis. *Ann. Neurol.* 8: 574–579.

Muir, S.R., Jones, R.D., Andreae, J.H., and Donaldson, I.M. 1995. Measurement and analysis of single and multiple finger tapping in normal and Parkinsonian subjects. *Parkinsonism Relat. Disord.* 1: 89–96.

Navon, D., Gopher, D., Chillag, N., and Spitz, G. 1984. On separability of and interference between tracking dimensions in dual-axis tracking. *J. Mot. Behav.* 16: 364–391.

Neilson, P.D. 1972. Speed of response or bandwidth of voluntary system controlling elbow position in intact man. *Med. Biol. Eng.* 10: 450–459.

Neilson, P.D. and Neilson, M.D. 1980. Influence of control-display compatability on tracking behaviour. *Quart. J. Exp. Psychol.* 32: 125–135.

Neilson, P.D., Neilson, M.D., and O'Dwyer, N.J. 1992. Adaptive model theory: application to disorders of motor control. In J.J. Summers, (Ed.), *Approaches to the Study of Motor Control and Learning*, pp. 495–548. Amsterdam, Elsevier Science.

Neilson, P.D., Neilson, M.D., and O'Dwyer, N.J. 1993. What limits high speed tracking performance? *Hum. Mov. Sci.* 12: 85–109.

Neilson, P.D., Neilson, M.D., and O'Dwyer, N.J. 1995. Adaptive optimal control of human tracking. In D.J. Glencross and J.P. Piek (Eds.), *Motor Control and Sensory-Motor Integration: Issues and Directions*, pp. 97–140. Amsterdam, Elsevier Science.

Neilson, P.D., Neilson, M.D., and O'Dwyer, N.J. 1998. Evidence for rapid switching of sensory-motor models. In J. Piek (Ed.), *Motor Control and Human Skill: A Multidisciplinary Perspective*, pp. 105–126. Champaign, IL, Human Kinetics.

Neilson, P.D., O'Dwyer, N.J., and Nash, J. 1990. Control of isometric muscle activity in cerebral palsy. *Dev. Med. Child Neurol.* 32: 778–788.

Notterman, J.M., Tufano, D.R., and Hrapsky, J.S. 1982. Visuo-motor organization: differences between and within individuals. *Percep. Mot. Skills* 54: 723–750.

O'Dwyer, N.J., Ada, L., and Neilson, P.D. 1996. Spasticity and muscle contracture following stroke. *Brain* 119: 1737–1749.

O'Dwyer, N.J. and Neilson, P.D. 1995. Learning a dynamic limb synergy. In D.J. Glencross and J.P. Piek (Eds.), *Motor Control and Sensory-Motor Integration: Issues and Directions*, pp. 289–317. Amsterdam, Elsevier Science.

O'Dwyer, N.J. and Neilson, P.D. 1998. Adaptation to a changed sensory-motor relation: immediate and delayed parametric modification. In J.P. Piek (Ed.), *Motor Behavior and Human Skill — A Multidisciplinary Approach*, pp. 75–104. Champaign, IL, Human Kinetics.

Sriharan, A. 1997. *Mathematical modelling of the human operator control system through tracking tasks.* Masters in Engineering thesis. University of New South Wales, Sydney, Australia.

Patrick, J. and Mutlusoy, F. 1982. The relationship between types of feedback, gain of a display and feedback precision in acquisition of a simple motor task. *Quart. J. Exp. Psychol.* 34A:171–182.

Pitrella, F.D. and Kruger, W. 1983. Design and validation of matching tests to form equal groups for tracking experiments. *Ergonomics* 26:833–845.

Potvin, A.R. and Tourtellotte, W.W. 1975. The neurological examination: advancement in its quantification. *Arch. Phys. Med. Rehabil.* 56:425–442.

Potvin, A.R., Albers, J.W., Stribley, R.F., Tourtellotte, W.W., and Pew, R.W. 1975. A battery of tests for evaluating steadiness in clinical trials. *Med. Biol. Eng.* 13:914–921.

Potvin, A.R., Doerr, J.A., Estes, J.T., and Tourtellotte, W.W. 1977. Portable clinical tracking-task instrument. *Med. Biol. Eng. Comput.* 15:391–397.

Potvin, A.R., Tourtellotte, W.W., Potvin, J.H., Kondraske, G.V., and Syndulko, K. 1985. *The Quantitative Examination of Neurologic Function*, CRC Press, Boca Raton, FL.

Poulton, E.C. 1964. Postview and preview in tracking with complex and simple inputs. *Ergonomics* 7:257–266.

Poulton, E.C. 1974. *Tracking Skill and Manual Control*, New York, Academic Press.

Riedel, S.A., Harris, G.F., and Jizzine, H.A. 1992. An investigation of seated postural stability. *IEEE Eng. Med. Biol. Mag.* 11:42–47.

Robertson, C. and Flowers, K.A. 1990. Motor set in Parkinson's disease. *J. Neurol. Neurosurg. Psych.* 53:583–592.

Roscoe, J.T. 1975. *Fundamental Research Statistics for the Behavioral Sciences*, 2nd ed. New York, Holt, Rinehart & Winston.

Schmidt, R.A. 1982. *Motor Control and Learning: A Behavioral Emphasis*, Champaign, IL, Human Kinetics.

Sheridan, M.R., Flowers, K.A., and Hurrell, J. 1987. Programming and execution of movement in Parkinson's disease. *Brain* 110:1247–1271.

Sheridan, T.B. 1966. Three models of preview control. *IEEE Trans. Hum. Factors Electron.* 7:91–102.

Siegel, D. 1985. Information processing abilities and performance on two perceptual-motor tasks. *Percep. Mot. Skills* 60:459–466.

Sittig, A.C., Denier van der Gon, J.J., Gielen, C.C., and van Wilk, A.J. 1985. The attainment of target position during step-tracking movements despite a shift of initial position. *Exp. Brain Res.* 60:407–410.

Stelmach, G.E. and Worrington, C.J. 1988. The preparation and production of isometric force in Parkinson's disease. *Neuropsychologica* 26:93–103.

Stern, Y., Mayeux, R., Rosen, J., and Ilson, J. 1983. Perceptual motor dysfunction in Parkinson's disease: a deficit in sequential and predictive voluntary movement. *J. Neurol. Neurosurg. Psychiatr.* 46:145–151.

Stern, Y., Mayeux, R., and Rosen, J. 1984. Contribution of perceptual motor dysfunction to construction and tracing disturbances in Parkinson's disease. *J. Neurol. Neurosurg. Psychiatr.* 47:983–989.

Thomas, J.S., Croft, D.A., and Brooks, V.B. 1976. A manipulandum for human motor studies. *IEEE Trans. Biomed. Eng.* 23:83–84.

van den Berg, R., Mooi, B., Denier van der Gon, J.J., and Gielen, C.C.A.M. 1987. Equipment for the quantification of motor performance for clinical purposes. *Med. Biol. Eng. Comput.* 25:311–316.

Vasta, P.J. and Kondraske, G.V. 1994. Performance prediction of an upper extremity reciprocal task using non-linear causal resource analysis. *Proc. Int. Conf. IEEE Eng. Med. Biol. Soc.* 16 (CD-ROM).

Vince, M.A. 1948. The intermittency of control movements and the psychological refractory period. *Brit. J. Psychol.* 38:149–157.

Viviani, P. and Mounoud, P. 1990. Perceptuomotor compatibility in pursuit tracking of two-dimensional movements. *J. Mot. Behav.* 22:407–443.

Warabi, T., Noda, H., Yanagisawa, N., Tashiro, K., and Shindo, R. 1986. Changes in sensorimotor function associated with the degree of bradykinesia of Parkinson's disease. *Brain* 109:1209–1224.

Watson, R.W. 1994. *Advances in zero-based consistent deconvolution and Evaluation of human sensory-motor function.* Ph.D. Dissertation, University of Canterbury, Christchurch, New Zealand.

Watson, R.W. and Jones, R.D. 1998. A comparison of two-dimensional and one-dimensional tracking performance in normal subjects. *J. Mot. Behav.* 30:359–366.

Watson, R.W., Jones, R.D., and Sharman, N.B. 1997. Two-dimensional tracking tasks for quantification of sensory-motor dysfunction and their application to Parkinson's disease. *Med. Biol. Eng. Comput.* 35:141–145.

Welford, A.T. 1968. *Fundamentals of Skill*, London, Methuen.

Further Information

The Quantitative Examination of Neurologic Function by Potvin et al. [1985], is a two volume book which provides a superb in-depth review of instrumentation and methods for measurement of both normal and abnormal neurologic function.

An excellent overview of "Control of Postural Stability" is contained in the theme section (edited by G. Harris) of the December 1992 issue of *IEEE Engineering in Medicine and Biology Magazine*.

78

Measurement of Information-Processing Subsystem Performance Capacities

George V. Kondraske
Paul J. Vasta
University of Texas-Arlington

78.1 Introduction

The human brain has been the subject of much scientific research. While a tremendous amount of information exists and considerable progress has been made in unlocking its many mysteries, many gaps in understanding exist. However, it is not essential to understand in full detail how a given function of the brain is mediated in order to accept that it (i.e., the function) exists, or to understand how to maximally isolate, stress, and characterize at least selected attributes of its performance quantitatively. In this chapter, a systems view of major functional aspects of the brain is used as a basis for discussing methods employed to measure what can be termed central processing performance capacities. Central processing capacities are distinguished from the information that is processed. In humans, the latter can be viewed to represent the contents of **memory** (e.g., facts, "programs," etc.). Clearly, both the information itself and the characteristics of the systems that process it (i.e., the various capacities discussed below) combine to realize what are commonly observed as skills whether perceptual, motor, cognitive, or other.

Investigations of how humans process information have been performed within various fields including psychology, cognitive science, and information theory with the primary motivation being to better understand how human information-processing works and the factors that influence it. On the basis that it provided a rigorous definition for the measurement of information, it can be argued that Shannon's information theory [Shannon, 1948] has been and continues to be one of the more important developments to influence both the science and engineering associated with human information processing. Several early attempts to apply it to human information processing [Hick, 1952; Hyman, 1953; Fitts, 1954] have stood the test of time and have provided the basis for subsequent efforts of both researchers and practitioners. These works are central to the material presented here. In addition, the work of Wiener [1955] is also noteworthy in that it began the process of viewing human and artificial information processing from a common perspective. Analogies between humans and computers have proven to be very useful up to certain limits.

While there is considerable overlap and frequent interchange, the roles of science and engineering are different. In the present context, the emphasis is on aspects of the latter. It has been necessary to engineer useful measurement tools and processes without complete science to serve a wide variety of purposes that have demanded **attention** in both clinical and nonclinical contexts. Whether purposeful or accidental, methods of systems engineering have been incorporated and have proven useful in dealing with the complexity of human brain structure and function. While scientific controversies continue to exist, much research has contributed to the now common view of separate (both in function and location) processing subsystems that make up the whole. Various versions of a general distributed, multiprocessor model of human brain function have been popularly sketched [Gazzaniga, 1985; Minsky, 1986; Ornstein, 1986]. For example, it is widely known that the occipital lobe of the brain is responsible for visual information processing while other areas have been found to correspond to other functions. It is not possible to do justice here to the tremendous scope of work that has been put forth and therefore to the brain itself. Nonetheless, this compartmentalistic or systems approach, which stresses major functional systems that must exist based on overwhelming empirical evidence, has proven to be useful for explaining many normal and pathologic behavioral observations. This approach is essential to the development of meaningful and practical performance measurement strategies such as those described.

78.2   Basic Principles

Many of the past efforts in which performance-related measurements have played a significant role have been directed toward basic research. Furthermore, much of this research has been aimed at uncovering the general operational frameworks of normal human information processing and not the measurement of performance capacities and their use, either alone or in combination with other capacity metrics, to characterize humans of various types (e.g., normal, aged, handicapped, etc.). However, representative models and theories provide direction for, and are themselves shaped by, subsequent measurement efforts. While there are many principles and basic observations that have some relevance, the scope of material presented later is limited to topics that more specifically support the understanding of human information-processing **performance capacity** measurement.

78.2.1   Functional Model of Central Information Processing

A simplified, although quite robust, model that is useful within the context of human information processing is illustrated in Figure 78.1. With this figure, attention is called to systems, their functions, and major interconnectivities. At a functional level that is relatively high within the hierarchy of the human

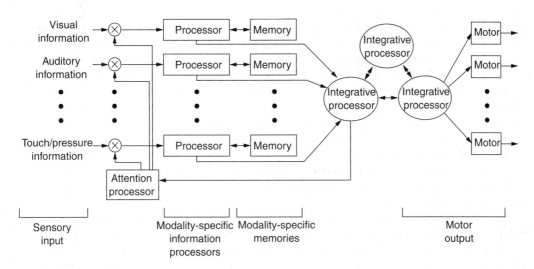

FIGURE 78.1   A functional systems-level block diagram of human information-processing description of the measurement of sybsystem performance capacities.

central nervous system, the central processing system can be considered to be composed of two types of subsystems (1) *information processors* and (2) *memories*. As can be seen from the diagram, information from the environment is provided to the information-processing subsystems through human sensor subsystems. These not only include the obvious sensors (e.g., the eyes) that receive input from external sources but also those specifically designed to provide information regarding the internal environment, including proprioception and state of being. The capacity to process information input from multiple sources at a conscious level is finite. Overload is prevented by limiting the amount of information simultaneously received; specific sensory information of high priority is controlled by what may be termed an *attention* **processor**. Information associated with a given sensor system is processed by a corresponding processor. The model further suggests that there are memory subsystems for each sensory modality in bidirectional communications with the associated processor. Thus, modality-specific information (e.g., visual, auditory, etc.) may be referenced and processed with new information. As information is received and processed at modality-specific levels it is combined at a higher level by integrative processors to generate situation-specific responses. These may be in the form of a musculoskeletal, cognitive, or attention-modifying events, as well as any combination of these.

General measurement issues of fidelity, validity, and reliability are natural concerns in measurement of information-processing performance capacities. Special issues emerge that increase the overall complexity of the problem when attempting to measure attributes that reflect *just* the information-processing subsystems. Unlike a computer where one may remove a memory module, place it in a special test unit, and determine its capacity, the accessibility of the subsystems within the human brain is such that it is impossible to perfectly isolate and directly measure any of the individual components. When measuring characteristics of human information-processing subsystems, it is necessary to address measurement goals that are similar to those applied to analogous artificial system within the constraint that human sensors and motoric subsystems must also be utilized.

78.2.2   Performance Capacities

In considering the performance of human information-processing systems, the resource-based perspective represented by the Elemental Resource Model [Kondraske, 2000] is adopted here. This model for human performance encompasses all types of human subsystems and is the result of the application of a general theoretical framework for system performance to the human system and its subsystems. A central idea incorporated in this framework, universal to all types of systems, is that of *performance capacity*.

This implies a finite availability of some quantity that thereby limits performance. A general two-part approach is used to identify unique performance capacities (e.g., visual information **processor speed**) (1) identify the system (e.g., visual information processor) and (2) identify the dimension of performance (e.g., speed). In this framework, system performance capacities are characterized by availability of performance resources along each of the identified dimensions. These *performance resources* are to be distinguished from less rigorously defined general processing resources described by others [e.g., Kahneman, 1973; Wickens, 1984]. However, many of the important basic constructs associated with the idea of "a resource" are employed in a similar fashion in each of these contexts. For processors, key dimensions of performance are speed and accuracy. *Processor speed* and **processor accuracy** capacities are thus identified. For memory systems, key dimensions of performance are storage capacity, speed (e.g., retrieval) and accuracy (e.g., retrieval). Other important attributes of performance capacities are discussed in other sections of this chapter.

Many aspects of information-processing performance have been investigated resulting in discoveries that have provided insight to the capacities of subsystems as well as refinement to both system structure and function definitions [Lachman et al., 1979]. One of the oldest studies in which the basic concept of information-processing performance capacity was recognized addressed "speed of mental processes" [Donders, 1868]. The basic idea of capacity has been a central topic of interest in human information-processing research [Moray, 1967; Posner and Boies, 1971; Schneider and Shiffrin, 1977; Shiffrin and Schneider, 1977].

78.2.3 Stimulus–Response Scenario

The *stimulus–response scenario*, perhaps most often recognized in association with behavioral psychology, has emerged as a fundamental paradigm in psychology experiments [Neel, 1977]. Aside from general utility in research, it is also an essential component of strategies for measurement of human information-processing performance capacities. A typical example is the well-known reaction time test in which the maximum speed (and sometimes accuracy) at which information can be processed is of interest. Here, a subject is presented a stimulus specific to some sensory modality (e.g., visual, auditory, and tactile) and is instructed to respond in a prescribed manner (e.g., lift a hand from a switch "as fast as possible" when the identified stimulus occurs). This general approach, which has become so popular and useful in psychology, can also be recognized as one that has been commonly employed in engineering to characterize artificial systems (e.g., amplifiers, motors, etc.). A specific known signal (stimulus) is applied to the system's input and the corresponding output (response) is observed. Specified, measurable attributes of the output, in combination with the known characteristics of the input, are used to infer various characteristics of the system under test. When the focus of interest is the performance limits of processing systems, these characteristics include processing speed, processing accuracy, memory storage capacity, etc.

In performance capacity tests, an important related component is the **prestimulus set**, or simply the way in which the system is "programmed to respond to the stimulus." This is usually accomplished by one or more components of the instructions given to the subject under test (e.g., respond "as quickly as possible," etc.) just prior to the execution of an actual test.

78.2.4 Measurement of Information (Stimulus Characterization)

Within a given sensory modality, it is easy to understand that different stimuli place different demands or "loads" on information-processing systems. Thus, in order to properly interpret results of performance tests, it is necessary to describe the stimulus. While this remains a topic of ongoing research with inherent controversies, some useful working constructs are available. At issue is not simply a qualitative description, but the *measurement* of stimulus content (or complexity). Shannon's information theory [1948], which teaches how to measure the amount of information associated with a generalized information source, has been the primary tool used in these efforts. Thus, a stimulus can be characterized in terms of the amount of information present in it. Simple stimuli (e.g., a light that is "on" or "off") possess less information than complex stimuli (e.g., a computer screen with menus, buttons, etc.). The best successes in attempts to quantitatively characterize stimuli have been achieved for simple discrete stimuli [Hick, 1952; Hyman, 1953]. From Shannon, the amount of information associated with a given symbol "i," selected from a source with "n" such symbols is given by:

$$I_i = \log_2(1/p_i) \tag{78.1}$$

where p_i is the probability of occurrence of symbol "i" (within a finite symbol set) and the result has the units of "bits." Thus, high probability stimuli contain less information than low probability stimuli. It is a relatively straightforward matter to control the probabilities associated with symbols that serve as stimuli in test situations. The application of basic information theory to the characterization of stimuli that are more complex (i.e., multiple components, continuous stimuli) is challenging both theoretically and practically (e.g., large symbol sets, different sets with different probability distributions that must be controlled, etc.).

If stimuli are not or cannot be characterized robustly in terms of a measure with units of "bits," operationally defined units are frequently used (e.g., "items," "chunks," "stimuli," etc.). In addition, as many stimulus attributes as possible are identified and quantified and others are simply "described." This at least maximizes the opportunity for obtaining repeatable measurements. However, the additional implication is that the number of "bits per item" or "bits per chunk" is waiting to be delineated and perhaps a conversion could be substituted at a later time. While this state leaves much to be desired from a rigorous measurement perspective, it is nonetheless quite common in the evolution of measurement for many physical quantities and allows useful work to be conducted.

78.2.5 Speed–Accuracy Trade-Off

Fundamental to all human information-processing systems and tasks is the so-called **speed–accuracy trade-off**. This basic limitation can be observed in relatively high-level everyday tasks such as reading, writing, typing, listening to a lecture, etc. Psychologists [Wicklegren, 1977] have studied this trade-off in many different contexts. Fitts [1966] demonstrated a relationship between measures reflecting actual performance (reaction time and errors) to incentive-based task goals (i.e., were subjects attempting to achieve high speed or high accuracy). As shown in Figure 78.2, relationships that have been found suggest an upper limit to the combination of speed and accuracy available for information-processing tasks. In this figure, original reaction time measures have been transformed by simple inversion to obtain true speed measures, which also conform to the resource construct used in modeling performance capacities, as described in Section 78.2.2. The result then defines a two-dimensional (e.g. speed–accuracy) performance envelope for information-processing systems. The area within this envelope, given that each dimensions represents a resource-based performance capacity, represents a higher level or composite performance capacity metric (with units of speed × accuracy), analogous in some respects to a gain–bandwidth product or work (force × displacement) metric.

78.2.6 Divided Attention and Time Sharing

An approach sometimes used in a variety of measurement contexts incorporates a *dual-task or divided attention scenario* that is designed to require use of attention resources in two different simultaneously executed tasks [e.g., Wickens, 1984]. For example, visual tracking (primary task) accuracy *and* speed of response to an embedded visual stimulus (secondary task) can be measured. Details of the potential time-sharing possibilities at play are quite complex [Schneider and Shiffrin, 1977; Shiffrin and Schneider, 1977].

In comparison to single-task performance test situations, in which the attention processor may not be working at capacity, the additional demand is designed to change (compared to a single-task baseline) and sometimes maximizes the stress on attention performance resources. Performance on both primary and secondary tasks, compared to levels attained when each task is independently performed, can provide an indirect measure of capacity associated with attention [Parasuraman and Davies, 1984]. This approach

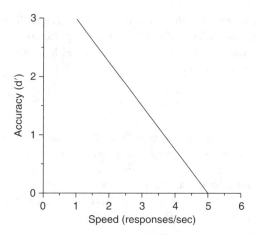

FIGURE 78.2 A typical information-processing performance envelope in two-dimensional speed–accuracy space. (Data from Wickelgren, W.A. 1977. *Acta Psychol.* 41, 67–85.)

has been useful in determining relative differences in demand imposed by two different primary tasks by comparison of results from respective tests in which a fixed secondary task is used with different primary tasks. Of more direct relevance to the present context, an appropriate secondary task can be used to control in part the conditions under which a given performance capacity (defined in a standard way and measured in association with the primary task) is measured, for example, visual information-processing speed can be measured with no additional attention load or with several different additional attention load levels. While it may be possible to rank order secondary tasks in terms of the additional load presented, there are no known methods to quantify attention load in absolute terms.

78.3 General Measurement Paradigms

Despite the complexity of human information-processing, a fairly small number of different measurement paradigms have emerged for quantification of the many unique human information-processing performance capacities. This is perhaps in part due to the limited number of system types (e.g., processors and memories). A good portion of the observed complexity can therefore be attributed to the number of different processors and memories, as well as the vastness and diversity of actual information that humans typically possess (i.e., facts, knowledge, skills, etc.). While most of the paradigms described below have been used for decades, it is helpful to recognize that they all conform to, or can be made to conform to, the more recently proposed [Kondraske, 1987, 1995] generalized strategy for measuring any aspect of performance for any human subsystem (1) maximally isolate first the system of interest, (2) maximally isolate the dimensions of performance of interest, and (3) maximally stress (tempered by safety considerations when appropriate) the system along those dimensions.

78.3.1 Information-Processing Speed

The paradigm for measuring information-processing speed is commonly referred to as a reaction time test since the elapsed time (i.e., the processing time) between the onset of a given stimulus and the occurrence of a prescribed response is the basic measurable quantity. To obtain a processing speed measure, the stimulus content in "bits," "chunks," or simply "stimuli" is divided by the processing time to yield measures with units of bits, chunks, or stimuli. Choice of stimulus modality isolates a specific sensory processor, whereas choice of a responder (e.g., index finger, upper extremity motion caused primarily by shoulder flexors, etc.) isolates a motoric processor associated with generation of the response. Much research has addressed the allocation of portions of the total processing time to various subsystem components (Sternberg, 1966).

TABLE 78.1   The Combination of the Human Sensor Subsystem (Determined by Stimulus Source) and Responder Isolates Unique Subsystems

Capacity types	Stimulus type(s)	Responder[a]	Measurements
Attention	Visual Auditory	Upper extremity Vocal system	Length of time that a task can be performed to specification and accuracy (if appropriate for task) when subject is instructed to perform for "as long as possible"
Processor speed	Visual Visual Visual Auditory Auditory Auditory Vibrotactile	Upper extremity Lower extremity Vocal system Upper extremity Lower extremity Vocal system Upper extremity	Inverse of time required to react to stimulus (i.e., stimuli/sec) when subject is instructed to respond "as quickly as possible"
Processor accuracy	Visual Visual Visual Auditory Auditory Auditory Vibrotactile	Upper extremity Lower extremity Vocal system Upper extremity Lower extremity Vocal system Upper extremity	Subject is asked to perform task (e.g., typically recognition of symbols from set with similar information content across symbols) "as accurately as possible" and without stress on speed of measures of accuracy. The correct percentage (out of a predetermined set size) is often used, although different accuracy measures have been proposed [Green and Swets, 1966; Wicklegren, 1977].
Processor speed–accuracy	Visual Visual Visual Auditory Auditory Auditory Vibrotactile	Upper extremity Lower extremity Vocal system Upper extremity Lower extremity Vocal system Upper extremity	Basically a combination of tests that stress speed and accuracy capacities individually, as well as both speed and accuracy measures are obtained as defined above to get off-axis data points in two-dimensional speed–accuracy space. Both speed and accuracy can be maximally stressed (e.g., by instructing subject to perform "as fast and accurately as possible") or accuracy can be measured at different speeds by varying time available for responses and stressing accuracy within this constraint
Memory storage capacity	Visual Visual Visual Auditory Auditory Auditory Vibrotactile	(Same options as above[b])	Maximum amount of information of type defined by stimulus that the subject is able to recall. Stimuli usually consist of sets of symbols of varying complexity in different sets (e.g., spatially distributed lights, alphanumeric characters, words, motions, etc.) but similar amount of information per symbol in a given set. Units of "bits" are ideal, but not often possible if number of bits per symbol is unknown. In such cases, units are often reported as "symbols," "chunks," or "items"

A number of representative, but not exhaustive combinations are illustrated for each information-processing capacity type. Depending on objectives of the test task (as communicated to the subject under test) and metrics obtained, many different unique capacities are defined. In some applications (e.g., in evaluating a subject who has suffered a stroke in very localized region of the brain) the specificity is important. In others (e.g., in evaluating a neurologic disease with widespread generalized effects) the responder may be chosen for convenience.

[a] General terms are used in table to illustrate combination options. Very specific definition that controls the motoric functional units involved as precisely as possible should be used for any given capacity test. For example (1) Upper extremity (shoulder flexor vs. elbow flexor vs. digit 2 flexor) and (2) Vocal system (lingua-dental "ta" vs. labial "pa" response), etc.

[b] Unless motor memory capacities are being tested, the responder is typically chosen to minimize stress on motoric processing and, compared to processor performance measures, not to isolate a unique motor memory system.

The system of primary interest as presented here is the sensory processor. Processing times associated with the motoric processor involved in the response are substantially less in normal systems. However, it is recommended that a given processor speed capacity be identified not only by the sensor subsystem stressed, but also by the responder (e.g., visual shoulder flexor information processor speed). This identifies not only the test scenario employed but also the complete information path.

78.3.2 Information-Processing Accuracy and Speed–Accuracy Combinations

In contrast to processor speed capacity that describes limits on information rate, accuracy relates to the ability to resolve content. In general, paradigms for tests that include accuracy measures typically involve a finite set of symbols with a corresponding set of responses. Various stimulus presentation–response scenarios can be used. For example, a stimulus can be randomly selected from the set with the subject required to identify the stimulus presented. Alternately, a subset of stimuli can be presented and the subject asked to select the response corresponding to the symbol not in the subset (size of subsets should be small if it is desired to minimize stress on memory capacities). A key element is that, within a poststimulus–response window, the subject is forced to select one of the available responses. This allows accuracy of the response to be measured in any of a number of ways ranging from relatively simple to complex [Green and Swets, 1966; Wicklegren, 1977]. The response window is either relatively open-ended, as short as possible and variable (based on the speed of the subject's response), or fixed at a given length of time. When only accuracy is stressed, subjects are instructed to perform as accurately as possible and the stress on speed is minimized (e.g., "take your time"). In a second type of speed–accuracy test, subjects are instructed to perform as fast and as accurately as possible, maximally stressing both dimensions while both accuracy and speed of responses are measured. In a variation of this general paradigm, a fixed-response window size is selected to challenge response speed. This provides a known point along the speed dimension of performance. In all three cases, measured response accuracy provides the second coordinate of a point in the two-dimensional speed–accuracy performance space. The combination of different paradigms can be used to determine the speed–accuracy performance envelope (see Section 78.2.5).

78.3.3 Memory Capacity

As used here, *memory capacity* refers to the amount of information that can be stored and recalled. It is well accepted that separate memory exists for different sensory modalities. Also, short-, medium-, and long-term memory systems have been identified [Crook et al., 1986]. Thus, separate capacities can be identified for each. Higher level capacities can also be identified with processes that utilize memory, such as scanning [Sternberg, 1966]. A comprehensive assessment of memory would require tasks that challenge the various memory systems to determine resources available, singly and along different combinations of their various modalities, most directly relevant to the individual's developmental stage (infant, youth, adolescent, young adult, middle aged adult, or older adult), and reflecting the diversity and depth of life experiences of that individual. No such comprehensive batteries are available. As noted by Syndulko et al. [1988], "Most typically, a variety of individual tests are utilized that evaluate selected aspects of memory systems under artificial conditions that relate best to college students." This general circumstance is in part due to the lack of generalized performance measurement strategies for memory. Despite such diversity, perhaps the most common variation of the many memory capacity tests involves providing a stimuli of the appropriate modality and requiring complete, accurate recall (i.e., a response) after some specified period of delay. The response window is selected to be relatively long so that processor speed is only minimally stressed. Typically, a test begins with a stimulus that has low information content (i.e., one that should be within capacity limits of the lowest one expects to encounter). If the response is correct, the information content of the stimuli is increased and another trial is administered. It is typically assumed that the amount of information added after each successful trial is fairly constant. Examples include: adding another light to a spatially distributed light pattern, adding another randomly selected digit (0–9) to a sequence of such digits, etc. By continuing this process of progressively increasing the amount of stimulus information until an inaccurate response is obtained, the isolated memory capacity is assumed to be maximally stressed. The result is simply the amount of information stored and recalled, in units of bits, chunks, or items.

78.3.4 Attention

Tests for basic attention capacity can be considered to be somewhat analogous to endurance capacity tests for neuromuscular systems. Simply put, the length of time over which a specified information-processing task can be executed provides a measure of attention capacity (or attention span). The test paradigm typically involves presentation at random time intervals of a randomly selected stimulus from a finite predefined symbol set for a relatively short, fixed time (e.g., 1 sec). Within a predefined response window (with a maximum duration that is selected so that processing speed resources are minimally stressed), the subject must generate a response corresponding to the stimulus that occurred. Attention is maximally stressed by continuing this process until the subject either (1) makes no response within the allocated response window, or (2) produces an incorrect response (i.e., a response associated with a stimulus that was not presented). These criteria thus essentially define the point at which the specified task (i.e., recognize stimuli and respond correctly within a generous period of time allotted) can no longer be completed. Once again, choice of stimulus modality isolates a specific sensory processor (e.g., visual, auditory, tactile, etc.). Clearly, stimulus complexity is also important. Stress on higher-level cognitive resources can be minimized by choice of simple stimuli (e.g., lights, tones, etc.). Motoric processors associated with response generation are also involved. However, these are minimally stressed and as long as basic functionality is present the choice of responder should have little influence on results compared to, for example, the influence occurring during processor speed capacity measurements.

78.4 Measurement Instruments and Procedures

Given the above functional systems model for human information-processing (Figure 78.1) and review of measurement paradigms for information-processing subsystems, a general architecture for instruments capable of measuring information-processing performance capacities can be defined (Figure 78.3). It is interesting to observe that this architecture parallels the human information-processing system (i.e., compare Figure 78.1 and Figure 78.3).

Most such instruments are computer based, allowing for generation of stimuli with different contents, presentation of stimuli at precisely timed intervals, measurement of processing times (from which processing speeds are derived) with high accuracy (typically, to within 1 msec), and accurate recording of responses and determination of their correctness.

A typical desktop computer system fits the general architecture presented in Figure 78.3 and, as such, it has been widely exploited "as is" physically with appropriate software to conduct information-processing tests. This is adequate for tests for higher level, complex cognitive processing tasks due to the longer processing times involved. That is, screen refresh times and keyboard response times are smaller fractions of total times measured and contribute less error. However, for measurement of more basic performance

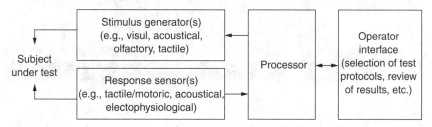

FIGURE 78.3   The general architecture for instruments used to measure human information-processing performance capacities.

capacities and to allow testing of subjects who do not possess normal physical performance capacities, custom test setups are essential. The general design goal for these stimuli generators and response sensors is to minimize the stress on human sensory, motor, and aspects of central processing resources that are not the target of the test. For example, the size of standard keyboard switches imposes demands on positioning accuracy when, for example, visual information-processing accuracy is being tested. According to Fitts' Law [Fitts, 1954], the task component involved with hitting the desired response key (i.e., the component that occurs after the visual information-processing component) requires longer processing times (associated with the motoric response task) for smaller targets. Thus, to minimize such influences, a relatively large target is suggested. Along the same lines of reasoning, these additional design guidelines are important (1) key stimulus attributes that are not related to information content should be well above normal minimum human sensing thresholds (e.g., relatively bright lights that do not stress visual sensitivity and large characters or symbols that do not stress visual acuity), (2) response speeds of stimulus generators and response sensors should be much faster than the fastest human response speed that is anticipated to be measured.

Even the many custom devices reported in the literature (as well as commercially available versions of some) have been devised to support research into fundamental aspects of information-processing and are used in studies that typically involve only healthy young college students. While such devices measure the stated or implied capacities well in this population, the often unstated assumption regarding other involved performance capacities (i.e., that they are available in "normal" amounts) is severely challenged when the subject under test is a member of a population with impairments (e.g., head injured, multiple sclerosis, Parkinson disease, etc.).

A representative instrument [Kondraske et al., 1984; Kondraske, 1990] is illustrated in Figure 78.4. This device incorporates 8 LEDs and 15 high-speed touch sensors ("home," A1–A8 and B1–B6) and a dedicated internal microprocessor to measure an array of different performance capacities associated with information-processing. Measures at the most basic hierarchical level (visual information-processing speed, visual–spatial memory capacity, visual attention span, etc.) and intermediate level (coordination tasks involving different sets of more basic functional units) are included.

For example, visual-upper extremity information-processing speed is measured in a paradigm whereby the test subject first places his/her hand on the "home" plate. A random time after an audible warning

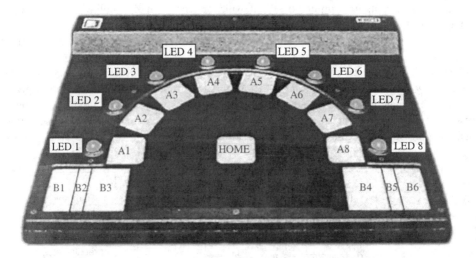

FIGURE 78.4 Major components of a specific microprocessor-based instrument (Human Performance Measurement, Inc. Model BEP I) for measurement of a selected subset of information-processing capacities incorporating high-intensity LEDs for visual stimuli and large contact area, fast touch sensors to acquire responses (made by the upper extremity) from the subject under test (semicircle radius is 15 cm).

cue, one out of eight LEDs (e.g., LED 4) stimulates the subject to respond "as quickly as possible" by lifting his/her hand off the home plate and touching the sensor (e.g., A4) associated with the lighted LED. Each LED represents a binary (ON or OFF) information source. Since an equiprobable selection scheme is employed, the $\log_2$ (# choices) represents the number of bits of information to be processed when determining which LED is lighted. In this example, the number of choices is eight; prior to the test the subject was informed that any one of eight LEDs would be selected. Modes reflecting different information loads (1, 2, 4, or 8 choices) are available. Processing speed (in stimuli per sec) is obtained as a result from each trial by inverting the total processing time, measured as the time from presentation of the stimulus until the subject's hand is lifted off the home plate. By combining time measures from two or more tests with different information loads, a more direct measure of true processing speed in bits per second is obtained. For example, results from an 8-choice (3 bit load) test and a 1-choice test (0 bit load) are combined as follows: $(3 \text{ bits} - 0 \text{ bits})/(t_3 - t_0)$, where t_n is the reaction time measured for an "n" bit information load. This method removes transmission and other time delays not associated with the primary visual information-processing task. Multiple trials are performed (typically, $3 \times$ number of choices, but no less than five trials for any mode) to improve test–retest reliability in the final measures, which are computed by averaging over a fraction (best 80%) of the trials. While even more trials might further improve repeatability of final capacity measures in some subjects, the overall test duration must be considered in light of the desire (from a test design perspective) to minimize stress on attention resources that could vary widely over potential test subjects. Careful trade-offs are necessary.

Visual–spatial memory capacity is measured using the same device. A random sequence of LEDs, beginning with a sequence length of "one," is presented to the subject. The subject responds by contacting (with their preferred hand) the subset of touch sensors (from A1 to A8) corresponding to the LEDs incorporated in a given stimulus presentation, in the same order as the LEDs sequence was presented. A correct response causes a new trial to be initiated automatically with the sequence length increased by one. The maximum length of this sequence (in items) that the subject can repeat without error is used as the measure of visual–spatial memory capacity. The better of two trials is used as a final score. The bright LEDs, relatively large contact area of the touch sensors (5×5 cm^2), and a relatively long poststimulus–response window (up to 10 sec) ensure that other performance resources are minimally stressed.

A measure of visual attention span is obtained with a task in which random LEDs are lighted for 1 sec at random intervals ranging from 4 to 15 sec. After each LED is lighted, a response window is entered (3 sec maximum) during which the subject is required to indicate that a lighted LED was observed by contacting the corresponding touch sensor. The task continues until either the wrong touch sensor is contacted or no response is received within the defined response window. The time (in seconds) from the beginning of the test until an "end of test" criterion is met is used as the measure of visual attention performance capacity. The simple stimuli ensure that higher level cognitive resources are minimally stressed. This allows a wide range of populations to be tested, including young children. Some normal subjects can achieve very long attention spans (e.g., hours) with this specific scenario, while some head-injured subjects (for example) produce times less than 60 sec.

One example of a more comprehensive, computer-based memory performance test battery is that developed by Crook and colleagues [1986]. This battery is directed at older adults, evaluates memory in the visual and auditory modalities at each of the three temporal process levels, and utilizes challenges that relate well to the daily activities of the target group. The challenges (i.e., stimulus sets) are computer generated and controlled, administered by means of a color graphics terminal, and, in some cases, played from a videodisc player to provide as realistic of a stimulus representation as possible outside of using actors in the everyday environment of the subject. The battery takes 60 to 90 min to administer, and provides a profile of scores across the various measurement domains. Extensive age and gender norms are available to scale the scores in terms of percentiles. Despite its scope, it does not provide, nor was it intended to provide, information about modalities other than visual and auditory (e.g., tactile, kinesthetic, or olfactory). It also does not address long-term memory storage beyond about 45 min. (Consider the test administration complexities in doing so.) Nonetheless, it represents one of the most sophisticated memory performance measurement and assessment systems currently available.

78.5   Present Limitations

General methods and associated tools do not exist to quantify the information content of any arbitrary stimulus within a given modality (e.g., visual, auditory, etc.). Success has only been achieved for relatively simple stimuli (e.g., lights which are on or off, at fixed positions spatially, etc.). It can be said, however, that serious attempts to quantify complex stimuli even in one modality appear to be lacking. To the practitioner, this prevents standardization that could occur across many information-processing performance capacity metrics. For example, information-processing speed capacities cannot yet universally be expressed in terms of bits. Perhaps more significantly, this limitation not only impacts looking toward the human and the measurement of intrinsic performance capacities, but also the analysis of information-processing tasks in quantitative terms. This, in turn, has limited the way in which information-processing performance capacity measures can be utilized. Whereas one can measure grip strength available in a subject (a neuromuscular capacity) and also the worst-case grip force required to support turning a door knob, it is not yet possible to determine how much visual information one must process to reach out and find the door knob.

As was also noted, one cannot ideally isolate the systems under test. The required involvement of human sensory and motoric systems also requires the use of ancillary performance tests that establish at least some minimal levels of performance availabilities in these systems (e.g., visual acuity, etc.) in order to lend validity to measures of information-processing performance capacities. New imaging techniques and advanced electroencephalographic and magnetoencephalographic techniques such as brain mapping may offer the basis for new approaches that circumvent in part this limitation. While the cost and practicality of using these techniques routinely is likely to be prohibitive for the foreseeable future, the use of such techniques in research settings to optimize and establish validity of simpler methods can be anticipated.

Moray [1967] was one of many to use the analogy to data and program storage in a digital computer to facilitate understanding of a "limited capacity concept" with regard to human information-processing. In the material presented, emphasis has been placed on the components analogous to those within the realm of computer hardware (i.e., processors and memories). These have been dealt with at their most basic operational levels for testing purposes, attempting to intentionally limit stresses on the test subject's acquired skill (i.e., stored information itself). It has been implied and is argued that knowledge of these hardware system capacities is in itself quite useful (e.g., it is helpful to know whether your desktop computer's basic information-processing rate is 800 MHz or 2 GHz). However, many tasks that humans perform daily, which involve information-processing require not only processing and storage capacities, but also the use of *unique information* acquired in the past (i.e., training or "programs"). These software components, which like processor and memory performance capacities also represent a necessary but not sufficient resource for completion of the specific task at hand, present even greater challenges to evaluation. If the analogy to computer programs is used (or even musical scores, plans, scripts, etc.), it can be observed that even the smallest "programming error" can lead to a failure of the total system in accomplishing its intended purpose with the intended degree of performance. Checking the integrity of human "programs" can be envisioned to be relatively easy if the desired functionality is in fact found to be present. However, if functionality is not present and diagnostic data points to a "software problem," a more difficult challenge is at hand. Methods which can be employed to reveal the source of the error in the basic information itself (i.e., the contents of memory) can be expected to be just as tedious as checking the integrity of code written for digital computers.

Defining Terms

Attention: A performance capacity representing the length of time that an information-processing system can carry out a prescribed task when maximally stressed to do so. This is analogous to endurance in neuromuscular subsystems.

Dual-task scenario: A test paradigm characteristic by a primary and secondary task and measurement of subject performance in both.

Memory: One of two major subsystem types of the human information-processing system that performs the function of storage of information for possible later retrieval and use.

Performance capacity: A quantity in finite availability that is possessed by a system or subsystem, drawn on during the execution of tasks, and limits some aspect (e.g., speed, accuracy, etc.), a system's ability to execute tasks; or, the limit of that aspect itself.

Processor: One of two major subsystems types within the human information-processing system that performs the general function of processing information. Multiple processors at different hierarchical levels can be identified (e.g., those specific to sensory modalities, integrative processors, etc.).

Processor accuracy: The aspect, quality, or dimension of performance of a processor that characterizes the ability to correctly process information.

Processor speed: The aspect, quality, or dimension of performance of an information processor that characterizes the rate at which information is processed.

Prestimulus set: The manner in which an human system is programmed to respond to an ensuing stimulus.

Speed–accuracy trade-off: A fundamental limit of human information-processing systems at any level of abstraction that is most likely due to a more basic limit in channel capacity; that is, channel capacity can be used to achieve more accuracy at the expense of speed or to achieve more speed at the expense of accuracy.

References

Crook, T., Salama, M., and Gobert, J. 1986. A computerized test battery for detecting and assessing memory disorders. In *Senile Dementia: Early Detection*. Eds. Bes, A. et al., pp. 79–85. John Libbey Eurotext.

Donders, F.C. 1868–1869. Over de snelheid van psychische processen. Onderzoekingen gedaan in het Psyiologish Laboratorium der Utrechtsche Hoogeschooll. In *Attention and Performance II*. Ed. W.G. Koster. translated by W.G. Koster. *Acta Psychol.* 30: 412–31.

Fitts, P.M. 1954. The information capacity of the human motor system in controlling the amplitude of movement. *J. Exp. Psychol.* 47: 381–391.

Fitts, P.M. 1966. Cognitive aspects of information processing: III. Set for speed versus accuracy. *J. Exp. Psychol.* 71: 849–857.

Gazzaniga, M.S. *The Social Brain*. Basic Books, Inc., New York.

Green, D.M. and Swets, J.R. 1966. *Signal Detection Theory and Psychophysics*. John Wiley and Sons, Inc., New York.

Hick, W. 1952. On the rate of gain of information. *Q. J. Exp. Psychol.* 4: 11–26.

Hunt, E. 1986. Experimental perspectives: theoretical memory models. In *Handbook for Clinical Memory Assessment of Older Adults*. Ed. Poon, L.W., pp. 43–54. American Psychological Assoc., Washington, D.C.

Hyman, R. 1953. Stimulus information as a determinant of reaction time. *J. Exp. Psychol.* 45: 423–432.

Kahneman, D. 1973. *Attention and Effort*. Prentice-Hall, Englewood Cliffs, NJ.

Kondraske, G.V. 1987. Human performance: science or art. In *Proceedings of 13th Northeast Bioengineering Conference*. Ed. Foster, K.R., pp. 44–47. Institute of Electrical and Electronics Engineers, New York.

Kondraske, G.V., Potvin, A.R., Tourtellotte, W.W. and Syndulko, K. 1984. A computer-based system for automated quantification of neurologic function. *IEEE Trans. Biomed. Eng.* 31: 401–414.

Kondraske, G.V. 1990. A PC-based performance measurement laboratory system. *J. Clin. Eng.* 15: 467–478.

Kondraske, G.V. 1995. A working model for human system–task interfaces. In *Handbook of Biomedical Engineering*. Ed. Bronzino, J.D., CRC Press, Inc., Boca Raton, FL.

Lachman, R., Lachman, J.L., and Butterfield, E.C. 1979. *Cognitive Psychology and Information Processing: An Introduction*. Lawrence Erlbaum Assoc., Hillsdale, NJ.

Minsky, M. 1986. *The Society of Mind*. Simon & Schuster, New York.

Moray N. 1967. Where is capacity limited? A survey and a model. *Acta Psychol.* 27: 84–92.

Neel, A. 1977. *Theories of Psychology: A Handbook*. Schenkman Publishing Co., Cambridge, MA.

Ornstein, R. 1986. *Multimind*. Hougton Mifflin Co., Boston.

Parasuraman, R. and Davies, D.R., Eds. 1984. *Varieties of Attention*. Academic Press, Inc., Orlando, FL.

Posner, M.I. and Boies, S.J. 1971. Components of attention. *Psychol. Rev.* 78: 391–408.

Sanders, M.S. and McCormick, E.J. 1987. *Human Factors in Engineering and Design*. McGraw-Hill, New York.

Schneider, W. and Shiffrin, R.M. 1977. Controlled and automatic human information processing: I. Detection, search, and attention. *Psychol. Rev.* 84: 1–66.

Shannon, C.E. 1948. A mathematical theory of communication. *Bell Syst. Tech. J.* 27: 379–423.

Shiffrin, R.M. and Schneider, W. 1977. Controlled and automatic human information processing: II. Perceptual learning, automatic attending, and a general theory. *Psychol. Rev.* 84: 127–190.

Squire, L.R. and Butters, N. 1992. *Neuropsychology of Memory*. The Guilford Press, New York.

Sternberg, S. 1966. High-speed scanning in human memory. *Science* 153: 652–654.

Syndulko, K., Tourtellotte, W.W., and Richter, E. 1988. Toward the objective measurement of central processing resources. *IEEE Eng. Med. Biol. Soc. Mag.* 7: 17–20.

Wickens, C.D. 1984. *Engineering Psychology and Human Performance*. Charles E. Merrill Publishing, Columbus, OH.

Wickelgren, W.A. 1977. Speed–accuracy tradeoff and information processing dynamics. *Acta Psychol. (North-Holland)* 41: 67–85.

Wiener, N. 1955. *Cybernetics; or, Control and Communications in the Animal and the Machine*. Wiley, New York.

Further Information

A particularly informative, yet concise historical review of the major perspectives in psychology leading up to much of the more recent work involving quantitative measurements of information processing and determination of information-processing capacities is provided in Neel, A. 1977. *Theories of Psychology: A Handbook*, Schenkman Publishing Co., Cambridge, MA.

Human information processing has long been and continues to be a major topic of interest of the U.S. military. Considerable in-depth information and experimental results are available in the form of technical reports, many of which are unclassified. *CSERIAC Gateway*, published by the Crew System Ergonomics Information Analysis Center (CSERIAC), is distributed free of charge and provides timely information on scientific, technical, and engineering knowledge. For subscription information contact AL/CFH/CSERIAC, Bldg. 248, 2255 H St., Wright-Patterson Air Force Base, Ohio, 45433. Also, the North Atlantic Treaty Organization AGAARD (Advisory Group for Aerospace Research & Development) Aerospace Medical Panel Working Group 12, has worked on standards for a human performance test battery for military environments (much of which addresses information processing) and has defined data exchange formats. Documents can be obtained through the National Technical Information Service (NTIS), 5285 Port Royal Road, Springfield, VA 22161, USA.

Information regarding the design, construction, and evaluation of instrumentation (including quantitative attributes of stimuli, etc.) are often embedded in journal articles with titles that emphasis the major question of the study (i.e., not the instrumentation). Most appear in the many journals associated with the fields of psychology, neurology, and neuroscience.

79

High-Level Task Analysis: Cognitive Components

Kenneth J. Maxwell
BMK Consultants

79.1 The Purpose of This Chapter

Effective and safe use of biomedical products requires, among other capabilities, knowledge, interpretive reasoning, attention, and memory. Biomedical products are not alone in these requirements. The integration of information technology (IT) into communications, manufacturing, transportation, power, and medical systems has shifted the predominant activities of many human-performed **tasks** from manual to cognitive. However, biomedical products support health systems and their successful use is often critical. Designers need to understand and accommodate the knowledge and cognitive abilities of users in product design. As a result, data, models, and metrics for describing and understanding **cognitive tasks** and the cognitive capabilities of persons performing them have become very important to engineering design.

Task analysis is a generic term that refers to methods for applying task data to improve engineering design decisions. This chapter presents a process and associated methods for analyzing cognitive tasks (or the **cognitive components** of high-level tasks). It further describes the role of cognitive task analysis along with human performance and machine models (as applicable) in product design, and presents a quantitative, performance-based framework for performing a unified human–machine–task analysis. This chapter is not intended as a review. Selected techniques are presented to familiarize the reader with different major approaches that are currently applied to solving real-world engineering problems.

79.2 Fundamentals

A task is a goal-directed pattern of activities or operations. High-level tasks refer to complex, composite activities or operations that entail performing many simpler but interrelated tasks in meaningful ways [Kirwan and Ainsworth, 1992]. Typically these combinations of low-level tasks are procedural in nature. Performing tasks imposes sensory–perceptual, motor, cognitive, and emotional demands on the agents, persons, or machines performing them that result from the combination of (1) the activities and operations being performed; and (2) the level of performance needed to be achieved.

Task analysis is a process for (1) identifying and breaking down high-level tasks into their constituent, mutually exclusive, lower-level tasks; (2) describing intertask relationships and dependencies; (3) determining task goals and procedures; and (4) specifying task performance and skill requirements.

To the degree that task descriptions are quantified in terms that can be related to models of human performance and skill and to models of machine performance, the design decisions based on the analysis will be better for at least two reasons. First, the designer will be better able to ensure that the performing agents collectively have sufficient performance and skill capabilities. Second, the designer can better control and optimize the distribution, also called allocation, of performance and skill requirements among the performing agents.

79.2.1 Task Levels

Tasks are performed in the context of and to fulfill human purposes. High-level tasks are defined in terms of an applied goal that contributes to satisfying an even higher-level purpose. Low-level tasks combine to accomplish high-level tasks. Figure 79.1 depicts two general tasks: an application task and an interaction task. The interaction task is the set of all interactions between the human and the product. For illustration purposes the figure includes one human interacting with one product, but the more complex systems with many humans interacting among themselves and with many products of various complexities are possible.

In Figure 79.1, the human and product both contribute to performing the application task, and they do this in concert by successfully interacting. The application task represents high-level tasks such as monitoring blood glucose level, retrieving and reviewing a patient's medical history, delivering medications to various hospital departments using a robot, or planning a surgical procedure using simulation systems.

The interaction task includes the set of lower-level interactions that are performed by the human and product to accomplish the application task that may also be at different levels. For example, the application-level goal of reviewing a medical record may involve the interaction-level task of retrieving the record from an electronic database. The retrieval task, in turn, entails lower-level interaction tasks of search that involves the still lower-level task of formulating a proper search query. Each level of tasks may impose cognitive demands.

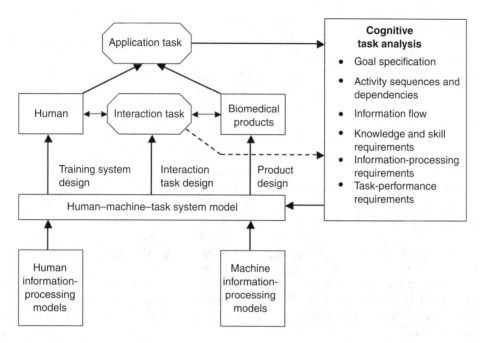

FIGURE 79.1 Task-to-design process flow.

79.2.2 General Analysis-to-Design Process Flow

In addition to the tasks, Figure 79.1 depicts the relationships between task analysis, human and machine models, and design activities. Design is iterative. However, prototyping and testing processes which are essential to the iteration of design are not depicted in Figure 79.1. Also absent are user-profiling activities that should be performed early in the design process and that would compliment the human performance models.

In Figure 79.1, a task analysis at both the application and interaction levels in conducted. The dashed line between the interaction task and the task analysis is meant to indicate that this can only be accomplished if there is an existing product to analyze. In some cases another similar product or product analogue may be useful to analyze.

Task data by themselves are of limited use in design because the task data address only requirements for resources. To be useful in design, task data must be analyzed along with the goals and performance capabilities of the agents (i.e., humans and machines) that will need to perform the tasks. The process of meeting particular task requirements with particular human, machine, and human–machine inter-action resources is called human–machine–task modeling. Design concepts need to be consistent with this model to be successful. As depicted in Figure 79.1, designs applicable for each element flow from this model.

To the degree that the human–machine–task system analysis is coordinated by consistent, or at least relatable, constructs across all elements its effectiveness in guiding good design concepts will increase. Further, the quality and precision of applied decisions are enhanced to the degree that these constructs are quantitative. Schweickart et al. [2003] present a means of generating a quantitative computer-based model of operators performing real-world tasks from the cognitive task analysis. This technique ensures relatedness between the analysis and the model. The **Elemental Resource** Model (ERM) framework [Kondraske, 1995] for human–machine–task system design described later combines the use of task analysis and resource requirement modeling techniques with human performance and machine per-formance models also producing a consistent set of constructs between analysis and models to guide design.

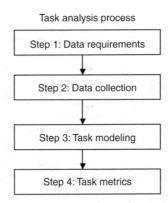

FIGURE 79.2   Task analysis as a four-step process.

79.3   Cognitive Task Analysis: Process and Methods

Figure 79.2 depicts the task-analysis process in four major steps. Before any data are collected, required data should be defined on the basis of the characteristics of the design decisions the analysis is to support. Selection and use of data-collection methods, task models, and task metrics are later informed by these data requirements.

79.3.1   Step 1: Data Requirements Definition

In Step 1, the task data required for the analysis are determined. The major factors involved in determining data needs are (1) the scope of design problems being addressed (i.e., the functional scope of the human–machine–task system being analyzed); (2) the point in the system design process at which the analysis is conducted; and (3) the extent to which the product is new or being revised. Task analysis can be applied to existing systems or to proposed systems for which tasks are in the process of being defined.

Task analysis is used through the different phases and iterations of product development. Different types of task data can be collected as the fidelity of system prototypes progresses and operational systems become available. These differences are apparent by examining three points in the system engineering process at which task analysis is of particular utility.

Predesign: Task data, together with data about human and technology availability and performance, are used to (1) define and allocate tasks, (2) develop procedures to accomplish the tasks, and (3) identify the needed human–machine interfaces. Note that the description of a task depends on the technology assumed. For example, a writing task would be accomplished differently with paper and pencil, a manual typewriter, or a computer with word processing software.

Design phase: During the design phase, task scenarios, prototypes, and simulations are used to detail and refine the task procedures, task requirements, allocation decisions, and human–machine interface design.

Postdevelopment: Analyzing well-defined tasks performed by an operational system provides a detailed description of task procedures and resource requirements that can be used to improve task performance and the system design. For example, Rogers et al. [2001] were able to reveal many sources of errors and design recommendations from their task analysis of a consumer blood glucose meter. Suri [2000] used task and user analyses of an existing defibrillator to identify errors and safety concerns, and as a basis for a new design. Morphew et al. [2001] used cognitive task analysis to understand the cognitive skills needed to safely and effectively maneuver a robotic arm.

The applied purpose of the task analysis has the greatest impact on what type of data are needed. Applications of task analysis vary greatly and include decisions that may or may not involve machines.

Applications include, but are not limited to, those described as follows:

Human–machine task allocation: Allocation of tasks is a major systems-engineering decision. Task analysis is used to identify task load and performance requirements and contributes to assessing workload. Workload assessment provides a basis for assigning task responsibilities to humans and machines such that performance requirements can be satisfied and workload levels are not excessively low or high. These assessments augment qualitative allocation strategies (e.g., Fitts' lists) in which tasks are assigned on judgments of the relative performance capacities of humans and machines on generic tasks. Allocating tasks requires that the resource demands associated with each lower-level task are assessed and that the human and machine resources available can be matched against these at comparable levels of analysis.

In modern human–machine systems, task assignments may be adaptive or blended rather than strictly allocated. The information-processing capabilities of modern machines often includes some form of task knowledge and reasoning capabilities that provide for an adaptive task allocation that shifts the task demands on the basis of contextual variables. Also, in many cases human performance is augmented by (blended with) machine performance to accomplish a given task.

Task–technology tradeoffs: Task analyses may be performed for systems that have yet to be developed but for which functional and performance requirements have been defined. In these cases, the analysis will be based on the defined requirements combined with data on human performance capacities and available machine technology. These analyses can be used to assess the workload, technology, and performance tradeoffs expected with different human–machine system configurations.

Human–machine interface design: Cognitive task analysis provides not only a basis for allocating task responsibilities to humans and machines but can also be used to define display and control requirements for the interface between humans and machines.

Job design: The roles humans satisfy in complex systems and organizations (e.g., manager, operator, maintainer) are generally designed to include many cognitive tasks. By identifying and describing the mental skills and resources required for task performance, task analysis provides a basis for optimizing job performance in new and existing systems.

Personnel selection and job fitness: Cognitive task analysis yields a specification of information-processing resources (e.g., speed, accuracy) required for task performance. This specification can be used in combination with measurements of the available resources an individual possesses. Assessing performance resource sufficiency provides a basis for selecting personnel and determining if injured, rehabilitated personnel are sufficiently recovered to safely return to work.

Training systems development: Task analysis identifies and characterizes the skills, knowledge, and mental capabilities that are necessary or sufficient for task performance. More specifically, it can be used to characterize differences in these abilities and in task performance between experts and novices. These differences serve as a basis for designing effective personnel training systems.

These applications of task analysis reduce to answering the following types of questions:

- What is the best way to structure the task procedures?
- Does a specific individual have the needed cognitive resources to perform the task?
- What knowledge or skills does an individual need to acquire to perform the task with a given technology?
- Can the task be modified to accommodate the special needs of individuals?

When biomedical products or other machines are involved:

- What human and machine combinations are most capable of performing the task?
- How should human and machine components interact in performing the task?

To answer these applied questions, the following data must be defined and described:

- The cognitive demands of the application task (e.g., knowledge, required information-processing activities, speed, and accuracy in performance actions)

- The cognitive capacities of humans in the system (e.g., knowledge, learning ability, processing speed, processing accuracy)

If machines are involved:

- The information-processing capacities of machine components (e.g., knowledge, artificial intelligence, processing speed, algorithms, and data)
- The cognitive demands of the human–machine interaction task
- The human–machine interaction capacities of the humans in the system
- The human–machine interaction capacities of applicable machines

79.3.2 Step 2: Data Collection

Once the required task data are determined, they need to be collected. Table 79.1 lists four generic categories of techniques for acquiring data about cognitive tasks. The categories are not mutually exclusive. For example, all techniques use some form of observation, and instrumented human-interface techniques and **protocol analysis** are used as **knowledge-acquisition** techniques. Each generic category is described in more detail here.

Knowledge-acquisition and elicitation techniques: Knowledge acquisition refers to the process of obtaining the knowledge and reasoning processes needed to perform tasks. **Knowledge elicitation** is the activity of eliciting from persons the knowledge they possess. Initially, elicitation techniques were applied to elicit knowledge from experts for the development of knowledge-based systems. The expert knowledge elicited is only as good as the expert from which it was elicited. Recently, Weiss and Shanteau [2003] have defined three categories of expertise; expert judges, prediction experts, and performance experts and an empirical assessment technique for determining experts. More generally, knowledge-acquisition techniques have been used as a means of analyzing the cognitive components of tasks [Lehto et al., 1992].

TABLE 79.1 Task Data-Collection Techniques

Technique	Data collected	Requirements	Application phase
Knowledge acquisition	Knowledge required to perform tasks	Task performers Interaction instruments, prototypes, and simulations (dependent on techniques used)	All
Protocol analysis	Procedures Strategies Knowledge	Task performers Task scenarios	Design Postdevelopment
Instrumented human interface	Overt human action (e.g., keys pressed)	Task performers Applicable hardware and software	Design Postdevelopment
Observation	Overt machine behaviors Overt human actions Situation state and state changes	Task performers Prototypes or developed systems Monitoring instruments	Design Postdevelopment
Ethnographic design studies	How humans currently perform tasks How humans relate to technology in real-world settings	Real-world contexts Task performers Documentation instruments (e.g., video recorder)	All

Knowledge-acquisition methods include:

- Interviewing techniques
- Event-based knowledge elicitation [Fowlkes et al., 2000]
- Automatic inductive methods that infer and specify knowledge
- Protocol analysis [Ericsson and Simon, 1984]
- Psychological scaling [Cooke and McDonald, 1988]
- Repertory grids from personal construct psychology theory [Boose, 1985]
- Observational techniques [Boy and Nuss, 1988]

See Cooke [1994] for a review of knowledge elicitation techniques.

Protocol analysis: Protocol analysis refers to various techniques for collecting data in the form of verbal reports. In this methodology, persons generate thinking-aloud protocols of the unobservable (i.e., mental) activities they perform while accomplishing a task [Ericsson and Simon, 1984]. The verbal reports represent behavioral descriptions from which task strategies, requirements, procedures, and problem areas can be derived. Protocols provide data on the sequence in which tasks are performed and thus can be used to identify the strategies used by humans in accomplishing tasks that can be accomplished in multiple ways.

There are several issues that need to be considered about the validity of using verbal reports as data and inferring thought processes from them. Ericsson and Simon [1984] address these concerns by demonstrating how verbal protocols are distinct from retrospective responses and classic introspection by trained observers and detailing the methods for collecting and analyzing protocols.

Instrumented human-interface techniques: These techniques are used to passively and unobtrusively collect objective data on task performance and the procedures by instrumenting human–machine interfaces. These techniques are used to record the timing, sequences, and frequencies of explicit actions. These can, for example, model navigation through a website using search and hyperlink actions or the low-level actions that are done to accomplish the navigation such as keystrokes, button pushes, mouse movements.

The data associated with actions can be used to infer workload and to study the frequency of actions, their temporal relationships, and human error. Although these data are objective, they are restricted to overt responses and, by themselves, do not provide a basis for analyzing cognitive components. Modeling the cognitive task components involves correlating these action data with data about the situations and system behavior that elicited the actions and the changes in the situations and system state caused by the actions, that is, knowledge of context is vital to properly interpreting interactions.

Observation techniques: Observation is a generic term referring to many techniques that can use a wide range of instruments to monitor situations and the behavior of systems and task performers. Two types of observation are distinguished. In direct observation, a human observer is with the task performer as he or she performs the task. In indirect observation, a human observer monitors the task performer remotely with audio and visual monitoring systems. Indirect observation can be done as the task is being performed or after the fact by using a recording. Observation techniques may be unobtrusive or invasive, record subjective or objective data, and may be used in controlled testing or real-world environments.

Ethnographic design studies: These are in-the-field studies that have been adopted from anthropology research. The researchers are embedded to some level with the users and garner data on how they interact in real life with the products or systems under study or similar products or systems or to identify the need for such products. In an ethnographic study of independent elders, Forlizzi et al. [2004] identified two groups of elders, (1) well and (2) declining, based in part by cognitive factors identified during the study.

79.3.3 Steps 3 and 4: Data Modeling and Metric Computation

Steps 3 and 4 are the actual analysis steps. In Step 3, the task data are modeled in accordance with a selected modeling method. This task model is employed in Step 4 to compute various task metrics that are

TABLE 79.2   Analytic Techniques for Modeling Tasks

Technique	Modeled dimensions/characteristics	Analysis
Task–time line analysis	Temporal onset, duration, and concurrences	Task-load estimates Task complexity
GOMS, NGOMSL, and keystroke-level analysis	Task and system knowledge required by task performers Overt low-level actions Procedures Temporal relationships	Task complexity Knowledge requirements Performance estimates from production rule simulation
Task-action grammar	Task and system knowledge required by task performers Observable low-level actions Action sequences	Task complexity Task consistency Knowledge requirements
Fleishman and Quaintance's cognitive task taxonomy	Identifies 23 cognitive abilities underlying task performance. Tasks are modeled in terms of required abilities	Cognitive ability requirements Performance requirements
Rasmussen's cognitive task analysis	Generic activities, knowledge states, and dependencies in cognitive task performance	Knowledge requirements Task complexity
Knowledge-representation techniques	Task and System knowledge required by task performers	Knowledge requirements
Elemental resource model	Mental resources needed to perform tasks Resources are defined in terms of function and performance requirements	Functional requirements Performance requirements

useful in solving the applied problem. Table 79.2 lists seven major approaches for analyzing the cognitive components of tasks. Each has been shown to be useful in applied decision making, and each is described here. For an extended review of techniques, see Linton et al. [1989].

Task–timeline analysis: Timeline analysis organizes and relates low-level tasks on the basis of their time of onset, duration, and concurrences in the context of performing a high-level task. Any **task taxonomy** or decomposition model can be used to define the lower-level tasks that will be mapped to the high-level **task timeline**. Generally, the task–timeline mapping is constructed by decomposing a high-level task in terms of specific scenarios because different scenarios can have very different task and time requirements.

This technique is useful for analyzing workload, allocating tasks, and determining human and system performance requirements. When the resource requirements for each lower-level task are mapped to the timeline, the result is a dynamic task-demand profile.

Wickens [1984] discusses two limitations of timeline analysis. First, the technique often does not account for time-sharing capabilities in which the performance of multiple tasks can be accomplished efficiently when resource demands are low. Second, the technique is most effective when analyzing forced-pace activities. The more freedom the human has to schedule activities, the harder it is to construct a useful timeline.

GOMS and NGOMSL analysis: GOMS, an acronym for goals, operators, methods, and selection rules [Card et al., 1983, 1986], is an analytic technique for modeling (1) the knowledge about a task and a machine that a task performer must possess and (2) the operations that a task agent must execute in order to accomplish the task using the machine. It is based on work by Newell and Simon [1972] in human problem solving. The model was extended by Kieras [1988] into NGOMSL (for natural GOMS language), which affords a more detailed analysis and specification of tasks. In both GOMS and NGOMSL goals represent what a human is trying to accomplish. Operators are elementary perceptual, cognitive, or motor acts that may be observable or unobservable. Methods are sequences of operations that accomplish a goal. Selection rules are criteria used to select one method to apply when many methods are available.

The NGOMSL analysis uses this model to predict quantitative measures of the complexity of the knowledge required to perform a task with a system. These measures include learning time, amount of transfer, and task execution time. To accomplish this, methods (i.e., procedural knowledge) are represented in the form of production rules. These are IF–THEN rules that describe knowledge in approximately equal-sized units. The number of rules needed to represent a task provides a measure of the complexity of that task. Time predictions are obtained by modeling the production rules in a computer program that stimulates the tasks being analyzed.

The keystroke-level task model is an abbreviated application of the GOMS analysis [Card et al., 1983] that models only the overt actions (i.e., the observable operators and methods) taken by the task performer. In this way it does not require the inferences about mental processes required by the full GOMS approach. The model was developed with regard to a computer system and defines six operators: a keystroke or mouse button push, pointing using a mouse, moving the mouse, moving hands between the mouse and keyboard, mental preparation, and system response. Tasks are modeled by identifying the sequence of operators needed to perform the task.

Task-action grammar analysis: Task-action grammar (TAG) [Payne and Green, 1986; Schiele and Green, 1990] is a formalism for modeling the knowledge required to perform simple tasks with a given system. Task knowledge is represented as sequences of simple acts. Similarities in the syntactic representation of simple tasks are used to derive higher-level schemas that apply across tasks possessing a family resemblance. The ability to derive schemas is used to assess the consistency of the tasks performed with a given user interface and has implications for ease of learning and overall usability. In similarity with NGOMSL, the number of grammatical rules and schemas provides a quantitative measure of task and interface complexity.

Rasmussen's cognitive task analysis: Rasmussen [1986] and Rasmussen and Goodstein [1988] define a framework for cognitive task analysis that was derived from an analysis of human–machine interaction in process-control tasks. One element of this framework is a schematic structure for describing cognitive tasks and information requirements. The schematic structure includes a sequence of (1) information-processing activities, (2) states of knowledge resulting from performing the information-processing activities, and (3) conditions (related to the experience of the human performing the task) that allow the processing sequence to be shortened. This structure constitutes a generic processing task model into which specific task data can be mapped. The information-processing activities are:

- Detecting a need for action
- Observing relevant data
- Identifying the present system state
- Interpreting the present system state
- Evaluating possible consequences of this state with reference to a goal
- Defining a desired target state
- Formulating procedures to achieve the desired state
- Executing the actions required by the procedures

Fleishman and quaintance's cognitive task taxomy: Task taxonomies classify tasks on the basis of various characteristics and properties. As such, they can serve a useful purpose in modeling tasks. Tasks of the same taxonomic classification will have similar characteristics and similar requirements. This inference provides a basis for efficiently creating models for analyzed tasks. Fleishman and Quaintance [1984] provide an extensive review of taxonomies of human performance and identify four classifications (1) behavior descriptions, (2) behavior requirements, (3) ability requirements, and (4) task characteristics. They further detail a taxonomy of human abilities that identifies 23 cognitive factors underlying task performance. These factors were derived from an analysis of empirical performance data collected from a large number of diversified tasks and individuals. The factors constitute a structure for modeling cognitive tasks. That is, these factors can be mapped onto specific tasks and thus specify the cognitive abilities needed to perform the task.

Knowledge-representation techniques: Knowledge representation is a generic term that refers to several formalisms for modeling knowledge about tasks, systems, and the physical environment. Major representation schemes include production rules, frames, scripts, and cases. Production rules represent knowledge as a set of condition–consequence (i.e., IF–THEN) associations. The Executive Process-Interactive Control (EPIC) cognitive architecture incorporates a cognitive processor implemented as a production rule system with an associated working memory [Kieras and Meyer, 1997; Hornoff, 2004]. Barnard & May [1999] present a unified cognitive architecture based on interacting cognitive subsystems. The architecture incorporates two approaches, one of which implements cognitive activity as a production rule system.

Frames, scripts, and cases are different forms of schemas that represent knowledge as typical stereotypical chunks. Rules and scripts generally represent procedural knowledge, while frames and cases represent declarative knowledge. By formally representing data acquired from knowledge-acquisition techniques, a model of the procedural and declarative knowledge required to perform a task is created.

Elemental resource analysis of tasks: The ERM [Kondraske, 1995] defines human performance in terms of the performance and skill resources (capacities) that a human or system possesses and which can be brought to bear in performing tasks. Elemental resources are defined at a low level such that many of them may be required to perform a high-level task. In addition, intermediate-level resources are defined to provide task-analysis targets at a less granular (i.e., higher hierarchical) level. In this model, a resource is defined as a paired construct consisting of a functional capability (e.g., visual–word recognition) combined with a performance capability (e.g., recognition speed). Thus, even though the functional capability is the same, visual–word-recognition speed and visual–word-recognition accuracy are defined as two distinct resources because they model two distinct dimensions of performance. This model can be applied in task analysis by decomposing the mental components of a task in terms of the resources that a human or system performing them is required to process.

79.4   Models of Human Cognitive Processing and Performance

The analysis of task data by themselves is of limited use in solving applied problems because task data address only one side of the design problem, that is, requirements. For example, a task–timeline analysis provides a model from which a measure of task demand can be computed. However, this analysis does not indicate whether the task load is acceptable or how it could be optimally distributed among humans and machines. Making these judgments requires consideration of human and machine capabilities. Similarly, using the NGOMSL and TAG models, a measure of task complexity can be computed, indicating that one task or procedure is more complex than another. However, these judgments are based solely on the number of task steps and the amount of information needed to perform each step and do not consider how difficult each step is for a human or machine to perform.

Using these task models without incorporating human and machine models forces a general assumption that task difficulty is a linear function of complexity (modeled as more task-steps or information requirements). Even with this assumption, the task model by itself provides no indication of the acceptability of the task complexity or expected human or machine performance. Both these judgments require considerations of human and machine processing and performance models.

Because of these issues, task analysis is used in combination with human and machine models to make design decisions. Using task, human, and machine models in concert requires that the cognitive components being modeled are described in consistent, or at least relatable, terms. Further, the quality and precision of the decision will be enhanced to the degree that the task model describes requirements quantitatively, while the human and machine models describe their capabilities quantitatively.

Five models of human cognitive processes and performance are listed in Table 79.3 and discussed below. These were selected because they (1) describe concepts that are generally applicable to a wide range

TABLE 79.3 Models of Human Cognitive Processes and Performance

Model	Description	Modeled components
Multiple resource model of attention and W/INDEX	Models attention as a collection of separable processing resources. W/INDEX is a computer model of workload that adopts the multiple-resource construct and accounts for resource conflict from concurrent processing	Identifies separable processing resources Time-sharing ability Automatic processing
Model human processor (HMP)	Models human information processing in terms of processing subsystems, memories, and performance parameters	Performance is modeled by assigning time values to the model's parameters Perceptual, cognitive, motor processing subsystems Long-term and working memories
Keystroke-level performance model	Models the performance (i.e., time) estimated for executing each of six defined actions, from which overall estimated task completion times can be computed	Performance is modeled by assigning time values to each of six modeled actions
Skills, rules, and knowledge model	Models human information processing in terms of three levels of behavioral control: skill based, rule based, and knowledge based	Models the processes and requirements for each level of behavior Can be used with quantitative models of human performance to estimate task time and errors
Technique for human error-rate prediction (THERP)	Structure methodology for modeling human error and task completion in terms of probabilities	Predicts human error and task completion probabilities using a human performance database and expert judgments
Elemental resource model of human and system performance (ERM)	Models human and system performance in terms of basic elements of performance and elemental resources	Performance is modeled in terms of elemental units that can be combined to provide estimates of high-level task performance and completability
ACT-R	Models perceptual and cognitive learning and performance. A set of parameters, each of which control a specific behavior, are set to match task data	Quantitative aspects of task learning and performance

of information-processing tasks and (2) are engineering-oriented models for use on applied problems. Connectionist (e.g., neural network) models [Rumelhart and McClelland, 1986; Schneider and Detweiller, 1987] and the optimal control model [Barron and Kleinman, 1969], which represent major but different approaches to modeling human processing, are intentionally not included due to space constraints.

79.4.1 Multiple-Resource Model of Attention and W/INDEX

In psychology, resource models of attention attribute the capability to perform the mental components of tasks to the capacity of applicable and available processing resources, time-sharing skills, and automatic processes. Attention is modeled as either a single processing resource or multiple, separable processing resources. In these models, the processing resource or resources afford a capacity to perform information-processing tasks (e.g., perception, cognition, and response selection) but have limited availability. The definition of resources here is different from that used in the ERM, which formally includes a specific performance dimension as part of the definition of a performance resource, which is distinguished from the system itself.

Norman and Bobrow [1975] adopted a single-resource model to examine the theoretical relationships between the application of the resource and performance on a single and multiple tasks. For a given task, performance may be limited by insufficient processing resources (resource-limited) or by insufficient data (data-limited). In multitask situations, a human performing the tasks is assumed to be capable of controlling the allocation of a portion of the processing resource to each task. Different allocation strategies result in different relative performance on each task. The relationship between allocation strategies and relative performance is plotted on a graph called the performance–operating characteristic. Automated processing (e.g., skill-based) is assumed not to require processing resources.

The multiple-resource model of attention [Navon and Gopher, 1979; Wickens, 1980, 1984] extends and specifies the resource concept by identifying several separate processing resources that are exclusive to a subset of activities. Results of numerous dual-task studies were used to distinguish separable resources. The model identifies different resource structures for verbal and auditory modalities, spatial and verbal codes, manual and vocal responses, and between (1) selection and execution of responses and (2) perceptual and central processing stages.

W/INDEX, for workload index [North and Riley, 1989], is a computer model for predicting operator workload that uses the multiple-resource construct and accounts for time-sharing skills. A task–timeline combined with a design model that differentiates different interface channels (e.g., visual or auditory, manual or verbal) is used to compile an interface activity matrix. This matrix specifies, by subjective ratings, the amount of attention the task demands for each channel. A conflict matrix is generated with respect to each design channel that specifies a penalty resulting when the operator must attend simultaneously to multiple channels. The W/INDEX algorithm is then applied to these data resulting in a workload profile.

79.4.2 The Model Human Processor

Model human processor (MHP) [Card et al., 1983, 1986] defines three interacting processing subsystems: perceptual, cognitive, and motor. The perceptual and cognitive subsystems include memories. Within each subsystem, processing parameters (e.g., perceptual processor, long-term memory, visual-image memory, and eye movements) and metrics (e.g., capacity, speed, and decay rate) are defined. Using data from numerous empirical studies, the MHP defines typical and range values for 19 parameters. To apply the model, processing parameters are associated with an analysis of the steps involved in accomplishing a task with a given system. Values for each parameter are assigned and summed, providing time estimates for task completion.

79.4.3 Skills, Rules, and Knowledge Model

Rasmussen [1983, 1986] developed a three-level model for describing qualitatively different modes of human information processing. Skill-based processing describes sensorimotor performance that is accomplished without conscious control. The behavior exhibited is smooth, automated, and integrated and only moderately based on feedback from the environment. Skill-based processes are generally simple automated behaviors, but they can be combined by higher-level conscious processes into long sequences to fit complex situations. Rule-based processing describes performance that is goal directed and consciously controlled in a feed-forward manner from stored rules that have been developed from experience. Rule-based processing does not use feedback control.

Knowledge-based processing is the highest level and applies to unfamiliar situations for which rules are available. Performance is goal controlled and conscious. The goal and plans need to be explicitly developed, and reasoning is accomplished with knowledge (i.e., a mental model) of the system and environment.

This three-level model can be directly related to Rasmussen's framework for cognitive task analysis. Knowledge-based processing requires performing all the activities in the framework. Rule-based processing provides a means to bypass activities by applying rules that have been stored from familiarity. Skill-based processing provides a means to go directly from detection to execution. Thus the processing required is a function of the experience of the task performer and the nature of the task.

79.4.4 Technique for Human Error-Rate Prediction

The technique for human error-rate prediction (THERP) [Swain and Guttmann, 1980] is a widely applied human reliability method [Meister, 1984] used to predict human error rates (i.e., probabilities) and the consequences of human errors. The method relies on conducting a task analysis. Estimates of the likelihood of human errors and the likelihood that errors will be undetected are assigned to tasks from available human performance databases and expert judgments. The consequences of uncorrected errors are estimated from models of the system. An event tree is used to track and assign conditional probabilities of error throughout a sequence of activities.

79.4.5 ACT-R

The ACT-R architecture developed by Anderson is the basis for much work in cognitive modeling. See Anderson and Matessa [1998] for an in depth discussion of the model. It uses both procedural and declarative representations and incorporates many parameters that can be set to optimize the fit to task data. ACT-R can be used to model individual task performance as well as average performance [Rehling et al., 2004].

79.4.6 Elemental Resource Model of Human Performance

Elemental resource model [Kondraske, 1995] was discussed briefly in the preceding section as a task-analysis technique. That discussion addressed how the ERM uses the same quantitative modeling construct (i.e., elemental performance resources) for task requirements and human capabilities. Major classes of resources include motor, environmental (i.e., sensing), central processing (i.e., perception and cognition), and skills (i.e., knowledge). Central processing and information (skill) resources are of interest in this chapter. When applied to humans or to machines (i.e., agents that perform tasks), the ERM describes the perceptual, cognitive, and knowledge resources available to the agent. If the agent has a deficiency in any of these elemental resources, a task requiring that resource cannot be completed by the agent. In this case, agents with sufficient resources need to be selected, agents with insufficient resources need to be trained, or the task goals or procedures need to be modified to accommodate the resources available to the agents targeted to perform the task. ERM derives from a broader theory of general systems performance theory (GSPT) developed by Kondraske.

Gettman et al. [2003] report an application of this performance model to laparoscopic surgery. In this study, the relationships between objective measures of human basic performance resources (BPRs) and laparoscopic performance were evaluated using Nonlinear Causal Resource Analysis (NCRA), a novel predictive and explanatory modeling approach based on GSPT. Results suggest promise in predicting laparoscopic performance, and thus the predictive power of applying such analysis and modeling strategies in design.

79.5 Models of Machine Processing Capabilities

Table 79.4 describes models of machine and performance. These models vary greatly in scope and detail. They are presented to illustrate that quantitative analysis of performance resources using the ERM extends to machine capabilities. These models are not elaborated further.

79.6 A Human–Machine–Task Analytic Framework

Making applied decisions involves performing a combined human–machine–task analysis of available and required mental capacities. This analysis (1) requires that the mental components of tasks, the mental capabilities of humans, and the information-processing capabilities of machines be modeled and analyzed in compatible and consistent terms and (2) is greatly enhanced if the terms are quantitative. From the

TABLE 79.4   Models of Machine Processes and Capabilities

Machine model	Description	Components/parameters
Process models	This refers to a category of models that describe the flow of information and the process performed on information through a system. It is useful for determining the consequences of failures in THERP	Flow Transformations Dependencies Normal performance
Principles of operation models	In this category machines are modeled in terms models of their operating principles. These are also useful for determining the consequences of failures needed to apply THERP	Physical properties Mathematic formulas Mathematic relationships Logical relationships Normal range of performance
Human interaction models	In this category the characteristics of the machine side of the human–machine interface are modeled	Physical properties Information content Information display format Performance metrics
Rasmussen's abstraction hierarchy	Developed for modeling process systems. Provides a task-independent description of systems at five levels	Hierarchy levels that include process, operation, and interaction descriptions
ERM	Models machines in terms of the performance resources they possess. Resource definition is consistent across task, human, and machine domains	Elemental information-processing performance resources available to the machine

techniques and models described above for task analysis and human and machine models, a methodology for a unified, quantitative human–machine–task analysis of mental components is described.

The approach first quantifies task requirements by combining techniques that produce detailed task-decomposition analyses of goals, actions, and required procedures (e.g., GOMS, NGOMSL, TAG, keystroke-level task model, or Rasmussen's cognitive framework) with timeline analysis, where applicable, and the elementary resource analysis of tasks. The task-decomposition models are used to specify tasks at a level at which the elemental mental resources required to perform the tasks can be specified. The timeline provides a basis for specifying performance requirements. Other performance dimensions too should be used depending on the task.

The next step employs quantitative models of human performance and technology to reach an applied decision that best satisfies the required resources if sufficient resources are available. If sufficient resources are not available, additional performance and skill resources need to be obtained to complete the task, or the task requirements need to be reduced. Quantitative models of human performance include MHP, THERP, and ERM. Using the MHP, the human processing parameters needed for each task operation are identified. The time values assigned to each parameter are used to compute task time estimates. This approach is limited to estimating performance in terms of time. THERP maps operations to the tasks included in human reliability databases to estimate human error probabilities. The ERM provides a framework for specifying performance and functional capacities at the resource level. It is the only model that (1) incorporates all required dimensions of performance and skills and (2) uses consistent modeling constructs across tasks, humans, and machines.

Using the approach outlined above establishes a basis for making applied decisions objectively. The task-analysis portion of this approach is illustrated by the following example.

79.7 Brief Example: Analysis of Supervisory Control Task

Supervisory control refers to the role a human plays in operating a semiautomatic process or system. Examples include control of large systems such as a nuclear power plant and specific instrumentation such as a robotic or assistive device. Performing supervisory control is high-level task that predominantly consists of mental components. This task is used to generically illustrate the use of analytic techniques to model a task.

79.7.1 High-Level Goals

Two major modes of operation are distinguished [Wickens, 1984]. In one mode (normal), the system is behaving as expected. The primary role of the human controller is to monitor system activity and modify performance parameters in accordance with planned output goals. In the second mode (fault), the system is faulty. The goal of the human controller, in this case, is to detect and diagnose the fault and intervene to bring the process back into normal performance.

79.7.2 Task Decomposition and Procedures

Sheridan [1987] identifies 10 functions performed by a supervisory controller within these modes of operation. Rasmussen's cognitive task framework, which was developed with regard to process-control tasks, includes 8 functions applicable to the fault mode of operation. Figure 79.3 depicts these 8 generic functions as a top-level breakdown of the supervisory-control task in fault mode. For this example, only selected tasks are decomposed to lower levels. At each level, the decomposition is not intended to be complete. Selected tasks at each level are intended to be illustrative and representative of increasingly specific and simple tasks. The arrow within each level provides procedural information. The goals of the lower-level tasks are defined by their titles (e.g., acquire data). Only the situation-interpretation task is decomposed. In reference to Rasmussen's human information-processing model, the task is assumed to be knowledge based. The lower-level tasks represent a hypothesis-testing strategy for knowledge-based diagnosis described by Rasmussen and Goodstein [1988]. However, other models of lower-level tasks could be used. Note that although a Rasmussen model is illustrated, the decomposition could be accomplished with other applicable models (e.g., GOMS).

79.7.3 Required Resources

Of the task-modeling techniques presented above, only Fleishman and Quaintance's cognitive abilities taxonomy and the ERM provide for explicit analysis of required resources. The approach defined by the ERM is illustrated in this example because it defines similar analyses for human and machine performance. As such, it is the only technique that models all three components of a human–machine–task system in the same way. For three of the lowest-level tasks, a set of elemental central processing resources is identified. Humans or machines responsible for performing each task are required to possess these resources to accomplish the task successfully. Four types of elemental mental resources are identified: knowledge, memory, perception, and reasoning. Resources are distinguished by their functional type and the performance dimension they specify. In the example, the performance dimensions are generically identified. In application, values should be assigned to these dimensions to the degree they are available or obtainable. Given time and cost constraints for the analysis, the ability to quantify all resources may not be practical. Task priorities can be used to selectively quantify resources, or the resource model can be used less rigorously as a guide to decision making if specific data are not available [Maxwell, 1995]. Once values are assigned, these required resources can be analyzed in concert with sets of available resources possessed by humans and machines. Available resources will have values that indicate a performance capability.

Although the MHP is a human processing and performance model, it can be adapted for use in a way analogous to the way the ERM is used in task analysis. The MHP would be applied as usual by identifying the processing parameters needed to accomplish each low-level task. However, instead of using the human

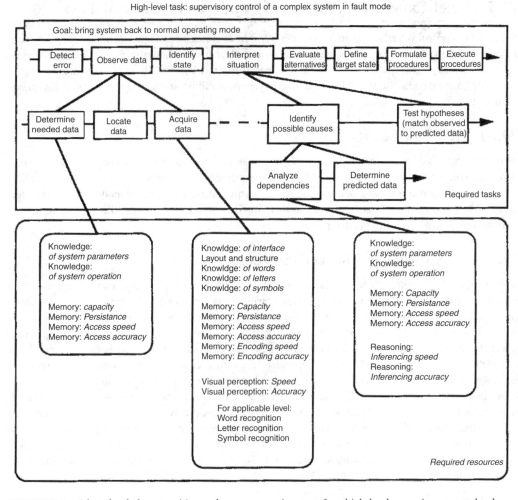

FIGURE 79.3   Selected task decomposition and resource requirements for a high-level supervisory control task.

performance values associated with these parameters, time values required by the task would be derived and assigned. These required times could then be compared with the estimated human performance times available for these low-level tasks to determine the sufficiency of human processing to meet the task's requirements.

79.7.4 Performance Assessment

After the task is specified, human and machine performance models can be applied to estimate task performance. The MHP and keystroke-level performance model can provide task performance estimates in terms of task completion time. THERP can be used to estimate human error probabilities for each task and task sequence. The ERM approach can be used to estimate performance along any required dimension and to compare required with available resources along any required dimension as long as the human performance data are available. The results of the ERM assessment would identify stress levels on capacities (e.g., resources stressed too long or beyond maximum capacity). These results indicate limiting factors to successful task performance. Limiting factors can be identified at elemental or intermediate performance resource levels. As such, the ERM represents a more comprehensive and internally consistent model than the others. It is more comprehensive in that it can be used to model any performance dimension. It is more consistent in that (1) all resources are defined in similar terms, (2) all resources are defined at the same level of description, and (3) resource requirements for tasks and resources available to humans and machines are all defined identically.

Defining Terms

Cognitive components: The perceptual, cognitive, and knowledge-processing components of a task.

Cognitive tasks: Tasks that consist predominantly of mental components and, in ERM terms, require mental performance and skill resources to perform.

Elemental resource: These consist of performance and skill resources. Performance resources are each defined as a couplet consisting of an elementary functional capability associated with a low-level unidimensional quantitative capacity, either available or required, to perform the function. Skill resources are defined in terms of the knowledge, either available or required, to perform an elemental function.

Knowledge acquisition and elicitation: Any of several techniques for obtaining knowledge about a task or system or eliciting it from a human.

Protocol analysis: Protocols are verbal reports generated contemporaneously by a person accomplishing a task that describe the unobservable (mental) processes being performed.

Task: A goal-directed, procedural activity that is defined with regard to the resources (i.e., capabilities) that performing agents (i.e., humans or machines) must possess to accomplish the goal.

Task analysis: The process of (1) decomposing high-level tasks into their constituent, mutually exclusive, lower-level tasks; (2) describing intertask relationships and dependencies; and (3) defining each task's goals, procedures, and performance and skill requirements.

Task taxonomy: A classification of tasks in accordance with a defined method, strategy, or set of criteria.

Task timeline: A time-based profile of a high-level task that maps its lower-level tasks by time-of-onset, duration, and concurrences onto a timeline.

References

Anderson, J.R. and Matessa, M. 1998. The rational analysis of categorization and the ACT-R architecture. In M. Oaksford and N. Chater (Eds.), *Rational Models of Cognition*, pp. 197–217. Oxford, Oxford University Press.

Barnard, P.J. and May, J. 1999. Representing cognitive activity in complex tasks. *Hum. Comput. Interact.* 14: 93–158.

Barron, S. and Kleinman, D.L. 1969. The human as an optimal controller and information processor. *IEEE Trans. Man-Mach. Syst.* MMS-10: 9.

Boose, J.H. 1985. A knowledge acquisition program for expert systems based on personal construct psychology. *Int. J. Man-Mach. Stud.* 23: 495.

Boy, G. and Nuss, N. 1988. Knowledge acquisition by observation: application to intelligent tutoring systems. In *Proceedings of the Second European Knowledge Acquisition Workshop* (EKAW-88), pp. 11.1–11.14.

Card, S.K., Moran, T.P., and Newell, A. 1983. *The Psychology of Human–Computer Interaction*. Hillsdale, NJ, Erlbaum.

Card, S.K., Moran, T.P., and Newell, A. 1986. The model human processor. In K.R. Boff, L. Kaufman, and J.P. Thomas (Eds.), *Handbook of Perception and Human Performance*, Vol. II, pp. 45-1–45-35.

Cooke, N.J. 1994. Varieties of knowledge elicitation techniques. *Int. J. Hum. Comput. Stud.* 41: 801–849.

Cooke, N.M. and McDonald, J.E. 1988. The application of psychological scaling techniques to knowledge elicitation for knowledge-based systems. In J.H. Boose and B.R. Gaines (Eds.), *Knowledge-Based Systems, Vol. 1: Knowledge Acquisition for Knowledge-Based Systems*, pp. 65–82. New York, Academic Press.

Ericsson, K.A. and Simon, H.A. 1984. *Protocol Analysis*. Cambridge, MA, MIT Press.

Fleishman, E.A. and Quaintance, M.K. 1984. *Taxonomies of Human Performance: The Description of Human Tasks.* Orlando, FL, Academic Press.

Forlizzi, J., DiSalvo, C., and Gemperle, F. 2004. Assistive robots and an ecology of elders living independently in their homes. *Hum. Comput. Interact.* 19: 25.

Fowlkes, J.E., Salas, E., Baker, D.P., Canon-Bowers, J.A., and Stout, R.J. 2000. The utility of event-based knowledge elicitation. *Hum. Factors* 42: 1.

Gettman, M.T., Kondraske, G.V., Traxer, O., Ogan, K., Napper, C., Jones, D.B., Pearle, M.S., and Cadeddu, J.A. 2003. Assessment of basic human performance resources predicts operative performance of laparoscopic surgery. *J. Am. Coll. Surg.* 197: 489–496.

Hornoff, A.J. 2004. Cognitive strategies for the visual search of hierarchical computer displays. *Hum.-Comput. Interact.* 19: 3.

Kieras, D.E. 1988. Towards a practical GOMS model methodology for user interface design. In M. Helander (Ed.), *Handbook of Human–Computer Interaction,* pp. 135–157. New York, Elsevier Science Publishers.

Kieras, D.E. and Meyer, D.E. 1997. An overview of the EPIC architecture for cognition and performance with application to human–computer interaction. *Hum. Comput. Interact.* 12: 4.

Kirwan, B. and Ainsworth, L.K. 1992. *A Guide to Task Analysis.* London, Taylor & Francis.

Kondraske, G.V. 1995. A working model of human–system–task interfaces. In J.D. Bronzino (Ed.), *The Biomedical Engineering Handbook.* Boca Raton, FL, CRC Press.

Lehto, M.R., Boose, J., Sharit, J., and Salvendy, G. 1992. Knowledge acquisition. In G. Salvendy (Ed.), *Handbook of Industrial Engineering,* 2nd ed. New York, Wiley.

Linton, P.M., Plamondon, B.D., Dick, A.O. et al. 1989. Operator workload for military system acquisition. In G.R. McMillan et al. (Eds.), *Applications of Human Performance Models to System Design,* pp. 21–46. New York, Plenum Press.

Maxwell, K.M. 1995. Human–computer interface design issues. In J.D. Bronzino (Ed.), *The Biomedical Engineering Handbook,* pp. 2263–2277. Boca Raton, FL, CRC Press.

Meister, D. 1984. Human reliability. In F.A. Muckler (Ed.), *Human Factors Review,* pp. 13–54. Santa Monica, CA, Human Factors and Ergonomics Society.

Morphew, M.E., Balmer, D.V., and Khourt, G.J. 2001. Human performance in space. *Ergon. Des.* 9: 4.

Navon, D. and Gopher, D. 1979. On the economy of the human processing system. *Psychol. Rev.* 86.

Newell, A. and Simon, H. 1972. *Human Problem Solving.* Englewood Cliffs, NJ, Prentice-Hall.

Norman, D. and Bobrow, D. 1975. On data-limited and resource-limited processing. *J. Cogn. Psychol.* 7: 44.

North, R.A. and Riley, V.A. 1989. W/INDEX: a predictive model of operator workload. In G.R. McMillan et al. (Eds.), *Applications of Human Performance Models to System Design,* pp. 81–90. New York, Plenum Press.

Payne, S.J. and Green, T. 1986. Task-action grammars: a model of mental representation of task languages. *Hum. Comput. Interact.* 2: 93.

Rasmussen, J. 1983. Skills, rules, and knowledge: signals, signs, and symbols and other distinctions in human performance models. *IEEE Trans. Syst. Man. Cybern.* SMC-13: 257.

Rasmussen, J. 1986. *Information Processing and Human–Machine Interaction.* New York, North-Holland.

Rasmussen, J. and Goodstein, L.P. 1988. Information technology and work. In M. Helander (Ed.), *Handbook of Human–Computer Interaction,* pp. 175–201. New York, Elsevier Science Publishers.

Rehling, J., Lovett, M., Lebiere, C., Reder, L.M., and Demiral, B. 2004. Modeling complex tasks: an individual difference approach. In *Proceedings of the 26th Annual Conference of the Cognitive Science Society,* pp. 1137–1142. August 4–7, Chicago, IL, USA.

Rogers, W.A., Mykityshyn, A.L., Cambell, R.H., and Fisk, A.D. 2001. Analysis of a "simple" medical device. *Ergon. Des.* 9: 1.

Rumelhart, D.E. and McClelland, J.L. 1986. *Parallel Distributed Processing, Explorations in the Microstructure of Cognition, Vol. I: Foundations.* Cambridge, MA, MIT Press.

Schiele, F. and Green T. 1990. HCI formalisms and cognitive psychology: the case of task-action grammar. In M. Harrison and H. Thimbleby (Eds.), *Formal Methods in Human–Computer Interaction*, pp. 9–62. Cambridge, U.K., Cambridge University Press.

Schneider, W. and Detweiller, M. 1987. A connectionist/control architecture for working memory. In G.H. Bower (Ed.), *The Psychology Learning and Motivation*, Vol. 21, pp. 53–119. Orlando, FL, Academic Press.

Schweickert, R., Fisher, D.L., and Proctor, R.W. 2003. Steps toward building mathematical and computer models from cognitive task analysis. *Hum. Factors* 45: 1.

Sheridan, T.B. 1987. Supervisory control. In G. Salvendy (Ed.), *Handbook of Human Factors*, New York, Wiley.

Suri, J.F. 2000. Saving lives through design. *Ergon. Des.* 8: 3.

Swain, A.D. and Guttmann, H.E. 1980. Handbook of Human Reliability Analysis with Emphasis on Nuclear Power Plant Applications. Report no. NUREG/CR-1278, Nuclear Regulatory Commission, Washington.

Weiss, D.J. and Shanteau, J. 2003. Emperical assessment of expertise. *Human Factors*, 45, 104–114.

Wickens, C.D. 1980. The structure of attentional resources. In R. Nickerson and R. Pew (Eds.), *Attention and Performance VIII*. Hillsdale, NJ, Erlbaum.

Wickens, C.D. 1984. *Engineering Psychology and Human Performance*. Columbus, OH, Charles E Merrill.

Further Information

Applications of Human Performance Models to System Design, edited by G.R. McMillan, D. Beevis, E. Salas, M.H. Strub, R. Sutton, and L. Van Breda, includes several chapters that describe task analysis and its relationship to human performance and workload analysis in the context of system design. *Behavioral Analysis and Measurement Methods*, by David Meister, provides a review and practical guide to applying task-analytic methods. *The Handbook of Perception and Human Performance*, Vols. I and II, edited by K.R. Boff, L. Kaufman, and J.P. Thomas, provides broad range of human factors and ergonomic data related to perceptual and cognitive task performance. *The Handbook of Human Factors*, edited by G. Salvendy, reviews task-analytic methods, workload and resource models of cognitive processing, and human performance models in detail. *The Handbook of Industrial Engineering*, edited by G. Salvendy, reviews task analytic techniques and human performance models in the context of industrial design applications. The journal *Human Factors*, published by the Human Factors and Ergonomics Society, is a source for new task-analytic techniques and application studies. *Cognitive Psychology* and *Information Processing*, by R. Lachman, J.L. Lachman, and E.C. Butterfield, presents an extensive discussion of the information-processing approach as applied to research in modern experimental and cognitive psychology.

80

Task Analysis and Decomposition: Physical Components

Sheik N. Imrhan
University of Texas-Arlington

A task can be viewed as a sequence of actions performed to accomplish one or more desired objectives. Task analysis and decomposition involve breaking down a task into identifiable elements or steps and analyzing them to determine the resources (human, equipment, and environmental) necessary for the accomplishment of the task. As indicated in earlier chapters, all human tasks require the interaction of mental and physical resources, but it is often convenient, for analytical purposes, to make a distinction between tasks that require predominantly physical resources of the person performing the tasks and tasks that require predominantly mental resources. These different types of tasks are often analyzed separately. Usually, in physical tasks, the mental requirements are described but are not analyzed as meticulously as the physical requirements. For example, a heavy-lifting task in industry requires musculoskeletal strength and **endurance**, decision making, and other resources, but the successful completion of such a task is limited by musculoskeletal strength. Decision-making and cognitive resources may be lightly tapped, and so the heavy-lifting task analysis will tend to focus only on those factors that modify the expression of musculoskeletal strength while keeping the other kinds of requirements at a descriptive level. The descriptions and analyses of manual materials handling tasks in Chaffin and Andersson [1991] and Ayoub and Mital [1991] exemplify this kind of focus. The degree with which a resource may be stressed depends on a number of factors, among which are the resource availabilities (capacities) of the person performing the task compared with the task demands.

This chapter deals with the analysis and decomposition of only the physical aspects of tasks. It is assumed that nonphysical resources are either available in nonlimiting quantities or are not crucial to task accomplishment. While the compartmentalization of task characteristics tends to blur the natural connections among the various human performance resources, it is still the most pragmatic method available for task analysis.

Physical task analysis first achieved scientific respectability in the early part of this century from the work of the industrial engineer Frederick Winslow Taylor [Taylor, 1911] and, shortly afterward, by Frank and Lillian Gilbreth [Gilbreth and Gilbreth, 1917]. Taylor and the Gilbreths showed how a task can be broken down into a number of identifiable, discrete steps that can be characterized by type of physical motions, energy expenditure, and time required to accomplish the task. By this method, they argued that many task steps, normally taken for granted, may contribute little or nothing to the accomplishment of the task and can therefore be eliminated. As a result of these kinds of analyses, Taylor and the Gilbreths were able to enhance productivity of individual workers on a scale that was considered unrealistic at that time. The basic approach to the highest level of physical task analysis today has evolved from the motion and time studies of Taylor and the Gilbreths (known as taylorism), both in the industrial and nonindustrial environments. The exact methods have become more sophisticated and refined, incorporating new technologies and knowledge accumulated about human-task interaction.

From its roots in time and motion studies, task analysis has become a very complex exercise. No longer is a single task considered in isolation, as shoveling was by Taylor and bricklaying by the Gilbreths. Today, different ideas in management and advanced data analytical methods have established the need for cohesion between physical tasks and (1) the more global processes, such as jobs and occupations encompassing them, and (2) the more detailed processes contained within them (the different types of subtasks and basic elements of performance). Campion and Medsker [1992] give examples of the first, and Kondraske [1995] gives examples of the second. This chapter describes physical task analysis, showing the approach for proceeding from higher-level tasks to lower-level ones. Figure 80.1 shows a summary of the overall approach.

80.1 Fundamental Principles

The fundamental principle of physical task analysis is the establishment of the work relationships between the person performing the task and the elements of the task under specified environmental and social conditions. The main driving forces are performance enhancement, protection from injuries and illnesses, and decision making. The order of importance depends on the particular context in which the task analysis is performed. Performance enhancement is a concern in all disciplines that deal with human performance, though the approaches and objectives may differ. In physical rehabilitation, for example, performance enhancement focuses on improving the performance of basic physical functions of the human body, such as handgrip, elbow flexion, etc., that have deteriorated from injury or illness. In athletics, it focuses on improving performance to the highest possible levels, such as the highest jump or the fastest 100-m run. In exercise and fitness, it aims at improving body functions to enhance health and quality of life. Finally, in the discipline of ergonomics, it aims at enhancing task performance as well as the health and safety of people at work.

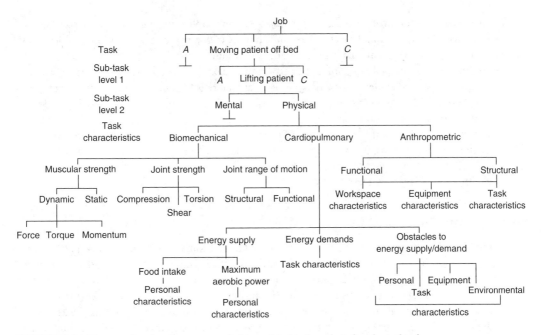

FIGURE 80.1   Diagram showing the concept of a hierarchical task analysis for physical tasks.

80.1.1 Speed–Accuracy Principle

Performance enhancement and protection from injuries and illnesses are not necessarily mutually exclusive. In performance enhancement, the aim is to complete a task as accurately and quickly as possible. Both accuracy and speed are important in the work environment, especially in manufacturing, and are influenced by other factors. When lack of accuracy or precision leads to dire consequences, as in air traffic control jobs, then a decision to sacrifice speed is usually made. The basic concept of Fitt's law [1954] is relevant to these situations. It is difficult to find examples of cases where gross inaccuracy is tolerable, but in many cases more speed is required and less accuracy is tolerable, and a different point on the speed–accuracy continuum is selected. In the manufacturing environment, speed translates into productivity and accuracy into quality, and both determine profitability of the production enterprise. Speed and accuracy are rarely attainable at the highest levels simultaneously. In practice, a certain amount of one may be sacrificed for the other. Thus, industrial engineers who set these tolerable limits talk of "optimum" speed instead of "fastest" speed and "optimum" quality instead of "perfect" quality. These facts must be borne in mind when analyzing physical tasks. A task analysis indicating that a person can increase his or her speed of performance should not necessarily imply that the task is being done inefficiently, because quality of performance may deteriorate with increased speed. This kind of flawed reasoning can occur when a variable is dealt with in isolation, without regard to its interaction with other variables.

80.1.2 Stress–Strain Concept

In task analysis, it is common practice to distinguish between stress and strain. However, these terms are sometimes used interchangeably and confusedly. In this chapter, stress refers to a condition that may lead to an adverse effect on the body, whereas strain refers to the effect of stress on the body. For example, working at a computer job in dim lighting often leads to headaches. The dim lighting is considered the stress, and the headache is the strain. The term stressor is also widely used as a synonym for stress. Strain has often been wrongly called stress. These terms must be clearly defined to determine which factors are causative ones (stresses) and which are consequences (strains). Stress is determined by task demands, while strain is determined by the amount of physical resources expended beyond some tolerable level, defined by the person's resource capacities. The stress–strain principle is pivotal to task analysis when one is concerned with errors, **cumulative traumas**, and injuries in the workplace and is applicable to task situations where task demands are likely to exceed human resource capacities.

Ayoub et al. [1987] developed a quantitative stress–strain index, called the **job severity index** (JSI), from empirical task analysis and epidemiologic data for manual materials handling tasks. This index computes the ratio of "job task physical demands to person physical capacities" from several interacting variables. The application of the JSI is also detailed in Ayoub and Mital [1991]. Also, Kondraske [1995] defines a quantitative measure of stress that can be applied to individual performance resources. In this measure, defined as the "ratio of resource utilization to resource availability," an adverse effect may be noted when the stress level exceeds a threshold, which may be different for different types of performance resources (e.g., strength, range of motion, etc.).

80.1.3 Cumulative Strains

The elimination of motions and other physical actions that do not contribute directly to task performance (tayloristic practice) has led to a concentration of work at specific localities in the body and to consequent overwork at those localities, but this concentration often leads to rapid consumption of the limited resources of the working systems. For example, VDT data entry is a highly repetitive task with very little variation; work is concentrated heavily on the hands (rapid finger motions for operating the keyboard) and in the neck and trunk (prolonged static muscular contraction), and this often leads to cumulative trauma disorders of the hands, wrists, neck, and shoulders. By comparison, traditional typists performed a variety of tasks in addition to using the keyboard — changing paper on the typewriter, filing documents, using the phone, etc. — and this helped to stem the depletion of physiologic resources caused by rapid finger work or sustained static muscular contractions in the neck and shoulder. Also, it is now recognized that some functions of the body that have not been considered "productive" under taylorism are highly stressed and may even be the limiting factors in task performance. In data processing, the muscles of the neck and back maintain prolonged static contractions that often result in muscular strains in the neck and back and limit work time. Traditional task analysis does not always consider this static muscular work as productive, even though it is absolutely necessary for steadying the arms (for keyboard and mouse use) and the head (for viewing the screen and documents). Likewise, **work pauses**, which have been considered wasteful, are now valued for their recuperative effects on the physical (and mental) working systems of the body. The increasing awareness of the causes of work-related cumulative trauma disorders will continue to influence the interpretation of data derived from task analyses.

80.2   Early Task-Analysis Methods

The history of physical task analysis does not show a trend toward the development of a single generalized model. The direction of physical task analysis has been influenced by Taylorism and by specific efforts in the military that were later adapted to the industrial and other nonmilitary environments. A list of influential methods, to which readers are referred, is given below:

1. Time studies of Fredrick Winslow Taylor [Taylor, 1911]
2. Time and motion studies of Frank and Lillian Gilbreth [Gilbreth and Gilbreth, 1917]
3. **Job analysis** developed by the U.S. Department of Labor in the 1930s [Drury et al., 1987]
4. The U.S. Air Force "method for man–machine task analysis" developed by R. Miller [1953]
5. Singleton's methods [Singleton, 1974]
6. **Hierarchical task analysis** (HTA) developed by Annette and Duncan [1974]
7. Checklist of worker activities developed by E.J. McCormick and others for the U.S. Office of Naval Research [Drury et al., 1987]
8. **Position analysis questionnaire** [McCormick et al., 1969]

9. The AET method (Arbeitswissenchaftliches Erhenbungsverfahen zur Tatigkeitsanalyse, or ergonomic job analysis) developed by Rohmert and Landau [Drury et al., 1987]

80.3   Methods of Physical Task Analysis

Methods of physical task analysis vary widely. Drury and colleagues [1987] point out that "the variation of task analysis format is the result of different requirements placed on the task analysis." While this is a pragmatic method for short-term results, a more general approach for long-term solutions is needed. Such an approach should aim to proceed from higher- to lower-level tasks, as discussed in other chapters [Kondraske, 1995]. The following general sequence of analysis is recommended:

1. Statement of the objectives of the task analysis
2. Description of the system within which the tasks reside
3. Identification of jobs (if relevant) within the system
4. Identification of the tasks
5. Identification of subtasks that can stand independently enough to be analyzed as separate entities
6. Determination of the specific starting point of each task
7. Determination of the specific stopping point of each task
8. Characterization of the task as discrete, continuous, or branching [Drury et al., 1987]
9. Determination of task resources (human, equipment, and environmental) required to perform the task (this step is the essence of task description)
10. Determination of other support systems (e.g., in work situations, managerial and supervisory help may be needed)
11. Determination of possible areas of **person–task conflicts**
12. Determination of possible consequences of conflict, for example, errors, slowing down of work rate, deterioration of quality of end product, decline in comfort, harm to health, and decline in safety

After the task analysis is performed and the resulting data analyzed, solutions for solving the associated problems are formulated then implemented; for example, repositioning of the mechanical hoist used for lifting and moving a patient at the beginning of the lift to minimize human muscular input. This is then followed by an evaluation period in which enough data is gathered to compare the task states before or after the changes. The evaluation criteria must be compatible with the stated objectives of the task analysis.

80.3.1   General Methods for Background Information

Many different techniques for gathering information in physical task analysis have evolved over the years, especially in the industrial and biomedical engineering environments. The quality and quantity of information that the techniques provide are limited by available equipment, and it seems that the quality and quantity of available equipment lag far behind the state of the art in technology. General data-gathering techniques, which are somewhat self-descriptive, include:

- Direct observation (predominantly visual)
- Indirect observation (e.g., replay of videotape)
- Document review
- Questionnaire survey
- Personal interview

80.3.2 Specific Techniques

Specialized data-gathering techniques [Winter, 1990; Chaffin and Andersson, 1991; Niebel, 1993] that have evolved into powerful tools in the industrial environment and which can be used for task analysis in other situations include:

- **Motion study** — details the motions made by the various segments of the body while performing the task
- **Time study** — details the time taken to perform each motion element
- Micromotion study — detailed description of motion using mainly videotapes
- Kinematic analysis — measures or estimates various motion parameters for specified body segments, for example, displacement, velocity, acceleration. (It involves micromotion studies.) The data are used for subsequent biomechanical analyses, for example, to determine mechanical strain in the musculoskeletal system [Chaffin and Andersson, 1991]
- Kinetic analysis — measures or estimates forces produced by body segments and other biomechanical parameters (e.g., center of mass, moment of inertia, etc.) and physical parameters of objects (e.g., mass, dimension, etc.) (the data are used for subsequent biomechanical analyses)

In the assessment of jobs in the occupational environment, two of the most useful motion-study methods are Rapid Upper Limb Assessment (RULA) and the Ovako Working Posture Analysis System (OWAS). These methods are used for assessing the risk to musculoskeletal cumulative strains from work postures. In RULA [McAtamney and Corlett, 1993], the geometric configurations of the upper arms, lower arms, wrists, neck, and trunk are estimated by visual observation and an overall score is calculated for posture. This score is then modified by incorporating data on the muscular forces exerted by the upper limbs and the frequency of exertion. Stressful postures and their contributing factors can therefore be identified and risk to injuries assessed. The OWAS method [Kahru et al., 1977] is similar to RULA but does not incorporate frequency of muscular force exertions.

Specialized data-analytic techniques include:

- Methods analysis — determines the overall relationships among various operations, the work force, and the equipment
- Operations analysis — determines the details of specific operations
- Worker–equipment relationship study — determines the interactions between people and their equipment

Examples of the above techniques that are frequently used for analyzing industrial jobs, but may also be used for other tasks involving people, are discussed in Gramopadhye and Thaker [1999]. Among the most useful are flow charts such as sequence diagrams, functional flow analysis, and decision diagrams, which depict the links among tasks and subtasks. These charts may also be used in conjunction with summary tables of the number of activities, duration of activities, and distance traveled by the human worker. They therefore facilitate improvements in system efficiency and identification of sources of possible operation errors. Examples of their applications are shown in Barnes [1980] for baking soda crackers and by Lock and Strutt [1985, in Gramopadhye and Thacker, 1999] for inspection in transport aircraft structures. Other techniques such as link analysis (Chapanis, 1962), critical incident technique [Meister, 1985], fault tree analysis [Green, 1983], and failure modes and effects analysis are not specific to physical task analysis but may be used in systems analysis involving physical tasks.

80.3.3 Decomposition of Physical Tasks

Physical tasks can be viewed as exchanges of energy within a system consisting of the human, the task, the equipment, and the environment. In task analysis and decomposition, we look at the human on one side and the other system components on the other side and then determine the nature of the exchange. The energy is transmitted by muscular action. Tasks are hierarchical, however, and for systematic decomposition, it is useful to identify the various levels and proceed in a top-down sequence (see Figure 80.1). The items in the various levels given here are self-explanatory, but there is considerable content within each. Detailed descriptions of each is beyond the scope of this chapter, and readers should consult the references [Singleton, 1974; Corlett et al., 1979; Meister, 1985; Winter, 1990; Niebel, 1993; Chaffin and Andersson, 1994] for standard measurement procedures and analyses.

Level I

Identifying general types of tasks according to levels of energy requirements:

- Tasks requiring great muscular forces
- Tasks requiring medium to low levels of muscular forces

Tasks requiring very low levels of muscular forces are not predominantly physical. Their successful accomplishment is strongly dependent on cognitive resources. The application of strong and weak muscular forces is not necessarily mutually exclusive. Such forces may be exerted simultaneously by different muscular systems or may even alternate within the same system. For example, a typing task may require strong back extensor forces while sitting bent forward (if the workstation is poorly designed) and weak finger flexion forces for activating the keyboard keys, and a weak index finger flexion may be required to activate a trigger on a hand drill while strong handgrip forces stabilize the drill.

Level II

Identifying the crucial subsystems involved in the generation and transference of forces of varying intensities involved in tasks:

- Musculoskeletal — for great forces
- Cardiopulmonary — for medium to low forces
- General body posture
- Body motion
- Local segmental motion
- Local segmental configuration
- **Anthropometry**
- Workplace and equipment dimensions

The last three subsystems modify directly the expression of muscular force.

Level III

Identifying environmental requirements and constraints. Environmental conditions influence performance and functional capacities in humans. They should therefore be measured or estimated in task analyses. Table 80.1 describes common environmental constraints.

TABLE 80.1 Environmental Factors in Task Analysis

Environmental factor	Constraint	Examples of effects
Illumination	Insufficient intensity	Errors
Heat	Excessive heat and humidity	Lowering of physiologic endurance
Cold	Excessive cold	Numbness of hands — inability to grasp hand tool properly
Vibration	Excessive amplitude	Loss of grip and control of vibrating tool
Noise	Excessive intensity	Inability to coordinate job with coworkers
Body supporting surface	Slipperiness	Difficulty in balancing body
Space	Insufficient workspace	Inability to position body properly

Level IV

Identifying body actions in relation to tasks. These actions can be decomposed into two major types:

1. Those which involve body motions. They are used for either changing body positions or moving objects
2. Those which do not involve body motions. They are used primarily for balancing and stabilizing the body for performing some task. Body posture is especially important here, especially when great muscular forces must be exerted

These actions are not mutually exclusive during task performance. One part of the body may move, while another part, involved in the task, may be still. For example, the fingers move rapidly when using a keyboard, but the rest of the hand is kept motionless while the fingers are moving. Table 80.2 through Table 80.5 depict practical decompositions of these actions as well as those requiring muscular forces.

Level V

Identifying anthropometric variables. Human anthropometry interacts with workplace and equipment dimensions. Tasks are performed better when the interaction defines a close "match" between human body size and task-related physical dimensions. Therefore, physical task analysis may be inadequate without measurements of the dimensions of people performing the task and the corresponding dimensions of other aspects of the system of which the task is a part. This kind of matching is one of the basic thrusts in the discipline of ergonomics. Grandjean [1988] and Konz [1990] discuss these issues in many types of human–task environments, and Pheasant [1986] gives numerous body dimensions related to task design. Some important examples of human–system dimensions that must be considered during task analysis are shown in Table 80.6.

TABLE 80.2 Representative Actions with Motions

Class of action	Subclass	Purpose of action	Examples
Whole body		Positioning body	Walking, crawling, running, jumping, climbing
		Transporting object	Lifting, lowering, carrying horizontally, pushing, pulling, rotating
Gross segmental	Arm movement	Applying forces to object	Reaching for object, twisting, turning, lifting, lowering, transporting horizontally, positioning, pressing down, pushing, pulling, rotating
	Leg movement	Applying forces	Rotating (e.g., foot pedal), pushing
	Trunk movement	Generating momentum	Sitting and bending forward, backward, and sideways to retrieve items on a table
Fine segmental	Finger movement	Applying forces	Turning, pushing, pulling, lifting

TABLE 80.3 Representative Actions with Motions

Class of action	Subclass	Purpose of action	Examples
Whole body		Balancing body	Standing while preparing meal in kitchen
		Supporting or stabilizing object	Bracing ladder while coworker climbs on it
Segmental	Arm		Holding food item with one hand while cutting it with other hand
	Leg	Supporting body	Forcing foot on ground while sitting in constrained posture

TABLE 80.4 Representative Actions Requiring Forces, for Different Types of Forces

Class of action	Subclass	Sub-subclass	Body–object contact	Purpose of action	Examples
Whole body	Whole body	Dynamic	One hand, two hands, or other contact	Generate great forces that must be transmitted over small localized area or large area. The effort produces motion of whole body	Lift, push, pull
		Static	One hand, two hands, or other contact	Generate great forces that must be transmitted over small localized area or large area. The effort does not produce motion	Lift, push, pull
	Segmental	Static	One hand, two hands, one foot, or two feet	Generate forces (over a wide range of magnitude) that must be transmitted over a relatively small localized area. The effort does not produce motion of the body segment	Gripping with whole hand, pinching, pressing down, twisting, turning, pushing, pulling, or combinations
		Dynamic	One hand, two hands, one foot, or two feet	Generate great forces that must be transmitted over small localized area or large area. The effort produces motion of the body segment	Pushing, pulling, pressing down

TABLE 80.5   Posture While Performing Tasks

Class	Subclass	Purpose	Examples
Whole body	Standing, sitting, kneeing, lying down, other	Optimize body leverage; position body for making proper contact with object; other	Squatting at beginning of a heavy lift to prevent excessive strain in the lower back
Segmental	Arms, legs, trunk, hands, other	Optimize segment leverage; position segment for making proper contact with object	Placing elbow at about right angles while using wrench to prevent excessive shoulder and muscle efforts

TABLE 80.6   Human Anthropometry and System Dimensions

Body dimensions	System dimensions
Height, arm length, shoulder width	Workspace — height of shelf, depth of space under work table, circumference of escape hatch
Leg length, knee height	Equipment size — distance from seat reference point to foot pedal of machine, height from floor to dashboard of vehicle
Hand length, grip circumference	Hand tool size — trigger length, handle circumference
Crotch height, arm length	Apparel size — leg length of pants, arm length of shirt
Face height, hand width	Personal protective equipment — height of respirator, width of glove

80.4   Factors Influencing the Conduct of Task Analysis

While task analysis traditionally focuses on what a person does and how he or she does it, other factors must be considered to complete the picture. In general, the characteristics of the task, the equipment used, and environmental conditions must all be accounted for. Human functional performance cannot be viewed in isolation because the person, the task, the equipment, and the environment form a system in which a change in one factor is likely to affect the way the person reacts to the others. For example, in dim lighting, a VDT operator may read from a document with marked flexion of the neck but with only slight flexion (which is optimal) when reading from the screen. Brighter ambient lighting may prevent sharp flexion when reading from documents but is likely to decrease contrast of characters on the screen. Screen character brightness must therefore be changed to maintain adequate reading performance to prevent sharp flexion of the neck again.

80.4.1   Knowing the Objectives of Task Analysis

Motion, speed, force, environment, and object (equipment) characteristics are common factors for consideration in task analysis. However, the reasons for performing a task are an equally important factor. Tasks that may involve the same equipment and which may seem identical may differ in their execution because of their objectives. Thus, a person opening a jar in the battlefield in the midst of enemy fire to retrieve medicines will not perform that task in exactly the same way as a person at home opening a similar jar to retrieve sugar for sweetening coffee. In the former case, speed is more important, and both the type of grasp used and the manual forces exerted are likely to be markedly different from the latter case. Napier [1980] recognized this principle, in relation to gripping tasks, when he wrote that the "nature of the intended activity influences the pattern of grip used on an object." These kinds of considerations in task analysis can influence the design of objects and other aids and the nature of education and training programs.

80.4.2 Levels of Effort

The level of required effort when performing similar tasks in different environments is not necessarily the same, and the interpretation of task-analysis data is influenced by these differences. Tasks in the workplace are designed so that human physical effort is minimized, whereas tasks in the competitive athletics environment are designed to tap the limits of human performance resources. There are other differences. An athlete paces himself or herself according to his or her own progress. He or she has greater freedom to stop performing a task should physical efforts become painful or uncomfortable. In the workplace, however, there is often little freedom to stop. Many workers often push themselves to the limits of their endurance in order to maintain (flawed) performance goals set by their employers. This is why cumulative strains are more prevalent in the workplace than in many other environments. These differences in performance levels may influence the way task analyses are performed among the different disciplines and the application of the data derived therefrom.

80.4.3 Criticality of Tasks

An inventory of task elements is necessary for describing the requirements of the task. It can tell us about the person, equipment, and environmental requirements for performing a job, but we must also be able to identify specific elements or factors that can prevent the successful completion of the task or that can lead to accidents and injuries. These critical elements are usually measured in detail or estimated and used for developing quantitative models for predicting success or failure in performance. One such widely researched element is the compression force on the L5/S1 disk in the human spine while performing heavy-lifting tasks [Chaffin and Andersson, 1984]. This force is being used by the National Institute of Occupational Safety and Health as a criterion for determining how safe a lifting activity is. If analysis of task-analysis data indicates that the **safety limit** (3400 N of compression) is exceeded then work redesign, based on task-analysis information, must be implemented [National Technical Information Service, 1991; NIOSH, 1981].

80.5 Measurement of Task Variables

During task analysis, variables must be measured for subsequent data summary and analysis. It is important to know not only what the inventory of task-related variables is but also to what degree the variables are related to or affect overall performance. The measurement of task-related variables allows for quantification of the overall system. For example, the NIOSH lifting equation [National Technical Information Service, 1991] shows how task variables such as the horizontal distance of the load from the body, the initial height of the load, the vertical height of lift, the frequency of lifting, the angular displacement of the load from the saggital plane during lifting, and the type of hand–handle coupling affect the maximal weight of the load that can be lifted safely by most people in a manual materials-handling task. The number of task-related variables measured should be adequate for describing the task and for representing it quantitatively. However, there are often constraints. These include:

1. The number of variables that can be identified
2. The number of variables that can be measured at an acceptable level of reliability and accuracy
3. The availability of measurement instruments

Merely summarizing individual measurements seldom yields the desired information. Task performance is essentially a multivariable operation, and variables often must be combined by some quantitative method that can yield models representative of the performance of the task. Sometimes a variable cannot be measured directly but can be estimated from other measured variables. The estimated variable may then be used in a subsequent modeling process. A good example of this is the intraabdominal pressure achieved during heavy lifting. Though it can be predicted by a cumbersome process of swallowing a pressure-sensitive pill, it also can be estimated from the weights of the upper body and load lifted and other variables related to lifting posture. Its estimate can then be used to estimate the compressive force in the L5/S1 disk and the tension in the erector spinae muscles during lifting. Imrhan and Ayoub [1988] also show how estimated velocity and acceleration of elbow flexion and shoulder extension can be used, with other variables, to predict linear pulling strength.

80.5.1 Task-Related Variables

Variables that are usually measured during physical task analysis include:

1. Those related to the physical characteristics of task objects or equipment:
   (a) Weight of load lifted, pushed, carried, etc.
   (b) Dimensions of load
   (c) Location of center of mass of load
2. Those related to the nature of the task:
   (a) The frequency of performance of a cycle of the task
   (b) The range of heights over which a load must be lifted
   (c) The speed of performance
   (d) The level of accuracy of performance
3. Those related to the capacities of various physical resources of the person:
   (a) Muscular strength
   (b) Joint range of motion
   (c) Joint motion (velocity and acceleration)
   (d) **Maximal aerobic power**
   (e) Anthropometry
4. Those related to the environment:
   (a) Temperature
   (b) Illumination
   (c) Vibration
5. Those related to workplace design:
   (a) Amount of space available for the task
   (b) Geometric and spatial relationships among equipment
   (c) Furniture dimensions
6. Those related to anthropometry:
   (a) Length, breadth, depth, or circumference of a body segment
   (b) Mass and mass distribution of a body segment
   (c) Range of motion of a skeletal joint

80.5.2 Instruments for Gathering Task-Analysis Data

A great number of instruments are available for measuring variables derived from task analyses. The choice of instruments depends on the type of variables to be measured and the particular circumstances. In general, there should be instruments for recording the sequence of actions during task, for example, videotape with playback feature, and instruments for measuring kinematic, kinetic, and anthropometric variables [Winter, 1990; Chaffin and Andersson, 1994]. The main kinematic variables include displacement (of a body part), velocity, and acceleration. Kinetic variables include force and torque. Anthropometric variables include body segment length, depth, width, girth, segment center of mass, segment radius of gyration, segment moment of inertia, joint axis of rotation, and joint angle. Some variables are measured directly, for example, acceleration (with accelerometers), force applied at a point of contact between the body and an object (with load cells), and body lengths (with anthropometers); some may be measured indirectly, for example, joint angle (from a videotape image) and intraabdominal pressure (using swallowed pressure pill); and others may be estimated by mathematic computations from other measured variables, e.g., compressive force on the lumbosacral (L5/S1) disk in the lower back. Posture targeting, a method for recording and analyzing stressful postures in work sampling [Corlett et al., 1979], is becoming popular.

The measurements of performance capacities associated with human functions should conform to certain criteria. Details can be found in Brand and Crownshield [1981] and Chaffin [1982]. A general set of psychometric criteria is also discussed by Sanders and McCormick [1993]. It includes measurement accuracy, reliability, validity, sensitivity, and freedom from contamination. Meeting these criteria depends not only on the instruments used but also on the methods of analysis and the expertise of the analyst. It is almost impossible to satisfy these criteria perfectly, especially when the task is being performed in its natural environment (as opposed to a laboratory simulation). However, the analyst must always be aware of them and must be pragmatic in measuring task variables. Meister [1985] lists the following practical requirements for measurements (1) objective, (2) quantitative, (3) unobtrusive, (4) easy to collect, (5) requiring no special data-collection techniques or instrumentation, and (6) of relatively low cost in terms of money and effort by the experimenter. However, these are not necessarily mutually exclusive.

80.6 Uses and Applications of Task Analysis

The uses of task-analysis information depend on the objectives of performing the task, which, in turn, depend on the environment in which the task is performed. Table 80.7 gives the different situations.

80.7 Future Developments

To date, there is no reliable quantitative model that can combine mental and physical resources. A general-purpose task-analysis method that uses active links between the various compartments of

TABLE 80.7 Uses and Applications of Task Analysis

Uses and applications	Examples of relevant situations
Modeling human performance and determining decision-making strategies	A model showing the sequence of the various steps required to perform a task and the type of equipment needed at each step
Predicting human performance	Using a quantitative model to predict whether an elderly person has enough arm strength to lift a pot full of water from a cupboard onto a stove
Redesigning of the existing tasks or designing of new tasks	Eliminating an unnecessary step in the packaging of production items into cartons; designing a different package for a new item based on task-analytic data gathered for a related item
Determining whether to use task-performance aids	The analysis may show that most elderly persons do not possess enough strength to open many food jars and may, therefore, need a mechanical torqueing aid
Personnel selection or placement	Matching personnel physical characteristics with task requirements can reveal which person may be able to perform a task and, hence, be assigned to it
Determining whether to use aids that enhance health or safety	Task analysis may show that too much dust always gets into the atmosphere when opening packages of a powered material and that workers should wear a respirator
Determining educational and training procedures	Identification of difficult task steps or the need for using mechanical aids, together with knowledge of workers' skills, may indicate the level of education and training needed
Allocating humans to machines and machines to humans	Matching people skills and capacities with the resource demands of machines
Determining emergency procedures	Task-analysis information may indicate which steps are likely to result in dangerous situations, and therefore, require contingency plans

human functions would be an ideal method, but our lack of knowledge about the way in which many of these "compartments" communicate precludes the development of such a method. The present approach to compartmentalization seems to be the most pragmatic approach. It offers the analyst access to paths from a gross task or job to the myriad of basic task elements of performance. Unfortunately, actual systems and subsystems used in practice seem to be loosely defined and inconsistent, often with confusing metrics and terminologies for important variables. Moreover, available task-analysis models deal only with specific classes of application [Drury, 1987]. A general-purpose model is badly needed for handling different mental and physical resources at the same time, dealing with wide ranges in a variable, and bridging the gaps across disciplines. Such a model should help us to perform task analyses and manipulate the resulting data from environments ranging from the workplace, the home (activities of daily living), athletics, exercise and fitness, and rehabilitation. Such a model can also help to eliminate the present trend of performing task analyses that are either too specific to apply to different situations or not specific enough to answer focused questions. Fleishman [1982] deals with the issue. At least one recent effort is active [Kondraske, 1995]. However, as Landau et al. [1998] points out, such generalizability has a cost in that the associated data is produced at a higher level of abstraction, which is likely to be difficult for a practitioner to apply to specific problems.

There is also a need for better quantification of performance. We need to know not only what kind of shifting in resources a person resorts to when one route to successful task accomplishment is blocked (e.g., insufficient strength for pressing down in a certain sitting posture) but also the quantity and direction of that shift. For example, we need to know not merely that a change in posture can increase manual strength for torqueing but also what the various postures can yield and what quantity of specific mental resources are involved in the change. The models today that answer the quantitative questions are mainly ones of statistical regression, and they are limited by the number of variables and the number of levels of each variable that they can deal with.

Defining Terms

Anthropometry: The science that deals with the measure of body size, mass, shape, and inertial properties.

Cumulative trauma: The accumulation of repeated insults to body structures over a period of time (usually months or years) often leading to "cumulative trauma disorders."

Endurance: The maximum time for which a person can perform a task at a certain level under specified conditions without adverse effects on the body.

Fitts' law: The equation, derived by P. Fitts, showing the quantitative relationship between the time for a human (body segment) to move from one specific point to another (the target) as a function of distance of movement and width of the target.

Hierarchical task analysis: The analysis of a task by breaking it down to its basic components, starting from an overall or gross description (e.g., lifting a load manually) and moving down in a series of steps in sequence.

Job analysis: Any of a number of techniques for determining the characteristics of a job and the interactions among workers, equipment, and methods of performing the job.

Job severity index: An index indicating the injury potential of a lifting or lowering job. It is computed as the ratio of the physical demands of the job to the physical capacities of the worker.

Local segment: A specific body segment, usually the one in contact with an object required for performing a task or the one most active in the task.

Maximal aerobic power: The maximal rate at which a person's body can consume oxygen while breathing air at sea level.

Motion study: The analysis of a task or job by studying the motions of humans and equipment related to its component activities.

Person–task conflict: The situation in which task demands are beyond a person's capacities and the task is unlikely to be performed according to specifications by that person.

Position analysis questionnaire: A checklist for job analysis, developed by the Office of Naval Research in 1969, requiring the analyst to rate or assess a job from a list of 187 job elements.

Safety limit: The maximum stress (e.g., load to be lifted) that most workers can sustain under specified job conditions without adverse effects (injuries or cumulative strains) on their bodies.

Time study: The study of a task by timing its component activities.

Work pause: A short stoppage from work.

References

Ayoub M.M., Bethea N.J., Deivanayagam S. et al. 1979. Determination and Modeling of Lifting Capacity. Final report, HEW (NIOSH), grant no. 5R01–OH–00545–02.

Ayoub M.M. and Mital A. 1991. *Manual Materials Handling*. London, Taylor & Francis.

Barnes R. 1980. *Motion and Time Study Design and Measurement of Work*. New York, John Wiley and Sons.

Campion M.A. and Medsker G.J. 1992. *Handbook of Industrial Engineering*. New York, Wiley.

Chaffin D.B. and Andersson G.D. 1991. *Occupational Biomechanics*. New York, Wiley.

Chapanis A. 1962. *Research Techniques in Human Engineering*. Baltimore, Johns Hopkins University Press.

Corlett E.N., Madeley S.J., and Manenica I. 1979. Postural targeting: a technique for recording work postures. *Ergonomics* 22: 357.

Drury G.D., Paramore B., Van Cott H.P. et al. 1987. Task analysis. In J. Salvendy (Ed.), *Handbook of Human Factors*, pp. 371–399. New York, Wiley.

Fleishman E.A. 1982. Systems for describing human tasks. *Am. Psychol.* 37: 821.

Fitts P. 1954. The information capacity of the human motor system in controlling the amplitude of movement. *J. Exp. Psychol.* 47: 381.

Gilbreth F.B. and Gilbreth F.M. 1917. *Applied Motion Study*. New York, Sturgis and Walton.

Gramopadhye A. and Thacker J. 1999. Task Analysis. In W. Karwowski and W.S. Marras (Eds.), *The Occupational Ergonomics Handbook*, pp. 297–329. Boca Raton, FL, CRC Press.

Grandjean E. 1988. *Fitting the Task to the Man*, 4th ed. New York, Taylor & Francis.

Imrhan S.N. and Ayoub M.M. 1988. Predictive models of upper extremity rotary and linear pull strength. *Hum. Factors* 30: 83.

Kondraske G.V. 1995. A working model for human system task interfaces. In J.D. Bronzino (Ed.), *Handbook of Biomedical Engineering*. Boca Raton, FL, CRC Press.

Kahru O., Kansi P., and Kuorinka I. 1977. Correcting working postures in industry. A practical method for analysis. *Appl. Ergon.* 8: 199–201.

Konz S. 1990. *Work Design: Industrial Ergonomics*. Worthington, Ohio, Publishing Horizon.

Landau K.L., Rohmert W., and Brauchler R. 1998. Task analysis: part I — guidelines for the practitioner. *Int. J. Indust. Ergon.* 22: 3–11.

McAtamney L. and Corlett E.N. 1993. RULA: a survey method for the investigation of work-related upper limb disorders. *Appl. Ergon.* 24: 91–99.

Meister D. 1985. *Behavioral Analysis and Measurement Methods*. New York, Wiley.

Napier J.R. 1980. *Hands*. New York, Pantheon.

National Technical Information Service. 1991. Scientific Support Documentation for the Revised 1991 NIOSH Lifting Equation. PB91-226274. U.S. Department of Commerce, Springfield, VA.

Niebel B.W. 1993. *Motion and Time Study*, 9th ed. Homewood, II, Richard D. Irwin.

NIOSH, 1981. Work Practices Guide for Manual Lifting. NIOSH technical report no 81–122, US Department of Health and Human Services, National Institute of Occupational Safety and Health, Cincinnati, OH.

Pheasant S. 1986. *Bodyspace*. London, Taylor & Francis.

Singleton. 1974. *Man–Machine Systems*. London, Penguin.

Taylor F.W. 1911. *The Principles of Scientific Management.* New York, Harper.
Winter D.A. 1990. *Biomechanics and Motor Control of Human Movement,* 2nd ed. New York, Wiley.

Further Information

For the design of equipment in human work environments where task analysis is employed, see *Human Factors Design Handbook*, by W.E. Woodson [McGraw-Hill, New York, 1981]. For human anthropometric data that are useful to task analysis, see NASA Reference Publication 1024: Anthropometric Source Book, vol 1: *Anthropometry for Designers* [Webb Associates, Yellow Springs, Ohio, 1978].

81

Human–Computer Interaction Design

Kenneth J. Maxwell
BMK Consultants

81.1 Purpose of This Chapter

The fields of Biomedical Engineering and Human–Computer Interaction (HCI) share a special reciprocity. On one hand, biomedical products, including instrumentation, devices, bioinformatics systems and robots, are becoming increasingly reliant on information technology (IT). HCI factors are principal determinants of the adoption, effectiveness, and safe use of these products. On another hand, biomedical research and data play an important role in human–computer interface technology. Biomedical factors will increasingly require consideration as HCI technology extends to incorporate alternative modalities of interaction.

This chapter provides the reader with fundamentals for addressing HCI design and highlights areas of particular interest to biomedical engineers. Work in HCI is abundant in academic, government, and commercial sectors. This chapter selects from this work essential and practical information needed to incorporate (a) human experience considerations into the engineering of biomedical products and

(b) biomedical considerations into the engineering of human–computer interface technology. References to broaden the reader's knowledge of HCI are provided in the Further Information section.

81.2 HCI Directions and Design Challenges

Since the second edition of this handbook, the field of HCI has matured and expanded in several new directions relevant to biomedical engineering. Much of this expansion is linked to dramatic changes in computing technology.

Computing is becoming both more social and more personal. The Internet enables electronic social networks and communities that are supplying needed support and resources for patients. Communication and network systems provide facilities for distant collaboration among physicians. At the same time, HCI and the information provided by systems are becoming increasingly personalized. For example, the ability to search or navigate large databases, websites, and networks for focused retrieval of information is increasingly tailored to individual needs.

Computing is becoming more mobile and ubiquitous. Data services including web browsing, e-mail, and text messaging are common on cell phone and personal data assistant (PDA) form factors and are integrated with voice services. From a physical interaction perspective, mobile form factors present HCI design challenges including restricted display space and input mechanisms, function integration, management of multiple communication channels, and reduced computing power. For biomedical applications, wearable devices that monitor and transmit data from a patient will become more commonplace. Wearable devices must be comfortable emotionally as well as physically for the wearer, similar to the impact of an accessory to clothing.

Computing is becoming more embedded in devices, instruments, and other products [Norman, 1998]. Such devices have special purpose interfaces, because of their specific and limited functionality. Due to this reduced complexity, the HCI design task may appear to not require much consideration. Although the scale of the HCI design effort may be smaller for devices than for large systems, attention to HCI factors should remain prominent. Rogers et al. [2001] in an analysis of a commonly used blood glucose meter found that although the instructions listed thee general steps these actually required a total of 52 sub-steps, many of which were sources of error in operating the device for the participants in the study. Many problems can sabotage the **usability** of simple products [Darnell, 2004]. These are unnecessary and can be avoided when proper methods are applied to understand users, identify potential problems, and design a quality user experience. Satisfying user needs represents value to customers and can present a competitive advantage.

To address these new computing paradigms, HCI has increasingly diversified. Interaction is tending toward becoming more multimodal. Alternative modes of interaction such as speech, gesture, and haptic feedback, for example, can provide the means for managing interaction across a variety of user needs, device form factors, and computing contexts.

Interfaces are tending to become visually richer. Greater computing power has enabled support of visualization and visual simulation techniques that enable a myriad of biomedical applications that were impractical not long ago.

HCI is also moving beyond what Maxwell [2002] calls basic usability concerns toward broader elements of human experience including social interaction and collaboration, motivations [Fogg, 2003; Shneiderman, 2002] emotions [Norman, 2004] context [Abowd et al., 2002] and integration with real-world interactions [Streitz et al., 2002].

81.3 HCI in Biomedical Products

81.3.1 Instrumentation and Biometrics

Biomedical instruments increasingly embed computing power, and to the extent they do, the instrument's interface involves HCI. These products include simple consumer devices for home use by the general public up through complex instruments used by researchers, physicians, and other professionals. Increasingly biometric data such as fingerprint recognition is being used to secure access to computers or devices.

81.3.2 Medical Information Systems, Bioinformatics, and Simulation

Advanced computing power and computational tools have made possible the collection and complex analysis of very large amounts of biomedical data, contributing to improvements in health care and understanding of biological processes. However, in many cases, these improvements can only be realized if researchers, practitioners, and patients themselves can effectively, satisfactorily, and safely operate equipment and systems.

One major area of large information systems in general and medical information systems in particular is search. Researchers are rapidly moving to find more efficient ways to do searches. Leroy et al. [2003] found that Genescene, a system that parses natural language text automatically using a rule-based system and which provides biological researchers with research findings was more useful and efficient than keyword searches. Wildemuth et al. [1998] although finding no performance difference between Boolean keyword searches and hypertext navigation, did report that users preferred the Boolean keyword searches. Miller et al. [2004] report findings that suggest that the quality of link labels in hypertext navigation through a website architecture has a great effect on search efficiency.

Visualization techniques have greatly improved many areas of biomedical research and practice [Johnson et al., 2004], including medical diagnosis, planning of surgical techniques, and simulation of biological behavior. Cavassa and Simo [2003] present work on a virtual patient system that provides a 3-D model of the patient and an ER room with a physiological model that can react to interventions.

81.3.3 Robotic Service Systems

Robots will be a part of our everyday lives in the near future. Biomedical applications of both professional and personal service robots are becoming increasingly common. A survey conducted by the United Nations Economic Comission for Europe (UNECE) in conjunction with the International Federation of Robotics (IFR) [2004] estimated that a stock of 21,000 professional service robots at the end of 2003 and projected 75,000 by the end of 2007. These include medical robots, underwater robots, surveillance robots, demolition robots, and many other types of robots for carrying out a multitude of tasks. Medical robots comprised 12% of the 2003 estimates.

On the professional side, robots will, among other tasks, autonomously deliver records and medicine throughout hospitals or extend a surgical team's performance. On the personal side, robots will play a role in assisting with many aspects of life, such as assisting elders in living independently or facilitating rehabilitation. For example, Forlizzi et al. [2004] reports an ethnographic study of elders living independently in their own homes for the purpose of exploring how assistive robotic products can help elders live independently longer.

Plaisant et al. [2000] developed a robotic toy with which children could interactively create and replay stories assisting with physical and developmental problems. Yanco et al. [2004] evaluated human–robot interaction at a robotics competition using a tailored set of usability criteria developed by Scholtz [2002] that can be applied to a broad range of robotic applications.

81.3.4 Biomedical Engineering and Interaction Technologies

The applications discussed above address the interaction between humans and biomedical products that embed or employ computers. However, as HCI technology develops to address new paradigms, new modes of interaction, such as haptic feedback, gestural, and speech interfaces will increasingly involve biomedical factors.

For example, early results from Keates et al. [2004] suggest that haptic-force feedback is very promising for providing significant interaction performance improvements for motion-impaired users.

Han et al. [2002] report that a 2-D force feedback device could be used to present 3-D shapes using a force-shading technique, a haptic analog to bump mapping in computer graphics. Bach-y-Rita et al. [2003] found that a system in which electrotactile stimuli were delivered to the tongue via flexible electrode arrays placed in the mouth provided a feasible means for tactile vision substitution.

81.4 Fundamentals

81.4.1 Human-Centered Design

Human-centered (also referred to as *user-centered*) is a modern design philosophy and methodology for deriving and allocating functional requirements, driving design concepts, and setting evaluation criteria from the perspectives of the person or persons that will use the products being developed. This philosophy was promoted as an alternative to design approaches that emphasized technology and market factors over user experience, resulting in designs that frequently and unnecessarily compromised the user's motivations, performance, safety, and emotional responses. **Human-centered design** does not and should not exclude technology and market factors, but is meant to ensure that along with these factors the realized products or systems satisfy human needs and desires [Norman, 1998]. Human-centered design is ubiquitous and is an enduring tradition toward achieving highly usable products. As testament an international standard [ISO 13407, 1999] provides a guide to its application.

Usability refers to the capacity of a machine or system to be used by intended persons for accomplishing intended purposes. It is a multifaceted concept that can include effectiveness, efficiency, time-to-learn, safety, and emotional satisfaction. International standard, ISO 9241-11 [1998] defines usability as, "the *effectiveness, efficiency,* and *satisfaction* with which specified users achieve specified goals in particular environments." Effectiveness is, "the accuracy and completeness with which specified users can achieve specified goals in particular environments." Efficiency is, "the resources expended in relation to the accuracy and completeness of goals achieved." Satisfaction relates specifically to the user and is, "the comfort and acceptability of the work system to its users and other people affected by its use." A human-centered methodology is the widely accepted path toward realizing a design that embodies usability qualities. Usability is a major factor affecting the operational performance, availability, maintainability, and reliability of a human–product system.

The following are some characteristics of human-centered design:

- The purposes of all users involved are identified.
- The product is viewed as a tool that users employ to accomplish their purpose.
- The user is always performing a higher-level task than the product.
- Tasks are allocated away from the users rather than to the users. This is not simply a matter of perspective but rather is fundamental to a human-centered approach. That is, the user is assumed to be performing a high-level task. Lower-level tasks that are better performed by the computer are allocated from the user to the computer. This approach is opposed to the one that considers the computer as the high-level task performer and allocates to the user lower-level tasks that the machine cannot do well.
- Tasks performed by users are meaningful.
- The user's responsibilities provide satisfaction and make use of the user's talents and skills.
- Intended users of the product participate in the design process.
- The user's skills and performance capabilities are explicitly considered in and accounted for in design decisions.

Many techniques, methods, and tools have been developed for the purpose of providing designers with information about users very early in the product and system development process. These approaches are employed to inform the specification of function and design requirements and the synthesis of design concepts, as well as forming a basis for test and evaluation criteria.

Of foremost concern to designers using the human-centered approach is human purpose. As computing technology and HCI has progressed, there has been a transition from focusing on what computers can do to what human can do [Shneiderman, 2003]. This transition is manifest in the evolution of human needs and wants that computer-based products are intended to satisfy [Maxwell, 2002]. The human purpose for a product or system may be broad or specific. Purpose can translate directly into the function of a product or system but not necessarily so. For example, the function of a consumer blood-pressure monitor is to measure a user's blood pressure, but its purpose is broader. It is to enable a convenient, frequent, and private monitoring of blood pressure, to inform the user, and toward the goal of keeping the user's blood pressure at a healthy level. In this broader sense the purpose fulfills not only the needs of the user of the monitor (the patient) but also the purposes of the user's doctor and more broadly of the user's health insurer. From a very different human perspective the monitor needs to serve the purposes of the people who make and sell it, and it is in this way that the human-centered approach can be used to consider user, market, and technology factors together.

A first step in employing a human-centered approach is to identify the intended users and to characterize them with attributes relevant to the product or system. This involves characterizing users along any number of relevant dimensions such as age, skill level, geographic location, context-of-use (e.g., home or work), The purpose of such an analysis is to determine the range of these characteristics and the extent to which users are similar and different. Similarities can be used to categorize users and to direct design decisions to address the needs of these categories. Design requirements can be very different across user groups. Differences within groups can be used to inform the degree of flexibility, personalization, and adaptability needed.

As part of a project to improve the usability of bioinformatics web sites, Javahery et al. [2004] report a user analysis of the biomedical research community. Their analysis described users with regard to seven characteristics: user's language, familiarity with the internet, bioinformatics background, education level, profession, experience with specific web sites, and the tasks performed on web sites. Of course, the specific characteristics that are relevant will vary with the product or system being developed or evaluated.

81.4.1.1 Ethnographic Studies

These are in-the-field studies that have been adopted from anthropology research. The researchers are embedded to some level with the users and garner data on how they interact in real life with the products or systems under study or similar products or systems or to identify the need for such products. In an ethnographic study of independent elders, Forlizzi et al. [2004] identified two groups of elders, well and declining, using characteristics of mobility, cognitive function, and household maintenance.

User groups can be defined along many different dimensions depending on the application. Two typical and general grouping criteria are function- and resource-needs-based. For biomedical applications functional user groups commonly include those identified below:

- *Practitioners and service providers*: This group includes, doctors, nurses, psychologists, social workers, paramedics, and other providers of medical care.
- *Biomedical science researchers*: This group uses biomedical instruments, simulation tools, data-analysis software, and data-mining software to conduct research and development in laboratories or in the field.
- *Administrators*: This group represents hospital administration, doctor's office, and insurance personnel that use biomedical records and data as part of their daily work.
- *Legal*: This group includes lawyers, paralegals, court and government representatives, expert witnesses, and insurance-industry representatives that employ biomedical products for legal purposes.
- *Analysts*: This group includes persons who perform data mining and other analyses of biomedical data using computer systems.
- *Patients*: This is a specific subset of the general public user group that is using biomedical products or systems under the advice of a doctor or during a period of care.

- *General public*: This group is maximally diverse and use a variety of consumer instruments and products as well as accessing a variety of online medical information belonging to online support networks.
- *Information technology support personnel*: This group includes persons that install, manage, configure, diagnose, and repair biomedical IT systems.
- *Biomedical engineers*: This group includes persons that use computer-based tools to design and build biomedical products.

Resource-needs-based groups typically are differentiated along the dimensions identified here. Users belonging to different groups along these dimensions will typically need different levels of assistance and training.

- *Age*: Elders and children make up especially important broad groups.
- *Disabilities*: These typically are further grouped by type such as vision, hearing, motor skills, and cognition.
- *Current medical condition*: Groups can be defined by any condition needing current care.
- *Current lifestyle*: Any number of cultural variables can be used to identify groups.
- *History*: Any number of medical, lifestyle, or family variables can be used to specify the relevant groups.
- *Expertise*: This dimension differentiates the level of knowledge and skill users have with a particular product or system or the functions they perform.

Another step in employing a human-centered approach is to describe what and how users will do interacting with the product or system. The methods discussed here can be employed to generate this needed information.

81.4.1.2 Use-Case Analysis

Use-case analysis is a part of the Unified Modeling Language (UML) development process [Booch et al., 1999]. This analysis is meant to specifically identify and characterize each use of a product or system by each user. UML calls these users "actors." Use-cases are valuable for identifying each functional type of user and the functions that they will perform.

81.4.1.3 Scenario-Based Analysis and Design

In this analysis a set of representative scenarios are defined and used to examine how the product or system will be used in the contexts of its use. Scenarios are especially useful for revealing and addressing highly critical, low-probability situations. Rosson [1999] develops a form of user-interaction scenarios that are an expansion of use-case scenarios. These are particularly useful for modeling a user's goals, expectations, and reactions and provide a means of tracing these user aspects through to design. See Carroll [2000] for more scenario-based design.

81.4.1.4 Participatory Design and Knowledge Acquisition

Participatory design is a cooperative approach that includes some users on the design team as active participants in the design process. This approach ensures that the design team includes domain expertise and as such represents the expectation that this expertise will translate into successful designs. Participatory design is very applicable to biomedical products because in many cases expert medical knowledge will need to be incorporated into the system and an understanding of the medical knowledge of the various user groups will be needed to inform the design. The various methods discussed in this section are not meant to be exclusive of one another and the use of more than one approach is encouraged. Carroll et al. [2002] provides a particularly good example of this, by combining participatory methods with a scenario-based design approach and ethnographic design techniques.

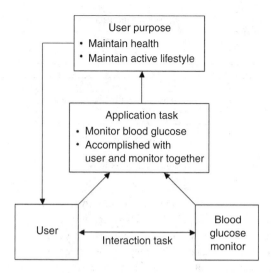

FIGURE 81.1 The user's purpose is served by the application task, which is accomplished through the interaction task.

81.4.1.5 Task Analysis, Allocation, and Modeling

Task analysis is a process of decomposing the activities and functions that need to be performed into their constituents. When humans interact with products or systems, two types of tasks are performed: an **interaction task** and an **application task**. The interaction task consists of the activities that the user performs to use the product or system. These activities include moving a mouse device, typing keyboard inputs, viewing displays, searching for and managing files, managing displays, setting preferences, and running programs.

The application task refers to the user's functional objectives that will in turn satisfy the user's purpose. These objectives vary widely and include planning a surgery, performing a statistical analysis, diagnosing a patient's condition, finding information in a database, monitoring blood pressure, and living independently. The application task is a higher-level task than the interaction task, meaning that the interaction tasks are subtasks that contribute to accomplishing the application task. Figure 81.1 illustrates the relationships between these two task levels and the greater purpose being satisfied for a user employing a blood glucose monitor. Note that the user and the monitor work together to accomplish the application task.

81.4.2 Quantifying Tasks

Tasks can be analyzed qualitatively and quantitatively. There are several methods for quantifying various aspects of HCI tasks. The GOMS (for goals, operators, methods, and selection rules) and keystroke-level models [Card et al., 1983, 1986], when used in combination with human-performance models such as the model human processor, provide task-performance estimates and knowledge requirements. The NGOMSL (for natural GOMS language) [Kieras, 1998] and TAG (task action grammar) [Payne and Green, 1986; Schiele and Green, 1990] models provide quantitative metrics for interaction task complexity and consistency.

Another effort to define quantitative usability metrics generated the metrics for usability standards in computing (MUSiC) methodology [Bevan and Macleod, 1994]. This methodology uses these metrics for specifying usability goals and intermittently testing to verify meeting the goals as part of the design process.

Kondraske [1995] has developed an elemental resource model (ERM) of human performance [Kondraske, 1995] that can be applied to quantify tasks in terms of the requirements for and availability of performance and skill resources. Each performance resource is defined in terms of a quantitative unidimensional capability to perform an elemental function. Skill resources are defined in terms of

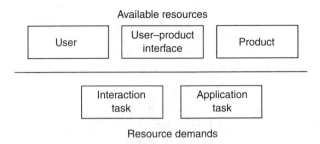

FIGURE 81.2   Designs must supply adequate resources to meet resource demands.

knowledge and experience. Adopting this model allows usability tradeoffs in design decisions to be stated in terms of the relationships between (1) available resources and the sources that possess them and (2) required resources and the sinks that expend them. Sources of resources include the user, the product, and the user–product interface. Sinks are the interaction and application tasks, Figure 81.2. The ERM is the only model that (1) incorporates all required dimensions of performance and skills, (2) provides a performance-modeling capability at elementary and intermediate levels, and (3) uses consistent modeling constructs across tasks, humans, and products.

Since, as in the example in Figure 81.1, the human and the biomedical product work together to satisfy the application task, the resources needed to accomplish both tasks are distributed between the human and the product. With this model, the design process can manage required and available resources to guide acceptable solutions. The usability of a given design concept can be predicted on the basis of this resource management. The designer has partial or full control over the resources required of the user to perform the interaction and application tasks by optimally off-loading (i.e., allocating) required resources to the product and user–product interface. Figure 81.3 illustrates the resource correspondence between the user, product, and interface between them. The arrows indicate the flow of information across the interface. The arrow between the cognitive–emotive resources is dashed to indicate that this level of information exchange is indirect and managed through input–output resources.

The designer has much control over the design of the interaction task. Although tempting, it is useful not to let HCI tasks to be defined by existing noncomputer-based ways of doing the task. Meaning, do not rely solely on existing task flows. The process of creating innovative task flows for new environments is what Kramer et al. [2000] calls "exploring the blue sky."

81.4.3 Minimal and Optimal Usability

Use of the ERM enables the designer to define and explore design boundaries. For example, the ERM would define an HCI design as minimally usable when all the user's performance and skill resources needed to accomplish the interaction and application tasks are exhausted in achieving a desired level of application-task performance. This means that the user can perform the task using the product only with maximal effort and expenditure of resources. Note that this definition of usability does not address the design of the HCI specifically. Rather, it addresses the relationship between the performance that can be obtained with a given HCI design and the effort a user needs to expend to achieve it. This means that different users will have different points at which an HCI for a given task will be minimally usable.

The concept of optimal usability is more complex. An optimized design will allow users maximal use of their performance and skill resources, allocated at their discretion to the application task, to maximize their performance on the application task. Thus an optimal design minimizes the resources required to perform the interaction task and enhances the utility of the user's resources in performing the application task. This means that the interface will support the user in performing the portion of the application task allocated to the user. This is accomplished through application-level design issues associated with the organization and level of objects, actions, and information.

User resources   Product/interface resources

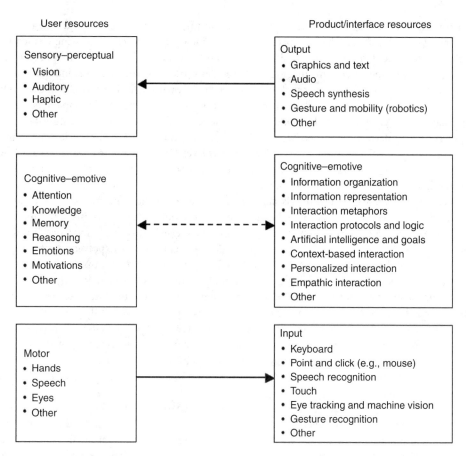

FIGURE 81.3 Resource correspondence between user resources and product/interface resources.

81.5 Performance-Based Usability Design Decisions

Successful HCI design decisions must be made on the basis of (1) knowledge about the user's performance and skill resources, (2) the performance and skill resource requirements of the application task, and (3) the performance capabilities of available technology.

Design strategies for achieving usability follows from an analysis of available and required resources and application of HCI design principles that act to reduce resource task demand on users. For example, usability will tend to increase as the resources required of the user to perform the interaction and application tasks decrease. Usability will tend to increase as interface resource availability of the resources increases.

A detailed discussion regarding performance resources is presented by Kondraske [1995] and in this Handbook. Different resource sources and tasks impose different design objectives. One performance-based design objective is to apply HCI resources to minimize the number of performance resources the user needs to perform the interaction task. This approach permits the user to allocate more resources to performing the application task. Achieving this objective includes (1) incorporating appropriate input and display devices to meet the user's sensory–motor resources and (2) use of organizations, representations, and levels of object, actions, and information that fit within the limits of the user's cognitive resources.

A second performance-based design objective is to apply HCI resources to optimize the resources the user needs to perform the application task. Many of the objects, actions, and information with which the user interacts are application-task-specific. Organization and representation decisions should be based on these task-specific requirements. For example, if the application task involves drawing, the user needs general software and hardware drawing tools and devices.

This consideration can be used to illustrate the relationship between application and interaction task-level design issues. A software-drawing package can provide different levels of drawing elements (e.g., having a tool to directly draw n-sided polygons vs. a line-drawing tool from which a polygon can be drawn segment by segment). Assume that the HCI provides a palette of drawing tools and that it includes primitive and complex tools. The user can draw an n-sided polygon using the line tool or using the polygon tool. Both tools are included in the palette. The issue here is how the decision to develop the polygon tool and include it in the product is made. The decision must be based on the user's application-task need to draw polygons. This need is established by an analysis of the application task. Thus the decision to include the polygon tool is an HCI decision at the application-task level. Once this applied need is established, the HCI design needs of how to represent, where to locate, and how to operate the tool are addressed. These are HCI design issues at the interaction-task level.

The decisions at these two task levels can be further used to illustrate interactions in assessing performance-based usability. A decision to include the polygon tool made on the basis of the application-task requirements will increase usability at the application-task level in that the user will need to use fewer sensory–motor resources to create a polygon. However, the inclusion of the polygon tool complicates the interaction-task level in that more items are added to the tool palette and that procedures need to be defined for drawing it. As discussed later, these complications are addressed by applying HCI design principles that reduce performance and skill-resource demands. Because the ERM defines performance resources at an elemental level, performance-based design can be conducted at the elemental level or at higher intermediate levels. Intermediate levels reduce the granularity of the analysis and provide for use of composite performance resources. For example, analyzing a menu-selection task performed with a mouse device at an elemental level would involve performance resources for speed, accuracy, and steadiness of positioning movements. An intermediate-level analysis could use pointing as a composite performance resource.

In exploring why users often have difficulty progressing from basic ways of doing a task to more efficient ways, Bhavnani and John [2000], conclude that there is an intermediate level of knowledge required that is not explicit in knowledge of the tool or the task. They discuss several reasons for inefficient use. Because, the ERM represents a systematic means of modeling resources at an intermediate level it provides a way to address this problem from a performance rather than from a knowledge perspective.

81.6 Heuristics for Reducing Task-Resource Demands

The ERM can be used in a rigorous way when performance data are obtainable or less rigorously as a set of principles to guide designing for enhanced usability. Rigorous application requires an analysis of available and required performance and skill resources and performance data associated with each resource. These data are usually not obtainable for all resources. Less rigorous application uses the principles of resource economics, resource stress, and analyses of the performance and skill resources involved in tasks to guide the design toward lower resource demands on the user. Usability can be improved by applying resource-demand-reducing HCI heuristics. Five major design heuristics that act to reduce task demands on performance and skill resources are described.

81.6.1 Naturalness and Familiarity of Interaction

Usability will be improved to the degree that the interaction is natural and familiar. Naturalness and familiarity reduce training requirements and increase available resources (e.g., available knowledge and sensory–motor performance). For physical components at a task level, this means that the user's sensory and effector modalities are properly matched to the required interactions, for example, keyboards used for typing, keypads for data entry, and mouse, pen, or touch-screen devices for pointing. For physical components at a feature level, this means that (1) user anthropometrics are employed in defining workstation and component configurations and dimensions and (2) that the physical characteristics of controls and displays (e.g., operating force, sensitivity, brightness, intensity, and size of displayed information) are congruous with the users and physical capabilities. For mental components at a task level, natural interaction means that the HCI models the user's tasks in accordance with the user's knowledge and experience. For mental components at a feature level, natural interaction means that the user's perceptual and cognitive capabilities and limitations are employed in defining HCI features (e.g., icons, names, screen layouts, and the behavior of window controls such as scroll bars). Direct manipulation interaction techniques (e.g., drag and drop) are a form of natural interaction in that they create a software mechanism with a physical analogy.

81.6.2 Simplicity of Interaction

Simplicity applies across a wide variety of design issues and must be incorporated in every architectural category. Applying this principle reduces training requirements, memory demands, perceptual demands, and the cognitive demands for inference. For the physical interface component, applying this principle reduces the number of physical steps needed to select and invoke actions and reduces movement precision requirements.

81.6.3 Consistency

Consistency reduces training requirements and memory requirements and promotes skill development. Consistency applies across a wide variety of design issues and must be incorporated in every architectural category. Examples include object, action, and information organizations, task flows, representations for objects and actions, and procedures. TAG [Payne and Green, 1986; Schiele and Green, 1990] provides a formal technique for analyzing consistency.

81.6.4 Robustness

Robustness refers to the ability of the design to tolerate user error and to span the functional requirements of the user. Error tolerance reduces resources needed to recover from errors and reduces initial accuracy requirements, allowing the user to increase operating speed. Users may commit errors because of a lack of knowledge. In this case, the user may be exploring the system to learn it. These are not errors. But this type of behavior should be expected, and the design should allow the user to do this exploration and to recover from anything he or she may do. Users may commit errors because of a misunderstanding or negative transfer from other systems. Thus a user may infer that a menu item will elicit a given behavior because it does so on another system that he or she has used. Or the user may feel that he or she understands what a given menu item or icon means and be wrong. Users may commit errors through unintentional commands. For example, a user may inadvertently click a wrong button, hit a wrong key, or select a wrong item from a menu. Ensuring adequate functional coverage reduces the functional demands on the user.

81.6.5 Accommodation of User Capabilities

In resource terms, applying this design principle increases the fit between an individual user's available mental and physical resources and those required by the interaction and application tasks. There are two major dimensions on which users vary: experience and capability.

Along the experience dimension users vary between experts and novices on either the interaction or application task. Thus a user could be very experienced with the applied task but not with doing that task on a computer. Similarly, a user may be very used to using computers but not skilled in the applied task. Novice users will (1) need more guidance and feedback, (2) require more structure to the task, (3) rely more on memory-aiding design features (e.g., menus), and (4) benefit more from online help facilities than expert users. Expert users (1) will want more flexibility in task control, (2) will want shortcut methods to do high-level actions, (3) will rely more on recall rather than memory aids, and (4) will benefit more from the use of preferences and tailored configurations than novice users [Brown, 1988; Galitz, 1993].

Along the capacity dimension users vary between healthy and impaired. In the ERM, impairments are not defined differently from any other performance or skill differences among users. All differences are defined in terms of the amount of specific performance resources available to an individual. Impaired users will vary greatly in capacity and experience. Only through an analysis of resources demanded by the task and resources available to the user can an adequate design for an impaired user be accomplished successfully.

81.7 Design Iteration

The methods described earlier generate the information needed by designers to develop design concepts. Early design concepts need not and should not be overly detailed. HCI design is an iterative process and the benefits of iteration are lost if too much detail is specified in early iterations. Generating quality designs requires imagination and unnecessary detail too early will tend to block innovations at more abstract levels of the design. Iteration guides a graceful narrowing that matches design solutions to the level of understanding of the users and the tasks available. Each cycle either corrects design problems or refines the detail of design areas that work.

After design concepts have been developed they need to be prototyped and evaluated. Prototypes are early forms of a product or system that incorporate partially or fully the functions and features of a system. Prototypes can be developed at any of a range of fidelities and are an essential tool in evaluating usability as well as engineering feasibility and marketability. Early prototypes will generally be of low fidelity and may only model part of the functionality of the product. As with the design, prototypes will evolve to greater fidelity and functionality.

Evaluation is a matter of testing, measuring, and validating the usability of the design. Usability evaluations are performed iteratively. Since the designs and their prototypes will be at evolving levels of specification their evaluations may be performed in fundamentally different ways. Relatively inexpensive and expedient evaluations include cognitive walkthroughs and expert heuristic inspections [Nielson, 1994]. More elaborate evaluations include format empirical studies that can collect objective task-performance data as well as subjective data.

Evaluations will lead to a reexamination of requirements, narrowing of the range of design concepts under consideration, and refinement of superior concepts in a subsequent design iteration.

Defining Terms

Application task: Refers to the objectives the user is employing the product to accomplish.

Human-centered design: Human-centered design refers to a philosophy of human-machine system design that places the focus of the design process on the needs of the human who uses the system to accomplish a task.

Interaction task: Refers to the activities that the user performs to use the product (e.g., moving a mouse device, typing keyboard inputs, viewing displays, searching for and managing files, managing displays, setting preferences, and executing programs).

Usability: Usability is a multidimensional quality that affords the user practical and convenient interaction with the product for achieving applied objectives. The concept of usability is fundamental to the design of any human system.

References

Abowd G.D. and Mynatt E.D. 2002. Charting past, present, and future research in ubiquitous computing. In J.M. Carroll (Ed.), *Human–Computer Interaction in the New Millennium*, pp. 513–535. ACM Press, New York.

Bach-y-Rita P., Tyler M.E., and Kaczmarek K.A. 2003. Seeing with the brain. *Int. J. Human–Computer Interaction* 15: 287–297.

Bental D. and Cawsey, A. Personalized and adaptive systems for medical consumer applications. *Commun. ACM* 45: 5.

Bevan N. and Macleod M. 1994. Usability measurement in context. *Behav. Inform. Technol.* 13: 132.

Bhavnani S.K. and John B.E. 2000. The strategic use of complex computer systems. *Human–Computer Interaction* 15: 2, 3.

Booch G., Rumbaugh J., and Jacobson I. 1999. *The Unified Modeling Language User Guide*. Addison-Wesley, Reading, MA.

Brown C.M. 1988. *Human–Computer Interface Design Guidelines*. Ablex Publishing, Norwood, NJ.

Card S.K., Moran T.P., and Newell A. 1986. The model human processor. In K.R. Boff, L. Kaufman, J.P. Thomas (Eds.). *Handbook of Perception and Human Performance*, Vol. II, pp. 45-1–45-35. John Wiley & Sons, New York.

Card S.K., Moran T.P., and Newell A. 1983. *The Psychology of Human–Computer Interaction*. Hillsdale, NJ, Erlbaum.

Carroll J.M. (Ed.). 2000. *Making Use: Scenario-Based Design of Human–Computer Interactions*. MIT Press, Cambridge, MA.

Carroll J.M., Chin G., Rosson M.B., and Neale D.C. 2002. The development of cooperation: five years of participatory design in the virtual school. In J.M. Carroll (Ed.), *Human–Computer Interaction in the New Millennium*, pp. 191–209. ACM Press, New York.

Cavazza M. and Simo A. 2003. A virtual patient based on qualitative simulation. IUI'03, January 12–15, Miami, FL.

Darnell M.J. 2004. Bad human factors designs. http://www.baddesigns.com/

Fogg B.J. 2003. *Persuasive Technology*. Morgan Kaufmann, San Francisco, CA.

Forlizzi J., DiSalvo C., and Gemperle F. 2004. Assistive robots and an ecology of elders living independently in their homes. *Human–Computer Interaction* 19: 1, 2.

Galitz W.O. 1993. *User-Interface Screen Design*. QED Publishing Group, Boston.

Han H., Yamashita J., and Fujishiro I. 2002. 3D haptic shape perception using a 2D device. *ACM SIGGRAPH*, p. 135.

ISO 13407. 1999. Human-centred design processes for interactive systems. International Organization for Standardization.

ISO 9241-11. 1998. Ergonomic requirements for office work with visual display terminals (VDTs) Part 11: Guidance on usability. International Organization for Standardization.

Javahery H., Seffah A., and Radhakrishnan T. 2004. Beyond power: making bioinformatics tools user-centered. *Commun. ACM* 47: 11.

Johnson C.R., MacLeod R., Parker S.G., and Weinstein D. 2004. Biomedical computing and visualization software environments. *Communications of the ACM* 47: 11.

Keates S., Clarkson P.J., and Robinson P. 2004. Computer assistance for motion-impaired users. Cambridge Engineering Design Centre. http://www.edc.eng.cam.ac.uk/inclusivedesign/computeraccess/

Kieras D.E. 1988. Towards a practical GOMS model methodology for user interface design. In M. Helander (Ed.), *Handbook of Human–Computer Interaction*, pp. 135–157. Elsevier Science Publishers, New York.

Kondraske G.V. 1995. A working model for human–system–task interfaces. In J.D. Bronzino (Ed.), *The Biomedical Engineering Handbook*, pp. 2157–2174. CRC Press, Boca Raton, FL.

Kramer J., Noronha S., and Vergo J. 2000. A user-centered design approach to personalization. *Commun. ACM* 43: 8.

Leroy G., Chen H., Martinez J.D., Eggers S., Falsey R.R., Kislin K.L., Huang Z., Li J., Xu J., McDonald D.M., and Ng G. 2003. Genescene: biomedical text and data mining, information retrieval and data mining. *JCDL'03: Proceedings of the 3rd ACM/IEEE-CS Joint Conference on Digital Libraries*, pp. 116–118.

Maxwell K. 2002. The maturation of HCI: moving beyond usability toward holistic interaction. In J.M. Carroll (Ed.), *Human–Computer Interaction in the New Millennium*, pp. 191–209. ACM Press, New York.

Miller C.S. and Remington R.W. 2004. Modeling information navigation: implications for information architecture. *Human–Computer Interaction* 19: 3.

Nielsen, J. and Mack, R.L. (Eds.). 1994. *Usability Inspection Methods*. John Wiley & Sons, New York, NY.

Norman D.A. 2004. Emotional design. *Basic Books*. Dept. of Perseus Book Group, Cambridge, MA.

Norman D.A. 1998. *The Invisible Computer*. MIT Press, Cambridge, MA.

Payne S.J. and Green T. 1986. Task-action grammars: a model of mental representation of task languages. *Human–Computer Interaction* 2: 93.

Plaisant C., Druin A., Lathan C., Dakhane K., Edwards K., Vice J.M., and Montemayor J. 2000. A storytelling robot for pediatric rehabilitation. *Assets '00*, November 13–15, Arlington, VA.

Raghupathi W. and Tan J. 2002. Startegic IT applications in health care. *Communications of the ACM* 45: 12.

Rogers W.A., Mykityshyn A.l., Cambell R.H., and Fisk A.D. 2001. Analysis of a "simple" medical device. *Ergonomics in Design* 9: 1.

Rosson M.B. 1999. Integrating development of task and object models. *Communications of the ACM* 42: 1.

Schiele F. and Green T. 1990. HCI formalisms and cognitive psychology: the case of task-action grammar. In M. Harrison and H. Thimbleby (Eds.), *Formal Methods in Human–Computer Interaction*, pp. 9–62. Cambridge University Press, Cambridge, UK.

Scholtz J. 2002. Evaluation methods for human-system performance of intelligent systems. *Proceedings of the 2002 Performance Metrics for Intelligent Systems (PerMIS) Workshop*. National Institute of Standards and Technology, Gaithersburg, MD.

Shneiderman B. 2002. *Leonardo's Laptop*. MIT Press, Cambridge, MA.

Streiz N.A., Tandler P., Muller-Tomfelde C., and Konomi S. 2002. Roomware: toward the next generation of human–computer interaction based on an integrated design of real and virtual worlds. In J.M. Carroll (Ed.), *Human–Computer Interaction in the New Millennium*, pp. 553–578. ACM Press, New York.

UNECE and IFR. 2004. United Nations Economic Commission for Europe and the International Federation of Robotics: World Robotics 2004. New York and Geneva, United Nations.

Yanco H.A., Drury J.L., and Sholtz J. 2004. Beyond usability evaluation: analysis of human–robot interaction at a major robotics competition. *Human–Computer Interaction* 19: 1, 2.

Wildemuth B.M., Friedman C.P., and Downs S.M. 1998. Hypertext versus boolean access to biomedical information: A comparison of effectiveness, efficiency, and user preferences. *ACM Transactions on Computer–Human Interaction* 5: 2.

Further Information

Human-centered design: www.upassoc.org/usability_resources/about_usability/what_is_ucd.html

Usability methods: usabilitynet.org/tools/methods.htm

Usability standards: www.usability.serco.com/trump/resources/standards.htm

General Information

Association for Computing Machinery, Special Interest Group in Computer–Human Interaction (ACM SIGCHI): www.acm.org/sigchi/

HCI Bibliography, suggested readings: www.hcibib.org/readings.html

Human Factors and Ergonomics Society: www.hfes.org/

Industrial Design Society of America: www.idsa.org/

Usability Net: usabilitynet.org

Usability Professionals' Association: www.upassoc.org/

82

Applications of Human Performance Measurements to Clinical Trials to Determine Therapy Effectiveness and Safety

Pamela J. Hoyes Beehler
University of Texas-Arlington

Karl Syndulko
UCLA School of Medicine

A **clinical trial** is a research study involving human subjects and an intervention (i.e., device, drug, surgical procedure, or other procedure) that is ultimately intended to either enhance the professional capabilities of physicians (i.e., improve the service delivered), improve the quality of life of patients, or contribute to the field of knowledge in those sciences which are traditionally in the medical field setting — for example, physiology, anatomy, pharmacology, epidemiology, neurology, cognitive psychology, etc. [Levin, 1986]. Clinical trials research is in the business of evaluating therapeutic interventions intended to benefit humans. Its value is directly related to the relevance of the questions "Do our treatments work?" "How well do our treatments work?" and "Are our treatments safe?" For example, drug A is designed and anticipated to relieve sinus congestion. Is there a drug interaction when drug A is taken with drug B and/or moderate levels of alcohol consumption such that while congestion is relieved (i.e., drug *A* is effective), human information processing capacities are reduced (i.e., is drug *A* safe?). And what is the time course of effects with regard to positive and negative (or adverse) effects? Thus it is clear that not only steady-state issues buy also dynamic questions are on interest in clinical trials research.

While clinical trials research incorporates many different components, the focus of this chapter is limited to study questions associated with human **performance capacity** variables and their measurement as they contribute to the determination of therapy effectiveness and safety. Such variables have been incorporated into trials since the use of controlled studies in the medical field began. However, the methodology employed to address human performance variables has been slowly but steadily shifting from mostly subjective to more objective instrumented methods [e.g., Tourtellotte et al., 1965] as both the understanding of the phenomena at play and the demand for improved quality of studies have increased. This chapter begins by briefly examining a classification of typical clinical trials study models, presents a summary of methods employed and key methodologic issues in both the design and conduct of studies (with special emphasis on issues related to the selection of measures and interpretation of results), and ends with a walk-through of a typical example that demonstrates the methods described. Brief discussion of the benefits that can be attributed to the use of objective, instrumented measures of human performance capacities as well as their current limitations in clinical trials research is also presented. While it is emphasized that most methods and issues addressed are applicable to any intervention, the use of human performance variables in pharmaceutical clinical trials has been most prevalent, and special attention has been given here to this application.

82.1 Basic Principles: Types of Studies

Depending on the set of primary and secondary questions to be addressed, considerable variety can exist with respect to the structure of a given trial and the analysis that is performed. Within the focus and scope of this chapter, clinical trials are classified into two categories for discussion: (1) safety-oriented and (2) efficacy-oriented. According to the Food and Drug Administration (FDA) [1977], four phases of research studies are required before a drug can be marketed in the United States. Phase I is known as *clinical pharmacology* and is intended to include the initial introduction of a drug into humans. These studies are safety-oriented; one issue often addressed is determination of the maximum tolerable dose. Phases II and III are known as *clinical investigation* and *clinical trials*, respectively, consisting of controlled and uncontrolled clinical trials research. Phase IV is the *postmarketing of clinical trials* to supplement premarketing data. Both safety and efficacy are addressed in phases II to IV investigations. As specified earlier, not all interventions studied are drugs. However, a similar phased approach is also characteristic of the investigation of therapeutic devices and treatments.

Safety-oriented trials usually involve vital sign measures (e.g., heart rate, blood pressure, respiration rate), clinical laboratory tests (e.g., blood chemistries, urinalysis, ECG), and adverse reaction tests (both mental and physical performance capacities) to evaluate the risk of the intervention. In this chapter we focus on the adverse reaction components, most of which historically have been addressed with subjective reporting methods. In the case of drug interventions, different doses (e.g., small to large) are administered within the trial, and the dose-related effects are examined. Thus the rate at which a drug is metabolized (**pharmacokinetics**), as evidenced by changes in drug concentrations in blood, cerebral spinal fluid, urine, etc., is usually addressed in safety-oriented drug studies, as well as the maximum dosage which subjects can tolerate [Baker et al., 1985; Fleiss, 1986; Tudiver et al., 1992; Jennison and Turnbull, 1993].

Efficacy-oriented trials are usually conducted after initial safety-oriented trials have established that the intervention has met safety criteria, but they will always have safety questions and elements as well. In this type of study, the goal is to objectively determine the therapeutic effect. Whatever the type of intervention, these studies are designed around the bottom-line question "Is the intervention effective?" In many cases (e.g., drugs for neurologic disorders, exercise programs for musculoskeletal injuries, etc.), *effectiveness* implies improvement or retarding the rate of deterioration in one or more aspects of mental and/or physical performance. With regard to disease contexts, it is necessary to distinguish performance changes that merely reflect treatment of systems as opposed to those which reflect the slowing or reversal of the basic disease process. Studies typically include pre- and postintervention measurement points and, whenever feasible, a control group that is administered a placebo intervention [Fleiss, 1986; Weissman, 1991; Tang and Geller, 1993]. The situation is complicated because there are many performance capacities that could be affected. In response to the intervention, some capacities may improve, some may remain unchanged, and some may be adversely affected. Thus efficacy-oriented studies typically include a number of secondary questions that address specificity of effects. When the intervention is a drug, both the pharmacokinetics and *pharmacodynamics* are often addressed. Pharmacodynamic studies attempt to relate physiologic and/or metabolic changes in the concentration of the agent over time to corresponding changes in the therapeutic effect. Thus repeated measurement of selected performance capacities are required over relatively short periods of time as part of these **protocols**.

Clinical trials involving human performance metrics generally use the **randomized clinical trial** (RCT) design. The RCT is a way to compare the efficacy and safety of two or more therapies or regimens. It was originally designed to test new drugs [Hill, 1963]; however, over the last 25 years, it has been applied to the study of vaccinations, surgical interventions, and even social innovations such as multiphasic screening [Levin, 1986]. Levin [1986] describes four key elements of RCTs: (1) the trials are "controlled," that is, part of the group of subjects receive a therapy that is tested while the other subjects receive either no therapy or another therapy; (2) the significance of its results must be established through statistical analysis; (3) a double-blind experimental design should be used whenever possible; and (4) the therapies being compared should be allocated among the subjects randomly. Levin [1986] further noted that "the RCT is the gold standard for evaluating therapeutic efficacy."

82.2 Methods

Studies are defined and guided by *protocols*, a detailed statement of all procedures and methods to be employed. Figure 82.1 summarizes the major steps in clinical trials in which human performance variables represent those of primary interest, although the general process is similar for most trial involving human subjects.

82.2.1 Selecting Study Variables

In many clinical trials, performance measurements must be focused on the specific disease or set of symptoms against which a medication or intervention is directed. The critical element is selection of an outcome assessment that will indicate directly whether the intervention can eliminate key signs or symptoms of the disease, improve function affected by the disease, or even simply delay further disease progression and loss of function. Economic and statistical constraints of such trials often indicate that a minimal set of measures must be used to provide valid, reliable, and sensitive indicators of changes in underlying disease activity related to the treatments. In many instances, there is considerable controversy about what constitutes a valid and reliable assessment of the underlying disease process, or there may be de facto standards adopted by clinicians, pharmaceutical companies, and the FDA as to the choice of outcome assessments. In many diseases, these standards may be physician rating scales of disease severity. Thus objective studies may be required in the case of specific diseases and disorders to delineate the most sensitive set of performance measures for clinical trial evaluations [Mohr and Prouwers, 1991]. Further, it often must be demonstrated to clinicians, drug companies, and the FDA that the objective performance measures selected as outcome assessments actually do provide equal or more sensitive indicators of disease progression (and improvement) than do existing rating scale measures traditionally utilized in clinical trials. Experience with human performance testing in multiple sclerosis clinical trials, discussed below, illustrates these issues.

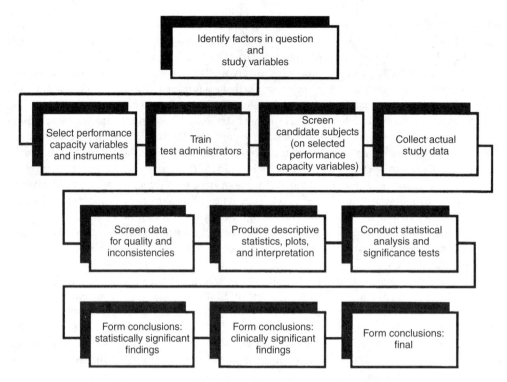

FIGURE 82.1 Summary of major steps in the conduct of a clinical trial involving human performance capacities.

When objective measurement of performance capacities has been incorporated into many clinical trials, concepts and tools from human performance engineering can facilitate the selection of variables and shed some light on issues noted above. In either safety- or efficacy-oriented studies, study variable selection can be characterized as a two-step process: (1) identification of the factors in question (Table 82.1) and (2) selection of the relevant *performance capacities* to be measured and associated measurement instruments. This link between these two steps often represents a challenge to researchers for a number of reasons. First, duality in terminology must be overcome. Concerns about an intervention are typically initially identified with "negative" terms such as "dizziness" and not in terms of performance capacities such as "postural stability." Human performance models based on systems engineering concepts [Kondraske, 1995] can be used to facilitate the translation of both formal and lay terms used to identify adverse effects to relevant performance capacities to be measured, as shown in Table 82.1.

In Kondraske's [1995] model, performance capacities are modeled as resources that a given system possesses and draws up to perform tasks. It also provides a basis for delineation of *hierarchical* human systems and their performance capacities as well as a basis to quantitatively explain the interaction of available performance capacities with demands of higher-level tasks (e.g., such as those encountered in daily living). The hierarchical aspect is particularly important in selecting performance capacities to be measured. It is generally good practice to include a combination of carefully selected lower-level and higher-level capacity measures. This combination allows careful tradeoffs between information content (i.e., specificity) and simplicity of the protocol (e.g., number of variables, time for test administration, etc.). Higher-level capacities (characterizing systems responsible for gait, postural stability, complex mental task, etc.) are dependent on the performance capacities of multiple lower-level subsystems. Thus a few higher-level performance capacities can reflect multiple lower-level capacities (e.g., knee flexor strength, visual information processing speed, etc.). However, lower-level capacity measures are typically less variable than higher-level capacities within individuals (i.e., on retest) and within populations. Therefore, small changes in performance can be more readily discriminated statistically if they exist and are attributable primarily to localized lower-level capacities (e.g., see data in Potvin et al. [1985]). Also, more specific

TABLE 82.1   Representative Examples of Linking Factors in Question to Specific Measurable Performance Capacities

Factor in question[a]	Selected relevant performance capacities[b]
General central nervous system effects (of drug)	Selected activity of daily living execution speed Postural stability Upper extremity neuromotor channel capacity Manual manipulation speed Visual-upper extremity information processing speed Visual attention span Visual-spatial memory capacity Visual-numerical memory capacity
Alcohol interaction (of drug)	Selected activity of daily living execution speed Postural stability Visual information processing speed Visual-spatial memory capacity
Dizziness	Postural stability
Drowsiness	Selected activity of daily living execution speed Visual attention span Visual-upper extremity information procession speed Bond-Lader visual analog scale
Slowness of movement, psychomotor retardation	Visual-upper extremity information processing speed Upper extremity random reach movement speed Index finger (proximal intercarpal phalangeal joint), flexion-extension speed
Mood	Emotional stability (e.g., with Hamilton anxiety scale, Bond-Lader analog scale and other similar tools)
Speed	Reaction time
Coordination	Finger tapping
Tremors, abnormal movements	Limb steadiness Postural stability Vocal amplitude and pitch steadiness
Joint stiffness or pain	Extremes and range of motion Isomeric strength (selected joins)
Weakness, strength	Postural stability (one leg, eyes open) Isometric grip strength Isometric strength (representative set of upper and lower extremity, proximal and distal muscle groups)
Sensation	Vibration sensitivity Thermal sensitivity

[a] Terms used include those often used by pharmaceutical companies to communicate adverse effects to general public.
[b] Lists are illustrative and not exhaustive. More or fewer items can be included depending on time available or willingness to expend for data collection, with commensurate tradeoffs between specificity and protocol simplicity.

information can provide valuable insights into physiologic effects if they are present. By combing both types, broad coverage can be achieved (so that aspects of human performance in which the expectation of an effect is less remain included), as well as a degree of specificity, while keeping the total number of study variables to a reasonable size. In addition, if an effect is found in both a higher-level capacity and a related lower-level capacity, an internal cross-validation of finding is obtained. Many early studies incorporated variables representing looks across different hierarchical levels but did not distinguish them by level during analysis and interpretation. While such logic begins to remove the guesswork, much work remains to refine variable-selection methodology.

To address the broad, bottom-line questions regarding safety and efficacy, the formation of **composite scores** (i.e., some combination of scores from two or more performance capacity challenges or "tests") is necessary. A resource model and the concept of hierarchical human systems also can be used to develop composite variables for practical use in clinical trials. Component capacities can be selected that are theoretically or empirically most sensitive to the disease or condition under study. The composite variable is then created by calculating a more traditional weighted arithmetic sum [Potvin et al., 1985] or product [Kondraske, 1989] of the component scores. In both cases, the definition of component scores is important (i.e., whether a smaller or larger number represents better performance). Treatments are not approved if only a small subset of individuals is helped. Composite measures provide the only objective means of integrating multidimensional information about an intervention's effects. The primary advantages of the composite variable is the creation of a single, global, succinct measure of the disease, condition, or intervention, which is often essential as the primary outcome assessment for efficacy. The major disadvantage is loss of detailed information about the unique profile of performance changes that each subject of a group as a whole may show. Such tradeoffs are to be expected. Thus both composite and component measures play important but different roles in clinical trials.

It is imperative that the selection of the study measures also consider a test's objectivity (nonbiased), reliability (consistency), and validity (measures what is intends to measure) to add to the quality of the measurements. Many complex issues, which are beyond the present scope, are associated with measuring and interpreting the quality of a measurement. (See Safrit [1990], Baumgartner and Jackson [1993], and Hastad and Lacy [1994] for more information.)

82.2.2 Formation of the Subject Pool

Clinical research investigations usually involve a *sample* group of subjects from a defined population. Selection of the study population so that generalizations from that sample accurately reflect the defined population is a dilemma that must be adequately addressed. If **probability sampling** is chosen, each subject in the defined population theoretically has an equal chance of being included in the sample. The advantage of this kind of sampling is that differences between treatment groups can be detected and the probability that these differences actually exist may be estimated. If **nonprobability sampling** is chosen, there is no way to ensure that each subject had an equal chance of being included in the sample. Conclusions of nonprobability sampling therefore have less merit (not as generalizable) than those based on probability sampling.

Studies with healthy subjects are believed to be necessary before exposing sick persons to some interventions because persons with disease or injuries commonly have impaired function of various organs that metabolize drugs and may take medications that can alter the absorption, metabolism, and/or excretion rates of the intervention. Gender issues also should be a concern in clinical trials because of new FDA regulations [Cotton, 1993; Merkatz et al., 1993; Stone, 1993].

All subjects selected as study candidates should be informed of the procedures that will be utilized in the clinical trials investigation by signing an informed consent document, as required by the Department of Health and Human Services *Code of Federal Regulations* [1985] and other federal regulations applicable to research involving human subjects. Using all or a subset of study measurement variables (in addition to medical history and examinations as necessary), a screening procedure is recommended to determine if each subject meets the minimum performance criteria established for subject inclusion. When patients are part of the sample group, this performance screening also can be used to establish that the sample includes the desired balance of subjects with different amounts of "room for improvement" on relevant variables. An added benefit of this screening process is that subjects and test administrators obtain experience with test protocols, equipment, an procedures that will add to the validity of the study.

Unless available from a previous similar study, it is typical for pilot data to be collected to estimate the expected size of outcome effects. With this information, the power of the statistical analysis (i.e., the likelihood that a significant difference will be detected) can be estimated so that sample size can be determined [Cohchran and Cox, 1957; Kepple, 1982; Fleiss, 1986]. Another concern is that some of the original subject pool will not complete the study or will have incomplete data. High attrition rates may damage the credibility of the study, and every effort should be made to not lose subjects.

DeAngelis [1990] estimates that attrition rates higher than 50% make the interpretation of clinical trial research very difficult. Some researchers believe that no attempt should be made to replace these subjects because even random selection of new subjects will not ensure bias caused by differential participation of all the subjects.

82.2.3 Data Collection

Investigators should seek to minimize sources of variability by careful control of the test conditions and procedures. Proper control can be attained by (1) using rooms that are reasonably soundproof or sound-deadened, well lighted, and of a comfortable temperature; (2) selecting chairs and other accessories carefully (e.g., no wheels for tests in which the subject is seated); (3) testing subjects one at a time without other subjects in the test room; (4) using standardized written instructions for each test to eliminate variability in what is stated; (5) allowing for familiarization with the test instruments and procedures; (6) not commenting about subject performance to avoid biased raising or lowering of expectations; (7) arranging a test order to offset fatigue (mental and physical) or boredom and to include rest periods; and (8) training test administrators and evaluating their training using healthy subjects, especially in multicenter studies, so that consistent results can be obtained.

82.2.4 Data Integrity Screening

Despite all good efforts and features incorporated to ensure high-quality data, opportunities exist for error. It is therefore beneficial to subject data obtained during formal test sessions to quality screenings. This is a step toward forming the official study data set (i.e., the set that will be subjected to statistical and other analyses). Several independent analyses used to screen data, which are typically computer-automated, are described below.

Screening of baseline measures against inclusionary criteria: If human performance study variables with specific performance criteria are used as part of the subject selection process as recommended above, each subject's baseline score can be compared with the score obtained during inclusionary testing. For most variables, baseline scores should not differ from inclusionary testing by more than 20% [Potvin et al., 1985]. Greater deviations point to examiner training, test procedure, or subject compliance problems.

Screening against established norms: For variables that are not included in inclusionary screenings or in studies where performance variables are not used as part of the subjects inclusionary criteria, baseline data can be screened against established reference data (e.g., human performance means and standard deviations). Data are considered acceptable if they fall within an established range (e.g., two standard deviation units of the reference population mean). From the perspective of risk associated with not identifying a data point that could be a potential problem, this is a fairly liberal standard that can still identify problems in data collection and management. Standards that lessen risk can, or course, be employed at the discretion of the investigator, but at the expense of the possible identification of a larger number of data points that require follow-up.

Screening against anticipated effects: It is more difficult to screen nonbaseline data for quality because of the possible influences of the intervention. However, criteria can be established based on (1) absolute level of variables (both maximums and minimums) and (2) rates and direction of change from one measurement period to the next. Even criteria that allow a rather wide range of data (or changes across repeated measures) can be useful in detecting gross anomalies and is recommended.

If anomalies are discovered using the screening methods described above, several outcomes are possible: (1) the anomaly can be traced and rectified (e.g., it may be attributable to a human or computer error with backup available); (2) the anomaly may be explainable as a procedural error, but it may not be possible to rectify; and (3) the anomaly may be unexplainable. Data anomalies that are explainable with supporting documentation could justify classification of the given data items as "missing data" or replacement of all data for the corresponding subject in the data set (i.e., the subject could be dropped from the study and replaced with another). There is no justification for eliminating or replacing data anomalies for which a documentable explanation does not exist.

82.2.5 Analysis and Interpretation of Results

Traditional inferential statistical analysis should be performed according to the statistical model and significance levels agreed on by the clinical research team when the study is designed. However, data also should be analyzed and interpreted from a clinical perspective as well.

In experimental research, tests of **statistical significance** are the most commonly used tools for assessing possible associations between independent and dependent variables as well as differences among treatment groups. The purpose of significance (i.e., statistical) tests is to evaluate the research hypothesis at a specific level of probability, or p value. For example, if a p value of .05 was chosen, the researcher is asking if the levels of treatment (for example) differ significantly so that these differences are not attributable to a chance occurrence more than 5 times out of 100. By convention, a p value of .01 (1%) or .05 (5%) is usually selected as the cutoff for statistical significance. Significance tests cannot accept a research hypothesis; all that significance tests can do is reject or fail to reject the research hypothesis [Thomas and Nelson, 1990]. Ultimately, significance tests can determine if treatment groups are different, but not why they are different. Good experimental design, appropriate theorizing, and sound reasoning are used to explain why treatment groups differ.

Exclusive reliance on tests of statistical significance in the present context can mislead the clinical researcher, and interpretation of **clinical significance** is required. The key issue here is the size of the observed effect; p values give little information on the actual magnitude of a finding (i.e., decrement or improvement in performance, etc.). Also, statistical findings are partially a function of sample size. Thus even an effect that is small in size can be detected with tests of statistical significance in a study with a large sample. For example, a mean difference in grip strength of 2 kg may be found in response to drug therapy. This difference is a quite small fraction of the variability in grip strength observed across normal individuals, however. Thus, although statistically significant, such a change would perhaps have a minimal impact on an individual's ability to function in daily activities which make demands on grip strength performance resources. Thus clinical significance addresses cause-and-effect relationships between study variables and performance in activities of daily life or other broad considerations such as the basic disease process. The danger of not defining clinical significance appropriately can be either that a good intervention is not used in practice (e.g., it may be rejected for a safety finding that is statistically significant but small) or that a poor intervention is allowed into practice (e.g., it may result in statistically significant improvements that are small).

Ideally, if empirical data existed that established what amount of a given performance capacity such as visual information processing speed (VIPS) was necessary to perform a task (e.g., driving safely on the highway), then it would be possible to interpret statistically significant findings (e.g., a decrement in VIPS of a known amount) to determine if the change would be a magnitude that would limit the individual from successfully accomplishing the given task. Unfortunately, while general cause–effect relationships between laboratory-measured capacities and performance in high-level tasks are evident, quantitative models do not yet exist, and completely objective interpretations of clinical significance are not yet possible. As such, the process by which clinical significance is determined is less well developed and structured. More recent concepts introduced by Kondraske [1988a,b, 1989] based on the use of **resource economic** principles (i.e., the idea of a threshold "cost" associated with lower-level variables typically employed in clinical trials for achieving a given level of human performance in any given high-level task) may be helpful in defining objective criteria for clinical significance. This approach directly addresses cause-and-effect relationships between performance capacities and high-level tasks with an approach much like that which an engineer would employ to design a system capable of performing a specified task.

Despite known limitations, interpretation of clinical significance is always incorporated into clinical trials in some fashion. Any change in human performance for a given variable should be first documented to be statistically significant before it is considered to be a candidate for clinical significance (i.e., a statistically significant difference is a necessary but not a sufficient condition for clinical significance). Objective determination of clinical significance can be based in part on previous methods introduced by Potvin et al. [1985] in clinical trials involving neuromotor and central processing performance tests. They advocate the use of an objective criteria whereby a decrease or increase in a human performance capacity (with healthy test subjects, for example) should be greater than 20% to be classified as "clinically significant." Kondraske [1989] uses a similar approach that uses z-scores (i.e., number of standard deviation units form a population mean) as the basis for determining criteria. This accounts for population variability which is different for different performance capacity variables. A recent approach is to assess effect size, a statistical metric that is independent of sample size and which takes into account data variability. This method provides an objective basis for comparison of the magnitude of treatment effects among studies [Cohen, 1988; Ottenbacher and Barrett, 1991].

82.3 Representative Application Examples

82.3.1 Safety-Oriented Example: Drug–Alcohol Interaction

In this section, selected elements of an actual clinical trial are presented to further illustrate methods and issues noted above. To maintain confidentialities, the drug under test is simple denoted as drug A.

Identify factors in question: Upper respiratory infections are among the most frequent infections encountered in clinical practice and affect all segments of the general population. The pharmacologic agent of choice for upper respiratory infections are the antihistamines (reference drug), which possess a wide margin of safety and almost no lethality when taken alone in an overdose attempt. Although quite effective, antihistamines can produce several troublesome side effects (i.e., general CNS impairment, sedation, and drowsiness) and have been incriminated in automobile accidents as well as public transportation disasters. New drugs (e.g., drug A) are being developed to have similar benefits but fewer side effects. From prior animal studies, drug A has been shown to have minimal effects on muscle relaxation and muscular coordination as well as less sedative and alcohol-potentiating effects than those associated with classical antihistamines. Based on drug A's history and concerns, the following factors in question were identified in this clinical trial: general CNS impairment, alcohol interaction, dizziness, drowsiness, mood, and slowness of movement/speed. The purpose of this investigation was to examine the effect of drug A on human performance capacity relative to a reference drug and placebo as well as the drug-alcohol potentiating interaction effects after multiple dose treatment.

Select performance capacity variables and instruments: With the factors in question identified, the following performance capacity variables and their testing instruments were selected for the clinical trial: visual information processing speed (VIPS), finger tapping speed (TS), visual arm lateral reach coordination (VALRC), visual spatial memory capacity (VSMC), postural performance (PP), digit symbol substitution task (DSST), and Bond-Lader Visual Analog Scale (BLS). These variables were collectively called the *human performance capacity test battery* (HPCTB) (Table 82.2). Due to space limitations, only one performance capacity variable (VMRS — visual information processing speed, i.e., VIPS) is discussed in this section.

Experimental design: The first primary objective of this investigation was to examine after 8 days of oral dosing the relative effects of drug A, reference drug, and placebo on the human performance capacity of healthy male and female adult volunteers (see Table 82.2). This effect was determined by examining the greatest decrease in human performance capacity from day 1 of testing (i.e., baseline at -0.5 h drug ingestion time) to day 8 of testing at drug ingestion times of 0.0, 1.0, 2.0, 4.0, and 6.0 h. The second primary objective was to examine after 9 days of oral dosing the relative effects of drug A, reference drug, and placebo in combination with a single dose of alcohol served immediately after drug administration (male alcohol dose 0.85 g/kg body weight, female alcohol dose 0.75 g/kg body weight) on the human performance capacity of healthy male and female adult volunteers (see Table 82.2). This effect was determined by comparing the greatest decrease in performance on the ninth day of study drug treatment (at drug ingestion times of 0.0, 1.0, 2.0, 4.0, and 6.0 h) to baseline on day one of

TABLE 82.2   Experimental Schedule for Human Performance Capacity
Test Battery (HPCTB)

	Drug ingestion times (h)					
Test day	−0.5	0.0	1.0	2.0	4.0	6.0
1[a]	HPCTB					
8[b]		HPCTB	HPCTB	HPCTB	HPCTB	HPCTB
9[b,c]		HPCTB	HPCTB	HPCTB	HPCTB	HPCTB

Note: The human performance capacity test battery (HPCTB) was
administered in the following order: VIPS, TS, VALRC, VSMC, PP, DSST,
and BLS.
[a] On day 1 of testing only, the −0.5 HPCTB was performed and utilized as the
baseline value for test days 8 and 9.
[b] The peak effect was determined by comparing baseline values (day 1) against
the greatest detriment in performance for the eighth and ninth testing days at
drug ingestion times of 0.0, 1.0, 2.0, 4.0, and 6.0 h.
[c] On day 9 of testing, an alcohol drink was served immediately after drug
administration and was ingested over a 15-min period.

testing (−0.5 h drug ingestion time) for the HPCTB (see Table 82.2). Independent variables were treatment
group (1 = drug A, 2 = reference drug, and 3 = placebo) and gender (male/female). The dependent
variable was maximum decrease in performance (peak effect) for each human performance capacity study
variable and was determined by comparing the baseline value (day 1) against the greatest decrease in performance at drug ingestion times of 0.0, 1.0, 2.0, 4.0, and 6.0 h for day 8 and day 9 of testing. Inferential
statistical analysis of the data was performed using a 3 (treatment group: reference drug, drug A, and
placebo) by 5 (hour; 0, 1, 2, 4, and 6) mixed factorial ANOVA with repeated measures on hour for each
dependent variable. Statistical tests of significance of all ANOVAs were conducted at the 0.05 level.

Data screening: For each dependent variable, baseline treatment data were compared against the criteria
established for subject inclusion using each subject's performance score from the HPCTB to identify
data anomalies. Then the expected increases/decreases in human performance capacity from baseline
treatment data were compared against the drug therapy-influenced data to determine if these changes
were within "reasonable" limits. Potential anomalies were detected in less than 5% of the data, with most
occurring within records for only a few subjects. These cases were investigated, and in consultation with
the principal investigator, decisions were made and documented to arrive at the official data set.

Descriptive statistical analysis: Figure 82.2 illustrates the visual information processing speed (VIPS) for
treatment groups reference drug, drug A, and placebo. On day 1 of testing (baseline), all treatment groups
had similar VIPSs, with means between 5.7 and 5.8 stimuli per second. On day 8 of testing and at drug
ingestion time of 2 h, VIPS decreased to 4.9 stimuli per second for drug A, to 5.1 stimuli per second for
reference drug and to 5.65 stimuli per second for the placebo. On day 8, the greatest group impairment of
VIPS occurred at drug ingestion time of 4 h. Drug A appeared to have the greatest impairment of VIPS
(4.6 stimuli per second), followed by the reference drug group (4.9 stimuli per second). This decrease in
performance was not present with the placebo group (5.61 stimuli per second). By the sixth hour after drug
ingestion on day 8, VIPS improved toward baseline for treatment groups reference drug (5.1 stimuli per
second) and drug A (5.3 stimuli per second), while the placebo group remained unchanged (5.58 stimuli
per second). One day 9 of testing, all treatment groups received their assigned drug and alcohol. By 1 h
after drug ingestion, all treatment groups' VIPSs were impaired from baseline, with drug A showing the
greatest impairment (4.3 stimuli per second), followed by reference drug (4.6 stimuli per second) and
placebo (4.9 stimuli per second). All treatment groups' VIPSs improved toward baseline values by the
second hour after drug ingestion (5.0 to 5.1 stimuli per second) and the fourth hour after drug ingestion
(5.4 to 5.5 stimuli per second), respectively. By the sixth hour after drug ingestion, reference drug and
drug A plateaued between 5.55 and 5.6 stimuli per second, respectively, while the placebo group improved
slightly above the baseline value (5.8 stimuli per second). The basic pattern observed (i.e., decrease from

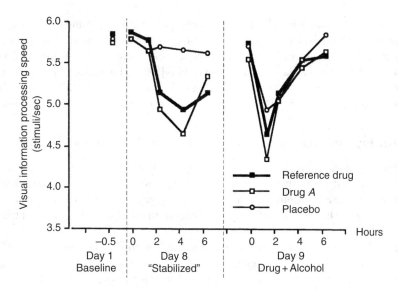

FIGURE 82.2 One performance capacity variable (visual information processing speed) for three treatment groups (drug *A* — the drug under test — reference drug, and placebo) taken from any actual efficacy-oriented study. Note changes from baseline to drug stabilization (day 8) and interaction with alcohol (day 9). See text for further explanation.

baseline, return to baseline, impairment of all groups, including placebo, with alcohol) lend validity to the overall study.

Statistical analysis and significance test results: On day 8 of testing, significant differences in VIPS for main effects treatment group and hour were observed. There was a significant interaction, however, between treatment group and hour of drug ingestion. Post hoc analysis demonstrated that treatment groups drug *A* and reference drug were significantly slower in VIPS than the placebo group at drug ingestion times of 2, 4, and 6 h, but there was no difference in VIPS between treatment groups drug *A* and reference drug. (Simple main effects and simple, simple main effects showed that the placebo group had faster VIPSs than both reference drug and drug *A* treatment groups at drug ingestion times of 2, 4, and 6 h.)

On day 9 of testing when the drug-alcohol potentiating interaction effect was of primary interest, significant differences in VIPS occurred for main effects treatment group and hour, but there were no interactions between treatment group and hour of drug ingestion. Post hoc analysis demonstrated that treatment groups drug *A* and reference group were significantly slower in VIPS than the placebo group at 1 h after drug ingestion only, but there was no statistically significant difference in VIPS between treatment groups drug *A* and reference group at any hour after drug-alcohol ingestion. Also, the drug-alcohol interaction was significant 1 h after drug-alcohol ingestion for all treatment groups.

Conclusions from statistically significant findings: After 8 days of oral dosing, while a significant difference was found for both drug treatment groups compared with the placebo group, there was no significant difference in VIPS between drug *A* and reference drug treatment groups. The effect was apparent at approximately the same drug ingestion time of 4 h. It was concluded that drug *A* had the same effect on safety as the reference drug in terms of CNS impairment as measured by VIPS.

After 9 days of oral dosing in combination with alcohol consumption, drug *A* and reference drug caused a greater decrease in VIPS compared with the placebo group. This effect was most apparent at 1 h after drug ingestion. The placebo group also decreased its VIPS at 1 h after drug ingestion at a statistically significant level. It was concluded after 9 days of oral dosing that drug *A* in combination with alcohol produced the same effect as the reference drug in combination with alcohol in terms of CNS impairment as measured by VIPS.

Conclusions from clinically significant findings. Since there was no statistically significant difference between drug *A* and the reference drug on either day 8 or day 9, the only findings requiring an interpretation of clinical significance are the statistically significant findings for both drug A and reference drug relative to the placebo group. On both day 8 and day 9, these findings are clinically significant using either the Potvin et al. [1985] percentage change or Kondraske [1989] z-score approach. Using the resource economic model for human performance [Kondraske, 1988a,b, 1989], it can be argued that, for example, during critical events during tasks such as driving, all of an individual's available VIPS resource is drawn on. Clearly, the substantial decrease in VIPS observed can compromise safety during such events.

82.3.2 Efficacy-Oriented Study: Experiences in Neurology

Performance testing in clinical trials in neurology has grown tremendously within the last decade [Mohr and Brouwers, 1991], but within specific disease areas there remains reluctance to accept the replacement of traditional rating-scale evaluations of disease presence and progression by objective performance testing [Syndulko et al., 1993]. The evolution of clinical evaluations in multiple sclerosis clinical trials illustrates this point.

Evaluation of disability change or deterioration in multiple sclerosis (MS) historically has been limited to physician rating scales that attempt to globally summarize some or most of the salient clinical features of the disease. General consensus in the use of rating scales for MS has been achieved in the specification of a minimal record of disability (MRD) for MS that incorporates several physician- and paramedical-administered rating scales for evaluating MS disease status and its effects on the patient's life (International Federation of Multiple Sclerosis Societies, 1984). However, there has been general dissatisfaction with the use of rating scales in MS clinical trials because of issues of lack or sensitivity to disease change, lack of interrater reliability, and simply the inherent reliance on subjective ratings of signs, symptoms, and unmeasured performance changes [Paty et al., 1992].

As an alternative to MS rating scales, comprehensive, quantitative evaluation of human performance was originally proposed and developed over 25 years ago for use in MS clinical trials [Tourtellotte et al., 1965]. The first application of performance testing in a major MS clinical trial was the multicenter cooperative ACTH study [Rose et al., 1968]. The study proved that human performance testing could be incorporated into a multicenter MS clinical trial and that examiners at multiple centers could be trained to administer the tests in a standardized, repeatable fashion. The results generally supported fairly comparable levels of sensitivity among the outcome measures, including performance testing [Dixon and Kuzma, 1974]. Subsequent analyses showed that a priori composites that provided succinct summary measures of disease change in key functional areas could be formed from the data and that these composite measures were sensitive to treatment effects in relapsing/remitting MS patients [Henderson et al., 1978]. Despite the favorable results of the ACTH study, performance testing did not achieve general acceptance in MS clinical studies. Comprehensive performance testing as conducted in the ACTH trial was considered time-consuming, the instrumentation was not generally available, and despite the use of composites, the number of outcome measures remained too large. In a recent double-blind, placebo-controlled collaborative study in 12 medical centers, the study design included both rating-scale and performance measures as outcome assessments in the largest sample of chronic progressive MS patients studied to date (The Multiple Sclerosis Study Group, 1990). Analyses of the change in performance composite scores from baseline over the 2-year course of the clinical trial showed that the drug-treated patients worsened significantly less than the placebo-treated patients. In contrast, the EDSS and other clinical rating scores did not show significant treatment effects for the subset of MS patients at the same center [Syndulko et al., 1993]. This indicated that the performance composites were more sensitive than the clinical disability measures to disease progression and treatment effects. A more recent comparative analysis of the full data set also supports the greater sensitivity of composites based on performance testing compared with rating scales to both MS disease progression and to a treatment effect [Syndulko et al., 1994a,b]. Although the biomedical community remains divided regarding the best outcome assessment in MS clinical trials, the accumulating evidence favors performance testing over clinical measures.

Another type of efficacy-oriented study of particular note in the context of this chapter involves the combination of pharmacodynamic models with instrumented, objective, and sensitive performance capacity measurements to optimize therapeutic effectiveness by fine-tuning dose prescription for individual subjects. For example, the results from a Parkinson's disease study by Hacisalihzade et al. [1989] suggest that performance capacity measurements, which would play a key role in a strategy to determine pharmacodynamics of a drug for the individual (i.e., not a population), could become a component in the management of some patients receiving long-term drug therapy.

82.4   Future Needs and Anticipated Developments

The field of clinical trials in which human performance variables are of interest has expanded at such a rapid rate in recent years that it has been difficult for researchers to keep up with all the new technologies, instrumentations, and methodologies. The type of evaluation employed has steadily shifted from mostly subjective to more objective, which can be argued to provide improved measurement quality. Increased standardization of human performance measurements has led to greater cost-effectiveness due to computer-based test batteries [Woollacott, 1983; Kennedy et al., 1993]. Thus, even if the quality of measurement were the same with methodologies that used less sophisticated methods, the initial investment would frequently be saved with newer data management techniques. This sentiment has not yet been accepted by all segments of the relevant communities. Also, the speed at which data can now be collected (which is especially important when changes over short time periods are of interest, as in pharmacodynamic studies) has led to greater cost-effectiveness. Furthermore, since instrumented devices are becoming commercially available and more widely used, it is not necessary nor desirable for researchers whose primary interest is the intervention of disease process to "reinvent" measurements (possibly with subtle but significant changes that ultimately inhibit standardization) for use in studies. Also, new measurements that may be different — but not necessarily better — must undergo long and expensive studies prior to their use in clinical trials. Although certain human performance measures are becoming standard in selected situations, more experience is needed before a substantial degree of standardization in human performance measurement is achieved in such situations.

The perfect research strategy in clinical trials involving human performance capacities to determine therapy effectiveness and safety may not be possible due to financial and/or ethical considerations. Thus the challenge of clinical trials research in the future is to maintain scientific integrity while conforming to legal mandates and staying within economic feasibility; i.e., an optimization is almost always necessary. Multidisciplinary research efforts can be useful in these circumstances.

Defining Terms

Clinical significance: An additional level of interpretation of a statistically significant finding that addresses the size of the effect found.

Clinical trial: A research study involving human subjects and an intervention (i.e., device, drug, surgical procedure, or other procedure) that is ultimately intended to either enhance the professional capabilities of physicians, improve the quality of life of patients, or contribute to the field of knowledge in those sciences which are traditionally in the medical field setting.

Composite score: A score derived by combining two or more measured performance capacities.

Efficacy-oriented clinical trial: A study that is conducted to objectively determine an intervention's effectiveness along with any pharmacokinetic or pharmacodynamic interactions.

Nonprobability sampling: A method of sampling whereby no subject in a defined population has an equal chance of being included in the sample.

Performance capacities: Dimensional capabilities or resources (e.g., speed, accuracy, strength, etc.) that a given human subsystem (e.g., visual, central processing, gait production, posture maintenance, etc.) possesses to perform a given task.

Pharmacodynamics: The physiologic and/or metabolic changes in the concentration of a drug over time to corresponding measurable performance capacity changes in the therapeutic effect.

Pharmacokinetics: The rate at which a drug is metabolized, as evidenced by changes in drug concentrations in blood, cerebral spinal fluid, urine, etc.

Probability sampling: A method of sampling whereby each subject in a defined population theoretically has an equal chance of being included in the sample.

Protocol: A detailed statement of all procedures and methods to be employed in a research investigation.

Randomized clinical trial (RCT): A study that uses controlled trials whereby part of the group of subjects receives a therapy that is tested, while the other subjects receive either no therapy or another therapy.

Resource economics: A cause-effect type of relationship between available performance resources (i.e., capacities) and demands of higher-level tasks in which the relevant subsystems are used.

Safety-oriented clinical trial: A study that usually involves vital sign measures (e.g., heart rate, blood pressure, respiration rate), clinical laboratory tests (e.g., blood chemistries, urinalysis, ECG), and adverse reaction tests (both mental and physical performance capacities) to evaluate the risk of an intervention.

Sample: A proportion of the defined population that is studied. When used as a verb (sampling), it refers to the process of subject selection.

Significance (statistical) test: A tool used for assessing possible associations between independent and dependent variables as well as differences among treatment groups.

Statistical significance: An evaluation of the research hypothesis at a specific level of probability so that any differences observed are not attributable to a chance occurrence.

References

Baker, S.J., Chrzan, G.J., Park, C.N., and Saunders, J.H. 1985. Validation of human behavioral tests using ethanol as a CNS depressant Model. *Neurobehav. Toxicol. Teratol.* 7: 257.

Baumgartner, T.A. and Jackson, A.S. 1993. *Measurement for Evaluation*, 4th ed. Dubuque, Iowa, Wm. C. Brown.

Cochran, W.G. and Cox, G.M. 1957. *Experimental Designs*, 2nd ed. New York, John Wiley & Sons.

Cohen, J. 1988. *Statistical Power Analysis for the Behavioral Sciences*. Hillsdale, NJ, Lawrence Erlbaum Associates.

Cotton, P. 1993. FDA lifts ban on women in early drug tests, will require companies to look for gender differences. *JAMA* 269: 2067.

DeAngelis, C. 1990. *An Introduction to Clinical Research*. New York, Oxford University Press.

Department of Health and Human Services. 1985. *Code of Federal Regulation of the Department of Health and Human Services*, title 45, part 46.

Dixon, W.J. and Kuzma, J.W. 1974. Data reduction in large clinical trials. *Commun. Stat.* 3: 301.

Food and Drug Administration. 1977. *General Considerations for the Clinical Evaluation of Drugs*. DHEW Publication No. (FDA) 77–3040. Washington.

Fleiss, J.L. 1986. *The Design and Analysis of Clinical Experiments*. New York, John Wiley & Sons.

Hacisalihzade, S.S., Mansour, M., and Albani, C. 1989. Optimization of symptomatic therapy in Parkinson's disease. *IEEE Trans. Biomed. Eng.* 36:363.

Hastad, D.N. and Lacy, A.C. 1994. *Measurement and Evaluation*, 2nd ed. Scottsdale, Ariz, Gorsuch Scarisbrick.

Henderson, W.G., Tourtellotte, W.W., Potvin, A.R., and Rose, A.S. 1978. Methodology for analyzing clinical neurological data: ACTH in multiple sclerosis. *Clin. Pharmacol. Ther.* 24: 146.

Hill, A.B. 1963. Medical ethics and controlled trials. *Br. Med. J.* 1: 1043.

Horne, J.A. and Gibbons, H. 1991. Effects of vigilance performance and sleepiness of alcohol given in the early afternoon (post lunch) vs early evening. *Ergonomics* 34: 67.

International Federation of Multiple Sclerosis Societies. 1984. Symposium on a minimal record of disability for multiple sclerosis. *Acta Neurol. Scand.* 70(Suppl): 101–217.

Jennison, C. and Turnbull, B.W. 1993. Group sequential tests for bivariate response: interim analyses of clinical trials with both efficacy and safety endpoints. *Biometrics* 49:741.

Jones, B. and Kenward, M.G. 1989. *Design and Analysis of Crossover Trials*. New York, Chapman and Hall.

Kennedy, R.S., Turnage, J.J., and Wilkes, R.L. 1993. Effects of graded doses of alcohol on nine computerized repeated-measures tests. *Ergonomics* 36:1195.

Kepple, G. 1982. *Design and Analysis a Researcher's Handbook*, 2nd ed. Englewood Cliffs, NJ, Prentice-Hall.

Kondraske, G.V. 1988a. Workplace design: an elemental resource approach to task analysis and human performance measurements. International Conference for the Advancement of Rehabilitation Technology, Montreal, Proceedings, pp. 608–611.

Kondraske, G.V. 1988b. Experimental evaluation of an elemental resource model for human performance. Tenth Annual IEEE Engineering in Medicine and Biology Society Conference, New Orleans, Proceedings, pp. 1612–1613.

Kondraske, G.V. 1989. Measurement science concepts and computerized methodology in the assessment of human performance. In T. Munsat (Ed.), *Quantification of Neurologic Deficit*. Stoneham, MA, Butterworth.

Kondraske, G.V. 1995. A working model for human system-task interfaces. In J.D. Bronzino (Ed.), *Handbook of Biomedical Engineering*. Boca Raton, FL, CRC Press.

Levin, R.J. 1986. *Ethics and Regulation of Clinical Research*, 2nd ed. Baltimore, Urban & Schwarzenberg.

Merkatz, R.B., Temple, R., and Sobel, S. 1993. Women in clinical trials of new drugs: a change in Food and Drug Administration policy. *N. Engl. J. Med.* 329:292.

Mohr, E. and Prouwers, P. 1991. *Handbook of Clinical Trials: The Neurobehavioral Approach*. Berwyn, PA, Swets and Zeitlinger.

Ottenbacher, K.J. and Barrett, K.A. 1991. Measures of effect size in the reporting of rehabilitation research. *Am. J. Phys. Med. Rehabil.* 70(suppl 1):S131.

Paty, D.E., Willoughby, E., and Whitakek, J. 1992. Assessing the outcome of experimental therapies in multiple sclerosis. In *Treatment of Multiple Sclerosis: Trial Design, Results, and Future Perspectives*, pp. 47–90. London, Springer-Verlag.

Potvin, A.R., Tourtellotte, W.W.T., Potvin, J.H. et al. 1985. *Quantitative Examination of Neurologic Function*, vols I and II. Boca Raton, FL, CRC Press.

Rose, A.S., Kuzma, J.W., Kurtzke, J.F. et al. 1968. Cooperative study in the evaluation of therapy in multiple sclerosis: ACTH vs placebo in acute exacerbations. Preliminary report. *Neurology* 18:1.

Safrit, M.J. 1990. *Evaluation in Exercise Science*. Englewood Cliffs, NJ, Prentice-Hall.

Salame, P. 1991. The effects of alcohol in learning as a function of drinking habits. *Ergonomics* 34:1231.

Stone, R. 1993. FDA to ask for data on gender differences. *Science* 260:743.

Syndulko, K., Ke, D., Ellison, G.W. et al. 1994a. Neuroperformance assessment of treatment efficacy and MS disease progression in the Cyclosporine Multicenter Clinical Trial. *Brain* (submitted).

Syndulko, K., Ke, D., Ellison, G.W. et al. 1994b. A comparative analysis of assessments for disease progression in multiple sclerosis: I. Signal to noise ratios and relationship among performance measures and rating scales. *Brain* (submitted).

Syndulko, K., Tourellotte, W.W., Baumhefner, R.W. et al. 1993. Neuroperformance evaluation of multiple sclerosis disease progression in a clinical trial. 7:69.

Tang, D. and Geller, N.L. 1993. On the design and analysis of randomized clinical trials with multiple endpoints. *Biometrics* 49:23.

The Multiple Sclerosis Study Group. 1990. Efficacy and toxicity of cyclosporine in chronic progressive multiple sclerosis: a randomized, double-blind, placebo-controlled clinical trial. *Ann. Neurol.* 27:591.

Thomas, J.R. and Nelson, J.K. 1990. *Research Methods in Physical Activity*, 2nd ed. Champaign, Il, Human Kinetics Publishers.

Tourtellotte, W.W., Haerer, A.F., Simpson, J.F. et al. 1965. Quantitative clinical neurological testing: I. A study of a battery of tests designed to evaluate in part the neurologic function of patients with multiple sclerosis and its use in a therapeutic trial. *Ann. NY Acad. Sci.* 122:480.

Tudiver, F., Bass, M.J., Dunn, E.V. et al. 1992. *Assessing Interventions Traditional and Innovative Methods.* London, Sage Publications.

Weissman, A. 1991. On the concept "study day zero." *Perspect. Biol. Med.* 34:579.

Willoughby, P.D. and Whitaker, J.E. 1992. Assessing the outcome of experimental therapies in multiple sclerosis. In R.A. Rudick and D.E. Goodkin (Eds.), *Treatment of Multiple Sclerosis: Trial Design, Results, and Future Perspectives*, pp. 47–90. London, Springer-Verlag.

Woollacott, M.H. 1983. Effects of ethanol on postural adjustments in humans. *Exp. Neurol.* 80:55.

Further Information

The original monograph, *Experimental and Quasi-Experimental Designs for Research*, by D.T. Campbell and J.C. Stanley [Boston: Houghton Mifflin, 1964], is a classic experimental design text. The book *Statistics in Medicine*, by T. Colton [Boston: Little, Brown, 1982], examines statistical principles in medical research and identifies common perils when drawing conclusions from medical research. The book *Clinical Epidemiology: The Essentials*, R.H. Fletcher, S.W. Fletcher, and E.H. Wagner (2nd ed., Baltimore: Williams and Wilkins, 1982), is a readable text with concise descriptions of various types of studies. *Clinical Trials: Design, Conduct, and Analysis*, by C.L. Meinert [New York: Oxford University Press, 1986], is a comprehensive text covering most details and provides many helpful suggestions about clinical trials research. R.J. Porter and B.S. Schoenberg, *Controlled Clinical Trials in Neurological Disease* [Boston: Kluwer Academic Publishers, 1990], is also a comprehensive text covering clinical trials with a special emphasis on neurologic diseases.

83

Applications of Quantitative Assessment of Human Performance in Occupational Medicine

Mohamad Parnianpour
Ohio State University

As early as 1700, Bernardino Ramazzini, one of the founders of occupational medicine, had associated certain physical activities with musculoskeletal disorders (MSD). He postulated that certain violent and irregular motions and unnatural postures of the body impair the internal structure [Snook et al., 1988]. Presently, much effort is directed toward a better understanding of work-related musculoskeletal disorders involving the back, cervical spine, and upper extremities. The World Health Organization (WHO) has defined occupational diseases as those work-related diseases where the relationship to specific causative factors at work has been fully established [WHO, 1985]. Other work-related diseases may have a weaker or unclear association to working conditions. They may be aggravated, accelerated, or exacerbated by workplace factors and lead to impairment of workers' performance. Hence obtaining the occupational history is crucial to proper diagnosis and appropriate treatment of work-related disorders. The occupational physician must consider the conditions of both the workplace and the worker in evaluation of injured workers. Biomechanical and ergonomic evaluators have developed a series of techniques for quantification of the task demands and evaluation of the stresses in the workplace. Functional capacity evaluation also has been advanced to quantify the maximum performance capability of workers. The motto of ergonomics is to avoid the mismatch between the task demand and functional capacity of individuals. A multidisciplinary group of physicians and engineers constitutes the rehabilitation team that will work together to implement the prevention measures. Through proper workplace design, workplace stressors could be minimized. It is expected that one-third of the compensatable low back pain in industry could be prevented by proper ergonomic workplace or task design. In addition to reducing the probability of both the initial and recurring episodes, proper ergonomic design allows earlier return to work of injured workers by keeping the task demands at a lower level. Unfortunately, ergonomists are often asked to redesign the task or the workplace after a high incidence of injuries has already been experienced. The next preventive measure that has been suggested is preplacement of workers based on the medical history, strength, and physical examinations [Snook et al., 1988]. Training and education have been the third prevention strategy in the reduction of musculoskeletal disorders. Some components of these educational packages such as "back schools" and the teaching of "proper body mechanics" have been used in the rehabilitation phase of injured workers as well.

Title I of the Americans with Disability Act [ADA, 1990] prohibits discrimination with regard to any aspect of the employment process. Thus the development of preplacement tests has been impeded by the possibility of discrimination against individuals based on gender, age, or medical condition. The ADA requires physical tests to simulate the "essential functions" of the task. In addition, one must be aware of "reasonable accommodations," such as lifting aids, that may make an otherwise infeasible task possible for a disabled applicant to perform. Healthcare providers who perform physical examinations and provide recommendations for job applicants must consider the rights of disabled applicants. It is extremely crucial to quantify the specific physical requirements of the job to be performed and to examine an applicant's capabilities to perform those specific tasks, taking into account any reasonable accommodations that may be provided. Hence task analysis and functional capacity assessment are truly intertwined.

Work-related disorders of the upper extremities, unlike low back disorders, can better be related to specific anatomic sites such as a tendon or compressed nerve. Examples of the growing number of cumulative trauma disorders of the upper extremities and the neck are **carpal tunnel syndrome (CTS)**, **DeQuervain's disease**, **trigger finger**, **lateral epicondylitis (tennis elbow)**, **rotator cuff tendinitis**, **thoracic outlet syndrome**, and **tension neck syndrome**. The prevalence of these disorders is higher among some specific jobs, such as meat cutters, welders, sewer workers, grinders, meat packers, and keyboard operators. Some of the common risk factors leading to pain, impairment, and physical damage in the neck and upper extremities are forceful motion, repetitive motion, vibration, prolonged awkward posture, and mechanical stress [Kroemer et al., 1994].

This chapter is intended to illustrate the application of some principles and practices of human performance engineering, especially quantification of human performance in the field of occupational medicine. I have selected the problem of low back pain to illustrate a series of concepts that are essential to evaluation of both the worker and the workplace, while realizing the importance of the disorders of the neck and upper extremities. By inference and generalization, most of these concepts can be extended to these situations.

83.1 Principles

Assessment of function across various dimensions of performance (i.e., strength, speed, endurance, and coordination) has provided the basis for a rational approach to clinical assessment, rehabilitation strategies, and determination of return-to-work potential for injured employees [Kondraske, 1990]. To understand the complex problem of trunk performance evaluation of low back pain (LBP) patients, the terminology of muscle exertion must first be defined. However, it should be noted that a number of excellent reviews of trunk muscle function have been performed [Andersson, 1991; Beimborn and Morrissey, 1988; Newton and Waddell, 1993; Pope, 1992]. I do not intend to reproduce this extensive literature here, since my motive is to provide a critical analysis that will lead the reader toward an understanding of the future of functional assessment techniques. A more extensive clinical application is provided elsewhere [Szpalski and Parnianpour, 1996; Parnianpour and Shirazi-adl, 1999].

83.1.1 Impairment, Disability, and Handicap

The tremendous human suffering and economic costs of disability present a formidable medical, social, and political challenge in the midst of growing healthcare costs and scarcity of resources. The WHO [1980] distinguished among impairment, disability, and handicap. Impairment is any loss or abnormality of psychological, physiologic, or anatomic structure or function — impairment reflects disturbances at the organ level. Disability is any restriction or lack of ability (resulting from impairment) to perform an activity in the manner or within the range considered normal for a human being — disability reflects disturbances at the level of person. Handicap is a disadvantage for a given individual, resulting from an impairment or a disability, that limits or prevents the fulfillment of a role that is normal (depending on age, sex, and social and cultural factors) for that individual. Since disability is the objectification of an impairment, handicap represents the socialization of an impairment or disability. Despite the immense improvement presented by the International Classification of Impairments, Disabilities, and Handicaps (ICIDH), the classification is limited from an industrial medicine or rehabilitation perspective. The hierarchical organization lacks the specificity required for evaluating the functional state of an individual with respect to task demands.

Kondraske [1990] has suggested an alternative approach using the principles of resource economics. The resource economics paradigm is reflective of the principal goal of ergonomics: fitting the demands of the task to the functional capability of the worker. The Elemental Resource Model (ERM) is based on the application of general performance theory that presents a unified theory for measurement, analysis, and modeling of human performance across all different aspects of performance, across all human subsystems, and at any hierarchical level. This approach uses the same bases to describe both the fundamental dimensions of performance capacity and task demand (available and utilized resources) of each functional unit involved in performance of the high-level tasks. The elegance of the ERM is due to its hierarchical organization, allowing causal models to be generated based on assessment of the task demands and performance capabilities across the same dimensions of performance [Kondraske, 1990].

83.1.2 Muscle Action and Performance Quantification

The details of the complex processes of muscle contraction in terms of the bioelectrical, biochemical, and biophysical interactions are under intense research. Muscle tensions is a function of muscle length and its rate of change and can be scaled by the level of neural excitation. These relationships are called the length–tension and velocity–tension relationships. From a physiologic point of view, the measured force or torque applied at the interface is a function of (1) the individual's motivation (magnitude of the neural drive for excitation and activation processes), (2) environmental conditions (muscle length, rate of change of muscle length, nature of the external load, metabolic conditions, pH level, temperature, and so forth), (3) prior history of activation (fatigue), (4) instructions and descriptions of the tasks given to the subject, (5) the control strategies and motor programs employed to satisfy the demands of the task, and (6) the biophysical state of the muscles and fitness (fiber composition, physiologic cross-sectional area of the muscle, cardiovascular capability). It cannot be overemphasized that these processes are complex and interrelated [Kroemer et al., 1994]. Other factors that may affect the performance of patients are misunderstanding of the degree of effort needed in maximal testing, test anxiety, depression, nociception, fear of pain and reinjury, as well as unconscious and conscious symptom magnification.

The following sections review some methods to quantify performance and lifting capability of isolated trunk muscles during a multilink coordinated manual materials handling task. Relevant factors that influence the static and dynamic strength and endurance measures of trunk muscles will be addressed, and the clinical applications of these assessment techniques will be illustrated.

The central nervous system (CNS) appropriately excites the muscle, and the generated tension is transferred to the skeletal system by the tendon to cause motion, stabilize the joint, and resist the effect of external forces on the body. Hence the functional evaluation of muscles cannot be performed without the characterization of the interfaced mechanical environment.

The four fundamental types of muscle exertion or action are isometric, isokinetic, isotonic, and isoinertial. In isometric exertion, the muscle length is kept constant, and there is no movement. Although mechanical work is not achieved, physiologic work, that is, static work, is performed, and energy is consumed. When the internal force exerted by the muscle is greater than the external force offered by the resistance, then concentric, that is, shortening, muscle action occurs, whereas if the muscle is already activated and the external force exceeds the internal force of the muscle, then eccentric, that is, lengthening, muscle action occurs. When the muscle moves, either concentrically or eccentrically, dynamic work is performed. If the rate of shortening or lengthening of the muscle is constant, the exertion is called isokinetic. When the muscle acts on a constant inertial mass, the exertion is called isoinertial. Isotonic action occurs when the muscle tension is constant throughout the range of motion.

These definitions are very clear when dealing with isolated muscles during physiologic investigations. However, terminology employed in the literature of strength evaluation is imprecise. The terms are intended to refer to the state of muscles, but they actually refer to the state of the mechanical interface, that is, the dynamometer. Isotonic exertion, as defined, is not as realizable physiologically because muscular tensions change as its lever arm changes despite the constancy of external loads. Special designs may vary the resistance level in order to account for changes in mechanical efficiency of the muscles. In addition, the rate of muscle length change may not remain constant even when the joint angular velocity is regulated by the dynamometer during isokinetic exertions. During isoinertial action, the net external resistance is not only a function of the mass (inertia) but also a function of the acceleration. The acceleration, however, is a function of the input energy to the mass. Hence, to fully characterize the net external resistance, we need to have both the acceleration and the inertial parameters (mass and moment of inertia) of the load and body parts. Future research should better quantify the inertial effects of the dynamometers, particularly during nonisometric and nonisokinetic exertions.

For any joint or joint complex, muscle performance can be quantified in terms of the basic dimensions of performance: strength, speed, endurance, steadiness, and coordination. Muscle strength is the capacity to produce torque or work by voluntary activation of the muscles, whereas muscle endurance is the ability to maintain a predetermined level of motor output — for example, torque, velocity, range of motion, work, or energy — over a period of time. Fatigue is considered to be a process under which the capability of muscles diminish. However, neuromuscular adjustments take place to meet the task demands (i.e., increase in neural excitation) until there is final performance breakdown — endurance time. Coordination, in this context, is the temporal and spatial organizations of movement and the recruitment patterns of the muscle synergies.

Despite the proliferation of various technologies for measurement, basic questions such as "What needs to be measured and how can it best be measured?" are still being investigated. However, there is a consensus on the need to measure objectively the performance capability along the following dimensions: range of motion, strength, endurance, coordination, speed, acceleration, etc. Strength is one of the most fundamental dimensions of human performance and has been the focus of many investigations. Despite the general consensus about the abstract definition of strength, there is no direct method for measurement of muscle tension *in vivo*. Strength has often been measured at the interface of a joint (or joints) with the mechanical environment. A dynamometer, which is an external apparatus onto which the body exerts force, is used to measure strength indirectly.

Different modes of strength testing have evolved based on different levels of technologic sophistication. The practical implication of contextual dependencies on the provided mechanical environment of the strength measures must be considered during selection of the appropriate mode of measurement. In this regard, equipment that can measure strength in different modes is more efficient in terms of both initial capital investment, required floor space in the clinics or laboratories, and the amount of time it takes to get the person in and out of the dynamometer.

83.2 Low Back Pain and Trunk Performance

The problem of LBP is selected to present important models that could be used by the entire multidisciplinary rehabilitation team for the measurement, modeling, and analysis of human performance [Kondraske, 1990]. The inability to relate LBP to anatomic findings and the difficulties in quantifying pain have directed much effort toward quantification of spinal performance. The problem is made even more complex by the increasing demand of the healthcare system to quantify the level of impairment of patients reporting back pain without objective findings.

There are three basic impairment evaluation systems, each having their merits and shortcomings: (1) anatomic, based on physical examination findings, (2) diagnostic, based on pathology, and (3) functional, based on performance or work capacity [Luck and Florence, 1988]. The earlier systems were anatomic, based on amputation and ankylosis. Although this approach may be more applicable to the hand, it is very inappropriate for the spine. The diagnostic-based systems suffer from lack of correspondence between the degree of impairment for a given diagnosis and the resulting disability and even more from the lack of a clear diagnosis. A large percentage of symptom-free individuals have anatomic findings detectable by the imaging technologies, while some LBP patients have no structural anomalies.

The function-based systems are more desirable from an occupational medicine perspective for the following reasons: they allow the rehabilitation team to rationally evaluate the prospect for return to light-duty work and the type of "reasonable accommodations" needed (such as assistive devices) that could reduce the task demand below the functional capability of the individual. By focusing on remaining ability and transferable skills rather than the disability or structural impairment of the injured worker, the set of feasible jobs can be identified. These points are extremely important, given the natural history of work disability after a single low back pain episode causing loss of work time: 40 to 50% of workers return to work by 2 weeks, 60 to 80% return by 4 weeks, and 85 to 90% return by 12 weeks. The small portion of disabled workers who become chronic are responsible for the majority of the economic cost of LBP. It is therefore the primary goal of the rehabilitation team to prevent the LBP, which is self-correcting in most cases, no matter what kind of therapy is used, from becoming a chronic disabling predicament. Injured workers should neither be returned to work too early nor too late, since both could complicate the prognosis. The results of functional capacity evaluation and task demand quantification should guide the timing for returning to work. It is clear that psychosocioeconomic factors become increasingly more important than physical factors as the disability progresses into "chronicity syndrome" and play a major role in defining the evolution of a low back disability claim. Future research should further establish the reliability and reproducibility of performance assessment tools to expedite their widespread use [Luck and Florence, 1988; Newton and Waddell, 1993].

83.2.1 Maximal and Submaximal Protocols

Biomechanical strength models of the trunk are usually based on static maximal strength measurement. In real-life work situations, individuals rarely exert lengthy or maximum static effort. In most clinical situations, submaximal protocols are recommended, especially in patients with pain or with cardiovascular problems. Also, submaximal testing is less susceptible to fatigue and injury. The activities of daily living also have a great deal of submaximal efforts at the self-selected pace. Hence it has been argued that testing at the preferred rate may be complementary to the maximal effort protocols. The preferred motion can be solicited by instructing the subject to perform repetitive movement at a pace and through the range of motion which he or she feels is the most comfortable. It has been shown that LBP patients and normal individuals have different resisted preferred flexion/extension motion characteristics. Having the subject perform against resistance is based on the hypothesis that, at higher resistance levels, the separation between the performance levels of patients and normal subjects becomes more evident. It has been shown, for example, that functional impairment of trunk extensors in LBP patients with respect to the normal population is larger at higher velocities during isokinetic trunk extension. However, the proponents of unconstrained testing have argued that separation of these groups can be performed based on the position, velocity, and acceleration profiles of the trunk during self-selected flexion/extension tasks. They have noted that pain and fear of reinjury may become the limiting factors. The sudden surge in acquiring performance measures of LBP patients during the initial rehabilitation process also underscores the validity of this concept.

83.2.2 Static and Dynamic Strength Measurements of Isolated Trunk Muscles

Weakness of the trunk extensor and abdominal muscles in patients with LBP was demonstrated using the cable tensiometer to measure isometric strength. The disadvantage of the cable tensiometer (which records applied force) is that it neglects to measure the lever arm distance from the center of trunk motion. It is also recommended that cable tensiometer be used to determine peak isometric torques rather than the stable average torque exerted over a 3-sec period. Dynamometers used for testing dynamic muscle performances contain either hydraulic or servo motor systems to provide constant velocity, for example, isokinetic devices, or constant resistance, for example, isoinertial devices. The isokinetic devices can be further categorized into passive and active types. The robotics-based dynamometers can actively apply force on the body and hence allow eccentric muscle performance assessments, while only concentric exertions can be measured by the passive devices. Eccentric muscle action can stimulate the lowering phase of a manual materials handling task. Based on sports medicine literature, eccentric action has been implicated for its significant role in the muscle injury mechanism. Using isokinetic dynamometers, the isometric and isokinetic strengths of trunk extensor and abdominal muscles were shown to be weaker in LBP patients compared with healthy individuals. Dedicated trunk testing systems have become the cornerstone of objective functional evaluation and have been incorporated in the rehabilitation programs in many centers.

Two issues of importance for future research are the role of pelvic restraints and the significance of using newly developed triaxial dynamometers as opposed to more traditional uniaxial dynamometers. Studies on healthy volunteers have shown that trunk motions occur in more than one plane — lateral bending accompanies the primary motion of axial rotation. Numerous attempts have been made to measure the segmental range of motion three-dimensionally in the lumbar spine with the purpose of quantifying abnormal coupling and diagnosing instabilities.

The effect of posture on the maximum strength capability can be described based on the length-tension relationship of muscle action. Marras and Mirka [1989] studied the effect of trunk postural asymmetry, flexion angle, and trunk velocity (eccentric, isometric, and concentric) on maximal trunk torque production. It was shown that trunk torque decreased by about 8.5% of the maximum for every 15° of asymmetric trunk angle. At higher trunk flexion angles, extensor strength increased. Complex, significant interaction effects of velocity, asymmetry, and sagittal posture were detected. The ranges of velocity studies were more limited (±30°/sec) than those used customarily in spinal evaluation. Tan et al. [1993] tested 31 healthy males for the effects of standing trunk-flexion positions (0, 15, and 35°) on triaxial torques and did **electromyograms** (EMGs) of 10 trunk muscles during isometric trunk extension at 30, 50, 70, and 100% of maximum voluntary exertions (MVE). Trunk muscle strength was significantly increased at a more flexed position. However, the accessory torques in the transverse and coronal planes were not affected by trunk postures. The recorded lateral bending and rotation accessory torques were less than 5 and 16% of the primary extension torque, respectively. The rectus abdominis muscles were inactive during all the tests. The EMGs of the erector spinae varied linearly with higher values of MVE, while the latissimus dorsi had a nonlinear behavior. The obliques were coactivated only during 100% MVE. The neuromuscular efficiency ratio (NMER) was constructed as the ratio of the extension torque over the processed (RMS) EMG of the extensor muscles. It was hoped that NMER could be used in clinical settings where generation of the maximum exertion are not indicated. However, the NMER proved to have a limited clinical utility because it was significantly affected by both exertion level and posture. The NMER of the extensor muscles increased at more flexed position. Studies that have combined the EMG activities and dynamometric evaluations have the potential of discovering the neuromuscular adaptation during different phases of injury and rehabilitation processes.

83.2.3 Static and Dynamic Trunk Muscle Endurance

The high percentage of type I fibers in the back muscles, in addition to the better vascularization of these muscle groups, contributes to their superior endurance. Physiologic studies indicate that at higher muscle utilization ratios (relative muscle loads), fatigue is detected earlier. Isometric endurance tests have been used to compute the median frequency (MF) of the myoelectrical activities of trunk muscles in both normal and LBP populations. The expected decline of the median frequency with fatigue is parameterized by the intercept (initial MF) and the slope of the fall. It has been shown that trunk range of motion (ROM) and isometric strength suffered from lower specificity and sensitivity than spectral parameters. Trunk muscle endurance does differ between healthy subjects and those reporting LBP. During isometric endurance testing, trunk flexors develop fatigue faster than extensors in symptom-free subjects. The flexor fatigability appeared significantly higher in patients with LBF as compared with controls. Chronicity also influences trunk muscle endurance. Chronic LBP patients showed reduced abdominal as well as back muscle endurance as compared with the healthy controls and lower back muscle endurance as compared with the intermittent LBP group. Individuals with a history of debilitating LBP demonstrated less isometric trunk extensor endurance than either normal individuals or patients with history of lesser LBP.

Soft tissues subjected to repetitive loading, due to their viscoelastic properties, demonstrate creep and load relaxation. The loss of precision, speed, and control of the neuromuscular system induced by fatigue reduces the ability of muscles to protect the weakened passive structure, which may explain many industrial, clinical, and recreational injury mechanisms. These results further indicate the necessity of relating clinical protocols to the job and show how short-duration maximal isometric testing alone cannot provide the complex functional interaction of strength, endurance, control, and coordination.

Parnianpour et al. [1988] studied the effect of isoinertial fatiguing of flexion and extension trunk movements on the movement pattern (angular position and velocity profile) and the motor output (torque) of the trunk. They showed that, with fatigue, there is a reduction of the functional capacity in the main sagittal plane. There is also a loss of motor control enabling a greater range of motion in the transverse and coronal planes while performing the primary sagittal task. Association of sagittal with coronal and transverse movements is considered more likely to induce back injuries; thus the effect of fatigue and reduction of motor control and coordination may be an important risk factor leading to injury-prone working postures. The endurance limit is a more useful predictor of incidence and recurrence of low back disorders than the absolute strength values. Although physiologic criteria used in the National Institute for Occupational Safety and Health Lifting Guide [NIOSH, 1981] considered cardiovascular demands of dynamic repetitive lifting tasks, the limits of muscular endurance were not explicitly addressed. Future research should fill this gap, since the maximum strength measures should not guide the design decisions. Maximum level of performance can only be maintained for short periods of time, and muscular fatigue should be avoided to prevent the development of MSD. This caveat should be applied to all dimensions of performance capability [Kondraske, 1990].

A prospective, randomized study among employees in a geriatric hospital showed that exercising during work hours to improve back muscle strength, endurance, and coordination proved cost-effective in preventing back symptoms and absence from work [Gundewall et al., 1993]. Every hour spent by the physiotherapist on the exercise group reduced the work absence by 1.3 days. In this study, both training and testing equipment were very modest. Endurance training is based on exercises with high repetition and low resistance, while strength training requires exercise with high resistance and low repetition.

83.2.4 Lifting Strength Testing

The National Institute for Occupational Safety and Health [NIOSH, 1981] recommended static, that is, isometric, strength measurements as its standard for lifting tasks. This was based on the evidence that associated LBP with inadequate isometric strength. The incidence of an individual's sustaining an on-the-job back injury increases threefold when the task-lifting requirements approached or exceed the individual's strength capacity. However, lifting strength is not a true measure of trunk function but is a global measure taking into account arm, shoulder, and leg strength as well as the individual's lifting technique and overall fitness. It has been shown that strength tests were more valid and predictive of risk of low back disorders if they simulated the demands of the job. The clinicians must be aided with easy-to-use and validated instruments or questionnaires to gather information about the task demands in order to decide what testing protocol best simulates the applicant's spinal loading conditions.

Static strength measurements have been reported to underestimate significantly the loads on the spine during dynamic lifts. Comparing static and dynamic biomechanical models of the trunk, the predicted spinal loads under static conditions were 33 to 60% less than those under dynamic conditions, depending on the lifting technique. The recruitment patterns of trunk muscles (and thus the internal loading of the spine) are significantly different under isometric and dynamic conditions. General manual materials handling tasks require a coordinated multilink activity that can be simulated using classic psychophysical techniques or the robotics-based lift task simulators. Various lifting tests, including static, dynamic, maximal, and submaximal, are currently available. The experimental results of correlational studies have confirmed the theoretical prediction that strength will be dependent on the measurement technique. Since muscle action requires external resistance, the effect of muscle action will depend on the nature of the resistance. These results refute the implicit assumption that a generic strength test exists that can be used for preplacing workers (preemployment) and predicting the risk of injury or future occurrence of LBP. The psychometric properties of isokinetic and isoresistive modes of strength testing were recently addressed. The quantification of the surface response of strength as a function of joint angle and velocity was only possible for isokinetic testing, while isoresistive tests yielded a very sparse data set. Figure 83.1 and Figure 83.2 illustrate these points graphically.

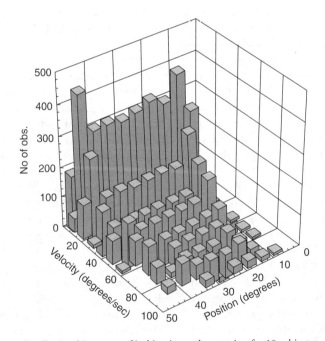

FIGURE 83.1 Bivariate distribution histogram of isokinetic trunk extension for 10 subjects.

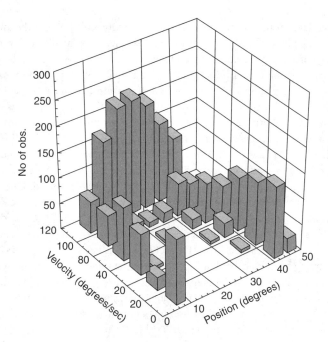

FIGURE 83.2 Bivariate distribution histogram of isotonic trunk extension for 10 subjects.

The wide conflicting results found in the literature regarding the relationship of an individual's strength to the risk of developing LBP may be due to inappropriate modes of strength measurements, that is, lack of job specificity. Isometric strength testing of the trunk is still widely used, especially in large-scale industrial or epidemiologic studies, because it has been standardized and studied prospectively in industry. Compared with trunk dynamic strength testing protocols, the trunk isometric strength testing protocols are simpler and less expensive.

One outstanding issue during dynamic testing is the unresolved problem of how the wealth of information can be presented in a succinct and informative fashion. One approach has been to compare the statistical features of the data with the existing normal databases. This is particularly crucial because one does not have the option of comparing the results to the "contralateral asymptomatic joint," as one has with lower or upper extremity joints. Given the large differences between individuals, I recommend comparison be made to job-specific databases. For example, it is more appropriate for the trunk strength of an injured construction worker to be compared with age- and gender-controlled healthy construction workers than with data from healthy college graduate students or office workers. However, given the scarcity of such data, I argue for comparison of performance capacity with job demand based on task analysis. The performance capacity evaluation is once again linked to task demand quantification.

83.2.5 Inverse and Direct Dynamics

A major task of biomechanics has been to estimate the internal loading of musculoskeletal structure and establish the physiologic loading during various daily activities. Kinematic studies deal with joint movement, with no emphasis on the forces involved. However, kinetic studies address the effect of forces that generate such movements. Using sophisticated experimental and theoretical stress/strain analyses, hazardous/failure levels of loads have been determined. The estimated forces and stresses are used to estimate the level of deformation in the tissues. This technique allows one to assess the risk of overexertion injury associated with any physical activity. Given repetitive motions and exertion levels much lower than the ultimate strength of the tissues, an alternative injury mechanism, the cumulative trauma model, has been used to describe much of the musculoskeletal disorders of the upper extremities.

The experimental data on the joint trajectories are differentiated to obtain the angular velocity and acceleration. Appropriate inertial properties of the limb segments are used to compute the net external moments about each joint. This mapping from joint kinematics to net moments is called inverse dynamics. Direct dynamics refers to studies that simulate the motion based on known actuator torques at each joint. The key issue in these investigations is understanding the control strategies underlying the trajectory planning and performance of purposeful motion. A highly multidisciplinary field has emerged to address these unsolved questions (see Berme and Cappozzo [1990] for a comprehensive treatment of these issues.)

It should be pointed out that determination of the external moments about different joints during manual materials-handling tasks is based on the well-established laws of physics (Figure 83.3). However, the determination of human performance and assessment of functional capacity are based on other disciplines, for example, psychophysics, that are not as exact or well developed. One can describe easily the job demand, in terms of the required moments about each joint, by analyzing the workers performing the tasks. However, one is unable to predict the ability to perform an arbitrary task based on the incomplete knowledge of functional capacities at the joint levels. A task is easily decomposed to its demands at the joint level; however, one cannot compose (construct) the set of feasible tasks based on one's functional capacity knowledge. The mapping from high-level task demands to the joint-level functional capacity for a given performance trial is unique. However, the mapping from joint-level functional capacity to the high-level task demand is one to many (not unique). The challenge to the human performance research community is to establish this missing link. Much of the integration of ergonomics and functional analysis depends on removal of this obstacle. The question of whether a subject can perform a task based on knowledge of his or her functional capacity at the joint level remains an area of open research. When ergonomists or occupational physicians evaluate the fitness of task demands and worker capability, the following clinical questions will be presented; (1) Which space should be explored for determining normalcy, fit, or equivalence? (2) Should we consider the performance of the multilink system in the joint space or end-effector (cartesian workspace)? These issues have profound effects on both the development of new technologies and the evaluation of trunk or lifting performance.

The enormous degrees of freedom existing in the neuromusculoskeletal system provide the control centers both the kinematic and actuator redundancies. The redundancies provide optimization possibility. Since one can lift an object from point A to point B with infinite postural possibilities, it can be suggested that certain physical parameters maybe optimized for the learned movements. The possible candidates for objective function to be optimized are movement time, energy, smoothness, muscular activities, etc. This approach, though still in its early stage, may be very important for spine functional assessment. One could compare the given performance with the optimal performance that is predicted by the model. This approach provides specific goals and gives biofeedback with respect to the individual's performance.

83.2.6 Comparison of Task Demands and Performance Capacity

The regression analysis was used to model the dynamic torque, velocity, and power output as a function of resistance level during flexion and extension using the B-200 Isostation [Parnianpour et al., 1990]. Results indicated that the measured torque was not a good discriminator of the tenth, fiftieth, and ninetieth percentile population. However, velocity and power were shown to effectively discriminate the three populations. Based on these data, it was suggested that during clinical testing, sagittal plane resistance should not be set at higher than about 80 N · m in order to minimize the internal loading of spine while taxing trunk functional capacity. This presentation of data may be useful to the physician or ergonomist in evaluating the functional capacity requirements of workplace manual materials-handling tasks. For example, a manual material-handling task that requires about 80 N · m (61 ft · lb) of trunk extensor strength could be performed by 90% of the population in the normal database if the required average trunk velocity does not exceed 40 degrees per second, while only 50% could perform the task if the velocity requirement exceeds 70 degrees per second. More important, only the top tenth percentile population could perform the task if the velocity requirement approaches 105 degrees per second (Figure 83.4). A few versions of lumbar motion monitors that can record the triaxial motion in the workplace have been used

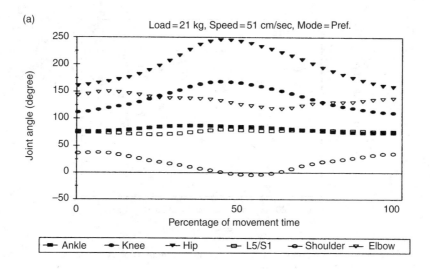

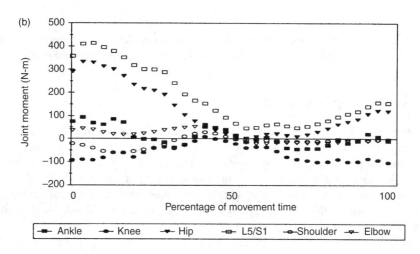

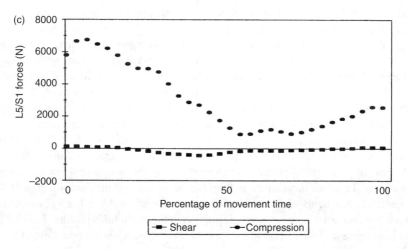

FIGURE 83.3 The dynamic analysis of a sagittal plane symmetrical isokinetic lift (load 21 kg, speed = 51 cm/sec, mode = preferred method of lifting): (a) joint angle; (b) net muscular joint moment; and (c) the joint reaction forces at L5/S1.

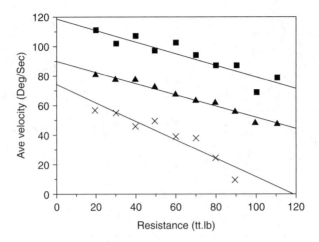

FIGURE 83.4   The average extension velocity measured during maximum trunk extension against a set resistance for 10th (×), 50th (▲), and 90th (■) percentile distribution.

to provide the trunk movement requirements. The preceding example also illustrates the importance of having the same bases for evaluation of both task and the functional capability of the worker.

83.3   Clinical Applications

Clinical studies have utilized quantitative human performance, that is, strength and endurance measures, to predict the first incidence or recurrence of LBP and disability outcome and also as a prognosis measure during the rehabilitation process. Training programs to enhance the endurance and strength of workers have been implemented in some industries. More studies on the effectiveness of these programs are needed. It can be hypothesized that these programs complement the stress-management programs to enhance both worker satisfaction and coping strategies with regard to physical and nonphysical stressors at the workplace.

Functional-based impairment evaluation schemes traditionally have used spinal mobility. Given the poor reliability of range of motion (ROM), its large variability among individuals, and the static psychometric nature of ROM, the use of continuous dynamic profiles of motion with the higher-order derivatives has been suggested. Dynamic performances of 281 consecutive patients from the Impairment Evaluation Center at the Mayo Clinic were used. As part of the comprehensive physical and psychological evaluation, 281 consecutive LBP patients underwent isometric and dynamic trunk testing using the B200 Isostation. **Feature extraction** and **cluster analysis** techniques were used to find the main profiles in dynamic patient performances. The middle three cycles of movements were interpolated and averaged into 128 data points; thus the data were normalized with respect to cycle time. This allowed for comparison between individuals. Figure 83.5 presents the main profiles of sagittal trunk angular position. The number of patients in each group is also noted on the graph. Patients in the first ($n = 48$) and second ($n = 55$) groups had similar flexion mobility; however, those in the first group had more limited extension mobility. The time to peak sagittal position also varied among the five groups. Forty-seven patients in the fifth group showed extreme impairment in both flexion and extension. The third group (26 patients) showed differential impairments with respect to direction of motion. A marked improvement over the use of ROM has been achieved by preserving information in the continuous profiles. The LBP patients in this study are heterogeneous with respect to their movement profile. Uniform treatment of these patients is questionable, and rehabilitation programs should consider their specific impairments. Future research should incorporate the clinical profiles with these movement profiles to further delineate the heterogeneity of LBP patients. Marras et al. [1993] used similar feature-extraction techniques to characterize the

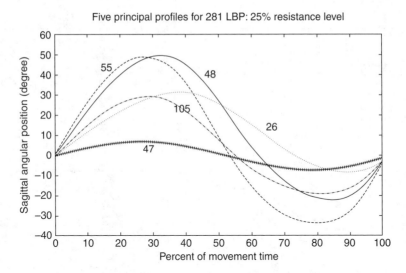

FIGURE 83.5 The five principal profiles of trunk sagittal movement for 281 low back pain patients.

movement profiles of 510 subjects belonging to normal ($n = 339$) and 10 LBP patient groups ($n = 171$). Subjects were asked to perform flexion/extension trunk movement at five levels of asymmetry, while the three-dimensional movement of the spine was monitored by the Lumbar Motion Monitor (an exoskeleton goniometer developed at the Biodynamics Lab of The Ohio State University). Trunk motions were performed against no resistance, and no pelvic stabilization was required. The quadratic discriminant analysis was able to correctly classify over 80% of the subjects. The same technology was used to develop logistic regression models to identify the high-risk jobs in industrial workplaces. Hence principles of human performance can be applied successfully to the worker and the task to avoid the mismatch between performance capability and task demand.

The key limitations in the development of the discriminate functions for classification purposes, are the data-driven nature of the algorithms and the lack of theoretical orientation in the process of development and validation of these models. It is suggested that the mathematical simulation of flexion or extension trunk movement may identify an objective basis for the evaluation and assessment of trunk kinematic performance. A catalog of movement patterns that are optimal with respect to physical and biomechanical quantities may contribute to the emergence of a more theoretically based computational paradigm for the evaluation of kinematic performance of normal subjects and patients. It must be emphasized that in this paradigm one has no intention to claim that the central nervous system actually optimizes any single or composite cost function.

To provide clinical insight for interpretation of the distinctive features in the movement profiles, Parnianpour et al. [1999] have suggested an optimization-based approach for simulation of dynamic point-to-point sagittal trunk movement. The effect of strength impairment on movement patterns was simulated based on minimizing different physical cost functions: Energy, Jerk, Peak Torque, Impulse, and Work. During unconstrained simulations, the velocity patterns of all models are predicted, while time to peak velocity is distinct for each cost function (Figure 83.6). Imposing an 80% reduction in extensor muscle strength diminished the significant differences between unimpaired optimal movement profiles (Figure 83.7). The results indicate that the search for finding the objective function being used by central nervous system is an ill-posed problem since we are sure if we have included all the active constraints in the simulation. The four application areas of these results are (1) providing optimized trajectories for biofeedback to patients during the rehabilitation process; (2) training workers to lift safely; (3) estimating the task demand based on the global description of the job; and (4) aiding the engineering evaluation to develop ergonomic and workplace interventions which are needed to accommodate individuals with prior disability.

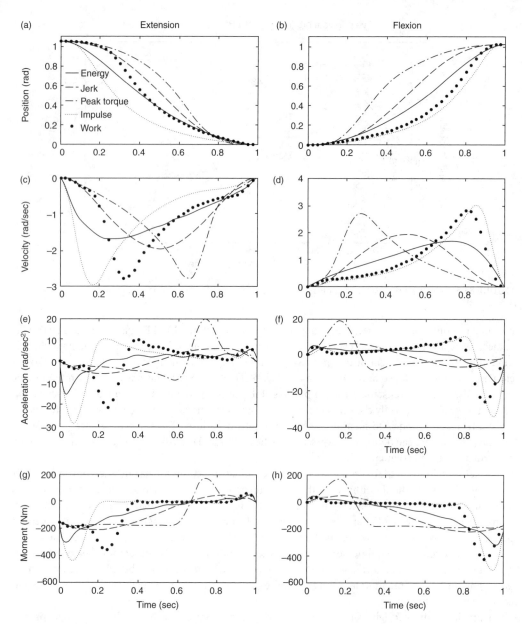

FIGURE 83.6 The optimized unconstrained trunk flexion and extension trajectories for the five cost functions: Energy, Jerk, Peak Torque, Impulse, and Work.

83.4 Conclusions

The outcome of trunk performance is affected by the many neural, mechanical, and environmental factors that must be considered during quantitative assessment. The objective evaluation of the critical dimensions of functional capacity and its comparison with the task demands is crucial to the decision-making processes in the different stages of the ergonomic prevention and rehabilitation process. Knowing the tissue tolerance limits from biomechanical studies, task demands from ergonomic analysis, and function capacities from performance evaluation, the rehabilitation team will optimize the changes to the workplace or the task that will maximize the functional reserves (unutilized resources) to reduce the occurrence of fatigue and overexertion. This will enhance worker satisfaction and productivity while reducing the risk of the MSD.

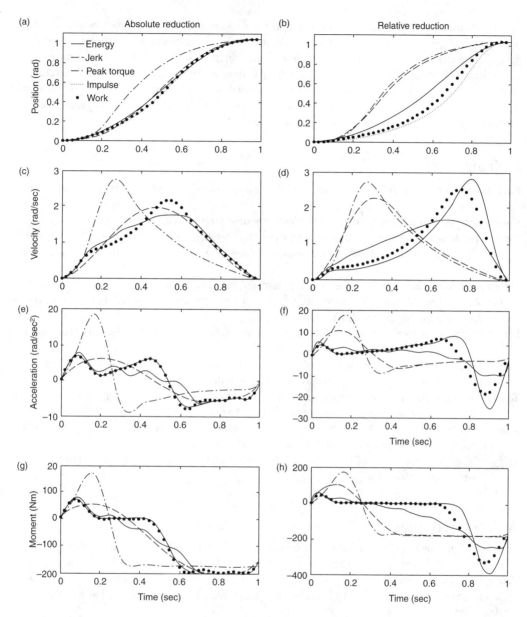

FIGURE 83.7   The optimized trunk flexion trajectories for the five cost functions with the relative and absolute peak extensor strength impairments. The relative strength reduction meant that the extensor strength was reduced to 80% of the peak extension moment required during unconstrained simulations. The absolute strength reduction meant that the extensor strength was set to 200 Nm.

Based on ergonomic and motor control literature, the testing protocols that best simulate the loading conditions of the task will yield more valid results and better predictive ability. Ergonomic principles indicate that the ratio of the functional capacity to the task demand (utilization ratio) is critical to the development of muscular fatigue, which may lead to more injurious muscle recruitment patterns and movement profiles due to loss of motor control and coordination. However, large prospective studies are still needed to verify this. The most promising application for these quantitative measures is to be used as a benchmark for the safe return to work of injured workers, given the enormous variations within the normal population. With the advent of technologies to monitor trunk performance in the workplace, one can obtain estimates of the injurious levels of task demands (kinematic and kinetic parameters), which can be used to guide preplacement and rehabilitation strategies. The more functional the clinical tests become, the more clinicians need a complex interpretation scheme. An increasingly complex interpretation scheme opens the possibility of using mathematical modeling with intelligent computer interfaces. The ability to identify subgroups of patients or high-risk individuals based on their functional performance will remain an open area of research to interested biomedical engineers within the multidisciplinary group of experts addressing neuromusculoskeletal occupational disorders.

Defining Terms

Carpal tunnel syndrome (CTS):   The result of compression of the median nerve in the carpal tunnel of the wrist.

Cluster analysis: A statistical technique to identify natural groupings in data.

DeQuervain's disease: A special case of tendosynovitis (swelling and irritation of the tendon sheath) which occurs in the abductor and extensor tendons of the thumb, where they share a common sheath.

Electromyogram: Recordings of the electric potentials produced by muscle action.

Feature extraction: A statistical technique to allow efficient representation of variability in the original signals while reducing the dimensions of the data.

Lateral epicondylitis (tennis elbow):   Tendons attaching to the epicondyle of the humerus bone become irritated.

Rotator cuff tendinitis: The irritation and swelling of the tendon or the bursae of the shoulder that is caused by continuous muscle or tendon effort to keep the arm elevated.

Tension neck syndrome: An irritation of the levator scapulae and trapezius group of muscles of the neck commonly occurring after repeated or sustained overhead work.

Thoracic outlet syndrome: A disorder resulting from compression of nerves and blood vessels between the clavicle and the first and second ribs at the brachial plexus.

Trigger finger: A special case of tendosynovitis where the tendon becomes nearly locked so that forced movement is not smooth.

Acknowledgments

The authors acknowledge the support from OSURF and NIDRR H133E30009. The authors would like to thank invaluable comments and contributions of Drs. George V. Kondraske, Margareta Nordin, Victor H. Frankel, Elen Ross, Jackson Tan, Robert Gabriel, Robert R. Crowell, William Marras, Sheldon R. Simon, Heinz Hoffer, Ali Sheikhzadeh, Jung Yong Kim, Sue Ferguson, Patrick Sparto, and Kinda Khalaf.

References

Andersson, G.B.J. 1991. Evaluation of muscle function. In J.W. Frymoyer (Ed.), *The Adult Spine: Principles and Practice*, p. 241. New York, Raven Press.

Beimborn, DS and Morrissey, MC. 1988. A review of literature related to trunk muscle performance. *Spine* 13: 655.

Berme, N. and Cappozzo, A. 1990. *Biomechanics of Human Movement: Applications in Rehabilitation, Sports and Ergonomics.* Worthington, Ohio, Bertec Corporation.

Gundewall, B., Liljeqvist, M., and Hansson, T. 1993. Primary prevention in back symptoms and absence from work. *Spine* 18: 587.

Kondraske, G.V. 1990. Quantitative measurement and assessment of performance. In R.V. Smith and J.H. Leslie (Eds.), *Rehabilitation Engineering*, Boca Raton, FL, CRC Press.

Kroemer, K.E., Kroemer, H., and Kroemer-Elbert, K. 1994. *Ergonomics: How to Design for the Ease & Efficiency.* Englewood Cliffs, NJ, Prentice Hall.

Luck, J.V. and Florence, D.W. 1988. A brief history and comparative analysis of disability systems and impairment evaluation guides. *Office Practice* 19: 839.

Marras, W.S. and Mirka, G.A. 1989. Trunk strength during asymmetric trunk motion. *Human Factors* 31: 667.

Marras, W.S., Parnianpour, M., and Ferguson, S.A. et al. 1993. Quantification and classification of low back disorders based on trunk motion. *Eur. J. Med. Rehabilit.* 3: 218.

National Institute for Occupational Safety and Health (NIOSH). 1981. Work practice guide for manual lifting (DHHS Publication No. 81122). Washington, DC: U.S. Government Printing Office.

Newton, M. and Waddell, G. 1993. Trunk strength testing with Iso-Machines, Part 1: review of a decade of scientific evidence. *Spine* 18: 801.

Parnianpour, M., Nordin, M., and Kahanovitz, N. et al. 1988. The triaxial coupling of torque generation of trunk muscles during isometric exertions and the effect of fatiguing isoinertial movements on the motor output and movement patterns. *Spine* 13: 982.

Parnianpour, M., Nordin, M., and Sheikhzadeh, A. 1990. The relationship of torque, velocity and power with constant resistive load during sagittal trunk movement. *Spine* 15: 639.

Parnianpour, M. and Shirazi-Adl, A. 1999. Quantitative assessment of trunk performance. In W. Karwowski and W.S. Marras (Eds.), *Handbook of Occupational Ergonomics*, pp. 985–1006, Boca Raton, FL, CRC Press.

Parnianpour, M., Wang, J.L., and Shirazi-Adl, A. et al. 1999. A computational method for simulation of trunk motion: Towards a theoretical based quantitative assessment of trunk performance. *Biomed. Eng. Appl. Basis Commun.* 11: 1–12.

Pope, M.H. 1992. A critical evaluation of functional muscle testing. In J.N. Weinstein (Ed.), *Clinical Efficacy and Outcome in the Diagnosis and Treatment of Low Back Pain*, p. 101, Ltd., New York, Raven Press.

Snook, S.H., Fine, L.J., and Silverstein, B.A. 1988. Musculoskeletal disorders. In B.S. Levy and D.H. Wegman (Eds.), *Occupational Health: Recognizing and Preventing Work-Related Disease*, pp. 345–370, Little, Brown and Co., Boston/Toronto.

Szpalski, M. and Parnianpour, M. 1996. Trunk performance, strength and endurance: measurement techniques and application. In S. Weisel and J. Weinstein (Eds.), *The Lumbar Spine*, 2nd ed., pp. 1074–1105, Philadelphia, W.B. Saunders.

Tan, J.C., Parnianpour, M., and Nordin M. et al. 1993. Isometric maximal and submaximal trunk exertion at different flexed positions in standing: triaxial torque output and EMG. *Spine* 18: 2480.

World Health Organization. 1980. *International Classification of Impairments, Disabilities, and Handicaps.* Geneva, WHO.

World Health Organization. 1985. Identification and Control of Work-Related Diseases. Technical report no. 174. Geneva, WHO.

84

Human Performance Engineering Design and Analysis Tools

Paul J. Vasta
George V. Kondraske
University of Texas-Arlington

84.1   Introduction

Computer software applications have been implemented in virtually every aspect of our lives and the field of human performance has not proven to be an exception. Due to the growing recognition of the role of human performance engineering in many different areas (e.g., clinical medicine, industrial design, etc.) and the resulting increase in requirements of the methods involved, having the "right tool for the job" is becoming of vital importance. Software developers bear the brunt of the responsibility of determining the qualities of a software application that define it as being "the right tool" for a specific job. In contrast, users of this class of tools must determine when their application extends a given tool beyond its intended scope. These abilities require a knowledge base spanning a number of different fundamental concepts and methods encompassing not only the obvious aspects of human performance and computer programming, but also many other less obvious issues related to database requirements, parameter standards, systems engineering principles, and software architecture. In addition, foresight of how specific components can best be integrated to fit the needs of a particular usage is also necessary.

This chapter addresses selected aspects of computer software tools specifically directed toward human performance design and analysis. The majority of tools currently available emphasize biomechanical models, and as such, this emphasis is reflected here. However, a much broader scope in terms of the body systems incorporated is anticipated, and an effort is made to consider the evolution of more versatile and integrated packages. Selected key functional components of tools are described and a representative sample of currently emerging state-of-the-art packages is used to illustrate not only a snapshot of the capabilities now available, but also those which are needed and options that exist in terms of the fundamental approach taken to address similar problems.

In general, the development of computer software applications, especially in maturing fields such as human performance engineering, serves multiple purposes. The most apparent is the relative speed and accuracy that can be achieved in computationally intensive tasks (e.g., dynamic analysis) compared to performing the processes by hand. In addition, computers can handle large amounts of data and help keep track of the multitude of parameters associated with the human architecture. This allows otherwise impossible procedures, such as the detailed analysis of a complex **human–task interface**, visualization of a human figure in a **virtual workspace**, or the computation of time-series multibody joint torques, to be realized. Perhaps more important, though, are the indirect benefits provided. For example, relatively complex analytic methods utilized in research facilities can be directly implemented in the field by practitioners, with the need for only a complete knowledge of how to effectively *use* the capability available (which is substantially different than the knowledge required to *create* that ability). Moreover, because the software environment demands rigor (e.g., coding structure requirements, data handling and storage, etc.) and since the potential scope of end-user needs in terms of functional and parametric components encompassed is broad, decisions are forced and rules must be clearly delineated. These characteristics thus serve as a motivation to develop standards for (or at least decide upon the use of) many items including methods, parameters, parameter definition conventions, and units of measure. Such efforts can expose and correct inadequacies inherent in current standards while successful software tools (i.e., those which make their way into everyday use) facilitate dissemination of key knowledge and standards to both researchers and practitioners alike.

It can be anticipated that most analysis or decision-making tasks required of practitioners will be made available in computer-based form, including some that are not currently feasible to perform at all except, perhaps, by using intuitive methods that are inconsistently applied and produce results of questionable validity. Given the extent of the possible list of tools within a given package, and considering the substantial overlap of various support functions, classification of packages is difficult. This has been seen already in the relatively modest number of those currently available.

84.2 Selected Fundamentals

It is typical to think of a software capability in terms of a high-level process, for example "gait analysis," where the end result is of primary interest since the underlying processes are performed "invisibly." Yet these supportive processes, many of which have common mathematical methodologies and modeling approaches, determine the ultimate usability and applicability of the software to a given problem and, therefore, deserve closer examination. It makes sense to consider these methods generically not only because they are common to several existing packages, but also because they will undoubtedly be important in others.

84.2.1 Physics-Based Models and Methods

Physics-based methods are implemented when direct analysis of the system or its resources is feasible. With regard to the human system, such methods are commonly applied in biomechanical analysis where unknown parameters, such as joint torque, are derived from known characteristics, such as segment lengths and reaction forces, based on established physical laws and relationships.

Given that relatively simple biomechanical analyses typically include multiple segments and degrees of freedom, the feasibility of employing such methods depends not only on the availability of the required input data, but on the capability to process large amounts of information as well. As the analytical complexity of the task increases, for example, with the inclusion of motion, the significance of implementing such processes within a computer software application becomes readily apparent.

Physical motion is common to most situations in which the human functions and is therefore fundamental to the analysis of performance. Parameters such as segment position, orientation, velocity, and acceleration are derived using kinematic or dynamic analysis or both. This approach is equally appropriate for operations on a single joint system or **linked multibody systems**, such as is typically required for human analysis. Depending on the desired output, foreword (direct) or inverse analysis may be employed to obtain the parameters of interest. For example, inverse dynamic analysis can provide joint torque, given motion and force data while foreword (direct) dynamic analysis uses joint torque to derive motion. Especially for three-dimensional analyses of multijoint systems, the methods are quite complex and are presently a focal point for computer implementation [Allard et al., 1994].

Physics models used to address biomechanical aspects of human performance are relatively well established and utilized in both research and applied domains. In contrast, concepts and methods directed toward other aspects of human performance, such as information processing (in purely perceptual contexts as well as in neuromotor control contexts), are based on strong science and have been incorporated into one-of-a-kind computer models, but to our knowledge have not been engineered into any general-purpose computer tools. It can be argued that Shannon's information theory provides the basis for a similar set of "physics-based" cause-and-effect models to support the incorporation of this aspect of human performance into computer-based modeling and analysis tools. Considerable work has gone into the application of information theory to human information processing [Lachman et al., 1979] within research domains. The definition of neuromotor **channel capacity** [Fitts, 1954] and metrics for the information content of a visual stimulus measured in bits [Hick, 1952; Hyman, 1953] are some examples of the influence of information theory that have become well established. Given the considerable science that now exists, useful computer-based analytic tools that use these ideas as basic modeling constructs are likely to emerge.

84.2.2 Inference-Based Models

Often, direct measurement of a **performance resource** or structural element is not feasible or practical and estimates must be inferred from models based on representative populations. Inferential-based methods, therefore, utilize derived relationships between parameters to provide an estimation (or prediction) of an unknown quantity based on other available measures. One type of modeling approach in such a situation is through statistical regression. This process utilizes data measured from a population of subjects with characteristics similar to the subject or population of interest, to derive a function which represents a "typical" relationship between the independent (measured) variable and the dependent (desired) variable. Specifically, this is achieved through the determination of the function that minimizes the error between the actual and the predicted value across all observations of the independent variable. This process results in an approximation of the desired parameter with a quantified standard error [Remington and Schork, 1985]. Applications of this method require that the dependent variable is distributed normally and with constant variance, and correspondingly, that an estimation of its typical value (for a given population) is desired. Applied to the human system, regression is often implemented to develop **data models**, which are then used to estimate unknown structural parameter values from known parameters, such as the estimation of body segment moments of inertia from stature and weight [McConville et al. 1980]. Regression has also been used to predict task performance from a wide variety of other variables (e.g., height, weight, age, other performance variables, etc.). A specific example is the determination of the maximum acceptable load during lifting tasks as a function of variables such as body weight and arm strength [Jiang and Ayoub, 1987].

A conceptually different and relatively new example of an inferential model, motivated by human performance problems specifically, is nonlinear causal resource analysis (NCRA) [Kondraske, 1988; Vasta and Kondraske, 1994]. Quantitative task demands, in terms of performance variables that characterize the involved subsystems, are inferred from a population data set that includes measures of subsystem performance resource availabilities (e.g., speed, accuracy, etc.) and overall performance on the task in question. This method is based on the following simple concept: Consider a sample of 100 people, each with a known amount of cash (e.g., a fairly even distribution from $0 to $10,000). Each person is asked to try to purchase a specific computer, the "cost" of which is unknown. In the subgroup that was able to make the purchase (some would not have enough cash), the individual who had the least amount of cash provides the key clue. That "amount of cash availability" provides an estimate of the computer's cost (i.e., the unknown value). Thus, in human performance, demand is inferred from resource availabilities.

84.2.3 Fidelity

An important principle that has not often received the scrutiny it deserves is that of the level of fidelity desired, or perhaps more critically, necessary for a particular application. This includes anything that affects the range of applicability or quality of the results provided in a given application. Fidelity can be characterized in terms of three distinctly different components: (1) model scope, (2) computational quality (e.g., resolution limits, compounding of errors, convergence limits of numerical methods, etc.), and (3) data quality (e.g., noise, intrinsic resolution limits, etc.). Model scope considers the extent to which major systems are incorporated (e.g., neuromuscular, sensory, cognitive, etc.) and, as a separate issue, the extent to which these major subsystems are represented (e.g., peak torque and angle limits vs. a three-dimensional torque-angle-speed envelope for neuromuscular systems of rotational joints).

84.2.4 Parameter Conventions

Often, the exact definition of parameters across (and even within) scientific disciplines varies, limiting communication of findings and inhibiting dissemination of knowledge. Careful selection and clear documentation of **parameter conventions** is an important principle in producing analytic software that can be understood, accepted, and used.

Within the broad scope of parameters that could possibly be incorporated in analytic and other software tools, there are many parameter convention challenges that arise. Due to the fact that of the reported analyses in which various parameters that appear have been of restricted scope and largely special purpose, more generalized situations where convention is important have escaped standardization in terms broad enough to support all application needs. As one example, consider the description of relative orientation between two object-attached coordinate systems in three dimensions (in the context of the human system, this specifies joint angle). There are two basic forms of angle set representations, each derived in terms of the method of rotation of one coordinate system (attached to a moving object) about a specific axis: (1) Fixed angle representation, which involves referencing each rotation of the moving system to some fixed reference frame and, (2) Euler angle representation, indicating that each consecutive rotation of the moving system is referenced to the coordinate axes of its present orientation. Given multiple degrees of freedom, multiple angles result representing the amount of rotation about a specific axis and at a defined position in the order of rotations. The specification of these parameters defines the associated angle set convention (i.e., fixed or Euler). Utilization of the terms "roll, pitch, and yaw" [Chao, 1980] in communicating this convention, originally used to describe ship and aircraft orientation, can also lead to confusion. This is not only due to the lack of similarity between the defined reference frame of an aircraft and that of a human segment, but also due to its altered definition within other disciplines (e.g., fixed angle representation [Spong and Vidyasagar, 1989]. Thus, depending on the "type" of Euler angle used and the sequence of axes about which the rotations occur, two entirely different orientations are likely to result. This discussion does not even consider the clinical perspective on joint angles, where only angles measured in three orthogonal planes [Panjabi et al., 1974] are considered. Despite the fact that the human architecture has remained constant (unlike many artificial systems), to our knowledge there is no standard convention that defines all angles in a total human link model for three-dimensional motion.

84.2.5 Data Formats

The utilization of data, especially within a software environment, involves both communication and manipulation not only within a single stand-alone application, but often across facilities, databases, and platforms. Data formats, in this light, can be considered among the most important of the components fundamental to analytic software. Problematic effects may result from aspects including inconsistent adoption of terminology (e.g., endurance vs. fatigue), units of measure specifications, file structures, parameter coding, and database structure. Computer-aided design (CAD) environments in traditional engineering disciplines (e.g., drafting, mechanical design, etc.) have confronted such issues with standardization such as the DXF file formats (used for two- and three-dimensional geometric drawings; even accepted by some numerical machining systems) and the Gerber format (used to communicate a printed circuit board specification to board manufacturers). Within the realm of human performance engineering, standards for data formats remain at the forefront of developmental needs. Some limited standards are emerging, such as the relatively consistent use of ASCII text files with either labeled or position-dependent parameters. However, there are currently no known, agreed upon, or de facto standards for positions, labels, units of measure, and so on.

84.3 Scope, Functionality, and Performance

As summarized in Figure 84.1, CAD-like human performance software depends on conceptual issues as well as decisions regarding fidelity, functionality, and implementation. There is also a great deal of interaction among these categories. Topics within each category were derived in part from a review of current packages (e.g., those described below) and an assessment of other issues and needs. These lists are intended to be illustrative and not exhaustive. While *every* major category applies to *any* given software tool, not all topics listed within a category will always be relevant.

Conceptual issues include taxonomies on which a given package is based (e.g., basic approaches to motor control, system performance, task categorizations and analysis, data estimation, etc.), parameter choices and codification (e.g., hierarchical level of representation, identification in structured input/output file formats), and compliance with or deviation from accepted standards with the varied communities that deal with human performance. They may well deserve special recognition given the impressionable developmental stage of the class of software tools addressed. Perhaps because developers are so familiar with a given perspective or body of knowledge, key conceptual issues are often overlooked or incorporated de facto from previous work (e.g., research studies) that is similar (but perhaps not identical) to the intended purpose of a given package, which is frequently broader and more general than the research efforts or projects that inspired it. Software packages impose on users the constructs on which they are based and this may result in conflicts within an already structured environment. Conceptual foundations and approaches are not yet as clearly defined in human performance as they are in disciplines such as electrical and mechanical engineering. This is further complicated by the wide variety of disciplines (and therefore educational backgrounds) represented by those with interest in participating in software development. Clear and complete disclosure of the conceptual foundation used by developers is thus helpful to both users (potential and actual) and developers.

The concept and scope of fidelity in the present context has been delineated in Section 84.2.3 and is further represented by the subtopics in Figure 84.1. We have chosen to apply it here in its broadest sense. In a fairly recent National Research Council panel on human performance modeling [Baron et al., 1990], recommendations were made toward problems regarding design and implementation issues. Though not specifically addressing computer software, the extension of the discussion is natural given present technology and implementation methods. While it was concluded that an all-inclusive model (i.e., high

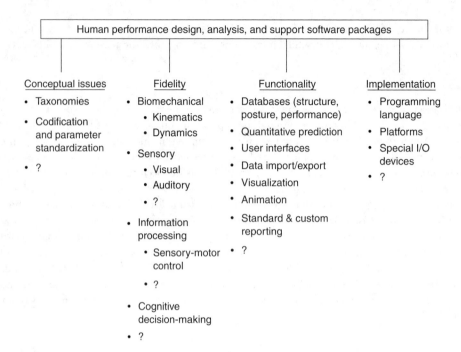

FIGURE 84.1   Related aspects of human design and performance software describe the diversity and scope of underlying issues.

fidelity, in the sense that biomechanical, information processing, sensory, and perceptual aspects, etc. are represented) might be desirable, it is highly unlikely that it could be achieved or would be useful, as the inherent complexity would impede effective usage. The basic recommendation made was to pursue more limited scope submodels. The implication is that two or more computer-based versions of such submodels could be integrated to achieve a wide range of fidelity, with the combination selected to meet the needs of particular situations. However, there is neither a general framework nor set of guidelines for developers of submodels (i.e., an **open-architecture concept**) that would facilitate integration of relatively independent software development efforts. Thus, integration is left to the end user and typically only cumbersome methods are available.

Fidelity should be considered in combination with productivity and both must be carefully assessed against needs. For example, a package that provides the user with control over a large number of parameters (e.g., joint stiffness, balance control, etc.) that define the human system under analysis, typically allows for greater intrinsic fidelity and can be valuable if the ability to specify parameters at that level of detail is an absolute user requirement. If not, this level of specificity only increases the number of prerequisite steps to achieve a given analysis and leads to a more complex program in terms of operation and function (which is perhaps most evident in the user interface). Furthermore, more accurate results are not necessarily obtained. Programs that are structured to automatically rely on default parameter values that can be inspected or changed when desired serve both types of needs. However, concern is typically raised that "lazy" users will forego the entry of values more appropriate to the situation at hand. Thus, while software developers can provide features that greatly simplify procedures and recommendations regarding their proper use, users bear the responsibility of choosing when to invoke such features. Fidelity issues are often viewed as "either" or "or" choices, when many times a "both" or "all" approach is quite feasible. This gives the user the decision-making power and responsibility for decisions that may affect quality of results. Such approaches also typically result in a greater user pool for a given package. The manner in how such flexibility is implemented, however, is critical. For example, if fidelity decisions are likely to be made once in a given installation, schemes that require decision making with each analysis can prove to be cumbersome and ineffective.

Functionality can be considered in terms of basic and special subcategories. Far too often, attention is given to special features while those that are more basic (such as import/export capabilities) are ignored. Most items listed in Figure 84.1 under the "functionality" category are self explanatory, although it should be noted that features such as importing and exporting are more complex in the present context than one might anticipate due in part to the lack of standards for parameters representation (see above). Developers must carefully select functionality and potential users must carefully evaluate the impact of those choices against their specific needs. For example, the processing power required to display and animate contoured multisegment human figures in real time and in three dimensions is substantial. Programs with this ability typically require high-end platforms and also require that a large fraction of the programming effort and user interface be used for this functionality. The addition of processes such as a dynamic analysis places even a greater stress on processing power and complexity. Visualization of human figures in three dimensions along with some environmental components is essential for some applications. For many applications, such as those in which numerical results are required and conveyed to others with simple printed reports, such visualization are not required, or contribute little, to achieving the desired end purpose (although they are almost always viewed as "attractive" by potential users). Functionality options are further developed and exemplified in the discussion of actual software packages below (Section 84.4).

The last of these four categories describes the support structure upon which the software packages are built. Software implementation in today's ever-changing computer market requires careful thought. In addition to host platform and standard accessories, special input/output interfaces are often necessary (e.g., to allow direct access to laboratory acquired kinematic data). Support software for such special hardware is not always available on all platforms, preventing operation with analytic software in the same environment. Choice of programming language (supporting modules and libraries, platform diversity) and the operating system (Macintosh®, Windows™, Unix, etc.) are also critical. As exemplified in Section 85.4, no existing packages run on all platforms and under all operating systems users who wish to employ multiple packages are left with cumbersome and often costly solutions.

As computing power at the single-user level (i.e., personal computer) increases, there is little doubt that a full set of state-of-the-art features covering a broad scope of human performance and data needs *could* be integrated into a single package. At present, though, limitations are real and necessary. These are the result of specific trade-offs that must be considered during development when determining target users. Operational costs include software acquisition, maintenance, basic platform acquisition and outfitting, and training costs. A large feature set and high performance are not always indicative of a software tool's value. Value is lost if a user's requirements are either unfulfilled or greatly exceed by the functionality and performance of a program. Unfortunately, general trade-offs that are acceptable within different groups of users have not yet become evident.

84.4 Functional Overview of Representative Packages

In this section, a selected set of different types of software packages intended specifically for human design and performance analysis applications are described. At least one example of each type exists and is noted for reference and to illustrate the types of functionality developers are addressing in response to perceived needs. No endorsement of any example cited is implied. The packages included vary widely in function and performance and should not be considered to be directly comparable. Operational costs reflect this diversity, ranging from relatively inexpensive (e.g., approximately $100.00 plus the price of a moderately equipped PC™) to the level defined by high-end workstations (e.g., thousands of dollars for software licenses plus the cost of a Unix-based workstation). As with desktop computer applications, such as word processors and spreadsheets, the packages used to illustrate functionality are under constant development, and changing feature-sets, performance, and cost are to be anticipated.

The types of packages included illustrate fundamental options with regard to general or dedicated analysis (e.g., user-defined tasks vs. gait), different levels of analysis (e.g., "muscle" vs. "joint" levels in biomechanical analyses), body-function-specific or general-purpose analysis (e.g., gait vs. user-defined function), fidelity in terms of scope (e.g., biomechanical, sensory, neuromotor control, etc.), and target user orientation (medical vs. nonmedical design; although overlap is possible). It should be noted that while particular packages are highlighted under certain categories, underlying features and functions are common across many applications.

84.4.1 Human Parameter Databases

The need for data is evident in all aspects of human-related CAD and the analysis of human performance. In certain situations, requirements may be for a specific individual or a representative population. In the former case, there are certain parameters that are not readily attainable (e.g., location of center of mass for a segment, inertia, etc.) and therefore must be estimated, as in the latter case, from normative values derived from studies. For a number of years, these estimates have been available in book form primarily as lookup tables. This format, however, does not take advantage of current technology and is not sufficient for use with software-based analytic tools. Some currently available packages, in addressing this need, have included data tables that are utilized exclusively within the program. Programs such as *MannequinPro* and *SafeWork* (detailed below) for example, each include a significant database of anthropometric measures for various populations. The user specifies design parameter values by choosing characteristics such as gender, ethnic origin, and morphology representative of the desired population. Various other stand-alone database software packages, for example, *PeopleSize* (targeted initially for clothing design), allow data to be exported, thereby providing at least an indirect support for external applications.

In addition to measures such as segment lengths, parameters including reach and range of motion for selected postures are frequently provided in databases (e.g., horizontal sitting reach, etc.). Because it is prohibitive (if not impossible) to measure and report all possible situations, this issue may be more adequately addressed through the use of parametric data models. Data derived from such models would provide estimates for all possible conditions as well as having the additional advantage of requiring lesser storage and management requirements. Caution is warranted with regard to issues such as model validity, statistical sample sizes and variations, combinatory effects of merging databases or data models, and traceability of data to original sources.

84.4.2 Biomechanical, Muscle-Level Modeling and Analysis

Software for interactive musculoskeletal modeling *SIMM* is a graphics-based tool for modeling and visualization of any human or animal musculoskeletal system and is directed at lower-level structures, that is, individual muscles. The program allows users to model any type of musculoskeletal system using files, which specify (1) the skeletal structure through polygonal surface objects, (2) the joint kinematics, and (3) the muscle architecture through specifications of a line of action for each muscle and isometric force data. *SIMM* contains various tools for observing and editing the model (see Figure 84.2). The user can visualize and animate the model, display or hide the individual muscles (shown as line segments), manipulate joint angles, muscle forces, and moment arms. Joint torques (static) can be analyzed via plots and graphs and all of the muscle parameters may be edited including visual alteration of muscle lines of action. Finally, the user also has control over joint kinematics by altering the cubic splines used to control the animated joint movements. Developers claim that *SIMM* is aimed at biomechanics researchers, kinesiologists, workspace designers, and students who can benefit from visual feedback showing muscle locations and actions.

Musculographics, the developers of *SIMM*, also produce a component as part of the SIMM suite specifically directed toward gait analysis that provides ground reaction force vectors and color-highlighted muscle activity through animation of the model. The software is designed to input data files written by movement analysis systems and can display plots of data such as muscle lengths and ground reaction forces. Another application, the *Dynamics Pipeline*, is a general-purpose package that provides forward and inverse dynamics to calculate motions resulting from forces or torques required to generate a given motion,

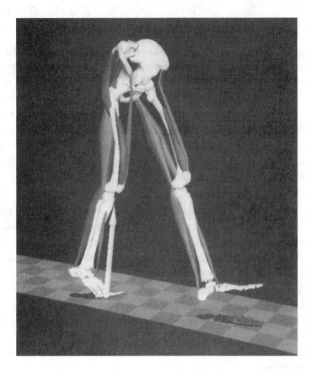

FIGURE 84.2   Muscle attachments and utilization (indicated by shading) for the lower extremities during gait, created and displayed using SIMM software.

respectively. *SIMM* was also made available for Microsoft Windows. However, the original Unix-based version is still available.

84.4.3 Body Function–Specific Tools

GaitLab is a Windows™-based software package that allows fundamental parameters of human gait to be derived, analyzed, and inspected. At this time it is available inexpensively ($49.95) as part of a larger package from Kiboho Publishers. The program is divided into two main sections (i.e., subprograms that run under the "shell" of the main application): (1) a mathematics section, which provides processes for generating text files representing various gait parameters throughout a gait cycle; and (2) a graphics section that creates plots of the parameters as well as a representation of gait through an animated stick figure. Documentation covers the gait parameters and equations associated with the software package as well as the underlying principles for their use in gait analysis. Software accepts different, custom-formatted data files (ASCII text) based on direct measurements of a human subject. These include anthropometric, kinematic (i.e., three-dimensional positions of anatomic landmarks), force plate, and electromyographic (EMG) measures. Sample files are included for a healthy adult male, female, and an adult male with cerebral palsy. From this data, text files are created for lower-extremity body segment parameters (mass, center of gravity position, and moment of inertia), linear kinematics (joint center, heel, and toe locations, segment reference frames), center of gravity (position, velocity, and acceleration), angular kinematics (joint angles, angular velocity, and acceleration), and dynamics (joint forces and torques). The package can also display up to three simultaneous plots of these parameters in any combination. Time, percent of gait cycle, and marker position scales are also available for plotting against any of the variables.

    GaitLab provides a useful function in its ability to generate the above mentioned parameters and is effective with its simplistic stick figure animation, allowing minimal processing power/speed requirements while providing the nuances of lower limb movement pertinent to gait analysis. It is just one of many examples of function-specific packages.

84.4.4 Biomechanical, Joint-Level, Total Human Analysis

ADAMS is a software package designed for mechanical design and system simulation in general. It is an extensive package incorporating specific components for both modeling and kinematic/dynamic analysis. What sets *ADAMS* apart from other nonperformance-based simulation/dynamics packages is the availability of a module, LifeMOD, specifically designed to allow the user to create a human model. The human model may be edited as needed but is provided in a default configuration of a 19 joint-body architecture with five anthropometric body size databases. Because the package focuses on mechanical systems in general, a great deal of control is provided to the user over the parameters of the model including contact forces, joint friction, damping, and nonlinear stiffness as well as control parameters. Having this capability, the human model is able to affect control over objects in its environment as well as responding biomechanically to contact. Supplemental toolsets may be (custom) developed to provide proper control over model parameters such as motion resistance relationships, joint strength and range of motion limits, and delays in neuromuscular response. For a given model, kinematic or dynamic simulations may be run and values for any parameter can be plotted on screen. Both forward and inverse dynamic analyses are available and graphics-based facilities such as the specification of trajectories via mouse input are available. The simulations may be used to generate detailed animation movie (.avi) files.

Because *ADAMS'* capabilities are so extensive, it has become one of the most widely used mechanical system simulation packages. Outside of the realm of human performance analysis, the package is targeted at engineers and scientists who require complete observation and control of the model parameters across many hierarchical levels. While this format affords great fidelity and specificity in the analysis, there is also a great deal of complexity and detail that must be addressed in every new simulation run. Though **performance assessment** is not an inherent or recognized feature in the package, custom modules may be incorporated, which would allow for direct comparison of system resource utilization and stress against the demands of the task.

84.4.5 Visualization for Low-End Computer Platforms

MannequinPro, while having inherent database functionality, is essentially a visualization tool that allows users to quickly create three-dimensional humanoid figures, which may be represented in stick-figure form, as a wireframe "robot" with polygonal segments, or as its name implies, a mannequin with higher-resolution segments. These figures may be postured within preset (i.e., noneditable) range-of-motion limits, as well as viewed from many different perspectives. They are created automatically by the program according to user-defined structural aspects chosen from a list of specifications for gender, population percentile, body type, age, and nationality. The package also provides a modest drawing (CAD-type) tool for creating various objects to be placed in the scene with the figure. Two additional features extend *MannequinPro* beyond the domain of a "simple" object rendering tool. The first is provided through animation effects, allowing the mannequin to walk via an internally generated gait sequence (a specific path may be defined through a virtual workspace), reach to a specific location, or move through any sequence of positions created on a frame-by-frame basis by the user. The second feature allows the user to specify forces acting on the mannequins hands or feet from which static torques are calculated for both left and right wrists, elbows, shoulders, neck, back, hips, knees, and ankles.

As a visualization tool, *MannequinPro* provides a needed capability for a modest price and requires only a personal computer to run. Figures are easily produced to the anthropometric specifications available and posing, reaching, and walking functions, though limited, are simple to control. The package is primarily operated from mouse input with standard point, click, and drag operations that should be familiar to most users of current commercial software. Once the scene is created with humans and objects in their workspace, it is up to the user to extract any information regarding function and performance from the visual images presented by the package. These features, as well as others, are also contained within the software package *Jack* and *SafeWork* (described below), which provide greater functionality but are targeted toward workstation environments. In sum, *MannequinPro*, with a good price-to-performance ratio, is an effective tool when human visualization with moderate graphics is required at the single-user platform level.

84.4.6 Extended Visualization for the High-End Workstations

Jack, developed within the University of Pennsylvania Center for Human Modeling and Simulation [Badler et al., 1993], and *SafeWork* are a high-end CAD-oriented design and visualization packages. Similar in function to *MannequinPro* (above), but with considerably more flexibility and detail, they are designed to allow human factors engineers to place a human in a virtual workstation environment while still in the design phase. Both extend far beyond the capabilities of *MannequinPro*, trading simplicity for specificity in that they provide users with control over a large range of variables regarding many aspects of the human figure and its virtual environment. Human models are fully articulated and preset or user-definable anthropometric parameters that include segment dimensions, joint limits, moments of inertia, and strength allow highly specific representation. The total functionality of these packages are far too great to list the individual aspects here, but examples include reach, hand gripping, balance (including reorientation behavior), collision detection, light and camera (view) manipulation, animation, and kinematic/dynamic analysis. *Jack* also allows for real-time posture tracking of a human operator through position and orientation sensors (see Figure 84.3).

Similar to the functionality of *ADAMS*, these packages provide a great deal of control over the design and manipulation of the human figure. Because of the large number of controllable parameters and the difficulty involved in providing an interface allowing three-dimensional manipulation of high-end graphics in a two-dimensional environment, the majority of users will require training. *Jack* and *SafeWork* require a Silicon Graphics workstation to run.

84.4.7 Total Human, Performance-Based, Human–Task Interface Analysis

While now under development, *HMT–CAD* represents yet a different perspective in that it is based primarily on performance modeling constructs [e.g., Kondraske, 2005] and is aimed at producing bottom-line assessments regarding human-to-task, human-to-machine, and eventually machine-to-task interfaces using a logic similar to that used by systems-level designers. In a joint effort between Photon Research Associates, Inc. and the University of Texas at Arlington Human Performance Institute, performance models and decision-making strategies are combined with advanced multibody dynamic analysis.

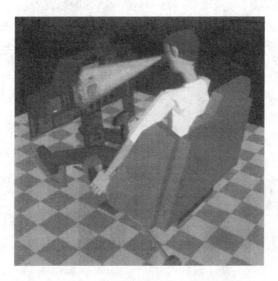

FIGURE 84.3   A human/workspace figure created and displayed using Jack software.

HMT-CAD's initial development emphasized a top-down approach that set out with the goal of realizing a shell that would allow systematic incorporation of increasingly higher fidelity in a modular, stepwise fashion. The initial modules encompass biomechanical and neuromuscular aspects of performance that bases analyses on knowledge of range/extremes of motion, torque, and speed capacities. Gross total human (23 links and 41 degrees of freedom) and hand link models (16 links and 22 degrees of freedom each) are included. The Windows™-based tool provides a predefined framework for specifying human structure and performance parameters (e.g., anthropometry, strength, etc.) for individuals or populations. A task library is included based on an object-oriented approach to task analysis. HMT–CAD attempts to help communicate information about many parameters via a custom graphical–button interface. For example, one analysis result screen shows a human figure surrounded by buttons connected to body joints. Button color (e.g., red or green) communicates whether an analysis found limiting factors for the specified person in the specified task associated with that joint system. Using computer mouse input, clicking on red buttons produces a new window showing a list of performance capacities and stress levels associated with systems of that joint. Maximally stressed performance resources are tagged. *HMT–CAD* uses the same systems of level modeling constructs for human and artificial systems. A novel technique that transparently draws upon a large set of data models as needed is used to provide "the best analysis possible" with the data provided by the user. This allows users to directly specify values for all parameters if desired, but does not require this for each analysis (see Figure 84.4).

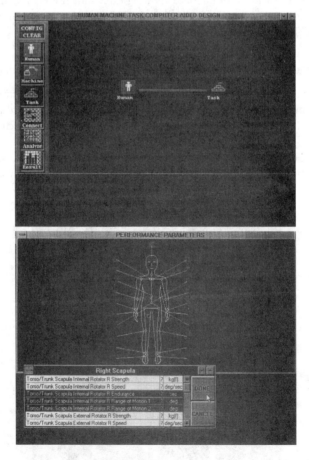

FIGURE 84.4   A desktop environment of the HMT-CAD performance assessment package including system model development and analysis result reporting.

In the present prototype, analysis scope is very limited (upper extremity, object moving tasks). Databases are being populated to allow a similar fidelity of analysis for trunk and lower-extremity analyses. Development of an optimization engine based on minimizing stress across performance resources [Kondraske and Khoury, 1992] to solve problems in which redundant approaches are possible is underway. No capability is currently provided for animation of human movement, as binary assessments (e.g., red and green buttons) and numerical results (stress levels on performance capacities) are emphasized. However, an interface to emerging general-purpose animation tools is planned. Long-term development will proceed to increase fidelity in a stepwise fashion by the inclusion of performance capacities for other major systems (e.g., information processing associated with motor control) as well as additional performance capacities for major systems represented at any given time (e.g., the inclusion of neuromuscular endurance limits).

The inferential NCRA methodology discussed earlier has recently been used to create a companion NCRA software package by the University of Texas at Arlington's Human Performance Institute. It is based on General System Performance Theory concepts and the Elemental Resource Model [Kondraske, 2005] and performs the following functions:

- *Perform Task Analyses (Build NCRA models):* Models consist of a set of Resource Demand Functions, each of which relates the amount of a given performance resource required to achieve a specific level of High Level Task (HLT) performance.
- *Predict HLT Performance:* Using an NCRA model and a set of measures representing basic performance resource availability (i.e., performance capacities) for a set of "n" subjects as "inputs" to the model (i.e., independent variables), individualized predictions of performance in the HLT are computed.
- *Identify Limiting Performance Resources:* In addition to a prediction of HLT performance, for each subject in a Prediction Source Data set, the performance resource that prevents that subject from "performing better" is identified.
- *Obtain Other Useful Performance-Related Measures:* Various options are available to explore the stress on the performance resources of individuals associated with a given level of HLT performance.

Importantly, NCRA allows models to be formulated that mix neuromuscular, information processing, sensory, and life-sustaining performance resources. It is anticipated that many existing data sets, which have been previously used to develop regression-based models, can be used with NCRA (see Figure 84.5).

84.5 Anticipated Development

While it is relatively easy to outline the functionality and unique aspects of the software discussed above, it is a great deal harder to describe the level of difficulty required to achieve a desired end result and to characterize how well functions are performed. Online "help" systems, multimedia components, associated software development tools, improved parameter measurement tools, and higher-fidelity models will no doubt impact these aspects.

As mundane as it may seem, perhaps nothing is more important to the overall advancement of this class of software tools than the development of standards for parameters used, parameter conventions, and data formats. It is likely that de facto standards will emerge from individual commercial endeavors. Due to the diversity of professionals involved, it is difficult to envision the evolution of "standards by committee." Observation of success stories in analogous efforts also supports this opinion. This, in turn, will enable progress to be made in database and data model development, which is vital to the many of the more routine functions such software will perform. Combined with modular object-oriented programming techniques, the emergence of true multitasking operating systems on desktop computers, and the support for interprocess communication (such as dynamic data exchange) will encourage developers. Many new tools, both similar to and completely different than those describe here, can be anticipated.

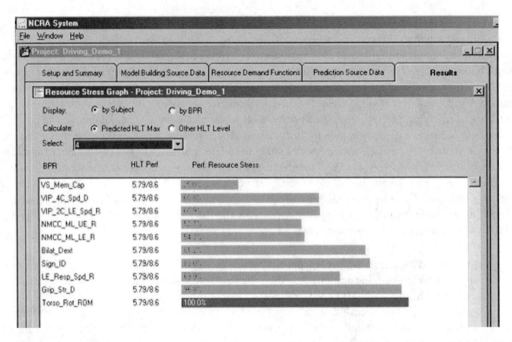

FIGURE 84.5   Screen capture from NCRA software illustrating results for one individual applied to a model of driving performance. Overall driving performance level (HLT performance) and limiting performance resources (in this case "torso rotation range of motion") are predicted based on a set of more basic performance resource measures (BPRs). BPR measures are lower-level performance capacities relative to the higher-level task modeled.

Defining Terms

Channel capacity: The maximum rate of information flow through a specific pathway from source to receiver. In the context of the human, a sensorimotor pathway (e.g., afferent sensory nerves, processors, descending cerebrospinal nerve and α-motoneuron) is an example of a channel through which motor control information flows from sensors to actuators (muscle).

Data model: A mathematical equation derived as a representation of the relationship between a dependent variable and one or more independent variables. Similar in function to a database, data models provide parameter values across conditions of other related parameters.

Human–task interface: The common boundary between the human and a task specified by the demands of a task on the respective resources of the human and the capacities of the human's resources involved in performing the task.

Linked multibody system: A system of three or more individual segments joined (as an open or closed chain) in some manner with the degree of freedom between any two segments defined by the characteristics of the corresponding hinge.

Open-architecture concept: A general methodology for the development of functional modules that may be readily integrated to form a higher-level system through well-defined design and interface constructs.

Parameter conventions: Aspects and usage of a parameter that are specifically defined with respect to general implementation.

Performance assessment: The process of determining the level or degree in which a system can perform a specific task given the demands required and the availabilities of the resources of the system which are involved in performing the task.

Performance resource: Defined as a functional unit and an associated dimension of performance (e.g., knee extensor strength) that is available to a system.

Virtual workspace: A representation of a three-dimensional physical workspace generated by computer software and displayed on a video monitor or similar device. This enables, for example, the inclusion and manipulation of computer-generated objects within the virtual workspace such that designs can be tested and modified prior to manufacturing.

References

Allard, P., Stokes, I.A.F., and Blanchi, J.P. (Eds.) 1994. *Three-Dimensional Analysis of Human Movement*, Human Kinetics, Champaign, IL.

Badler, N.I., Phillips, C.B., and Webber, B.L. 1993. *Simulating Humans: Computer Graphics Animation and Control*, Oxford University Press, New York.

Badler, N.I. 1989. Task-oriented animation of human figures. In *Applications of Human Performance Models to System Design*, G.R. McMillan, D. Beevis, and E. Salas, (Eds.), Plenum Press, New York.

Baron, S., Kruser, D.S., and Huey, B.M. (Eds.) 1990. *Quantitative Modeling of Human Performance in Complex, Dynamic Systems*, National Academy Press, Washington, DC.

Chao, E.Y.S. 1980. Justification of triaxial goniometer for the measurement of joint rotation. *Biomechanics*, 13: 989–1006.

Craig, J.J. 1989. *Introduction to Robotics Mechanics and Control*, 2nd ed., Addison-Wesley, New York.

Delp, S.L., Loan, J.P., Hoy, M.G., Zajac, F.E., Topp, E.L., and Rosen, J.M. 1990. An interactive graphics-based model of the lower extremity to study orthopaedic surgical procedures. *IEEE Trans. Biomed. Eng.*, 37: 757–767.

Fitts, P. 1954. The information capacity of the human motor system in controlling the amplitude of movement, *J. Exp. Psychol.*, 47: 381–391.

Hick, W. 1952. On the rate of gain of information, *Quart. J. Exp. Psychol.*, 4: 11–26.

Hyman, R. 1953. Stimulus information as a determinant of reaction time, *J. Exp. Psychol.*, 45: 423–432.

Jiang, B.C. and Ayoub, M.M. 1987. Modelling of maximum acceptable load of lifting by physical factors. *Ergonomics*, 30: 529–538.

Khan, C. 1991. Humanizing AutoCAD. *Cadence*, June.

Kondraske, G.V. 2005. The elemental resource model for human performance. In *Handbook of Biomedical Engineering*. J.D. Bronzino (Ed.) CRC Press Inc., Boca Raton, FL.

Kondraske, G.V. 1988. Experimental evaluation of an elemental resource model for human performance. In *Proceedings, Tenth Annual IEEE Engineering in Medicine and Biology Society Conference*, New Orleans, pp. 1612–1613.

Kondraske, G.V. and Khoury, G.J. 1992. Telerobotic system performance measurement: motivation and methods. In *Cooperative Intelligent Robotics in Space III* (*Proceedings of the SPIE 1829*), J.D. Erickson (Ed.), pp. 161–172, SPIE.

Lachman, R., Lachman, J.L., and Butterfield, E.C. 1979. *Cognitive Psychology and Information Processing: An Introduction*, Lawrence Erlbaum Assoc., Hillsdale, NJ.

McConville, J.T., Churchill, T.D., Kaleps, I., Clauser, C.E., and Cuzzi, J. 1980. *Anthropometric Relationships of Body and Body Segment Moments of Inertia*, Air Force Aerospace Medical Research Laboratory, AFAMRL-TR-80-119, Wright-Patterson Air Force Base, Ohio.

Panjabi, M.M, White III, A.A., and Brand, R.A. 1974. A note on defining body parts configurations. *J. Biomech.*, 7: 385–387.

Pheasant, S.T. 1986. *Bodyspace: Anthropometry, Ergonomics and Design*, Taylor & Francis, Philadelphia, PA.

Remington, R.D. and Schork, M.A. 1985. *Statistics with Applications to the Biological and Health Sciences*, Prentice-Hall, NJ.

Spong, M.W. and Vidyasagar, M. 1989. *Robot Dynamics and Control*, John Wiley & Sons, New York.

Vaughan, C.L., Davis, B.L., and O'Connor, J.C. 1992. *Dynamics of Human Gait*, Human Kinetics, Champaign, IL.

Vasta, P.J. and Kondraske, G.V. 1994. Performance prediction of an upper extremity reciprocal task using non-linear causal resource analysis. In *Proceedings, Sixteenth Annual IEEE Engineering in Medicine and Biology Society Conference*, Baltimore, MD, pp. 305–306.

Winter, D.A. 1990. *Biomechanics and Motor Control of Human Movement*, 2nd ed. John Wiley & Sons, New York.

Further Information

For explicit information regarding the software packages included in this chapter, the developers may be directly contacted as follows:

ADAMS: Mechanical Dynamics, 2301 Commonwealth Blvd., Ann Arbor, MI 48105, USA, 800-88-ADAMS, http://www.adams.com.

GaitLab: originally published by Human Kinetics,1607 N. Market St., Box 5076, Champaign, IL 61825, (217) 351-5076, Now available from Kiboho Publishers, http://www.kiboho.co.za/GaitCD/.

HMT-CAD: Human Performance Institute, The University of Texas at Arlington, P.O. Box 19180, Arlington, TX 76019, (817) 272-2335.

Jack: Center for Human Modeling and Simulation, The University of Pennsylvania, 200 South 33rd St., Philadelphia, PA 19104-6389, (215) 573-9463, http://www.cis.upenn.edu/~hms/jack.html.

s MannequinPro: HumanCAD, a division of Biomechanics Corporation of America, 1800 Walt Whitman Road, Melville, NY, 11747, (516) 752-3568, http://www.humancad.com.

Nonlinear Causal Resource Analysis (NCRA): Human Performance Institute, The University of Texas at Arlington, P.O. Box 19180, Arlington, TX 76019, (817) 272-2335.

PeopleSize: Open Ergonomics Ltd., Loughborough Technology Centre, Epinal Way, Loughborough, LE11 3GE, UK, +44 (0) 1509 218 333, http://www.openerg.com/psz.htm.

SafeWork: Genicom Consultants Inc., 3400 de Maisonneuve Blvd. West, 1 Place Alexis Nihon, Suite 1430, Montreal, Quebec, CANADA, H3Z 3B8, (514) 931-3000, http://www.safework.com.

SIMM: Musculographics, Inc. c/o Motion Analysis. Corp., 3617 Westwind Blvd., Santa Rosa, CA 95403, (707) 579-6500, ww.musculographics.com.

Readers are also encouraged to simply perform web searches on the relevant package keywords or acronyms to discover a wide range of application examples, use issues, and discussions relevant to specific packages.

A broad perspective of issues related to those presented here may be found in: Matilla, M. and Karwowski, W., eds. 1992. Computer applications in ergonomics, occupational safety, and health, In: *Proceedings of the International Conference on Computer-Aided Ergonomics and Safety '92*, Tampere, Finland, North-Holland Publishers, Amsterdam.

Additionally, periodic discussions of related topics may be found in the following publications: CSERIAC Gateway, published by the Crew System Ergonomics Information Analysis Center. For subscription information contact AL/CFH/CSERIAC, Bldg. 248, 2255 H St., Wright-Patterson Air Force Base, Ohio, 45433; IEEE Transactions on Biomedical Engineering or IEEE Engineering in Medicine & Biology Magazine. For further information contact: IEEE Service Center, 445 Hoes Lane, P.O. Box 1331, Piscataway, NJ, 08855-1331.

Numerous other related sites can be found on the internet. Among those of interest are:

Biomechanics World Wide: includes a very thorough listing of various topics related to biomechanics inlcuding links to educational, corporate, and related sites of interest. http://www.per.ualberta.ca/biomechanics/bwwframe.htm.

Biomch-L: an internet list-server supporting discussions regarding topics relating to biomechanics. http://isb.ri.ccf.org/isb/biomch-l/.

Motion Lab Systems, Inc.: a collection of information and links to a variety of Internet sites focused on Electromyography, Biomechanics, Gait Analysis, and Motion Capture. Includes both commercial and non-commercial sites. http://www.emgsrus.com/links.htm.

85

Human Performance Engineering: Challenges and Prospects for the Future

George V. Kondraske
University of Texas-Arlington

85.1 Introduction

Human Performance Engineering is a dynamic area with rapid changes in many facets and constantly emerging developments that affect application possibilities. Materials presented in other chapters of this section of the text illustrate the breadth and depth of effort required as well as the variety of applications in this field. At the same time, the field is relatively young and as is often the case in such instances, some "old" issues remain unresolved and new issues emerge with new developments. With the other material in this section as background, this chapter focuses on selected issues of a general nature (i.e., cutting across various human subsystem types and applications) in three major areas vital to the future of the field (1) human performance modeling; (2) measurement; and (3) data-related topics. In addition to the identification of some key issues, some speculation is presented with regard to the lines along which future work may develop. Awareness of the specific issues raised is anticipated to be helpful to practitioners who must operate within the constraints of the current state-of-the-art. Moreover, the issues selected represent scientific and engineering challenges for the future that will require not only awareness but also the collaboration of researchers and practitioners from the varied segments of the community to resolve.

85.2 Models

It is important to distinguish various types of models encountered in human performance. They include conceptual, statistically-based predictive models, predictive models based on cause-and-effect [Kondraske et al., 1997], and data models [Vasta and Kondraske, 1995]. Issues related to data models are described in Section 85.4 of this chapter, while those related to the remaining types are discussed in this section.

Traditionally, a tremendous amount of activity in various segments of the human performance community has been directed toward development of statistically-based predictive models (e.g., regression models). This remains the most popular approach. By their very nature, each of these is very application specific. Even within the intended application, success of these models has mostly ranged from poor to marginal, with a few reports of models that look "very good" in the populations in which they were tested. However, the criteria for "good" has been skewed by the early performance achieved with these methods and statistically significant "r" values of 0.6 have come to be considered "good." Even if predictive performance was excellent, the long-term merit of statistically-based prediction methods can be questioned on the basis that this approach is intrinsically inefficient. A unique and time-consuming modeling effort, requiring new data collection with human subjects, is required for every situation. At the same time, powerful computer-based tools are commonly available that facilitate the generation of what is estimated to be hundreds and perhaps thousands of these regression models on an annual basis. It appears that many researchers and practitioners have forgotten that one purpose of such statistical methods is to provide insight into the cause-and-effect principles at play and into generalizations that might be more broadly applied. Statistically-based regression models will continue to serve useful purposes within the specific application contexts for which they are developed. However, the future of predictive modeling in human performance engineering must be based on cause-and-effect principles. The sentiment for the need to shift from statistical to more physically based models is present and growing in several of the related application disciplines as evidenced by a sampling of quotations from the literature presented in Table 85.1.

A National Research Council panel on human performance modeling [Baron et al., 1990] conducted one of the more broad-looking investigations regarding complex human performance models; that is, those that consider one or more major attributes (e.g., biomechanical, sensory, cognitive, structural details, etc.) of a total or near-total human. The convening of this panel itself underscored the interest in and need for human performance models. As an interesting aside, while the panel's focus was on modeling, a large fraction of the efforts cited as background represented major software packages, most of which were developed to support defense industry needs. A major application for such models is in computer simulation of humans in various circumstances, which could be used to support prediction and

TABLE 85.1 Representative Quotations Illustrating the Need for a Shift Toward the Development of Causal Models

Quote	Field	References
…there has been little advancement of the science of ergonomics…the degree of advancement is so low that, in my opinion, ergonomics does not yet qualify as a science…There has been no progress in the accumulation of general knowledge…because nearly all studies have not been general studies.	Human factors	Smith, 1987
…experiments are performed year after year to answer the same questions, those questions — often fundamental ones — remain unanswered…the methodology employed today is a hodgepodge of quick fixes that evolved over the years into a paradigm that is taught and employed as sacrosanct, when in fact it is woefully inadequate and frequently incompetent…	Human factors	Simmon, 1987
…authors and users of these instruments lacked a conceptual model…lack of a well-developed conceptual model is unfortunately characteristic of the entire history of the field…	Rehabilitation	Frey, 1987

other analysis needs. A series of useful recommendations were included in panel's report regarding the direction that should be taken in future work. However, recommendations were quite general in nature and no specific plans were outlined regarding how some of these objectives might actually be achieved. Nonetheless, it was clear from the choice of the previous works cited and from the recommendations that development of cause-and-effect, general-purpose models should receive priority. The elemental resource model presented at the beginning of this section of the text [Kondraske, 2005] is one example of a causal, integrative model that reflects an initial attempt to incorporate many of this panel's recommendations.

Whether primarily statistical or causal in nature, frustration with what has been characterized or perceived as "limited success" achieved to date in efforts to unlock and formalize the underpinnings of complex human functions such as speech, gait, lifting, and memory have led to attacks in recent years on the basic reductionistic approach that has been pursued most aggressively. In fact, reductionism has been characterized as a "dead end" methodology — one that has been tried and has failed [Gardner, 1985; Bunge, 1977], as further evidenced by the following somewhat representative quote [Weismer and Liss, 1991]:

[T]his view held the scientific community spellbound until people started looking past the technological issues, and asking how well the reductionist observations were doing at explaining behavior, and the answer was, miserably. Many microscopic facts had been accumulated, and incredible technological advances had been made, but the sum of all of these reductionist observations could not make good sense of macroscopic levels of movement behavior.

Prior to total abandonment, it is perhaps wise not only to characterize the performance of reductionism, but also to question why it might have failed *thus far*. For example, it may be prudent to entertain the proposition that reductionism may be "a correct approach" that has failed to date because of a problem with one or more components associated with its implementation. Are we certain that this is not the case?

One potential explanation for an apparent failure of reductionism is simply the manner in which manpower has been organized (i.e., the research infrastructure) to attack problems of the magnitude of those considered, for example, by the National Research Council panel noted earlier. With some exceptions, the majority of funded research efforts is short term and involve very small teams. Is it possible that the amount of information "to reduce" is too much to produce results that would be characterized as "success" (i.e., does the equivalent of an undercapitalized business venture exist?)? It is further observed that the value of *reduction* is often only demonstrable by the ability to *assemble*. As noted, the prime tool of assembly thus far has been statistical in nature and relatively few causal models have been seriously entertained. With regard to human systems, it is clear that there are many such "items" to assemble and many details to consider if "assembly" — with high fidelity — is to result. Furthermore, it is clear that tools (i.e., special computer software) are needed to make such assembly efforts efficient enough to consider undertaking. Has the data management and analytic power of computers, which have only been readily available in convenient-to-use forms and with required capacities for less than a decade, been fully exploited in a "fair test" of reductionism?

Reductionism is clearly a methodology for understanding "that which is." Drawing by inference from engineering design in general, a close relationship can be observed to systems engineering synthesis methods used to define "that which will be." In artificial systems (as opposed to those which naturally occur, like humans), reverse engineering (basically, a reductionistic method) has been used quite successfully to create functionally equivalent replicas of products. The methodology employed is guided by knowledge of the synthesis process. The implementation of reductionism in human performance modeling can possibly benefit from the reverse mental exercise of "building a human," which may not be so abstract given current efforts and achievements in rehabilitation engineering. In looking toward the future, it is fair to ask, "To what extent have those who have attempted to apply reductionism, or who have dismissed it, attempted to bring to bear methods of synthesis?" The real support for reductionism is success obtained with methods based on this concept; new findings of an extremely encouraging nature are beginning to come forth [Kondraske et al., 1997].

The issue of biological variability is also frequently raised in the context of the desire to develop predictive models of human performance. It is perhaps noteworthy that variability is an issue with which one must deal in the manufacture of man-made products (i.e., particularly with regard to quality assurance in manufacturing), which are designed almost exclusively using causal principles. Taguchi methods [Bendell et al., 1988], a collection of mathematics and concepts, have been used in widespread fashion with remarkable success in modeling and controlling variability in the characteristics of a final product, which is based on the combination of many components, each of which has multiple characteristics, which also range within tolerance bands. Similarity of these circumstances suggests that Taguchi methods may also be valuable in human performance engineering. Investigations of this nature are likely to be a part of future work.

85.3 Measurements

85.3.1 Standardization of Variables and Conditions

Human performance literature is replete with different measures that characterize human performance. Despite the number and magnitude of efforts where human performance is of interest, a standard set of measurement variables has yet to emerge. Relatively loose, descriptive naming conventions are used to identify variables reported leading to the perception of differences when, upon careful inspection, the variables used in two different studies or modeling efforts are the same. In other cases, the names of variables are the same, but conditions under which measures are acquired are different or not reported with enough detail to evaluate if numerical data is comparable (across the reports in question) or not.

The needs of science and engineering are considerably different. Although standardization is generally considered to be desirable in both arenas, the former stresses that only those methods used be accurately reported so that they may be replicated. There has been, unfortunately, little motivation to achieve standardization in any broad sense in the human performance research world. In traditional areas of engineering, it is the marketplace that has forced the development of standards for naming of variables such as performance characteristics of various components (e.g., sensors, actuators, etc.) and for conditions under which these variables are measured. In more recent years, product databases (e.g., for electronic, mechanical, and electromechanical components) and systems level modeling software (i.e., computer-aided design and computer-aided manufacturing), along with the desire to reduce concept-to-production cycle times, have further increased the levels of standardization in these areas.

Despite the somewhat gloomy circumstance at present, there are some signs of potential improvement. An increasing number of research groups are beginning to attack problems of larger scale and interest is growing with regard to the ability to exchange data and models. Several small standards development efforts have surfaced recently in specific areas such as biomechanics to develop, for example, standards for kinematic representation of various body joints. The advent of an increasing number of commercially available measurement tools has also driven a trend to similarity in conventions used in some specific subareas. However, the quest for standardization in measurement that is often heard voiced is still a distant vision. A willingness to suffer the inconvenience of "standardizing" in the short run in exchange for a greater convenience and "power" over the long run must be recognized by a critical mass of researchers, instrument manufacturers, and practitioners before a significant breakthrough can occur. The large number of different professional bodies and societies that may potentially become involved in promulgating an official set of standards will most likely contribute to slow progress in this area.

85.3.2 New Instruments

Instruments to acquire measures of both human structure and performance have been improving at a rapid pace, commensurate with the improvement of base technologies (e.g., sensors, signal conditioning, microprocessors, and desktop computer systems, etc.). Compared to one decade ago, a practitioner or researcher can today assemble a relatively sophisticated and broad-based measurement laboratory with commercially available devices instead of facing the burden of fabricating his or her own instruments. However, a considerable imbalance still exists across the profile of human performance with regard to commercial availability of necessary tools. This imbalance extends to the profile of tools seen in use in contexts such as rehabilitation and sports training. In particular, devices that measure sensory performance capacities are not nearly as commonplace or well developed as those which measure, for example, strength and range of motion. Likewise, there are few commercially available instruments that measure aspects of neuromotor control in any general sense other than, for example, in a selected task such as maintaining stable posture. The complexity and diversity of higher-level human cognitive processes has also hindered development of measurement instruments in this domain that possess any true degree of commonality in content across products. A wide variety of computer-based test batteries have been proliferating that are more or less implementations of the great number of tests formerly administered in paper–pencil format.

From a practitioner's perspective, prospects for the future are both good and bad. There is some evidence that suppliers of instruments that cover areas of the performance where there has been vigorous competition (e.g., dynamic strength) are experiencing market saturation and uncertainty on the part of consumers regarding what is "the best way" to acquire necessary information. This may force some groups to drop product lines, while others are expressing subtle interests in expanding measurement instrument product lines to fill empty niches. This latter behavior is good in that it will likely increase the scope of measurement tools that is commercially available. However, problems associated with standardization often confuse potential users and this, in general, has slowed progress in the adoption of more objective measurement instruments (compared to subjective methods) in some application areas. This, in turn, has inhibited product providers from taking the risk associated with the introduction of new products.

Compared to the commercial availability of tools that characterize the performance of various human subsystems, instruments that quantify task attributes are much less prevalent. However, the perception that increased emphasis on this area will increase the utility of measures that characterize the human will likely motivate a substantial increase in the number and variety of products available for task characterization. In addition, factors such as the Americans with Disabilities Act (ADA), which encourages worksite evaluations and modifications to facilitate employment of individuals with disabilities and the increase in work-site related injuries such as carpal tunnel syndrome have led to an increased demand for such tools.

There has been a subtle but noticeable developing sense of awareness in the various communities that there is room for more than one kind of instrument to measure a given variable. Thus, debates regarding "the correct approach," which were commonplace, are beginning to be replaced with debates concerned with determining "the best approach for a given situation." A prime example is in the area of strength measurement. Devices range from relatively inexpensive handheld dynamometers that provide rapid measurements and meaningful results with neurologic patients to expensive devices with electric or hydraulic servomotor systems that are more suited, for example, for use in sports medicine contexts. This trend is quite healthy and is likely to spread too though it has been driven by different constraints in different circumstances.

85.3.3 Measuring the Measurements

Reliability and validity have been the keywords associated with characterizing the quality of measures of human structure and performance [Potvin et al., 1985]. Often, these terms are used in a manner that implies that a given test "has it" or "does not have it" (i.e., reliability or validity) when in fact both should be recognized as continuums.

There are traditional, well-known methods used in academic circles to quantify reliability. The result produced implies an interpretation of "how much" reliability a given test has, but there is no corresponding way to determine how much is needed (in the same terms that reliability of a test is measured) so that one could determine if one has "enough." Other aspects of the academic treatment of human performance measurement quality are similarly troublesome with regard to the implications for widespread, general use of measurements. For example, there is an inherent desire (and need) to generalize the results of a given reliability study for a given instrument and, at the same time, a reluctance on the part of those who conduct such studies to do so in writing. The strictly academic position is that one can *never* generalize a reliability study; that is, it applies only to a situation which is identical to that reported (i.e., that instrument, those subjects, that examiner, that room, that time of day, etc.). So, one may ask, what is the value of reporting any such study? The purely academic view may be the most correct, but strict interpretation is completely useless to a practitioner who needs to reach a conclusion regarding the applicability of a given instrument in given application. The mere fact that reliability studies are reported implies that there is an expectation of generalization to *some* degree. The question is, "How much generalization can one make? This issue has not been adequately addressed from a general methodological standpoint. However, awareness of this issue and the need for improved methods are growing.

What is the general "quality" of measurement available today? The following is offered as a reasonably "healthy" perspective on this complex issue:

1. Technology has advanced to the point where it is now possible to measure many of the basic physical variables employed measurement such as time, force, torque, angles, linear distance, etc. very accurately, with high repeatability, and with high resolution without significant difficulty.
2. Most of the difference on test–retest is due to limitations in how well one can reasonably control procedures and actual variability of the parameter measured — even in the most ideal test subjects.
3. Many studies have been conducted on the reliability of a wide variety of human performance capacities. Some true generalization can be achieved by looking at this body of work as a whole and not from attempts to generalize from only single studies.
4. Across the many types of variables investigated, results of such studies are amazingly quite similar. Basically, they say that if your instrumentation is good, and if you carefully follow established, optimal test administration procedures, then it should be possible to obtain results on repeat testing that are within a range of 5 to 20% of each other. The exact location achieved in this range depends in large part on the particular variable in question (e.g., repeated measures associated with complex tasks with many degrees of freedom such as lifting or gait will differ more than repeated measures of hinge joint range of motions). In addition, the magnitude of the given metric will influence such percentage characterizations since errors are often fixed amounts and independent of the size of the quantity measured. Thus, when measuring quantities with small magnitudes, a larger variability (i.e., more like 20%) should be anticipated. One can usually determine an applicable working value in these straightforward, usable terms (e.g., 5 or 20%) that allow direct comparison to an evaluation of needs by careful review of the relevant reliability studies.

A major point of this discussion is to illustrate that traditional methods used to "measure the measurements" do not adequately communicate the information that current and potential users of measurements often need to know. Traditional methods were valuable to some degree in providing relative indicators within the context of academic group studies. However, methods that are more similar to those used to characterize measurement system performance in physics and other traditional engineering areas (e.g., accuracy, signal-noise-ratio concepts, etc.) are needed. This will help practitioners who must make single measurements on individual subjects (i.e., not populations) to support clinical decision making [Mayer et al., 1997]. As the manner in which measurements are used continues to change to include more of the latter, new interest and methods for quantifying the quality of measurements can be anticipated.

85.4 Databases and Data Modeling

Much research has been conducted to define measurements of human structure and performance and to collect and characterize data as basis to increase understanding and make inferences in different contexts. A wide variety of problems of major medical and other societal significance require the use of such data:

1. For diagnostic purposes (i.e., when assessing measures obtained from a subject-under-test, such as to determine the efficacy of an intervention or treatment in a medical context).

2. for modeling and simulation (e.g., analyses for return-to-work decisions of injured employees, to support job-site modifications for individuals with disabilities, design specifications for virtual reality systems).

3. Status/capacity evaluations (e.g., disability determinations for insurance settlements, worker's compensation claims, etc.).

4. To obtain a better understanding of disease and aging processes (e.g., associated with such problems as falls in elderly populations, etc.).

5. To gain insight into the impact of environmental and occupational factors (e.g., as in epidemiologic studies, such as in lead toxicity or carpal tunnel syndrome).

6. To support ergonomic design of consumer products and living environments for use by the public in general. Despite such a diverse range in needs for basically the same information, there has been little — if any — attempt to organize, integrate, and represent available data in a compact, accessible form that can serve the cited needs.

Figure 85.1 illustrates the scope of the general problem and infers a potential approach to integration. At the most basic level, individual measurements for a given variable must be collected and databased. In addition, databases of data from published studies are required to identify specific gaps that limit either analytic functionality or fidelity in the types of tasks, which data must support. Data from the literature is typically available only in summary form, that is, in terms of means and standard deviations for defined populations. Future research is required to define and validate methods for integrating data, for example, from multiple studies to form a single, more robust data model for a given performance or structure parameter. This will involve testing data models developed from databases of individual measures and databases of studies against each other. Development of data warping methods (e.g., to adapt predictions of

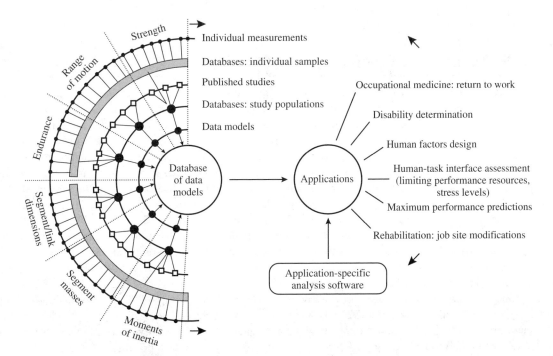

FIGURE 85.1 Schematic summary of proposed integration of human structural and performance data to realize compact representations (i.e., parametric data models) to support analyses in multiple application areas. Only several types of performance resources and aspects of structure are represented. The problem of realizing a complete array of such models in a form generally useable by multiple analysis tools is complex.

expected performance levels to subjects of different body sizes and ages) is required to provide models that would be transparent operationally and would allow analyses to proceed in data-limited situations with predictable tradeoffs in fidelity. In many areas, especially with regard to practitioners such as occupational and physical therapists, performance characterization has been viewed only unidimensionally. More multidimensional perspectives are needed for an adequate representation of fidelity [e.g., Kondraske, 2000]. Another major aspect of data modeling therefore involves the development of multivariate models of performance envelopes [Vasta and Kondraske, 1997] for individual human subsystems (e.g., knee flexors, visual information processors, etc.). Such models would support, for example, prediction of available torque production capacity under different specified conditions (e.g., joint angle, speed, etc.). In summary, a basic strategy is required for harvesting the vast amount of previously collected data to obtain compact, accessible representations. Means must be incorporated in this strategy to allow for integration of data from multiple sources and continuous update as new data are collected to enhance fidelity and range of applicability of composite models.

As previously noted, individuals within the human performance community typically adopt a variety of terms or identification schemes for structures and parameters employed in both the execution and communication of their work. The sheer number of parameters and variety of combinations in which they may be required to meet analysis needs may be sufficient to justify a more formal approach [e.g., Kondraske, 1993], thereby facilitating the development of common data structures. The engineering contexts in which data models can be envisioned to be used require more rigor and stability. Computer-based models and analyses beg for codification of terms and parameters (i.e., for databases, etc.). In this regard, these emerging applications bring to light the lack of precision in terminology and confusion in definitions. Moreover, the ability to integrate models and analysis modules developed independently within more narrow subsets of the field to address more complex problems requires standardized notation if for no other reason than for efficiency. Development of a standardized systematic notation is compelling; it is postulated that without such a notation, progress to the next level of sophistication cannot occur.

85.5 Measure or Predict?

The large number of different human performance parameters discussed in this section of the text motivates an often-heard question from practitioners: "What is the most important thing to measure?" Clearly, the interest behind such questions is efficiency; it takes time to measure and practitioners are generally under many pressures to be efficient. Figure 85.2 casts the issue in a way that reflects a hierarchical organization of parameters, where each box can represent many different parameters. It can generally be argued that in many situations the "need to know" exists at multiple levels in this hierarchy. Thus, this presents a somewhat bleak outlook for practitioners that generally results in the use of only the most gross level of measurement (e.g., subjective rating scales) because it is "quick." Significant advancement in applications beyond the research lab demands that this problem be addressed.

One possibility that could contribute to solving this dilemma is to utilize models to estimate performance at a given hierarchical level using measurements obtained at lower hierarchical levels. It is argued that this may be an optimal long-term strategy. Methods such as Nonlinear Causal Resource Analysis and other discussed in Chapter 156 [Vasta and Kondraske, 2005], and promising results that have been obtained thus far in limited contexts, provide a basis for believing in the promise of this strategy. In the ideal situation, many different laboratories could contribute to building and evaluating high-quality models for many different "higher-level tasks" (emphasizing that "higher level" is a relative concept). Independently developed models could be integrated into computer-based tools available to practitioners. A reasonable set of measurements made at selected levels could then be used with such tools to obtain a huge "added value" by having performance in a number of different higher-level tasks estimated through use of the models. In essence, one would obtain the equivalent of measurements that would otherwise require hours of measurement time in an instant.

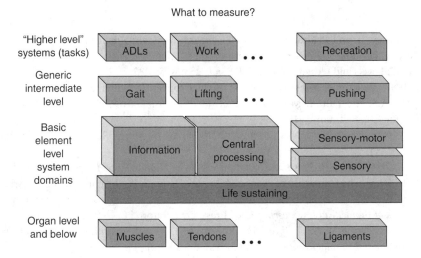

FIGURE 85.2 Performance capacity and related parameters are of interest at many hierarchical levels, posing the problem of deciding what to measure in any given application and presenting a problem of complexity for which solutions must be defined.

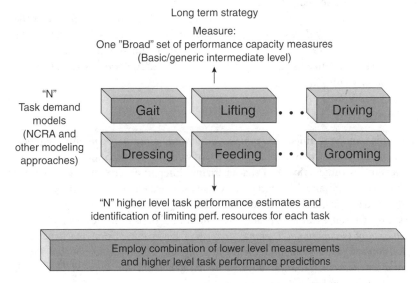

FIGURE 85.3 Summary of a long-term strategy in which models are used to predict performance capacities at higher levels using measurements obtained at lower levels to provide the required scope of information that is generally of interest.

85.6 Summary

A relatively high degree of sophistication currently exists with regard to the science, engineering, and technology of human performance. The field is, nonetheless, relatively young and undergoing natural maturation processes. Remaining needs in terms of both conceptual underpinnings and tools (which are not independent) are enormous. Future progress, however, is likely to be more dependent on collaborative efforts of different types. The magnitude and nature of problems that are at the forefront demand the achievement of agreement among a critical mass of researchers and practitioners. Both the challenges and prospects for the future are significant.

References

Bendell, A., Disney, J., and Pridmore W.A. 1988. *Taguchi Methods: Applications in World Industry*, IFS Publishing, London.

Bunge, M. 1977. Levels and reduction. *Am. J. Physiol.*, 233: R75–R82.

Frey, W.D. 1987. Functional assessment in the '80's: a conceptual enigma, a technical challenge. In: Halpern, A.S. and Fuhrer, M.J. (Eds.), *Functional Assessment in Rehabilitation*, Paul H. Brookes Publishing Co., Baltimore, MD.

Gardner, H. 1985. *The Mind's New science: A History of Cognitive Revolution*. Basic Books, Inc., New York, NY.

Kondraske, G.V. 1993. *The HPI Shorthand Notation System for Human System Parameters, (Technical Report 92-001R V1.5)*, The University of Texas at Arlington, Human Performance Institute, Arlington, TX.

Kondraske, G.V. 1995. A working model for human system–task interfaces. In: Bronzino, J.D. (Ed.), *Handbook of Biomedical Engineering*. CRC Press, Boca Raton, FL.

Potvin, A.R. , Tourtellotte, W.W. , Potvin, J.H. , Kondraske, G.V. and Syndulko, K. 1985. *The Quantitative Examination of Neurologic Function*. CRC Press, Boca Raton, FL.

Simmon, C.W. Will egg-sucking ever become a science? *Human Factors Soc. Bull.*, 30: 1.

Smith, L.L. 1987. Whyfore human factors. *Human Factors Soc. Bull.*, 30: 1.

Vasta, P.J. and Kondraske, G.V. 1992. *Standard Conventions for Kinematic and Structural Parameters for the "Gross Total Human" Link Model*, Technical Report 92-003R V1.0, The University of Texas at Arlington Human Performance Institute.

Vasta, P.J. and Kondraske, G.V. 2005. Human Performance Engineering: Design and Analysis Tools. In: Bronzino, J.D. (Ed.), *Handbook of Biomedical Engineering*. CRC Press, Boca Raton, FL.

Weismer, G. and Liss, J.M. 1991. Reductionism Is a dead-end in speech research, In: Moore, C.A., Yorkston, K.M., and Beukelman, D.R. (Eds.) *Dysarthria and Apraxia of Speech*, Paul H. Brookes Pub Co., Baltimore, MD.

Further Information

The section of this handbook titled "*Human Performance Engineering*" contains chapters that address human performance modeling and measurement in considerably more detail.

Manufacturers of instruments used to characterizing different aspects of human performance often provide technical literature and bibliographies of studies related to measurement quality, technical specifications of instruments, and application examples.

Future articles of relevance can be expected on a continuing basis in the following journals:

American Journal of Occupational Therapy; Archives of Physical Medicine and Rehabilitation; Human Factors; IEEE Transactions on Rehabilitation Engineering and IEEE Transactions on Biomedical Engineering; Journal of Biomechanics; Journal of Occupational Rehabilitation; Physical Therapy; Rehabilitation Management; Rehabilitation Research and Development.

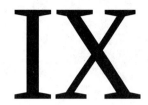

Ethics

Joseph D. Bronzino
Trinity College

86

Beneficence, Nonmaleficence, and Medical Technology

86.1 Introduction

Two moral norms have remained relatively *constant across* the various moral codes and oaths that have been formulated for health-care deliverers since the beginnings of Western medicine in classical Greek civilization, namely beneficence — the provision of benefits — and nonmaleficence — the avoidance of doing harm. These norms are traced back to a body of writings from classical antiquity known as the *Hippocratic Corpus.* Although these writings are associated with the name of Hippocrates, the acknowledged founder of Western medicine, medical historians remain uncertain whether any, including the *Hippocratic Oath,* were actually his work. Although portions of the Corpus are believed to have been authored during the sixth century BC, other portions are believed to have been written as late as the beginning of the Christian Era. Medical historians agree, though, that many of the specific moral directives of the *Corpus* represent neither the actual practices nor the moral ideals of the majority of physicians of ancient Greece and Rome.

Nonetheless, the general injunction, *"As to disease, make a habit of two things — to help or, at least, to do no harm,"* was accepted as a fundamental medical ethical norm by at least some ancient physicians. With the decline of Hellenistic civilization and the rise of Christianity, beneficence and nonmaleficence became increasingly accepted as the fundamental principles of morally sound medical practice. Although beneficence and nonmaleficence were regarded merely as concomitant to the craft of medicine in classical Greece and Rome, the emphasis upon compassion and the brotherhood of humankind, central to Christianity, *increasingly made* these norms the only acceptable motives for medical practice. Even today the provision of benefits and the avoidance of doing harm are stressed just as much in virtually all contemporary Western codes of conduct for health professionals as they were in the oaths and codes that guided the health-care providers of past centuries.

Traditionally, the ethics of medical care have given greater prominence to nonmaleficence than to beneficence. This priority was grounded in the fact that, historically, medicine's capacity to do harm far exceeded its capacity to protect and restore health. Providers of health care possessed many treatments that posed clear and genuine risks to patients but that offered little prospect of benefit. Truly effective therapies were all too rare. In this context, it is surely rational to give substantially higher priority to avoiding harm than to providing benefits.

The advent of modern science changed matters dramatically. Knowledge acquired in laboratories, tested in clinics, and verified by statistical methods has increasingly dictated the practices of medicine. This *ongoing alliance* between medicine and science became a critical source of the plethora of technologies that now pervades medical care. The impressive increases in therapeutic, preventive, and rehabilitative capabilities that these technologies have provided have pushed beneficence to the forefront of medical morality. Some have even gone so far as to hold that the old medical ethic of *"Above all, do no harm"* should be superseded by the new ethic that *"The patient deserves the best."* However, the rapid advances in medical technology capabilities have also produced great uncertainty as to what is most beneficial or least harmful for the patient. In other words, along with increases in ability to be beneficent, medicine's technology has generated much debate about what actually counts as beneficent or nonmaleficent treatment. To illustrate this point, let us turn to several specific moral issues posed by the use of medical technology [Bronzino, 1992; 1999].

86.2 Defining Death: A Moral Dilemma Posed by Medical Technology

Supportive and resuscitative devices, such as the respirator, found in the typical modern intensive care unit provide a useful starting point for illustrating how technology has rendered medical morality more complex and problematic. Devices of this kind allow clinicians to sustain respiration and circulation in patients who have suffered massive brain damage and total permanent loss of brain *function.* These technologies force us to ask: precisely when does a human life end? When is a human being indeed dead? This is not the straightforward factual matter it may appear to be. All of the relevant facts may show that the patient's brain has suffered injury grave enough to destroy its functioning forever. The facts may show that such an individual's circulation and respiration would permanently cease without artificial support. Yet these facts do not determine whether treating such an individual as a corpse is morally appropriate. To know this, it is necessary to know or perhaps to decide on those features of living persons that are essential to their status as "living persons." It is necessary to know or decide which human qualities, if irreparably lost, make an individual identical in all morally relevant respects to a corpse. Once those qualities have been specified, deciding whether total and irreparable loss of brain function constitutes death becomes a straightforward factual matter. Then, it would simply have to be determined if such loss itself deprives the individual of those qualities. If it does, the individual is morally identical to a corpse. If not, then the individual must be regarded and treated as a living person.

The traditional criterion of death has been irreparable cessation of heartbeat, respiration, and blood pressure. This criterion would have been quickly met by anyone suffering massive trauma to the brain prior to the development of modern supportive technology. Such technology allows indefinite artificial maintenance of circulation and respiration and, thus, forestalls what once was an inevitable consequence of severe brain injury. The existence and use of such technology therefore challenges the traditional criterion of death and forces us to consider whether continued respiration and circulation are in themselves sufficient to distinguish a living individual from a corpse. Indeed, total and irreparable loss of brain function, referred to as "brainstem death," "whole brain death," and, simply, "brain death," has been widely accepted as the legal standard for death. By this standard, an individual in a state of brain death is legally indistinguishable from a corpse and may be legally treated as one even though respiratory and circulatory functions may be sustained through the intervention of technology. Many take this legal standard to be the morally appropriate one, noting that once destruction of the brain stem has occurred, the brain *cannot function* at all, and the body's regulatory mechanisms will fail unless artificially sustained. Thus, mechanical sustenance of an individual in a state of brain death is merely postponement of the inevitable and sustains nothing of the personality, character, or consciousness of the individual. It is merely the mechanical intervention that differentiates such an individual from a corpse and a mechanically ventilated corpse is a corpse nonetheless.

Even with a consensus that brainstem death is death and thus that an individual in such a state is indeed a corpse, hard cases remain. Consider the case of an individual in a persistent vegetative state, the condition known as "neocortical death." Although severe brain injury has been suffered, enough brain function remains to make mechanical *sustenance* of respiration and circulation unnecessary. In a persistent vegetative state, an individual exhibits no purposeful response to external stimuli and no evidence of self-awareness. The eyes may open periodically and the individual may exhibit sleep–wake cycles. Some patients even yawn, make chewing motions, or swallow spontaneously. Unlike the complete unresponsiveness of individuals in a state of brainstem death, a variety of simple and complex responses can be elicited from an individual in a persistent vegetative state. Nonetheless, the chances that such an individual will regain consciousness virtually do not exist. Artificial feeding, kidney dialysis, and the like make it possible to sustain an individual in a state of neocortical death for decades. This sort of condition and the issues it raises were exemplified by the famous case of Karen Ann Quinlan. James Rachels [1986] provided the following description of the situation created by Quinlan's condition:

> In April 1975, this young woman ceased breathing for at least two 15-minute periods, for reasons that were never made clear. As a result, she suffered severe brain damage, and, in the words of the attending physicians, was reduced to a "chronic vegetative state" in which she "no longer had any cognitive function." Accepting the doctors' judgment that there was no hope of recovery, her parents sought permission from the courts to disconnect the respirator that was keeping her alive in the intensive care unit of a New Jersey hospital.
> The trial court, and then the Supreme Court of New Jersey, agreed that Karen's respirator could be removed. So it was disconnected. However, the nurse in charge of her care in the Catholic hospital opposed this decision and, anticipating it, had begun to wean her from the respirator so that by the time it was disconnected she could remain alive without it. So Karen did not die. Karen remained alive for ten additional years. In June 1985, she finally died of acute pneumonia. Antibiotics, which would have fought the pneumonia, were not given.

If brainstem death is death, is neocortical death also death? Again, the issue is not a straightforward factual matter. For, it too, is a matter of specifying which features of living individuals distinguish them from corpses and so make treatment of them as corpses morally impermissible. Irreparable cessation of respiration and circulation, the classical criterion for death, would entail that an individual in a persistent vegetative state is not a corpse and so, morally speaking, must not be treated as one. The brainstem death criterion for death would also entail that a person in a state of neocortical death is not yet a corpse. On this criterion, what is crucial is that brain damage be severe enough to cause failure of the body's regulatory mechanisms.

Is an individual in a state of neocortical death any less in possession of the characteristics that distinguish the living from cadavers than one whose respiration and circulation are mechanically maintained? Of course, it is a matter of what the relevant characteristics are, and it is a matter that society must decide. It is not one that can be settled by greater medical information or more powerful medical devices. Until society decides, it will not be clear what would count as beneficent or nonmaleficent treatment of an individual in a state of neocortical death.

86.3   Euthanasia

A long-standing issue in medical ethics, which has been made more pressing by medical technology, is euthanasia, the deliberate termination of an individual's life for the individual's own good. Is such an act ever a permissible use of medical resources? Consider an individual in a persistent vegetative state. On the assumption that such a state is not death, withdrawing life support would be a deliberate termination of a human life. Here a critical issue is whether the quality of a human life can be so low or so great a liability to the individual that deliberately taking action to hasten death or at least not to postpone death is morally defensible. Can the quality of a human life be so low that the value of extending its quantity is totally negated? If so, then Western medicine's traditional commitment to providing benefits and avoiding harm would seem to make cessation of life support a moral requirement in such a case.

Consider the following hypothetical version of the kind of case that actually confronts contemporary patients, their families, health-care workers, and society as a whole. Suppose a middle-aged man suffers a brain hemorrhage and loses consciousness as a result of a ruptured aneurysm. Suppose that he never regains consciousness and is hospitalized in a state of neocortical death, a chronic vegetative state. He is maintained by a surgically implanted gastronomy tube that drips liquid nourishment from a plastic bag directly into his stomach. The care of this individual takes 7 and 1.5 h of nursing time daily and includes (1) shaving, (2) oral hygiene, (3) grooming, (4) attending to his bowels and bladder, and so forth.

Suppose further that his wife undertakes legal action to force his caregivers to end all medical treatment, including nutrition and hydration, so that complete bodily death of her husband will occur. She presents a preponderance of evidence to the court to show that her husband would have wanted this result in these circumstances.

The central moral issue raised by this sort of case is whether the quality of the individual's life is sufficiently compromised by neocortical death to make intentioned termination of that life morally permissible. While alive, he made it clear to both family and friends that he would prefer to be allowed to die rather than be mechanically maintained in a condition of irretrievable loss of consciousness. Deciding whether the judgment in such a case should be allowed requires deciding which capacities and qualities make life worth living, which qualities are sufficient to endow it with value worth sustaining, and whether their absence justifies deliberate termination of a life, at least when this would be the wish of the individual in question. Without this decision the traditional norms of medical ethics, beneficence and nonmaleficence, provide no guidance. Without this decision, it cannot be determined whether termination of life support is a benefit or a harm to the patient.

An even more difficult type of case was provided by the case of Elizabeth Bouvia. Bouvia, who had been a lifelong quadriplegic sufferer of cerebral palsy, was often in pain, completely dependent upon others, and spent all of her time bedridden. Bouvia, after deciding that she did not wish to continue such a life, entered Riverside General Hospital in California. She desired to be kept comfortable while starving to death. Although she remained adamant during her hospitalization, Bouvia's requests were denied by hospital officials with the legal sanction of the courts.

Many who might believe that neocortical death renders the quality of life sufficiently low to justify termination of life support, especially when this agrees with the individual's desires, would not arrive at this conclusion in a case like Bouvia's. Whereas neocortical death completely destroys consciousness and makes purposive interaction with the individual's environment impossible, Bouvia was fully aware and mentally alert. She had previously been married and had even acquired a college education. Televised interviews with her portrayed a very intelligent person who had great skill in presenting persuasive arguments to support her wish not to have her life continued by artificial means of nutrition. Nonetheless, she judged her life to be of such low quality that she should be allowed to choose to deliberately starve to death. Before the existence of life-support technology, maintenance of her life against her will might not have been possible at all and at least would have been far more difficult.

Should Elizabeth Bouvia's judgment have been accepted? Her case is more difficult than the care of a patient in a chronic vegetative state because, unlike such an *individual, she* was able to engage in meaningful interaction with her environment. Regarding an individual who cannot speak or otherwise meaningfully interact with others as nothing more than living matter, as a "human vegetable," is not especially difficult. But to regard Bouvia this way is not easy. Her awareness, intelligence, mental acuity, and ability to interact with others means that although her life is one of discomfort, indignity, and complete dependence, she is not a mere "human vegetable."

Despite the differences between Bouvia's situation and that of someone in a state of neocortical death, the same issue is posed. Can the quality of an individual's life be so low that deliberate termination is morally justifiable? How that question is answered is a matter of what level of quality of life, if any, is taken to be sufficiently low to justify deliberately acting to end it or deliberately failing*teK"rt"ifd it. If there is such a level, the conclusion that it is not always beneficent or even nonmalefkent to use life-support technology must be accepted.

Another important issue here is respect for individual autonomy. For the cases of Bouvia and the hypothetical instance of neocortical death discussed earlier, both concern voluntary euthanasia, that is, euthanasia voluntarily requested by the patient. A long-standing commitment, vigorously defended by various schools of thought in Western moral philosophy, is the notion that competent adults should be free to conduct their lives as they please as long as they do not impose undeserved harm on others. Does this commitment entail a right to die? Some clearly believe that it does. If one owns anything at all, surely one owns one's life. In the two cases discussed earlier, neither individual sought to impose undeserved harm on anyone else, nor would satisfaction of their wish to die do so. What justification can there be then for not allowing their desires to be fulfilled?

One plausible answer is based upon the very respect of individual autonomy at issue here. A necessary condition, in some views, of respect for autonomy is the willingness to take whatever measures necessary to protect it, including measures that restrict autonomy. An autonomy-respecting reason offered against laws that prevent even competent adults from voluntarily entering lifelong slavery is that such an exercise of autonomy is self-defeating and has the consequence of undermining autonomy altogether. By the same token, an individual who acts to end his own life thereby exercises his autonomy in a manner that places it in jeopardy of permanent loss. Many would regard this as justification for using the coercive force of the law to prevent suicide. This line of thought does not fit the case of an individual in a persistent vegetative state because his/her autonomy has been destroyed by the circumstances that rendered him/her neocortically dead. It does fit Bouvia's case though. Her actions indicate that she is fully competent and her efforts to use medical care to prevent the otherwise inevitable pain of starvation is itself an exercise of her autonomy. Yet, if allowed to succeed, those very efforts would destroy her autonomy as they destroy her. On this reasoning, her case is a perfect instance of limitation of autonomy being justified by respect for autonomy and of one where, even against the wishes of a competent patient, the life-saving power of medical technology should be used.

86.3.1 Active vs. Passive Euthanasia

Discussions of the morality of euthanasia often distinguish active from passive euthanasia in light of the distinction made between killing a person and letting a person die, a distinction that rests upon the difference between an act of commission and an act of omission. When failure to take steps that could effectively forestall death results in an individual's demise, the resultant death is an act of omission and a case of letting a person die. When a death is the result of doing something to hasten the end of a person's life (giving a lethal injection, e.g.) that death is caused by an act of commission and is a case of killing a person. When a person is allowed to die, death is a result of an act of omission, and the motive is the person's own good; the omission is an instance of passive euthanasia. When a person is killed, death is the result of an act of commission, and the motive is the person's own good; the commission is an instance of active euthanasia.

Does the difference between passive and active euthanasia, which reduces to a difference in how death comes about, make any moral difference? It does in the view of the American Medical Association. In a statement adopted on December 4, 1973, the House of Delegates of the American Medical Association asserted the following [Rachels, 1978]:

> The intentional termination of the life of one human being by another — mercy killing — is contrary to that for which the medical profession stands and is contrary to the policy of the American Medical Association (AMA).
>
> The cessation of extraordinary means to prolong the life of the body where there is irrefutable evidence that biological death is imminent is the decision of the patient and immediate family. The advice of the physician would be freely available to the patient and immediate family.

In response to this position, Rachels [1978; 1986] answered with the following:

> The AMA policy statement isolates the crucial issue very well, the crucial issue is "intentional termination of the life of one human being by another." But after identifying this issue and forbidding "mercy killing," the statement goes on to deny that the cessation of treatment is the intentional termination of a life. This is where the mistake comes in, for what is the cessation of treatment in those circumstances (where the intention is to release the patient from continued suffering), if it is not "the intentional termination of the life of one human being by another?"

As Rachels correctly argued, when steps that could keep an individual alive are omitted for the person's own good, this omission is as much the intentional termination of life as taking active measures to cause death. Not placing a patient on a respirator due to a desire not to prolong suffering is an act intended to end life as much as the administration of a lethal injection. In many instances the main difference between the two cases is that the latter would release the individual from his pain and suffering more quickly than the former. Dying can take time and involve considerable pain even if nothing is done to prolong life. Active killing can be done in a manner that causes death painlessly and instantly. This difference certainly does not render killing, in this context, morally worse than letting a person die. Insofar as the motivation is merciful (as it must be if the case is to be a genuine instance of euthanasia) because the individual is released more quickly from a life that is disvalued than otherwise, the difference between killing and letting one die may provide support for active euthanasia. According to Rachels, the common rejoinder to this argument is the following:

> The important difference between active and passive euthanasia is that in passive euthanasia the doctor does not do anything to bring about the patient's death. The doctor does nothing and the patient dies of whatever ills already afflict him. In active euthanasia, however, the doctor does something to bring about the patient's death: he kills the person. The doctor who gives the patient with cancer a lethal injection has himself caused his patient's death; whereas if he merely ceases treatment, the cancer is the cause of death.

According to this rejoinder, in active euthanasia someone must do something to bring about the patient's death, and in passive euthanasia the patient's death is caused by illness rather than by anyone's conduct. Surely this is mistaken. Suppose a physician deliberately decides not to treat a patient who has a routinely curable ailment and the patient dies. Suppose further that the physician were to attempt to exonerate himself by saying, "I did nothing. The patient's death was the result of illness. I was not the cause of death." Under current legal and moral norms, such a response would have no credibility. As Rachels noted, "*it would be no defense at all for him to insist that he didn't do anything. He would have done something very serious indeed, for he let his patient die.*"

The physician would be blameworthy for the patient's death as surely as if he had actively killed him. If causing death is justifiable under a given set of circumstances, whether it is done by allowing death to occur or by actively causing death is morally irrelevant. If causing someone to die is not justifiable under a given set of circumstances, whether it is done by allowing death to occur or by actively causing death is also morally irrelevant. Accordingly, if voluntary passive euthanasia is morally justifiable in the light of the duty of beneficence, so is voluntary active euthanasia. Indeed, given that the benefit to be achieved is more quickly realized by means of active euthanasia, it may be preferable to passive euthanasia in some cases.

86.3.2 Involuntary and Nonvoluntary Euthanasia

An act of euthanasia is involuntary if it hastens the individual's death for his own good but against his wishes. To take such a course would be to destroy a life that is valued by its possessor. Therefore, it is no different in any morally relevant way from unjustifiable homicide. There are only two legitimate reasons for hastening an innocent person's death against his will: self-defense and saving the lives of a larger number of other innocent persons. Involuntary euthanasia does not fit either of these justifications. By definition, it is done for the good of the person who is euthanized and for self-defense or saving innocent others. No act that qualifies as involuntary euthanasia can be morally justifiable. Hastening a person's death for his own good is an instance of nonvoluntary euthanasia when the individual is incapable of agreeing or disagreeing. Suppose it is clear that a particular person is sufficiently conscious enough to be regarded a person but cannot make his wishes known. Suppose also that he is suffering from the kind of ailment that, in the eyes of many persons, makes one's life unendurable. Would hastening his death be permissible? It would be if there was substantial evidence that he has given prior consent. This person may have told friends and relatives that under certain circumstances efforts to prolong his life should not be undertaken or continued. He might have recorded his wishes in the form of a Living Will (provided later) or on audio- or videotape. Where this kind of substantial evidence of prior consent exists, the decision to hasten death would be morally justified. A case of this scenario would be virtually a case of voluntary euthanasia.

To My Family, My Physician, My Clergyman, and My Lawyer:

If the time comes when I can no longer take part in decisions about my own future, let this statement stand as testament of my wishes: If there is no reasonable expectation of my recovery from physical or mental disability. I, _____, request that I be allowed to die and not be kept alive by artificial means or heroic measures. Death is as much a reality as birth, growth, maturity, and old age — it is the one certainty. I do not fear death as much as I fear the indiginity of deterioration, dependence, and hopeless pain. I ask that drugs be mercifully administered to me for the terminal suffering even if they hasten the moment of death.

This request is made after careful consideration. Although this document is not legally binding, you who care for me will, I hope, feel morally bound to follow its mandate. I recognize that it places a heavy burden of responsibility upon you, and it is with the intention of sharing that responsibility and of mitigating any feelings of guild that this statement is made.

Signed:_____
Date: _____

Witnessed by:

_____

_____

But what about an instance in which such evidence is not available? Suppose the person at issue has never had the capacity for competent consent or dissent from decisions concerning his life. It simply cannot be known what value the individual would place on his life in his present condition of illness. What should be done is a matter of what is taken to be the greater evil — mistakenly ending the life of an innocent person for whom that life has value or mistakenly forcing him to endure a life that he radically disvalues.

Living Will statutes have been passed in at least 35 states and the District of Columbia. For a Living Will to be a legally binding document, the person signing it must be of sound mind at the time the will is made and shown not to have altered his opinion in the interim between the signing and his illness. The witnesses must not be able to benefit from the individual's death.

86.3.3 Should Voluntary Euthanasia be Legalized?

Recent events have raised the question: "Should voluntary euthanasia be legalized?" Some argue that even if voluntary euthanasia is morally justifiable, it should be prohibited by social policy nonetheless. According to this position, the problem with voluntary euthanasia is its impact on society as a whole. In other words, the overall disutility of allowing voluntary euthanasia outweighs the good it could do for its beneficiaries. The central moral concern is that legalized euthanasia would eventually erode respect for human life and ultimately become a policy under which "socially undesirable" persons would have their deaths hastened (by omission or commission). The experience of Nazi Germany is often cited in support of this fear. What began there as a policy of euthanasia soon became one of eliminating individuals deemed racially inferior or otherwise undesirable. The worry, of course, is that what happened there can happen here as well. If social policy encompasses efforts to hasten the deaths of people, respect for human life in general is eroded and all sorts of abuses become socially acceptable, or so the argument goes.

No one can provide an absolute guarantee that the experience of Nazi Germany would not be repeated, but there is reason to believe that its likelihood is negligible. The medical moral duty of beneficence justifies only voluntary euthanasia. It justifies hastening an individual's death only for the individual's benefit and only with the individual's consent. To kill or refuse to save people judged socially undesirable is not to engage in euthanasia at all and violates the medical moral duty of nonmaleficence. As long as only voluntary euthanasia is legalized, and it is clear that involuntary euthanasia is not and should never be, no degeneration of the policy need occur. Furthermore, such degeneration is not likely to occur if the beneficent nature of voluntary euthanasia is clearly distinguished from the maleficent nature of involuntary euthanasia and any policy of exterminating the socially undesirable. Euthanasia decisions must be scrutinized carefully and regulated strictly to ensure that only voluntary cases occur, and severe penalties must be established to deter abuse.

References

Bronzino, J.D. Chapter 190. Beneficence, nonmaleficence and technological progress. In *The Biomedical Engineering Handbook.* CRC Press, Boca Raton, FL, 1995; 2000.

Bronzino, J.D. Chapter 10. Medical and Ethical Issues in Clinical Engineering Practice. *Management of Medical Technology.* Butterworth, 1992.

Bronzino, J.D. Chapter 20. Moral and Ethical Issues Associated with Medical Technology. *Introduction to Biomedical Engineering.* Academic Press, New York, 1999.

Rachels, J. Active and passive euthanasia. In *Moral Problems,* 3rd ed., Rachels, J. (Ed.), Harper and Row, New York, 1978.

Rachels, J. *Ethics at the End of Life: Euthanasia and Morality,* Oxford University Press, Oxford, 1986.

Further Information

Dubler, N.N. Nimmons D. *Ethics on Call.* Harmony Books, New York, 1992.

Jonsen, A.R. *The New Medicine and the Old Ethics.* Harvard University Press, Cambridge, MA, 1990.

Seebauer, E.G. and Barry, R.L. *Fundamentals of Ethics for Scientists and Engineers.* Oxford University Press, Oxford, 2001.

87

Ethical Issues Related to Clinical Research

Joseph D. Bronzino
Trinity College

87.1   Introduction

The Medical Device Amendment of 1976, and its updated 1990 version, requires approval from the Food and Drug Administration (FDA) before new devices are marketed and imposes requirements for the clinical investigation of new medical devices on human subjects. Although the statute makes interstate commerce of an unapproved new medical device generally unlawful, it provides an exception to allow interstate distribution of unapproved devices in order to conduct clinical research on human subjects. This investigational device exemption (IDE) can be obtained by submitting to the FDA *"a protocol for the proposed clinical testing of the device, reports of prior investigations of the device, certification that the study has been approved by a local institutional review board, and an assurance that informed consent will be obtained from each human subject"*[Bronzino et al., 1990a, b, 1992, 1995, 1999, 2000].

With respect to clinical research on humans, the FDA differentiates devices into two categories: those devices that pose significant risk and those that involve insignificant risk. Examples of the former include orthopedic implants, artificial hearts, and infusion pumps. Examples of the latter include various dental devices and daily-wear contact lenses. Clinical research involving a significant-risk device cannot begin until an institutional review board (IRB) has approved both the protocol and the informed consent form and the FDA itself has given permission. This requirement to submit an IDE application to the FDA is waived in the case of clinical research where the risk posed is insignificant. In this case, the FDA requires only that approval from an IRB be obtained certifying that the device in question poses only insignificant risk. In deciding whether to approve a proposed clinical investigation of a new device, the IRB and the FDA must determine the following:

1. Risks to subjects are minimized
2. Risks to subjects are reasonable in relation to the anticipated benefit and knowledge to be gained

3. Subject selection is equitable
4. Informed consent materials and procedures are adequate
5. Provisions for monitoring the study and protecting patient information are acceptable

The FDA allows unapproved medical devices to be used without an IDE in three types of situations: emergency use, treatment use, and feasibility studies. However, in each instance there are specific ethical issues.

87.2   Ethical Issues in Feasibility Studies

Manufacturers seeking more flexibility in conducting investigations in the early developmental stages of a device have submitted a petition to the FDA, requesting that certain limited investigations of significant-risk devices be subject to abbreviated IDE requirements. In a feasibility study, or "limited investigation," human research on a new device would take place at a single institution and involve no more than ten human subjects. *The sponsor of a limited investigation would be required to submit to the FDA a "Notice of Limited Investigation," which would include a description of the device,* a summary of the purpose of the investigation, the protocol, a sample of the informed consent form, and a certification of approval by the responsible IRB. *In certain circumstances, the FDA could require additional information, or require the submission of a full IDE application, or suspend the investigation* [Bronzino et al., 1990a, b].

Investigations of this kind would be limited to certain circumstances *(1) investigations of new uses of existing devices, (2) investigations involving temporary or permanent implants during the early developmental stages, and (3) investigations involving modification of an existing device.*

To comprehend adequately the ethical issues posed by clinical use of unapproved medical devices outside the context of an IDE, it is necessary to utilize the distinctions between practice, nonvalidated practice, and research elaborated in the previous pages. How do those definitions apply to feasibility studies?

Clearly, the goal of this sort of study, that is, generalizable knowledge, makes it an issue of research rather than practice. Manufacturers seek to determine the performance of a device with respect to a particular patient population in an effort to gain information about its efficacy and safety. Such information would be important in determining whether further studies (animal or human) need to be conducted, whether the device needs modification before further use, and the like. The main difference between use of an unapproved device in a feasibility study and use under the terms of an IDE is that the former would be subject to significantly less intensive FDA review than the latter. This, in turn, means that the responsibility for ensuring that use of the device is ethically sound would fall primarily to the IRB of the institution conducting the study.

The ethical concerns posed here are best comprehended with a clear understanding of what justifies research. Ultimately, no matter how much basic research and animal experimentation has been conducted on a given device, the risks and benefits it poses for humans cannot be adequately determined until it is actually used on humans.

The benefits of research on humans lie primarily in the knowledge that is yielded and the generalizable information that is provided. This information is crucial to medical science's ability to generate new modes and instrumentalities of medical treatment that are both efficacious and safe. Accordingly, for necessary but insufficient condition for experimentation to be ethically sound, it must be scientifically sound [Capron, 1978, 1986].

Although scientific soundness is a necessary condition of ethically acceptable research on humans, it is not of and by itself sufficient. Indeed, it is widely recognized that the primary ethical concern posed by such investigation is the use of one person by another to gather knowledge or other benefits where these benefits may only partly or not at all accrue to the first person. In other words, the human subjects of such research are at risk of being mere research resources, as having value only for the ends of the research. Research upon human beings runs the risk of failing to respect them as people. The notion that human beings are not mere things but entities whose value is inherent rather than wholly instrumental is one of the most widely held norms of contemporary Western society. That is, human beings are not valuable wholly or solely for the uses to which they can be put. They are valuable simply by being the kinds of entities they are. To treat them as such is to respect them as people.

Respecting individuals as people is generally agreed to entail two requirements in the context of biomedical experimentation. First, since what is most generally taken to make human beings people is their autonomy — their ability to make rational choices for themselves — treating individuals as people means respecting that autonomy. This requirement is met by ensuring that no competent person is subjected to any clinical intervention without first giving voluntary and informed consent. Second, respect for people means that the physician will not subject a human to unnecessary risks and will minimize the risks to patients in required procedures.

Much of the ethical importance of the scrutiny that the FDA imposes upon use of unapproved medical devices in the context of an IDE derives from these two conditions of ethically sound research. The central ethical concern posed by use of medical devices in a feasibility study is that the decreased degree of FDA scrutiny will increase the likelihood that either or both of these conditions will not be met. This possibility may be especially great because many manufacturers of medical devices are, after all, commercial enterprises, companies that are motivated to generate profit and thus to get their devices to market as soon as possible with as little delay and cost as possible. These self-interested motives are likely, at times, to conflict with the requirements of ethically sound research and thus to induce manufacturers to fail (often unwittingly) to meet these requirements. Note that profit is not the only motive that might induce manufacturers to contravene the requirements of ethically sound research on humans. A manufacturer may sincerely believe that its product offers great benefit to many people or to a population of especially needy people and so from this utterly altruistic motive may be prompted to take shortcuts that compromise the quality of the research. Whether the consequences being sought by the research are desired for reasons of self-interest, altruism, or both, the ethical issue is the same. Research subjects may be placed at risk of being treated as mere objects rather than as people.

What about the circumstances under which feasibility studies would take place? Are these not sufficiently different from the "normal" circumstances of research to warrant reduced FDA scrutiny? As noted above, manufacturers seek to be allowed to engage in feasibility studies in order to investigate new uses of existing devices, to investigate temporary or permanent implants during the early developmental stages, and to investigate modifications to an existing device. As also noted earlier, a feasibility study would take place at only one institution and would involve no more than ten human subjects. Given these circumstances, is the sort of research that is likely to occur in a feasibility study less likely to be scientifically unsound or to fail to respect people in the way that normal research upon humans does in "normal" circumstances?

Such research would be done on a very small subject pool, and the harm of any ethical lapses would likely affect fewer people than if such lapses occurred under more usual research circumstances. Yet even if the harm done were limited to a failure to respect the ten or fewer subjects in a single feasibility study, the harm would still be ethically wrong. To wrong ten or fewer people is not as bad as to wrong in the same way more than ten people but it is to engage in wrongdoing nonetheless. In either case, individuals are reduced to the status of mere research resources and their dignity as people is not properly respected.

Are ethical lapses more likely to occur in feasibility studies than in studies that take place within the requirements of an IDE? Although nothing in the preceding discussion provides a definitive answer to this question, it is a question to which the FDA should give high priority in deciding whether to allow this type of exception to IDE use of unapproved medical devices. The answer to this question might be quite different when the device at issue is a temporary or permanent implant than when it is an already approved device being put to new uses or modified in some way. Whatever the contemplated use under the feasibility studies mechanism, the FDA would be ethically advised not to allow this kind of exception to IDE use of an unapproved device without a reasonably high level of certainty that research subjects would not be placed in greater jeopardy than in "normal" research circumstances.

87.3 Ethical Issues in Emergency Use

What about the mechanism for avoiding the rigors of an IDE for emergency use?

The FDA has authorized emergency use where an unapproved device offers the only alternative for saving the life of a dying patient, but an IDE has not yet been approved for the device or its use, or an IDE has been approved but the physician who wishes to use the device is not an investigator under the IDE [Bronzino et al., 1990a, b].

Because the purpose of emergency use of an unapproved device is to attempt to save a dying patient's life under circumstances where no other alternative is at hand, this sort of use constitutes practice rather than research. Its aim is primarily benefit to the patient rather than provision of new and generalizable information. Because this sort of use occurs prior to the completion of clinical investigation of the device, it constitutes a nonvalidated practice. What does this mean?

First, it means that while the aim of the use is to save the life of the patient, the nature and likelihood of the potential benefits and risks engendered by use of the device are far more speculative than in the sort of clinical intervention that constitutes validated practice. In validated practice, thorough investigation, including preclinical studies, animal studies, and studies on human subjects of a device has established its efficacy and safety. The clinician thus has a well-founded basis upon which to judge the benefits and risks such an intervention poses for his patients.

It is precisely this basis that is lacking in the case of a nonvalidated practice. Does this mean that emergency use of an unapproved device should be regarded as immoral? This conclusion would follow only if there were no basis upon which to make an assessment of the risks and benefits of the use of the device. The FDA requires that a physician who engages in emergency use of an unapproved device must *"have substantial reason to believe that benefits will exist. This means that there should be a body of preclinical and animal tests allowing a prediction of the benefit to a human patient."*

Thus, although the benefits and risks posed by use of the device are highly speculative, they are not entirely speculative. Although the only way to validate a new technology is to engage in research on humans at some point, not all nonvalidated technologies are equal. Some will be largely uninvestigated and assessment of their risks and benefits will be wholly or almost wholly speculative. Others will at least have the support of preclinical and animal tests. Although this is not sufficient support for incorporating use of a device into regular clinical practice, it may, however, represent sufficient support to justify use in the desperate circumstances at issue in emergency situations. Desperate circumstances can justify desperate actions, but desperate actions are not the same as reckless actions; hence, the ethical soundness of the FDA's requirement that emergency use be supported by solid results from preclinical and animal tests of the unapproved device.

A second requirement that the FDA imposes on emergency use of unapproved devices is the expectation that physicians *"exercise reasonable foresight with respect to potential emergencies and make appropriate arrangements under the IDE procedures. Thus, a physician should not 'create' an emergency in order to circumvent IRB review and avoid requesting the sponsor's authorization of the unapproved use of a device."*

From a Kantian point of view, which is concerned with protecting the dignity of people, it is a particularly important requirement to create an emergency in order to avoid FDA regulations which prevent the patient being treated as a mere resource whose value is reducible to a service of the clinician's goals. Hence, the FDA is quite correct to insist that emergencies are circumstances that reasonable foresight would not anticipate.

Also especially important here is the nature of the patient's consent. Individuals facing death are especially vulnerable to exploitation and deserve greater measures for their protection than might otherwise be necessary. One such measure would be to ensure that the patient, or his legitimate proxy, knows the highly speculative nature of the intervention being offered. That is, to ensure that it is clearly understood that the clinician's estimation of the intervention's risks and benefits is far less solidly grounded than in the case of validated practices. The patient's consent must be based upon an awareness that the particular device has not undergone complete and rigorous testing on humans and that estimations of its potential are based wholly upon preclinical and animal studies. Above all the patient must not be lead to believe that there is complete understanding of the risks and benefits of the intervention. Another important point here is to ensure that the patient is aware that the options he is facing are not simply life or death but may include life of a severely impaired quality, and therefore that even if his life is saved, it may be a life of significant impairment. Although desperate circumstance may legitimize desperate actions, the decision to take such actions must rest upon the informed and voluntary consent of the patient, especially when he/she is an especially vulnerable patient.

It is important here for a clinician involved in emergency use of an unapproved device to recognize that these activities constitute a form of nonvalidated practice and not research. Hence, the primary obligation is to the well-being of the patient. The patient enters into the relationship with the clinician with the same trust that accompanies any normal clinical situation. To treat this sort of intervention as if it were an instance of research and hence justified by its benefits to science and society would be to abuse this trust.

87.4   Ethical Issues in Treatment Use

The FDA has adopted regulations authorizing the use of investigational new drugs in certain circumstances where a patient has not responded to approved therapies. This "treatment use" of unapproved new drugs is not limited to life-threatening emergency situations, but rather is also available to treat "serious" diseases or conditions.

The FDA has not approved treatment use of unapproved medical devices, but it is possible that a manufacturer could obtain such approval by establishing a specific protocol for this kind of use within the context of an IDE.

The criteria for treatment use of unapproved medical devices would be similar to criteria for treatment use of investigational drugs (1) the device is intended to treat a serious or life-threatening disease or condition, (2) there is no comparable or satisfactory alternative product available to treat that condition, (3) the device is under an IDE, or has received an IDE exemption, or all clinical trials have been completed and the device is awaiting approval, and (4) the sponsor is actively pursuing marketing approval of the investigational device. The treatment use protocol would be submitted as part of the IDE, and would describe the intended use of the device, the rationale for use of the device, the available alternatives and why the investigational product is preferred, the criteria for patient selection, the measures to monitor the use of the device and to minimize risk, and technical information that is relevant to the safety and effectiveness of the device for the intended treatment purpose.

Were the FDA to approve treatment use of unapproved medical devices, what ethical issues would be posed? First, because such use is premised on the failure of validated interventions to improve the patient's condition adequately, it is a form of practice rather than research. Second, since the device involved in an instance of treatment use is unapproved, such use would constitute nonvalidated practice. As such, like emergency use, it should be subject to the FDA's requirement that prior preclinical tests and animal studies have been conducted that provide substantial reason to believe that patient benefit will result. As with emergency use, although this does not prevent assessment of the intervention's benefits and risks from being highly speculative, it does prevent assessment from being totally speculative. Here too, although desperate circumstances can justify desperate action, they do not justify reckless action. Unlike emergency use, the circumstances of treatment use involve serious impairment of health rather than the threat of premature death. Hence, an issue that must be considered is how serious such impairment must be to justify resorting to an intervention whose risks and benefits have not been solidly established.

In cases of emergency use, the FDA requires that physicians not use this exception to an IDE to avoid requirements that would otherwise be in place. This particular requirement would be obviated in instances of treatment use by the requirement that a protocol for such use be previously addressed within an IDE.

As with emergency use of unapproved devices, the patients involved in treatment use would be particularly vulnerable patients. Although they are not dying, they are facing serious medical conditions and are thereby likely to be less able to avoid exploitation than patients under less desperate circumstances. Consequently, it is especially important that patients be informed of the speculative nature of the intervention and of the possibility that treatment may result in little or no benefit to them.

87.5 The Safe Medical Devices Act

On November 28, 1991, the Safe Medical Devices Act of 1990 (Public Law 101-629) went into effect. This regulation requires a wide range of health-care institutions, including hospitals, ambulatory-surgical facilities, nursing homes, and outpatient treatment facilities, to report information that "reasonably suggests" the likelihood that the death, serious injury, or serious illness of a patient at that facility has been caused or contributed to by a medical device. When a death is device related, a report must be made directly to the FDA *and* to the manufacturer of the device. When a serious illness or injury is device related, a report must be made to the manufacturer *or* to the FDA in cases where the manufacturer is not known. In addition, summaries of previously submitted reports must be submitted to the FDA on a semiannual basis. Prior to this regulation, such reporting was voluntary. This new regulation was designed to enhance the FDA's ability to quickly learn about problems related to medical devices. It also supplements the medical device reporting (MDR) regulations promulgated in 1984. MDR regulations require that reports of device-related deaths and serious injuries be submitted to the FDA by manufacturers and importers. The new law extends this requirement to users of medical devices along with manufacturers and importers. This act represents a significant step forward in protecting patients exposed to medical devices.

References

Bronzino, J.D. Flannery, E.J. and Wade, M.L. "Legal and Ethical Issues in the Regulation and Development of Engineering Achievements in Medical Technology," Part I *IEEE Engineering in Medicine and Biology*, 1990a.

Bronzino, J.D. Flannery, E.J. and Wade, M.L. "Legal and Ethical Issues in the Regulation and Development of Engineering Achievements in Medical Technology," Part II *IEEE Engineering in Medicine and Biology*, 1990b.

Bronzino, J.D. Chapter 10 "Medical and Ethical Issues in Clinical Engineering Practice." *Management of Medical Technology*. Butterworth. 1992.

Bronzino, J.D. Chapter 20 "Moral and Ethical Issues Associated with Medical Technology." *Introduction to Biomedical Engineering*. Academic Press, New York, 1999.

Bronzino, J.D. Chapter 192. "Regulation of Medical Device Innovation." *The Biomedical Engineering Handbook*. CRC Press, Bocaraton, FL, 1995; 2000.

Capron, A. "Human Experimentation: Basic Issues." *The Encyclopedia of Bioethics*, Vol. II. The Free Press, Glencoe, II. 1978.

Capron, A. "Human Experimentation." (J.P. Childress et al., Eds.) University Publications of America.

Further Information

Dubler, N.N. and Nimmons, D. *Ethics on Call*. Harmony Books, New York, 1992.

Jonsen, A.R. *The New Medicine and the Old Ethics*. Harvard University Press, Cambridge, MA, 1990.

Index

Note: Page numbers in *italics* refer to illustrations.

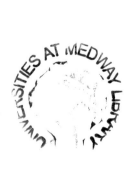